Handbook of
OBESITY

Handbook of OBESITY

edited by

GEORGE A. BRAY
Pennington Biomedical Research Center
Louisiana State University
Baton Rouge, Louisiana

CLAUDE BOUCHARD
Physical Activity Sciences Laboratory
Laval University
Ste.-Foy, Quebec, Canada

W. P. T. JAMES
Rowett Research Institute
Aberdeen, Scotland

MARCEL DEKKER, INC.

NEW YORK • BASEL

Library of Congress Cataloging-in-Publication Data

Handbook of obesity/edited by George A. Bray, Claude Bouchard,
   W. P. T. James.
      p.   cm.
   Includes bibliographical references and index.
   ISBN 0-8247-9899-6 (hardcover: alk. paper)
   1. Obesity.   I. Bray. George, A.   II. Bouchard, Claude.
III.   James, W. P. T. (William Philip Trehearne)
   [DNLM: 1. Obesity.   WD 210 H236 1997]
RC628.H29   1997
616.3' 98—dc21
DNLM/DLC
for Library of Congress
                                                                        97-34402
                                                                         CIP

The publisher offers discounts on this book when ordered in bulk quantities. For more information, write to Special Sales/Professional Marketing at the address below.

This book is printed on acid-free paper.

MARCEL DEKKER, INC.
270 Madison Avenue, New York, New York 10016
http://www.dekker.com

Current printing (last digit):
10 9 8 7 6 5

PRINTED IN THE UNITED STATES OF AMERICA

Preface

This volume has been designed to provide up-to-date coverage of the range of subjects that make up the field of obesity research. The chapters have been written by many of the leading scientists and clinicians in the field.

We have divided the book into four sections. Part one deals with the history, definitions, and prevalence of obesity. The first of these nine chapters outlines the history of obesity using a series of timelines to put the important events in the development of obesity research into the historical context. This is followed by a chapter written by the three editors on definitions that can be used to frame the subject matter of obesity. Chapters on the measurement of body composition follow. The global prevalence of obesity in children and in the elderly is then presented in three separate chapters. This section ends with a discussion of the behavioral and psychological correlates of obesity, and the cultural context in which obesity is viewed by different ethnic groups.

The second section focuses on the etiological factors involved in the development of this problem. The first chapter is a detailed presentation of the genetics of human obesity. A genetic approach has proved particularly important since the discovery of leptin and the rapid mapping of genetic loci that are associated with the development of obesity. A great deal has been learned about obesity from the study of animals models, a variety of which are presented by two of the experts in the field. The third chapter deals with the rise of genetic approaches to obesity, which has been aided by advances in molecular biology. There follow three chapters on the intake of food. One of these deals with this problem in humans, the second with the problem in animals, and the third with the neural basis for the intake of food in both humans and animals. Together these chapters provide a vivid view of the current standing of the field of nutrient intake.

Our understanding of the importance of adipose tissue has steadily increased, from regarding it as a simple storage organ to recognizing it as a secretory organ as well. The important differences between white and brown adipose tissue have also been elucidated, and their role in the development and maintenance of human obesity defined. These concepts are developed in the next four chapters. The final group of chapters in the second section deals with energy expenditure. There is a chapter on energy expenditure and thermogenesis during test, and one on physical activity and its relation to obesity and food intake. Finally, the roles of the endocrine system, the autonomic nervous system, and substrate handling are discussed. From this second section the reader should obtain a detailed understanding of the genetic basis of obesity; the role and control of food intake in the development of obesity; the way fat cells function as a storage, thermogenic, secretory organ; and, finally, the way in which energy expenditure is controlled and involved in the development of obesity.

The fourth section deals with the pathophysiology of obesity, that is, the mechanisms by which obesity produces damaging effects on health. The first two chapters in this section deal with the role of central fat and the metabolic syndrome. This is followed by a detailed discussion of the effects of obesity on a variety of individual organ systems. Three chapters are devoted to problems of the cardiovascular system and lipoprotein abnormalities, which are important consequences of obesity. Diabetes is one of the most frequent problems associated with obesity, as explained in one chapter. The ways in which obesity enhances the risk of gall bladder disease are developed in another chapter. This is followed by a clear discussion of the pulmonary problems arising from obesity, one of which (the Pickwickian syndrome, or sleep apnea) is named after the famous fat boy, Joe, in Dickens' *Pickwick*

Papers. Obesity has important effects on the risk for gout and arthritis and this is discussed in a separate chapter. Two chapters in this section deal with the effects of obesity on endocrine function and pregnancy. Finally, the problem of weight cycling and the risks of intentional and unintentional weight loss are discussed in two chapters that have picked up important themes of obesity research and put them into a valuable new perspective.

The final section deals with prevention and treatment. Since an ounce of prevention is worth a pound of cure, the section begins with a chapter on prevention. This is followed by a clinically useful set of guidances for the evaluation of the overweight patient. The cornerstones for treatment of obesity—behavior therapy, diet, and exercise—are presented in three separate chapters. These are followed by three important chapters on the management of diabetes, hypertension, and hyperlipidemia in the obese individual. Finally, there is a chapter on the current status of pharmacological treatment of obesity and a chapter on the surgical approaches that can be used for a individual for whom other approaches to treatment have failed.

The preparation of this volume has required the work of many people. First, we want to thank the authors and their secretarial assistants for submitting the chapters so promptly. This will make the entire volume timely. Several individuals in the editors' officer have also played a key role in moving this volume forward. We want to thank especially Ms. Millie Cutrer and Terry Hodges in Baton Rouge, Ms. Karen Horth and Ms. Diane Drolet in Quebec City, and Ms. Jean James in Aberdeen. The guiding hand at Marcel Dekker, Inc., who has been so valuable in nudging and cajoling us along when we needed, is Ms. Lia Pelosi. We thank you all and hope that the readers appreciate the important role each of you, and others we have not mentioned, including especially our long-suffering families, has made to the success of this volume.

George A. Bray
Claude Bouchard
W. P. T. James

Contents

PART III   PATHOPHYSIOLOGY

Contributors

Gérard Ailhaud, Ph.D. Professor, Center of Biochemistry, Faculty of Sciences, University of Nice-Sophia Antipolis, Nice, France

Jeanine Albu, M.D. Assistant Professor, Division of Endocrinology, Diabetes and Nutrition, Department of Medicine, St. Luke's–Roosevelt Hospital and Columbia University College of Physicians and Surgeons, New York, New York

David B. Allison, Ph.D. Associate Research Scientist, Obesity Research, St. Luke's–Roosevelt Hospital and Columbia University College of Physicians and Surgeons, New York, New York

Peter Arner, M.D., Ph.D. Doctor, Department of Medicine, Unit of Endocrinology, Karolinska Institute and Huddinge Hospital, Huddinge, Sweden

Arne Astrup, M.D., Ph.D. Director and Professor, Research Department of Human Nutrition, Royal Veterinary and Agricultural University, Frederiksberg, Denmark

Richard L. Atkinson, M.D. Professor, Departments of Medicine and Nutritional Sciences, University of Wisconsin–Madison, Madison, Wisconsin

Douglas L. Ballor, Ph.D. Tacoma, Washington

Richard N. Baumgartner, Ph.D. Associate Professor and Assistant Director, Clinical Nutrition Program, Division of Epidemiology, Department of Medicine, University of New Mexico School of Medicine, Albuquerque, New Mexico

Peter N. Benotti, M.D. Chief, Department of Surgery, Englewood Hospital and Medical Center, Englewood, New Jersey, and Professor of Surgery, Mt. Sinai School of Medicine, New York, New York

Vicki K. Bentley-Condit, Ph.D. Assistant Professor, Department of Anthropology, Grinnell College, Grinnell, Iowa

Per Björntorp, M.D., Ph.D., F.R.C.P., Edin. Professor, Department of Heart and Lung Diseases, Sahlgren's Hospital, University of Gothenburg, Gothenburg, Sweden

Steven N. Blair, P.E.D. Director of Research and Director, Epidemiology and Clinical Applications, The Cooper Institute for Aerobic Research, Dallas, Texas

John E. Blundell, Ph.D., F.B.Ps.S Professor, Department of Psychology, University of Leeds, Leeds, England

Claude Bouchard, Ph.D. Professor, Physical Activity Sciences Laboratory, Laval University, Ste.-Foy, Quebec, Canada

George A. Bray, M.D., M.A.C.P. Executive Director and Professor, Pennington Biomedical Research Center, Louisiana State University, Baton Rouge, Louisiana

Peter J. Brown, Ph.D. Professor, Departments of Anthropology and International Health, Emory University, Atlanta, Georgia

Ian D. Caterson, M.B., B.S., B.Sc(Med), Ph.D., F.R.A.C.P. Director Clinical Endocrinology, University of Sydney, Sydney, New South Wales, Australia

Flavia M. Cicuttini, M.Sc, MB.BS, F.R.A.C.P., Ph.D. Doctor, Department of Epidemiology and Preventive Medicine, Monash University, Victoria, Australia

Jean-Pierre Després, Ph.D. Professor and Scientific Director, Departments of Medicine, Food Science and Nutrition, and Lipid Research Center, Laval University and Medical Research Center, Ste.-Foy, Quebec, Canada

William H. Dietz, M.D., Ph.D.   Professor of Pediatrics, Tufts University School of Medicine and Boston Floating Hospital, Boston, Massachusetts

Madeleine L. Drent, M.D., Ph.D.   Doctor, Department of Endocrinology, Free University Hospital, Amsterdam, The Netherlands

Robert H. Eckel, M.D.   Professor, Division of Endocrinology, Metabolism, and Diabetes, Department of Medicine, University of Colorado Health Sciences Center, Denver, Colorado

Janis S. Fisler, Ph.D.   Research Cardiologist, Department of Medicine and Division of Cardiology, University of California at Los Angeles School of Medicine, Los Angeles, California

Jean-Pierre Flatt, Ph.D.   Professor, Department of Biochemistry and Molecular Biology, University of Massachusetts Medical School, Worcester, Massachusetts

Susan K. Fried, Ph.D.   Associate Professor, Department of Nutritional Sciences, Cook College, Rutgers University, New Brunswick, New Jersey

Ehud Grossman, M.D.   Associate Professor of Medicine, Hypertension Unit, The Chaim Sheba Medical Center, Tel-Hashomer, Israel

Barbara Hansen, Ph.D.   Professor, Department of Physiology, Obesity and Diabetes Research Center, University of Maryland School of Medicine, Baltimore, Maryland

Hans Hauner, M.D.   Professor, Clinical Department, Diabetes Research Institute at the Heinrich-Heine-University Dusseldorf, Dusseldorf, Germany

Magda M. I. Hennes, Ph.D.   Assistant Professor, Department of Medicine, Medical College of Wisconsin, Milwaukee, Wisconsin

Steven B. Heymsfield, M.D.   Professor, Department of Medicine and Obesity Research Center, St. Luke's–Roosevelt Hospital and Columbia University College of Physicians and Surgeons, New York, New York

James O. Hill, Ph.D.   Professor, Center for Human Nutrition, University of Colorado Health Sciences Center, Denver, Colorado

Jean Himms-Hagen, D.Phil.   Professor, Department of Biochemistry, University of Ottawa, Ottawa, Ontario, Canada

Bartley G. Hoebel, Ph.D.   Professor, Department of Psychology, Princeton University, Princeton, New Jersey

W. P. T. James, M.D., D.Sc, F.R.C.P., F.R.C.P.(E), F.R.S.E.   Professor and Director, Rowett Research Institute, Aberdeen, Scotland

Robert W. Jeffery, Ph.D.   Professor, Division of Epidemiology, University of Minnesota School of Public Health, Minneapolis, Minnesota

Eric Jéquier, M.D.   Professor, Director, Institute of Physiology, Faculty of Medicine, University of Lausanne, Lausanne, Switzerland

Kaoru Kameda-Takemura, M.D., Ph.D.   Assistant Professor, The Second Department of Internal Medicine, Osaka University Medical School, Suita, Osaka, Japan

David E. Kelley, M.D.   Associate Professor, Division of Endocrinology and Metabolism, University of Pittsburgh School of Medicine, Pittsburgh, Pennsylvania

Ahmed H. Kissebah, M.D., Ph.D., F.A.C.P.   Professor and Chief, Division of Endocrinology, Metabolism and Clinical Nutrition, Medical College of Wisconsin, Milwaukee, Wisconsin

Cynthia W. Ko, M.D.   Department of Medicine, University of Washington and Veterans Administration Puget Sound Health Care System, Seattle, Washington

Henry S. Koopmans, Ph.D.   Professor, Department of Physiology and Biophysics, University of Calgary, Calgary, Alberta, Canada

Peter G. Kopelman, M.D., F.R.C.P.   Reader in Medicine, Department of Diabetes and Metabolism, St. Bartholomew's and The Royal London · School of Medicine and Dentistry at Queen Mary and Westfield College, London, England

Glenn R. Krakower, Ph.D.   Lab Director, Clinical Research Center, Department of Medicine, Medical College of Wisconsin, Milwaukee, Wisconsin

John G. Kral, M.D., Ph.D.   Professor, Department of Surgery, State University of New York Health Science Center at Brooklyn, Brooklyn, New York

Ronald M. Krauss, M.D.   Senior Scientist and Department Head, Department of Molecular and Nuclear Medicine, Ernest Orlando Lawrence Berkeley National Laboratory, University of California at Berkeley, Berkeley, California

I-Min Lee, M.B., B.S., Sc.D.   Assistant Professor, Department of Medicine, Brigham and Women's Hospital and Harvard Medical School, Boston, Massachusetts

Sum P. Lee, M.D., Ph.D.   Professor and Chief, Department of Medicine, University of Washington and Veterans Administration Puget Sound Health Care System, Seattle, Washington

Sarah F. Leibowitz, Ph.D.   Associate Professor, Department of Neurobiology, The Rockefeller University, New York, New York

Ian Andrew MacDonald, Ph.D.   Professor, Department of Physiology and Pharmacology, University of Nottingham Medical School, Nottingham, England

Yuji Matsuzawa, M.D., Ph.D.   Professor and Chairman, The Second Department of Internal Medicine, Osaka University Medical School, Suita, Osaka, Japan

Franz H. Messerli, M.D.   Director, Hypertension Laboratory, Alton Ochsner Medical Foundation, New Orleans, Louisiana

Patrick Mahlen O'Neil, Ph.D.   Professor, Department of Psychiatry and Behavioral Sciences, Medical University of South Carolina, Charleston, South Carolina

Richard A. Parisi, M.D.   Associate Professor, Department of Medicine, University of Medicine and Dentistry of New Jersey and Robert Wood Johnson Medical School, New Brunswick, New Jersey

Louis Pérusse, Ph.D.   Research Scholar, Physical Activity Sciences Laboratory, Laval University, Ste.-Foy, Quebec, Canada

F. Xavier Pi-Sunyer, M.D.   Professor of Medicine, Director, Division of Endocrinology, Diabetes, and Nutrition, St. Luke's–Roosevelt Hospital and Columbia University College of Physicians and Surgeons, New York, New York

Eric P. Poehlman, Ph.D.   Professor, Department of Medicine, University of Vermont, Burlington, Vermont

D. C. Rao, Ph.D.   Professor and Director, Division of Biostatistics, Washington University School of Medicine, St. Louis, Missouri

Peter J. Reeds, Ph.D.   Professor, Department of Pediatrics, USDA/ARS Children's Nutrition Research Center and Baylor College of Medicine, Houston, Texas

Treva Rice, Ph.D.   Research Assistant Professor, Division of Biostatistics, Washington University School of Medicine, St. Louis, Missouri

Daniel Ricquier, Sc.D., Ph.D.   Research Investigator and Laboratory Director, Research Center for Endocrinology and Development, National Center of Scientific Research, Meudon, France

Áila M. Rissanen, M.D.   Associate Professor, Department of Psychiatry, Helsinki University, Helsinki, Finland

Albert P. Rocchini, M.D.   Director, Department of Pediatrics, Children's Memorial Hospital and Northwestern University, Chicago, Illinois

Robert Ross, Ph.D.   Assistant Professor, School of Physical and Health Education, Queen's University, Kingston, Ontario, Canada

Stephan Rössner, M.D., Ph.D.   Professor, Department of Health Behavior Research and Obesity Unit, Karolinska Institute, Stockholm, Sweden

Colleen D. Russell, B.S.   Department of Nutritional Sciences, Rutgers University, New Brunswick, New Jersey

Edward Saltzman, M.D.   Instructor, Division of Clinical Nutrition, Tufts University School of Medicine, New England Medical Center and the Jean Mayer USDA Human Nutrition Research Center on Aging at Tufts University, Boston, Massachusetts

Wim H. M. Saris, M.D., Ph.D.   Professor, Nutrition Research Institute, NUTRIM, University of Maastricht, Maastricht, The Netherlands

Yves Schutz, Ph.D., M.P.H.   Lecturer in Human Nutrition, Institute of Physiology, University of Lausanne, Lausanne, Switzerland

Robert S. Schwartz, M.D.   Professor, Department of Medicine, University of Washington and Harborview Medical Center, Seattle, Washington

Jacob C. Seidell, Ph.D.   Head, Department of Chronic Diseases and Environmental Epidemiology, National Institute of Public Health and the Environment, Bilthoven, The Netherlands

Jean-Aimé Simoneau, Ph.D.   Associate Professor, Physical Activity Sciences Laboratory, Laval University, Ste.-Foy, Quebec, Canada

Gabriele E. Sonnenberg   Associate Professor, Division of Endocrinology, Metabolism, and Clinical Nutrition, Clinical Research Center, Medical College of Wisconsin, Milwaukee, Wisconsin

Tim D. Spector, M.D., M.Sc., M.R.C.P.   Consultant Rheumatologist, Department of Rheumatology, St. Thomas' Hospital, Guys' and St. Thomas' Trust, London, England

Judith S. Stern, Sc.D.   Professor, Department of Nutrition and International Medicine, University of California at Davis, Davis, California

Richard J. Strobel, M.D.   Assistant Professor, Department of Medicine, University of Medicine and Dentistry of New Jersey and Robert Wood Johnson Medical School, New Brunswick, New Jersey

Kingman P. Strohl, M.D.   Professor, Department of Medicine, Case Western Reserve University, Cleveland, Ohio

R. James Stubbs   Rowett Research Institute, Bucksburn, Aberdeen, Scotland

Michael J. Toth, Ph.D.   Research Associate, Department of Medicine, University of Vermont, Burlington, Vermont

Angelo Tremblay, Ph.D.   Professor, Physical Activity Sciences Laboratory, Laval University, Ste.-Foy, Quebec, Canada

Luc F. Van Gaal, M.D., Ph.D.   Professor of Medicine, Departments of Endocrinology, Metabolism, and Clinical Nutrition, University of Antwerp, Antwerp, Belgium

Zi-Mian Wang, M.S.   Research Associate, Obesity Research Center, St. Luke's–Roosevelt Hospital and Columbia University College of Physicians and Surgeons, New York, New York

Craig H. Warden, Ph.D.   Assistant Professor, Departments of Medicine, Rowe Genetics, and Pediatrics, University of California at Davis, Davis, California

Donald A. Williamson, Ph.D.   Professor, Department of Psychology, Pennington Biomedical Research Center, Louisiana State University, Baton Rouge, Louisiana

Rena R. Wing, Ph.D.   Professor of Psychiatry, Psychology, and Epidemiology, Department of Psychiatry, University of Pittsburgh School of Medicine, Pittsburgh, Pennsylvania

Shizuya Yamashita, M.D., Ph.D.   The Second Department of Internal Medicine, Osaka University Medical School, Suita, Osaka, Japan

Susan Zelitch Yanovski, M.D.   Director, Obesity and Eating Disorders Program, National Institute of Diabetes and Digestive and Kidney Diseases, National Institutes of Health, Bethesda, Maryland

David A. York, Ph.D.   Professor and Chief of Basic Sciences, Pennington Biomedical Research Center, Louisiana State University, Baton Rouge, Louisiana

Paul Zimmet, M.D., Ph.D., FRACP   Professor, Departments of Biochemistry and Molecular Biology, Monash University and International Diabetes Institute, Melbourne, Australia

Handbook of
OBESITY

1

Historical Framework for the Development of Ideas About Obesity

George A. Bray
Pennington Biomedical Research Center, Louisiana State University, Baton Rouge, Louisiana

I. INTRODUCTION

We do not live in our own time alone; we carry our history within us.

Gaarder (1, p. 152)

He who cannot draw on three thousand years is living from hand to mouth.

Goethe (1, p. 231)

The goal of historical scholarship is said to be to reconstruct the past, but the only past available from reconstruction is that which we can see from the present. The nature of science as an analytical discipline, involved at one and the same time in the uncertainties of discovery and in the accumulation of a body of objective knowledge, raises some special problems of historical reconstruction.

Crombie (2, p. 4)

These quotes apply admirably to this chapter on this history of obesity. All of the chapters except this one examine "the nature of science as an analytical discipline. . . . and the accumulation of a body of objective knowledge." This chapter is left to explore the historical framework in which this accumulation of a body of objective knowledge about obesity has occurred. I am not an historian, and thus, lack the perspective of someone trained in this field. I am, rather, a practicing scientist who has tried to understand the processes of experimental science to apply them to improving my own. In an earlier review (3) I covered a number of concepts in the history of obe-

sity. Other historical milestones for obesity have been examined in the selections made for "Classics in Obesity," published in the journal *Obesity Research*. This chapter will build on these earlier papers and attempt to place these contributions to the field of obesity into a broader historical context (4,5).

This chapter is divided into three sections. The first will review the limited data on obesity in prehistoric times. The second will consider obesity from the beginning of recorded history (ca. 3600 B.C.) to the onset of the scientific era (ca. A.D. 1500). The third will cover the development of concepts about obesity in the scientific era from A.D. 1500 to the present. Although these divisions are arbitrary, they provide the framework that will be used here.

To facilitate placing the scientific events discussed in this chapter into a broader historical context, I have prepared a series of timelines, each covering one century, which place historical developments in the fields of science and other events in relation to obesity. Although the discussion will range into fields prior to the beginning of the period called the "scientific era" (A.D. 1500 to the present), the timeline begins with the period I have called the scientific era (around A.D. 1500) and continues to the present. The prescientific era is defined here as prior to the development of the printing press by Gutenberg in 1456, but for convenience, it will be dated at A.D. 1500.

Clearly, there were many important scientific and mathematical advances before 1500 (6,7). However, the advent of printing with moveable type and the appearance of the scientific method led to an accelerating rate of scientific advance after A.D. 1500. The time line consists of 11 separate lines, showing developments in science and technology, anatomy and histology, physiology, chemistry/biochemistry, genetics, pharmacology, neuroscience, and clinical medicine. Observations in clinical medicine related to obesity antedate 1500, but the impact of many discoveries on scientific medicine was delayed until the beginning of the 19th century. If one wanted a demarkation line for the beginning of modern medicine, it might well be the French Revolution (1789–1800) (8,9).

II.   PREHISTORIC MEDICINE (to 3000 B.C.)

A.   Paleomedicine

The study of medicine prior to written history can be done from artistic representations and from skeletal finds and related artifacts. Among the earliest evidence of man's therapeutic efforts were those aimed at the relief of fevers and burns, attempts to relieve pain and to stop bleeding. Trepanning, or drilling holes in the skull to let out "evil spirits," to treat "epilepsy," or to relieve skull fractures, was practiced in many parts of the world up to the 19th century. The medicine man and the relation of magic and religion to healing and disease are prominent features of prehistoric medicine and in some rural cultures, even today. That obesity was known in this early period is evident from Stone Age artifacts.

B.   Stone Age Obesity

1.   Paleolithic Artifacts

Table 1 is a list of several artifacts from the paleolithic Stone Age that depict obesity. These artifacts were found across Europe from Southwestern France to Russia, north of the Black Sea. The location in which they were found

and their appearance is shown in Figure 1. They occur during a fairly narrow period in the early upper paleolithic period (upper periogordian or gravettian) some 23,000–25,000 years ago (10). They are distributed over more than 2,000 km from west to east. Their composition is ivory, limestone, or baked clay. The most famous of these is the Venus of Willendorf, a small statuette measuring 11 cm in height with evidence of abdominal obesity and pendulous breasts (11). The similarity in design of these artifacts, as shown in Figure 2, suggests that there may have been communication across Europe during this period of glaciation. This and the other paleolithic female figurines are frequently viewed as primordial female deities, reflecting the bounty of the earth (12). In a review of historical ideas published as a thesis in 1939, Hautin (13) concludes that these figures prove the existence of obesity in the paleolithic era and that they also symbolize the expression and possible aesthetic ideals of the period. "The women immortalized in stone age sculpture were fat; there is no word for it. . . . obesity was already a fact of life for paleolithic man—or at least for paleolithic woman" (12).

2.   Neolithic Artifacts

The Neolithic period spans the time from 8000 B.C. to 5500 B.C. This period saw the introduction of agriculture and establishment of settlements. The Neolithic Age along with the Chalcolithic or Copper Age, which continued to 3000 B.C., were notable for numerous "Mother Goddesses" artifacts found primarily in Anatolia. The richest finds are from the excavations at Catalhoyuk and Hacilar and are from the period between 5000 and 6000 B.C. Most of these figurines are made of baked clay, but a few are of limestone or alabaster. Their corpulence is abundantly evident in the pendulous breasts and large abdominogluteal areas. They range in height from 2.5 to 24 cm, but most are between 5 and 12 cm. They are seated, standing, or lying.

Table 1   Paleolithic Venus Figurines with Prominent Obesity

Name and place found	Number found	Height	Composition
Willendorf, Austria	1	11 cm	Limestone
Dolni Vestonice, Czechoslovakia	Many	11.4 cm	Terracotta
Savignano, Italy	1	24 cm	Serpentine
Grimaldi, France	Many		Terracotta
Laussel, France	Many		Terracotta
Lespugue, France	1	14.7 cm	Ivory
Gagarino, Russia	Many		Ivory
Kostenki, Russia	Many	47 cm	Ivory
Catal Huyak, Turkey	Many		Terracotta

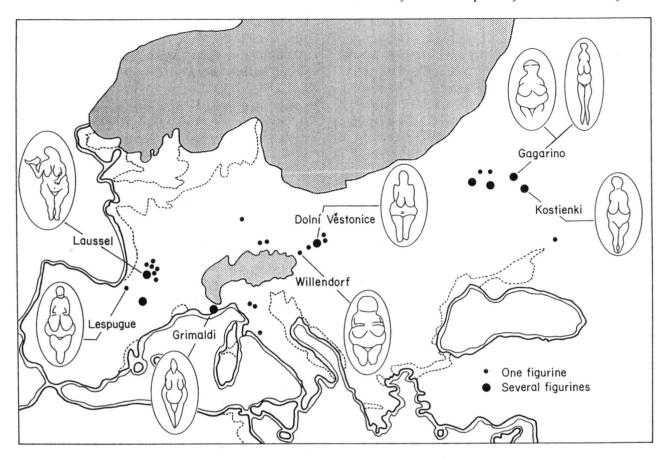

Figure 1   Location of the paleolithic "Venus" figurines. Obese figurines have been found throughout Europe and in the middle East.

One of the most famous from Catalhoyuk is 20 cm tall. She sits on a leopard throne with two lions serving as her armrests. The figurines from this period show exaggeration of hips, bellies, and breasts, with genital areas indicated by triangular decoration, symbolizing motherhood and womankind, attributes shared by later Mother Goddess figurines from Kybele to Artemis. It is important to note that no diety or mythological figure has ever borne as many different names as the Mother Goddess. On the Kultepe tablets (1800 B.C.) she is known as Kubaba, the Lydians called her Kybebe, the Phrygians Kybele, and the Hittites Hepat. In ancient Pontic Comana (near Tokat) and Cappadocian Comana (Kayseri) she was known by the ancient Anatolian name of Ma. She was Marienna and Lat to the Sumerians, Arinna to the people of the Late Hittite period, Isis to the Egyptians, Rhea to the Greeks, Artemis to the Ephesians, and Venus to the Romans. The name Kybele has even survived into modern times as the Anglo-Saxon Sybil and its variants, and Turkish Sibel. At Catalhoyuk she is depicted as giving birth to a child; at Hacilar

she is holding a child. This child is represented in later myth by gods such as Attis, Adonis, and Tammuz (14).

III.   MEDICINE AND OBESITY FROM THE BEGINNING OF RECORDED HISTORY TO A.D. 1500 (PRESCIENTIFIC MEDICINE)

Medical traditions have developed in all cultures. Several of these are described below. Evidence for obesity has been identified in all of these medical traditions and geographic regions, suggesting that, independent of diet, the potential to store nutrients as fat was selected for by evolution at an early period in human development.

A.   Mesopotamian Medicine

The Tigris and Euphrates River basin was the land of healers and astrologers. Cuneiform writing, libraries, sanita-

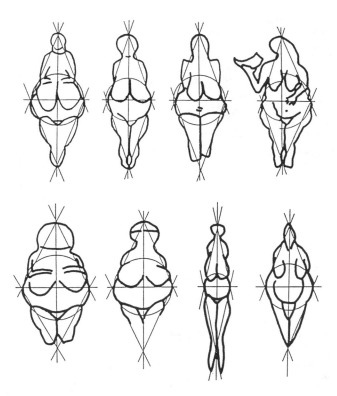

Figure 2   Similarity in design of the "Venus" figurines. All of the figures identified have similar structural features, although they were composed of several different materials. This similarity suggests that there may have been communication or migration between these sites during the upper Paleolithic period.

tion, and medical knowledge are evident by 3600 B.C. Of the 30,000 clay tablets with cuneiform writing that were recovered in the library at Nineveh from approximately 2000 B.C., 800 are related to medical matters. The medical armamentarium of Sumerian physicians consisted of more than 120 minerals and 250 herbs including cannabis, mustard, mandragora, belladonna, and henbane (15). A terracotta statuette showing enormously fat thighs and arms was found at Susa in the middle Elamite period in the 12th century B.C.E. (16,17), indicating the continuing representation of obesity in artifacts of the female body.

B.   Egyptian Medicine

Paralleling the Mesopotamian medical tradition were the traditions of medicine in Egypt where the relationship between priests and physicians was very close. Imhotep, who became the god of healing, began as a Viser to King Zoser (2900 B.C.). Imhotep was a man of great accomplishment who in addition to being a physician was also an architect, a poet, and a statesman. Two major archeo-

logical finds, the Edwin Smith papyrus (18), written between 2500 and 2000 B.C. and the Ebers papyrus, written approximately 1550 B.C., provide major knowledge about medicine in Egypt. Obesity was known to the Egyptians. A study of royal mummies showed that both stout women (Queens Henut-Tawy and Inhapy) and stout men were not uncommon in Egypt, at least not among the higher classes, although "obesity was regarded as objectionable" (19). Several examples of obesity are also seen in the stone reliefs that were the principal artistic medium: a doorkeeper in the temple of Amon-Ra Khor-en-Khonsu; a cook in Ankh-ma-Hor's tomb (6th dynasty) (20); a fat man enjoying food presented to him by his lean servants in Mereruka's tomb; the local yeoman, the famed Sheikh et Balad (19); and the grossly obese harpist playing before the prince Aki (Middle Kingdom) (21). Studies of the skinfolds of mummies such as Amenophis III and Ramsses III show that they were fat (21). One of the most interesting figures is that of the Queen of Punt from the temple of Queen Hatshepsut, Deir el-Bahri (18th dynasty). She has marked steatopygia and appears to have shortening of the lower extremities suggesting dyschondroplasia or dislocated hips (19–22).

C.   Chinese and Tibetan Medicine

The early Chinese believed that disease was sent by the gods or by demons. Bone inscriptions indicate the presence of leprosy, typhoid fever, cholera, and plague. Anatomical dissection was not permitted because of ancestor worship. The Yellow Emperor (Huang Di) and the Divine Farmer (Shen Nong Bencaojing) are the legendary founders of Chinese medicine (23), which contains 365 drugs and the Hung Tu Hei Ching (Yellow Emperor's Inner Canon), dates from 200 B.C., and is a dialogue on bodily functions and disease. In China, Zhang Zihongjing was considered the Father of Medicine, the equivalent of Hippocrates in Greece. Zhang described symptoms and treatment for many diseases. Hua Toh (3rd century A.D.) is the only known surgeon from ancient China. Acupuncture, the art of treatment by inserting sharp needles into the body, was developed and reached its zenith in China. Thus, technique of placing sharp objects in the pinna of the ear to reduce "appetite" has been used to treat obesity.

  The Tibetan offspring of the Chinese Tradition is beautifully illustrated in the 17th-century treatise entitled *The Blue Beryl* composed by Sangye Gyamtso, the scholar and regent of Tibet. It is an erudite yet practical commentary on the ancient text entitled *The Four Tantras* (24). In this text obesity is described as a condition requiring catabolic treatment. It also notes that "overeating . . . causes illness and shortens life span. It is a contraindication of the use of compresses or mild enemas." For treatment of obesity two suggestions are made; "The vigorous massage of the body with pea flour counteracts phlegm diseases and obesity. . . . The gullet, hair compress and flesh of a wolf remedy goiters, dropsy and obesity" (24).

D. Indian Medicine

The fourth great medical tradition is that of Indian medicine (23). In the sacred medical texts of Ayurvedic medicine, sin was viewed as the cause of disease and medical knowledge was closely interwoven with religion and magic. The Caraka Samhita was the first document on Indian medicine and the Susruta Samhita was the second great medical Sanskrit text. In the Caraka Samhita, which described 20 sharp and 101 blunt instruments as well as an operating table, at least 500 drugs are listed along with 700 medical herbs. Included, among others, are cinnamon, borax, castor oil, ginger, and sodium carbonate. The Ayurveda recommended the administration of testicular tissue (organo therapy) as a cure for impotence as well as for obesity (25).

E. Meso-American Medicine

Prior to the "discovery" of the New World by Columbus in 1492, there were three high cultures in the Meso-American world. The Incas occupied the highlands along the west coast of what is now Peru. The Mayan culture occupied the Yucatan peninsula and surrounding areas of central America, and the Aztecs were the occupants of the central plateaus of central America. When Columbus, Cortez, and their compatriots arrived in the new world, the Meso-American cultures were exposed to several devastating diseases, including measles, smallpox, and chickenpox, which were more lethal than the arms the invaders brought. The cultures of pre-Columbian Americans were still "stone-age" cultures, but were highly sophisticated in their knowledge of mathematics, astronomy, and language. Among the most useful drugs discovered in the new world was the cinchona bark (quinine), which was used to treat fevers, including malaria. Diseases were believed to be caused by supernatural, magical, and natural causes. Treatment was related to the cause (26). One of the sources of information about disease in pre-Columbian societies is their sculptural artifacts. These figurines represent malnutrition, deformity, and physical illness (27). Some of the individuals represent people suffering from various diseases including spinal defects, endemic goiter, obesity, eye diseases, and skin ailments (27).

F. Greco-Roman Medicine

From the vantage point of Western Civilization, Greco-Roman medicine has been the major source of our medical tradition. The health hazards associated with obesity were clearly noted in the medical writings of Hippocrates, who stated that "sudden death is more common in those who are naturally fat than in the lean" (28). These traditions also note that obesity was a cause of infertility in women and that the frequency of menses was reduced in the obese.

Galen was the leading physician of Roman times. His influence on medicine and medical teaching lasted more than 1000 years. He identified two types of obesity, one he called "moderate" and the other "immoderate." The former is regarded as natural and the other as morbid.

Descriptions of obesity and sleep apnea also date from Roman times. Dionysius, the tyrant of Heracleia of Pontius who reigned about 360 B.C., is one of the first historical figures afflicted with obesity and somnolence. This enormously fat man frequently fell asleep. His servants used long needles that were inserted through his skin and fat to awaken him when he fell asleep. Kryger cites a second case of Magas, King of Cyrene, who died in 258 B.C. He was a man "weighted down with monstrous masses of flesh in his last days; in fact he choked himself to death" (29,30).

G. Arabic Medicine

With a decline of Roman influence after A.D. 400, scholarly activity shifted from Rome to Byzantium and then to the broader Arabic World following the rise of Islam in the 8th century. One of the leading figures of this medical tradition was Ibn Sina, or Avicenna in its westernized form. Like Galen, he was an influential author who published more than 100 books. Obesity was well known to the Arabic physician. His approach to treating obesity is described later.

With increasing trade and travel, the European culture gradually reestablished contact with Arabian medicine and the Roman traditions that it absorbed. Both the crusades and the invasions by the Arabs of the Peloponessus and southern Spain brought an infusion of classical knowledge from which came the Renaissance and the beginning of the "scientific era" (2,31).

IV. SCIENTIFIC MEDICINE (A.D. 1500 TO THE PRESENT)

The remainder of this chapter will focus on science and medicine since 1500. Medieval science (1150–1450) was constrained by the earlier Greek paradigm of Aristotelian Science. With the introduction of instruments such as the mechanical watch, the magnetic compass, and the magnifying glass, it became possible to critically examine some features of experience and the underlying philosophical tradition. Out of this interaction grew the experimental method of verification and falsification that provides the basis of the Scientific Era (32).

In the following sections, I will review each of the major areas that affect the development of the "science of obesity." To put this in the broader context, the reader is referred again to the timeline Fig. 3).

A. Anatomy

The date 1543 is pivotal in the story of anatomy and for scientific thought in general. That was the year that Vesalius published his treatise on human anatomy (33), the first truly modern anatomy based on his own dissections. Andreas Vesalius was only 28 years old when he published his masterpiece. Also in 1543, Copernicus (34) published his book on the solar system, arguing that planets revolved around the sun. In his accurate and careful dissections, Vesalius showed that the human body could be directly explored by appropriate experimental methods. In so doing, he applied the concept of direct verification and experimental manipulation and identified a number of inaccuracies in the anatomy of Galen, which appears to have been based only on animal dissections. A key element in communicating his discoveries was the process of movable type and printing, invented by Gutenberg. This technical development spawned the distribution of printing presses throughout Europe over the next 50 years. This made classic literature widely available and made it possible to communicate original observations to an ever-growing audience in a relatively short time as contrasted with handwritten books. The revolution in communication had begun, and the age of anatomy ushered in at the beginning of the 16th century expanded rapidly. This was also the peak of the Renaissance. Up to the 16th century, Galen and his writings from Roman times had been the main source of information about anatomy, physiology, and clinical medicine. Although there is no clear evidence that Galen ever dissected a human cadaver, his influence was only broken by the application of direct observation and verification 1500 years later.

The first anatomical dissections of obese individuals are attributed to Bonetus (35). Other descriptions appear in the publications by Morgagni (36), by Haller (37,38) and most particularly by Wadd (39). Of the 12 cases presented in Wadd's book *Comments on Corpulency, Lineaments of Leanness*, two had been examined at postmortem and had been found to have enormous accumulations of fat. This was the first instance of a monograph devoted to obesity that contained anatomical dissections.

B. Microscopic Anatomy (Histology)

The invention of the microscope in the 17th century moved anatomy to the next level. By the middle decades of the 17th century, early microscopists had begun to publish the results of their histological investigation using simple microscopes. The important initial observations by Malpighi (40), Hooke (41), and Leeuwenhoek (42) identified the pulmonary circulation, the fine structure of small animals, and red blood cells, among others.

Gradually, the sophistication of the microscope improved first with the introduction of the compound microscope and then with achromatic lenses. These developments made microscopes sufficiently powerful to define intracellular structure, and thus, the concept of the "cell" as the basic unit of life came to fruition in the middle of the 19th century. It was the combination of the achromatic microscope, which allowed sufficient resolution to distinguish the multiple intracellular components of cells, coupled with the intellectual genius of Schwann (43) and of Schleiden (44), which recognized the unifying principles of the cell wall, nucleus, and an area of structures surrounding this nucleus as the basic elements of cell biology. Shortly afterward, the first substantial textbooks of microscopic anatomy were published (45,46), and shortly after that, the recognition of the fat cell as the member of this group. A description of the growth and development of fat cells was published in 1879 by Hoggan and Hogan (47). In his early observations on the development of the fat vesicle, Hassall (48), suggested that certain types of obesity might result from an increased number of fat cells. It was more than a century later that the work of Hirsch (49) and Björntorp (50) elaborated this important concept as the "hyperplastic" form of obesity. Within 20 years following the promulgation of the cellular theory of biology (43,44), Virchow (51,52) provided a cellular interpretation of pathology. The next advance in microscopic anatomy was the introduction of the electron microscope by Knoll and Ruska in 1932 (53), which provided a detailed look at the fat cell (54).

C. Physiology

The application of experimental methods is nowhere better illustrated than in the discovery of the circulation of the blood by Harvey in 1616, which he published in 1628 (55). His theory is a monumental example of the way in which experimental observations and human reason were

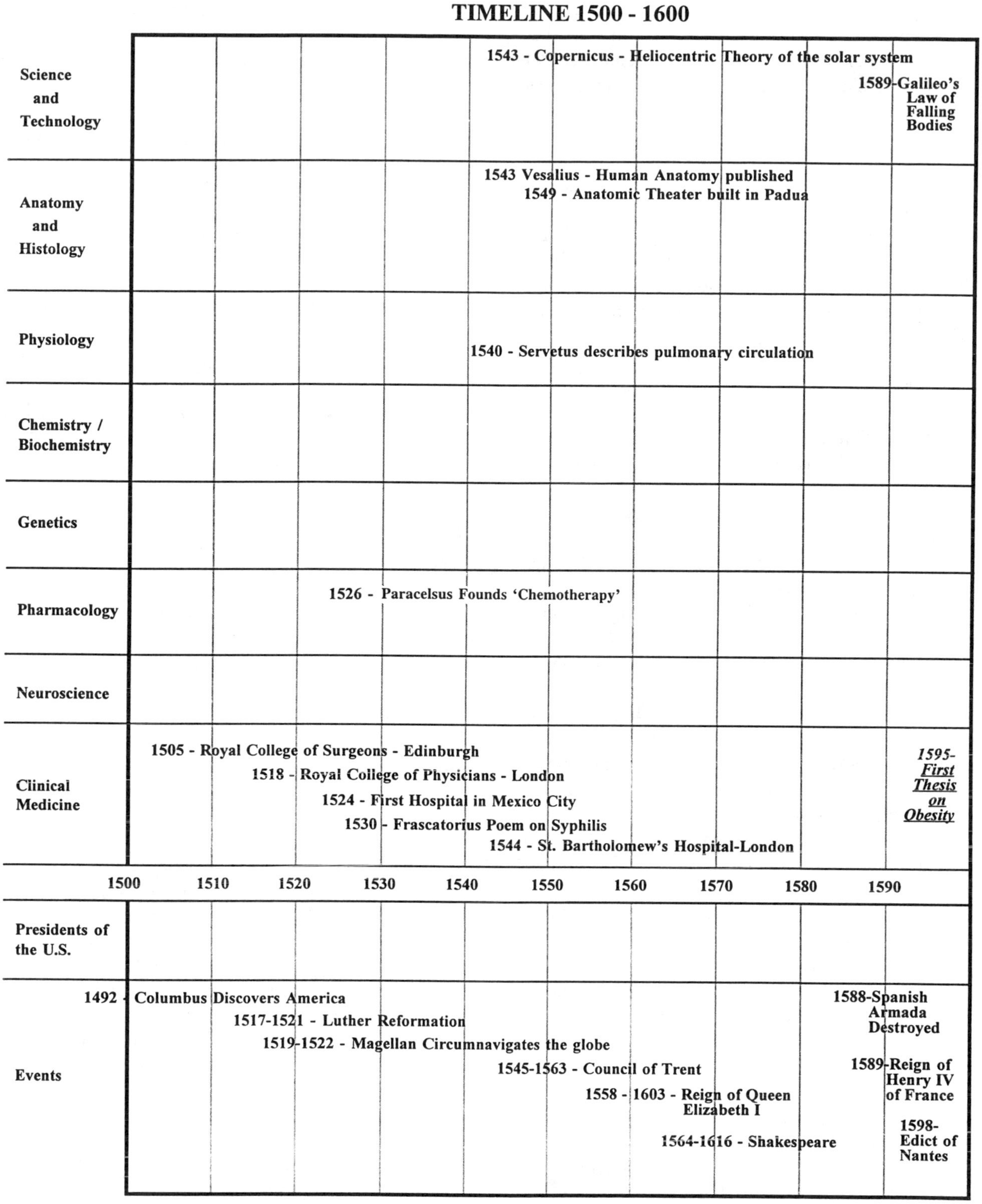

TIMELINE 1500 - 1600

Science and Technology					1543 - Copernicus - Heliocentric Theory of the solar system					1589-Galileo's Law of Falling Bodies
Anatomy and Histology					1543 Vesalius - Human Anatomy published 1549 - Anatomic Theater built in Padua					
Physiology					1540 - Servetus describes pulmonary circulation					
Chemistry / Biochemistry										
Genetics										
Pharmacology		1526 - Paracelsus Founds 'Chemotherapy'								
Neuroscience										
Clinical Medicine	1505 - Royal College of Surgeons - Edinburgh 1518 - Royal College of Physicians - London 1524 - First Hospital in Mexico City 1530 - Frascatorius Poem on Syphilis 1544 - St. Bartholomew's Hospital-London									*1595- First Thesis on Obesity*
	1500	**1510**	**1520**	**1530**	**1540**	**1550**	**1560**	**1570**	**1580**	**1590**
Presidents of the U.S.										
Events	1492 - Columbus Discovers America 1517-1521 - Luther Reformation 1519-1522 - Magellan Circumnavigates the globe 1545-1563 - Council of Trent 1558 - 1603 - Reign of Queen Elizabeth I 1564-1616 - Shakespeare									1588-Spanish Armada Destroyed 1589-Reign of Henry IV of France 1598- Edict of Nantes

Figure 3   Timeline for developments in science, obesity, and contemporary events in the 16th century. (Copyright ©1996 George A. Bray.)

brought together. His theory of the circulation of the blood was published before the presence of capillaries that connect the arterial and venous circulations had been described (40). While in medical school in Padua, Harvey had seen his professor, Realdo Colombo d'Aquapendente, demonstrate the presence of valves in the veins, which only allowed blood to flow one way. At some point between his graduation from Padua in 1596 and his anatomical dissections at the Royal College of Physicians in London in 1616, he realized their importance (56). He presented his "discovery" to the Royal College of Physicians in 1616 to a "ho-hum" reception. Gradually, the importance of the discovery and of the method by which he argued its cogency became apparent. He demonstrated experimentally that the valves in the veins allowed blood to travel in only one direction. From the limited quantity of blood in the body, he argued that the blood must circulate and be reused. It was, however, not for another 50 years that the capillary circulation was demonstrated by Malpighi (40).

The early physiological studies by Harvey on the circulation of the blood set the stage for further work in physiology. Two of these themes are of particular relevance to obesity. The first is metabolism and the second digestion. In 1614, Santorio (57,58) described his metabolic balance, a pulse watch for measuring the pulse and way of measuring temperature. He was following the dictum of his contemporary, Gallileo, who said: "Measure what can be measured, and make measurable what cannot be measured." The balance that Santorio constructed consisted of a platform on which he could sit, counterbalanced by a bean to which weight could be added or subtracted to record changes in his weight and bodily functions. With this system, he could measure his food intake and his excretory losses. In more recent times, Newburgh and Johnston (59) used a similar method to record the loss of water with respiration and showed that it accounted for about 24% of the heat produced by the body.

The second group of physiological studies that relate to obesity were those on the gastrointestinal tract and digestion. In 1752, Reamur (60) succeeded in isolating the gastric juice from a bird, his pet kite, and showing that it digested food. Later in the 18th century, Spallanzani (61,62) showed that gastric juice would digest food and prevent putrefaction outside the body. The American Beaumont (63) published his direct observation of digestion made possible by studies of his patient, Alexis St. Martin, who suffered a bullet wound in his abdomen that healed with a fistula allowing direct observation of the stomach and its contents (63). The understanding of the way food was digested and absorbed was advanced by

Magendie and his distinguished pupil Claude Bernard, the leaders of the French physiological school. It was Bernard who demonstrated the digestive function of the pancreas (64).

These 19th-century observations on digestion were followed in the early 20th century by the seminal and long-lasting theory that hunger resulted from gastric contractions. This theory was based on direct measurements of the association of gastric contraction with hunger by Cannon and Washburn (65) and independently by Carlson (66).

D. Chemistry and Biochemistry

Modern chemistry might be traced to the 17th-century work of Rober Boyle, who established the concept of chemical elements (67). By the late 17th century, Boyle (6) recognized that when a lighted candle went out, a mouse living in the same environment rapidly died. It was clear that some important element was present in the air that was essential for life and for the candle to burn. At the beginning of the 18th century, George Stahl (69) postulated that this substance was phlogiston. It was not until the work of Priestley (70), of Scheele who simultaneously discovered what we now call oxygen (71), and particularly of Lavoisier (72) that the phlogiston theory was replaced by the oxygen theory of combustion.

The Oxygen Theory culminated from the research of Lavoisier in the last three decades of the 18th century. Lavoisier recognized from his work that oxidation meant combining with oxygen. His experimental work showed that metabolism was similar to combustion (72). Lavoisier's death at the hands of Revolutionary French government in 1794 deprived humanity of one of its great intellects.

The legacy of Lavoisier from the 18th century served as the basis for the laws of the conservation of mass and energy (73) and formed the basis for the work of Rubner (74,75), who formulated the law of surface area based on the observation of a linear relationship between metabolic expenditure of animals of many sizes and their surface area [body weight]$^{0.7}$. This law of surface area and the work of Pettenkofer and Voit (76) in Germany were the framework on which Atwater and Rosa constructed the first functional human calorimeter at Wesleyan College in Middletown, Connecticut in 1896 (77). The instrument served as a tool for extensive studies on metabolic requirements during food intake and on the effects of starvation by Atwater (78) and by Benedict (79,80).

Following the work of Atwater and Benedict in the early 20th century, studies using metabolic chambers languished until after World War II. The earliest of these post–World War II chambers were built in Paris, France, and at the National Institutes of Health in Bethesda, Maryland. However, it was the chamber built in Lausanne, Switzerland, by Jequier (81) that has provided the most extensive and continuing series of studies on energy expenditure in human subjects in the post–World War II period. This chamber and the ones built in Phoenix, Arizona, patterned after the one in Lausanne and the one in London built by Garrow (82), have shown that for human beings, fat-free mass provides a slightly better relationship between energy expenditure than surface area. Utilizing this information, several predictors of obesity have developed including a low metabolic rate, a high rate of carbohydrate oxidation as indicated by a high respiratory quotient (RQ), and insulin sensitivity (83).

The study of energy expenditure in human beings and animals has advanced rapidly in the past two decades following the introduction of doubly labeled water as a technique for measuring total energy expenditure in free-living subjects (84). Doubly labeled water measures energy expenditure by following the path of deuterium and oxygen through the metabolic pathways in the body compartments. Deuterium can only be excreted as water while ^{18}O can be excreted as urinary water or as carbon dioxide following respiratory combustion of carbon containing compounds. Thus, the ratio of deuterium to ^{18}O gradually diverges following the administration of these isotopic forms of water and this rate of diversion can be used to calculate energy expenditure if the respiratory quotient is known. Application of this technique to human beings shows that overweight people underestimate their dietary intake more than normal-weight people (81,85). This tool has provided a new paradigm by which to assess energy needs and questions the validity of data obtained from dietary records.

The chemistry of biological systems was the natural outgrowth of chemistry. The term "biology" as the study of living things with the "cell" as its base unit was a 19th-century concept. Biological chemistry, or biochemistry, is also a 19th-century concept, which may be dated from the demonstration by Wohler (86) in 1828 that urea, an organic molecule, could be synthesized from inorganic materials.

The study of body composition was also an important 19th-century contribution to the biochemistry of obesity. Chemical analysis of human cadavers was conducted, and the fat stores in adipose tissue were demonstrated to be primarily triglyceride (86).

Biological chemistry in the mid-19th century was dominated by Claude Bernard (diabetes) and his teacher Magendie (87) in France and by Liebig and his studies of food chemistry in Germany (88). Magendie was a leader in the application of the experimental method to the study of living animals. His pupil, Claude Bernard, discovered liver glycogen as the source of blood glucose (89). He also showed that damage (*piqure*) to the hypothalamus could produce glycosuria. His scientific philosophy was one of "gradualism." Scientific theory would naturally lead to step-by-step progress, a concept that was a dominant element in the 19th-century philosophy of science. This concept of gradualism is in sharp contrast to the concept of paradigm shifts (90) and scientific revolutions (91) (see below).

Claude Bernard's contemporary in Germany was Liebig. His concept that the macronutrients, carbohydrates, proteins, and fat were all that were needed for nutrition served as the basis for nutritional science during much of the 19th century. Overthrow of this theory by the discovery of vitamins at the turn of the 20th century gave birth to the field of nutrition (92). The development of nutrition through the first last half of the 20th century is epitomized by the discovery of vitamins and their function. This era closed in 1948 with the elucidation of the structure of vitamin B_{12}. With the closing of this era, the impact of macronutrients again took center stage through the recognition of the role of dietary fats and obesity as "causes" of chronic disease (93,94).

The 20th century has seen an explosion in the application of chemical and biochemical techniques to the study of obesity. Sophistication in the measurement of body components has greatly expanded. The work by Behnke, Feen, and Welham applied the techniques of density for quantitating the fat and nonfat compartments of the body (95). This methodology has been followed by the application of radioactive isotopes (96) to the study of body composition by many workers after World War II (97). New techniques have continued to provide ever better ways of characterizing the human body. Radioactive isotopes have largely been replaced by stable isotopes. The introduction of ultrasound for measuring fat thickness, of computed axial tomographic (CT) scans and magnetic resonance imaging (MRI) scans to measure regional fat distributions, the use of dual energy X-ray absorptiometry to measure body fat, lean body compartments, and bone mineral, and the use of whole body neutron activation have provided sophisticated techniques for accurate and detailed determination of body composition in vivo (98).

E.   Genetics and Molecular Biology

The setting for the biological revolution of the last quarter of the 20th century had its roots in the mid-19th century with the publication by Darwin of the *Origin of the Species* (99) and by Mendel of the unitized inheritable traits subsequently called genes (100). In the early 20th century, Garrod suggested the concept of "metabolic" disorders in a classic monograph (100). Genetic work was greatly aided by the use of the fruitfly, *Drosophilia*, with their giant chromosomes, and of mice, whose breeding cycle was relatively short. Gradually genetic material was traced to the nucleus and to deoxyribonucleic acid (DNA). A new field of molecular biology was born from the seminal work of Watson and Crick (101), who proposed the double-helix model for the structure of this DNA leading to the "cracking" of the genetic code and the development of the tools of molecular biology. With these techniques it became possible to identify and isolate the genes underlying the rare forms of inherited obesity in animals (102–104).

The first breakthrough came in 1992 with the identification of the genetic defect in an obese mouse called the yellow obese mouse. The agouti gene, which produces this defect, provides the information to make a 133-amino-acid peptide (102). In the yellow obese mouse, the agouti gene is expressed in many tissues where it is not normally expressed. The resulting agouti protein serves as a competitor for melanocyte stimulating hormone (MSH) receptors and through this mechanism can account for the yellow coat color and hyperphagia present in these animals.

Shortly after the discovery of the agouti gene, the genetic defect in the *ob/ob* mouse was identified (103). The *ob* gene is altered with a stop message (codon) at amino acid 105. This truncates the normal 167-amino-acid protein leptin. In the normal animal leptin appears to signal the brain about the state of peripheral fat stores and their adequacy for reproduction. Leptin is also involved in modulating a number of other steroid messages. In the obese (*ob/ob*) mouse, leptin will reverse the obesity and correct the other defects.

The third obesity gene to be cloned was for the recessively inherited FAT mouse (104). The nature of this gene defect was suspected from the high levels of proinsulin in these animals. Cleavage of insulin to proinsulin requires the enzyme carboxypeptidase E. It was subsequently determined that this gene was defective, resulting in defective synthesis of hormones and neuromediators, from prothormones and proneuromediators.

Genetic susceptibility for human obesity has also benefitted from the advances in genetics and molecular biology. Beginning with the work of Davenport (105) on the inheritance of body mass index in families and the work of Verschuer on identical twins (106), a growing body of data argues that important components of total-body fat mass and fat distribution are inherited (107,108). From this basis in epidemiological data, a search has begun for the genes that are involved in human (109) and animal forms of obesity. From the studies of responsiveness to

dietary fat in animals, at least 12 different genes have been identified as playing a role (110,111). In human beings, a large and growing number of candidate genes have been explored for their possible relationship with the development of obesity and several have been shown to contribute in small ways to this syndrome (109).

F. Pharmacology

The field of pharmacology, the study of drugs and their biological effects, grew from a base in chemistry (112) and the early findings in biology. Its early successes included the isolation of morphine, strychnine, emitine, and quinine and the publication of the first *Pharmacopeia* by Magendie in 1822 (13). One of the major advances in this field in the 19th century was the introduction of anesthesia, which was discovered almost simultaneously by three Americans, Crawford Long, W. T. G. Morton, and Horace Wells, between 1842 and 1846 (114–116). The first effective public demonstration was given in the Ether Dome of the Massachusettes General Hospital in Boston, Massachusetts in October 1846. This was followed by the introduction of carbolic acid to reduce infection in the operating room by Sir Joseph Lister in 1865 (117,118).

The 19th century also saw a number of efforts at "pharmacological" treatment of obesity. Among these were the use of hydrotherapy and various laxatives and purgatives. Thyroid extract was also initially used to treat obesity in the late 19th century, beginning in 1893.

A key element in the entire field of pharmacology was the discovery of aniline in the 19th century (119). Developed by the dye industry, aniline served as the base for synthesizing numerous drugs in the 20th century and for the "magic bullet" concept of Ehrlich (120). Dinitrophenol was one of these aniline products. It was introduced for treatment of obesity, when weight loss was noted in workers in the chemical industry who handled dinitrophenol. This drug was subsequently abandoned after it produced cataracts and neuropathy. This tragedy of treatment shows the need for careful clinical evaluation of drugs before they are made available for general clinical use.

Amphetamine was a second product of the synthetic organic chemical industry that was used for treatment of obesity. In the 1930s, dextroamphetamine, which was synthesized in 1887 (121), was shown to produce weight loss in individuals being treated for narcolepsy (122). Because amphetamine is addictive, it fell into disrepute and lead to a negative view of all drugs with a similar chemical structure. However, the similarity of chemical structure on paper proved misleading pharmacologically. The β-phenethylamine chemical structure is the backbone of amphetamine (alpha-methyl β-phenethylamine). Amphetamine affects two neurotransmitter, dopamine and norepinephrine. Modifying the β-phenethylamine structure can completely change the effect on neurotransmitter. Phentermine is a β-phenethylamine cousin of amphetamine that affects only norepinephrine. Fenfluramine, another β-phenethylamine cousin, is pharmacologically unrelated to amphetamine since it affects only serotonin.

G. Neuroscience

A neural basis for some kinds of obesity became evident at the beginning of the 20th century. The case reports by Babinski (123) and by Frohlich (124) were preceded by a case reported by Mohr (125). Each report described single individuals who developed obesity in association with a tumor at the base of the brain. This important clinical finding opened a new field of research and heralded the development of techniques to produce obesity by injection of toxic material such as chromic oxide at the base of the brain (126) or, more specifically, by localized electrolytic or thermal damage to specific hypothalamic nuclei (127). Such a specific anatomical localization of hypothalamic centers where damage would produce either increased food intake (damage to ventromedial hypothalamus) or decreased food intake (damage to lateral hypothalamus) (128) led, in 1954, to the dual-center hypothesis of Stellar (129), which served as the basis for thinking about hunger and satiety for the next 20 years.

It soon became clear that hyperphagia was not essential for the development of obesity after a hypothalamic lesion (130) or in genetically obese mice (131). An alternative explanation for the development of obesity was provided by the autonomic hypothesis (132) based on the observations of increased activity of the vagus nerve and parasympathetic nervous system (133) and reduced activity of the sympathetic nervous system (134). This insight, coupled with the role of brown adipose tissue and the thermogenic component of the sympathetic nervous system in heat generation in small animals and in inhibiting food intake, have been central to the development of β-adrenergic drugs as potential agents for treating obesity (135).

The discovery of peptides that are usually present in the brain and in the gastrointestinal tract has brought together the areas of neuroscience and physiology in the control of body fat and obesity. Secretin was the first GI hormone found (136). Subsequently, cholecystokinin was found to stimulate contraction of the gall bladder and then to reduce food intake (137). Of the many peptides now known, neuropeptide Y is among the most interesting because it will stimulate food intake and produce obesity when given continuously (138).

H. Clinical Medicine and Obesity

Well before the scientific era, which I have dated as beginning in A.D. 1500, individuals with massive obesity have been noteworthy. Table 2 lists some of the largest individuals on record. Cases of monstrous obesity have been noted since antiquity (29,30,139,140). In the 19th century, Dubourg (141) discussed 25 cases, Schindler (142) identified 17 such cases, and a Maccary 11 (143). Individual cases have also been reported by many other authors (144–153). These individuals were frequently noted for their "odd" or "monstrous" appearance. The outlook for this group was particularly bleak, from both a clinical and social perspective.

These case reports beg a very important question, which has only recently begun to be answered. That is, are all cases of obesity the same? Classification of obesity can be viewed as one component of the more general ef-

Table 2 Cases of Extraordinary Obesity

Name	Gender	Age at death	Maximum weight (kg)	Ref.
Lambert	M	39	335	1
Bright	M		280	Coe
Darden	M	59	462	3
Campbell	M	22	332	Gould
Valenzuela	M	39	385	3
Titman	—	36	318	2
Zadina	M	29	332	2
Raggio	M	27	381	2
—	F		385	Gould
Maguire	M	31	367	2
Karns	F	28	338	2
Nunez	F	23	343	2
Hall	M	37	318	2
Pontico	F	35	350	2
Hughes	M	32	485	3
Craig	M	38	411	3
Knorr	M	46	408	3
King	F	35	381	3

Sporadic cases of obesity have been noted since antiquity. Gould and Pyle (140) describe a large number of cases of massive obesity in children and adults. They cite the writings of Athenaeus, who described Darius, the tyrant of Heraclea, as so enormous that he was in constant danger of suffocation, which was treated by putting needles in the back of his chair. Several other very fat people identified by Gould and Pyle are William the Conqueror; Charles le Gros; Louis le Gros; Humbert II, Count of Maurienne; Henry I, King of Navarre; Henry III, Count of Champagne; Conan III, Duke of Brittany; Sancho I, King of Leon; Alphonse II, King of Portugal; the Italian poet Bruni, who died in 1635; Vivonne, a General under Louis XIV; Frederick I, King of Wurtemberg; and Louis XVII.

forts to classify diseases. Although many classifications of disease exist, one of the most interesting was the effort to classify disease based on the classification of plants and animals introduced by Linnaeus (154). His system involved giving each individual a genus and species name and categorizing the genera more generally into classes, orders, and phyla. Although Sydenham began such a systematic classification of disease, the two best-known efforts to classify diseases in this way were published by Sauvages (155) and Cullen (156). In both of them obesity was called "polysarcie." In the English translation of Cullen's work obesity is in class III, "The Cachexieas." It is listed under the second order called Intumescentiae with a genus name of *Polysarcia* (corporis pinguedinosa intumescentia molesta). Obesity, as a word to describe increased fatness, gradually replaced polysarcie, embonpoint, and corpulence during the 19th century. A more detailed discussion of the classifications of obesity, beginning with the division into endogenous and exogenous by von Noorden, can be found in this chapter.

The first book to deal entirely with this problem is the book by Wadd entitled *Comments on Corpulency, Lineaments of Leanness* (39). In this book he reports a series of clinical cases, many with illustrations of morbidly obese individuals presented both descriptively and graphically. Most of the cases were from correspondence, a characteristic way of evaluating patients by "consulting physicians" since the physical examination was not a part of the usual examination. Of the 12 cases he presents, all patients but one were men. Weights were noted in five and ranged from 106 kg (16 st 10 lb, or 234 lb) to 146 kg (23 st 2 lb, or 324 lb). Two of the patients examined at postmortem had enormous accumulations of fat. Although autopsy observations of obese individuals had been made previously, this is the first instance in which they are included in a monograph devoted to obesity.

Wadd notes that sudden death is not uncommon in the corpulent, thus revalidating Hippocrates. "A sudden palpitation excited in the heart of a fat man has often proved as fatal as a bullet through the thorax." In several of the cases, corpulent patients were seeking specific pills to treat their obesity. Wadd makes a distinction between the therapeutic activists and those favoring less aggressive therapy, with the homeopathists being at the far extreme with minimal dosage of medication. "Truly it has been said—some Doctors let the patient die, for fear they should kill him; while others kill the patient, for fear he should die."

One important lesson from these massively obese individuals was the association of obesity with sleep apnea, a disease often referred to as the Pickwickian syndrome (157,158). Patients with alveolar hypoventilation, which produces this syndrome, date back to Greco-Roman times (29,30). The earliest published report of hypoventilation and its consequences was by Russel in 1866 (159).

Other clinical subtypes of obesity, in addition to the massively obese, have been gradually recognized. Cases of hypothalamic injury with obesity have been identified since 1840 (125), and received particular attention following the reports by Babinski (123) and by Frohlich (124). Also, in the early 20th century Cushing recognized (160) that obesity was associated with basophilic adenomas of the pituitary gland (161). Cushing's syndrome can also be caused by medication with adrenal steroids and has been associated with the use of a number of other drugs, including phenothiazines, some antidepressants (amitriptyline), some anticonvulsants (valproate), and antiserotonin drugs (cyproheptadine). Other endocrine diseases such as hypogonadism and isolated growth hormone deficiency are also associated with increased fat deposits. Several rare genetic disorders have obesity as a finding (109). Finally, a sedentary life-style and a high-fat diet, particularly in animals, have been reported to produce obesity.

Besides the lessons from individual patients that have been provided by these case reports are the lessons that come from evaluation of collective data. Quetelet (162) was one of the leaders in developing "mathematical" methods to evaluate populations. He developed the concept of the "average man" and used the ratio of weight divided by the square of stature (kg/m^2) as a measure of an individual's fatness. This unit, the body mass index, might be termed the Quetelet Index (QI) after the man who developed what has become a widely used way of evaluating weight status.

A second important population based view of clinical medicine came from the life insurance industry (94). As early as 1901, data began to appear showing that both excess amounts of weight and central distribution of this weight were associated with shortened life expectancy. Because of the financial need to relate risk to policy costs, the insurance industry has continued to provide data showing these relationships. This information was responsible for stimulating evaluation of the association of weight status with mortality risks in a variety of population-based studies (163–167). In all of these studies, a curvilear increase in risk of mortality is associated with rising weight or body mass (Quetelet) index.

Although the relationship of central fat to increased mortality could be discerned in these early insurance studies, it remained for Vague (168) to bring this concept to the attention of professionals. Although Vague's data is clear, the measurement of the adipomuscular ratio that he used was a complex one and it remained for the simpler measurement of waist-to-hip circumference ratio and the subscapular skinfold measurement to provide the wide recognition for the risk that centrally located fat poses. With better methods of measuring fat distribution with CT and MRI scans, it is now clear that increased visceral fat is the principal culprit.

I. Treatment of Obesity

1. Treatment with Diet and Exercise

> In America there are fewer cures for obesity undertaken than abroad . . . because . . . there are fewer obese people here.
>
> Carter et al. (169)

This statement was made in 1917, but time and the tides have overcome America, which now has an epidemic of obesity.

The clinical approach to treatment of obesity long antedates the scientific era. From the time of Hippocrates (170) and Galen (171) in the prescientific era, diet and exercise were an integral part of the therapeutic regimen for obese patients. Hippocrates, the "father of medicine," suggested in the 5th century B.C. that:

> Obese people and those desiring to lose weight should perform hard work before food. Meals should be taken after exertion and while still panting from fatigue and with no other refreshment before meals except only wine, diluted and slightly cold. Their meals should be prepared with a sesame or seasoning and other similar substances and be of a fatty nature as people get thus, satiated with little food. They should, moreover, eat only once a day and take no baths and sleep on a hard bed and walk naked as long as possible (170).

Nearly 2,000 years ago, Galen outlined his approach to treatment of the obese as follows:

> I have made any sufficiently stout patient moderately thin in a short time, by compelling him to do rapid running, then wiping off his perspiration with very soft or very rough muslin and then massaging him maximally with diaphoretic inunctions, which the younger doctors customarily call restoratives, and after such massage leading him to the bath after which I give him nourishment immediately but bade him rest for a while and do nothing to which he was accustomed, then lead him to a second bath and then gave him abundant food of little nourishment so as to fill him up but distribute little of it to the entire body (171).

From this Greco-Roman beginning, dietary treatment can be traced to the Arabic tradition in medicine. In the

first book of Avicenna's Cannon he describes how to reduce the overweight individual.

> The regimen which will reduce obesity. (1) Produce a rapid descent of the food from the stomach and intestines, in order to prevent completion of absorption by the mesentery. (2) Take food which is bulky but feebly nutritious. (3) Take the bath before food, often. (4) Hard exercise . . . (172).

When the Western medical tradition moved to Europe in the 11th–13th centuries, so did the concepts of hygiene, diet, and exercise. These were embodied in the "institutes of medicine," a major component of medical education for centuries. One of the most widely used guides was the *Regimen Sanitatis* (173) developed at Salerno in the 12th century, which did not specifically provide advice for obesity. Chaucer, the 14th-century poet, did reiterate the advice flowing from Hippocrates when he said: "Agonys glotonye, the remedie is abstinence." ("Against gluttony the remedy is abstinence").

Dietary treatment in the 18th century was summarized by Tweedie:

> In attempting its cure, when the habit is threatened with any morbid effects, from the plethora existing either in the head or lungs, this must be removed by a bleeding or two; and as corpulent people do not bear blood-letting well, purging is most to be depended upon for the removal of the plethora (174).
>
> He also says that the diet should be sparing. They should abstain from spirits, wines, and malt liquors, drinking in their stead, either spring water, toast and water, or else water agreeably acidulated by any pure vegetable acids.

Finally he increases exercise gradually.

The 18th-century Italian layman Cornaro (175) was a champion of dietary moderation after he successfully conquered his own obesity. At the beginning of his book he says:

> O wretched, miserable Italy! Does not though plain see, that gluttony deprives [us] of more soul years, than either war, or the plague itself could have done? (p. 5).

Cornaro's doctor's advice was to eat or drink nothing that was not wholesome and that only in small quantities.

Comments on obesity have occasionally come from the field of gastronomy with the classic work by Brillat-Savarin in 1825 being the best known. This masterpiece has been published in many attractive and beautifully illustrated editions (176). He attributes obesity to two causes.

> The first is the natural temperament of the individual. . . . The second principal cause of obesity lies in the starches and flours which man uses as the base for his daily nourishment. . . . A double cause of obesity results from too much sleep combined with too little exercise. . . . The final cause of obesity is excess, whether in eating or drinking.

From this, Brillat-Savarin moves to treatment. He says:

> Any cure of obesity must begin with the three following and absolute precepts: discretion in eating, moderation in sleeping, and exercise on foot or on horseback.

Having said this much he goes on to say:

> Such are the first commandments which science makes to us: nevertheless I place little faith in them.
> . . .

He then goes on to recommend a diet low in grains and starches.

In spite of the long history of dietary recommendations for treatment of obesity, it wasn't until 1863 that the first "popular" diet book appeared. This was a small, 21-page pamphlet by Mr. William Banting entitled *A Letter on Corpulence Addressed to the Public* (177). In this pamphlet, he recounted his successful weight loss experience using a diet prescribed by his ear surgeon, Dr. William Harvey (178). The immediate success of this pamphlet led to reprinting worldwide and a popularization of the term "Bantingism" to refer to his diet.

Banting's cure (very severe) was as follows:

Breakfast, 8 A.M.: 150–180 g 5–6 oz) meat or broiled fish (not a fat variety of either); a small biscuit or 30 g (1 oz) dry toast; a large cup of tea or coffee without cream, milk, or sugar

Dinner, 1 P.M.: Meat or fish as at breakfast, or any kind of game or poultry, same amount; any vegetable except those that grow underground, such as potatoes, parsnips, carrots, or beets; dry toast, 30 g (1 oz); cooked fruit without sugar; good claret, 300 cc (10 oz), Madeira, or sherry

Tea, 5 P.M.: Cooked fruit, 60–90 g (2–3 oz); one or two pieces of zwieback; tea, 270 cc (9 oz) without milk, cream, or sugar

Supper, 8 P.M.: Meat or fish, as at dinner, 90–120 cc (3–4 oz); claret or sherry, water, 210 cc (7 oz)

Fluids restricted to 1050 cc (35 oz)/day.

From these humble beginnings, diet books by professionals, self-styled professionals, and lay people have continued to appear, particularly as the concerns about obesity as a health and cosmetic problem have increased (5).

I have summarized two diets from the early 20th century to show the approaches that were used at that time (169).

Von Noorden's Diet. Von Noorden, one of the leading scholars of obesity at the beginning of the 20th century, based his dietary approach on an estimate of the caloric requirement. Basal calorie needs were estimated from ideal weight. For this he assumed that a 70-kg individual would require 37 kcal/kg, or 2590 calories. If the individual weighed an extra 30 kg, he or she would need 1110 extra calories to feed his extra 30 kg. Von Noorden's first-degree reduction diet reduced energy to 80% of the basal needs, or for the 70-kg individuals to 2000 kcal/day. His second-degree reduction diet reduced intake to 60%, or 1500 kcal/day for the individual requiring 2500 kcal/day. His third-degree reduction, which was infrequently used, lowered calories to 40%, or 1000 kcal/day. His dietary approach also reduced fat to 30 g/day. His protein allowance was 120–180 g/day with carbohydrate intake around 100 g/day. His menu plan, adapted from Carter et al. (169), is summarized as follows:

	Minimal	Maximal
Protein	120 g (4 oz) = 492 cal	180 g (6 oz) = 738 cal
Fat	30 g (1 oz) = 280 cal	30 g (1 oz) = 280 cal
Carbohydrate	100 g (3⅓ oz) = 410 cal	120 g (4 oz) = 492 cal
	1182 cal	1510 cal

A sample of the Von Noorden Diet is shown below:

Breakfast: Lean meat, 80 g (2⅔ oz); bread, 25 g (1 oz); tea, one cup with milk, no sugar

Midmorning: One egg

Luncheon: Soup, 1 small portion; lean meat, 160 g (5⅓ oz); potatoes, 100 g (3⅓ oz); fruit, 100 g (3⅓ oz)

Afternoon:
3 P.M. Cup of black coffee
4 P.M. Fruit, 200 g (6⅔ oz)
6 P.M. Milk, 250 cc (8 oz)

Dinner: Meat, 125 g (3⅙ oz); bread (graham), 30 g (1 oz); fruit, small portion as sauce without sugar; salad, vegetable or fruit, radishes, pickles

Ebstein's Diet. At the other extreme is the high-fat diet illustrated by Ebstein's diet. Ebstein modified existing diets by allowing a considerable amount of fat and restricting the carbohydrates by forbidding all sugar, sweets, and potatoes, but allowing 180–210 g (6–7 oz) of bread. Vegetables that grow above ground are allowed and all sorts of meat, especially fat, is permitted. Fats are allowed at 120–180 g (4–6 oz)/day. He used a three-meal plan with the largest meal at midday.

> Breakfast: One large cup of black tea, without cream or milk, or sugar; white or brown bread, 60 g (2 oz) with plenty of butter
>
> Dinner, 2 P.M.: Clear soup, meat 120–180 g (4–6 oz) with gravy, especially fat meat, is recommended; vegetables in abundance (as noted above); small amount of fresh or stewed fruit (without sugar) or salad; two or three glasses of light white wine; shortly after dinner a cup of tea is allowed with sugar or milk
>
> Supper, 7:30 P.M.: Large cup of tea, without sugar or milk; one egg with or without a small portion of meat, preferably fat; occasionally a little cheese or fresh fruit
>
> Total values: Protein, 100 g (3⅓ oz); fat, 85 g (3 oz); carbohydrate, 50 g (2⅔ oz)

These two approaches, the low-fat–high-protein–high-carbohydrate diet and the high-fat–low-carbohydrate diet, have been repeating themes throughout the 20th century but their origins were in the late 19th century. Had either of these approaches "cured" obesity, as their proponents suggested, there would have been no need for the continual supply of new diets that we have seen throughout the 20th century (5).

As a prelude to its clinical application, the metabolic features of starvation were explored by Benedict using metabolic chambers (79,80), and the suggestion that calories could be dissipated by "luxuskonsumption," or burning off of unneeded calories, was promulgated by Gulick (179) and Neumann (180) but challenged by the critical studies of Wiley Newburgh (181).

A practical application of the work on starvation was published by Evans (182), who showed the potential benefits of a very low calorie food diet. Although Evans continued to publish on this approach to diet until the beginning of World War II (182), this idea was lost sight of until "fasting" was reintroduced as a treatment for obesity by Bloom in 1959 (183). Following this enthusiastic report, the field gradually moved to the use of liquid formula diets, which were initially popularized from the Rockefeller University metabolic ward and reached a major crisis with the report of 17 deaths following a formula diet compounded from gelatin (184), proving again that gelatin protein is inadequate for human nutrition

(92,185). New diets subsequently appeared using high-quality protein, and sales reached another peak with the hospital-based programs of the late 1980s. When the U.S. Government raised concerns about these diets and other "commercial weight control" programs (186), there was a rapid and sudden decrease in public interest and a loss of commercial profitability.

2. Behavior Modification

One of the central developments in the treatment of obesity in the 20th century has been in the behavioral field. Following the introduction of psychoanalytic techniques by Freud and his colleagues (187), several theories were proposed, suggesting that obesity might result from "personality" disorders. These were carefully tested and found to be wanting (188). That obesity had important social components, however, became clear from its relation to socioeconomic status (189). The prevalence of obesity was found to be much higher in the lower social and economic groups than in the higher social and economic groups in this seminal Manhattan study.

Although psychoanalytic approaches were unproductive as a basis for treatment, other streams of behavioral research were productive. One of these approaches stems from the work on conditioned reflexes by Pavlov and his followers (190) and the other from the work on operant behavior by Skinner (191,192). It was an adaptation of these latter techniques that was used by Stuart (193) in his classic study in 1967. Stuart treated 11 patients, eight of whom were available for follow-up at the end of the year. In this group, weight losses using techniques of monitoring food intake and manipulating the environment in which it was eaten were indeed striking. Subsequent to this seminal work, the principles of behavior modification have been widely applied, and some would consider them to be central to the treatment of obesity in the late 20th century.

3. Pharmacotherapy

As the understanding of pharmacology has increased, so too has its application to treatment of obesity become more focused. Although one might call Withering the "Father of Pharmacology" because he published his findings on digitalis (194) in 1785, the first chemical work was in the early 19th century and during the important period of French hegemony in medicine (8). A summary of 19th-century treatments is provided by Sajous (195).

> Besides the familiar dietetic treatment, thyroid gland to enhance catabolism, but not in the large doses

usually prescribed, which provide hypercatabolism and greatly weaken the patient. From 2 to 3 grains t.i.d. are enough to increase gradually the lipolytic power of the blood. Potassium iodide in increasing doses can be used instead, when thyroid extract cannot be obtained. Hyoscine hydrobromate 1/100 grain t.i.d. assists the reducing process by increasing the propulsive activity of the arterioles and causing them to drive an excess of blood into the fat-laden areas. Carlsbad, Homburg, and Marienbad waters owe their virtues mainly to the alkaline and purgative salts they contain, especially sodium sulphate. As a beverage alkaline Vichy water is advantageous to enhance the osmotic properties of the blood and facilitate the elimination of wastes (p. 1867).

Shortly after the discovery of endocrine organ extracts in the 19th century, they were used for the treatment of obesity, as early as the 1890s (195).

The fact that thyroid preparations in sufficient doses promote the rapid combustion of fats has caused them to be used extensively in this disorder. . . . In large doses [thyroid gland] . . . imposes hyperoxidation upon all cells . . . we behold gradual emaciation beginning with the adipose tissues, which are the first to succumb. Hence the use of thyroid preparations in obesity.

Sajous goes on to say that small doses (66 mg or 1 grain) are indicated in all cases to begin with.

Briefly, in all cases of obesity in which thyroid gland is rationally indicated, the feature to determine is whether directly or indirectly hypothyroidia underlies the adiposis (195).

Sajous also describes the use of testicular extracts: "Testicular preparations, including spermine, have been recommended in a host of disorders, particularly . . . obesity . . . but others again have failed to obtain any favorable results" (195).

The first serendipitous observation on the use of aniline-derived drugs was the discovery by Lesses and Myerson (122), in 1937, that amphetamines might be useful in the treatment of obesity. This molecule underwent many chemical medications including the synthesis of fenfluramine, a drug that was shown to act on serotonergic mechanisms. Realizing that both serotonergic and noradrenergic receptors were involved in modulating food intake, Weintraub et al. in 1992 published a 4-year study showing that combination therapy might be better than monotherapy (196). This classic series of papers has opened a whole new pharmacological approach to obesity.

4. Surgery

Surgical intervention for excess fat can be dated from Talmudic times. According to Preuss (197), Rabbi Eleazar was given a sleeping potion and taken into a marble chamber where his abdomen was opened and many basketfuls of fat were removed. "Plinius also describes a very similar 'heroic cure for obesity': the son of the Consul L. Apronius had fat removed and thus his body was relieved of a disgraceful burden." More recently, in A.D. 1190, a surgeon cut open the abdomen of Count Dedo II of Groig "to remove the excessive fat from him" (p. 215). Following the introduction of anesthesia in 1846, this procedure was revived.

The historical review of gastrointestinal function in relation to obesity may be perceived to have reached its zenith (or nadir, depending on one's perspective) with the introduction of gastrointestinal operations for obesity. Three operative approaches have been developed to treat obesity. The first procedure, reported by Kremen et al. (198), was a jejunoileal bypass on a single patient. Believing that if weight were lost, patients would be able to maintain the weight loss, Payne and DeWind performed a series of 11 jejunocolic anastomoses, which produced significant diarrhea and weight loss (199). When the patients were reanastomosed, they regained weight. Against this background, these authors and many others carried out jejunoileal bypass operations, which were associated with numerous metabolic and infectious complications and were largely discontinued as a surgical approach to obesity in the 1970s.

An alternative approach to altering gastrointestinal function to treat obesity was developed by Mason and Ito (200), who performed the first gastric reduction operation. These procedures have now become the dominant operative procedures for the treatment of obesity and are the subject of a major clinical trial in Sweden.

V. TOWARD A SCIENCE OF OBESITY

Toward the end of the Middle Ages, two historical and philosophic traditions, one of Indo-European origin with Greco-Roman philosophy as its base, and the other of Semitic origin with the Hebrew and Christian traditions as its base, reached a form of resolution synthesis in the Hegelian sense (201) from which the Renaissance and modern science both took their roots (1,202).

The modern scientific tradition is the tradition of "experimental" science. That is, progress was made by designing "experiments" to test hypotheses and applying mathematical analysis to the results. The fruitfulness of this tradition is everywhere around us. Its application to

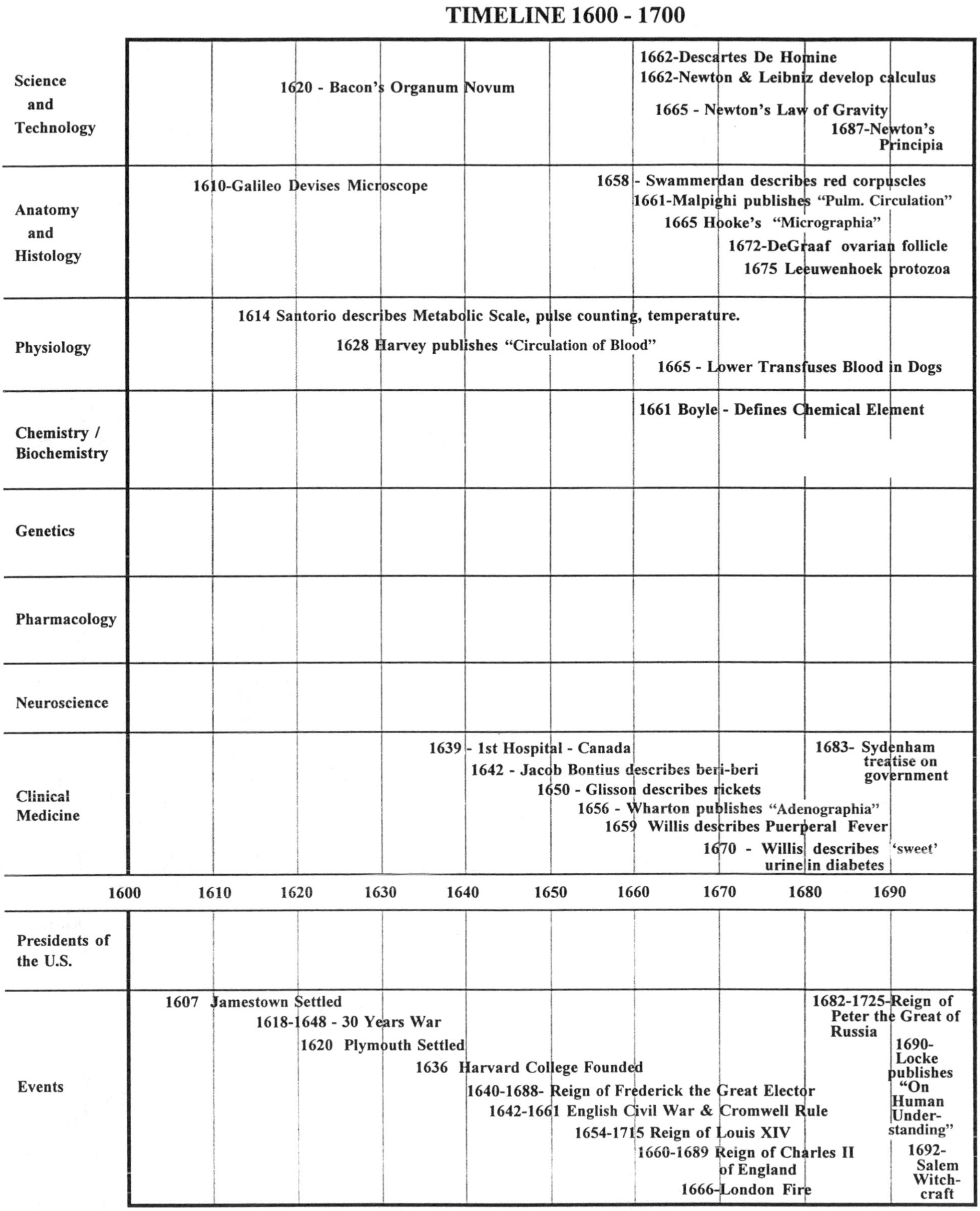

TIMELINE 1600 - 1700

Science and Technology		1620 - Bacon's Organum Novum			1662-Descartes De Homine 1662-Newton & Leibniz develop calculus 1665 - Newton's Law of Gravity 1687-Newton's Principia	
Anatomy and Histology	1610-Galileo Devises Microscope			1658 - Swammerdan describes red corpuscles 1661-Malpighi publishes "Pulm. Circulation" 1665 Hooke's "Micrographia" 1672-DeGraaf ovarian follicle 1675 Leeuwenhoek protozoa	
Physiology	1614 Santorio describes Metabolic Scale, pulse counting, temperature. 1628 Harvey publishes "Circulation of Blood" 1665 - Lower Transfuses Blood in Dogs	
Chemistry / Biochemistry				1661 Boyle - Defines Chemical Element	
Genetics						
Pharmacology						
Neuroscience						
Clinical Medicine			1639 - 1st Hospital - Canada 1642 - Jacob Bontius describes beri-beri 1650 - Glisson describes rickets 1656 - Wharton publishes "Adenographia" 1659 Willis describes Puerperal Fever 1670 - Willis describes 'sweet' urine in diabetes	1683- Sydenham treatise on government

1600	1610	1620	1630	1640	1650	1660	1670	1680	1690

Presidents of the U.S.	
Events	1607 Jamestown Settled 1618-1648 - 30 Years War 1620 Plymouth Settled 1636 Harvard College Founded 1640-1688- Reign of Frederick the Great Elector 1642-1661 English Civil War & Cromwell Rule 1654-1715 Reign of Louis XIV 1660-1689 Reign of Charles II of England 1666-London Fire 1682-1725-Reign of Peter the Great of Russia 1690-Locke publishes "On Human Understanding" 1692-Salem Witchcraft

Figure 4 Time line for developments in science, obesity, and contemporary events in the 17th century. (Copyright ©1996 George A. Bray.)

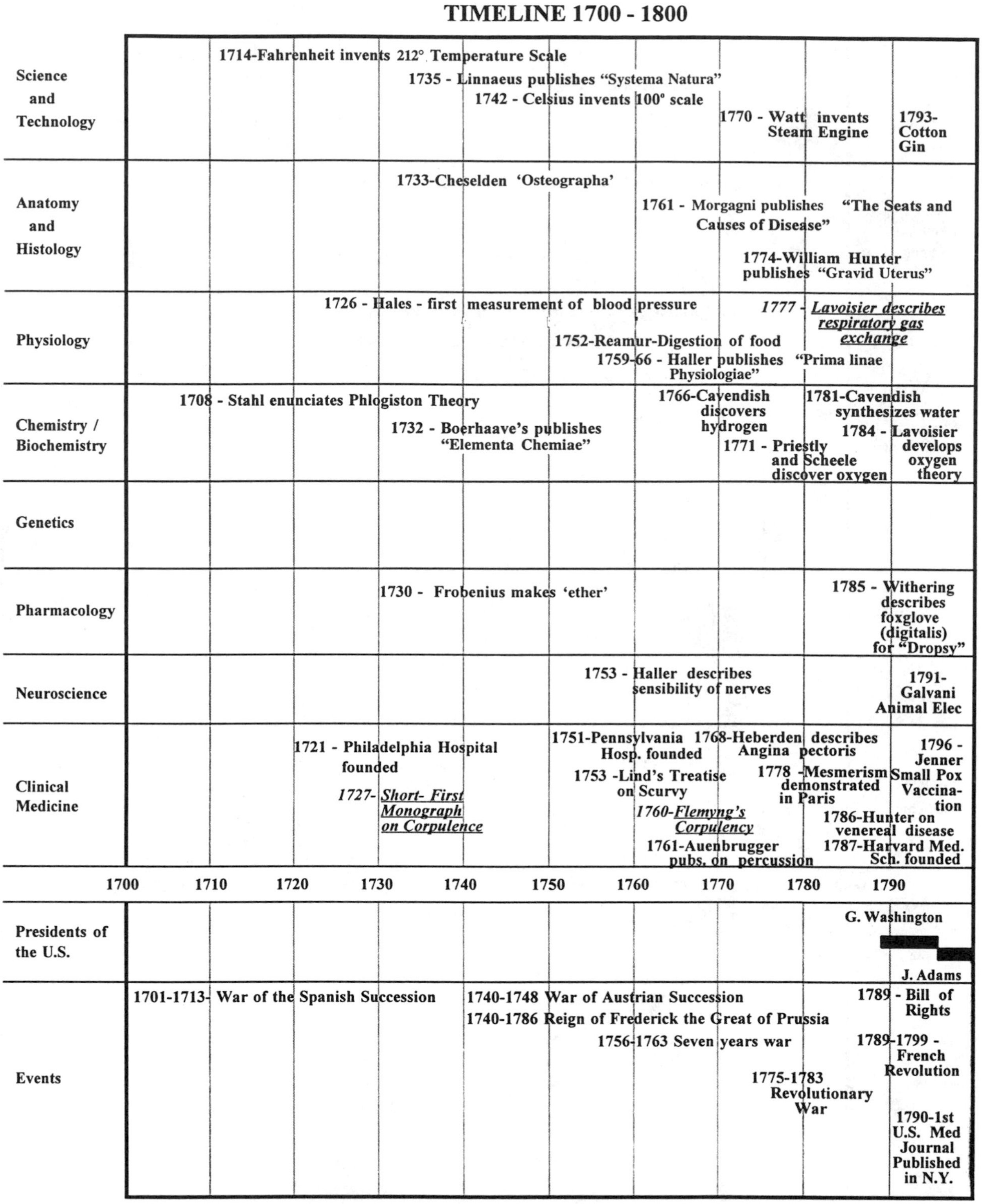

TIMELINE 1700 - 1800

	1700	1710	1720	1730	1740	1750	1760	1770	1780	1790
Science and Technology		1714-Fahrenheit invents 212° Temperature Scale		1735 - Linnaeus publishes "Systema Natura" — 1742 - Celsius invents 100° scale				1770 - Watt invents Steam Engine		1793-Cotton Gin
Anatomy and Histology				1733-Cheselden 'Osteographa'			1761 - Morgagni publishes "The Seats and Causes of Disease"	1774-William Hunter publishes "Gravid Uterus"		
Physiology			1726 - Hales - first measurement of blood pressure			1752-Reamur-Digestion of food — 1759-66 - Haller publishes "Prima linae Physiologiae"		1777 - *Lavoisier describes respiratory gas exchange*		
Chemistry / Biochemistry	1708 - Stahl enunciates Phlogiston Theory			1732 - Boerhaave's publishes "Elementa Chemiae"			1766-Cavendish discovers hydrogen — 1771 - Priestly and Scheele discover oxygen	1781-Cavendish synthesizes water — 1784 - Lavoisier develops oxygen theory		
Genetics										
Pharmacology				1730 - Frobenius makes 'ether'				1785 - Withering describes foxglove (digitalis) for "Dropsy"		
Neuroscience							1753 - Haller describes sensibility of nerves		1791-Galvani Animal Elec	
Clinical Medicine			1721 - Philadelphia Hospital founded — 1727- *Short- First Monograph on Corpulence*			1751-Pennsylvania Hosp. founded — 1753 -Lind's Treatise on Scurvy — 1760-*Flemyng's Corpulency* — 1761-Auenbrugger pubs. on percussion	1768-Heberden describes Angina pectoris — 1778 -Mesmerism demonstrated in Paris — 1786-Hunter on venereal disease — 1787-Harvard Med. Sch. founded	1796 - Jenner Small Pox Vaccination		
Presidents of the U.S.									G. Washington ▬▬ J. Adams	
Events	1701-1713- War of the Spanish Succession				1740-1748 War of Austrian Succession — 1740-1786 Reign of Frederick the Great of Prussia	1756-1763 Seven years war		1775-1783 Revolutionary War	1789 - Bill of Rights — 1789-1799 - French Revolution — 1790-1st U.S. Med Journal Published in N.Y.	

Figure 5 Time line for developments in science, obesity, and contemporary events in the 18th century. (Copyright ©1996 George A. Bray.)

TIMELINE 1800 - 1900

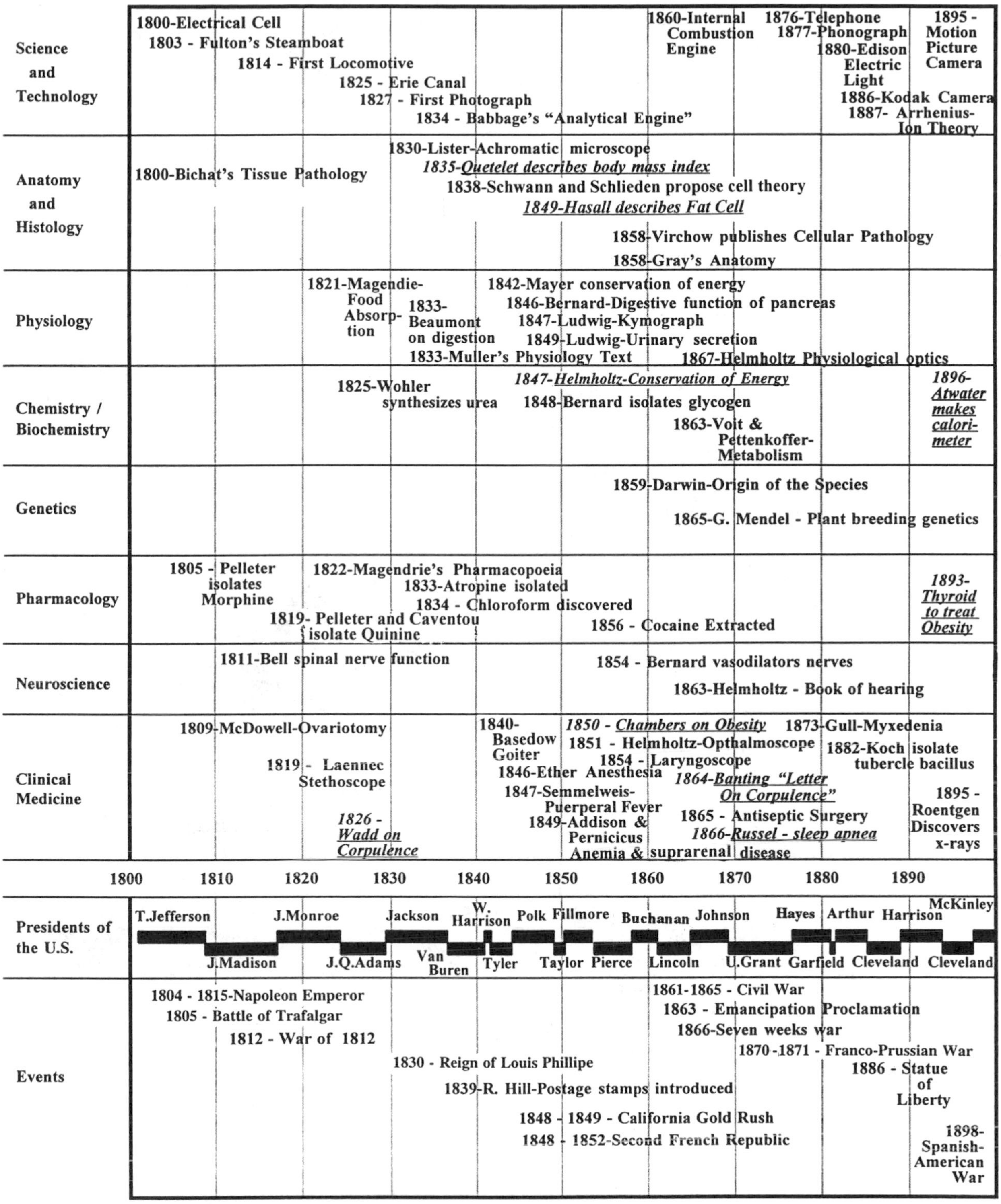

Science and Technology	1800-Electrical Cell · 1803 - Fulton's Steamboat · 1814 - First Locomotive · 1825 - Erie Canal · 1827 - First Photograph · 1834 - Babbage's "Analytical Engine" · 1860-Internal Combustion Engine · 1876-Telephone · 1877-Phonograph · 1880-Edison Electric Light · 1886-Kodak Camera · 1887- Arrhenius-Ion Theory · 1895 - Motion Picture Camera
Anatomy and Histology	1800-Bichat's Tissue Pathology · 1830-Lister-Achromatic microscope · *1835-Quetelet describes body mass index* · 1838-Schwann and Schlieden propose cell theory · *1849-Hasall describes Fat Cell* · 1858-Virchow publishes Cellular Pathology · 1858-Gray's Anatomy
Physiology	1821-Magendie-Food Absorption · 1833-Beaumont on digestion · 1833-Muller's Physiology Text · 1842-Mayer conservation of energy · 1846-Bernard-Digestive function of pancreas · 1847-Ludwig-Kymograph · 1849-Ludwig-Urinary secretion · 1867-Helmholtz Physiological optics
Chemistry / Biochemistry	1825-Wohler synthesizes urea · *1847-Helmholtz-Conservation of Energy* · 1848-Bernard isolates glycogen · 1863-Voit & Pettenkoffer-Metabolism · *1896-Atwater makes calorimeter*
Genetics	1859-Darwin-Origin of the Species · 1865-G. Mendel - Plant breeding genetics
Pharmacology	1805 - Pelleter isolates Morphine · 1819- Pelleter and Caventou isolate Quinine · 1822-Magendrie's Pharmacopoeia · 1833-Atropine isolated · 1834 - Chloroform discovered · 1856 - Cocaine Extracted · *1893-Thyroid to treat Obesity*
Neuroscience	1811-Bell spinal nerve function · 1854 - Bernard vasodilators nerves · 1863-Helmholtz - Book of hearing
Clinical Medicine	1809-McDowell-Ovariotomy · 1819 - Laennec Stethoscope · *1826 - Wadd on Corpulence* · 1840-Basedow Goiter · 1846-Ether Anesthesia · 1847-Semmelweis-Puerperal Fever · 1849-Addison & Pernicicus Anemia & suprarenal disease · *1850 - Chambers on Obesity* · 1851 - Helmholtz-Opthalmoscope · 1854 - Laryngoscope · *1864-Banting "Letter On Corpulence"* · 1865 - Antiseptic Surgery · *1866-Russel - sleep apnea* · 1873-Gull-Myxedenia · 1882-Koch isolate tubercle bacillus · 1895 - Roentgen Discovers x-rays

Decade axis: 1800 · 1810 · 1820 · 1830 · 1840 · 1850 · 1860 · 1870 · 1880 · 1890

Presidents of the U.S.	T.Jefferson · J.Madison · J.Monroe · J.Q.Adams · Jackson · Van Buren · W. Harrison · Tyler · Polk · Taylor · Fillmore · Pierce · Buchanan · Lincoln · Johnson · U.Grant · Hayes · Garfield · Arthur · Cleveland · Harrison · Cleveland · McKinley
Events	1804 - 1815-Napoleon Emperor · 1805 - Battle of Trafalgar · 1812 - War of 1812 · 1830 - Reign of Louis Phillipe · 1839-R. Hill-Postage stamps introduced · 1848 - 1849 - California Gold Rush · 1848 - 1852-Second French Republic · 1861-1865 - Civil War · 1863 - Emancipation Proclamation · 1866-Seven weeks war · 1870-1871 - Franco-Prussian War · 1886 - Statue of Liberty · 1898-Spanish-American War

Figure 6   Time line for developments in science, obesity, and contemporary events in the 19th century. (Copyright ©1996 George A. Bray.)

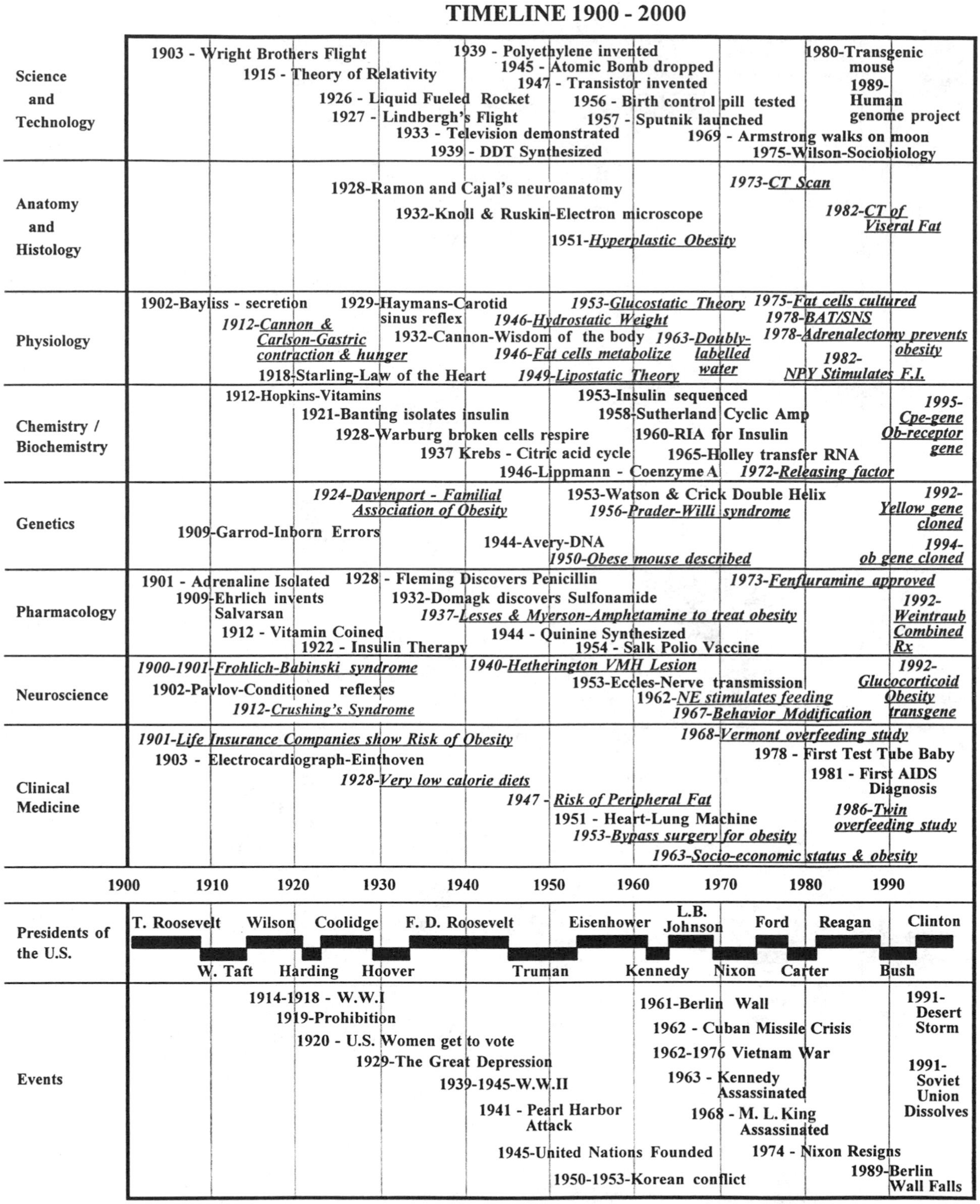

TIMELINE 1900 - 2000

Science and Technology

1903 - Wright Brothers Flight
1915 - Theory of Relativity
1926 - Liquid Fueled Rocket
1927 - Lindbergh's Flight
1933 - Television demonstrated
1939 - DDT Synthesized
1939 - Polyethylene invented
1945 - Atomic Bomb dropped
1947 - Transistor invented
1956 - Birth control pill tested
1957 - Sputnik launched
1969 - Armstrong walks on moon
1975-Wilson-Sociobiology
1980-Transgenic mouse
1989-Human genome project

Anatomy and Histology

1928-Ramon and Cajal's neuroanatomy
1932-Knoll & Ruskin-Electron microscope
1951-*Hyperplastic Obesity*
1973-*CT Scan*
1982-*CT of Viseral Fat*

Physiology

1902-Bayliss - secretion
1912-*Cannon & Carlson-Gastric contraction & hunger*
1918-Starling-Law of the Heart
1929-Haymans-Carotid sinus reflex
1932-Cannon-Wisdom of the body
1946-*Hydrostatic Weight*
1946-*Fat cells metabolize*
1949-*Lipostatic Theory*
1953-*Glucostatic Theory*
1963-*Doubly-labelled water*
1975-*Fat cells cultured*
1978-*BAT/SNS*
1978-*Adrenalectomy prevents obesity*
1982-*NPY Stimulates F.I.*

Chemistry / Biochemistry

1912-Hopkins-Vitamins
1921-Banting isolates insulin
1928-Warburg broken cells respire
1937 Krebs - Citric acid cycle
1946-Lippmann - Coenzyme A
1953-Insulin sequenced
1958-Sutherland Cyclic Amp
1960-RIA for Insulin
1965-Holley transfer RNA
1972-*Releasing factor*
1995-*Cpe-gene Ob-receptor gene*

Genetics

1909-Garrod-Inborn Errors
1924-*Davenport - Familial Association of Obesity*
1944-Avery-DNA
1950-*Obese mouse described*
1953-Watson & Crick Double Helix
1956-*Prader-Willi syndrome*
1992-*Yellow gene cloned*
1994-*ob gene cloned*

Pharmacology

1901 - Adrenaline Isolated
1909-Ehrlich invents Salvarsan
1912 - Vitamin Coined
1922 - Insulin Therapy
1928 - Fleming Discovers Penicillin
1932-Domagk discovers Sulfonamide
1937-*Lesses & Myerson-Amphetamine to treat obesity*
1944 - Quinine Synthesized
1954 - Salk Polio Vaccine
1973-*Fenfluramine approved*
1992-*Weintraub Combined Rx*

Neuroscience

1900-1901-*Frohlich-Babinski syndrome*
1902-Pavlov-Conditioned reflexes
1912-*Crushing's Syndrome*
1940-*Hetherington VMH Lesion*
1953-Eccles-Nerve transmission
1962-*NE stimulates feeding*
1967-*Behavior Modification*
1992-*Glucocorticoid Obesity transgene*

Clinical Medicine

1901-*Life Insurance Companies show Risk of Obesity*
1903 - Electrocardiograph-Einthoven
1928-*Very low calorie diets*
1947 - *Risk of Peripheral Fat*
1951 - Heart-Lung Machine
1953-*Bypass surgery for obesity*
1963-*Socio-economic status & obesity*
1968-*Vermont overfeeding study*
1978 - First Test Tube Baby
1981 - First AIDS Diagnosis
1986-*Twin overfeeding study*

	1900	1910	1920	1930	1940	1950	1960	1970	1980	1990

Presidents of the U.S.

T. Roosevelt — W. Taft — Wilson — Harding — Coolidge — Hoover — F. D. Roosevelt — Truman — Eisenhower — Kennedy — L.B. Johnson — Nixon — Ford — Carter — Reagan — Bush — Clinton

Events

1914-1918 - W.W.I
1919-Prohibition
1920 - U.S. Women get to vote
1929-The Great Depression
1939-1945-W.W.II
1941 - Pearl Harbor Attack
1945-United Nations Founded
1950-1953-Korean conflict
1961-Berlin Wall
1962 - Cuban Missile Crisis
1962-1976 Vietnam War
1963 - Kennedy Assassinated
1968 - M. L. King Assassinated
1974 - Nixon Resigns
1989-Berlin Wall Falls
1991-Desert Storm
1991-Soviet Union Dissolves

Figure 7 Time line for developments in science, obesity, and contemporary events in the 20th century. (Copyright ©1996 George A. Bray.)

obesity has come, as it has come to all other areas, but progress has been slow. From the beginning of the "scientific era" (A.D. 1500) to the beginning of "modern medicine" (A.D. 1800), only a few scholarly theses with obesity as the subject matter had been published (203–208). In general, these theses reflected the Hippocratic and Galenic traditions, or the more contemporary traditions provided by the iatrochemical and iatromechanical views of the world originating in the mechanical and chemical explanations of life. As interest in obesity increased, a much larger number of these were published in the 18th century (209–242), which also saw publication of the first monographs on the subject (243,244). Table 3 lists most English, French, and German monographs up to 1950 (243–294). Two works were published in English before 1800 (Table 3). The first of these was by Thomas Short. He begins by saying, "I believe no age did ever afford more instances of corpulency than our own." From Short's perspective, treatment of obesity required restoring the natural balance and removal of the secondary causes. One should, if possible, pick a place to live where the air is not too moist or too soggy and one should not reside in flat, wet countries or in the city or the woodlands. He thought that exercise was important and that the diet should be "moderate spare and of the more detergent kind."

A second monograph, by Flemyng (244), listed four causes of corpulency. The first cause is "the taking in of too large a quantity of food, especially of the rich and oily kind." He went on to note that not all obese people were big eaters. The second causes of obesity is "too lax a texture of the cellular or fatty membrane . . . whereby its cells or vesicles are liable to be too easily distended." The third cause was an abnormal state of the blood that facilitated the storage of fat in the vesicles. Finally, defective evacuation was also an important cause. Since Flemyng believed sweat, urine, and feces all contained "oil," he believed that the treatment for obesity was to increase the loss of "oil" by each of these three routes. Thus, laxatives and diuretics could be used for treatment.

From the beginning of the 19th century, the base of medical literature relating to obesity increased. Corpulency and polysarcy were the terms most in use at the beginning of the 19th century, but by the end of the century, the term obesity had replaced both of them. Additional monographs on obesity appeared in English, French, and German (Table 3). The cell theory was proposed and fat cells identified. The laws of thermodynamics were developed and tested in animals and human beings by the first part of the 20th century.

I have picked the year 1850 as a dividing line for the beginning of a modern science of obesity (245). This was the time when the French clinical school, which began with the French Revolution, went into its long decline and the German laboratory school began its rapid ascent. This was after the fat cell had been described, the Quetelet Index had been published, and the conservation of energy had been published (246). From 1850 to the beginning of World War II, the hegemony of German laboratory science in the field of obesity and elsewhere was evident (245).

With the advent of the 20th century, concerns about the relationship of obesity to health risks gradually replaced concerns about being underweight (5). As this century has progressed, four themes have coalesced to form the basis of a modern science of obesity: the behavioral or psychological aspects of obesity, the physiological approach to a controlled system of food intake, the cellular basis for obesity centered in the growing diversity of cellular functions for the fat cell, and the genetic and molecular biological approaches to understanding the problem.

From the beginning of World War II and the publication of the monograph by Rony (246), a period of Amer-

Table 3 Monographs on Obesity

English	French	German
18th century		
Short (243)		
Flemyng (244)		
19th century		
Wadd (39, 270)	Maccary (143)	Kisch (276)
Chambers (271)	Dancel (274)	Ebstein (277)
Harvey, J. (272)	Worthington (275)	
Harvey, W. (273)		
20th century		
Williams (278)	Leven (287)	Noorden (292)
Christie (279)	Heckel (288)	Pfaundler (263)
Rony (280)	Le Noir (289)	Gries & Berchtold (294)
Rynearson & Gastineau (281)	Boivin (290)	
Craddock (282)	Cref & Herschberg (291)	
Bruch (283)		
Mayer (284)		
Bray (121)		
Garrow (285)		
Stunkard (286)		

ican hegemony began. In the post–World War II period, the growth of the National Institutes of Health has served as a major stimulus for research in obesity (247). Several important events occurred that brought the scientific threads of obesity together. The first was the formation of many associations for the study of obesity. The first of them was in the United Kingdom, which held its first meeting in 1968 (248). This was followed in 1972 by the first Fogarty Center Conference on Obesity (249), and one year later by the First International Congress on Obesity (250). Following this Congress, it was clear that a journal devoted to obesity was needed, and the *International Journal of Obesity* began publication in 1976 under the editorship of Dr. Alan Howard and Dr. George Bray. Subsequent International Congresses were held in 1977 in Washington, DC (251), in 1980 in Rome, Italy (252), in 1983 in New York City (253), in 1986 in Jerusalem (254), in 1990 in Kobe, Japan, in 1994 in Toronto, Canada, and in 1998 in Paris. A meeting is planned for 2002 in São Paulo, Brazil. In 1986 the International Association for the Study of Obesity was formed under the leadership of Dr. B. Hansen. As growth continued, a second journal appeared in 1980, titled *Obesity and Weight Regulation*. This journal, like so many others, succumbed, in part, because it was not affiliated with one of the national associations. *Obesity Surgery* was the third journal to be founded and was followed in 1993 by *Obesity Research*, published by the North American Association for the Study of Obesity (255). This rapid growth of scientific institutions surrounding a scientific discipline is characteristic of developments that have occurred throughout the scientific sphere to provide a way of focusing the activities of scientists in a manageable way (256–269).

REFERENCES

1. Gaarder J. Sophie's World. A Novel about the History of Philosophy (translated by P. Moller). London: Phoenix House, 1995, paperback.
2. Crombie AC, ed. Scientific Changes. Historical Studies in the Intellectual, Social and Technical Conditions for Scientific Discovery and Technical Investigation, from Antiquity to the Present. New York: Basic Books, 1963.
3. Bray GA. Obesity: historical development of scientific and cultural ideas. Int J Obes 1990; 14:909–926.
4. Mardinie, Notes sur l'histoire de l'obesitè. Thesis de Paris, 1934. Paris: Les Presses Universitaires de France, 1934.
5. Schwartz H. Never Satisfied. A Cultural History of Diets, Fantasies and Fat. New York: Doubleday, 1986.
6. Needham J. Science and Civilization in China. Cambridge: Cambridge University Press, 1988, 6 vol.
7. Singer C. Homyard EJ, Hall AR, Williams TI. A History of Technology. New York: Oxford University Press, 1954–1958, 5 vol.
8. Ackerknecht EH. Medicine at the Paris Hospital. Baltimore: Johns Hopkins University Press, 1967.
9. Foucault M. The Birth of the Clinic. An Archaeology of Medical Perception. New York: Vintage Books, 1973.
10. Gamble C. The Palaeolithic Settlement of Europe. Cambridge: Cambridge University Press, 1986.
11. Chauvet S. La medecine chez les peuples primitifs. Paris: Librairie Maloine, 1936.
12. Beller AS. Fat and Thin: A Natural History of Obesity. New York: Farrar, Straus and Giroux, 1977.
13. Hautin RJR. Obesity. Conceptions actuelle. These pour le Doctorat en Medecine. Bordeaux: Imprimerie Bier, 1939.
14. Kulacoglu, B. Gods and Goddesses (translated by J. Ozturk). Anhura: Museum of Anatolian Civilizations; 1992.
15. Garrison F. An Introduction to the History of Medicine. Philadelphia: WB Saunders, 1914.
16. Contenau G. La medecine en Assyrie et en Babylonie. Paris: Librairie Maloine, 1938.
17. Spycket A. Kassite and middle Elamite sculpture. In: Later Mesopotamia and Iran. Tribes and Empires 1600–538 B.C. London: British Museum Press, 1995: 30, plate 18.
18. Smith E. The Edwin Smith Surgical Papyrus. Published in facsimile and hieroglyphic transliteration with translation and commentary in two volumes by James Henry Breasted. Chicago: University of Chicago Press, 1930. Classics of Medicine, Special Edition, 1984.
19. Darby WJ, Ghalioungui P, Grevetti L. Food: The Gift of Osiris. London: Academic Press, 1977.
20. Nunn JF. Ancient Egyptian Medicine. London: British Museum Press, 1996.
21. Reeves C. Egyptian Medicine. London: Shire Publications, 1992.
22. Filer J. Egyptian Bookshelf Disease. London: British Museum Press, 1995.
23. Alphen JV, Aris A. Oriental Medicine: An Illustrated Guide to the Asian Arts of Healing. Boston: Shambhala, 1996.
24. Tibetan Medical Paintings. Illustrations to the Blue Beryl Treatise of Sangye Gyamtso. (1635–1705). New York: Harry N Abrams, 1992.
25. Iason AH. The Thyroid Gland in Medical History. New York: Frobin Press, 1946.
26. Ortiz de Montellano BR. Aztec Medicine, Health and Nutrition. New Brunswick: Rutgers University Press, 1990, paperback.
27. Vogel VJ. American Indian Medicine. Norman: University of Oklahoma Press, 1970; 7th paperback printing, 1990.
28. Hippocrates. Oeuvres completes d'Hippocrate. Traduction nouvelle avec le texte grec en ragard . . . par E. Littre. Paris; JB Balliere, 1839.
29. Kryger MH. Sleep apnea. From the needles of Dionysius to continuous positive airway pressure. Arch Intern Med 1983; 143:2301–2303.

30. Kryger, MH. Fat, sleep, and Charles Dickens: literary and medical contributions to the understanding of sleep apnea. Clin Chest Med 1985; 6:555–562.

31. Campbell D. Arabian medicine and its influence on the middle ages. London: Kegan Paul, Trench, Trubner, 1926.

32. Beaujouan G. Motives and opportunities for science in the medieval universities. In: Crombie AC, ed. Scientific Change. Historical Studies in the Intellectual, Social and Technical Conditions for Scientific Discovery and Technical Invention, from Antiquity to the Present. New York: Basic Books, 1963:232–234.

33. Vesalius A. De humani corporis fabrica. Basil: ex off. Joannis Oporini, 1543.

34. Copernicus N. De revolutionibus orbium colestium. Libri VI. Nuremberg: Apud Ioh. Petrium; 1543.

35. Bonetus T. Sepulchretum, sive anatomia practica, ex cadaveribus morbo denatis, proponens historias omnium humani corporis affectum. Geneva: Sumptibus Leonardi Chouet, 1679 2 vol.

36. Morgagni GB. De sedibus, et causis morborum per anatomen indagatis Libri Quinque. Venice: typog. Remordiniana, 1761.

37. Haller A. Corpulence ill cured; large cryptae of the stomach (etc). Path Observ 1756; 44–49.

38. Haller A. Elementa physiologiae corporis humani. Lausanne: Marci-Michael Boursquet & Sociorum, 1757.

39. Wadd W. Comments on Corpulency, Lineaments of Leanness Mems on Diet and Dietetics. London: John Ebers, 1829.

40. Malpighi M. Opera omnia. London: R Scott, 1686.

41. Hooke R. Micrographia, or Some Physiological Descriptions of Minute Bodies Made by Magnifying Glasses; with Observations and Inquiries Thereupon. London: J Martyn & J Allestry, 1665–1667.

42. Leeuwenhoek van A. The Select Works of Antony van Leeuwenhoek, Containing his Microscopial Discoveries in Many of the Works of Nature (translated from the Dutch and Latin editions published by the author Samual Hoole). London: G Sidney, 1800.

43. Schwann T. Mikroscopische Untersuchungen uber di Ubereinstimmung in der Struktur un dem Wachstum der Thiere und Pflanzen. Berlin: Sander, 1839.

44. Schleiden MJ. Beitrage zur Phytogenesis. Arch Anat Physiol Wiss Med 1839; 137–176.

45. Henle FGJ. Allgemeine Anatomie. Leipzig: L Voss, 1841.

46. Hassall A. The Microscopic Anatomy of the Human Body, in Health and Disease. London: Samuel Highley, 1849.

47. Hoggan G, Hogan FE. On the development and retrogression of the fat cell. J R Microscope Soc 1879; 2:353.

48. Hassall A. Observations on the development of the fat vesicle. Lancet 1849; 1:63–64.

49. Kirsch J, Kittle JL. Cellularity of obese and nonobese human adipose tissue. Fed Proc 1970; 29:1516–1521.

50. Björntorp P, Sjostrom L. Number and size of adipose tissue fat cells in relation to metabolism in human obesity. Metabolism 1971; 20:703–713.

51. Virchow R. Die Cellularpathologie in inrer Begrundung auf physiologische und pathologische Gewebelehre. Berlin: August Hirschwald, 1858.

52. Virchow R. Cellular Pathology (translated from the second edition of the original by Frank Chance). London: J Churchill, 1860.

53. Knoll M, Ruska E. Beitrag zur geometrischen Electronenoptik. Ann Physik 1932; 12;607–661.

54. Renold AE, Cahill GF, eds. Handbook of Physiology. Section 5. Adipose Tissue. Behesda, MD: American Physiological Society, 1965.

55. Harvey W. The Anatomical Exercises of Dr. William Harvey. De Motu Cordis 1628: De circulatione sanguinis 1649: The first English text of 1653 now newly edited by Geoffrey Keynes. London: Nonesuch Press, 1928.

56. Osler W. The Evolution of Modern Medicine. New Haven, CT: Yale University Press, 1921.

57. Santorio S. Medicina Statica: or, Rules of Health, in Eight Sections of Aphorisms. English'd by J.D. London: John Starkey, 1676.

58. Santorio, Santorio. Medicina Statica: Being the Aphorisms of Sanctorius, translated into English with large explanations. The second edition. To which is added Dr. Keil's Medicina Statica Britannica, with Comparative Remarks and Explanations. As also Medic-physical Essays . . . by John Quincy. London: W and J Newton, A Bell, W Taylor, and J Osborne, 1720.

59. Newburgh LH, Johnston MW. The Exchange of Energy Between Man and the Environment. Springfield, IL: Charles C Thomas, 1930.

60. Reamur RAF. Sur la digestion des oiseaux. Hist Acad Roy Sci 1756; 266–307, 461–495.

61. Spallanzani L. Opusculi di fiscia animale e vegetabile. Moedena: Soc. tipografica, 1776, 2 vols.

62. Spallanzani L. Dissertations Relative to the Natural History of Animals and Vegetables (translated from the Italian). London: J Murray and S Highley, 1796, 2 vol.

63. Beaumont W. Experiments and Observations on the Gastric Juices and the Physiology of Digestion. Plattsburgh: FP Allen, 1833.

64. Bernard C. De l'origine du sucre dans l'economie animale. Arch Gen Med 1848; 18 (4th ser): 303–319.

65. Cannon WB, Washburn AL. An explanation of hunger. Am J Physiol 1912; 29:441–454.

66. Carlson AJ. The Control of Hunger in Health and Disease. Chicago: University of Chicago Press, 1916.

67. Partingon JR. A Short History of Chemistry, 2nd ed. London: Macmillan, 1951.

68. Boyle R. The Works of the Honourable Robert Boyle. London: A Millar, 1764.

69. Stahl GE. Theoria medica vera. Physiologiam & pathologiam. Halae, Literis Ophanotrophei, 1708.

70. Priestley J. Experiments and Observation on Different Kinds of Air. London: J Johnson, 1775.

71. Scheele CW. The Discovery of Oxygen Part 2. Edinburgh: William F. Clay, 1894 (Alembic Club Reprint No. 8)

(From Chemische Abhandlung von der Luft und dem Feuer, Uppsala und Leipzig, 1777).

72. Lavoisier AL. Traite elementiare de chemie, presente dans un order nouveau et d'apres les couvertes modernes . . . Paris: Chez Cuchet, 1789.

73. Helmholtz HLF. Uber die Erhaltung der Kraft, eine physikalische Abhandlung. Berlin: G Reimer, 1847.

74. Rubner M. Die gesetze des Energieverbrauches bei der Ernahrung. Leipzig: Franz Deuticke, 1902.

75. Rubner M. The Laws of Energy Consumption in Nutrition. New York: Academic Press, 1982.

76. Pettenkofer MJ, Voit C. Untersuchuingen uber die Respiration. Ann Chem Pharm (Heidelberg) 1862–1863; Suppl 2:52–70.

77. Atwater WO, Rosa EB. Description of a New Respiration Calorimeter and Experiments on the Conservation of Energy in the Human Body. US Department of Agriculture, Office of Experimental Station, 1899: 63.

78. Atwater WO, Benedict FG. Experiments on the metabolism of matter and energy in the human body. 1900–1902. Office of the Experiment Station-Bulletin no. 136. Washington, DC: Government Printing Office, 1903.

79. Benedict FG. A Study of Prolonged Fasting. 1915. Report No. 203. Washington, DC: Carnegie Institution of Washington.

80. Benedict FG, Miles WR, Roth P, Smith HM. Human vitality and efficiency under prolonged restricted diet. Washington DC: Carnegie Institution, 1919; 280.

81. Jequier E, Schultz Y. Long-term measurements of energy expenditure in humans using a respiration chamber. Am J Clin Nutr 1983; 38:989–998.

82. Garrow J. Energy Balance and Obesity in Man, 2nd ed. Amsterdam; Elsevier/North Holland Biomedical Press, 1978.

83. Ravussin E, Swinburn BA. Pathophysiology of obesity. Lancet 1992; 340:404–408.

84. Schoeller DA, Van Santen E, Peterson DW, Dietz W, Jaspan J. Klein PD. Total body water measurement in humans with O and H labeled water. Am J Clin Nutr 1980; 33: 2686–2693.

85. Lichtman SW, Pisarska K, Berman ER, et al. Discrepancy between self-reported and actual caloric intake and exercise in obese subjects. N Engl J Med 1992; 327: 1893–1898.

86. Wohler F. Ueber kunstliche Bildung des Harnstoffs. Ann Phys Chem (Leipzig) 1828; 12:253–256.

87. Magendie F. Precis elementaire de physiologie. Paris: Mequignon-Marvis, 1816.

88. Liebeg JV. Chemistry and Its Application to Agriculture and Physiology (translated by Lyon Playfair). London: Taylor and Walton, 1842.

89. Bernard C. Memoire sur le pancreas et sur le role du suc pancreatique dans les phenomenes digestif. Suppl CR Acad Sci (Paris), 1856; 1:379–563.

90. Kuhn TS. The Structure of Scientific Revolutions. Chicago: The University of Chicago Press; 1962.

91. Cohen IB. Revolution in Science. Cambridge, MA: Belknap Press of Harvard University Press; 1985.

92. McCollum EV. A History of Nutrition. The Sequence of Ideas in Nutrition Investigations. Boston: Houghton Mifflin, 1957.

93. Select Committee on Nutrition and Human Needs (hearing) of the United States Senate 95th Congress. Diet Related to Killer Diseases. Washington, DC: U.S. Government Printing Office, 1977. Vol. VI–VII (2VI, 2VII).

94. Society of Actuaries. Build Study of 1979. City Recording and Statistical Corp, 1980.

95. Behnke AR Jr, Feen BG, Welham WC. The specific gravity of healthy men. Body weight divided by volume as an index of obesity. JAMA 1942; 118;495–498.

96. Hevesy G. Radioactive Indicators. Their Application in Biochemistry, Animal Physiology, and Pathology. New York: Interscience Publishers, 1948.

97. Moore FD, Oleson KH, McMurrey JD, Parker HV, Ball MR, Boyden CM. The Body Cell Mass and Its Supporting Environment. Philadelphia: WB Saunders, 1963.

98. Wang Z, Pierson RN, Heymsfield SB. The five-level model: a new approach to organizing body composition. Am J Clin Nutr 1992; 56(1):19–28.

99. Darwin C. On the Origin of Species by Means of Natural Selection or the Preservation of Favoured Races in the Struggle for Life. London: John Murray, 1859.

100. Garrod AE. Inborn Errors of Metabolism. The Coonian Lectures delivered before the Royal College of Physicians of London, in June, 1908. London: Henry Frowde; Hodder & Stoughton; Oxford University Press, 1909.

101. Watson JD, Crick FH. Molecular structure of nucleic acids: A structure for deoxyribose nucleic acid. Nature 1953; 171(4356):737–738.

102. Bultman SJ, Michaud EJ, Woychik RP. Molecular characterization of the mouse agouti locus. Cell 1992; 71: 1195–1204.

103. Zhang YY, Proenca R, Maffei M, Barone M, Leopold L, Friedman JM. Positional cloning of the mouse obese gene and its human homolog. Nature 1994; 372:425–432.

104. Naggert JK, Fricker LD, Varlamov O, et al. Hyperproinsulinaemia in obese fat/fat mice associated with a carboxypeptidase-e mutation which reduces enzyme-activity. Nature Genet 1995; 10:135–142.

105. Davenport CB. Body Build and Its Inheritance. Washington DC: Carnegie Institution, 1923; 329:37.

106. Vershuer OV. Die Verebungsbiologishe Zwillingsforschung. Ihre Biologischen Grundlagen. Mit 18 Abbildungen. Ergebnisse der Inneren Medizin und Kinderheilkunde. 31th 3d. Berlin: Verlag Von Julius Springer, 1927.

107. Vogler GP, Sorensen TI, Stunkard AJ, Srinivassen MR, Rao DC. Influences of genes and shared family environment on adult body mass index assessed in an adoption study by a comprehensive path model. Int J Obes 1995; 19: 40–45.

108. Bouchard C, Despres J, Mauriege P. Genetic and nongenetic determinants of regional fat distribution. Endocr Rev 1993; 14(1):72–93.

109. Bouchard C, Perusse L. Current status of the human obesity gene map. Obes Res 1997; 5:81–90.

110. Warden CH, Fisler JS, Shoemaker SM, et al. Identification of 4 chromosomal loci determining obesity in a multifactorial mouse model. J Clin Invest 1995; 95:1545–1552.

111. West DB, Goudey-Lefevre J, York B, Truett GE. Dietary obesity linked to genetic-loci on chromosome-9 and chromosome-15 in a polygenic mouse model. J. Clin Invest 1994; 94:1410–1416.

112. Paracelsus. Wunder artzney, vonn allerley leibs gebruchen, unnd zu fallende Krankheiten, ohn sondere Beschwerung, Unlust unnd Verdrusz, kurtzlich zu heilen, unnd die Gesundheit widerumb mit geringem Kosten zun Wegen zubringen . . . Basel: Sebastian Henricpetri, 1573.

113. Magendie F. Formulary for the preparation and employment of several new remedies, namely, resin of nux vomica, strychnine, morphine, hydrocyanic acid, preparations of cinchona . . . (translated from the Formulaire of M. Magendie, published in Paris, October 1827). London: T and G Underwood, 1828.

114. Wells H. A History of the Discovery of the Application of Nitrous Oxide Gas, Ether, and Other Vapors to Surgical Operations. Hartford, CT: J Gaylord Wells, 1847.

115. Warren E. Some Accounts of the Letheon: Or, Who Is the Discoverer of Anesthesia. Boston: Dutton and Wentworth, 1847.

116. Bowditch NL. The Ether Controversy. Vindication of the Hospital Report of 1848. Boston: John Wilson, 1848.

117. Lister J. On the effects of the antiseptic system of treatment upon the salubrity of a surgical hospital. Lancet 1870; 1:4–6, 40–42.

118. Lister JB. The Collected Papers of Joseph, Baron Lister, Member of the order of merit, fellow, and sometime president of the Royal Society, Knight Grand Cross of the Danish Order of the Danebrog Knight of the Prussian Order pour le Merite Associe Etranger de l'Institut de France. Oxford: Clarendon Press, 1909.

119. Canguilhem G. Ideology and Rationality in the History of the Life Sciences (translated by A. Goldhammer). Cambridge, MA: MIT Press, 1988.

120. Ehrlich P, Hata S. Die experimentelle Chemotherapie der Spirillosen. Berlin: Julius Springer, 1910.

121. Bray GA. The Obese Patient, 9th ed. Philadelphia: WB Saunders, 1976.

122. Lesses MF, Myerson A. Human Autonomic pharmacology. XVI. Benzedrine sulfate as an aid in the treatment of obesity. N Engl J Med 1938; 218:119–124.

123. Babinski MJ. Tumeur du corps pituitaire sans acromegalie et avec de development des organes genitaux. Rev Neurol 1900; 8:531–533.

124. Frohlich A. Ein fall von tumor der hypophysis cerebri ohne akromegalie. Wiener Klin Rdsch 1901; 15:883–886.

125. Mohr B. Hypertrophie der Hypophysis cerebri und dadurch bedingter Druck auf die Hirngrundflache, insebesondere auf die Sehnerven, das Chiasma derselben und den linkseitigen Hirnschenkel. Wschr ges heilk 1840; 6: 565–571.

126. Smith PE. The disabilities caused by hypophysectomy and their repair. The tuberal (hypothalmic) syndrome in the rat. JAMA 1927; 88:159–161.

127. Hetherington AW, Ranson SW. Hypothalamic lesions and adiposity in the rat. Anat Rec 1940; 78:149–172.

128. Anand BK, Brobeck JR. Hypothalamic control of food intake in rats and cats. Yale J Biol Med 1951; 24:123–146.

129. Stellar E. The physiology of motivation. Psychol Rev 1954; 5:22.

130. Han PW. Hypothalamic obesity in rats without hyperphagia. Ann NY Acad Sci 1967; 30:229–242.

131. Coleman DL. Obese and Diabetes: Two mutant genes causing diabetes-obesity syndromes in mice (review). Diabetologia 1978; 14:141–148.

132. Powley TL, Opsahl CA. Ventromedial hypothalamic obesity abolished by subdiaphragmatic vagotomy. Am J Physiol 1974; 226:25–33.

133. Bray GA, York DA. Hypothalamic and genetic obesity in experimental animals: an autonomic and endocrine hypothesis. Physiol Rev 1979; 59:719–809.

134. Nishizawa Y, Bray GA. Ventromedial hypothalamic lesions and the mobilization of fatty acids. J Chem Invest 1978; 61(3):714–721.

135. Rothwell NJ, Stock MJ. A role for brown adipose tissue in diet-induced thermogenesis. Nature 1979; 281:31–35.

136. Bayliss WM. Principles of General Physiology, 2nd ed revised. London: Longmans, Green, 1918.

137. Gibbs J, Young RC, Smith GP. Cholecystokinin elicits satiety in rats with open gastric fistulas. Nature 245(5424): 323–325, 1973.

138. Stanley BG, Kyrkouli SE, Lampert S, Leibowitz SF. Neuropeptide Y chronically injected into the hypothalamus: a powerful neurochemical inducer of hyperphagia and obesity. Peptides 1986; 7:1189–1192.

139. Celsus AAC. De Medicina (with an English translation by WG Spencer). London: Heinemann, 1935–1938; 3 vol.

140. Gould GM, Pyle WL. Anomalies and Curiosities of Medicine. New York: Julian Press, Inc., 1956, original copyright, 1896.

141. Doubourg L. Recherches sur les causes de la polysarcie. Paris: A Parent, quarto, 1864:54.

142. Schindler CS. Monstrose Fettsucht. Wiener Med Presse 1871; 12:410–412, 436–439.

143. Maccary A. Traite sur la polysarcie. Paris: Gabon, 1811.

144. Glais J. De la grossesse adipeuse. Paris: A Parent, 1875; 1–36.

145. Dupytren. Observation sur un cas d'obesite, suivie de maladie du coeur et de la mort. J. Med Chir Pharm 1806; 12:262–273.

146. Anonymous. The Life of That Wonderful and Extraordinarily Heavy Man, Daniel Lambert, from His Birth to the

Moment of His Dissolution; with an Account of Men Noted for Their Corpulency, and Other Interesting Matter. New York: Samuel Wood & Sons, 1818.

147. Barkhausen. Merkwurdige allgemeine Fettablagerung bei einem Knaben von 5 1/4 Jahren. Hannov Ann f ges Heilk. 1843; 8:200–203 (case report).

148. Coe T. A letter from Dr. T. Coe, Physician at Chelmsford in Essex, to Dr. Cromwell Mortimer, Secretary R.S. concerning Mr. Bright, the Fat man at Malden in Essex. Phil Trans 1751–1752; 47:188–193.

149. Don WG. Remarkable case of obesity in a Hindoo boy aged twelve years. Lancet 1859; 1:363.

150. Eschenmeyer. Beschreibung eines monstrosen fett Madchen, das in einem Alter von 10 jahren starb, nach dem es eine hohe van 5 fuss 3 zoll und ein Gewicht von 219 pfund erreicht hatte. Tubing Bl Naturw Arznk 1815; 1:261–285.

151. Gordon S. Art. XV. Reports of rare cases. IV. Case of extensive fatty degeneration in a boy 14 years of age. Death from obstructed arterial circulation. Dublin Q J Med Sci 1862; 33:340–349.

152. McNaughton J. Cases of polysarcia adiposa in childhood. New York Medical and Physical Journal No XXX July 1829 New Series—No II. New York: CS Francis, 1829: 317–322.

153. Wood T. A sequel to the case of Mr. Thomas Wood, of Billericay, in the Country of Essex, by the same. Med Trans (Coll Physicians, Lond) 1785; 3:309–318.

154. Linnaeus Cv. Species plantarum. Stockholm: Salvius, 1753.

155. Sauvages FB. Nosologia methodica sistens morborum classes juxta Sydenhami menten and botanicorum ordinem. Amstelodami; Fratrum de Tournes, 1768, 2 vol.

156. Cullen W. First Lines of the Practice of Physic, by William Cullen, M.D., Late Professor of the Practice of Physic in the University of Edinburgh, and Including the Definitions of the Nosology; with Supplementary Notes Chiefly Selected from Recent Authors, Who Have Contributed to the Improvement of Medicine by Peter Reid, M.D. Edinburgh: Abernethy and Walker, 1810, 2 vol.

157. Burwell CS, Robin ED, Whaley RD, Bickelman AG. Extreme obesity associated with alveolar hypoventilation; a Pickwickian syndrome. Am J Med 1956; 21;811–818.

158. Robin ED. (Ed). Claude Bernard and the Internal Environment. A Memorial Symposium. New York: Marcel Dekker, 1979.

159. Russel J. A case of polysarka, in which death resulted from deficient arterialization of the blood. Br Med J 1866; 1:220–221.

160. Cushing H. The Pituitary Body and Its Disorders. Clinical States Produced by Disorders of the Hypophysis Cerebri. Philadelphia: JB Lippincott, 1912.

161. Cushing H. The basophil adenomas of the pituitary body and their clinical manifestations. Pituitary basophilism. Bull Johns Hopkins Hosp 1932; L:137–195.

162. Quetelet A. Sur l'homme et le developpement de ses facultes, ou essai de physique sociale. Paris: Bachelier, 1835.

163. Dawber TR. The Framingham Study: The Epidemiology of Atherosclerotic Disease. Cambridge, MA: Harvard University Press, 1980.

164. Keys A, Aravanis C, Blackburn HW, et al. Epidemiological studies related to coronary heart disease: characteristics of men aged 40–59 in seven countries. Acta Med Scand 1966; 460(Suppl):1–392.

165. Lew EA, Garfinkel L. Variations in mortality by weight among 750,000 men and women. J Chronic Dis 1979; 32:563–576.

166. Waaler HT. Height, weight and mortality: the Norwegian experience. Acta Med Scand 1984; 679:1–56.

167. Manson JE, Willett WC, Stampfer MJ, et al. Body weight and mortality among women. N Engl J Med 1995; 333: 677–685.

168. Vague J. La differentiation sexuelle. Facteur determinant des formes de l'obesite. Presse Med 1947; 55:339–340.

169. Carter HS, Howe PE, Mason HH. Nutrition and Clinical Dietetics. Philadelphia: Lea & Febiger, 1917.

170. Precope J. Hippocrates on Diet and Hygiene. London: Zeno, 1952.

171. Green RM. A Translation of Galen's Hygiene (De Sanitate Tuenda). Springfield, IL: Charles C Thomas, 1951.

172. Gruner OC. A Treatise on the Canon of Medicine of Avicenna Incorporating a Translation of the First Book. London: Luzac, 1930.

173. Harington J. The School of Salernum Regimen Sanitatis Salernitanum. New York: Paul B Hoeber, 1920.

174. Tweedie J. Hints on Temperance and Exercise, Shewing Their Advantage in the Cure of Dyspepsia, Rheumatism, Polysarcia, and Certain States of Palsy. London: T Rickaby, 1799.

175. Cornaro L. Sure and Certain Methods of Attaining a Long and Healthful Life: With Means of Correcting a Bad Constitution, 5th English ed. London: D Midwinter, 1737; p. 11.

176. Brillat-Savarin JA. The Physiology of Taste or, Meditations on Transcendental Gastronomy (translated from the French by MFK Fisher; drawings and color lithographs by Wayne Thiebaud). San Francisco: Arion Press, 1994.

177. Banting W. A Letter on Corpulence Addressed to the Public. London: Harrison and Sons, 1863.

178. Harvey W. On Corpulence in Relation to Disease: With Some Remarks on Diet. London: Henry Renshaw; 1872.

179. Gulick A. A study of weight regulation in the adult human body during over-nutrition. Am J Physiol 1922; 60: 371–395.

180. Neumann RO. Experimental Beitrage zur Lehre von dem taglichen Nahrungsbedarf des Menschen unter besonderer Berucksichtigung der notwendigen Eiweifsmenge. Arch Hyg 1902; 45:1–87.

181. Wiley FH, Newburg LH. The doubtful nature of "luxuskonsumption." J Clin Invest 1931; 10:733–744.

182. Evans FA. A radical cure of simple obesity by dietary measures alone. Atlantic Med J 1926; 30:140–141.

183. Bloom WL. Fasting as an introduction to the treatment of obesity. Metabolism 1959; 8:214–220.

184. Sours HE, Frattali VP, Brand CD, Feldman RA, Forbes AL, Swanson RC, Paris AL. Sudden death associated with very low calorie weight reduction regimens. Am J Clin Nutr 34:453–461, 1981.

185. Carpenter KF. Protein and Energy: A Study of Changing Ideas in Nutrition. Cambridge: Cambridge University Press, 1994.

186. U.S. House of Representatives. Hearing before the Subcommittee on Regulation, Business opportunities, and energy of the Committee on Small Business. Deception and Fraud in the Diet Industry, Part I of II. Washington, DC: U.S. Government Printing Office, 1990.

187. Freud S. The Interpretation of Dreams (authorized translation of third edition with introduction by AA Brill, PhD, MD). New York: Macmillan, 1913.

188. Stunkard AJ, Mendelson M. Obesity and the body image. I. Characteristics of disturbances in the body image of some obese persons. Am J Psychiatry 123: 1296–1300, 1967.

189. Moore ME, Stunkard AJ, Srole L. Obesity, social class, and mental illness. JAMA 1962; 181:962–966.

190. Pavlov IP. Conditioned Reflexes: An Investigation of the Physiological Activity of the Cerebral Cortex (translated by GV Anrep). London: Oxford University Press, 1928.

191. Skinner BF. Science and Human Behavior. New York: Macmillan; 1953.

192. Ferster CB, Nurenberger JI, Levitt EB. The control of eating. J Math 1962; 1:87–109.

193. Stuart RB. Behavioral control of overeating. Behav Res Ther 1967; 5:357–365.

194. Withering W. An Account of the Foxglove and Some of Its Medical Uses: With Practical Remarks on Dropsy and Other Diseases. Birmingham: M. Swinney, 1785.

195. Sajous CE de M. The Internal Secretion and the Principles of Medicine, 7th ed. Philadelphia: FA Davis Company, 1916:710, 724, 782.

196. Weintraub M, Sundaresan PR, Schuster B, *et al*. Long term weight control: The National Heart, Lung and Blood Institute funded multimodal intervention study. I–VII. Clin Pharmacol Ther 1992; 51:581–646.

197. Preuss J. Biblical and Talmudic Medicine (translated and edited by F Rosner, MD). New York: Hebrew Publishing Company, 1978.

198. Kremen AJ, Linner JH, Nelson CH. Experimental evaluation of nutritional importance of proximal and distal small intestine. Ann Surg 140; 439–448, 1954.

199. Payne JH, DeWind LT, Commons RR. Metabolic observations in patients with jejunocolic shunts. Am J Surg 1963; 106:273–289.

200. Mason EE, Ito C. Gastric bypass. Ann Surg 1970; 170: 329–339.

201. Sarton G. The History of Science and the New Humanism. New York: Henry Holt, 1931.

202. Sarton G. A History of Science. Ancient Science Throughout the Golden Age of Greece. Cambridge, MA: Harvard University Press, 1952.

203. Schenkio MM. De pinguedinis in animalibut generatione et concretione. In: Erastus, Th. Philosophi et medici celeberrimi disputationum et episolarum medicnalium, volumen doctissimum. Tiguri: Johan Wolphium, 1595.

204. Ettmueller M. Pratique de medicine speciale . . . sur les maladies propres des hommes, des femmes & des petits enfans, avec des Dissertations . . . sur l'epilepsie, l'yvresse, le mal hypochondriaque, la douleur hypochondriaque, la corpulence, & la morsure de la vipere (trad. nouv). Lyon: Thomas Amaulry, 1691.

205. Gosky AU. Disputatio solennis de marasmo, sive marcore: macilentia item & gracilitate sanorum; macilentia & gracilitate aegrotatium; crassitie & corpulentia sanorum naturali; crassitie & magnitudine corporis morbosa aegrorum. Argentina: Typis Eberhardii Welperi, 1658.

206. Held JF. Disputationem medica de corpulentia nimia. Publicae . . . censurae . . . submittit. Jena; Nisianis, 1670.

207. Leisner KC. Dissertatio medica de obesitate exsuperante. Jena: Typ Gollnerianis, 1683.

208. Widemann GM. Disputatio medica de corpulaentia nimia. Lipsia: Typ Krugerianus, 1681.

209. Vaulpre JM. De obesitate, comodis et noxis. Montepellier: Joannem-Franciscum Picot, 1782.

210. Fecht EH. Disputatio medica inauguralis de obesitate nimia. Rostochi: J Wepplingii, 1701.

211. Triller DW. De pinguedine seu succo nutritio superfluo. Halae: Type C Henklii, 1718.

212. Bass G. Dissertationem inauguralem medicam de obesitate nimia. Erfordiae: Preolo Heringii, 1740.

213. Bertram JW. Dissertatio inauguralis medica de pinguedine. Halae Magdeb: JC Hilligeri, 1739.

214. Bon J. Dissertatio medica inauguralis. De mutatione pinguedinis. Harderovici: Apud Johannem Moojen, 1742.

215. Bougourd O. An obesis somnus brevis salubrior? Paris: In Heerkens, Quaes Paris 1754:88–93.

216. Dissertatio inauguralis medica de obesitate. Vienna: Typis Joan Thomae Nobil de Trattnern, 1776.

217. Ebart FCW. Dissertatio inauguralis medica de obesitate nimia et morbis inde orindus. small quarto ed. Gottingen: Lit JH Schulzii, 1780.

218. Hoelder FB. Obesitatis corporis humani nosologia. Tubingae: Lit Schrammianis, 1775.

219. Homeroch CF. De pinguidine ejusque sede tam secundum quam preaeter naturam constitutis. Lipsiae: Ex Offician Langenhemiana, 1738:37.

220. Hulsebusch JF. Dissertatio inauguralis medica sistens pinguedinis corporis humani, sive panniculi adiposi veterum, hodie membranae cullulosae dictae fabricam, ejusque, & contenti olei historiam, usum, morbos. Lugduni Batavorum: Joh Arnold Langerak, 1728.

221. Jansen WX. Pinguedinis animalis consideratio physiologica et pathologica. Lugduni Batavorum: J Hazebroek, A van Houte et Andream Koster, 1784.

222. Kroedler JS. Theses inauguralis medicae de eo quod citius moriantur obesi, quam graciles secundum Hippocratis aphorismum XLIV. Sect II. Erfordiae: Typis Groschianis, 1724.

223. La Sone JMF. An in macilentis liberior quam in obesis circulatio. Paris: Quillau, 1740.

224. Locke SCJ. De celeri corporum incremento causa debilitatis in morbis. Lipsiae: Ex Officina Langenhemia, 1760.

225. Lohe AW. Exhibens de morbis adipis humani principia generalia, Duisburg, 1772.

226. Muller PA. Dissertatio physiologica de pinguedine corporis. Hafniae; Typis Andreae Hartvigi Godiche, 1766.

227. Oswald JH. Obesitatis corporis humani therapia. Tubingae: Litteris Schrammianis, 1775.

228. Person C. An parcior obesis, quam macilentis sanguinis missio. Paris: Quillau, 1748.

229. Pohl JC. Dissertationem inauguralem de obesis et voracibus eorumque vitae incommodis ac morbis. Lipsiae: JC Langenhemii, 1734.

230. Polonus SI. Dissertatio medica inauguralis de pinguedine. Harderovici: Typis Everardi Tyhoff, 1797.

231. Quabeck KJ. Dissertatio inauguralis medica de insolito corporis augmento frequenti morborum futurorum signo. Halae Magdeb: JC Hendelii, 1752.

232. Redhead J. Dissertatio physiologica-medica, inauguralis, de adipe, quam annuente summo numine. Edinburgh; Balfour et Smellie, 1789.

233. Riegels ND. De usu glandularum superrenalium in animalibus nec non de origine adipis. Hafniae, 1790.

234. Reussing HCT. Dissertatio inauguralis medica de pinguedine sana et morbosa. Jena: Ex Officina Fiedleriana, 1791.

235. Riemer JA. De obesitatis causis praecipuis. Halae and Salem: Stanno Hendeliano, 1778.

236. Schroeder PG. Dissertatio inauguralis medica de obesitate vitanda. Rintelii: JG Enax, 1756.

237. Schulz C. Disputatio medica inauguralis de obesitate quam, annuente summo numine. Lugduni Batavorum: Conradum Wishoff, 1752.

238. Seifert PDB. Dissertatio phyiologico-pathologico de pinguedine. Gryphiswaldiae: IH Eckhardt, 1794.

239. Steube JS. Dissertatio medica de corpulentia nimia. Jena: Litteris Mullerianus, 1716.

240. Tralles BL. Dissertatio de obesorum ad morbos mortemque declivitte. Halae Magdeb: Litteris Hilligerianis, 1730.

241. Trouillart G. Dissertatiio physiologico-practica inauguralis de pinguedine, et morbis ex nimia ejus quantitate. Harderovici: Apud Joannem Moojen, 1767.

242. Verdries JM. Dissertatio medica inauguralis de pinguedinis usibus et nocumentis in corpore humano, 8th ed. Giessae Hassorum: JR Vulpius, 1702.

243. Short T. A Discourse Concerning the Causes and Effects of Corpulency Together with the Method for Its Prevention and Cure. London: J Roberts, 1727.

244. Flemyng M. A Discourse on the Nature, Causes and Cure of Corpulency. Illustrated by a remarkable case, read before the Royal Society, November 1757 and now first published. London: L Davis and C Reymers, 1760.

245. Bray GA. Commentary on paper by Chambers. Obes Res 1993; 1;85–86.

246. Bray GA. Quetelet: quantitative medicine. Obes Res 1994; 2:68–71.

247. Harden VA. Inventing the NIH. Federal Biomedical Research Policy, 1887–1937. Baltimore: Johns Hopkins University Press, 1986.

248. Baird IM, Howard AN. Obesity: Medical and Scientific Aspects. Proceedings of the First Symposium of the Obesity Association of Great Britain. Edinburgh & London: E & S Livingstone, Ltd., 1961.

249. Bray GA. (ed) Obesity in perspective. Fogarty International Center Series on Preventive Med. Washington, DC: U.S. Government Printing Office. Publication #75-708. DHEW Publication 176. Parts 1 and 2.

250. Howard AN. Recent Advances in obesity research. Proceedings of the 1st International Congress on Obesity. London: Newman Publishing, 1975.

251. Bray GA. Recent Advances in Obesity Research: II. Proceedings of the 2nd International Congress on Obesity 23–26 October 1977, Washington DC. London: Newman Publishing 1978.

252. Björntorp P, Cairella M, Howard AN, eds. Recent Advances in Obesity Research. III. Proceedings of the 3rd International Congress on Obesity. London: John Libbey, 1981:374–387.

253. Hirsch J, Van Itallie TB, eds. Recent Advances in Obesity Research. IV. Proceedings of the 4th International Congress on Obesity 5–8 October, 1983 New York, USA. London: John Libbey, 1985.

254. Berry EM, Blondheim SH, Eliahou E, Shafrir E, eds. Recent Advances in Obesity. V. Proceedings of the 5th International Congress on Obesity. London: John Libbey, 1987:290–292.

255. Bray GA. Obesity research and medical journalism. Obes Res 1995; 3:65–71.

256. Bray GA. Commentary on Banting letter. Obes Res 1993; 1(2):148–152.

257. Bray GA. Commentary on Atwater classic. Obese Res 1993; 1(3):223–227.

258. Bray GA. Commentary on classics in obesity. 4. Hypothalamic obesity. Obes Res 1993; 1(4):325–328.

259. Bray GA. Commentary on classics in obesity. 5. Fat cell theory and units of knowledge. Obes Res 1993; 1(5): 403–407.

260. Bray GA. Commentary on classics in obesity. 6. Science and politics of hunger. Obes Res 1993; 19(6):489–493.

261. Bray GA. Letter on corpulence. Obes Res 1993; 1: 153–163.

262. Bray GA. Lavoisier and scientific revolution: the oxygen theory displaces air, fire, earth and water. Obes Res 1994; 2:183–188.

263. Bray GA. What's in a name? Mr. Dickens' "Pickwickian" fat boy syndrome. Obes Res 1994; 2:380–383.

264. Bray GA. Harvey Cushing and the neuroendocrinology of obesity. Obes Res 1994; 2:482–485.

265. Bray GA. The inheritance of corpulence. Obes Res 1994; 2:601–605.

266. Bray GA. Life insurance and overweight. Obes Res 1995; 3:97–99.

267. Bray GA. From very-low-energy diets to fasting and back. Obes Res 1995; 3:207–209.

268. Bray GA. Laurence, Moon, Bardet, Biedl: reflections on a syndrome. Obes Res 1995; 3:383–386.

269. Bray GA. Luxusconsumption—myth or reality? Obes Res 1995; 3:491–494.

270. Wadd W. Cursory Remarks on Corpulence; or Obesity Considered as a Disease: With a Critical Examination of Ancient and Modern Opinions, Relative to Its Causes and Cure. London: Callow, 1816.

271. Chambers TK. Corpulence; or, Excess of Fat in the Human Body; Its Relation to Chemistry and Physiology, Its Bearings on Other Diseases and the Value of Human Life and Its Indications of Treatment. London: Longman, Brown, Green and Longmans, 1850.

272. Harvey J. Corpulence, Its Diminution and Cure Without Injury to Health. London: John Smith & Co, 1864.

273. Harvey W. On Corpulence in Relation to Disease: With Some Remarks on Diet. London: Henry Renshaw, 1872.

274. Dancel JF. Traite theorique et pratique de l'obesite (trop grand embonpoint). Avec plusieurs observations de guerison de maladies occasionees ou entretienues par cet etat anormal. Paris: J.B. Bailliere et fils, 1863; 1–357.

275. Worthington LS. De l'obesite. Etiologie, therapeutique et hygiene. Paris: E. Martinet, 1875:188 pp.

276. Kisch EH. Die fettleibigkeit (lipomatosis universalis. Auf gurndlage Zahlreicher beobachtungen klinisch Dargestellt. Stuttgart: Ferdinand Enke, 1988.

277. Ebstein W. Die Fettleibigkeit (Korpulenz) un ihre Behandulung nach physiologicschen Grundsatzen. Weisbaden: Bergmann, 1882.

278. Williams LLB. Obesity. London: Milford, 1926.

279. Christie WF. Obesity: A Practical Handbook for Physicians. London: William Heinemann; 1937.

280. Rony HR. Obesity and Leanness. Philadelphia: Lea & Febiger, 1940.

281. Rynearson EH, Gastineau CF. Obesity. Springfield, IL: Charles C Thomas, 1949.

282. Craddock D. Obesity and Its Management. Edinburgh and London: E and S Livingstone, 1969.

283. Bruch H. The Importance of Overweight. New York: WW Norton, 1957.

284. Mayer J. Overweight: Causes, Cost and Control. Englewood Cliffs, NJ: Prentice-Hall, 1968.

285. Garrow JS. Treat Obesity Seriously. A Clinical Manual. Edinburgh and London: Churchill Livingstone, 1981.

286. Stunkard AJ. The Pain of Obesity. Palo Alto, CA: Bull Publishing Co., 1976.

287. Leven G. Du obésité. Paris: G Steinheil, 1901.

288. Heckel F. Grandes et petites obésité. Cure Radicale. Paris: Masson, 1911.

289. LeNoir P. L'obésité et son traitement. Paris: JB Bailliere, 1907.

290. Boivin F. La cure physiologique de l'obésité. Paris: Jules Rousset, 1911; 1–191.

291. Cref AF, Heschberg AD. Abrege d'obésité. Paris: Masson, 1979.

292. Von Noorden C. Obesity: The indications for reduction cures being Part I of several clinical treatises on the pathology of Disorders of Metabolism and Nutrition. Bristol: John Wright & Co., 1903.

293. Pfaundler M. Korpermass-studien an Kindern. Berlin: Springer, 1916.

294. Gries FA, Berchtold P, Berger M. Adipositas, pathophysiologie, klinik und therapie. Berlin: Springer-Verlag, 1976.

2

Definitions and Proposed Current Classification of Obesity

George A. Bray
Pennington Biomedical Research Center, Louisiana State University, Baton Rouge, Louisiana

Claude Bouchard
Laval University, Ste.-Foy, Quebec, Canada

W. P. T. James
Rowett Research Institute, Aberdeen, Scotland

I. INTRODUCTION

Excessive body mass for stature, and more specifically an excessive body fat content, is a condition of concern because it is in and of itself socially and physically debilitating and it represents a risk factor for increased morbidity and mortality rate. In this chapter, the various types of human obesity, their assessment, their prevalence in various nations, and their etiologies will be described. Subsequently, the health consequences of being obese and the various contemporary treatment options will be discussed.

For more than 100 years, the life insurance industry has pointed out that increased body weight is associated with excess mortality (1). This has been one stimulus for including measures of body weight, stature, and occasionally skinfolds in epidemiological studies on the factors associated with the development of cardiovascular diseases and cancer (2). In recent years, fat distribution has also been included (3). It is now clear that a high body mass for height or a high body fat level and upper body obesity plus weight gain in adult life are associated with the risk of developing several chronic diseases. As a transition from the historical review of obesity, this chapter will review some approaches to defining obesity as a prelude.

II. THE TYPES OF HUMAN OBESITY

The perception that not all obese individuals are alike and that it would be useful to distinguish several types of obesity is an ancient one (4). More than 40 years ago, Professor Jean Vague from Marseille suggested that the topography of fat storage and body type were of prime importance in interpreting the health consequences of an obese state (Vague, 1947, 1956). He concluded that the male pattern of fat distribution (android obesity) carried a greater health risk than the female profile (gynoid obesity). However, the importance of Vague's work was not fully appreciated until the 1980s.

It was left primarily to Professors Ahmed Kissebah, in Milwaukee, Wisconsin, and Per Björntorp, in Göteborg, Sweden, to document, in the early 1980s, in a variety of animal and human studies that indeed android obesity was a greater risk for cardiovascular disease and type II diabetes mellitus and to identify some of the potential mechanisms responsible for these deleterious effects (10, 13, 36, 37). Following the work of their laboratories, the topic of regional fat distribution is one that has dominated the field of obesity research for the last 10 years (3).

Several hundred papers and many national and international meetings on this topic have provided evidence that three main adipose tissue features are of particular importance from a health perspective (3). First, increased morbidity and higher mortality rates are seen in those with an excessive proportion of body fat or a high body mass relative to stature. Second, the risk profile tends to be more dangerous when the excess fat is mainly stored on the upper body and less on the buttocks and lower limbs, i.e., when fat topography is typically male-like. Finally, recent research has suggested that the most atherogenic fat depot of the human body is within the abdominal cavity around the viscera, particularly the fat depots with small blood vessels draining into the portal vein carrying blood back to the liver. The amount of abdominal visceral fat appears to be critical in determining whether obesity is going to have major or minor health implications for a given individual (10).

These three types of human obesity are derived from anatomical considerations as well as degrees of health risk. Other systems of classification have also been used. For instance, human obesity can be defined on the basis of fat cell characteristics, genetic syndromes, neuroendocrine mechanisms, etiological factors, and other approaches. However, none of these classification systems enjoys the level of popularity in clinical and scientific circles the world over than the anatomical-health-risk approach currently does.

Overweight, obesity, and adiposity are the commonly used expressions for increased body fat and have replaced the older terms such as corpulence, polysarcie, and embonpoint (4). Overweight can be expressed as relative weight or ratios of weight to height. Relative weight is the ratio of actual to standard weight as determined from a table of reference body weights expressed relative to height, frequently as a percentage. Weight-to-height ratios can also be expressed as the body mass index (BMI) or Quetelet index, which is body weight (in kilograms) divided by the square of the height (in meters), i.e., weight/(height)^2 (5). The BMI is more highly correlated with body fat than with other indices of height and weight (6). The nomogram in Figure 1 allows rapid determination of BMI for given levels of height and weight.

III. ASSESSMENT OF HUMAN OBESITIES

To assess obesity properly, one must theoretically measure body fat content and fat topography and compare the

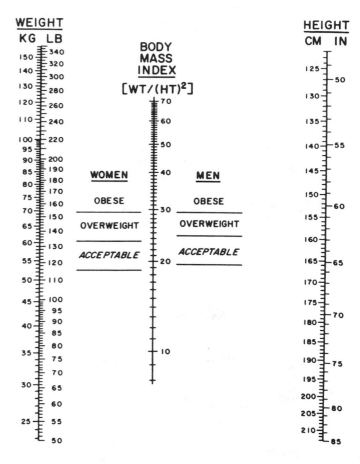

Figure 1 Nomogram for determining body mass index. To use this nomogram, place a ruler or other straightedge between the body weight in kilograms or pounds (without clothes) located on the left-hand line and the height in centimeters or in inches (without shoes) located on the right-hand line. The body mass index is read from the middle of the scale and is in metric units. (Copyright 1978, George A. Bray. Used with permission.)

numbers obtained for an individual of a given age and gender class with valid sets of reference values. Although the procedure seems to be quite simple and straightforward, it has proven to be one of the most difficult tasks in both research and clinical settings. Indeed, at least three body fat phenotypes are of prime interest (total body fat content, upper body fat, abdominal visceral fat), and they need to be evaluated in a laboratory environment, in the physician's office, and in the field for large-scale population studies.

Table 1 lists the methods currently available to obtain a direct or a predicted measure of total body fat content. All of the laboratory-based methods provide estimates of body fat that are in relatively good agreement and are reproducible. Traditionally, body density derived from un-

Table 1 Classification of Desirable Weight Levels as Assessed by the BMI

Classification	Sex	Age group (years)	Recommended BMI (kg/m²)
U.S. Departments of Agriculture and Health and Human Services (USDA/DHHS)	Both	19–34	19–25
National Academy of Sciences (NAS)	Both	19–24	
		25–34	
		35–44	
		45–54	
		55–64	
		≥65	
		19–24	
		20–25	
		21–26	
		22–27	
		23–28	
		24–29	
National Center for Health and Statistics (NCHS)	Male	20–74	20.7–27.8
	Female	20–74	19.1–27.3
World Health Organization (WHO)	Both	Adults	20–25
Minister of National Health and Welfare Canada (Canadian)	both	20–65	20–27

derwater weighing and converted to a proportion of fat in the body has been considered the gold standard procedure. The method assumes that a two-compartment model of body composition is adequate for the purpose of obtaining a valid measure of body fat content. It is a reasonable assumption provided that the density of fat-free tissues does not vary widely. Unfortunately, it does fluctuate with disease (e.g., osteoporosis), growth, aging, exercise, training, and malnutrition. Erroneous estimates of body fat content can thus be reached under a variety of circumstances although the magnitude of the errors introduced remains relatively small (in terms of percentage of body fat). But it is important to note that the underwater-weighing-derived measured of body density is not in error; rather it is the conversion of body density to body fat content that is vulnerable to deviations from the basic postulate.

Other methods can be used to arrive at an estimate of body fat content, and they do not require that the density of fat free tissues be constant from person to person. Most notable among these methods is the dual emission X-ray absorptiometer (DEXA), which exposes the body to a very small dose of radiation but is thought to provide a highly accurate measure of total body fat content. Several other techniques are commonly used in a few laboratories with the aim of estimating total body fat. They include isotopic dilution to assess body water, body potassium content to assess skeletal muscle mass, CT scanning and MRI examination at a large number of sites or over the whole body, and other complex procedures. All these methods are expensive and require elaborate instrumentation; they are therefore confined to the laboratory and are used almost exclusively for research purposes.

Simple approaches include the use of the BMI or the Quetelet index defined as body weight (kg) divided by the square of the height (m) as surrogate for body fat content, the prediction of body fat from simple anthropometric measurements such as skinfolds and circumferences, and, more recently, bioelectric impedance (BIA). The BMI is typically used in large scale population studies. BIA has considerable merit but more research is needed on its limitations and on the conditions under which it is best used in a variety of circumstances. In general, these methods are best suited for the physician's office or the epidemiological research environment; they provide reasonably good estimates of mean total body fat for a group of subjects or patients but they are less accurate for a given individual.

Assessment is also quite complex when it comes to upper body fat or abdominal visceral fat. Since these markers of regional fat distribution should ideally be monitored along with total body fat content, the overall measurement issue is indeed not a simple one. At this time, abdominal visceral fat can only be measured by CT scan or MRI. Again, the anthropometric prediction of visceral fat from simple anthropometric measurements (waist circumference, sagittal diameter, or others) gives reasonable mean values for a group but is not very accurate for a given individual. Hopefully, new and less costly procedures will become available soon to assess abdominal visceral fat in a noninvasive manner and without radiation exposure.

A variety of methods have been brought to bear on the problem of assessing upper body fat. Circumferences and skinfolds can provide data to index the amount of upper body fat as well as the amount of fat on the upper body relative to the lower body. Thus, waist circumference or the ratio of waist to hip circumferences (WHR) have been commonly used in both clinical research and epidemiological study settings. Similar indications about regional fat distribution can be derived from the sum of several skinfolds obtained from truncal sites or from the sum of trunk skinfolds relative to a lower limb sum of skinfolds. Regional fat distribution can also be assessed from data derived from CT or MRI examinations. It is expected that the same analysis will eventually be possible from a DEXA examination. A nomogram can be used to make rapid assessment of the BMI (Fig. 1) and of the WHR (Fig. 2), as reproduced here.

Table 1 shows the recommended BMI ranges from several expert committees (7). Obesity refers to an excess of total body fat, which can be assessed by a variety of techniques (see Chapter 3). A summary of these methods and their relative cost and ease of use is shown in Table 2. This also identifies those methods that can be used to estimate visceral fat. Table 3 provides the ranges of body fat for men and women.

Adiposity refers to both the distribution and the size of the adipose tissue depots. Since half or more of the body fat is subcutaneous, measurement of skinfold thickness has frequently been used to estimate fat and its distribution. Other techniques involve the use of soft tissue X-rays, ultrasound, electrical conductivity, electrical impedance, CT scans, and MRI scans. From a practical point of view, the circumference of the waist is the simplest method to evaluate upper body obesity, but the ratio of waist circumference divided by the hip circumference, the subscapular skinfold, the ratio of triceps-to-subscapular skinfolds, and the ratio of thigh circumference to abdominal girth have also been used.

Fat cells in specific depots an be measured by needle biopsies of adipose tissue followed by osmium fixation of the fat cell (8) or separation of isolated fat cells by collagenase digestion and then measuring their size under a microscope (9). Because these procedures are invasive they are commonly limited to laboratory studies.

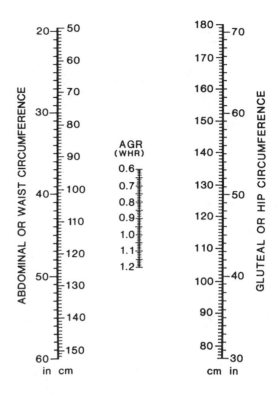

Figure 2   Abdominal (waist) to gluteal (hips) ratio (WHR) can be determined by placing a straightedge between the column for waist circumference and the column for hip circumference and reading the ratio from the point where this straightedge crosses the WHR line. The waist or abdominal circumference is the smallest circumference below the rib cage and above the umbilicus, and the hips or gluteal circumference is taken as the largest circumference at the posterior extension of the buttocks.

IV. FAT CELL SIZE AND NUMBER

The number of fat cells can be estimated from measurements of total body fat and the average size of a fat cell. A reliable estimate of the total number of fat cells should be based on the average size of fat cells from more than one location, because fat cells differ in size from one region to another. Normally, there are no more than 60 billion fat cells. In general, cells proliferate most rapidly from birth to 2 years of age and during late childhood and puberty. In some types of obesity, they can increase 3–5 times more than the normal number. In hypercellular obesity, the number of fat cells is dramatically increased. This type of obesity usually occurs in early or middle childhood but may also occur in adult life.

A higher-than-normal number of fat cells is usually present in people more than 75% above their desirable weight (10,11). when obesity begins during adult life, it often involves enlargement of adipose tissue cells. Hyper-

Table 2   Methods of Estimating Body Fat and Its Distribution

Method	Cost	Ease of use	Accuracy	Measures regional fat
Height and weight	$	Easy	High	No
Skin folds	$	Easy	Low	Yes
Circumferences	$	Easy	Moderate	Yes
Ultrasound	$$	Moderate	Moderate	Yes
Density				
Immersion	$	Moderate	High	No
Plethysmograph	$$$	Difficult	HIgh	No
Heavy Watr				
Tritiated	$$	Moderate	High	No
Deuterium oxide, or heavy oxygen	$$$	Moderate	High	No
Potassium isotope (40K)	$$$$	Difficult	HIgh	No
Total body electrical conductivity (TOBEC)	$$$	Moderate	High	No
Bioelectric impedance (BIA)	$$	Easy	High	No
Fat-soluble gas	$$	Difficult	High	No
Absorptiometry- (Dual energy x-ray absorptiometry = DEXA; Dual photon absorptiometry = DPA)	$$$	Easy	High	Yes
Computed tomography (CT)	$$$$	Difficult	High	Yes
Magnetic resonance imaging (MRI)	$$$$	Difficult	High	Yes
Neutron activation	$$$$	Difficult	High	No

$ = low cost; $$ = moderate cost; $$$ = high cost; $$$$ = very high cost.
Source: Bray & Gray, West J Med, 1988.

trophic obesity tends to correlate with an android or truncal fat distribution and is often associated with metabolic disorders such as glucose intolerance, hyperlipidemia, hypertension, and coronary artery disease (12–15).

V. WEIGHT STANDARDS

A. Body Weight

The generation of national weight standards requires information on a large group of subjects. In the United States, for most of the 20th century, the life insurance industry has provided the data base for the most widely used tables of desirable body weight. In 1959 and again in 1983 the Metropolitan Life Insurance Company published tables of "ideal" or "desirable" weights for Americans based on data obtained from the pooled experience of the life insurance industry in the United States (16,17). Although these surveys of weight and stature among insured individuals provide data on nearly 5 million people, they suffer from a self-selection bias; i.e., they provide data only on people who choose to take out life insurance. The insured tend to have a longer life expectancy, to be healthier, and, on average, to weigh less than the general pop-

ulation and to have few minorities in the database. They are thus no longer appropriate for general use.

A second database has been generated by the National Center for Health Statistics (NCHS), which in the past 20 years performed five surveys, including measurements of weight and stature of a representative sample of Americans from census tracts in the United States (18–20). These surveys include between 10,000 and 20,000 people. As interest in the health implications of obesity has increased, the number of nationally representative surveys has also increased. Good survey data are available from Australia (21), Canada (22), The Netherlands (23), the United Kingdom (24), Japan, and many other countries.

Table 3   Criteria for Obesity in Males and Females

Category	Body fat (%)	
	Males	Females
Normal	12–20	20–30
Borderline	21–25	31–33
Obesity	>25	>33

Source: Adapted from Lohman (45).

Using the nationally representative database of the United States, appropriate weight standards might be determined in one of two ways. First, the normal distribution of weight in relation to height could be arbitrarily divided into overweight and severely overweight groups. This approach has been used by the American NCHS. They define overweight as those above the 85th percentile of weight for height using as a reference the values of 20–29-year-olds obtained in the surveys conducted between 1976 and 1980. With this technique, a BMI higher than 27.8 kg/m² for men and above 27.3 kg/m² for women is considered overweight. Severe overweight or obesity is defined as the 95th percentile of 20–29-year-olds in the same survey. The latter BMI values correspond to 31.1 kg/m² for men and 32.3 kg/m² for women. This approach was used in the Surgeon General's Report on Nutrition and Health but not by the National Institute of Aging, the Dietary Guidelines, or the Diet and Health Report (25).

The NCHS approach has several drawbacks. First, the standards could change as the weight distribution of the population changes. Second, the values for BMI of 27.8 kg/m² for men and 27.3 kg/m² for women for the 85th percentile will be very difficult for health professionals and the public to remember and work with. Third, and most important, is the underlying assumption that average weight is a healthy or preferred weight. Moreover, it is assumed in this approach that optimal weights remain constant at different ages—an assumption that may not be justified (26,27). Finally, such cutoff values are arbitrary.

Weight standards can also be based on the BMI associated with the lowest overall risk to health. The minimal death rate in several prospective studies is associated with a BMI of 22–25 kg/m². Andres et al. (26) reanalyzed the Build and Blood Pressure Study of 1979 (16,17) and showed that the BMI associated with the lowest mortality increased with age. A similar increase in the BMI distribution curve with age is evident from a study conducted in Norway (28). On the basis of these collated data, adjustment of BMI in relation to age may seem reasonable. One proposal would have a BMI range of 19–25 kg/m² for men of all ages and women 18–35 years of age. Women over 35 years would have a value of 21–27 kg/m². In contrast, BMI above 25 kg/m² was associated with increased risk of death in 78,612 young women followed for 32 years (29). In the Nurses Health Trial, BMI values above 27 kg/m² were associated with increased risk of heart disease, cancer, and other diseases. The risk for non-insulin-dependent diabetes mellitus (NIDDM) begins to increase significantly at a BMI above 22 kg/m².

Table 4 Modified WHO Classification of Overweight and Obesity

	BMI
Normal range	18.50–24.99
Grade I overweight	25.00–29.99
Grade IIa overweight	30.00–34.99
Grade IIb overweight	35.00–39.99
Grade III overweight	≥40.00

Alternative to selecting a BMI cutpoint based on specific diseases is to adopt a single set of cutpoints at 5 BMI unit intervals, as suggested by Garrow (30). This has been adapted by the World Health Organization and is shown in Table 4. Table 5 shows the percentage of people in several countries who are overweight or obese by these criteria.

B. Fat Distribution

Fat distribution can be estimated by skinfolds, by waist circumference, by waist-to-hip circumference ratio, or by such sophisticated techniques as ultrasound, DEXA, CT, or MRI. Fat distribution can also be estimated from subscapular skinfold thickness (31,32), which has shown important relationships to risk of disease. Skinfold measurements on the trunk and extremities can be used for principal component analysis, which generally yields a first component for total fat and a second component with loading on upper versus lower body fat (33, 34, and 35).

Databases for circumferences have been developed from Swedish studies in Göteborg (35,36), from studies in Milwaukee, Wisconsin (13,37), and from the Canadian Fitness Survey (38). A nomogram for determining the waist (abdominal) to hip (gluteal) circumference ratio (WHR) is shown in Figure 2. The percentile distribution of these values for men and women in relation to age is plotted in Figure 3 from data obtained in the Canadian Fitness Surveys (38).

VI. ADIPOSITY STANDARDS

Quantitative estimates of total fat have only been determined in relatively small samples compared to data on height and weight (39–42). the available data on body fat have used three main methods: skinfolds, hydrodensitometry, and dual-energy X-ray absorptiometry.

Table 5 Percentage of Overweight and Obese Persons in Several Affluent Countries

	Age (years)	% overweight[a]		% obese[b]	
		Men	Women	Men	Women
Austraia	25–64	44	25	12	13
Canada	18–74	41	23	15	15
Germany	25–69	49	45[c]	16	16
Sweden	16–84	35	26	7	8
United States[d]	>20	39	25	18	23

[a]Overweight = BMI 25–29.
[b]Obese = BMI ≥ 30.
[c]BMI 20–24.
[d]R. Kuczmarski (personal communication).

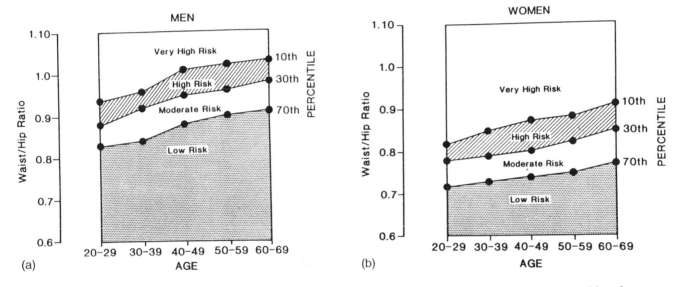

Figure 3 Percentiles for the ratio of abdominal circumference to guteal circumference (WHR) are shown for men (a) and women (b) by age groups. The relative risk for the percentiles is indicated based on the available information. (Plotted from tabular data in the Canadian Standardized Test of Fitness, Third Edition 1986. Available from Fitness and Amateur Sport Canada, 365 Laurier Ave. W., Ottawa, Ontario, K1A OX6.)

A. Skinfolds

Durnin and Womersley (44) provided tables for estimating body fat from skinfolds measured at four different sites. Several other groups have also provided equations for estimating body fat for men and women of various ages, using skinfolds from selected sites (45,46). Triceps and subscapular skinfolds were measured in the surveys conducted by the NCHS; however, these measurements cannot be used to establish standards for determining fatness because no data were collected on the relationship of these skinfolds to other measures of body fat. It is nonetheless possible to divide the population into percentiles of body fat by determining skinfold measurements from triceps and the subscapular region. It should be kept in mind, however, that the standard error of estimate of the prediction of percent body fat from skinfolds reaches about 3–4 percentage units, which results in wide confidence intervals for the predicted value. However, when BMI is above 30 kg/m², the estimates of overweight and obesity are more congruent.

B. Hydrodensitometry

No large databases are available.

C. Dual-Energy X-Ray Absorptiometry

DEXA has almost supplanted densitometry as the gold standard for measuring body fat. The percent of body fat estimated from DEXA varies with age, gender, ethnicity, and level of physical activity. The technique can be used to quantify the absolute amount of fat on the trunk, the

abdominal area, or any body segment. However, DEXA cannot distinguish between subcutaneous and intra-abdominal (visceral) fat.

VII. IS OBESITY A DISEASE?

Much of the previous discussion has been about the definition of weight, body fat, and fat distribution standards and their relations to disease risk. Obesity, hypercholesterolemia, and high blood pressure are similar in this re-

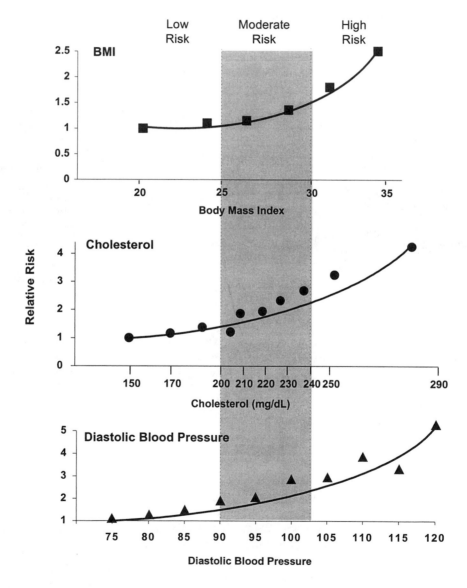

Figure 4   Relationship of BMI, cholesterol, and blood pressure to risk of ill health. The vertical lines reflect accepted subdivisions for low, moderate, and high risk. All three curves show a curvilinear increase with increasing level of risk factor. (Copyright 1995, George A. Bray.)

gard. Figure 4 shows the relationship between each of these in relation to risk of death. It is clear that as each of these risk factors increases along its continuum, relative risk increases. High blood pressure per se is not a risk, but rather the damage it does to vessels in the brain, heart, eye, and kidney. Similarly, high cholesterol is not a risk per se, but rather through the damage it does to vessels that occlude or provide a nidus for coagulation and the development of atherosclerosis. The same argument applies to obesity. It is not the increased fat per se, but its consequences on other systems. Flemyng caught this distinction clearly more than 200 years ago when he said: "corpulency, when in an extraordinary degree, may be reckoned a disease, as it in some measure obstructs the free exercise of the animal functions; and hath a tendency to shorten life, by paving the way to dangerous distempers" (47).

REFERENCES

1. Bray GA. Commentary on classics in obesity. Life insurance and overweight. Obes Res 1995; 3:97–99.
2. Dawber TR. The Framingham Study: The Epidemiology of Atherosclerotic Disease. Cambridge: Harvard University Press, 1980.
3. Bouchard C, Despres J, Mauriege P. Genetic and nongenetic determinants of regional fat distribution. Endocr Rev 1993; 14(1):72–93 (review).
4. Bray GA. Obesity: historical development of scientific and cultural ideas. Int J Obes Relat Metab Disord 1990; 14(2):6.
5. Quetelet A. Sur l'homme et le developpement de ses facultes, ou essai de physique sociale. Paris: Bachelier, 1835.
6. Benn RT. Some mathematical properties of weight-for-height indices used as measures of adiposity. Br J Prev Soc Med 1971; 25:42–50.
7. Sichieri R, Everhart JE, Hubbard VS. Relative weight classifications in the assessment of underweight and overweight in the United States. Int J Obes Relat Metab Disord 1992; 16:303–312.
8. Hirsch J, Gallian E. Methods for the determination of adipose cell size in man and animals. J Lipid Res 1968; 9:110–119.
9. Sjostrom L, Björntorp P. Body composition and adipose tissue cellularity in human obesity. Acta Med Scand 1974; 195:201–211.
10. Björntorp, P. Adipose tissue in obesity (Wellendorf lecture). In: Hirsch J, Van Itallie TB, eds. Recent Advances in Obesity Research, 4th ed. London: John Libbey, 1985:163–170.
11. Hirsch J, Batchelor B. Adipose tissue cellularity in human obesity. J Clin Endocrinol Metab 1976; 5:299–311.
12. Feldman R, Sender AJ, Sieglaub AB. Difference in diabetic and nondiabetic fat distribution patterns by skin fold measurements. Diabetics 1969; 18:478–486.
13. Kissebah AH, Vydelingm N, Murray R, et al. Relation of body fat distribution to metabolism complications of obesity. J Clin Endocrinol Metab 1982; 54:254–260.
14. Krotkiewski M, Björntorp P, Sjostrom L, Smith U. Impact of obesity on metabolism in men and women. Importance of regional adipose tissue distribution. J Clin Invest 1983; 72:1150–1162.
15. Vague J. Degree of masculin differentiation of obesities: factor determining predisposition to diabetes, atherosclerosis, gout, and uric calculous disease. Am J Clin Nutr 1956; 4:20–34.
16. Society of Actuaries. Build and Blood Pressure Study, Vol 1. Chicago: Society of Actuaries, 1959.
17. Society of Actuaries. Build Study of 1979. Chicago: Society of Actuaries/Assoc Life Ins Med Directors of AM, 1980.
18. Troiano RP, Flegal KM, Kuczmarski RJ, Campbell SM, Johnson CL. Overweight prevalence and trends for children and adolescents. The National Health and Nutrition Examination Surveys, 1963 to 1991. Arch Pediatr Adolesc Med 1995; 149:1085–1091.
19. Kuczmarski RJ, Flegal KM, Campbell SM, Johnson CL. Increasing prevalence of overweight among US adults: the National Health and Nutrition Examination Surveys, 1960 to 1991. JAMA 1994; 272:205–211.
20. Najjar MF, Rowland M. Anthropometric reference data and prevalence of overweight, United States, 1976–1980. Vital Health Statist 1987; 238(11):87–1688.
21. Australia's Health 1992. The third biennial report of the Australian Institute of Health and Welfare. Canberra: Australian Government Publishing Service, 1992.
22. Reeder BA, Angel A, Ledux M, et al. Obesity and its relation to cardiovascular disease risk factors in Canadian adults. Can Med Assoc J 1992; 146(11):2009–2019.
23. Seidell JC, Verschuren WMM, Kromhout D. Prevalence and trends of obesity in The Netherlands 1987–1991. Int J Obes 1995; 19:924–927.
24. United Kingdom
25. Surgeon Generals Report DD. The Surgeon General's Report on Nutrition and Health. DHHS (PHS) Publ. No. 88-50210. Public Health Service, US Department of Health and Human Services. Washington DC: US Government Printing Office, 1988:1–712.
26. Andrews R, Elahi D, Tobin J, Muller D, Brant L. Impact of age on weight goals. Ann Intern Med 1985; 10:1030–1033.
27. Diet and Health, Implications for Reducing Chronic Disease Risk. Washington, DC: National Research Council, National Academy Press, 1989.
28. Waaler HT. Height, weight and mortality: the Norwegian experience. Acta Med Scand 1984; 679:1–56.
29. Hoffmans MDAF, Kromhout D, de Lezenne Coulander C. The impact of body mass index of 78,612 18-year-old Dutch mean on 32-year mortality from all causes. J Clin Epidemiol 1988; 41:749–756.
30. Garrow JS. Treat Obesity Seriously: A Clinical Manual. London: Churchill Livingstone, 1981.

31. Donahue RP, Abbott RD, Bloom E, Reed DM, Yano K. Central obesity and coronary heart disease in men. Lancet 1987; 1:821–824.

32. Stokes J, III, Garrison RJ, Kannel WB. The independent contributions of various indices of obesity to the 22-year incidence of coronary heart disease: the Framingham Heart Study. In: Vague J, Björntorp P, Guy-Grand B, Rebuffe-Scrive M, Vague P, eds. Metabolic Complications of Human Obesities. Amsterdam: Excerpta Medica, 1985:49–57.

33. Ducimetiere P, Richard J, Cambien F. The pattern of subcutaneous fat distribution in middle-aged men and the risk of coronary heart disease: the Paris Prospective Study. Int J Obes 1986; 10:229–240.

34. Mueller WH. The genetics of human fatness. Yearbook Phys Anthropol 1983; 26:215–230.

35. Liz, Rice T, Perusse L, Bouchard E, Rar D. E. Farribal aggregation of subcutaneous fat patterning: principal components of skinfolds in the Quebec Farruly Study. Am J Hum Biol 1996; 8:535–542.

36. Lapidus L, Bengtsson C, Larsson B, Pennert K, Rybo E, Sjostrom L. Distribution of adipose tissue and risk of cardiovascular disease and death: a 12 year follow-up of participants in the population study of women in Gothenburg, Sweden. Br Med J 1984; 289:1257–1261.

37. Larsson B, Svardsudd K, Welin L, Wilhelmsen L, Björntorp P, Tibblin G. Abdominal adipose tissue distribution, obesity, and risk of cardiovascular disease and death: 13 year follow-up of participants in the study of men born in 1913. Br Med J 1984; 288:1401–1404.

38. Hartz AJ, Rupley CC, Rimm AA. The association of girth measurements with disease in 32,856 women. Am J Epidemiol 1984; 119:71–80.

39. Fitness and Amateur Sport. Canadian Standardized Test of Fitness (For 15 to 69 Years of Age). Operation Manual. 3rd ed. Ottawa, Ontario Canada: Minister of State, Fitness and Amateur Sport, Govt Canada, 1986.

40. Cheek DB. Human Growth. Philadelphia: Lea & Febiger, 1968.

41. Cohn SH, Vaswani AN, Yasumura S, Yuen K, Ellis KJ. Improved models for determination of body fat by in vivo neutron activation. Am J Clin Nutr 1984; 40:255–259.

42. Ashwell M, Chinn S, Stalley S, Garrow JS. Female fat distribution—a photographic and Cellularity study. Int J Obes Relat Metab Disord 1978; 2(3):289–302.

43. Segal KR, Gutin B, Presta E, Wang J, Van Itallie TB. Estimation of human body composition by electrical impedance methods: a comparative study. J Appl Physiol 1985; 58:1565–1571.

44. Durnin JV, Womersley J. Body fat assessed from total body density and its estimation from skinfold thickness: measurements on 481 men and women aged from 16 to 72 years. Br J Nutr 1974; 32:77–97.

45. Lohman TG. Skinfolds and body density and their relation to body fatness: a review. Hum Biol 1981; 53:181–225.

46. Lukaski HC. Methods for the assessment of human body composition: traditional and new. Am J Clin Nutr 1987; 46:537–556.

47. Flemyng M. A discourse on the nature, causes and cure of corpulency. Illustrated by a remarkable case, read before the Royal Society, November 1757 and now first published. London: L. Davis and C. Reymers, 1760.

3

Evaluation of Total and Regional Body Composition

Steven B. Heymsfield, David B. Allison, and Zi-Mian Wang
St. Luke's–Roosevelt Hospital and Columbia University College of Physicians and Surgeons, New York, New York

Richard N. Baumgartner
University of New Mexico School of Medicine, Albuquerque, New Mexico

Robert Ross
Queen's University, Kingston, Ontario, Canada

I. OVERVIEW

Quantifying the amount and distribution of adipose tissue and its related components is integral to the study and treatment of human obesity. Body composition research is a field devoted specifically to the development and extension of methods for the in vivo quantification of adipose tissue, as well as other biochemical and anatomical components of the body. This field has progressed during the last 40 years from the whole-body, "somatic," or organism level, to anatomical dissections, to biophysical approaches for the in vivo estimation of components, and most recently to underlying genetic and molecular mechanisms determining variability in composition. In this chapter we focus on methods of estimating body composition components in the context of evaluating human obesity and its associated risks.

This chapter first describes the organization of human body composition with an emphasis on body fatness. A general overview is then provided on approaches to measuring body composition components, especially fat mass, adipose tissue, and related components. The concepts developed in this section are then used to describe each of the available whole-body and regional methods for as-

sessing adipose tissue and related body composition components in the study of obesity.

II. BODY COMPOSITION LEVELS

The human body may be considered to consist of multiple components distributed across five basic levels of organization: atomic, molecular, cellular, anatomical, or, more precisely, "tissue-system," and whole-body (Fig. 1). The 35–40 primary components at the five levels of organization are summarized in Table 1. Each component is considered discrete without overlap with other components at the same level. Components, however, may overlap across levels. The sum of the components at a level equals body weight or mass. These facts allow the formulation of explicit body composition equations for estimating unknown components from measured ones and body weight. Some of these are given in Table 2.

A complete assessment of the disordered body composition known clinically as "obesity" involves the quantification of components at all five levels of body composition. The following sections consequently review our model of the five body levels of composition organization as a prelude to a more detailed discussion of contemporary methods for assessing body composition in obesity.

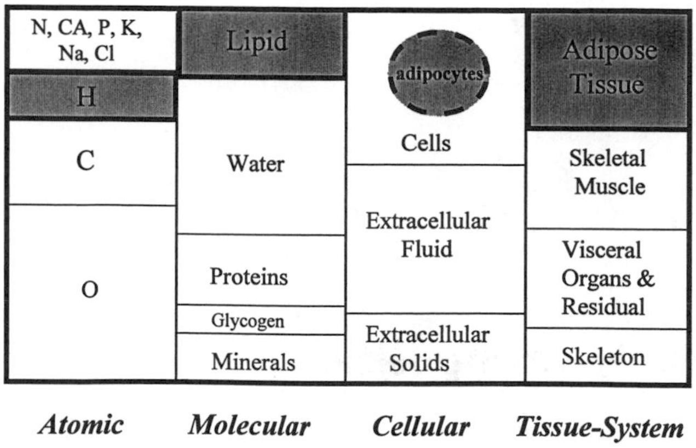

N, CA, P, K, Na, Cl	Lipid	adipocytes Cells	Adipose Tissue
H			Skeletal Muscle
C	Water	Extracellular Fluid	
O	Proteins		Visceral Organs & Residual
	Glycogen	Extracellular Solids	Skeleton
	Minerals		
Atomic	**Molecular**	**Cellular**	**Tissue-System**

Figure 1 The first four of the five levels of human body composition. Components related to "fatness" are enclosed in bold.

This includes the merits and limitations of various in vivo methods when applied to obese patients in both clinical and epidemiological settings and issues related to the use of the measured variables in evaluating effects of treatment, prognosis, and risk of morbidity and mortality.

A. The Five-Level Model of Body Composition

As shown in Figure 1, we conceive of human body composition as organized into discrete components at five basic levels of organization. An understanding of the theoretical and empirical bases of these levels, and of the interrelationships among the components at different levels, is essential for correct application of contemporary body composition methodology.

I. Atomic

The human body is comprised of 11 elements that account for over 99.5% of body weight (1). Three of these

elements, carbon, hydrogen, and oxygen, are found in storage triglycerides (3). The elemental stoichiometry of some common triglycerides found in humans (see Table 3). The average proportions of these are carbon, hydrogen, and oxygen are considered stable at approximately 76.7%, 12.0%, and 11.3%, respectively (3,4). These stable elemental proportions of triglycerides allow the development of methods for deducing total body fat from total body carbon and other elements (5).

2. Molecular

The above elements, including trace elements that occur in low, but essential concentrations, combine to form various chemical compounds that may be grouped into the broad classes that define the molecular level of body composition. The main components of the molecular level are shown in Table 1, and include water, lipids, proteins, minerals, and carbohydrates. Each of the nonaqueous components represents many different, but closely related chemical compounds. For example, the "protein" component consists of several hundred different compounds of protein.

The major molecular level components can be formulated into various models as summarized in Table 2. Generally, it is not feasible to measure all components at the molecular level. The direct quantification of body "fat" or lipid, in particular, has proven difficult historically. As a result, a variety of methods have been developed for estimating this component indirectly using measurements of other components in various models. Two-, three-, and four-component models are widely used in body composition research and these will be presented in later sections. Given the introduction of new methods of quantifying body fat directly, some of these models have been reoriented in recent years toward estimating other components that are difficult to measure, for example total-body protein.

Table 1 Main Body Composition Components

	Level				
	Atomic	Molecular	Cellular	Tissue-system	Whole-body
Components	O, C, H, N, Ca, P, S, K, Na, Cl, Mg	Fat, water, protein bone mineral, non–bone tissue mineral, glycogen, fat-free body mass, fat-free solids	Fat cells, cell mass, intracellular fluid, extracellular fluid, extracellular solids, body cell mass	Adipose tissue (AT), subcutaneous AT, visceral AT, bone, skeletal muscle, skeleton	Head, neck, arms, trunk, legs
Number of components	11	8	6	6	5

Source: From Ref. 2, with permission.

Table 2 Body Composition Equation at Different Body Composition Levels

Level	Equation	Model
Atomic	BW = O + C + H + N + Ca + P + S + Na + Cl + Mg	11-component
Molecular	BW = F + A + Pro + Ms + Mo + G	6-component
	BW = F + A + Pro + M	4-component
	BW = F + A + solids	3-component
	BW = F + Mo + residual	3-component
	BW = F + FFM	2-component
Cellular	BW = CM + ECF + ECS	
	BW = F + BCM + ECF + ECS	
Tissue-system	BW = AT + SM + bone + other tissues	

A, water; AT, adipose tissue; BCM, body cell mass; BW, body weight; CM, cell mass; ECF, extracellular fluid; ECS, extracellular solids; F, fat; FFM, fat-free body mass; G, glycogen; M, mineral; Mo, bone mineral; Ms, soft tissue mineral; Pro, protein; SM, skeletal muscle.
Source: From Ref. 1, with permission.

Lipid is the main molecular level component of interest in the study of human obesity. The term "lipid" refers to all chemical compounds that are insoluble or weakly soluble in water, but are soluble in organic solvents such as chloroform and diethyl ether (6,7). Lipids isolated from human tissues include triglycerides, sphyngomyelin, phospholipids, steroids, fatty acids, and terpenes. Triglycerides, commonly referred to as "fats," are the primary storage lipids in humans and comprise the largest fraction of the total lipid component (3,4) (Table 3). At present there is limited information on the exact proportion of total lipids as triglycerides, or the amount of within- and between-person variability. The "reference man," however, is considered to consist of 13.5 kg of total lipid of which 12.0 kg, or 89%, is "fat" (4).

A summary of molecular level component characteristics is presented in Table 4. These characteristics are used in developing body composition methods and their application will be presented in later sections.

Table 3 Stoichiometry and Elemental Composition of Representative Triglycerides

Formula	Chemical Carbon (%)	Hydrogen (%)	Oxygen (%)
$C_{57}H_{104}O_6$	77.4	11.8	10.9
$C_{51}H_{98}O_6$	75.9	12.2	11.9
$C_{55}H_{102}O_6$	76.9	11.9	11.2
$C_{55}H_{104}O_6$	76.7	12.1	11.2
"Average" triglyceride	76.7	12.0	11.3

Source: Data from Refs. 3 and 4.

3. Cellular

The cellular level includes three main components, cell mass, extracellular fluid, and extracellular solids. Cells can be divided into specific types such as connective, epithelial, nervous, and muscular. Adipocytes or fat cells serve as the primary storage site for triglycerides. It is often desirable to exclude inert, storage triglycerides in the estimation of "body cell mass." This component may be grouped separately as "fat mass" or combined with "extracellular solids" as a "metabolically inert" component. The concept of body cell mass was originated by Moore and refers to the mass of materials composing cells that are actively involved in energy consumption and heat production (8). This concept has considerable clinical and physiological significance, but the exact definition and measurement of body cell mass are usually difficult in practice.

4. Tissue-System

The main components at this level are adipose tissue, skeletal muscle, bone, and visceral organs (e.g., liver, kidneys, heart, etc.). The adipose tissue component includes adipocytes with collagenous and elastic fibers, fibroblasts, capillaries, and extracellular fluid. Adipose tissue can be classified by distribution into four types, subcutaneous, visceral, interstitial, and yellow marrow (4). The introduction of computerized axial tomography (CT) over the past decade allowed the first accurate quantification of visceral adipose tissue (VAT) (9). More recently, magnetic resonance imaging (MRI) has been developed for this purpose, as described below.

Human adipose tissue is often assumed to have an approximate average composition consisting of 80% lipid, 14% water, 5% protein, and <1% mineral, and a density

Table 4 Characteristics of Molecular Level Components

Component	Density (g/cm³)	Elemental stoichiometry
Water	0.99371 at 36°C	0.111 H; 0.889 O.
	0.994 at 37°C	
Protein	1.34 at 37°C	0.532 C; 0.070 H; 0.161 N; 0.227 O; 0.01 S.
Glycogen	1.52 at 37°C	0.444 C; 0.062 H; 0.494 O.
Minerals	3.042 (weighted avg of bone and nonbone)	
Bone[a]	2.982 at 36–36.7°C	0.398 Ca; 0.002 H; 0.185 P; 0.414 O.
Nonbone	3.317 at approx. 40°C	
Lipid	0.9007 at 36°C	0.767 C; 0.120 H; 0.113 O.

[a]Calculated from the largest component of bone mineral, calcium hydroxyapatite $[Ca_3(PO_4)_2]_3Ca(OH)_2$. Other small elemental contributions to bone, such as Na, are recognized.
Source: Data from Ref. 8.

of 0.92 g/cm³ at body temperature (10). Adipocytes, however, range in lipid content from a negligible amount in connective tissue precursors to a high lipid content in mature adipocytes observed in morbidly obese subjects. According to Martin and colleagues, for every 10% increase in relative adiposity there is a corresponding rise in adipose tissue lipid fraction of 0.124 (11). Variation in adipocyte fat content is shown for the rat in Figure 2. As the rat matures, there is a progressive increase in adipose tissue fat content and a corresponding relative reduction in water. The change in fat content with age in the rat result is a lowering of adipose tissue density, a phenomenon that is important to consider when attempting to convert measured adipose tissue volume to mass.

A notable feature of adipose tissue is the relatively large extracellular fluid compartment relative to cell mass. Of

the 14% of average adipose tissue samples as water, 11% is extracellular water (11).

5. Whole Body

Skinfolds, circumferences, and linear dimensions are all measurements at the whole-body level. These measurements are often used with prediction equations to estimate components at the other four body composition levels (1).

The human body can thus be divided into discrete components that are distributed into five increasingly complex levels. The study of human obesity involves investigation of many components at all five body composition levels. In the sections that follow our main emphasis will be on methods that are used to quantify "fatness" or "adiposity."

III. BODY COMPOSITION METHODS

A. Organization

Body composition methods can be organized as outlined in Figure 3 (12). Methods can be broadly divided into in vivo and in vitro. This chapter will focus only on in vivo body composition methods.

In vivo body composition methods can be classified into six categories as outlined in Figure 3. These categories are based on the basic body composition methodology formula (12):

$$C = f(Q) \qquad (1)$$

where C is unknown component, Q is a measurable quantity, and f is the mathematical function that links Q to C. All body composition methods share this basic formula in common. The formula indicates that body composition

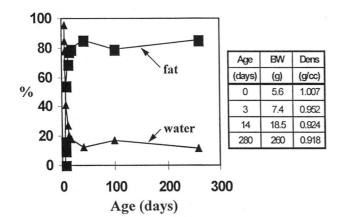

Figure 2 Inguinal fat pad composition in the rat. Fat and water content are expressed as a percent of fat pad weight. Adipose tissue density was calculated from composition data (3).

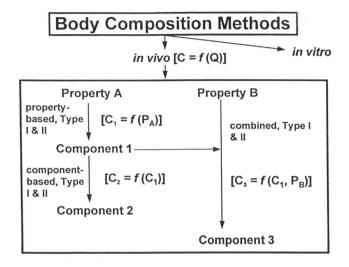

Figure 3 Organization of body composition methods. (From Ref. 12, with permission.)

methods can be organized according to measurable quantity and mathematical function (12).

I. Measurable Quantities

Property-Based Methods. Property-based methods all apply the general formula $C = f(P)$, where P is a measurable property. A relatively small number of physical, chemical, and biological properties are used in body composition assessment. These include anthropometric dimensions, electrical resistance, radioactive decay profiles, weight, volume, oxygen consumption, infrared interactance, fat soluble gas uptake, and X-ray attenuation.

Examples of property-based methods include estimation of total body fat from measured skinfold thicknesses (13,14), body volume (by underwater weighing) (15), and X-ray attenuation (by dual-energy X-ray absorptiometry) (16).

All property-based methods ultimately rely on the measurement of one or more properties. Property-based methods are the foundation of body composition methodology.

Component-Based Methods. Component-based methods all apply the general formula $C_u = f(C_k)$, where C_u is an unknown component and C_k is a known component. The known component must first be derived using a property-based method.

An example of a component-based method is estimation of total-body fat from total-body carbon and other elements (5).

Combined Methods. Some methods are based on both a measurable property and known component. These combined methods all apply the general formula $C_u = f(P, C_k)$.

Examples of combined methods include estimation of total body fat from (1) body volume (a measurable property) and total body water (a known component), and (2) body weight (a measurable property) and total body potassium (a known component) (12).

2. Mathematical Functions

Mathematical functions applied in the fundamental body composition equation can be broadly classified into two types (Figure 3). The creation of these two function types is somewhat arbitrary, although in practice we found the distinction between various mathematical functions useful in understanding method development and errors.

Descriptive (Type I) Methods. Descriptive or type I methods are all based on statistically derived regression equations (12). These methods share in common three characteristics: a reference method for measuring the component of interest, a well-characterized subject group, and the application of statistical methods to derive the function for predicting the component from the measured properties or components. Because they are developed on discrete subject groups, type I prediction equation methods are often "population specific." This means that an equation does not necessarily provide accurate estimates when applied to people who differ in terms of sex, ethnicity, age, or health status from those included in the sample from which the equation was derived. As a result, estimates from prediction equations should be validated against those from an established laboratory-based method in a random subsample of participants or patients before the equation is applied to the entire study population. Some approaches that may be used in the development of prediction equations and the potential errors that might arise were reviewed recently by Roche and Guo (17).

An example of a type I prediction method is the estimation of total body water (TBW) using the bioelectric impedance approach, as found in Lukaski et al. (18). Bioelectric resistance, stature, and TBW by deuterium dilution were measured in a group of subjects. Simple linear regression analysis was used to derive an equation for predicting TBW (kg) from the two measurable properties height (H, cm) and bioelectric resistance (R, ohm): TBW $= 0.63 \times H^2/R + 2.03$, $r = 0.95$, $p < 0.0001$. Although the general formula for relating body water volume to height and resistance is based on a theoretical model that relates conductive volume to length (L) and resistance (V = rL^2/R), the coefficient r cannot be derived a priori and must be estimated statistically. This contrasts with the approach taken in type II methods.

Mechanistic (Type II) Methods. Mechanistic or type II methods are all formulated from what we generally refer to as biological models. A "model" in this context denotes the a priori specification of the function relating a component to a property or another component based on the assumption of one or more constant physical, biochemical, physiological, anatomical, or other structural relationships between components (12) in many cases a clear underlying mechanism can be found to support the observed stable relationships. Most models specify functions in the form of proportions or ratios. Some examples include TBW/FFM (0.73 kg/kg), carbon/fat (0.767 kg/kg), total-body potassium/FFM (0.00266 kg/kg), and nitrogen/protein (0.16 kg/kg) (1). In contrast to type I methods, the values for the ratios or proportions used in these models are formulated a priori based on data from chemical analyses of human tissues or animal experiments and do not require statistical methods in their development. Nevertheless, type II methods may be population-specific also and their application to a new group sometimes requires validation of the assumptions made in the underlying model.

An example of a classic type II method is estimation of FFM (kg) from TBW (kg): FFM = 1.37 × TBW. This method was first popularized by Pace and Rathbun (19), who observed a relatively constant hydration of FFM in animals (0.73), and others subsequently observed similar hydration in humans (20) (Fig. 4). The method gained

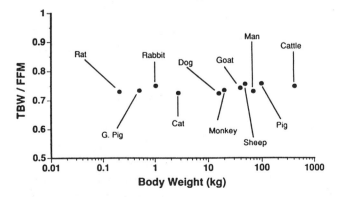

Figure 4 Total-body water to FFM ratio in animals and humans plotted as a function of the logarithm of body weight. (Data from Refs. 19 and 20.)

widespread clinical use due to the ease and low cost of isotope dilution methods for TBW measurement.

3. Errors of Estimation

In summary, all in vivo body composition methods attempt to estimate or predict the size, volume or mass of an unknown component from measurements of associated properties or other components using various equations or models. An important area of body composition methodology is quantitative analysis of the magnitude and directions of the different types of errors that may occur. A variety of previous efforts have been made to address this complicated area, and it would not be appropriate to provide a detailed review in this chapter (21–23). The following paragraphs provide a general overview of basic concepts.

Error in in vivo body composition research can arise from several different sources. Most of these can be considered in terms of the following modification of our general model:

$$C_u = f(Q) = a + b\,C_T + e_b + e_m, \qquad (2)$$

where C_u is the unknown component's estimated value, C_T is the unknown component's "true" value, a and b jointly describe any biases associated with misspecification of the function (f) for estimating C_u, e_b is "biological error," and e_m is "measurement error" of Q. For simplicity, it is assumed that the function relating the "true" value to the estimate is linear and that e_b and e_m are random and independent.

Random measurement errors (e_m) are the easiest to consider and can be quantified from two or more repeated estimates derived using the same instrumentation, observers, equations, or models. This type of error is referred by a variety of names, including "reliability," "reproducibility," and "precision," and can be expressed in variety of ways, such as the standard error of the repeated estimates ("technical error"), the coefficient of variation, or the intraclass correlation (24). An important aspect in analyzing these errors is to establish that they are truly random. A simple approach is to plot the differences between the repeated estimates against the mean of the two estimates (25). The errors should neither increase nor decrease in relation to the mean of the estimates, and the average of the errors should equal zero. If this is not found, then one or more problems need to be considered with regard to the specification of the function (type I equation or type II model) used to derive the estimates.

In Eq. (2), the parameters a and b can be interpreted as describing "constant bias" (or "offset") and "relative bias," respectively (24). If the function relating Q to C_u

were completely "unbiased," the expectation would be that $a = 0$ and $b = 1$. These biases can arise for a variety of reasons in both type I and type II methods and these reasons can often be very difficult to identify. Clearly, bias occurs when the function is valid for some individuals but not others, differs systematically according to age, gender, race, health status, or other characteristics, or is influenced by some other, unidentified variable. Bias is the main reason many type I equations are often found to be "population-specific" and type II methods are sometimes constrained due to the "limited validity" of the a priori assumptions made in the underlying models. The detection of and correction for "bias" actually preoccupy much of the literature on body composition methodology where new methods are assessed for "accuracy." It is important to recognize that this work usually assumes one selected method represents a "gold standard" defining "accurate" estimates.

The biological error component in Eq. (2) can be considered in at least two ways, both of which may have more or less importance depending on the type of study. In one context, this error can be considered the part of within-subject variability that is not due to measurement errors. Habicht (26, see also 22) defined this error as "undependability" to capture the fact that most biological variables fluctuate within individuals over time. For example, body weight fluctuates on a day-to-day basis independent of errors in the measurement of weight. This type of error can be seen to be important mainly with regard to quantifying changes in body composition over time, where it may be difficult to separate errors due to measurement "unreliability" from those due to biological "undependability."

Biological errors can be considered in the context of type II methods as random, biological variability both within and between subjects that is not incorporated in or fully captured by the model used to estimate the unknown component. An example might be the type II equation used to estimate FFM from TBW. Assume that the constant value, 0.732, converts TBW into an unbiased estimate of FFM. That is, there is no evidence that age, gender, race, obesity, disease, or other characteristics and factors affect this value so that it is appropriate for some groups but not others. Thus, this type II formula will provide an accurate estimate of the true mean value for the group of study subjects. However, individual estimates may contain error due in part to the fact that random biological variability may still exist between subjects in the amount of water in the FFM.

Finally, an important aspect in the consideration of errors in body composition research is the concept of "propagated errors." This is important because most methods estimate unknown components based on properties or other components that contain errors. In other words, biases and/or errors in the estimation of TBW from isotope dilution analysis will be propagated to estimates of FFM, regardless of issues related to misspecification of the fluctuation relating TBW to FFM. It is not unusual for propagated errors to become magnified by the type I or II method used. In addition, errors are compounded when combined methods are applied or prediction equations are used that required several variables. It has been argued that the application of "multicomponent" or combined methods can provide more accurate estimates for individuals since false assumptions regarding functional relationships and biological variability can be reduced or even eliminated. This is true only if the multiple components and/or properties are measured with high precision. If they are not, the compounded propagated errors of measurement may become so great as to "swamp" any reduction in biological errors to be derived from the multicomponent approach.

It should be recognized that our schema of body composition methods makes some implicit assumptions regarding the relative accuracy's of different methods. Clearly, those classified as type I are, on the whole, considered less accurate because they are based on equations that are usually derived by statistical calibration against components measured using type II methods. Hence, the estimates provided by type I approaches cannot be more accurate than the "criterion" type II estimate they are calibrated against. Any errors in the type II criterion estimates will be propagated to and often magnified in the type I method. There is a wide range of opinion as to the relative accuracy of type II methods. We avoid the use of the term "gold standard" in reference to any of these. The choice of a "criterion" or "reference" method depends on consideration of a variety of factors, including: the level of the component to be estimated, the precision of the instrumentation used and technical expertise of the user, the validity of any assumptions made, and the types of subjects measured.

IV. APPLICATIONS TO THE STUDY OF OBESITY

Most body composition research related to obesity is based on the molecular level (fat and FFM) and tissue-system level (adipose tissue, adipose tissue-free body mass, and skeletal muscle). Measurements of interest include whole-body and regional components. The main available methods are outlined in Table 5. We have selected methods for review that are in current use and that

Table 5 Whole-Body (W) and Regional (R) Measurement Methods Used in Assessing Adiposity-Related Components

Method	Adiposity-related component					
	Fat	FFM	SAT	VAT	ATFM	SM
Type I						
Body weight	W	W				
Anthropometry	W, R	W, R	W, R	W	W, R	W, R
Bioimpedance and conductivity	W, R	W, R				W, R
Ultrasound	W, R	W, R	W, R	W	W, R	W, R
Type II						
Isotope dilution (total body water)	W	W				
Hydrodensitometry	W	W				
Dual-energy X-ray absorptiometry	W, R	W, R	R			R
Whole-body counting/IVNA	W	W				W
Imaging (CT, MRI)			W, R	W, R	W, R	W, R

ATFM, adipose tissue-free body mass; CT, computed tomography; FFM, fat-free body mass; IVNA, in vivo neutron activation analysis; MRI, magnetic resonance imaging; SAT, subcutaneous adipose tissue; SM, skeletal muscle; VAT, visceral adipose tissue.

are considered appropriate for clinical and research applications. The table is divided into type I and type II methods, and the range of whole-body and regional estimates at molecular and tissue-system levels is shown for each method. An important feature of type I methods is that they are generally capable of providing predictions of a wide range of components using relatively simple, inexpensive measurements. As a result, they are preferred "field methods" for large-population studies. Their accuracy, as noted above, depends in part on that of the more cumbersome and expensive type II, or "laboratory-based," methods they are usually calibrated against. The following sections describe each of the methods in Table 5 in detail with specific reference to their relative merits and limitations in the assessment of obesity.

A. Descriptive (Type I) Methods

I. Anthropometry

Anthropometry is the least expensive, most widely used method of assessing human body composition. Anthropometric measurements are used in clinical and epidemiological studies to grade the degree of adiposity in individuals and groups and to estimate the prevalence of overweight and obesity in populations. The measurements are also used to describe the anatomical distribution of adipose tissue and to classify individuals and groups with regard to the "type" of obesity—"centralized" or "peripheral." The various measures, and the ratios or indices derived from them, are important for evaluating the health risks associated with excess body fatness or obesity and any changes that occur during treatment of obese patients (27).

The anthropometric measurements considered as most useful in assessing obesity include weight, stature, skinfold thicknesses, circumferences of the trunk and limbs, and sagittal trunk thickness. Ultrasound is considered in this section as a "quasi-anthropometric" method that is being applied increasingly in clinical studies to quantify adipose tissue distribution. It is placed here, instead of in the section on imaging, because of the limited nature of the regional body composition information provided.

Anthropometric variables do not correspond directly to body composition components but are superficial, somatic measures that are influenced by and, consequently, correlated with variation in the underlying, or "latent," components. Anthropometric variables therefore can be used either as "proxy variables" for the latent components or as the "measurable quantity" in type I property-based methods. The following sections will consider the merits and limitations of these two different approaches to using weight, stature, skinfold thicknesses, circumferences, and sagittal trunk thickness to grade or predict body fatness, classify individuals or groups as "obese," and describe adipose tissue distribution.

Weight, Stature, and Body Mass Indices. Standardized methods have been described for measuring weight and stature, as well as other anthropometric variables (28). For most clinical research purposes, it is desirable to measure body weight to the nearest ±0.1 kg using a beam-balance scale. Spring scales or electronic scales may be used but generally require more frequent and careful calibration. Subjects should be measure either nude or wearing standardized light clothing of known weight. If other, heavier clothing is worn it is necessary to estimate and record the additional weight of this clothing. The presence of edema, a common problem in severely obese subjects, should be noted. A variety of practical problems may be encountered when measuring the weight of obese subjects. Severely obese patients may have difficulty standing on standard scales, which may be too narrow or too high above the floor for an individual with balance problems. Specifically designed chair or sling scales may be used.

The preferred method of measuring stature is to the nearest ± 1 cm using a wall-mounted stadiometer. Inexpensive, plastic stadiometers are available for clinical use that have acceptable accuracy. Close attention should be paid to standardized positioning of the subject when making the measurement (28). As for weight, a variety of practical problems may be encountered when measuring the stature of obese subjects. For example, the standard method requires the subject to stand erect with the head, shoulders, and buttocks against the stadiometer board. This positioning may be difficult to achieve for obese individuals with large, protruding buttocks.

It is sometimes considered difficult and expensive to measure weight and stature in very large epidemiological surveys, and it is usually not possible to obtain measurements of past weight or stature for retrospective studies. In these settings many investigators have relied on self-reported weight and stature. This assumes that the subjects know and can report their weight and stature both accurately and reliably. It is possible to verify this assumption in a subsample of participants with measured values in a cross-sectional survey, but this is difficult in retrospective studies where recalled weight or stature may be many years in the past.

Among adults, self-reported weight and height are generally highly correlated with measured weight and height. Correlations for reported stature range from 0.53 (29) to 0.99 (30); and those for weight range from 0.89 to 0.99 (30). The magnitudes of the correlations vary somewhat across studies and in relation to age and sex. In any event, high correlations do not necessarily reflect accuracy, since systematic differences (constant and relative biases) between self-reported and measured values may exist regardless of the strength of the correlations. Biases in the self-reporting of weight and height have been documented. Obese people tend to underreport their weight more than nonobese people. Women consistently underreport their weight and men tend to underreport it when they are overweight and overreport it when they are underweight. Thus, with regard to weight at least, men would appear to be the more fickle sex. A review of such biases can be found in Bowman and DeLucia (31) and Cameron and Evers (32).

Recall of weight and height at earlier ages, reports by surrogates (e.g., parents, spouses, children, siblings), and records from driver's licenses (33) can also be used in place of measured variables. These can be expected generally to have less reliability and accuracy than self-reported current weight, and correlations with measured weight are considerably less. There is at present little evidence that self-measurements are any more accurate or reliable than simple self-reported estimates.

Body weight and stature can be used to estimate "relative weight." This requires the calculation of the percent difference between the measured weight for an individual and an "ideal" weight for stature found in standard tables such as those published by the Metropolitan Insurance Company (34). A common criticism of this approach is that the tables are not really representative of the general population, only of insurance policy holders. Additionally, the current tables attempt to adjust for "frame size," which adds a third required measurement of elbow breadth that is of doubtful value. A more common approach is to calculate "body mass index" (weight/stature^2) and to compare this value to percentiles for the distribution of this index by sex, age, and race tabulated from the large surveys conducted by the National Center for Health Statistics, such as the National Health and Nutrition Surveys (35). The prevalence of "overweight" or "obese" in population is defined as the percent of individuals with body mass indices greater than a specified cutoff value. The convention established by the National Center for Health Statistics is to define "overweight" as BMIs greater than the value at the 85th percentile, and "obese" as greater than the 95th percentile value, for young adults (20–29 years). Although this approach provides a common basis for comparing populations for the prevalence of overweight and obesity, there are a number of serious limitations due to the imperfect nature of weight/stature^2 as an index of body fatness. A full appreciation of these limitations requires a brief review of the concepts underlying weight-stature indices.

The general objective of weight stature indices is to obtain a measure of body weight (W) that is independent of stature (S). An example of such an index is given in Eq. (1), which is based on the assumed relationship implied in Eq. (2).

$$\frac{W}{S^b} = a \qquad \text{and} \qquad (3)$$

$$W = aS^b \qquad (4)$$

In Eqs. (3) and (4), a and b are constants. These equations indicate that for any increment in S^b, body weight changes in a proportional manner so as to keep the W/S^b ratio constant. The great statistician, astronomer, epidemiologist, and anthropometrist Lambert-Adolphe-Jacques Quetelet first observed that among adults weight in kilograms seemed to increase in proportion to the square of stature in meters (36). Quetelet's Index, W/S^2, was further established to be a useful index for grading adiposity in population studies by Keys, who appears to have been responsible for renaming it the "Body Mass Index" (37). It is now conventional to refer to W/S^2 as the "Body Mass Index," or "BMI," but the reader should be aware that an infinite number of weight-structure indices can be constructed using different powers of stature, as well as weight (38). Historically, various investigators have presented arguments for the merits of different values of b in W/S^b, based on the influence of age, gender, and race, and even disease risk on the association between weight and stature (39–43). Benn even suggested that the power coefficient, b, should be established empirically within a population rather than applying a common coefficient across all populations (44).

It is important to keep in mind that the underlying assumption in the use of body mass indices is that they reflect variation among people in body fatness (45). Garn et al. (46) cogently reminded us of three limitations to this assumption: (1) the correlation of BMIs with stature may be influenced by age; (2) BMIs may be influenced by body proportions, specifically leg length relative to trunk size; and (3) BMIs may be correlated with lean as well as fat mass. Quetelet's Index, or BMI, is not perfectly correlated with body fatness: r's with percent body fat range widely from about 0.40 to 0.90 across various studies. Moreover, the association of BMI with percent body fat may be nonlinear, especially at higher levels of adiposity (47). This suggests that the index can vary in sensitivity for grading body fatness among populations. Abdel-Malek and associates (38) presented a method for empirically determining powers for both weight and stature that would maximize the association between total body fat or percent body fat and weight-stature indices in a group or subsample of a population. As for the approach of Benn (44), this method had not been widely applied.

A potentially more troublesome problem is the fact that body mass indices are also associated with FFM. This is due to fact that weight includes FFM and stature is not correlated perfectly with FFM. As result, body mass indices tend to retain significant correlations with FFM even when powers of b are found that minimize the correlation between weight and stature. The net result is that there may be a considerable range of body fatness (or leanness) among individuals with the same body mass index (48,49). The magnitudes of the associations of body mass indices with fat and fat-free components are also influenced by age, gender, and racial differences in body com-

position and by variation in body proportions. Substantial misclassification bias can result when cutoff values are used to classify people as "overweight" or "obese" that do not take these factors into consideration (49,50). For example, differential misclassification with age would occur if the 85th percentile for BMI corresponded systematically to a greater percent body fat in elderly than in young adults, which is likely to occur because older people lose muscle mass with age while maintaining or increasing body fat. As a result, the prevalence of "obesity" (e.g., percent body fat > 30% in women) in the elderly would be underestimated relative to that in the young adults. It follows that estimates of risk for diseases associated with obesity would be biased in the elderly compared to young age groups since a greater percentage of "obese" individuals would be misclassified as nonobese (i.e., more "false negatives" in elderly than young age groups).

Body weight and stature, or indices such as BMI, can also be used in equations to estimate body composition. As a simple example, percent body fat can be calculated using the following equations (50):

Subjects	n	Equation	R^2	SE	p
Men	214	$1.402 \times$ BMI $+ 0.177$ $\times$ age $- 22.519$	0.52	5.54	<0.001
Women	290	$1.591 \times$ BMI $+ 0.096$ $\times$ age $- 11.666$	0.56	5.75	<0.001

SE, standard error of model.

A four-compartment method based on body volume, TBW, and bone mineral mass was used to derive percent fat in healthy Caucasian adults with BMI < 35 kg/m². The equations were then developed by statistical regression of the criterion fat estimate on BMI and age. A good practice is to cross-validate such equations if they are to be used to predict subject body composition.

Skinfold Thicknesses. These are measurements of a double thickness or "fold" of skin, underlying fascia, and subcutaneous adipose tissue that are taken using calipers at standardized locations on the body. The essential technique is to pinch and elevate a skinfold at specific anatomical sites using the thumb and fingers and to measure the thickness of the fold with specially designed calipers. These measurements are therefore correlated with, but are not directly representative of, the actual thickness of subcutaneous adipose tissue. This has been illustrated by comparisons of skinfold thickness measurements with radiographic and ultrasound measurements of subcutaneous adipose tissue thickness at different anatomical sites (51–53). Because about 70–90% of total adipose tissue is subcutaneous, skinfold thickness can be used to grade or predict total-body fat (27,45). In addition, since the thickness of subcutaneous adipose tissue varies among different anatomical locations, skinfold thicknesses are useful for describing subcutaneous body fat distribution or "fat patterning" (54). They are not useful, however, for predicting amounts of intra-abdominal adipose tissues.

Carefully standardized methods of measuring skinfold thicknesses have been developed and it is important to adhere strictly to these to ensure reliable measurements that are comparable with published tables of reference data, and that can be used in appropriate equations for predicting body fat (27,28). A variety of skinfold calipers are available and measurements may differ systematically between brands depending on quality and the control of pressure between the jaws of the calipers. Jaw pressure is important because skinfolds vary within and between individuals in compression when measured (27,55). Variability in compression is a major factor affecting the reliability of skinfold thickness measurements. Calipers with different jaw pressures will produce systematically different readings, and those with manually controlled jaw pressures will be less reliable than those with built-in spring mechanisms. As a result, the use of different brands of skinfold calipers within a study is not recommended unless their systematic differences are known. Research-quality calipers (e.g., Holtain, Lange, Harpenden) exert constant pressure between the jaws (10 g/cm^3) and have a finer scale of measurement (0.1-mm intervals) than the inexpensive, plastic calipers marketed for clinical use (27).

In theory, skinfold thicknesses can be measured anywhere on the body that a double fold of skin and subcutaneous adipose tissue can be pinched and elevated. In practice, only a few standard sites are commonly measured based on their accessibility, ease of measurement, and high correlation with measures of total-body fat. The triceps and subscapular sites meet these criteria best in most sex, ethnicity, and age groupings, and are used widely for grading fatness (27,28). Extensive reference data are available for skinfold thickness at these sites that are stratified by sex, ethnicity, and age (28). Additional skinfolds that may be useful for grading adiposity or describing adipose tissue distribution include suprailiac and paraumbilical (for abdominal adipose tissue), and medial thigh and medial (or lateral) calf (for leg adipose tissue). Fewer reference data, however, are available for these sites, which limits their usefulness in some contexts.

The most common way to use skinfold thickness data is to compare individual values or group means to tabulated reference values for appropriate sex, ethnic, and age groupings. An implicit assumption is that the reference data are "representative," in the sense of being collected from a randomly selected sample of well-defined population. In the United States, data collected in the National Health and Nutrition Examinations Surveys (NHANES) are most commonly used for this purpose (35). As for BMI, a "cutpoint" is chosen from the distribution of the reference data for a skinfold variable (e.g., >85th percentile for triceps at age 20–29 years), and individuals in the study sample with values greater than the cutpoint are classified as "obese." The prevalence of obesity in the study sample is defined as the percentage with values greater than the cut off point. This approach to using skinfold thicknesses has the same merits and limitations as described above for estimating prevalence of "overweight" or "obesity" using BMI.

Skinfold thicknesses can also be used as continuous variables grading adiposity or adipose tissue distribution within a study population. This approach works well if the study population is relatively homogeneous. It works less well if the study population is heterogeneous and the association of the selected skinfold thickness with total fat mass or percent body fat varies by sex, ethnicity, age, or characteristics. As a result, stratification on sex, ethnicity, and age is generally recommended when skinfold thicknesses are used as continuous measures of grading levels of body fatness or obesity in analyses of relative risks or correlations with risk factors.

Skinfold thicknesses are also used in equations that predict body density, total body fat mass, or percent body fat. The most widely used equations are those of Jackson and Pollock (13) and Durnin and Womersely (14). When applied with close attention to proper measurement technique, these equations can predict percent body fat with errors between 3.5 and 5% (21). An advantage to the use of skinfold thickness prediction equations is that they estimate rather than grade the underlying variables of interest (e.g., body density, total body fat, percent body fat). Subsequent analyses can then deal directly with associations between the estimates and the various outcomes of interest, rather than with indirect associations with imperfect proxy variables or indices. This can greatly facilitate interpretation of some associations as long as the predicted values can be considered accurate. A disadvantage is that type I equations for predicting body composition from skinfold thicknesses are "population specific." Therefore, they must always be cross-validated in at least a subsample of a study population before general application. This clearly adds to the expense and difficulty of using these equations. Lohman (21), and others (17) have developed explicit criteria for evaluation of the accuracy of prediction equations in cross-validation studies.

An important problem is the simple feasibility of obtaining reliable data for very obese subjects. Skinfold calipers can accurately measure skinfolds only up to 40 mm (Holtain) or 60 mm (Lange) in thickness. This may limit the ability to measure skinfolds at some sites and in obese subjects. In addition, the reliability of the measurements may decrease with increasing thickness (55). As a result of these limitations, some may prefer the use of circumference measurements for grading or predicting body fatness, or quantifying adipose tissue distribution in obese subjects.

Ultrasound. Ultrasonic measurements of subcutaneous adipose tissue thickness have been explored as an alternative to skinfolds (53,56,57). The benefits to ultrasound are: (1) the measurements theoretically have greater validity in relation to actual subcutaneous adipose tissue thickness; (2) they are not affected by variation within and between persons for tissue compressibility; (3) greater thickness can be measured than with currently available skinfold calipers; and (4) sites can be measured that are inaccessible to calipers, for example paraspinal adipose tissue in the lumbar region. There are also two major drawbacks: (1) the measurements are obtained at considerably increased cost; and (2) reliable measurements can only be made using B-mode, imaging ultrasound by highly trained technicians (27). B-mode imaging ultrasound provides a real-time two-dimensional image of skin and subcutaneous adipose tissue and underlying interface with muscle. The image can be frozen and printed, providing a permanent record, and the subcutaneous adipose tissue thickness can be measured using a ruler or digitizer. Considerable skill may be needed in obtaining the images, depending on the ultrasound equipment used, and in identifying correctly the adipose tissue-muscle interface on the image. At some sites, this interface may be easily confused with other fibrous tissue interfaces and bone reflections.

Ultrasound has also been explored as a method of quantifying the amount of intra-abdominal adipose tissues (58,59). This approach appears promising and merits further development since the alternatives are either very expensive (e.g., CT or MRI) or inaccurate (e.g., circumference ratios or prediction equations).

Circumferences. Body circumferences are useful in that, unlike skinfold thicknesses, they can always be measured, even in extremely obese subjects. Circumferences reflect internal as well as subcutaneous adipose tissue, but are also influenced by variation in muscle and bone. As a result, the interpretation of circumference measurements, and especially circumference ratios, is often not straightforward. As for all anthropometric variables, body circumferences should be measured with close attention to stan-

dardized procedures (28). Flexible, inelastic cloth or steel tapes are recommended.

The most useful circumferences for grading or predicting body fat and for describing adipose tissue distribution are upper arm, chest, waist or abdomen, hip or buttocks, thigh (proximal or midthigh), and calf (27,28). Waist or abdomen circumferences are usually very highly correlated with total fat mass and percent body fat in men (r values > 0.85); in women, hip or thigh circumferences may have slightly higher correlations. Correlations of upper arm, thigh, and calf circumferences with measures of body fat are somewhat lower, and these circumferences tend to be more strongly influenced by variation in appendicular skeletal muscle. Nationally representative reference data are available for abdominal, hip, and midthigh circumferences from the Third U.S. National Health and Nutrition Examination Survey (35).

Adipose Tissue Distribution. Numerous epidemiological and clinical studies have established that centralized obesity, in which fat is stored preferentially in adipocytes on and within the trunk rather than the extremities, represents the obesity phenotype that conveys the largest risk for morbidity and mortality from the major chronic diseases: heart disease, cancer, and diabetes (49,60). A variety of anthropometric approaches have been developed to grade or classify centralized adipose tissue distribution. Recent efforts have been focused on developing type I equations for predicting the amount of VAT, which is believed to be the main aspect of centralized obesity associated with risk. The following section reviews the merits and limitations of these anthropometric approaches.

Skinfold thicknesses have been used to describe primarily the distribution of subcutaneous adipose tissues. This aspect of the adipose tissue distribution has been called "fat patterning," to distinguish it from the more general form that includes the amounts and distribution of internal adipose tissues (54,60). Historically, three main approaches have been used to describe fat patterning: pattern-profile, ratio, and principal components methods. The pattern-profile method was first applied by Garn (54) and compares two or more groups graphically for mean values of skinfold thicknesses across several anatomical sites. It provides a useful, visual comparison of differences or similarities between groups for anatomical variation in subcutaneous fat thickness. Cluster analysis provides a more sophisticated, statistical approach to defining pattern profiles (61).

A variety of skinfold thickness ratios have been used to index fat patterning. The ratio of the subscapular to triceps skinfolds is one of simplest and most widely used. Some consider it to be important to include a skinfold on the leg, such as the lateral calf or medial thigh skinfold (62). The advantages of the ratio approach are that it requires few variables, simple computation, and provides a single continuous variable for grading subjects. Three problems can be identified, however, with ratio indices of fat patterning: (1) they tend to be correlated with total fat mass or percent body fat; (2) they may have poor sensitivity and validity with regard to the latent variable, subcutaneous adipose tissue distribution; and (3) it may be difficult to determine whether a correlation with another variable (e.g., serum HDL cholesterol) is due to variation in the numerator or denominator of the ratio. The use of a greater number of skinfolds, and the sum of all skinfolds in the denominator, may partly alleviate these problems. Principal-components analysis is a more sophisticated statistical approach to constructing fat pattern indices. This approach summarizes the information in several skinfold variables in a smaller number of new, statistically independent indices that are not correlated with total body fat (63). When this method is applied to data for several skinfold variables, it provides the best "criterion" measures for judging the validity and sensitivity of simpler ratio indices.

The main criticism of skinfold thickness methods in the study of obesity is that they do not capture variation in the amounts of internal adipose tissues, especially those surrounding the viscera. "Visceral adipose tissue" has been recognized as the main aspect of body fat distribution that is associated with increased risk for chronic disease (60). As a result, many prefer indices based on circumferences that are believed to include variation in visceral adipose tissues. The most popular circumference index is the "waist/hip ratio" (WHR), followed by the "waist/thigh ratio" (WTR). The waist/hip ratio was the first used to assess the associations between adipose tissue distribution and chronic disease morbidity and mortality (64–68). Numerous studies have now shown that WHR is an independent predictor of metabolic disturbances including insulin resistance, hyperlipidemia, hypertension, and atherosclerosis (67–70). Similar associations have been also been reported for WTR, as well as for skinfold thickness indices and some other circumference indices such as the "conicity index" (71–75). In general, the association of risk factors, as well as morbidity and mortality, with circumference indices tends to be somewhat stronger than with skinfold thickness indices of adipose tissue distribution. This is generally thought to be due to either the increased measurement error in skinfold thicknesses or the influence of VAT volume on waist circumference. As for BMI or skinfolds, cutoff values for the WHR have been recommended for defining "upper body obesity" (70). The recommended values generally used are >0.95 in men and >0.80 in women. It is important to recognize that these values were selected based on the increase in risks with increasing WHR and not on the association with adipose tissue distribution.

There are several problems in the use of circumference ratios as indices of adipose tissue distribution. First, standard definitions of the circumferences are not always followed, making it difficult to compare results across studies (76). For example, the "waist" circumference has been defined variously as at the level of the smallest circumference on the torso below the sternum; the umbilicus; the lower margin of the ribs; and the iliac crests. The "hip" circumference has been defined as at the level of: the iliac crests; the anterior iliac spines; the greater trochanters; or the maximum posterior protrusion of the buttocks. There may be considerable differences among circumferences measured at these locations. Some may vary between subjects in relation to bone landmarks (e.g., smallest circumference on torso below the sternum) or may be difficult to identify in obese subjects. There is scarcely any difference between a "waist" circumference measured at the level of the umbilicus and a "hip" circumference measured at the level of the iliac crests in most subjects. Obviously, "waist" circumference in one study may be the same as "hip" circumference in another when both are defined as at the level of the iliac crests.

In obese subjects, the identification of the "waist" may be extremely subjective, if not impossible, and the measurement is more correctly defined as an abdominal circumference. The location of the abdominal circumference in relation to a soft-tissue landmark, such as the umbilicus, is not recommended because many obese subjects will have an extremely pendulous abdominal adipose panniculus. The umbilicus may be directed downward and located well below the horizontal, transverse plane of the midabdomen. This may lead to considerable variation among subjects in the definition of this measurement. In addition, a pendulous panniculus may result in overlapping of abdominal and hip circumferences or interfere with the standard measurement of hip circumference.

A second problem is that circumferences are influenced by variation in muscle and bone as well as adipose tissues, as noted previously. These influences may be particularly difficult to sort out when ratio indices are used. It has been assumed conventionally that increased WHRs mainly reflect increased VAT, based on studies that report significant correlations between WHR and VAT area, as measured using imaging methods (see below). Some studies, however, have reported significant correlations with measures of cross-sectional muscle area also, in particular those for the pelvis or hips (77,78). Thus, variation in WHR may reflect the effects increased VAT on waist circumference (numerator) as well as decreased gluteofemoral muscle on hip circumference (denominator). This influence of muscle has been recognized increasingly and may be important in understanding the relationship of WHR to chronic disease risk. Larsson et al. (66) reported that risk of heart disease was greatest in those with lower BMIs and high WHRs. Filipovsky et al. (72) reported that all-cause and cancer mortality over 20 years of follow-up in the Paris Prospective Study was greatest in those with low BMIs but high WTRs. The low BMIs in these study might reflect low muscle mass, rather than fat; subsequently, the high WHRs or WTRs might reflect a combination of increased VAT and muscle loss (49). It should be remembered that the phenotype originally described by Vague (79), who first drew attention to the association of body composition and metabolic disease, consisted of an expanded abdominal fat mass in conjunction with thin legs. The latter might reflect muscle atrophy associated with disease as much as lack of subcutaneous adipose tissue on the extremities. This potentially important association between visceral adiposity and skeletal muscle was recently reemphasized by Björntorp (60).

A third problem is the strong correlation of circumferences and circumference ratios with total adiposity. This makes it difficult statistically to separate the effects of centralized adipose tissue distribution from obesity. This confounding is further exacerbated by the moderate positive correlations of body fatness and centralized adipose tissue distribution with age. Many early studies that reported significant correlations between WHR and VAT did not control for the confounding influences of age and BMI. Seidell et al. (80) reported that WHR did not correlate significantly with ratio of visceral to subcutaneous adipose tissue, as measured using CT, after adjustment for age and BMI. Similarly, Ross et al. (81) reported that, after controlling for both age and adiposity, WHR explained only 12% of the variation in absolute levels of VAT in men. Furthermore, the observed relationship between WHR and relative VAT was nonexistent. Thus, while WHR is an independent predictor of numerous metabolic aberrations, its association with risk may not be attributed simply to its association with the amounts of either absolute or relative VAT.

Several investigators have argued that simple waist circumference is a better index of variation in VAT than WHR (82,83). It is important to note, however, that waist circumference is very highly correlated with total adiposity (r values > 0.90) in most populations. Also, the error of prediction of VAT from waist circumference, alone or in combination with other variables, is large (49,80,81,84–87). Ross et al. (88) recently reported that the sensitivity and specificity of waist circumference for

predicting absolute values of VAT was poor. These observations are explained in large measure by the intraindividual variation in the visceral-to-subcutaneous adipose tissue ratio.

It is important to establish whether reductions in VAT are related to concurrent reductions WHR or waist circumference. Some have reported that WHR changes with weight loss, but others have not (89–95). Ross et al. (96,97) recently reported that diet- and exercise-induced reductions in VAT (kg) were significantly associated with reduced waist circumferences in obese male ($r = 0.69$) and female ($r = 0.47$) subjects. For the two groups combined, a 1-cm reduction in waist circumference was associated with a 4% reduction in VAT ($p < 0.01$). The standard deviation associated with the 4% reduction in VAT per centimeter reduction in waist circumference, however, was also 4%. This suggests that the ability to quantify small changes in VAT volume from waist circumference is limited by interindividual variations in the reduction of abdominal subcutaneous and lean tissue. Thus, whereas changes in visceral obesity are clearly associated with changes in waist circumference, it is not possible to accurately predict small changes in VAT.

Efforts to develop equations for predicting VAT have not generally been successful. The errors associated with these equations tend to be large: 25–40% (80–88). This level of accuracy is clearly insufficient for estimating changes in individuals and may be inadequate for comparing groups. Few of these equations have been cross-validated in independent samples. Future efforts to develop this approach have value, however, given the inadequacies described above for skinfold and circumference indices. At present, it would appear that new or different anthropometric measurements will be needed to increase the accuracy of prediction equations to acceptable levels. One measure that has been suggested is the sagittal thickness of the trunk or abdomen.

Sagittal Thickness. Several studies have suggested that sagittal trunk thickness correlates more highly than other anthropometric variables with the volume of visceral adipose tissue quantified by imaging methods (83,87). As a result, it may be useful both as a simple index, like waist circumference, or as an independent variable in equations for predicting VAT. There is at present no standardized technique for measuring sagittal trunk thickness and, to date, its use has been limited mostly to clinical studies.

Sagittal trunk thickness may be defined as the maximum diameter of the abdomen in the sagittal plane. As for circumferences, this measurement may be obtained technically in all subjects regardless of obesity level. Bony landmarks for the standard location of this measurement have not been identified: alternative possibilities include the xiphoid process of the sternum, the fourth lumbar vertebrae, or the iliac crests. It is important to note that the choice between these landmarks will result in measurements at very different levels on the trunk or abdomen. Sliding calipers with long, parallel blades are necessary for this measurement.

Although sagittal trunk thickness may be taken with the participant standing, measurement in the supine recumbent position may be preferred to maximize the association with the latent variable, intra-abdominal adipose tissue volume. Theoretically, when a person with an enlarged intra-abdominal adipose tissue mass lies supine, the mass shifts cranially causing anterior projection of the abdomen, which is measured as increased sagittal thickness (87). When a person is standing, gravity pulls the intra-abdominal adipose tissue mass downward and the maximum sagittal thickness may be located somewhat lower. It is important to keep in mind that the level of the maximum measurable diameter, either supine or standing, will likely vary among some subjects. The extent to which these measurements are influenced by the amount of subcutaneous abdominal adipose tissue, and shifts in its distribution between supine and standing measurements, is not well established.

Results for the use of sagittal thickness to grade or predict visceral adipose tissue volume in several Swedish studies have been summarized by Sjöstrom (87). Visceral adipose tissue volume was estimated using seven cross-sectional CT scans of the abdomen. Sagittal thickness was measured on the CT image at the level of L4–5. Visceral adipose tissue (VAT) volume was regressed on sagittal thickness (ST) in 17 men, producing an equation, VAT (L) = 0.731 × ST (cm) − 11.5, (R^2 = 0.81). This equation was later cross-validated in two independent samples of seven and 13 men, respectively, with virtually indistinguishable results. A similar regression equation was developed using data for 10 women and cross-validated in nine independently selected women: VAT (L) = 0.370 × ST(cm) − 4.85, (R^2 = 80). Sjöstrom also showed that changes in VAT volume were accurately tracked by changes in sagittal thickness in six patients with Cushing's disease during treatment.

Pouliot et al. (83) analyzed associations of sagittal thickness with visceral adipose tissue area on CT images at L4–5 in 81 men and 70 women, 30–42 years of age. Sagittal thickness correlated better with VAT area than waist/hip ratio in both sexes; however, it also correlated strongly with subcutaneous abdominal adipose tissue area. Taken together, the results of the studies by Sjöstrom (87)

and Pouliot et al. (83) indicate that sagittal thickness is somewhat more sensitive than conventional indices such as waist/hip ratio for grading or predicting the amounts of visceral adipose tissue.

The measurements of sagittal thickness in these studies were taken from the CT scans, rather than anthropometrically. Sjöstrom, however, reported that the squared difference between sagittal thicknesses measured anthropometrically and on the CT images in his studies was only 1.7%. In an independent study, Van der Kooy et al. (98) reported a high correlation (r = 0.94) between sagittal thickness measured with the subject standing and from MRI images at the same level. It may be important to consider that the errors of estimation for VAT averaged about 20% in these studies, which could allow for considerable misclassification when subjects are grouped by sagittal thickness. Finally, the strong correlation with abdominal subcutaneous adipose tissue areas reported by Pouliot et al. (83) is bothersome because it suggests that sagittal thickness may not accurately discriminate visceral from subcutaneous abdominal adipose tissue.

We have examined the association of sagittal diameter with VAT volume in elderly participants in the New Mexico Aging Process Study (unpublished data). Visceral adipose tissue volume was quantified using an MRI protocol developed by Ross et al. (81). Sagittal diameter was measured using sliding calipers while the participant was supine at a level of L4–5. The R^2 for the regression of VAT volume on sagittal diameter was 0.75 in nine elderly men, similar to that reported by Sjöstrom. The corresponding R^2 for nine women, however, was only 0.09. In contrast, the R^2 for the regression of sagittal thickness on subcutaneous adipose tissue volume for the trunk in the women was 0.33. This suggestion that while sagittal diameter, measured anthropometrically, is a moderately sensitive index of VAT in elderly men, it may not be useful in elderly women. The mean sagittal diameter in our women was 20.8 ± 2.9 cm, which is similar to the mean for women reported by Sjöstrom (87). The corresponding mean VAT volume, however, was 1.51 ± 0.59 L, which is about one-half that reported by Sjöstrom. The difference between studies for mean VAT volume is partly attributable to a different definition of VAT in our study. This difference could explain the lack of correlation between sagittal diameter and VAT in the women in our study and highlights issues related to definition and measurement of VAT that are addressed in greater detail below in a section on measuring VAT from CT and MRI methods.

Whereas establishment of the association of sagittal diameter with the latent variable of interest, VAT, is important, it is also important to examine the sensitivity of this measure in relation to risk factors associated with visceral obesity. Richelsen and Pedersen (99) recently analyzed associations of sagittal thickness and other indices of VAT with serum total cholesterol, triglyceride, LDL and HDL, fasting insulin, and glucose concentrations in 58 middle-aged men. They concluded that sagittal thickness was slightly better correlated with an adverse lipid, insulin, and glucose risk profile than waist/hip ratio. Similar findings were also reported in the study by Pouliot et al. (83). Taken together, these studies suggest that sagittal diameter may be preferable to other indices of VAT as a risk factor in epidemiological studies of obesity-associated chronic diseases. In this regard, Seidell et al. (100) reported that abdominal sagittal thickness was a strong predictor of mortality in younger adult men enrolled in the Baltimore Longitudinal Study.

Further studies are needed to establish the usefulness of sagittal thickness for grading or predicting visceral adipose tissue and as a risk factor in different age, sex, and ethnic groups.

2. Bioimpedance and Conductivity

Bioelectric impedance (BIA) and total-body electrical conductivity (TOBEC) are techniques of predicting body composition based on the electrical conductive properties of the human body. The ability of the body to conduct an electric current is due to the presence of free ions, or electrolytes, in the body water. The amount of electricity that can be conducted is determined mainly by the total volume of electrolyte-rich fluid in the body. Measures of bioelectric conductivity are therefore proportional to TBW and to body composition components with high water concentrations such as the fat-free and skeletal muscle mass. As a result, these methods do not estimate body fatness, but instead they predict FFM and fat must be derived secondarily as the difference between predicted FFM and body weight (101).

Many factors other than the amount and electrolyte concentration of body water, however, influence measurements of electrical conductivity. These include body temperature, distribution of fluids between intra- and extracellular spaces, body proportions or "geometry," the amounts and structures of different conductive, as well as nonconductive, tissues, and technical issues such as correct calibration and application of the equipment. The complex effects of these factors on measurements of bioelectric conductivity have been reviewed elsewhere (102–105). The net result, however, is that exact functional relationships between measurements of bioelectric conductivity and TBW and other fat-free components cannot be derived from either physicochemical models or ex-

perimentally. Thus, relationships between conductivity measurements and body composition components must be established indirectly by statistical calibration against criterion measures (e.g., estimates of TBW from tritium dilution analysis) in a sample of subjects. Bioimpedance analysis and TOBEC are therefore type I property-based methods.

Although the underlying principles are shared, BIA and TOBEC differ completely in the approach taken to measuring bioelectric conductivity. In TOBEC, an electrical current is induced in the body by insertion into a large electric coil that is generating an electromagnetic field. The amount of whole-body conductivity is quantified from the energy loss in the coil, which is proportional to the strength of surrounding magnetic field, the specific conductivity, cross-sectional area, and length of the body. Complex calibration equations are necessary for converting the measures of conductivity (phase changes due to energy absorption) to estimates of TBW or FFM. TOBEC devices have been shown to have high precision (<1%) and accuracy (0.7–1.6 L) when estimating TBW (104). Errors for estimates of FFM are slightly larger (1.4–2.9 kg) (105). Unfortunately, the equipment for in vivo measurement of adults is large, cumbersome, and expensive. In addition, TOBEC is not applicable to severely obese patients who will not fit inside the electric coil. As a result, TOBEC devices for body composition analysis of adults have not been successful commercially and are no longer manufactured.

Bioimpedance analysis is technically simpler, much less expensive, and only marginally less precise and accurate than TOBEC. Because it is portable, it is suitable for field use and is being applied increasingly as an adjunct to anthropometry. The most commonly used BIA method injects a high-frequency, low-amplitude alternating electric current (50 kHz at 500–800 mA) into the body using distally placed electrodes and measures the voltage drop due to resistance with proximal electrodes. Conventionally, surface electrodes are used with standardized placements on the right ankle and hand, although other electrode arrangements have been described (106). The amount of resistance measured (R) is inversely proportional to the volume of electrolytic fluid in the body. It is also dependent on the proportions or "geometry" of this volume (i.e., ratio of length (L) to cross-sectional area (A), or $R = \rho \cdot L/A$). These relationships have led to the use of the simple formula $V = \rho L^2/R$ as the theoretical basis of most BIA applications, where V is conductive volume (e.g., TBW), L is a measure of body length (usually stature), R is measured resistance, and ρ is an estimate of the "specific resistivity" of the conductive material (103).

There are a number of limitations to the validity of this simple formula, some of which seem obvious. The formula is accurate only for a cylindrical conductor with uniform cross-sectional area and homogenous composition (e.g., a wire). The human body could be described as a series of roughly cylindrical conductors with variable cross-sectional area and heterogenous, highly structured composition. The value of ρ is influenced by all of these factors and consequently cannot be deduced directly. As a result, equations for predicting body composition must be developed based on independent measurements of resistance, stature and other anthropometric variables, and TBW or FFM in a sample of subjects. Least-squares regression techniques are applied to the data to derive an equation of the basic form:

$$V \text{ (i.e., TBW or FFM)} = a + b(S^2/R) + e \quad (5)$$

where a is intercept, b is slope, and e is residual error or unexplained variation in V due to random measurement errors and/or misspecification of the parameters (a and b) in the equation. It is not possible to interpret the parameter b in this equation as an estimate of r in the formula $V = rL^2/R$, unless the intercept (a) and residual error (e) approach zero. These conditions are rarely, if ever, met for the reasons given above. The equation may contain body circumferences and skinfold thickness also, although the inclusion of these additional variables reduces the main benefit of BIA relative to anthropometric prediction equations. The reason BIA is becoming increasingly popular is that only a few, simple, highly reproducible measurements are needed.

As for most type I, property-based methods, BIA prediction equations tend to lose accuracy when applied to subjects who do not resemble those included in the sample from which the equations were developed. Thus, their "generalizability" may be limited and all BIA equations must be cross-validated in independent samples to verify their applicability. Several published and widely used equations for estimating FFM in populations with various characteristics are presented in Table 6. Few, if any, equations have been developed that can be demonstrated to be applicable to all individuals without regard to age, gender, ethnicity, or obesity. Our experience is that the performance of a particular equation can be unpredictable, even when applied with close attention to measurement techniques and equipment to a sample with characteristics closely similar to those of the source sample. As a result, it is recommended that *any* externally developed BIA equation be cross-validated in a random subsample against estimates from a type II method (e.g., DXA or underwater weighing) before general extension to an entire study population.

Several investigators have reported that BIA equations tend to overestimate FFM (and underestimate % fat) in obese subjects that the amount of overestimation increases with increasing body fatness (107–113). As a result, equations have been developed specifically for obese subjects that reputedly reduce this effect (Table 6). Several factors, however, may even limit the accuracy of these equations. First, resistance as measured conventionally from the ankle to the wrist is mainly determined by the part of the body with the smallest cross-sectional area. Studies using segmental measurements of resistance have shown that the resistance of the limbs are considerably greater than that of the trunk, and that whole-body resistance is dominated by the resistance of the arm and, secondarily, the leg (106). Thus, BIA may be relatively insensitive to changes in the composition of the trunk that occur in obesity. Second, it is generally assumed that fat and bone, because of their low conductivity, do not affect measured resistance. However, it is theoretically possible for fat to affect resistance if it is present in sufficient quantity, particularly on the limbs (103). Both of these factors may reduce the accuracy of BIA methods when applied to obese individuals with either extreme trunkal (android) or peripheral (gynoid) fat distributions. Finally, obesity may alter the composition of the FFM, and few published equations have been developed using criterion estimates that accurately quantify these changes. It must always be considered that errors in the criterion methods used to statistically calibrate BIA equations will be propagated to and reflected in the equations.

B. Mechanistic (Type II) Methods

1. Isotope Dilution

Dilution methods include a group of body composition methods designed to quantify fluid compartments (e.g., TBW, extracellular fluid, and plasma volume) and the components that exist entirely within body fluid compartments, such as exchangeable potassium, sodium, and chlorine. Dilution methods are based on the use of a labeled tracer with three properties.: (1) it has the same or similar distribution space as the component analyzed; (2) it has a distinct property (e.g., radioactivity or color) that can be quantitatively measured; and (3) it is nontoxic in the amounts used.

A dose of tracer (T) is administered to the subject, and after an equilibration interval, a portion of the tracer exchanges with other molecules or is excreted; any excreted tracer can be measured in urine. The tracer that remains in the body (T') then homogeneously distributes within the unknown component (C) volume. The following model then applies:

Table 6   Some Commonly Used Equations for Predicting FFM From Bioelectric Impedance Analysis

Study	Subject number (codes)	Formula	R^2	SEE (kg)
Lukaski et al. (111)	151 (men = 1, women = 0)	FFM (kg) = 0.734 × S^2/R + 0.096 × Xc + 0.116 × W + 0.878 × Sex − 4.03	0.98	2.1
Van Loan and Mayclin (107)	188 (men = 0, women = 1)	FFM (kg) = 0.00085 × S^2 + 0.3736 × W − 0.02375(R) − 0.1531 × Age − 4.291 × Sex + 17.7868	0.97	3.1
Segal et al. (110)	472 Men (<20% fat)	FFM (kg) = 0.00066 × S^2 − 0.02117 × R + 0.62854 × W − 0.1238 × Age + 9.3329	0.89	2.5
	597 Men (>20% fat)	FFM (kg) = 0.00089 × S^2 − 0.02999 × R + 0.42688 × W − 0.070 × Age + 14.5243	0.88	3.0
	323 Women (<30% fat)	FFM (kg) = 0.00065 × S^2 − 0.01397 × R + 0.42087 × W + 10.43485	0.82	2.0
	175 Women (>30% fat)	FFM (kg) = 0.00091 × S^2 − 0.01466 × R + 0.2999 × W − 0.07012 × Age + 9.37938	0.92	2.0
Deurenberg et al. (113)	661 (men = 1, women = 0)	FFM (kg) = 0.340 × S^2/R + 0.1534 × S + 0.273(W) − 0.127 × Age + 4.56 × Sex − 12.44	0.95	2.6

R, resistance; S, stature; W, weight; Xc, reactance.

$$P^* = R \times (C + T'), \qquad (6)$$

where T' represents the known amount of tracer in the body at equilibrium, P^* is the known measured distinct tracer property, and R is the ratio of P^* to the sum of C and T'. Because T' is much smaller than C, the model can be simplified to

$$P^* = R \times C \qquad (7)$$

One can analyze a sample of the unknown component such as blood or a piece of tissue. Because the tracer is homogeneously distributed in the unknown component,

$$\Delta P^* = R \times \Delta C \qquad (8)$$

where ΔC and ΔP^* are the measured unknown component mass and tracer property, respectively. Combining this formula with the above equation, a dilution model is derived:

$$C = [P^* \times \Delta C]/\Delta P^* \qquad (9)$$

In the model, P^* (distinct measured property of the tracer at equilibrium) is known, and ΔC and ΔP^* can be measured in samples. The unknown component (C) volume can thus be calculated.

Total Body Water.   Although dilution methods are widely used in the measurement of extracellular fluid, plasma volume, and exchangeable electrolytes (K_e, Na_e, and Cl_e) (114), the most important use is measurement of TBW.

This is because water is the largest component at the molecular body composition level in normal adults and also because water occupies a relatively constant fraction (73.2%) of FFM (19–21).

Water labeled with either two isotopes of hydrogen (deuterium, ^2H_2O; tritium, ^3H_2O) or oxygen ($H_2^{18}O$) has been used to quantitate TBW by the dilution method in healthy and diseased individuals (115–126). The use of deuterium, a stable isotope, is safe and preferred for children and pregnant women (118,125,126). The assay for deuterium in biological fluids relies on labor-intensive techniques such as fixed-filter infrared absorption, mass spectrometry, gas chromatography, or magnetic resonance spectroscopy (122,126). Tritium is radioactive and should not be used in children or in pregnant women. On the other hand, it is somewhat easier to measure with widely available scintillation counters (115).

Once the dilution volume is known, TBW volume and mass can be calculated from isotope exchange fraction and water density. Each of the three isotopes measures a specific dilution volume that is somewhat larger than actual TBW volume. For the two hydrogen isotopes, tritium and deuterium, the dilution volume is larger than actual TBW because the H atoms in the tracer fluid exchange with H atoms bound to carboxyl, hydroxyl, and amino groups (116,119,121). Similarly, the ^{18}O tracer exchanges with oxygen atoms in carboxyl and phosphate groups (116,120). Exchange of labeled atoms with unlabeled atoms from molecular components may vary owing to a number of factors (121), but most investigators assume a stable exchange of approximately 4–5% for tritium and deuterium and ~1% for ^{18}O (120,127). Thus, TBW is calculated as the product of isotope dilution volume and a correction factor that accounts for isotope exchange (e.g., ^{3}H$_2$O and ^{2}H$_2$O dilution volumes $\times$ 0.95–0.96; H$_2$^{18}O dilution volume $\times$ 0.98–0.99). At present, there does not appear to be a universally accepted, fully valid method of estimating isotope exchange. Total body water volume is converted to mass using the density of water at body temperature (0.994 g/cc at 36°C or 0.993 g/cc at 37°C).

Total body water can be used in a series of type II methods to estimate total body fat and FFM. For example:

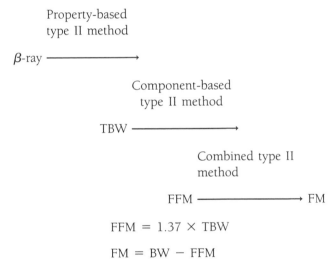

Property-based
type II method

β-ray $\longrightarrow$

Component-based
type II method

TBW $\longrightarrow$

Combined type II
method

FFM $\longrightarrow$ FM

FFM = 1.37 $\times$ TBW

FM = BW $-$ FFM

In the first step the measurable property is a specific isotope decay profile (0.018 MeV β-ray) and the mathematical function is based on the dilution model. In the second step it is assumed that the proportion of FFM as water is constant at 0.732 (20). Although there is substantial support for this proportion throughout many animal species, including humans (see Fig. 4), it should be recognized that this value represents a physiological steady state with some degree of "undependability." That is, individuals may fluctuate about this value over time. At any moment in time, some will be in steady state while others will not. The effects of this type of "biological error" on the use of this type II approach were reviewed in a previous section. In any event, this proportion is used in the model shown above to calculate FFM from TBW. In the last step a property (body weight) and an estimated component (FFM) are used to further estimate total body fat. These steps are similar for the other isotopes of water.

The TBW method is widely used and the specific isotope selected depends on available funds, analytical facil-

ities, and subjects. In addition to error associated with "biological error" or "undependability," the most important concern is bias due to systematic variation in TBW/FFM ratio with age, gender, race, obesity, disease, or other factors. As an example, TBW/FFM is known to be higher in infants and young children than in adults (21,129). Some have speculated that TBW/FFM is decreased in obesity and elevated in elderly people (128,130). Certain disease (e.g., renal disease, congestive heart failure) clearly result in alterations of TBW/FFM. Finally, the early phase of weight loss (first 1–2 weeks) with obesity treatment may be associated with relatively greater water loss than of other FFM components and thus the assumed TBW/FFM ratio may not be constant with dynamic weight change (131).

2. Hydrodensitometry

Two-Compartment Method. Underwater weighing is one of the oldest in vivo methods of analyzing human body composition as a two-component (fat and FFM) model. It held the status of being the "gold standard" for body composition analysis for many years, but this has been challenged increasingly in the last decade as questions are raised regarding the underlying assumptions.

Underwater weighing is based on the Archimedean principle that a solid object submerged in water is subject to a buoyant force that is equal to the weight of the water displaced by the object, or the loss in weight of the object when it is weighed while submerged in the water. Thus, the specific gravity or "density" of the object can be determined from the weight of the object divided by the loss in weight when submerged in water. The human body generally has a density close to that of water (1.0 g/cm^3). Individual deviations from this value are mainly due to the amount of fat in the body. Because fat is less dense than water, the lower the body density the greater the amount of body fat. Behnke and Wilmore were the first to show that this method could be used to deduce the percentage of weight that is fat from body density using a simple two-component model that assumes specific densities for fat and fat-free fractions of body weight (132; Table 4).

Lipid extracts of human adipose tissue, which are mostly triglycerides, have a mean density of 0.9007 g/cm^3 at body temperature (133). The mean density of FFM has been estimated to be 1.100 g/cm^3 based on data from cadaver studies (134). Fat-free body mass is assumed to be composed of constant proportions of water (73.2%), minerals (6.8%), and protein (19.5%) with residual amounts (<1%) of other chemical components (e.g., glycogen). The densities of these individual chemical components are also considered to be constants at body temperature (Tables 4 and 7). Body densities generally vary between 1.08 g/cm³ (very lean) and 1.03 g/cm³ (moderately obese). Obese subjects will have body densities less than 1.03 g/cm³, and severely obese people may have densities less than 1.00 g/cm³.

The most commonly used two-component model for estimating body composition from body density measured by underwater weighing was derived originally by Siri (135) using the basic formula:

$$\frac{1}{D} = \frac{F}{d_f} + \frac{FFM}{d_{ffm}}, \qquad (10)$$

where D is body density, F is the fraction of body weight that is fat, FFM is the fraction that is fat-free, and d_f and d_{ffm} are the densities of the fat (0.9007 g/cc) and fat-free (1.1000 g/cc) components, respectively. This equation is then solved for F:

$$\%Fat = \left[\frac{d_f \cdot d_{ffm}}{D(d_{ffm} - d_f)} - \frac{d_f}{d_{ffm} - d_f} \right] \times 100 \qquad (11)$$

Substituting in the assumed densities for fat and fat-free components yields the equation:

$$\%Fat = 495/D - 450 \qquad (12)$$

A revised model proposed by Brozek et al. (134) (%Fat = 457/D − 414.2) gives slightly lower estimates in obese subjects due to somewhat different underlying assumptions regarding the densities of fat (0.8888 g/cc) and fat-free (1.1033 g/cc) components. Further revised models have been proposed that adjust the coefficients in two-component equations for systematic differences in the composition of the FFM association with age, sex, ethnicity, and level of fatness (129,130). An example is the equation proposed by Deurenberg that assumes a decreased density of FFM due to increased water content in the adipose tissue of obese subjects:

$$\%Fat = \frac{509.9}{D} - 466.6 \qquad (13)$$

This equation gives slightly lower estimates in obese subjects than both the Siri and the Brozek equations. These

Table 7   Some Multicomponent Methods for Measuring Total Body Fat

Author	Measurable property	Known component	Simultaneous equation	Fat mass equation
Siri (135)	BW, BV	Water	BW = FM + water + protein + mineral BV = FM/0.900 + water/0.994 + protein/1.34 + mineral/3.04 protein = 2.40 × mineral	FM = 2.057 × BV − 0.786 × water − 1.286 × BW
Lohman (129)	BW, BV	Mineral	BW = FM + water + protein + mineral BV = FM/0.9007 + water/0.994 + protein/1.34 + mineral/3.04 Water = 4.00 × protein	FM = 6.386 × BV + 3.961 × mineral − 6.09 × BW
Baumgartner et al. (23)	BW, BV	Water, TBBM	BW = FM + water + protein + TBBM + Ms BV = FM/0.9007 + water/0.994 + protein/1.34 + TBBM/2.982 + Ms/3.317 Ms = 0.235 × TBBM	FM = 2.75 × BV − 0.714 × water + 1.148 × mineral − 2.05 × BW
Selinger (142)	BW, BV	Water, TBBM	BW = FM + water + protein + TBBM + Ms BV = FM/0.9007 + water/0.994 + protein/1.34 + TBBM/2.982 + Ms/3.317 Ms = 0.0105BW	FM = 2.75 × BV − 0.714 × water + 1.129 × TBBM − 2.037 × BW
Heymsfield et al. (127)	BW, BV	Water, TBBM	BW = FM + water + TBBM + residual BV = FM/0.9907 + water/0.99371 + TBBM/2.982 + residual/1.404	FM = 2.513 × BV − 0.739 × water + 0.947 × TBBM − 1.79 × BW

BV, body volume (L); BW, body weight (kg); FM, fat mass (kg); Ms, soft tissue mineral (kg); TBBM (kg) = ashed bone from DXA × 1.0436.
Source: From Ref. 10. See text and original citations for assumed component densities at body temperatures.

adjusted equations should not be applied without verifying in a random subsample of a study population that the assumed deviations in fat-free composition actually occur. None of these equations consider human individuality or variability in the composition of FFM that may occur independent of age, sex, ethnicity, or obesity. Because the composition of FFM may change with weight loss, two-component models based on body density alone may provide inaccurate estimates of the amount of fat lost (136).

A limitation of underwater weighing is that accurate measurements require active participation and effort by the subject being measured. In the conventional approach, the subject must submerge his body completely while exhaling maximally, and then hold his breath and body position for several seconds until a weight measurement is obtained. Some individuals cannot perform adequately, and underwater weighing is not feasible in young children, frail elderly, or those with serious cardiovascular or pulmonary disease. In those who can perform the procedure, errors may occur due to body movement and the buoyant effects of air in the gastrointestinal tract and lungs. Errors due to movement during submersions may be reduced by the use of electronic load cells and stable, chair systems, rather than spring scales and body slings. It is not feasible to measure the amount of air and gas in the stomach and intestinal tract, and a fixed value is usually assumed (~100 ml). The large air volume in the lungs can be adjusted for if accurate measurements are available, and predicted values or constants should not be used. Residual lung volume can be measured when the subject is out of the water using a spirometer with the He dilution or N washout, or during weighing with systems designed for this purpose. The simultaneous measurement of residual lung volume and underwater weight may be preferred because it controls for the effects of the increased pressure of water on the thorax during immersion. Some studies suggest, however, that these effects are small and result in only a slight reduction in residual volume in normal subjects (137). Maximum effort and compliance by the subject during spirometry, whether in or out of the water, and repeated measurements of residual volume may be more important. Inaccurate measurements of air in the lungs can be a major source of error when estimating body density from underwater weighing.

Although feasible, underwater weighing of obese subjects may present special problems. Obesity is often association with respiratory problems and reduced lung function, which may make it more difficult to obtain accurate measurements of residual lung volume. Because obese subjects have a strong tendency to float, it is necessary to use a weight belt, or other tare weight system, to completely submerge the body. The tare weights must be measured and recorded carefully to obtain an accurate underwater weight. Despite the various limitations reviewed above, high levels of precision can be achieved with underwater weighing. Moreover, underwater weighing may be the only practical method of measuring body fat in very obese subjects who cannot be evaluated by other methods. The minimum possible error from all sources (technical and biological) for percent body fat by underwater weighing has been estimated to be about ±2.5% (21). This represents an ideal, however, that can be achieved only if very careful attention is given to optimizing the performance of subjects and the quality of the equipment, and if all assumptions are valid.

Multicomponent Methods. An alternative approach to the two-component underwater weighing method is to use multicomponent methods that include measures of TBW and bone mineral masses in addition to body density, assuming flexible densities for each component (Table 7) (138–141). Table 7 shows selected examples of three- and four-component type II combined methods of estimating fat mass along with the measurable quantities and simultaneous equations upon which they are based. The equations in Table 7 are based on component densities at body temperature, which ranges between 36°C and 37°C. In certain groups, such as children, the elderly, African-Americans, or sick patients, these type II combined methods may provide more accurate estimates of body fatness than the simpler, two-component models. Precise measures of TBW and bone mineral masses are required, however, to avoid swamping the gain in accuracy with increased, propagated errors of the additional measurements. In addition, the benefit in terms of improved accuracy should always be evaluated in relation to the increased cost associated with obtaining the additional measurements of TBW or total body bone mineral. These costs may be justified when the goal is to estimate changes in body fat over time, as in clinical weight loss studies.

3. Dual-Energy X-Ray Absorptiometry

Dual-energy X-ray absorptiometry (DXA) is primarily designed for measuring the amount of mineral within bone, but can also be used to estimate the amount of fat in soft tissues (143). DXA systems were introduced in the early 1990s as faster, more accurate substitutes for dual-photon absorptiometric (DPA) systems that had been used over the previous decade. The difference is that DXA uses an X-ray tube and a switch or filter to generate a collimated beam of photons at two energy levels, whereas DPA produces the beam using a radioisotope. The use of an X-ray source provides a higher energy flux, resulting in reduced scan times and increased precision (143). The X-ray systems, on the other hand, are also more susceptible to errors associated with thickness-related beam-hardening effects than the older isotope-based systems. The principles of analyzing bone mineral and soft-tissue compositions are otherwise the same in both types of systems (143,144).

The foundations of DXA and the methods used to obtain estimates of soft-tissue body composition have been described in detail elsewhere (144,145). In brief, the method is based on the differential attenuation of a collimated beam of photons at two, effective energy levels as it passes through the body. The ratio of the mass attenuation coefficients (R value) at the two energy levels is used to estimate soft-tissue and bone mineral masses, and the concentration of fat (lipid) in the soft tissues on a pixel-by-pixel basis as the beam traverses or scans the body in raster pattern. These estimates require specific assumptions regarding the minimum attenuation of bone minerals in order to separate bone from soft tissues, and a calibration curve for estimating the amount of fat from the R values for soft tissues (Rst). The compositional estimates for each pixel are summed to provide total-body estimates. For pixels that contain both soft and bone tissues, the composition of the soft-tissue component is interpolated from the nearest pixels that do not contain bone (143,145). Fat estimates by DXA are based on a measured property (Rst, the relative X-ray attenuation at the two main effective energies) and a "model" (the assumed known and constant Rst values for fat and bone-mineral free lean). DXA is thus a type II property-based method.

DXA estimates bone mineral, fat, and fat-free soft-tissue masses for the whole body and separately for the arms, legs, and trunk. The body segment estimates are somewhat less precise and accurate than those for the whole body (143). Although DXA has been demonstrated to have very high precision, there are some outstanding questions as to its accuracy, particularly in obese subjects. The accuracy of DXA systems is influenced by the thickness of the energy-absorbing tissues in the path of the X-ray beam, and accuracy decreases with increasing thickness due to beam hardening. The estimation of fat in soft tissue appears to be affected to a greater extent than the estimation of bone mineral content (146). The range of body thickness for optimal accuracy is 10–25 cm. Most men have sagittal trunk thickness >25 cm, and many obese individuals are >27 cm thick. The square root of weight/stature is correlated highly with sagittal trunk thickness and can used as a substitute for this measure: scans of individuals with values > 0.72 (corresponding approximately to trunk thickness > 27 cm) should be

expected to contain increased error (147). Manufacturers of DXA systems have included correction algorithms in their operating software for effects of body thickness, but the effectiveness of these has not been independently established. Different versions of software may provide somewhat different estimates of fat and fat-free soft-tissue masses that may be increased in obese subjects (148).

Efforts to validate the accuracy of DXA may be divided into three groups, as reviewed recently by Kohrt (149). Several studies have compared DXA with physicochemical analyses of pig carcasses, and generally show better results for larger animals (150–152). DXA has also been evaluated using experimental models composed of measured amounts of biological tissues or nonbiological tissue-equivalent materials (153,154). These studies suggest that errors in estimating the composition of soft-tissue equivalent materials increase when the thickness of the X-ray–absorbing materials are either <10 cm or >20 cm. Laskey et al. (154) tested the Lunar DPX using a phantom consisting of a plastic tank, with a spine phantom and aluminum block representing the head in the bottom, that was filled with variable amounts of lard and tap water to simulate soft tissue. Between 10 and 20 cm depth, DPX overestimated the amount of lard by 3% and for depths >22 cm the amount was overestimated by up to 25%. In vivo studies of DXA accuracy can be separated into experimental versus observational groups. In experimental studies, packets of lard have been placed on lean subjects to simulate increased amounts of adipose tissues (152, 155). These studies have produced mixed results that seem to depend on where the additional lard was placed on the body (trunk vs. legs), the type of scanner, and the version software used. Other experiments have tested effects of changes in hydration of the FFM using either patients undergoing hemodialysis or volunteers ingesting large amounts of water. Generally, DXA has been shown to measure changes in body fluids accurately and to correctly attribute these changes to the fat-free soft-tissue mass (156). Observational studies have compared DXA to estimates from hydrodensitometry or TBW in cross-sectional samples of subjects over wide ranges of body fatness (147,157–159). As Kohrt has pointed out, it is not possible in these studies to attribute any differences to either DXA or the comparison method since neither method is without error (149). It is important to note that few studies were specifically designed to test the accuracy of DXA in obese subjects.

In summary, most studies show that DXA estimates of body composition are highly reproducible. This has been evaluated in a variety of experiments. Reported technical errors for estimates of percent fat range from 0.3 to 1.4%; errors for FFM range from 0.3 to 0.9 kg (143,147,160).

Reported coefficients of variation range from 0.5 to 4% for percent body fat, 1 to 1.7% for fat mass, and 0.7 to 1.0% for FFM (156,161). Although there is substantial evidence that DXA estimates lose accuracy with increasing thickness, reports are conflicting as to whether thickness results in a systematic bias toward either over- or underestimation of body fatness (154,158). These conflicting results might be attributable to the use of different scanners and versions of software incorporating different calibration standards and thickness corrections. In any event, it is reasonable to expect that DXA estimates will lose both accuracy and precision in thicker, obese subjects.

The application of DXA to body composition analysis of obese patients is subject to additional practical limitations. Many obese individuals will simply be too wide for the scan field (~190 by 60 cm): the soft tissue falling outside of the scan field will not be included in the body composition analysis, resulting in biased estimates. As a result, DXA manufacturers generally do not recommend scanning individuals >100 kg body weight. The represents a serious limitation to the application of DXA body composition analysis to obese men. In addition, it may be difficult to obtain accurate regional body composition data. For example, it may not be possible to abduct the arms sufficiently from the trunk, or to separate the legs sufficiently at the thighs, in obese subjects to obtain accurate estimates of separate arm and leg soft-tissue masses. Recently, Tatarrani and Ravussin (161) described an approach that combines information from two DXA scans taken for each side of the body in obese subjects. This approach appeared to provide reasonably accurate estimates, compared to those from hydrodensitometry, but required careful attention to subject positioning in the scan field and added significantly to total scan and data analysis time also. As a more economical alternative, the authors suggest multiplying body weight by % fat estimates from one half-body scan to estimate whole fat and fat-free masses. This method is likely to be accurate, however, only in subjects with little anatomical asymmetry between the right and left halves of the body.

4. Whole-Body Counting/Neutron Activation

A group of methods referred to as whole-body counting/ in vivo neutron activation analysis can be used to estimate adiposity-related components. The methods share in common the ability to quantify all main elements at the atomic body composition level in vivo including H, C, N, O, P, Ca, Cl, K, and Na (162–164). Once these elements are known, it is possible to then calculate, using simultaneous equations, the main molecular level components such as fat, protein, water, and minerals. Components at other lev-

els, such as body cell mass, extracellular fluid, intracellular fluid, and skeletal muscle, can also be calculated using models based on measured elements (165,166). Only a few centers throughout the world are capable of measuring all of the major elements, while several additional centers are capable of measuring one or two elements. Whole-body counting alone can measure naturally occurring potassium 40 (115). When subjects are activated with a neutron source first and then placed back in a whole-body counter, additional elements such as Na, Cl, Ca, and P can be quantified by "delayed-gamma" neutron activation (164). Two other methods, prompt-gamma and inelastic neutron scattering neutron activation, are used to measure elements such as N, H, C, and O. Each neutron activation system is unique and many alternative methods have been advanced over the years.

In this section we provide a selective review of two methods, whole-body counting for potassium 40 and the multicomponent total-body carbon method of estimating fat mass. These representative methods provide the main concepts related to all in vivo neutron activation methods.

Total Body Potassium Method. Whole-body ^{40}K counting is a classic and widely used technique for evaluating adiposity (167). The natural abundance of potassium 40 in the human body is constant at 0.0118% of total body potassium (167). Potassium 40 is radioactive and emits a characteristic 1.46-MeV γ-ray that can be counted by detection systems with appropriate shielding (115,167). The procedure is to first measure ^{40}K in a whole-body counter and then calculate total body potassium from ^{40}K.

Potassium is an atomic level component that forms different relationships with components at high body composition levels. For example, a "subordinate" relationship exists between total body potassium and FFM at the molecular level (i.e., all of the potassium is within FFM), and there is an "overlapping" relationship between total body potassium and body cell mass at the cellular level (i.e., potassium is distributed in both body cell mass and the extracellular compartment). Once total-body potassium is known, FFM can be estimated by assuming a constant relationship between total body potassium and FFM,

$$FFM = \frac{TBK}{ratio} \quad (14)$$

where "ratio" is the assume constant proportion of FFM as potassium. Previous investigators have suggested a series of TBK/FFM ratios. Behnke reported a TBK/FFM ratio of 2.46 and 2.28 g/kg for men and women, respectively (3,132). Lukaski et al. suggested 2.46 and 2.50 g/ kg for the TBK/FFM ratios in men and women, respectively (168). Pierson et al. (169) suggested 2.65 g/kg and

2.26 g/kg for the TBK/FFM ratio in men and women, respectively. Forbes et al., based on a small number a cadaver analyses, reported TBK/FFM ratios of 2.66 and 2.50 g/kg in men and women, respectively (170). Recent studies indicate that the TBK/FFM ratio is sex and age dependent (171). Fat mass can be calculated as the difference between body weight and total-body potassium-derived FFM.

The total-body potassium method of estimating FFM and fat mass is of great historical significance. Many early obesity studies were carried out with total-body potassium measured by whole-body counting as the reference method for fat and FFM. Whole-body counters are costly and there are important technical issues that require attention to achieve accurate results. Today there are methods of equivalent, if not greater, accuracy for quantifying fat and FFM that are more readily available to research laboratories and of equal or lower cost.

Total-body potassium can also be measured using dilution of the radioactive isotope ^{42}K (117). This method is useful in specialized whole-body counter calibration studies, but has not practical application in the study of human obesity. The short half-life of ^{42}K (12.4 hr) and the radiation exposure involved preclude the routine use of this isotope. Exchangeable potassium (K_e), which is accounts for most of total body potassium, can also be measured using a combination of exchangeable sodium and TBW measurements (114) and this might be a useful approach at centers in which whole-body counters are unavailable.

Although the application of total body potassium as a measure of adiposity in human obesity research is limited, total-body and exchangeable potassium provide useful measures of body cell mass. The body cell mass compartment is often considered a measure of metabolically active tissue. The measurement and interpretation of body cell mass is discussed in detail by Moore and his colleagues (117).

Total-Body Carbon Method.   The total-body carbon method is a useful example of how total-body fat mass can be estimated from the combined measurement of elements in vivo. The method represents an evolution of methods at the Brookhaven National Laboratory in Upton, New York. The initial model for estimating fat mass developed by Cohn and colleagues at Brookhaven was relatively simple (172). Two measured elements, N and Ca, were used to calculate total-body protein and mineral, respectively. Tritium dilution volume was used to estimate TBW, and fat mass was then calculated as the difference between body weight and the sum of total-body protein, water, and mineral. Additional improvements in the model were made as

new information became available by Heymsfield and colleagues (127,141). The most recent advance occurred when Kehayias and colleagues introduced inelastic neutron scattering for measuring total-body carbon (163,173).

The total-body carbon method provides fat estimates that are independent of the two-component total-body potassium, water, and underwater weighing methods. This method can be used as a reference method for evaluating other body composition methods.

The total-body carbon method is based on the observation that almost all body carbon is incorporated into four components at the molecular level of body composition, fat, protein, glycogen, and bone mineral.

Kyere and colleagues (162) first proposed a model in which fat could be calculated from total-body carbon. The model was later improved upon by Kehayias and colleagues (5,173).

The total-body carbon method for measuring fat was derived from four simultaneous equations,

$$TBC = 0.77 \times fat + 0.532 \times protein + 0.444 \times glycogen + carbon\ in\ bone\ mineral \quad (15)$$

$$TBN = 0.16 \times protein \quad (16)$$

$$Glycogen = 0.044 \times protein \quad (17)$$

$$Carbon\ in\ bone\ mineral = 0.05 \times TBCa \quad (18)$$

where all units are in kg, and TBC, TBN, and TBCa represent total-body carbon, nitrogen, and calcium, respectively. Solving the simultaneous equations for fat mass:

$$Fat = 1.30 \times TBC - 4.45 \times TBN - 0.06 \times TBCa. \quad (19)$$

This equation indicates that the TBC method measures total-body fat as a function of three elements, C, N, and Ca. There are two important issues to consider with respect to Eq. (19): whether or not the coefficients are constant and whether total-body carbon, nitrogen, and calcium be measured accurately. We now discuss each of these points in detail.

Equation (15) includes the proportions of total-body carbon as fat, protein, glycogen, and bone mineral. Equations 16–18 further indicate the ratios between protein and nitrogen, between glycogen and protein, and between carbon and calcium in bone mineral. All of the coefficients in Eqs. (16)–(18) are assumed constant.

Although triglycerides extracted from human tissues vary in fatty acid composition, their carbon/triglyceride ratios (C/TG) are very close to 0.77. The following are some of the main human triglycerides: $C_{51}H_{98}O_6$ (C/TG = 0.759); $C_{55}H_{104}O_6$ (0.767); $C_{57}H_{102}O_6$ (0.769); and

$C_{57}H_{104}O_6$ (0.774). These various stoichiometries indicate that the C/TG ratio varies within a narrow range (0.759–0.774). It is therefore reasonable to assume a constant C/TG ratio of 0.77 in Eq. (15).

Total-body protein can be calculated from total-body nitrogen, and nitrogen can be measured by prompt-gamma neutron activation analysis. This calculation is based on the assumption that a constant ratio (0.16) exists between nitrogen and protein [Eq. (16)]. Protein includes almost all compounds containing nitrogen, varying from simple amino acids to complex nucleoproteins (174). The current suggested chemical formula for protein is $C_{100}H_{159}N_{26}O_{32}S_{0.7}$. The C/protein and N/protein ratios in this widely accepted formula are 0.532 and 0.16, respectively. Chemical analysis confirmed the validity of the ratios for most proteins analyzed, although a few specific proteins have N contents that are different from 0.16 (e.g., 0.137 and 0.172 for albumin and collagen, respectively) (174). The chemical analysis of two cadavers, however, yielded whole-body N/protein rations of 0.156 and 0.158, close to the assumed value of 0.16 (175).

Glycogen is not included in most body composition models owing to its small amount. In the total-body carbon method for estimating fat, glycogen content was included because of the high C/glycogen ratio of 0.444. In the model of Kehayias et al. the glycogen/protein ratio was assumed constant at 0.044 (5). This consideration must be approximate because the concentrations of glycogen in liver, skeletal muscle, and heart vary significantly with fasting and feeding. Total-body glycogen content is about 0.3–0.5 kg and thus the total amount of carbon in glycogen is thus only ~0.2 kg. The model error from the assumed constant glycogen/protein ratio therefore has only a small effect on the accuracy of total-body fat estimates.

The main compound of bone mineral, calcium hydroapatite $[Ca_3(PO_4)_2]_3$ $Ca(OH)_2$, does not contain carbon. Biltz and Pellegrino found that the ratio of carbon to bone calcium is 0.05 g/g (176). It is known that almost all body calcium is incorporated into bone mineral. The total-body carbon method estimates carbon in bone mineral, presumably incorporated as carbon in bicarbonate, from total-body calcium [Eq. (18)]. Although the carbon/calcium ratio is an approximation, errors in this proportion have only small effect on fat estimates as with glycogen.

The total-body carbon method does not consider the carbon in soft-tissue minerals as HCO_3^-. This is because the very small amount of carbon in soft tissue minerals has almost no impact on fat estimates.

From the above discussion it is clear that many assumptions are needed in developing the total-body carbon method for measuring total body fat. The main assumptions, however, appear to be highly stable.

Returning to the second aspect of the total-body carbon method, measurement of C, N, and Ca, all three elements are quantified by neutron activation analysis.

Total body carbon ins measured by inelastic scattering, which is based on the reaction $^{12}C + n \rightarrow {}^{12}C^* + n' \rightarrow {}^{12}C + n' + \gamma$ (4.44 MeV) (163,173). Total-body nitrogen is measured using prompt–γ-neutron activation analysis, and its reaction is $^{14}N + n \rightarrow {}^{15}N^* \rightarrow {}^{14}N + \gamma$ (10.83 MeV) (177). Delayed–γ-neutron activation is used to measure total-body calcium based on the reaction: $^{48}Ca + n \rightarrow {}^{49}Ca^* \rightarrow {}^{49}Ca + \gamma$ (3.10 MeV) (164).

All three of the neutron activation analysis methods involve radiation exposure, and this is the main disadvantage of the total-body carbon method. The average exposure is 0.26, 2.5, and 0.16 for prompt-γ, delayed-γ, and inelastic scattering neutron activation analysis, respectively.

The between-measurement coefficients of variations for total-body carbon, nitrogen, and calcium are 3.0%, 2.7%, and 0.8%, respectively (163,164,173). The propagated error in the TBC method of measuring total body fat is 3.4–4.0% (5).

The TBC method is not widely used in the study of body composition since only a few laboratories in the world have the necessary three neutron activation systems. However, the TBC method is important because it is based on highly stable models that are not effected to an appreciable degree by age, sex, and ethnicity. In some respects, at least conceptually, the TBC method approaches the potential accuracy in estimating total body fat afforded by lipid extraction of human cadavers.

5. Imaging

Imaging methods, such as CT and MRI, are considered the most accurate means available for in vivo quantification of body composition on the tissue-system level. These approaches are not used extensively owing to the high cost and expertise needed. They are the only methods available, however, for accurate quantification of internal adipose tissue, which is recognized increasingly as the key aspect of obesity associated with chronic metabolic disease risk. As a result, data from CT or MRI are considered necessary for the development and calibration of simpler, less expensive approaches to the estimation or prediction of absolute and relative amounts of visceral adipose tissues.

Computed Tomography. Heymsfield and colleagues were among the first to explore the use of CT in body composition research. They initially used CT to quantify the cross-sectional area of arm muscle in 1979 (178); subsequent reports described methods of estimating visceral organ volumes (179) and VAT (9). Borkan and colleagues were the first to systematically evaluate VAT, in 1982 (180). Sjostrom and his colleagues introduced whole-body imaging and multicomponent analysis to quantify total-body and regional adipose tissue, skeletal muscle, bone, and other organ/tissue volumes (181).

The basic CT system consists of an X-ray tube and receiver that rotate in a perpendicular plane to the subject. The measurable properties of CT are 0.1–0.2 Å, 60–120 kVp X-rays that are attenuated as they pass through tissues (182). Attenuation is expressed as the linear attenuation coefficient, or CT number. The CT number is a measure of attenuation relative to air and water. The CT numbers of air and water are defined as −1000 and 0 Hounsfield number (HU), respectively. The X-ray beam attenuation is related to three factors; coherent scattering, photoelectric absorption, and Compton interactions (182). Physical density is the main determinant of attenuation and, therefore, CT number. There is a linear correlation between CT number and tissue density (183,184). Each of the image pixels or voxels has a CT number that gives contrast to the image. Image reconstruction is usually done with mathematical techniques based on either two-dimensional Fourier analysis, filtered back-projection, or a combination of the methods.

CT body composition methods are designed to quantify components at the tissue-system level of body composition. The main components are adipose tissue, skeletal muscle, bone, visceral organs, and brain. The adipose tissue component is further divided into subcutaneous, visceral, yellow marrow, and the interstitial adipose tissue that occurs between muscle fibers (4). Cross-sectional images are composed of picture elements or pixels, usually 1 mm by 1 mm squares. Slice thicknesses vary, and when considered in three dimensions the image consists of volume elements or voxels. Each pixel/voxel is assigned a value on a gray scale that reflects the composition of the tissue.

Quantifying tissue volume by CT requires two steps. First, the tissue area (cm^2) on each cross-sectional CT image is determined using one of two methods (178,181,185–188). In one technique, the investigator traces the perimeter of the target tissue with a light pen or track-ball controlled cursor. The area of the circumscribed tissue is then calculated, usually with software installed on the CT scanner console. The second approach employs an computerized edge-detection procedure that identifies the area of the target tissue by selecting pixels within a given HU range, for example −190 to −30 HU for adipose tissue (187).

Once the tissue areas (cm^2) are quantified for a series of images, the total volume can be calculated by integrating data from multiple contiguous slices. The tissue mass can be then calculated if a value for the density of the tissue is assumed. A formula for estimating mass would be:

$$C = d \times \sum_{i=1}^{n} [A_i \times (B_i + C_i)/2], \qquad (20)$$

where C is the mass of the target tissue (g), d is the assumed density for the tissue (e.g., 0.92 g/cm^3 for adipose tissue), A_i is the distance (cm) between scans, and B_i and C_i are the tissue areas (cm^2) in adjacent images (181).

CT tissue area and volume measurements have been shown to be highly reproducible. Kvist et al. (187) reported an average error of ±0.6% for whole-body adipose tissue volume for duplicate measures in four subjects. Chowdhury et al. (185) reported intraobserver errors for a large number of CT-measured body composition components. Some examples are for skin = 2.4%, total adipose tissue = 0.4%, and heart = 3.4%. An earlier report by Brummer et al. (189) indicated interobserver errors of 0.7%, 0.4%, and 2.1% for total adipose tissue, skeletal muscle, and visceral organs, respectively.

Several studies have established the accuracy of area and volume measurements from CT. Heymsfield et al. (179) reported that organ masses estimated using CT were highly reproducible and agreed with actual mass to within 5–6%. Rossner and colleagues (190) found good agreement between CT and cadaver adipose tissue areas and ratios (r's ranged from 0.77 to 0.94). Chowdhury and colleagues (185) reported that the average difference between body weight and mass determined from CT measured tissue volumes was 0.024 ± 0.65 kg and the coefficient of variation was 0.85%. Wang and colleagues (191) reported that body volume calculated from 22 CT slices was highly correlated with body volume from underwater weighing in 17 men ($r = 0.990$, $p = 0.0001$, SEE = 1.9 L, $n = 17$), although there was a statistically significant difference between mean values (CT = 74.8 ± 13.9 L vs. UWW = 73.6 ± 13.7 L, $p < 0.02$). This difference between mean volumes may be due to difficulty in accurately estimating residual lung volumes and in quantifying lung parenchymal volume by CT.

Magnetic Resonance Imaging. The estimation of body composition components on the tissue-system level using MRI is essentially the same as for CT. The two methods differ mainly in the manner in which the images are acquired, which has subsequent bearing on practical considerations of costs and applicability, as well as technical aspects of image analysis, relative accuracy, and reliability.

MRI does not use ionizing radiation. Instead, it is based on the interaction between hydrogen nuclei (protons), which are abundant in all biological tissues, and the magnetic fields generated and controlled by the MRI system's instrumentation. Hydrogen protons have a nonzero magnetic moment, which causes them to behave like tiny magnets. When a subject is placed inside the magnet of a magnetic resonance imager, where the field strength is typically 10,000 times stronger than the Earth's, the magnetic moments of the protons align themselves with the magnetic field. After the H protons have been aligned in a known direction, a pulsed radio-frequency field (RF) is applied to the body tissues causing a number of hydrogen protons to absorb energy. When the RF is turned off, the protons gradually return to their original positions, releasing in the process the energy that they absorbed in the form of an RF signal. It is this signal that is used to generate the magnetic resonance images by computer.

Foster et al (192) were among the first to illustrate the applicability of MRI to body composition analysis. Hayes et al. (193) first demonstrated the quantification of subcutaneous adipose tissue distribution in human subjects using MRI. A variety of studies have subsequently used MRI to quantify adipose tissue and/or lean tissue areas or volumes in children (194), normal males and females (195–198), obese males and females (199), diabetics (200), and elderly people (201). To date, three groups have employed MRI to evaluate whole-body adipose tissue and lean tissue distribution in human subjects (198,199,202–205).

Historically, an important problem with the application of MRI to body composition analysis has been the substantial time needed to obtain images of sufficient quality and resolution for reliable measurements. For example, depending on the pulse sequence used, the acquisition of a set of MRI images for the abdomen could require between 8 (197) and 16 min (206). Recent advances in MRI technology have reduced the time needed to obtain the same quality images of the abdomen to approximately 25 sec, and a series of images for whole-body analysis can be acquired in less than 30 min (96,97). These advances should make MRI a much more accessible instrument for body composition studies in the future.

A multislice MRI protocol for whole body analysis is illustrated in Figure 5 (96). The pulse sequence used to obtain images of the abdomen in this protocol requires 26 sec. During this time the subject must hold his or her breath to reduce the effects of respiratory motion on the images.

A factor that has impeded the use of MRI in body composition analysis has been the availability of appropriate image analysis software. In contrast to CT, this software is not generally included on most MRI control consoles. As a result, MRI image data usually must be translated and downloaded to a separate workstation with image analysis software. Once this is accomplished, the approach to the analysis of MRI images is similar to that used for CT images. The perimeter of the tissue of interest can be traced using a light pen or mouse-controlled pointer and the area within the perimeter can be calculated by multiplying the number of pixels in the highlighted region by their known area (207,28). Alternatively, image segmentation algorithms can be used that highlight all pixels within a selected range of intensities believed to be representative of a specific tissue. The latter approach, however, is considered more problematic when applied to MRI than to CT images for three reasons: (1) the distribution of pixel intensity (gray-scale) values for different tissues overlap more for MRI than for CT images; (2) noise due to respiratory motion blurs the borders between tissues in the abdomen to a greater extent in MRI than in CT; and (3) inhomogeneity in the magnetic field can produce "shading" at the peripheries of MRI images.

Once tissue areas have been quantified from MRI images, volumes (cm^3) and masses may be calculated in a manner similar to that described above for CT. Ross et al. (197), however, have defined a somewhat different mathematical formula for deriving tissue volumes from measurements of a series of axial MRI images. This formula recognizes that each image has a slice thickness and that the pixels identified for a tissue are actually volume elements, or voxels. Thus, the formula is based on volumes of truncated cones defined by pairs of consecutive images as follows:

$$V_{AB} = (h/3)[A_1 + B_2) + (A_1 \times B_2)^{1/2}] \qquad (21)$$

where V is total tissue volume, A and B are the two consecutive images, and h is the distance between slices.

Overall, the reported reliability of body composition estimates from MRI is somewhat less than that for CT. For example, Seidell et al. (80) reported CV%'s for repeated measurements of total, visceral, and subcutaneous adipose tissue areas for the abdomen of 5.4, 10.6 and 10.1%, respectively. Baumgartner et al. (78) reported CV%'s of <5% for total and subcutaneous adipose tissue and 16% for VAT, which were calculated from two repeated measurements by two independent observers on 25 sets of images. The large CV for VAT was attributed to difficulty in consistently identifying cutoff values for discriminating adipose from non-adipose-tissue pixels due to noise associated with magnetic field inhomogeneity and blurring due to intestinal movement.

It is important with MRI to distinguish error association with repeated analyses of the same image from that

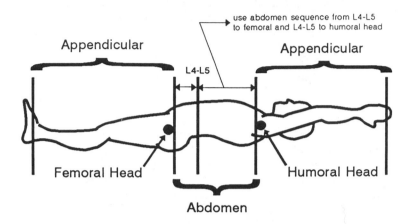

Figure 5 Multislice, whole-body MRI data acquisition protocol including examples of T1-weighted MRI pulse sequences, which provide good tissue contrast between adipose and lean tissues. These sequences were developed using a GE Signa Advantage 1.5 Tesla magnet with software version 5.4.2.

associated with repeated acquisition of the image. At least four studies report reliability data for repeated image acquisitions (198,206,209,210). The CVs for measurements of subcutaneous abdominal adipose tissue areas measured for two images taken at the same level range from 2% to 6%. The reported CVs for VAT are somewhat higher, ranging from 6% to 12%. Overall, these reported CVs for MRI are about 2–3 times greater than those for studies using CT.

Recently, Ross et al. (197) described special, interactive image analysis software that allows the analyst to correct misclassified pixels. Although considerable training and experience are needed to use of this software, reliability equivalent to those for CT can be achieved. Decreased scan times and other improvements in imaging techniques should further increase the reliability of future MRI body composition analyses. A more detailed review of the procedures used to determine body composition using MRI can be found elsewhere (186,211).

Several studies support the accuracy of MRI estimates of human adipose tissue and skeletal muscle. Using a rat model, Ross et al. (94) reported that whole-carcass chem-

ically extracted lipid was highly correlated with MRI–adipose tissue mass ($r = 0.97$, $p < 0.01$) and that the standard error of estimate was 10.5%. Fowler et al. (207) compared MRI–adipose tissue measurements to those obtained by dissection in a group of lean and obese pigs. The authors observed that the distribution of MRI–adipose tissue correlated strongly with adipose tissue distributed by dissection ($r = 0.98$), and that the mean square error was 2.1%. Engstrom et al. (212) compared the cross-sectional area measurements of skeletal muscle determined from the proximal thigh in cadavers to the corresponding MRI-measured cross-sectional areas and reported that the correlation coefficient between the two approached unity ($r = 0.99$). Recently, Abate et al. (208) compared MRI measures of abdominal subcutaneous and visceral adipose tissue to that obtained by direct weighing of the same adipose tissue compartments after dissection in three human cadavers. In this study the authors subdivided VAT into intraperitoneal and retroperitoneal depots. For the various compartments the mean difference between the two methods was 0.076 kg, or 6%.

Visceral Adipose Tissue. Perhaps the most important use of CT and MRI imaging methods in body composition studies is the measurement of VAT. No other methods are presently available that accurately quantify this component, which is strongly associated with the development of insulin resistance and hyperlipidemias in obese subjects.

Although comparisons to cadaver data suggest that CT and MRI provide accurate estimates of VAT, the best way to apply these methods to the in vivo measurement of VAT has not been fully established. Several important issues need to be resolved. First, there is little consensus regarding the definition of VAT. It is unclear what anatomical landmarks or boundaries should be used to identify VAT. For example, should VAT include both intra- and retroperitoneal adipose tissues? The distinction between adipose tissue depots is important because omental adipose tissue releases free-fatty acids (FFAs) directly into the liver through the portal vein. An increased flux of FFAs to the liver in those with enlarged VAT is suspected to be one factor leading to deranged hepatic insulin and lipoprotein metabolism.

From a pathophysiological perspective, VAT might be best defined as those adipose tissues that drain into the liver through the portal vein. Strict application of this definition would exclude retroperitoneal adipose tissues. This definition, however, may be neither technically nor clinically practical. The peritoneum is not visible on either CT or MRI images. As a result, attempts to separate VAT into intra- and retroperitoneal components have relied on arbitrary criteria (199,213–215). In any case, it has not been established whether the separate estimation of intraperitoneal or omental adipose tissue improves associations with metabolic variables or disease risk (199). At present, it seems appropriate to recommend that the definition of VAT include both intra- and retroperitoneal adipose tissues.

In addition, anatomical landmarks defining the boundaries for VAT volume are not well established. There is considerable variation among studies using multiple-image protocols for both the number and location of the images (CT or MRI) used to determine VAT volume (197,202,205,215). This may partly explain large differences among studies for estimated VAT volumes in apparently similar populations. To be consistent with the definition of VAT as adipose tissues that are portally drained, it is suggested that the T9–10 and S2–3 intervertebral spaces be used to define the upper and lower VAT landmarks. The T9–10 space corresponds to an anatomical position marginally above the hilar region of the spleen, whereas the S2–3 space corresponds anatomically to the rectosigmoid junction. These two landmarks define

a region within which the majority of VAT is portally drained.

It is not clear whether single or multiple images are needed to accurately estimate VAT. The area of VAT from a single L4/L5 image correlates highly with VAT volume (180,187,197). In addition, VAT area determined from a single slice appears to correlate as strongly with metabolic variables as do volumes from multiple images (199). On the other hand, it may be preferable to quantify VAT volumes in studies designed to develop anthropometric prediction equations. Sjöström (216) presented data suggesting that the error associated with VAT prediction by anthropometry can be reduced if VAT volume is measured using multiple images.

Lean Tissues. It may also be important to consider measurements of lean tissue volume or mass using CT or MRI methods in conjunction with those for adipose tissue due to the role of skeletal muscle in the development of insulin resistance and glucose intolerance. At present, there are few data for the reliability or accuracy of measurements of lean tissues by MRI. Baumgartner et al. (78) reported CV%'s of <5% for repeated measurements of lean tissue areas (skeletal muscle plus bone) on MRI images of the midarm and midthigh. Ross et al. (199) recently reported a CV of 1.2% for repeated measurements of lean tissue on a single image of the proximal thigh and 3.9% for the total lean tissue volume of the leg. The availability of a noninvasive method for measuring lean tissue, without the approximations of anthropometric techniques, represents a significant advance. The results reported here suggest that MRI may serve as a criterion method for skeletal muscle measurement, thereby providing reference data for anthropometric comparison.

Summary. Several factors should be considered when choosing a study imaging method. Both CT and MRI produce high-resolution scans of all major tissue-system-level body composition components. Both methods are very expensive and require high techical skill for application. In general, CT has been shown to provide more reliable data than MRI, although this is changing rapidly with the introduction of new imaging techniques and image analysis software. A major advantage of MRI is the lack of ionizing radiation. At present no known health risks are associated with MRI at the current magnet field strengths of about 1.5 T. Newer scanning protocols are rapid and cost is usually reduced. The small-bore magnets create a problem for claustrophobic patients and very obese patients cannot usually fit within the magnet core. An important advantage of CT is that instruments are widely available. A second advantage of CT is the high resolution of images and the consistency of tissue attenuation values from scan to scan. Within reasonable limits, water, skeletal muscle, adipose tissue, and other components have similar HU distributions within and between scans. The consistency of attenuation data allows development of standardized protocols for reading scans and separating various tissues from each other.

The cost of CT scanning is variable and access during peak patient hours may be limited. The major disadvantage of CT is the associated radiation exposure. This limits study of children and women in childbearing years. Regional studies with appropriate scanner settings substantially lowers radiation dose compared to whole-body studies. Radiation exposure is still a concern in long-term longitudinal studies with repeated measurements over time. Finally, some very obese patients may be too large to fit within the scanner and our experience is that CT study is limited to patients below about BMI 35 kg/m².

V. CONCLUSIONS

There are many methods of estimating body composition components, particularly those components related to obesity. Today practically all major body composition components can be quantified in vivo. Our review has focused on widely available methods or those of special conceptual interest.

The selection a component assessment method depends largely on the specific purpose for body composition assessment. The question posed will dictate the requirement for method accuracy and precision. Additional relevant factors include method cost, safety, practically, and availability. These are important considerations as most research centers now have multiple available methods ranging from CT and MRI to DXA, BIA, and anthropometry.

Like many other areas of scientific endeavor, the study of human body composition has emerged over the past decade as a distinct research area with powerful investigative tools. These modern resources should aid in establishing pathogenesis and quantifying risk and treatment response of today's most serious nutritional disorder in industrialized countries, human obesity.

ACKNOWLEDGMENTS

This work was supported by National Institutes of Health Grants P01-DK 42618, R01-AG 13021 (SBH), and R01-AG 10149 (RNB), and Grant 951R057 from the Canadian Fitness and Lifestyle Research Institute (RR).

REFERENCES

1. Wang ZM, Pierson RN Jr, Heymsfield SB. The five level model: a new approach to organizing body composition research. Am J Clin Nutr 1992; 56:19–28.
2. Heymsfield SB, Wang ZM, Visser M, Gallagher D, Pierson RN. Techniques used in the measurement of body composition: an overview with emphasis on bioimpedance analysis. Am J Clin Nutr 1996; 64:S478–S484.
3. Behnke AR. Role of fat in gross body composition and configuration. In: Rodahl K, ed. Fat as a Tissue. New York: McGraw-Hill, 1964:285–313.
4. Snyder WS, Cook MJ, Nasset ES, et al. Report of the Task Group on Reference Man. Oxford: Pergamon Press, 1975.
5. Kehayias JJ, Heymsfield SB, LoMonte AF, Wang J, Pierson RN Jr. In vivo determination of body fat by measuring total body carbon. Am J Clin Nutr 1991; 53:1339–1344.
6. Diem K, ed. Documental Geigy Scientific Tables. Ardsley, NY: Geigy Pharmaceuticals, 1962.
7. Gurr MI, Harwood JL. Lipid Biochemistry, 4th ed. London: Chapman and Hall, 1991.
8. Moore FD, Olsen KH, McMurray JD, Parker HV, Ball MR, Boyden CM: The Body Cell Mass and Its Supporting Environment: Body Composition in Health and Disease. Philadelphia: WB Saunders, 1963.
9. Heymsfield SB, Noel R. Radiographic analysis of body composition by computerized axial tomography. Nutr Cancer 1981; 17:161–172.
10. Heymsfield SB, Wang ZM, Withers R. Multicomponent molecular-level models of body composition analysis. In: Roche A, Heymsfield SB, Lohman T, eds. Human Body Composition. Champaign IL: Human Kinetics, 1996: 129–148.
11. Martin AD, Daniel MZ, Drinkwater DT, Clarys JP. Adipose tissue density, estimated adipose lipid fraction and whole body adiposity in male cadavers. Int J Obes 1994; 18: 79–83.
12. Wang ZM, Heshka S, Pierson RN Jr, Heymsfield SB. Systematic organization of body composition methodology: overview with emphasis on component-based methods. Am J Clin Nutr 1995; 61:457–465.
13. Jackson AS, Pollock ML. Generalized equations for predicting body density of women. Med Sci Sports Exerc 1980; 12:175–182.
14. Durnin JVGA, Womersely J. Body fat assessment from total body density and its estimation from skinfold thickness: measurements on 481 men and women aged 16 to 72 years. Br J Nutr 1974; 32:77–97.
15. Behnke AR, Feen BG, Welham WC. The specific gravity of healthy men. JAMA 1942; 118:495–498.
16. Mazess RB, Barden HS, Bisek JP, Hanson J. Dual-energy X-ray absorptiometry for total-body and regional bone-mineral and soft-tissue composition. Am J Clin Nutr 1990; 51:1106–1112.
17. Roche AF, Guo S. Development, testing and use of predictive equations for body composition measures. In: Kral

JG, VanItallie TB, eds. Recent developments in Body Composition Analysis: Methods and Applications. London: Smith-Gordon, 1993:1–16.

18. Lukaski HC, Johnson PE, Bolonchuk WW, Lykken GI. Assessment of fat-free mass using bioelectrical impedance measurement of the human body. Am J Clin Nutr 1985; 41:810–817.

19. Pace N, Rathbun EN. Studies on body composition. III. The body water and chemically combined nitrogen content in relation to fat content. J Biol Chem 1945; 158: 685–691.

20. Sheng HP, Huggins RA. A review of body composition studies with emphasis on total body water and fat. Am J Clin Nutr 1979; 32:630–647.

21. Lohman TG. Advances in Body Composition Assessment. Champaign, IL: Human Kinetics, 1992.

22. Mueller SH, Martorell R. Reliability and accuracy of measurement. In: Lohman TB, Roche AF, Martorell R, eds. Anthropometric Standardization Reference Manual. Champaign, IL: Human Kinetics 1988:83–87.

23. Lohman TG, Going SB. Multicomponent models in body composition research: opportunities and pitfalls. In: Ellis KJ, Eastman JD, eds. Human Body Composition. New York: Plenum Press, 1993:53–58.

24. Dunn G. Design and Analysis of Reliability Studies: The Statistical Evaluation of Measurement Errors. London: Arnold Edward, 1989.

25. Habicht J-P, Yarbrough C, Martorell R. Anthropometric field methods: criteria for selection. In: Jelliffe DB, Jelliffe EFP, eds. Nutrition and Growth. New York: Plenum Press, 1979:365–387.

26. Bland JM, Altman DG. Statistical methods for assessing agreement between two methods of clinical measurement. Lancet 1986; 8:307–310.

27. Roche AF, Baumgartner RN, Guo S. Anthropometry: classical and modern approaches. In: Whitehead RG, Prentice A, eds. New Techniques in Nutritional Research. New York: Academic Press, 1991:242–260.

28. Lohman TG, Roche AF, Martorell R. Anthropometric Standardization Reference Manual. Champaign, IL: Human Kinetics, 1988.

29. Kuskowska-Wolk A, Karlsson P, Stolt M, Rossner S. The predictive validity of Body Mass Index based on self reported weight and height. Int J Obes 1989, 13:441–453.

30. Lass NJ, Andes SR, McNair CD, Cline AL, Pecora MC. Correlational study of subjects' self-reported and measured heights and weights. Percept Motor Skills 1982; 54: 102.

31. Bowman RL, DeLucia JL. Accuracy of self-reported intake: A meta-analysis. Behav Ther 1992; 23:637–655.

32. Cameron R, Evers SE. Self-report issues in obesity and weight management: state-of-the art and future directions. Behav Assess 1990; 12:91–106.

33. Le Marchand L, Yoshizawa CN, Nomura AMY. Validation of body size information on driver's licenses. Am J Epidemic 1988; 128:874–877.

34. Metropolitan Life Insurance Company. 1983 Metropolitan height and weight tables. Stat Bull 1983; 64:9.

35. Najjar MF, Rowland M. Anthropometric Reference Data and Prevalence of Overweight. Washington, DC: U.S. Govt. Printing Office. Vital and Health Statistics, Series 11, No 238. (DHEW publication no. (PHS) 7-1688), 1987.

36. Quetelet LAJ. Anthropometric ou misure des differentes facultes de l'homme. Brussels: C Marquardt, 1871:479.

37. Keys A, Aravanis C, Blackburn H, Van Buchem FSP, Buzina R, Djordjevic BS, Fidanza F, Karvonen MJ, Menotti A, Puddu V, Taylor HL. Coronary heart disease: overweight and obesity as risk factors. Ann Intern Med 1972; 77: 15–27.

38. Abdel-Malek AK, Mukherjee D, Roche AF. A method of constructing an index of obesity. Hum Biol 1985; 57:415.

39. Billewicz WZ, Kemsley WFF, Thomson AM. Indices of adiposity. Br J Prev Soc Med 1962; 16:183–188.

40. Khosla T, Lowe CR. Indices of obesity derived from body weight and height. Br J Prev Soc Med 1967; 21:122–128.

41. Florey CD. The use and interpretation of ponderal index and other weight-height ratios in epidemiological studies. J Chronic Dis 1970; 23:93.

42. Lee J, Kolonel LN, Hinds MW. The use of an inappropriate weight-height derived index of obesity can produce misleading results. Int J Obes 1982; 6:233–239.

43. Lee J, Kolonel LN. Are body mass indices interchangeable in measuring obesity-disease associations? Am J Public Health 1984; 74:376–377.

44. Benn RT. Some mathematical properties of weight-for-height indices used as measures of adiposity. Br J Prev Soc Med 1971; 25:42–50.

45. Roche AF, Siervogel RM, Chumlea WC, Webb P. Grading body fatness from limited anthropometric data. Am J Clin Nutr 1981; 34:2831–2838.

46. Garn SM, Leonard WR, Hawthorne VM. Three limitations of the body mass index. Am J Clin Nutr 1986; 44: 996–997.

47. Garrow JS, Webster J. Quetelet's index (W/H2) as a measure of fatness. Int J Obes 1985; 9:147–153.

48. Bouchard C. Genetics of human obesities: introductory notes. In: Bouchard C, ed. The Genetics of Obesity. Boca Raton, FL: CRC Press, 1994:1–16.

49. Baumgartner RN, Heymsfield SB, Roche AF. Human body composition and the epidemiology of chronic disease. Obes Res 1995; 3:73–95.

50. Gallagher D, Visser M, Sepulveda D, Pierson RN Jr, Harris T, Heymsfield SB. How useful body mass index for comparison of body fatness across age, gender, and ethnic groups? Am J Epidemiol 1996; 143:228–239.

51. Himes JH, Bouchard C. Validity of anthropometry in classifying youths as obese. Int J Obes 1989; 13:183–193.

52. Garn SM, Gorman EL. Comparison of pinch-caliper and teleroentgenogrammetric measurements of subcutaneous fat. Hum Biol 1956; 28:407–411.

53. Kuczmarski RJ, Fanelli MT, Koch GG. Ultrasonic assessment of body composition in obese adults: overcoming the limitations of the skinfold caliper. Am J Clin Nutr 1987; 45:717–724.

54. Garn SM. Relative fat patterning: an individual characteristics. Hum Biol 1955; 27:75–89.

55. Himes JH, Roche AF, Siervogel RM. Compressibility of skinfolds and the measurement of subcutaneous fatness. Am J Clin Nutr 1979; 32:1734–1740.

56. Weits T, Van Der Beek EJ, Wedel M. Comparison of ultrasound and skinfold caliper measurements of subcutaneous fat tissue. Int J Obes 1985; 10:161–168.

57. Bellisari A. Sonographic measurement of adipose tissue. J Ultr Med 1993; 9:11–18.

58. Armellini F, Zamboni M, Rigo L, Tedesco T, Bergamo-Andreis IA, Procacci C, Bosello O. The contribution of sonography to the measurement of intra-abdominal fat. J Clin Ultrasound 1990; 18:563–567.

59. Bellisari A, Roche AF, Siervogel RM. Reliability of B-mode ultrasonic measurements of subcutaneous adipose tissue and intra-abdominal depth: comparisons with skinfold thicknesses. Int J Obes 1993; 17:475–480.

60. Björntorp P. Visceral obesity: a "civilization syndrome." Obes Res 1993; 1:206–222.

61. Bouchard C. Introductory notes on the topic of fat distribution. In: Bouchard C, Johnston F, eds. Fat Distribution During Growth and Later Health Outcomes. New York: Alan R Liss, 1988:1–8.

62. Bailey SM, Garn SM, Katch VL, Guire KE. Taxonomic identification of human fat patterns. Am J Phys Anthrop 1982; 59:361–366.

63. Mueller WH, Stallones L. Anatomical distribution of subcutaneous fat: skinfold site choice and construction of indices. Hum Biol 1981; 53:321–335.

64. Baumgartner RN, Roche AF, Guo S, Lohman TG, Boileau RA, Slaughter M. Adipose tissue distribution: the stability of principal components by sex, ethnicity and maturation stage. Hum Biol 1986; 58:719–735.

65. Lapidus L, Bengtsson C, Larsson B, Pennart K, Rybo E, Sjöström L. Distribution of adipose tissue and risk of cardiovascular disease and death: a 12 year follow up of participants in the population study of women in Gothenburg, Sweden. Br Med J 1984; 289:1257–1261.

66. Larsson BK, Svardsudd L, Welin L, Wilhelmsen L, Björntorp P, Tibblin G. Abdominal adipose tissue distribution, obesity and risk of cardiovascular disease and death: 13 year follow up of participants in the study of men born in 1913. Br Med J 1984; 288:1401–1404.

67. Ohlson LO, Larsson B, Svardsudd K, et al. The influence of body fat distribution on the incidence of diabetes mellitus, 13.5 years of follow-up of the participants of the study of men born in 1913. Diabetes 185; 34;1055–1058.

68. Seidell JC, Deurenberg P, Hautvast JGAJ. Obesity and fat distribution in relation to health—current insights and recommendations. World Rev Nutr Diet 1987; 50:57–91.

69. Kissebah AH. Insulin resistance in visceral obesity. Int J Obes 1991; 15:109–115.

70. Després JP. Lipoprotein metabolism in visceral obesity. Int J Obes 1991; 15:45–52.

71. Bray GA. Pathophysiology of obesity. Am J Clin Nutr 1992; 55(Suppl):488S–494S.

72. Filipovsky J, Ducimetiere P, Darne B, Richard JI. Abdominal body mass distribution and elevated blood pressure are associated with increased risk of death from cardiovascular diseases and cancer in middle-aged men. The results of a 15-20-year follow-up in the Paris prospective study I. Int J Obes 1993; 17:197–203.

73. Valdez R, Seidell JC, Ahu UI, Weiss U. A new index of abdominal adiposity as an indicator of risk for cardiovascular disease: a cross-population study. Int J Obes 1993; 17:77–82.

74. Jakicic JM, Donnelly JE, Jaward AF, Jacobson SC, Gunderson R, Pasquale. Association between blood lipids and different measures of body fat distribution. Int J Obes 1993; 17:131–137.

75. Ducimetière P, Richard J, Cambien F. The pattern of subcutaneous fat distribution in middle-aged men and the risk of coronary disease. The Paris prospective study. Int J Obes 1986; 10:229–240.

76. Houmard JA, Wheeler WS, McCammon MR, Wells JM, Truitt N, Hamad SF, Holbert D, Israel RG, Barakat HA. An evaluation of waist to hip ratio measurement methods in relation to lipid and carbohydrate metabolism in men. Int J Obes 1991; 15:181–188.

77. Seidell JC, Björntorp P, Sjöstrom L, Sannerstedt R, Krotkiewski M, Kvist H. Regional distribution of muscle and fat mass in men—new insight into the risk of abdominal obesity using computed tomography. Int J Obes 1989; 13:289–304.

78. Baumgartner RN, Rhyne RL, Garry PJ. Body composition in the elderly from MRI: association with cardiovascular disease risk factors. In: Ellis K, Eastman J, eds, Human Body Composition: In Vivo Methods, Models, and Assessment. New York: Plenum Press, 1993:35–38.

79. Vague J. The degree of masculine differentiation of obesities: a factor determining predisposition to diabetes, atherosclerosis, gout and uric calculous diseases. Am J Clin Nutr 1956; 4:20–34.

80. Seidell JC, Oosterlee A, Thijssen M, Burema J, Deurenberg P, Hautvast J, Josephus J. Assessment of intra-abdominal and subcutaneous abdominal fat: relation between anthropometry and computed tomography. Am J Clin Nutr 1987; 45:7–13.

81. Ross R, Léger L, Morris D, De Guise J, Guardo R. Quantification of adipose tissue by MRI: relationship with anthropometric variables. J Appl Physiol 1992; 72:787–795.

82. Kekes-Szabo T, Hunter GR, Nyikos I, Nicholson C, Snyder S, Lincoln B. Development and validation of computed tomography derived anthropometric regression equations for estimating abdominal adipose tissue distribution. Obes Res 1994; 2:450–457.

83. Pouliot MC, Després JP, Lemieux S, Moorjani S, Bouchard C, Tremblay A, Nadeau A, Lupien PJ. Waist circumference and abdominal sagittal diameter: best simple anthropometric indexes of abdominal visceral adipose tissue accumulation and related cardiovascular risk in men and women. Am J Cardiol 1994; 73:460–468.

84. Després JP, Prud'homme D, Pouliot MC, Tremblay A, Bouchard C. Estimation of deep abdominal adipose tissue accumulation simple anthropometric measurements in men. Am J Clin Nutr 1989; 49:33–36.

85. Kvist H, Chowdury B, Grangard U, Tylén U, Sjöstrom L. Total and visceral adipose tissue volumes derived from measurements with computed tomography in adult men and women: predictive equations. Am J Clin Nutr 1988; 48:1351–1361.

86. Koester RS, Hunter GR, Snyder S, Khaled MA, Berland LL. Estimation of computerized tomography derived abdominal fat distribution. Int J Obes 1992; 50:444–447.

87. Sjöstrom L. Body composition studies with CT and with CT-calibrated anthropometric techniques. In: Kral JG, VanItallie TB, eds. Recent Developments in Body Composition Analysis: Methods and Applications. London: Smith-Gordon, 1993:17–34.

88. Ross R, Rissanen J, Hudson R. Sensitivity associated with the identification of visceral adipose tissue levels using waist circumference in men and women: effects of weight loss. Int J Obes 1996; 20:533–538.

89. Wadden TA, Stunkard AJ, Johnson FE, et al. Body fat deposition in adult obese women. II. Changes in fat distribution accompanying weight reduction. Am J Clin Nutr 1988; 47:229–234.

90. Pasquali R, Antenucci, D, Casimirri, F, et al. Clinical and hormonal characteristics of obese amenorrheic hyperandrogenic women before and after weight loss. J Clin Endocrinol Metab 1989; 68:173–179.

91. Fujioka K, Colletti PM, Kim H, Devine W, Cuyegkeng T, Pappas T. Magnetic-resonance imaging used for determining fat distribution in obesity and diabetes. Am J Clin Nutr 1991; 54:623–628.

92. Ashwell MA, McCall SA, Cole TJ, Dixon AK. Fat distribution and its metabolic complications: interpretations. In: Human Body Composition and Fat Distribution. Wageningen: EURO-NUT NG Norgan, 1986:227–242.

93. Presta E, Leibel RL, Hirsh J. Regional changes in adrenergic receptor status during hypocaloric intake do not predict changes in adipocyte size or body shape. Metabolism 1990; 39:307–315.

94. Ross R, Léger L, Marliss EB, Morris DV, Geougeon R. Adipose tissue distribution changes during rapid weight loss in obese adults. Int J Obes 1991; 15:733–739.

95. Zamboni M, Armellini F, Turcato E, Todesto T, Bissoli L, Bergamo-Andreis IA, Bosselo O. Effect of weight loss on regional body fat distribution in premenopausal women. Am J Clin Nutr 1993; 58:29–34.

96. Ross, R, Pedwell H, Rissanen J. Effects of energy restriction and exercise on skeletal muscle and adipose tissue in women as measured by magnetic resonance imaging. Am J Clin Nutr 1995; 61:1179–1185.

97. Ross R, Pedwell H, Rissanen J. Response of total and regional lean tissue and skeletal muscle to a program of energy restriction and resistance exercise. Int J Obes 1995; 19:781–787.

98. Van der Kooy K, Leenen R, Seidell JC, Deurenberg P, Visser M. Abdominal diameters as indicators of visceral fat: comparison between magnetic resonance imaging and anthropometry. Br J Nutr 1993; 70:47–58.

99. Richelsen B, Pedersen SB. Associations between different anthropometric measurements of fatness and metabolic risk parameters in non-obese, healthy, middle-aged men. Int J Obes 1995; 19:169–174.

100. Seidell JC, Andres R, Sorkin JD, Muller DC. The sagittal waist diameter and mortality in men: the Baltimore Longitudinal Study on Aging. Int J Obes 1994; 18:61–67.

101. Baumgartner RN, Chumlea WC, Roche AF. Impedance for body composition. In: Pandolf KB ed. Exerc Sport Sci Rev, Vol 18. Baltimore: Williams & Wilkins, 1990: 193–224.

102. Kushner RF. Bioelectric impedance analysis: a review of principles and applications. J Am Coll Nutr 1992; 11: 199–209.

103. Baumgartner RN. Electrical Impedance and TOBEC. In: Roche AF, Lohman TG, Heymsfield SB, eds. Human Body Composition: Methods and Findings. Champaign, IL: Human Kinetics, 1996.

104. VanLoan M, Mayclin P. A new TOBEC instrument and procedure for the assessment of body composition: use of Fourier coefficients to predict lean body mass and total body water. Am J Clin Nutr 1987; 45:131–137.

105. Boileau RA. Utilization of total body electrical conductivity in determining body composition. In: Designing Foods: Animal Product Options in the Marketplace. National Research Council. Washington, DC: National Academy Press, 1988:251–257.

106. Baumgartner RN, Chumlea WC, Roche AF. Estimation of body composition from segmental impedance. Am J Clin Nutr 1989; 50:221–225.

107. VanLoan M, Mayclin P. Bioelectrical impedance analysis: Is it a reliable indicator of lean body mass and total body water? Hum Biol 1987; 59:299–309.

108. Hodgdon JA, Fitzgerald PI. Validity of impedance predictions at various levels of fatness. Hum Biol 1987; 59: 281–298.

109. Lukaski H. Applications of bioelectric impedance analysis: a critical review. In: Yasumura S, Harrison JE, McNeill KE, Woodhead AD, Dilmanian FA, eds. In Vivo Body Composition Studies: Recent Advances. New York: Plenum Press, 1989: 365–374.

110. Segal KR, VanLoan M, Fitzgerald P, Hodgdon J, VanItallie TB. Lean body mass estimation by bioelectrical impedance analysis: a four-site cross-validation study. Am J Clin Nutr 1988; 47:7–14.

111. Lukaski H, Bolonchuk W, Hall C, Siders W. Validation of tetrapolar bioelectric impedance method to assess human body composition. J Appl Physiol 1986; 60:1327–1332.

112. Gray DS, Bray GA, Gemayel N, Kaplan K. Effect of obesity on bioelectrical impedance. Am J Clin Nutr 1989; 50: 255–260.

113. Deurenberg P, Vanderkooy K, Leenan R, Westrate J, Seidell JC. Sex and age specific population prediction formulas for estimating body composition from bioelectrical impedance: a cross-validation study. Int J Obes 1991; 15: 17–25.

114. Shizgal HM, Spanier AH, Humes J, Wood CD, Indirect measurement of total exchangeable potassium. AM J Physiol 1977; 233:F253–259.

115. Pierson RN Jr, Wang J, Colt E, Neumann P. Body composition measurements in normal men: the potassium, sodium, sulfate, and tritium space in 58 adults. J Chronic Disease, 1982; 35:419–428.

116. Culebras JM, Moore FD. Total body water and the exchangeable hydrogen. I. Theoretical calculation of nonaqueous exchangeable hydrogen in Man. Am J Physiol 1977; 232:R54–59.

117. Moore FD, Oleson KH, McMurray JD, Parker HV, Ball MR, Boyden CM. The Body Cell Mass and Its Supporting Environment. Philadelphia: WB Saunders, 1963.

118. Lukaski HC. Method for the assessment of human body composition: traditional and new. Am J Clin Nutr 1987; 46:537–556.

119. Scholler DA, Van Santer E, Petersen DW, Dietz W, Jaspan J, Klein PD. Total body water measurements in humans with ^{18}O and ^{2}H labeled water. Am J Clin Nutr 1980; 33: 2686–2693.

120. Wong WW, Cochran WJ, Klish WJ, et al. In vivo isotope-fractionation factors and the measurement of deuterium- and oxygen-18 dilution spaces from plasma, urine, saliva, respiratory water vapor, and carbon dioxide. Am J Clin Nutr 1988; 47:1–6.

121. Goran MI, Poehlman ET, Nair KS, et al. Effect of gender, body composition, and equilibration time on the ^{3}H-to-^{18}O dilution space ratio. Am J Physiol 1992; 263: E1119–1124.

122. Wang J, Pierson RN, Kelly WG. A rapid method for the determination of deuterium oxide in urine: application to the measurement of total body water. J Lab Clin Med 1973; 82:170–178.

123. Matthews DE, Heymsfield SB. ASPEN 1990 Research Workshop on Energy Metabolism. J Parent Ent Nutr 1991; 15:3–14.

124. Schoeller DA, Jones PJH. Measurement of total body water by isotope dilution: a unified approach to calculations. In: Ellis KJ, Yasumura S, Morgan WD, eds. In Vivo Body Composition Studies. London: Institute of Physical Sciences in Medicine, 1987;131–137.

125. Schoeller DA, Van Santen E, Petersen DW, et al. Total body water measurement in humans with ^{18}O and ^{2}H labeled water. Am J Clin Nutr 1980; 33:2686–2693.

126. Schoeller D. Isotope dilution methods. In: Björntorp P, Brodoff BN, eds. Obesity. New York: JB Lippincott, 1992; 80–88.

127. Heymsfield SB, Lichtman S, Baumgartner RN, et al. Body composition of humans: comparison of two improved four-compartment models that differ in expense, technical complexity, and radiation exposure. Am J Clin Nutr 1990; 52:52–58.

128. Waki M, Kral JG, Mazariegos M, Wang J, Pierson RN Jr, Heymsfield SB. Relative expansion of extracellular fluid in obese vs. nonobese women. Am J Physiol 1991; 261: E199–E203.

129. Lohman TG. Applicability of body composition techniques and constants for children and youths. Exerc Sport Sci Rev 1986; 14:325–357.

130. Deurenberg P, Leenen R, Van der Kooy K, Hautvast JGAJ. In obese subjects the body fat percentage calculated with Siri's formula is an overestimate. Eur J Clin Nutr 1989; 43:569–575.

131. Kooy KVD, Leenen R, Deurenberg P, Seidell JC, Westerterp KR, Hautvast JGAJ. Changes in fat-free mass in obese subjects after weight loss: a comparison of body composition measures. Int J Obes 1992; 16:675–683.

132. Behnke AR, Wilmore JH. Evaluation and Regulation of Body Build and Composition. Englewood Cliffs, NJ: Prentice-Hall, 1974.

133. Fidanza F, Keys A, Anderson JT. Density of body fat in man and other mammals. J Appl Physiol 1953; 6: 252–256.

134. Brozek J, Grande F, Anderson T, Keys A. Densitometric analysis of body composition: a revision of some assumptions. Ann NY Acad Sci 1963; 110:113–140.

135. Siri WE. Body composition from fluid spaces and density. In: Brozek J, Henschel A, eds. Techniques in the Measurement of Body Composition. Washington, DC: National Academy of Sciences, 1961:223–244.

136. Murgtroyd PR, Coward WA. An improved method for estimating changes in whole-body fat and protein mass in man. Br J Nutr 1989; 62:311–314.

137. Sawka MN, Weber H, Knowlton RG. The effect of total body submersion on residual lung volume and body density measurements in man. Ergonomics 1978; 21:89–94.

138. Friedl KE, DeLuca JP, Marchitelli LJ, Vogel JA. Reliability of body-fat estimations from a four-component model by using density, body water, and bone mineral measurements. Am J Clin Nutr 1992; 55:764–770.

139. Fuller NJ, Jebb SA, Laskey MA, Coward WA. Four compartment model for the assessment of body composition in humans; comparison with alternative methods, and evaluation of the density and hydration of the fat-free mass. Clin Sci 1992; 82:687–693.

140. Heymsfield SB, Waki M. Body composition in humans: advances in the development of multicompartment chemical models. Nutr Rev 1991; 49:97–108.

141. Heymsfield SB, Waki M, Kehayias J, et al. Chemical and elemental analysis of humans in vivo using improved

body composition models. Am J Physiol (Endocrine Metab) 1991; 261:E190–198.

142. Selinger A. The body as a three component system. Unpublished doctoral dissertation, University of Illinois, Urbana, 1977.

143. Mazess RB, Chestnut CH, McClung M, Genant H. Enhanced precision with dual-energy X-ray absorptiometry. Calcif Tissue Int 1992; 51;14–17.

144. Peppler WW, Mazess RB. Total body mineral and lean body mass by dual-photon absorptiometry. Calcif Tissue Int 1981; 33:353–359.

145. Gotfredsen A, Jensen J, Borg J, Christiansen C. Measurement of lean body mass and total body fat using dual photon absorptiometry. Metabolism 1986; 35:88–93.

146. Goodsitt MM. Evaluation of a new set of calibration standards for the measurement of fat content via DPA and DXA. Med Phys 1992; 19:35–44.

147. Wellens R, Chumlea WC, Guo S, Roche AF, Neo NV, Siervogel RM. Body composition in white adults by dual-energy X-ray absorptiometry, densitometry, and total body water. Am J Clin Nutr 1994; 59:547–555.

148. Van Loan MD, Keim NL, Berg K, Mayclin PL. Evaluation of body composition by dual energy X-ray absorptiometry and two different software packages. Med Sci Sport Exerc 1995; 27:587–591.

149. Kohrt W. Body composition by DXA: tried and true? Med Sci Sports Exerc 1995; 27:1349–1353.

150. Brunton JA, Bayley HS, Atkinson SA. Validation and application of dual-energy X-ray absorptiometry to measure bone mass and body composition in small infants. Am J Clin Nutr 1993; 58:839–845.

151. Ellis KJ, Shypailo RJ, Pratt JA, Pond WG. Accuracy of dual energy X-ray absorptiometry for body-composition measurements in children. Am J Clin Nutr 1994; 60:660–665.

152. Svendsen OL, Haarbo J, Hassager C, Christiansen C. Accuracy of measurements of body composition by dual-energy X-ray absorptiometry. J Appl Physiol 1993; 74:770–775.

153. Heymsfield SB, Wang J, Heshka S, Kehayias JJ, Pierson RN. Dual-photon absorptiometry: comparison of bone mineral and soft tissue mass measurements in vivo with established methods. Am J Clin Nutr 1989; 49:1283–1289.

154. Laskey MA, Lyttle KD, Flaxman ME, Barber RW. The influence of tissue depth and composition on the performance of the Lunar dual-energy X-ray absorptiometer whole-body scanning mode. Eur J Clin Nutr 1992; 46:39–45.

155. Snead DB, Birge SJ, Kohrt WM. Age-related differences in body composition by hydrodensitometry and dual-energy X-ray absorptiometry. J Appl Physiol 1993; 74:770–775.

156. Going SB, Massett MP, Hall MC, Bare LA, Root PA, Williams DP, Lohman TG. Detection of small changes in body composition by dual-energy X-ray absorptiometry. Am J Clin Nutr 1993; 57:845–850.

157. Clark RR, Kuta JM, Sullivan JC. Prediction of percent body fat in adult males using dual energy X-ray absorptiometry, skinfolds, and hydrostatic weighing. Med Sci Sport Exerc 1993; 528–535.

158. Van Loan MD Mayclin PL. Body composition assessment: dual-energy X-ray absorptiometry (DEXA) compared to reference methods. Eur J Clin Nutr 1992; 46:125–130.

159. Pritchard JE, Nowson CA, Strauss BJ, Carlson JS, Kaymakci B, Wark JD. Evaluation of dual energy X-ray absorptiometry as a method of measurement of body fat. Eur J Clin Nutr 1993; 47:216–228.

160. Hansen N, Lohman TG, Going SB, Hall MC, Pamenter RW, Bare LA, Boyden TW, Houtkooper LB. Prediction of body composition in premenopausal females from dual-energy X-ray absorptiometry. J Appl Physiol 1993; 75:1637–1641.

161. Tatarrani PA, Ravussin E. Use of dual-energy X-ray absorptiometry in obese individuals. Am J Clin Nutr 1995; 62:730–734.

162. Kyere K, Oldroyd B, Oxby CB, Burkinshaw L, Ellis RE, Hill GL. The feasibility of measuring total body carbon by counting neutron inelastic scatter gamma rays. Phys Med Biol 1982; 27:805–817.

163. Kehayias JJ, Heymsfield SB, LoMonte AF, Wang J, Pierson RN Jr. In vivo determination of body fat by measuring total body carbon. Am J Clin Nutr 1991; 53:1339–1344.

164. Dilmanian FA, Weber DA, Yasumura S, et al. The performance of the BNL delayed-gamma neutron activation system. In: Yasumura S, Harrison JE, McNeill KG, et al, eds. Advances in In Vivo Body Composition Studies. New York: Plenum Press, 1990:309–315.

165. Ryde SJS, Birks JL, Morgan WD, et al. A five-compartment model of body composition of healthy subjects assessed using in vivo neutron activation analysis. Eur J Clin Nutr 1993; 47:863–874.

166. Heymsfield SB, Waki M, Kehayias J, Lichtman S, Dilmanian FA, Kamen Y, Wang J, Pierson RN Jr. Chemical and elemental analysis of human in vivo using improved body composition models. Am J Physiol 1991; 261:E190–198.

167. Forbes GB. Human Body Composition; Growth, Aging, and Activity. New York: Springer-Verlag, 1987.

168. Lukaski HC, Mendez J, Buskirk ER, Cohn SH. A comparison of methods of assessment of body composition including neutron activation analysis of total body nitrogen. Metabolism 1981; 30:777–782.

169. Pierson RN, Lin DHY, Phillips RA. Total-body potassium in health: Effects of age, sex, height, and fat. Am J Physiol 1974; 226:206–212.

170. Forbes RM, Mitchell HH, Cooper AR. Further studies on the gross composition and mineral elements of the adult human body. J Biol Chem 1956; 223:969–975.

171. Pierson RN, Wang J, Thornton JC, Van Itallie TB, Colt EWD. Body potassium by four-pi ^{40}K counting: an anthropometric correction. Am J Physiol 1984; F234–F239.

172. Cohn SH, Vaswani AN, Yasumura S. Improved model for determination of body fat by in vivo neutron activation. Am J Clin Nutr 1984; 40:255–259.

173. Kehayias JJ, Ellis KJ, Cohn SH, et al. Use of a pulsed neutron generator for in vivo measurement of body carbon. In: Ellis KJ, Yasumura S, Morgan WD, eds. In Vivo Body Composition Studies. London: Institute of Physical Sciences in Medicine, 1987:427–435.

174. Cunningham J. N × 6.25: recognizing a bivariate expression for protein balance in hospitalized patients. Nutrition 1994; 10:124–127.

175. Knight GS, Beddoe AH, Streat SJ, Hill GL. Body composition of two human cadavers by neutron activation and chemical analysis. Am J Physiol 1986; 250:E179–185.

176. Biltz RM, Pellegrino ED. The chemical anatomy of bone. J Bone Joint Surg 1969; 51A:456–466.

177. Vartsky D, Ellis KJ, Cohn SH. In vivo measurement of body nitrogen by analysis of prompt gammas from neutron capture. J Nucl Med 1979; 20:1158–1165.

178. Heymsfield SB, Olafson RP, Kutner MH, Nixon DW. A radiographic method of quantifying protein-calorie undernutrition. Am J Clin Nutr 1979; 32:693–702.

179. Heymsfield SB, Fulenwider T, Nordlinger B, Balow R, Sones P, Kutner M. Accurate measurement of liver, kidney, and spleen volume and mass by computerized axial tomography. Ann Intern Med 1979; 90:185–187.

180. Borkan GA, Gerzof SG, Robbins AH, et al. Assessment of abdominal fat content by computerized tomography. Am J Clin Nutr 1982; 36:172–177.

181. Sjostrom L, Kvist H, Cederblad A, Tylen U. Determination of total adipose tissue and body fat in women by computed tomography, ^{40}K, and tritium. Am J Physiol 1986; 250:E736–E745.

182. Sprawls P. The Physical Principles of Diagnostic Radiology. Baltimore: University Park Press, 1977:101–117.

183. Wang ZM, Heshka S, Heymsfield SB. Application of computerized axial tomography in the study of body composition: evaluation of lipid, water, protein, and mineral in healthy men. In: Ellis KJ, Eastman JD, eds. In: Human Body Composition: In Vivo Methods, Models, and Assessment. New York: Plenum Press, 1993:3–4.

184. Heymsfield SB, Noel R, Lynn M, Kutner M. Accuracy of soft tissue ensity predicted by CT. J Comput Assist Tomogr 1979; 3:859–860.

185. Chowdhury B, Sjöström L, Alpsten M, Kostanty J, Kvist H, Löfgren R. multicompartment body composition technique based on computerized tomography. Int J Obes 1994; 18:219–234.

186. Heymsfield SB, Ross R. Imaging Techniques of Body Composition: Advantages of Measurement and New Uses. National Academy of Sciences Press (in press).

187. Kvist H, Sjöstrom L, Tylen U. Adipose tissue volume determination in women by computed tomography; technical considerations. Int J Obes 1986; 10:53–67.

188. Seidell JC, Bakker CJC, Van Der Kooy K. Imaging techniques for measuring adipose-tissue distribution—a comparison between computed tomography and 1.5-T magnetic resonance. Am J Clin Nutr 1990; 51:953–957.

189. Brummer RJM, Lonn L, Grangard UI, Bengtsson BA, Kvist H, Sjostrom L. Adipose tissue and muscle volume determinations by computed tomography in acromegaly, before and one year after adenectomy. Eur J Clin Nutr 1993; 23:199–205.

190. Rossner S, Bo WJ, Hiltbrandt E, Hinson W, Karstaedt N, Santago P, Sobol WT, Crouse JR. Adipose tissue determinations in cadavers—a comparison between cross-sectional planimetry and computed tomography. Int J Obes 1990; 14:893–902.

191. Wang ZM, Visser M, Ma R, Baumgartner RN, Kotler D, Gallagher D, Heymsfield SB. Skeletal muscle mass: evaluation of neutron activation and dual-energy x-ray absorptiometry methods. J Appl Physiol 1996; 80:824–831.

192. Foster MA, Hutchinson JMS, Mallard JR, Fuller M. Nuclear magnetic resonance pulse sequence and discrimination of high- and low-fat tissues. Mag Res Imaging 1984; 2:187–192.

193. Hayes PA, Sowood PJ, Belyavin A, Cohen JB, Smith FW. Sub-cutaneous fat thickness measured by magnetic resonance imaging, ultrasound, and calipers. Med Sci Sports Exerc 1993; 20(3):303–309.

194. De Ridder CM, De Boer RW, Seidell JC, Nieuwenhoff CM, Jeneson JAL, Bakker CJG, Zonderland ML, Erich WBM. Body fat distribution in pubertal girls quantified by magnetic resonance imaging. Int J Obes 1992; 16:443–449.

195. Staten MA, Totty WG, Kohrt WM. Measurement of fat distribution by magnetic resonance imaging. Invest Radiol 1989; 24:345–349.

196. Fowler PA, Fuller MF, Glasby CA, Foster MA, Cameron GG, McNiel G, Maughan RJ. Total and subcutaneous adipose tissue distribution in women: the measurement of distribution and accurate prediction of quantity by using magnetic resonance imaging. Am J Clin Nutr 1991; 54:18–25.

197. Ross R, Léger L, Morris DV, de Guise J, Guardo R. Quantification of adipose tissue by MRI: relationship with anthropometric variables. J Appl Physiol 1992; 72(2):787–795.

198. Sohlstöm A, Wahlund LO, Forsum E. Adipose tissue distribution and total body fat by magnetic resonance imaging, underwater weighing, and body-water dilution in healthy women. Am J Clin Nutr 1993; 58:830–838.

199. Ross R, Shaw KD, Rissanen J, Martel Y, De Guise J, Avruch L. Sex differences in lean and adipose tissue distribution by magnetic resonance imaging: anthropometric relationships. Am J Clin Nutr 1994; 59:1277–1285.

200. Gray D, Fujioka K, Colletti PM, Kim H, Devine W, Cuyegkeng T, Pappas T. Magnetic-resonance imaging used for determining fat distribution in obesity and diabetes. Am J Clin Nutr 1991; 54:623–627.

201. Baumgartner, RN, RL Rhyne C, Troup S, Wayne, Garry PJ. Appendicular skeletal muscle areas assessed by mag-

netic resonance imaging in older persons. J Gerontol 1992; 47:M67–72.

202. Fowler PA, MF Fuller CA, Glasby MA, Foster GG, Cameron G, McNiel, Maughan RJ. Total and subcutaneous AT distribution in women: the measurement of distribution and accurate prediction of quantity by using magnetic resonance imaging. Am J Clin Nutr 1991; 54:18–25.

203. Ross R, Rissanen J. Mobilization of visceral and subcutaneous adipose tissue in response to caloric restriction and exercise. Am J Clin Nutr 1994; 60:695–703.

204. Ross R, Pedwell H, Rissamen J. Effects of energy restriction and exercise on skeletal muscle and adipose tissue in women as measured by magnetic resonance imaging. Am J Clin Nutr 1995; 61:1179–1185.

205. Sohlström A, Wahlund LO, Forsum E. Adipose tissue distribution as assessed by magnetic resonance imaging and total body fat by magnetic resonance imaging, underwater weighing, and body-water dilution in healthy women. Am J Clin Nutr 1993; 58:830–838.

206. Seidell JC, Bakker CJC, Van Der Kooy K. Imaging techniques for measuring adipose-tissue distribution–a comparison between computed tomography and 1.5-T magnetic resonance. Am J Clin Nutr 1990; 51:953–957.

207. Fowler PA, Fuller MF, Glasbey CA, Cameron GG, Foster MA. Validation of the in-vivo measurement of adipose tissue by magnetic resonance imaging of lean and obese pigs. Am J Clin Nutr 1992; 56:7–13.

208. Abate N, Burns D, Peshock RM, Garg A, Grundy SM. Estimation of adipose tissue means by magnetic resonance imaging: validation against dissection in human cadavers. J Lipid Res 1994; 35:1490–1496.

209. Ross R, Léger L, Guardo R, De Guise J, Pike BG. Adipose tissue volume measured by magnetic resonance imaging and computerized tomography in rats. J Appl Physiol 1991; 70(5):2164–2172.

210. Gerard EL, Snow RC, Kennedy DN, et al. Overall body fat and regional fat distribution in young women: Quantification with MR imaging. American Journal of Radiology, 1991; 157:97–104.

211. Ross R. Magnetic resonance imaging provides new insights into the characterization of adipose and lean tissue distribution. Can J Physiol Pharmacol. 1996; 74: 778–785.

212. Engstrom CM, Loeb GE, Reid JR, Forrest WJ, Avruch L. Morphometry of the human thigh muscles. A comparison between anatomical sections and computer tomographic and magnetic resonance images. J Anat 1991; 176: 139–156.

213. Ashwell M, Cole TJ, Dixon AK. Obesity: new insight into the anthropometric classification of fat distribution shown by computed tomography. Br Med J 1985; 290: 1692–1694.

214. Baumgartner RN, Heymsfield SB, Roche AF, Bernardino M. Abdominal composition by computed tomography. Am J Clin Nutr 1988; 48:936–945.

215. Kvist H, Sjöstrom L, Tylen U. Adipose tissue volume determinations in women by computed tomography: technical considerations. Int J Obes 1986; 10:53–67.

216. Sjöström L. A computer-tomography based multicomponent body composition technique and anthropometric predictions of lean body mass, total and subcutaneous adipose tissue. Int J Obes 1991; 15:19–30.

4

Time Trends in the Worldwide Prevalence of Obesity

Jacob C. Seidell
National Institute of Public Health and the Environment, Bilthoven, The Netherlands

Áila M. Rissanen
Helsinki University, Helsinki, Finland

I. INTRODUCTION

The World Health Organization has recently proposed a classification based on three degrees of overweight expressed in terms of the body mass index (BMI) (kg/m^2) (1)

Normal range: BMI 18.50–24.99 kg/m^2
Grade I overweight: BMI 25.00–29.99 kg/m^2
Grade II overweight: BMI 30.00–39.99 kg/m^2
Grade III overweight: BMI $\geq$ 40.00 kg/m^2

These cutoff points for classification of overweight are identical to those proposed by Bray (2) as "functional classification based on the degree of risk estimates from BMI" and agree with most definitions of obesity around the world. A notable exception is the United States where obesity is defined on the bases of the distribution of the BMI in the NHANES I study: 27.8 kg/m^2 in men and 27.3 kg/m^2 in women. In some American definitions, cutoff points are dependent on age, implying that Americans are allowed to weigh more (and thus gain weight) when getting older. In addition, in some countries a single cutoff point of 27 kg/m^2 is used to define obesity. Needless to say, such differences in cutoff points have great impact on the estimates of the prevalence of obesity in a given population (2). For meaningful epidemiological comparisons between populations it is necessary to apply a single cutoff point. In the majority of studies reviewed in this chapter,

the prevalence of obesity was based on the cutoff point of 30 kg/m^2 (corresponding with grade II overweight as defined by the WHO). The prevalence of grade overweight is usually very high, with the majority of adult populations having BMIs exceeding 25 kg/m^2.

Because surveys based on self-reported height and weight may give biased estimates of the obesity prevalence, they are excluded from the data presented in this chapter. There are limitations to the use of BMI in ascertaining the degree of obesity in adult populations, and health risks are known to be particularly related to increased abdominal fat. A chapter on worldwide prevalence of obesity should ideally contain comparisons and time trends in abdominal fat distribution. Unfortunately, there is limited material on indicators of fat distribution, such a body circumferences, that have applied similar and standardized methodology.

II. PREVALENCE OF OBESITY IN EUROPE

Obesity, defined as a BMI greater than 30 kg/m^2, is a common condition in Europe (3). To make a comparison possible between countries, it is necessary to compare population-based data on measured height and weight in which identical protocols for measurement were applied and which were collected in the same period. The most comprehensive data on the prevalence of obesity in Europe are from the WHO MONICA study (4). The majority of these data were collected between 1983 and 1986. The populations are not necessarily representative of the countries in which they are located.

Table 1 shows the age-standardized prevalence of obesity in 38 European centers participating in this study (5). Only in three centers was the prevalence slightly lower than 10% [Gothenburg in Sweden (men and women);

Toulouse in France (men); Catalonia in Spain (men)] and, on the average, the prevalence of obesity was about 15% in men and 22% in women. Given the large within- and between-country estimates of the prevalence of obesity, it is difficult to derive an overall prevalence figure for Europe as a whole from these data. It is fairly safe to assume that such an overall prevalence figure would be in the range of 10–20% in men and 15–25% in women.

Table 1 Prevalence of Obesity (BMI $\geq$ 30 kg/m^2) in European WHO MONICA (first round) Populations

Area of Europe	Country	Center	Prevalence	
			Men	Women
Northern	Denmark	Glostrup	11	10
	Finland	Kuopio Province	18	19
	Finland	North Karelia	17	24
	Finland	Turku-Loima	19	17
	Iceland	Iceland	11	11
	Sweden	Gothenburg	7	9
	Sweden	Northern Sweden	11	14
Western	U.K.	Glasgow	11	16
	U.K.	Belfast	11	14
	Germany	Bremen	14	18
	Germany	Rhein-Neckar	13	12
	Germany	Augsburg	18	15
	Germany	Augsburg (rural)	20	22
	Belgium	Luxembourg Province	13	18
	Belgium	Ghent	11	15
	France	Lille	14	19
	France	Toulouse	9	11
	France	Strasbourg	22	23
	Switzerland	Ticino	20	15
	Switzerland	Vaud-Fribourg	13	13
Eastern	Russia	Novosibirsk	14	44
	Russia	Moscow	13	33
	Lithuania	Kaunas	22	45
	E. Germany	Halle County	18	27
	E. Germany	Karl-Marx-Stadt	14	19
	E. Germany	Cottbus County	17	23
	E. Germany	"Rest of DDR MONICA"	17	21
	Poland	Warsaw	18	26
	Poland	Tarnobrzeg Voivodship	13	32
	Czech Rep.	Czech Republic	21	32
	Romania	Bucharest	20	31
	Serbia	Novi Sad	17	29
Southern	Spain	Catalonia	9	24
	Italy	Area Brianza	11	15
	Italy	Friuli	16	19
	Mean ± SD		14.8 ± 3.9	22.0 ± 9.6

Source: Adapted from Ref. 5.

The study of explanations for the large diversity in prevalence data, on the other hand, could give important clues to the understanding of the origins of common obesity. Striking, for example, are the very high BMI in the women from Eastern European countries. Figure 1 illustrates that the variation in obesity is much larger in women than in men. It also shows that there is only a moderate association ($r = 0.39$, $p = 0.02$) of the prevalence between men and women. The distributions of the BMI values in men seem to be rather homogeneous throughout Europe despite large socioeconomic and cultural differences between the countries. In addition, it is clear that there are major differences in the mortality rates of cardiovascular disease, which, at least in men, cannot be explained by differences in BMI (6).

III. TRENDS IN OBESITY PREVALENCE IN EUROPE

Table 2 shows some of the available recent trend data on obesity in Europe. The prevalence has increased by about 10–40% in most countries in the past decade. It escalated in the United Kingdom where the prevalence doubled

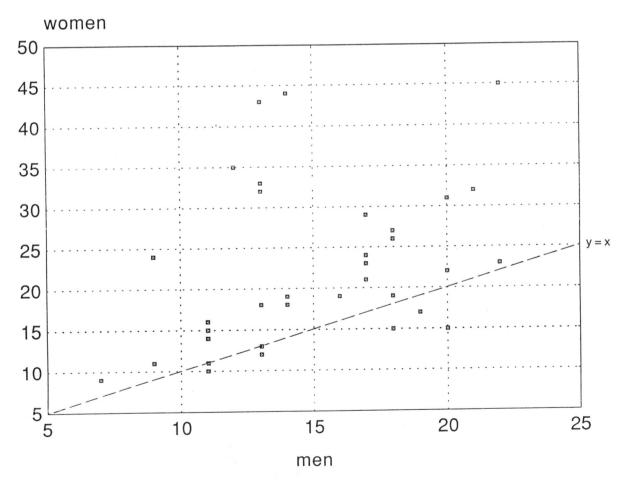

Figure 1 Plot of age-standardized prevalence of obesity (BMI $\geq$ 30 kg/m^2) in men and women participating in the WHO MONICA study. (Adapted from Ref. 5.)

Table 2 Trends in Obesity Prevalence in Some European Countries in the 1980s

Country (Ref.)	Obesity definition (BMI cutoff point)	Year	Ages (years)	Men (%)	Women (%)
England (7)	30 kg/m²	1980	16–64	6	8
		1986/7		7	12
		1991		13	15
Sweden (8,9)	Men: 30 kg/m² Women: 28.6 kg/m²	1980/1	16–84	4.9	8.7
		1988/9		5.3	9.1
Finland (10)	30 kg/m²	1978/9	20–75	10	10
		1985/7		12	10
		1991/3		14	11
Germany (11)	30 kg/m²	1985	25–69	15.1	16.5
		1988		14.7	17.2
		1990		17.2	19.3
East Germany (12)[a]	30 kg/m²	1985	25–65	13.7	22.2
		1989		13.4	20.6
		1992		20.5	26.8
West Germany (12)[a]	30 kg/m²	1986	25–65	14.7	15.2
		1988		13.7	15.0
		1991		16.0	21.4
Netherlands (13–15)	30 kg/m²	1987–1991	20–59	7	9
		1993	20–59	8	10
		1994	20–59	10	11

[a]Data supplied by Prof. Dr. L. Heineman, Zentrum für Epidemiologie und Gesundheitsforschung Berlin, Zepernick, Germany. Age-standardized to Segis: *World Population*. Data from East-Germany from MONICA surveys 1985 and 1989, 1992 data from Health Interview and Examination Survey. Information for West Germany is from the three population surveys in the context of the German Cardiovascular Prevention Study.

during this period. There is some evidence that this increasing trend is leveling off among women, at least in some Scandinavian countries (16,17).

In most countries an increasing prevalence was observed. Preliminary data from Denmark (16) showed that the obesity prevalence increased in men and decreased in women in the period 1960–1980. In a Finnish study based on data accumulated in three regions (17), a strong increase in the prevalence of obesity was noted in men in the period 1972–1992 (Fig. 2b) In women a decrease was observed in the 1970s followed by a leveling off or an increase, depending on the region (Fig. 2b). In The Netherlands, the prevalence remained lower than in Finland but a considerable increase was observed in both men and women over the period 1987–1994 (Fig. 3).

Subgroup analyses by sex, age, and educational level with regard to time trends yielded different results in different countries. In some studies the increase in the prevalence of obesity was most pronounced in young adults whereas in others it was more pronounced in older subjects. Usually, there was a stronger increase in the prevalence of obesity in those with relatively low educational levels compared to those with higher education. Figure 4a and 4b (18) illustrates with data from eastern Finland (18)

that changes in BMI may be different between levels of education. In men in 1972 there was no clear association between educational level and BMI whereas this association was clearly an inverse one by 1987. In women, the inverse association between educational level and BMI became more pronounced over time and decrease in average BMI was seen in women with the highest educational level while no change was observed in those with low education levels (Fig. 4a and 4b).

Although some people have attempted to explain the secular changes in the prevalence of obesity by changes in some life-style factors on a population basis (19,20) the causes of this increase are uncertain. Diminished physical activity, high-fat diets, and inadequate adjustments of energy intakes to the diminished energy requirements are likely to be major determinants of the observed changes. Prentice and Jebb (20) have proposed that, on a population level, limited physical activity may be more important than energy or fat consumption in explaining the time trends of obesity in the United Kingdom. Their analysis was based on aspects of physical activity (such as number of hours spent watching television) and household consumption survey data. Although such data may be indicative, such analyses may also be biased. Particularly, en-

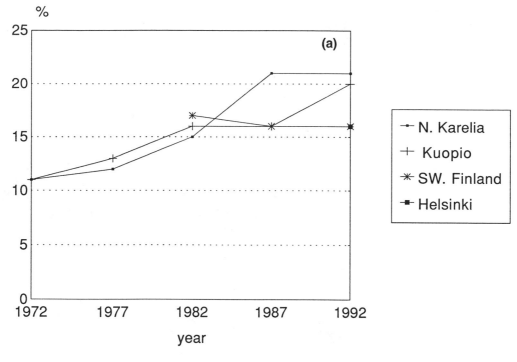

Men

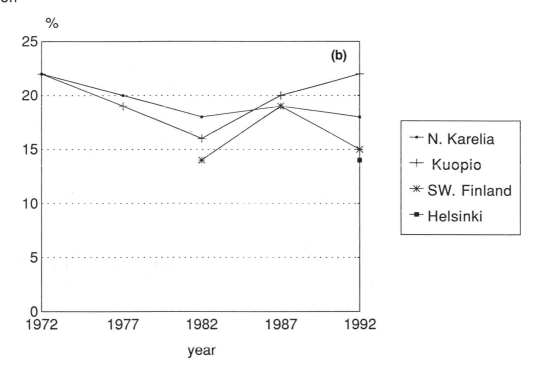

Women

Figure 2   Trends in obesity prevalence in different regions in Finland in men (a) and women (b). (Data adapted from Ref. 17.)

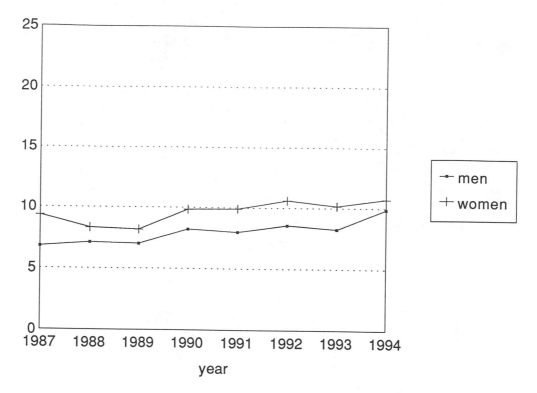

Figure 3   Trends in obesity prevalence in The Netherlands in men and women. (Adapted from Refs. 13–15.)

ergy and fat consumption are underreported with increasing degrees of overweight (21). Changes in smoking behavior may also contribute to changes in body weight on a population level. Data from the United States demonstrated that widespread smoking cessation could explain a quarter in men and a sixth in women of the increase in prevalence of overweight (22). In other studies, it was shown that the increase in the obesity prevalence may be independent of smoking status (19).

Epidemiological methods that can be used to assess energy intake and energy expenditure may be subject to bias but, in addition, they also have considerable ratio of within- to between-subject variation. Only small changes in energy balance are needed to increase average BMI by one unit. Depending on the distribution of BMI in the population, this may greatly increase the prevalence of obesity (see below). These small changes in energy balance may not be detectable by epidemiological measures of energy expenditure and intake.

A. Example

The prevalence of obesity in The Netherlands in 1994 was 6.1% in men aged 30–34 and 10.0% in men aged 35–39 (15). Average BMI increased from 24.9 to 25.3 kg/m². Let

us assume that this is the result of weight gain consisting of pure fat. With an average height of about 1.8 m, such a dramatic increase in BMI can be produced by a weight increase of 1.3 kg in 5 years, or about 0.7 g/day. It is clear that disturbances in energy balance in the range of 5–10 kcal/day cannot be picked up by any method. Thus, changes in BMI in a population are an extremely sensitive indicator of small and persistent changes in energy balance.

IV. OBESITY IN NON-EUROPEAN INDUSTRIALIZED COUNTRIES

Table 3 shows data from affluent countries outside Europe. The prevalence rates in adults in New Zealand, Australia, and Canada are all in the range of 10–15%. It is difficult to compare data from the United States with these data because, as mentioned earlier, U.S. studies present prevalence data based on different cutoff points for BMI (i.e., 27.8 kg/m² for men and 27.3 kg/m² for women). Based on these criteria, about a third or more of U.S. adults can be considered obese (23). Studies in minority populations in Australia (aboriginals) show either much higher or much lower prevalence compared to the white

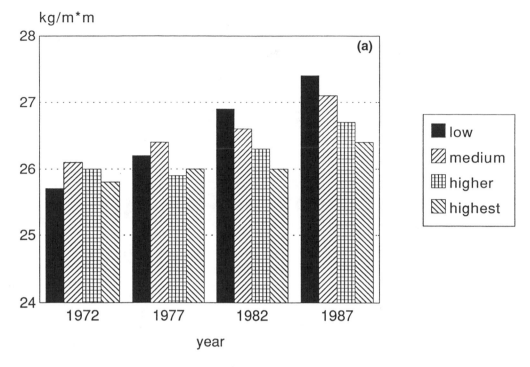

men

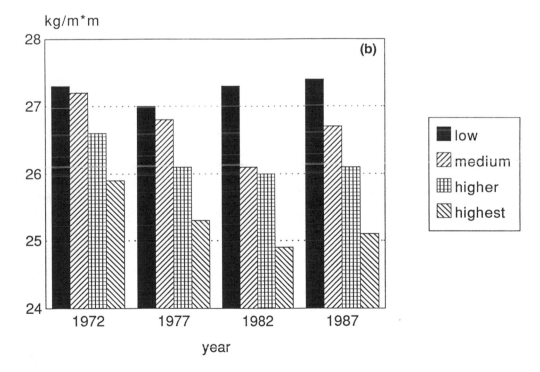

women

Figure 4 Trends in average body mass index in eastern Finland by educational level. Stratification of educational level (years of education) using birth-cohort-specific cutoff points (see Ref. 18 for more details). (Adapted from Ref. 18.)

Table 3 Prevalence of Obesity in Non-European Industrialized Countries

Country (Ref.)	Sample	BMI cutoff	Year	Ages (years)	Men (%)	Women (%)
USA (whites) (23)	Representative	27.8 (♂) 27.3 (♀)	1988/91	20–74	32.0	33.5
USA (blacks) (23)	Representative	27.8 (♂) 27.3 (♀)	1988/91	20–74	31.8	49.2
Canada (24)	Representative	30	1991	18–74	15	15
New Zealand (25)	Random Sample	30	1989	18–64	10	13
Australia (26)	Adults in capital cities	30	1990	20–69	9.3	11.1
Australia (5)	Newcastle Perth Auckland (NZ)	30	1986	35–65	15 9 8	16 11 9
Australia (26)	Melbourne Chinese	30	1989	25–69	0.8	2.3
Australia (27)	Southeastern Australia	30	1990?	25–64 Aboriginals Europids	24.6 17.4	38.0 17.8
Australia (28)	Vietnamese-born Southwestern Sidney	25	1991?	18+	15	13
Australia (29)	Nonaboriginal Australian Central Australian aboriginal West Kimberley aboriginal Yologu (Arnhem Land)	30	1980 1985 1986 1991		6 22 n.d. 2	9 51 17 4

population. Obesity seems to be very prevalent in aboriginal from southeastern and central Australia but very uncommon in northern Australia. This may reflect the degree of "westernization" of these aboriginals.

Among Chinese and Vietnamese immigrants, obesity is also rare but reportedly more common than in their countries of origin. Bennett made an extensive analysis of BMI in immigrants to Australia (30). Compared to people born in Australia, immigrants, particularly women, from southern Europe and the Middle East, as well as men from eastern Europe, had higher average BMIs. Men and women from Asia and the United Kingdom had low BMIs. In immigrants who lived longer than 16 years in Australia, differences in BMI compared to people born in Australia were usually much less pronounced. Table 4 shows that in most non-European industrialized countries the prevalence of obesity is increasing. The data from Australia show that, just as in Sweden, the increasing prevalence of obesity could not be explained by increased smoking cessation (31).

Table 5 shows that obesity is quite common in minority populations in the United States with very high prevalences in people living in Hawaii. Table 6 shows that obesity is also quite common in populations living on Pacific islands. Dramatic increases have also been shown in Mauritius, Western Samoa, and New Guinea (34,37,38).

V. OBESITY IN THE MIDDLE EAST

Table 7 shows that obesity is common among women from Arabic countries such as Saudi Arabia and Kuwait. Obesity is less common among parents of schoolchildren in southern Iran.

VI. OBESITY IN DEVELOPING COUNTRIES

Table 8 shows that when relatively low cutoff points (e.g., 25 or 27 kg/m^2) are used, obesity exists in countries such

Table 4 Trends in Obesity in Non-European Industrialized Countries

Country (Ref.)	Obesity definition (BMI cutoff point)	Year	Ages (years)	Men (%)	Women (%)	
Australia (smokers) (31)	All: 25 kg/m²	1980	25–64	44	18[a]	35[b]
		1983		46	25	36
		1986		50	34	52
Australia (ex-smokers) (31)	All: 25 kg/m²	1980	25–64	60	18[a]	40[b]
		1983		58	24	46
		1986		63	29	45
Australia (nonsmokers) (31)	All: 25 kg/m²	1980	25–64	48	22[a]	43[b]
		1983		45	26	47
		1986		49	29	52
Brazil (32)	All: 30 kg/m²	1975	25–64	3.1	8.2	
		1989		5.9	13.3	
Canada (33)	All: 27 kg/m²	1985	25–64	20	14	
		1991		30	20	
Mauritius (ethnic groups combined) (34)	All: 30 kg/m²	1987	25–74	3.4	5.3	
		1992		10.4	15.1	
USA (whites) (23)	Men: 27.8 kg/m² Women: 27.3 kg/m²	1962	20–74	23.0	23.6	
		1971/4		23.8	24.0	
		1976/80		24.2	24.4	
		1988/91		32.0	33.5	
USA (blacks) (23)	Men: 27.8 kg/m² Women: 27.3 kg/m²	1962	20–74	22.1	41.6	
		1971/4		23.9	43.1	
		1976/80		26.2	44.5	
		1988/91		31.8	49.2	

[a]Women younger than 50 years.
[b]Women older than 50 years.

as China and India. Obesity is more common in urban than in rural areas. Figure 5 shows that the relationship between obesity and income may be inverse in urban areas (just as in other industrialized countries) but positive in rural areas in China.

Popkin et al. showed that obesity in China (BMI $\geq$ 27 kg/m²) increased from 1.7% to 2.9% in men and remained 4.3% in women in the short period from 1989 to 1991 (48). The increase was particularly pronounced in men with a relatively high income (from 1.5% in 1989 to 3.8% in 1991). At the same time, however, there were increases in the prevalence of undernutrition (BMI < 18.5 kg/m²). Also, in Brazil there were profound changes in the relationship between income and female obesity in the period 1974–1989 (32). The increase in the prevalence of obesity occurred in all income groups but was relatively largest in the poorest groups. In 1974 the women with the highest income were heaviest whereas in 1989 the

women with the middle income were heaviest. There were strong positive correlations between family income in the poorest and middle-income families but no relationship in the richest families (32).

Data from Africa are fragmentary at best and suggest that obesity is relatively uncommon but more prevalent in urban areas than in rural areas. A study in urban Zulus with low socioeconomic status (49) showed that 3.7% of the men and 22.6% of the women could be considered to be obese (no definition of obesity was given, however).

VII. CONCLUSIONS

In this overview we used BMI $\geq$ 30 kg/m² as a cutoff point for defining obesity, as proposed by the WHO. It can be generally safely assumed that individuals with BMIs of 30 kg/m² or higher have an excess fat mass in their

Table 5 Obesity in Minority Populations in the United States

Population description	Men (%)	Women (%)
Non-Hispanic white	24	24
Non-Hispanic black	26	44
Mexican American	31	42
Puerto Rican	26	40
Cuban American	28	32
American Indian, Alaska	34	40
Native Hawaiian	66	63
Western Samoan	33	48
Hawaii Samoan	75	80
San Antonio:		
Barrio Mexican American	49	65
Transitional Mexican American	52	54
Non-Hispanic white	40	36
Suburbs, Mexican American	45	34
Suburbs, non-Hispanic white	31	21

Obesity defined as BMI ≥ 27.8 kg/m^2 for men and 27.3 kg/m^2 for women.
Source: Adapted from Ref. 35.

Table 6 Prevalence of Obesity (BMI $\geq$ 30 kg/m^2) in Adults Aged 25–69 Years in Various Pacific and Indian Populations[a]

Population description	Year	Men (%)	Women (%)
Nauru (Micronesia)	1987	65	70
Western Samoa (Polynesia)	1991		
Urban		58	77
Rural		42	59
Papua New Guinea (Melanesia)	1991		
Urban coastal		36	54
Rural coastal		24	19
Highlands		5	5
Mauritius	1992		
Asian Indian		5	16
Creole		8	21
Chinese		2	6

[a]Only most recent figures (after 1987).
Source: Adapted from Ref. 36.

body. It has been repeatedly shown, however, that BMIs may not correspond to the same degree of fatness across populations. As an example, Swinburn et al. demonstrated fat percentages derived from biological impedance measurements were different at identical BMI and were lower in Polynesians compared to Caucasian Australians (50). For cross-sectional comparisons, BMI values should be in-terpreted with caution. For trend analyses, such issues are of no concern. In many countries around the world the prevalence of obesity seems to have been increasing during the last 10–20 years. As Stamler stated, "The emergence in the 20th century of obesity as a mass problem of ever-increasing proportions is an unprecedented phenomenon" (51). The increase in obesity may be partly responsible for the worldwide epidemic of (non-insulin-dependent) diabetes mellitus as described by the WHO (52). Only small changes in life-style (energy intakes, physical activity) may be responsible for (individually) relatively minor weight increases, thereby shifting the distribution of BMI in the population a little to the right. This

Table 7 Prevalence of Obesity (BMI $\geq$ 30 kg/m^2) in the Middle East

Country (Ref.)	Sample	Year	Ages (years)	Men (%)	Women (%)
Saudi Arabia (39)	Female medical students	1990	18–25	—	4.5
Saudi Arabia (39)	Women attending primary care clinic	?	18–35	—	20.2
Saudi Arabia (39)	Women attending King Fahd Clinic	?	15–25	—	11.4
Saudi Arabia (40)	Women attending clinic in Riyadh	1992	Adult	—	47
Kuwait (39)	Adult females	?		—	42
Kuwait (41)	Adults attending primary health care	1994	18+	32.3	43.8
Iran (42)	Parents of schoolchildren, southern Iran	1989	20–59	5	5

Table 8 Prevalence Data from Developing and Transitional Countries

Country (Ref.)	Sample	BMI cutoff	Year	Ages (years)	Men (%)	Women (%)
Asia						
India (43)	Rural Thiruvaran, Thapuram	27	1991	25–34	1.7	4.3
				35–4	4.2	9.8
				45–54	4.3	13.3
				55–64	?	11.1
				65+	4.9	2.5
India (44)	Residents of Bombay middle class	30	1991	15–30	0.3	3.1
				31–50	6.5	9.6
				50+	8.1	9.8
China (5)	Beijing	30	1986	35–65	3	9
China (45)	Chinese HANES	27	1991	20–45	2.9	4.3
				rural	1.9	3.8
				urban	5.2	5.6
China (46)	Yi farmers (rural)	25	1989		1.8	5.4
	Yik immigrants (urban)				7.7	11.8
	Han chinese (urban)				6.5	10.5
Africa						
Tunisia (47)	Suburban adult Tunisian's Sahel	30	1991	20+	12	26
Congo (♀)	Cited by WHO	30	1986/7		3.4	
Ghana			1987/8		0.9	
Mali			1991		0.8	
Morocco			1984/5		5.2	
Tunisia (1)			1990		8.6	
South America						
Brazil	Cited by WHO	30	1989	adults	8.9	
Cuba			1982	adults	9.5	
Peru (1)			1975/6		9.0	

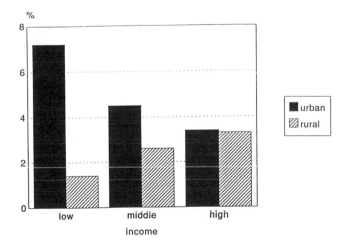

Figure 5 Obesity (body mass index ≥ 27 kg/m²) in China (Chinese health and nutrition examination survey in 1989) by urbanization and income. (Adapted from Ref. 45.)

may have important consequences for the percentage of obese individuals in a population. It is unlikely that such changes in life-style can be readily identified. These data also imply that only small increases in physical activity or reductions in energy intake may be sufficient to decrease the prevalence of obesity in the coming decades. Reducing the prevalence of obesity in society cannot be solved by putting all obese subjects on a slimming diet. Prevention of obesity in individuals not yet overweight may also have an important contribution in reducing the prevalence of obesity (53).

REFERENCES

1. WHO Expert Committee. Physical Status: The Use and Interpretation of Anthropometry. WHO Technical Report Series no. 854. Geneva: WHO, 1995.

2. Bray GA, Etiology and prevalence of obesity. In: Bouchard C, ed. Boca Raton, FL: CRC Press, 1994:17–33. Genetics of Obesity.

3. Seidell JC. Obesity in Europe–scaling an epidemic. Int J Obes 1995 19(Suppl 3):S1–S4.

4. WHO MONICA Project: risk factors. Int J Epidemiol 1989; 18(Suppl 1):S46–S55.

5. Molarius A, Seidell JC, Kuulasmaa K, Dobson A, Sans S. Smoking and body weight: WHO MONICA Project J Epidemiol Comm Health 1996 (in press).

6. Seidell JC. Obesity in Europe–some epidemiological observations. In: Ailhaud G, et al, eds. Obesity in Europe 91. John Libbey, London, UK 1992:109–112.

7. Department of Health. The Health of the Nation: One Year On . . . A Report on the Progress of the Health of the Nation, Department of Health, 1993.

8. Kuskowska-Wolk A, Bergström R. Trends in body mass index and prevalence of obesity in Swedish women 1980–89. J Epidemiol Commun Health 1993; 47:195–199.

9. Kuskowska-Wolk A, Bergström R. Trends in body mass index and prevalence of obesity in Swedish men 1980–89. J Epidemiol Commun Health 1993; 47:103–108.

10. Berg AM, Rissanen A. Secular trends in obesity in the Finnish population (unpublished manuscript).

11. Hoffmeister H, Mensink GBM, Stolzenberg H. National Trends in risk factors for cardiovascular disease in Germany. Prev Med 1994; 23:197–205.

12. Heineman L, Barth W, Hoffmeister H. Trend of cardiovascular risk factors in the east German population 1968–1992. J Clin Epidemiol 1995; 48:787–795.

13. Seidell JC, Verschuren WMM, Kromhout D. Levels and trends of obesity in The Netherlands 1987–1991. Int J Obes 1995; 19:924–927.

14. Smit HA, Verschuren WMM, Bueno de Mesquita HB, Seidell JC. Monitoring of Risk Factors and Health in The Netherlands (MORGEN-project). RIVM report no 263200002, 1994.

15. Seidell JC, Blokstra, Smit HA, Verschuren WMM, Janssen A, Bueno de Mesquita HB. Monitoring of Risk Factors and Health in The Netherlands (MORGEN-project). RIVM report no 263200003, 1995.

16. Mikkelsen KL, Heitmann BL, Sörensen TIA. Secular changes in mean body mass index and its prevalence of obesity—three Danish population studies of 31,000 subjects. Int J Obes 1995; 19(Suppl 2):30 (abstract).

17. Pietinen P, Vartiainen E, Männisto S. Trends in body mass index and obesity among adults in Finland from 1972 to 1992. Int J Obes 1996; 20:114–120.

18. Pekkanen J, UUtela A, Valkonen T, Vartiainen E, Toumilehto J, Puska P. Coronary risk factor levels: differences between educational groups in 1972–87 in eastern Finland. J Epidemiol Commun Health 1995; 49:144–149.

19. Wolk A, Rössner S. Effects of smoking and physical activity on body weight: developments in Sweden between 1980 and 1989. J Intern Med 1995; 237:287–291.

20. Prentice AM, Jebb SA. Obesity in Britain: gluttony or sloth? Br Med J 1995; 311:437–439.

21. Heitmann BL, Lissner L. Dietary underreporting by obese individuals—is it specific or non-specific? Br Med J 1995; 311:986–989.

22. Flegal KM, Troiano RP, Pamuk ER, Kuczmarski RJ, Campbell SM. The influence of smoking cessation on the prevalence of overweight in the United States. N Engl J Med 1995; 333:1165–1170.

23. Kuczmarski RJ, Flegal KM, Campbell SM, Johnson CL. Increasing prevalence of overweight among US adults. The National Health and Nutrition Examination Surveys 1960 to 1991. JAMA 1994; 272:205–211.

24. Reeder BA, Angal A, Ledoux M, et al. Obesity and its relation to cardiovascular risk factors in Canadian adults. Can Med Assoc J 1992; 146:2009–2019.

25. Ball MJ, Wilson BD, Robertson IK, Russel DG. Obesity and fat distribution in New Zealanders: a pattern of coronary heart disease risk. NZ Med J 1993; 106:69–72.

26. Hsu-Hage BH-H, Wahlqvist ML. Cardiovascular risk in adult Melbourne Chinese. Aust J Public Health 1993; 17: 306–313.

27. Guest CS, O'Dea K, Hopper JL, Larkins RG. Hyperinsulinemia and obesity in aborigines of south-eastern Australia, with comparisons from rural and urban Europid populations. Diab Res Clin Pract 1993; 20:155–164.

28. Rissel C, Russel C. Heart disease risk factors in the Vietnamese community of southwestern Sydney. Aust J Public Health 1993; 17:71–73.

29. Jones COH, White NG. Adiposity in aboriginal people from Arnhem Land, Australia, variation in degree and distribution associated with age, sex, and lifestyle. Ann Hum Biol 1994; 21:207–227.

30. Bennett SA. Inequalities in risk factors and cardiovascular mortality among Australia's immigrants. Aust J Public Health 993; 17:251–261.

31. Boyle CA, Dobson AJ, Egger C, Magnus P. Can the increasing weight of Australians be explained by the decreasing prevalence of cigarette smoking? Int J Obes 1994; 18: 55–60.

32. Moreiro CA, Mondini L, Medeiros de Souza AL, Popkin BM. The nutrition transition in Brazil. Eur J Clin Nutr 1995; 49:105–113.

33. Millar WJ, Stephens I. Social status and health risks in Canadian adults: 1985 and 1991. Health Rep 1993; 5: 143–156.

34. Hodge AM, Dowse GK, Gareeboo H, Tuomilehto J, Alberti KGMM, Zimmet PZ. Incidence, increasing prevalence, and predictors of change in obesity and fat distribution over 5 years in the rapidly developing population of Mauritius. Int J Obes 1996; 20:137–146.

35. Kumanyika SK. Obesity in minority populations: an epidemiological assessment. Obes Res 1994; 2:166–182.

36. Hodge AM, Zimmet PZ. The epidemiology of obesity. Ballieres Clin Endocrinol Metab 1994; 8:577–599.

37. Hodge AM, Dowse GK, Toelupe P, Collins VR, Imo T, Zimmet PZ. Dramatic increase in the prevalence of obesity in Western Samoa over the 13 year period 1978–1991. Int J Obes 1994; 18:419–428.

38. Hodge AM, Dowse GK, Koki G, Mavo B, Alpers MP, Zimmet PZ. Modernity and obesity in coastal and highland papua New Guinea. Int J Obes 1995; 19:154–161.

39. Rasheed P, Abou-Hozaifa BM, Khan A. Obesity among young Saudi female adults: a prevalence study on medical and nursing students. Public Health 1994; 108:289–294.

40. Al-Shammari SA, Khoja TA, Al-Maatouq MA, Al-Nuaim LA. High prevalence of clinical obesity among Saudi females: a prospective, cross-sectional study in the Riyadh region. J Trop Med Hyg 1994; 97:183–188.

41. Naser Al-Isa A. Prevalence of obesity among adult Kuwaitis: a cross-sectional study. Int J Obes 195; 19:431–433.

42. Ayatollah SMT, Carpenter RG. Height, weight, BMI and weight-for-height of adults in southern Iran: how should obesity be defined? Ann Hum Biol 1993; 20:13–19.

43. Kutty VR, Balakrishan KG, Jayasree AK, Thomas J. Prevalence of coronary heart disease in the rural population of Thiruvananthapuram district Kerala, India. Int J Cardiol 1993; 39:59–70.

44. Dhurandar NV, Kulkarni PR. Prevalence of obesity in Bombay. Int J Obes 1992; 16:367–375.

45. Popkin BM, Keyou G, Fengying Z, Guo X, Haijiang M, Zohoori N. The nutrition transition in China: a cross-sectional analysis. Eur J Clin Nutr 1993; 47:333–346.

46. He J, Klag MJ, Whelton PK, Cheng J-Y, Qian M-C, He G-Q. Body mass index and blood pressure in a lean population in Southwestern China. Am J Epidemiol 1994; 139: 380–389.

47. Ghannem H, Maarouf R, Tabka A, Haj Frej A, Marzouki M. La triade obesite, hypertension et troubles de la glycoregulation dans une population semi-urbaine du Sahel Tunesien. Diab Metab 1993; 19:310–314.

48. Popkin BM, Paeratakul S, Ge K, Fengying Z. Body weight patterns among the Chinese: results from the 1989 and 1991 China Health and Nutrition Surveys. Am J Public Health 1995; 85:690–694.

49. Seedat YK, Mayet FGH, Ltaiff GH, Joubert G. Study of risk factors leading to coronary heart disease in Zulus. J Hum Hypertens 1993; 7:529–532.

50. Swinburn B, Craig P, Strauss B, Daniel R. Body mass index: is it an appropriate measure of obesity in Polynesians? Int J Obes 1995; 19:213 (abstract).

51. Stamler J. Epidemic obesity in the United States. Arch Intern Med 1993; 153:1040–1044.

52. King H, Rewers M. Diabetes in adults is now a third world problem. Bull WHO 1991; 69:643–648.

53. Russel CM, Williamson DF, Byers T. Can the year 2000 objective for reducing overweight in the United States be reached? A simulation study of the required changes in body weight. Int J Obesity 1995; 19:149–53.

5

Prevalence of Obesity in Children

William H. Dietz
Tufts University School of Medicine and Boston Floating Hospital, Boston, Massachusetts

I. INTRODUCTION

Childhood obesity is among the most prevalent nutritional problems that affect children in developed countries. In this chapter, we will review the identification, prevalence, environmental associations, and consequences of childhood obesity. The data reviewed support the assertion that the effective prevention and treatment of childhood obesity will have a major impact on the prevalence of adult obesity and its complications.

II. IDENTIFICATION

The diagnosis of obesity connotes a state of ill health. However, in children, pathological consequences of obesity are rare. Psychosocial dysfunction is one of the most prevalent consequences. Therefore, one definition of obesity in childhood could be based on the appearance of excess adiposity. However, the appearance of obesity is a highly subjective judgment that varies by ethnicity. For example, among African-Americans, women rank ideal body weight at levels that are significantly higher than the levels provided by Caucasian women (1). As expected, the concern about excess adiposity also varies by ethnic group. Those groups that rank excess adiposity at lower body weights tend to have an increased anxiety about excessive body fat and a higher frequency of eating disorders.

The ideal measure of body fatness should be a measure that correlates well with body fat, can be measured easily, and has a reasonable predictive value for morbidity and mortality. Specificity in the diagnosis of childhood obesity is probably of greater importance than sensitivity (2), because of the great concern associated with the diagnosis, and the high prevalence of eating disorders among subsets of the pediatric population, such as adolescent girls. Therefore, a cutoff that minimizes false positives will be more appropriate, even if it does not detect all children who are obese.

In children, pediatricians commonly use weight for height to determine whether the child's body weight is appropriate for height. Among children and adolescents 6–18 years of age, the correlation coefficient of weight for height with percentage body weight as fat compared favorably with the correlation coefficients for both the body mass index (BMI) and triceps skinfold (3), suggesting that any of the measures provided a reasonable assessment of body fat. Both the triceps skinfold thickness and BMI greater than the 85th percentiles for age and gender appear to have comparable low sensitivities and high specificities (2). Triceps skinfold thickness and the weight and height measurements necessary for the calculation of body mass index are easily measured. However, measurement of the triceps skinfold thickness requires calipers that are not generally available in pediatricians' offices. Reliable measurements of the triceps skinfold thickness requires practice, and between-observer measurements are not as reproducible as measurements of height and weight. Furthermore, although the triceps skinfold thickness provides a direct measurement of body fat, the measurement may be a less reliable measure as body fatness increases. Therefore, relative weight or BMI may represent more useful and reliable measurements for comparisons between surveys.

The low prevalence of aftereffects other than psychosocial difficulties in children and adolescents makes it difficult to establish a definition of obesity based on pathological consequences or physiological alterations. Among the consequences of greatest concern is the persistence of obesity into adulthood. In this context, use of weight for height (4) or BMI (5) appears equally well suited to estimate the risks of persistent obesity or long-term sequelae.

These observations led us to suggest (6) that the 95th percentile of the body mass index be used to screen adolescents for obesity. If an adolescent's BMI exceeds the 95th percentile for adolescents of the same age and gender, the diagnosis of excess adipose tissue should be confirmed by measurement of the triceps skinfold thickness, and the adolescent should be screened for the presence of additional risk factors, including family history, blood pressure, cholesterol, and concern about weight (Fig. 1). This approach has not yet been considered for pediatric populations other than adolescents.

III. CHANGES IN ADIPOSITY WITH AGE

Adiposity changes dramatically in childhood and adolescence. In an early and substantial series of studies of body composition of children and adolescents, Cheek described the changes in body fat, determined from the measurement of body composition with deuterium oxide (7). Cheek's estimates were not corrected for either the exchange of deuterium with body hydrogen or the change in the hydration factor with age (8). Because the lack of correction for the equilibrium of deuterium with body hydrogen will underestimate total body fat, and lack of correction of the hydration factor with age will underestimate body fat, these errors will tend to cancel. Based on Cheek's data, body fat as a percentage of body weight in males increases in the prepubertal phase of growth and declines coincident with the growth spurt. In contrast, fat as a percentage of body weight in girls remains relatively constant prior to adolescence, but increases during the adolescent growth spurt. Between the ages of 10 and 15 years in boys and girls, Cheek estimated that body fat as a percentage of body weight declines from 17.8% to 11.2% in boys, but rises from 16.6% to 23.5% in girls. Similar changes were subsequently described by other investigators (9).

Studies of adipocyte size and number in infancy and childhood demonstrate substantial age-dependent variations in their contribution to body fat mass (10,11). Cross-sectional and longitudinal studies of adipocyte numbers indicate that adipocyte numbers increase modestly throughout infancy and childhood, but that a pronounced and significant increase occurs after age 10. Obese children have increased numbers of adipocytes, regardless of the age at which they are studied.

Fat cell size increases to adult levels in late infancy and then decreases back to the level observed in early infancy (10). Thereafter, fat cell size remains constant until early adolescence. Among obese children, increases in fat cell size to adult levels occur coincident with the development of obesity, and do not increase further until late adolescence. These data indicate that in late infancy, increases in body fat in nonobese children are primarily attributable to increases in adipocyte size, whereas after age 10, increases in body fat reflect an increase in both adipocyte size and number. Among obese children, both adipocyte size and number are increased. Weight loss reduces adipocyte size, but does not affect adipocyte number (12).

Changes in the triceps skinfold thickness parallel the changes in body fat described by Cheek (13). Beginning at age 4–5 years, the triceps skinfold begins to increase slightly in girls, and subsequently increases even more rapidly coincident with the increases in body fat that accompany the female adolescent growth spurt. In boys, the triceps skinfold thickness decreases around age 4 years, begins to increase again 1 or 2 years before adolescence, and subsequently decreases coincident with the increase in fat free mass and decrease in fat mass that accompanies the male adolescent growth spurt.

The BMI decreases over the first year of life in both males and females, and reaches a nadir at 4–5 years of age. Thereafter, in a phase of growth that has been called the period of adiposity rebound (14), the BMI begins to increase in both males and females. Because changes in body fat characterized by the triceps skinfold are not reflected by changes in the BMI, the triceps skinfold must be used clinically to clarify whether an increased BMI reflects an increase in frame size and muscle mass or an increase in body fat.

Changes in the distribution of body fat begin immediately prior to adolescence and continue to change throughout this period of rapid growth (15,16). In both genders, body fat shifts from a peripheral distribution to central distribution. For example, in cross-sectional studies of girls, ratios of trunk to extremity skinfold thicknesses begin to increase at approximately 8 years of age and plateau by about age 12 years. In cross-sectional studies of boys, the increase in the trunk: extremity ratio begins between 10 and 11 years of age, perhaps coincident

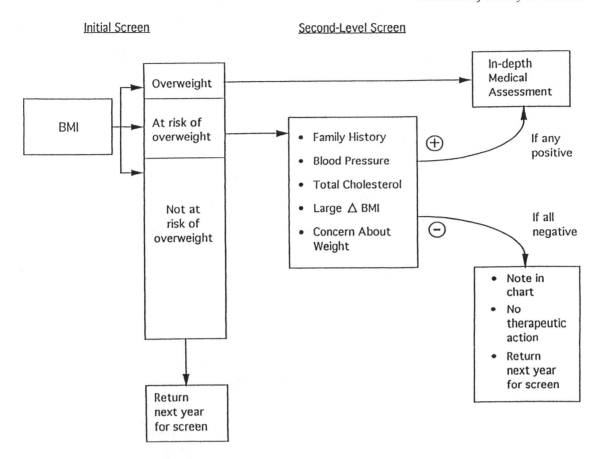

Figure 1 Screening criteria for the identification of adolescent obesity. Children are considered at overweight if their BMI is equal to or greater than the 95th percentile for age and gender. Children between the 85th and 95th percentiles are considered at risk. If children at risk have a positive family history or are positive for other criteria indicated here, they require an in-depth medical assessment. If the second-level screening criteria are negative, these patients should be seen again for reevaluation in 1 year. (From Ref. 6.)

with the preadolescent increase in fatness. In contrast to females, no plateau appears to occur in boys. Furthermore, body fat distribution becomes more centralized in males than in females. Longitudinal data demonstrate the same increase in males, but minimal changes in fat distribution in girls. The canalization of fatness in males during adolescence appears more pronounced than in females.

The limited studies that have been done suggest that visceral fat deposition also changes substantially through childhood and adolescence. In young children, visceral fat occupies approximately 50% of the cross-sectional visceral fat area in 11–13-year-old children (17–19). Between adolescence and adulthood the cross-sectional area increases four- to fivefold (20). However, cross-sectional area measurements of fatness are probably not as relevant meta-

bolically as the ratio of intra-abdominal adipose tissue to total body fat. As Goran et al. have pointed out, the ratio of intra-abdominal adipose tissue to total body fat increases almost threefold (17) from early childhood to adulthood. However, longitudinal and cross-sectional studies that have examined the interrelationships between visceral fat and total body fat in adolescents and the relationship of changes in the ratio of intra-abdominal to total body fat to the timing of puberty have not yet been done.

Although these studies do not encompass the entire range of childhood and adolescence, they suggest that the most rapid increases in visceral fat occur in late adolescence. In adults, body fatness relates directly to the quantity of visceral fat deposition, although the relationship between total and visceral fat differs by gender (20). No such data are yet available for adolescents, although a similar relationship would be expected. The mechanisms that control the location and quantity of fat deposited, as well as those that control the changes in body fat that occur at adolescence, remain unclear.

Few long-term studies have examined the degree to which excess adiposity present in childhood predicts obesity in adulthood. Fatness and fat distribution determined by anthropometric measures in early childhood do not correlate well with fatness and fat distribution present at puberty (16). Retrospective data suggested that approximately 30% of obese women were obese in adolescence, whereas only 10% of obese men were obese during the same period (4). A recent review suggested that almost one third of obese preschool children became obese adults, whereas obesity persists in almost one-half of obese school-age children (21). However, because the review included studies that differed widely in design, populations considered, definition of obesity, the age at which subjects were measured, and the duration of follow-up, the reliability and validity of this conclusion are questionable.

IV. PREVALENCE

Prevalence estimates based on triceps skinfold thickness and BMI have both shown substantial increases in the prevalence of obesity in the United States over the last three decades. A series of national studies performed in the United States enabled us to estimate changes in the prevalence of obesity (22). These data are shown in Table 1. Using as reference data skinfold thicknesses measured during the second and third National Health Examination Surveys (NHES Cycles 2 and 3), we examined changes in the prevalence of obesity in the first and second National Health Examination Survey data. Over the 20-year period between 1963 and 1980, we showed that the prevalence of childhood obesity had increased by 54% in children aged 6–11 years and by almost 40% in adolescents aged 12–17 years. During the same period, comparisons of changes in the BMI failed to confirm the observations based on triceps skinfold thickness (23). At least two possibilities could account for this discrepancy. First, as indicated above, the standardization of measures such as height and weight across surveys is considerably easier than the standardization of skinfold thickness. However, an alternate possibility is that if activity declined over the same period that adiposity increased, reductions in muscle mass might be counterbalanced by increases in body fat. Decreased muscle mass and increased body fat could produce changes in skinfold thickness that are not accompanied by changes in BMI. The latter interpretation now

Table 1 Changes in the Prevalence of Obesity Based on Triceps Skinfold Thickness Between 1963 and 1980 in U.S. Children Aged 6–11 Years and Adolescents Aged 12–17 Years

	Prevalence		
Group	NHES	NHANES I	NHANES II
White boys	19.5%	25.0%	31.5%
Black boys	8.1%	9.6%	16.6%
White girls	18.6%	22.8%	26.0%
Black girls	9.5%	20.0%	20.9%
White male adolescents	16.7%	17.6%	19.5%
Black male adolescents	7.5%	8.9%	12.7%
White female adolescents	16.6%	24.5%	25.5%
Black female adolescents	12.8%	20.4%	25.1%

NHES, National Health Examination Survey Cycle 2, 1963–1965; NHANES, National Health Examination Survey. NHANES I was performed between 1971 and 1974, and NHANES II was performed between 1976 and 1980.
Source: Data from Ref. 22.

appears vindicated by comparisons of the prevalence of obesity, defined as a BMI greater than the 85th percentiles for age and gender from the NHANES II, between NHANES II and NHANES III, completed in 1991 (24,25). These data suggest that the prevalence of obesity in adolescents aged 12–17 years has increased by over 30% in males and by over 45% in females. Similar changes in prevalence occurred among younger children. In both genders, and among children 6–11 years old and adolescents 12–17 years old, the increase in the prevalence of obesity defined as a BMI greater than the 95th percentile appeared even greater than the increase in prevalence, defined by a BMI greater than the 85th percentile. These data indicate that the distribution of fatness in the population has become increasingly skewed toward increased body fat. We observed similar changes in earlier surveys using the triceps skinfold thickness.

Based on the earlier skinfold data, the patterns of fatness within the pediatric population appear to differ from those among adults. In all of the surveys except NHANES III, which is not available for analysis, the prevalence of obesity was greater among Caucasian children than among other ethnic groups. Furthermore, in contrast to adults, the prevalence of obesity varied directly with socioeconomic class in both genders. Nonetheless, the prevalence of obesity appeared to increase more rapidly among African-American children and adolescents than among Caucasians. These data suggested that the ethnic differences in obesity were narrowing. Native American children appear at particularly high risk for the development of obesity (26). No data from NHANES III are yet available to examine changes in the prevalence of obesity across ethnic groups or by socioeconomic class.

In adults, the prevalence of obesity appears greater among residents of the United States than among individuals in France or the United Kingdom (27). Although similar comparisons of children have not been made, the changes observed in the U.S. pediatric population appear paralleled by changes elsewhere in the world. The prevalence of obesity estimated by skinfold thickness in Canada appears to be increasing as rapidly as it has among children in the United States (28). Mean BMI appears to be increasing rapidly among children and adolescents in Denmark (29), Italy (30), Bahrain (31), and Brazil (32), even among poorer populations (33). Few other countries have provided survey data that permit the assessment of prevalences in the pediatric age group.

V. ASSOCIATIONS

A variety of environmental and behavioral variables are associated with childhood and adolescent obesity. These variables can be categorized as variables within the physical and behavioral environment.

A. The Physical Environment

Within the physical environment in the United States, obesity is associated with region, season, and population density (34). Each of the variables within the physical environment exerts a two- to threefold effect on risk. Obesity is more prevalent in the Northeast United States, followed by the Midwest, South, and West. Within each region, obesity is increased in the winter and spring, and decreased in the summer and fall. Furthermore, within each region, obesity is more prevalent in highly urbanized areas than in areas in which the population is less dense.

The mechanism that accounts for the environmental associations is not clear. Each of the physical variables alters the availability or costs of low-caloric-density foods like fruits and vegetables. Each of the variables also affects the facilities or opportunities for exercise or activity. Each of the variables may also reflect ethnicity, as well as social norms related to increased body weight.

B. The Behavioral Environment

Dietary intake and the energy spent on activity represent the only discretionary components of energy intake and expenditure. Behavior contributes significantly to both. For example, parental intakes of carbohydrate, fat, and calories appear to account for 23–97% of the variance of children's intakes of the same nutrients (35). However, weights in these studies were not considered in the analyses. Therefore, family resemblances of nutrient intake may only reflect familial resemblances in size. This possibility is strengthened by the observation that the relationship between parent and child preferences for specific sets of foods does not differ substantially from the relationship between the preferences of children and unrelated adults (36). Resemblances in nutrient intake, when they occur, appear to reflect a common environment rather than a genetically mediated preference for macronutrients (37).

Children appear quite capable of self-regulation of dietary intake under unsupervised settings. Although meal-to-meal variation in caloric intake is substantial among children, the variation between day-to-day caloric intake is considerably lower (38). The degree of parental control of a child's food intake appears to affect adversely the child's capacity to regulate his own food intake. In a setting in which the capacity of children to adjust their food intake in response to the caloric density of the diet was measured, children whose mothers were more controlling of their child's food intake were less capable of self-regulating their own intake (39). Interestingly, lack of knowledge about a child's intake may also impair the regulation of intake. As a recent Danish study showed (40), the risk of subsequent overweight among 9–10-year-old children was not increased by the frequency with which children consumed sweets, or when the mother accepted the child's consumption of sweets, but the risk of overweight was significantly increased if the mother lacked knowledge about her offspring's sweet-eating habits.

Additional observations have suggested that psychosocial stress was associated with rapid rates of weight gain (41,42). The increased effects of stress on weight gain in girls emphasize both the biological susceptibility to obesity in early puberty and the increased adverse social effects of obesity in females. In the studies cited, the retrospective collection of data represents a potential source of bias. Furthermore, these observations do not eliminate the possibility that rapid weight gain caused an increase in psychological problems rather than the reverse.

Both activity and inactivity appear to affect the risk of obesity and its complications in childhood and adolescence. As shown in Table 2, the quantity of energy spent on activity, expressed as a percentage of total energy expenditure, appears to increase from infancy and early childhood to adolescence. Although young children appear more active than adults, the reduced nonbasal energy expenditure that occurs in early childhood may reflect the increased time spent sleeping, rather than a decrease in the energy spent on activity. The energy spent on activity

Table 2 Mean (SD) Energy Costs of Activity for Children and Adolescents Determined from the Doubly Labeled Water Method and Resting Metabolic Rate

Age group (Ref.)	Males	Combined[a]	Females
Infants (43)		1.35 (.29)[b]	
Five years (44)	1.36 (.13)		1.40 (.17)
Nine to twelve years (45)	1.61 (.23)		1.53 (.28)
Twelve to eighteen years (46)	1.79 (.20)		1.69 (.28)

Data are expressed as total energy expenditure/resting or sleeping metabolic rate.
[a]Data not differentiated by gender.
[b]Study measured total energy expenditure/sleeping metabolic rate.

also appears inversely related to fatness (47). Whether decreased nonbasal energy expenditure increases the risk for the development of childhood or adolescent obesity has not been established.

Activity reflects a strong familial component. The observation that familial correlations of activity appeared higher within generations than across generations suggests that levels of activity may reflect an environmental rather that a genetic influence (48). However, more intensive analyses of a large cohort representing almost 400 families confirmed the observation that stronger correlations of physical activity occurred within the same generation, but also demonstrated a heritability of 29% for the level of habitual physical activity. No genetic effect was found for exercise participation (49). In recent studies in which we compared parent and child patterns of activity (50), measures of vigorous activity were better correlated between spouses than between mother-daughter or father-daughter pairs. In contrast, time spent watching television was better correlated within families. These results suggest that patterns of inactivity rather than patterns of activity are correlated within families. As we have previously demonstrated, television time is significantly related to the prevalence of obesity (51). Whether the association of obesity with television viewing reflects the effect of television on food intake or inactivity remains unclear.

Sedentary activity tracks better than physical activity from adolescence into young adulthood (52). Skinfold thickness was reduced among active individuals in late adolescence, but BMI did not differ, suggesting that the reduction in fatness associated with physical activity was counterbalanced by an increase in fat-free mass. Increases in physical activity appear to improve health-related behaviors whereas increases in sedentary activity appear associated with a deterioration in the same behaviors.

Changes in physical activity were independently associated with changes in insulin and triglycerides among boys, but not girls.

The multiple factors that affect the prevalence of obesity vary substantially within populations. For example, multivariate analyses of data from the National Longitudinal Survey of Youth failed to demonstrate behavioral or sociodemographic variables that operated similarly across all ethnic and both gender groups (53). Therefore, the linkage of demographic or behavioral variables to obesity must be evaluated separately in different ethnic groups and emphasizes that interventions must be population-specific.

VI. CRITICAL PERIODS FOR THE DEVELOPMENT OF OBESITY

Recent data suggest that the likelihood of persistence of obesity, and therefore the likelihood of adverse consequences of obesity in adulthood, may be related to the age of onset (54). Several periods appear to constitute specific periods of increased risk. These include the prenatal period, the period of adiposity rebound, and the period of adolescence. Although the mechanisms that are entrained at these periods to promote the increased risk of persistence of obesity or its complications are poorly understood, obesity present at each of these periods appears to be associated with an increased risk of persistence and subsequent disease.

The most compelling data that suggest that the prenatal period constitutes a period of increased risk for persistent adiposity derives from studies of infants of diabetic mothers. Infants of mothers with diabetes during pregnancy, regardless of whether their mother's diabetes is gestational, insulin-dependent, or non-insulin-dependent, tend to be fatter at birth than infants whose mothers were nondiabetic or prediabetic during pregnancy. Long-term follow-up studies of infants of mothers who were diabetic during pregnancy suggest that the prevalence of obesity is increased at later ages that extend through adolescence (55). Shorter-term studies further suggest that body weight in such infants normalizes by about 1 year of age and subsequently begins to diverge from the norm between 5 and 7 years of age (56).

The suggestion that fetal life represents a critical period for adiposity has recently been disputed by a long-term follow-up study (57) that demonstrated an effect of differences in birthweight between monozygotic twins on adult weight and height, but not BMI. However, because birth length was not measured, these analyses only permitted the assessment of differences in weight, rather than the effect of weight relative to height. Furthermore, the analyses as performed do not exclude the possibility of an effect at the extremes of weight differences at birth.

Other data suggest that a variety of other factors associated with an increased risk of cardiovascular disease may also begin to operate at this time. For example, lower-birthweight babies have been shown to have an increased risk of syndrome X and later heart and pulmonary disease in adulthood (58). Furthermore, low birthweight is also associated with an increase in intra-abdominal fat deposition that may in turn account for an increased likelihood of risk factors for cardiovascular disease, including hypertension, diabetes, and hyperlipidemia (59). These data suggest that both obesity and its sequelae in adults may have their onset in utero.

The second period of childhood that appears to constitute a period of increased risk for later obesity is the period known as adiposity rebound. Early acceleration of the BMI after its nadir at 4–5 years of age appears associated with an increased risk of later obesity (60,61). However, as indicated above, infants of mothers with gestational or insulin-dependent diabetes during pregnancy also appear to have onset of their obesity during this period (56).

Several possibilities may explain the association of early adiposity rebound and later obesity. First, those children who experience early adiposity rebound may be those in whom intrauterine exposure to maternal diabetes or maternal glucose intolerance entrained factors that increase body fat during this stage of childhood. Alternatively, both genetic and intrauterine factors that operate to produce obesity may be activated at this time.

The final developmental stage in which the onset of obesity constitutes an increased risk for the development of adult obesity appears to be the period of female adolescence. As indicated above, adolescence in the female represents a period of increased risk for the development of adult obesity. Approximately 30% of obesity in 36-year-old women may begin at this time, whereas in males, only approximately 10% of obesity present at 36 years of age begins at adolescence (4).

VII. ADVERSE CONSEQUENCES IN ADULTHOOD FOR CHILDHOOD-ONSET OBESITY

Despite the lower likelihood that obesity present at adolescence will persist in males, adult mortality is significantly increased among men who were obese as adolescents. For example, we completed a 55-year follow-up study of adults who were obese as adolescents, defined as

a BMI greater than the 75th percentile in subjects of the same age and sex studied in NHANES I (62). The results of these studies demonstrated a significantly greater risk of all-cause mortality and death from coronary heart disease, atherosclerotic cerebrovascular disease, and colorectal cancer in men but not women.

However, in both genders, the risk of coronary heart disease and atherosclerosis was increased relative to adults who had not been overweight during adolescence. In men, the risk of mortality did not change substantially when adjusted for weight at approximately 55 years of age. Likewise, in both genders, the risks of morbidity did not change substantially when adjusted for weight in midlife.

These data suggest that the effect of obesity present in adolescence has a profound influence on morbidity and mortality in adult life that is independent of the effect of adolescent-onset obesity on adult weight. The effect of adolescent obesity on adult morbidity and mortality may be due either to direct effects of adolescent obesity or to other mechanisms including genetic factors that entrain both body fatness and adult morbidity. The changes in body fat distribution that occur at adolescence represent a logical mechanism to explain the effects of adolescent fatness on adult morbidity and mortality.

In a second study, we demonstrated that obesity present in older adolescents and young adults had a substantial adverse impact on a variety of psychosocial outcomes (63). As shown in Table 3, obesity present in young women was associated with an adverse impact on household income, education, and rates of marriage, poverty, and college completion. The persistence of these effects after control for a variety of baseline measures, including self-esteem, household income, parental education, and the income of the family of origin, suggests that obesity

Table 3 Effects of Obesity in Young Women on Psychological Outcomes

Outcome	Adjusted difference (CI)
School	−0.3 year (−0.1 year, −0.6 year)
Marriage	−20% (−13%, −27%)
Household income	−$6710 (−$3942, −$9478)
Poverty	+10% (+4%, +16%)

Obesity was defined as a BMI greater than the 95th percentile for women of the same age studied in NHANES I. The data represent the differences in the outcomes and the confidence intervals of the differences between obese and nonobese women.

Results controlled for baseline income, parents education, chronic health condition, height, self-esteem, age, ethnicity.

Source: Data from Ref. 63.

is an important determinant rather than a consequence of socioeconomic status in women. No significant effects of obesity in men were found on any of the variables examined. However, stature in men appeared to play a role comparable to the role of obesity in women on the social and economic indicators examined.

These results suggest that discrimination against obese women is widespread and has grave social and economic consequences. Although we anticipated that the effects of discrimination would have an adverse impact on the self-esteem of the women included in the study, no effect could be demonstrated.

VIII. SUMMARY

In the last two decades, obesity has become the most prevalent nutritional disease among children and adolescents in North America. Although comparable data from other countries are lacking, the prevalence of obesity appears to be increasing rapidly in other developed countries. The effects of childhood obesity on morbidity and mortality indicate that effective prevention and therapy for childhood obesity are likely to have a significant impact on adult disease. Furthermore, programs aimed at treatment of overweight children appear to have a substantially better long-term success rate than similar programs in adults (64). However, the bias against the obese reflected in the allocation of health care resources, the lack of political power accorded children, limited reimbursement for the treatment of obesity, and the direction of resources to treatment or secondary prevention of adults rather than primary prevention of disease in childhood suggests that effective national programs directed at childhood obesity will continue to be neglected. In the interim, efforts must be directed toward the identification and propagation of successful treatment and prevention strategies.

REFERENCES

1. Rucker CE, Cash TF. Body images, body-size perceptions, and eating behaviors among African-American and White college women. Int J Eating Disord 1992; 12:291–299.
2. Himes JH, Bouchard C. Validity of anthropometry in classifying youths as obese. Int J Obes 1989; 13:183–193.
3. Roche AF, Siervogel RM, Chumlea WC, Webb P. Grading body fatness from limited anthropometric data. Am J Clin Nutr 1981; 34:2831–2838.
4. Braddon FEM, Rodgers B, Wadsworth MEJ, Davies JMC. Onset of obesity in a 36 year birth cohort. Br Med J 1986; 293:299–303.
5. Must A, Dallal GE, Dietz WH. Reference data for obesity: 85th and 95th percentiles of body mass index (wt/ht^2)—a correction. Am J Clin Nutr 1991; 54:773.
6. Himes JH, Dietz WH. Guidelines for overweight in adolescent preventive services: recommendations from an expert committee. Am J Clin Nutr 1994; 59:307–316.
7. Cheek DB. Human Growth. Philadelphia: Lea & Febiger, 1968.
8. Boileau RA, Lohman TG, Slaughter MH, Ball TE, Going SB, Hendrix MK. Hydration of the fat-free body in children during maturation. Hum Biol 1984; 56:651–666.
9. Malina RM, Bouchard C. Models and methods for studying body composition. In: Malina RM, Bouchard C. Growth, Maturation, and Physical Activity. Champaign, IL: Human Kinetics, 1991.
10. Knittle JL, Timmers K, Ginsberg-Fellner F, Brown RE, Katz DP. The growth of adipose tissue in children and adolescents. Cross-sectional and longitudinal studies of adipose tissue cell number and size. J Clin Invest 1979; 63:239–246.
11. Poissonnet CM, LaVelle M, Burdi AR. Growth and development of adipose tissue. J Pediatr 1988; 113:1–9.
12. Knittle JL, Ginsberge-Fellner F. Effect of weight reduction on in vitro adipose tissue lipolysis and cellularity in obese adolescents and adults. Diabetes 1972; 21:754–761.
13. Garn SM, Clark DC. Trends in fatness and the origins of obesity. Pediatrics 1976; 57:443–455.
14. Rolland-Cachera M-F, Deheeger M, Guilloud-Bataille M, Avons P, Patois E, Sempe M. Tracking the development of adiposity from one month of age to adulthood. Ann Hum Biol 1987; 14:219–229.
15. Malina RM, Bouchard C. Subcutaneous fat distribution during growth. In Bouchard C, Johnston FE, eds. Fat Distribution During Growth and Later Health Outcomes. New York: Alan R Liss, 1988.
16. Roche AF, Baumgartner RN. Tracking in fat distribution during growth. In: Bouchard C, Johnston FE, eds. Fat Distribution During Growth and Later Health Outcomes. New York: Alan R Liss, 1988.
17. Goran MI, Kaskoun M, Shuman WP. Intra-abdominal adipose tissue in young children. Int J Obes 1995; 19:279–283.
18. Fox K, Peters D, Armstrong N, Sharpe P. Bell M. Abdominal fat deposition in 11-year old children. Int J Obes 1993; 17:11–16.
19. de Ridder CM, de Boer RW, Seidell JC, Nieuwenhoff CM, Jeneson JAL, Bakker CJG, Zonderland ML, Erich WBM. Body fat distribution in pubertal girls quantified by magnetic resonance imaging. Int J Obes 1992; 16:443–449.
20. Lemieux S, Prud'homme D, Bouchard C, Tremblay A, Despres' J-P. Sex differences in the relation of visceral adipose tissue to total body fatness. Am J Clin Nutr 1993; 58:463–467.
21. Serdula MK, Ivery D, Coates RJ, Freedman DS, Williamson DF, Byers T. Do obese children become obese adults? A review of the literature. Prev Med 1993; 22:167–177.

22. Gortmaker SL, Dietz, WH, Sobol AM, Wehler CA. Increasing pediatric obesity in the United States. Am J Dis Child 1987; 141:535–540.

23. Harlan WR, Landis JR, Flegal KM, Davis CS, Miller ME. Secular trends in body mass in the United States. Am J Epidemiol 1988; 128:1065–1074.

24. Division of Health Examination Statistics, National Center for Health Statistics, Centers for Disease Control. Prevalence of overweight among adolescents—United States, 1988–91. Morbid Mortal Weekly Rep 1994; 43:818–820.

25. Troiano RP, Flegal KM, Kuczmarski RJ, Campbell SM, Johnson CL. Overweight prevalence and trends for children and adolescents. Arch Pediatr Adolesc Med 1995; 149:1085–1091.

26. Broussard BA, Sugarman JR, Bachman-Carter K, Booth K, Stephenson L, Strauss K, Gohdes D. Toward comprehensive obesity prevention programs in Native American communities. Obes Res 1995; 3(Suppl 2):289s–297s.

27. Laurier D, Guiguet M, Chau NP, Wells JA, Valleron A-J. Prevalence of obesity a comparative survey in France, the United Kingdom and the United States. Int J Obes 1992; 16:565–572.

28. Limbert J, Crawford SM, McCargar LJ. Estimates of the prevalence of obesity in Canadian children. Obes Res 1994; 2:321–327.

29. Thomsen BL, Ekstrom C, Sorensen TIA. Changes in the distribution of weight, height and body mass index (BMI=W/H^2) at ages 7 to 14 years in a population of Danish boys born 1930 through 1966. Int J Obes 1995; 19(Suppl 2):52.

30. Marelli G, Colombo E. Six years of epidemiological monitoring of childhood obesity. Int J Obes 1995; 19(Suppl 2):52.

31. Musaiger AO, Matter AM, Alekri SA, Mahdi AR. Obesity among secondary school students in Bahrain. Nutr Health 1993; 9:25–32.

32. Sichieri R, Recine E, Everhart JE. Growth and body mass index of Brazilians ages 9 through 17 years. Obes Res 1995; 3(Suppl 2):117s–121s.

33. Sawaya AL, Dallal G, Solymos G, Sousa MH, Ventura ML, Roberts SB, Sigulem DM. Obesity and malnutrition in a shantytown population in the city of São Paulo, Brazil. Obes Res 1995; 3(Suppl 2):107s–115s.

34. Dietz WH, Gortmaker SL. Factors within the physical environment associated with childhood obesity. Am J Clin Nutr 1984; 39:619–624.

35. Laskarzewski P, Morrison JA, Khoury P, Kelly K, Glatfelter L, Larsen R, Glueck CJ. Parent-child nutrient intake interrelationships in school children ages 6 to 19: the Princeton School District Study. Am J Clin Nutr 1980; 33:2350–2355.

36. Birch LL. The relationship between children's food preferences and those of their parents. J Nutr Ed 1980; 12:14–18.

37. Perusse L, Tremblay A, LeBlanc C, Cloninger CR, Reich T, Rice J, Bouchard C. Familial resemblance in energy intake:

contribution of genetic and environmental factors. Am J Clin Nutr 1988; 47:629–635.

38. Birch LL, Johnson SL, Andresen G, Peters JC, Schulte MC. The variability of young children's intake. N Engl J Med 1991; 324:232–235.

39. Johnson SL, Birch LL. Parents' and children's adiposity and eating style. Pediatrics 1994; 94:653–661.

40. Lissau I, Breum L, Sorensen TIA. Maternal attitude to sweet eating habits and risk of overweight in offspring: a ten-year prospective population study. Int J Obes 1993; 17:125–129.

41. Mellbin T, Vuille JC. Rapidly developing overweight in school children as an indicator of psychosocial stress. Acta Paediatr Scand 1989; 78:568–575.

42. Mellbin T, Vuille JC. Further evidence of an association between psychosocial problems and increase in relative weight between 7 and 10 years of age. Acta Paediatr Scand 1989; 78:576–580.

43. Davies PSW, Wells JCK, Fieldhouse CA, Day JME, Lucas A. Parental body composition and infant energy expenditure. Am J Clin Nutr 1995; 61:1026–1029.

44. Fontvieille AM, Harper IT, Ferraro RT, Spraul M, Ravussin E. Daily energy expenditure by five-year-old children, measured by doubly labeled water. J Pediatr 1993; 123:200–207.

45. Livingstone MBE, Coward WA, Prentice AM, Davies PSW, Strain JJ, McKenna PG, Mahoney CA, White JA, Stewart CM, Kerr M-JJ. Daily energy expenditure in free-living children: comparison of heart rate monitoring with the doubly labeled water (^{2}H$_2$^{18}O) method. Am J Clin Nutr 1992; 56:343–352.

46. Bandini LG, Schoeller DA, Dietz WH. Energy expenditure in obese and non-obese adolescents. Pediatr Res 1990; 27:198–203.

47. Davies PSW, Gregory J, White A. Physical activity and body fatness in pre-school children. Int J Obes 1995; 19:6–10.

48. Perusse L, LeBlanc C, Bouchard C. Familial resemblance in lifestyle components: results from the Canada Fitness Survey. Can J Public Health 1988; 79:201–205.

49. Perusse L, Tremblay A, LeBlanc C, Bouchard C. Genetic and environmental influences on level of habitual physical activity and exercise participation. Am J Epidemiol 1989; 129:1012–1022.

50. Must A, Ching PLYH, Dietz WH. Like parent, like daughter? Patterns of physical activity and inactivity within families (submitted).

51. Dietz WH, & Gortmaker SL. Do we fatten our children at the TV set? Television viewing and obesity in children and adolescents. Pediatrics 1984; 75:807–812.

52. Raitakari OT, Porkka KVK, Taimela S, Telama R, Rasanen L, Viikara JSA. Effects of persistent physical activity and inactivity on coronary risk factors in children and young adults. The Cardiovascular Risk in Young Finns Study. Am J Epidemiol 1994; 140:195–205.

53. Must A, Gortmaker SL, Dietz WH. Risk factors for obesity in young adults: Hispanics, African Americans and whites

in the transition years, age 16–28 years. Biomed Phama-cother 1994; 48:143–156.

54. Dietz WH. Critical periods in childhood for the development of obesity. Am J Clin Nutr 1994; 59:955–959.

55. Pettit DJ, Baird HR, Aleck KA, Bennett PA, & Knowler WC. Excessive obesity in offspring of Pima Indian women with diabetes during pregnancy. N Engl J Med 1983; 308: 242–245.

56. Vohr BR, Lipsitt LP, Oh W. Somatic growth of children of diabetic mothers with reference to birth size. J Pediatr 1980; 97:196–199.

57. Allison DB, Paultre F, Heymsfield SB, Pi-Sunyer FX. Is the intra-uterine period really a critical period for the development of adiposity? Int J Obes 1995; 19:397–402.

58. Barker DJP, Hales CN, Fall CHD, Osmond C, Phipps K, Clark PMS. Type 2 (non-insulin-dependent) diabetes mellitus, hypertension and hyperlipidemia (syndrome X): relation to reduced fetal growth. Diabetologia 1993; 36: 62–67.

59. Law CM, Barker DJP, Osmond C, Fall CHD, Simmonds SJ. Early growth and abdominal fatness in adult life. J Epide-miol Commun Health 1992; 46:184–186.

60. Rolland-Cachera M-F, Deheeger M, Bellisle F, Sempe M, Guilloud-Batouille M, Patois E. Adiposity rebound in children: A simple indicator for predicting obesity. Am J Clin Nutr 1984; 39:129–135.

61. Siervogel RM, Roche AF, Guo S, Mukherjee D, Chumlea WC. Patterns of change in weight/stature^2 from 2 to 18 years: findings from long-term serial data for children in the Fels Longitudinal Growth Study. Int J Obes 1991; 15: 479–485.

62. Must A, Jacques PF, Dallal GE, Bajema CJ, Dietz WH. Long-term morbidity and mortality of overweight adolescents; a follow-up of the Harvard Growth Study of 1922 to 1935. N Engl J Med 1992; 327:1350–1355.

63. Gortmaker SL, Must A, Perrin JM, Sobol AM, Dietz WH. Social and economic consequences of overweight in adolescence and young adulthood. N Engl J Med 1993; 329: 1008–1012.

64. Epstein LH, Valoski A, Wing RR, McCurley J. Ten-year follow-up of behavioral, family based treatment for obese children. JAMA 1990; 264:2519–2523.

6

Obesity in the Elderly

Robert S. Schwartz
University of Washington and Harborview Medical Center, Seattle, Washington

I. INTRODUCTION

In young and middle-aged individuals obesity is an important metabolic and cardiovascular risk factor that is associated with highly prevalent disorders such as hypertension, diabetes, hyperinsulinemia, dyslipidemia, and atherosclerosis (1). While older individuals do not necessarily appear to be obese, it is clear that they frequently suffer from similar obesity-related disorders. This had led some investigators in the field of aging to consider many older individuals as having a "covert" form of obesity. Because the elderly are the fastest-growing segment of our population, and contribute greatly to overall health care utilization and cost (2), the problem of obesity in this older population will have staggering repercussions to our health care system as well as to the lives of many older individuals (3).

This chapter will discuss the scope of the problem of obesity in the elderly, define the body composition and fat distribution changes that usually occur with aging, outline possible etiological factors in aging-associated obesity, and, finally, consider potential treatments.

II. PREVALENCE OF OBESITY IN THE ELDERLY

A. Age-Related Changes in Weight and Body Composition

Cross-sectional data from the NHANES III study demonstrate that the prevalence of overweight, reaches a maximum for both men [42%, with a mean body mass index (BMI) of 27.6] and women (52%, with a mean BMI of 28.5) between the ages of 50 and 59 (4). In this study, which had no upper age limit for subject entry and specifically oversampled older individuals, the prevalence of overweight and the mean BMI both tended to drop in oldest age groups, falling to 18% in men (mean BMI 24.7) and 26% in women (mean BMI 24.6) over age 80. There were notable differences in the effects of age on obesity in different racial/ethnic groups. African-American men had the highest prevalence of overweight in the 20–29-year age range, but this rate tended to increase relatively less in the older age cohorts when compared to either Caucasians or Hispanics. Hispanic subjects had the highest prevalence of obesity in the males (between ≈50 and 55%) in the groups spanning 40–69 years old. In women yet a different picture emerged. Caucasian women had the lowest prevalence of obesity in each age group, with a peak (≈50%) at 50–59 years. Hispanic women had their highest prevalence of obesity (≈55%) at a younger age (40–49 years). African-American women had their peak prevalence of obesity later (≈60%; 60–69 years) and overall had the highest prevalence of obesity when compared to the other racial/ethnic groups.

However, these findings reflect a common problem in the interpretation of cross-sectional data, a bias due to the disproportionately higher death rate in obese subjects during middle age (5,6). A truer understanding of the complex age-related changes in weight or BMI requires longitudinal data. Indeed, a 15-year follow-up study of seven different age cohorts of men (21–80 years old at entry) demonstrated a significant difference in the effect of aging on weight or BMI in the different cohorts (7). The cohorts of men who were the oldest at entry weighed the least and tended to remain stable or lose a small amount of weight over the period of follow-up, while the younger cohorts were heavier at baseline and continued to gain weight with time. Thus, there seemed to be substantial cohort effect of aging on body weight. More consistent were the changes observed in fat distribution, with all cohorts showing increments in central distribution of fat during the period of follow-up (see below).

The observed changes in BMI with aging were also accompanied by profound changes in body composition that can substantially influence the interpretation of such data. Studies have consistently demonstrated clinically important losses of fat-free mass (FFM) with age in both men and women. This phenomenon has recently received the appellation "sarcopenia" (8). While the loss of FFM influences many aspects of clinical geriatric care, such as strength, endurance, and overall functional ability (8–12), here we will consider only how it may affect the determination of obesity in older individuals. Thus, because FFM declines by as much as 40% between the ages of 30 and 70 (13–18), at any given body weight or BMI, older persons will be considerably fatter (19). Even the content of fat within lean tissues such as muscle is greater with aging. Therefore, the measurements of body composition by methods such as computed tomography (CT), magnetic resonance imaging (MRI), and dual energy X-ray absorptiometry (DEXA) might underestimate total adiposity.

Stature frequently declines (0.5–1.5 cm/decade) with age (13) owing to decrements in the height of the vertebral bodies and shrinkage of intervertebral disk spaces, and the use of present height commonly overestimates BMI in the elderly. This can be corrected by using maximal historical height, but one must be concerned with the usual caveats regarding recalled data. A preferred method is the use of knee height as suggested by Chumlea et al. (20). Skinfold thickness correlates less well with total adiposity in older individuals (21), making assessment of adiposity by skinfold measurements difficult to interpret. Well-known age-related changes in the composition of FFM can significantly affect the determination of body density and, therefore, body composition using the "gold standard" hydrodensitometry method (22). While the density of fat changes little with aging (0.9 g/ml), variation in hydration state and in bone mineral can distort the actual density of FFM from the value usually assumed in prediction equations (1.10 g/ml). Tissue dehydration would increase the true density of FFM while loss of bone mineral would

produce the opposite affect. The loss of water would probably have the more profound affect and for any given total body density measure, the established prediction equations would underestimate the amount of adiposity (23). However, studies are not consistent in finding a decline in the hydration state of lean tissue in older subjects (24,25). Whereas one study found no significant change in hydration of lean tissue between young and older women (24), another found that not correcting for measured total body water produced a 4% underestimation of percent body fat (%BF) in older women but no significant difference in older men when compared to multicompartmental methods (25). In the latter study, the variation in the measurement of %BF between the two- and four-compartmental models was inversely related to the hydration state of the FFM. A recent cross-sectional study found that while total body water declined in both men and women between ages 60 and 80, the decline was significant only in the women (13). The loss of water appeared to be mainly from intracellular fluid. This study also found that men lost FFM twice as quickly as women (0.22 vs 0.10 kg/year), and that men lost more mass from the upper extremities while women lost equally from the upper and lower extremities. Only women had a significant age-related decline in fat mass (−0.28 kg/yr) and %BF (−0.21%). Any observed changes in body water with aging may also affect estimates of body composition using total body water or bioelectrical impedance, the latter being a measure that is exquisitely sensitive to hydration state (26).

While there is some disagreement, it appears that the changes in hydration state in healthy older persons are small and probably do not have a major affect on estimates of adiposity. Nevertheless, the direction of the changes that have been observed would tend to produce an underestimate of body fat.

B. Age-Related Changes in Fat Distribution

It has been well demonstrated that many of the metabolic abnormalities associated with obesity are strongly and independently related to a central distribution of adiposity (27–32). However, what is less well recognized is that aging is associated with an increasingly more central distribution of adiposity in both men and women (7,33–36). At any given level of adiposity, more fat will be centrally distributed in older individuals. While this is apparently a slowly progressive change with age in men, in women the accumulation of central fat may begin to increase only after menopause (37–40). Other studies suggest that the increase in central adiposity after menopause can, for the most part, be accounted for merely by age (41,42). Of interest, a recent cross-sectional study found no age-related change in fat distribution in men or women between the ages of 60 and 80, suggesting this accumulation may reach its maximum in middle age and early old age (13).

Intra-abdominal fat accumulation, known to be independently related to the metabolic concomitant of obesity (43–48), has also been demonstrated to be greater at any given BMI or %BF in older individuals (49–51). Again, while the accumulation of intra-abdominal fat with aging may be progressive in men, it appears to occur to a greater extent in women following menopause (40,52). One study (53), using magnetic resonance imaging, found no increase in visceral adiposity with age.

While there are differences in fat distribution which appear to be related to racial/ethnic groups, relatively little is known about how this is affected by aging. It appears that African-American women have greater central fat distribution than Caucasian women before menopause (54) but that the slope of the increase with age is not different between the two groups. Of interest, NHANES I also noted that central adiposity conferred relatively less risk for cardiovascular disease in black women (55). This finding agrees with earlier reports that central adiposity was not a strong risk factor for the development of non-insulin-dependent diabetes (NIDDM) or atherosclerotic cardiovascular disease in black women (56). In addition, the Charleston Heart Study determined that central fat distribution did not predict all-cause or coronary heart disease deaths in black women (57). Other studies found that while Hispanics have a greater central distribution of fat, this was not associated with excess all-cause mortality in subjects over age 45 (58). Studies by Fujimoto et al. in Japanese-Americans have demonstrated relatively greater amounts of central and intra-abdominal fat when compared to Caucasians and a strong relationship between intra-abdominal fat and the development of insulin resistance and NIDDM frequently observed in this population (47,48,59).

C. Menopause and Obesity in Women

There are relatively few data on changes in adiposity and fat distribution associated with menopause in women. This is an important issue because of the relationships that have been noted between obesity and cardiovascular disease (5), and obesity and certain cancers (60,61) in postmenopausal women. As noted above, body weight reaches its maximum in women very near the time of menopause and there is an increase in relative adiposity for any given

weight or BMI. While some studies find that the increase in weight accompanying menopause is more related to age than menopause itself (41,62), other have noted specific menopause-related increases in BMI (42), overall adiposity (39), central adiposity (37,39), and intra-abdominal adiposity (40). A recently published longitudinal study that followed 35 women aged 44–48 for 6 years found that those women who experienced menopause during the period of follow-up lost significantly more fat-free mass (FFM; −3 vs. −0.5 kg), and had greater increase in fat mass (FM; 2.5 vs 1.0 kg), waist-to-hip ration (WHR; 0.04 vs. 0.01) and insulin (11 vs −2 pmol/L). The changes were associated with greater reductions in physical activity and resting energy expenditure in the postmenopausal women. It is also noteworthy that in one randomized, placebo-controlled study in which early postmenopausal women were prospectively studied for 2 years, hormone replacement therapy prevented the accumulation of abdominal adiposity while having no effect on FFM (63).

III. CAUSES OF OBESITY IN OLDER PERSONS

A. Intake Versus Expenditure

The accumulation of excess calories stored as adipose tissue requires an imbalance in the usually tight relationship between caloric intake and expenditure. While adiposity has a tendency to increase with age, caloric intake is either unchanged (64) or declines (65) when assessed in longitudinal studies. Furthermore, the increment in adiposity with aging cannot be blamed on increased relative fat intake in the diet (66) since this too appears to decline with aging (64,65). Therefore, it is most likely that the age-related increase in obesity is in some way related to deficits in energy expenditure. This supports older studies that have noted a decline in energy expenditure with age (17) and is consistent with studies that have found a relationship between the tendency to gain weight and a lower rate of energy expenditure. Recently, this topic has been carefully reviewed (67). The relationship between resting metabolic rate (RMR) and age appears to be curvilinear if a sufficient number of older individuals are included. While three-fourths of this decline in RMR can be accounted for by decrements in FFM, one-quarter remains unexplained. Poehlman et al. have suggested that this decline in RMR may be related to inactivity and have demonstrated normalization in older men after endurance training (68). Others have not been able to demonstrate an endurance training-related improvement in RMR in older subjects (69). While the thermic effect of feeding

(TEF) may decline with age (70), this may be more related to inactivity than to age itself (67). Furthermore, variability in TEF does not predict subsequent weight gain (71).

B. Inactivity

The component of daily energy expenditure that is most variable between individuals is the thermic effect of exercise (TEE), the energy expended with physical activity. Older individuals are more inactive than their younger counterparts (72,73), and several investigators have proposed that this difference in activity level may account for much of the age-associated gain in adiposity (74). This is supported by 10-year follow-up data from the NHANES-I study which looked at the relationship between recreational physical activity and subsequent weight gain (75). Both at baseline and at follow-up, physical activity was inversely related to body weight. Low physical activity at follow-up was strongly associated with major weight gain (more than 13 kg), and the relative risk of major weight gain, comparing the low- and high-activity groups, was 3.1 in men and 3.8 in women. This activity component can best be measured by evaluating free-living energy expenditure using the doubly labeled water technique (76). Using this method, reduced physical activity levels are associated with increased %BF (77).

IV. METABOLIC CONSEQUENCES OF OBESITY IN OLDER PERSONS

Many of the common obesity-related metabolic abnormalities found in young and middle-aged individuals appear to be related to insulin resistance and hyperinsulinemia, what has come to be called the "insulin resistance" or "metabolic" syndrome (78). While the exact components of this syndrome may be somewhat variable in certain populations (79,80), in general it is made up of central obesity (43,81), insulin resistance and hyperinsulinemia (82), abnormal glucose metabolism (83), dyslipidemias (45,84) such as high triglycerides, reduced high-density-lipoprotein cholesterol and small dense low-density lipoprotein particles (85), hypertension (78), and atherosclerosis (86).

These same metabolic disorders are extremely prevalent in older populations. For example, it is well known that glucose tolerance worsens with age, with a 1–2 mg/dl increase in fasting glucose and a 10–20 mg/dl increase in postprandial glucose for each decade after age 30 (87). NIDDM is the fifth most common chronic disease in the elderly, affecting about 20% of individuals over age 65, with approximately half of these being undiagnosed (88).

Diabetes has profound effects on health care utilization and costs, with up to one-seventh of all health care dollars being spent caring for diabetic patients (89). While in the past this high frequency of diabetes and glucose intolerance has been considered attributable to aging, more recent studies strongly suggest that most, if not all, of the "age-related" changes in insulin sensitivity and glucose tolerance can be accounted for by changes in body composition, fat distribution, and inactivity (49,90–94). Similarly, there is an exceedingly high prevalence of hypertension in elderly populations (95). It is estimated that between 30% and 50% of all persons over age 65 have hypertension (either systolic-diastolic or isolated systolic), with somewhat lower prevalence rates in studies that require multiple readings to make the diagnosis and higher rates in African-Americans.

Dyslipidemia is commonly noted in obese individuals, especially those with a central or intra-abdominal distribution of fat (45,96). The most commonly described abnormalities include elevations in triglyceride and reductions in high-density-lipoprotein cholesterol (HDL-C) levels. While similar abnormalities have been detected in older subjects (97,98), these abnormalities occur in both obese and nonobese older individuals (99). In two prospective studies, plasma insulin level was found to predict the development of dyslipidemia after either 3.5 or 8 years of follow-up. Apolipoprotein abnormalities have also been described in older subjects, such as increases in Apo B, reductions in Apo AI, and the development of small dense LDL particles (100). These abnormalities are all similar to those noted with central adiposity (96) and are associated with an elevated risk for atherosclerosis (86).

Many studies demonstrate that obesity is related to increased mortality in young and middle-aged individuals. While the relationship between body weight and mortality was initially noted to be U-shaped, with excess mortality at both extremes of the body weight range, it now seems likely that this was due to confounders such as excess cigarette smoking and illness-related weight loss in the lowest weight group. More recent analyses have found no increase in mortality in the lowest weight group (5,6). The relationship between obesity and overall mortality in older individuals has been a point of major controversy for a number of years and continues still. Andres has suggested that the weight associated with the lowest mortality increases with age (101), while others suggest this is not the case when the data are corrected for smoking and early deaths (102,103). There are few data on ethnic differences in the relationship between obesity and mortality in older individuals, but one large prospective study noted the lowest mortality in the 60–84th percentiles for weight in white men compared to the 40–59th percentiles in black men (104). The opposite was true for women, with the lowest mortality in the 40–59th percentiles for weight in white women and in the 60–84th percentiles for the black women. This study demonstrated a U-shaped curve, with excess mortality at both the lowest and highest percentiles for body weight, even when corrected for smoking or when only nonsmokers were included. It is suggested that the added mortality at very low weights in these older subjects might be accounted for by excess hip fractures.

V. TREATMENT OF OBESITY IN OLDER PERSONS

A. Effects of Voluntary Weight Fluctuation on Mortality

There is compelling evidence supporting the association of obesity and weight gain with heart disease (105), diabetes (106), and excess all-cause mortality (5). It is less clear, however, whether there is a significant impact associated with losing excess weight or, indeed, whether the impact is positive or negative. Several large studies in both middle-aged and older adults find that weigh fluctuations, either up or down, are associated with excess cardiovascular and all-cause mortality (107–109), with similar findings in two separate Asian populations (110,111). Together, these studies strongly suggest that the lowest mortality is found in subjects with the most stable weights. These studies have been rightfully criticized because they often did not distinguish between intentional and unintentional weight loss (112), or failed to take into account important preexisting disease (113). An important recent study by Williamson et al (114), has specifically attempted to obviate these problems by evaluating the effects of intentional weight loss in over 43,000 nonsmoking middle-age (40–64 years) Caucasian women followed prospectively for 12 years. Early deaths, within the first 3 years, were excluded. The data were stratified by preexisting obesity-related illness, and adjusted for age, starting BMI, alcohol use, physical activity, and overall health. This study demonstrated that any amount of weight loss in subjects with obesity-related illness was associated with a 20% decrement in all-cause mortality, which was due to both a 40–50% fall in cancer deaths and a 30–40% reduction in diabetes-related deaths. The data were much less clear in women without preexisting obesity-related disease who intentionally lost weight.

While it appears that there are potential long-range benefits to weight loss especially in those with obesity-related disorders, a caveat must be emphasized for the elderly. Weight loss is frequently part of the "failure to thrive syndrome" seen in very old patients (115). Recent work by Wallace et al. demonstrated in a group of outpatient Veterans over age 65 that involuntary weight loss of ≥4% in one year was associated with a 2.5-fold greater risk of dying within the next 2 years of follow-up when compared to non-weight-losers. This was despite a significant decrement in WHR in the weight losers. These results were not affected by adjusting for age, BMI, tobacco use, and health status. Surprisingly, the relative risk of dying was the same in subjects whose weight loss was voluntary. These data suggest that while dietary weight loss in patients with obesity-related illness may positively impact outcomes, physicians should be cautious in prescribing weight loss in otherwise healthy obese older patients. In addition, rapid or relatively easy loss of weight should be investigated.

B. Dietary Weight Loss Studies in Older Individuals

There have been few published reports of dietary weight loss interventions specifically in older subjects. While the study by Williamson et al. (114) supports a benefit to intentional weight loss in middle-aged subjects, it is possible that exacerbation of the usual age-related loss of lean mass could be worsened by a weight loss diet. In a recently published study of obese older men (mean of 60 years) who underwent a 10-month calorie restriction, only 23% of the 9.3 kg of weight that was lost was lost as FFM (116). This is similar to preliminary studies in our laboratory (117) in which 16 older men (mean 66 years) lost 10 kg on a 1200-kcal dietary restriction (American Heart Association Diet, Phase I). In this study only 20% of weight loss was as FFM. The percentages of weight loss as FFM in these relatively healthy older individuals are consistent with those found in younger subjects (117). In both of the above studies, weight loss produced a small, but significant improvement in the waist-to-hip ratio. However, in our study, despite a decrement WHR and in intra-abdominal adiposity measured by CT, there was no preferential loss of intra-abdominal fat as compared to fat from more peripheral depots (117).

A recent randomized controlled study compared the effect of a 9-month hypocaloric (AHA, Phase I) diet on insulin action and glucose tolerance in middle-aged and older subjects (mean age 60 ± 8 years) with either normal or impaired glucose tolerance (118). After an average weight loss of 9 kg, there was a significant fall in the glucose area (~22%) following an oral glucose challenge. This reduction in glucose area was related to the decrease in waist circumference. In fact, almost half of the subjects who initially had impaired glucose tolerance normalized following weight loss. In a subgroup of eight subjects the weight loss was found to induce a fall in both the first- and second-phase insulin response to a hyperglycemic clamp and an improvement in insulin action.

In a study by Dengel et al., weight loss was associated with improvement in the lipoprotein profile, reductions in the LDL/HDL-C ratio and triglyceride concentration, and increments in the HDL$_2$-C (119). We have noted similar improvements in HDL and triglyceride concentrations but no change in the concentration of total or LDL cholesterol (120). However, there was a 22% decline in hepatic lipase, consistent with less dense and less atherogenic LDL particles. Six of the seven subjects who initially had the more atherogenic, small, dense LDL phenotype pattern B reverted to a more favorable LDL pattern A following weight loss (121). No change was noted in the subjects with pattern A at baseline. Thus, while the concentration of LDL failed to change with weight loss, the size and composition of the LDL particles became more favorable.

C.   Exercise Training in Older Individuals

Many important benefits of exercise training for older persons have now been documented (122). Exercise alone is not associated with large reductions in adipose tissue mass in intervention studies (123), and it has been estimated that a 6-month period of exercise training alone would reduce fat mass by only 2.6 kg and % body fat by only 3%. However, in large population studies greater physical activity is associated with lower body weight and higher fitness levels are inversely related to all-cause mortality in subjects at any BMI level (124). Interestingly, the most impressive effect on mortality occurs in subjects with BMIs $\geq$ 30. There is also good evidence that physical activity is associated with lower blood pressure (125), as well as less diabetes (126), dyslipidemia, and atherosclerosis (127), all disorders that are common in obesity. In addition, exercise has been demonstrated to help in the maintenance of weight loss after dietary restriction (128,129).

There is much less data on the metabolic effects of an exercise intervention in older subjects but this has become an area of great interest in recent years. As in other groups, endurance exercise training in older subjects is associated with only modest losses in weight and fat (130,131), consistent with the estimates by Wilmore (123). However, recent studies strongly suggest that the fat that is lost comes preferentially from intra-abdominal depots (128,129). This appears to be different from the more general loss of adipose mass with caloric restriction (117). Associated with this preferential loss of central adipose tissue following exercise are improvements in lipid, glucose, and insulin metabolism (91,132,133). For example, after 6 months of intensive endurance exercise subjects

lost only 2.5 kg of weight and a similar amount of fat. This was associated with a 20% loss of intra-abdominal adipose tissue area on CT. With these changes, insulin sensitivity improved by more than 33% despite no improvement in oral glucose metabolism (91). There was a 23% reduction in triglyceride and an almost 70% increment in HDL$_2$ cholesterol (132). Recent evidence suggests that most if not all of the metabolic effects of exercise require weight loss and that metabolic improvements are greatly lessened if body weight is purposely maintained (134). Since energy intake has been noted to be increased in free-living subjects who are training (68,130), weight loss is felt to be due to enhanced energy expenditure. While both the thermic effect of exercise and RMR are increased with exercise training (68), it is of interest that 24-hr energy expenditure may not increase in older men with endurance training (135). This suggests that they were more sedentary at other times of the day when they were not exercising. Therefore, the true etiology of the fat loss is unclear but may be related to enhancement of sympathetic nervous system activity (136) or lipid oxidation (137).

There is considerably less data on the effects of resistance training on adiposity and metabolism in older subjects. While it is now well known that the elderly can increase both their FFM and strength with resistance training (8,138), only recently has it been demonstrated that there are also reductions in both fat mass and intra-abdominal fat mass (139). Newer studies suggest that resistance training may also have positive effects, similar to endurance training, on insulin action (140,141) but little or no improvements in lipoprotein profile seems to occur (142).

Both endurance and resistance exercise are beneficial in the elderly. Although the amount of weight loss associated with training is small, it may preferentially come from the most critical intra-abdominal depots and, thus, be associated with substantial metabolic improvement. In addition, exercise is associated with the maintenance or an increment in lean body mass.

D.   Drug Treatment for Obesity in the Elderly

The use of appetite suppressants to treat obesity in older patients will not be discussed here. However, because of the great interest in the use of trophic factors in the elderly, it is reasonable to discuss briefly how these factors may affect adiposity and fat distribution. This area has recently been thoroughly reviewed and the reader is referred to Ref. 143 for more details on this growing field. While age-related decrements in the growth hormone (GH)/insulin-like growth factor-I (IGF-I) axis have been implicated in the decline in FFM with aging, some data now indicate that changes in this axis might also account for the increase in central adiposity noted in the elderly. Indeed, studies in both growth-hormone-deficient adults replaced with GH and healthy older subjects supplemented with GH demonstrate reductions in both total and central adiposity. However, supplementation of older subjects with GH is not without significant side effects and long-term positive effects on lean mass, bone mass, fat mass, and, most important, strength and function remain unproved (144). There is no consensus about the effects of testosterone supplementation on adiposity in older men. While one study found no change in weight, body fat, or WHR, another found no change in total fat but a 10% decline in intra-abdominal adiposity after 9 months of testosterone supplementations. As noted above, there are also some data that suggest that estrogen replacement in women can prevent the postmenopausal accumulation of central fat.

ACKNOWLEDGMENTS

The author is supported by: NIH Grant RO-1 AG 10943, NIH Grant RO-1 DK 48152, NIH Grant UO-1 DK 48413, and NIH Grant P-30 DK 35816.

REFERENCES

1. Pi-Sunyer FX. Medical hazards of obesity. Ann Intern Med 1993; 119:655–660.
2. Mittelmark MB. The epidemiology of aging. In: Hazzard WR, Bierman EL, Blass JP, Ettinger WHJ, Halter JB, eds. The Principles of Geriatric Medicine and Gerontology. New York: McGraw-Hill, 1994:135–152.
3. Colditz GA. Economic costs of obesity. Am J Clin Nutr 1992; 55:503S–507S.
4. Kuczmarksi RJ, Flegal KM, Campbell SM, Johnson CL. Increasing prevalence of overweight among US adults. The National Health and Nutrition Examination Surveys, 1960 to 1991 [see comments]. JAMA 1994; 272: 205–211.
5. Manson JE, Willett WC, Stampfer, MJ, Colditz GA, Hunter DJ, Hankinson SE, Hennekens CH, Speizer FE. Body weight and mortality among women [see comments]. N Engl J Med 1995; 333:677–685.
6. Lee IM, Manson JE, Hennekens CH, Paffenbarger RS, Jr. Body weight and mortality. A 27-year follow-up of middle-aged men [see comments]. JAMA 1993; 270: 2823–2828.
7. Grinker JA, Tucker K, Vokonas PS, Rush D. Body habitus changes among adult males from the normative aging study: relations to aging, smoking history and alcohol intake. Obes Res 1995; 3:435–446.
8. Evans WJ, Campbell WW. Sarcopenia and age-related changes in body composition and functional capacity. J Nutr 1993; 123:465–468.
9. Frontera WR, Meredith CN, O'Reilly KP, Knuttgen HG, Evans WJ. Strength conditioning in older men: skeletal muscle hypertrophy and improved function. J Appl Physiol 1988; 64:1038–1044.
10. Fiatarone MA, Marks EC, Ryan ND, Meredith CN, Lipsitz LA, Evans WJ. High-intensity strength training in nonagenarians. Effects on skeletal muscle. JAMA 1990; 263: 3029–3034.
11. Buchner DM, Beresford SA, Larson EB, LaCroix AZ, Wagner EH. Effects of physical activity on health status in older adults. II. Intervention studies. Annu Rev Public Health 1992; 13:469–488.
12. Buchner DM, Cress ME, Wagner EH, de Lateur BJ, Price R, Abrass IB. The Seattle FICSIT/Movelt study: the effect of exercise on gait and balance in older adults. J Am Geriatr Soc 1993; 41:321–325.
13. Baumgartner RN, Stauber PM, McHugh D, Koehler KM, Garry PJ. Cross-sectional age differences in body composition in persons 60+ years of age. J Gerontol 1995; 50A:M307–M316.
14. Evans WJ. What is sarcopenia? J Gerontol 1995; 50A:5–8.
15. Flynn MA, Nolph GB, Baker AS, Martin WM, Krause G. Total body potassium in aging humans: a longitudinal study. Am J Clin Nutr 1989; 50:713–717.
16. Novak LP. Aging, total body potassium, fat-free mass, and cell mass in males and females between ages 18 and 85 years. J Gerontol 1972; 27:438–443.
17. Tzankoff SP, Norris AH. Longitudinal changes in basal metabolism in man. J Appl Physiol 1978; 45:536–539.
18. Cohn SH, Vartsky D, Yasumura S, Savitsky A, Zanzi I, Vaswani A, Ellis KJ. Compartmental body composition based on total-body potassium and calcium. Am J Physiol 1980; 239:E524–E530.
19. Baumgartner RN, Heymsfield SB, Roche AF. Human body composition and the epidemiology of chronic disease. Obes Res 195; 3:73–95.
20. Chumlea WC, Guo SS, Steinbaugh ML. Prediction of stature from knee height for black and white adults and children with application to mobility-impaired or handicapped persons. J Am Diet Assoc 1994; 94:1385–1388.
21. Chumlea WC, Roche AF, Webb P. Body size, subcutaneous fatness and total body fat in older adults. Int J Obes 1984; 8:311–317.
22. Baumgartner RN, Stauber PM, McHugh D, Wayne S, Garry PJ, Heymsfield SB. Body composition in the elderly using multicompartmental methods. Basic Life Sci 1993; 60:251–254.
23. Baumgartner RN, Heymsfield SB, Lichtman S, Wang J, Pierson RN Jr. Body composition in elderly people: effect of criterion estimates on predictive equations. Am J Clin Nutr 1991; 53:1345–1353.

24. Mazariegos M, Wang ZM, Gallager D, Baumgartner RN, Allison DB, Wang J, Pierson RN Jr, Heymsfield SB. Differences between young and old females in the five levels of body composition and their relevance to the two-compartment chemical model. J Gerontol 1994; 49: M201–208.

25. Hewitt MJ, Going SB, Williams DP, Lohman TG. Hydration of the fat-free body mass in children and adults: implications for body composition assessment. Am J Physiol 1993; 265:E88–95.

26. Chumlea WC, Guo SS. Bioelectrical impedance and body composition: present status and future directions [see comments]. Nutr Rev 1994; 52:123–131.

27. Lapidus L, Bengtsson C, Hallstrom T, Björntorp P. Obesity, adipose tissue distribution and health in women—results from a population study in Gothenburg, Sweden. Appetite 1989; 13:25–35.

28. Larsson B, Seidell J, Svardsudd K, Welin L, Tibblin G, Wilhelmsen L, Björntorp P. Obesity, adipose tissue distribution and health in men—the study of men born in 1913. Appetite 1989; 13:37–44.

29. Ohlson LO, Larsson B, Svardsudd K, Welin L, Eriksson H, Wilhelmsen L, Björntorp P, Tibblin G. The influence of body fat distribution on the incidence of diabetes mellitus. 13.5 years of follow-up of the participants in the study of men born in 1913. Diabetes 1985; 34: 1055–1058.

30. Larsson B, Svardsudd K, Welin L, Wilhelmsen L, Björntorp P, Tibbin G. Abdominal adipose tissue distribution, obesity, and risk of cardiovascular disease and death: 13 year follow-up of participants in the study of men born in 1913. Br Med J Clin Res Ed 1984; 288:1401–1404.

31. Krotkiewski M, Björntorp P, Sjostrom L, Smith U. Impact of obesity on metabolism in men and women. Importance of regional adipose tissue distribution. J Clin Invest 1983; 72:1150–1162.

32. Kissebah AH, Vydelingum N, Murray R, Evans DJ, Hartz AJ, Kalkhoff RK, Adams PW. Relation of body fat distribution to metabolic complications of obesity. J Clin Endocrinol Metab 1982; 54:254–260.

33. Stevens J, Knapp RG, Keil JE, Verdugo RR. Changes in body weight and girths in black and white adults studied over a 25 years interval. Int J Obes 1991; 15:803–808.

34. Carmelli D, McElroy MR, Rosenman RH. Longitudinal changes in fat distribution in the Western Collaborative Group Study: a 23-year follow-up. Int J Obes 1991; 15: 67–74.

35. Shimokata H, Tobin JD, Muller DC, Elahi D, Coon PJ, Andres R. Studies in the distribution of body fat. I. Effects of age, sex, and obesity. J Gerontol 1989; 44:M66–73.

36. Vague J. The degree of masculine differentiation of obesities: a factor determining predisposition to diabetes, atherosclerosis, gout and uric calculous disease. Am J Clin Nutr 1956; 4:20–34.

37. Svendsen OL, Hassager C, Christiansen C. Age- and menopause-associated variations in body composition and fat distribution in healthy women as measured by dual-energy X-ray absorptiometry. Metabolism 1995; 44: 369–373.

38. Poehlman ET, Toth MJ, Gardner AW. Changes in energy balance and body composition at menopause: a controlled longitudinal study. Ann Intern Med 1995; 123:673–675.

39. Ley CJ, Lees B, Stevenson JC. Sex- and menopause-associated changes in body-fat distribution. Am J Clin Nutr 1992; 55:950–954.

40. Kotani K, Tokunaga K, Fujioka S, Kobatake T, Keno Y, Yoshida S, Shimomura I, Tarui S, Matsuzawa Y. Sexual dimorphism of age-related changes in whole-body fat distribution in the obese. Int J Obes Relat Metab Disord 1994; 18:207–212.

41. Wang Q, Hassanger C, Ravn P, Wang S, Christiansen C. Total and regional body-composition changes in early postmenopausal women: age-related or menopause-related? Am J Clin Nutr 1994; 60:843–848.

42. Pasquali R, Casimirri F, Labate AM, Tortelli O, Pascal G, Anconetani B, Gatto MR, Flamia R, Capelli M, Barbara L. Body weight, fat distribution and the menopausal status in women. The VMH Collaborative Group. Int J Obes Relat Metab Disord 1994; 18:614–621.

43. Despr'es JP. Abdominal obesity as important component of insulin-resistance syndrome. Nutrition 1993; 9: 452–459.

44. Bouchard C, Despr'es JP, Mauriege P. Genetic and nongenetic determinants of regional fat distribution. Endocr Reve 1993; 14:72–93.

45. Pouliot MC, Despr'es JP, Nadeau A, Moorjani S, Prud'Homme D, Lupien PJ, Tremblay A, Bouchard C. Visceral obesity in men. Associations with glucose tolerance, plasma insulin, and lipoprotein levels. Diabetes 1992; 41: 826–834.

46. Matsuzawa Y, Shimomura I, Nakamura T, Keno Y, Tokunaga K. Pathophysiology and pathogenesis of visceral fat obesity. Ann NY Acad Sci 1995; 748:399–406.

47. Boyko EJ, Leonetti DL, Bergstrom RW, Newell Morris L, Fujimoto WY. Visceral adiposity, fasting plasma insulin, and blood pressure in Japanese-Americans. Diabetes Care 1995; 18:174–181.

48. Fujimoto WY, Bergstrom RW, Leonetti DL, Newell Morris LL, Shuman WP, Wahl PW. Metabolic and adipose risk factors for NIDDM and coronary disease in third-generation Japanese-American men and women with impaired glucose tolerance. Diabetologia 1994; 37:524–532.

49. Cefalu WT, Wang ZQ, Werbel S, Bell Farrow A, Crouse Jr, Hinson WH, Terry JG, Anderson R. Contribution of visceral fat mass to the insulin resistance of aging. Metabolism 1995; 44:954–959.

50. Schwartz RS, Shuman WP, Bradbury VL, Cain KC, Fellingham GW, Beard JC, Kahn SE, Stratton JR, Cerqueira MD, Abrass IB. Body fat distribution in healthy young and older men. J Gerontol 1990; 45:M181–185.

51. Borkan GA, Hults DE, Gerzof SG, Robbins AH, Silbert CK. Age changes in body composition revealed by computed tomography. J Gerontol 1983; 38:673–677.

52. Lemieux S, Prud'homme D, Bouchard C, Tremblay A, Despr'es JP. Sex differences in the relation of visceral adipose tissue accumulation to total body fatness. Am J Clin Nutr 1993; 58:463–467.

53. Baumgartner RN, Rhyne RL, Garry PJ, Chumlea WC. Body composition in the elderly from magnetic resonance imaging: associations with cardiovascular disease risk factors. Basic Life Sci 1993; 60:35–38.

54. Gasperino JA, Wang J, Pierson RN Jr, Heymsfield SB. Age-related changes in musculoskeletal mass between black and white women. Metabolism 1995; 44:30–34.

55. Freedman DS, Williamson DF, Croft JB, Ballew C, Byers T. Relation of body fat distribution to ischemic heart disease. The National Health and Nutrition Examination Survey I (NHANES I) Epidemiologic Follow-up Study. Am J Epidemiol 1995; 142:53–63.

56. Dowling HJ, Pi Sunyer FX. Race-dependent health risks of upper body obesity. Diabetes 193; 42:537–543.

57. Stevens J, Keil JE, Rust PF, Tyroler HA, Davis CE, Gazes PC. Body mass index and body girths as predictors of mortality in black and white women [see comments]. Arch Intern Med 1992; 152:1257–1262.

58. Stern MP, Patterson JK, Mitchell BD, Haffner SM, Hazuda HP. Overweight and mortality in Mexican Americans. Int J Obes 990; 14:623–629.

59. Fujimoto WY, Newell Morris LL, Grote M, Bergstrom RW, Shuman WP. Visceral fat obesity and morbidity: NIDDM and atherogenic risk in Japanese American men and women. Int J Obes 1991; 2:41–44.

60. Colditz GA. Epidemiology of breast cancer. Findings from the nurses' health study. Cancer 1993; 71:1480–1489.

61. Austin H, Austin JM Jr, Partridge EE, Hatch KD, Singleton HM. Endometrial cancer, obesity, and body fat distribution. Cancer Res 1991; 51:568–572.

62. Wing RR, Matthews KA, Kuller LH, Meilahn EN, Plantinga PL. Weight gain at the time of menopause. Arch Intern Med 1991; 151:97–102.

63. Haarbo J, Marslew U, Gotfredsen A, Christiansen C. Postmenopausal hormone replacement therapy prevents central distribution of body fat after menopause. Metabolism 1991; 40:1323–1326.

64. Garry PJ, Hunt WC, Koehler KM, VanderJagt DJ, Vellas BJ. Longitudinal study of dietary intakes and plasma lipids in healthy elderly men and women. Am J Clin Nutr 1992; 5:682–688.

65. Hallfrisch J, Muller D, Drinkwater D, Tobin J, Andres R. Continuing diet trends in men: The Baltimore Longitudinal Study of Aging (1961–1987). J Gerontol 1990; 45: M186–M191.

66. Swinburn B, Ravussin E. Energy balance or fat balance? Am J Clin Nutr 1993; 57:766S–770S.

67. Poehlman ET. Regulation of energy expenditure in aging humans. J Am Geriatr Soc 1993; 41:552–559.

68. Poehlman ET, Gardner AW, Goran MI. Influence of endurance training on energy intake, norepinephrine kinetics, and metabolic rate in older individuals. Metabolism 1992; 41:941–948.

69. Schultz LO, Nyomba BL, Alger S, Anderson TE, Ravussin E. Effect of endurance training on sedentary energy expenditure measured in a respiratory chamber. Am J Physiol 1991; 260:E257–261.

70. Schwartz RS, Jaeger LF, Veith RC. The thermic effect of feeding in older men: the importance of the sympathetic nervous system. Metabolism 1990; 39:733–737.

71. Tataranni PA, Larson DE, Snitker S, Ravussin E. Thermic effect of food in humans: methods and results from use of a respiratory chamber. Am J Clin Nutr 1995; 61: 1013–1019.

72. Wagner EH, LaCroix AZ, Buchner DM, Larson EB. Effects of physical activity on health status in older adults. I. Observational studies. Annu Rev Public Health 1992; 13: 451–468.

73. Poehlman ET, Copeland KC. Influence of physical activity on insulin-like growth factor-I in healthy younger and older men. J Clin Endocrinol Metab 1990; 71: 1468–1473.

74. Vaughan L, Zurlo F, Ravussin E. Aging and energy expenditure. Am J Clin Nutr 1991; 53:821–828.

75. Williamson DF, Madans J, Anda RF, Kleinman JC, Kahn HS, Byers T. Recreational physical activity and ten-year weight change in a US national cohort. Int J Obes Relat Metab Disord 1993; 17:279–286.

76. Goran MI, Calles-Escandon J, Poelman ET, O'Connell M, Danforth E Jr. Effects of increased energy intake and/or physical activity on energy expenditure in young healthy men. J Appl Physiol 1994; 77:366–372.

77. Rising R, Harper IT, Fontvielle AM, Ferraro RT, Spraul M, Ravussin E. Determinants of total daily energy expenditure: variability in physical activity. Am J Clin Nutr 1994; 59:800–804.

78. DeFronzo RA, Ferrannini E. Insulin resistance. A multifaceted syndrome responsible for NIDDM, obesity, hypertension, dyslipidemia, and atherosclerotic cardiovascular disease. Diabetes Care 1991; 14:173–194.

79. Chaiken RL, Banerji MA, Huey H, Lebovitz HE. Do blacks with NIDDM have an insulin-resistance syndrome? Diabetes 1993; 42:444–449.

80. Morales PA, Mitchell BD, Valdez RA, Hazuda HP, Stern MP, Haffner SM. Incidence of NIDDM and impaired glucose tolerance in hypertensive subjects. The San Antonio Heart Study. Diabetes 1993; 42:154–161.

81. Björntorp P. Abdominal obesity and the metabolic syndrome. Ann Med 1992; 24:465–468.

82. Ferrannini E. The insulin resistance syndrome. Curr Opin Nephrol Hypertens 1992; 1:291–298.

83. Lemieux S, Despr'es JP. Metabolic complications of visceral obesity: contribution to the aetiology of type 2 diabetes and implications for prevention and treatment. Diabetes Metab 1994; 20:375–393.

84. Mitchell BD, Haffner SM, Hazuda HP, Valdez R, Stern MP. The relation between serum insulin levels and 8-year changes in lipid, lipoprotein, and blood pressure levels. Am J Epidemiol 1992; 136:12–22.

85. Austin MA, Mykkanen L, Kuusisto J, Edwards KL, Nelson C, Haffner SM, Pyorala K, Laakso M. Prospective study of small LDLs as a risk factor for non-insulin dependent diabetes mellitus in elderly men and women. Circulation 1995; 92:1770–1778.

86. Despr'es JP, Marette A. Relation of components of insulin resistance syndrome to coronary disease risk. Curr Opin Lipidol 1994; 5:274–289.

87. Kahn SE, Schwartz RS, Porte DJ, Abrass IB. The glucose intolerance of aging: implications for intervention. Hosp Pract 1991; 26:29–38.

88. Harris MI. Epidemiology of diabetes mellitus among the elderly in the United States. Clin Geriatr Med 1990; 6: 703–719.

89. Rubin RJ, Altman WM, Mendelson DN. Health care expenditures for people with diabetes mellitus. J Clin Endocrinol Metab 1992; 78:809A–809F.

90. Meyers DA, Goldberg AP, Bleecker ML, Coon PJ, Drinkwater DT, Bleecker ER. Relationship of obesity and physical fitness to cardiopulmonary and metabolic function in healthy older men. J Gerontol 1991; 46:M57–65.

91. Kahn SE, Larson VG, Beard JC, Cain KC, Fellingham GW, Schwartz RS, Veith RC, Stratton JR, Cerqueira MD, Abrass IB. Effect of exercise on insulin action, glucose tolerance, and insulin secretion in aging. Am J Physiol 1990; 258: E937–943.

92. Coon PJ, Rogus EM, Drinkwater D, Muller DC, Goldberg AP. Role of body fat distribution in the decline in insulin sensitivity and glucose tolerance with age. J Clin Endocrinol Metab 1992; 75:1125–1132.

93. Shimokata H, Muller DC, Fleg JL, Sorkin J, Ziemba AW, Andres R. Age as independent determinant of glucose tolerance. Diabetes 1991; 40:44–51.

94. Kohrt WM, Kirwan JP, Staten MA, Bourey RE, King DS, Holloszy JO. Insulin resistance in aging is related to abdominal obesity. Diabetes 1993; 42:273–281.

95. Applegate WB. High blood pressure treatment in the elderly. Clin Geriatr Med 1992; 8:103–117.

96. Despr'es JP. Dyslipidaemia and obesity. Baillieres Clin Endocrinol Metab 1994; 8:629–660.

97. Katzel LI, Busby Whitehead MJ, Goldberg AP. Adverse effects of abdominal obesity on lipoprotein lipids in healthy older men. Exp Gerontol 1993; 28:411–420.

98. Chumlea WC, Baumgartner RN, Garry PJ, Rhyne RL, Nicholson C, Wayne S. Fat distribution and blood lipids in a sample of healthy elderly people. Int J Obes Relat Metab Disord 1992; 16:125–133.

99. Mykkanen L, Laakso M, Pyorala K. Association of obesity and distribution of obesity with glucose tolerance and cardiovascular risk factors in the elderly. Int J Obes Relat Metab Disord 1992; 16:695–704.

100. Mykkanen L, Kuusisto J, Haffner SM, Pyorala K, Laakso M. Hyperinsulinemia predicts multiple atherogenic changes in lipoproteins in elderly subjects. Arterioscler Thromb 1994; 14:518–526.

101. Andres R. Mortality and obesity: the rationale for age-specific height-weight tables. In: Hazzard WR, Bierman EL, Blass JP, Ettinger WHJ, Halter JB, eds. Principles of Geriatric Medicine and Gerontology. New York: McGraw-Hill, 1994:847–853.

102. Harris T, Cook EF, Garrison R, Higgins M, Kannel W, Goldman L. Body mass index and mortality among nonsmoking older persons. The Framingham Heart Study. JAMA 1988; 259:1520–1524.

103. Garrison RJ, Castelli WP. Weight and thirty-year mortality of men in the Framingham Study. Ann Intern Med 1985; 103:1006–1009.

104. Cornoni Huntley JC, Harris TB, Everett DF, Albanes D, Micozzi MS, Miles TP, Feldman JJ. An overview of body weight of older persons, including the impact on mortality. The National Health and Nutrition Examination Survey I—Epidemiologic Follow-up Study. J Clin Epidemiol 1991; 44:743–753.

105. Willett WC, Manson JE, Stampfer MJ, Colditz GA, Rosner B, Speizer FE, Hennekens CH. Weight, weight change, and coronary heart disease in women. Risk within the "normal" weight range [see comments]. JAMA 1995; 273: 461–465.

106. Colditz GA, Willett WC, Rotnitzky A, Manson JE. Weight gain as a risk factor for clinical diabetes mellitus in women [see comments]. Ann Intern Med 1995; 122: 481–486.

107. Blair SN, Shaten J, Brownell K, Collins G, Lissner L. Body weight change, all-cause mortality, and cause-specific mortality in the Multiple Risk Factor Intervention Trial [see comments]. Ann Intern Med 1993; 119:749–757.

108. Lee IM, Paffenbarger RS Jr. Change in body weight and longevity [see comments]. JAMA 1992; 268:2045–2049.

109. Andres R, Muller DC, Sorkin JD. Long-term effects of change in body weight on all-cause mortality. A review [see comments]. Ann Intern Med 1993; 119:737–743.

110. Ho SC, Woo J, Sham A. Risk factor change in older persons, a perspective from Hong Kong: weight change and mortality. J Gerontol 1994; 49:M269–272.

111. Iribarren C, Sharp DS, Burchfiel CM, Petrovitch H. Association of weight loss and weight fluctuation with mortality among Japanese American men [see comments]. N Engl J Med 1995; 333:686–692.

112. Williamson DF, Pamuk ER. The association between weight loss and increased longevity. A review of the evidence. Ann Intern Med 1993; 119:731–736.

113. Pamuk ER, Williamson DF, Serdula MK, Madans J, Byers TE. Weight loss and subsequent death in a cohort of U.S. adults. Ann Intern Med 1993; 119:744–748.

114. Williamson DF, Pamuk E, Thun M, Flanders D, Byers T, Heath C. Prospective study of intentional weight loss and

mortality in never-smoking overweight US white women aged 40–64 years [published erratum appears in Am J Epidemiol 1995 I; 142(3):369]. Am J Epidemiol 1995; 141:1128–1141.

115. Verdery RB. Failure to thrive in the elderly. Clin Geriatr Med 1995; 11:653–660.

116. Dengel DR, Hagberg JM, Coon PJ, Drinkwater DT, Goldberg AP. Effects of weight loss by diet alone or combined with aerobic exercise on body composition in older obese men. Metabolism 1994; 43:867–871.

117. Schwartz RS, Barsness S. Effect of moderate dietary restriction (MDR) on body composition in older men. Gerontologist 1993; 33:139.

118. Colman E, Katzel LI, Rogus E, Coon P, Muller D, Goldberg AP. Weight loss reduces abdominal fat and improves insulin action in middle-aged and older men with impaired glucose tolerance. Metabolism 1995; 44: 1502–1508.

119. Dengel DR, Hagberg JM, Coon PJ, Drinkwater DT, Goldberg AP. Comparable effects of diet and exercise on body composition and lipoproteins in older men. Med Sci Sports Exerc 1994; 26:1307–1315.

120. Abrass IB, Barsness S, Schwartz RS. Effect of moderate dietary restriction (MDR) on lipid profiles in older men. Gerontologist 1993; 33:43.

121. Nevin DN, Schwartz RS, Brunzell JD. Evidence that central obesity modulates genetic expression of low density lipoprotein subclass phenotype B. Diabetes 1994; 43(Suppl 1):35A.

122. Schwartz RS, Buchner DM. Exercise in the elderly: physiologic and functional effects. In: Hazzard WR, Bierman EL, Blass JP, Ettinger WHJ, Halter JB, eds. Principles of Geriatric Medicine and Gerontology, Vol 3. New York: McGraw-Hill, 1994:91–105.

123. Wilmore JH. Variations in physical activity habits and body composition. Int J Obes Metab Dis 1995; 19: S107–S112.

124. Barlow CE, Kohl HW, Gibbons LW, Blair SN. Physical fitness, mortality and obesity. Int J Obes Metab Dis 1995; 19:S41–S44.

125. Schwartz RS, Hirth VA. The effects of endurance and resistance training on blood pressure. Int J Obes Metab Dis 1995; 19:S52–S57.

126. Helmrich SP, Ragland DR, Leung RW, Paffenbarger RS Jr. Physical activity and reduced occurrence of non-insulin-dependent diabetes mellitus [see comments]. N Engl J Med 1991; 325:147–152.

127. Despres JP, Lamarche B, Bouchard C, Tremblay A, Prud'homme D. Exercise and the prevention of dyslipidemia and coronary heart disease. Int J Obes Metab Dis 1995; 19:S45–S51.

128. Pavlov KN, Krey S, Steffee WP. Exercise as an adjunct to weight loss and maintenance in moderately obese subjects. Am J Clin Nutr 1989; 49:1115–1123.

129. Ewbank PP, Darga LL, Lucas CP. Physical activity as a predictor of weight maintenance in previously obese subjects. Obes Res 1995; 3:257–263.

130. Schwartz RS, Shuman WP, Larson V, Cain KC, Fellingham GW, Beard JC, Kahn SE, Stratton JR, Cerqueira MD, Abrass IB. The effect of intensive endurance exercise training on body fat distribution in young and older men. Metabolism 1991; 40:545–551.

131. Kohrt WM, Obert KA, Holloszy JO. Exercise training improves fat distribution patterns in 60- to 70-year-old men and women. J Gerontol 1992; 47:M99–105.

132. Schwartz RS, Cain KC, Shuman WP, Larson V, Stratton JR, Beard JC, Kahn SE, Cerqueira MD, Abrass IB. Effect of intensive endurance training on lipoprotein profiles in young and older men. Metabolism 1992; 41:649–654.

133. Kirwan JP, Kohrt WM, Wojta DM, Bourey RE, Holloszy JO. Endurance exercise training reduces glucose-stimulated insulin levels in 60- to 70-year-old men and women. J Gerontol 1993; 48:M84–90.

134. Katzel LI, Bleecker ER, Colman EG, Rogus EMS JD, Goldberg AP. Effects of weight loss vs. aerobic exercise training on risk factors for coronary disease in healthy, obese, middle-aged and older men. JAMA 1995; 274:1915–1921.

135. Goran MI, Poehlman ET. Endurance training does not enhance total energy expenditure in healthy elderly persons. Am J Physiol 1992; 263:E950–957.

136. Poehlman ET, Danforth E Jr. Endurance training increases metabolic rate and norepinephrine appearance rate in older individuals. Am J Physiol 1991; 261:E233–239.

137. Poehlman ET, Gardner AW, Arciero PJ, Goran MI, Calles-Escandon J. Effects of endurance training on total fat oxidation in elderly persons. Am J Physiol 1994; 76: 2281–2287.

138. Treuth MS, Ryan AS, Pratley RE, Rubin MA, Miller JP, Nicklas BJ, Sorkin J, Harman SM, Goldberg AP, Hurley BF. Effects of strength training on total and regional body composition in older men [published erratum appears in J Appl Physiol 1994; 77(6):following table of contents]. J Appl Physiol 1994; 77:614–620.

139. Treuth MS, Hunter GR, Kekes Szabo T, Weinsier RL, Goran MI, Berland L. Reduction in intra-abdominal adipose tissue after strength training in older women. J Appl Physiol 1995; 78:1425–1431.

140. Miller JP, Pratley RE, Goldberg AP, Gordon P, Rubin M, Treuth MS, Ryan AS, Hurley BF. Strength training increases insulin action in healthy 50- to 65-yr-old men. J Appl Physiol 1994; 77:1122–1127.

141. Smutok MA, Reece C, Kokkinos PF, Farmer C, Dawson P, Shulman R, DeVane Bell J, Patterson J, Charabogos C, Goldberg AP, et al. Aerobic versus strength training for risk factor intervention in middle-aged men at high risk for coronary heart disease. Metabolism 1993; 42: 177–184.

142. Kokkinos PF, Hurley BF, Smutok MA, Farmer C, Reece C, Shulman R, Charabogos C, Patterson J, Will S, Devane-Bell J, et al. Strength training does not improve

lipoprotein-lipid profiles in men at risk for CHD [see comments]. Med Sci Sports Exerc 1991; 23:1134–1139.

143. Schwartz RS. Trophic factor supplementations: effect on age-associated changes in body composition. J Gerontol 1995; 50A:151–156.

144. Papadakis MA, Grady D, Black D, Tierney MJ, Gooding GAW, Schambelan M, Grunfeld C. Growth hormone replacement in healthy older men improved body composition but not functional ability. Ann Intern Med 1996; 124:708–716.

7

Obesity and Eating Disorders

Susan Zelitch Yanovski

National Institute of Diabetes and Digestive and Kidney Diseases, National Institutes of Health, Bethesda, Maryland

I. INTRODUCTION

Eating disorders are psychophysiological disturbances characterized by abnormalities in affects, cognitions, and behaviors regarding food intake and body image. While predominantly affecting adolescent and young adult women, these illnesses affect individuals of both genders and a wide range of ages. Eating disorders are also found across the spectrum of weights, from the emaciated individual with anorexia nervosa to the severely obese patient with binge eating disorder. Left untreated, eating disorders can result in severe functional disability, or even death, in individuals at an otherwise healthy time of life.

Disordered eating may manifest itself through dietary restriction, binge eating, or both. Other inappropriate compensatory behaviors used to control weight include vomiting, abuse of diuretics, laxatives, anorexiant medications, or thyroid hormones, and excessive exercise.

Binge eating is defined as eating, in a discrete period of time (e.g., within any 2-hr period), an amount of food that is definitely larger than most people would eat in a similar period of time *plus* a sense of lack of control over eating during the episode (e.g., a feeling that one cannot stop eating or control what or how much one is eating) (1). Note that both consumption of an objectively large amount of food and sense of loss of control are necessary for the definition of a binge episode. Loss of control in the absence of consumption of a large amount of food (e.g., a self-described "binge" consisting of two cookies) is considered a "subjective" bulimic episode. Conversely, an

objectively large amount of food consumed without a concomitant feeling of loss of control is considered an "objective" overeating episode (2).

II. DIAGNOSTIC CHARACTERISTICS

Anorexia nervosa is characterized by refusal to maintain a normal body weight, along with a fear of gaining weight. Diagnostic criteria for anorexia nervosa are shown in Table 1A. The *Diagnostic and Statistical Manual of Mental Disorders*, 4th Edition (DSM-IV) (1) criteria divide anorexia into the restricting and binge-eating/purging subtypes. Approximately 50% of patients with anorexia nervosa experience binge eating and/or purging at some point in their illness.

Bulimia nervosa is characterized by frequent episodes of binge eating accompanied by emotional distress, plus the presence of frequent compensatory behaviors to avoid weight gain (Table 1, B.) (1). The DSM-IV further classifies patients as belonging to the purging or nonpurging subtypes. Purging is common in bulimia nervosa, and includes vomiting (80–90%) and laxative use (38–75%) (4). Less common forms of purging include diuretic abuse, abuse of thyroid hormone or anorexiant medications, induction of vomiting through use of ipecac, and use of enemas. Diabetics have been known to withhold insulin to avoid weight gain (5).

Binge eating disorder is a newly described eating disorder characterized by frequent episodes of binge eating accompanied by emotional distress, but without the regular

115

Table 1 Diagnostic Criteria for Eating Disorders

A. Anorexia Nervosa
A. Refusal to maintain body weight at or above a minimally normal weight for age and height
B. Intense fear of gaining weight or becoming fat, even though underweight
C. Disturbance in the way in which one's body or shape is experienced.
D. In postmenarchal females, amenorrhea
E. Type:
  Restricting type
  Binge-eating/purging type

B. Bulimia Nervosa
A. Recurrent episodes of binge eating
B. Recurrent inappropriate compensatory behaviors to prevent weight gain
C. The binge eating and inappropriate compensatory behaviors both occur, on average, at least twice a week for 3 months
D. Self-evaluation is unduly influenced by body weight and shape
E. Type:
  Purging type
  Nonpurging type

C. Binge Eating Disorder[a]
A. Recurrent episodes of binge eating
B. The binge eating episodes are associated with at least three behavioral indicators of loss of control
C. Marked distress regarding binge eating
D. The binge eating occurs, on average, at least 2 days a week for 6 months
E. The binge eating is not associated with the regular use of inappropriate compensatory behaviors and does not occur exclusively during the course of anorexia nervosa or bulimia nervosa

[a]Diagnostic criteria for binge eating disorder are listed in the Appendix of the DSM-IV as an example of eating disorder, not otherwise specified (p. 729).
Source: Summary of the DSM-IV Criteria. Washington, DC: American Psychiatric Association, 1994.

use of compensatory behaviors (Table 1, C.). Binge eating disorder is listed in the DSM-IV in an appendix as an example of an Eating Disorder Not Otherwise Specified (EDNOS). A diagnosis of EDNOS is also used for disordered eating that does not meet criteria for one of the established eating disorders (e.g., purging only once weekly, weight loss without amenorrhea, etc.)

III. EPIDEMIOLOGY

Anorexia nervosa, as categorized by the DSM-IV, is relatively uncommon, affecting 0.5–1% of adolescent and young adult women (6), although a much larger percentage experience subthreshold symptoms. Approximately 5–10% of patients with anorexia nervosa are male (7). There is some evidence that the incidence of anorexia nervosa is increasing among adolescents, but not adults (8). Although most individuals with anorexia nervosa are adolescents or young adults, onset has been reported in prepubertal children and postmenopausal women (9). It is more common in industrialized societies where food is plentiful and thinness is valued, but anorexia nervosa is found in individuals from all cultures and social strata (10,11).

The prevalence of bulimia nervosa has been estimated at 1–3% of high school and college-age women (6,12), although a much greater percentage engage in bulimic behaviors, such as binge eating and/or purging, that are not of sufficient frequency or duration to meet criteria for the disorder (13,14). Ten to fifteen percent of patients with bulimia nervosa are male (15), and it is more frequent in homosexual men (16) and athletes who must "make weight" for competition, such as wrestlers (17). Bulimia nervosa is found in all racial, ethnic, and socioeconomic groups (18). A substantial subset of patients with bulimia nervosa have previously met criteria for anorexia nervosa, with some studies reporting such a history in up to 60% (19).

Binge eating disorder is the most common eating disorder, affecting 2–3% of the general population (20–22). Its prevalence increases with increasing severity of adiposity, affecting about 5% of obese individuals in the community, 10–15% of mildly obese individuals in commercial weight-loss programs, and about 30% of obese individuals seeking specialized treatment, such as very low calorie diet programs (23). The prevalence of binge eating disorder among severely obese individuals undergoing bariatric surgery may exceed 50% (24). Unlike anorexia nervosa and bulimia nervosa, a large proportion of individuals with binge eating disorder are men, estimated at 40% in the original field studies (20,21). The age at diagnosis of binge eating disorder is older than that seen in anorexia nervosa or bulimia nervosa, averaging in the mid- to late thirties; however, age of onset of significant binge eating is often a decade or more earlier (23). An age-matched study of patients with bulimia nervosa and binge eating disorder showed a younger age of onset of binge eating behavior among those with binge eating disorder (14.3 vs 19.8 years), although both groups reported first dieting at similar ages (15.0 vs. 16.2 years) (25).

IV. PATHOPHYSIOLOGY

A. Individual and Familial Psychological Factors

A number of psychological factors have been described in patients with eating disorders, including difficulties in self-esteem and self-regulation, along with a sense of ineffectiveness and helplessness. Eating disorders, in this view, represent the attempt of the patient to gain control in the arena of eating and weight. Girls who are conflicted about maturation and sexuality are felt to be particularly prone to the development of anorexia nervosa. There are limitations in determining the premorbid psychological factors that may predispose to the development of eating disorders, primary among which is that this information has generally been obtained retrospectively, after the eating disorder has developed.

B. Sociocultural Factors

It has been proposed that "dieting disorders," is a more proper term than "eating disorder" because the underlying essential feature of anorexia nervosa, bulimia nervosa, and associated conditions is "the inappropriate and excessive pursuit of thinness" (26). For individuals with either anorexia nervosa or bulimia nervosa, attempts at weight loss and dietary restriction (often severe) almost invariably precede the development of the significant symptoms of disordered eating. The current cultural milieu, in which thinness, fitness, and body shapes that are impossible for most women to obtain are prized, no doubt contribute to the dissatisfaction with body size and shape that is normative among women. While most women have tried to lose weight, relatively few develop eating disorders (27), leading some investigators to suggest that dieting may be a "necessary, but insufficient" condition for the development of eating disorders (28). The relationship between *dietary restraint* and binge eating is complex, and many factors, including the type and degree of dietary restraint, individual psychological and biological predispositions, and the sociocultural milieu, may contribute to binge eating in the susceptible individual.

The link between dieting and the development of disordered eating is even less in binge eating disorder than in anorexia or bulimia nervosa (29). Studies to date have indicated that binge eating precedes or occurs at approximately the same time as first attempts of weight loss in about half of all subjects (21,30); however, these studies have the disadvantage of being retrospective. Berkowitz et al. (31), have evaluated obese adolescent girls, many of whom had not previously attempted weight loss, and found a significant percentage who nonetheless reported

serious difficulties with binge eating. Some studies suggest that, rather than being "restrained" eaters, obese binge eaters exhibit high levels of disinhibition, or loss of control due to affective, pharmacological, or cognitive stimuli (32,33). Marcus et al. have found that, when compared to bulimia nervosa patients, obese binge eaters report less dietary restraint, but score similarly on other measures of eating disorders psychopathology regarding weight and shape (34). This finding has implications for the modification of treatments developed for bulimia nervosa to address the special needs of nonpurging obese binge eaters.

C. Affective Disorders

Affective disorders are common among patients with eating disorders, leading some researchers to postulate that eating disorders are a variant of affective disorders. Comorbid major depression is frequent among patients with eating disorders (35–37), occurring in over half of all patients in some series. In addition, family history of affective disorders is often more frequent among patients than controls. The response of symptoms to antidepressant treatment, in both bulimia nervosa and binge eating disorder, has been proposed as further evidence of this link. However, it is unknown if the depression seen in bulimia nervosa and binge eating disorder is primary, secondary to the eating disorder, or due to an underlying common pathogenesis. Dysfunction of the serotonergic pathways, which could affect both appetite and mood, has been postulated as one such possible mechanism (38). While depression is common in patients with anorexia nervosa, at least some of these symptoms may be secondary to the accompanying starvation, as similar affective symptoms have been produced in normal volunteers undergoing long-term semistarvation (39). Therefore, the relationship between eating disorders and affective disorders remains unclear.

D. Other Comorbid Psychiatric Conditions

Obsessive-compulsive disorder is reportedly more frequent in both anorexia nervosa and bulimia nervosa (40), and some researchers have speculated that disturbances in neurally active substances, such as central arginine vasopressin, may contribute to the perpetuation of compulsive behaviors in patients these disorders (41). Among individuals with binge eating disorder, no increase in either obsessive-compulsive disorder or obsessive-compulsive personality disorder has been noted (36). Other anxiety and related disorders, such as generalized anxiety disorder and phobias, are also common in eating disorders (42,43).

Personality disorders involving impulsivity (including borderline personality disorder), are found more frequently in those with eating disorders involving binge eating than among controls, across the weight spectrum. For example, one study found that obese individuals with binge eating disorder have a 14 percent prevalence of borderline personality disorder versus only 1 percent of obese individuals without binge eating disorder (36). Avoidant personality disorder has also been reported to be more prevalent among these subjects with than without binge eating disorder (36,44).

Binge eating is also associated with a higher likelihood of substance abuse than is seen in control populations, in both the binge eating subtype of anorexia nervosa (45), bulimia nervosa (46), and binge eating disorder (21). Among obese individuals, a family history of substance abuse is more likely among individuals with than without binge eating disorder (36). Similarly, studies of patients with bulimia nervosa and the purging subtype of anorexia nervosa have found high rates of substance abuse in among relatives of patients compared with controls (47,48).

To summarize, psychiatric comorbidity is common in patients with eating disorders. Among obese individuals, the presence of binge eating disorder may explain the increased levels of psychopathology previously attributed to the presence of obesity per se (36,49,50).

E. Biological Predisposition

Biological predisposition to eating disorders has been proposed. Twin studies have indicated that anorexia nervosa is more likely in identical than in fraternal twins, supporting a genetic predisposition for the disorder (51). Although abnormalities in numerous neuroendocrine and metabolic systems have been described in eating disorders, it is often difficult to sort out the effects of semistarvation or purging behaviors from disturbances that might be primary (52). Few data are available to support preexisting neuroendocrine or other physiological differences among those who will later develop eating disorders, but the possibility exists that a biological vulnerability to eating disorders interacts with environmental factors to increase the likelihood of their development.

F. Sexual Abuse

The contribution of sexual abuse to the development of eating disorders remains controversial. While some authors have cited sexual abuse as a major causal factor in eating disorders (53), others have found that the prevalence of sexual abuse is no greater in eating disordered patients than in patients being treated for other psychiatric disorders (54). It has been suggested that some types of sexual abuse, such as earlier and more persistent abuse, may predispose to eating disorders, and that it is binge eating, rather than dietary restriction that is associated with sexual abuse (55). Although sexual abuse may play a direct role in the development of eating disorders for some patients, it appears to be a risk factor for psychiatric disorders in general, rather than specific for eating disorders (56).

G. Addiction

Addiction has been postulated to play a role in disordered eating, with some individuals addicted to certain foods or combinations of foods. Although substance abuse and other impulse control disorders are associated with binge eating in some studies, there is no evidence that "addiction" to foods such as refined flour, simple sugars, or carbohydrates occurs or triggers binge episodes (57). A recent, and interesting, finding, however, is that both lean and obese female binge eaters, women with binge eating disorder, who prefer to binge on foods that are both sweet and high in fat, may decrease their intake of these foods selectively when given naloxone (58). The role of β-endorphins and other endogenous opioids in the development or maintenance of binge eating, while unknown, is intriguing.

V. SIGNS AND SYMPTOMS

Eating disorders are often "hidden disorders" and will not be recognized without gentle probing by the clinician. Both anorexia nervosa and bulimia nervosa, however, are associated with a host of medical complications, affecting virtually every organ system.

A. Anorexia Nervosa

In patients with anorexia nervosa, emaciation will be obvious. Often, the patient is brought to the clinician's attention by the family, who are concerned about weight loss. The patient frequently tries to minimize concerns about her intake and low body weight, and may resort to subterfuge, such as wearing heavy clothing while being weighed.

Although physical complaints are remarkably few given the degree of emaciation (59), patients present with a variety of signs and symptoms referable to low body weight.

These including constipation, abdominal pain, cold intolerance, hypothermia, hypotension, bradycardia, edema, lanugo, and dry skin (59). Hypercarotenemia, with its resultant yellow-orange discoloration of skin, may result from excessive ingestion of orange fruits and vegetables, or from abnormalities in vitamin A absorption or metabolism (60). Amenorrhea, as one of the necessary criteria for diagnosis, is present in all women, but men also show evidence of a hypgoonadal state. Laboratory abnormalities, particularly in patients who purge, are frequent, and include electrolyte abnormalities, elevation of liver enzymes, elevated blood urea nitrogen, hypercholesterolemia, and normochromic normocytic anemia (61).

Anorexia nervosa, with its resultant hypoestrogenemic state, predisposes patients to osteoporosis, which may be severe. The best predictors of bone loss are low body weight, early onset and long duration of amenorrhea, low calcium intake, and hypercortisolism (62). The role of estrogen replacement in anorexia nervosa in order to prevent osteoporosis is controversial, with studies yielding mixed results (63,64). Bone density does improve with weight recovery and resumption of menses, although it usually remains significantly below control levels many years later (65,66).

B. Bulimia Nervosa

Patients with bulimia nervosa frequently show no abnormalities on physical examination. In one study, the most frequent reason for presentation to a general practitioner of the bulimic patient was to request a weight loss diet (67). Other common presenting complaints include gastrointestinal symptoms, such as bloating or constipation, amenorrhea, or irregular cycles (68). Rarely, patients may present with palpitations or cardiac arrhythmias secondary to electrolyte imbalance. Pathognomonic signs in bulimia nervosa include a "chipmunk" cheek appearance, due to non-inflammatory stimulation of the salivary glands, particularly the parotids (69) (Fig. 1). Erosions of the lingual surface of the teeth and multiple dental caries are seen, due to the exposure to acid from repeated vomiting (70). Russell's sign (71) (scarring and abrasions on the dorsum of the hands during self-induced vomiting) can also be seen (Fig. 2). Laboratory abnormalities, which may be frequent in purging patients, include metabolic alkalosis and hypokalemia (72).

Hyperamylasemia is seen in about one-third of actively binge eating/purging patients and is due to elevation of the salivary isoenzyme, secondary to vomiting (73). Rare, but serious complications of bulimia nervosa include

Mallory-Weiss tears of the esophagus due to forceful vomiting, and cardiomyopathy secondary to ipecac abuse.

C. Binge Eating Disorder

Patients with binge eating disorder are frequently obese and may present with obesity-associated disorders. Patients with binge eating disorder are also more likely than obese nonbinge eaters to present with signs of gastrointestinal disturbance, such as nausea, vomiting, abdominal pain, and bloating (74).

VI. TREATMENT

A. Anorexia Nervosa

Anorexia nervosa is treated through a combination of nutritional rehabilitation and psychotherapy, with the goals of weight restoration, development of healthy eating habits, improvement in moods/behaviors, reduction in obsessions with thinness, and amelioration of concomitant physical and psychiatric symptoms (6).

1. Nutritional Rehabilitation

Nutritional rehabilitation is crucial and should be accomplished either prior to or concomitant with psychotherapy. The involvement of a dietician for meal planning is helpful. Refeeding should be slow and cautious, to prevent edema and cardiac failure (75). Use of enteral or parenteral feeding is generally unnecessary, unless life-threatening inanition is present and the patient refuses oral feeding (6). Behavioral modification, in which privileges are tied to specified weight gain, may be useful in the initial stages for promoting increased intake.

2. Psychotherapy

Psychotherapy may be provided individually or in groups. In younger patients with anorexia nervosa, who frequently live with their family of origin, family therapy is also used. Individual psychological therapies include cognitive-behavioral psychotherapy, in which faulty cognition regarding eating and weight are examined, and psychodynamic or interpersonal psychotherapy, in which the patient's current interpersonal relationships with others are explored. Cognitive behavioral psychotherapy is described in more detail below. In patients undergoing inpatient or partial hospitalization, the therapeutic milieu is also an integral part of treatment.

In the current climate of managed care, inpatient treatment is increasingly being replaced by less expensive and

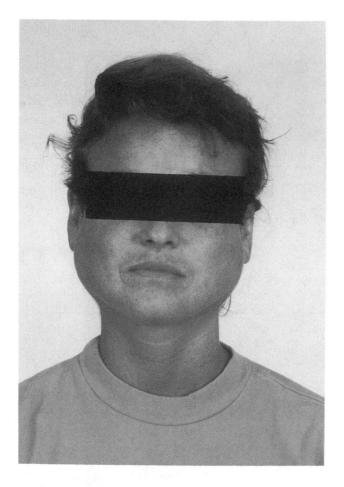

Figure 1 Bilateral parotid gland swelling associated with bulimia nervosa. (Reprinted from Yanovski SZ. Bulimia nervosa: the role of the family physician. Am Fam Physician 1991; 44:1234.)

orexia nervosa. Short-term administration of *anxiolytics* before meals is sometimes useful in helping patients who have a great deal of anxiety during refeeding, but has little role in long-term management (78). While *antidepressant medications* can be useful in patients with concomitant depression, it is generally preferable to reassess mood after nutritional rehabilitation, as semistarvation can produce both cognitive and affective changes. However, a few open-label trials suggest that fluoxetine may have efficacy in preventing relapse in the subset of patients with anorexia nervosa who have achieved their goal weight (79,80). *Cyproheptadine*, a serotonin antagonist, is an antihistamine known to increase appetite and cause weight gain. Thus, it has been tried as a therapeutic agent to promote weight gain in anorexia nervosa. While studies of its efficacy have been equivocal, Halmi and colleagues have found a small benefit in the subgroup of restricting anorectics, while worsening symptoms in the subgroup of anorexics with bulimic symptoms (81).

To summarize, the role of medication in the treatment of anorexia nervosa is limited at present. While some reports suggest the potential for modest improvements in selected subgroups of patients with certain medications, more research is needed to further characterize the optimal use of these agents.

B. Bulimia Nervosa

Bulimia nervosa is generally treated in an outpatient setting. Both psychotherapy and medication have been shown to be efficacious in the treatment of bulimia nervosa.

1. Cognitive-Behavioral Psychotherapy (CBT)

CBT is the most well-studied psychological treatment for bulimia nervosa and is generally considered first-line treatment for this disorder (82). Originally developed by Fairburn (83), CBT is based on the premise that central to the disorder are maladaptive cognitions regarding the fundamental importance of weight and shape. In this model, the extremes of dietary restraint that are used to control weight lead to compensatory binge eating. Thus, the modification of these abnormal attitudes and behaviors of weight and shape may be expected to ameliorate the consequent dietary restriction, binge eating, and purging (84). While modifications of the technique are frequent, the original program consisted of time-limited, individual treatment given over 20 weeks (85).

Studies of treatment efficacy show very good short-term outcomes for CBT. Reviews have shown mean re-

intensive therapies, including outpatient care and partial hospitalization. One randomized study has shown good outcomes in anorexic patients assigned to outpatient treatment (76). However, many experts believe that inpatient treatment is preferable for all but the most mild forms of anorexia nervosa (6). While anorexia nervosa is the diagnosis most likely to require hospitalization, there are indications for hospitalization in patients with any of the eating disorders (Table 2).

3. Medications

Medications are less often used in the treatment of anorexia nervosa than in bulimia nervosa. Few medications have proven effective in long-term studies. *Antipsychotic medications* show no benefit in long-term weight recovery (77,78) and are now rarely used in the treatment of an-

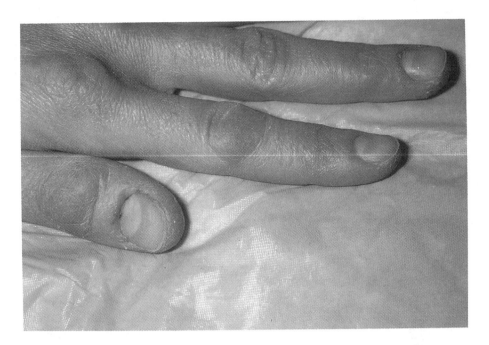

Figure 2 Scarring on the dorsum of the hand due to self-induced vomiting.

ductions in binge eating and purging of from 79 to 86%, with about half of patients "abstinent" from binge eating or purging at the end of treatment (86).

2. Interpersonal Psychotherapy (IPT)

IPT has also been shown to improve symptoms in bulimia nervosa. This type of psychotherapy, originally developed for the treatment of depression, has been adapted for the treatment of eating disorders. In contrast to CBT, which

Table 2 Indications for Hospitalization in Eating Disorders

Medical
   Extreme emaciation (<70% of ideal body weight)
   Dangerous medical complications (e.g., renal failure, hypokalemia, arrhythmias)
   Intercurrent infection
   Suicidal tendencies or attempts
Psychosocial
   Marked family disturbance inaccessible to treatment
   Inability to function at work or school
Psychotherapeutic
   Previous treatment failures
   Nonavailability of specialized treatment in the community
   Failure to respond to optimal outpatient care

focuses on the elimination of dietary restriction and distorted cognitions about weight and shape, IPT focuses on improving negative moods and low self-esteem that may trigger binge eating, through the mastery of social and interpersonal relationships (87). IPT has been shown to have similar efficacy to CBT in reducing binge eating in bulimia nervosa, although it is somewhat less effective in reducing purging, dietary restraint, and dysfunctional attitudes toward weight and shape at the end of treatment (88). At longer-term follow-up, up to 6 years, both treatments appear to be equally efficacious (89).

3. Antidepressant Medications

Antidepressants, including tricyclics, monoamine oxidase inhibitors, and selective serotonin reuptake inhibitors (SSRI), are frequently used in the treatment of bulimia nervosa and have been proven effective in numerous studies (90). Monoamine oxidase inhibitors (MAOI) have the disadvantage of requiring restriction of certain foods, which may be difficult for some bulimic patients. SSRI, such as fluoxetine, have fewer adverse effects than tricyclics and MAOI, and have the additional advantage of not causing weight gain. While trials with a variety of antidepressant agents of different classes have shown short-term efficacy in reduction of binge eating, there are a number of limitations to these studies. Most were conducted using fixed dosages over relatively short periods of time and involved populations of normal-weight, purging women. Thus, the optimal dose ranges, duration of treatment, and treatment response in the nonpurging bulimic patient are not clear. In a dose-response study of fluoxetine for bulimia nervosa, the most effective dose was 60 mg/day, significantly higher than that used for depression (91). There is no evidence that history of physical abuse predicts responsiveness of bulimic symptoms to fluoxetine, although a greater response to nonspecific symptoms such as depression has been noted in one study (92).

Antidepressant treatment, while more effective than placebo, is not a "magic bullet." Walsh et al. (93) found that while antidepressant treatment reduced frequency of binge eating in bulimic patients, many were still symptomatic at the end of the 8-week treatment period, and only a small minority completely abstinent from binge eating and purging. In addition, almost half of patients who showed initial improvement relapsed over the subsequent 4 months, despite continued use of the drug. Most experts do not recommend medication alone in the treatment of bulimia nervosa (90). There is some support for switching antidepressant medications if a patient fails to respond to one drug (90,94).

4.   Other Pharmacotherapeutic Agents

Other pharmacotherapeutic agents that have been evaluated for bulimia nervosa include *anticonvulsants* (95), *lithium carbonate* (96), L-*tryptophan* (97), and naltrexone (98). However, none of these agents has been consistently shown to be useful for treatment of his disorder. One trial evaluating the efficacy of *fenfluramine* versus desipramine in 22 patients with bulimia nervosa found decreases in binge eating and improvement in depression over the 15-week trial period with both agents (99). While both drugs reduce binge eating and vomiting, only fenfluramine produced a small weight loss. However, a larger placebo-controlled study of *dexfenfluramine* in 42 patients found no antidepressant effect for dexfenfluramine and a slight weight gain (100). In addition, patients who experienced the most symptomatic improvement in binge eating/purging showed a paradoxical tendency to drop out of the study. Another controlled trial of *dexfenfluramine* versus placebo found no advantage over brief psychotherapy alone in the treatment of bulimia nervosa (101).

5.   Combined Medication and Psychotherapy

Medications and psychotherapy are often used in combination. Studies have found that CBT added to medication is more efficacious than medication alone (90). While one study found that medication added to CBT provided little additional benefit (102), study patients received state-of-the-art CBT in an intensive outpatient setting, and the results may not be applicable to patients receiving less intensive psychotherapeutic treatment. It is reasonable to add an antidepressant medication (such as an SSRI or tricyclic) to psychotherapy if a patient does not have an adequate response to psychotherapy.

6.   Support/Self-help Groups

Support/self-help groups are commonly used in bulimia nervosa. These may be led by professionals or laypersons. Twelve-step programs, such as Overeaters Anonymous (103), are helpful for some patients, although controlled studies of their efficacy are not available.

C.   Binge Eating Disorder

Binge Eating Disorder is generally treated with similar therapies to bulimia nervosa, including cognitive behavioral and interpersonal psychotherapy and antidepressant medications.

I.   Psychotherapy and Weight Loss Treatment

Both CBT (104,105) and IPT (87) have been shown to promote reductions in binge eating for up to 12 months following treatment. Treatment is generally similar to that used for bulimia nervosa, with some modifications. It has been hoped that, as these psychotherapies may work through differing mechanisms, patients failing to improve with one form of psychotherapy might respond favorably to another. However, a study using IPT as "salvage" therapy for patients who failed to respond to CBT found no additional benefit of IPT in this group (106).

Many patients who undergo eating disorders treatment do not lose weight, and some even gain weight (107). Because many patients with binge eating disorder are obese, weight loss is often an additional goal of treatment. Most studies find that, in the short term, binge eaters can lose weight well in standard weight loss treatment programs (108,109), although some studies have found a greater risk of dropping out of treatment or earlier regain of lost weight (110–112). One study, however, has found less frequent treatment attrition among obese women with binge eating disorder than among those without the disorder (113), while another has found episodic overeaters, who do not experience feelings of loss of control, to be at risk for attrition (109).

A frequent concern in using calorie-restricted diets in obese patients is that such dietary restriction will trigger the onset of binge eating in those who have not previously experienced this problem and will worsen binge eating in those already affected. Although one study found that a third of nonbinge eaters reported episodes they labeled as "binges" after a very low calorie diet program (114), others have found that weight loss treatment actually improves binge eating and associated psychopathology over the short-term (32,33,107) and does not induce binge eating in obese subjects who previously reported no difficulties in this area (33).

2. Medication

Antidepressant medication is frequently used in the treatment of binge eating disorder, although few studies of its efficacy have been published (107,115,116). Agras et al. (107) found that adding desipramine to a combination of cognitive-behavioral therapy and behavioral weight loss treatment did not provide any additional benefit in reduction of binge eating. However, those on medication did maintain a significantly larger weight loss at 3-month post-treatment follow-up, as well as favorable reductions in disinhibition.

Fluoxetine has been evaluated as a weight loss agent in a group of obese individuals that included binge and nonbinge eaters (117). That study demonstrated significant weight loss in both groups while medication was continued, but no differential advantage was found for binge eaters. The effects of fluoxetine on binge eating frequency or severity were not measured.

A report of an 8-week, double-blind, placebo-controlled trial using *dexfenfluramine* in obese individuals with binge eating disorder found significant decreases in binge frequency in the active treatment group compared with placebo, although neither group lost weight during the treatment period (118). A few preliminary studies have suggested that opiate antagonists such as *naltrexone* (119,120) or *naloxone* (58) may eventually play a role in the treatment of binge eating disorder, but such approaches are still experimental.

The ideal sequence for treatment of binge eating disorder (i.e., treating the eating disorder before, concomitant with, or after attempts at weight loss) is not yet known. Because patients who stop binge eating during CBT lose more weight than those who do not (107), it does appear that many individuals with binge eating disorder may benefit from treatment for their eating disorder to maximize the chances for successful adherence to a weight loss treatment program.

VII. PROGNOSIS

A. Anorexia Nervosa

Anorexia nervosa is a condition with severe morbidity and a high mortality, estimated at up to 20% over 20 years, although most studies show considerably lower rates, closer to 5% (121). The major reasons for death include starvation, suicide, and cardiac arrhythmias due to fluid and electrolyte imbalance (121). A 10-year follow-up study of 76 severely ill anorexics found high rates of chronicity, with 41% experiencing bulimic episodes 10 years after initial treatment, and a 13-fold increase in mortality (122). Less than one-quarter of patients in that series were considered fully recovered. In a review of 14 outcome studies, Herzog et al. (121) report that 22–70% of patients were within the normal weight range at follow-up, while 15–43% were considered underweight. Overweight is not common among patients with a history of anorexia nervosa. Even when overweight is defined as 10% above "standard" weight, studies report a prevalence of only 2–10% (121). The same review reported that abnormal eating behaviors remain common over the long term in anorexia nervosa, with 23–67% reporting continued dieting, and up to half reporting binge eating and/or purging. Thus, while about half of all patients report normal weight over the long term, reproductive function, psychological well-being, and attitudes towards food and weight remain abnormal for the majority of patients with anorexia nervosa. While these studies are often of patients hospitalized at tertiary referral centers and may reflect the "worst-case scenario," it is clear that for many patients anorexia nervosa remains a chronic and persistent disorder.

Predictors of poor outcome in anorexia nervosa include long duration of illness, comorbid personality disorder, low body weight, and the presence of bulimic symptoms (6,121).

B. Bulimia Nervosa

Mortality due to bulimia nervosa does not appear to be as common as in anorexia nervosa, although few studies have been published. One study of 96 bulimic patients did find an increased standardized mortality ratio, with three patients dying during follow-up, two of whom died in accidents, and one of whom died after falling to a low body weight (123).

Specific prognostic indicators for treatment outcome are few. No relationship has been found between pretreatment levels of binge eating or vomiting and treatment response (124), although laxative abuse has been reported to be a predictor of poor prognosis (4). Some studies have found that poor prognosis is associated with a history of anorexia nervosa or with large weight fluctuations (125). History of substance abuse has been linked to poor treatment outcome in some (126,127) but not all (128), studies. Family history of drug abuse, while associated with an increased likelihood of drug abuse in the patient, is not associated with severity of bulimic symptoms (48). Bulimic patients with a family history of substance abuse are more likely to have a personal history of having been overweight (48). Fairburn et al. found that high premorbid weight predicted poor outcome to psychotherapeutic treatment (89).

Most studies do not find a link between depression at presentation and treatment outcome, although improvement in bulimic symptoms leads to a reduction in depressive symptoms (129). In fact, much of the generalized psychological distress seen in standardized tests administered to patients with bulimia nervosa appears to improve with reduction in bulimic symptoms (125). The coexistence of personality disorders in the bulimic patient has frequently been found to predict poor response to treatment (130,131).

While psychotherapy and pharmacotherapy lead to significant reductions in binge eating and purging behaviors, success, defined as complete "abstinence" from symptomatic behaviors, is much more variable. For example, one study evaluating treatment response of hospitalized bulimic patients between 2 and 5 years after the initial hospitalization found an 84% reduction in binge eating and 76% reduction in vomiting; however, only 13% reported no binge eating of vomiting at follow-up (132). In addition, most patients with bulimia report some additional treatment between initial evaluation and follow-up one or more years later (133). A study of 30 women followed for up to 42 months found high rates of chronicity, relapse, and recurrence, with a 63% probability of relapse by 78 weeks after recovery (134). Therefore, bulimia nervosa may be best thought of as a chronic, relapsing illness, in which symptoms tend to improve, but not disappear, over time. Without treatment, some studies report no change in symptoms over time (135), while others report modest improvement (136). Because bulimia nervosa has only been identified in the past decade, longer-term (i.e., 10- or 20-year follow-up) is not available.

C. Binge Eating Disorder

Binge eating disorder has only recently been described, and little is known about its long-term outcome or prognostic indicators. One longitudinal study with 3 years of follow-up found that patients with binge eating disorder showed significant improvement in both specific and general psychopathology over time, while improvement in body weight was not maintained over the 3-year period (137). Both early onset of binge eating (107,138) and more severe binge eating at baseline (107) have been associated with poorer response to treatment.

REFERENCES

1. American Psychiatric Association. Diagnostic and Statistical Manual of Mental Disorders, 4th ed. Washington, DC: American Psychiatric Association. 1994:539–550.
2. Fairburn CG, Cooper Z. The Eating Disorder Examination, 12th ed. In: Fairburn CG, Wilson GT, eds. Binge Eating: Nature, Assessment, and Treatment. New York: Guilford Press, 1993:317–360.
3. Casper RC, Eckert ED, Halmi KA, Goldberg SC, Davis JM. Bulimia: its incidence and clinical importance in patients with anorexia nervosa. Arch Gen Psychiatry 1980; 37:1030–1035.
4. Gwirtsman HE. Laxative and emetic abuse in bulimia nervosa. In: Yager J, Gwirtsman H, Edelstein CK, eds. Special Problems in the Management of Eating Disorders. Washington, DC: American Psychiatric Press, 1991.
5. Griffith JP. Eating disorders among diabetics: a case report and literature review. West Virginia Med J 1992; 88: 276–278.
6. American Psychiatric Association. Practice guidelines for eating disorders. Am J Psychiatry 1993; 150:212–228.
7. Hoeck HW. The incidence and prevalence of anorexia nervosa and bulimia nervosa in primary care. Psychol Med 1991; 21:455–460.
8. Lucas AR, Beard CM, O'Fallon WM, Kurland LT. 50-year trends in the incidence of anorexia nervosa in Rochester, Minnesota: a population-based study. Am J Psychiatry 1991; 148:917–922.
9. Garner DM. Pathogenesis of anorexia nervosa. Lancet 1993; 341:1631–1635.
10. Rastam M, Gillberg C. The family background in anorexia nervosa: a population-based study. J Am Acad Child Adolesc Psychiatry 1991; 30:283–289.
11. Pate JE, Pumariega AJ, Hester C, Garner DM. Cross-cultural patterns in eating disorders: a review. J Am Acad Child Adolesc Psychiatry 1992; 31:802–809.
12. Drewnowski A, Hopkins SA, Kessler RC. The prevalence of bulimia nervosa in the US college student population. Am J Public Health 1988; 78:1322–1325.
13. Halmi KA, Falk JR, Schwartz E. Binge eating and vomiting: a survey of a college population. Psychol Med 1981; 11:697–706.
14. Fairburn CG, Beglin SJ. Studies of the epidemiology of bulimia nervosa. Am J Psychiatry 1990; 147:401–408.
15. Carlat DJ, Camargo CA. Review of bulimia nervosa in males. Am J Psychiatry 1991; 148:831–843.

16. Heffernan K. Sexual orientation as a factor in risk for being eating and bulimia nervosa: a review. Int J Eating Disord 1994; 16:335–347.

17. Woods ER, Wilson CD, Masland RP. Weight control methods in high school wrestlers. J Adolesc Health Care 1988; 9:394–397.

18. Rand CSW, Kuldau JM. Epidemiology of bulimia and symptoms in a general population: sex, age, race, and socioeconomic status. Int J Eating Disord 1992; 11:37–44.

19. Sharp CW, Freeman CPL. The medical complications of anorexia nervosa. Br J Psychiatry 1993; 162:452–462.

20. Spitzer RL, Devlin M, Walsh BT, et al. Binge eating disorder: a multisite field trial of the diagnostic criteria. Int J Eating Disord 1992; 11:191–203.

21. Spitzer RL, Yanovski S, Wadden T, et al. Binge eating disorder: its further validation in a multisite study. Int J Eating Disord 1993; 13:137–153.

22. Gotestam KG, Agras WS. General population-based epidemiological study of eating disorders in Norway. Int J Eating Disord 1995; 18:119–126.

23. Yanovski SZ. Binge eating disorder: current knowledge and future directions. Obes Res 1993; 1:306–324.

24. Adami GF, Gandolfo P, Bauer B, Scopinaro N. Binge eating in massively obese patients undergoing bariatric surgery. Int J Eating Disord 1995; 17:45–50.

25. Raymond NC, Mussell MP, Mitchell JE, de Zwaan M, Crosby RD. An age-matched comparison of subjects with binge eating disorder and bulimia nervosa. Int J Eating Disord 1995; 18:135–143.

26. Beumont PJV, Garner DM, Touyz SW. Diagnoses of eating or dieting disorders: what may we learn from past mistakes? Int J Eating Disord 1994; 16:349–362.

27. Drewnowski A, Yee DK, Kurth CL, Krahn DD. Eating pathology and DSM-III-R bulimia nervosa: a continuum of behavior. Am J Psychiatry 1994; 151:1217–1219.

28. Wilson GT. Relationship of dieting and voluntary weight loss to psychological functioning and binge eating. Ann Intern Med 1993; 119(7, pt 2):727–730.

29. Yanovski SZ. The chicken or the egg: binge eating disorder and dietary restraint. Appetite 1995; 24:258.

30. Wilson GT, Nonas CA, Rosenblum GD. Assessment of binge eating in obese patients. Int J Eating Disord 1993; 13:23–34.

31. Berkowitz R, Stunkard AJ, Stallings VA. Binge-eating disorder in obese adolescent girls. Ann NY Acad Sci 1993; 699:200–206.

32. Marcus MD. Binge eating in obesity. In: Fairburn CG, Wilson GT, eds. Binge Eating: Nature, Assessment, and Treatment. New York: Guilford Press, 1993:77–96.

33. Yanovski SZ, Sebring N. Recorded food intake of obese women with binge eating disorder before and after weight loss. Int J Eating Disord 1994; 15:135–150.

34. Marcus MD, Smith D, Santelli R, Kaye W. Characterization of eating disordered behavior in obese binge eaters. Int J Eating Disord 1992; 12:249–256.

35. Marcus MD, Wing RR, Ewing L, Kern E, Gooding W, McDermott M. Psychiatric disorders among obese binge eaters. Int J Eating Disord 1990; 9:69–77.

36. Yanovski SZ, Nelson JE, Dubbert BK, Spitzer RL. Association of binge eating disorder and psychiatric comorbidity in obese subjects. Am J Psychiatry 1993; 150:1472–1479.

37. Hudson JI, Pope HG, Yurgelun-Todd D, Jonas JM, Frankenburg FR. A controlled study of lifetime prevalence of affective and other psychiatric disorders in bulimic outpatients. Am J Psychiatry 1987; 144:1283–1287.

38. Weltzin TE, Fernstrom MH, Kaye WH. Serotonin and bulimia nervosa. Nutr Rev 1994; 52:399–408.

39. Keys A, Brozek J, Henschel A, Mickelson O, Taylor HL. The Biology of Human Starvation. Minneapolis: University of Minnesota Press, 1950.

40. Hsu LKG, Kaye W, Weltzin T. Are the eating disorders related to obsessive compulsive disorder? Int J Eating Disord 1993; 14:305–318.

41. Altemus M, Pigott TA, Kalogeras K, et al. Elevations in arginine vasopressin and corticotropin-releasing hormone secretion in obsessive compulsive disorder. Arch Gen Psychiatry 1992; 49:9–20.

42. Laessele R, Wittchen H, Fichter M, et al. The significance of subgroups of bulimia and anorexia nervosa: lifetime frequency of psychiatric disorders. Int J Eating Disord 1989; 8:569–574.

43. Halmi KA, Eckert E, Marchi P, et al. Comorbidity of psychiatric diagnoses in anorexia nervosa. Arch Gen Psychiatry 1991; 48:712–718.

44. Specker S, deZwaan M, Raymond N, Mitchell J. Psychopathology in subgroups of obese women with and without binge eating disorder. Compr Psychiatry 1994; 35:185–190.

45. Garner DM. Binge eating in anorexia nervosa. In: Fairburn CG, Wilson GT, eds. Binge Eating: Nature, Assessment, and Treatment. New York: Guilford Press, 1993:50–76.

46. Mitchell JE, Hatsukami D, Eckert ED, Pyle RL. Characteristics of 275 patients with bulimia. Am J Psychiatry 1985; 142:482–485.

47. Hudson JI, Pope HG, Jonas JM, Yurgeluen-Todd D. Family history of anorexia nervosa and bulimia. Br J Psychiatry 1983; 142:133–138.

48. Mitchell JE, Hatsukami D, Pyle R, Eckert E, Bulimia with and without a family history of drug abuse. Addict Behav 1988; 13:245–251.

49. Telch CF, Agras WS. Obesity, binge eating, and psychopathology: are they related? Int J Eating Disord 1994; 15:53–61.

50. Antony MM, Johnson WG. Carr-Nangle RE, Abel JL. Psychopathology correlates of binge eating and binge eating disorder. Compr Psychiatry 1994; 35:386–392.

51. Holland A, Sicotte N, Treasure J. Anorexia nervosa: evidence for a genetic basis. J Psychosom Res 1988; 32:561–571.

52. Yanovski SZ. Biological correlates of binge eating. Addictive Behaviors. 1995; 20:705–712.

53. Hall RCW, Tice L, Beresford TP, Wooley B, Hall AK. Sexual abuse in patients with anorexia nervosa and bulimia. Psychosomatics 1989; 30:73–69.

54. Connors ME, Morse W. Sexual abuse and eating disorders: a review. Int J Eating Disord 1993; 13:1–11.

55. Everill JT, Waller G. Reported sexual abuse and eating psychopathology: a review of the evidence for a causal link. Int J Eating Disord 1995; 18:1–11.

56. Welch SL, Fairburn CG. Sexual abuse and bulimia nervosa: three integrated case control comparisons. Am J Psychiatry 1994; 151:402–407.

57. Wilson GT. Binge eating and addictive disorders. In: Fairburn CG, Wilson GT, eds. Binge Eating: Nature, Assessment, and Treatment. New York: Guilford Press, 1993: 97–120.

58. Drewnowski A, Krahn DD, Demitrack MA, Nairn K, Gosnell BA. Naloxone, an opiate blocker, reduces the consumption of sweet high-fat foods in obese and lean female binge eaters. Am J Clin Nutr 1995; 61:1206–1212.

59. Mitchell JR. Medical complications of anorexia nervosa and bulimia. Psychiatr Med 1984; 1:229–255.

60. Robboy MS, Sato AS, Schwabe AD. The hypercarotenemia in anorexia nervosa: a comparison of vitamin A and carotene levels in various forms of menstrual dysfunction and cachexia. Am J Clin Nutr 1974; 27:362–367.

61. Sharp CW, Freeman CPL. The medical complications of anorexia nervosa. Br J Psychiatry 1993; 162:452–462.

62. Salisbury JJ, Mitchell JE. Bone mineral density and anorexia nervosa in women. Am J Psychiatry 1991; 148: 768–744.

63. Kreipe RE, Hicks DG, Rosier RN, Puzas JE. Preliminary findings of the effects of sex hormones on bone metabolism in anorexia nervosa. J Adolesc Health. 1993; 14: 319–324.

64. Klibanski A, Biller BM, Schoenfeld DZ, Herzog DB, Saxe VC. The effects of estrogen administration on trabecular bone loss in young women with anorexia nervosa. J Clin Endocrinol Metab 1995; 80:898–904.

65. Herzog W, Minne H, Deter C, et al. Outcome of bone mineral density in anorexia nervosa patients 11.7 years after first admission. J Bone Miner Res 1993; 8:597–605.

66. Rigotti NA, Neer RM, Skates SJ, Herzog DB, Nussbaum SR. The clinical course of osteoporosis in anorexia nervosa. A longitudinal study of cortical bone mass. JAMA 1991; 6:1133–1138.

67. King MB. Eating disorders in a general practice population. Prevalence, characteristics, and follow-up at 12 to 18 months. Psychol Med 1989; 14:1–34.

68. McClain CJ, Humphries LL, Hill KK, Nickl NJ. Gastrointestinal and nutritional aspects of eating disorders. J Am Coll Nutr 1993; 12:466–474.

69. Levin PA, Falko JM, Dixon K, Gallup EM, Saunders W. Benign parotid enlargement in bulimia. Ann Intern Med 1980; 93:827–889.

70. Roberts MW, Li SH. Oral findings of anorexia nervosa and bulimia nervosa: a study of 47 cases. J Am Dent Assoc 1987; 115:407–410.

71. Russell G. Bulimia nervosa: an ominous variant of anorexia nervosa. Psychol Med 1979; 9:429–448.

72. Mitchell JE, Pyle RL, Eckert ED, Hatsukami D, Lentz R. Electrolyte and other physiological abnormalities in patients with bulimia. Psychol Med 1983; 13:273–278.

73. Gwirtsman HE, Kaye WH, George DT, Carosella NW, Greene RC, Jimerson DC. Hyperamylasemia and its relationship to binge-purge episodes: development of a clinically relevant laboratory test. J Clin Psychiatry 1989; 50: 196–204.

74. Crowell MD, Cheskin LJ, Musial F. Prevalence of gastrointestinal symptoms in obese and normal weight binge eaters. Am J Gastroenterol 1994; 89:387–391.

75. Solomon SM, Kirby DF. The refeeding syndrome: a review. J Parenter Enter Nutr 1990; 14:90–97.

76. Gowers S, Norton K, Halek C, Crisp AH. Outcome of outpatient psychotherapy in a random allocation treatment study of anorexia nervosa. Int J Eating Disord 1994; 15:165–177.

77. Vandereycken W. Neuroleptics in the short-term treatment of anorexia nervosa: a double-blind placebo controlled study with sulpiride. Br J Psychiatry 1984; 144: 288–292.

78. Kennedy SH, Goldbloom DS. Current perspectives on drug therapies for anorexia nervosa and bulimia nervosa. Drugs 1991; 41:367–377.

79. Gwirtsman HE, Guze BH, Yager J, Gainsley, B. Fluoxetine treatment of anorexia nervosa: an open clinical trial. J Clin Psychiatry 1990; 51:378–382.

80. Kaye WH, Weltzin TE, Hsu LKG, Bulik CM. An open trial of fluoxetine in patients with anorexia nervosa. J Clin Psychiatry 1991; 52:464–471.

81. Halmi KA, Eckert ED, LaDu TJ, et al. Anorexia nervosa: treatment efficacy of cyproheptadine and amitriptyline. Arch Gen Psychiatry 1986; 43:177–181.

82. Wilson GT. Treatment of bulimia nervosa; when CBT fails. Behav Res Ther 1996; 34:197–212.

83. Fairburn CG. A cognitive-behavioral approach to the management of bulimia. Psychol Med 1981; 11:707–711.

84. Fairburn CG. Cognitive-behavioral treatment for bulimia. In: Garner DM, Garfinkle PE, eds. Handbook of Psychotherapy for Anorexia Nervosa and Bulimia. New York: Guilford Press, 160–192.

85. Wilson GT, Fairburn CG. Cognitive treatments for eating disorders. J Consult Clin Psychol 1993; 61:261–269.

86. Craighead LW, Agras WS. Mechanisms of action in cognitive-behavioral and pharmacological interventions for obesity and bulimia nervosa. J Consult Clin Psychol 1991; 59:115–125.

87. Wilfley DE, Agras WS, Telch CF, et al. Group cognitive-behavioral therapy and group interpersonal psychotherapy for the non-purging bulimic individual: a controlled comparison. J Consult Clin Psychol 1993; 61:296–305.

88. Fairburn CG. Jones R, Peveler RC, et al. Three psychological treatments for bulimia nervosa a comparative trial. Arch Gen Psychiatry 1991; 48:463–469.

89. Fairburn CG, Norman PA, Welch SL, O'Connor MR, Doll HA, Peveler RC. A prospective study of outcome in bulimia nervosa and the long-term effects of three psychological treatments. Arch Gen Psychiatry 1995; 52: 301–312.

90. Walsh BT, Devlin MJ. The pharmacologic treatment of eating disorders. Psychiatr Clin North Am 1992; 15: 149–160.

91. Fluoxetine Bulimia Nervosa Collaborative Study Group. Fluoxetine in the treatment of bulimia nervosa: a multicenter, placebo-controlled double-blind trial. Arch Gen Psychiatry 1992; 49:139–147.

92. McCarthy MK, Goff DC, Baer L, Cioffi J, Herzog DB. Dissociation, childhood trauma, and the response to fluoxetine in bulimic patients. Int J Eating Disord 1994; 15: 219–226.

93. Walsh BT, Hadigan CM, Devlin MJ, Gladis M, Roose SP. Long-term outcome of antidepressant treatment for bulimia nervosa. Am J Psychiatry 1991; 148:1206–1212.

94. Mitchell JE, Pyle RL, Eckert ED, Hatsukami D, Pomeroy C, Zimmerman R. Response to alternative antidepressants in imipramine nonresponders with bulimia nervosa. J Clin Psychopharmacol 1989; 9:291–293.

95. Kaplan AS, Garfinkel PE, Darby PL, Garner DM. Carbamazapine in the treatment of bulimia. Am J Psychiatry 1986; 47:339–345.

96. Hsu LK, Clement L, Santhouse R, Ju ES. Treatment of bulimia nervosa with lithium carbonate. A controlled study. J Nerv Ment Dis 1991; 179:351–355.

97. Sandy R. L-Tryptophan in neuropsychiatric disorders: a review. Int J Neurosci 1992; 67:127–144.

98. de Zwaan M, Mitchell JE. Opiate antagonists and eating behavior in humans: a review. J Clin Pharmacol 1992; 32: 1060–1072.

99. Blouin AG, Blouin JH, Perez EL, et al. Treatment of bulimia with fenfluramine and desipramine. J Clin Psychopharmacol 1988; 8:261–269.

100. Russell GFM, Checkley SA, Feldman J, Eisler I. A controlled trial of d-fenfluramine in bulimia nervosa. Clin Neuropharmacol 1988; 11:S146–S159.

101. Fahy TA, Eisler I, Russell GF. A placebo-controlled trial of d-fenfluramine in bulimia nervosa. Br J Psychiatry 1993; 162:597–603.

102. Mitchell JE, Pyle RL, Eckert ED, et al. A comparison study of antidepressants and structured intensive group psychotherapy in the treatment of bulimia nervosa. Arch Gen Psychiatry 1990; 47:149–157.

103. The Twelve Steps of Overeaters Anonymous. Los Angeles: Overeaters Anonymous, 1990.

104. Telch CF, Agras WS, Rossiter EM, Wilfley D, Kenardy J. Group cognitive-behavioral treatment for the non-purging bulimic: an initial evaluation. J Consult Clin Psychol 1990; 58:629–635.

105. Smith DE, Marcus MD, Kaye W. Cognitive-behavioral treatment of obese binge eaters. Int J Eating Disord 1992; 12:257–262.

106. Agras WS, Telch CF, Arnow B, et al. Does interpersonal therapy help patients with binge eating disorder who fail to respond to cognitive behavioral therapy? J Consult Clin Psychol 1995; 63:356–360.

107. Agras WS, Telch CF, Arnow B, Eldredge K, Wilfley D, Raeburn SD, Henderson J, Marnell M. Weight loss, cognitive-behavioral, and desipramine treatments in binge eating disorder: an additive design. Behav Ther 1994; 25: 225–238.

108. LaPorte DJ. Treatment response in obese binge eaters: preliminary results using a very low calorie diet (VLCD) and behavior therapy. Addict Behav 1992; 17:247–257.

109. Wadden TA, Foster GD, Letizia KA. Response of obese binge eaters to treatment by behavior therapy combined with very low calorie diet. J Consult Clin Psychol 1992; 60:808–811.

110. Yanovski SZ, Gormally JF, Leser MS, Gwirtsman HE, Yanovski JA. Binge eating disorder affects outcome of comprehensive very low calorie diet treatment. Obes Res 1994; 2:205–212.

111. Marcus MD, Wing RR, Hopkins J. Obese binge eaters: affect, cognitions, and response to behavioral weight control. J Consult Clin Psychol 1988; 56:433–439.

112. Loro AD, Orleans CS. Binge eating in obesity: preliminary findings and guidelines for behavioral analysis and treatment. Addict Behav 1981; 6:155–166.

113. Ho KSI, Nichaman MZ, Taylor WC, Lee ES, Foreyt JP. Binge eating disorder, retention, and dropout in an adult obesity program. Int J Eating Disord 1995; 18:291–294.

114. Telch CF, Agras WS. The effects of a very low calorie diet on binge eating. Behav Ther 1993; 24:177–193.

115. McCann UD, Agras WS. Successful treatment of nonpurging bulimia with desipramine: a double blind placebo controlled study. Am J Psychiatry 1990; 147:1509–1513.

116. Gardiner HM, Freeman CP, Jesinger DK, Collins SA. Fluvoxamine: an open pilot study in moderately obese female patients suffering from atypical eating disorders and episodes of bingeing. In J Obes 1993; 17:301–305.

117. Marcus MD, Wing RR, Ewing L, Kern E, McDermott M, Gooding W. A double-blind placebo-controlled trial of fluoxetine in the treatment of obese binge eaters and nonbinge eaters. Am J Psychiatry 1990; 147:876–881.

118. Stunkard AJ, Berkowitz RI, Tanrikut C, Reiss E, Young L. D-Fenfluramine treatment of binge eating disorder. Am J Psychiatry 1996; 153:1455–1459.

119. Alger SA, Shwalberg MD, Bigaouette JM, Michalek AV, Howard LJ. Effect of a tricyclic antidepressant and opiate antagonist on binge-eating behavior in normoweight bulimic and obese binge eating subjects. Am J Clin Nutr 1991; 53:865–871.

120. Marrazzi MA, Markham KM, Kinzie J, Luby ED. Binge eating disorder: response to naltrexone. Int J Obes 1995; 19:143–145.

121. Herzog DB, Keller MB, Lavori PW. Outcome in anorexia nervosa and bulimia nervosa: a review of the literature. J Nerv Ment Dis 1988; 176:131–142.

122. Eckert ED, Halmi KA, Marci P, Grove W, Crosby R. Ten-year follow-up of anorexia nervosa: clinical course and outcome. Psychol Med 1995; 25:143–156.

123. Patton GC, Mortality in eating disorders. Psychol Med 1988; 18:947–951.

124. Fairburn CG, Kirk J, O'Connor M, Anastasaides P, Cooper PJ. Prognostic factors in bulimia nervosa. Br J Clin Psychol (in press).

125. Garner DM. Psychotherapy outcome research with bulimia nervosa. Psychother Psychosom 1987; 48:129–140.

126. Hatsukami D, Mitchell JE, Eckert E, Pyle R. Characteristics of patients with bulimia only, bulimia with affective disorder, and bulimia with substance abuse problems. Addict Behav 1986; 11:399–406.

127. Lacey JH. Bulimia nervosa, binge eating, and psychogenic vomiting: a controlled treatment study and long-term outcome. Br Med J 1983; 286:1609–1613.

128. Abraham SF, Mira M, Llewellyn-Jones D. Bulimia: a study of outcome. Int J Eating Disord 1983; 2:175–180.

129. Wilson GT, Rossiter E, Kleifield EI, Lindholm L. Cognitive-behavioral treatment of bulimia nervosa: a controlled evaluation. Behav Res Ther 1986; 24:277–288.

130. Fairburn CG, Peveler RC, Jones R, Hope RA, Doll HA. Predictors of 12-month outcome in bulimia nervosa and the influence of attitudes to shape and weight. J Consult Clin Psychol 1993; 61:696–698.

131. Rossiter EM, Agras WS, Telch CF, Schneider JA. Cluster B personality disorder characteristics predict outcome in the treatment of bulimia nervosa. Int J Eating Disord 1993; 13:349–357.

132. Swift WJ, Ritholz M, Kalin NH, Kaslow N. A follow-up study of thirty hospitalized bulimics. Psychosom Med 1987; 49:45–55.

133. Mitchell JE, Davis L, Goff G, Pyle R. A follow-up study of patients with bulimia. Int J Eating Disord 1986; 5:441–450.

134. Keller MB, Herzog DB, Lavori PW, Bradburn IS, Mahoney EM. The naturalistic history of bulimia nervosa: extraordinarily high rates of chronicity, relapse, recurrence, and psychosocial morbidity. Int J Eating Disord 1992; 12:1–9.

135. King MB. The natural history of eating pathology in attenders to primary medical care. Int J Eating Disord 1991; 10:379–387.

136. Yager J, Landsverk J, Edelstein CK. A 20-month follow-up study of 628 women with eating disorders. I. Course and severity. Am J Psychiatry 1987; 144:1172–1177.

137. Fichter MM, Quadflieg N, Brandl B. Recurrent overeating: an empirical comparison of binge eating disorder, bulimia nervosa, and obesity. Int J Eating Disord 1993; 14:1–16.

138. Marcus MD, Moulton, MM, and Greeno CG. Binge eating onset in obese patients with binge eating disorder. Addict Behav 1995; 20:747–755.

8

Behavioral and Psychological Correlates of Obesity

Donald A. Williamson
Pennington Biomedical Research Center, Louisiana State University, Baton Rouge, Louisiana

Patrick Mahlen O'Neil
Medical University of South Carolina, Charleston, South Carolina

I. OVERVIEW OF RESEARCH EVIDENCE

A. General Psychopathology and Obesity

Obesity is not a psychiatric diagnosis (1). Among nonclinical samples, rates of general psychopathology do not appear to be significantly greater in obese groups than in nonobese groups (2–5). However, in the overall population, the lifetime prevalence rates of certain psychiatric disorders are substantial; similar rates among obese samples are thus not necessarily attributable to obesity.

On the other hand, obese people seeking treatment for their obesity often display higher prevalence rates of psychiatric diagnoses and other evidence of psychopathology than does the general population. Three studies found lifetime prevalence rates of Axis I (noncharacterological, e.g., anxiety or depression) psychiatric disorders of 48–57% for obese persons applying for outpatient or surgical weight loss treatments (6–8). Comparable lifetime Axis I rates for the general population are 26–35% (9). One study reported lifetime Axis II (personality disorder) rates of 57% among applicants for outpatient treatment (6). It has been noted that the extent of psychological distress seen among treatment-seeking obese groups is similar to that observed among other groups of medical or surgical patients (5).

Significantly, direct comparisons of treatment-seeking obese samples with nonclinical obese samples have also provided some indication of higher rates of psychopathology and/or distress among the treatment seekers. Prather and Williamson (10) found that samples of obese females seeking treatment were more depressed and histrionic than a group of obese women from a nonclinical sample. Fitzgibbon et al. (2) compared obese people applying for weight loss treatment, obese persons not seeking treatment, and a nonobese, nonclinical control group. They found that treatment seekers reported more symptoms of borderline personality disorder than did the nonclinical obese or the nonobese controls, who did not differ, and that only treatment-seeking obese subjects showed more overall psychiatric symptomatology than the nonobese controls.

It has been argued that it is premature to conclude from the published literature that obesity does not increase the risk of psychiatric problems, but that certain psychological factors may render some obese people more vulnerable to psychological disturbance (11). We will address this issue below.

B. Personality Profiles of Obese Persons

Personality traits represent psychological/behavioral dimensions along which there is a broad range of variation across members of the normal population, but on which a given individual is generally consistent over time and across situations. Examples of personality traits are:

extraversion/introversion, obsessive-compulsive tendencies, rigidity/flexibility, masculinity/femininity, dominance/submission, etc.

In general, there is little evidence that obese persons differ from the nonobese on such general dispositional traits; differences, when found, have not been replicated (12,13). An earlier view concluded that there are very few personality characteristics that are unique to obese persons (13).

Personality *type* can be thought of as the relative configuration of several individual traits. If the obese population can be characterized uniquely on the basis of personality type(s), then it should display, relative to the nonobese population, greater homogeneity of personality types and/or different types.

Neither sign of an "obese personality" has been found. For example, scores on the Minnesota Multiphase Personality Inventory of 170 female applicants for obesity surgery were examined using cluster analysis. The five derived cluster profiles that emerged were similar to those found in similar studies with other populations; furthermore, only 55% of the obese sample had individual profiles that fit one of these prototypes (14).

Because similar studies with obesity surgery applicants have also demonstrated the heterogeneity of personality types among even this small, extreme segment of the obese population (4), it is unlikely that the broader and much more numerous population of all obese persons is any more homogeneous. It appears that the obese differ from each other as much as they differ from nonobese persons, on psychological characteristics and traits not explicitly concerned with weight and eating. Indeed, given the vast numbers of obese people, it would be naïve to expect otherwise. Considering these findings, researchers have turned their attention to variables that are more specific to weight concerns and eating habits.

C. Weight- and Eating-Related Variables

Obese persons have been found consistently to differ from nonobese persons on a number of psychological factors and behavioral patterns related specifically to weight and eating. For example, Klesges (12) compared overweight and nonoverweight college students on general measures of depression, assertiveness, and self-consciousness, and also on measures of these characteristics as they applied to weight and eating (e.g., dysphoria concerning weight control, self-consciousness about body size). Although there were no group differences on the general measures, the overweight subjects were more depressed and self-conscious and less assertive on the weight and eating measures.

Relative to nonoverweight persons, obese people have been found to have self-defeating, pessimistic thoughts about weight and eating more frequently and with more conviction, and to react to dietary transgressions with more absolutistic, perfectionistic self-statements (15,16). Clinical and nonclinical obese groups have also reported more difficulty in controlling negative emotional eating, food temptations, and overeating (2). They also score higher on the Perceived Hunger scale of the Three Factor Eating Questionnaire (TFEQ), which appears to measure awareness of and susceptibility to hunger (17,18). The following subsections review this research literature.

1. Dietary Restraint and Overeating

Earlier research found that overeating often occurs when control of eating is threatened or disrupted or when self-imposed limits on dietary intake are exceeded (19,20). Such self-imposed limits upon dietary intake have been referred to as "dietary restraint." Several measures of dietary restraint have been developed and they are reviewed below. Central to theories that connect dietary restraint and overeating is the notion that negative emotion, positive emotion, stress, alcohol consumption, and other psychosocial variables disrupt or "disinhibit" the person's control over eating. This "disinhibition effect" has been reported in numerous laboratory studies of obese and "nonobese" restrained eaters (e.g., 19–21). In most of these studies, restrained eaters were compared with unrestrained eaters (based on responses to questionnaires described later) and half of the subjects were asked to eat a preload (e.g., pudding or ice cream) or negative emotion was induced (22). Restrained eaters receiving the "disinhibition" (preload or negative mood induction) were found to eat more food in a subsequent eating test relative to unrestrained eaters and to restrained eaters who were not administered the "disinhibitor." This finding was counterintuitive since it suggested that under certain circumstances, overeating could be provoked by eating small amounts of food or by negative emotion. Over the course of the past 15–20 years, disinhibition of dietary restraint became a highly regarded psychological explanation for the binge eating and overeating that is common in obesity and in bulimia nervosa (23).

Recent research on this topic has suggested that the psychological phenomena of dietary restraint and overeating may be somewhat independent (24–26). The results of these studies suggest that for some persons, dietary restraint may be a precursor for overeating, but in others, overeating may occur in the relative absence of dietary restraint. "Unrestrained" overeaters are generally very obese (25,26). Lowe (27) has suggested that these "unrestrained" overeaters may have tried to manage body weight by dieting in the past, but gave up in response to the failure of dieting and subsequent weight gain. One implication of this recent research is that a subset of previously obese persons are successful at weight reduction without significant psychological disturbance (24,26).

2. Body Image/Dissatisfaction

Body image is defined as the cognitive perception (or evaluation) of one's body size and appearance, and the emotional response to that perception (28–30). The personal significance of these perceptions and their affective consequences vary greatly from individual to individual; for some, body image is a minor influence on psychological well-being while for others it is the preeminent determinant.

Regarding perceptual aspects of body image, obese adults have been found to be less accurate than average weight adults in judging their body size, tending to see themselves as bigger than they are. Average estimates by obese subjects have been found to be 6–12% larger than actual, compared to average estimates within 1–2% by average-weight subjects; relative to average-weight subjects, obese subjects have been found three times as likely to overestimate their size (31–33). It should be noted that these are averages and that estimation errors in both directions occur among all weight groups. Further, the finding of obesity-associated impairment in body size estimation is not universal (11). Obesity in childhood may have lingering effects on body perception; average-weight adults who were obese as children have been found to be much more likely than never-obese adults to overestimate their body size (33).

Whether the cognitive representation of the body is accurate or not, the emotional response to that representation may be positive, neutral, or negative. An extreme example of the latter possibility is seen in body image disparagement, which includes "overwhelming preoccupation with one's obesity, often to the exclusion of any other personal characteristics" and "appraisal of one's own body as grotesque and even loathsome, and the consequent feeling that others can look on him/her only with horror and contempt" (34). While body image disparagement is not seen among most persons above recommended weight, it is thought to be far more common among the severely obese (4,35). Other risk factors may be preadult onset of obesity, disturbed childhood family environment including parental criticism of weight, and neurotic symptoms (34,36).

Negative body self-esteem without the severity of body image disparagement may be seen among some adults at all levels of obesity, especially treatment seekers and women (37,38). In a review, French et al. (39) found consistent evidence (five of six studies) that body esteem was lower among obese children and adolescents than among their nonobese peers.

D. Obesity and Quality of Life

There has been considerable research on the quality of life experienced by obese persons. The results of these studies have suggested that there is considerable diversity in the quality of life associated with obesity in childhood, adolescence, and adulthood. Generally, increased adiposity has been associated with decreased quality of life. The following sections review this research literature.

1. Self-Esteem

There is inconsistent evidence that among preteen children, obesity is associated with somewhat lower overall self-esteem, though still in the normal range. Among adolescents and young adults, evidence for this inverse relationship is more consistent (11,39). Among adult treatment seekers, obesity is generally associated with impaired self-esteem (40).

Finding of impaired self-esteem among obese samples is not necessarily proof that obesity is the cause and decreased self-esteem the result. Two prospective studies, one of black girls and boys in middle school and one of white adolescent girls, found that higher self-esteem scores were associated with lower weight gain over the next 1–3 years (39). The results of the studies on self-esteem and obesity suggest that obesity is associated with moderately lowered self-esteem, which may in part motivate efforts to lose weight.

2. Interpersonal Consequences of Obesity

It has been noted (4,5,11,41) that, at least in the United States, obese people live in a world that often receives them with notable antipathy. Numerous studies have documented overt discrimination against obese people in employment and educational settings, and the likely effects of such discrimination (42,43). Negative attitudes against the obese are found among children and adults, and even among health care professionals (41,44–47).

Given that the obese person frequently interacts with persons so negatively disposed, it is somewhat surprising that there is such scant evidence of profoundly impaired overall self-esteem and higher rates of depression among the nonclinical obese population. However, one result of repeated interactions with a somewhat unrewarding world may be reduced opportunities to develop certain social skills. Miller et al. (48) had obese and nonobese women converse on the telephone with anonymous partners. Ratings of the interaction were made by the telephone partner and by persons hearing tapes of the telephone conversations, in all cases unaware of each subject's weight status. Relative to the nonoverweight women, the obese women were rated (solely on the basis of the conversation) as less friendly, less likable, less attractive, and less socially skilled.

However, the same research team later found that obese women, relative to nonobese women, showed no impairment in social relationships, whether rated by themselves or others (48). Perhaps the social skill deficits indicated in the earlier study may be most apparent in casual interactions and may not extend to difficulties in establishing and maintaining relationships. It should be noted that both of these studies were limited to obese women.

3. Overall Quality of Life

The cumulative effects of obesity within psychosocial, physical, and professional domains appear to lower overall quality of life as perceived by the obese person, with greater decrements at greater degrees of obesity (40,49). Obesity at age 16–24 years has been found to predict impaired quality of life 7 years later on such objective indicators as likelihood of marriage and, for women, education, income, and poverty rate; it is noteworthy that these decrements were relative to comparable measures on persons with other chronic health problems (43). Heavier women are more likely than leaner women to marry men with less education (a major indicator of socioeconomic status) than their own (50).

The impact of obesity on perceived quality of life is seen most clearly in the improvements reported by formerly morbidly obese persons who have lost substantial weight (4). In one study, gastric bypass patients who had lost 45 kg (100 lb) or more indicated they would rather be blind, deaf, dyslexic, diabetic, or an amputee than return to their former morbidly obese status, and stated unanimously they would decline multimillionaire status if it also required them to be obese (35).

II. RISK FACTOR MODELS OF PSYCHOLOGICAL DISTURBANCE AND OBESITY

From the previous review, it should be clear that there is considerable heterogeneity in the psychological characteristics of obese individuals. Just as obesity's impact on physical health is influenced by such variables as degree

overweight, fat distribution, and personal and family health histories, the psychological effects of obesity seem to be moderated by numerous other variables. That is, some subgroups of obese people may experience certain psychological sequelae not reflected in studies of the vast, heterogeneous obese population (11). Certainly, the consistent findings that treatment-seeking obese are more likely to demonstrate psychological impairment indicate that there are groups of people who may be psychological casualties of the condition. We next note a few demonstrated moderators of the relations between obesity and certain psychological variables.

A. Gender

Although men tend to experience more physical health risk from obesity, women disproportionately suffer its psychological and social consequences. This is seen especially with such variables as body image, self-esteem, quality of life, marriage prospects, and education (11,40,43,50).

B. Ethnicity

Dieting and dissatisfaction with weight and body size are observed less frequently among African-American women than among Caucasian women. This racial difference has been demonstrated with overweight and nonoverweight females ranging in age from teenagers to the elderly (51,52). Overweight African-American women may possess a more positive body image than is seen among overweight Caucasian women (53). African-American men, relative to Caucasian men, are less likely to rule out dating an overweight woman (54). It appears that obesity may be somewhat less stigmatized, by the obese person and others, in African-American culture.

C. Binge Eating

There is substantial, consistent evidence that the rates of psychopathology are higher among obese binge eaters than among obese nonbingers (3,55,56). Further, obese binge eaters report more restrictive and perfectionistic dieting standards, less dieting, lower self-efficacy, more hunger, and a higher tendency toward disinhibition of restrained eating (57–60). Among clinical samples, they may also be more likely to report victimization histories (61), although this was not found in one population study comparing women with binge eating disorder to bulimics and non-eating-disordered women (62).

D. Severity of Obesity

Many of the psychosocial correlates of obesity appear to relate to degree of obesity. For example, the intrapersonal and interpersonal agony of obesity is described most acutely by the data from applicants for obesity surgery, the morbidly obese (4,35,47). A national survey of women found that women with a body mass index of 36 kg/m² or more were more likely to report histories of rape, sexual molestation, and posttraumatic stress disorder than were less overweight or nonoverweight women (63). Binge eaters, with their greater collection of psychological difficulties, tend to be more obese than nonbinging overweight persons (56).

E. Risk Factor Model

Friedman and Brownell (11) have argued that it is now clear that only a minority of obese persons experience significant psychological disturbances that appear to stem from their obesity. They have recommended that future research should attempt to identify psychosocial risk factors, e.g., gender, ethnicity, presence of binge eating, severity of obesity, body dysphoria, etc., that are predictive of increased psychological disturbance, e.g., depression, lowered self-esteem, and impaired quality of life. By identifying these risk factors, treatment interventions could target those individuals who are most at risk for the development of adverse psychological reactions to obesity.

III. PSYCHOLOGICAL EFFECTS OF DIETING AND WEIGHT LOSS

Efforts to achieve weight loss entail physiological readjustments, major life-style changes, and restriction of appetitive behavior. In the case of surgery, physiological functioning and food consumption are greatly altered beyond the control of the patient.

Weight loss attempts thus are potentially quite significant psychologically. When these attempts are successful, the results may include improved health, increased functional capacity, altered stimulus value to others and self, and expanded evidence of capacity for self-improvement. Thus, weight loss itself is also likely to have profound psychological impact.

In this section, we will briefly review some of the psychological effects of weight loss and dieting. Unfortunately, it is frequently difficult to segregate effects of weight loss efforts per se from those of weight loss. Unless specifically or contextually indicated, the findings reported should be assumed to refer to both the process of losing weight and its resultant weight loss.

A. Effects Upon Mood

The notion that dieting has adverse psychological consequences is frequently held by the lay public. A few early, uncontrolled studies suggested that this was the case (64). However, a large number of subsequent, more highly controlled studies have found that dieting by obese persons has, at worst, neutral psychological effects and that weight loss frequently results in improvement on many psychological parameters. As one review summarized, "More recent studies that describe treatments for obesity introduced since the early 1970s—such as behavior therapy, very low calorie diets, and surgery—report few negative and many positive psychological effects" (65).

Reductions in depression and trait anxiety are frequently observed among obese patients who have undergone moderate caloric restriction, very-low-calorie diets (VLCDs), or weight loss surgery (3,4,66). With moderate caloric restriction or VLCD, these improvements are more consistently seen when behavior therapy accompanies the diet (3,67). It has been suggested that pretreatment psychological status may influence psychological response to dieting and weight loss (65). During VLCDs, anxiety and depression do not appear to be influenced by degree of ketogenesis (68) or whether the diet is food- or formula-based (69).

It is noteworthy that improvements in mood are seen in many methods of weight loss despite certain dieting-related physiological changes suggestive in other circumstances of mood impairment. For example, among obese patients, serum triiodothyronine (T_3) is reduced substantially during VLCD (70), but the degree of reduction is unrelated to changes in depression. Nonoverweight volunteers undergoing a 3-week low-calorie diet (VLCD) showed reductions in total plasma tryptophan and in the ratio of tryptophan to competing amino acids, both indicators of reduced availability of tryptophan for serotonin synthesis (71). Whether this effect applies to obese dieters remains to be demonstrated, however.

B. Hunger During Dieting

Hunger might be thought to be a natural consequence of decreased caloric intake below weight maintenance needs. However, with VLCDs, after the first week or two, hunger and preoccupation with food either decrease or remain at pretreatment levels (68,69,72,73). Hunger and preoccupation with food seem to be lower during weight loss on a VLCD or following surgery than during moderate caloric restriction (4,69,72,73), although at least one study, with obese type II diabetic subjects, found no difference in hunger between VLCD and low-caloric conditions (74).

C. Body Image/Dissatisfaction

Few studies have systematically examined the effects of weight loss on body image measures. Adolescent boys completing a weight loss camp and women completing a VLCD program have been found to underestimate their resultant body sizes (3,75). Positive changes in affective responses to body image, including reductions in body image disparagement, have been seen consistently among patients who have lost weight via weight loss surgery (4,35,47).

D. Overall Quality of Life

Weight loss appears to improve perceived quality of life along many dimensions, for weight loss surgery patients and for patients undergoing more traditional treatment with smaller losses (4,35,40,47,49). Patients often report improvements in occupational functioning and success, marital and other relationships, self-esteem, and physical functioning, and note reductions in perceived discrimination. Thus, there is now a clear consensus that weight loss is generally associated with improved mood and quality of life. As noted earlier, dieting is not necessarily associated with binge eating or overeating. Therefore, many of the earlier concerns voiced about voluntary efforts to lose weight appear to have been overstated.

IV. PSYCHOLOGICAL ASSESSMENT METHODS

This section reviews methods for assessing psychological factors associated with obesity. The methods selected for review measured: (1) general psychopathology, (2) eating behavior, (3) physical activity, and (4) body image dissatisfaction. Each of the methods has been used in research relevant to obesity. Also, the reliability and validity of each method have been established. Much of the research described in the preceding section used the methods described below.

A. General Psychopathology

I. Minnesota Multiphase Personality Inventory

The Minnesota Multiphase Personality Inventory has recently been updated and revised (MMPI-2; 76). The MMPI is one of the most widely used psychological tests ever developed. It has been validated for use in many psychiatric and medical disorders, including obesity (77). The MMPI-2 has 567 questions that are answered true or false. The MMPI-2 has three validity scales and 10 clinical scales, which have received considerable attention from researchers and clinicians. In addition, hundreds of supplemental scales have been developed (78,79). Scale scores have been standardized to provide norms for comparison to an individual's MMPI profile. A t-score greater than 65 or less than 35 is regarded as statistically abnormal, as defined by 1.5 standard deviations above or below the mean. The average MMPI profile for obese samples does not generally include any scale elevations (77,80). Persons diagnoses with an eating disorder, e.g., binge eating disorder, generally have higher scores on most MMPI scales, indicating higher levels of psychopathology in these populations (10,80). Therefore, the primary use of the MMPI with obesity is to screen for significant psychiatric problems associated with some obese individuals.

2. Symptom Checklist-90

The Symptom Checklist-90 (SCL-90) asks subjects to respond to 90 physical and psychiatric complaints by rating the distress they experience on a five-point rating scale ranging from *not at all* to *extremely* (81). From these ratings, three global measures and nine symptom subscales are derived (77). Two studies (10,82) reported no differences between obese and nonobese samples on the subscales of the SCL-90. Prather and Williamson (10) distinguished between obese binge eaters and nonbinge eaters and found no differences between these two subgroups on the SCL-90 subscales. Marcus et al. (59) found the two subgroups to differ on all of the SCL-90 subscales, which is consistent with the general consensus that persons diagnoses with binge eating disorder report greater psychopathology than persons with simple cases of obesity (56). Therefore, like the MMPI, the SCL-90 may have some utility for screening general psychopathology in obese persons.

3. Beck Depression Inventory

The Beck Depression Inventory (BDI) was developed to measure the symptoms of depression using 21 items with four levels of severity associated with each symptom (83). The BDI has been studied extensively and its reliability and validity are well established (84). A number of studies have found obese binge eaters to have higher scores on the BDI in comparison to obese nonbinge eaters (10,59). Also, Prather and Williamson (10) reported that obese nonbinge eaters seeking weight loss therapy scored higher on the BDI relative to obese persons in the general population. Thus, the BDI is well suited for measuring the symptoms of depression associated with obesity.

4. State-Trait Anxiety Inventory

The State-Trait Anxiety Inventory (STAI) measures the severity of situational (state) and generalized (trait) anxiety (85). The STAI instructs the person to rate 40 anxiety symptoms on a four-point rating scale ranging from *not at all* to *very much so*. The STAI has been studied for over 25 years and its reliability and validity are well established. Current evidence suggests that the STAI may be useful for the measurement of generalized anxiety that is associated with obese binge eaters (80).

B. Eating Behavior: Self-Report Inventories

I. Restraint Scale

The Restraint Scale was originally developed by Herman and Mack (19) to measure chronic dieting. Over a number of years, the Restraint Scale was revised to a 10-item questionnaire with two subscales: (1) Weight Fluctuation and (2) Concern for Dieting (86). The reliability and validity of the Restraint Scale has been established by many studies (87). It has been used frequently in laboratory studies of eating behavior. As noted earlier, a common finding in these studies is that persons scoring high on the Restraint Scale overeat when dietary restraint is disinhibited by the availability of a preload or by the induction of positive or negative affect (27). High scores on the Restraint Scale have been associated with a pattern of dieting, overeating, and fluctuation of body weight.

2. Three Factor Eating Questionnaire

The Three Factor Eating Questionnaire (TFEQ) is a 51-item self-report inventory with three subscales: (1) Dietary Restraint, (2) Disinhibition, and (3) Perceived Hunger (88). Reliability of the scales has been established. The scales were originally derived using factor analysis to separate the behaviors associated with dieting and overeating. Subsequent studies have reported relatively weak correlations between the Dietary Restraint scale and the other two scales, but strong positive correlations between the Disinhibition and Perceived Hunger scales (25,26). Validity studies of the TFEQ have supported the validity of the Dietary Restraint scale as a measure of the intent to diet as well as a measure of actual dieting behavior (24,26,89). Two recent studies have supported the validity of the Disinhibition scale as a measure of overeating (24,26). Validation of the Perceived Hunger scale has received less attention.

3. Dutch Eating Behavior Questionnaire

The Dutch Eating Behavior Questionnaire (DEBQ) is a 33-item questionnaire with three subscales: (1) Emotional Eating, (2) Restrained Eating, and (3) External Eating (90). The DEBQ was developed to separate the measurement of dieting and overeating in response to emotions or external cues for eating, e.g., availability of foods or the smell of food. Subsequent research has established the reliability and validity of the subscales of the DEBQ (87). Allison et al. (89) concluded that the Restrained Eating scale of the DEBQ may be the most pure measure of dietary restraint that is available.

4. Eating Behavior Inventory

The Eating Behavior Inventory (EBI) was developed by O'Neil, et al. (91) to assess behaviors prescribed by behavioral weight loss programs. Behaviors sampled by the EBI include: self-monitoring of food intake and body weight, refusing offers of food, eating at only one place, shopping from a list, and eating in response to emotions. The EBI has 26 items answered on a five-point rating scale. Factor analysis of the EBI yielded three factors: (1) control over eating, (2) use of behavioral weight control methods, and (3) use of stimulus control procedures (92). Tests of the reliability and validity of the EBI have yielded positive results. The EBI has been found to be sensitive to treatment effects (91); therefore, it may be most useful as a measure of behavior change as a function of treatment.

5. Binge Scale Questionnaire

The Binge Scale Questionnaire is a brief (nine-item) self-report inventory for measuring binge eating and vomiting (93). The Binge Scale has been used in studies of binge eating and bulimia nervosa. Scores on the nine items are summed to form a total score. A score greater than 15 is associated with a clinically significant problem with binge eating (94). Research has supported the reliability and validity of the Binge Scale as a measure of the severity of bulimia.

6. Binge Eating Scale

The Binge Eating Scale (BES) was developed by Gormally et al. (95) as a measure of binge eating. The BES has 16 items, which are individually weighted to provide a total score. The test-retest reliability of the BES has not been established. The validity of the BES as a measure of binge eating has been reported (95). Many of the initial studies of binge eating associated with obesity used scores on the BES to define binge eaters (94). With the specification of more specific diagnostic criteria for binge eating disorder (1), this approach for defining binge eating in obesity is probably inadequate (96). Current research suggests that structured interviews may be the most valid method for defining binge eating disorder and/or binge eating (96,97).

7. Bulimia Test-Revised

The Bulimia Test (98) was revised by Thelen et al. (99) to reflect changes in the diagnostic criteria for bulimia nervosa (100). The Bulimia Test-Revised (BULIT-R) has 28 items that are summed to form a single score. The reliability and validity of the BULIT-R has been established in a number of studies (101). Scores on the BULIT-R are highly correlated with scores on the original BULIT ($r =$ .99); therefore, the two forms of the test can be regarded as comparable. Williamson et al. (102) found obese binge eaters to score higher on the BULIT than obese subjects without significant binge eating.

8. Emotional Eating Scale

Arnow et al. (103) developed the Emotional Eating Scale to measure the desire to eat in response to three emotions, which form three subscales: (1) anger/frustration, (2) anxiety, and (3) depression. The EES has 25 items that are answered on a five-point scale. Support for the reliability and validity of the EES has been reported (103). All three subscales were found to be correlated with measures of binge eating. The EES is a relatively new measure of eating behavior. It would appear to be useful for studies of binge eating and could also be used as a measure of treatment outcome in studies of weight loss and/or modification of binge eating or overeating.

9. Eating Questionnaire-Revised

The Eating Questionnaire-Revised (EQ-R) was developed as a symptom checklist to screen for a diagnosis of bulimia nervosa (104). The EQ-R has 15 items, which can be summed to yield a total score or to yield a symptom profile. The EQ-R has been found to be a single factor test that has adequate reliability and validity as a measure of binge eating (101,104). Obese binge eaters have been found to score higher on the EQ-R relative to obese subjects without binge eating problems. Normative data for obesity, binge eating disorder, bulimia nervosa, anorexia nervosa, and normal-weight subjects have been reported (101).

10. Forbidden Food Survey

The Forbidden Food Survey (FFS) was designed to evaluate a person's emotional reaction to eating different types of food (195). The FFS is constructed by grouping 45 common foods into five food groups (milk, meat, grains, fruits/vegetables, and beverages) by three caloric levels (high, medium, and low). Subjects are asked to rate how they would feel about themselves after eating each food, using a five-point rating scale. The FFS has been found to be reliable and valid as a measure of anxiety about eating different types of foods (105,106).

C.   Eating Behavior: Nutrient Intake

1.   Self-Monitoring of Eating

Behavioral diaries are often used to evaluate the interaction of environment and emotions upon eating behavior (106). This assessment approach requires the subject to monitor the events surrounding eating behavior, e.g., situational variables, mood, and the availability of foods. This approach has been validated in numerous studies of binge eating and overeating associated with obesity (102,107–109). These studies have generally instructed subjects to monitor eating behavior for 2 weeks. There are some problems associated with this approach. Compliance with the procedure is a common problem for about 30% of research participants (106). If self-monitoring is extended beyond 2 weeks, compliance usually becomes an even greater problem. Also, the accuracy and validity of nutrient intake data derived from behavioral diaries have been questioned, especially in obese persons (110). For these reasons, self-monitoring of eating may be most useful for evaluating the self-perception of overeating and binge eating (107,109).

2.   Food Frequency Questionnaires

Food frequency questionnaires are often designed for the aims of a particular project. They are typically constructed by arranging essential foods in food groups of comparable nutrient content or additives, e.g., dietary fat, carbohydrates, or vitamins. Subjects are generally asked to specify how often they consume each food and in what quantities or portion size (111). The two most commonly used standardized food frequency questionnaires were developed by Rimm et al. (121) and Block et al. (113). The reliability and validity of these food frequency questionnaires have been established and they are frequently used to assess nutrient intake in large population-based studies (111).

D.   Eating Behavior: Structured Interviews

1.   Eating Disorder Examination

The Eating Disorder Examination (EDE) was developed as a semistructured interview for measuring five aspects of anorexia and bulimia nervosa (114). The five subscales of the EDE are named: dietary restraint, bulimia, eating concern, weight concern, and shape concern. The EDE has been revised 12 times (96). Interrater reliability for the EDE has been found to be satisfactory over several studies (101). The EDE was developed as a measure of treatment outcome for bulimia nervosa. It has been found to be sensitive to behavior change during treatment and to be a valid indicator of bulimic and anorexic symptoms (96). One of the greatest strengths of the EDE is its method for defining overeating. Four types of overeating are distinguished using the EDE based on the presence or absence of loss of control over eating and the objective amount of food that was eaten. The four forms of overeating are described as: (1) objective bulimic episodes, (2) subjective bulimic episodes, (3) objective overeating, and (4) subjective overeating.

2. Interview for Diagnosis of Eating Disorders

Williamson (80) published the original version of the Interview for Diagnosis of Eating Disorders (IDED). Since that time the IDED has been revised four times (97). The IDED was developed specifically for the diagnosis of eating disorders. The IDED-IV has been validated for the diagnosis of binge eating disorder, anorexia nervosa, bulimia nervosa, and eating disorder not otherwise specified, as defined by the American Psychiatric Association (1). Interrater reliability of the IDED-IV has been found to be satisfactory, especially for the purpose of differential diagnosis. The validity of the IDED-IV has also been established. These findings are of special relevance to the field of obesity because the IDED-IV is one of the few methods that have been validated for diagnosing binge eating disorder association with obesity. Given the problems associated with the validity of questionnaire methods for diagnosing binge eating disorder, the development of the IDED-IV is of considerable important to this area of obesity research.

E. Physical Activity

1. Questionnaires and Interviews

In a recent review, Shelton and Klesges (115) reported five questionnaire and interview methods that have been developed for the measurement of physical activity: (1) Baecke Questionnaire, (2) Harvard Alumni Activity Survey, (3) Lipid Research Clinics Prevalence Study Questionnaire, (4) Minnesota Leisure Time Physical Activity Questionnaire (MLTPAQ), and (5) Stanford Seven-Day Physical Activity Recall Questionnaire. Of these methods, the MLTPAQ has been most extensively researched and vali-

dated. The MLTPAQ is administered via interview and, consequently, is somewhat labor- and time-consuming. The other methods can be administered by questionnaire. Each of these questionnaire methods has certain advantages and disadvantages, which requires the researcher to match the instrument to the particular needs of the project.

2. Activity Monitors

Mechanical monitors of activity have improved considerably over the past 10 years, moving from simple pedometers to computerized devices that measure the quantity and intensity of movement. One of the newer activity monitors is the Caltrac accelerometer (manufactured by Muscle Dynamics, Inc.; Torrance, CA). It has been validated as a measure of energy expenditure via exercise (116). Lawson et al. (24) tested the Caltrac accelerometer as one measure of energy expenditure. They found that obese subjects who reported overeating expended less energy per kilogram of body weight in comparison to a leaner comparison group. These preliminary data suggest that the potential for using the newer activity monitors to measure physical activity is quite good.

F. Body Image/Dissatisfaction

1. Body Silhouette Methods

One approach for measuring body image and dissatisfaction has used different types of body figural stimuli, which vary from very thin to very obese (117). Stunkard et al. (118) created the first set of body silhouettes for men and women. Williamson et al. (82) reported a similar set for women. In most of the studies of body silhouettes as a measure of body image and dissatisfaction, researchers have instructed subjects to first select the body silhouette that best matches their current body size and then to select the silhouette that matches their ideal body size. Recent research has validated the discrepancy between current and ideal body size as a measure of body dissatisfaction (119,120). One disadvantage of the body figural stimuli that are currently available for use is that they were not designed for use with extremely obese persons, i.e., above about 250 lb, which has limited their use in obesity research.

2. Questionnaires

Many questionnaires have been developed for the measurement of body dissatisfaction or body dysphoria (117). A recent factor analytic study (121) found many of the more commonly used questionnaires to form a single factor. These questionnaires were: (1) the body dissatisfaction scale of the Eating Disorder Inventory-2 (122), (2) the Body Shape Questionnaire (123), and (3) the Body Image Automatics Thoughts Questionnaire (124). These questionnaires may be used to evaluate body dissatisfaction associated with obesity and the reduction of body dissatisfaction that would be expected to accompany weight loss.

V.   SUMMARY AND CONCLUSIONS

Research pertaining to behavioral and psychological correlates of obesity is now a well-developed research area. Earlier studies attempted to establish personality types and psychopathology specific to obesity. This approach started with the assumption that there was a psychological basis for obesity. Research on obesity ran a similar course to research pertaining to other "psychosomatic" disorders, e.g., asthma, headache, and ulcers; i.e., no consistent personality profile specific to obesity was established. Instead, this research found that only a minority of obese persons were significantly distressed and that these distressed persons were overrepresented in samples seeking weight loss treatment. In response to these earlier findings, behavioral researchers turned their attention to the psychological factors that were more specific to eating and body weight, e.g., overeating, binge eating, dieting, and body image/dissatisfaction. From this research effort, many assessment methods for measuring behavioral and psychological correlates of obesity were developed. Using these methods, behavioral scientists have begun to identify risk factors that are predictive of psychological distress associated with obesity. We believe that this research effort should be continued. Also, behavioral research has found that weight loss is generally associated with beneficial psychological effects. This set of findings is very encouraging since it suggests that the psychological distress associated with obesity is, in principle, reversible.

REFERENCES

1.   Diagnostic and Statistical Manual of Mental Disorders, 4th ed. Washington, DC: American Psychiatric Association, 1994.
2.   Fitzgibbon ML, Stolley, MR, Kirschenbaum DS. Obese people who seek treatment have different characteristics than those who do not seek treatment. Health Psychol 1993; 12:342–345.
3.   O'Neil PM, Jarrell MP. Psychological aspects of obesity and dieting. In: Wadden TA, Van Itallie TB, eds. Treatment of the Seriously Obese Patient. New York: Guilford Press, 1992.
4.   Stunkard AJ, Wadden TA. Psychological aspects of severe obesity. Am J Clin Nutr 1992; 55:524S–532S.
5.   Wadden TA, Stunkard JJ. Social and psychological consequences of obesity. Ann Intern Med 1985; 103: 1062–1067.
6.   Berman WH, Berman ER, Heymsfeld S, Fauci M, Ackerman S. The effect of psychiatric disorders on weight loss in obesity clinic patients. Behav Med 1993; 18:167–162.
7.   Goldsmith SJ, Anger-Friedfeld K, Beren S, Rudolph D, Boeck M, Aronne L. Psychiatric illness in patients presenting for obesity treatment. Int J Eating Disord 1992; 12:63–71.
8.   Halmi KA, Long M, Stunkard AJ, Mason E. Psychiatric diagnosis of morbidly obese gastric bypass patients. Am J Psychiatry 1980; 137:470–472.
9.   Robins LN, Helzer JE, Weissman MM, Orvaschel H, Gurenberg E, Burke JD, Regier DA. Lifetime prevalence of specific psychiatric disorders in three sites. Arch Gen Psychiatry 1984; 41:949–958.
10.   Prather RC, Williamson, DA. Psychopathology associated with bulimia, binge eating, and obesity. Int J Eating Disord 1988; 7:177–184.
11.   Friedman MA, Brownell KD. Psychological correlates of obesity: moving to the next research generation. Psychol Bull 1995; 117:3–20.
12.   Klesges RC. Personality and obesity: global versus specific measures. Behav Ther 1984; 6:347–356.
13.   Leon GR, Roth L. Obesity: Psychological causes, correlations, and speculations. Psychol Bull 1977; 84:117–139.
14.   Blankmeyer BL, Smylie KD, Price DC, Costello RM, McFee AS, Fuller DS. A replicated five cluster MMPI topology of morbidly obese female candidates for gastric bypass. Int J Obes 1990; 14:235–247.
15.   O'Connor J, Dowrick PW. Cognition in normal weight, overweight, and previously overweight adults. Cognit Ther Res 1987; 11:315–326.
16.   Paine PM. Investigation of the abstinence violation effect in an obese population. Dissertation Abstr Int 1982; 42: 3434B–3435B.
17.   Bjorvell H, Rossner S, Stunkard AJ. Obesity, weight loss, and dietary restraint. Int J Eating Disord 1986; 5: 727–734.
18.   Stunkard AJ, Wadden TA. Restrained eating and human obesity. Nutr Rev 1990; 48(Suppl 2):78–86.
19.   Herman CP, Mack D. Restrained and unrestrained eating. J Personality 1975; 43:647–660.
20.   Herman CP, Polivy J. Anxiety, restraint, and eating behavior. J Abnorm Psychol 1975; 84:666–672.
21.   Polivy J, Herman CP. Dieting and binging: a causal analysis. Am Psychologist 1985; 40:193–201.
22.   Cools J, Schotte DE, McNally RJ. Emotional arousal and overeating in restrained eaters. J Abnorm Psychol 1992; 101:348–351.
23.   Polivy J, Herman CP. Etiology of binge eating: psychological mechanisms. In: Fairburn CG, Wilson GT, eds. Binge

Eating: Nature, Assessment and Treatment. New York: Guilford Press, 1993:173–205.

24. Lawson OJ, Williamson DA, Champagne CM, DeLany JP, Brooks ER, Howat PM, Wozniak PJ, Bray GA, Ryan DH. The association of body weight, dietary intake, and energy expenditure with dietary restraint and disinhibition. Obes Res 1995; 3:433–439.

25. Westenhoefer J. Dietary restraint and disinhibition: is restraint a homogeneous construct? Appetite 1991; 16: 45–55.

26. Williamson DA, Lawson OJ, Brooks ER, Wozniak PJ, Ryan DH, Bray GA, Duchmann EG. Association of body mass with dietary restraint and disinhibition. Appetite 1995; 25:31–41.

27. Lowe MR. The effects of dieting on eating behavior: a three-factor model. Psychol Bull 1993; 114:100–121.

28. Rosen JC. Body image disorder: Definition, development, and contribution to eating disorders. In: Crowther JH, Tennenbaum DL, Hobfoll SE, Stephens MAP, eds. The Etiology of Bulimia: The Individual and Family Context. Washington, DC: Hemisphere Publishers, 1992:157–177.

29. Thompson JK. Body image: Extent of disturbance, associated features, theoretical models, assessment methodologies, intervention strategies, and a proposal for a new DSM-IV diagnostic category—Body Image Disorder. In: Hersen M, Eisler RM, Miller PM, eds. Progress in Behavior Modification. Sycamore, IL: Sycamore Publishers, 1992: 3–54.

30. Williamson DA. Body image disturbances in eating disorders: a form of cognitive bias? Eating Disord J Treat Prev 1996; 4:47–58.

31. Collins JK. Methodology for the objective measurement of body image. Int J Eating Disord 1987; 6:393–399.

32. Collins JK, Beaumont PJV, Touyz SW, Krass J, Thompson P, Philips T. Variability in body shape perception in anorexic, bulimic, obese, and control subjects. Int J Eating Disord 1987; 6:633–638.

33. Counts CR, Adams HE. Body image in bulimic, dieting, and normal females. J Psychopathol Behav Assess 1985; 7:289–300.

34. Stunkard AJ, Mendelson M. Disturbances in body image of some obese persons. J Am Diet Assoc 1961; 38: 328–331.

35. Rand CSW, MacGregor AMC. Successful weight loss following obesity surgery and the perceived liability of morbid obesity. Int J Obes 1991; 15:577–579.

36. Stunkard AJ, Burt V. Obesity and the body image. II. Age at onset of disturbances in the body image. Am J Psychiatry 1967; 123:1443–1447.

37. Cash TF. Body-image attitudes among obese enrollers in a commercial weight-loss program. Percept Motor Skills 1993; 77:1099–1103.

38. Rosen JC, Orosan P, Reiter J. Cognitive behavior therapy for negative body image in obese women. Behav Ther 1995; 26:25–42.

39. French SA, Story M, Perry CL. Self-esteem and obesity in children and adolescents: A literature review. Obes Res 1995; 3:479–490.

40. Kolotkin RL, Head S, Hamilton M, Tse C-KJ. Assessing impact of weight on quality of life. Obes Res 1995; 3: 49–56.

41. Allon N. The stigma of overweight in everyday life. In: Wolman BB, ed. Psychological Aspects of Obesity: A Handbook. New York: Van Nostrand Reinhold, 1982.

42. Klesges RC, Klem ML, Hanson CL, Eck LH, Ernst J, O'Laughlin D, Garrott A, Rife R. The effects of applicant's health status and qualifications on simulated hiring decisions. Int J Obes 1990; 14:527–535.

43. Gortmaker SL, Must A, Perrin JM, Sobol AM, Dietz WH. Social and economic consequences of overweight in adolescence and young adulthood. N Engl J Med 1993; 329: 1008–1012.

44. Blumberg P, Mellis PP. Medical students' attributes toward the obese and the morbidly obese. Int J Eating Disord 1985; 4:169–175.

45. Oberrieder H, Walker R, Monroe D, Adeyanju M. Attitude of dietetics students and registered dietitians toward obesity. J Am Diet Assoc 1995; 95:914–916.

46. Price JH, Desmond SM, Krol RA, Snyder FF, O'Connell JK. Family practice physician's beliefs, attitudes, and practices regarding obesity. Am J Prev Med 1987; 3:339–345.

47. Rand CSW, MacGregor AMC. Morbidly obese patients' perceptions of social discrimination before and after surgery for obesity. South Med J 1990; 83:1390–1395.

48. Miller CT, Rothblum ED, Barbour L, Brand PA, Felicio DM. Do obese women have poorer social relationships than nonobese women? Reports by self, friends, and co-workers. J Personality 1990; 58:365–380.

49. Kral JG, Sjostrom LV, Sullivan MEE. Assessment of quality of life before and after surgery for severe obesity. Am J Clin Nutr 1992; 55:611S–614S.

50. Garn SM, Sullivan TV, Hawthorne VM. Educational level, fatness, and fatness differences between husbands and wives. Am J Clin Nutr 1989; 50:740–745.

51. Kumanyika S. Obesity in black women. Epidemiol Rev 1987; 9:31–50.

52. Stevens J, Kumanyika SK, Keil JE. Attitudes toward body size and dieting: Differences between elderly black and white women. Am J Public Health 1994; 84:1322–1325.

53. Kumanyika S, Wilson JF, Guilford-Davenport M. Weight-related attitudes and behaviors of black women. J Am Diet Assoc 1993; 93:416–422.

54. Powell AD, Kahn AS. Racial differences in women's desires to be thin. Int J Eating Disord 1995; 17:191–195.

55. Kolotkin RL, Revis ES, Kirkley B, Janick L. Binge eating in obesity: Associated MMPI characteristics. J Consult Clin Psychol 1987; 55:872–876.

56. Yanovski SZ, Nelson JE, Dubbert BK, Spitzer RL. Association of binge eating disorder and psychiatric comorbidity in obese subjects. Am J Psychiatry 1993; 150: 1472–1479.

57. Cook VL, O'Neil PM, Hedden CE, Brewerton TD, Cochrane CE. Psychological correlates of binge-eating disorder in obese persons. Obes Res 1993; 1:86S (abstract).

58. Marcus MD, Wing RR, Lamparski DM. Binge eating and dietary restraint in obese patients. Addict Behav 1985; 10: 163–168.

59. Marcus MD, Wing RR, Hopkins J. Obese binge eaters: Affect, cognition, and response to behavioral weight control. J Consult Clin Psychol 1988; 5:433–439.

60. Yanovski SZ. Binge eating disorder: Current knowledge and future directions. Obes Res 1993; 1:306–324.

61. Kanter RA, Williams BE, Cummings C. Personal and parental alcohol abuse, and victimization in obese binge eaters and nonbingeing obese. Addict Behav 1992; 17: 439–445.

62. Dansky BS, Brewerton TD, Kilpatrick DG, O'Neil PM. The National Women's Study: Relationship of victimization and PTSD to bulimia nervosa. Int J Eating Disord (in press).

63. Danksy BS, O'Neil PM, Brewerton TD, Kilpatrick DG. The nature of the relationship between obesity and victimization in a national sample of U.S. women. Ann Behav Med 1993; 15:S67 (abstract).

64. Stunkard AJ, Rush J. Dieting and depression reexamined: a Critical review of reports of untoward responses during weight reduction for obesity. Ann Intern Med 1974; 81: 526–533.

65. French SA, Jeffery RW. Consequences of dieting to lose weight: effects on physical and mental health. Health Psychol 1994; 13:195–212.

66. Wilson GT. Relation of dieting and voluntary weight loss to psychological functioning and binge eating. Ann Intern Med 1993; 119:727–730.

67. Wing RR, Epstein LH, Marcus MD, Kupfer DJ. Mood changes in behavioral weight loss programs. J Psychosom Res 1984; 28:189–196.

68. Rosen JC, Leitenberg H. Bulimia nervosa: Treatment with exposure and response prevention. Behav Ther 1982; 13: 117–124.

69. Wadden TA, Stunkard AJ, Brownell KD, Day SC. A comparison of two very-low-calorie diets: protein-sparing modified fast versus protein-formula-liquid diet. Am J Clin Nutr 1985; 41:533–539.

70. Wadden TA, Mason G, Foster GD, Stunkard AJ, Prange AJ. Effects of a very low calorie diet on weight, thyroid hormones, and mood. Int J Obes 1990; 14:249–258.

71. Anderson IM, Parry-Billings M, Newsholme EA, Fairburn CG, Cowen PJ. Dieting reduces plasma tryptophan and alters brain 5-HT function in women. Psychol Med 1990; 20:785–791.

72. Lappalainen R, Sjoden PO, Hursti T, Vesa V. Hunger/craving responses and reactivity to food stimuli during fasting and dieting. Int J Obes 1990; 14:679–688.

73. Wadden TA, Stunkard AJ, Day SC, Gould RA, Rubin CJ. Less food, less hunger: reports of appetite and symptoms in a controlled study of a protein-sparing modified fast. Int J Obes 1987; 11:239–249.

74. Wing RR, Marcus MD, Blair EH, Burton LR. Psychological responses of obese type II diabetic subjects to very-low-calorie diet. Diabetes Care 1991; 14:596–599.

75. Speaker JG, Schultz C, Grinker JA, Stern JS. Body size estimation and locus of control in obese adolescent boys undergoing weight reduction. Int J Obes 1983; 7:73–83.

76. Butcher JN. MMPI-2 in Psychological Treatment. New York: Oxford University Press, 1990.

77. Morey LC, Kurtz JE. Assessment of general personality and psychopathology among persons with eating and weight-related concerns. In: Allison DB, ed. Handbook of Assessment Methods for Eating Behaviors and Weight-Related Problems. Thousand Oaks, CA: Sage Publications, 1995:1–22.

78. Wiggins JS. Substantive dimensions of self-report in the MMPI item pool. Psychol Monogr 1966; 80:22 (whole no. 630).

79. Graham JR. The MMPI: A Practical Guide, 2nd ed. New York: Oxford University Press, 1987.

80. Williamson DA. Assessment of Eating Disorders: Obesity, Anorexia, and Bulimia Nervosa. New York: Pergamon Press, 1990.

81. Derogatis L. Manual for the Symptom Checklist-90, Revised. Baltimore: Johns Hopkins Press, 1977.

82. Williamson DA, Kelley ML, Davis CJ, Ruggiero L, Blouin DC. Psychopathology of eating disorders: a controlled comparison of bulimic, obese, and normal subjects. J Consult Clin Psychol 1985; 53:161–166.

83. Beck AT, Rush AJ, Shaw BR, Emery G. Cognitive Therapy for Depression. New York: Guilford Press, 1979.

84. Beck AT, Steer RA, Garbin MG. Psychometric properties of the Beck Depression Inventory: twenty-five years of evaluation. Clin Psychol Rev 1988; 8:77–100.

85. Spielberger CD, Gorsuch RL, Lushene RE. Manual for the State Trait Anxiety Inventory. Palo Alto, CA: Consulting Psychologists Press, 1970.

86. Polivy J, Herman PH, Howard KI. Restraint Scale: assessment of dieting. In: Hersen M, Bellack AS, eds. Dictionary of Behavioral Assessment Techniques. New York: Pergamon Press, 1988:377–380.

87. Gorman BS, Allison DB. Measures of restrained eating. In: Allison DB, ed. Handbook of Assessment Methods for Eating Behaviors and Weight-Related Problems. Thousand Oaks, CA: Sage Publications, 1995:149–184.

88. Stunkard AJ, Messick S. The Three-Factor Eating Questionnaire to measure dietary restraint, disinhibition, and hunger. J Psychosom Res 1985; 29:71–83.

89. Allison DA, Kalinsky LB, Gorman BS. A comparison of the psychometric properties of three measures of dietary restraint. Psychol Assess 1992; 4:391–398.

90. Van Strein T, Frijters JER, Bergers GPA, Defares PB. The Dutch Eating Behavior Questionnaire (DEBQ) for assessment of restrained, emotional, and external eating behavior. Int J Eating Disord 1986; 5:295–315.

91. O'Neil PM, Currey HS, Hirsh AA, Malcolm RJ, Sexauer JD, Riddle FE, Tayor CT. Development and validation of the Eating Behavior Inventory. J Behav Assess 1979; 1 (Suppl 2):123–132.

92. Currey HS, O'Neil PM, Malcolm R, Riddle FE. Factor analysis of the eating behavior inventory, 4th International Congress on Obesity, New York, October 1983.

93. Hawkins RC, Clement PF. Development and construct validation of a self-report measure of binge eating tendencies. Addict Behav 1980; 5:219–226.

94. Pike KM, Loeb K, Walsh BT. Binge eating and purging. In: Allison DB, ed. Handbook of Assessment Methods for Eating Behaviors and Weight-Related Problems. Thousand Oaks, CA: Sage Publications, 1995:303–346.

95. Gormally J, Black S, Daston S, Rardin D. The assessment of binge eating severity among obese persons. Addict Behav 1982; 7:47–55.

96. Fairburn CG, Cooper Z. The eating disorder examination. In: Fairburn CG, Wilson GT, eds. Binge Eating: Nature, Assessment, and Treatment, 12th ed. New York: Guilford Press, 1993:3–14.

97. Williamson DA, Anderson DA, Gleaves DH. Anorexia and bulimia nervosa: structured interview methodologies and psychological assessment. In: Thompson K, ed. Body Image, Eating Disorders, and Obesity: A Practical Guide for Assessment and Treatment. Washington, DC: American Psychological Association Books 1996:205–223.

98. Smith MC, Thelen MH. Development and validation of a test for bulimia. J Consult Clin Psychol 1984; 52: 863–872.

99. Thelen MH, Farmer J, Wonderlich S, Smith M. A revision of the Bulimia Test: The BULIT-R. Psychol Assess 1991; 3:119–124.

100. Diagnostic and Statistical Manual of Mental Disorders, 3rd ed-rev. Washington, DC: American Psychiatric Association, 1987.

101. Williamson DA, Anderson DA, Jackman LP, Jackson SR. Assessment of eating disordered thoughts, feelings, and behaviors. In: Allison DB, ed. Methods for the Assessment of Eating Behaviors and Weight Related Problems. Newbury Park, CA: Sage Publications, 1995:327–386.

102. Williamson DA, Prather RC, McKenzie SJ, Blouin DC. Behavioral assessment procedures can differentiate bulimia nervosa, compulsive overeater, obese, and normal subjects. Behav Assess 1990; 12:239–252.

103. Arnow B, Kenardy J, Agras WS. The Emotional Eating Scale: The development of a measure to assess coping with negative affect by eating. Int J Eating Disord 1995; 18 (Suppl 1):79–90.

104. Williamson DA, Davis CJ, Goreczny AJ, McKenzie SJ, Watkins PC. The Eating Questionnaire-Revised: a new symptom checklist for bulimia. In: Keller PA, Ritt LG, eds. Innovations in Clinical Practice: A Sourcebook. Sarasota, FL: Professional Resource Exchange, 1989:321–326.

105. Ruggiero L, Williamson DA, Davis CJ, Schlundt DG, Carey MP. Forbidden food survey: measure of bulimic's an-

ticipated emotional reactions to specific foods. Addict Behav 1988; 13:267–274.

106. Schlundt DG. Assessment of specific eating behaviors and eating style. In: Allison DB, ed. Handbook of Assessment Methods for Eating Behaviors and Weight-Related Problems: Measures, Theory, and Research. Thousand Oaks, CA: Sage Publications, 1995:241–302.

107. Gleaves DH, Williamson DA, Barker SE. Additive effects of mood and eating forbidden foods upon the perceptions of overeating and binging in bulimia nervosa. Addict Behav 1993; 18:299–309.

108. Schlundt DG, Johnson WG, Jarrell MP. A naturalistic functional analysis of eating behavior in bulimia and obesity. Adv Behav Res Ther 1985; 7:149–162.

109. Williamson DA, Gleaves DH, Lawson OJ. Biased perception of overeating in bulimia nervosa and compulsive binge eaters. J Psychopathol Behav Assess 1991; 13: 257–268.

110. Bandani LG, Schoeller DA, Cyr HN, Dietz WH. Validity of reported energy intake in obese and nonobese adolescents. Am J Clin Nutr 1990; 52:421–425.

111. Wolper C, Heshka S, Heymsfield SB. Measuring food intake: an overview. In: Allison DB, ed. Handbook of Assessment Methods for Eating Behaviors and Weight-Related Problems: Measures, Theory, and Research. Thousand Oaks, CA: Sage Publications, 1995:215–240.

112. Rimm EB, Giovannucci EL, Stampfer MJ, Colditz GA, Litin LB, Willet WC. Reproducibility and validity of an expanded self-administered semiquantitative food frequency questionnaire among male health professionals. Am J Epidemiol 1992; 135:1114–1126.

113. Block G, Hartman A, Naughton D. A reduced dietary questionnaire: development and validation. Epidemiology 1990; 1:58–64.

114. Cooper Z, Fairburn CG. The Eating Disorder Examination: A semi-structured interview for the assessment of the specific psychopathology of eating disorders. Int J Eating Disord 1987; 6:1–8.

115. Shelton ML, Klesges RC. Measures of physical activity and exercises. In: Allison DB, ed. Handbook of Assessment Methods for Eating Behaviors and Weight-Related Problems: Measures, Theory, and Research. Thousand Oaks, CA: Sage Publications, 1995:185–214.

116. Pambianco G, Wing RR, Robertson R. Accuracy and reliability of the Caltrac accelerometer for estimating energy expenditure. Med Sci Sports Exerc 1990; 22:858–862.

117. Thompson JK. Assessment of body image. In: Allison DB, ed. Handbook of Assessment Methods for Eating Behaviors and Weight-Related Problems: Measures, Theory, and Research. Thousand Oaks, CA: Sage Publications, 1995: 119–148.

118. Stunkard A, Sorenson T, Schlusinger F. Use of the Danish Adoption Register for the study of obesity and thinness. In: Kety S, Rowland LP, Sidman RL, Matthysse SW, eds. The Genetics of Neurological and Psychiatric Disorders. New York: Raven Press, 1983:115–120.

119. Gleaves DH, Williamson DA, Eberenz KP, Sebastian SE, Barker SE. Clarifying body-image disturbance; analysis of a multidimensional model using structural modeling. J Personality Assess 1995; 64:478–493.

120. Williamson DA, Gleaves DH, Watkins PC, Schlundt DG. Validation of a self-ideal body size discrepancy as a measure of body size dissatisfaction. J Psychol Behav Assess 1993; 15(Suppl 1):57–68.

121. Williamson DA, Barker SE, Berman LE, Gleaves DH. Body image, body dysphoria, dietary restraint: factor structure in nonclinical subjects. Behav Res Ther 1995; 33(Suppl 1):85–93.

122. Garner DM. Eating Disorder Inventory-2 Manual. Odessa, FL: Psychological Assessment Resources, 1991.

123. Cooper PJ, Taylor MJ, Cooper Z, Fairburn CG. Development and validation of the Body Shape Questionnaire. Int J Eating Disord 1987; 6:485–494.

124. Brown TA, Johnson WG, Bergeron KC, Keeton WP, Cash TF. Assessment of body-related cognitions in bulimia: the Body Image Automatic Thoughts Questionnaire. Unpublished manuscript, 1990.

9

Culture, Evolution, and Obesity

Peter J. Brown
Emory University, Atlanta, Georgia

Vicki K. Bentley-Condit
Grinnell College, Grinnell, Iowa

I. INTRODUCTION: AN ANTHROPOLOGICAL APPROACH

This chapter uses an anthropological perspective to examine the relationship between evolution, culture, and obesity. This approach can add significantly to our understanding of obesity in the broad context of history and human behavior. We suggest that the modern epidemic of obesity is rooted in our evolutionary past. This is because both genetic and cultural predispositions to obesity are shaped by an interaction of internal (e.g., biological, psychological, perceptual) and external (e.g., environmental, cultural) forces. The first goal of this chapter is to examine three factors that affect the individual's propensity toward, and interpretation of, his or her own obesity: gender, ethnicity, and socioeconomic status. The social epidemiological distribution of obesity can be best explained in reference to the evolution of human genetic traits and the cultural creation of group and personal identities. The second goal is to describe social science research on the negative consequences of being obese in a culture that values slenderness and often interprets fatness as a sign of moral failing. Finally, we advocate a biocultural approach to understanding obesity. By incorporating both cultural and evolutionary views, such an approach may yield an integrated understanding of the variation in both incidence and interpretation of obesity in different social and ethnic groups.

The etiology of obesity is complex. Excess adiposity is caused by the interaction of genetic predispositions operating under necessary environmental conditions. In recent years, the evidence for the existence of genes that enable individuals to store energy reserves in the form of fat has been increasingly impressive; those individuals with "fat phenotypes" are likely to develop adult obesity (1–6). These genes, and their metabolic processes of fat deposition, are part of our species' evolutionary heritage dating back at least 20,000 years.

Cultural practices are also involved in obesity etiology. While cultural predispositions to obesity are changeable, genetic predispositions resulting from evolution are not—at least not in the short run. As such, culture (which affects both diet and exercise patterns) is the key to obesity prevention. Moreover, it is important that the existing beliefs and practices of populations at risk for obesity be understood. It is impossible to completely separate cultural/behavioral from genetic/evolutionary factors. While cultural practices and beliefs can offer insight into the "how" of obesity, an evolutionary perspective can help us to understand "why." Combining these perspectives has the potential to offer a deeper understanding of this condition.

This chapter is organized in four parts: first, it considers the basic concepts of evolution, culture, and obesity; second, it reviews evolutionary factors in terms of gender, class, and ethnic differences; third, it examines cultural factors with regard to gender, ethnic, and socioeconomic interpretations; and fourth, it outlines the benefits of taking a biocultural approach to understanding the effects of obesity.

II. BASIC CONCEPTS: DEFINING THE COMPONENTS

A. Evolution Defined

To understand why obesity has become a problem in contemporary developed societies, it is necessary to be cognizant of both human evolution and the basic tenets of evolutionary process. The three primary principles of Darwinian evolution are: (1) there must be variation, (2) this variation must be heritable, and (3) this heritable variation must lead to differential reproductive success (7). The interaction of these principles results in natural selection, the principle mechanism of evolution. Selection occurs through the reproductive advantages afforded to those individuals better adapted to their environment. Thus, evolution (and hence natural selection) is not just a matter of survival but also of reproduction (8).

So, why should obesity have evolved? What reproductive advantage could have been afforded to individuals with "obese phenotypes" in human evolutionary history? Before addressing these questions, we should point out that any evolutionary advantages of obesity would not necessarily have to be evident in current society. Evolution is a long, slow process. There is often a lag time between environmental change and organism evolution. The changes that most societies have undergone in just the past 200 years far outpace any possible evolutionary adjustments.

The environmental conditions necessary for a high prevalence of obesity are quite new. Throughout most of human history, obesity was neither a common problem nor a realistic possibility for the majority of individuals, as humans were regularly subjected to food shortages in the process of their evolution. Chronic food shortages, which continue to plague humanity, have been powerful agents of natural selection for both genes and cultural traits. It is only in the context of relative affluence and constant food surpluses that obesity and overweight have become such widespread and intractable health problems.

B. Culture

From an anthropological perspective, culture plays a fundamental role in causing the social epidemiological distribution of obesity. Culture refers to the learned patterns of behavior and beliefs characteristic of a society or social group. Those who share a cultural system of thought and behavior range from isolated tribes (traditionally studied by anthropologists) to subunits of complex societies, like social classes. Culture includes directly observable material aspects, like diet or productive economy, as well as important ideological components, such as aesthetic standards of ideal body type.

Cultural behaviors and beliefs are learned in childhood, are often deeply held, and are seldom questioned by adults who pass this "obvious" knowledge to their offspring. As such, cultural beliefs and values are largely unconscious factors in the motivations of individual behaviors. Cultural beliefs define what is normal, and because of this, constrain the individual's behavioral choices. The concept of culture is clearly related to social categories like ethnicity that are characterized by particular beliefs and practices. Ethnicity refers to the cultural commonalities of group members who claim reference to common origins and who operate in the context of a wider social system.

Brown (9) has shown that three levels of a cultural system (i.e., the productive economy, the social organization, and the belief system) play a role in the etiology of obesity. The productive economy must produce a food surplus that is distributed through the social system. Both the productive economy and the social system had adaptive functions in the context of food shortages, particularly for the privileged classes. Cultural beliefs can function as predisposing factors to obesity.

In terms of overall human history, culture represents *Homo sapiens'* primary mechanism of evolutionary adaptation. The capacity for culture is the primary reason for the evolutionary success of humans because of its distinct advantages of greater speed and flexibility over genetic evolution (10). Anthropologists believe that all cultural variations in the world today are derived from the original human life-style of hunting and gathering. Contemporary human biology was largely shaped by this prehistoric past, and current chronic diseases are the result of a discordance between our paleolithic biology and the modern culture of affluence (11).

C. Obesity is Defined by Culture

Definitions of obesity and overweight have been the subject of substantial medical debate, in part because they must be based on inferred definitions of normality or "ideal" body proportions. In this regard, it is important to remember that culture defines normalcy, and scientific debates about the definition of obesity thus contain an often unrecognized cultural component. Complicating the matter of defining obesity is the point that obesity also appears to be a state of mind (12). Once the label is assigned by the individual to his/herself, it is difficult to remove—even following weight loss. "Feeling fat" is a common complaint today, even among individuals who are not. Thus obesity is both a physiological and a psychological condition (13).

The sociocultural history of height and weight standards in the United States, and the historical changes in the moral meanings of different body types, and scales, have been the subject of recent books (14,15). From 1943 to 1980 definitions of "ideal weights" for height for women were consistently lowered, while those for men remained approximately the same (16). A debate followed the 1983 upward revision of ideal weights for women (based on new mortality statistics), which revealed that many experts saw the revision as "backsliding." In other words, definitions of ideal and normal body size reflected cultural and cosmetic standards, as well as medical issues. In contemporary American and Western European societies, the cosmetic ideal of body size for women is thinner than the medical ideal.

A critically important dimension to the definition of obesity involves the distribution of fat around the body trunk (central body fat) or on the limbs (peripheral body fat). This important distinction is of such importance that measures of fat distribution like waist-to-hips ratio may be more useful measures of mortality risk associated with obesity than the traditional percent over "ideal body weight." In fact, Björntorp has argued that only abdominal obesity should be distinguished as obesity, and that peripheral accumulation of fat should receive less emphasis in the same way that muscle enlargement, large ears, or large feet are not distinguished by medical terminology (17). Given the cultural emphasis on body weight in American society, it is not likely that the definition of medical obesity will be changed in this way, despite its powerful medical logic. For the purposes of this chapter, we accept the traditional biomedical definitions of obesity. However, we insist that these definitions are culturally mediated.

III. EVOLUTION AND SOCIAL-EPIDEMIOLOGICAL CONTEXT OF OBESITY

Like most diseases, obesity exhibits a nonrandom historical and social distribution. What social groupings are most at risk for obesity and why the condition is distributed that way are important issues. There are three facts about this social distribution that are particularly cogent: (1) a gender difference in the total percent, site distribution, and prevalence of obesity; (2) the concentration of

obesity in certain ethnic groups; and (3) a powerful and complex relationship between social class and obesity. Since these three factors are inextricably linked, there is some overlap in the discussion that follows.

Because of their commonness and inevitability in human prehistory and history, food shortages have been a powerful force in both biological and cultural evolution. Whiting's cross-cultural ethnographic survey of 118 nonindustrial societies (with hunting and gathering, pastoral, horticultural, and agricultural economies) found some form of food shortages for *all* of the societies in the sample (18). Seasonal availability of food results in a seasonal cycle of weight loss and gain with greater fluctuation among agriculturists (19,20). The threat of hunger still plagues a large proportion of the world's population, including an estimated 20 million Americans (21).

Given the frequency of food shortages under natural conditions, selection favored individuals who could effectively store calories in times of surplus. For most individuals, such fat stores would be called on at least every 2–3 years. In this evolutionary context the usual range of human metabolic variation would have produced many individuals with a predisposition to become obese, yet they would never have the opportunity to do so. Furthermore, in this context there could be little or no natural selection *against* such a tendency. Selection could not provide for the eventuality of continuous surplus because it had simply never existed.

In archaeological terms, the current epidemic of overweight and obesity is very recent. For 99% of the genus *Homo*'s history, humans were hunters and gatherers. There are no reported cases of obesity among current peoples following a hunting and gathering way of life. We believe obesity was so rare as to be virtually nonexistent until the invention of farming (approximately 10,000 years ago) and the subsequent Industrial Revolution (9).

The genetic components of obesity have been clearly demonstrated by Stunkard and colleagues (22). As such, the difficulty which most individuals have in *permanently* losing weight can be best understood in an ultimate evolutionary context. More than 20 years ago, researchers were reporting diet 5-year failure rates of more than 98% (23). Because humans evolved in environmental contexts of chronic food shortages, our bodies have an evolutionary predisposition to store energy in the form of fat in preparation for the inevitability of bad times. Humans tend to utilize fat stores relatively slowly; in conditions of energy deficit, muscle loss and even organ shrinkage occur before all fat stores are used. This is a major reason why the process of weight loss tends to be slow. In addition, evidence suggests an improvement in the physiological efficiency of extracting and storing fat from food in the context of food storages (24). From the point of view of the body, there is no difference between purposeful dieting and unintended famine. When given access to excess calories, the "starved body" is an even more efficient hoarder than it was in the prefamine condition. Consequently, a dieter may experience the "yo-yo" phenomenon of not only easily regaining the previously lost weight but, potentially, to return to a heavier equilibrium point than before dieting.

A.   Ethnic Differences

Obesity is more common in certain *kinds* of socioeconomic systems rather than in societies located in particular geographic zones (25). This indicates that culture plays a central etiological role in obesity and that simple-minded geographic determinism has no explanatory power. Worldwide, the highest reported prevalence of obesity is among Micronesians on the island of Nauru; the age-standardized adult obesity prevalence is 84.7% of males and 92.8% of females (26). Inhabitants of Nauru have remarkable access to Western foods and trade goods because of the exportations of particularly valuable mineral deposits from the island. In Europe, there is a higher prevalence of obesity among southern groups than northern groups within the same countries; there is also a higher risk of obesity in rural than urban dwellers (27). This distribution probably also reflects relative levels of economic development. However, within the United States where there is generally high overall prevalence of overweight and obesity (28), the behavioral risk factor surveys coordinated by the Centers for Disease Control indicate that the geographic distribution of obesity in the white majority population is generally higher in the northern Midwest, with Wisconsin having the highest prevalence (29). To date, we know of no adequate explanation for this geographic distribution.

From an evolutionary point of view, genetic selection would have been particularly intense in particular historical-ecological contexts affecting small populations; wherein particular conditions may act as population "bottlenecks" combining the evolutionary forces natural selection and genetic drift (including founder effect). This scenario has been suggested for both Native Americans and Pacific Islanders. In the modern context of complex multiethnic societies, genes that predispose for obesity may be maintained within ethnic groups because of the widespread social practice of endogamy (marriage within the group). In the United States, marriage partner correlations for ethnic minorities are extremely high (30), and this social practice may concentrate the genetic predispositions to obesity in particular subpopulations. In other words, a

pattern of "assortative mating" by social class as well as physical attributes (particularly stature) may also be related to the genetic etiology of obesity. U.S. ethnic groups with elevated rates of obesity include: African-Americans (particularly in the rural south) (31), Southwestern Native Americans (55), Hispanic Americans and Puerto Ricans (32), Gypsies (33), and Pacific Islanders (26). Genetic admixture with American Indian groups of the southwest has been suggested as a cause of elevated obesity rates among Mexican-Americans (34). The high prevalence of obesity in these ethnic groups reflects the interaction of genes, social class, and culture; it is a difficult task to disentangle the relative effects of these factors.

B.   Gender Differences

It is difficult to underestimate the importance of gender in understanding both the social epidemiology and sociological consequences of obesity. The greatest amount of sexual dimorphism (morphological differences between men and women) in humans is in the site of distribution of fat tissue. Women have more overall fat and much more peripheral body fat in the legs and hips (35) than men; men have, proportionally, much more central body fat. This gender difference pattern appears to be universal in our species. Since it is found in contemporary hunting and gathering groups like the !Kung San as well as in complex industrial countries (9), this gender dimorphism has clear evolutionary roots.

In the environment of human evolution, females with greater energy reserves in fat would have a selective advantage over their lean counterparts in withstanding the stress of food shortage, not only for themselves, but for their fetuses or nursing children. Humans have evolved to "save up" food energy for the inevitability of food shortages through the synthesis and storage of fat. Females have been selected for more peripheral body fat because that type of adipose tissue is mobilized after being endocrine-primed during late pregnancy and lactation (36). A minimal level of female fatness increases reproductive success because of its association with regular cycling and earlier menarche (37). Thus, the gender differences in fat deposition sites and obesity prevalence are a part of human evolutionary history.

IV.   CULTURAL FACTORS IN THE SOCIAL EPIDEMIOLOGY OF OBESITY

Cultural explanations are concerned with the direct, proximate, mechanisms that bring something about (7). Cultural explanations occur at a level distinct from that of evolutionary, or ultimate, explanations. In their own right, cultural explanations do not deal with adaptive significance and reproductive consequences. Thus, cultural explanations do not compete with evolutionary ones; these two anthropological approaches are, in fact, complementary.

Cultural explanations of obesity subsume aspects which are traditionally thought of as "learned behaviors." For example, it is not unusual among the mainstream white American culture for parents to encourage their children to eat particular foods by rewarding them with other food items. Many a parent has "bribed" a child with dessert in order to encourage the eating of vegetables. Recent research has shown that this culturally sanctioned pattern of rewards actually contributes to a dislike of the "good" foods and a preference for the "bad" foods (38). Thus, an evolutionary preference for high-fat foods is *reinforced* through learning; the difficulty that most individuals have in avoiding fattening foods has both evolutionary and cultural foundations.

A. Ethnicity and Culture

Ethnicity is an important variable for understanding the distribution of obesity, but it brings with it the danger of stereotyping—the mistaken notion that all members of a group are alike. While it is valuable to describe the *range* of variation in behaviors and beliefs among ethnic groups in the United States with high prevalence of obesity, it is important to remember that these ethnic groups are heterogeneous and that upwardly mobile ethnics more closely resemble mainstream American culture in attitudes about obesity and ideal body shape. However, obesity studies have shown that even when socioeconomic status was controlled as a factor, particular ethnic groups have significantly higher rates of obesity (39). Additionally, nutritionists have indicated that, even within mainstream U.S. culture, ethnic groups maintain dietary conventions meaningful to their own background (40).

Culturally defined standards of a beautiful body vary between societies and across historical epochs (41). In a preliminary cross-cultural survey using the Human Relation Area File data, Brown (9) found that 81% of the societies for which there were sufficient data rated "plumpness" or being "filled out" as an attribute of beauty in females, particularly fat deposits on the hips and legs. Among the Havasupai of the American Southwest, a fat woman "stands" for a thin pubertal girl by placing her foot on the girl's back. The Havasupai consider fat legs and arms essential to beauty and this practice "makes" the girl attractively plump (42). The Amhara of the Horn of Africa refer to thin hips in a woman as "dog hips," a typical insult

(43). Cross-cultural research also reveals that the male body ideal is most often bigness (large stature and muscularity), but not necessarily fatness (9,121).

In a more comprehensive cross-cultural comparison of ethnographic date from the Human Relations Area Files, Anderson and colleagues (44) show that cultural ideals of a plump body shape for women is correlated with five variables: the reliability of food supply; climate; the status of women; the value of women's work; and the adverse consequences of adolescent sexual expression for girls. These socioecological variables appear to be clearly linked to biocultural evolutionary processes.

American ideals of thinness occur in a setting where it is easy to become fat, and the preference for plumpness occurs in settings where it is easy to remain lean. Each in its own particular cultural context, these standards of beauty require the investment of individual effort and economic resources. There are particular cultural behaviors and beliefs about obesity that characterize the dominant white culture. Mainstream obesity ideology can be summarized as: (1) obesity is always bad for your health; (2) obesity is primarily due to uncontrolled individual behaviors, particularly overeating and underexercising; and (3) anyone who wants to be can be slim (45). The idea that anyone can be slim is an important assumption in both the social stigmatization of overweight and the commercialization of the weight-loss industry. There is also evidence that men are less concerned with the social meaning of fatness in comparison to women.

Especially for women, slenderness signifies an individual's self-control over the power of food and the temporary conquest of the body's natural tendency to decline. Exercise classes and dieting foods are commodities with salient cultural meanings for such control of culture over nature. The dominant American ideology is that some approximation of the "perfect body" can be acquired, given sufficient physical and financial investment (46). As the following examples show, members of ethnic minorities do not necessarily share the cultural beliefs of the white cultural majority.

I. Hispanic Americans

There has been substantial research on social and cultural factors related to obesity among Hispanic Americans, the second largest ethnic minority in the United States (47). The Centers for Disease Control survey of this broad category of diverse ethnic subgroups (Mexican-Americans, Puerto Ricans, Cuban Americans) reported high prevalences of overweight and obesity (32). The subgroup with the highest prevalence was Mexican-American women for whom, traditionally, the concept of fatness (*gordura*) has had positive cultural connotations meaning prosperity and health. This group does not believe that everyone can be slim, nor are they optimistic about the prospects of successful dieting. This fatalistic interpretation appears to be an important proximate mechanism affecting the obesity rate in this ethnic group (48).

There are also positive associations and a lack of social stigma of obesity to be found in Puerto Rican communities on both the island and the U.S. mainland (49). For Puerto Rican women, weight gain after marriage is a positive reflection on the husband as a good provider and on the woman as wife, cook, and mother. Even though some degree of plumpness in women is a marker of sexual attractiveness, weight gain after marriage also reflects a woman's marital fidelity, since it is not proper for a mother to be too concerned with her physical appearance (49). As such, weight loss is socially discouraged. This group also has a widespread fatalistic concept concerning the possibility of successful weight loss for the obese. Massara (50) has presented quantitative evidence suggesting significant differences in ideal body preferences between this ethnic community and mainstream American culture. Body types that are considered obese by biomedical standards are judged as "not too heavy" by Puerto Ricans for whom the folk definition of obese is 82% heavier than the medical ideal weight for height.

2. African-Americans

Studies over the past three decades have indicated that African-American women have great risk of overweight and obesity (51). The ratio of obesity prevalences for African-American to white women is nearly 2:1, even when controlling for social and socioeconomic class (52). As in the general population, there is an inverse correlation of obesity and social class for women in this ethnic group. Collectively, African-Americans appear to have a more relaxed attitude toward weight and weight gain than people in the mainstream culture (52). Among African-American adolescent girls, obesity is not correlated with low self-esteem as it is among whites (53). Obesity in this age group increased by 96% from 1963/65 to 1976/80 (54). African-American males are less likely to reject a female based on her weight than are white males (61). Gillum (31) reports ethnic differences in the definition of overweight for African-Americans compared to biomedical standards; less than half of the obese African-American women in one sample classified themselves as being much overweight (55). Styles (56) argues that African-American women view plumpness and bigness as signs of health, prosperity, and a "job well done" especially in the domestic arena. In this cultural context, the advantages of a large

body include being given respect and reduced chances of being bothered by young men in the neighborhood. Fatness is a component of a positive self-identity (121). The perceived risk of a food shortage—not for the society as a whole but for the immediate family—may be very important, especially if food shortages were personally experienced in the past.

3. Native Americans

Despite remarkable cultural diversity among Native American groups in the United States, these ethnic groups tend to be poor, rural, medically underserved, and characterized by elevated rates of obesity. The Pima Indians of central Arizona have the highest reported rates of obesity (and associated chronic diseases) in the country. Over one-half of all young adults in this group exceed the 90th percentile of weight/height standards (57). Such obesity prevalence in Native Americans is a historically recent phenomenon. For both the Pima and Navajo from the Southwest, obesity was extremely rare 40 years ago, although among Navajo obesity was absent in children of traditional families but reported for children of acculturated families (58). In many Native American groups, central body fatness does not carry negative social connotations. For example, Weidman reports that the Oklahoma Cherokee have an "obese body image" which includes the idea that for successful men the stomach should overhang the large Western-style belt (59).

4. Pacific Islanders

Obesity tends to be a serious problem among Pacific Islanders both in their native countries and among immigrants to the United States. According to Collins and colleagues (26), the prevalence of obesity is highest among Polynesians (males 44%, females 72%) and Micronesians (males 54%, females 68%). Samoans, a Polynesian group, are the most numerous Pacific Islands ethnic group currently residing in the United States. Samoans who migrate and become acculturated are at elevated risk of obesity and related chronic diseases. The traditional cultural values of Samoans idealize fatness as a sign of social power and prosperity (60). Food has great social and symbolic importance in these cultures. In many migrant Pacific Island populations, adult body size is viewed as unchangeable and inevitable.

B. Gender, Culture, and Fat

Because the ethnic, gender, and socioeconomic aspects of obesity are closely intertwined, there is unavoidable overlap in these discussions. In most traditional societies, fatness has frequently been a symbol of motherhood and maternal nurturance in adult women. In societies where women attain status primarily through successful motherhood, this symbolic association increases the cultural acceptability of obesity. The symbolic association links gender and well-being since a fat woman, symbolically, is well taken care of, and she in turns takes good care of her children. In contrast, the cultural ideal of thinness is found in relatively few developed societies where motherhood is not the primary means of female status attainment (44). This transformation is a modern historical one, and anthropologists have described the coinciding cultural changes in ecology, domestic gender relations, and cultural ideals of body type (121). In rural Spain, this social and physical change of the ideal female image is described as "from the Virgin Mary to the modern woman" (61); in Africa, it has been described as a change from the woman's role as "mother" to that of "mate" (62). This historical change is probably relative to the "epidemiological and demographic transitions," and because these processes have not equally affected all class groupings, it may help explain the relationship with socioeconomic class.

In mainstream U.S. culture, being overweight or obese is generally viewed as a more serious social problem for females than for males (63). Since this cultural fact includes both self-perceptions of attractiveness and feelings of well-being (or health), it influences biomedical reporting of prevalence rates, therapy-seeking behavior, and the overall interpretation of fatness as a problem. In this social context, females worry more about their weight, are more critical about their bodies, and, in general, desire to weigh less (64–67). Although these tendencies are more pronounced from adolescence onward, recent research indicates significant body shape dissatisfaction among girls as young as 9 years of age (68,69). Males and females have very different attitudes about gaining and losing weight. Women's concerns with these issues are reflected in body image distress, dieting patterns, desire to lose weight, and consumption of low-fat and low-calorie products (70,71). In general, men tend to be satisfied with their weight, and possibly because of this, men's self-reports of weight tend to be more accurate with a bias toward overestimating their weight. Conversely, because women tend to be dissatisfied with their weight, their self-reports tend to be underestimates (72,73). These cultural attitudes about gender and weight are further reflected in self-perception of "body image"; significantly more females than males perceive themselves as heavier than they really are (74,75). The same pattern holds for others' perceptions since females are more likely to be described by others as overweight than males with the same degrees of fatness (76). Despite these differences in interpretation and perception

by sex, a 1994 Behavioral Risk Factor Survey of approximately 30,000 individuals revealed very similar proportions of "overweight" and "very overweight" by gender (i.e., overweight: male = 15.8%, female = 15.9%; very overweight: male = 6.3%, female = 7.8%) (77).

C. Socioeconomic Class and Fat

Obesity is a serious problem primarily in those societies characterized by economic modernization, affluence, food surplus, and social stratification. Numerous studies of traditional societies undergoing the process of economic modernization demonstrate rapid increases in the prevalence of obesity (78–82). Trowell and Burkitt's volume of 15 case studies of epidemiological change in modernizing societies concludes that obesity is the first of the "Western diseases" (so-called "diseases of civilization") to appear (83).

The relationship between the risk of obesity and social class has received substantial attention by many researchers. Social class is a powerful predictor of the prevalence of obesity in both modernizing and affluent societies, although the direction of the association varies with the type of society. This relationship is the subject of Sobal and Stunkard's (84) comprehensive meta-analysis of more than 100 separate studies. In developing countries, there is a strong and consistent positive association of social class and obesity for men, women, and children; correspondingly, there is an inverse correlation between social class and protein-calorie malnutrition (85). This is a logical and expected pattern in that socially dominant groups with better access to strategic resources should have better nutrition and better health.

In heterogeneous and affluent societies like the United States, there is a strong inverse correlation of social class and obesity, particularly for females (86–89). Because of the association between obesity and socioeconomic status (SES, a social consensus component of social class), some researchers have suggested that SES may actually be a causal factor (90). For a general U.S. sample, children of both sexes tend to be associated with the obesity status of their mothers, and these mother-child dyads demonstrate an inverse correlation between SES and obesity (91). For women in affluent societies like the United States, the association of obesity and social class is not constant through the life cycle. Garn and Clark (92) have demonstrated a pattern of reversal in which economically advantaged girls are initially fatter than their poor counterparts, but as adults they show less overweight and obesity. The inverse correlation of obesity and social class for females in affluent societies is extremely strong and carries with it important socially symbolic associations. As with developing countries, again we see that the socially dominant have better access to strategic resources. However, these resources are more likely to include fat-free and low-calorie products as well as access to personal trainers and fitness programs.

Numerous proximate factors potentially affect the obesity and SES relationship. Among these are nutritional knowledge, access to resources, the media, and perception regarding locus of weight control (93). Each of these factors has the ability to exacerbate genetic tendencies. Among middle- and upper-class women in the United States, thinness represents the moral success of self-control over one's body (44,45) and there is, as well, a reported inverse relationship between perception of ideal body weight and SES (94). Thinness has been associated with high social status in the United States for most of this century and is typified by the statement "you can never be too rich or too thin" (44,95).

V. CULTURAL REACTIONS TO OBESITY

A. Stigmatization

Fatness is symbolically linked to psychological dimensions such as "self-worth" and sexuality in many societies of the world, but the nature of that symbolic association is not constant. Whereas in mainstream U.S. cultures, obesity is socially stigmatized (96,97), for most cultures of the world, fatness is viewed as a welcome sign of health and prosperity (98). In preindustrial societies thinness is stigmatized as a symptom of starvation [like among the !Kung San of Botswana (99)] or in contemporary central Africa as a sign of AIDS.

In dominant American society, overweight and obesity are viewed as obvious symbols of an individual's moral failings in self-control. Social reactions to obesity fit well with Goffman's concept of stigmatized condition, like a physical deformity always apparent to others (100). As a body type thought to be an index of moral character, "fatness" carries a definite negative connotation in the United States in a way that "thinness" does not. Unlike a physical handicap, however, obesity is viewed as intentional and obese individuals are held accountable and personally responsible for their condition (101). The expectation of accountability for the physical condition is a key element in the stigmatization. The well-documented stigma of obesity in American culture may be tied to the value system of the "Protestant ethic" and its emphasis on the need for individuals to control their animal impulses. Stigmatization lies not in the condition, but in others' reactions to the condition and has led to stereotype of the obese per-

son as "lazy, unkempt, less intelligent, unhealthy, and insecure" (102,103).

The stigmatization and attitudes regarding obesity are not easily rectified. Harris and colleagues (104) found that providing test subjects with factual knowledge about obesity did not lead to a change in attitudes. In fact, obese individuals are, in general, disliked and discriminated against by members of the mainstream U.S. culture (105). While this relates to a social pattern of victim blaming for the obese, it is remarkable how very few social sanctions there are *against* the expression of antiobese attitudes. "Fat-ism" is a socially tolerated prejudice of the 1990s, much as racism was prior to the civil rights movement of the 1960s. Prejudice against the obese appears to be associated with social conservatism and beliefs in authoritarian values. Because some obese individuals share these overarching cultural attitudes, this can exacerbate problems with low self-esteem (106); these outlooks are further complicated by the retention of a negative (distorted) body image interpretation even after significant weight loss (107). According to Allon, the core American cultural value expressed in these prejudices and beliefs is that people get what they deserve (96). Therefore, the sociological issues of blame, the struggle for status, and the added cultural burdens of being a woman are all symbolically linked to the dominant ideal of thinness for women.

B. Discrimination and Downward Social Mobility

Both prejudices and discrimination accompany the stigmatization of obesity. Obese individuals are routinely charged higher insurance rates than are thin individuals. Overweight individuals have difficulty finding stylish clothes in their size, despite the fact that this group represents a significant market. Many aspects of our lives that the nonobese take for granted, from airplane seats to car interiors, are not accommodating to persons of size (70). Because of cultural values, this physical attribute is thought to be more than an inconvenience but a matter of personal shamefulness.

For more than two decades, researchers have reported a continued social bias against obese persons ranging from admission to colleges (108) and job discrimination (109,110) to renting an apartment (111). Such discrimination may have direct bearings on the socioeconomic status of obese persons. There appears to be a negative-feedback loop linking obesity, stigma, discrimination, low self-esteem, and increased obesity. Social researchers have demonstrated that easily observable characteristics that are correlates of social status in the United States (e.g., race, gender, physical appearance) influence how individuals are evaluated (112). Physical attractiveness generates positive perceptions and expectations and leads to a self-fulfilling prophecy. Physical unattractiveness, including obesity, generates negative social-psychological perceptions, expectations, and hence, outcomes (97).

There are few reports available regarding the direct effects of obesity on socioeconomic status. Early work by Stunkard (113) reviewed the effects of obesity on social class in women. He found that while 22% of women who dropped in social class over their lifetimes were obese, only 12% of women who were upwardly mobile in terms of social class were obese; this evidence supported the conclusion that the experience of obesity has a negative impact on social class. More recently, Sobal (114) examined the issue of "obesity as a causal factor in socioeconomic status." Across cultures, he argues, societal body-type preferences tend to be reflected among people in the higher social ranks. Consequently people with the "preferred" body types are more likely to move up in social status than individuals with an undesirable body type. Having the nonpreferred body type can lead to an individual being the recipient of behaviors (e.g., prejudice, discrimination) that negatively influence components of socioeconomic status such as education, occupation, and marriage partners. Discriminatory behaviors reduce the social mobility of these individuals and thus result in obesity influencing socioeconomic status. There is a need for more social science research on this topic.

VI. CONCLUSIONS: THE BIOCULTURAL APPROACH

Human obesity is the result of two distinct, but interacting, processes—biological and cultural evolution. Biological evolution involves change in the frequency of particular genes over time, primarily because of the action of natural selection on individuals. Cultural evolution involves systematic changes in the configurations of cultural systems, ideologies, and behaviors over time. The anthropological record has many examples of genetic and cultural evolution enhancing each other in a pattern that may be called biocultural evolution or coevolution (115).

A. Where Evolution and Culture Converge

In the case of obesity, Stunkard (116) has described models of the possible interaction of genes and environment. Sobal and Stunkard (84) identified mediating variables affecting the obesity and socioeconomic status relationship, two of which were genetic and cultural inheritance. The

significant progress in recent years in clarifying the genetic contribution to obesity has, to a significant degree, highlighted our ignorance about the role of culture or environment. The genes that today predispose individuals to obesity are the result of the operation of natural selection through food shortages. At the same time, it was the invention of agriculture, and particularly industrial agriculture, which allowed for the production of a reliable surplus of food. The technological changes associated with cultural evolution reduced the energy requirements of human labor. For example, the statistical association of television watching and obesity in children (117) is the result of both lower activity levels and the strong and sometimes contradictory symbolic messages about eating and ideal body types (118).

Cultural evolution has affected other human biological functions such as patterns of human reproduction and infant feeding that may play a role in female obesity. In traditional societies, pregnancy and lactation represent serious and continuing energy demands. One cultural solution to this problem has been the custom of "fattening huts" for elite pubescent girls in traditional West Africa, particularly among the Annang, Efik, and Ibibio of Nigeria (119–121), as well as in parts of Oceania (122). A girl spent up to 2 years in seclusion during which she was well fed and not allowed to work. At the end of this rite of passage, girls publicly displayed symbols of womanhood and marriageability, particularly fatness. The health benefit of this custom is that elite women start their reproductive careers with an energy surplus in the form of peripheral fat. Poorer women in these traditional societies suffer a significantly greater risk of protein-energy malnutrition. Correspondingly, the fact that women in economically developed societies have fewer pregnancies and are less likely to breast-feed means that they also have less opportunity to mobilize peripheral fat stores and suffer greater risk of obesity. The inverse correlation between social class and bottle feeding in the United States, in this way, contributes to the inverse relation of social class and obesity.

B. Conclusions

Each social and cultural factor discussed here influences obesity; however, it is the multiplicative nature of these factors that makes etiology and treatment such a complicated issue. It is overly simplistic to postulate that obesity is strictly a biological phenomenon, resulting from surplus energy intake. It is also overly simplistic to argue that obesity is merely the by-product of socioeconomic and cultural conditions of poverty and poor nutritional knowledge. Rather, the research community must recognize that obesity is the result of biological predispositions that can be exacerbated by particular cultural factors.

We believe that the principles outlined here can benefit both the understanding and treatment of obesity. Recognition of obesity's long evolutionary history offers insight into why weight loss is so difficult to maintain; it also points to the absurdity of ideas that failure to lose weight is a reflection of moral weakness or a failure of will. The evolutionary process has programmed our bodies, particularly our fat cells, to behave in a certain manner when faced with starvation. In evolutionary terms, this is a sound reproductive strategy ensuring survival, reproduction, and the individual's continued representation in the gene pool.

In terms of understanding obesity, recognition of the roles played by gender, ethnicity, and social class should help both the practitioner and the layperson in comprehending the attitudes toward obesity and self-perceptions of obese individuals. Incorporating these factors into a treatment plan is likely to improve treatment success.

REFERENCES

1. Bouchard C, Tremblay A, Despres J, et al. The response of long-term overfeeding in identical twins. N Engl J Med 1990; 322:1477–1482.
2. Price RA, Cadoret FJ, Stunkard AJ, Troughton E. Genetic contributions to human fatness: an adoption study. Am J Psychiatry 1987; 144:1003–1008.
3. Ravussin E, Lillioja S, Knowler WC, et al. Reduced rate of energy expenditure as a risk factor for body-weight gain. N Engl J Med 1988; 318:467–472.
4. Stunkard AJ, Foch TT, Zdenek H. A twin study of human obesity. JAMA 1986; 256:51–54.
5. Stunkard AJ, Sorenson TIA, Hanis C, et al. An adoption study of obesity. N Engl J Med 1986; 314:193–198.
6. Stunkard AJ, Harris JR, Pedersen NL, McClearn G. The body-mass index of twins who have been reared apart. N Engl J Med 1990; 322:1483–1487.
7. Trivers R. Social Evolution. Menlo Park, CA: Benjamin/Cummings Publishing Co. 1985.
8. Daly M, Wilson M. Sex, Evolution, and Behavior. Boston: Willard Grant Press, 1983.
9. Brown PJ. Culture and the evolution of obesity. Hum Nature 1991; 2:31–57.
10. Brown PJ. Cultural and genetic adaptations to malaria: problems of comparison. Hum Biol 1986; 14:311–332.
11. Eaton SB. Shostak M, Konner M. The Paleolithic Prescription. New York: Harper & Row, 1988.
12. Cash TF. Hicks K. Being fat versus thinking fat: relationships with body image, eating behaviors, and well-being. Cogn Ther Res 1990; 14:327–341.
13. Kreitler S, Chemerinski A. Body-image disturbance in obesity. Int J Eating Disord 1990; 9:409–418.
14. Schwartz H. Never Satisfied: A Cultural History of Diets, Fantasies and Fat. New York: Free Press, 1986.
15. Seid RP. Never Too Thin: Why Women Are at War with Their Bodies. New York: Prentice-Hall, 1989.
16. Ritenbaugh C. Obesity as a culture-bound syndrome. Cult Med Psychiatry. 1982; 6:347–361.
17. Björntorp P. How should obesity be defined? J Intern Med 1990; 227:147–149.
18. Whiting MG. A cross-cultural nutrition survey. Doctoral thesis, Harvard School of Public Health, Cambridge, MA, 1958.
19. Wilmsen E. Seasonal effects of dietary intake in the Kalahari San. Fed Proc 1978; 37:65–71.
20. Hunter JM. Seasonal hunger in a part of the West African savanna: a survey of body weights in Nangodi, North-East Ghana. Trans Inst Bri Geogra 1967; 41:167–185.
21. Physician Task Force on Hunger in America. Hunger in America: The Growing Epidemic. Boston: Harvard School of Public Health, 1985.
22. Stunkard AJ, Harris JR, Pedersen NL, McClearn GE. The body-mass index of twins who have been reared apart. N Engl J Med 1990; 322:1483–1487.
23. Feinstein A. How do we measure accomplishment in weight reduction? In: Lasagna A, ed. Obesity: Causes, Consequences and Treatment. New York: Medcom Pres, 1974:81–87.
24. Rodin J. Obesity: why the losing battle? In: Wolman B, ed. Psychological Aspects of Obesity: A Handbook. New York: Van Nostrand Reinhold, 1982:30–87.
25. Baba S, Zimmet P. eds. World Data Book on Obesity. New York: Elsevier Science Publishers, 1990.
26. Collins V, Dowse G, Zimmet P. Prevalence of obesity in Pacific and Indian Ocean populations. In: Baba S, Zimmet P, eds. World Data Book on Obesity. New York: Elsevier Science Publishers, 1990.
27. Kluthe R, Shubert A. Obesity in Europe. Ann Intern Med 1985; 103:1037–1042.
28. Gurney M, Gornstein J. The global prevalence of obesity—an initial view of available data. World Health Stat Q 1988; 41:251–254.
29. Lantz P, Remington PL. Obesity in Wisconsin. Wisconsin Med J 1990 (April):172–176. See also: Centers for Disease Control. Prevalence of overweight-behavioral risk factor surveillance system, 1987. MMWR 1989; 38:421–423.
30. Carlson EA. Human Genetics. Lexington, MA: DC Health, 1984.
31. Gillum RF. Overweight and obesity in black women. J Natl Med Assoc 1987; 79:865–871.
32. Centers for Disease Control. Prevalence of overweight for hispanics—United States, 1982–1984. MMWR 1989; 38:838–842.
33. Thomas JD, Douchette MM, Thomas DC, Stoeckle JD. Disease, lifestyle and consanguinity in 58 American Gypsies. Lancet 1987; 2:377–379.

34. Gardner LI, Stern MP, Haffner SM, et al. Prevalence of diabetes in Mexican Americans. Diabetes 1984; 33:86–92.

35. Kissebah AH, Freedman DS, Peiris AN. Health risks of obesity. Med Clin North Am 1989; 73:111–138.

36. Huss-Ashmore R. Fat and fertility: demographic implications of differential fat storage. Yrbk Phys Anthropol 1980; 23:65–91.

37. Frisch RE. Body fat, menarche, fitness and fertility. Hum Reprod 1987; 2:521–533.

38. Birch LL. Obesity and eating disorders: a developmental perspective. Bull Psyche Soc 1991; 29:265–272.

39. Stern MP, Pugh JA, Gaskill SP, Hazuda HP. Knowledge, attitudes, and behavior related to obesity and dieting in Mexican Americans and Anglos: the San Antonio heart study. Am J Epidemiol 1982; 115:917–927.

40. Kittler PG, Sucher K. Food and Culture in America: A Nutrition Handbook. New York: Van Nostrand Reinhold, 1989.

41. Bray GA. Obesity: Historical development of scientific and cultural ideas. Int J Obes 1990; 14:909–926.

42. Smithson CL. The Havasupai Woman. Salt Lake City; University of Utah Press, 1958.

43. Messing SD. The highland plateau Amhara of Ethiopia. Doctoral dissertation (anthropology), University of Pennsylvania, 1957.

44. Anderson JL, Crawford CB, Nadeau J, Lindberg T. Was the Duchess of Windsor right? A cross-cultural review of the socioecology of ideals of female body shape. 1992; Ethol Sociobiol 13:197–227.

45. Ritenbaugh C. Body size and shape: a dialogue of culture and biology. Med Anthropol 1991; 13:173–180.

46. Glassner B. Bodies: Why We Look the Way We Do. New York: GP Putnam's Sons, 1988.

47. Ross CE, Mirowsky J. The social epidemiology of overweight: a substantive and methodological investigation. J Health Soc Behav 1983; 24:288–298.

48. Stern M, Pugh J, Gaskill S, Hazuda H. Knowledge, Attitudes and behavior related to obesity and dieting in Mexican Americans and Anglos: the San Antonio heart study. Am J Epidemiol 1982; 115:917–927.

49. Massara EB. Que gordita! A Study of Weight Among Women in a Puerto Rican Community. New York: AMS Press, 1989.

50. Massara EB. Obesity and cultural weight evaluations. Appetite 1980; 1:291–298.

51. Kumanyika S. Obesity in black women. Epidemiol Rev 1987; 9:31–50.

52. Rand CSW, Kuldau JM. The epidemiology of obesity and self-defined weight problem in the general population: gender, race, age, and social class. Int J Eating Disord 1990; 9:329–343.

53. Kaplan KM, Wadden TA. Childhood obesity and self-esteem. J Pediatr 1986; 109:367–370.

54. McAraney ER, Stevens-Simon C. First, do no harm. Low birth weight and adolescent obesity. Am J Dis Child 1993; 147:983–984.

55. McGee M, Hale H. Social factors and obesity among black women. Free Inquiry 1980; 8:83–87.

56. Styles MH. Soul, black women and food. In: Kaplan JR, ed. A Woman's Conflict: The Special Relationship Between Women and Food. Englewood Cliffs, NJ: Prentice-Hall, 1980:161–176.

57. Knowler WC, Pettitt DJ, Savage PJ, Bennett PH. Diabetes incidence in Pima Indians: contribution of obesity and parental diabetes. Am J Epidemiol 1981; 113:144–156.

58. Garb JL, Garb JR, Stunkard AJ. Social factors and obesity in Navajo Indian children. In: Howard A, ed. Recent Advances in Obesity Research. London, Newman, 1975: 37–39.

59. Wiedman DW. Diabete mellitus and Oklahoma Native Americans: a case study of culture change in Oklahoma Cherokee. PhD dissertation (anthropology), University of Oklahoma, 1979.

60. Fitzpatrick-Nietchmann, J. Pacific islanders—migration and health. West J Med 1983; 139:44–49.

61. Collier J. From Mary to modern woman: the material basis of marianismo and its transformation in a spanish village. Am Ethnol 1986; 13:100–107.

62. Powdermaker H. An anthropological approach to the problem of obesity. Bull NY Acad Sci 1960; 36:286–295.

63. Harris MB, Walters LC, Waschull S. Gender and ethnic differences in obesity-related behaviors and attitudes in a college sample. J Appl Soc Psyc 1991; 21:1545–1566.

64. Clifford E. Body satisfaction in adolescence. Percept Mot Skills 1971; 33:119–125.

65. Dwyer JT, Feldman JJ, Seltzer CC, Mayer J. Adolescent attitudes toward weight and appearance. J Nutr Educ 1969; 1:14–19.

66. Drewnowski A, Yee DK. Men and body image: are males satisfied with their body weight. Psychosom Med 1987; 49:626–634.

67. Wadden TA, Stunkard AJ. Psychopathology and obesity. Ann NY Acad Sci 1987; 499:55–65.

68. Hill AJ, Draper E, Stack J. A weight on children's minds: body shape dissatisfaction at 9 years old. Int J Obes 1994; 18:383–389.

69. Hill AJ, Bhatti R. Body shape perception and dieting in preadolescent British Asian girls; links with eating disorders. Int J Eating Disord 1995; 17:175–183.

70. Jasper CR, Klassen ML. Stereotypical beliefs about appearance: implications for retailing and consumer issues. Percept Mot Skills 1990; 71:519–528.

71. Grilo CM, Wilfley DE, Brownel KD, Rodin J. Teasing, body image, and self-esteem in a clinical sample of obese women. Addict Behav 1994; 19:443–450.

72. Cash TF, Counts B, Hangen J, Huffine CE. How much do you weigh? Determinants of validity of self-reported body weight. Percept Mot Skills 1989; 69:248–250.

73. Cash TF, Grant JR, Shovlin JM, Lewis RJ. Are inaccuracies in self-reported weight motivated distortions? Percept Mot Skills 1992; 74:209–210.

74. Connor-Greene PA. Gender differences in body weight perception and weight-loss strategies of college students. Women Health 1988; 14:27–42.

75. Rodin J, Silberstein L. Striegel-Moore R. Women and weight: a normative discontent. In: Dienstbier RA, Sonderegger TB, eds. Psychology and Gender. Lincoln: University of Nebraska Press, 1985:267–307.

76. White DR, Schliecker E, Dayan J. Gender differences in categorizing adolescents' weight status. Psych Rep 1991; 68:978.

77. Simones EJ,k Byers T, Coates RJ, Serdula MK, Mokdad AH, Health GW. The association between leisure-time physical activity and dietary fat in American adults. Am J Public Health 1995; 85:240–244.

78. Page LB, Damon A, Moellering RC. Antecedents of cardiovascular disease in six solomon island societies. Circulation 1974; 49:1132–1146.

79. Zimmet P. Epidemiology of diabetes and its microvascular manifestations in pacific populations: the medical effects of social progress. Diabetes Care 1979; 2:144–153.

80. West K. Diabetes in American Indians. Adv Metabol Disord 1978; 9:29–48.

81. Christakis G. The prevalence of adult obesity. In: Bray G, ed. Obesity in Perspective. Bethesda; MD: Fogarty International Center Series on Preventive Medicine, 1975; 2: 209–213.

82. Phillips M, Kubisch D. Lifestyle diseases of aborigines. Med J Aust 1985; 143:218.

83. Trowell HC, Burkitt DP. Western Diseases: Their Emergence and Prevention. Cambridge, MA: Harvard University Press, 1981.

84. Sobal J, Stunkard AJ. Socioeconomic status and obesity: a review of the literature. Psychol Bull 1989; 105: 260–275.

85. Arteaga P, Dos Santos JE, Dutra de Oliveira JE. Obesity among schoolchildren of different socioeconomic levels in a developing country. Int J Obes 1982; 6:291–297.

86. Goldblatt PB, Moore ME, Stunkard AJ. Social factors in obesity. JAMA 1965; 192:1039–1044.

87. Burnight RG, Marden PG. Social correlates of weight in an aging population. Milbank Mem Fund Q 1967; 45: 75–92.

88. Rolland-Cachera MF, Bellisle F. No correlation between adiposity and food intake: why are working class children fatter? Am J Clin Nutr 196; 44:779–787.

89. Sobal J. Obesity and socioeconomic status: a framework for examining relationships between physical and social variables. Med Anthropol 1991; 13:231–248.

90. Noppa H, Hallstrom T. Weight gain in adulthood in relation to socioeconomic factors, mental illness and personality traits: a prospectivity study of middle-aged women. J Psychosom Res 1981; 25:83–89.

91. Golden MP, Saltzer EB, DePaul-Snyder L, Reiff M. Obesity and socioeconomic class in children and their mothers. J Dev Behav Pediatr 1993; 4:113–118.

92. Garn SM, Clark DC. Trends in fatness and the origin of obesity. Pediatrics 1976; 57–443–456.

93. Bowen DJ, Tomoyasu N, Cauce AM. The triple threat: a discussion of gender, class, and race differences in weight. Women Health 1991; 17:123–143.

94. Furnham A, Baguma P. Cross-cultural differences in the evaluation of male and female body shapes. Int J Eating Disord 1994; 15:81–89.

95. Levenstein H. Revolution at The Table: The Transformation of the American Diet. New York: Oxford University Press, 1988.

96. Allon N. The stigma of obesity in everyday life. In: Wolman BJ, ed. Psychological Aspects of Obesity: A Handbook. New York: Van Nostrand Reinhold, 1981; 130–174.

97. Cahnman WJ. The stigma of obesity. Soc Q 1968; 9: 294–297.

98. Furnham A, Alibhai N. Cross-cultural differences in the perception of female body shapes. Psychol Med 1983; 13: 829–837.

99. Lee R. The !Kung San: Men, Women, and Work in a Foraging Society. Cambridge, MA: Harvard University Press, 1979.

100. Goffman E. Stigma: Notes on the Management of a Spoiled Identity. New York: Simon & Shuster, 1963.

101. Wooley SC, Wooley OW, Dyrenforth SR. Obesity and women. II. A neglected feminist topic. Women Stud Int Q 1979; 2:81–92.

102. Harris MB, Harris RJ, Bochner S. Fat, four-eyed, and female: stereotypes of obesity, glasses, and gender. J Appl Soc Psyc 1982; 12:503–516.

103. Crocker J. Cornwell B, Major B. The stigma of overweight: affective consequences of attributional ambiguity. J Person Soc Psych 1993; 64:60–70.

104. Harris MB, Walters LC, Waschull S. Altering attitudes and knowledge about obesity. J Soc Psych 1991; 131: 881–884.

105. Crandall C, Biernat M. The ideology of anti-fat attitudes. J Appl Soc Psyc 1990; 20:227–243.

106. Cash TF, Counts B, Huffine C. Current and vestigial effects of overweight among women: fear of fat, attitudinal body image, and eating behaviors. J Psychopathol Behav Assess 1990; 12:157–167.

107. Powers PS. Obesity—The Regulation of Weight. Baltimore: Williams & Wilkins, 1980.

108. Canning H, Mayer J. Obesity—its possible effect on college acceptance. N Engl J Med 1966; 275:1172–1174.

109. Louderback L. Fat Power: Whatever You Weigh Is Right. New York: Hawthorn Books, 1970.

110. Rothblum ED, Brand PA, Miller CT. The relationship between obesity, employment discrimination, and employment-related victimization. J Vocat Behav 1990; 37:251–266.

111. Karris L. Prejudice against obese renters. J Soc Psych 1977; 101:159–160.

112. Umberson D, Hughes M. The impact of physical attractiveness on achievement and psychological well-being. Soc Psych Q 1987; 50:227–236.

113. Stunkard AJ. The Pain of Obesity. Palo Alto, CA: Bull Publishing Co. 1976.

114. Sobal J. Obesity and socioeconomic status: a framework for examining relationships between physical and social variables. Med Anthropol 1991; 13:231–247.

115. Durham WH. Coevolution: Genes, Culture and Human Diversity. Palo Alto, CA: Stanford University Press, 1991.

116. Stunkard AJ. Some perspectives on human obesity: its causes. Bull NY Acad Med 1988; 64:902–923.

117. Dietz WH. You are what you eat—what you eat is what you are. J Adolesc Health Care 1990; 11:76–81.

118. Nichter M, Nichter M. Hype and weight. Med Anthropol 1991; 13:249–284.

119. Brink PJ. The fattening room among the Annang of Nigeria. Med Anthropol 1989; 12:131–143.

120. Malcolm LW. Note on the seclusion of girls among the Efik at Old Calabar. Man 1925; 25:113–114.

121. Cassidy C. The good body: when big is better. Med Anthropol 1991; 13;181–214.

122. Marshall DS. Sexual behavior on Mangaia. In: Marshall D, Suggs RE, eds. Human Sexual Behavior; Variations in the Ethnographic Spectrum. New York: Basic Books, 1971.

10

The Genetics of Human Obesity

Claude Bouchard and Louis Pérusse
Laval University, Ste.-Foy, Quebec, Canada

Treva Rice and D. C. Rao
Washington University School of Medicine, St. Louis, Missouri

I. INTRODUCTION

The genetics of human obesity is receiving increasing attention as exemplified by the number of papers published on the subject since 1980. The growth has been particularly remarkable in the 1990s. The interest in the causes of the present epidemic of obesity in the Western world and the promise of finding potentially new prophylactic and therapeutic means are largely responsible for this trend.

Several lines of research are currently being explored in the effort to identify the genes involved in causing obesity, rendering someone susceptible to obesity, or determining the metabolic response to an obese state. Animal research includes the study of single-gene rodent models of obesity, the identification and characterization of loci contributing to obesity by the quantitative trait locus (QTL) method based on cross-breeding of informative inbred rodent strains, and mouse transgenic or knockout models designed to study the effects of variation in expression of candidate or other specific genes. Molecular methods and animal models are reviewed in other chapters and will not be dealt with here except as they pertain to the human putative equivalents of the rodent genes.

This chapter will cover six major topics: (1) the definition of the obesity phenotypes; (2) an overview of the evidence from Mendelian genetic syndromes having obesity as a feature; (3) the findings from genetic epidemiology studies; (4) the evidence from experimental interventions designed to understand the contribution of specific genotype-environment interaction effects; (5) the current status of the role of specific genes and relationship or linkage with molecular markers; and (6) a discussion of the useful strategies in future studies on the genetics of human obesity. The evidence for a role of genetic factors in energy and macronutrient intake as well as in the various energy expenditure components (resting metabolic rate, thermic response to food, and energy expenditure associated with physical activity) will not be reviewed here. The interested reader is referred to recent reviews on these topics (1,2). Even though we have made notable progress during the last decade, we still have a long way to go. For instance, the risk of becoming obese when one or two of the parents are overweight or obese, or when both parents are of normal weight, is not even properly understood. It has been suggested that severely obese persons generally have one or two parents who are obese, but there are a good number of such persons who have two normal-weight parents (3). Much research is needed on this basic issue that would essentially provide us with valid population estimates of the lambda coefficient (4) for various degrees of severity of obesity. In the present context, the lambda coefficient could be defined as the probability of being affected (i.e., being overweight or obese) given that a biological relative (for instance a parent or sibling) is affected.

A word of caution to the reader: this chapter is being written in a period characterized by rapid accretion of new evidence. It is therefore likely that the chapter will be outdated to a significant extent by the time this book is finally published, a most frustrating experience for the authors!

II. THE PHENOTYPES

Interest in the genetics of human obesity has increased considerably during the last decade partly because of the realization that some forms of obesity were associated with high risks for various morbid conditions and mortality rate. Obesity can no longer be seen as a homogenous phenotype. However, a commonly agreed-upon classification of the obesity phenotypes does not exist yet. Nonetheless, based on the topography of the adipose tissue and its association with a variety of metabolic characteristics, four different types of human obesity can be recognized (5–7). We are not referring to the heterogeneity of the clinical manifestations of obesity or their determinants, but only to the phenotypes of body fat.

These four types of obesities are outlined in Table 1. Type I is characterized by excess body mass or body fat without any particular concentration of fat in a given area of the body. The other types have to do with excessive accumulation of fat in some areas of the body; that is, they are based on the anatomical distribution of body fat. Type II is defined as excess subcutaneous fat on the trunk, particularly in the abdominal area, and is equivalent to the so-called android or male type of fat deposition. Type III is characterized by an excessive amount of fat in the abdominal visceral area and can be labeled abdominal visceral obesity. The last type (type IV) is defined as gluteofemoral obesity and is observed primarily in women (gynoid obesity). Thus, excess fat can be stored primarily in the truncal-abdominal area or in the gluteal and femoral area. This implies that a given body fat content, say 30% or 50 kg, may exhibit different anatomical distribution characteristics.

Strictly speaking, one should therefore talk about the obesities rather than obesity. But the situation is even more complex as the phenotypes are not of the simple Mendelian kind. Segregation of the genes is not readily perceived, and whatever the role of the genotype in the etiology, it is generally attenuated or exacerbated by nongenetic factors. In other words, variation in human body fat is caused by a complex network of genetic, nutritional, metabolic, energy expenditure, psychological, and social variables.

The evidence accumulated over the last decade indicates that it is useful to distinguish several obesity phe-

Table 1 The Types of Obesity Phenotypes in an Anatomical Perspective

Type I obesity	Excess body mass or percent fat
Type II obesity	Excess subcutaneous truncal-abdominal fat (android)
Type III obesity	Excess abdominal visceral fat
Type IV obesity	Excess gluteofemoral fat (gynoid)

Source: From Ref. 171.

notypes for the evaluation of the relationships between excess body fat and the etiology of cardiovascular diseases and non-insulin-dependent diabetes mellitus (NIDDM) or the other risk factors for these diseases. However, it is important to recognize that these phenotypes are not fully independent of one another, as shown by the data of Figure 1. The level of covariation among the various body fat phenotypes ranges from about 30 to 50% and perhaps more in some circumstances. One implication of the above is that studies designed to investigate the causes of the individual differences in the various body fat phenotypes, including genetic causes, should control for these levels of covariation.

In clinical settings, the body mass index (BMI) is commonly used to assess the normality of body weight in patients. The correlation between the BMI and total body fat or percent body fat is high in large and heterogeneous samples. The predictive value of the BMI is, however, much less impressive in a given individual especially when the BMI is below 30 kg/m^2 or so. Thus, the BMI is an indicator of heaviness and only indirectly of body fat (7,8). Any estimate of the genetic effect on BMI is bound to be influenced in unknown proportions by the contri-

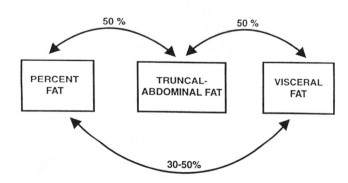

Figure 1 Common variance between three body fat phenotypes. Fat mass estimated from underwater weighing: truncal-abdominal fat assessed from skinfolds or CT scans; abdominal visceral fat estimated by CT scan at the L4/L5 vertebrae. (From Ref. 171.)

bution of the genotype to fat mass, muscle mass, skeletal mass, and other components. Nevertheless, the BMI is worth considering because of its clinical use, simplicity to measure, and reasonable correlation with body composition. However, the most appropriate indicator of obesity remains the percentage of body fat or fat mass adjusted for body stature in the case of heterogeneous samples.

A properly assessed phenotype is a *sine qua non* for a valid and productive genetic study. The data summarized in Table 2 indicate why the BMI is only a partially acceptable surrogate measure of body fat content. The variance explained by BMI in percent body fat derived from underwater weighing in large samples of adult men and women, 35–54 years of age, attains only about 40%. At the extremes of body fat content distribution, BMI is more closely associated with percent body fat; that is, the variance explained may reach 60% and more. This is not entirely satisfactory as genetic studies deal with individual differences in the phenotype of interest, and for them to be successful, the phenotype of complex multifactorial trait must be measured with a reasonable degree of precision.

The fact that percent body fat remains quite heterogeneous at any level of BMI is further illustrated in Table 3, which is based on data from middle-age adult males. For instance, in 27 men with a BMI of 28–30, the mean percent body fat was 28, but the range varied from 15 to 41%. We have observed the same phenomenon and with as much heterogeneity in women at all levels of BMI.

The same point can be made for regional fat distribution phenotypes. Thus the correlation between the waist-to-hip circumferences ratio (WHR) and abdominal visceral fat is positive and generally significant in various populations, but the association is characterized by a wide scatter of scores. For instance, in a study of 51 adult obese women, the correlation between WHR and CT-assessed

Table 3 Heterogeneity of Body Fat Content for a Given BMI Class in Males, 35–54 Years of Age

		Percent body fat[a]		
n	BMI	Mean	Min	Max
27	20–22	17	8	32
76	23–25	22	11	35
46	26–27	26	16	40
27	28–30	28	15	41

[a]From underwater weighing.
Source: From Ref. 171.

abdominal visceral fat reached 0.55 (9). However, for a WHR of about 0.80, the visceral fat area at the L4–L5 level ranged from a low of about 50 cm^2 to a high of approximately 200 cm^2. Even though the covariation between total body fat and abdominal visceral fat is statistically significant, the relationship is also characterized by a high degree of heterogeneity. As shown in Table 4, when BMI and percent body fat are constrained to narrow ranges, one generally finds a threefold range for the amount of CT-assessed abdominal visceral fat in adult males. Thus in 16 men with BMI values of 30 or 31 and a percentage of body fat ranging from 30 to 33, mean abdominal visceral fat was 153 cm^2 with a range of 77–261 cm^2. Again, the same lack of coupling between BMI, percent body fat, and abdominal visceral fat was observed in adult women.

The above data suggest that even though it may be necessary to use the BMI, WHR, or a prediction of abdominal visceral fat in clinical settings, such practice is not desirable in the context of scientific research designed to understand the causes and metabolic consequences of variation in body fat content or in fat topography.

III. MENDELIAN GENETIC DISORDERS

Although it is well established that obesity runs in families, the vast majority of cases do not segregate in families with a clear pattern of Mendelian inheritance. However, some rare Mendelian disorders with obesity as a clinical feature have been identified in humans (10), suggesting that single genes could cause obesity in humans. A list of these disorders, categorized by the mode of inheritance, is given in Table 5. These disorders were identified from the On line Mendelian Inheritance in Man (OMIM) computerized data base by searching for syndromes in which the word "obesity" appeared in the field "clinical synopsis." A total of 34 entries (syndromes) were recovered from

Table 2 Percent Variance ($r^2 \times 100$) Explained by BMI in Body Composition in Adults, 35–54 Years of Age

	BMI in 342 males	BMI in 356 females
Percent fat	41	40
Fat-free mass	37	25
Sum of 6 skinfolds	58	67
TER	10	8

Percent fat and fat-free mass were derived from underwater weighing assessment of body density. TER = ratio of trunk to extremity skinfolds. Trunk skinfolds are the sum of subscapular, suprailiac, and abdominal skinfolds. Extremity skinfolds are the sum of triceps, biceps, and medial calf skinfolds.
Source: From Ref. 171.

Table 4 Variation in Amount of Abdominal Visceral Fat for Given BMI and Percent Body Fat Classes in Males, 35–54 Years of Age

n	BMI	% fat (range)	Visceral fat in cm²		
			Mean	Min	Max
15	21–22	14–18	58	31	84
19	24–25	19–24	89	50	140
18	27–28	25–29	133	63	199
16	30–31	30–33	153	77	261

Abdominal visceral fat measured by CT scan at the L4–L5 level. Percent fat derived from underwater weighing.
Source: From Ref. 171.

this search. However, not all were included in the table either because only a few cases have been reported, or because obesity was not a primary feature of the disorder.

These disorders share several clinical features. Hypogenitalism, various dysmorphic features affecting the facies and the limbs, delayed growth and maturation, and mental retardation are common features. These similarities have often led to misclassifications. For example, the Laurence-Moon and the Bardet-Biedl syndromes have long been considered as a single syndrome (Laurence-Moon-Bardet-Biedl syndrome) because of the presence of hypogenitalism, pigmentary retinopathy, and mental retardation in both syndromes. However, the Laurence-Moon syndrome could not be considered as an obesity syndrome as obesity is not observed in all cases, whereas it is a common feature of the Bardet-Biedl syndrome. Another example is the Carpenter syndrome (MIM = 201000), which shares similarities with the Summit syndrome (MIM = 272350) but for which obesity is observed only in older patients.

Among the disorders listed in Table 5, the Prader-Willi syndrome (PWS) represents the most common (estimated prevalence of 1:25,000) and the best characterized human obesity syndrome. In addition to obesity, the PWS is characterized by reduced fetal activity, hypotonia at birth, short stature, hypogonadism, small hands and feet, and hyperphagia that usually develops between 12 and 18 months. Patients with PWS rarely survive beyond 30 years of age and diabetes or cardiac failure is the main cause of death. Although familial inheritance of PWS has sometimes been described, the vast majority of cases are sporadic. It has been established that PWS is most often caused by a deletion of the paternal 15q11.2–12 segment. The inheritance of PWS is characterized by the presence of imprinting; i.e., the differential expression of the disease depends on whether the deletion is inherited from the mother or from the father. When the deletion is on the paternal chromosome, the resulting phenotype is PWS. Absence of the same region in the maternal chromosome 15 results in another syndrome, called the Angelman syndrome, with includes a severe motor and mental retardatio, ataxia, and hypotonia, but not obesity.

For most of the syndromes listed in Table 5 the specific genetic or molecular defect is not known. About a third of them, mainly autosomal dominant and X-linked syndromes, have been mapped. Although individuals affected with these disorders represent a very small fraction of the obese population, they represent examples that single genes could be important in the development of human obesity and that these genes have considerable pleiotropic effects. The evidence for the contribution of single genes to these disorders will be summarized later.

IV. GENETIC EPIDEMIOLOGY OF HUMAN OBESITY

Several problems are associated with genetic epidemiology studies of obesity (11). First, as discussed earlier, obesity is not a simple Mendelian trait. For example, whether or not genetic propensities are expressed may depend on appropriate environmental stimulation (i.e., gene by environment interaction), or developmental stage (i.e., age dependency), or sex (i.e., sex-limited). Second, obesity is not a homogeneous trait stemming from a unique gene or set of genes. For example, there is generalized obesity, as well as preferential deposition of fat in localized sites (see Table 1), and each type of obesity may have its own genetic determinants, as well as other determinants that are shared with other traits. Third, excess body fat is seldom measured by direct methods. For example, relative weight and BMI are only indirect or partial measures. As such, they may index other traits such as bone and muscle mass, which also may have separate genetic determinants.

However, genetic epidemiology methods remain useful for addressing specific questions in human obesity, such as in determining if there are genetic factors underlying an obesity phenotype, in characterizing the source of the genetic influence through maternal versus paternal transmission, and whether the trait is sex-limited or age-dependent, or if there is assortative mating, and so forth. Other strategies include documenting the presumptive causes of obesity (e.g., energy intake or energy expenditure) and considering their complex biological and behavioral interactions in a network design (i.e., multivariate genetic epidemiology studies). Here, we first describe the types of data and analytical methods commonly used by genetic epidemiologists and then review the findings for

Table 5 Mendelian Disorders with Obesity as Clinical Feature

MIM no.	Disorder	Mapping	Comments
Autosomal dominant			
100800	Achondroplasia (ACH)	4p16.13	Caused by mutations in the fibroblast growth factor receptor-3 gene; obesity aggravates the joint problems and contributes to early cardiovascular mortality.
103200	Adiposis dolorosa (Dercum disease)	NA	Characterized by subcutaneous lipomas and obesity
103580	Albright Hereditary osteodystrophy		Autosomal recessive and X-linked varieties also exist; caused by defects in G protein; obesity secondary to unresponsiveness of fat cells to lipolytic messages
122000	Posterior polymorphous Corneal dystrophy (PPCD)	20q11	Obesity observed in 3 affected persons of 2-generation pedigree
144800	Morgani-Stewart-Morel syndrome	NA	Thickening of the inner table of the frontal bone with obesity and hypertrichosis
157980	Momo syndrome	NA	Overgrowth syndrome characterized by macrosomia, obesity, macrocephaly, and ocular (MOMO) abnormalities
176270	Prader-Willi syndrome (PWS)	15q11.2–12	The most common Mendelian obesity disorder; caused by deletion of the paternal 15q11.2–12 segment
181450	Schinzel syndrome	NA	Major features include hand malformations, delayed growth and maturation, and obesity
184700	Polycystic ovarian syndrome	NA	Obesity, hirsutism, amenorrhea, and insulin resistance are clinical features of the polycystic ovaries
Autosomal recessive			
203800	Alstrom syndrome	NA	In addition to obesity, features include retinitis pigmentosa, deafness, insulin resistance, and diabetes
	Badet-Biedl		Previously and incorrectly called Laurence-Moon-Bardet-Biedl syndrome; carriers are at increased risk of obesity; linkage with markers on 11q13 (BBS1), 3p13–12 (BBS3) and 15q22.3–23 (BBS4) also reported
209900	BBS2	16q21	
209901	BBS1	11q13	
600151	BBS3	3p13–12	
600374	BBS4	15q22.3–23	
210350	Biemond syndrome	NA	In addition to obesity, features include mental retardation, hypogenitalism, polydactyly, and malformation of the iris
216550	Cohen syndrome (CHS1)	8q22–23	Connective tissue disorder characterized by hypotonia, obesity, prominent incisors, and short stature
219080	Cushing disease	NA	Could be of adrenal or pituitary origin; central obesity is a characteristic feature of this disease
248100	Macrosomia Adiposa congenita	NA	One Danish kindred in which 7 infants developed gross obesity soon after birth; adrenocortical adenomas found at autopsy
257500	Pickwickian syndrome	NA	Fat boy syndrome characterized by marked obesity and somnolence (see Ref. 172)

Table 5   Continued

MIM no.	Disorder	Mapping	Comments
264010	Urban-Rogers-Meyer syndrome	NA	Disorder described in 3 male children and characterized by genital anomalies, mental retardation, obesity, short stature, osteoporosis, and contractures of fingers
269870	Short stature-obesity syndrome	NA	Short stature, obesity, and brachydactyly in brother and sister born to consanguineous parents
272350	Summit syndrome	NA	3 cases reported with skull malformation and obesity; share similarities with the Carpenter syndrome
X-linked			
301900	Borjeson-Forssman-Lehmann syndrome (BFLS)	Xq26–q27	Clinical features include severe mental retardation, hypogonadism, marked obesity; may be caused by mutation in the SOX3 gene (of the family of genes related to SRY, the testis-determining factor)
303110	Choroideremia with deafness and obesity	Xq21	Chromosomal deletion in Xq21
309400	Chudley mental retardation syndrome	NA	Mental retardation, short stature, mild obesity, and hypogonadism reported in 5 individuals of a pedigree
309585	Wilson-Turner syndrome (WTS)	Xq21.1–22	Mental retardation syndrome including obesity, gynecomastia, and limb abnormalities
312870	Simpson-Golabi-Behmel syndrome (SGBS)	Xq25–27	Prenatal and postnatal overgrowth syndrome with slight obesity

MIM = Mendelian inheritance in man; NA = not available.

several human obesity traits. Finally, recommendations for future studies are proposed.

A.   Review of Methods

I.   Multifactorial

Genetic epidemiology studies of human obesity use a variety of family data designs and a variety of statistical methods to partition the underlying phenotypic variance of a trait into genetic and/or environmental sources. In multifactorial studies (i.e., investigating polygenic and common environmental causes), the basic model is: $V_P = V_G + V_C + V_E$, where the phenotypic variance (V_P) is due to the additive genetic variance (V_G), common (shared) environmental variance (V_C), and the residual or non-shared environmental variance (V_E). These factors can be partitioned into more specific environmental (sibling vs. spouse vs. between generations) and genetic (gene-by-environment interactions, or G × E, dominance deviations, and gene-by-gene interactions, or epistasis) components. The specificity in parameterizing a model depends on the type of data collected. The genetic heritability of a trait is expressed as the percent of total phenotypic variance due to the additive genetic effects ($h^2 = V_G/V_P$) and the common environmental component is the percent due to common environments ($c^2 = V_C/V_P$).

Family Studies. In traditional nuclear families (i.e., parents and their biological offspring, which characterizes many human obesity studies), family members generally share both genes and environments to some degree, so it is difficult to separate the G and C components. Therefore, a transmissibility or familiarity is usually reported, which includes both sources of shared variance [$t^2 = (V_G + V_C)/V_P$]. One may simply compute t^2 by doubling the average familial correlation (i.e., parent-offspring and sibling), or more rigorously using maximum likelihood path analysis (e.g., the TAU model; 12), which yields information on how well the model fits the data. The major advantage of using path (or variance components) analysis in general is that additional sources of familial resemblance may be isolated (e.g., spouse resemblance and additional sibling resemblance). Simple correlation methods fail to account for these sources and thus may provide biased estimates of the familialities. The only difference between the familial correlations approach and the method of path analysis is that while familial correlations provide an aggregate measure of familial aggregation, path analysis attempts to decompose the aggregate measure into separate genetic and environmental effects (heritabilities).

To separate the effects due to G and C, at least two types of strategies are used. First, in the context of path analysis, an "environmental index" (which is computed by regressing the phenotype on relevant environmental measures and retaining the predicted score; 13) can be used to estimate C (e.g., PATHMIX; 14), such that the remaining familial resemblance is due to genetic determinants. While this remaining component is entirely genetic, some of the total genetic effect may have been included in the effect of C. If so, the remainder may be more appropriately regarded as "residual" genetic heritability. Familial correlations of the residual phenotype, adjusted for the environmental measures by regression analysis, may also be used to estimate the "residual" genetic contribution. The second strategy for separating G and C is to use additional familial relationships (i.e., twins, adoptees, longitudinal data), although each of these additional family types brings with it further assumptions, as outlined below.

Twin Studies. Twin studies allow for separation of the genetic component of variance since monozygotic twins (MZ) share 100% of their genes while dizygotic twins (DZ) share half on the average. However, the major problems with twin data are that MZ twins may share more common environmental effects (c^2_{MZ}) and dominance deviations (nonadditive genetic effects) than do DZ twins (c^2_{DZ}), thus inflating the genetic component. In fact, heritability estimates derived from twin data are usually much higher than those derived from other family designs, and at times are unrealistically high. Under reasonable assumptions, the expected MZ and DZ twin correlations are: $r_{MZ} = h^2 + d^2 + c^2_{MZ}$ and $r_{DZ} = h^2/2 + d^2/4 + c^2_{DZ}$, where d^2 represents the variance component due to dominance deviations. The most commonly used estimates are: $2(r_{MZ} - r_{DZ}) = h^2 + 1.5d^2 + 2(c^2_{MZ} - c^2_{DZ})$ and $2r_{DZ} - r_{MZ} = (2c^2_{DZ} - c^2_{MZ}) - d^2/2$, which show clearly that $2(r_{MZ} - r_{DZ})$ overestimates h^2 always (unless $d^2 = 0$ and $c^2_{MZ} = c^2_{DZ}$) and that $2r_{DZ} - r_{MZ}$ involves an unpredictable bias in the estimation of c^2. The correlation between MZ twins reared apart (r_{MZA}) is a relatively unbiased estimate of the broad-sense heritability (additive + dominance genetic effects). However, such samples are rare.

As previously noted with family data, twin data can also be analyzed using model-fitting approaches, which basically involve solving a series of simultaneous equations in order to estimate the underlying genetic and environmental parameters that best fit the observed familial correlations. The most commonly used maximum-likelihood computer program is LISREL (15); special LISREL applications to twin data are found in Boomsma et al. (16). A more simple model-fitting approach using twin data was described by DeFries and Fulker (17). Multiple linear regression is used to predict one twin's score from the other twin's score as well as additional variables (e.g., age and gender), including the coefficient of relationship (1.0 for MZs and 0.5 for DZs) and a dummy interaction term that is the product of the twin's score and the coefficient of relationship. The partial regression coefficient for the interaction term provides a direct estimate of h^2, while the partial regression of one twin's score on the other represents the shared environmental influence.

Adoption Studies. Full adoption studies are useful in separating the common environmental effects, since adoptive parents and their adopted offspring (and adopted sibling pairs) share only environmental sources of variance, while the adoptees and their biological parents share only genetic sources of variance. There are several potential problems with adoption data. For example, selective placement and late placement in the adoptive home may result in inflated common environmental estimates if placement is due in part to genetic similarity between the biological and adoptive parents. This effect is often unmeasured since it is difficult to obtain measures on the biological parents of the adoptees, especially the biological father. Furthermore, interpreting the results from some adoption studies is complicated by the fact that some of the "adopted" children may be natural children from one parent and stepchildren of the other. Such a partial adoption design inflates the common environmental effect to the degree there is assortative mating (due to genetic causes) between the natural and stepparents. Another consideration with adoption data as compared to intact nuclear families is that adoption studies fail to account for the possible influence of gene by environment correlations. Heritabilities are derived from adoption data similarly to the family studies (i.e., doubling the average familial correlations, or more rigorously using path analysis).

Longitudinal Studies and Temporal Trends. It is generally recognized that fat accumulates with time, so obesity phenotypes are usually adjusted for age prior to analysis. This procedure corrects for age trends in the mean and variance (i.e., heteroscedasticity), but temporal trends may still be evident in the covariance among family members. Trends in the familiality may arise through secular environmental effects, or through age-limited developmental effects of genes as reflected, for instance, in the growth spurt at puberty (18). Correlation methods for tracking the familiality estimates across time involve comparisons at different ages using either longitudinal measurements or cross-sectional data. Mueller (19) suggested that if the age effects were due to genes and not environmental factors, then sibling correlations should diminish as a function of increased age difference in young siblings, but not adult siblings. Bouchard (20) proposed partialing out environmental indicators from correlations between siblings who were measured at the same chronological age. Path analysis also allows for exploration of temporal trends (e.g., TAUTREND; 21) by modeling parameters as functions of age (i.e., heritability, spouse resemblance) or age differences (e.g., residual sibling resemblance), or by modeling separate familial estimates for parent and offspring generations (e.g., PATHMIX; 14).

There is another, and even more critical, implication of the fact that overweight and obesity are conditions that become established over time as body fat accumulates. With body fat accretion up to a new body mass level (e.g., a given obesity level), the causes of the positive energy balance that led to obesity become progressively masked. For instance, an apparent deficit in resting energy expenditure is compensated by an increase in the metabolic mass associated with weight gain (22), similarly for an apparent deficit in lipid oxidation rate that is eliminated when the gain in fat mass has been large enough to ensure a greater reliance on lipid oxidation (23). This adds a dimension to the complexity of the task of understanding the causes of obesity and defining the role of genes. To unmask the true susceptibilities to be in positive energy balance, one has to rely on longitudinal data that will make it possible to define the relevant predictors of obesity and to specify their genetic and molecular bases.

2. Multivariate (Genetic Pleiotropy)

For many obesity traits, especially indirect measures such as the BMI, there may be several unique determinants underlying the observed phenotype. Moreover, when considering a clinical syndrome or a network of interactions involving multiple traits, there are likely several underlying genetic and/or environmental etiologies. Multivariate genetic epidemiology studies are designed to simultaneously examine several traits and determine the extent to which the separate measures may be influenced by unique and common genes and environments. Multivariate studies may be conducted under both the multifactorial and major gene models.

The fundamental concept underlying multifactorial multivariate studies is cross-trait resemblance between pairs of relatives, for example trait 1 in parents with trait 2 in offspring. See Volger and Fulker (24) for detailed methods using different family types. In general, cross-trait heritability is computed by adapting the methods previously outlined for the univariate methods and represents the degree to which the two traits share common genetic (i.e., genetic pleiotropy) and environmental determinants. Similarly, pleiotropy in the major gene component may be assessed using bivariate segregation models (i.e., multilocus-multitrait; 25). These methods are useful in documenting the complex behavioral and biological interactions in a network design.

3. Major Gene (Commingling and Segregation)

The additive genetic component (multifactorial) results from the effects of many genes, each with a small influence on the phenotype (i.e., polygenic). There are other types of genetic effects that are not necessarily additive in nature. For example, major gene models are characterized as a single locus having a large impact on the phenotype. While the frequency distribution of a multifactorial trait is usually represented as a single normal distribution, a major gene trait is characterized as a mixture of distributions. Commingling analysis (e.g., SKUMIX; 26) is often used to determine whether there is distributional admixture. While the finding of commingled distributions is consistent with the hypothesis of a major gene, commingling can also arise from other sources, including environmental, and can be induced by pooling potentially heterogeneous subgroups. Therefore, commingling analysis is useful for (1) screening likely phenotypes for more rigorous testing using segregation analysis, and (2) determining whether the form of the distribution is heterogeneous across subgroups (male vs. female and/or parent vs. offspring). Such subgroup heterogeneity has implications for the expected segregation patterns.

Segregation analysis (e.g., POINTER; 27) is used whether the trait is segregating in families according to Mendelian expectations. In the mixed model (28), the phenotype is assumed to be composed of the independent and additive contributions from a major gene effect, a multifactorial background, and a unique environmental component (residual). The major effect is assumed to result from the segregation at a single locus having two alleles (i.e., **A** and **a**), where the **A** allele is defined as decreasing the quantitative phenotype. The transmission pattern from parents to offspring is tested to verify if the gene is segregating according to Mendelian expectations. The transmission pattern is generally characterized by three parameters representing the probabilities that individuals with genotypes **AA**, **Aa**, and **aa**, transmit allele **A** to the offspring (which are 1, 1/2, and 0 under Mendelian expectations). More recently, further refinements in the segregation models have been presented that allow for covariate effects to be genotype-dependent (e.g., PAP; 29, 30; and REGREES; 31). For example, the effect of the major gene may depend on the age of the individual (i.e., genes turning on or off over time), or may have different effects in males and females, or may depend on environmental (life-style) conditions. Once a putative major gene has been identified using these methods, verification is motivated through linkage studies. The segregation studies may be helpful in identifying families that appear to have a similar segregating putative gene.

4. Combined Path, Segregation, and Linkage

All obesity phenotypes are complex and are multifactorial in the sense that there are a number of genetic and/or nongenetic determinants. Therefore, it is highly unlikely that we will discover anything close to "the gene" that explains most of the variation for the phenotype and solves the whole puzzle. Instead, we expect the genetic component of many traits to be in the oligogenic (few genes) to polygenic (many genes) range, with an elaborate interplay between many factors, including gene-gene and gene-environmental interactions. While a lot of analytic progress can be and has been made using the standard genetic epidemiological tools discussed so far, and we are firm believers in the principle of never using a complex model when a simple one will do, we also believe that a combined approach is potentially much more powerful and holds great promise for these traits. Indeed, a combined approach may be the only way to disentangle the interplay of the multiple underlying processes.

One of the most useful combined genetic epidemiological modeling tools is a general-purpose model and a flexible computer program called SEGPATH (32). SEGPATH is a user-friendly computer program that can be used to generate programs to implement linear models for pedigree data, based on a flexible, model-specification syntax. All programs generated by SEGPATH produce maximum likelihood estimates of the model parameters from a family dataset. Within the confines of linear models, SEGPATH models can perform segregation analysis, path analysis, or combined segregation and path analysis. In fact, any user-specified path model can be structured to analyze any number of multivariate phenotypes, environmental indices, and/or measured covariate fixed effects (including measured genotypes). Population heterogeneity models, repeated-measures models, longitudinal models, autoregressive models, developmental models, and gene by en-

vironment interaction models can all be created under SEGPATH.

The general model implemented in SEGPATH includes both a segregation component ($\mathbf{g}$) and a multifactorial path model component ($\mathbf{m}$), as well as the fixed-effect covariates ($\mathbf{f}$), so that the phenotype ($\mathbf{P}$), univariate or multivariate, is determined by:

$$\mathbf{P} = \mathbf{g} + \mathbf{m} + \mathbf{f} + \mathbf{r} \tag{1}$$

where $\mathbf{r}$ is the residual. In this formulation, $\mathbf{g}$ can denote any number of unlinked major genes, with whatever pleiotropic effects they may have on the (multivariate) phenotype(s), and $\mathbf{m}$ denotes an arbitrary path model so that $\mathbf{m}$ may be a linear expression with many terms containing multiple heritable components. Likewise, $\mathbf{f}$ represents any number of fixed covariate effects. Equation (1) defines a set of regression equations for each person in a pedigree, which are linked, via the general, user-specific path model part, $\mathbf{m}$, as well as the major gene part, $\mathbf{g}$. In the current version of SEGPATH, however, $\mathbf{g}$ denotes only a single, biallelic major gene, with transmission characterized as in the unified mixed model. Fixed effects of covariates (e.g., measured genotypes) and genotype-specific covariate effects ($\mathbf{g} \times \mathbf{f}$) are also included.

Combined path and regressive models provide another alternative. Regressive models have been extended by incorporating a simple path model (the so-called TAU model) (33). This was achieved for both class A and class D regressive models by expressing the residual correlations in the regressive models in terms of parameters of the path model. Explicit solutions were presented for path coefficients in terms of the residual correlations. The estimate of the transmissibility appears to be robust under class A and class D models. Additionally, the combined modeling was further extended by incorporating the BETA path model of polygenic and familial environmental transmission into the more realistic class D regressive model (34). This was done by expressing correlations among the residuals from major genotype (RMGs) of family members under the class D regressive model as functions of path coefficients under the BETA path model. The likelihood function under the combined model was factorized into a product of conditional densities, which is dominated by bivariate normal densities. Statistical inference under the combined model is analogous to that under the class D regressive model.

In yet another approach, segregation and linkage analyses were combined. Quantitative traits for which evidence of a major gene effect has been found via segregation analysis can be tested for linkage to markers by using parametric methods in addition to the nonparametric sibpair approach described later. Parametric methods in general are more powerful when good information is available on the parameters of the major gene model (e.g., gene frequency and genotypic means). Thus, a test of linkage can be evaluated by fixing the major gene parameters to their maximum likelihood estimates and contrasting the hypothesis that the recombination fraction (θ) is zero versus the model where θ is 1/2. This test can be carried out in the context of the mixed model in PAP (29) or, alternatively, in the context of regressive models using the computer program REGRESS (31,35). For those markers exhibiting significant lod scores, the maximum likelihood estimate of the recombination fraction can be obtained, along with those for the parameters of the genetic model in REGRESS. In other words, when a genuine linkage relationship is detected, it is possible to simultaneously maximize over all parameters of the model, thereby using all possible information. Parametric linkage analysis is very powerful when the underlying trait model is known. However, it would be more robust to use the nonparametric sibpair linkage whenever the underlying genetic model is unknown.

B. Review of Findings

I. Excess Body Mass or Body Fat

While most multifactorial studies of the BMI show significant familial resemblances, the relative importance of genes and common familial environment varies. Some studies place more importance on the familial environment as compared to polygenic effects (36–40), and others suggest that genetic effects outweigh those of the familial environment (41–49). Recent studies suggest that genetic effects are relatively stronger. For example, in MZ twins reared apart (45,48,50) the correlations were very similar to those for MZ twins reared together, suggesting that the shared familial environment had little or no effect. Two of the larger studies of the BMI [Norwegian sample of about 75,000 individuals (51) and over 9000 individuals in Tecumseh, Michigan (40)] suggest that the total familiality of the BMI may be between 30% to 40% in families. A somewhat higher estimate (69%) was reported in the large Virginia study of adult twins and their families (nearly 30,000 individuals); both common environment and gene-environment interactions were also significant, but accounted for a relatively small percentage of the variance (52).

The genetic epidemiology features of excess body mass or body fat have been summarized recently (53). Table 6 describes the trends in the heritability levels based on a large number of studies. The results are generally quite heterogeneous. The heritability level is highest with twin studies, intermediate with nuclear family data, and lowest

Table 6 Overview of the Genetic Epidemiology of Human Body Fat/Obesity

	Heritability/ transmission	Maternal/ paternal	Familial environment
Nuclear families	30–50	No	Minor
Adoption studies	10–30	Mixed results	Minor
Twin studies	50–80	No	No
Combined strategies	25–40	No	Minor

Based on the trends in about 50 different studies. In most of these studies, the BMI was the phenotype considered. In some cases, skinfolds or estimates of percentage body fat or fat mass were used.
Source: From Ref. 53.

when derived from adoption data. When several types of relatives are used jointly in the same design, the heritability estimates typically cluster around 25–40% of the age- and gender-adjusted phenotype variance. There is no clear evidence for a specific maternal or paternal effect, and the common familial environment effect is marginal.

Temporal trends (or age effects) in the familial resemblance for BMI have also been explored (see Ref. 54 for a more complete review). Recent studies suggest that age trends in the familial effects of BMI may be primarily genetic, and that the trends diverge in different directions between childhood and adulthood. Two studies using path analysis techniques (21,55) suggested that the familiality increased from birth to adulthood, which Cardon (55), using adoptive and biological families, measured longitudinally, attributed to genetic (rather than environmental) factors. In studies assessing familiality in adults (56–59), there was a general decrease in the genetic heritability during adulthood. Fabsitz et al. (58) suggested that there were two major genetic effects, one increasing at or prior to age 20, and the other decreasing after age 20.

A common observation is that the obese person in familial studies of obesity is, on the average, 10–15 BMI units heavier than his or her mother, father, brothers, or sisters (3,60,61). Such a large difference between a proband and his or her first-degree relatives is suggestive of the contribution of a recessive gene having a large effect. This hypothesis can be tested by complex segregation analysis. Major gene effects have been reported for the BMI (or some measure of height-adjusted weight) using segregation analysis (see Table 7). In general, support for a major gene resulted when studies incorporated very large sample sizes (62–64), used samples selected for obe-

Table 7 Segregation Studies of Obesity

Source	Sample	Individuals (families)	Phenotype	% variance for major gene	% variance for multifactorial	Notes
			BMI or Body Fat			
Karlin et al. (68)	LRC	1167(123)	BMI	No		Ascertained[a]
Zonta et al. (69)	Italian	(179)	BMI	No		Ascertained[b]
Price et al. (62)	LRC	2935(961)	BMI[d]	14	34	Ascertained[a]
Province et al. (63)	Tecumseh	9226(3281)	BMI	20	41	Offspring
					20	Parents
Ness et al. (64)	LRC	3925(861)	BMI	14	34	White
		231(60)		No	50	Black (Marginal)
Moll et al. (65)	Muscatine	1302(284)	BMI	35	42	Ascertained[c]
Tiret et al. (70)	French	2534(629)	BMI[e]	No	35–40	
Rice et al. (72)	QFS	619(175)	%BF	45	22	
			FM	45	26	
Rice et al. (71)	QFS	1223(301)	BMI	No	42	
Borecki et al. (66)	QFS	1223(301)	BMI	[f]	30	
Commuzzie et al. (73)	Mexican Americans	543(26)	FM	35	20	Males
				42	35	Females
Feitosa et al. (75)	India	1691(432)	BMI	37	53	Offspring
					8	Parents
			BMI[g]	No	80	Offspring
					14	Parents
			Upper Body Fat			
Paganini-Hill (173)	S-leut	784(89)	Triceps SF	83		
			Subscapular SF	26		
Zonta et al. (69)	Italian	(179)	Discriminant score[h]	Yes		Ascertained[b] Dominant mode
Hasstedt et al. (95)	Utah	774(59)	RFPI	42	9.5	Ascertained[i]
Province et al. (63)	Tecumseh	(3281)	TER	No		
Borecki et al. (94)	QFS	1223(301)	TER-fm	37	29	
			SF6-fm	34	36	
			TSF3-fm	No		
			Abdominal Visceral Fat			
Bouchard et al. (97)	QFS	382(100)	AVF	51	21	
			AVF-fm	No	44	
			Type 4?			
Borecki et al. (94)	QFS	1223(301)	TER-fm	37	29	

[a]Both random sample and ascertained (for high lipid value of proband) sample.
[b]Ascertained for obese and nonobese schoolchildren.
[c]Four ascertained groups: random, lean, heavy, and gain groups of schoolchildren. The gain group includes families of students who gained at least two quartiles of relative weight between two surveys.
[d]BMI adjusted for social class and LRC clinic.
[e]BMI is height (linear and quadratic)-adjusted weight using regression analysis.
[f]Multifactorial effect was inferred by doubling the average residual familial (sibling and parent-offspring) correlations; the major gene effect is genotype-dependent on age and sex, and the percent of variance accounted for was not reported.
[g]BMI adjusted for energy intake and energy expenditure of activities.
[h]Discriminant score (obese vs. nonobese) of weight, subscapular skinfold, chest depth, and adjusted for age, sex, height.
[i]Ascertained through pedigrees with various cardiovascular, coronary heart, and hypertensive diseases.

sity (65), or allowed for genotype-dependent effects in the major gene component (66). In addition, somewhat different models result among the different studies. For example, several studies reported no evidence for a major gene (67–71), while a majority of the studies suggested a recessive locus accounted for 35–45% of the variance (between 30 and 50% was multifactorial) or less (14–20%; 62–64).

The mixed evidence for a major gene for BMI may be related to several factors. First, there are likely to be gene by environment interactions, where some genotypes are more susceptible than others. In other words, whether the phenotype of obesity is expressed may depend on having an "obesity" gene and exposure to the relevant environmental conditions. Evidence of this is suggested in the experiments on MZ twins (see next section). Second, the major gene effect may depend on the ethnicity, as suggested by Ness et al.'s (64) study of black and white Lipid Research Clinic (LRC) families. While the major gene evidence was marginal for the black families (but significant in the white families), the multifactorial effect was higher in the black (50% of the variance) than white families (34%). Third, the effect of the major gene may vary depending on developmental stage (age) or sex, as suggested by Borecki et al. (66). Fourth, there may be more than one major gene for the BMI (accounted for by variability in correlated phenotypes such as percent body fat), with different frequencies among the different samples. Evidence of this is suggested by the different models among the positive results studies and the suggestion by Tiret et al. (70) that either a recessive or a codominant major gene fits the data depending on the method used. This latter hypothesis is also appealing given the nature of the BMI measurement. That is, the BMI is a general measure of body build and incorporates fat mass, muscle mass, and skeletal mass. Recent evidence suggests that there may be major gene effects for fat mass (e.g., 72,73) and skeletal tissue (e.g., 74), so the major gene detected for BMI may be the one that is most correlated with skeletal tissue. Moreover, one recent study (75) suggests that the major effect of the gene for BMI may be mediated by energy intake and energy expenditure of activity; another energy expenditure component, resting metabolic rate, may also have a major gene component (e.g., 76). Mitchell et al. (77) and Kaplan et al. (78) suggested that exercise or activity levels had the potential to suppress the (polygenic) heritability of BMI. Whether the same major gene affects both traits (i.e., genetic pleiotropy), or whether the gene primarily affects one trait (e.g., fat mass or energy metabolism) which in turn affects the BMI remains to be investigated.

Relatively less is known about direct measures of general obesity (i.e., fat mass, FM, and % body fat, %BF). In Utah families, Ramirez (79) reported that the familiality for %BF (measured with bioelectrical impedance) was about 25%. In the QFS, the familiality for %BF (measured with underwater weighing) was 40%, but dropped to 36% after adjusting for energy intake and energy expenditure (80,81). In Quebec twins and adopted and biological families, the genetic heritability for each of %BF and FM was about 25%, with an additional 30% due to familial environment effects (82). Together, these studies suggest that between 25 and 40% of the variance in total fat mass may be genetic in origin.

Only two segregation studies for fat mass and/or percent body fat have been reported to date; one conducted on the QFS (72) using underwater weighing techniques, and another on Mexican American families in San Antonio (73) using bioelectrical impedance techniques. The results were very similar for both studies. A recessive locus accounting for up to 45% of the variance (and affecting 6% of the sample) was detected, with an additional 22–26% of the phenotypic variance due to multifactorial effects (72). In addition, Comuzzie et al. (73) reported that the effect of the major gene component depended on sex and accounted for slightly more variance in females (42%) than males (35%). Both studies also were in agreement that no major gene was evident for fat-free mass (FFM), although a major non-Mendelian effect accounting for 60% of the variance was reported by Rice et al. (72). Such types of effects may be due to major environmental factors, or even gene by environment interactions.

2. Upper Body Fat (Android Obesity)

The major phenotypes examined are the waist-to-hip ratio (WHR) (79,83–87) and ratios of subcutaneous skinfold thicknesses reflecting an android or a gynoid profile of subcutaneous fat topography. For the WHR familiality estimates varied from 28% in adoptive and biological families (83) to 40–50% in traditional nuclear families (84,86) to over 60% in longitudinal family data (Fels Longitudinal Study; 85). In two other studies (79,87) the familial correlations were either nonsignificant or inconsistent across different family pairs. No major gene studies were reported for WHR.

Comparison of results across studies for fat distribution using skinfold measures is complicated by the fact that different skinfolds are measured across different studies. One of the more widely used measures of fat distribution is the trunk-to-extremity subcutaneous skinfold ratio (TER). Most often, the simple ratio of trunk sum to extremity sum is used, although a few studies use principal components analysis to extract the relevant factors underlying a set of skinfolds. The first component derived from such analysis is generalized fat with nearly equal loading across all skinfold measures. The second component is usually a trunk to extremity contrast, and the third (not often reported) is an upper-to-lower contrast. The familiality for the 2nd (33–52%) and 3rd (31–49%) components (88,89) was likely to be due to genetic factors since spouse correlations were not significant. Path analysis of the 2nd principal component in French-Canadian biological and adoptive families (90) accounted for about 40% of the familial variance, of which 18% was genetic in origin. After adjusting the second component for BMI, the genetic heritability increased to 30%. The genetic heritability increased to as high as 50% when the second principal component or other indicators of android or gynoid fat distribution was adjusted for total body fat content (91). The phenotypic, genetic, and nongenetic correlation matrices extracted from an analysis of eight skinfold measures in Mexican American families were analyzed using principal component analysis (92). The results suggested that the pattern of central versus peripheral fat distribution was largely a function of the genetic correlation structure and was interpreted as evidence for global genetic pleiotropy among the skinfold traits. Familial estimates for the TER using the ratio of simple skinfold sums is about 37% (83) in a large survey of the Canadian population (over 18,000 individuals from more than 11,000 households). After adjusting for percent body fat, the total familiarity increased to over 63%, of which 28% was genetic in origin. Similar results were obtained in the sample of twins and adoptive and biological families of QFS (82).

These results for regional fat distribution suggest that there is a significant familial influence on the pattern of subcutaneous fat distribution and that adjusting for total body fat usually results in an increased familiality. This implies that for a given level of fatness, some individuals store more fat on the trunk or abdominal area (android) while others store primarily on the lower body (gynoid). This pattern is consistent with an hypothesis of both genetic pleiotropy (i.e., similar genes affecting both fat distribution and total body fat) and oligogenic (an additional major genetic system specific to fat distribution). This question was more specifically addressed in the QFS using a trivariate familial correlation model (93). In that study, cross-trait familial resemblance (e.g., trait 1 in parents with trait 2 in offspring, or interindividual cross-trait correlations) was examined among %BF, BMI, and TER. The results suggested that although all three measures were significantly correlated within individuals, the interindi-

vidual (familial) cross-trait resemblance was significant for BMI with each of %BF and TER (bivariate heritabilities of 10% and 18%, respectively), but %BF and TER showed no cross-trait familial resemblance. This supported the hypothesis that there may be entirely different underlying genes and/or environmental factors influencing the adiposity phenotypes of total body fat and regional fat distribution.

Relatively few segregation studies have been reported for fat distribution measures. For the TER, no support for a major gene was found in the large Tecumseh sample (63), or in the QFS (94). However, after adjusting the fat distribution measure for overall level of fatness using multiple regression (94), a recessive locus accounted for 37% of the variance with an additional 29% due to a multifactorial component. This supports the previous multifactorial studies, which suggest that the some of the genetic determinants for fat distribution are independent from those for total fat mass. A putative major locus was also reported in the Utah pedigrees (95) for a relative fat pattern index [RFPI = subscapular / (subscapular + suprailiac)]. The recessive locus accounted for 42% of the variance, with 9.5% due to the multifactorial effect. The authors interpreted this effect as a tendency for individuals with the recessive genotype to have small suprailiac rather than large subscapular skinfolds.

3. Abdominal Visceral Fat

We are aware of only one family study investigating abdominal visceral fat. Familial correlations in the Quebec Family Study (96) for abdominal total, abdominal visceral, and abdominal subcutaneous fat tissue were about 0.35, with somewhat lower spouse correlations for total (0.30) and subcutaneous (0.21) and higher spouse correlations for abdominal visceral fat (0.36). The heritability (twice the average familial correlations) was about 70% for each of the three measures. The effect of adjusting each of these measures for total body fat was to reduce the magnitude of the familial correlations and thus the heritability estimates (greater than 55% for total and visceral abdominal fat and 42% for subcutaneous abdominal fat). This suggests that some of the same multifactorial factors (polygenic and/or familial environment) impact similarly on total body fat and visceral fat.

A major gene hypothesis for abdominal visceral fat was examined in the QFS (97). A putative recessive locus accounted for 51% of the variance, with 21% due to a multifactorial component. However, after adjusting for fat mass, support for a major gene was reduced; although the major effect was significant, the Mendelian and no transmission (i.e., environmental) models were not resolved. It was suggested that the major gene previously noted for fat mass in these data (72) was also responsible for the major gene detected for abdominal visceral fat. In other words, genetic pleiotropy was inferred, where the same major gene affected both fat mass and the abdominal visceral fat traits. A cross-trait study conducted between fat mass and abdominal visceral fat (98) supported the pleiotropy hypothesis. The bivariate (cross-trait) familiarity was 29–50% (with sex differences). Moreover, since the univariate familiarities for each trait were even higher (55–77% for fat mass and 55–65% for abdominal visceral fat), each trait was assumed to be influenced by additional familial factors that were specific to each. Given the significant spouse cross-trait correlations, at least some of the bivariate familial effect may be environmental in origin.

4. Lower Body Fat (Gynoid Obesity)

All studies reviewed in the section on android obesity as assessed from WHR, TER, or principal components of sets of skinfolds apply equally well to the evaluation of the genetic components of gynoid obesity. In addition, one other study purported to measure gluteofemoral fat. In a study based on the Danish Adoption Register, participants were asked to match their (and other relatives) body type to one of nine silhouette pictures, which ranged from very thin to obese (99). While this measure correlated with the BMI (ranging from 0.63 to 0.88) and with the sum of several skinfolds (ranging from 0.39 to 0.66), the authors suggested that it favored the gynoid type of fat distribution. Relatives were placed in four classes as determined by weight of the adoptee. The mean silhouette score of the adoptees' biological mothers and siblings increased significantly across weight classes, while no mean differences were observed for adoptive relatives, suggesting primarily a genetic control for this measure.

5. Summary: Relationship Between Total Fat and Fat Topography

The genetic epidemiological studies reported in this chapter regarding total fat and fat topography suggests a complex relationship underlying the etiological causes of their covariation. Most of the evidence comes from studies comparing the multifactorial and major gene evidence for topographical fat both prior to and after adjusting for total fat (using multiple regression). In general, total fat adjustment alters the familial inferences for topographical measures. These studies suggest substantial shared major gene and multifactorial determinants between total fat and abdominal visceral fat, but only the major gene compo-

nent for total fat mass appears to influence subcutaneous fat distribution.

Regarding the major gene component for subcutaneous fat distribution, prior to adjustment for total fat there was evidence for a major (non-Mendelian) effect for TER, but only after adjustment did the transmission appear to be Mendelian. In other words, the TER may be both a pleiotropic and oligogenic trait, in that removal of the effects due to a putative major locus for total fat leads to the deletion of a secondary locus specific to fat distribution. In contrast, adjusting abdominal visceral fat for total fat reduces the evidence for a putative major locus. Together, these results suggest at least two putative major loci underlying obesity phenotypes, one determining total and abdominal visceral fat, and the other determining how subcutaneous adipose tissue is distributed.

Regarding the multifactorial (polygenic and/or common environmental) causes of the covariation between the traits, similar patterns are noted. For subcutaneous fat distribution, the generalized heritabilities increase after total fat adjustment, while bivariate studies find no evidence for a genetic correlation. Together, these results suggest that there are entirely different multifactorial causes for the variations in total fat and subcutaneous fat distribution. For abdominal visceral fat, however, total fat adjustment leads to decreased generalized heritability estimates, with bivariate studies suggesting a substantial bivariate heritability. Thus, total fat and abdominal visceral fat may share many of the same polygenic and/or common environmental factors.

In summary, the common etiologies of total fat and fat topography involve complex relationships. The exact nature of these relationships vary according to the source (major and multifactorial) and specific topographical measure.

C. Recommendations for Future Studies

Many questions remain to be addressed concerning the genetic epidemiology of obesity. First, temporal trends have been extensively explored only for the BMI. Age effects perhaps operate in both the multifactorial and major gene components, which has not been pursued for obesity (including fat distribution, primary measures of body fat, and abdominal visceral fat). Second, more attention should be paid to sex differences in the genetic and environmental components for obesity phenotypes. Although sex differences are often noted in familial correlations, few attempts have been made to estimate the familial influences by sex. Comuzzie et al. (100), using a variance decomposition method to examine the genetic architecture of sexual dimorphism, found evidence for a sex by genotype interaction for several obesity measures, including the BMI and several skinfolds. Third, only one family study has been reported for measures of visceral fat, which may be one of the more important obesity components as regards overall morbidity and mortality. Confirmation from other sources is needed. Fourth, many of the obesity phenotypes appear to be influenced by both major gene and multifactorial sources of variance. In the context of segregation models, further decomposition of the multifactorial effect into separate polygenic and common environmental sources may be useful. Development of new models that combine path analysis and segregation analysis can be useful for this (33,34). In all these pursuits, particular attention should be paid to gene-gene and gene-environment interactions.

The major unexplored area that genetic epidemiology can address, however, involves multivariate associations among the different obesity phenotypes, and between obesity types and other physiological and metabolic parameters. For example, we reviewed some studies that suggest that the cross-trait relationship between total body fat and each of fat distribution and abdominal visceral fat measures is in part familial. However, the degree to which those relationships are due to shared genes remains to be disentangled. Similarly, the relationship between fat mass and fat-free mass with resting metabolic rate has been shown to be familial (76,101), but the relative contributions from major genes, polygenes, and common environments has not been delineated. These patterns suggest a network of multiple causes underlying the degree and form of adiposity. Evaluation of these questions, however, needs some further methodological work. For example, more complex models incorporating multiple phenotypes (total fat, fat distribution, visceral fat, metabolic measures, etc), and multiple sources of familial resemblance, including multiple major loci, may be useful (25). Moreover, since many of these measures have been shown to be influenced by developmental and sex-specific factors, such multivariate models should allow for genotype-dependent covariate effects. Linkage investigations will also benefit from incorporating interactions with the covariates. Models combining both linkage analysis and segregation analysis (31) and also incorporating genotype-dependent covariate effects may allow for clearer localization of relevant obesity genes to specific chromosomal sites.

V.   GENE-ENVIRONMENT INTERACTIONS

Genotype-environment interaction (G × E) arises when the response of a phenotype (e.g., fat mass) to environ-mental changes (e.g., dietary restriction) depends on the genotype of the individual. Although it is well known that there are interindividual differences in the responses to various dietary interventions, whether in terms of serum cholesterol changes to high-fat diet (102) or in terms of body weight gains following chronic overfeeding (103), very few attempts have been made to test whether these differences are genotype-dependent. Most of the genetic epidemiology studies of human obesity have assumed the absence of genotype-environment interaction simply because of the difficulty in handling such interaction effects in quantitative genetic models. Methods from both genetic epidemiology (unmeasured genotype approach) and from molecular epidemiology (measured genotype approach) can now be used to detect G × E effects in humans. These methods will first be briefly reviewed followed by a summary of our current knowledge about the importance of G × E effects for phenotypes related to obesity.

A.   Review of Methods

An epidemiological approach was proposed by Ottman (104) to investigate the relationship between genetic predisposition and associated risk factors and determine if there is support for a G × E interaction, and if so, the form it may take. For example, Figure 2 illustrates five plausible models as described by Ottman (104). These models are not path diagrams, but rather are more similar to metabolic paths, and the direction of the arrows denotes direction of causality. The model in Figure 2A posits that the genotype increases the expression of the risk factor. In Figure 2B, the genotype exacerbates the effect of the risk factor. In both cases, only the presence of the risk factor is necessary for disease expression, although the genotype will have some additional effect. Figure 2C is the reverse of 2B, where the risk factor exacerbates the effect of the genotype; only the latter is "required" for disease expression. In Figure 2D, both the genotype and the risk factor are required to raise risk, and in Figure 2E, the genotype and the risk factor each influences risk of disease individually.

The basic approach involves classifying individuals into four groups based on the presence or absence of genetic susceptibility and presence or absence of the risk factor (104). Genetic susceptibility can be measured directly if the susceptibility gene is known or if there are closely linked markers. Even in the absence of any molecular data, however, family history of the disease can be used to develop indicators of genetic susceptibility. In the most simplistic analysis, the pattern of hits and misses in the four groups (assessed with odds ratios) suggests whether or not a particular type of G × E interaction (as illustrated

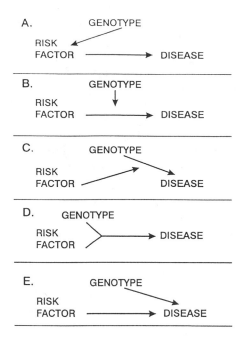

Figure 2 Five hypothetical relationships between genetic susceptibility to disease and risk factors for disease. The genetic susceptibility may be either polygenic or due to a dominant, recessive, or X-linked major locus. The risk factor may be only one of many factors associated with disease risk and may itself have either genetic or nongenetic origins. (From Ref. 104.)

in Fig. 2) is consistent. The basic method has been expanded to include assessing relative risks in affected twin pairs with known exposure (105), and in assessing the preventive effects of targeted environmental exposures to genetically susceptible persons in population studies (106). Familial aggregation of disease was also examined within strata based on classifying probands with respect to their relative risks (107). However, none of these methods have been applied to the study of obesity.

Several other genetic approaches can be used to detect G × E effects. Two of these strategies are of the unmeasured-genotype approach type. The first one would be to incorporate G × E effects in the statistical genetic models (108–111). Ignoring such interaction effects when they exist has been shown to reduce the power to detect major gene effects (66,112). Second, using intervention studies we have proposed that one way to test for the presence of a G × E effect in humans was to challenge several genotypes in a similar manner by submitting both members of monozygotic (MZ) twin pairs to a standardized treatment (environment) and compare the within- and the between-pair variances of the response to the treatment

(113). This comparison can be done using a two-way analysis of variance (ANOVA) for repeated measures on one factor (the treatment effect), in which the genotype effect is random, the treatment effect is fixed, and twins are nested within pairs. Using this ANOVA, F-ratios for the treatment effect and for genotype-treatment effect can easily be obtained. The intraclass correlation can be computed from the within- and between-pairs means of squares. The finding of a significantly higher variance in the response between pairs than within pairs suggests that the changes induced by the treatment are more heterogeneous in genetically dissimilar individuals, which will translate into a higher intrapair resemblance in the response.

Some of the conditions that are important to fulfill in this intervention design include (113): (1) determine the twin zygosity as precisely as possible; (2) keep age variation at a minimum; (3) use same-sex twin pairs or control for sex differences if both male and female twin pairs are involved; (4) apply the treatment in exactly the same manner to all twins under rigorously controlled conditions; and (5) select phenotypes that are not greatly influenced by prior exposure to the treatment used in the study. In a series of experiments conducted by male MZ twins over the last 10 years in our laboratory, we used either exercise training or overfeeding as treatments to investigate G × E effects in obesity-related phenotypes (results described below). Although the design is useful to detect G × E effects, there are some important limitations associated with it. First, for obvious ethical reasons, there are limitations regarding the experimental treatments that can be undertaken with human subjects regarding the severity of the nutritional stress imposed and the duration of the treatment. Second, even though it is possible to exert a satisfactory experimental control and reach full standardization over energy intake, it is not possible to fully standardized energy expenditure in positive or negative energy balance studies. Indeed, because of individual differences in resting metabolic rate, thermic effect of food, fidgeting, or variations in the energy cost of weight maintenance associated with changes in body mass, subjects will invariably differ in their levels of energy expenditure. Third, such intervention studies, in addition to being very expensive to undertake, are very difficult to conduct over a long period of time on a large number of subjects.

Four methods can be used to provide evidence for G × E effect in humans when molecular markers are available. The first is to compare the influence of a gene on a given phenotype between populations of different ethnic and cultural backgrounds. An example of this approach is provided by the study of Hallman et al. (114), who showed that the effect of apolipoprotein E polymorphism on total cholesterol levels varied among populations with different amounts of fat in their diet. The cholesterol-raising effect of the ϵ_4 allele, for example, was found to be highest in populations on high-fat diets like Tyrolea and Finland, and lowest in populations on low-fat diets like Japan and Sudan, which provides evidence of gene-diet interaction. The second method consists of comparing the effect of a gene between subgroups of individuals within the same population, but categorized on the basis of variables that can potentially affect the phenotype under study (e.g., sex, age, race, disease status, etc.). An example of this approach can be found in the results of Zee et al. (115), who reported an association between a polymorphism in the LDL-receptor gene and hypertension, but only in overweight or obese subjects. In the third method, the response to an environmental stimulus (diet, exercise training, medication, or others) is investigated among individuals with different genotypes at a given gene or marker locus. For example, using an approach similar to the MZ twin experimental design described above, but with singletons instead of twins, it would be possible to study the response to chronic alterations in energy balance as a function of genetic characteristics at specific candidate genes or marker loci. A fourth method is based on the "variability gene" concept introduced by Berg (116). Compared to a "level gene" that influences the level of a phenotype, a "variability gene" is a gene that contributes to the framework within which environmental factors cause phenotypic variation, or in other words, to the susceptibility to changes in the environment. To detect this G × E effect it has been proposed that phenotypic differences between members of MZ twins of various genotypes at the genetic locus be compared (117). An important advantage of the measured genotype approach over the unmeasured genotype approach in the study of G × E is that it makes possible the identification of the responsible genes, thereby providing means of recognizing individuals at higher risk of disease because of differences in susceptibility to risk factors.

B. Review of Findings

Evidence from both the unmeasured and measured genotype approaches is available regarding the presence of G × E effects in obesity-related phenotypes. Using appropriate statistical modeling, three studies reported major gene effects for measures of height-adjusted weight, but only after accounting for age and/or gender effects in the model (66,70,72), suggesting that the·effect of this putative gene on body mass is dependent on the sex and the age of the individual, which is a special case of genotype-environment effect.

Using the unmeasured genotype approach, we studied the role of the genotype in determining the response to changes in energy balance by submitting both members of MZ twin pairs either to positive energy balance induced by overfeeding (118,119) or to negative energy balance induced by exercise training (120,121). The objective of these studies was to determine whether the sensitivity of individuals to gain fat when exposed to positive energy balance or to lose fat when exposed to negative energy balance was modulated by the genotype. The results of these studies (reviewed below) revealed the presence of significant genotype-energy balance interaction effects for body weight, body fat, and fat distribution phenotypes, suggesting that generic factors are important in determining how an individual will respond to alterations in energy balance.

I. The Positive Energy Balance Experiments

It is generally recognized that there are some individuals prone to excessive accumulation of fat, for whom losing weight represents a continuous battle, and others who seem relatively well protected against such a menace. We have tried to test whether such differences could be accounted for by inherited differences. In other words, we asked whether there were differences in the sensitivity of individuals to gain fat when chronically exposed to short- and long-term positive energy balance and whether such differences were dependent or independent of the genotype.

The Short-Term Experiment.   In a first study, we exposed six pairs of male MZ twins to a 2.4 MJ/day (1000 kcal/day) energy intake surplus for 22 consecutive days (82,118). Individual differences in body weight, fat mass, subcutaneous fat, and site of fat deposition gains were observed with this short-term overfeeding protocol but these differences were not randomly distributed. Indeed, significant intrapair resemblance was observed for the changes in most body composition and fat distribution variables despite the fact that the treatment was of short duration and that the changes induced by the treatment were not large. The intrapair resemblance in the response to overfeeding, as assessed by the intraclass coefficient computed with the individual changes, reached 0.88 for total fat mass and 0.76 for fat-free mass. Subjects gained body weight and body fat but there was a nonsignificant 7% increase in resting metabolic rate (122).

The Long-Term Experiment. Twelve pairs of male MZ twins ate a 2.4 MJ/day (1000 kcal/day) caloric surplus, 6 days a week, for 100 days (119). Significant increases in body weight and fat mass were observed after the period of overfeeding. Data showed that there were considerable interindividual differences in the adaptation to excess calories and that the variation observed was not randomly distributed, as indicated by the significant within-pair resemblance in response. For instance, there were at least 3 times more variance in response between pairs than within pairs for the gains in body weight, fat mass, and fat-free mass (Fig. 3, left). These data, and those on the response to short-term overfeeding, demonstrate that some individuals are more at risk than others to gain fat when energy intake surplus is clamped at the same level for everyone and when all subjects are confined to a sedentary life-style. The within-identical-twin-pair response to the standardized caloric surplus suggests that the amount of fat stored is likely influenced by the genotype.

The long-term overfeeding study also revealed that there was 6 times more variance between pairs than within pairs for the changes in upper body fat and in CT-determined abdominal visceral fat when both were adjusted for the gain in total fat mass. These observations indicate that some individuals are storing fat predominantly in selected fat depots primarily as a result of undetermined genetic characteristics. It also suggests that variations in regional fat distribution are more closely related to the genotype of the individuals than variations in body mass and in overall body composition.

At the beginning of the overfeeding treatment, almost all the daily caloric surplus was recovered as body energy gain, but the proportion decreased to 60% at the end of the 100-day protocol (123). The weight gain pattern followed an exponential with a half-duration of about 86 days. We have estimated that the weight gain attained in the experiment reached about 55% of the anticipated maximal weight gain had the overfeeding protocol been continued indefinitely (123). The mean body mass gain for the 24 subjects of the 100-day overfeeding experiment was 8.1 kg, of which 5.4 kg was fat mass and 2.7 kg was fat-free-mass increases. Assuming that the energy content of body fat is about 22 MJ/kg (9300 kcal/kg) and that of fat free tissue is 2.42 MJ/kg (1020 kcal/kg) then about 63% of the excess energy intake was recovered on the average as body mass changes. This proportion is of the same order as that reported by other investigators (124,125), i.e., between 60% and 75% of total excess energy intake. There were, however, individual differences among the 24 subjects with respect to the amount of fat and fat free tissues gained.

Resting metabolic rate in absolute terms increased by about 10% with overfeeding. However, the increase was only marginal when it was expressed per unit of fat-free

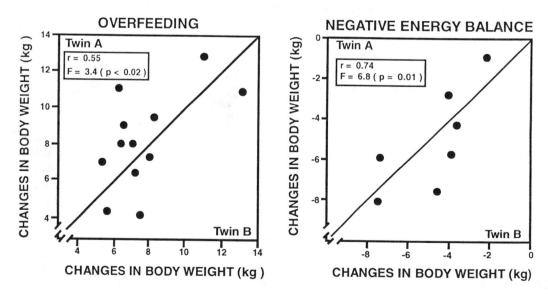

Figure 3 Intrapair resemblance in the response of identical twins to long-term changes in energy balance. (Left) Twelve pairs of identical twins were submitted to an 84,000-kcal energy intake surplus over 100 days. (Right) Seven pairs were subjected to a negative energy balance protocol caused by exercise. The energy deficit was 58,000 kcal over 93 days. (From Refs. 119, 121 with permission.)

mass (126,127). The intrapair resemblance for the changes in resting metabolic rate brought about by overfeeding was significant but it became nonsignificant when the changes in body mass or body composition were taken into account. The thermic response to food, as assessed by indirect calorimetry for a period of 4 hr following the ingestion of a 2.4-MJ (1000-kcal) meal of mixed composition, did not increase with overfeeding when resting metabolic rate was subtracted from postprandial energy expenditure (126). In contrast, postprandial energy expenditure and the total energy cost of weight maintenance increased significantly but the increments were mostly due to the gain in body mass.

2. The Negative Energy Balance Experiment

A short-term negative energy balance experiment was also undertaken with 6 pairs of MZ twins. The energy deficit was achieved by exercise performed twice a day, for 22 consecutive days, for about 50 min/session, on the cycle ergometer. The exercise prescription was precisely controlled for each subject, during each exercise session, and was designed to induce an extra energy expenditure of 2.4 MJ/day (1000 kcal/day) over resting metabolic rate while baseline energy intake was maintained throughout (128). The changes in body composition were generally small and not related to the twin lines. The only exception was for the fat-free-mass changes, which were more similar within pairs in comparison to the between-pairs variance.

Seven pairs of young adult male identical twins completed a negative energy balance protocol during which they exercised on cycle ergometers twice a day, 9 out of 10 days, over a period of 93 days while being kept on a constant daily energy and nutrient intake (121). The mean total energy deficit caused by exercise above the estimated energy cost of body weight maintenance reached 244 MJ. Baseline energy intake was estimated over a period of 17 days preceding the negative energy balance protocol. Mean body weight loss was 5.0 kg and it was entirely accounted for by the loss of fat mass. Fat-free mass was unchanged. Body energy losses reached 191 MJ, which represented about 78% of the estimated energy deficit. Decreases in metabolic rates and in the energy expenditure of activity not associated with the cycle ergometer protocol must have occurred to explain the difference between the estimated energy deficit and the body energy losses. Subcutaneous fat loss was slightly more pronounced on the trunk than on the limbs as estimated from skinfolds, circumferences, and CT. The reduction in abdominal visceral fat area was quite striking, from 81 cm^2 to 52 cm^2. At the same submaximal power output level, subjects oxidized more lipids than carbohydrates after the program as indicated by the changes in the respiratory exchange ratio. Intrapair resemblance was observed for the changes in body weight (Fig. 3, right), fat mass, percent fat, body energy content, sum of 10 skinfolds, abdominal visceral fat, and respiratory exchange ratio during submaximal work. Even though there were large individual differences in response to the negative energy balance and exercise protocol, subjects with the same genotype were more alike in responses than subjects with different genotypes particularly for body fat, body energy, and abdominal visceral fat changes. High lipid oxidizers and low lipid oxidizers during submaximal exercise were also seen despite the fact that all subjects had experienced the same exercise and nutritional conditions for about 3 months.

Thus, changes in body mass, body fat, and body energy content were characterized by more heterogeneity between twin pairs than within pairs. These results are remarkably similar to those that we reported earlier for body mass, body fat, and body energy gains with 12 pairs of twins subjected to a 100-day overfeeding protocol.

C. Recommendations for Future Studies

The results reviewed above clearly show that gene-environment interaction is an important factor to consider in the study of the genetic basis of obesity. However, the genetic determinants of the response of body fat to changes in energy intake and/or energy expenditure are poorly understood. The development of genetic models and statistical methods of analysis incorporating G × E effect would certainly be useful to increase our understanding of the way genes modulate the response of complex phenotypes such as those related to obesity. By using genetic polymorphism at candidate genes, interaction can be tested at different levels, such as the polygenic level in addition to the major gene level (111). These candidate genes could be identified from animal models such as the dietary obese mice and tested for association and linkage in human studies.

Intervention studies involving manipulation of one of the two components of the energy balance equation and conducted on a large number of individuals should be undertaken to increase our knowledge on the genetic determinants of the susceptibility to obesity. Although difficult to realize, these types of studies offer a unique opportunity to understand the physiological and metabolic mechanisms responsible for changes in body composition. Moreover, if conducted on pairs of biologically related individuals, such as sib-pairs, these studies have the potential to lead to the identification of genes associated with either a susceptibility or a resistance in the response to the environmental stressor imposed by the intervention.

VI. MOLECULAR MARKERS OF HUMAN OBESITY

A. Review of Methods

Support for a role of a gene in human obesity or variation in body fat content has been obtained from the six lines of evidence in Table 8. All of them will be addressed in turn with the exception of the evidence accumulated from transgenic rodent models and gene knockout experiments, which are reviewed in another chapter. Although the latter studies provide support for the potential role of a gene in body fat content fluctuation when it is overexpressed in some or all tissues or when the genes is inactivated or results in a nonfunctional peptide, the true contribution of these genes to human obesity remains to be clarified.

B. Review of Findings

1. Mendelian Disorders

Genetic syndrome characterized by the presence of obesity (see Table 5) could be useful in the identification of loci contributing to obesity. Among the disorders listed in Table 5, nine have been mapped to eight different chromosomes (3, 4, 8, 11, 16, 20, and X). With Bardet-Biedl syndrome alone having been linked to four different chromosomal regions, a total of 12 loci are linked to these Mendelian disorders. Although these disorders account for a very small fraction of the obese population, they illustrate that single gene defects could lead to the development of human obesity.

To determine whether these loci contribute to obesity in otherwise clinically normal people, Reed et al. (129) tested for linkage relationships between 17 genetic markers spanning the regions of the Prader-Willi, the Bardet-Biedl (BBS1, 2 and 3), the Cohen, the Borjeson, and the Wilson-Turner syndromes and the BMI measured in subjects from 44 families with obese probands. Analyses based on a total of 207 pairs of siblings revealed no evi-

Table 8 Human Obesity Genes: Lines of Evidence

Mendelian disorders (MIM)
Single-gene Rodent Models
QTL from cross-breeding experiments
Transgenic and knockout models
Association studies
Linkage studies

dence of linkage between any of the markers and obesity in these families. These results suggest that the genetic loci contributing to obesity in these families are not the same as those involved in the Mendelian disorders reported above. However, before excluding these chromosomal regions as potential carriers of loci predisposing to obesity in clinically normal subjects, other studies with a larger number of genetic markers will have to be performed. Furthermore, these negative results do not exclude the possibility that individuals carrying one copy of a gene responsible for an autosomal recessive disorders are at a greater risk of becoming obese than individuals with no copy of the defective gene. For example, it has recently been shown that the prevalence of obesity was significantly higher among heterozygous carriers (parents of affected individuals) of a gene responsible for the Bardet-Biedl syndrome compared to age- and sex-matched normal noncarriers, suggesting that this gene may predispose to obesity in the general population (130).

2. Single-Gene Rodent Models

Because of the high degree of homology in the genomes of mammalian species, it is possible to use rodent models of obesity to identify genes potentially involved in the etiology of human obesity. Several different single-gene mutations have been shown to cause obesity in rodents: diabetes (*db*), fat (*fat*), obese (*ob*), tubby (*tub*), adipose (*Ad*), and Yellow (A^y) in the mouse, and fatty (*fa*) in the rat (131). Although all these mutations result in obesity in the animals, the time of onset and the severity of obesity vary among the various mutations. Furthermore, the obesity phenotype is frequently associated with metabolic abnormalities including insulin resistance, hyperinsulinemia, NIDDM, hyperglycemia, hypertension, and hyperlipidemias (132). All the mutations, listed in Table 9, were found to have homologous regions in the human genome. A more extensive treatment of these rodent models is presented in other chapters. None of these regions have yet been found to be related to obesity in humans. Recently, 16 markers located on chromosome 20 in a region homologous to the Yellow mutation in the mouse (20q12–13.11) were tested for linkage with BMI and percent body fat assessed by bioelectrical impedance in a maximum of 210 sib-pairs from 45 obese families (133). No evidence of linkage was found, suggesting that this gene does not contribute to obesity in humans.

3. QTL from Cross-Breeding Experiments

Another method originally developed for plant genetics is now commonly used with rodents to identify loci that influence quantitative phenotype such as obesity. It is

Table 9 Single-Gene Rodent Models of Obesity, Gene Products, and Possible Synteny Between Rodent Obesity Genes and Human Chromosome Regions

Locus	Gene product	Transmission	Mouse chromosome	Human chromosome
Mouse				
Diabetes (*db*)	Leptin receptor (OB-R)	Recessive	4	1p35–31
Fat (*fat*)	Carboxypeptidase E (CPE)	Recessive	8	4q21
Obese (*ob*)	Leptin	Recessive	6	7q31.3
Tubby (*tub*)	Cloned, but not identified	Recessive	7	11p15.1
Yellow (A^y)	Agouti signaling protein (ASP)	Dominant	2	20q11.2
RAT				
Fatty (*fa*)	Leptin receptor (OB-R)	Recessive	5	1p35–31

known as the quantitative trait locus mapping method or the QTL. The method is fully described in another chapter.

Briefly, QTL mapping requires two key resources: two inbred strains and a detailed genetic map of the animal genome. The procedure requires the following steps (134): (1) two inbred strains divergent for the phenotype under consideration are crossed to produce F_1 and then F_2 or backcross progeny; (2) the animals are individually genotyped for markers to span the entire genome at close intervals; (3) the animals are appropriately phenotyped; and (4) QTLs are located by an interval mapping approach such as that provided by the program MAPMAKER (135). MAPMAKER uses genetic markers and quantitative phenotypes to identify QTLs with a LOD score method. Because of the density of the genetic map of the mouse genome, mice are at present the preferred species for QTL studies. Moreover, regions of homology between mouse and human chromosomes have been extensively defined and this allows quite often for the identification of the approximate location of a putative gene linked to the phenotype of interest on the human gene map.

To date, eight QTLs have been identified by this method; they are summarized in Table 10. Fisler et al. (136) obtained a backcross between the strains *Mus spretus* and C57BL/6J, which they called the BSB mouse. BSB exhibits a wide range of carcass lipid, from 1 to 50% and more. On the basis of the QTL approach with a large number of markers, Warden et al. (137,138) identified four "multigenic obesity" (Mob) loci on four different mouse chromosomes. A first locus (Mob-1) on BSB chromosome 7 determines the lipid content of the carcass (LOD score of 4.2). A second locus (Mob-2), on chromosome 6, affected only subcutaneous fat pads (LOD = 4.8). A third locus (Mob-3), encoded on chromosome 12, was linked to percentage lipid in the carcass (LOD = 4.8), while Mob-4 (chromosome 15) was linked primarily to

mesenteric fat (LOD = 3.4). Syntenic regions with these four mouse QTLs are on human chromosomes 10q21–26, 11p14-ter and 16p13–11 for Mob-1, 7q22–36 for Mob-2, 14q13–32 for Mob-3, and 5q11–13 for Mob-4 (Table 10).

A mouse polygenic model of differential susceptibility to dietary fat has been developed by crossing a dietary-lipid-sensitive strain (AKR/J) with a resistant strain (SWR/J). After 12 weeks of feeding on a moderately high-fat diet, the AKR/J strain had approximately six-fold higher carcass fat than the SWR/J strain (139). F_2 animals and backcross data were used and, to date, three QTLs have been identified (140,141). Do1 (chromosome 4), Do2 (chromosome 9), and Do3 (chromosome 15) are linked to the level of adiposity and, in the case of Do2, also to mesenteric fat. Although regions of homology in the human genome have not been described, it appears likely that syntenic areas can be found on human chromosome 1p36–32 for Do1, 3p21 for Do2, and 5p14–12 for Do3.

Finally, one QTL on mouse chromosome 2 was uncovered in a cross between mouse NZB/B1NJ and SM/J strains (142). The human equivalent of this locus appears to be on human chromosomes 20p11.2–q13.2. Other loci have been reported recently for the various QTL experiments defined above but they are unpublished at this time and are not reported here.

QTLs have also been uncovered for fat distribution phenotypes. Thus, Mob-2, Mob-4, and Do2 have been shown to be linked with specific fat depots, including mesenteric fat for Do2 (137,138,140,141). Mob-2 accounted for 7% of femoral fat while Mob-4 was associated with about 6% of mesenteric fat. The strongest linkage was between Do2 and mesenteric fat, with the QTL accounting for 47% of the variance in this fat depot. The syntenic regions of these QTLs are thought to be recovered on human 7q22–q36, 5q11–13 and 3p21.

Table 10   Quantitative Trait Loci (QTL) Linked to Body Fat Phenotypes

Mouse cross	Locus	LOD score	Effect on adiposity	Mouse chromosome	Human location	Ref.
AKR/J	Do1	4.5	NA	4	1p36–32	West et al. (140)
X	Do2	4.8	7% adiposity 47% mesenteric fat	9	3p21	West et al. (141)
SWR/J	Do3	3.9	4% adiposity	15	5p14–12	West et al. (141)
C57BL/6J	Mob-1	4.2	7% percent fat	7	10q21–26	Warden et al. (138)
X	Mob-2	4.8	7% femoral fat	6	11p14–ter	Warden et al. (138)
Mus Spretus	Mob-3	4.8	7% percent fat	12	16p13–11	Warden et al. (138)
	Mob-4	3.4	6% mesenteric fat	15	7q22–36 14q13–32 5q11–13	Warden et al. (138)
NZB/B1NJ X SM/J	D2Mit22 D2Mit28		36% percent fat	2	20p11.2–q13.2	Fisler et al. (142)

Do = dietary obese; Mob = multigenic obesity; NA = not available.

4. Association Studies

Association and linkage studies are important tools for the delineation of the genetic basis of overweight and obesity. The concept of association refers to a situation in which the correlation of a genetic polymorphism with a phenotype is investigated. Such studies are generally carried out on samples of unrelated individuals. They may take several forms including comparison of cases versus controls (e.g., obese vs. lean subjects), analysis of variance across genotypes for the locus under consideration, and comparison of carriers versus noncarriers of a given allele. Association studies are most useful when confined to candidate genes. If a significant association is observed with a polymorphism at a candidate gene locus, there are three likely explanations: (1) the locus is causally related to the phenotype; (2) the locus is in linkage disequilibrium with the trait locus as a result of natural selection or chance; or (3) this is an artifact due to population admixture. Association studies may provide important information on genes with a major or a minor contribution to a phenotype; the method is particularly useful for the identification of genes that make only a minor contribution (143).

It is important to recognize that the strength of an association is critical in the appraisal of its relevance as a marker for the susceptibility to obesity. Although there are no commonly agreed upon standards, one may regard an association as strong when the p value is less than 0.001 or when the mutation accounts for at least 10% of the phenotypic variance adjusted for the proper concomitants. In contrast, a weak association may be characterized by a p value < 0.05 or with the locus associated with less than 5% of the phenotype variance. In all cases, replication studies are highly desirable.

The evidence for the presence of a significant association between a candidate gene and BMI or body fat phenotypes is summarized in Table 11, which reveals that only five markers had an association that reached a p value of 0.01 or better. These are Apo B, Apo D, TNF-α (a closely linked marker of the gene), DRD2, and LDLR. Among those genes, only one (Apo B) was confirmed in an independent study albeit at a lower p value (0.05). In the case of the dopamine D2, receptor (DRD2), an independent study found no relationship with BMI (144). On the other hand, the weak associations observed with HSD3B1 or UCP were only with the changes in fatness over time in the Quebec Family Study adults and not with body fat content at a given point in time (145,146). As for fat distribution phenotypes, significant associations have been reported with HSD3B1 and specific skinfold sites among unrelated adults (146).

Table 11 does not include the significant associations reported previously with the ABO (9q34) blood group and the human leukocyte antigen (HLA) systems. A review of these studies (147) suggests that the results are rather ambiguous, some studies finding association of ABO with body weight, while others did not. The few studies that used BMI or skinfold thicknesses as phenotypes reported negative results. In an attempt to further clarify the issue, the association between ABO blood type and body weight was recently investigated in four culturally distinct pop-

Table 11 Evidence for the Presence of an Association with BMI or Body Fat Phenotypes

Gene	Location	No. of cases	Phenotype	p value	Ref.
			Evidence		
HSD3B1	1p13.1	132	12-year changes in sum of 6 skinfolds	0.04	Vohl et al. (146)
ATP1A2	1q21–23	122	Percent fat	0.05	Dériaz et al. (174)
Apo B	2p24–23	132	BMI	0.005	Rajput-Williams et al. (175)
		181	BMI	0.05	Saha et al. (176)
ACP1	2p25	75	BMI in children	0.02	Lucarini et al. (177)
Apo D	3q26–ter	114	BMI	0.006	Vijayaraghavan et al. (178)
UCP	4q28–31	123	High fat gainers over 12 years	˙0.05	Oppert et al. (145)
TNF-α	6p21.3	304	BMI but not percent fat	0.01	Norman et al. (179)
LPL	8p22	24	Gains in fat mass with overfeeding	0.05	Bouchard et al. (180)
		236	BMI	0.05	Jemaa et al. (181)
DRD2	11q23.1	392	Relative weight	0.002	Comings et al. (182)
LDLR	19p13	84	BMI in hypertensive	0.004	Zee et al. (115)

Gene abbreviations and their chromosomal location are from the Human Genome Data Base.
HSD3B1 = 3-beta hydroxysteroid dehydrogenase; ATP1A2 = sodium potassium adenosine triphosphatase alpha-2 subunit; Apo B = apolipoprotein B; ACP1 = acid phosphatase; Apo D = apolipoprotein D; UCP = uncoupling protein; TNF-α = tumor necrosis factor alpha; LPL = lipoprotein lipase; DRD2 = Dopamine D₂ receptor; LDLR = low-density lipoprotein receptor.

ulation samples and it was concluded that there is no evidence to support an association between ABO blood types and body weight (148). A few studies have also looked at association between obesity and class I HLA markers. Although frequencies of the HLA B18, Bw35, and Cw4 antigens were found to be significantly higher in obese subjects compared to controls in some reports (149,150), no association between HLA antigens and percent body fat or subcutaneous fat could be found in a larger population (151).

5. Linkage Studies

Linkage refers to the cosegregation of a marker and a trait locus together in families. Linkage analysis can be performed with candidate gene markers or with a variety of other anonymous polymorphic markers such as microsatellites. Evidence for linkage becomes more apparent as the marker loci get closer to the true trait locus that cosegregates with the marker(s). The procedure can be undertaken with large pedigrees or with panels of nuclear families. It is commonly used for complex multifactorial phenotypes that are characterized by the presence of a segregating major gene. However, it is not always appropriate to use a parametric LOD score approach, especially when the genetic model for the phenotype cannot be specified.

An alternative and practical method is the nonparametric sib-pair linkage method, which allows screening for potential linkage relationships between a quantitative phenotype and a genetic marker (152). The method is based on the notion that sibs who share a greater number of alleles (at a given locus) identical by descent at a linked marker locus should also share more alleles at the phenotypic locus. Thus these sibs should have more similar phenotypes than pairs of sibs who share fewer marker alleles. The slope of the regression of squared sibpair phenotype differences on the proportion of genes identical by descent is expected to be negative when linkage is present. An important advantage of the method is that it does not need a trait model; i.e., it is not necessary to specify the mode of inheritance for the phenotype being considered. The method can be used to include the information at all loci available in a multipoint linkage strategy (e.g., 153). No linkage results have been reported to date for obesity with the multipoint sib-pair linkage strategy and very few with the parametric approach based on pedigrees or nuclear families.

Since most of the results summarized in Table 12 were derived using one marker at a time, it is useful to consider the issue of the strength of evidence for such data. Usually, evidence for linkage is considered strong if the p value attains 0.001 and less but still requires replication. A weak or suggestive linkage ($p < 0.05$) may be regarded as important for motivating replication studies. From Table 12, it is obvious that only a few of the linkages reported have relatively strong evidence. ACP1 (2p25), TNF-α (closely linked marker) (6p21.3), KEL (7q33), and ADA (20q12-13.11) are the only markers exhibiting such a linkage relationship. The others are supported by weaker evidence at this time. One marker on 1q31-32 was shown to be linked to BMI with a LOD score of 3.6 at a recombination fraction of 0.05 in a three-generation pedigree in which the prevalence of obesity was high (154). Since these findings are sensitive to the assumptions made about mode of transmission, penetrance, and other characteristics, we need more information before concluding the presence of a linkage with a marker on 1q.

Three markers have been found to be weakly linked with TER adjusted for total body fat content in the Quebec Family Study. The MN (GYPA) (4q28-31) and the KEL (7q33) were both found to be linked ($p = 0.03$ and 0.04) with TER based on a minimum of 160 pairs of sibs of the QFS (54). Another linkage was reported by Oppert et al. (155) between the α_{2a}-adrenergic receptor gene (ADRA2A; 10q24-26) and the same phenotype.

Association and linkage studies that have generated negative results are numerous and have been summarized elsewhere (156). Most of the negative results were reported once and replication studies are needed to ensure that the findings are not false negative. The only clear case appears to be that of the β_3-adrenergic receptor (ADRB3) gene for which the same mutation was shown to be independent of BMI in three different studies (also percent fat in one study) (157–159). Note also that most association studies are based on small sample sizes.

This overview reveals that several genes can cause obesity or are linked with body fat content in animals. Table 13 lists those genes, loci, or markers for which the evidence of an association or a linkage with obesity, BMI, or body fat content is strongest. The list includes the loci

Table 12 Evidence for the Presence of Linkage with BMI or Body Fat Phenotypes Based on the Sib-Pair Method

Gene or marker	Location	Evidence			
		No. of pairs	Phenotype	p value	Ref.
D1S202	1q31–32	3-generation pedigree	BMI	LOD = 3.6 at θ = .05	Murray et al. (154)
ACP1	2p25	>300	BMI	.004	Bailey-Wilson et al. (183)
BF	6p21	>168	Triceps, subscapular, and suprailiac skinfolds	$.01 < p < .03$	Wilson et al. (184)
GLO1	6p21	>168	Suprailiac skinfold relative weight	$.004 < p < .05$	Wilson et al. (184)
TNF-α	6p21.3	304	% body fat	.002	Norman et al. (179)
KEL	7q33	402	BMI and sum of 6 skinfolds	<.0001	Borecki et al. (54)
ESD	13q14.1–14.2	194	% body fat and sum of skinfolds	<.04	Borecki et al. (54)
ADA	20q13.11	428	BMI and sum of 6 skinfolds	$.02 < p < .001$	Borecki et al. (54)
P1	22q11	>168	Relative weight	.03	Wilson et al. (184)

See previous tables for abbreviations of loci already referred to.
Gene abbreviations and their chromosomal location are from the Human Genome Data Base.
BF = properdin factor B; GLO1 = glyoxylase I; KEL = blood group Kell; ESD = esterase D; ADA = adenosine deaminase; P1 = blood group P.

Table 13 Summary of the Rodent (Human Homologous Regions) and Human Loci Potentially Associated or Linked with Obesity or Body Fat

Human chromosome	Locus	Human chromosome	Locus
1p36–32	Mouse Do1	11p15.1	Mouse Tubby
1p35–31	Mouse Db	11p14-ter	Mouse Mob-1
1p35–31	Rat Fa	11q13	BBS1
1q31–32	D1S202	13q14.1–14.2	ESD
2p24–23	Apo B	14q13–32	Mouse Mob-3
2p25	**ACP1**	15q11.2–12	PWS
3p21	Mouse Do2	15q22.3–23	BBS4
3p13–12	BBS3	16p13–11	Mouse Mob-1
4p16.3	ACH	16q21	BBS2
4q21	Mouse Fat	20	NZB QTL
5p14–12	Mouse Do3	20q11	PPCD
5q11–13	Mouse Mob-4	20q11.2	Mouse Yellow
6p21	BF	**20q13.1**	**ADA**
6p21	GLO1	22q11	P1
6p21.3	**TNF-α**	Xq21	Choroideremia
7q31	Mouse Ob	Xq21.1–22	WTS
7q22–36	Mouse Mob-2	Xq25–27	SGBS
7q33	**KEL**	Xq26–27	BFLS
8q22–23	CHS1		
10q21–26	Mouse Mob-1		

See previous tables for abbreviations. Loci in bold type are those showing the strongest evidence of association or linkage in human studies.

from single-gene rodent models, QTL from cross-breeding experiments, Mendelian disorders exhibiting obesity as one of the clinical features, and genes supported by robust evidence from association and linkage studies conducted on human populations. Four chromosomal arms (2p, 6p, 7q, and 20q) are of particular interest as strong evidence for association or linkage with a marker in each of these regions has been reported. However, to date, no study has replicated the linkage for any of the four chromosomal areas. Other regions of considerable interest include 1p, 3p, 11p, 15q, and perhaps Xq. The compendium of markers and genes related to obesity or body fat is likely to grow significantly in the coming years.

C. Recommendations for Future Studies

The search for the molecular causes of the susceptibility to obesity is well on its way to be successful. The reliance on a variety of strategies and technologies is a characteristic of the field and it should continue to be so. There has been a notable cross-fertilization between the animal model research and the human studies with respect to the

genes and chromosomal areas to target. This spirit of collaboration needs to be extended in the future. Indeed, the task is so complex that a single laboratory or institution is not likely to be in a position to develop the necessary data base and master all the technologies to make major contributions to the goal of defining the genes and molecular markers of the susceptibility to obesity.

A major recommendation then is to promote collaborative research. The establishment of networks of laboratories and institutions would be one way to augment the probability of making major advances soon in this field. The tools are available. What is needed is better concentration of minds and resources on well-defined tasks. However, single and team-initiated research is and will remain an essential element of the overall effort to understand the molecular and genetic aspects of the etiology of obesity. Some of the theoretical issues are addressed in the next section.

VII. OPTIMUM STRATEGIES FOR EVALUATION OF THE GENETIC DETERMINANTS OF HUMAN OBESITY

Overwhelming evidence reviewed so far suggests a significant and substantial genetic component in human obesity. However, as we have seen earlier, the nature of the evidence and the magnitude of the genetic component varied a great deal depending on the phenotype studied and the particular type of genetic epidemiological method used. A picture that is clearly emerging from the diverse findings is that multiple genetic loci are involved in human obesity, just as is evident in animal models.

A. Primary and Secondary Obesity Genes

It is helpful to distinguish between two types of obesity genes, *primary* and *secondary*, all of which collectively contribute to and determine the variability in obesity. The primary genes are those whose primary contribution is to human obesity (and which may, and likely do, influence other correlated traits perhaps to a lesser extent), and whose effect sizes are large enough to be detected through appropriate studies. Likewise, the secondary genes for human obesity are those whose primary effects are on other traits with pleiotropic effects on obesity that are likely much smaller and whose detection in the context of obesity is difficult at best. The combined effects of the primary genes may be characterized as oligogenic (few genes, each with a large enough effect), and the aggregate effects of the secondary obesity genes may be regarded as polygenic (many genes, each with a small effect). Regardless of the terminology suggested here, there can be little disagreement that human obesity involves multiple genes, some with large and some with small effects.

B. Inadequacy of Current Approaches

While the model-fitting approaches in genetic epidemiology have been largely successful in demonstrating the underlying complexity in the transmission of human obesity, there are limitations in such studies that necessitate alternatives. One limitation arises because of the fact that most model-fitting approaches are based on largely untestable assumptions. However realistic some of these assumptions may be, there is always some degree of uncertainty. Second, analysis of multilocus traits like obesity requires more advanced and complex models that are mostly lacking or highly specialized (see Ref. 25). For example, when segregation analysis based on single-locus models is applied to a trait determined by two genes, it fails to characterize either gene accurately (even though it can sometimes succeed in inferring a gene with a large effect) (160). Finally, such model-fitting approaches alone are inadequate for evaluating the specific genetic determinants of human obesity, although they are useful in suggesting possible genetic mechanisms. Marker studies are essential.

C. Optimum Strategy

We believe that an optimum strategy should combine the strengths of four companion methods to maximize our chances of finding the primary genes of human obesity. Only after finding the primary genes can specialized methods be fruitful in finding the secondary genes.

1. Genetic Epidemiological Model-Fitting Approach

While this approach alone is unlikely to yield major findings, the results can guide our subsequent inquiries. It is even more so when the power of multivariate models and longitudinal studies is exploited, the former to evaluate possible pleiotropic gene effects (same gene contributing to multiple correlated phenotypes) and the later to detect genes at varying stages of expression and thus to investigate the stable genetic components. This approach would be even more useful after finding specific obesity genes using the molecular approaches discussed below. They will aid in evaluating gene-gene and gene-environment interactions and in characterizing the gene effects. They will also enable us to investigate if any additional familial (ge-

netic) component exists, after accounting for all known obesity genes, something that can motivate the search for additional genes.

2. Association Studies Using Candidate Genes

Association studies provide perhaps one of the simplest and most appealing ways to find genes for complex traits. It is useful to recall here that a significant association implies one of three things: (1) we found one of the functional variants; (2) there is linkage disequilibrium between the marker and an obesity gene, or (3) there is population admixture. Unfortunately, a high rate of false positives may result when there is admixture; however, association studies can still be useful especially to evaluate the role of markers at candidate gene loci, and in generating hypotheses for further evaluation. We believe that association studies using anonymous markers are not appealing.

3. Genome-Wide Search Using Anonymous Markers

Perhaps the single most promising method involves nonparametric sibpair linkage using evenly spaced anonymous markers. Such a search should ideally include all known candidate gene markers, in addition to a sufficiently large number of anonymous markers that are as evenly spaced throughout the genome as possible.

To maximize the power of the study design, we specifically propose that full sibships be used for this purpose. Each sibship should contain at least two sibs, and at least one of them must be very obese (say, from the upper 10th percentile of the distribution of BMI, which is approximately 28). Sampling this way from the upper tail is known to be more powerful, and hence requires much smaller sample sizes (161). Efficient quantitative trait locus (QTL) methodology can then be used to exploit the full variability within sibships. Particularly promising here is the interval mapping method of Fulker and Cardon (162), which builds on the strengths of the basic method of Haseman and Elston (152), and the interval mapping concept of Goldgar (163), which examines larger chromosomal regions.

In terms of marker density, it would be best to use a two-phase approach (164–166). In the first phase, one may use about 300–400 markers, roughly evenly spaced, which yields a 10-cM map. For the few significant linkages found in this phase, which will necessarily include some false positives, denser marker maps should be used in a second phase, say, 2 markers on either side of each "hit." Thus, for example, if 10 significant hits were detected in the first phase, the second phase could involve up to 40 additional markers to be typed. This way, the "candidate regions" containing obesity genes can be identified and narrowed. In fact, the Fulker-Cardon method can suggest the most likely locations of the obesity genes. The large number of linkage tests performed will inevitably yield false positives. Therefore, careful balance must be maintained between type I and type II errors. Fortunately, type I error is less critical in phase I, since phase II can help refute false hits, especially if a separate replicate sample is used in phase II. Hence, one may use relatively larger significance levels in phase I than in phase II. However, type II error is much more critical in phase I, since gene locations missed in phase I cannot be recovered in phase II. Use of independent replicate sample in phase II is our best insurance against false positives. Therefore, a very powerful study design is essential in phase I. This is achieved by sampling from the upper tail and by using large number of sibships. Based on preliminary calculations, it appears that about 300 sibships will provide enough power for detecting the primary obesity genes (167).

For example, for a trait with a sibling correlation of 0.25, to detect a gene with 80% power that explains 27% of phenotypic variance, one needs a sample of 110 sibpairs (220 subjects) where each pair contains at least one sib whose BMI is in the upper decile (BMI $\geq$ 28). One can attain 90% power with 146 much sibpairs (292 subjects). One can also attain 80% power with 47 triplets (141 subjects) or 90% power with 64 triplets (192 subjects), where each triplet contains at least one sib whose BMI is in the upper decile. These calculations are based on single-gene models and zero recombination between the trait and marker loci. Multiple-trait loci and nonzero recombination both require considerably larger samples. A sample of about 300 sibships of varying sizes, each with at least two sibs and at least one of them above the 90th percentile, provides a favorable design.

Since the gene effects are quite likely mediated by a host of life-style and other metabolic factors, it is desirable to obtain as much information on each subject as possible, including detailed phenotypic characterizations. That way, the possible role of these covariates can be incorporated in the data analysis. Also, even though the sampling may be based on BMI, the QTL analysis could/should be performed for each of the correlated phenotypes (e.g., BMI, sum of skinfolds, percent body fat, etc.). This will maximize the yield, since different genes may primarily contribute to different components of obesity.

Two additional thoughts are germane. First, while sampling from the upper tail of BMI or %BF will likely yield "obesity" genes (for type I obesity, see Table 1), one may need to devise different sampling strategies to detect the primary genes for fat patterning. Second, the recent methodology of Risch and Zhang (168), using extremely discordant sibpairs, appears to be even more powerful in that it requires a much smaller number of sibpairs, provided they are selected to be extremely discordant, i.e., one sib from the upper 10th percentile and another from the bottom 10th percentile. The sampling design proposed above, involving about 300 sibships each with at least one very obese sib, may include some extremely discordant sibpairs. However, it would be desirable to sample an additional 100 extremely discordant sibpairs, which would provide a reasonable sample size for applying the Risch and Zhang methodology. Whenever this is feasible, we strongly recommend that the original 300 sibship sample be used in the first phase, and the extremely discordant sibpairs be used in the second phase. This will provide replication using an independent sample, which is perhaps the best way of controlling false positives. We believe that samples for replication studies should be drawn from the same underlying population on which the original study was based. This is our best insurance against population heterogeneity.

Finally, when some obesity genes are found, it would be very useful to type these genes in a random sample of about 200 subject. This will enable estimation of the relevant gene frequencies in the underlying population. More important, detailed phenotypic characterization and studies of additional covariates will enable characterization of the gene effects and investigations of gene-gene and gene-environment interactions. This can be achieved through one of several means, for example, by regression of a phenotype (say % body fat) on all covariates, measured genotypes, and interactions among them.

4. Parametric Linkage Studies in Extended Families

After some obesity genes, or even markers in their close vicinity, are found, it would be desirable to type these genes/markers together with their flanking markers in extended families. Parametric linkage analysis by the LOD score method (169,170) will enable fine-tuning of the map locations. The resulting information can then be used for early detection of individuals at risk, which is efficacious for early intervention, and provide mapping information that could allow isolation and metabolic characterization of the gene(s).

VIII. SUMMARY AND CONCLUSIONS

The aim of this chapter was to provide a review of the current state of knowledge regarding the genetics of human obesity. Other chapters cover the animal model research in detail. The emphasis has been, therefore, on the results obtained in human studies but incorporating the evidence from animal studies, particularly with respect to the molecular markers.

This chapter summarizes the data pertaining to the heritability and the contribution of major genes for phenotypes of total body fat and fat topography based on the genetic epidemiology methods. The evidence for a contribution of genetic-environment interaction effects to variation in body mass, body fat, and fat distribution was also considered. The current status of the obesity gene map was described based on the evidence obtained from Mendelian disorders having obesity as a clinical feature, single-gene rodent models, cross-breeding experiments with inbred mouse strains, and association and linkage studies conducted on human samples. Finally, the chapter highlights some of the limitations of the conventional approaches and suggests a variety of strategies to optimize the search for the genes associated with the susceptibility to obesity and to define the inheritance patterns. The successes of the last few years in the effort to achieve these goals explain the present level of enthusiasm in the obesity research community regarding its ability to meet these challenges.

This overview of the available evidence highlights the needs for a better quantification of the lambda coefficient for various degrees of obesity, for the development of longitudinal data base that will increase the chance of untangling causes and effects of positive energy balance, and for a greater concertation among laboratories so that phenotypic data base and DNA markers can be pooled to address complex questions with the necessary statistical power.

GLOSSARY

ACH	Achondroplasia
ACP1	Acid phosphatase
ADA	Adenosine deaminase
Apo B	Apolipoprotein B
Apo D	Apolipoprotein D
ASP	Agouti signaling protein
ATP1A2	Sodium potassium adenosine triphosphatase α_2-subunit
BF	Properdin factor B
BFLS	Borjeson-Forssman-Lehmann syndrome
CHS1	Cohen syndrome
CPE	Carboxypeptidase E
Do	Dietary obese
DRD2	Dopamine D_2 receptor
ESD	Esterase D
GLO1	Glyoxalase I
HSD3B1	3-β hydroxysteroid dehydrogenase
KEL	Blood group Kell

LDLR	Low-density lipoprotein receptor
LPL	Lipoprotein lipase
MIM	Mendelian inheritance in man
Mob	Multigenic obesity
OB-R	Leptin receptor
P1	Blood group P
PPCD	Posterior polymorphous corneal dystrophy
PWS	Prader-Willi syndrome
SGBS	Simpson-Golabi-Behmel syndrome
TER	Ratio of trunk to extremity skinfolds
TNF-α	Tumor necrosis factor alpha
UCP	Uncoupling protein
WTS	Wilson-Turner syndrome

REFERENCES

1. Bouchard C, Dériaz O, Pérusse L, Tremblay A. Genetics of energy expenditure in human. In: Bouchard C, ed. The Genetics of Obesity. Boca Raton, FL: CRC Press, 1994; 135–145.
2. Pérusse L, Bouchard C. Genetics of energy intake and food preferences. In: Bouchard C. ed. the Genetics of Obesity. Boca Raton, FL: CRC Press, 1994:125–134.
3. Reed DR, Bradley EC, Price RA. Obesity in families of extremely obese women. Obes Res 1993; 1:167–172.
4. Risch N. Linkage strategies for genetically complex traits. Am J Hum Genet 1990; 46:222–228.
5. Bouchard C. Variation in human body fat: The contribution of the genotype. In: Bray G, Ricquier D, Spiegelman B, eds. Obesity: Towards a Molecular Approach. New York: Alan R Liss, 1990:17–28.
6. Bouchard C. La génétique des obésités humaines. Ann Med Interne 1992; 143:463–471.
7. Bouchard C. Human obesities: chaos or determinism? In: Ailhaud G, Guy-Grand B, Lafontane M, Ricquier C, eds. Obesity in Europe 91. Proceedings of the 3rd European Congress on Obesity. Paris: John Libbey 1992:7–14.
8. Garn SM, Leonard WR, Hawthorne VM. Three limitations of the body mass index. Am J Clin Nutr 1986; 44:996–997.
9. Ferland M, Després JP, Tremblay A, Pineault S, Nadeau A, Moorjani S, Lupien PJ, Thériault G, Bouchard C. Assessment of adipose tissue distribution by computed axial tomography in obese women: association with body density and anthropometric measurements. Br J Nutr 1989; 61:139–148.
10. McKusick VA. Catalogs of Autosomal Dominant, Autosomal Recessive, X-Linked, Y-Linked and Mitochondrial Phenotypes, OMIM (Online Mendelian Inheritance in Man). Baltimore: Johns Hopkins University Press, 1993.
11. Bouchard C. Genetics of body fat, energy expenditure and adipose tissue metabolism. In: Berry EM, Blondheim SH, Eliahou HE, Shafrir E, eds. Recent Advances in Obesity Research. London: John Libbey, 1987:16–25.
12. Rice J, Cloninger CR, Reich T. Multifactorial inheritance with cultural transmission and assortative mating. I. De-

scription and basic properties of the unitary model. Am J Hum Genet 1978; 30:618–643.

13. Rao DC, Wette R. Environment index in genetic epidemiology: an investigation of its role, adequacy, and limitations. Am J Hum Genet 1990; 46:168–178.

14. Rao DC, McGue M, Wette R, Glueck CJ. Path analysis in genetic epidemiology. In: Chakravarti A, ed. Human Population Genetics. The Pittsburgh Symposium. Stroudsburg, PA: Van Nostrand-Reinhold, 1984:35–81.

15. Jöreskog KG, Sörbom D. LISREL: Analysis of Linear Structural Relationships by the Method of Maximum Likelihood. Chicago, National Educational Resources, 1986.

16. Boomsma DI, Martin NG, Neale MC. Genetic analysis of twin and family data: structural modeling using LISREL. Behav Genet 1989; 19:5–161.

17. DeFries JC, Fulker DW. Multiple regression analysis of twin data. Behav Genet 1985; 15:467–473.

18. Malina RM, Bouchard C. Subcutaneous fat distribution during growth. In: Bouchard C, Johnston FE, eds. Fat Distribution During Growth and Later Health Outcomes. Current Topics in Nutrition and Disease. New York: Alan R Liss, 1988; 17:63–84.

19. Mueller WH. Transient environmental changes and age-limited genes as causes of variation in sib-sib and parent-offspring correlations. Ann Hum Biol 1978; 5:395–398.

20. Bouchard C. Transient environmental effects detected in sibling correlations. Ann Hum Biol 1980; 7:89–92.

21. Province MA, Rao DC. Path analysis of family resemblance with temporal trends: applications to height, weight, and Quetelet index in Northeastern Brazil. Am J Hum Genet 1985; 37:178–192.

22. Ravussin E, Lillioja S, Knowler WC, Christin L, Freymond D, Abbott WGH, Boyce V, Howard BV. Reduced rate of energy expenditure as a risk factor for body-weight gain. N Engl J Med 1988; 318:467–472.

23. Zurlo F, Lillioja S, Esposito-Del Puente A, Nyomba BL, Raz I, Saad MF, Swinburn BA, Knowler WC, Bogardus C, Ravussin E. Low ratio of fat to carbohydrate oxidation as predictor of weight gain: study of 24-h RQ. Am J Physiol 1990; 259:E650–E657.

24. Vogler GP, Fulker DW. Human behavior genetics. In Nesselroade JR, Cattell RB, eds. Handbook of Multivariate Experimental Psychology, 2nd ed. New York: Plenum Press, 1988:475–503.

25. Blangero J, Konigsberg LW. Multivariate segregation analysis using the mixed model. Genet Epidemiol 1991; 8:299–316.

26. Morton NE, Rao DC, Lalouel JM. Methods in Genetic Epidemiology. New York: Karger, 1983.

27. Lalouel JM, Rao DC, Morton NE, Elston RC. A unified model for complex segregation analysis. Am J Hum Genet 1983; 35:816–826.

28. Lalouel JM, Morton NE. Complex segregation analysis with pointers. Hum Hered 1981; 31:312–321.

29. Hasstedt SJ. PAP; Pedigree Analysis Package, Rev. 3, Department of Human Genetics University of Utah, Salt Lake City, 1989.

30. Konigsberg LW, Blangero J, Kammerer CM, Mott GE. Mixed model segregation analysis of LDL-C concentration with genotype-covariate interaction. Genet Epidemiol 1991; 8:69–80.

31. Bonney GE, Lathrop GM, Lalouel JM. Combined linkage and segregation analysis using regressive models. Am J Hum Genet 1988; 43:29–37.

32. Province MA, Rao DC. General purpose model and a computer program for combined segregation and path analysis (SEGPATH): Automatically creating computer programs from symbolic language model specifications. Genet Epidemiol 1995; 12:203–219.

33. Li Z, Bonney GE, Lathrop GM, Rao DC. Genetic analysis combining path analysis with regressive models: the TAU model of multifactorial transmission. Hum Hered 1994; 44:305–311.

34. Li Z, Bonney GE, Rao DC. Genetic analysis combining path analysis with regressive models: the BETA path model of polygenic and familial environmental transmission. Genet Epidemiol 1994; 11:431–442.

35. Borecki IB, Lathrop GM, Bonney GE, Yaouanq J, Rao DC. Combined segregation and linkage analysis of genetic hemochromatosis using affection status, serum iron, and HLA. Am J Hum Genet 1990; 47:542–550.

36. Hartz A, Giefer E, Rimm A. Relative importance of the effect of family environment and heredity on obesity. Ann Hum Genet 1977; 41:185–193.

37. Garn SM, Bailey SM, Cole PE. Similarities between parents and their adopted children. Am J Phys Anthrop 1977; 45:539–544.

38. Khoury P, Morrison J, Laskarzewski PM, Glueck CJ. Parent-offspring and sibling body mass index associations during and after sharing of common household environments: the Princeton School District Family Study. Metabolism 1983; 32:82–89.

39. Annest JL, Sing CF, Biron P, Mongeau JG. Familial aggregation of blood pressure and weight in adoptive families. III. Analysis of the role of shared genes and shared household environment in explaining family resemblance for height, weight, and selected weight/height indices. Am J Epidemiol 1983; 117:492–506.

40. Longini IM Jr, Higgins MW, Hinton PC, Moll PP, Keller JB. Genetic and environment sources of familial aggregation of body mass in Tecumseh, Michigan. Hum Biol 1984; 56:733–757.

41. Biron P, Mongeau J-G, Bertrand D. Familial resemblance of body weight and weight/height in 374 homes with adopted children. J Pediatrics 1977; 91:555–558.

42. Heller R, Garrison RJ, Havlik RJ, Feinleib M, Padgett S. Family resemblances in height and relative weight in the Framingham Heart Study. Int J Obes 14; 8:399–405.

43. Stunkard AJ, Foch TT, Hrubec Z. A twin study of human obesity. JAMA 1986; 256:51–54.

44. Stunkard AJ, Sørensen TIA, Hanis C, Teasdale TW, Chakraborty R, Schull WJ, Schulsinger F. An adoption study of human obesity. N Engl J Med 1986; 314:193–198.

45. Stunkard AJ, Harris JR, Pedersen NL, McClearn GE. The body-mass index of twins who have been reared apart. N Engl J Med 1990; 322:1483–1487.

46. Price RA, Cadoret RJ, Stunkard AJ, Troughton E. Genetic contributions to human fatness: an adoption study. Am J Psychiatry 1987; 144:1003–1008.

47. Sørensen TIA, Price RA, Stunkard AJ, Schulsinger F. Genetics of obesity in adult adoptees and their biological siblings. Br Med J 1989; 298:87–90.

48. Price RA, Gottesman II. Body fat in identical twins reared apart: roles for genes and environment. Behav Genet 1991; 21:1–7.

49. Vogler GP, Sørensen TIA, Stunkard AJ, Srinivasan MR, Rao DC. Influences of genes and shared family environment on adult body mass index assessed in an adoption study by a comprehensive path model. Int J Obes 1995; 19: 40–45.

50. MacDonald A, Stunkard J. Body mass indexes of British separated twins. N Engl J Med 1990; 322:1530.

51. Tambs K, Moum T, Eaves L, Neale M, Midthjell K, Lund-Larsen PG, Ness S, Holmen J. Genetic and environmental contributions to the variance of the body mass index in Norwegian sample of first- and second-degree relatives. Am J Hum Biol 1991; 3:257–267.

52. McLaughlin JA. The inheritance of body-mass index in the Virginia 30,000. Behav Genet 1991; 21:581 (abstract).

53. Bouchard C. Genetics of obesity: Overview and research directions. In: Bouchard C. ed. The Genetics of Obesity. Boca Raton, FL: CRC Press, 1994:223–233.

54. Borecki IB, Rice T, Pérusse L, Bouchard C, Rao DC. An exploratory investigation of genetic linkage with body composition and fatness phenotypes; the Quebec Family Study. Obes Res 1994; 2:213–219.

55. Cardon LR. Developmental analysis of the body mass index in the Colorado Adoption Project. Behav Genet 1991; 21:563–564 (abstract).

56. Korkeila M, Kaprio J, Rissanen A, Koskenvuo M. Effects of gender and age on the heritability of body mass index. Int J Obes 1991; 15:647–654.

57. Fabsitz R, Feinleib M, Hrubec Z. Weight changes in adult twins. Acta Genet Med Gemellol 1980; 29:273–279.

58. Fabsitz RR, Carmelli D, Hewitt JK. Evidence for independent genetic influences on obesity in middle age. Int J Obes 1992; 16:657–666.

59. Fabsitz RR, Sholinksy P, Carmelli D. Genetic influences on adult weight gain and maximum body mass index in male twins. Am J Epidemiol 1994; 140:711–720.

60. Lissner L, Sjöström L, Bengtsson C, Bouchard C, Larsson B. The natural history of obesity in an obese population and associations with metabolic aberrations. Int J Obes 1994; 18:441–447.

61. Adams TD, Hunt SC, Mason LA, Ramirez ME, Fisher AG, Williams RR. Familial aggregation of morbid obesity. Obes Res 1993; 1:261–270.

62. Price RA, Ness R, Laskarzewski P. Common major gene inheritance of extreme overweight. Hum Biol 1990; 62: 747–765.

63. Province MA, Arnqvist P, Keller J, Higgins M, Rao DC. Strong evidence for a major gene for obesity in the large, unselected, total Community Health Study of Tecumseh. Am J Hum Genet 1990; 47(Suppl):A143 (abstract).

64. Ness R, Laskarzewski P, Price RA. Inheritance of extreme overweight in black families. Hum Biol 1991; 63:39–52.

65. Moll PP, Burns TL, Lauer RM. The genetic and environmental sources of body mass index variability: the Muscatine Ponderosity Family Study. Am J Hum Genet 1991; 49:1243–1255.

66. Borecki IB, Bonney GE, Rice T, Bouchard C, Rao DC. Influence of genotype-dependent effects of covariates on the outcome of segregation analysis of the body mass index. Am J Hum Genet 1993; 53:676–687.

67. Fain PR. Characteristics of simple sibship variance tests for the detection of major loci and application to height, weight and spatial performance. Ann Hum Genet 1978; 42:109–120.

68. Karlin S, Williams PT, Jensen S, Farquhar JW. Genetic analysis of the Stanford LRC Family Study data. I. Structured exploratory data analysis of height and weight measurements. Am J Epidemiol 1981; 113:307–324.

69. Zonta LA, Jayakar SD, Bosisio M, Galante A, Pennetti V. Genetic analysis of human obesity in an Italian sample. Hum Hered 1987; 37:129–139.

70. Tiret L, André J-L, Ducimetière P, Herberth B, Rakotovao R, Guegen R, Spyckerelle Y, Cambien F. Segregation analysis of height-adjusted weight with generation- and age-dependent effects: the Nancy Family Study. Genet Epidemiol 1992; 9:389–403.

71. Rice T, Borecki IB, Bouchard C, Rao DC. Segregation analysis of body mass index in an unselected French-Canadian sample: the Quebec Family Study. Obes Res 1993; 1:288–294.

72. Rice T, Borecki IB, Bouchard C, Rao DC. Segregation analysis of fat mass and other body composition measures derived from underwater weighing. Am J Hum Genet 1993; 52:967–973.

73. Comuzzie AG, Blangero J, Mahaney MC, Mitchell BD, Hixson JE, Samollow PB, Stern MP, MacCluer JW. Major gene with sex-specific effects influences fat mass in Mexican Americans. Genet Epidemiol 1995; 12:475–488.

74. Jouanny P, Guillemin F, Kuntz C, Jeandel C, Pourel J. Environmental and genetic factors affecting bone mass: similarity of bone density among members of healthy families. Arthritis Rheum 1995; 38:61–67.

75. Feitosa M, Rice T, Nirmala-Reddy A, Reddy PC, Rao DC. Is the major gene effect on body mass index mediated by energy intake and energy expenditure of activity? (submitted).

76. Rice T, Tremblay A, Dériaz O, Pérusse L, Rao DC, Bouchard C. A major gene for resting metabolic rate unassociated with body composition: Results from the Quebec Family Study. Obes Res 1996; 4:441–449.

77. Mitchell LE, Nirmala A, Rice T, Reddy PC, Rao DC. The impact of energy intake and energy expenditure of activity on the familial transmission of adiposity in an Indian population. Am J Hum Biol 1993; 5:331–339.

78. Kaplan RM, Patterson TL, Sallis JF Jr, Nader PR. Exercise suppresses heritability estimates for obesity in Mexican-American families. Addict Behav 1989; 14:581–588.

79. Ramirez ME. Familial aggregation of subcutaneous fat deposits and the peripheral fat distribution pattern. Int J Obes 1993; 17:63–68.

80. Savard R, Bouchard C, Leblanc C, Tremblay A. Familial resemblance in fatness indicators. Ann Hum Biol 1983; 10:111–118.

81. Bouchard C. Inheritance of fat distribution and adipose tissue metabolism. In: Vague Björntorp P, Guy-Grand B, Rebuffé-Scrive M, Pague P, eds. Metabolic Complications of Human Obesities. Amsterdam: Elsevier Science Publishers, 1985:87–96.

82. Bouchard C, Pérusse L, Leblanc C, Tremblay A, Thériault G. Inheritance of the amount and distribution of human body fat. Int J Obes 1988; 12:205–215.

83. Pérusse L, Leblanc C, Bouchard C. Inter-generation transmission of physical fitness in the Canadian population. Can J Sport Sci 1988; 13:8–14.

84. Donahue RP, Prineas RJ, Gomez O, Hong CP. Familial resemblance of body fat distribution: the Minneapolis children's blood pressure study. Int J Obes 1992; 16:161–167.

85. Towne B, Roche AF, Chumlea WC, Guo S, Siervogel RM. No evidence of pleiotropy for either body mass index or waist/hip circumference ratio and plasma cholesterol concentration. Obes Res 1993; 1:1105 (abstract).

86. Sellers A, Drinkard C, Rich SS, Potter JD, Jeffery RW, Hong C-P, Folsom AR. Familial aggregation and heritability of waist-to-hip ratio in adult women: the Iowa Women's Health Study. Int J Obes 1994; 18:607–613.

87. Esposito-Del Puente A, Scalfi L, De Filippo E, Peri MR, Caldara A, Caso G, Contaldo F, Valerio G, Franzese A, Di Maio S, Rubino A. Familial and environmental influences on body composition and body fat distribution in childhood in Southern Italy. Int J Obes 1994; 18:596–601.

88. Mueller WH, Reid RM. A multivariate analysis of fatness and relative fat patterning. Am J Phys Anthrop 1979; 50:199–208.

89. Li Z, Rice T, Pérusse L, Bouchard C, Rao DC. Familial aggregation of subcutaneous fat patterning: principal components of skinfolds in the Quebec Family Study. Am J Hum Biol 1996; 8:535–542.

90. Bouchard C. Inheritance of human fat distribution. In: Bouchard C, Johnston FE, eds. Fat Distribution During Growth and Later Health Outcomes. Current Topics in Nutrition and Disease. Vol 17. New York: Alan R Liss, 1988:103–125.

91. Bouchard C. Genetic and environmental influences on regional fat distribution. In: Oomura Y, Tarui S, Inoue S, Shimazu T, eds. Progress in Obesity Research 1990. London: Libbey, 1991:303–308.

92. Comuzzie AG, Blangero J, Mahaney MC, Mitchell BD, Stern MP, MacCluer JW. Genetic and environmental correlations among skinfold measures. Int J Obes 1994; 18:413–418.

93. Rice T, Bouchard C, Pérusse L, Rao DC. Familial clustering of multiple measures of adiposity and fat distribution in the Quebec Family Study: a trivariate of percent body fat, body mass index, and trunk-to-extremity skinfold ratio. Int J Obes 1995; 19:902–908.

94. Borecki IB, Rice T, Pérusse L, Bouchard C, Rao DC. Major gene influence on the propensity to store fat in trunk versus extremity depots; evidence from the Quebec Family Study. Obes Res 1995; 3:1–8.

95. Hasstedt SJ, Ramirez ME, Kuida H, Williams RR. Recessive inheritance of a relative fat pattern. Am J Hum Genet 1989; 45:917–925.

96. Pérusse L, Després JP, Lemieux S, Rice T, Rao DC, Bouchard C. Familial aggregation of abdominal visceral fat level: results from the Quebec Family Study. Metabolism 1996; 45:378–382.

97. Bouchard C, Rice T, Lemieux S, Després L, Rao DC. Major gene for abdominal visceral fat area in the Quebec Family Study. Int J Obes 1996; 20:420–427.

98. Rice T, Pérusse L, Bouchard C, Rao DC. Familial clustering of abdominal visceral fat and total fat mass: the Quebec Family Study. Obes Res 1996; 4:253–261.

99. Sørensen TIA, Stunkard AJ. Does obesity run in families because of genes? An adoption study using silhouette as a measure of obesity. Acta Psychiatr Scand 1993; 370(Suppl):67–72.

100. Comuzzie AG, Glangero J, Mahaney MC, Mitchell BD, Stern MP, MacCluer JW. Quantitative genetics of sexual dimorphism in body fat measurements. Am J Hum Biol 1993; 5:725–734.

101. Rice T, Tremblay A, Dériaz O, Pérusse L, Rao DC, Bouchard C. Genetic pleiotropy for resting metabolic rate with fat-free mass and fat mass: the Quebec Family Study. Obes Res 1996; 4:125–131.

102. Beynen AC, Katan MB, Van Zutphen LF. Hypo- and hyperresponders: individual differences in the response of serum cholesterol concentration to changes in diet. Adv Lipid Res 1987; 22:115–171.

103. Sims EAH, Goldman RF, Gluck CM, Hortin ES, Kelleher PC, Rowe DW. Experimental obesity in man. Trans Assoc Am Phys 1968; 81:153.

104. Ottman R. An epidemiologic approach to gene-environment interaction. Genet Epidemiol 1990; 7:177–185.

105. Ottman R. Epidemiologic analysis of gene-environment interaction in twins. Genet Epidemiol 1994; 11:75–86.

106. Khoury MJ, Wagener DK. Epidemiological evaluation of the use of genetics to improve the predictive value of disease risk factors. Am J Hum Genet 1995; 56:835–844.

107. Ottman R, Susser E, Meisner M. Control for environment risk factors in assessing genetic effects on disease familial aggregation. Am J Epidemiol 1991; 134:298–309.

108. Plomin R, DeFries JC, Loehlin JC. Genotype-environment interaction and correlation in the analysis of human behavior. Physiol Behav 1977; 84:309–322.

109. Eaves LJ. The resolution of genotype-environment interaction in segregation analysis of nuclear families. Genet Epidemiol 1984; 1:215–228.

110. Eaves LJ. Including the environment in models for genetic segregation. J Psychiatr Res 1987; 21:619–647.

111. Blangero J. Statistical genetic approaches to human adaptability. Hum Biol 1993; 65:941–966.

112. Tiret L, Abel L, Rakotovao R. Effect of ignoring genotype-environment interaction on segregation analysis of quantitative traits. Genet Epidemiol 1993; 10:581–586.

113. Bouchard C, Pérusse L, Leblanc C. Using MZ twins in experimental research to test for the presence of genotype-environment interaction effect. Acta Genet Med Gemellol 1990; 39:85–89.

114. Hallman DM, Boerwinkle E, Saha N, Sandholzer C, Menzel HJ, Csazar A, Utermann G. The apolipoprotein E polymorphism: a comparison of allele frequencies and effects in nine populations. Am J Hum Genet 1991; 49:338–349.

115. Zee RYL, Griffiths LR, Morris BJ. Marked association of a RFLP for the low density lipoprotein receptor gene with obesity in essential hypertensive. Biochem Biophys Res Commun 1992; 189:965–971.

116. Berg K. Twin studies of coronary heart disease and its risk factors. Acta Genet Med Gemellol 1984; 33:349–361.

117. Magnus P, Berg K, Borresen AL, Nance WE. Apparent influence of marker genotypes on variation in serum cholesterol in monozygotic twins. Clin Genet 1981; 19:67–70.

118. Poehlman ET, Tremblay A, Després JP, Fontaine E, Perusse L, Theriault G, Bouchard C. Genotype-controlled changes in body composition and fat morphology following overfeeding in twins. Am J Clin Nutr 1986; 43:723–731.

119. Bouchard C, Tremblay A, Després JP, Nadeau A, Lupien PJ, Theriault G, Dussault J, Moorjani S, Pineault S, Fournier G. The response to long-term overfeeding in identical twins. N Engl J Med 1990; 322:1477–1482.

120. Poehlman ET, Tremblay A, Nadeau A, Dussault J, Thériault G, Bouchard C. Heredity and changes in hormones and metabolic rates with short-term training. Am J Physiol 1986; 250:E711–E717.

121. Bouchard C, Tremblay A, Després JP, Thériault G, Nadeau A, Lupien PJ, Moorjani S, Prudhomme D, Fournier G. The response to exercise with constant energy intake in identical twins. Obes Res 1994; 2:400–410.

122. Poehlman ET, Després JP, Marcotte M, Tremblay A, Thériault G, Bouchard C. Genotype dependency of adaptation

123. Dériaz O, Tremblay A, Bouchard C. Non linear weight gain with long term overfeeding in man. Obes Res 1993; 1:179–185.

124. Norgan NG, Durmin JVGA. The effect of 6 weeks of overfeeding on the body weight, body composition, and energy metabolism of young men. Am J Clin Nutr 1980; 33:978–988.

125. Ravussin E, Schutz Y, Acheson KJ, Dusmet M, Bourquin L, Jéquier E. Short-term, mixed-diet overfeeding in man: no evidence for "luxuskonsumption." J Physiol 1985; 249: E470–E477.

126. Tremblay A, Després JP, Thériault G, Fournier G, Bouchard C. Overfeeding and energy expenditure in humans. Am J Clin Nutr 1992; 56:857–862.

127. Dériaz O, Fournier G, Tremblay A, Després JP, Bouchard C. Lean body mass composition and resting energy expenditure before and after long-term overfeeding. Am J Clin Nutr 1992; 56:840–847.

128. Poehlman ET, Tremblay A, Marcotte M, Pérusse L, Thériault G, Bouchard C. Hereditary and changes in body composition and adipose tissue metabolism after short-term exercise training. Eur J Appl Physiol 1987; 56: 398–402.

129. Reed DR, Ding Y, Xu W, Cather C, Price RA. Human obesity does not segregate with the chromosomal regions of Prader-Willi, Bardet-Biedl, Cohen, Borjeson or Wilson-Turner syndromes. Int J Obes 1995; 19:599–603.

130. Croft JB, Morrell D, Chase CL, Swift M. Obesity in heterozygous carriers of the gene for the Bardet-Biedl syndrome. Am J Med Genet 1995; 55:12–15.

131. Friedman JM, Leibel RL, Bahary N. Molecular mapping of obesity genes. Mamm Genome 1991; 1:130–144.

132. Johnson PR, Gregoire F. Animal models of genetic obesity: peripheral tissue changes. In: Bouchard C, ed. The Genetics of Obesity. Boca Raton, FL: CRC Press, 1994: 161–179.

133. Xu W, Reed DR, Ding Y, Price RA. Absence of linkage between human obesity and the mouse Agouti homologous region (20q11.2) or other markers spanning chromosome 20q. Obes Res 1995; 3:559–562.

134. Warden CH, Daluiski A, Lusis AJ. Identification of new genes contributing to atherosclerosis: the mapping of genes contributing to complex disorders in animal models. In: Lusis AJ, Rotter JI, Sparkes RS, eds. Molecular Genetics of Coronary Artery Disease. Monographs in Human Genetics. Basel: Karger, 1992:419–441.

135. Lander ES, Botstein D. Mapping Mendelian factors underlying quantitative traits using RFLP linkage maps. Genetics 1989; 121:185–199.

136. Fisler JS, Warden CH, Pace MJ, Lusis AJ. BSB: a new mouse model of multigenic obesity. Obes Res 1993; 1: 271–280.

137. Warden CH, Fisler JS, Pace MJ, Svenson L, Lusis AJ. Coincidence of genetic loci for plasma cholesterol level and

in adipose tissue metabolism after short-term overfeeding. Am J Physiol 1986; 250:E480–E485.

obesity in a multifactorial mouse model. J Clin Invest 1993; 92:773–779.

138. Warden CH, Fisler JS, Shoemaker SM, et al. Identification of four chromosomal loci determining obesity in a multifactorial mouse model. J Clin Invest 1995; 95: 1545–1552.

139. West DB, Boozer CN, Moody DL, Atkinson RL. Dietary obesity in nine inbred mouse strains. Am J Physiol 1992; 262:R1025–R1032.

140. West DB, Waguespack J, York B, Goudey-Lefevre J, Price RA. Genetics of dietary obesity in AKR/J × SWR/J mice: segregation of the trait and identification of a linked locus on chromosome 4. Mamm Genome 1994; 5:546–552.

141. West DB, Goudey-Lefevre J, York B, Truett GE. Dietary obesity linked to genetic loci on chromosomes 9 and 15 in a polygenic mouse model. J Clin Invest 1994; 94: 1410–1416.

142. Fisler JS, Purcell-Huynh DA, Cuevas M, Luis AJ. The agouti gene may promote obesity in a polygenic mouse model. Int J Obes 1994; 18:104.

143. Greenberg DA. Linkage analysis of "necessary" disease loci versus "susceptibility" loci. Am J Hum Genet 1993; 52: 135–143.

144. Noble EP, Noble RE, Ritchie T, et al. D2 dopamine receptor gene and obesity. Int J Eating Disord 1994; 15: 205–217.

145. Oppert JM, Vohl MC, Chagnon M, et al. DNA polymorphism in the uncoupling protein (UCP) gene and human body fat. Int J Obes 1994; 18:526–531.

146. Vohl MC, Dionne FT, Pérusse L, Dériaz O, Chagnon M, Bouchard C. Relation between BglII polymorphism in 3β-hydroxysteroid dehydrogenase gene and adipose tissue distribution in humans. Obes Res 1994; 2:444–449.

147. Kelso AJ, Siffert T, Maggi W. Association of ABO phenotypes and body weight in a sample of Brazilian infants. Am J Hum Biol 1992; 4:607–611.

148. Kelso AJ, Maggi W, Belas KL. Body weight and ABO blood types: are AB females heavier? Am J Hum Biol 1994; 6: 385–387.

149. Digy JP, Raffoux C, Pointel JP, et al. HLA and familial obesity evidence for a genetic origin. In: Hirsch J, Van Itallie TB, eds. Recent Advances in Obesity Research IV. London: John Libbey, 1983:171–175.

150. Fumeron F, Apfelbaum M. Association between HLA-B18 and the familial obesity syndrome. N Engl J Med 1981; 305:645.

151. Bouchard C, Pérusse L, Rivest J, Roy R, Morissette J, Allard C, Thériault G, Leblanc C. HLA system body fat and fat distribution in children and adults. Int J Obes 1985; 9:411–422.

152. Haseman JK, Elston RC. The investigation of linkage between a quantitative trait and a marker locus. Behav Genet 1972; 2:3–19.

153. Kruglyak L, Lander ES. High-resolution genetic mapping of complex traits. Am J Hum Genet 1995; 56:1212–1223.

154. Murray JD, Bulman DE, Ebers GC, Lathrop GM, Rice GPA. Linkage of morbid obesity with polymorphic microsatellite markers on chromosome 1q31 in a three-generation Canadian kinbred. Am J Hum Genet 1994; 55: A197 (abstract).

155. Oppert JM, Tourville J, Chagnon M, Mauriège P, Dionne FT, Pérusse L, Bouchard C. DNA polymorphisms in the α_2- and β_2-adrenoceptor genes and regional fat distribution in humans: association and linkage studies. Obes Res 1995; 3:249–255.

156. Bouchard C, Pérusse L. Current status of the human obesity gene map. Obes Res 1996; 4:81–90.

157. Clément K, Vaisse C, Manning BSJ, et al. Genetic variation in the β_3-adrenergic receptor and an increased capacity to gain weight in patients with morbid obesity. N Engl J Med 1995; 333:352–354.

158. Walston J, Silver K, Bogardus C, et al. Time of onset of non-insulin-dependent diabetes mellitus and genetic variation in the β_3-adrenergic-receptor gene. N Engl J Med 1995; 333:343–347.

159. Widén E, Lehto M, Kanninen T, Walston J, Shuldiner AR, Groop LC. Association of a polymorphism in the β_3-adrenergic-receptor gene with features of the insulin resistance syndrome in Finns. N Engl J Med 1995; 333: 348–351.

160. Dizier MH, Bonaïti-Pellié C, Clerget-Darpoux F. Conclusions of segregation analysis for family data generated under two-locus models. Am J Hum Genet 1993; 53: 1338–1346.

161. Cardon L, Fulker DW. The power of interval mapping of quantitative trait loci, using selected sibpairs. Am J Hum Genet 1994; 55:825–833.

162. Fulker DW, Cardon LR. A sibpair approach to interval mapping of quantitative trait loci. Am J Hum Genet 1994; 54:1092–1103.

163. Goldgar DE. Multipoint analysis of human quantitative genetic variation. Am J Hum Genet 1990; 47:957–967.

164. Elston RC. Designs for the global research of the human genome by linkage analysis. Proceedings of the XVIth International Biometric Conference, Hamilton, New Zealand, 1992:39–51.

165. Elston RC. Hoch Award Lecture. P values, power, and pitfalls in the linkage analysis of psychiatric disorders. In: Gershon ES, Cloninger CR, eds. Genetics Approaches to Mental Disorders. American Psychiatric Press, Washington, DC, 1994.

166. Brown DL, Gorin M, Weeks DE. Efficient strategies for genomic searching using the affected pedigree-member methods in linkage analysis. Am J Hum Genet 1994; 54: 544–553.

167. Todorov AA, Borecki IB, Province M, Rao DC. Power of ascertained sibships for QTL linkage Hum Hered (in press).

168. Risch N, Zhang H. Extreme discordant sib pairs for mapping quantitative trait loci in humans. Science 1995; 268: 1584–1589.

169. Morton NE. Sequential tests for the detection of linkage. Am J Hum Genet 1955; 7:277–318.

170. Ott J. Analysis of Human Genetic Linkage. Baltimore: Johns Hopkins University Press, 1991.

171. Bouchard C. Genetics of human obesities: Introductory notes. In: Bouchard C. ed. The Genetics of Obesity. Boca Raton, FL: CRC Press, 1994:1–15.

172. Bray GA. What's in a name? Mr. Dickens' "Pickwickian" fat boy syndrome. Obes Res 1994; 2:380–383.

173. Paganini-Hill A, Martin AO, Spence MA. The S-leut anthropometric traits: genetic analysis. Am J Phys Anthrop 1981; 55:55–67.

174. Dériaz O, Dionne F, Pérusse L, et al. DNA variation in the genes of the Na,K-adenosine triphosphatase and its relation with resting metabolic rate, respiratory quotient, and body fat. J Clin Invest 1994; 93:838–843.

175. Rajput-Williams J, Knott TJ, Wallis SC, et al. Variation of apolipoprotein-B gene is associated with obesity, high blood cholesterol levels, and increased risk of coronary heart disease. Lancet 1988; 31:1442–1446.

176. Saha N, Tay JSH, Heng CK, Humphries SE. DNA polymorphisms of the apolipoprotein B gene are associated with obesity and serum lipids in healthy Indians in Singapore. Clin Genet 1993; 44:113–120.

177. Lucarini N, Finocchi G, Gloria-Bottini F, et al. A possible genetic component of obesity in childhood. Observations on acid phosphatase polymorphism. Experientia 1990; 46:90–91.

178. Vijayaraghavan S, Hitman GA, Kopelman PG. Apolipoprotein-D polymorphism: a genetic marker for obesity and hyperinsulinemia. J Clin Endocrinol Metab 1994; 79: 568–570.

179. Norman RA, Bogardus C, Ravussin E. Linkage between obesity and a marker near the tumor necrosis factor-α locus in Pima Indians. J Clin Invest 1995; 96:158–162.

180. Bouchard C, Dionne FT, Chagnon M, Moreel JF, Pérusse L. DNA sequence variation in the lipoprotein lipase (LPL) gene and obesity. FASEB J 1994; 8:923 (abstract).

181. Jemaa R, Tuzet S, Portos C, Betoulle D, Apfelbaum M, Fumeron F. Lipoprotein lipase gene polymorphisms: association with hypertriglyceridemia and body mass index in obese people. Int J Obes 1995; 19:270–274.

182. Comings DE, Flanagan SD, Dietz G, Muhleman D, Knell E, Gysin R. The dopamine D_2 (DRD2) as a major gene in obesity and height. Biochem Med Metab Biol 1993; 50: 176–185.

183. Bailey-Wilson JE, Wilson AF, Bamba V. Linkage analysis in a large pedigree ascertained due to essential familial hypercholesterolemia. Genet Epidemiol 1993; 10: 665–669.

184. Wilson AF, Elston RC, Tran LD, Siervogel RM. Use of the robust sib-pair method to screen for single-locus, multiple-locus, and pleiotropic effects: application to traits related to hypertension. Am J Hum Genet 1991; 48: 862–872.

11

Animal Models of Obesity

David A. York
Pennington Biomedical Research Center, Louisiana State University, Baton Rouge, Louisiana

Barbara Hansen
Obesity and Diabetes Research Center, University of Maryland School of Medicine, Baltimore, Maryland

I. INTRODUCTION

Until the recent past, the animal models that were available for the study of obesity either were of spontaneous origin or were the result of experimental manipulation of the environment or the hypothalamic centers that regulate food intake and energy balance (1,2). These models have mainly been focused on rodent species, but the more limited studies in other species, particularly nonhuman primates, have also yielded important new knowledge. Through study of these animal models we have achieved substantive insight into the physiological disturbances that can lead to obesity and into those disturbances that are consequent to the obese state. Studies of animal models have provided detailed knowledge on the developmental sequence of obesity and its associated abnormalities and on the anatomical, neurochemical, and endocrine systems that regulate food intake and energy expenditure. Above all, they have indicated the importance of the interactions between genetic inheritance and environmental factors in determining the susceptibility to develop obesity. Only recently however, have we begun to understand the precise biochemical abnormalities that can initiate the obese state. This understanding has come from two directions; first, through identification of the gene defects in three mouse obesities that are inherited as single gene defects, the Yellow (A^y/a) (3), the obese (*ob/ob*) (4), and the fat (Cpe^{fat}/Cpe^{fat}) (5) mice, and, second, through the use of trans-genic technologies to either cause, prevent, or reverse obesity (6–8). These recent advances signal the beginning of an exciting new era in which we shall begin to understand how body fat levels are regulated and how specific gene products affect the neuroendocrine systems that regulate food intake and energy expenditure. This information will lead to the development of new approaches for the treatment and prevention of the obesity disease in humans.

For classification purposes, the animal models may be subdivided into three groups, genetic, dietary and neuroendocrine, although it should be recognized that there is considerable overlap between them (Table 1). Indeed, some of the spontaneous obesities may involve all three components. The first group comprises several types of genetic models (Table 2). Single-gene rodent models are those in which the obesity is inherited either as a dominant (Yellow, A^y/a) or recessive (obese ob/ob, diabetes db/db, fatty fa/fa, fat or tub tb/tb) characteristics. The polygenic forms of obesity, which are normally of later onset and sometimes are less severe, are often associated with dietary manipulations. Finally, the transgenic approaches (Table 3) are providing a rapidly expanding group of models in which gene manipulations may either be targeted to a specific tissue, e.g., uncoupling protein knockout in brown adipose tissue or to more ubiquitous expression, e.g., Glut 4 overexpression or G-protein knockouts.

Table 1 Animal Models of Obesity

1. Genetic	a. Single genes
	b. Multigenic
	c. Transgenic
2. Dietary	a. High fat
	b. High fat/high carbohydrate (sucrose)
	c. High carbohydrate (sucrose)
	d. Cafeteria diets
	e. Chow to desert rodents
	f. Force-fed
3. Neuroendocrine	a. Lesions
	i. Electrolyte (VMH, PVN, amygdala)
	ii. Knife cut (hypothalamus, midbrain)
	iii. Chemical (GTG, MSG, BPM, 6-OHDA, IA, KA)
	iv. Viral (scrapie or Coxsackie virus)
	b. Chemical infusions
	i. NPY to PVN
	ii. NE to VMH
	c. Electrical stimulation of LH
	d. Ovariectomy
	e. Peripheral insulin
	f. Antidepressants
	g. Hibernation/migration

VMH, ventromedial hypothalamus; PVN, paraventricular nucleus; LH, lateral hypothalamus; GTG, goldthioglucose; MSG, monosodium glutamate; BMP, bipiperidyl mustard; IA, ibotenic acid; KA, kainic acid; NPY, neuropeptide Y; NE, norepinephrine; 6-OHDA, 6-hydroxydopamine.

The second group includes various dietary models of obesity (9). These encompass a wide variety of dietary manipulations ranging from forced overfeeding to provision of laboratory chow in desert rodents. Dietary obesity can also be induced by feeding high fat or high carbohydrate–high fat cafeteria diets to susceptible animals, and modest weight gains can be achieved with sucrose drinking solutions. The obesities associated with manipulation of dietary composition illustrate the strong association that exists between genetic inheritance and environmental influences. Rat and mouse strains vary greatly in their sensitivity to this form of obesity (10). Likewise within primate colonies there are wide-ranging individual differences in responses (11). The multigenic factors that predispose animals to this form of obesity make them probably the closest models for the study of human obesity.

The final group of models are those related to neuroendocrine and endocrine manipulations. Lesions of the ventromedial (VMH) and paraventricular (PVN) nuclei will induce obesity in a wide range of animal species including mouse, rat, and nonhuman primates (1,2,12). Conversely, damage to the lateral hypothalamus (LH) causes aphagia and loss of body fat. Studies with these models have illustrated the inextricable links between regulation of feeding behavior and autonomic regulation of peripheral metabolism and endocrine activity. These central regulatory systems may also be perturbed by chronic or acute infusions of neuropeptides [e.g., neuropeptide Y (NPY)] (13,14), neurotransmitters (e.g., norepinephrine) (15), antibodies, or antisense messages. Endocrine manipulations that affect body composition have focused primarily on insulin, glucocorticoids, and growth hormone. Finally, the natural seasonal and migratory changes observed in several species provide excellent models for the study of normal regulation of feeding behavior and body fat content (16).

Spontaneous, naturally occurring obesity is also common both in free-ranging and in laboratory or zoo-maintained nonhuman primates and has been described in a wide range of primate species. In addition, primate models of obesity have been experimentally induced. Previous reviews have described the various measures used to produce experimental obesity in primates (12,17), including the production of hypothalamic lesions to induce weight gain and diabetes-like syndromes, drug and hormonal approaches, and diet manipulations or forced overfeeding to produce weight gain. These methods have received little use in the past 10 years, probably due to the fact that, as monkeys have been held longer under laboratory conditions, well into middle age, more and more spontaneously obese animals have been identified, negating the necessity to experimentally create obese primate models. The present review will, therefore, focus on spontaneous obesity in both free-ranging and laboratory-maintained monkeys.

II. ADVANTAGES AND DISADVANTAGES OF ANIMAL MODELS FOR THE STUDY OF HUMAN OBESITY

There are many advantages to the use of animal models for the study of human obesity and these provide the basis for the preeminent contribution that animal studies have made to our understanding of the causes and consequences of obesity and the metabolic, endocrine, and neuroendocrine factors that underlie these changes. First, because of inbreeding and the ability to control the environment, the phenotype of rodent species can be controlled and more easily defined. This can be coupled with

Table 2 Genetically Inherited Forms of Obesity

Species	Name	Gene symbol	Inheritance	Alleles	Chromosome #	Gene product	Comment
Single gene							
Mice	Obese	ob	Recessive	ob²⁾	6	Leptin	
	Diabetes	db	Recessive	db²⁾, db³⁾, db^ad	4	Leptin receptor	Intracellular signaling domain
	Fat	Cpe^fat	Recessive		8	Carboxypeptidase E (H)	
	Tubby	Tub	Recessive		7	?	
	Yellow	A^y/a	Dominant		2	Agouti protein	Ubiquitous expression of agouti protein
	KK	K	Dominant		?	?	Gene has low (25%) penetrance
Rats	Zucker fatty	fa	Recessive	SHR/N-CP LA/N-CP SHHF/Mcc-Cp Koletsky	5	Leptin Receptor	Extracellular domain
Multigenic							
Mice	New Zealand obese	NZO			?	?	
	BSB				6, 7, 12, 15	?	Body fat varies 1–50%
	Acomys cahirinus						Obesity on lab chow diet
	AKR				4, 9, 15		High-fat diet
Rats	Osborne Mendel	OM			?	?	High-fat diet
							Obesity on lab chow diet
Gerbils	Sand rat (*Psammomys obesus*)	?			?	?	
Primates	Rhesus monkey	?			?	?	Spontaneous, adult onset
	Other primates	?			?	?	In many species in captivity

Table 3 Transgenic Models of Obesity

Gene	Overexpression or knockout	Promotor of construct	Tissue expression	Comment
Glut 4 transporter	Overexpression	aP2	Adipose	Obesity—hyperplasia but not hypertrophy of adipose tissue
				Does not prevent glucose intolerance
Glut 4 transporter	Overexpression	7kb 5′ 3T3-L2 Glut 4 gene	Adipose tissue, muscle	No effect on obesity but abolishes insulin resistance
Glucocorticoid type II receptor	Antisense expression	Human neuroflament gene		Severe reduction in central glucocorticoid type II receptors
CRF	Overexpression	Metallothionin	CNS, testis, heart, adrenal	Cushingoid features
Agouti	Ectopic expression	Human β-actin or mouse phosphoglycerate kinase	Ubiquitous	Reproduced phenotype of A^y/a
Diphtheria toxin A chain	Expression	aP2	Adipose	Destroys adipose tissue Prevents obesity
Diphtheria toxin A chain	Expression	Uncoupling protein	Brown adipose tissue	Destroys BAT Obesity with hyperphagia
β_3-adrenergic receptor	Knockout	aP2	White and brown adipose tissue	Modest obesity
Gq alpha protein	Knockout		Adipose tissue Liver	Obesity by 5 weeks of age

the ability to measure end points directly and precisely whether this be food intake, body composition, or the levels of a particular neuropeptide within the central nervous system (CNS). Such measures are often indirect, subject to large error, or impossible in humans. These advantages of animal models are well illustrated by the understanding we have gained of the neuroanatomical and neurochemical system within the CNS that are responsive to nutrient status and which regulate both feeding behavior and the autonomic responses to food intake. The ability to induce obesity in animals and the ability to study young preobese animals have helped to define the temporal sequence of events in the development of obesity. Finally, the availability of genetic models and the use of transgenics are providing insight into gene products that cause or reverse obesity and into the mechanisms of these effects.

The major concerns in the use of animal models relate to their relevance to human obesity. In humans, multiple genes are probably important in the susceptibility to develop obesity in a facilitative environment (18). The genes identified to date from animal studies may or may not be of major importance for the development of human obesity, but they may provide new avenues for defining the obesity phenotype and new approaches to the treatment of obesity. The environmental features regulating feeding may in some cases be different and more complex in humans than in rodents, but an understanding of the physiological systems that regulate ingestive behavior in animals will provide the basic framework upon which human feeding behavior can be modeled and understood. Finally, we should recognize that despite the major differences in metabolism between the rodent models and humans, significant insight can still be obtained from these animal models as well as from the primate animal models. Thus, the study of sympathetic control of brown adipose tissue metabolism in response to diet in rodents provided the basis for studies of the interactions between nutrient status and the sympathetic nervous system in man. The ability to express genes on differing background strains substantially increases the phenotypic variations and provides a wide range of models, which vary in the severity of their associated disorders (1). Additionally, the study of animal models of obesity has yielded new insights into the role of adipose tissue as a secretory organ and signaling system, secreting proteins such as adipsin, tumor necrosin factor-α (TNF-α), and leptin (4,19–21).

In this chapter, we shall review the understanding of obesity that has been obtained through the study of the wide range of animal models. The chapter will not be a comprehensive review of the literature in this field, but rather a synopsis of the characteristics of the models and the current understanding that we have achieved from these studies. In the final sections of the chapter, we review some of the common features that link the various models and the implications of the knowledge of animal obesities for the causes, treatment, and prevention of human obesity.

III. GENETIC MODELS OF OBESITY

A. Single Genes

1. The Obese (*ob/ob*) Mouse

The obese mouse inherits its obesity as a result of an autosomal recessive mutation on chromosome 6, which has now been identified as the leptin gene (4). Like the diabetes (*db/db*) mouse and the Zucker fatty (*fa/fa*) rat, the obesity of the *ob/ob* mouse begins to develop soon after birth and is associated with a decrease in brown adipose tissue (BAT) thermogenesis and an enhanced insulin secretory activity. The obesity rapidly develops after weaning, at which time the parallel development of hyperphagia exaggerates the degree of obesity attained. Prevention of hyperphagia by food restriction, pair feeding, or yoke feeding to lean controls does not prevent the obesity in *ob/ob* mice or the other single-gene mutations (22–24). Hyperinsulinemia, associated with hyperplasia and hypertrophy of islet tissue, is an early phenomenon and progressively increases with age as insulin resistance develops (25). Insulin resistance develops rapidly after weaning, but the severity of the hyperglycemia and diabetes is dependent upon the background strain of mouse upon which the *ob* gene is expressed. The obesity of adult *ob/ob* mice is severe with large excess deposits of adipose tissue in the intra-abdominal, subcutaneous, and intrathoracic compartments. The relative concentration of fat to the inguinal and axial regions gives the mice a characteristic pear shape.

Many neuroendocrine abnormalities have been described, including impaired sympathetic stimulation of BAT thermogenesis, enhanced parasympathetic stimulation of insulin secretion, overactivity of the hypothalamic-pituitary-adrenal axis, decreased growth hormone secretion, impaired thyroid hormone metabolism, and infertility (1,2; and see below). Similar changes have been described in several models of obesity (1,2).

Recently, Friedman and colleagues (4) were successful in cloning the obese *ob* gene. The gene is uniquely expressed in white adipose tissue, and possibly brown adipose tissue, and codes for a 4.5-kb mRNA containing a 167-amino-acid open reading frame. The obese C57BL/6J *ob/ob* mouse has a C-to-T mutation in codon 105, which changes an arginine code (CGA) to a stop codon

(TGA). A second mutation, ob^{2j}/ob^{2j}, has been mapped 7 kb upstream of the 4.5-kb ob RNA start site and is assumed to be the result of a structural alteration or a mutation in the promotor region.

The mouse ob gene is highly homologous with human, monkey, and rat ob genes (4,26–28). The protein product of this gene has been given the name leptin. The presence of a signal peptide sequence and the hydrophilic nature of the protein are consistent with a secreted protein, and leptin-like immunoreactivity has been identified in the serum of rodents, nonhuman primates, and humans. Despite very high levels of expression of the ob gene in adipose tissue of the ob/ob mouse, no leptin immunoreactivity can be detected in the serum of these mice, suggesting either that the truncated protein is not secreted or that it is not detected by the currently available antibodies. Similarly, increased levels of ob gene expression have been reported in a range of obese models, including the Zucker fa/fa rat (26,29), the diabetes db/db mouse (4), rats made obese by VMH lesions (27), rats fed a high-fat diet (30), and nonhuman primates (28). Despite the relationship of leptin gene expression to body fat level, it is evident that gene expression may be regulated by a number of signals. Streptozotocin diabetes reduces and insulin increases gene expression (31,32). Glucocorticoids enhance expression of leptin mRNA in adipocyte cultures (33). In contrast, adrenalectomy of obese fa/fa rats greatly attenuated the elevated levels of leptin mRNA, an effect that was reversed by corticosterone (29). In this case the changes in gene expression with adrenal status occurred in the absence of significant changes in body weight or fat at a time when food intake and insulin levels were reduced. Similarly, cold exposure of mice caused a very rapid reduction in leptin mRNA that appeared to be mediated directly or indirectly by the sympathetic system (34). We can anticipate rapid advances in our understanding of the factors that regulate leptin gene expression and leptin synthesis and secretion as well as in our knowledge of the site and mechanisms of action of this circulating protein.

Indeed, the putative leptin receptor was initially cloned and identified (35). Surprisingly, the highest concentrations and highest receptor mRNA levels were evident in lung, kidney, and the choroid plexus. Only low levels of receptor mRNA were evident in the hypothalamus. This distribution profile suggests that the receptor identified may be associated with excretion or transport of the protein and possibly not with its biological activity. However, as it is located on the choroid plexus, it could conceivably affect food intake through an inhibitory action on insulin transport (36).

The classic parabiotic studies of Coleman (37) and Hervey et al. (38) predicted the presence of a circulating factor that was secreted in response to increased body fat stores and that would regulate feeding behavior. Coleman (37) further suggested that ob/ob mice did not produce this factor and that db/db mice and fa/fa rats produced the factor but were unresponsive to it. The early studies of leptin suggest that it may have the characteristics of such a circulating signaling factor. First, as mentioned above, leptin gene expression increases with body fat in a range of animal models; second, both peripheral and central administration of leptin to ob/ob mice reduce food intake and body weight, and body fat content falls dramatically (39–41). In contrast, leptin has only moderate effects in milder forms of obesity such as that induced by high-fat feeding in mice (39) and is without effect in the diabetes db/db mouse (40) as predicted from the parabiosis experiments.

Leptin is also less effective when given to lean mice requiring approximately a 10-fold increase in does from that which is effective in ob/ob mice (39–41). This may reflect a substantial up-regulation of leptin-receptor activity in the ob/ob mouse in the absence of circulating leptin protein. Alternatively, it might indicate that an additional signal is required for leptin activity to be expressed. If gene transcription is paralleled by leptin synthesis and secretion, and only future studies will show if this is the case, the high leptin gene transcription rates reported in other forms of animal and human obesity suggest that resistance to leptin activity is a common, although not universal or uniform, feature of obesity.

There are numerous metabolic and endocrine abnormalities in the ob/ob mouse that cannot be related to hyperphagia. Thus leptin must also affect autonomic activity and most probably will also affect sexual maturation through effects on gonadotropic hormone secretion. While initial excitement about leptin has focused on the possibility of its action as a feedback signal to regulate central feeding and metabolic responses, it probably also has effects directly or indirectly on peripheral tissues such as the pancreas, to regulate insulin secretion and muscle, to regulate glucose transport and metabolism (42), and on the autonomic nervous system to enhance sympathetically mediated BAT thermogenesis and to reduce vagally mediated pancreatic insulin secretion (Fig. 1). The increase in rectal temperature of ob/ob mice treated with leptin is suggestive of a restoration of sympathetic drive to BAT (41). It is also likely that the glucocorticoid dependence of obesity will be closely associated with leptin-activated signaling pathways in the CNS and other tissues. Of particular significance is the observation that blood glucose of ob/ob mice was more sensitive to leptin administration

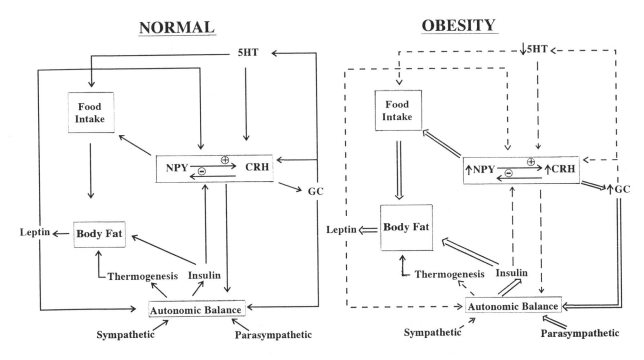

Figure 1 Peripheral and central signals that regulate body fat, food intake, and autonomic activity. In the normal animal, the balance between NPY and CRH is seen to be critical for the control of food intake and autonomic balance modulating insulin secretion and brown fat thermogenesis. Leptin probably is an important signal to regulate the NPY-CRH axis. In obesity, absence of appropriate leptin signaling leads to increased NPY activity. Increased activity of the HPA axis results in excessive glucocorticoid influences on the autonomic system. These effects are exacerbated by the development of central insulin resistance and loss of central serotoninergic activity. Dotted lines indicate reduced activity; thin lines, normal activity; double lines, excessive activity.

than food intake, body fat, or body weight (41). This might indicate that leptin acts on the glucose transport system.

2. The Diabetes (*db/db*) Mouse

The diabetes mouse (*db/db*) inherits its obesity as an autosomal recessive trait that results from a mutation on mouse chromosome 4 (43). It is phenotypically indistinguishable from the obese (*ob/ob*) mouse when both genes are expressed on the same background strain (44). On the C57B1/6J background, the obesity is severe and maintained throughout life; the hyperphagia is moderate, the diabetes also is moderate, with transient hyperglycemia, and the hyperinsulinemia is marked but maintained throughout life. In contrast, on the C57B1/Ks background, the hyperphagia and obesity are more extreme but there is moderate weight loss before early death associated with islet atrophy and pancreatic β-cell failure. The putative mouse leptin receptor that was initially cloned and identified (35) was subsequently shown to be one of several splice variants that coded for a short form of the receptor. Subsequently the long form of the receptor

was cloned by RT-PCR from mouse brain RNA using primers designed from the human long-form leptin receptor that was cloned from a fetal brain cDNA library. The receptor has a large extracellular region with a single membrane-spanning domain and either a short or long intracellular chain. This long intracellular domain, which is thought to be important for signalling mechanisms, is not translated in *db/db* mice since a G-to-T mutation (45,46) introduces a novel consensus splice donor site (AGGGAAA sequence to an AGGTAAA sequence). As a result of this mutation, a 106-base sequence of the terminal exon of the short form of the receptor is spliced into the long form of the receptor mRNA. This introduces a stop codon that prevents translation of the long intracellular domain of the receptor. A similar mutation is thought to be present in the *fa/fa* rat. Thus the original hypothesis proposed from the results of parabiosis experiments (37) that *db* coded for the receptor to the *ob* gene product leptin was correct. The short form of the receptor may be a transport protein. Further, the expression of the leptin receptor gene in multiple tissues suggests that leptin may have both central and peripheral sites of action.

3. The Zucker Fatty (fa/fa) Rat

Since its original description by Zucker and Zucker in 1961 (47), the *fa/fa* rat has become increasingly popular as a model for studying metabolic, endocrine, neurochemical, and behavioral aspects of obesity. The larger size of rats compared to mice provides distinct technical advantages over the mouse models. In contrast, the greater information available on the mouse genome makes the mouse models preferable for genetic studies. The *fa* gene has been mapped to chromosome 5 of the rat and is thought from linkage analysis to be syntenic with the *db* gene on mouse chromosome 4 (48). Although it is regarded as a recessive gene, the effects of *fa* on body fat and serum insulin may be dominant in the suckling pup during the first 20 days of life (49).

As would be expected from this information, the phenotypic expression of the *fa* gene in homozygous animals is similar to that of the *ob/ob* and *db/db* mice with the exception that this rat model is rarely hyperglycemic. Nevertheless, there are a number of allelic variants of the *fa/fa* rat (see Table 2). By introducing the corpulent (*fa^cp*) or Koletzky gene onto an inbred strain of rats derived from the hypertensive Okamoto strain (SHR/N) and further crossing onto other strains, e.g., LA/N, a variety of strains exhibiting various aspects of the syndrome X metabolic profile have been developed (50). The corpulent (*fa^cp*) SHR/N-*cp* and LA/N-*cp* rats display both pronounced hyperglycemia and hypertension. These have been used as models for syndrome X in humans. The SHR/n-*cp* rat also develops nephropathy, the Jcr:LA-*cp* rat has cardiovascular disease, and the SMHP/Mcc-*cp* rat has both hypertension and congestive heart failure. When the *fa* gene is transferred from its Brown-Norway background strain, on which diabetes is normally absent, to other backgrounds, long-lasting, severe diabetes may become characteristic, e.g., diabetic fatty (ZDF/Drt-*fa*), Wistar Kyoto fatty (WKY/NDrt-*fa*), or Wistar Kyoto diabetic (WDF/TA-*fa*).

The temporal sequence for the development of obesity in the *fa/fa* rat is similar to that of the *ob/ob* and *db/db* mice. Excess fat deposition is evident by 3 days of age (51), and impaired BAT thermogenesis (52) and excess insulin secretion are evident between days 5 and 10 (49,52). Indeed, the early onset of obesity may be prevented by treatment with sympathomimetic drugs or housing at high environmental temperatures (49,51–53). Excess fat is deposited at all sites and is particularly rapid after weaning. It cannot be prevented by restriction of food intake (54).

4. The Fat Mouse (fat/fat or Cpe^fat/Cpe^fat)

The fat mouse, unlike the *ob/ob* and *db/db* mice and the *fa/fa* rat, is an example of a late-onset form of obesity. The obesity may be severe (60–70 g body weight at 24 weeks) and is expressed in all adipose depots. In this mutant the obesity is not normally evident until 8–12 weeks of age and is not pronounced until 16–20 weeks of age. It arose out of an inbred HRS/J strain of mice and has been crossed onto the C57BLKS/J background strain to facilitate comparison with the obese and diabetes mutations. The fat mouse is characterized by massive hyperinsulinemia without significant hyperglycemia from weaning suggestive of extreme insulin resistance but does not display the pancreatic failure and severe diabetes that are evident in older *ob/ob* and *db/db* mice (55). When the mutation is transferred to the C57BLKS/J(HKS) background strain, the *fat/fat* mouse is diabetic but the diabetes is still less severe than that seen with *ob/ob* or *db/db* mice on the same background. Indeed, the mouse remains extremely sensitive to exogenous insulin. This apparent paradox has been explained by the recent identification of the fat gene and the demonstration that the apparent hyperinsulinemia was in fact a hyperproinsulinemia (5). The fat gene, located on chromosome 8, has been shown to code for carboxypeptidase E (5). A single base mutation that results in a serine202proline substitution severely reduces the activity of carboxypeptidase E in both the pancreatic islet and pituitary. This was confirmed by site-specific mutagenesis of the Cpe gene and its expression in a baculovirus system. Indeed immunoreactive carboxypeptidase E protein is undetectable in pancreas and pituitary of *fat/fat* mice, suggesting that the mutation affects either transcriptional or transational activity or stability of the mRNA or protein.

Carboxypeptidase E (also known as carboxypeptidase H) is required for cleavage of two arginine residues from the B chain of insulin during its processing from proinsulin. The impairment in processing of proinsulin in mice homozygous for the Cpe^fat allele is reflected in the 10-fold increase in proinsulin to insulin ratios in the pancreas that was present before development of obesity. The absence of carboxypeptidase E activity in the pancreas explains the very high level of proinsulin rather than insulin in the circulation and pancreas of the *fat/fat* mouse and its responsiveness to exogenous insulin. It is difficult to explain the development of obesity on the basis of the defect in proinsulin processing since proinsulin has little biological activity. In addition to proinsulin, a number of prohormones and proneuropeptides also require cleavage of paired dibasic residues from their C-terminal ends to yield the biologically active peptides, including the proopiomelanocortin peptides ACTH, MSH, β-endorphin and β-lipotropin, proenkephalins, preproNPY, vasopressin, oxytocin, and CCK. Naggert et al. (5) suggest that the obesity of the *fat/fat* mouse is thus likely to result from a complex pattern of alterations in neuropeptide activity and secretion within the hypothalamic-pituitary system rather than the hyperproinsulinemia.

5. The Tubby (*tub/tub*) Mouse

This mutation was first reported by Coleman and Eicher in 1990 (55). It is an autosomal recessive mutation on chromosome 7 distal to the hemoglobin β-chain complex gene (Hbb). On the C57BL/6J background, tubby mice are phenotypically very similar to fat mice except that the obesity develops more slowly, not being visually apparent until 9–12 weeks of age. All fat depots are enlarged. The *tub* mutation is associated with distinct sexual dimorphism in blood glucose, serum insulin, islet hypertrophy and hyperplasia, and β-cell degranulation, all changes being more pronounced in male mice. The hyperinsulinemia, mild at weaning, progressively increases with age. Morphological changes in the pancreatic islets occur earlier and are more pronounced in males. However, the *tub* mice remain mildly hypoglycemic, indicating the absence of the pronounced insulin resistance common to other mouse models of obesity. Infertility is also a feature of this mouse when severe obesity develops.

6. The Yellow (A^y/a) Obese Mouse

The agouti gene of the Yellow (A^y/a) obese mouse was the first single gene mutation for obesity to be identified in mice (see Ref. 56 for review). The Yellow (A^y/a) obese mouse and the KK mouse (57) discussed below are the only models of dominant inheritance of obesity so far described. The obesity of the yellow mouse is inherited as a mutation in the agouti protein coded on chromosome 2 and is associated with a moderate obesity and a high incidence of tumor growth. Although the homozygous (A^y/A^y) mouse is lethal in utero, there are a number of different alleles (A^vy/A^vy, A^iy/A^iy) at the agouti locus in which the defects are less severe and in which the degree of obesity is linked directly to the level of yellow pigmentation in the coat (58). The obesity of the yellow mice is less pronounced than in the obese and diabetes mice and is of later onset (8–12 weeks of age). While these animals share many of the characteristics common to all rodent obesities, they do differ in the clear sexual dimorphism of the associated hyperglycemia (59) (see below) and in the apparently normal activity of the hypothalamic-pituitary-adrenal axis (59,60).

The agouti (*a*) gene encodes a 131-amino-acid protein that is normally uniquely expressed in the hair follicle where it acts to inhibit eumelanin synthesis in response to stimulation by α-melanophore-stimulating hormone (α-MSH). In the Yellow mouse, exon 1 of the agouti gene is replaced by a unique sequence but exons 2–4, which contain the full coding sequence, are normal. The result of this mutation is the ubiquitous expression of the agouti gene in a wide range of tissues including white adipose tissue and brain (3). Transgenic mice expressing agouti unregulated and ubiquitously driven by the human β-actin promoter also develop yellow coat color and become obese (61–63), confirming that ectopic expression of normal agouti protein results in the obese yellow phenotype.

Two potential actions of agouti protein have been identified. Its ability to increase intracellular calcium levels may promote insulin resistance (64). Intracellular calcium levels are related to the level of expression of agouti protein and to body weight and degree of coat color. Using a murine melanoma cell line, Lu et al. (65) were able to demonstrate that agouti protein inhibited the stimulation of adenylyl cyclase by β-MSH, shifting the dose required for half-maximal stimulation from 1.7 to 13.4 nM by acting as a potent antagonist of the melancocortin-4 receptor (MC4-R). However, agouti had no effects on MC1, MC2, MC3, or MC5 receptors. Since MC4-R is primarily expressed in the hypothalamus and other brain regions that regulate neuroendocrine function, it is possible that the agouti effects on MC4 receptors mediate the development of obesity. Although the function of the MC4 receptor system in relation to the development of obesity is unclear, it could be related to the decreased acetylation of MSH present in the pituitary of A^y/a mice (66,67). Desacetyl and acetyl MSH vary in their biological effects. Acetyl MSH (αMSH) regulates eumelanin production and darkens the coat color but has little effect on food intake and body weight whereas desaceytl MSH has no effect on coat color but increases food intake and body fat deposition (68). These disparate hypotheses for the development of obesity in A^y/a mice may be connected if the MC4 receptor activity regulates calcium flux and either directly or indirectly acetylation of MSH during the processing of proopiomelanocortin (POMC) into its constituent neuropeptides.

7. KK Mice

Since the original description of the KK mouse (69), several different strains have been identified (see 50,57 for review). While the obesity and diabetes were originally thought to be inherited as a polygenic trait, the KK gene is now regarded as a dominant gene with low (25%) penetrance (57). The obesity and hyperinsulinemia are relatively mild although the hyperglycemia may be severe. The KK mice are, however, very sensitive to diet, and obesity may be prevented by dietary restriction. The temporal changes in this mouse are also very different from the other mouse models in that changes to or toward normality of body composition, insulin secretion, and insulin resistance may be evident in older (>6 months) animals. In these mice the pancreas appears to have the ability to increase insulin secretion without the subsequent necrosis seen in *ob/ob* and *db/db* mice. Once again, there are major variations across the different strains of KK mice.

B. Transgenic Models of Obesity

Transgenic techniques are now being used extensively to explore the role of specific gene products and a number of new models relevant to the study of obesity have resulted (Table 3). While these have not yet been extensively characterized, they have provided a number of illuminating, and sometimes confusing, insights into the mechanisms underlying the development of obesity. Barden and colleagues (70,71) incorporated type II glucocorticoid receptor antisense RNA construct into mice and focused s expression primarily to neural tissues by linking the construct to a human neurofilament gene promoter sequence 4. All transgenic offspring, whether homozygous or heterozygous for the construct, developed obesity (~2-fold increase in body weight) by 6 months of age despite clear evidence for reduced glucocorticoid receptor activity (72). Other evidence (see below), from a wide range of animal models, has indicated the dependence of all obesities on the presence of adrenal glucocorticoids and suggests that obesity is characterized by an overactivity of type II GR receptors. The explanation of these very divergent results is not clear. The type of obesity produced by antisense GR expression differs from other obesities in that energy intake and oxygen consumption during the dark phase were reduced and insulin levels were not significantly increased. Hypertriglyceridemia was evident and this may result from the substantial reduction in muscle lipoprotein lipase activity in the transgenic animal.

The antisense transgene for GR results in a mouse that probably has an excess peripheral GR activity and subnormal central GR activity and it may be this imbalance that promotes the obesity. Similarly, transgenic mice overexpressing the CRF gene express elevated levels of activity of the hypothalamic-pituitary adrenal systems and the mice become obese (72).

Of the several forms of glucose transporters that have been identified, Glut 4 is found in many tissues and is responsive to insulin. Overexpression of Glut 4 in white

adipose tissue (6–9-fold) and brown adipose tissue (2–4-fold) using the aP2-promoter/enhancer increased total body lipid 2–3-fold (8). This was associated with a massive increase in the basal transport of glucose into adipocytes and, interestingly, a twofold increase in fat cell number, but no increase in fat cell size. If this can be substantiated, it would provide the first model of obesity associated with hyperplastic growth of adipose tissue in the absence of cell hypertrophy. Of further significance is the observation that overexpression of the Glut 4 gene prevented the reduction of glycemic control in high-fat-fed obesity but did not prevent the development of obesity (8,73).

Targeted expression of a diphtheria toxin A chain gene has been used to selectively knock out tissue functional activity. By coupling the gene to uncoupling protein gene expression, brown adipose tissue thermogenic function was abolished and mice became obese (6) and developed hyperphagia. This model not only illustrates the importance of BAT thermogenesis to energy balance in rodents but also emphasizes that BAT may reciprocally affect food intake (74) probably through a sympathetically mediated signal, e.g., heat (75). This approach appears to be more successful than knockout of the β_3-adrenergic receptor gene in white and brown adipose tissue (76) as this yields only a moderate form of obesity in which BAT remained morphologically normal and responded normally to cold acclimation. This questions the relationship between BAT thermogenesis and feeding behavior proposed by Himms-Hagen (75).

When the diphtheria toxin A chain gene is targeted to adipose tissue with the promoter region of the aP2 gene and there are low levels of transgene expression, body fat levels are normal but the mice become resistant to monosodium glutamate (MSG)-induced obesity (77). The hyperlipidemia normally observed in MSG-induced obesity was still present in the transgenic mice, but unlike the nontransgenic MSG mice, they also remain fertile. Gαq protein knockouts in adipose tissue and liver expressed from birth also produced obesity that was associated with impaired lipolytic activity (78). A fuller description of this transgenic awaits publication of a full manuscript.

C. Polygenic Obesity

I.   The Sand Rat (*Psammomys obesus*)

When this rat is transferred from its herbivorous desert diet to a high-carbohydrate laboratory chow it rapidly develops obesity and diabetes (79). This may be prevented by severe restriction of chow intake (80). However, there is considerable individual variation in the response within and between colonies. It may range from normoglycemic/

normoinsulinemic through severe obesity, hyperinsulinemia, and syndrome X-like changes to a syndrome similar to the diabetes mouse in which there is severe diabetes and pancreatic failure. Shafrir (50) has recently reviewed the variability of the diabetes in this strain.

A similar murine obesity and diabetes has been reported in the spiny mouse (*Acomys caharinus*) (81). There is a relatively low frequency of diabetes and large variance in the severity of the syndrome in those animals affected.

2. New Zealand Obese (NZO) Mice

The NZO mouse, originally described by Bielschowsky and Bielschowsky (82) develops a moderate form of obesity from early life. This strain was developed by extensive brother X sister matings over 17 generations from parents initially selected for their agouti coat color. They become hyperinsulinemic and insulin resistant but have only moderate hyperglycemia (83). The increased deposition of visceral fat relative to other sites in NZO mouse could provide a suitable model of abdominal obesity in humans. This model is also somewhat unique in that insulin secretion in response to glucose, glucagon, and tolbutamide is impaired whereas there is an exaggerated response to arginine and a normal response to glyceraldehyde. The impaired glucose stimulation of insulin appears to be related to a defect in the uptake or glycolytic conversion of glucose into triose sugars.

3. BSB Mice

These mice, derived from a backcross of *Mus spretus* and C57BL/6J strains, have a body fat content that shows individual variation from 1 to 50% (84,85). They provide an excellent model for identification of gene linkages (see below).

4. Spontaneous Obesity in Primates

Within the class Mammalia, obesity has been identified in a number of orders, including the Rodentia as discussed above, the Carnivora (e.g., dogs, bear), the Artiodactyla (pigs, cattle), and the order Primates (which includes, for example, lemurs, monkeys, apes, and humans, a total of about 200 primate species), as well as in other orders, which include such mammals as the whale, walrus, manatee, hedgehog, and rhinoceros. Within the suborder Anthropoidea, obesity has been described in two of three superfamilies: Cercopithecoidea (Old World monkeys, including many species of macaques) and Hominoidea (including orangutans, chimpanzees, and gorillas—with specimens of the latter weighed in at over 180 kg, 400 lb). Obesity may also occur in the third superfamily Ce-

boidonea (New World monkeys); however, to date this has not been well documented. Most commonly, within the genus *Macaca*, obesity has been described in the species *Macaca fascicularis* (cynomolgus), *Macaca nigra* (misnomered the celebes ape), and most of all, in *Macaca mulatta* (rhesus) (11,86).

Age and the Prevalence of Obesity in Primates. One of the first surveys aimed at identifying the prevalence of obesity in a colony of group-housed monkeys examined the medical records of more than 800 pig-tailed macaques (*M. nigra*) in a large breeding facility (87). Tritiated water was then used to determine the relative body composition of those selected on the basis of heavy body weight for age. Several spontaneously obese individuals were identified; however, the incidence appeared to be very low. Retrospective consideration of this study, based on further understanding of obesity in primates gained over the past 20 years, suggests that the reason for the finding of a very low number of obese animals was the relatively young age distribution of the colony.

The obesity of nonhuman primates is clearly the adult-onset form, with no cases of obesity having yet been identified in an animal under the age of 7 years. Sexual maturity is reached in the female between 3 and 5 years, with completion of growth at 6–7 years of age, while in males, the corresponding ages are 4–6 years, and 8 years (88). The obese animals surveyed on the island of Cayo Santiago ranged in age from 9 to 16 years (89,90). Peak body weight on average is reached around the age of 15 years in *M. mulatta*. No early markers for the propensity to develop obesity at a later age have yet been identified.

Obesity: Contribution of Sex to Incidence and Fat Distribution. Obesity has been described both in male and in female monkeys. No study has been designed to examine clearly the incidence by sex. However, from observations such as those of the free-ranging monkeys on the island of Cayo Santiago (91), there does not appear to be a significant difference between the sexes in the development of obesity, nor in the distribution of body fat, which, for both sexes, is typically upper body or central. Using total body fat as determined by tritiated water distribution, together with anthropometric assessments of fat distribution, Bodkin et al. (92) have characterized the abdominal distribution of fat in *M. mulatta*. Fat distribution has been further examined used computed tomographic methods, with the finding of significant correlations between body mass index, intra-abdominal fat, abdominal subcutaneous fat, and total abdominal fat in female cynomologous monkeys (93). The body mass index used was calculated as the weight in kilograms divided by the length in centimeters from the suprasternal notch to the pubic symphysis, squared ($\times$ 100).

D. Measurement of Adiposity in Monkeys

The assessment of obesity in monkeys can be made by body weight alone, since, in adult animals, body weight and percent fat are highly correlated (within each sex) (94). The body mass index, or Quetelet index (weight/height²), was adapted for use in monkeys by substitution of the crown-rump length (in cm²) for height² (95). This body mass index, termed the Obesity Index Rh (for rhesus monkeys), was shown to be highly correlated with percent weight as fat, midgirth circumference, and body weight, but not with height, and is therefore the best simple measurement of body fatness in monkeys. Total height is not readily or accurately measured in monkeys, particularly as they age, and thus the usual body mass index used for humans is not sufficiently reliable. The tritiated water dilution method has also been reliably used to estimate total body fat content, and is highly correlated with the body mass index for monkeys.

IV. DIET-RELATED OBESITIES

A. Rodent Models

A wide range of dietary manipulations has been used to induce the development of obesity (see 1,2,69 for reviews). These include forced changes in the quantity of food eaten (force feeding) (95,96), changes in nutrient availability (sucrose drinking or polycose drinking solutions) (97,98), and changes in the composition of diet (high fat, high sucrose, cafeteria diets provided to laboratory rodents) (99–102) or normal chow diet fed to desert rodents as described above. A prominent feature of all these manipulations is their variability across individuals and strains of rodents (10,103,104) indicating a strong interaction between genotype and diet. This characteristic may be particularly relevant to the current epidemic of obesity in humans. The strain variability also provides the experimental opportunity for genetic analysis of these differences (105,106).

High-fat diets have been used in several forms to induce obesity (9,99). The diets normally consist of 30–60% fat energy. Weight gain and fat deposition vary with fat content and fat composition of the diet. Generally, weight gain increases with the percentage dietary fat and is also greater with highly saturated fat sources rather than the more unsaturated oils. Feeding fat as an individual micronutrient source will also enhance fat deposition in susceptible animals. High-fat diets or energy-dense diets increase

energy intake but obesity may still develop in the absence of hyperphagia (107).

Rats display a marked preference for sucrose, other disaccharides, and sweet monosaccharides. This characteristic has been used to promote the development of obesity. The degree of hyperphagia induced is greater if the carbohydrate (e.g., sucrose, fructose, or polycose) is presented as a drinking solution rather than incorporated into the food (99). Although there is considerable variability in the response to carbohydrate solutions with rat strain, age, and sex, increases in energy intake of between 10 and 20% and moderate increases in body fat can be attained (97,98).

In many experimental diets the high fat content is combined with high carbohydrates (9,102). The effect of adding sugar to the high-fat diets is variable and may depend on the precise carbohydrates and fats used. In contrast, the cafeteria diet, in which rats are provided with several human foods in addition to rat chow, has been very successful in producing obesity, even in strains of rat that are resistant to other forms of dietary obesity (108–110). This dietary regime, originally described by Sclafani and Springer (108), induces pronounced hyperphagia. This may be attributed to a variety of factors including the dietary composition, the variety of foods and flavors that enhance the hedonic qualities of the food in comparison to rat chow.

The response to a cafeteria diet is age-dependent, older rats being more sensitive and young rats more resistant to this form of obesity (111). Adrenalectomy increases the resistance of old rats to develop obesity when fed a cafeteria diet (112). Young rats may regain their original body weight after termination of cafeteria feeding whereas older rats are more prone to maintain the excess adiposity. Increased brown adipose tissue thermogenesis has been related to the resistance to cafeteria-diet-induced obesity in younger rats (111,112). Maintenance of high BAT thermogenesis and reduced food intake are both components that contribute to the restoration of normal weight after the termination of cafeteria feeding (113).

B. Diet, Food Intake, Activity, and Energy Expenditure in Nonhuman Primate Obesity

In spontaneously obese male rhesus monkeys ranging from 10 to 17 kg, no differences in food intake were observed between the most obese and the least obese groups, suggesting that differences in energy expenditure may contribute principally to the development of obesity (114). Obese animals showed reduced physical activity, however, although it has not been possible to document reduced activity in advance of the development of obesity.

Prevention of obesity by restraint of calories neither increased nor decreased physical activity relative to similar-weight animals. Energy expenditure per kilogram lean body mass was significantly reduced by calorie restriction and prevention of obesity (86).

Although several studies have involved dietary manipulations thought to facilitate the development of obesity, when these dietary regimen have been tested in young animals, obesity has not developed. For example, extremely high fat diets (60%) have been found to produce weight gain in monkeys. The usual dietary regimen of laboratory monkeys, primate chow, would be expected to be optimal in the prevention of obesity as it is high in fiber, low in fat (17%), and relatively low in caloric density (4 kcal/g). In colonies where the calorie allocation to each monkey is strictly controlled, obesity does not develop. Under conditions of ad libitum feeding (food continuously available for 8–24 hr/day), obesity will eventually develop in perhaps 50% or more of the animals, despite the presumed optimal diet composition. Long-term experimental limitation of calories adjusted on a individual basis can prevent the development of this middle-age-onset obesity.

C. Metabolic and Endocrine Responses to Diets that Induce Obesity

Differences in the metabolic and endocrine responses to the introduction of high-fat diets have been reported both within (115,116) and between (10,103,104,117) strains of rodents. Osborne-Mendel (OM) rats become obese on a high-fat (HF) diet whereas S5B/PI rats are resistant and remain thin (104,117). The variation in susceptibility to HF-diet-induced obesity between individual rats of a specific strain provides another model for determining the metabolic differences that predicate the susceptibility to dietary obesity. Hill and colleagues (115,118) have used the weight gain after 7 days' feeding of a semipurified high-fat diet as an index to identify obesity-prone (highest tertile of weight gain) and obesity-resistant (lowest tertile) rats.

Although numerous differences have been described between these strains, the physiological basis for their differing sensitivities to HF diets remains obscure. These differences include central responses to neuropeptides and hormones, alterations in autonomic activity, changes in peripheral metabolism, and the responses to peripheral metabolic signals.

1. Neuroendocrine Changes

Rodents that are obesity-prone have been characterized by an increased 24-hr urinary norepinephrine secretion (119), an increased glucose-induced norepinephrine secretion (120), a higher cephalic phase insulin release to saccharin (121), a higher 24-hr respiratory quotient (increased carbohydrate oxidation) (122), and a lower proportion of type I fibers in muscle (123). Activity of the α_2-adrenergic system within the ventromedial nucleus (VMN) may also be an important determinant of dietary obesity. Levin et al. (124,125) have shown that the individual response of a rat to the introduction of HF/high-carbohydrate diets can be predicted from the level of α_2-adrenergic receptors; rats with low α_2-adrenergic receptor (AR) activity become obese, those with high α_2-AR activity remain lean. Urinary catecholamine excretion was shown to be increased in a group of seven obese monkeys (126). These data suggest that an increased autonomic activity involving both increased sympathetic tone and enhanced afferent vagal activity might be markers for susceptibility to dietary obesity.

This general increase in sympathetic activity in rats susceptible to dietary obesity should be contrasted with the reduced sympathetic drive to BAT and its attenuated sympathetic response to the introduction of a high-fat diet in susceptible rats (127). This suggests that there are major differences in the central regulation of the autonomic system between animals that are sensitive or resistant to dietary obesity.

Several neuropeptide, endocrine, and metabolic signals that normally modulate feeding behavior are attenuated or absent in diet-resistant S5B/PI rats. The orexigenic effects of NPY, galanin, and 2-deoxy-D-glucose are greatly reduced and the anorectic responses to central insulin and enterostatin are attenuated or absent (128–130). In contrast, the inhibitory effect of corticortropin-releasing hormone (CRH) in feeding is normal (130). Reduced levels of norepinephrine and 5HT have been identified in the VMN of obesity-prone OM rats. These are increased on feeding a high-fat diet to the levels observed in obesity-resistant S5B/PI rats in which diet has no influence on these monoamines (131). The increased levels of ketone bodies and their increased uptake into the brain in S5B/PI (132) rats could underlie these abnormalities of feeding behavior and propensity to develop obesity through their regulation of serotoninergic pathways.

2. Lipid and Carbohydrate Metabolism in Dietary Obesity

An increased circulating level of ketone bodies has been identified in both S5B/PI (132) and Wistar rats (115) that are resistant to dietary obesity. This suggests that either the production or utilitization of ketone bodies is altered. The higher respiratory quotient of diet-sensitive rats (122) suggests that there may be both higher utilization and production of ketone bodies. However, the increased utilization of lipogenic substrates in obesity-resistant rats does not result from any increase in oxidative capacity of muscle (118) despite the changes in fiber type (123), heart, or liver (102). Lipid deposition is promoted by the parallel increase in adipose tissue and reduction in muscle lipoprotein lipase activities in obesity-prone rats (118). The relatively lower insulin levels in obesity-resistant compared to obesity-prone rats may be an important determinant of these metabolic differences.

In contrast to ketone bodies, the clearance of pyruvate in the obesity-resistant S5B/PI rats may be attenuated (134,135). The combined effects of elevated ketone bodies and the absence of pyruvate-induced insulin secretion may be responsible for the reduced hepatic pyruvate dehydrogenase activity. These abnormalities may explain the failure of pyruvate to inhibit food intake in the rat (133). Since daily turnover of carbohydrate stores may be an important determinant of food intake in rodents (135), the increased ratio of lipid to carbohydrate oxidation in diet-resistant rats may be a major factor in reducing food intake of resistant rats when high-fat diets are presented.

D. Genetics of Polygenic Obesities

Two groups have made progress in identifying genes that contribute to the development of polygenic obesity in rodents (84,85,105,106). Both have used the technique of quantitative trace locus (QTL) mapping to identify chromosomal locations that are linked to phenotypic differences in body fat. Warden and colleagues (84,85) have used BSB mice (see above), and West and colleagues (103,105,106) have used crosses of two strains of mice that were either sensitive (AKR/J) or resistant (SWR/J) to developing obesity by feeding a high fat/condensed mild diet for 12 weeks. These two models have both identified loci on proximal chromosome 15 (MOB4 and DOB3) that are linked to either mesenteric fat (BSB mouse) or total adiposity (AKR × SWR cross). In the BSB mouse MOB1 on chromosome 7 close to *tub* is linked to carcass lipid and MOB2 on chromosome 6 close to *ob* is linked to subcutaneous fatpad weight. Other linkages MOB3 (chromosome 12) and DOB3 (chromosome 15) for body fat and MOB4 (chromosome 15) and DOB2 (chromosome 9) for mesenteric fat are not close to known obesity genes.

While none of these linkages have yet to be proven to be allelic variants of known obesity genes, these data do suggest that there may only be a limited number of genes that have a major influence on body composition and that various mutations of known obesity genes might increase the sensitivity to dietary obesity.

E. Genetics of Nonhuman Primate Obesity

As in humans, several studies of nonhuman primates have documented a familial association in the development of obesity. A mother-daughter pair were identified in the 1977 survey of *M. nigra* mentioned above (87), and Schwartz et al. (91) noted several primary familial relationships among the obese animals of the Cayo Santiago colony. Environmental factors, probably principally ready access to food, also influence the incidence of obesity, which has been reported to be 7% among the free-ranging Cayo Santiago colony (up to age 16), to 50% or more in individually housed animals in an age range up to 33 years.

Further support for a genetic basis to nonhuman primate obesity comes by inference from studies of groups of *M. mulatta* held under identical environmental and dietary conditions, in which some animals have become obese, while others have remained lean throughout their lives.

To date, no single gene-induced cases of obesity have been reported in nonhuman primates. Several candidate genes have, however, recently received special attention for their possible roles in obesity. With the discovery of the gene responsible for obesity in the *ob/ob* mouse, and the identification of the circulating protein leptin that it encodes, exploration of its possible role in the spontaneous obesity of monkeys has been initiated. Leptin has been hypothesized to be an adipocyte-derived circulating factor involved in body weight regulation. The *ob* cDNA of the monkey has been cloned from adipose tissue and shown to have at least 47 bp of 5′ noncoding region, 501 bp of coding region, and 219 bp of 3′ noncoding region (28). The ob mRNA is 0.8 kb long, which is shorter than that for rodents or humans due principally to a shorter 3′ noncoding region. The ob protein is 167 amino acids in length, as in humans and rodents, and has 93% amino acid similarity to human ob protein. Among a group of normal-weight 7-year-old monkeys, the level of ob mRNA in adipose tissue was correlated to body weight and body fat. In a larger group of older monkeys, ob mRNA was also correlated to body weight and to fasting plasma insulin (28). There was a tendency for ob mRNA to be increased in the hyperinsulinemic obese group of monkeys and reduced relative to normals in a group of diabetic animals that had previously lost body weight. In a larger group of older monkeys, ob mRNA tended to be increased in the hyperinsulinemic obese group of monkeys and reduced relative to normals in a group of diabetic animals that had previously lost body weight. In a larger group of older animals, plasma leptin levels were correlated to obesity; however, this association was found to be reduced due to a subgroup of animals showing no relation between body weight and leptin. In 10 of 13 older monkeys examined during the development of increasing body weight and increasing adiposity, an increase in circulating leptin was positively associated with the increase in body weight (136) as illustrated by the example of one monkey in Figure 2. Thus, leptin levels, and possibly the activity of the leptin receptor in the brain and more importantly its postreceptor signaling mechanism, are attractive targets for further examination of therapeutic potential in obesity.

The β_3-adrenergic receptor, which is specifically expressed in adipose tissue, has been sequenced in the rhesus monkey (137). It shows 95% amino acid identity with the human β_3-receptor, differing between species in 22 of 408 amino acids. The rhesus monkey receptor contains an arginine at position 64, producing an amino acid variant that has been found in greater frequency in several groups of humans with a high propensity to obesity. Further studies of the β_3-adrenoreceptor axis should be fruitful in determining the possible therapeutic potential of β_3-agonists in obesity.

Defects in the insulin molecule, the insulin receptor, and/or its variants have long been considered possible candidates for the underlying cause of insulin resistance and obesity. The insulin molecule of the monkey is identical in structure to that of human, and the proinsulin differs in only one amino acid (138). The monkey insulin

receptor has been cloned and sequenced and found to have 99% amino acid identity to that of human (139). The two identified nonconservative amino acid changes have been examined by site-directed mutagenesis of the human insulin receptor and found to have no effect on insulin receptor affinity or autophosphorylation, thus indicating that these are not responsible for the heightened insulin resistance of monkeys relative to humans (140).

Since obesity has not been shown to be associated with any defect in the insulin receptor structure, nor with a defective insulin molecule in most humans or monkeys (although there are a few well-documented cases of each of these defects in extreme cases of insulin resistance in humans), the possibility of a defect in expression of the major insulin receptor variants was considered. Recently, differential expression of the two primary naturally occurring variants of the insulin receptor has been proposed to be involved in insulin resistance. Huang et al. (141) studied the relative expression of the type A insulin receptor isoform lacking exon 11 and of the type B isoform containing exon 11 in muscle of monkeys. Increased expression of the type A (higher affinity) isoform was shown in obese hyperinsulinemic monkeys compared to either normal or to diabetic animals, indicating that alterations in the insulin receptor mRNA splicing may be involved in the mechanisms of insulin resistance.

Other candidate genes are being identified, and their study in spontaneously obese primates should offer insights into their potential roles in human obesity.

V. HYPOTHALAMIC OBESITY

It has long been recognized that destruction of or damage to the VMH is associated with the development of obesity in a wide range of animal species including mice, rats, dogs, nonhuman primates, and humans (1,2). The original studies suggested that the hyperphagia associated with major lesions in this area was the primary cause of the obesity, but subsequent studies in weanling rats (142) and with chemically induced lesions (143–145) (see below) indicated that the hyperphagia was not necessary. This was confirmed by Parkinson and Weingarten (146), who showed that discrete lesions localized to the VMN would cause obesity without hyperphagia and that hyperphagia was evident only when the lesions extended beyond the VMN, probably damaging the ventral noradrenergic bundle (VNAB) input to the paraventricular nucleus. Lesions to the VNAB cause mild hyperphagia (147) but none of the other changes in feeding behavior normally associated with VMH lesions (148).

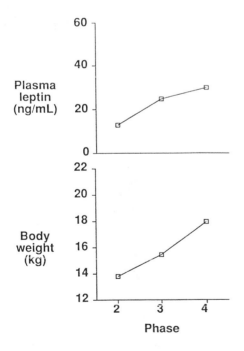

Figure 2 Change in plasma leptin with body weight (adiposity) in a single monkey.

VMH lesions can be caused by electrical, chemical (gold thioglucose, bipiperidyl mustard, monosodium glutamate, ibotenic acid), or viral (scrapie and Coxsackie virus) routes. Bipiperidyl mustard damages the VMH and dorsal vagal complex to produce obesity without hyperphagia (142,149), whereas monosodium glutamate, which damages the arcuate nucleus, induces hyperinsulinemia and obesity without hyperphagia (149,150). When these drugs are combined, the full hypothalamic syndrome of hyperphagia, hyperinsulinemia, and obesity is produced (150). However, ibotenic acid, which damages only neuronal cell bodies, does produce the full syndrome of hyperphagia and obesity after injection into the VMH (151). Thus, there appear to be two distinct syndromes of hypothalamic obesity. Damage restricted to the VMN normally produces obesity without hyperphagia as a result of changes in autonomic control of thermogenesis and insulin. In contrast, damage to neural pathways innervating the PVN or to the PVN itself predominantly causes a hyperphagic syndrome that may be related to changes in NPY and CRH activity (see below).

Electrical lesions of the paraventricular nucleus (PVN) or selective knife cuts in the hypothalamus may also induce an immediate increase in food intake and rapid development of severe obesity (1,2,152,153). Unlike VMH obesity, PVN obesity is prevented by restriction of food intake (152). These studies suggest that damage to the neuropeptide Y arcuate-PVN axis and the autonomic VMH center are required for development of the full hypothalamic obesity syndrome including hyperphagia, hyperinsulinemia, impaired sympathetic drive to BAT, and obesity. The involvement of these centers is further supported by the observations that chronic infusions of norepinephrine into the VMH but not the PVN and repeated injections of NPY into the PVN induce the rapid development of obesity (13–15,154). Indeed, overexpression and secretion of NPY may be a major stimulus to the development of obesity that is common to several models (155) (Fig. 1). Blockade of serotonin receptors (156) and damage to the ventral noraderenergic bundle by 6-hydroxydopamine (147,157) will also induce obesity.

Changes in autonomic activity that result from VMH lesions are primarily responsible for the alterations in peripheral metabolism (1,2,155). After VMH lesions, there is an increase in the activity of the afferent vagus innervation from the gastrointestinal tract (121) and the efferent vagal drive to the endocrine pancreas (121). The increase in insulin secretion that occurs within minutes of a VMH lesion is prevented by atropine (158) and prior subdiaphragmatic vagotomy prevents the hyperinsulinemic response to VMH lesions (159).

Initially a VMH-lesioned rat is very sensitive to this hyperinsulinemia, and both hepatic and adipose tissue lipogenesis and fat deposition are increased substantially (155,160). This, together with the reduced sympathetic drive to BAT and the consequent reduced level of thermogenesis (74,155,161,162), leads to a rapid increase in fat deposition and body weight. This is followed by the development of insulin resistance, initially in muscle and subsequently in adipose tissue and liver, that slows the weight gain until body weight plateaus at a much higher level (160).

VMH lesions reduce and VMH stimulation increases the sympathetic drive to BAT as assessed by a variety of methods, including direct electrical recording, norepinephrine turnover, and GDP binding by BAT mitochondria (1,2,163,164). The lesion apparently blocks selectively the ability of BAT to respond to signals associated with feeding and nutrient status since, like the obesity (165) of the fa/fa rat but not the ob/ob mouse (166), the BAT thermogenic response to hypothermia remains intact (162). However, the sympathetic drive to other tissues, e.g., liver and adrenal, may also be impaired since VMH-lesioned rats show a blunted increase in NEFA after glucoprivation and stress (161,167).

The metabolic, anthropometric, endocrine, and CNS changes observed in obesity that develops after VMH lesions are very similar to those observed in the genetic obesities of the fa/fa rat and ob/ob and db/db mice (1,2,155). These similarities have provided strong support for the belief that the gene defects of these models must affect hypothalamic function.

VI. ENDOCRINE OBESITY

Obesity can result from a number of endocrine manipulations, including peripheral injections of insulin (168) and excessive glucocorticoid activity resulting directly from hormone administration (72) or indirectly through transgenic overexpression of CRH (72). The most studied endocrine obesity is the result of ovariectomy, which will induce rapid weight gain and fat deposition in a number of species (169–172). This obesity may develop with hyperphagia, as in rats (169,173), or may develop without any increase in food intake, as in hamsters (171). The increase in food intake reflects the loss of the anorectic effect of estradiol, an effect mediated through the action of CRH (174). Estrogens also have direct effects on adipose tissue that favor fat deposition. Excessive secretion of epidermal growth factor (EGF) from salivary glands might also contribute to the development of this form of obesity (175). In the absence of hyperphagia, ovariectomy-induced obesity may result from reduction in BAT thermogenesis (173) or hepatic thermogenesis (171).

VII. FEATURES COMMON TO MANY MODELS OF OBESITY

A. Insulin Secretion

An enhanced secretion of insulin is a common characteristic of all the rodent obesities with the possible exception of the high-fat-fed dietary obesity (1,2) and the obesity that develops after surgical production of hypothalamic islands (176). This increase in insulin appears to be essential for the development of obesity (177) and, together with the excessive glucocorticoid stimulation, is responsible for the excessive fat deposition (178). In the single-gene mutations of *fa/fa* rat and *ob/ob* and *db/db* mice, increased insulin secretion is one of the earliest detectable abnormalities. In contrast, obesity may develop in monkeys without hyperinsulinemia (11).

The β-cells of both young *ob/ob* mice and *fa/fa* rats appear to have a normal secretory response to glucose and arginine but show both an increased sensitivity and increased responsiveness to the cholecystokinin (CCK) and acetylcholine (ACh) potentiation of glucose-induced insulin secretion (179,180). Since both CCK and ACh activate the phospholipase C signaling pathway, this may indicate some abnormality in this system that might be consequent to the enhanced vagal drive to the tissue. With increasing age, the pancreatic β-cells also show a reduced threshold to glucose stimulation, which leads to hyperinsulinemic response at low glucose levels. Adrenalectomy reduces insulin levels of obese animals and normalizes the glucose threshold for response. Since the direct effect of glucocorticoids in β-cells is to increase glucose cycling and reduce insulin secretion (181,182), it would appear that the glucocorticoid stimulation of insulin secretion that is evident in obese models is affected through the central regulation of autonomic drive to the pancreas. This has been confirmed in both *fa/fa* rats (183) and *ob/ob* mice (184). However, adrenalectomy does not normalize the response of perfused islets of *ob/ob* mice to ACh, suggesting that a factor other than vagal drive affects this signaling pathway. The identity of such a factor is unclear at present. Sympathetic drive to the pancreas is impaired in both VMH obesity (185) and genetic obesity (186,187), and removal of this β2-adrenergic inhibition might contribute to the enhanced insulin secretion. Alternatively, it is possible that a circulating factor such as leptin might modulate the sensitivity of β-cells to neural signals. This possibility will, no doubt, be investigated in the near future. Evidence for the importance of blood flow changes

in the pancreas has been presented by Atef et al. (188), who showed that the increased blood flow to islets of *fa/fa* and VMH rats was reversed by either vagotomy or treatment with the α2-adrenergic agonist clonidine. Other peptides might also be important modulators of the hyperinsulinemia. The pancreas from both Zucker obese (*fa/fa*) and the corpulent allele (*fa^{cp}/fa^{cp}*) shows exaggerated insulin secretory responses to the gastric inhibitory peptide GIP (189).

Obese monkeys, followed longitudinally, show a gradual slow decline in glucose tolerance, a decline that begins many years before the development of overt diabetes (190). This deterioration takes place at the same time as pancreatic insulin output is increased both basally and under stimulated conditions. β-Cell hyperresponsiveness to a glucose load has been shown to be a very early defect in obesity, possibly preceding the development of significant insulin resistance and hyperinsulinemia (191). The sequence of these progressive changes in body weight, glucose tolerance, pancreatic function and insulin sensitivity is shown in Figure 3. In obese monkeys, prior to

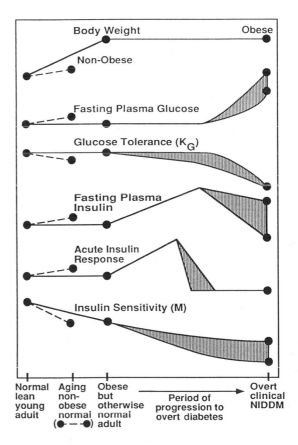

Figure 3 Progression of the development of glucose intolerance and diabetes with age and body weight in monkeys.

the development of overt diabetes, de Koning et al. (192) have found beginning changes in pancreatic β-cells, with proliferation of β-cell mass, and small deposits of islet-associated polypeptide as islet amyloid.

The insulin resistance is not a requirement for the development of obesity in rodents or primates. Furthermore, the hepatic insulin resistance as evidenced by the failure of insulin to suppress hepatic glucose production is not associated with obesity per se, but has been directly related to the subsequent development of overt NIDDM in monkeys (193) and insulin hypersecretion in Zucker *fa/fa* rats (194).

Reduced hepatic extraction of insulin has also been shown to be involved in sustaining hyperinsulinemia (92). Nevertheless, this reduction does not appear to be primary, occurring only as insulin levels increase above a portal insulin level of 700–1000 pmol/L (peripheral insulin level of greater than 350 pmol/L). Thus at the early stages in the development of both obesity and hyperinsulinemia, there appears to be no defect in hepatic insulin uptake (proportionate removal of ~34% of portal insulin across a range of insulin levels), while in severe hyperinsulinemia, hepatic insulin uptake is increased, but not sufficiently to prevent hyperinsulinemia (195).

B. Sexual Dimorphism of Diabetes

The incidence and severity of diabetes between the obese animal models shows large variations between the models, with background strain upon which a gene is expressed, and is often sexually dimorphic. Obese *ob/ob* and diabetes *db/db* mice have pronounced hyperglycemia and diabetes on the C57Bl/KsJ background strain but relatively mild diabetes on the C57Bl/6J background (37). In Yellow A^y/*a* mice, only the males are hyperglycemic although both sexes are hyperinsulinemic compared to their lean littermates (59). A similar sexual dimorphism in the expression of diabetes is observed in the Wistar Kyoto diabetic (WDF-TA-*fa*) rat (50). This variability in the diabetes is thought to reflect pleiotropic interactions of the obesity genes with other genes. Androgens potentiate stroptozotocin-induced diabetes whereas estrogens attenuate the diabetes (196). More recent work has suggested that differential hepatic metabolism of steroids is an important factor determining the diabetic status (Fig. 4). Sulfuration of androgenic and estrogenic steroids by specific sulfotransferase enzymes in the liver renders the steroids more hydrophilic and unable to bind to their appropriate receptor. The development of diabetes has been linked to the presence of high ratios of hepatic estrogen sulfotransferase (EST) to dehydroepiandrosterone androgen sulfo-

transferase (DST) activities, i.e., to androgenization of the liver. This ratio is high in male mice and in female mice that develop diabetes, but not in female obese mice that have normoglycemia in both the diabetes (*db/db*) (191) and Yellow (A^y/*a*) (59) mice. It is also elevated in both male and female *ob/ob* mice that develop severe diabetes (198). Other sulfurotransferases do not appear to be modified in obese-diabetic animals (199).

Temporal studies of the development of diabetes suggest that the hyperinsulinemia associated with obesity is not responsible for the hepatic androgenization of metabolism (197). The absence of any changes in sulfurylation activity in *fat/fat* mice despite their hyperinsulinemia supports this conclusion (198). However, there is substantial evidence to link the changes in hepatic metabolism of steroids to the hypersecretion of adrenal glucocorticoids.

Dexamethasone treatment of normoglycemic female obese viable Yellow (A^{vy}/*a*) mice induced severe hyperglycemia associated with induction of EST gene transcription and a large increase in enzyme activity (59). This effect was reversible on termination of the dexamethasone treatment. In *db/db* mice, hepatic EST gene transcription was elevated in both sexes and there was an additional suppression of DST gene transcription in females (199) that was reflected in parallel changes in enzyme activity. Indeed, in lean mice, Leiter and Chapman (199) were unable to detect any EST mRNA transcripts in the liver RNA although the gene is expressed constitutively in the testes where it is unaffected by the *db/db* genotype (200). Thus the interaction of hypercorticosteronemia, an appropriate background genome, and the obesity genes appears to determine hepatic glucose metabolism and diabetes through their effects in modulating sulfurylation of androgens and estrogens.

Obesity in male monkeys has been associated with abnormal androgen metabolism, with obese males having lower serum testosterone and lower dihydrotestosterone than lean males (201). Females had lower serum androgen levels than males, but there were no differences between obese and lean females. Gonadectomy in male and in female monkeys reduced body weight relative to intact animals; however, replacement therapy with testosterone propionate or dihydrotestosterone propionate resulted in an increase in lean body mass, but not in adiposity (202).

C. Insulin Resistance

In obesity, defects in insulin action, whole-body insulin resistance, and hyperinsulinemia are characteristic. Intracellularly, insulin insensitivity is selectively expressed on specific pathways, e.g., gluconeogenesis but not lipoge-

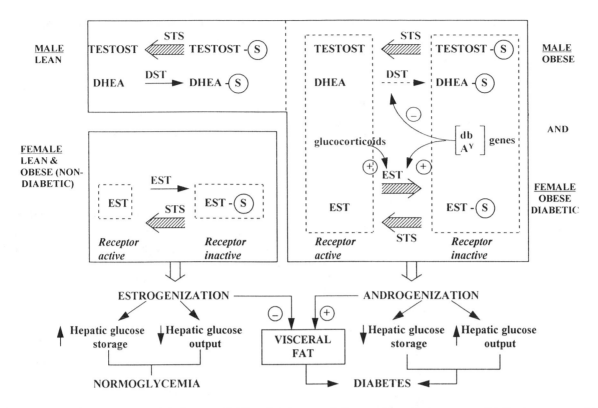

Figure 4 Hepatic androgenization and diabetes in *db/db* and A^y/*a* mice. Sulfation of steroids increases solubility but prevents binding to the steroid receptor. High levels of sex steroid transferase (STS) and low dehydroepiandrosterone (DHEA) sulfotransferase (DST) activity in males and estrogen sulfotransferase (EST) activity in females maintain the androgenic and estrogenic states, respectively, in males and females. In obese males and obese females that become diabetic, inhibition of DST and activation of EST promote androgenization. This alters the balance between hepatic glucose storage and output, promotes the deposition of visceral fat, and leads to the development of diabetes. S, sulfate; EST, estrogen; TESTOST, testosterone.

nesis in liver (203,204). The temporal sequence of these changes has been well documented, the hyperinsulinemia preceding the insulin resistance in rodents, although this sequence is less clear in nonhuman primates (see 1,2,155 for reviews). Insulin resistance appears initially in muscle although neither glucose transport levels nor glucose transporter 4 (Glut 4) levels change unless there is accompanying diabetes (205–207). Adipocytes are initially hyperresponsive to insulin, but insulin insensitivity develops later when a reduction in Glut 4 transporters and mRNA is common (208–210). The reduction in Glut 4 levels in BAT at an early age may be an important factor contributing to the impaired thermogenesis (207). Despite the similarity of the responses between different obese models, the mechanisms underlying the changes may not be identical. Thus the muscle insulin resistance of high-fat-fed rats is associated with a reduction in the intrinsic activity of the Glut 4 transporter (211), whereas that in the obese *fa/fa* rat has been liked to a failure to translocate the Glut

4 transporters to the plasma membrane after insulin stimulation (212), although this has subsequently been distributed (213,214). The excess production of TNF-α by adipose tissue (19), which represses Glut 4 gene transcription (215), has been proposed to be a causative factor in the development of insulin resistance and diabetes. However, it is clear that insulin resistance is secondary to the obese state and does not cause obesity (216).

D. In Vivo Metabolic and Endocrine Defects Associated with Obesity and Diabetes in Primates

Abdominal obesity in humans, as well as in monkeys, has been shown to be associated with diabetes mellitus. Monkeys with central or abdominal obesity could be classified as insulin-sensitive or insulin-resistant and showed a strong linear relationship between abdominal circumference and fasting plasma insulin and an inverse relationship with insulin resistance. Within the obese group there was, however, a diversity of degrees of insulin resistance (92).

In primates, spontaneous obesity has been shown to be associated with an increased frequency of dyslipidemia. Monkeys, like humans, show individual variability in susceptibility to diet-induced or spontaneous atherosclerosis (217), and these primates develop atherosclerotic lesions similar to humans (218). There was, however, in this study no significant relationship between abdominal circumference and the various lipoprotein fractions. Hannah et al. (219) showed that obese hyperinsulinemic normoglycemic monkeys have beginning increases in VLDL triglycerides, small reductions in HDL cholesterol, and no change in LDL cholesterol. This dyslipidemia was significantly exacerbated in those monkeys with NIDDM, as shown in Figure 5.

As previously described, many, but not all, obese monkeys go on to develop impaired glucose tolerance and then progress to overt NIDDM (12,86). This longitudinal process was first described by Hamilton and Ciaccia (220) as a period of middle-aged obesity and normal glucose tolerance associated with hyperinsulinemia, followed by glucose intolerance and frank diabetes. The progressive process was further defined as a series of successive phases leading from normal lean young animals to older monkeys with or without obesity (221). Among the obese, some then progress through successive phases of increasing hperinsulinemia and insulin resistance, progressive impairment of glucose tolerance, and finally, overt diabetes (221). Glucose tolerance, one measure of this progressive process, has been calculated using a number of different formulas, the optimal of which is defined by the slope of the decline of the $\log_e$ plasma glucose per minute between the time points 5 and 20 min of an intravenous glucose tolerance test using a glucose load of 0.25 g/kg body weight. This time period was determined to be optimally applicable to monkeys across the entire range of tolerance from young normal to severe diabetic (89). Kemnitz et al. (201,202) showed that during pregnancy, a deterioration of glucose tolerance and an increase in fasting plasma insulin levels occur in the monkeys in the highest preconception tertile of adiposity.

E. Hyperphagia/Autonomic Dysfunction

All animal obesities appear to be characterized by an imbalance between food intake and specific components of autonomic activity (1,2). Extensive literature now documents the close reciprocal integration between food intake and the sympathetic components (brown adipose tissue and heart) that regulate thermogenesis (74,222). This relationship holds constant over a wide range of experimental manipulations and pathological changes, including the response to various drugs, hormones, and neuropeptides, to metabolites and antimetabolites, and in comparisons of obese animals with their lean littermates. Indeed, Himms-Hagen has recently reemphasized the thermogenic regulation of feeding by relating changes in heat production resulting from the sympathetically mediated brown adipose tissue thermogenesis to initiation and termination of feeding (75). This hypothesis proposes that heat production (or the resulting temperature of a specific tissue, e.g., hypothalamus) acts as the afferent signal to regulate feeding. The attenuation of the CRF inhibition of food intake by the ganglionic blocker chlorisondamine (223) also supports this hypothesis. However, our studies of the dose-response relationship on the acute effects of β-adrenergic subtype agonists on food intake and metabolic rate do not support the proposal that a feedback relationship between that heat production on food intake can explain the reciprocal control of feeding and sympathetic drive to BAT (224). Rather they suggests that effectors may separately modulate these two pathways, or that this reciprocal control is modulated over a longer time frame.

F. Glucocorticoid Regulation of CNS Function in Obesity

The critical requirement for the presence of glucocorticoids for the development of obesity has been demonstrated in a wide range of the rodent models of obesity (1,2,225). Adrenalectomy will prevent the further development of the obese state in the genetic obesities (fa/fa, ob/ob, db/db, A^y/a), in hypothalamic obesity (VMH and PVN damage), and in dietary, viral, and endocrine forms of obesity (112,169,226–232). The effect may be reversed by glucocorticoid replacement. This effect can be observed at a number of levels; at the level of the animal food intake, body weight gain and fat deposition are normalized; at the system level, both the attenuated sympathetic and elevated parasympathetic activities are normalized (182,226,233); at the tissue level, hepatic and adipose tissue lipogenesis, hepatic gluconeogenesis, muscle glucose uptake, and insulin sensitivity are restored (234–236); at the molecular level, the expression of a range of genes [e.g., the overexpression of NPY mRNA in the hypothalamus (237), and tyrosine aminotransferase in the liver (238)]. The majority, but not all, of the physiological and metabolic changes associated with obesity are corrected by removal of adrenal steroids.

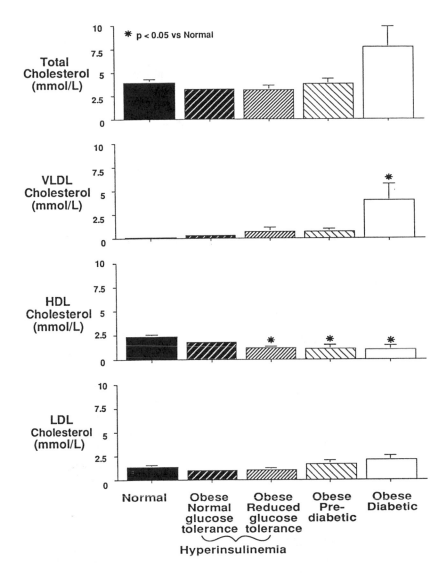

Figure 5 The development of dyslipidemia in monkeys.

Within the CNS, glucocorticoids may bind to both type I (mineralocorticoid) and type II (glucocorticoid) receptors. Although type I receptor activity may be important for regulation of food intake and growth in lean rats, type II receptor activity is required for energy storage as fat (239). This is consistent with the ability to block the development of both genetic and dietary obesity with the type II glucocorticoid receptor antagonist RU38-486 (117,240) and by the maintenance of hyperphagia, hyperinsulinemia, and weight gain of adrenalectomized VMH-lesioned rats with a type II receptor agonist (241).

The central effects of glucocorticoids have been shown to regulate the autonomic imbalance and hyperphagia common to obese rodents (Fig. 1). Adrenalectomy normalizes autonomic activity and food intake. Chronic central administration of the type II agonist dexamethasone to adrenalectomized *fa/fa* rats restores the vagally dependent hypersecretion of insulin to a glucose load (183). In *ob/ob* mice, glucocor0toids acutely (within 30 min) suppress sympathetic drive to BAT and enhance insulin secretion (184), suggesting that these responses are nongenomic and possibly mediated through the reciprocal regulation of CRH secretion. CRH is a potent stimulator of sympathetic drive to BAT and inhibits vagally mediated insulin secretion and food intake (183,186,242,243). Chronic administration of CRH intracerebroventricularly prevents or reverses the development of obesity, the hyperphagia, and the autonomic imbalance in *fa/fa* rats and in VMH-lesioned obese rats (186,244,245) at doses of CRH too low to activate the pituitary-adrenal axis (246).

Despite the attraction of this neuroendocrine hypothesis (247), the evidence for a diminished secretion of CRF in obese animals is not compelling. Indeed, the hypothalamic-pituitary-adrenal axis appears to be activated in several models of obesity, particularly in response to stress (225,248), and the normal diurnal cycle of serum corticosterone is frequently absent (1,2). Neither CRF nor arginine vasopressin levels are altered in the hypothalamus or pituitary of obese *fa/fa* rats (225,249). PVN-lesioned obese rats are also responsive to adrenalectomy (230) although the PVN is the only central site in which CRH production is sensitive to glucocorticoid levels (250). Nevertheless, excessive secretion of CRF into the hypophyseal-portal circulation of obese rats in comparison to lean rats after adrenalectomy (248) is suggestive of an attenuated glucocorticoid inhibition of CRH production in this form of obesity. The excessive levels of NPY and NPY mRNA that have been described in the PVN-arcuate axis of several obese models (251–254) are also consistent with excessive glucocorticoid activity that may be mediated indirectly through CRH or by the promotion of central insulin insensitivity (255; Woods S. and Chavez M., personal communication) since insulin and CRH appear to be physiological signals that can acutely regulate NPY production and secretion (256–260). Leptin also appears to inhibit NPY release and reduce prepro-NPY mRNA levels (254), although the mechanism of this effect is not yet clear. The high levels of NPY mRNA in diabetes *db/db* mice, which have a leptin receptor defect, are not reduced by chronic peripheral administration of leptin. Hence, the absence of leptin or the inability to respond to leptin because of receptor defects or other signaling factors might be the primary cause of the enhanced NPY activity that is common to the genetic obesities (Fig. 4). In contrast, the hyperphagia and obesity associated with feeding highly palatable diets may not be related to increased NPY synthesis and secretion (261).

There is also increasing evidence for elevated genomic responses to glucocorticoids in the CNS and in peripheral tissues. The activities of a number of glucocorticoid responsive enzymes are elevated (64,262,263), and this may well reflect an increase in gene transcription. This increase in sensitivity and responsiveness to glucocorticoids appears to be a characteristic of all obesities (1,2,225), but the causes of this have been unclear until recently. Increased levels of glucocorticoid type II (GR) receptors or altered affinity (K_d) of receptors has been reported for some brain regions of *fa/fa* rats (261,264). However, the

decreased level of cytosolic GR receptors in peripheral tissues of *ob/ob* mice and *fa/fa* rats (265,266) was not consistent with an exaggerated response to glucocorticoid stimulation. This apparent anomaly may have been clarified by recent observations on the liver of *fa/fa* rats (263) that suggest that GR gene transcription is increased and that increased synthesis of GR protein is associated with a concentration of GR in the hepatic nuclei rather than in the cytosol fraction. These data suggest that an abnormality in GR protein cycling between cytosol and nuclear compartments may play a role in the glucocorticoid sensitivity of all obese models.

G. Prevention of Obesity in Nonhuman Primates Having a High Propensity to Develop Obesity

Obesity is well recognized to be closely associated with the development of type II non-insulin-dependent diabetes mellitus in humans and in nonhuman primates. A long-term study, still ongoing, has attempted to prevent the development of adult-onset obesity in a group of monkeys through a calorie titration regimen in which calories have been adjusted weekly on an individual animal basis to prevent the development of obesity or weight gain. Thus, under this protocol, any gain of weight was met with a reduction in allocated calories, and conversely, weight loss was the trigger for increasing the calories allowed to each adult animal. Primary prevention of obesity in adult rhesus monkeys has been shown to powerfully and completely prevent the development of NIDDM (264). At the least, the onset of overt diabetes has been indefinitely delayed. Chronic long-term restriction of calories to prevent the development of obesity appears to have major effects on several metabolic pathways and on insulin action. The development of insulin resistance has been shown to be mitigated (267), and plasma insulin levels were reduced by calorie restriction (256). Basal glycogen synthase activity was greatly increased above the levels of normal lean young monkeys, and the normal effect of insulin to activate glycogen synthase was absent in the calorie-restricted monkeys. The change in glycogen synthase activity was inversely related to the change in glycogen phosphorylase activity. Nevertheless, despite prevention of the development of obesity, calorie restriction appeared to unmask some early defects potentially associated with the propensity to ultimately develop obesity.

REFERENCES

1. Bray GA, York DA, Fisler JS. Experimental obesity: a homeostatic failure due to defective nutrient stimulation of

the sympathetic nervous system. Vitamins Hormones 1990; 45:1–125.

2. Bray GA, Fisler JS, York DA. Neuroendocrine control of the development of obesity: understanding gained from studies of experimental models of obesity. Prog Neuroendocrinol 1990; 4:128–181.

3. Bultman SJ, Michaud EJ, Woychik RP. Molecular characterization of the mouse agouti locus. Cell 1992; 71: 1195–1204.

4. Zhang Y, Proenca R, Maffei M, Barone M, Leopold L, Friedman JM. Positional cloning of the mouse obese gene and its human homologue. Nature (Lond) 1994; 372: 425–432.

5. Naggert JK, Fricker LD, Varlamov O, Nishina PM, Rouille Y, Steiner DF, Carroll RJ, Paigen BJ, Leiter EH. Hyperproinsulinaemia in obese fat/fat mice associated with a carboxypeptidase E mutation which reduces enzyme activity. Nature Genet 1995; 10:135–142.

6. Lowell BB, S-Susulic V, Hamann A, Lawitts JA, Himms-Hagen J, Boyers BB, Kozak LP, Flier JS. Development of obesity in transgenic mice after genetic ablation of brown adipose tissue. Nature (Lond) 1993; 366:740–742.

7. Pepin M-C, Pothier F, Barden N. Impaired type II glucocorticoid-receptor function in mice bearing antisense RNA transgene. Nature (Lond) 1992; 355:725–727.

8. Shepherd PR, Gnudi L, Tozzo E, Yang H, Leach F, Kahn BB. Adipose cell hyperplasia and enhanced glucose disposal in transgenic mice overexpressing GLUT 4 selectively in adipose tissue. J Biol Chem 1993; 268: 22243–22246.

9. Sclafani A. Dietary obesity models. In: Björntorp P, Brodoff BN, eds. Obesity. Philadelphia: JB Lippincott, 1992: 241–248.

10. Schemmel R, Mickelson O, Gill J. Dietary obesity in rats: body weight and fat accretion in seven strains of rat. J Nutr 1970; 100:1041–1048.

11. Hansen BC, Bodkin NL, Jen K-LC, Ortmeyer HK. Primate models of diabetes. In: H Rifkin, Colwell JA, Taylor SI, eds. Diabetes. Amsterdam, The Netherlands: Elsevier Science, 1991:587–590.

12. Hansen BC. Obesity and diabetes in monkeys. In: Björntorp P, Brodoff BN, eds. Obesity. Philadelphia: JB Lippincott 1992:256–265.

13. Beck B, Sticker-Krongrad A, Nicolas JP, Burlet C. Chronic and continuous intracerebroventricular infusion of neuropeptide Y in Long-Evans rats mimics the feeding behavior of obese Zucker rats. Int J Obes 1992; 16: 295–302.

14. Zarjevskin, Cusin I, Vettor R, Rohner-Jeanrenaud F, Jeanrenaud B. Chronic intracerebroventricular neuropeptide-Y/administration to normal rats mimics hormonal and metabolic change of obesity. Endocrinology 1993; 133: 1753–1758.

15. Shimazu T, Noma M, Saito M. Chronic infusion of norepinephrine ito the ventromedial hypothalamus induces obesity in rats. Brain Res 1986; 369:215–223.

16. Morrison P, Galster W. Patterns of hibernation in the arctic ground squirrel. Can J Zool 1975; 53:1345–1355.

17. Kemnitz JW, Goy RW, Filtsch TJ, Lohmiller JJ, Robinson JA. Obesity in male and female rhesus monkeys: fat distribution, glucoregulation, and serum androgen levels. J Clin Endocrinol Metab 1989; 69:287–293.

18. Bouchard C, Perusse L. Current status of the human obesity gene map. Obes Res 1997 (in press).

19. Hotamisligil GS, Shargill NS, Spiegelman BM. Adipose expression of tumor necrosis factor-*a*: direct role in obesity-linked insulin resistance. Science 1993; 259:87–91.

20. Yamakawa T, Tanaka S, Yamakawa Y, Kiucchi Y, Isoda F, Kawamoto S, Okuda K, Sekihara H. Augmented production of tumor necrosis factor-*a* in obese mice. Clin Immunol Immunopathol 1995; 75:51–56.

21. Flier JS, Cook KS, Usher P, Speigelman BM. Severely impaired adipsin expression in genetic and acquired obesity. Science 1987; 237:405–408.

22. Cox CE, Powley TL. Development of obesity in diabetic mice pair fed with lean siblings. J Comp Physiol Psychol 1977; 91:347–358.

23. Dubuc P. Effects of limited food intake in the obese-hyperglycemic syndrome. Am J Physiol 1976; 230: 1474–1479.

24. Bray GA, York DA, Swerdloff RW. Genetic obesity in rats: I. The effects of food restriction on body composition and hypothalamic function. Metabolism 1973; 22:435–442.

25. Tomita T, Doull V, Pollock HG, Krizsan D. Pancreatic islets of obese hyperglycemic mice (*ob/ob*). Pancreas 1992; 7: 367–375.

26. Murakami T, Shima K. Cloning of rat obese cDNA and its expression in obese rats. Biochem Biophys Res Commun 1995; 209:944–952.

27. Funahashi T, Shimomura I, Hiracka H, Arai T, Takahashi M, Nakamura T, Nozaki S, Yamashita S, Takemura K, Tokunaga K, Matsuzawa Y. Enhanced expression of rat obese (*ob*) gene in adipose tissues of ventromedial hypothalamus (VMH)-lesioned rats. Biochem Biophys Res Commun 1995; 211:469–475.

28. Hotta K, Gustafson TA, Ortmeyer HK, Bodkin NL, Hansen BC. Structure and expression of the monkey obese (*ob*) mRNA. Exp Biol 1996 (in press).

29. Lin X, York DA, Harris RBS, Bray GA, Bruch RL. The effect of adrenalectomy and glucocorticoid replacement on Ob mRNA levels in adipose tissue of obese Zucker *fa/fa* rats. Obes Res 1995; 3:339s.

30. Lin X, York DA, Harris RBS, Bruch RL. The effect of high fat diets on expression of OB mRNA in a model of diet-induced obesity. Obes Res 1995; 3:389s.

31. Smith SR, Ramsay TG, Harris RB. Ob mRNA is responsive to insulin status in diabetic rats. Obes Res 1995; 3:389s.

32. Saladin R, De Vos P, Guerre-Millo Leturque A, Girard J, Staels B, Auwerx J. Transient increase in obese gene expression after food intake or insulin administration. Nature (Lond) 1995; 377:527–529.

33. De Vos P, Saladin R, Auwerx J, Staels B. Induction of ob gene expression by corticosteroids is accompanied by body weight loss and reduced food intake. J Biol Chem 1995; 270:15958–15961.

34. Trayhurn P, Duncan JS, Rayner DV. Acute cold-induced suppression of ob (obese) gene expression in white adipose tissue of mice: mediation by the sympathetic system. Biochem J 1995; 311:729–733.

35. Tartaglia LA, Dembski M, Weng X, Dang N, Culpepper J, Devos R, Richards GJ, Campfield LA, Clark FT, Deeds J, Muir C, Sanker S, Moriarty A, Moore KJ, Smutko JS, Mays GG, Woolf EA, Monroe CA, Tepper RI. Identification and expression cloning of a leptin receptor, Ob-R. Cell 1995; 83:1–20.

36. Schwartz MW, Figlewicz DP, Baskin DG, Woods SC, Porte Jr D. Insulin in the brain: a hormonal regulator of energy balance. Endocr Rev 1992; 13:387–414.

37. Coleman DL. Obesity and diabetes: two mutant genes causing diabetes-obesity syndromes in mice. Diabetologia 1978; 14:141–148.

38. Harris RB, Hervey E, Hervey GR, Tobin G. Body composition of lean and obese Zucker rats in parabiosis. Int J Obes 1987; 11:275–283.

39. Campfield LA, Smith FJ, Guisez Y, Devos R, Burn P. Recombinant mouse ob protein: evidence for a peripheral signal linking adiposity and central neural networks. Science 1995; 269:546–549.

40. Halaas JL, Gajiwala KS, Maffei M, Cohen SL, Chait BT, Rabinowitz D, Lallone RL, Burley SK, Friedman JM. Weight-reducing effects of the plasma protein encoded by the obese gene. Science 1995; 269:543–546.

41. Pelleymounter MA, Cullen MJ, Baker MB, Hecht R, Winters D, Boone T, Collins F. Effects of the obese gene product on body weight regulation in ob/ob mice. Science 1995; 269:540–543.

42. Ohshima K, Shargill NS, Cham TM, Bray GA. Effect of dexamethasone on glucose transport by skeletal muscles of obese (ob/ob) mice. Int J Obes 1989; 13:155–163.

43. Friedman JM, Leibel RL, Bahary N. Molecular mapping of obesity genes. Mamm Genome 1991; 1:130–144.

44. Coleman DL, Hummel KP. The influence of genetic background on the expression of the obese (ob) gene in the mouse. Diabetologia 1973; 9:287–293.

45. Lee G-H, Proenca R, Montez JM, Carol KM, Darvishzadeh JG, Lee JI, Freidman JM. Abnormal splicing of the leptin receptor in diabetic mice. Nature (Lond) 1996; 379:632–635.

46. Chen H, Charlat O, Tartaglia LA, Woolf EA, Weng X, Ellis SJ, Lakey ND, Culpepper J, Moore KJ, Breitbart RE, Duyk GM, Tepper RI, Morgenstern JP. Evidence that the diabetes gene encodes the leptin receptor: identification of a mutation in the leptin receptor gene in db/db mice. Cell 1996; 84:491–495.

47. Zucker LM, Zucker FT. Fatty, a new mutation in the rat. J Hered 1961; 52:275–278.

48. Truett GE, Bahary N, Friedman JM. Rat obesity gene fatty (fa) maps to chromosome 5: evidence for homology with the mouse gene diabetes (db). Proc Natl Acad Sci USA 1991; 88:7806–7809.

49. Truett, GE, Tempelman RJ, Walker JA. Codominant effects of the fatty (fa) gene during early development of obesity. Am J Physiol 1995; 168:E15–E20.

50. Shafrir E. Animal models of non-insulin-dependent diabetes. Diabetes Metab Revs 1992; 8:179–208.

51. Bazin R, Eteve D, Lavau M. Evidence for decreased GDP binding to brown adipose tissue mitochondria of obese (fa/fa) Zucker rats in the very first days of life. Biochem J 1984; 221:241–245.

52. Kortner G, Petrova O, Vogt S, Schmidt I. Sympathetically and nonsympathetically mediated onset of excess fat deposition in Zucker rats. Am J Physiol 1994; 267:E947–953.

53. Markewicz B, Kuhmichel G, Schmidt I. Onset of excess fat deposition in Zucker rats with and without decreased thermogenesis. Am J Physiol 1993; 265:E478–E486.

54. Bray GA, York DA, Swerdoff RW. Genetic obesity in rats. I. The effects of food restriction on body composition and hypothalamic function. Metabolism 1973; 22:435–442.

55. Coleman DL, Eicher EM. Fat (fat) and Tubby (tub): Two autosomal recessive mutations causing obesity syndromes in the mouse. J Hered 1990; 81:424–427.

56. Bray GA, York DA. Hypothalamic and genetic obesity in experimental animals. Physiol Rev 1979; 59:719–809.

57. Butler L, Gerritsen GC. A comparison of the modes of inheritance of diabetes in the Chinese hamster and KK mouse. Diabetologia 1970; 6:163–167.

58. Wolff GC. Body composition and coat color correlation in different phenotypes of "viable yellow" mice. Science 1965; 147:1145–1147.

59. Gill AM, Leiter EH, Powell JG, et al. Dexamethasone-induced hyperglycemia in obese A^{vy}/a (viable yellow) female mice entails preferential induction of hepatic estrogen sulfotransferase. Diabetes 1994; 43:999–1004.

60. Wolff GL, Flack JD. Genetic regulation of plasma corticosterone concentration and its response to castration and allogenic tumor growth in the mouse. Nature New Biol 1971; 232:181–182.

61. Perry W, Hustad C, Swing D, Jenkins N, Copeland N. A transgenic mouse assay for agouti protein activity. Genetics 1995; 140:267–274.

62. Klebig ML, Wilkinson JE, Geisler JG, Woychik RP. Ectopic expression of the agouti gene in transgenic mice causes obesity, features of type II diabetes, and yellow fur. Proc Natl Acad Sci USA 1995; 92:4728–4732.

63. Wilson BD Ollman MM Kany L, Stoffer M, Bell GI, Barsch GS. Structure and function of ASP, the human homolog of the mouse agouti gene. Hum Mol Genet 1995; 4:223–230.

64. Zemel MB, Kim JH, Woychik RP, et al. Agouti regulation of intracellular calcium: role in the insulin resistance of viable yellow mice. Proc Natl Acad Sci USA 1995; 92:4733–4737.

65. Lu D, Willard D, Patel IR, Kadwell S, Overton L, Kost T, Luther M, Chen W, Woychik RP, Wilkison WO, Cone RD. Agouti protein as an antagonist of the melanocyte-stimulating-hormone receptor. Nature (Lond) 1994; 371: 799–802.

66. Shimizu H, Shimomura Y, Uekara Y, et al. Reduced pituitary acetylation and possible role of hypothalamic monoamines in the yellow obese mouse. Neuroendocrinol Lett 1990; 12:31–42.

67. Tsujii S, Bray GA. Acetylation alters the feeding response to MSH and beta-endorphin. Brain Res Bull 1989; 23: 165–169.

68. Shimizu H, Shargill NS, Bray GA, Yen FT, Geselchen PD. Effects of MSH on food intake, body weight and coat color of the yellow obese mouse. Life Sci 1989; 45: 543–552.

69. Nakamura M, Yamada K. Studies on a diabetic (KK) strain in the mouse. Diabetologia 1967; 3:212–221.

70. Pepin M-C, Barden N. Decreased glucocorticoid receptor activity following glucocorticoid receptor antisense RNA gene fragment transfection. Mol Cell Biol 1991; 1647–1653.

71. Richard D, Chapdelaine S, Deshaies Y, Pepin M-C, Barden N. Energy balance and lipid metabolism in transgenic mice bearing an antisense GCR gene construct. Am J Physiol 1993; R146–R150.

72. Stenzel-Poore MP, Cameron VA, Vaughan J, Sawchenko PE, Vale W. Development of Cushing s syndrome in corticotropin-releasing factor transgenic mice. Endocrinology 1992; 130:3378–3386.

73. Ikemoto S, Thompson KS, Takahashi M, Itakura H, Lane MD, Ezaki O. High fat diet-induced hyperglycemia: prevention by low level expression of a glucose transporter (GLUT4) minigene in transgenic mice. Proc Natl Acad Sci USA 1995; 92:3096–3099.

74. Bray GA. Reciprocal relation between the sympathetic nervous system and food intake. Brain Res Bull 1991; 27: 517–520.

75. Himms-Hagen J. Role of brown adipose tissue termogenesis in control of thermoregulatory feeding in rats. A new hypothesis that links thermostatic and glucostatic hypotheses for control of food intake. Proc Soc Exp Biol Med 1995; 208:159–169.

76. Ross SR, Graves RA, Spiegelman BM. Targeted expression of a toxin gene to adipose tissue: transgenic mice resistant to obesity. Genes Dev 1993; 7:1318–1324.

77. Susalic VS, Ito M, Grujick D, Frederich RC, Lawitts JA, Tozzo E, Kahn BB, Harper ME, Himms-hagen J, Flier J, Lowell BB. Knockout of β_3-adrenergic receptor gene. Obes Res 1995; 3 Suppl 3:319s.

78. Galvin-Parton PA, Chen X, Moxham CM, Malbon CC. Induction of Gq alpha specific antisense RNA in vivo causes obesity and hyperadiposity. Obes Res 1995; 3(Suppl 3): 313s.

79. Schmidt-Neilsen K, Haines HB, Haskel DB. Diabetes mellitus in the sand rat induced by standard laboratory diets. Science 1964; 143:689–690.

80. Hackel DB, Frohman L, Mikat E, Lebovitz HE, Schmidt-Neilsen K, Kinney TD. Effect of diet on the glucose tolerance and plasma insulin levels of the sand rat (*Psammomys obesus*). Diabetes 1966; 15:105–114.

81. Gonet AE, Stauffacher W, Pictet R, Renold AE. Obesity an diabetes mellitus with striking congenital hyperplasia of the islets of Langerhans in spiny mice (*Acomys cahirinus*). I. Histological findings and preliminary metabolic observations. Diabetologia 1965; 1:162–171.

82. Bielschowsky M, Bielschowsky F. A new strain of mouse with hereditary obesity. Proc Univ Otago Med School 1953; 31:29–31.

83. Proietto J, Larkins RG. A perspective on the New Zealand obese mouse. In: Shafrir E, ed. Lessons from Animal Diabetes. London: Smith-Gordon, 1992:65–74.

84. Warden CH, Fisler JS, Shoemaker SM, Ping-Zi W, Svenson KL, Pace M, Lusis AJ. Identification of four chromosomal loci determining obesity in a multifactorial mouse model. J Clin Invest 1995; 95:1545–1552.

85. Warden CH, Fisler JS, Pace MJ, Svenson L, Lusis AJ. Coincidence of genetic loci for plasma cholesterol levels and obesity in a multifactorial mouse model. J Clin Invest 1993; 92:773–779.

86. Hansen BC. Primate animal models of NIDDM. In: Le Roith D, Olefsky JM, Taylor S, eds. Diabetes Mellitus: A Fundamental and Clinical Text. Philadelphia: JB Lippincott, 1995.

87. Walike C, Goodner CJ, Koerker DJ. Assessment of obesity in pigtailed monkeys (*Macaca nemestrina*). J Med Primatol 1977; 6:1515–1562.

88. Bercovitch FB, Goy RW. The socioendocrinology of reproductive development and reproductive success in macaques. In: Ziegler T, Bercovitch FB, eds. Socioendocrinology of Primate Reproduction. New York: Wiley-Liss, 1990:59–93.

89. Howard CF, Kessler MJ, Schwartz S. Carbohydrate impairment and insulin secretory abnormalities among Macaca mulatta. J Med Primatol 1986; 11:147–148.

90. Schwartz SM, Kenmitz JW. Age- and gender-related changes in body size, adiposity, and endocrine and metabolic parameters in free-ranging rhesus macaques. Am J Phys Anthro 1992; 89:109–121.

91. Schwartz SM, Kemnitz JW, Howard CF. Obesity in free-ranging rhesus macques. Int J Obes 1993; 17:1–9.

92. Bodkin NL, Hannah JS, Ortmeyer HK, Hansen BC. Central obesity in rhesus monkeys: association with hyperinsulinemia, insulin resistance, and hypertriglyceridemia. Int J Obes 1993; 17:53–61.

93. Laber-Laird K, Shively CA, Karstaedt N, Bullock BC. Assessment of abdominal fat deposition in female cynomolgus monkeys. Int J Obes 1990; 15:213–220.

94. Jen K-LC, Hansen BC, Metzger BL. Adiposity, anthropometric measures, and plasma insulin levels of rhesus monkeys. Int J Obes 1985; 9:213–224.

95. Cohn C, Joseph D. Changes in body composition with force feeding. Am J Physiol 1959; 196:965–968.

96. Rothwell NJ, Stock MJ. Regulation of energy balance in two models of reversible obesity in rats. J Comp Physiol Psychol 1979; 93;1024–1034.

97. Sclafani A. Carbohydrate induced hyperphagia and obesity in the rat: Effects of saccharide type, form and taste. Neurosci Biobehav Rev 1987; 11:155–161.

98. Kanarek RB. Orthen-Gambil N. Differential effects of sucrose, fructose and glucose on carbohydrate-induced obesity. J Nutr 1982; 112:1546–1554.

99. Ramirez I. High-fat diets stimulate transient hyperphagia whereas wet diets stimulate prolonged hyperphagia in Fischer rats. Physiol Behav 1991; 49:1223–1228.

100. Corbett SW, Stern JS, Keesey RE. Energy expenditure in rats with diet-induced obesity. Am J Clin Nutr 1986; 44:173–180.

101. Rothwell NJ, Stock MJ. The cafeteria diet as a tool for studies of thermogenesis. J Nutr 1988; 118:925–928.

102. Lucas F, Sclafani A. Hyperphagia in rats produced by a mixture of fat and sugar. Physiol Behav 1990; 47:51–55.

103. West DB, Boozer CN, Moody DC, Atkinson RL. Dietary obesity in nine inbred mouse strains. Am J Physiol 1992; 262:R1025–1032.

104. Fisler JS, Bray GA. Dietary obesity: Effects of drugs on food intake in S5B/PI and Osborne-Mendel rats. Physiol Behav 1985; 34:225–231.

105. West DB, Waguespack J, York B, Goudey-Lefevre J, Price RA. Genetics of dietary obesity in AKR/J × SWR/J mice: segregation of the trait and identification of a linked locus on chromosome 4. Mamm Genome 1995; 5:546–552.

106. West DB, Goudey-Lefevre J, York B, Truett GE. Dietary obesity linked to genetic loci on chromosomes 9 and 15 in a polygenic mouse model. J Clin Invest 1994; 94;1410–1416.

107. Jen K-LC, Greenwood MRC, Brasel JA. Sex differences in the effects of high fat feeding on behavior and carcass composition. Physiol Behav 1981; 27:161–166.

108. Sclafani A., Springer D. Dietary obesity in adult rats: Similarities to hypothalamic and human obesity syndromes. Physiol Behav 1976; 17:461–471.

109. Rothwell NJ, Saville ME, Stock MJ. Effects of feeding a "cafeteria" diet on energy balance and diet-induced thermogenesis in four strains of fat. J Nutr 1982; 112:1515–1524.

110. Fisler JS, Wood RD, Lupien JR, Bray GA. Weight gain and indexes of brown adipose tissue thermogenesis do not differ between S5B/PII and Osborne-Mendel rats feed cafeteria diets. Fed Proc 1985; 44:1162.

111. Rothwell NJ, Stock MJ. Effects of age on diet-induced thermogenesis and brown adipose tissue metabolism in the rat. Int J Obes 1983; 7:583–589.

112. Rothwell NJ, Stock MJ, York DA. Effects of adrenalectomy on energy balance, diet-induced thermogenesis and brown adipose tissue in adult cafeteria fed rats. Comp Physiol Biochem 1984; 78A:565–569.

113. Rothwell NJ, Stock MJ. A role for brown adipose tissue in diet-induced themogenesis. Nature (Lond) 1979; 281:31–35.

114. Kemnitz J, Francken G. Characteristics of spontaneous obesity in male rhesus monkeys. Physiol Behav 1986; 38:477–483.

115. Pagliassotti MJ, Knobel SM, Shahrokhi KA, Manzo AM, Hill JO. Time course of adaptation to a high-fat diet in obesity-resistant and obesity-prone rats. Am J Physiol 1994; 267:R659–R664.

119. Wilmot CA, Sullivan AC, Levin BE. Effects of diet and obesity on brain a_1- and a_2-noradrenergic receptors in the rat. Brain Res 1988; 453:157–166.

117. Okada S, York DA, Bray GA. Mifepristone (RU 486), a blocker of type II glucocorticoid and progestin receptors, reverses a dietary form of obesity. Am J Physiol 1992; 262:R1106–R1110.

118. Pagliassotti MJ, Pan DA, Prach PA, Koppenhafer TA, Storlein LH, Hill JO. Tissue oxidative capacity, fuel stores and skeletal muscle fatty acid composition in obesity-prone and obesity-resistant rats. Obes Res 1995; 3:459–464.

119. Levin BE. Sympathetic activity, age, sucrose preference, and diet-induced obesity. Obes Res 1993; 1:281–287.

120. Levin BE, Sullivan AC. Glucose induced norepinephrine levels and obesity resistance. Am J Physiol 1987; 253:R475–R481.

121. Berthoud H-R. Cephalic phase insulin response as a prediction of body weight gain and obesity induced by a palatable cafeteria diet. J Obes Weight Regul 1985; 4:120–128.

122. Chang S, Graham B, Yakubu F, Lin D, Peters JC, Hill JO. Metabolic differences between obesity prone and obesity resistant rats. Am J Physiol 1990; 259:R1103–R1110.

123. Abou Mrad J, Yakubu F, Lin D, Peters JC, Atkinson JB, Hill JO. Skeletal muscle composition in dietary obesity susceptible and dietary obesity resistant rats. Am J Physiol 1992; 262:R684–R688.

124. Levin BE. Obesity prone and resistant rats differ in their brain [^{3}H]-para-aminoclonidine binding. Brain Res 1990; 512:54–59.

125. Levin BE, Planas B. Defective glucoregulation of brain a_2-adrenoreceptors in obesity prone rats. Am J Physiol 1993; 264:R305–R311.

126. Wolden-Hansen T, Davis GA, Baum ST, Kemnitz JW. Insulin levels, physical activity, and urinary catecholamine excretion of obese and non-obese rhesus monkeys. Obes Res 1993; 1:5–17.

127. Yoshida T, Fisler JS, Fukushima M, Bray GA, Schemmel RA. Diet, lighting, and food intake affect norepinephrine turnover in dietary obesity. Am J Physiol 1987; 2542:R402–R408.

128. Okada S, York DA, Bray GA, Erlanson-Albertsson C. Differential inhibition of fat intake in two strains of rat by the peptide enterostatin. Am J Physiol 1992, 262:R1111-R1116.

129. Arase K, Fisler JS, Shargill NS, York DA, Bray GA. Intracerebroventricular infusions of 3-OHB and insulin in a rat model of dietary obesity. Am J Physiol 1988; 255: R974–R981.

130. Lin L, Bray GA, York DA. Comparison of Osborne-Mendel and S5B/PL strains of rat: central effects of galanin, NPY, β-casomorphin and CRH on intake of high fat and low fat diets. Obes Res 1996; 4:117–124.

131. Shimizu H, Fisler JS, Bray GA. Extracellular hypothalamic monoamines measured by in vivo microdialysis in a rat model of dietary fat-induced obesity. Obes Res 1994; 2: 100–109.

132. Bray GA, Teague RJ, Lee CK. Brain uptake of ketones in rats with differing susceptibility to dietary obesity. Metabolism 1987; 30:27–30.

133. Nagase H, York DA, Bray GA. The effects of pyruvate and lactate on food intake in rat strains sensitive and resistant to dietary obesity. Physiol Behav 1996; 59:555–560.

134. Nagase H, Bray GA, York DA. Pyruvate and hepatic pyruvate dehydrogenase levels in rat strains sensitive and resistant to dietary obesity. Am J Physiol 1996; 270: R489–R495.

135. Flatt JP. Opposite effects of variations in food intake on carbohydrate and fat oxidation in ad libitum fed mice. J Nutr Biochem 1991; 2:186–192.

136. Hansen BC, Bodkin NL, Ortmeyer HK, Hotta K, Nicolson MA. Longitudinal changes in plasma leptin levels (Ob gene protein) during the progression of overt non-insulin-dependent diabetes (NIDDM). Am Diabetes Assoc 1997 (in press).

137. Walston J, Lowe A, Berkowitz D, Silver K, Bodkin NL, Hansen BC, Shuldiner AR. The β-3-adrenergic receptor in the obesity and diabetes prone rhesus monkeys is highly homologous to the human receptor and contains arginine at codon 64. Endocr Soc 1997.

138. Naithani VK, Steffens GJ, Tager HS. Isolation and amino-acid sequence determination of monkey insulin and proinsulin. Hoppe-Seylers Z Physiol Chem 1984; 365: 571–575.

139. Huang Z, Ortmeyer HK, Hansen BC, Shuldiner AR. Insulin receptor mRNA splicing in adipose tissue of rhesus monkeys with non-insulin dependent diabetes mellitus (NIDDM). Endocrine Society Annual Meeting Program, 1995; p. 179.

140. Fan Z, Kole H, Bernier M, Huang Z, Accili D, Hansen BC, Shuldiner AR. Molecular mechanism of insulin resistance in the spontaneously obese and diabetic rhesus monkey: site directed mutagenesis of the insulin receptor. Endocrine Society Annual Meeting Program 1995; p. 180.

141. Huang Z, Bodkin N, Ortmeyer HK, Hansen BC, Shuldiner AR. Hyperinsulinemia is associated with altered insulin receptor mRNA splicing in muscle of the spontaneously obese diabetic rhesus monkey. J Clin Invest 1994; 94; 1289–1296.

142. Bernardis LL. Ventromedical and dorsomedial hypothalamic syndromes in the weanling rat: is the "center" concept really outmoded? Brain Res Bull 1985; 14:537–549.

143. Laughton W, Powley TL. Bipiperidyl mustard produced brain lesions and obesity in the rat. Brain Res 1981; 221: 415–420.

144. Brecher G, Waxler SH. Obesity in albino mice due to single injections of gold thioglucose. Proc Soc Exp Biol Med 1949; 70:498–501.

145. Rutman RJ, Lewis FS, Bloomer WD. Bipiperidyl mustard, a new obesifying agent in the mouse. Science 1966; 153: 1000–1002.

146. Parkinson WL, Weingarten HP. Dissociative analysis of ventromedial hypothalamic syndrome. Am J Physiol 1990; 259:R829–R835.

147. Ahlskog JE, Randall PK, Hoebel BG. Hypothalamic hyperphagia: dissociation from hyperphagia following destruction of noradrenergic neurons. Science 1975; 190: 399–401.

148. Sahakian BJ, Winn P, Robbins TW, Deeley RJ, Everitt BJ, Dunn LT, Wallace M, James WPT. Changes in body weight and food-related behavior induced by destruction of the ventral or dorsal noradrenergic bundle in the rat. Neuroscience 1983; 10:1405–1420.

149. Scallet AC, Olney JW. Components of hypothalamic obesity: bipiperidyl-mustard lesions add hyperphagia to monosodium glutamate-induced hyperinsulinemia. Brain Res 1986; 374:380–384.

150. Tanaka K, Shimada M, Nakao K, Kusonoki T. Hypothalamic lesion induced by injection of monosodium glutamate in suckling period and subsequent development of obesity. Exp Neurol 1978; 62:191–199.

151. Shimizu N, Oomura Y, Plata-Salam < n CR, Morimoto M. Hyperphagia and obesity in rats with bilateral ibotenic acid-induced lesions of the ventromedial hypothalamic nucleus. Brain Res 1987; 416:153–156.

152. Weingarten HP, Change PK, McDonald TJ. Comparison of the metabolic and behavioral disturbances following paraventricular and ventromedial hypothalamic lesions. Brain Res Bull 1985; 14:551–559.

153. Sclafani A, Grossman SP. Hyperphagia produced by knife cuts between the medial and lateral hypothalamus in the rat. Physiol Behav 1969; 4:533–537.

154. Stanley BG, Kyrkouli SE, Lampert S, Leibowitz SF. Neuropeptide Y chronically injected into the hypothalamus; a powerful neurochemical inducer of hyperphagia and obesity. Peptides 1986; 7:1189–1192.

155. Rohner-Jeanrenaud F. A neuroendocrine reappraisal of the dual-center hypothesis: its implications for obesity and insulin resistance. Int J Obes 1995; 19:517–534.

156. Breisch ST, Zemlan FP, Hoebel BG. Hyperphagia and obesity following serotonin depletion by intraventricular p-chlorophenylalanine. Science 1976; 192:382–385.

157. Ahlskog JE, Hoebel BG. Overeating and obesity from damage to a noradrenergic system in the brain. Science 1982; 182:166–169.

158. Rohner-Jeanrenaud F, Jeanrenaud B. Possible involvement of the cholinergic system in hormonal secretion by the perfused pancreas from ventromedial hypothalamic lesioned rats. Diabetologia 1981; 20:217–222.

159. Berthoud H-R, Jeanrenaud B. Acute hyperinsulinemia and its reversal by vagotomy after lesions of the ventromedial hypothalamus in anesthetized rats. Endocrinology 1979; 105:146–151.

160. Penicaud L, Rohner-Jeanrenaud F, Jeanrenaud B. In vivo metabolic changes as studied longitudinally after ventromedial lesions. Am J Physiol 1986; 250:E662–E668.

161. Assimiacopoulos-Jeannet F, Jeanrenaud B. The hormonal and metabolic basis of experimental obesity. Clin Endocrinol Metab 1976; 5:337–365.

162. Rohner-Jeanrenaud F, Seydoux J, Chiner A, Bas S, Giacobino JP, Assimiacopoulos-Jeannet F, Jeanrenaud B, Girardier L. Defective diet-induced but normal cold-induced brown adipose tissue adaptation in hypothalamic obesity in rats. J Physiol (Paris) 1983; 78:833–837.

163. Niijima A, Rohner-Jeanrenaud F, Jeanrenaud B. Role of the ventromedial hypothalamus on sympathetic efferents of brown adipose tissue. Am J Physiol 1984; 247:R650–R654.

164. Holt SJ, Wheal H, York DA. Response of brown adipose tissue to electrical stimulation of hypothalamic centers in intact and adrenalectomized Zucker rats. Neurosci Lett 1988; 84:63–67.

165. Holt S, York DA, Fitzsimons JTR. The effects of corticosterone, cold exposure and overfeeding with sucrose on brown adipose tissue of obese Zucker rats (fa/fa). Biochem J 1983; 214:215–223.

166. Hogan S, Himms-Hagen J. Abnormal brown adipose tissue in obese (ob/ob) mice: response to acclimation to cold. Am J Physiol 1980; 239:E301–E309.

167. Nishizawa Y, Bray GA. Ventromedial hypothalamic lesions and mobilization of fatty acids. J Clin Invest 1978; 61:714–721.

168. Lotter FC, Wards SC. Injections of insulin and changes of body weight. Physiol Behav 1977; 18:293–297.

169. Mook DG, Kenney NJ, Robert S, Nussbaum Al, Rodier WI III. Ovarian-adrenal interactions in regulation of body weight by female rats. J Comp Physiol Psychol 1972; 81:198–211.

170. Beatty WW, Briant DA, Vilberg TR. Effect of ovariectomy and estradiol injections on food intake and body weight in rats with hypothalamic lesions. Pharmacol Biochem Behav 1975; 3:539–544.

171. Jones AP, McElroy JF, Crnic L, Wades GN. Effects of ovariectomy on thermogenesis in brown adipose tissue and liver in Syrian hamsters. Physiol Behav 1991; 50:41–45.

172. Hausberger FX, Hausberger BC. Castration-induced obesity in mice. Body composition, histology of adrenal cortex and islets of Langerhans in castrated mice. Acta Endocrinol 1966; 53:571–583.

173. Yoshioka K, Yoshida T, Wakabayashi Y, Nishioka H, Kondon M. Reduced brown adipose tissue thermogenesis of obese rats after ovariectomy. Endocrinol Jpn 1988; 35:537–543.

174. Dagnault A, Ouerghi D, Richard D. Treatment with a-helical-CRF$_{(9-41)}$ prevents the anorectic effect of 17-β-estradiol. Brain Res Bull 1993; 32:689–692.

175. Kurachi H, Adachi H, Ohtsuka S, Morishige K, Amemiya K, Miyake A, Tokunaga K, Keno Y, Matsuzawa Y, Tanizawa O. Involvement of epidermal growth factor in inducing obesity in ovariectomized mice. Am J Physiol 1993; 265:E323–E331.

176. Ohsima K, Okada S, Onai T. The characteristics of obese rats induced by medial-basal hypothalmic deafferentation. Proc 5th. Congress of Japanese Association for the Study of Obesity, Tokyo, 1985:114–115.

177. York DA, Bray GA. Dependence of hypothalamic obesity on insulin, the pituitary and the adrenal gland. Endocrinology 1972; 90:885–893.

178. Strack AM, Sebastian RJ, Schwartz MW, Dallman MF. Glucocorticoids and insulin: reciprocal signals for energy balance. Am J Physiol 1995; 268:R142–R149.

179. Chen N-G, Romsos DR. Enhanced sensitivity of pancreatic islets from preobese 2-week-old ob/ob mice to neurohormonal stimulation of insulin secretion. Endocrinology 1995; 136:505–511.

180. Atef N, Brule C, Bihoreau M, Ktorza A, Picon L, Penicaud L. Enhanced insulin secretory response to acetylcholine by perifused pancreas of 5-day-old preobese Zucker rats. Endocrinology 1991; 129:2219–2224.

181. Khan A, Stenson C-G, Berggren P-O, Efendic S. Glucocorticoid increases glucose cycling and inhibits insulin release in pancreatic islets of ob/ob mice. Am J Physiol 1992; 263:E663–E666.

182. Khan A, Hong-Lie C, Landau BR. Glucose-6-phosphatase activity in islets from ob/ob and lean mice and the effect of dexamethasone. Endocrinology 1995; 136:1934–1938.

183. Stubbs M, York DA. Central glucocorticoid regulation of parasympathetic drive to pancreatic β-cells in the obese fa/fa rat. Int J Obes 1991; 15:547–553.

184. Okuda T, Romsos DR. Adrenalectomy suppresses insulin secretion from pancreatic islets of ob/ob mice. Int J Obes 1994; 18:801–805.

185. Sakaguchi T, Arase K, Bray GA. Sympathetic activity and food intake of rats with ventromedial hypothalamic lesions. Int J Obes 1988; 12:43–49.

186. Holt SJ, York DA. The effects of adrenalectomy, corticotropin releasing factor and vasopressin on the sympathetic firing rate of nerves to interscapular brown adipose tissue in the Zucker rat. Physiol Behav 1989; 45:1123–1129.

187. Van Zeggeren A, Li Ets. Food intake and choice in lean and obese Zucker rats after intragastric carbohydrates preloads. J Nutr 1990; 120:309–316.

188. Atef N, Korza A, Picon L, Pericand L. Increased islet blood flow in obese rats: role of the autonomic nervous system. Am J Physiol 1992; 262:E736–E740.

189. Pederson RA, Campos RV, Buchan AMJ, Chisholm CB, Russell JC, Brown JC. Comparison of the enteroinsular axis in two strains of obese rat, the fatty Zucker and the JCR:LA-corpulent. Int J Obes 1991; 15:461–470.

190. Metzger BL, Hansen BC, Speegle LM, Jen K-LC. Characteristics of glucose intolerance in obese monkeys. J Obes Weight Regul 1985; 4:153–167.

191. Hansen BC, Bodkin NL. Beta-cell hyperresponsiveness: earliest event in development of diabetes in moneys. Am J Physiol 1990; 259:R612–R617.

192. de Koning EJP, Bodkin NL, Hansen BC, Clark A. Diabetes mellitus in *Macaca mulatta* monkeys is characterized by islet amyloidosis and reduction in beta-cell population. Diabetologia 1993; 36:378–384.

193. Bodkin NL, Metzger BL, Hansen BC. Hepatic glucose production and insulin sensitivity preceding diabetes in monkeys. Am J Physiol 1989; 256:E676-E681.

194. de Soua CJ, Yu JH, Robinson DD, Ulrich RG, Meglasson MD. Insulin secretory defect in Zucker fa/fa rats is improved by ameliorating insulin resistance. Diabetes 1995; 44:984–991.

195. Hansen BC, Bodkin NL. Primary prevention of diabetes mellitus by prevention of obesity in monkeys. Diabetes 1993; 42:1809–1814.

196. Paik SG, Michelis MA, Kin YT, Shin S. Induction of insulin-dependent diabetes by streptozotocin. Inhibition by estrogens and potentiation by androgens. Diabetes 1982; 31:724–729.

197. Leiter EH, Chapman HD, Coleman DL. The influence of genetic background on the expression of mutations at the diabetes locus in the mouse. V. Interaction between the db gene and the hepatic sex steroid sulfotransferases correlates with gender-dependent susceptibility to hyperglycemia. Endocrinology 1989; 124:912–922.

198. Borthwick EB, Burchell A, Coughtrie MW. Differential expression of hepatic oestrogen, phenol and dehydroepiandrosterone sulphotransferases in genetically obese diabetic (ob/ob) male and female mice. J Endocrinol 1995; 144: 31–37.

199. Leiter EH, Chapman HD. Obesity-induced diabetes (diabesity) in C57BL/KsJ mice produces aberrant transregulation of sex steroid sulfotransferase genes. J Clin Invest 1994; 93:2007–2013.

200. Song W-C, Moore R, McLachlan JA, Negishi M. Molecular characterization of a testes-specific estrogen sulfotransferase and aberrant liver expression in obese and diabetogenic C57BL/KsJ-db/db mice. Endocrinology 1995; 136: 2477–2484.

201. Kemnitz JW, Goy RW, Flitsch TJ, Lohmiller JJ, Robinson JA. Obesity in male and female rhesus monkeys: fat distribution, glucoregulation, and serum androgen levels. J Clin Endocrinol Metab 1989; 69:287–293.

202. Kemnitz JW, Sladky KK, Flitsch TJ, Pomerantz SM, Gory RW. Androgenic influences on body size and composition of adult rhesus monkeys. Am J Physiol 1988; E857–E864.

203. Sanchez-Gutirrez JC, Sanchez-Arias JA, Lechuga CG, Valle JC, Samper B, Felru JE. Decreased responsiveness of basal gluconeogenesis to insulin action in hepatocytes isolated from genetically obese (fa/fa) Zucker rats. Endocrinology 1994; 134:1868–1873.

204. Godbole V, York DA. Lipogenesis in situ in the genetically obese "Zucker" fatty rat: role of hyperphagia and hyperinsulinaemia. Diabetologia 1978; 14:191–197.

205. Koranyi L, James D, Mueckler M, Permutt MA. Glucose transporter levels in spontaneously obese (db/db) insulin-resistant mice. J Clin Invest 1990; 85:962–967.

206. Slieker LJ, Sundell KL, Heath WF, Osborne HE, Bue J, Manetta J, Sportman JR. Glucose transporter levels in tissues of spontaneously diabetic Zucker fa/fa rat (ZDF/drt) and viable yellow mouse (A^{vy}/a). Diabetes 1992; 41: 187–193.

207. Ferresas L, Kelada ASMK, McCoy M, Proietto J. Early decrease in GLUT4 protein levels in brown adipose tissue of New Zealand obese mice. Int J Obes 1994; 18: 760–765.

208. Le Marchand-Brustel Y, Olichon-Berthe C, Gremeaux T, Tanti JF, Rochet N, Van Obberghen E. Glucose transporter in insulin sensitive tissues of lean and obese mice—Effect of the thermogenic agent BRL-26830A. Endocrinology 1990; 127:2687–2695.

209. Pedersen O, Kahn CRE, Kahn BB. Divergent regulation of the Glut-1 and Glut-4 glucose transporters in isolated adipocytes from Zucker rats. J Clin Invest 1992; 89: 1964–1973.

210. Pedersen O, Kahn CR, Flier JS, Kahn BB. High fat feeding causes insulin resistance and a marked decrease in the expression of glucose transporters (Glut 4) in fat cells of rats. Endocrinology 1991; 129:771–777.

211. Rosholt MN, King PA, Horton ES. High-fat diet reduces glucose transporter responses to both insulin and exercise. Am J Physiol 1994; 266:R95–R101.

212. King PA, Horton ED, Horton ES. Insulin resistance in obese (fa/fa) skeletal muscle is associated with a failure of glucose transporter translocation. J Clin Invest 1992; 90:1568–1575.

213. Zaninetti D, Greco-Perotto R, Assimiacopoulos-Jeannet F, Jeanrenaud B. Dysregulation of glucose and transporters in perfused hearts of genetically obese (fa/fa) rats. Diabeteologia 1989; 32:56–60.

214. Galante P, Maereker E, Scholz R, Rett K, Herberg L, Mosthaf L, Häring HU. Insulin-induced translocation of GLUT 4 in skeletal muscle of insulin-resistant Zucker rats. Diabetologia 1994; 37:3–9.

215. Stephens JM, Pekala PH. Transcriptional repression of Glut-4 and C/EBP genes in 3T3-L1 adipocytes by TNF. J Biol Chem 1991; 266:21839–21845.

216. Zarjevski N, Doyle P, Jeanrenaud B. Muscle insulin resistance may not be a primary etiological factor in the ge-

netically obese *fa/fa* rat. Endocrinology 1992; 130: 1564–1570.

217. Kritchevsky D. Animal models of lipoprotein metabolism. In: Schettler G, Habenicht AJR, eds. Handbook of Experimental Pharmacology, Principles and Treatment of Lipoprotein Disorders. Berlin: Springer-Verlag, 1994; 109: 207–218.

218. Williams JK, Clarkson TB. Nonhuman primate atherosclerotic models. In: White RA, ed. Atherosclerosis and Arteriosclerosis: Human Pathology and Experimental Animal Methods and Models. Boca Raton, FL: CRC Press, 1989: 261–285.

219. Hannah JS, Verdery RB, Bodkin NL, Hansen BC, Le N-A, Howard BV. Changes in lipoprotein concentrations during the development of noninsulin dependent diabetes mellitus in obese rhesus monkeys (*Macaca mulatta*). J Clin Endocrinol Metab 1991; 72:1067–1072.

220. Hamilton CL, Ciaccia P. The course of development of glucose intolerance in the monkey (*Macaca mulatta*). J Med Primatol 1978; 7:165–173.

221. Hansen BC, Brodkin NL. Heterogeneity of insulin responses: phases in the continuum leading to non-insulin-dependent diabetes mellitus. Diabetologia 1986; 29: 713–719.

222. York DA. Neuroendocrine and metabolic derangements. In: Stock M, Rothwell N, eds. Obesity and Cachexia. A Biological Council Symposium. London: Wiley, 1991: 103–118.

223. Britton DR, Indyke E. Effects of ganglionic blocking agents on behavioral responses to centrally administered CRF. Brain Res 199; 478:205–210.

224. Yamashita Junko, Onai T, York DA, Bray GA. Relationship between food intake and metabolic rate in rats treated with β-adrenoceptor agonists. Int J Obes 1994; 18:429-433.

225. York DA. CRF and glucocorticoids: central regulation of appetite autonomic activity by CRH, glucocorticoid and stress. Prog Neuroendocr Immunol 1992; 5:153–165.

226. Allars J, Holt SJ, York DA. Energetic efficiency and brown adipose tissue uncoupling protein of obese Zucker rats fed high carbohydrate and high fat diets: the effect of adrenalectomy. Int J Obes 1987; 11:591–607.

227. Saito M, Bray GA. Adrenalectomy and food restriction in the genetically obese (*ob/ob*) mouse. Am J Physiol 1984; 246:R20– .

228. Shimizu H, Shargill NS, Bray GA. Adrenalectomy and response to corticosterone and MSH in the genetically obese yellow mouse. Am J Physiol 1989; 256:R494–R500.

229. King BM, Banta AR, Tharel GN, Bruce BK, Frohman LA. Hypothalamic hyperinsulinemia and obesity: role of adrenal glucocorticoid. Am J Physiol 1093; 245:E194–199.

230. Tokunaga K, Fukushima M, Lupien JR, Bray GA, Kemnitz JN, Schemmel R. Adrenalectomy and food restriction in PVN and VMH lesioned rats. FASEB J 1988; A422.

231. Tokuyama K, Himms-Hagen J. Adrenalectomy prevents obesity in glutamate-treated mice. Am J Physiol 1989; 257:E139–E144.

232. Kim YS, Carp RI, Callahan SM, Wisniewski HM. Adrenal involvement in scrapie induced obesity. Proc Soc Exp Biol Med 1988; 189:21–27.

233. York DA, Holt SJ, Allars J, Payne J. Glucocorticoid and the central control of sympathetic activity in the obese *fa/fa* rat. In: Björntorp P, Rossner S, eds. Obesity in Europe. London: John Lippey, 1988:219–224.

234. York DA, Godbole V. Effect of adrenalectomy on obese "fatty" rats. Hormone Metab Res 1979; 11:646.

235. Ohshima, K, Shargill NS, Chan TM, Bray GA. Adrenalectomy reverses insulin resistance in muscle from obese (*ob/ob*) mice. Am J Physiol 1984; 246:E193–E197.

236. Freedman MR, Stern JS, Reaven GM, Mondon CE. Effect of adrenalectomy on in vivo glucose metabolism in insulin resistant Zucker obese rats. Hormone Metabol Res 1986; 18:296–298.

237. Akabayashi A, Watanabe Y, Wahlestedt C, McEwen BS, Paez X, Leibowitz SF. Hypothalamic neuropeptide Y, its gene expression and receptor activity relation to circulating corticosterone in adrenalectomized rats. Brain Res 1994; 665:201–212.

238. Shargill NS, York DA, Marchington D. Regulation of hepatic tyrosin aminotransferase in genetically obese rats. Biochim Biophys Acta 1983; 756:297–307.

239. Santana P, Akana SF, Hanson ES, Strack AM, Sebastian RJ, Dallman MF. Aldosterone and dexamethasone both stimulate energy acquisition whereas only the glucocorticoid alters energy storage. Endocrinology 1995; 136: 2214–2222.

240. Langley S, York DA. The effects of the antiglucocorticoid RU-486 on the development of obesity in the obese *fa/fa* Zucker rat. Am J Physiol 1990; 259:R539–R544.

241. Thomas TL, Devenport LD, Smith RD. Relative contribution of type I and II corticosterone receptors in VMH lesion-induced obesity and hyperinsulinemia. Am J Physiol 1994; 35:R1623–R1629.

242. Rohner-Jeanrenaud F, Jeanrenaud B. Vagal mediation of corticotropin-releasing-factor-induced increase in insulinemia in lean and genetically obese fa/fa rats. Neuroendocrinology 1990; 52:52–56.

243. Arase K, York DA, Shimizu H, Shargill N, Bray GA. Effects of corticotropin releasing factor on food intake and brown adipose tissue. Am J Physiol 1988; 255:E255–E259.

244. Arase K, Shargill NS, Bray GA. Effect of corticotropin releasing factor on genetically obese (fatty) rats. Physiol Behav 1989; 45:565–570.

245. Arase K, Shargill NS, Bray GA. Effects of intraventricular infusion of corticotropin-releasing factor on VMH-lesioned obese rats. Am J Physiol 1989; 256:R751–756.

246. Rohner-Jeanrenaud F, Walker C-D, Greco-Perotto R, Jeanrenaud B. Central corticotropin-releasing factor administration prevents the excessive body weight gain of genet-

ically obese (*fa/fa*) rats. Endocrinology 1989; 124: 733–739.

247. Jenrenaud B. Neuroendocrine and metabolism basis of type II diabetes as studied in animal models. Diabetes Metab Rev 1988; 4:603–614.

248. Guillame-Gentil C, Rohner-Jeanrenaud F, Abramo F, Bestetti GE, Rossi GL, Jeanrenaud B. Abnormal regulation of the hypothalamo-pituitary-adrenal axis in the genetically obese fa/fa rat. Endocrinology 1990; 126:1873–1881.

249. Bestetti GE, Abramo F, Guillaume-Gentil C, Rohner-Jeanrenaud F, Jeanrenaud B, Rossi GL. Changes in the hypothalamo-pituitary-adrenal axis of genetically obese fa/fa rats: a structural, immunocytochemical, and morphometrical study. Endocrinology 1990; 126:1880–1887.

250. Beyer HS, Matta SG, Sharp BM. Regulation of the messenger ribonucleic acid for corticotropin-releasing factor in the paraventricular nucleus and other brain sites of the rat. Endocrinology 1988; 123:2117–2123.

251. Sanacora G, Kershaw M, Finkelstein JA. Increased hypothalamic content of preproneuropeptide Y messenger ribonucleic acid in genetically obese Zucker rats and its regulation by food deprivation. Endocrinology 1990; 127: 730–737.

252. Chua Jr SC, Brown AW, Kim J, Hennessey KL, Leibel RL, Hirsch J. Food deprivation and hypothalamic neuropeptide gene expression: effects of strain background and the diabetes mutation. Mol Brain Res 1991; 11:291–299.

253. Wilding JP, Gilbey SG, Bailey CJ, Batt RA, Williams G, Ghatei MA, Bloom SR. Increased neuropeptide-Y messager ribonucleic acid (mRNA) and decreased neurotensin mRNA in the hypothalamus of the obese (*ob/ob*) mouse. Endocrinology 1993; 132:1939–1944.

254. Stephens TW, Basinski M, Bristow PK, Bue-Valleskey JM, Burgett SG, Craft L, Hale J, Hoffmann J, Hsiung HM, Krlauclunas A, MacKellar W, Rosteck Jr PR, Schoner B, Smith D, Tinsley FC, Zhang X-Y, Helman M. The role of neuropeptide Y in the antiobesity action of the obese gene product. Nature (Lond) 1995; 377:530–532.

255. Schwartz MW, Marks JL, Sipols AJ, Baskin DG, Woods SC, Kahn SE, Porte Jr D. Central insulin administration reduces neuropeptide Y mRNA expression in the arcuate nucleus of food-deprived lean (*fa/fa*) but not obese (*fa/fa*) Zucker rats. Endocrinology 1991; 1285:2645–2647.

256. Kemnitz JW, Roecker EB, Weindruch R, Elson DF, Baum ST, Bergman RT. Dietary restriction increases insulin sen-

sitivity and lowers blood glucose in rhesus monkeys. Am J Physiol 1994; 266:E540–E547.

257. Schwartz MW, Sipols AJ, Marks JL, Sanacora G, White JD, Scheurink A, Kahn SE, Baskin DG, Woods SC, Figlewicz, Porte D Jr. Inhibition of hypothalamic neuropeptide Y gene expression by insulin. Endocrinology 1992; 130: 3608–3616.

258. Behini-Hooft van Huijsduijnen OB, Rohner-Jeanrenaud F, Jeanrenaud B. Hypothalamic neuropeptide Y messenger ribonucleic acid levels in preobese and genetically obese (*fa/fa*) rats: potential regulation thereof by corticotropin-releasing factor. J Neuroendocrinal 1993; 5:381–386.

259. White BD, Dean RG, Martin RJ. Adrenalectomy decreases neuropeptide Y mRNA levels in the arcuate nucleus. Brain Res Bull 1990; 25:711–715.

260. Sahu A, Dube MG, Phelps CP, Sninsky CA, Kalra PS, Kalra SP. Insulin and insulin-like growth factor II suppress neuropeptide Y release from the nerve terminal in the paraventricular nucleus: a putative hypothalmic site for energy homeostasis. Endocrinology 1995; 136:5718–5724.

261. Wilding JPH, Gilbey SG, Mannan M, Aslam N, Ghatei MA, Bloom SR. Increased neuropeptide Y content in individual hypothalamic nuclei, but not neuropeptide Y mRNA, in diet-induced obesity in rats. J Endocrinol 1992; 132:299–304.

262. Langley S, York DA. Increased type II glucocorticoid receptor numbers and glucocorticoid sensitive enzyme activities in the brain of the Zucker rat. Brain Res 1990; 533:268–274.

263. Jensen M, Kilroy G, York DA, Braymer HD. Abnormal regulation of hepatic glucocorticoid receptor mRNA and receptor protein distribution in the obese Zucker rat. Obes Res 1996; 4:133–143.

264. White BD, Davenport WD, Porter JR. Responsiveness of isolated adrenocortical cells from lean and obese Zucker rats to ACTH. Am J Physiol 1988; 255:E229–E235.

265. Tsai HJ, Romsos DR. Glucocorticoid and mineralocorticoid receptor-binding characteristics in obese (*ob/ob*) mice. Am J Physiol 1988; 61:E495–499.

266. Shargill NS, Al-Baker I, York DA. Serum corticosterone and hepatic glucocorticoid receptors in obese Zucker rats. BioSci Rep 1988; 7:843–851.

267. Bodkin NL, Ortmeyer HK, Hansen BC. Long-term dietary restriction in older-aged rhesus monkeys: effects on insulin resistance. J Gerontol Biol Sci 1995; 50A: B142–B147.

12

Molecular Genetics of Obesity

Craig H. Warden
University of California at Davis, Davis, California

Janis S. Fisler
University of California at Los Angeles School of Medicine, Los Angeles, California

I. INTRODUCTION

The evidence for a genetic basis for obesity is compelling (1,2) and, in humans, comes from studies of adoptees (3), twins (4,5), and families (6). Genetic epidemiology studies suggest that the heritability of human obesity may be as low as 10% (adoption studies) to as high as 80% (twin studies) (7). These studies also indicate that familial environment has little impact on obesity (7,8). The number of genes involved in obesity has not been estimated from human studies primarily because such estimates are complicated by the conclusion that genes implicated in obesity may have major, minor, or polygene effects. Furthermore, more than one major gene may be present in the whole population. Minor genes would each account for less variance in any individual than major genes, while polygenes might each determine several percent of population variance. Genetic epidemiology studies suggest that the percentage of multifactorial (minor gene) transmission for obesity ranges from 25 to 42%, and five of seven studies suggest that there are major gene effects (7). However, the specific identity of major and minor genes remains unclear.

Some of the most compelling evidence for a genetic basis of obesity comes from the discovery of five mutations that cause spontaneous obesity and diabetes in mice fed chow diets (A^y, db, ob, tub, and fat) (9). The agouti (A^y) (10,11), obese (ob) (12), fat (13), diabetes (db) (14–16), and tubby (tub) genes have been cloned. As discussed below, studies of the physiology and biochemistry of obesity with these genes and their protein products are proving interesting.

II. APPROACHES TO IDENTIFY GENES CAUSING OBESITY

There are two broadly contrasted approaches to identify genes causing obesity (Fig. 1). They depend on the quality of the clues available about the trait being studied. In principle, all genes causing human obesity could be identified based on physiological or biochemical understanding of their roles. Such a candidate gene approach has been very productive for many diseases. Nevertheless, the candidate gene approach has clearly failed to find major genes involved in obesity. This difficulty has not been due to a lack of candidates; indeed, there are dozens, including genes controlling differentiation of adipocytes, adipocyte-specific adrenergic receptors, factors produced by adipocytes, such as tumor necrosis factor-α, and serotonin receptors (Fig. 1). It is now clear that part of the difficulty with candidate gene approaches has been that some genes important in regulating body weight were part of pathways that were unknown until the isolation by positional cloning efforts of the agouti, obese, and diabetes genes. In spite of these problems, some candidate genes likely to be important in body weight regulation have been identified

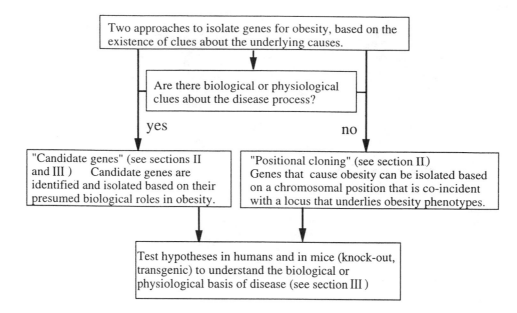

Figure 1 Methods to identify genes causing complex diseases, such as obesity. A biochemical or physiological approach with clues about the cause of obesity corresponds to the "top down" or "genotype down" approaches that have been described previously (30). The genetic approach without clues corresponds to the "bottom up" or "genotype up" methods.

by construction of transgenic or knockout mice, or by association studies in humans (Fig. 1).

Isolation of genes by positional cloning is the major alternative to the candidate gene approach. Positional cloning is based on finding chromosomal coincidence of a trait (obesity) with genetic markers in pedigrees. Positional cloning works without reference to any existing candidate genes. It has been accomplished for at least 40 genes causing monogenic diseases, including the mouse tubby, obese and diabetes genes (Fig. 1) (17). Positional cloning might work for genes producing human monogenic syndromes that include obesity as a phenotype, but little progress has been made.

Positional cloning has proven difficult in multifactorial traits primarily because of genetic locus heterogeneity (18). Thus, genes causing multifactorial traits such as obesity must to be isolated using more circuitous methods. Whole genome searches identifying chromosomal loci including genes causing obesity can be conducted without any previous knowledge of underlying causes, as is the situation for positional cloning (19). Unfortunately, these whole genome searches will not provide the precise chromosomal position needed to initiate positional cloning (20). Whole genome searches can, however, identify candidate genes based on position. A positional candidate gene is an expressed gene present in a chromosomal locus underlying a trait that shows some preliminary character-

istics consistent with a role in the trait being examined (17). Further tests can be used to prove a role of a positional candidate gene in the trait. Another way to overcome difficulties with positional cloning is to do positional cloning in animal models, followed by studies in humans. For instance, tools such as congenic mouse strains can provide a source of monogenic models that can be used for positional cloning.

A. Contrast, Comparison, and Evaluation of Methods for Genetic Studies

Genetics is troubled by more false positive and negative results than most fields of biological science. Difficulties arise from several distinct causes. The first difficulty in evaluating genetic studies is that there has been no standard for the description of linkage claims for complex disease. While it has been suggested that specific terminology should be used to describe the varying degrees of statistical certainty that can be observed in genetic studies (21), these standards have yet to be applied. It has been suggested that statistical significance of linkage results be described by a classification scheme providing increasing certainty that a gene underlying a complex disease has been identified. If one looks at sib-pair family studies, the descriptions, p values and LOD scores would be as follows: suggestive linkage would apply to results with a p

value of 7.4×10^{-4} and a LOD score of 2.2, significant linkage would describe results with a p value of 2.2×10^{-5} or a LOD score of 3.6, and highly significant linkage would describe results with a p value of 3×10^{-7} and a LOD score of 5.4. Suggestive linkage values would be expected to occur once at random per genome scan, while significant linkage values would be expected to occur 0.05 times at random in a genome scan. Highly significant linkage would then describe results expected to occur 0.001 times in a genome scan. Application of these criteria for reporting results will aid investigators in their evaluation of linkage claims, while still providing for the publication of results that need to be extended or replicated (21).

Additional problems with the evaluation of genetic studies result from the comparative strengths and weaknesses of association and linkage studies. Association studies examine population frequency of alleles, where linkage studies examine correlated inheritance in pedigrees. Significant linkage may be detected at a locus without significant association when many distinct alleles produce obesity in a population. Significant association may be detected without linkage when an allele explains a small percentage of variance so that the allele may occur more frequently in obese subjects but provide only insignificant evidence for linkage in family pedigrees (18).

The basic principle of association studies is that one uses appropriate genetic and statistical methods to search for alleles that are enriched in people with obesity or other disorders. If one has a specific mutation in a specific candidate gene to examine, association studies can be used to identify alleles with functional effects on obesity. This technique was used for studies of the β_3-adrenergic receptor, which is primarily involved in diabetes (22–24). Chromosomal regions, or loci, that contain genes influencing obesity can even be identified if one does not have functional alleles of candidate genes to test, since additional alleles that chance to be near the functional mutation can be used to identify that it is nearby. The additional, or random, alleles measured do not have to directly give rise to functional effects. One important limitation of association studies is that these measured alleles need to be relatively close to the functional allele (within 100–200 kb).

Many association studies have not been reproducible. While there are several explanations for this problem, population admixture is one reason for failure to reproduce association studies. Population admixture is problematic if obesity, or any other trait, is more prevalent in one ethnic group in an admixed population. Thus, any allele that happens to be more common in that group will be associated with obesity. An example occurred in studies of diabetes in Pima Indians, where association was found

to the Gm locus. However, each Pima has differing amounts of Caucasian ancestry, such that the presence of a Caucasian allele at the Gm locus is correlated with the presence of Caucasian alleles at loci anywhere in the genome, which is independently correlated with the risk of non-insulin-dependent diabetes mellitus (25).

In contrast to association studies, linkage studies in families provide the opportunity to survey the whole genome for genes causing complex traits, since linked alleles tend to be inherited together in pedigrees. Thus, even without any prior biochemical or physiological understanding of obesity, one can survey the whole genome of mice or humans to identify chromosomal loci influencing obesity. A 10-centimorgan (cM) map would require between 200 and 400 evenly distributed markers. Linkage studies can identify positional candidate genes present in obesity chromosomal loci or can guide positional cloning efforts. However, genetic locus heterogeneity, where mutations in two or more genes cause obesity, complicates identification of obesity chromosomal loci, since an individual locus may be linked with obesity in some families but not in others (18). Thus, contradictory results from different families will tend to cancel each other out, since evidence for linkage frequently needs to be summed from several families to reach statistical significance. However, although whole genome searches are laborious, they provide a robust method to identify genes causing obesity.

B. Cloning and Study of Genes Producing Monogenic Syndromes that Include Obesity as a Phenotype

Existing monogenic disorders that exhibit obesity, such as Prader-Willi, Bardet-Biedl, Carpenter, and Cohen syndromes, have unknown etiologies. While it has been difficult to determine if the underlying genes contribute to common forms of obesity, there has been one published hypothesis that people who are heterozygotes for Bardet-Biedl syndrome may make up 1–2% of the severely obese (26). Considerable effort has been given to learning about the Prader-Willi syndrome since it is associated with severe obesity and since it exhibits an unusual kind of inheritance involving maternal imprinting. The small nuclear ribonucleoprotein polypeptide N (*SNRPN*) gene maps to the Prader-Willi critically deleted region and is not expressed from maternal alleles in mice or humans, consistent with a role as the imprinted gene causing Prader-Willi (27,28). Although the function of *SNRPN* is unknown, it is expressed predominantly in brain, and it interacts with pre-mRNAs, implying that it may influence splicing of transcripts in the brain. At least two additional paternally expressed transcripts have been isolated from

300-kb telomeric to human *SNRPN*, suggesting the existence of an imprinting control region flanking *SNRPN* (29). No current evidence exists that variants at the Prader-Willi syndrome locus contribute to common forms of human obesity. A mouse model displaying imprinting influences on fatpad weights, which may be produced by alleles of the *Snrpn* gene, has been described and may furnish a model to test hypotheses about the origin of obesity in Prader-Willi (see below). Cloning of the genes for Bardet-Biedl, Carpenter, and Cohen syndromes should be pursued since these may provide novel insights into obesity (1).

C.   Use of Animal Models to Identify Genes of Body Weight Regulation

As compared to genetic studies of humans, investigations in animals are faster and often allow a more detailed and careful description of phenotype (18,30). Possible roles of cloned mouse genes can then be examined in humans (31). Mice will often be the animal model of choice for genetic studies, primarily owing to the availability of hundreds of inbred and congenic strains and the utility of a dense genetic linkage map and positional cloning tools. Moreover, the homologous regions of mouse and human chromosomes are so well defined that it is frequently possible to know the chromosomal location of a gene in humans by mapping it in mice, sometimes with more precision than is possible with human mapping studies (32). Other advantages of mouse or other animal models include the ability to manipulate diet and to obtain any tissue at various times during development. Thus, many investigations are more practical in mice than in humans, including studies of diet responsiveness, longitudinal studies, and analyses of critical periods in the development of obesity.

The rat has been used extensively in physiological and biochemical studies of energy homeostasis. A number of phenotypically well-characterized strains are available (33,34) and will, as a result of the rapidly expanding rat genetic map, be very useful in identifying candidate genes in the system of body weight regulation.

D.   Whole Genome Approaches

Procedures for whole genome scans and quantitative trait locus (QTL) mapping are available for animal models and humans. QTL mapping in animal models, which uses parametric statistical methods to identify genes that segregate with quantitative traits in genetic crosses, has been reviewed previously (18,30,35). Newer techniques include nonparametric QTL mapping of animal model backcrosses

for traits exhibiting nonnormal distribution, and the use of biometrical genome searches to describe the multigenic basis of quantitative traits (34). Examples of traits that are not normally distributed include survival times in an experiment of limited duration and qualitative data such as grades assigned by histological data.

A study of the multigenic basis of blood pressure illustrates a four-step biometrical approach to QTL mapping (34). The first step was to identify 17 loci with suggestive linkage to salt-loaded systemic blood pressure (NaSBP, $p < 0.05$). The second step included the simultaneous assessment of the effects of the 17 loci to identify five loci with significant effects on NaSBP. The third stage involved refining the location of each QTL that advanced to the second step. The fourth step determined the significance of each QTL when considered together with the other QTLs. The overall process thus identifies and locates multigenic loci with significant effects on NaSBP that might not be identified with the more typical QTL approach that identifies loci one at a time.

I.   QTL Mapping of Spontaneous and Diet-Induced Obesity in Animals

QTL mapping has been used to identify chromosomal loci linked to spontaneous obesity in at least three published mouse crosses. As discussed below, QTL mapping has been applied to spontaneous obesity in a cross of *Mus spretus* with C57BL/6J. QTL mapping has also been applied to crosses involving lines of mice that have been divergently selected for body weight or fat content (36) and to dietary-induced obesity (37,38). The pig has also been used as an animal model for QTL mapping of fat deposition genes (39). It is hard to determine the number of new obesity genes identified by animal model approaches since candidate genes are present in many of the QTLs. Nevertheless, it is clear that novel genes influencing spontaneous obesity have been located. The problem with these studies is that one must clone these genes to increase the physiological understanding of obesity.

QTL Mapping in BSB Mice.   During the course of genetic studies involving crosses between the strains *M. spretus* (SPRET/Pt) and C57BL/6J, we noticed varying degrees of obesity among backcross animals, which we call BSB mice, although both parental strains are relatively lean (40). The parental strains differ slightly in the percentage of body fat: the mean ($\pm$ SE) percent body fat for 3–4-month-old C57BL/6J mice is 7.5 ($\pm$ 1.0), whereas that for the *M. spretus* parent is 2.2 ($\pm$ 0.5) ($p < 0.05$). However, neither parent could be considered obese. The (C57BL/6J $\times$ *Spretus*) F_1 progeny are similar to the C57BL/6J parent with a mean percent body fat of 10.8 ($\pm$ 1.7) in 4–6-month-old mice. In contrast, BSB backcross progeny range from less than 1% to more than 60% body fat, far outside the range observed in either parent or in the F_1 mice. The simplest model for this outcome is that obesity results from the interactions of two genes, and that one locus must be homozygous for C57BL/6J alleles (BB), while the other locus is heterozygous (SB), since this is the only combination of two genes that is unique to backcross mice. We have identified four chromosomal loci that promote obesity in BSB mice: obesity is caused by heterozygous SB genotypes at three loci and a homozygous BB genotype at one locus.

BSB mice were examined for measures of obesity including percentage of body fat, body mass index (BMI), weight of fat pads, and for biochemical parameters related to obesity, including plasma triglycerides, glucose, insulin, corticosterone, glycerol, nonesterified fatty acids, and total and HDL cholesterol. Although the percentage of body fat is correlated with body weight and BMI, it is not correlated with body length.

We searched for genetic loci underlying quantitative traits using the MAPMAKER/QTL program (41), which calculates the strength of associations between genotypes and phenotypes as the log 10 of the likelihood of the odds ratio (LOD) score. It has been calculated that in a mouse backcross a LOD score of 3.3 is the threshold for statistically significant linkage (21). We noticed that *D7Mit8* on distal mouse chromosome 7 was significantly linked with total plasma cholesterol (LOD score 5.4), hepatic lipase (HL) activity (LOD score 5.1), and percentage of body fat (LOD score 3.2) (Fig. 2 and 3) (42,43). The locus was designated *Mob1*, for multigenic obesity-1. The *Mob1* locus explains 6.5% of the variance in the percentage of body fat. Mice that were heterozygous for *M. spretus* and C57BL/6J alleles at the *D7Mit8* marker had 28% more body fat than mice that were homozygous for C57BL/6J alleles at that locus ($p < 0.0003$). Several good candidate genes, including insulin-like growth factor 1 receptor (*Igf1r*), the Prader-Willi candidate gene (*Snrpn*), and tubby (*tub*) occur within the *Mob1* locus. A second locus, on mouse chromosome 6 near the marker *D6Mit1*, designated *Mob2*, exhibited a LOD score of 4.8, explaining 7.1% of the variance in femoral fatpad weight (Fig. 3) (42,43). Mice that were heterozygous at the *D6Mit1* locus had about twofold heavier femoral fatpads than mice that were homozygous C57BL/6J at that locus ($p < 0.0001$). This locus is very close to the mouse *ob* gene. Thus, alleles of the *ob* gene may underlie some of the variance in obesity in BSB mice. A third locus resides on mouse chromosome 12 near the marker *D12Mit27* (*Mob3*) (Fig. 3). It exhibits a LOD score of 4.8 for percentage body fat and explains

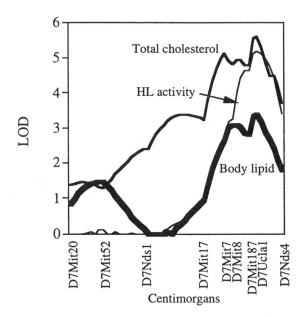

Figure 2 Coincidence of QTLs for total cholesterol, percent body fat, and hepatic lipase activity on chromosome 7 in BSB mice. BSB mice were typed for total plasma cholesterol, hepatic lipase activity, and percent body fat (total lipid) as described (42). Genetic markets typed on chromosome 7 were analyzed for linkage to these traits by the Mapmaker/QTL program.

7% of the variance. Mice that were heterozygous at the *D12Mit27* locus had 44% greater body fat than mice homozygous for C57BL/6J alleles at that locus ($p < 0.0002$). The fourth locus identified in BSB mice resides on mouse chromosome 15 near *D15Mit13* (*Mob4*) (Fig. 3). It exhibits a LOD score of 3.4 and explains 5.9% of the variance in mesenteric fat. Mice heterozygous at this locus had 32% *smaller* mesenteric fat pads than mice that were homozygous for C57BL/6J alleles ($p < 0.0001$). There was also suggestive linkage for percentage body fat at the chromosome 15 locus. An attractive candidate gene, growth hormone receptor (*Ghr*), is located within the *Mob4* locus.

Each of the four *Mob* loci does not appear to be additive with the other three (Fig. 4). *M. spretus* alleles promote obesity at the chromosome 6, 7, and 12 loci, whereas C57BL/6J alleles promote obesity at the chromosome 15 locus. Furthermore, the chromosome 15 locus appears to promote obesity only if the homozygous C57BL/6J genotype occurs on a background where the chromosome 6, 7, and 12 loci are all heterozygous.

QTL Mapping in Mice Selected for Body Weight. Four mouse lines were selected over 20 generations for high or low body weight and for high or low body fat content

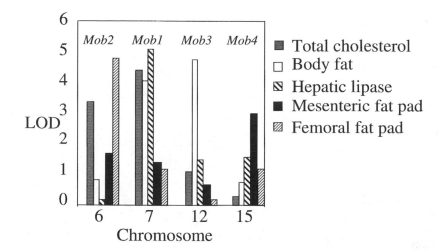

Figure 3 LOD scores for obesity and associated phenotypes at the four loci from the BSB backcross (see text). Peak LOD scores are shown for hepatic lipase activity, plasma total cholesterol, percent body fat, mesenteric and femoral fatpads on chromosomes 7, 6, 12, and 15. These correspond, respectively, to the *Mob1-4* loci. The peak LOD scores were calculated by the Mapmaker/QTL program for each of the traits in BSB mice. (Modified from Ref. 42, Fig. 6.)

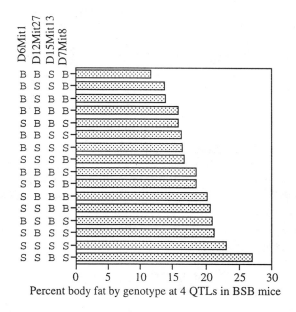

Figure 4 Genotypic interactions of *Mob* genes in multifactorial BSB obesity. For each QTL the market closest to the peak LOD score was used to determine genotype of the BSB mice. BSB mice were then grouped and body fat % plotted based on these genotypes. S, mice heterozygous for *Mus spretus* and C57BL/6J alleles; B, mice homozygous for C57BL/6J alleles. (Modified from Ref. 42, Fig. 5.)

(36). F_2 populations of crosses of the low × high body weight and low × high body fat lines were mapped for X chromosome markers. They revealed a QTL on the proximal X chromosome for body weight but not for body fat (44). QTLs for body fat have also been identified in a cross of M16i and CAST. M16i is the result of long-term selection for postweaning weight gain (45). Several markers were identified with significant effects for 12-week body weight and body fat. One marker on distal chromosome 2 revealed a *p* value of 0.001 (45).

QTL Mapping in a Diet-Induced Mouse Model. QTL mapping has been used to identify loci underlying diet-induced obesity in an F_2 cross between mouse strains SWR/J and AKR/J. These strains differ in their susceptibility to gain weight when fed a high-fat, high-sucrose diet (37,38). Whole genome mapping of this cross revealed loci on chromosomes 4, 9, and 15 that were linked to adiposity. It is possible that the chromosome 15 locus in the SWR/J × AKR/J cross is identical with that in BSB mice since it is located on the proximal portion of the chromosome with the peak LOD score at *D15Nds2*, 8.6 cM distal to *D15Mit13*, the peak marker in *Mob4*.

QTL Mapping for Growth and Fatness in Pigs. The European wild boar was crossed with a domestic pig to identify genes underlying growth and fat deposition (39). The most important effects were clustered on chromosome 4. It is probable that the corresponding human gene is located on chromosome 1 and may be in the region of chromosome 1 that includes the diabetes (*db*) homolog (39). This study was also interesting in that it used divergent outbred populations to start the QTL analysis. This demonstrated that QTL mapping can be applied to any cross where parental strain alleles and traits differ significantly.

2. QTL Mapping in Humans

Approaches to whole genome mapping in humans have undergone a rapid evolution. A number of potentially overlapping sampling designs are applicable to complex phenotypes such as weight regulation and obesity. These have been reviewed (18). Sibling designs are generally powerful and relatively insensitive to assumptions about mode of inheritance. Thus, they may be the method of choice for a systematic search of the human genome for an obesity gene or mapping of specific chromosomal regions. The methods include affected sibling pairs and triplets, sibships, and nuclear families built around affected sibling pairs. The latter method of sib-pair analysis (identity by descent) is arguably the most efficient (48). Until recently, the nonparametric sib-pair approach was the most generally useful, since one did not have to know the mode of inheritance of the trait. However, these sib-pair approaches suffer from several limitations: they examine linkage data at single markers and they cannot use all available alleles. A complete multipoint sib-pair analysis could overcome these limitations (19).

Once a chromosomal region linked to obesity has been identified, further mapping in nuclear and extended families may be used if a clear pattern of segregation can be identified (20). Parent-offspring and affected-control samples will be useful in screening candidate genes for possible linkage and for fine regional mapping of new genus through the identification of genetic disequilibrium.

A problem in identifying genes involved in body weight regulation is that for moderate obesity the familial relative risk (where λ = familial risk:population risk) is likely to be low, a situation that makes nonparametric linkage analysis difficult. Thus, a more stringent approach is to ascertain families through individuals with extreme obesity. These individuals should show an excess of major obesity genes, which could facilitate isolation of underlying genes by positional cloning (20). Families ascertained with extremely discordant sib-pairs will both avoid bilineal in-

heritance and will maximize the information gained from each person genotyped (49). Another approach is to produce whole genome maps in families enriched for obesity. Several such studies, including the Quebec Family Study (50), a study of Pima Indians (51,52), and a study of extremely discordant sib-pairs (53), are currently underway.

Two separate whole genome studies have reported suggestive evidence for linkage of obesity or obesity phenotypes to markers near the *ob* gene locus on human chromosome 7 (53,54). Although results of neither study could be described as producing significant evidence for linkage to the *ob* locus, taken together they do provide evidence that *ob* or a closely linked gene affects body weight regulation. While these initial studies have not reported any mutations in the *ob* coding sequence (55), these two results certainly suggest that further investigation of *ob* mutations is warranted.

E. Isolation of Genes Underlying Obesity

I. Positional Candidate Approaches to Isolate Genes

Coincidence of a candidate gene and a QTL suggests that the candidate gene may be the underlying basis of the QTL. For example, description of carboxypeptidase E (*Cpe*) as causing the *fat* mutation is an illustration of the positioned candidate approach applied to a monogenic mutation (see below for a more detailed discussion). The identification of the gene underlying a QTL affecting multiple intestinal neoplasia (*Min*) is another example of the positional candidate approach (56,57). Tumor phenotypes and incidence of mice bearing the *Min* mutation are strongly modified by mouse strain genetic background. A cross of mouse strains with different tumor incidences was used to identify the *Mom1* (modifier of *Min1*) locus on distal chromosome 4 that controls 50% of tumor number variation (56). The gene for secretory type II phospholipase A2 (*Pla2s*) was identified as a positional candidate since it mapped to the same region that contains *Mom1*. Further study revealed that allele type and tumor susceptibility of *Pla2s* show 100% concordance. Final proof of the role of *Pla2s* in tumor incidence of *Min* mice came from sequencing of *Pla2s*, which revealed that *Mom1*-susceptible mouse strains are spontaneous knockouts for *Pla2s*, thus altering cellular environment within the intestinal crypt (57).

A summary of obesity QTLs and candidate genes is provided in Figure 5 to simplify identification of positional candidates that are coincident with existing and future QTLs. QTLs shown are those identified for spontaneous and diet-induced obesity. One concept that may help to

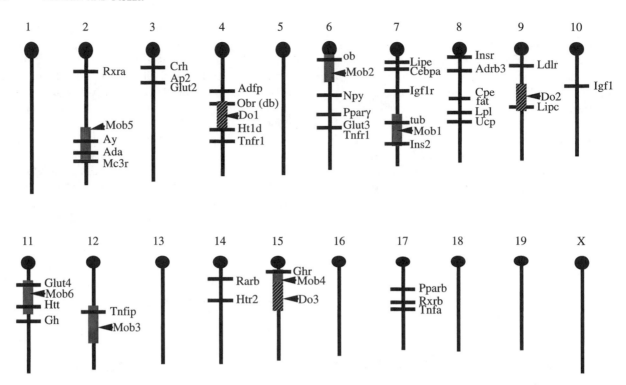

Figure 5 Chromosomal locations of obesity QTLs and positional candidate genes in mice. QTLs are those derived for spontaneous obesity in BSB (42) and NZB × SM mice (47) and diet-induced obesity in an AKR × SWR cross (37,38). Positions are shown as covering the 90% confidence intervals. Positional candidate genes include retinoic acid X receptor α (Rxrα, β), retinoic acid receptor β (Rarβ), peroxisome proliferator receptor β, γ (Pparβ, γ), agouti (A^y), tubby (tub), CCAATT enhancer-binding protein-α (C/EBPα, Cebpa), obese receptor (diabetes, db), carboxypeptidase E (Cpe, fat), obese mutation (ob or leptin), adenosine deaminase (Ada), melanocortin receptor 3 (Mc3r), corticotropin-releasing hormone (Crh), adipocyte specific fatty acid binding protein 2 (Ap2), glucose transporter 1-4 (Glut1-4), serotonin receptors (Htlr, Htt), tumor necrosis factor receptor 1 (Tnfr1), tumor necrosis factor α (Tnfα), tumor necrosis factor inhibitory protein (Tnfip), hormone-sensitive lipase (Lipe), lipoprotein lipase (Lpl), hepatic lipase (Lipc), insulin-like growth factor receptor (Igflr), insulin (Ins), insulin receptor (Insr), insulin growth factor (Igr1), uncoupling protein (Ucp), low-density-lipoprotein receptor (Ldlr), growth hormone (Gh), and growth hormone receptor (Ghr). [Positional candidate gene locations are derived from the committee maps of the Mouse Genome Database (MGD, The Jackson Laboratory) or from Ref. 144.]

explain differing results of the various crosses is that QTLs do not have to be invariable among distinct crosses, since only those genes regulating body weight that differ between any one pair of parental strains are revealed. Thus, four obesity QTLs were detected in the BSB cross (Mobl-4), and three others for diet-induced obesity in a cross of AKR × SWR (Dol-3). While there is some overlap, it would be remarkable to find identical QTLs in each cross, particularly since the effect of various alleles can fluctuate greatly depending on mouse strain background.

The severity of diabetes is remarkably influenced by whether the ob or db mutations are bred onto the C57BL/6J background (obesity and insulin resistance uncomplicated by diabetes) or whether they are bred onto the C57BL/KsJ background (obesity and insulin resistance complicated by severe diabetes) (58–60). It appears prob-

able that mapping and identification of genes modifying diabetes severity will reveal QTLs and positional candidates important in producing diabetes. C57BL/KsJ is an accidental congenic with C57BL/6J background and DBA donor strains, since it has been shown that C57BL/KsJ strain is an admixture of 84% C57BL/6J and 16% DBA/2J (61). This admixture will expedite identification of genes modifying diabetes severity (see next section). In Figure 5 we show a selective set of candidate genes that are either discussed in this review or for which some genetic evidence exists confirming their role in the regulation of body weight.

2. Uses of Congenic Strains to Study Complex Traits

Congenic mouse strains are a rich source for the more rapid identification of genes causing complex diseases. Congenic strains are produced by a regimen of crossing that moves a selected gene from a donor source onto a standard inbred-strain background. The resulting congenic strain contains the selected donor gene and surrounding donor chromosomal DNA equal to approximately 1–2% of the mouse genome (62,63). Thus for any one trait, one can study the effects of singe genes derived from the donor strain, isolated from effects of other donor strain genes, by comparison of phenotypes in background and congenic strains. Examinations of congenic strains have been helpful for corroboration of obesity QTLs (42). They can also be used to investigate the biochemistry and physiology of single loci causing complex traits, whether or not the underlying genes are known. For instance, congenic mouse strains have been useful in the study of atherosclerosis by showing that the *Apoa2* gene cannot be *Ath-1* (64). Also, congenics should exhibit monogenic Mendelian segregation of the trait in crosses of background and congenic strains and thus be useful tools for positional cloning.

We reasoned that the genetic variations influencing obesity in BSB mice may be relatively common, since many inbred strains of laboratory mice vary in body fat content and other traits related to obesity (65). Therefore, where possible, we examined previously created congenic strains whose donor chromosomal regions contain the *Mob* genes (42). Chromosome 7 is the site of several histocompatibility genes. These include the *H1*, *H22*, *H24*, *H4* (composed of the *H46* and *H47* loci), and *H19* loci. Positions are shown in Figure 6. These loci are present in existing congenic strains available from the Jackson Laboratory. One problem with comparison of data from the several chromosome 7 congenic strains is that they were created using two different background strains, C57BL/6ByJ and C57BL/10SnJ, and two different donor strains, 129/SnJ and BALB/cByJ (Fig. 6). However, overlapping donor regions from these congenics include most of chromosome 7, making these strains ideal for a chromosome survey.

Two of these congenic strains, B10.129(5M)/nSn and B10.C(41N)/Sn, contain a region of chromosome 7 flanking the *H1* minor histocompatibility gene (Fig. 7A) (62). The two congenic strains differed from the background C57BL/10SnJ strain in several parameters related to obesity (Fig. 7B). As compared to strain C57BL/10SnJ mice, the two congenic strains exhibited only about 25% of the retroperitoneal fatpad weight, about 60% of the body fat, and 110% of the plasma cholesterol. Total body weight and hepatic lipase activity were also decreased in the B10.129(5M)/nSn congenic strain. Thus, the characteristics of the locus isolated in these congenic strains are strikingly similar to the *Mob1* locus identified in BSB mice. We mapped the breakpoints between the background strain-derived and donor strain-derived chromosomes. Both congenic strains contain approximately 27–29 cM of donor strain DNA on chromosome 7. The *SNRPN* gene that underlies Prader-Willi syndrome, the insulin-like growth factor I receptor (*Igf1r*), and the *tubby* gene, a single gene mutant causing obesity in mice, are present in both congenic strains (42).

We have started a cross of the B10.129(5M)/nSn congenic with the C57BL/10SnJ background strain to fine-map and test the *Mob1* QTL. We crossed both males and females of both strains, since the donors strain region contains the imprinted *SNRPN* gene that is a candidate gene for the Prader-Willi syndrome (28). Body weight and fat-pad data (Table 1) in the F_1 mice are consistent with the hypothesis that a gene underlying differences in weight between the B10.129(5M)/nSn congenic and C57BL/10SnJ is imprinted and, thus, may be *SNRPN* (Prader-Willi).

3. Positional Cloning

The mammalian genome contains approximately 100,000 genes (70), but the functions of only a few percent are known (71–73). Some of the unknown genes are likely to be of great importance in obesity. How can we identify these genes? Biochemical studies will continue to provide new candidate genes, but with the notable exception of the *fat* (13) and β_3-adrenergic receptor genes (22–24), biochemical studies have not been very productive for studies of obesity.

Positional cloning is a powerful approach for identification and characterization of genes for monogenic disorders in which no biochemical or candidate gene can be identified. Unfortunately, positional cloning approaches are difficult to use in human studies of multifactorial disorders (20). The primary difficulty is mapping the responsible genetic loci, because multiple independently segregating loci contribution to the disorders. It has been calculated that 700 sib-pairs are needed to localize a gene to 1 cM that causes a twofold increase in risk (20). In contrast, for loci with relative risks exceeding 40 the situation resembles the case for single Mendelian traits. Unfortunately, there is no current evidence for obesity loci with high relative risks, nor have there been any reports of direct positional cloning in humans of genes underlying complex disease.

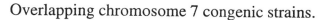

Overlapping chromosome 7 congenic strains.

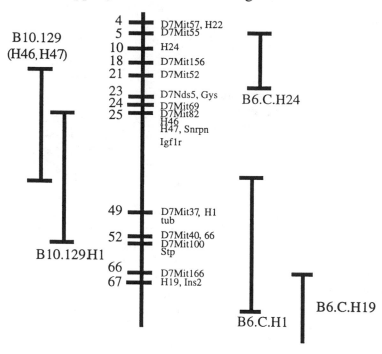

Figure 6 Overlapping congenic donor regions on mouse chromosome 7. The chromosome 7 map, with Mit SSLP markers typed, histocompatibility loci, and candidate genes, is shown in the center. Congenic donor regions are shown for five congenic strains. Borders mapped to within 1 cM are shown with a cross bar at the top or bottom of the line, while donor regions that are not mapped are shown open.

The tools of positional cloning are improving rapidly. A yeast artificial chromosome (YAC) contig covering the entire human genome has been constructed (71). More than 87,000 expressed human genes have been identified and chromosomal locations are being identified for many (70,72). While more than 40 genes have been identified by positional cloning, this strategy is being replaced by the more rapid positional candidate approach that involves identification of disease genes by searching for coincidence of disease gene chromosomal positions with expressed gene maps (17). Usefulness of the positional candidate approach will grow exponentially as the number of mapped expressed genes increases. Thus, mapping of a human obesity locus to a 1–2-cM interval may identify a group of 50–200 positional candidate genes that can be examined for their roles in body weight regulation. While still a considerable chore, this would at least provide a method for isolation of genes causing obesity.

Expressed genes isolated, sequenced, and mapped by the Human Genome Project will aid isolation of genes influencing murine obesity. Expressed human genes can be used to identify expressed mouse genes, in the same way that mouse and human chromosome homology can be used to identify corresponding chromosomal loci (32,74). Thus, information from QTL, mapping studies in mice or other animal models could be used to identify human obesity candidate genes. These genes, or the corresponding mouse genes, could be isolated and examined for their roles in body weight regulation.

III. WHAT HAS BEEN LEARNED ABOUT BODY WEIGHT REGULATION FROM STUDIES WITH CLONED GENES?

Molecular studies using cloned genes have provided fresh information about pathways causing obesity. For this review, the biochemical and physiological studies of cloned obesity genes are divided up based on the method used to show that the gene causes obesity. Thus, we will discuss in turn investigations using genes isolated by cloning of mouse single-gene modulations, candidate genes identified by a variety of procedures, and then candidate genes expressed by adipose tissue.

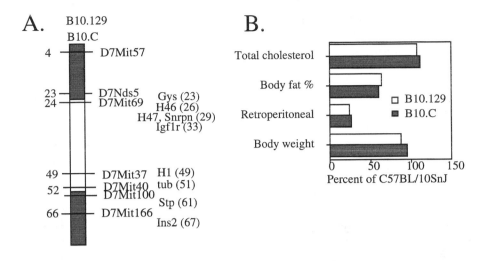

Figure 7 (A) Molecular mapping of chromosomal breakpoints showed that the B10.129(5M0)/nSn and the B10.C(41N)/Sn congenics were essentially identical. Polymorphisms were identified and typed in the parental and congenic strains by PCR (145). The distances in cM between markers are derived from the MGD consensus maps. (Modified from Ref. 42, Fig. 4.) (B) Effect on the *Mob1* gene on obesity-related traits in B10.129(5M)/nSn and B10.C(41N)/Sn congenic strains. Body weight, retroperitoneal fatpad, percent body fat, percent body water, and total plasma cholesterol found in the congenic strains are given as percent of the C57BL/10SnJ background strain. All animals were maintained on a chow diet and were between 135 and 175 days old at sacrifice. (Modified from Ref. 42, Fig. 3.)

A. Genes Causing Mouse Monogenic Mutations that Have Been Cloned Provide Tools for Studies of Obesity

This chapter will provide only brief descriptions of the biological effects of the cloned mouse monogenic obesity mutants, *ob*, *diabetes*, *agouti*, and *fat*, since they are discussed in another chapter. Studies of leptin (the *ob* protein product) have aided the identification of its receptor (*db*). Investigations continue on the role of leptin in the regulation of body weight, and on questions such as: What physiological actions does leptin have? And what are the signals that regulate leptin expression?

The recent proof that the *diabetes* mutation is indeed the leptin receptor (also named the obese receptor, OBR) brings to a close years of speculation about the nature of this mutation. It has been shown that the *db* gene product binds leptin with high affinity (14–16). A variety of splice variants of the leptin receptor are expressed in many tissues (15). The hypothalamus normally expresses a form with a long cytoplasmic tail involved in signal transduction. The original *db* mutation results from a splicing error in the hypothalamic form of the leptin receptor that produces a stop codon in the cytoplasmic segment of the protein, creating a receptor with a truncated intracellular tail lacking the signal transducing portion (14,15). Linkage and molecular studies in mice and rats have shown

that the *db* gene is the mouse homolog of the *fa* mutation in obese Zucker rats (75). Thus, it has been shown that plasma levels of leptin are increased in *db/db* mice and in obese Zucker rats (76). The many tissue-specific forms of the leptin receptor will provide a rich beginning for additional investigations.

Studies of the physiological actions of leptin showed that peripheral and central administration of microgram doses of leptin reduced food intake by 60% and body fat by 50% in *ob/ob* mice but did not affect food intake of

Table 1 Comparison of Summed Fat Pad Weights for 5–7-Month-Old Mice Derived from Crosses of Both Male and Female B10.129(5M)/nSn and C57BL/10SnJ Strains

Cross	No. of mice	Sex	Sum of four dissected fat pads (g) ± SE
B10.129(5M)/nSn (f) × C57BL/10SnJ (m) (Cross 1)	17	Male	5.0 ± 0.37
	17	Female	4.5 ± 0.47
C57BL/10SnJ (f) × B10.129(5M)/nSn (m) (Cross 2)	10	Male	5.0 ± 0.34
	12	Female	2.7 ± 0.55

Fisher PLSD post-hoc test: Female F_1 mice from cross 2 significantly different from cross 1, $p < 0.03$.

db/db mice (77–80). Injections of recombinant leptin also increased metabolic rate, body temperature, and activity in *ob/ob* mice. Leptin injections also inhibited neuropeptide Y (NPY) synthesis and release (80), perhaps providing one mechanism by which leptin could regulate body weight since NPY promotes food intake (81).

Several factors are known to regulate leptin mRNA levels in white adipose tissue. Elements regulating leptin expression include fasting and feeding, hormones, and lesions of the hypothalamus. Evidence that leptin expression is regulated as a function of energy balance comes from the observation that *ob* mRNA levels are decreased by starvation for 1–3 days and are increased by refeeding (82,83). Similarly, *ob* mRNA levels increase during the night when mice feed and decrease during the daytime fast (84). Hormonal factors may partially influence body weight regulation through control of leptin expression. Insulin injections in fasted animals increased *ob* mRNA to levels of fed controls (84), while corticosteroids induce *ob* mRNA in adipose tissue (85). Both mice with lesions of the hypothalamus and *db/db* mice express 20-fold higher *ob* mRNA in adipose tissue (82,86), providing additional evidence for the existence of a pathway regulating *ob* RNA.

While lack of leptin causes obesity in *ob* mice, studies in humans have shown that levels of leptin mRNA and plasma protein are increased rather than decreased in obese subjects (87–90), leading to the suggestion that human obesity may result from resistance to leptin, rather than lack of leptin protein. Additional evidence that leptin resistance is common in many forms of obesity comes from the observation that leptin levels are increased in a wide variety of mouse obesity models (91). As is the case for insulin in type II diabetes, resistance to leptin could be due to mutations in several to many genes.

Mutations at the *agouti* locus cause yellow fur, obesity, and diabetes (10,11). The agouti protein is normally expressed in skin and functions as a panacrine hormone regulating production of melanin by blocking the ability of α-melanocyte-stimulating hormone to activate its receptor (92). Ectopic expression of the normal *agouti* gene in transgenic mice causes obesity, features of type II diabetes, and yellow fur (66). Comparisons of the agouti coding sequence reveal similarity to Ca^{2+} blocking toxins produced by cone snails and a hunting spider (93). Indeed, it has been demonstrated that Ca^{2+} influx of soleus muscle correlates with obesity in mice with varying ectopic expression of the *agouti* gene (94).

Studies of the *fat* gene demonstrated that a mutation of carboxypeptidase E (*Cpe*) is responsible for the obesity (13). Genetic mapping showed that the obesity phenotype had a chromosomal position coincident with the positional candidate gene *Cpe*. This mutation reduces proinsulin processing in pancreatic islets. While the *fat* mutation represents an obesity-diabetes syndrome caused by a defective prohormone processing pathway, it is not clear that the hyperproinsulinemia of *fat* mice causes obesity, since hyperproinsulinemia is not associated with obesity in humans. Rather, the carboxypeptidase of *fat* mice is also defective in pituitary and brain, suggesting that obesity may develop as a result of defective prohormone processing for other neuroendocrine hormones (13).

B. Genetically Altered Mice Can Be Used to Test Hypotheses About the Role of Specific Genes in Obesity

Various methods are available for testing hypotheses about obesity-causing genes. These include transgenic mice expressing added genes and mice whose natural genes are deleted or altered by homologous recombination. Examples of methods feasible with transgenic mice include overexpression of genes in normal tissues, overexpression of genes in specific tissues (95), expression of mouse or human genes (96,97), expression of genes with inducible promoters (98,99), or expression of novel proteins designed to test specific hypotheses (for example, chimeric proteins or proteins with specific mutations) (100). The moderate overexpression of lipoprotein lipase (LPL) in skeletal muscle is one example of a hypothesis test performed using tissue-specific transgene expression. LPL overexpression decreased body lipid by approximately 20% (95). Essentially the same experiment was performed by another laboratory, which found that muscle specific overexpression of LPL led to myopathy, in addition to weight loss, in three independent transgenic lines (101). Studies of the overexpression of mouse (96) or human (97) apolipoprotein A-II (apoA-II) genes provide an example of species-specific influences of transgenes. Overexpression of mouse apoA-II protein resulted in elevated HDL cholesterol and promoted spontaneous atherosclerosis, while expression of human apo-A-II had very little influence on these traits. Tetracycline-responsive promoters are an example of inducible promoters for transgenic construction (98,99). An example of combining site-specific mutagenesis with transgenic mice comes from a study of the interaction of apolipoprotein B (apoB) with apolipoprotein (a) (apo(a)). Mouse, but not human, apoB binds covalently to apo(a) forming lipoprotein (a) (Lp(a)). The human (102) apoB gene was cloned into a yeast artificial chromosome (YAC) where site-directed mutagenesis was used to mutate the putative apo(a) binding site Cys-4057 to a Gly (100). This mutated human apoB gene was then used to construct transgenic mice where the human apoB did not bind to apo(a), thus demonstrating the essential role of Cys-4057 in the formation of Lp(a).

Homologous recombination in embryonic stem cells can be used in a wide variety of experiments, including testing the effects of complete absence of a specific protein (103), testing effects of the absence of a specific protein in a specific tissue (104,105), or introduction of targeted mutations into the germline of mice. Transgenic and knockout methods can be combined to eliminate expression of the endogenous mouse protein, which can then be replaced by the homologous human protein to "humanize" the mouse, or the missing protein can be replaced by transgenic constructs that are used to test specific hypotheses about in vivo structure and function.

At least six genes can cause obesity when overexpressed as transgenes or when knocked out. Examples of transgenes or knocked-out genes that affect body weight regulation include type II glucocorticoid receptor (106), transforming growth factor-α (107), GLUT4 (103,108), glycerol 3-phosphate dehydrogenase (109), the 5-HT2c serotonin receptor (110), and mitochondrial uncoupling protein (UCP) (111). The most remarkable feature of these six transgenic or knockout models is that each influences body weight through widely different pathways. Decreased type II glucocortoid receptor function caused by an antisense RNA transgene resulted in moderately overweight mice (106). The type II glucocortoid receptor may be important for terminating the stress response, as it is increased in animals exhibiting increased sensitivity to the negative feedback effects of corticosteroids. While previous studies have shown the requirement for corticosteroids for the expression of many forms of obesity (112), this was the first demonstration of obesity in transgenic mice with altered glucocorticoid feedback effect on the hypothalamus. Transgenic mice overexpressing TGF-α had epididymal fatpads reduced 40–80% and total body fat reduced 50% relative to control animals. When the insulin-responsive glucose transporter (GLUT4) was overexpressed in transgenic mice there was a two- to three-fold increase of total body fat (108). Fat cell size was not altered whereas fat cell number was increased twofold. Consistent with these results, knockout of the GLUT4 gene resulted in mice that were leaner than littermate controls (103). Mice overexpressing glycerol 3-phosphate dehydrogenase (GPDH) in brown fat exhibited severely reduced subcutaneous and peritoneal white fat depots, as well as brown fat hypertrophy (109). GPDH catalyzes the reduction of dihydroxyacetone phosphate to glycerol 3-phosphate, a precursor for triglyceride and phospholipid synthesis. GPDH is expressed most abundantly in brown fat. A role for serotonin in eating disorders has been demonstrated in mice lacking the 5-HT2c receptor. Serotonin

is believed to modulate numerous behavioral processes. Mice lacking the 5-HT2c serotonin receptor are overweight as a result of abnormal control of feeding behavior (110). Finally, mice expressing UCP in white and brown fat were made using a transgene with the fat-specific aP2 promoter linked to a UCP minigene (111). Female transgenic A^{vy} mice had body weights comparable with nontransgenic controls suggesting that UCP overexpression reduces fat stores. The diversity of genes now known to influence obesity indicates that more will be discovered, including genes in known and unknown pathways.

Transgenic mice can also be used to explore the biological consequences of ablating specific tissues. Such an approach was used to test the hypothesis that brown adipose tissue may function to promote or inhibit obesity depending on its size or metabolic activity. Brown adipose tissue is an important site for regulating thermogenesis due to the presence of brown fat–specific uncoupling protein (UCP) that promotes mitochondrial respiration (113–115). Respiration rates might influence the partitioning of calories into adipose tissue. A transgenic toxigene has been used to create lines of mice deficient in brown adipose tissue. The promoter from UCP was used to drive the expression of diphtheria toxin, resulting in the ablation of brown adipose tissue (116). In one transgenic line, brown fat deficiency persists and obesity develops with age. Obesity develops in these mice in the absence of hyperphagia, indicating increased metabolic efficiency. This study nicely confirmed the role of brown adipose tissue in body weight regulation of mice.

C. Candidate Genes Expressed by Adipose Tissue

Candidate genes can be tested for association with obesity. The candidate gene approach involves examining whether or not variations in body weight are accompanied by increased allele frequencies of genes that mechanistically may influence body weight. This involves comparison of allele frequencies in populations with those of the obese. This chapter will focus on recently cloned candidate genes produced by adipose tissue since obesity candidate genes have been extensively reviewed before (7,117). Adipose tissue is a rich source of candidate genes. We provide a brief review here to focus attention on several candidates that may explain the connections between body fat and plasma cholesterol levels in BSB mice.

A candidate gene approach was recently used to show that the β_3-adrenergic receptor (β_3-AR) is associated with non-insulin-dependent diabetes mellitus (NIDDM) and is associated with increased capacity to gain weight and higher waist-to-hip circumferences. RNA encoding β_3-AR is expressed in intra-abdominal or visceral adipose depots and in brown adipose tissue but not in subcutaneous adipose depots in humans (118,119). The β_3-AR is the major receptor mediating catecholamine-stimulated thermogenesis in brown adipose tissue and mediates the stimulation of lipolysis by catecholamines in white adipose tissue. Thus, low β_3-AR activity could promote obesity through several pathways. mRNA for the atypical β_3-AR subtype is dramatically reduced in adipose tissue from obese (ob/ob) mice relative to lean controls that, along with reduced expression of β_1-AR, results in impaired adenylyl cyclase response to β-agonists (120). Decreased expression of β_1- and β_3-AR is also associated with the diminution of adrenergic responsiveness of adipose tissue in the aging rat (121). Thus, the β_3-AR was examined as a candidate gene for obesity in several human populations. A missense mutation in codon 64 of the gene for the β_3-AR that results in a tryptophan substitution by arginine was detected with allelic frequency of 0.31 in Pima Indians, approximately three times higher than observed in Caucasians or African Americans (23). When Pima Indians were genotyped for this mutation, no linkage was observed between the mutation and obesity or NIDDM, but there was linkage with age of onset of NIDDM, and subjects homozygous for the mutation tended to have lower adjusted metabolic rates (23). The same Trp64Arg mutation is found in the Finnish population, with no difference in allelic frequency between diabetic and nondiabetic subjects (approximately 0.12) (24). In the Finnish subjects the Trp64Arg allele of the β_3-AR was associated with higher waist-to-hip circumference in women and with early onset of NIDDM. Finally, the Trp64Arg allele was associated with increased capacity to gain weight in a French group of morbidly obese subjects (22). Thus, the β_3-adrenergic receptor may be involved in susceptibility to weight gain, higher waist-to-hip circumference, and age of onset of NIDDM.

Overexpression of tumor necrosis factor-alpha (TNF-α) in adipose tissue contributes to the insulin resistance of obese animals (122,123) through down-regulation of the insulin-regulatable glucose transporter (GLUT4) (122,124) and inhibition of insulin receptor tyrosine kinase in adipose tissue and muscle (125). TNF-α also decreases the activity of lipoprotein lipase (126–128) and increases hormone-sensitive lipase in adipose tissue (129). In humans, adipose tissue TNF-α mRNA levels are higher in obese than lean subjects and are decreased with weight loss (128,130). Adipose tissue TNF-α mRNA is also strongly correlated with fasting insulin levels, a surrogate for insulin resistance in humans (130). Thus, TNF-α was examined as a candidate gene for obesity in Pima Indians. Pima Indians families were scored for three simple sequence length polymorphism (SSLP) markers near the

TNF-α gene. Sib-pair analysis revealed that a marker 10 kb from TNF-α was linked to percent body fat ($p = 0.002$) (51). The same marker was also associated with BMI ($p = 0.01$). In the entire coding region, only a single polymorphism in the proximal promoter was identified, and it was not associated with percent body fat. Thus, linkage could be due to undetected TNF-α variants or to variants of a closely linked gene. These results are consistent with the suggestion that TNF-α plays a role in development of human obesity but will require confirmation in additional families.

A possible connection between TNF-α and insulin resistance is provided by an experiment where mice with a null mutation of the adipocyte specific fatty acid binding protein (A-FABP) were created (131). Mice carrying the null mutation in A-FABP are developmentally normal; however, they do not express TNF-α or develop insulin resistance when obesity is induced by a high-fat diet (131). It is not clear how A-FABP is involved in the regulation of TNF-α expression.

Genes involved in the differentiation of adipose tissue provide a productive resource for analysis of body weight regulation candidate genes. The volume of lipid that an individual adipocyte can accumulate is fixed, while the capacity of adipose tissue to expand is without obvious limit. Thus, significant expansion of adipose tissue mass requires de novo differentiation of adipocytes from precursor cells (132). This process can occur at any time throughout life and may be contingent on nutritional status. Several transcription factors that promote differentiation of preadipocytes into adipose cells have been identified, with different expression patterns in several tissues and at various times of adipocyte differentiation. Development of adipose tissue is discussed at greater length in another chapter. Transcription factors affecting adipocyte differentiation include CCAATT enhancer-binding protein-α (C/EBPα), peroxisome proliferator-activated receptor $\gamma2$ (PPAR$\gamma2$) and the fatty acid activated receptor (FAAR) (133–135). A role for C/EBPα in obesity has been confirmed by the observation that hepatocytes and adipocytes of mice lacking C/EBPα fail to accumulate lipid (136). PPAR$\gamma2$, an adipocyte-specific nuclear hormone receptor, stimulates adipose differentiation of cultured fibroblasts (133). 15-Deoxy-$\Delta^{12,14}$-prostaglandin J2 is both an endogenous ligand for PPARγ and an inducer of adipogenesis (137,138). As a lipid-activated transcription factor, PPARγ represents a potential molecular link between cellular or systemic lipid metabolism and adipocyte differentiation. A number of clinical reagents are directed against nuclear hormone receptors. Examples include the estrogen receptor antagonist tamoxifen and RU-486, which is a progesterone and type II glucocortoid receptor antagonist. The antidiabetic thiazolidinediones also bind to PPARγ and regulate adipocyte differentiation. Thus, it may be possible to regulate adipocyte differentiation using activators or inhibitors of adipocyte-specific transcription factors. Indeed, it has already been shown that RU 486 stops fat deposition in obese *fa/fa* rats (139).

D. Speculations About Transcription Factors that May Affect Both Body Weight Regulation and Plasma Cholesterol Levels

BSB mice have coincident QTLs for plasma cholesterol, hepatic lipase activity, and body lipid percentage on chromosome 7 (see above and Fig. 2). It is unknown whether this coincidence results from random chance or from co-ordinated regulation. In principle, a transcription factor that influenced body obesity and plasma cholesterol levels could cause the coincidence of QTLs. Two such candidate genes have been described.

The adipocyte determination- and differentiation-dependent factor 1 (ADD1) is elevated in determined preadipocytes and is further increased during adipocyte differentiation (140). ADDI was cloned from a mouse adipocyte library, but the human homolog was cloned independently during a search for the sterol regulatory element-binding protein 1 (SREBP1) gene. SREBP1 regulates the transcription of several cholesterol responsive genes, including the low-density-lipoprotein receptor, 7-OH hydroxylase, and 3-hydroxy-3-methyl glutaryl coenzyme A reductase (HMG-CoA reductase) (141). The identity of ADD1 and SREBP1 proves that a single transcription factor influences both plasma cholesterol and obesity. Although SREBP1/ADD was an attractive candidate gene for *Mob1*, it has been mapped to mouse chromosome 8 (unpublished data) and thus cannot account for *Mob1*. However, other transcription factors may also affect both plasma cholesterol and obesity.

Two transcription factors have been shown to affect both apo A-II expression and adipocyte differentiation. PPARγ and retinoic acid X receptor-α (RXRα) promote adipocyte differentiation (see above). The apo A-II gene has been shown to include a functional peroxisome proliferator responsive element. Cotransfection assays showed that PPARγ and RXRα act to increase the transcription and translation of apo A-II in primary cultures of human hepatocytes, which will tend to increase levels of high-density-lipoprotein (HDL) cholesterol (142). These results may explain the observation that apoA-II levels are strongly correlated with body fat percentage in BSB mice ($r^2 = 0.223$). This correlation does not appear to result from nonspecific correlation of obesity with plasma cholesterol levels, since other apolipoproteins, including apoA-I and apoA-IV, are less well correlated with percent body fat ($r^2 = 0.018$ and 0.076, respectively). It is also interesting that studies in both mice and humans have found positive correlations of apoA-II levels with free fatty acid levels (96,143). Studies with PPARγ are consistent with this correlation since the fatty acid eicosatetraynoic acid (ETYA) promotes both adipocyte differentiation and apoA-II expression (133).

IV. SUMMARY

The tools of molecular genetics provide two complementary approaches that can be used to define the mechanisms of body weight regulation. On the one hand, genetic procedures can be used to identify chromosomal locations and then to isolate genes that cause obesity. This identification and isolation of genes causing obesity relies on linkage studies of human families or genetic crosses of mice (or other experimental animals) and subsequent positional cloning. The second general way that molecular genetics can be used to study body weight regulation is by testing hypotheses. This approach includes the production of transgenic or knockout animals starting with hypotheses about candidate genes. Thus, the tools of molecular genetics allow for the identification, isolation, and testing of genes that regulate body weight.

We believe that an overall examination of the current knowledge of body weight regulation provides the framework for several hypotheses about the pathways for body weight regulation. Regulation of corticosterone levels by adrenocorticotropic hormone (ACTH) may be part of a pathway for feedback regulation of leptin levels that is influenced by the central nervous system (CNS), since corticosterone regulates leptin mRNA levels. Another hypothesis derived from novel observations is that alteration of GLUT4 levels in transgenic and knockout mice may affect body weight regulation by influencing leptin mRNA expression. This hypothesis would be consistent with the regulation of leptin levels by glucose and insulin levels that has been demonstrated.

Finally, the results presented here provide great hope for the future, both that the basic biology of body weight regulation will be clarified and that safe and effective therapies will result from this increased understanding.

REFERENCES

1. Warden CH, Bouchard C, Friedman JM, Hebebrandt J, Hitman GA, Kozak LP, Leibel RL, Price RA, Zechner R. Group report: How can we best apply the tools of genetics to study body weight regulation? In: Bouchard C, Bray

GA, eds. Regulation of Body Weight: Biological and Behavioral Mechanisms. Vol. Life Science Research Report LS 57. West Sussex: Wiley 196:285–305.

2. Bouchard C. The genetics of obesity: from genetic epidemiology to molecular markers. Mol Med Today 1995; 1:45–50.

3. Vogler GP, Sorenson TIA, Stunkard AJ, Srinivasan MR, Rao DC. Influences of genes and shared environment on adult body mass index assessed in an adoption study by a comprehensive path model. Int J Obes 1995; 19:40–45.

4. Stunkard AJ, Harris JR, Pedersen NL, McClearn GE. The body-mass index of twins who have been reared apart. N Engl J Med 1990; 322:1483–1487.

5. Bouchard C, Tremblay A, Després J-P, Nadeau A, Lupien PJ, Thériault G, Dussault J, Moorjani S, Pineault S, Fournier G. The response to long-term overfeeding in identical twins. N Engl J Med 1990; 322:1477–1482.

6. Tambs K, Moum T, Eaves L, Neale M, Midthjell K, Lund-Larsen PG, Naess S, Holmen J. Genetic and environmental contributions to the variance on the body mass index in a Norwegian sample of first- and second-degree relatives. Am J Hum Biol 1991; 3:257–267.

7. Bouchard C. Genetics of obesity: overview and research directions. In: Bouchard C, ed. The Genetics of Obesity. Boca Raton, FL: CRC Press, 1994:223–233.

8. Stunkard AJ, Foch TT. Hrubec Z. A twin study of human obesity. JAMA 1986; 256:51–54.

9. Friedman JM, Leibel RL, Bahary N. Molecular mapping of obesity genes. Mamm Genome 1991; 1:130–144.

10. Bultman SJ, Michaud EJ, Woychik RP. Molecular characterization of the mouse *agouti* locus. Cell 1992; 71: 1195–1204.

11. Miller MW, Duhl DMJ, Vrieling H, Cordes SP, Ollmann MM, Winkes BM, Barsh GS. Cloning of the mouse *agouti* gene predicts a secreted protein ubiquitously expressed in mice carrying the lethal yellow mutation. Genes Dev 1993; 7:454–467.

12. Zhang Y, Proenca R, Maffel M, Barone M, Leopold L, Friedman JM Positional cloning of the mouse obese gene and its human homologue. Nature 1994; 372:425–432.

13. Naggert JK, Fricker LD, Varlamov O, Nishina PM, Rouille Y, Steiner DF, Carroll RJ, Paigen BJ, Leiter EH. Hyperproinsulinaemia in obese *fat/fat* mice associated with a carbohypeptide E mutation which reduces enzyme activity. Nature Genet 1995; 10:135–141.

14. Chen H, Charlat O, Tartaglia LA, Woolf EA, Weng X, Ellis SJ, Lakey ND, Culpepper J, Moore KJ, Breitbart RE, Duyk GM, Tepper RI, Morgenstern JP. Evidence that the diabetes gene encodes the leptin receptor: identification of a mutation in the leptin receptor gene in *db/db* mice. Cell 1996; 84:491–495.

15. Lee G-H, Proenca R, Montez JM, Carroll KM, Darvishzadeh JG, Lee JI, Friedman JM. Abnormal splicing of the leptin receptor in *diabetic* mice. Nature 1996; 379: 632–635.

16. Tartaglia LA, Dembski M, Weng X, Deng N, Culpepper J, Devos R, Richards GJ, Campfield LA, Clark FT, Deeds J, Muir C, Sanker S, Moriarty A, Moore KJ, Smutko JS, Mays GG, Woolf EA, Monroe CA, Tepper RI. Identification and expression cloning of a leptin receptor, OB-R.Cell 1995; 83:1263–1271.

17. Collins FS. Positional cloning moves from perditional to traditional. Nature Genet 1995; 9:347–350.

18. Lander ES, Schork NJ. Genetic dissection of complex traits. Science 1994; 265:2037–2048.

19. Kruglyak L, Lander ES. Complete multipoint sib-pair analysis of qualitative and quantitative traits. Am J Hum Genet 1995; 57:439–454.

20. Kruglyak L, Lander ES. High resolution genetic mapping of complex traits. Am J Hum Genet 1995; 56:1212–1223.

21. Lander ES, Kruglyak L. Genetic dissection of complex traits: guidelines for interpreting and reporting linkage results. Nature Genet 1995; 11:241–247.

22. Clement K, Vaisse C, Manning BSJ, Basdevant A, Guy-Grand B, Ruiz J, Silver KD, Shuldiner AR, Froguel P, Strosberg AD, Genetic variation in the beta3-adrenergic receptor and an increased capacity to gain weight in patients with morbid obesity. N Engl J Med 1995; 333: 352–354.

23. Walston J, Silver K, Bogardus C, Knowler WC, Celi FS, Austin S, Manning B, Strosberg AD, Stern MP, Raben N, Sorkin JD, Roth J, Shuldiner AR. Time of onset of non-insulin-dependent diabetes mellitus and genetic variation in the beta3-adrenergic-receptor gene. N Engl J Med 1995; 333:343–347.

24. Widen E, Lehto M, Kanninen T, Walston J, Shuldiner AR, Groop LC. Association of a polymorphism in the beta3-adrenergic-receptor gene with features of the insulin resistance syndrome in Finns. N Engl J Med 1995; 333: 348–351.

25. Weiss KM. Genetic Variation and Human Disease. Cambridge: Cambridge University Press, 1993.

26. Croft JB, Morrell D, Chase CL, Swift M. Obesity in heterozygous carriers of the gene for Bardet-Biedl syndrome. Am J Med Genet 1995; 55:12–15.

27. Reed ML, Leff SE. Maternal imprinting of human SNRPN, a gene deleted in Prader-Willi syndrome. Nature Genet 1994; 6:163–167.

28. Cattanach BM, Barr JA, Evans EP, Burtenshaw M, Beechy CV, Leff SE, Brannan CI, Copeland NG, Jenkins NA, Jones J. A candidate mouse model for Prader-Willi syndrome which shows an absence of *Snrpn* expression. Nature Genet 1992; 2:270–274.

29. Buiting K, Saitoh S, Gross S, Dittrich B, Schwartz S, Nicholls RD, Horsthemke B. Inherited microdelections in the Angelman and Prader-Willi syndromes define an imprinting center on human chromosome 15. Nature Genet 1995; 9:395–400.

30. Warden CH, Fisler JS. Identification of genes underlying polygenic obesity in animal models. In: Bouchard C, ed.

The Genetics of Obesity. Boca Raton, FL: CRC Press, 1994:181–197.

31. Friedman JM, Leibel RL, Bahary N, Siegel DA, Truett G. Genetic analysis of complex disorders: molecular mapping of obesity genes in mice and humans. Ann NY Sci 1991; 630:100–115.

32. Copeland NG, Jenkins NA, Gilbert DJ, Eppig JT, Maltais LJ, Miller JC, Dietrich WF, Weaver A, Lincoln SE, Steen RG, Stein LD, Nadeau JH, Lander ES. A genetic linkage map of the mouse: current applications and future prospects. Science 1993; 262;57–66.

33. Schemmel R, Mickelson O, Gill JL. Dietary obesity in rats: body weight and body fat accretation in seven strains of rats. J Nutr 1970; 100:1041–1048.

34. Schork NJ, Krieger JE, Trolliet MR, Franchini KG, Koike G, Kreiger EM, Lander ES, Dzau VJ, Jacob HJ. A biometrical genome search in rats reveals the multigenic basis of blood pressure variation. Genome Res 1995; 5:164–172.

35. Lander ES, Botstein D. Mapping Mendelian factors underlying quantitative traits using RFLP linkage maps. Genetics 1989; 121:185–199.

36. Hastings IM, Veerkamp RF. The genetic basis of response in mouse lines divergently selected for body weight or fat content. I. The relative contributions of autosomal and sex-linked genes. Genet Res 1993; 62:169–175.

37. West DB, Waguespack J, York B, Goudey-Lefevre J, Price RA. Genetics of dietary obesity in AKR/J X SWR/J mice: segregation of the trait and identification of a linked locus on chromosome 4. Mamm Genome 1994; 5:546–552.

38. West DB, Goudey-Lefevre J, York B, Truett GE. Dietary obesity linked to genetic loci on chromosome 9 and 15 in a polygenic mouse model. J Clin Invest 1994; 94: 1410–1416.

39. Andersson L, Haley CS, Ellegren H, Knott SA, Johansson M, Andersson K, Andersson-Eklund L, Edfors-Lilja I, Fredholm M, Hansson I, Håkansson J, Lundström K. Genetic mapping of quantitative trait loci for growth and fatness in pigs. Science 1994; 263:1771–1774.

40. Fisler JS, Warden CH, Pace MJ, Lusis AJ. BSB: a new mouse model of multigenic obesity. Obes Res 1993; 1: 271–280.

41. Paterson AH, Lander ES, Hewitt JD, Peterson S, Lincoln SE, Tanksley SD. Resolution of quantitative traits into Mendelian factors by using a complete linkage map of restriction fragment length polymorphisms. Nature 1988; 335:721–726.

42. Warden CH, Fisler JS, Shoemaker SM, Wen P-Z, Svenson KL, Pace MJ, Lusis AJ. Identification of four chromosomal loci determining obesity in a multifactorial mouse model. J Clin Invest 1995; 95:1545–1552.

43. Warden CH, Fisler JS, Pace MJ, Svenson KL, Lusis AJ. Coincidence of genetic loci for plasma cholesterol levels and obesity in a multifactorial mouse model. J Clin Invest 1993; 92:773–779.

44. Rance KA, Hastings IM, Hill WG, Keightley PD. Mapping of putative QTL influencing body weight on the X chromosome in mice. 5th World Congress on Genetics Applied to Livestock Production. Guelph: University of Guelph, 1994:268–269.

45. Pomp D, Cushman MA, Foster SC, Drudik DK, Fortman M, Eisen EJ. Identification of quantitative trait loci for body weight and body fat in mice. 5th World Congress on Genetics Applied to Livestock Production: University of Guelph, 1994:209–212.

48. Haseman JK, Elston RC. The investigation of linkage between a quantitative trait and a marker locus. Behav Genet 1972; 2:3–19.

49. Risch N, Zhang H. Extreme discordant sib pairs for mapping quantitative trait loci in humans. Science 1995; 268: 1584–1589.

50. Bouchard C. Genetic epidemiology, association, and sib-pair linkage: results from the Québec Family Study. In: Bray GA, Ryan DH, eds. Molecular and Genetic Aspects of Obesity. Baton Rouge; Louisiana State University Press, 1996; 5:470–481.

51. Norman RA, Bogardus C, Ravussin E. Linkage between obesity and a marker near the tumor necrosis-alpha locus in Pima Indians. J Clin Invest 1995; 96:158–162.

52. Norman R, Leibel RL, Bogardus C, Ravussin E. Genome scan for linkages of obesity to polymorphic DNA markers in Pima Indians. Obes Res 1995; 3(Suppl 3):353s–350.

53. Reed DR, Ding Y, Xu W, Cather C, Green ED, Price RA. Extreme, early-onset obesity is linked to markers flanking the human ob gene. Obes Res 1995; 3(Suppl 3): 353s–350.

54. Duggirala R, Blangero J, Leibel R, O'Connell P, Stern M. Linkage of markers on human chromosome 7 with obesity related traits in Mexican Americans. Obes Res 1995; 3(Suppl 3):360s–360.

55. Considine RV, Considine EL, Williams CJ, Nyce MR, Magosin SA, Bauer TL, Rosato EL, Colberg J, Caro JF. Evidence against either a premature stop codon or the absence of obese gene mRNA in human obesity. J Clin Invest 1995; 95:2986–2988.

56. Dietrich WF, Lander ES, Smith JS, Moser AR, Gould KA, Luongo C, Borenstein N, Dove W. Genetic identification of Mom-1, a major modifier locus affecting Min-induced intestinal neoplasia in the mouse. Cell 1993; 75:631–639.

57. MacPhee M, Chepenik KP, Liddell RA, Nelson KK, Siracusa LD, Buchberg AM. The secretory phospholipase A2 gene is a candidate for the Mom 1 locus, a major modifier of ApcMin-induced intestinal neoplasia. Cell 1995; 81: 957–966.

58. Hummel KP, Coleman DL, Lane PW. The influence of genetic background on expression of mutations at the diabetes locus in the mouse. 1 C57BL/KsJ and C57BL/6J strains. Biochem Genet 1972; 7:1–3.

59. Coleman DL, Hummel KP. Influence of genetic background on the expression of mutations at the diabetes locus in the mouse. II. Studies on background modifiers. Isr J Med 1975; 11:708–718.

60. Leiter EH, Chapman HD, Coleman DL. The influence of genetic background on the expression of mutations at the

diabetes locus in the mouse. V. Interaction between the db gene and hepatic sex steroid sulfotransferases correlates with gender-dependent susceptibility to hyperglycemia. Endocrinology 1989; 124:912–924.

61. Naggert JK, Mu J-L, Frankel W, Bailey DW, Paigen B. Genomic analysis of the C57BL/Ks mouse strain. Mamm Genome 1995; 6:131–133.

62. Graff RJ, Snell GD. Histocompatibility genes of mice: VIII. The alleles of the H-1 locus. Transplantation 1968; 6: 598–617.

63. Bailey DW. Genetics of histocompatibility in mice: I. New loci and congenic lines. Immunogenetics 1975; 2: 249–256.

64. Mehrabian M, Qiao J-H, Hyman R, Ruddle D, Laughton C, Lusis AJ. Influence of the ApoA-II gene locus on HDL levels and fatty streak development in mice. Arterioscler Thromb 1993; 13:1–10.

65. West DB, Boozer CN, Moody DL, Atkinson RL. Dietary obesity in nine inbred mouse strains. Am J Physiol Regul Integr Comp Physiol 1992; 262:R1025–R1032.

66. Klebig ML, Wilkison JE, Geisler JG, Woychik RP. Ectopic expression of the agouti gene in transgenic mice causes obesity, features of type II diabetes, and yellow fur. Proc Natl Acad Sci USA 1995; 92:4728–4732.

70. Adams MD, Kerlavage AR, Fleischmann RD, Fuldner RA, Bult CJ, Lee NH, Kirkness EF, Weinstock KG, Gocayne JD, White O, et al. Initial assessment of human gene diversity and expression patterns based upon 83 million nucleotides of cDNA sequence, Nature 1995; 377:3–174.

71. Goodfellow P. A big book of the human genome. Nature 1995; 377:25–286.

72. Little P. Navigational progress. Nature 1995; 377: 286–387.

73. Fields C, Adams MD, White O, Venter JC. How many genes in the human genome? Nature Genet 1994; 7: 345–346.

74. Nadeau JH, Davisson MT, Doolittle DP, Grant P, Hillyard AL, Kosowsky MR, Roderick TH. Comparative map for mice and humans. Mamm Genome 1992; 3:480–536.

75. Chau SC, Chung WK, Wu-Peng XS, Zhang Y, Liu S-M, Tartaglia L, Leibel RL. Phenotypes of mouse *diabetes* and rat *fatty* due to mutations in the OB (Leptin) receptor. Science 1996; 271:994–996.

76. Ogawa Y, Masuzaki H, Isse N, Okazaki T, Mori K, Shigemoto M, Satoh N, Tamura N, Hosoda K, Yoshimasa Y, Jingami H, Kawada T, Nakao K. Molecular cloning of rat Obese cDNA and augmented gene expression in genetically obese Zucker fatty (*fa/fa*) rats. J Clin Invest 1995; 96:1647–1652.

77. Pelleymounter MA, Cullen MJ, Baker MB, Hecht R, Winters D, Boone T, Collin F. Effects of the obese gene product on body weight regulation on *ob/ob* mice. Science 1995; 269:540–543.

78. Halaas JL, Gajiwala KS, Maffei M, Cohen SL, Chair BT, Rabinowitz D, Lallone RL, Burley SK, Friedman JM.

Weight-reducing effects of the plasma protein encoded by the obese gene. Science 1995; 269:543–546.

79. Campfield LA, Smith FJ, Guisez Y, Devos R, Burn P. Recombinant mouse OB protein; evidence for a peripheral signal linking adiposity and central neural networks. Science 1995; 269:546–549.

80. Stephens TW, Basinski M, Bristow PK, Bue-Valleskey JM, Burget SG, Craft L, Hale J, Hoffman J, Hsiung HM, Kriauciunas A, MacKellar W, Rosteck PR, Schoner B, Smith D, Tinsley FC, Zhang X-Y, Heiman M. The role of neuropeptide Y in the antiobesity action of the obese gene product. Nature 1995; 377:530–532.

81. Stanley BG, Anderson KC, Grayson MH, Leibowitz SF. Repeated hypothalamic stimulation with neuropeptide Y increases daily carbohydrate and fat intake and body weight gain in female rats. Physiol Behav 1989; 46: 173–177.

82. Fredrich RC, Löllmann B, Hamann A, Napolitano-Rosen A, Khan BB, Lowell BB, Flier JS. Expression of ob mRNA and its encoded protein in rodents. Impact of nutrition and obesity. J Clin Invest 1995; 96:1658–1663.

83. MacDougald OA, Hwang CS, Fan HY, Lane MD. Regulated expression of the obese gene product (leptin) in white adipose tissue and 3T3-L1 adipocytes. Proc Natl Acad Scie USA 1995; 92:9034–9037.

84. Saladin R, De Vos P, Guerre-Millo M, Leturque A, Girard J, Staels B, Auwerx J. Transient increase in obese gene expression after food intake or insulin administration. Nature 1995; 377:527–529.

85. Vos PD, Saladin R, Auwerx J, Staels B. Induction of ob gene expression by corticosteroids is accompanied by body weight loss and reduced food intake. J Biol Chem 1995; 270:15958–15961.

86. Maffei M, Fei H, Lee G-H, Dani C, Leroy P, Zhang Y, Proenca R, Negrel R, Ailhaud G, Friedman JM. Increased expression in adipocytes of ob RNA in mice with lesions of the hypothalamus and with mutations at the *db* locus. Proc Natl Acad Scie USA 1995; 92:6957–6960.

87. Considine RV, Sinha MK, Heiman ML, Kriauciunas A, Stephens TW, Nyce MR, Ohannesian JP, Marco CC, McKee LJ, Bauer TL, Caro JF. Serum immunoreactive-leptin concentrations in normal-weight and obese humans. N Engl J Med 1996; 334:292–295.

88. Hamilton BS, Paglia D, Kwan AYM, Deitel M. Increased *obese* mRNA expression in omental fat cells from massively obese humans. Nature Med 1995; 1:953–956.

89. Lönnqvist F, Amer P, Nordfors L, Schalling M. Overexpression of the obese (*ob*) gene in adipose tissue of human obese subjects. Nature Med 1995; 1:950–953.

90. Maffei M, Halaas J, Ravussin E, Pratley RE, Lee GH, Zhang Y, Fei H, Kim S, Lallone R, Ranganathan S, Kern PA, Friedman JM. Leptin levels in human and rodent: measurement of plasma leptin and ob RNA in obese and weight-reduced subjects. Nature Med 1995; 1: 1155–1161.

91. Friedrich RC, Hamann A, Anderson S, Löllmann B, Lowell BB, Flier JS. Leptin levels reflect body lipid content in mice: evidence for diet-induced resistance to leptin action. Nature Med 1995; 1:1311–1314.

92. Lu D, Willard D, Patel IR, Kadwell S, Overton L, Kost T, Luther M, Chen W, Woychik RP, Wilkinson WO, Cone RD. Agouti protein in an antagonist of the melanocyte-stimulating hormone receptor. Nature 1994; 371: 799–802.

93. Manne J, Argeson AC, Siracusa LD. Mechanisms for the pleiotropic effects of the agouti gene. Proc Natl Acad Sci USA 1995; 92:4712–4724.

94. Zemel MB, Kim JH, Woychik RP, Michaud EJ, Kadwell SH, Patel IR, Wilkinson WO. Agouti regulation of intracellular calcium: role in the insulin resistance of viable yellow mice. Proc Natl Acad Scie USA 1995; 92: 4733–4737.

95. Jensen DR, Morin CL, Schlaepfer IR, Pennington DS, Marcell T, Gutierrez-Hartman A, Eckel RH. Transgenic mice with overexpression of skeletal muscle lipoprotein lipase: divergent effects of differential overexpression on body lipid. Obes Res 1995; 3(Suppl 3):361s–360.

96. Warden CH, Hedrick CC, Qiao J-H, Castellani LW, Lusis AJ. Atherosclerosis in transgenic mice overexpressing apolipoprotein A-II. Science 1993; 261;469–472.

97. Schultz JR, Gong EL, McCall MR, Nichols AV, Clift SM, Rubin EM. Expression of human apolipoprotein A-II and its effect on high density lipoproteins in transgenic mice. J Biol Chem 1992; 267:21630–21636.

98. Furth PA, St-Onge L, Boger H, Gruss P, Gossen M, Kistner A, Bujard H, Hennighausen L. Temporal control of gene expression in transgenic mice by tetracycline-responsive promoter. Proc Natl Acad Sci USA 1994; 91:9302–9306.

99. Gossen M, Bujard H. Tight control of gene expression in mammalian cells by tetracycline-responsive promoters. Proc Natl Acad Sci USA 1992; 89:5547–5551.

100. McCormick SPA, Ng JK, Taylor S, Flynn LM, Hammer RE, Young SG. Mutagenesis of the human apolipoprotein B gene in a yeast artificial chromosome reveals the site of attachment for apolipoprotein(a). Proc Natl Acad Sci USA 1995; 92:10147–10151.

101. Levak-Frank S, Radner H, Walsh A, Stollberger R, Knipping G, Hoefler G, Sattler W, Weinstock PH, Breslow JL, Zechner R. Muscle-specific overexpression of lipoprotein lipase causes a severe myopathy characterized by proliferation of mitochondria and peroxisomes in transgenic mice. J Clin Invest 1995; 96:976–986.

102. Lawn RM, Wade DP, Hammer RE, Chiesa G, Verstuyft JG, Rubin EM. Atherogenesis in transgenic mice expressing human apoliproprotein(a). Nature 1992; 360:670–672.

103. Katz EB, Stenbit AE, Hatton K, DePinho R, Charron MJ. Cardiac and adipose tissue abnormalities but not diabetes in mice deficient in GLUT4, Nature 1995; 377:151–155.

104. Chambers CA. TKO'ed; Lox stock and barrel. BioEssays 1994; 16:865–868.

105. Gu H, Marth JD, Orban PC, Mossmann H, Rajewsky K. Deletion of a DNA polymerase beta gene segment in T cells using a cell type-specific gene targeting. Science 1994; 265:103–106.

106. Pepin M-C, Pothier F, Barden N. Impaired type II glucocorticoid-receptor function in mice bearing antisense RNA transgene. Nature 1992; 355:725–728.

107. Luetteke NC, Lee DC, Palmiter RD, Brinster RL, Sandgren EP. Regulation of fat and muscle development by transforming growth factor alpha in transgenic mice and in cultured cells. Cell Growth 1993; 4:203–213.

108. Gnudi L, Tozzo E, Shepherd PR, Bliss JL, Khan BB. High level overexpression of glucose transporter-4 driven by an adipose-specific promoter is maintained in transgenic mice on a high fat diet, but does not prevent impaired glucose tolerance. Endocrinology 1995; 136:995–1002.

109. Kozak LP, Kozak UC, Clarke GT. Abnormal brown and white fat development in transgenic mice overexpressing glycerol 3-phosphate dehydrogenase. Genes Dev 1991; 5: 2256–2264.

110. Tecott LH, Sun LM, Akana SF, Strack AM, Lowenstein DH, Dallman MF, Jullus D. Eating disorder and epilepsy in mice lacking 5-HT2c serotonin receptors. Nature 1995; 374:542–546.

111. Kopecky J, Clarke G, Enerbäck S, Spiegelman B, Kozak LP. Expression of the mitochondrial uncoupling protein from the aP2 gene promoter prevents genetic obesity. J Clin Invest 1995; 96:2914–2923.

112. Bray GA, Fisler JS, York D. Neuroendocrine control of the development of obesity: understanding gained from studies of experimental animal models. Frontiers Neuroendocrinol 1990; 11:128–181.

113. Himms-Hagen J. Brown adipose tissue thermogenesis: interdisciplinary studies. FASEB J 1990; 4:2890–2898.

114. Nichols DG. Brown adipose tissue mitochondria. Biochim Biophys Acta 1979; 549:1–29.

115. Rothwell NJ, Stock MJ. A role for brown adipose tissue in diet-induced thermogenesis. Nature 1979; 281:31–35.

116. Lowell BB, S-Susulic V, Hamann A, Lawitts JA, Himms-Hagen J, Boyer BB, Kozak LP, Flier JS. Development of obesity in transgenic mice after genetic ablation of brown adipose tissue. Nature 1993; 366:740–742.

117. Johnson PR, Greenwood MR, Horwitz BA, Stern JS. Animal models of obesity: genetic aspects. Annu Rev Nutr 1991; 11:325–353.

118. Giacobino J-P. Beta$_3$-adrenoceptor: an update. Eur J Endocrinol 1995; 132:377–385.

119. Emorine L, Blin N, Strosberg AD. The human beta$_3$-adrenoceptor; the search for a physiological function. Trends Pharmacol Sci 1994; 15:3–7.

120. Collins S, Daniel KW, Rohlfs EM, Ramkumar V, Taylor IL, Gettys TW. Impaired expression and functional activity of the beta$_3$- and beta1-adrenergic receptors in adipose tissue of congenitally obese (C57BL/6J *ob/ob*) mice. Mol Endocrinol 1994; 8:518–527.

121. Gettys TW, Rohlfs EM, Prpic V, Daniel KW, Taylor IL, Collins S. Age-dependent changes in beta-adrenergic receptor subtypes and adenylyl cyclase activation in adipocytes from Fischer 344 rats. Endocrinology 1995; 136: 2022–2032.

122. Hotamisligil GS, Shargill NS, Spiegelman BM. Adipose expression of tumor necrosis factor-alpha: direct role in obesity-liked insulin resistance. Science 1993; 259:87–91.

123. Hofmann C, Lorenz K, Braithwaite SS, Colca JR, Palazuk BJ, Hotamisligil GS, Spiegelman BM. Altered gene expression for tumor necrosis factor-alpha and its receptors during drug and dietary modulation of insulin resistance. Endocrinology 1994; 134:264–270.

124. Stephens JM, Pekala PH. Transcriptional repression of the GLUT4 and C/EBP genes in 3T3-L1 adipocytes by tumor necrosis factor-alpha. J Biol Chem 1991; 266: 21839–21845.

125. Hotamisligil GS, Budavari A, Murray D, Spiegelman BM. Reduced tyrosine kinase activity of the insulin receptor in obesity-diabetes: central role of tumor necrosis factor-alpha. J Clin Invest 1994; 94:1543–1549.

126. Fried SK, Zechner R. Cachectic/tumor necrosis factor decreases human adipose tissue lipoprotein lipase mRNA levels, synthesis, and activity. J Lipid Res 1989; 30: 1917–1923.

127. Grunfeld C, Gulli R, Moser AH, Gavin LA, Feingold KR. Effect of tumor necrosis factor administration in vivo on lipoprotein lipase activity in various tissues of the rat. J Lipid Res 1989; 30:579–585.

128. Kern PA, Saghizadeh M, Ong JM, Bosch RJ, Deem R, Simsolo RB. The expression of tumor necrosis factor in human adipose tissue: regulation by obesity, weight loss, and relationship to lipoprotein lipase. J Clin Invest 1995; 95: 2111–2119.

129. Patton JS, Shepard HM, Wilking H, Lewis G, Aggarwal BB, Eessalu TE, Gavin LA, Grunfeld C. Interferons and tumor necrosis factors have similar catabolic effects on 3T3-L1 cells. Proc Natl Acad Sci USA 1986; 83: 8313–8317.

130. Hotamisligil GS, Arner P, Caro JF, Atkinson RL, Spiegelman BM. Increased adipose tissue expression of tumor necrosis factor-alpha in human obesity and insulin resistance. J Clin Invest 1995; 95:2409–2415.

131. Hotamisligil GS, Peraldi P, Distel R, Jonhnson R, Papaloannou V, Arner P, Atkinson RL, Caro JF, Budavari A, Donovan A, Murray D, Ellis R, Spiegelman BM. Molecular basis of insulin resistance in obesity. Obes Res 1995; 3(Suppl 3):319s–310.

132. Ailhaud GP, Grimaldi PA, Negrel RL. Genetics and molecular biology of adipose cell characteristics. In: Bouchard C, ed. The Genetics of Obesity. Boca Raton, FL: CRC Press, 1994:199–212.

133. Tontonoz P, Hu E, Spiegelman BM. Stimulation of adipogenesis in fibroblasts by PPARgamma2, a lipid-activated transcription factor. Cell 1994; 79:1147–1156.

134. Hu ED, Tontonoz P, Spiegelman BM. Transdifferentiation of myoblasts by the adipogenic transcription factors PPARgamma and C/EBRalpha. Proc Natl Acad Sci USA 1995; 92:9856–9860.

135. Amri E-Z, Ailhaud G, Grimaldi PA. Fatty acids as signal transducing molecules: involvement in the differentiation of preadipose to adipose cells. J Lipid Res 1994; 35: 930–937.

136. Wang N-D, Finegold MJ, Bradley A, Ou CN, Abdelsayed AV, Wilde MD, Taylor LR, Wilson DR, Darlington GJ. Impaired energy homeostasis in C/EBPalpha knockout mice. Science 1995; 269:1108–1112.

137. Forman BM, Tontonoz P, Chen J, Brun RP, Spiegelman BM, Evans RM. 15-Deoxy-Δ 12,14-Prostaglandin J2 is a ligand for the adipocyte determination factor PPARγ. Cell 1995; 83:803–812.

138. Kliewet SA, Lenhard JM, Willson TM, Patel I, Morris DC, Lehmann JM. A Prostaglandin J2 metabolite binds peroxisome proliferator-activated receptor γ and promotes adipocyte differentiation. Cell 1995; 83:813–819.

139. Langley SC, York DA. Effects of antiglucocorticoid RU 486 on development of obesity in obese *fa/fa* Zucker rats. Am J Physiol 1990; 259:R539–R544.

140. Kim JB, Spotts GD, Halvorsen Y-D, Shih H-M, Ellenberger T, Towle HC, Spiegelman BM. Dual DNA binding specificity of ADD1/SREBP1 controlled by a single amino acid in the basic helix-loop-helix domain. Mol Cell Biol 1995; 15:2582–2588.

141. Yokoyama C, Wang X, Briggs MR, Admon A, Wu J, Hua X, Goldstein JL, Brown MS. SREBP-1, a basic-helix-loop-helix-leucine zipper protein that controls transcription of the low density lipoprotein receptor gene. Cell 1993; 75: 187–197.

142. Doolittle MH, LeBoeuf RC, Warden CH, Bee LM, Lusis AJ. A polymorphism affecting apoliprotein A-II transnational efficiency determines high density lipoprotein size and composition. J Biol Chem 1990; 265: 16380–16388.

143. Warden CH, Daluiski A, Bu X, Purcell-Huynh DA, De Meester C, Shieh B-H, Puppione DL. Gray RM, Reaven GM, Chen Y-DI, Rotter JI, Lusis AJ. Evidence for linkage of the apolipoprotein A-II locus to plasma apolipoprotein A-II and free fatty acid levels in mice and humans. Proc Natl Acad Sci USA 1993; 90:10886–10890.

144. Jones PS, Savory R, Barratt P, Bell AR, Gray TJB, Jenkins NA, Gilbert DJ, Copeland NG, Bell DR. Chromosomal localization, inducibility, tissue-specific expression and strain differences in three murine peroxisome-proliferator-activated-receptor genes. Eur J Biochem 1995; 233: 219–226.

145. Dietrich WF, Miller JC, Steen RG, Merchant M, Damron D, Nahf R, Gross A, Joyce DC, Wessel M, Dredge RD, Marquis A, Stein LD, Goodman N, Page DC, Lander ES. A genetic map of the mouse with 4,006 simple sequence length polymorphisms. Nature Genet 1994; 7:220–245.

13

Diet Composition and the Control of Food Intake in Humans

John E. Blundell
University of Leeds, Leeds, England

R. James Stubbs
Rowett Research Institute, Bucksburn, Aberdeen, Scotland

I. INTRODUCTION: THE STUDY OF HUMAN FOOD INTAKE

A. Context

We live in a society that is virtually obsessed with the influence of food on health, energy intake, and body weight regulation. While much of life in preindustrial societies has been concerned with locating, obtaining, or cultivating adequate quantities of appropriate foods, many people living in industrialized societies spend considerable time and effort in attempting to avoid excess food intake. For many individuals this has become an active process. The food industry in any Western society is worth billions of dollars per annum. In addition, consumers spend several billion dollars on products they hope will help them avoid excess food intake or remedy the consequences of overconsumption. Feeding and food are central to our health and well-being. Food characterizes cultural groupings and identifies social and religious occasions. The composition of the diet we eat is now considered a primary cause of morbidity and mortality [e.g., obesity, coronary heart disease (1)]. Our growing knowledge of the effects of the diet on health offer a potential means of preventing certain illnesses or alleviating the effects of others through nutritional support. The market economy has recognized the potential in this area and now "functional foods" and "nutraceuticals" are available with the promise of increased consumer longevity, health, and well-being.

A key problem, particularly for the layperson, is that it appears difficult to pinpoint the major facts that scientists have discovered about food intake. What are the salient discoveries in the area of appetite and energy balance? Researchers often find this a very difficult question to deal with. Why is this so? Is it because there are no facts (universally agreed statements)? Or is it because we are dealing with a form of *behavior*, which operates according to probabilistic rather than deterministic principles? There is a further reason why facts about food intake appear to be relatively rare. Reliable quantitative and qualitative facts about food intake appear difficult to obtain since the act of measurement may influence what is being measured. Even more frustrating to both the scientist and the general public is the problem of communicating the results of research to a population eager to understand how to regulate body weight and improve health and fitness. As soon as the media reduces research results to readily digested "sound bytes" deemed fit for public consumption, the information being relayed to the public has become distorted. This is often so in science. However, the field of ingestive behavior, energy balance, and obesity is constantly the subject of media interest, so this problem of media misrepresentation of our results is more acute.

It should be kept in mind that food intake is a form of behavior commonly believed to be under voluntary control. This behavior can be described by terms such as amount of energy ingested, structure of dietary pattern, or macronutrient profile. But all of these terms are the consequences of behavior (food being seized by the hands and transported to the mouth). Therefore, a study of food intake should concentrate on the way in which environmental, cognitive, or biological events can be translated into effects upon the act of behavior. It is also worth mentioning that not eating [one aspect of which is postingestive (PI) satiety] is also a form of behavior. Consequently, events that prevent eating are also important. Since prevention of weight gain or promotion of weight loss by noneating has become an active process and food intake is often under voluntary control, it might be suggested that energy intake is not always under total voluntary control. Understanding how energy balance is maintained requires an understanding of the forms of behavior that promote weight stability. Understanding the etiology of obesity and developing strategies for its treatment requires an elucidation of the mechanisms that influence the behaviors leading to weight gain and those that can bring about a sustained weight loss, respectively.

It is also important to recognize that certain environmental contexts favor or constrain specific forms of behavior. For example, a calorimeter environment constrains the ability of a subject to move about and select food. In a given environmental context, eating behavior bridges the gap between the nutritional environment and the physiological/biochemical mechanisms of weight control. One view of appetite regulation is that it may be seen as the adoption of forms of behavior that ensure an appropriate supply of energy and nutrients for the optimal performance of the organism in a given environment. It follows that strategies of appetite regulation appropriate to a hunter gatherer are not necessarily the same behavioral strategies as those of a bank clerk.

B. Eating Behavior or Fuel Intake?

Food consumption is the target of scientific research for a number of different researchers including physiologists, nutritionists, psychologists, biochemists, endocrinologists, and many others. All of these researchers share, as one of their primary goals, the attempt to understand the mechanisms responsible for human food consumption. However, the terminology that refers to this end-point may appear discordant. For one group of researchers, the phenomenon usually measured is called eating, human feeding, or food intake. In other scientific domains, the phenomenon is called dietary intake, energy intake, or, more commonly, spontaneous energy intake. Differences are also apparent at the level of scientific practice. The first group is often concerned with qualitative aspects of eating such as food choice, food preferences, and the sensory aspects of food together with subjective phenomena such as hunger, fullness, and hedonic sensations that accompany eating and are sometimes regarded as causal agents. The second group is primarily concerned with quantitative aspects of consumption and with the energetic value of food; at present, particular importance is attached to the macronutrient composition of food and its impact on energy balance (2).

The identification of food consumption as either a form of behavior or fuel intake is not just a semantic issue, and the study of human appetite should attempt to reconcile these different approaches. What is the relationship between the pattern of intake of meals and snacks (behavioral profile), the tastes and other sensory attributes of the foods consumed (qualitative pattern), and the total food consumed over a 24-hr period (spontaneous energy intake) together with the proportions of macronutrients (fuel balance)? How do the physiological consequences of nutrient ingestion influence subsequent feeding behavior? Is obesity brought about by enhanced feelings of hunger, weakened PI satiety, sensorily induced overconsumption, or hedonically mediated maladaptive food choices? Or is obesity a result of errors in processes governing energy balance such as inappropriate oxidation of fuels or different neurendocrine responses to varying dietary intakes? What is the relationship between these domains of explanation? If appetite research is to explain the mechanisms responsible for human food consumption, it must be multidisciplinary. The outcomes of studies on feeding behavior are probabilistic rather than absolute and therefore not as empirically reproducible as, for example, the behavior of molecules in solutions. This means that the experimental environment can be particularly important in determining the outcome. A specific issue or factor thought to be important in influencing feeding behavior needs to be examined in different groups of subjects and in different environments. If this factor is thought to be fundamental to biological regulation, it should be shown to operate in a number of different species.

II. METHODOLOGICAL APPROACHES TO STUDIES OF HUMAN FOOD INTAKE

A number of key methodological issues should be borne in mind when designing and interpreting studies of human feeding behavior.

A. Precision Versus Naturalness

Since the experimental environment itself can affect the outcome of experiments, workers involved in the study of human feeding behavior are faced with a major methodological problem. Feeding behavior can be studied either in free-living people where errors are large but subjects are behaving naturally in their usual environment, or factors affecting feeding behavior can be examined in the laboratory with great precision and accuracy but there is a danger of creating artifacts due to the artificiality of the experimental environment. This relationship is illustrated in Figure 1.

There has been a general shift in emphasis in recent years from qualitative studies examining factors such as eating style, rate, and duration as potential determinants of intake to more quantitative work based on the effects of controlled nutrient interventions on energy and nutrient intakes. A number of excellent reviews have discussed experimental techniques and methods associated with the study of feeding behavior (3–5). Various methods have their own inherent strengths and weaknesses. It is probably worth keeping in mind that neither calorimeter/cubicle environments nor free-living systems have a monopoly on scientific truth. The eating that goes on (and the nutrient and energy computations subsequently made) will be closely related to the nature of the research environment. For example, Shepherd (6) notes that sensory attributes of foods associated with salt, sugar, and fat may be important in influencing food choice when specific sensory measures of foods are related to nutrient intake or food consumption in the laboratory. In the real world the picture is much less clear. There is little convincing evidence that the same sensory attributes determine salt, sugar, and fat intake in free-living people. Other factors, such as convenience, price, nutritional beliefs, availability, brand image, and cultural and social influences, are likely to be more important. Thus the "noise" created by environmental influences in the real world obscures the relationships observed in the laboratory. This "noise" is, however, important because it influences food choice in the natural environment of the subjects.

Studies are therefore measuring not how the biobehavioral system functions, but how it functions under different circumstances. Is any of this relevant to how the system functions when it is not in an experiment and not being measured? Currently we favor (where possible) a methodological approach that attempts to bridge the gap between the laboratory and the real world by overlapping protocols that explore the same issue in different environmental contexts. Few individual studies are likely to unequivocally resolve major issues in appetite research.

B. Demand Characteristics

Although, as scientists, we may suppose that we can investigate the food intake of human subjects as if it were a piece of tissue in a test tube, this is unlikely to be the case. In any experimental circumstances subjects bring with them their past history of eating, beliefs about food,

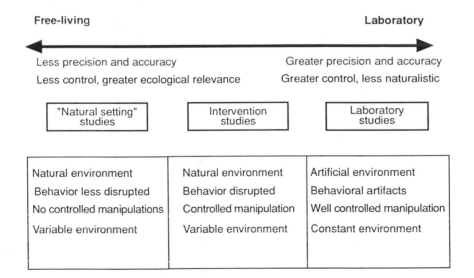

Figure 1 Constraints and limitations that the experimental environment places on studies of human feeding. In general, the environment ranges from totally free-living, which is realistic but very difficult to make measurements in, to the laboratory, where measurements are easy but may be contaminated by artifacts due to the artificiality of the laboratory surroundings.

and also their beliefs about what they are supposed to do to be a "good subject." These beliefs that will influence the volitional control over responses (namely eating) are often referred to as demand characteristics and are widely ignored (by researchers).

Demand characteristics, which obviously differ according to the experimental environment (see above), are also potently influenced by the instructions given to subjects. For example, instructions such as "eat as you normally would" and "eat to comfortable fullness" are likely to induce quite different controls over the food consumed. The first would suggest that the subject eats an appropriate perceived amount of food, and the second that the subject responds to internal signals. Such apparently small methodological differences may go unnoticed but could have significance effects on the measured outcome.

C. Power, Sensitivity, and Effect Size

These issues are, of course, relevant to all research but may assume special importance where a form of behavior is the measured variable. This is because there is likely to be large intersubject variability. As an example, attention can be drawn to short-term studies on appetite using some variant of the preload test meal paradigm. The problem concerns negative outcomes, i.e., where manipulations produce no significant effect (on the test meal intake). Negative outcomes may obviously arise from experiments conducted under low power (the type II error). This could be brought about by small numbers of subjects, small manipulations (at the border of detection threshold), and noise in the system. In certain cases an effect size of 10% may not be statistically significant. This can be contrasted with an epidemiological-type study using hundreds of subjects in which an effect size of 0.05% may be statistically significant. In these cases different arguments apply to achieve the optimum interpretation.

For those small-scale studies that fail to detect a change in the dependent variable a problem of interpretation arises. Is the manipulated (independent) variable truly without effect, or is the experimental system insensitive? Most scientists could design a legitimate-looking experiment, whose methodology could pass peer-review scrutiny, but that would inevitably lead to a negative outcome. It has been pointed out that the major problem to be overcome in biobehavioral experiments is the type II error (not the type I, which most scientists dread because they can be accused of fudging the data). The preload paradigm is vulnerable to type II errors from a number of sources, such as small quantity of nutrient given, small number of subjects, or the test meal consumed at a time when the effects of the preload have decayed to the point where

they are no longer significant. Studies conducted in the clinical setting are vulnerable to both type I and type II errors, often because of small sample sizes. Type I errors can occur due to confounding factors such as secondary complications of disease or medication.

D. Relevance of Questions Asked and Veridicality of Results

Research strategies should be formulated to address key theoretical or practical issues that are important to the study of human feeding behavior. The research question asked will, in part, influence the interpretation of results. For example, high-fat, energy-dense diets promote higher energy intakes than lower-fat, less energy-dense diets (7–9). The common interpretation of this result is that fat is poorly recognized by the body and that dietary fat per se promotes excess energy intakes. Other studies show isoenergetically dense high- and low-fat diets to produce similar energy intakes (10,11). Is the excess energy intake due to fat, energy density, or an interaction between these factors? Furthermore, what happens when subjects are allowed to select between high- and low-fat items that vary in energy density?

There is relatively little standardization of definitions and approaches in this area of research and this often makes comparisons of studies difficult. Furthermore, the problems of precision versus naturalness, demand characteristics, and sensitivity mean that the literature is awash with studies that provide conflicting results about the same issue. It is often only possible to gain a clearer view of an issue by examining all of the studies that have addressed that issue after careful consideration has been given to methodologies employed. The literature on the influence of sweetness on appetite, publications on the influence of dietary fat on PI satiety, and the role of CCK as a PI-satiety hormone are three clear examples where a number of conflicting results can be obtained from various studies in the literature. At present, there is a considerable degree of selective presentation of research results by interested parties who aim to use the scientific literature to market products that may or may not influence human feeding behavior or energy balance. It is important to consider all of the literature on a given area. Researchers have a responsibility to acknowledge the limitations of their own experimental designs and to avoid overgeneralizing results or drawing premature conclusions from individual studies conducted in specific experimental environments, on small numbers of subjects. Since the majority of positive results usually provide indirect support for a hypothesis, the limitations of that support should be acknowledged. The perfect experimental protocol to study human feeding behavior does not exist.

E. Bottom-up or Top-down Research?

There is currently a tendency to view the interest in biological science in terms of its ability to explain biological systems at the molecular and biochemical level. However, for any mechanism to be important to feeding behavior and body weight regulation it must operate under physiological conditions in the intact animal. We believe that it is useful to study human feeding by considering the way that feeding behavior operates as a system within the intact person. In addition, an understanding of how the intact system operates can be used as a reference when attempting to interpret the mechanisms underlying the development of obesity and pathological disturbances of feeding behavior. It is equally important to examine how changes in key features of the system may affect its overall functioning, for example, by understanding the role of CCK in meal termination and the maintenance of PI satiety. However, these components should always be viewed as parts of a more complex system, rather than the prime movers in a simple feedback loop. It is therefore necessary to attempt to understand the nature of the system and how it responds to changes in the environment.

III. THE NATURE OF THE APPETITE SYSTEM

A. Behavior of the Appetite System

Feeding is determined by a redundant biological system that operates through changes in behavior (by redundant we mean the system is actually a series of overlapping subsystems, which do not all need to be fully operational or intact for the whole system to function appropriately). The physiology of appetite is therefore the physiology of feeding behavior. Anatomically this system can be divided into the central nervous system and the neural pathways that communicate with peripheral physiology and metabolism (Fig. 2). The whole system operates through changes in behavior in response to changes in the internal or external environment. Both central and peripheral factors operate together, to evaluate and reinforce "appropriate" responses and to avoid inappropriate forms of behavior. The adaptability of this system lies in its redundancy. The fact that changes in plasma profiles of metabolites or stores of nutrients do not translate directly into feeding behavior is an important feature of a flexible system capable of adjusting to changes in the environment by learning about the sensory and physiological consequences of

feeding-related actions. In spite of the fact that there are few clear facts about food intake, there do appear to be a number of well-understood ways in which this system usually behaves—or probabilistic outcomes.

1. Feeding behavior is governed by a redundant system that has numerous afferent inputs. Not all of these inputs are necessary for the system to function. Feeding behavior can change in a number of measurable ways, such as meal size, frequency, and the composition of foods selected, or the rate and manner in which foods are ingested.

2. The system uses multiple sensory cues to learn about the consequences of ingesting certain foods. Mimicking the cues associated with certain foods can therefore, transiently at least, "mislead" the system.

3. The system is sensitive to certain changes in the external and internal environment (e.g., temperature or pregnancy, respectively) and to changes in the environmental supply of energy and nutrients. With respect to energy and nutrients, the sensitivity of the system (i.e., the capacity of the system to recognize changes in the environment) can often be greater than its responsiveness (i.e., its tendency to alter behavior in order to maintain the constancy of the internal environment). This may in part be due to the plasticity of intermediary metabolism in response to changes in energy and nutrient intake.

4. Evolution has selected our physiology and behavior to favor overconsumption rather than underconsumption. This means that the system is more responsive to deficits in energy and nutrients than to increments.

5. The system tends to exist in an equilibrium between energy intake and expenditure that maintains a stable body weight. This equilibrium can be disrupted in such a way that shifts body weight upward. A new equilibrium may then be achieved at a higher body weight.

6. The system is interconnected with other biological systems that influence motivation and behavior. Other external and internal influences can greatly perturb the system in such a way that food, (energy and nutrient) intake patterns become maladaptive. Other biobehavioral drives can override and distort the cues associated with feeding. This is especially so in the genesis of eating disorders.

The orientation set out above can be translated into basic questions concerning controlling mechanisms. Why does energy intake rise above energy expenditure? Why is it

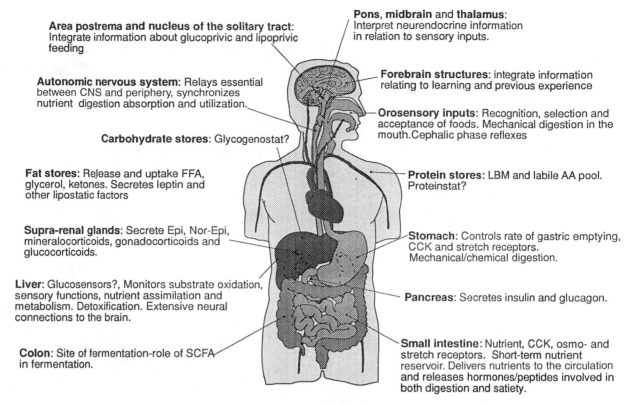

Area postrema and nucleus of the solitary tract: Integrate information about glucoprivic and lipoprivic feeding

Autonomic nervous system: Relays essential between CNS and periphery, synchronizes nutrient digestion absorption and utilization.

Carbohydrate stores: Glycogenostat?

Fat stores: Release and uptake FFA, glycerol, ketones. Secretes leptin and other lipostatic factors

Supra-renal glands: Secrete Epi, Nor-Epi, mineralocorticoids, gonadocorticoids and glucocorticoids.

Liver: Glucosensors?, Monitors substrate oxidation, sensory functions, nutrient assimilation and metabolism. Detoxification. Extensive neural connections to the brain.

Colon: Site of fermentation-role of SCFA in fermentation.

Pons, midbrain and thalamus: Interpret neurendocrine information in relation to sensory inputs.

Forebrain structures: integrate information relating to learning and previous experience

Orosensory inputs: Recognition, selection and acceptance of foods. Mechanical digestion in the mouth.Cephalic phase reflexes

Protein stores: LBM and labile AA pool. Proteinstat?

Stomach: Controls rate of gastric emptying, CCK and stretch receptors. Mechanical/chemical digestion.

Pancreas: Secretes insulin and glucagon.

Small intestine: Nutrient, CCK, osmo- and stretch receptors. Short-term nutrient reservoir. Delivers nutrients to the circulation and releases hormones/peptides involved in both digestion and satiety.

Figure 2 Anatomy of the human appetite system as represented by the relationship between peripheral physiology and the central nervous system. Only the main sites of physiological signals thought to be important in producing feedback signals that affect feeding are outlined. It is of note that all putative signals identified operate along the sequence of ingestion, absorption, metabolism, and storage. All such putative satiety signals have other primary functions.

that a decrease energy expenditure does not exert a restraining effect over food intake? (Are these the same question?) When and why does a positive energy balance fail to generate a negative signal to suppress food intake? Does the body contain a mechanism capable of detecting a positive energy balance (or positive nutrient balances)?

When energy intake continuously exceeds energy expenditure is this due to (1) the presence or potency of mechanisms that stimulate or facilitate intake, or (2) the weakness or failure of mechanisms that could prevent or inhibit intake? In other words, are the facilitatory influences too strong or the inhibitory influences too weak to maintain a stable body weight under a given set of environmental circumstances? In the event of a positive energy (or nutrient) balance, why do the negative signals not become stronger in the short term in order to suppress intake and restore balance? What are the signals that reestablish a new equilibrium at a higher body weight? What is the evidence concerning the operation of these signals?

B. Satiety Signals

Some physiological responses that follow food consumption are believed to terminate eating and/or maintain inhibition over further intake. These responses are usually referred to as "satiety signals." What are the features of foods that are believed to be monitored and that give rise to "satiety" signals? What is the status of the putative "satiety" signals?

It has been assumed or claimed that volume, weight, energy content, macronutrient proportion, and energy density may all be monitored and constitute the source of specific satiation or PI-satiety signals. These may be divided into general factors (e.g., weight, volume) that apply to all foods and specific factors (nutrient content, taste, and smell) that depend on the particular food consumed. Why should weight and volume appear as important features that affect food intake in some studies? (A liter of water would have weight and volume but would provide no energy or nutrients.) The ultimate function of satiation and PI signals is to monitor the biological value of foods and to play a role in the processing of ingested nutrients (all physiological signals involved in satiation, e.g., rate of gastric stretch, release of CCK, or PI satiety, including gastric emptying, nutrient oxidation, etc., have functions in addition to their role in a negative feedback system). A satiety signal is a function assumed by some underlying physiological property. Given a history of food seeking and consumption, it is inevitable that weight and volume of food will have become associated with (conditioned to) the important biological components of food, namely energy value and nutrient composition. The system has learned how to operate in a real environment and the objective of the system is to produce a veridical response. Brunswik's theory of perception provides a model for understanding this (12). Weight and volume are learned cues with high functional validity (proximal cues that correlate well with more distal cues such as hormone release, contact with gastrointestinal receptors, etc.). This is why weight and volume often appear to be important monitored variables (rather than energy or nutrient content) when nutritional composition of food has been surreptitiously manipulated. The system is operating sensibly according to its previous experience, but this does not mean that weight is fundamentally more important than energy content. Indeed, in one study by Kendall et al. (13) subjects were given medium- or low-fat foods to eat for 11 weeks. The low-fat foods were lower in energy density than the higher-fat foods. Subjects gradually tended to increase their energy intake on the low-fat diet in a partially compensatory manner over the 11 weeks. This suggests that subjects were gradually changing their perception of weight and volume cues, according to the physical and nutritional properties of the diet.

C. Satiation and Satiety

In discussing the function of "satiety signals" it is useful to specify what aspect of eating behavior they are supposed to inhibit. Some authors have distinguished between intrameal and intermeal satiety (14); others, such as Blundell (15), have called these processes satiation and PI satiety. They distinguish between events that (1) bring eating to a halt and (2) maintain inhibition over further eating after consumption—so-called postingestive satiety. For the purposes of this work "satiation" refers to intrameal satiety or the process that brings a meal to an end, "postingestive satiety" (PI satiety) refers to the inhibition of eating between meals (intermeal satiety), and "satiety"

is used to refer more collectively to the general use of the term, be the intention specific or colloquial.

In considering the control of patterns of food intake, it would seem important to distinguish between those factors (in food, in the biological system, or in the mind) that operate to adjust either the size of an eating episode or the interval between episodes. For example, CCK is often referred to as a satiety hormone; is this correct? The original studies carried out by Smith and colleagues indicated that CCK terminated eating in sham-feeding rats (16). Subsequent studies indicated that CCK reduced meal size but did not influence the frequency of meals (17). Therefore, CCK should more correctly be termed a satiation hormone or a hormone that prolongs intrameal satiety.

This analysis draws attention to those factors that influence food (1) while it is being eaten and (2) after it has been consumed. It would be expected that weight and volume would influence satiation but not PI satiety. Additionally, the palatability of food (and variety) would exert a major influence during consumption but less influence afterward. It may be inferred that cognitions would be markedly different during and after ingestion. Consequently, biological, environmental, and cognitive influences differ during the operation of satiation (intrameal satiety) and (intermeal) satiety.

How important is this? What are the implications?

1. Theoretical—Is it possible to differentiate biological factors that separately influence either satiation or PI satiety? Do some factors influence both?
2. Procedural—Any claim that an experimental manipulation influences satiety should be accompanied by an explanation as to whether it affects eating (while it is going on) or the aftereffects of eating.
3. Functional—Claims that a particular treatment causes overconsumption over the course of a day (hyperphagia) should specify whether the effect is operating during or after eating, and whether it affects meal size, frequency, or both. Is overeating in humans (leading to weight gain) due primarily to events that influence satiation or PI satiety (or both)? This specification has implications for feeding behavior therapy.
4. Therapeutic applications—Should the development of treatments for overweight and obesity (at the level of public health measures or clinical practice), via nutritional, behavioral, cognitive, surgical, or pharmacological strategies, be aimed at strengthening PI or satiety (or both)?

It follows that speaking about satiety "in general" can be confusing. Conceptual understanding would be improved by an increase in semantic precision. A scheme illustrating the relationship between hunger, appetite, satiation, and PI satiety and their purported influence on feeding behavior is illustrated In Figure 3.

D. The "Hunger State"

In 1955 Mayer pointed out that one of the key features of a short-term model of food intake is that it should be able to account for the hunger state (18). As mentioned above, this does not just have theoretical significance. There is at present an immense interest in pharmacological agents as tools that can be used to manipulate the hunger state (19). Parenthetically, it is of academic, and perhaps applied, interest to consider whether hunger and satiety can be dissociated. Being able to blunt the drive to eat should enhance compliance on weight-reducing programs. Being able to increase the drive to eat may increase longevity and quality of life in patients experiencing cachexia. Understanding how to increase and manage hunger and satiety also has important implications for the nutritional support of a number of clinical conditions. One of the great benefits of using human subjects is that they can be asked about their sensations and motivations. Un-

derstanding the profile of physiological changes that attend and underlie changes in the hunger state offers key sites for intervention and manipulation of the hunger state. Both indices of carbohydrate oxidation (20) and a preprandial drop in plasma glucose have been shown to predict the onset of feeding in rats (21) and humans (22). Furthermore, in animals abolition of the small but reproducible preprandial drop in blood glucose, by a small intravenous infusion, has been shown to inhibit eating for several hours (23). Under these conditions satiety is maintained and hunger is inhibited. The plateau in hunger that starving subjects feel after 1–2 days occurs at around the time that ketogenesis significantly replaces glucose oxidation as a major metabolic fuel for the brain. There is evidence that ketones can act to suppress appetite (24,25). Understanding how the intact system operates and which physiological events underlie changes in motivation to eat and feeding behavior can help unravel and manipulate the mechanisms that influence meal size, frequency, and composition. By doing this it may become possible to explore how these mechanisms are perturbed in disease states. Conversely, specific disease states can shed light on the normal functioning of intact processes involved in feeding behavior. Determining the mechanisms that influence feeding behavior necessarily entails understanding how parts of the system interact (1) with the environment (es-

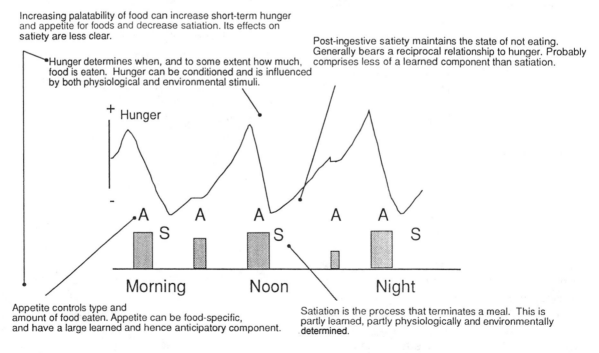

Figure 3   Schematic representation (not to scale) of the relationship between the subjectively expressed constructs of motivation in relation to feeding and their relationship to quantitative and qualitative feeding behavior.

pecially the food component) and (2) with each other to facilitate or inhibit eating and selection of foods.

IV. COMPARTMENTS OF THE APPETITE CONTROL SYSTEM

Figure 1 illustrates the anatomy of the system, its components, and their main functions. Figure 4 illustrates the way in which physiology and behavior interact in their response to food and food-related environmental stimuli. Together, these two figures outline the nature of the system. The biobehavioral system controlling feeding can be artificially divided into the following components:

1. Orosensory components
2. Gastrointestinal components
3. Circulating factors such as hormones, peptides, cytokines, and nutrients
4. Nutrient stores—gut contents, glycogen, muscle, and adipose tissue
5. Nutrient metabolism—whole-body ATP turnover, cellular mechanisms that are associated with the oxidation of the major metabolic fuels, e.g., sodium pump activity
6. The central and peripheral nervous systems including neurotransmitters, peptides, and other centrally acting compounds

These components of the system interact to produce facilitatory or inhibitory contributions to overall feeding patterns. Most components of the diet that are ingested are likely to act at multiple sites. Simply drinking a glass of water will influence gut motility, osmoreceptors, hormones (e.g., ADH), and the central nervous system.

A. Orosensory Components

Orosensory components are generally believed to provide facilitatory signals that increase food intake. However, it is of interest that removal of the sense of smell barely inhibits the intake of readily available food in pigs, presumably because the animals will learn to use other cues (26). Clearly, for many animals olfaction is critical to the location and acquisition of foods. When combined with learning, olfaction is a primary cue for identifying foods as being acceptable or not. As Le Magnen (27) puts it, " . . . the particular property of the olfactory system, compared to taste, is to individualise practically all active molecules by a discriminable odour . . ." Taste, texture, and smell of foods warn against toxins and other damaging components of food. The strength of this mechanism is indicated by the phenomenon of conditioned aversion to

foods that have produced subsequent illness (28–30). Rozin and colleagues suggest that rats learn sensory preferences/aversions for diets that are adequate/deficient in micronutrients in this way only after a trial-and-error period during which they sample a variety of diets offered to them (31,32). During this time they learn to associate the nutrient quality of the diet with its particular smell, flavor, or appearance. The same mechanisms are likely to operate in relation to dietary macronutrients. Increasing the sensory qualities and variety of these diets can lead to obesity in some strains of rats and may also be important for the maintenance of the obese state in humans (27). However, it is important to note that while people obviously select what they like this does not necessarily suggest that increasing the sensory quality or the variety of sensory attributes of a diet will lead to obesity. There is at present little hard evidence that increasing only the sensory variety of the diet in humans leads to sustained weight gain. This may simply be due to the difficulty of conducting such an experiment. Sensory factors may interact with other factors such as diet composition or genetic predisposition to precipitate hyperphagia. Internal cues interact with sensory information to help formulate appropriate food (nutrient) selection and foraging strategies (33–37). Aspects of sensory experience have been rated by healthy, free-living adults among the top three determinants that guide their food detection and ingestion (38,39). The extent to which subjects can accurately recall quantitative relationships between sensory experience and food intake is, however, very limited. Furthermore, these effects do not appear to be related to the nutrient-specific sensory qualities of the diet per se. Mattes (4) suggests that in the clinical setting where many environmental considerations are less prominent, pathologically induced sensory disturbances can be important, particularly in affecting the acceptability of specific foods, e.g., clinical supplements.

B. Gastrointestinal Components

The gut is thought to play an important role in the short-term regulation of feeding behavior. Initially it was believed that hunger sensations arose in the stomach (40). It is now accepted that a major role of the stomach is to regulate the flow of energy and nutrients into the small intestine. The stomach also places a physical constraint on the amount of food that can be consumed at a given meal. This fact has been applied, in extremis, during gastroplasty surgery as a means of obesity treatment. Stomach size adapts to the amount of food habitually eaten. This effect means that previously undernourished people have to eat small frequent meals, during the initial stages of

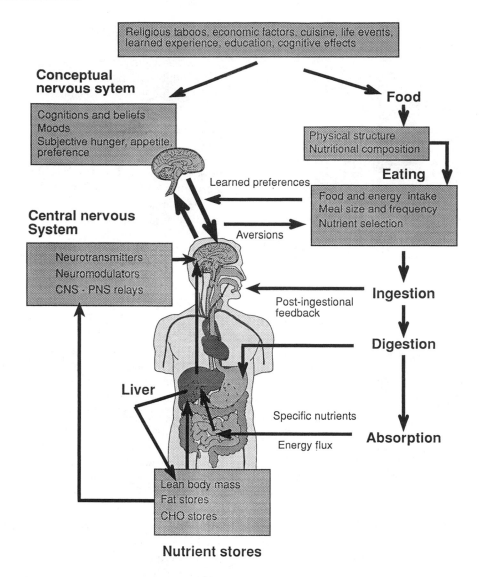

Figure 4 Interaction between physiology and behavior in the response to food and food-related environmental stimuli. Food elicits potent cognitive, learned behavioral, and physiological responses, which together determine the feeding strategies of an individual.

nutritional rehabilitation, although as refeeding progresses energy intakes can reach spectacular levels (41,42). Stretch and CCK receptors inform the CNS of the status of the stomach. The small intestine itself places a further constraint on the amount of food that can be ingested since a certain time is taken to complete digestion and absorption. Both processes appear to be particularly important in releasing cascades of signals (hormones, peptides, action potentials along gastrointestinal nerves) including the nutrients themselves to the postabsorptive circulation. It is interesting that patients with short intestines (and few secondary complications) attempt to eat to energy requirements. This means they are hyperphagic,

presumably to compensate for the decreased absorptive capacity of the shortened small intestine (Elia M, personal communication). In addition, stretch, CCK receptors, and osmoreceptors all appear to play some role in affecting short-term feeding.

C. The Liver

The liver is the main organ that receives and deals with the digestion products of a meal, except for chylomicrons, which initially bypass the liver, since they are absorbed through the lymphatic system. Parenthetically it has been suggested that this effect contributes to the delayed effects of fat in suppressing appetite (46). It has been suggested from preference conditioning experiments using portal infusions of fructose (43) that the liver also functions as a sensory organ. This is because rats learn to prefer flavors that are paired with a glucose infusion into the hepatic portal vein. The liver possesses extensive neural connections to the brain that appear to be involved in glucoprivic and lipoprivic feeding, at least in rodents (44). A detailed discussion of these links between nutrient metabolism and the CNS is given below. The liver is the main site of assimilation, metabolism, and distribution of nutrients subsequent to ingestion. Pharmacological impairment of nutrient oxidation in the liver stimulates intake (45). The liver is the most likely candidate as the central organ that communicates information about peripheral fuel status to the brain (46).

D. Circulating Factors

The circulation and the nervous system together inform the brain of the overall status of energy and nutrients that are (1) in the circulation, (2) moving into the circulation from the gut (and hence indirectly of their concentration in the gut), and (3) available nutrient stores. While the gut provides important cues that probably alert the brain to the likely influx of energy and nutrients, failure to reinforce this message by actual delivery of energy and nutrients will lead to diminished sensations of satiation and PI satiety. Thus sham-feeding dogs (47) and rats are hyperphagic (48,49). On the other hand, nutrient infusions as lipid or glucose fail to elicit the same degree of caloric compensation as oral loads of nutrients (50). These observations again attest to the redundancy of individual parts of the system.

E. Nutrient Stores

What is the role of nutrient stores in generating appetite-influencing signals? For carbohydrate do glycogen stores per se influence satiety? In view of the redundancy of the appetite system, this would seem unlikely. Since carbohydrate oxidation is related to the state of glycogen stores, it is possible that the process of regulating these stores is important for influencing eating behavior. This may also be true of protein stores.

It is also possible that changes in body size and composition can influence satiation, PI satiety, and the hunger state. Energy intake is clearly elevated after significant loss of body mass (41,42). Furthermore, during weight gain, body weight does not increase monotonically but usually plateaus at higher levels. This infers that some process limits the monotonic increase in body weight. Part of this

decrease in the rate of weight gain may be attributable to the increase in lean body mass (and the attendant increase in energy expenditure) that occurs as the fat mass expands. However, this increase in energy expenditure is unlikely to be the sole cause of the restabilization of body weight at a higher level. In some cases where subjects have been obligatorily overfed, they have shown a tendency to return to original body weight (51,52). These changes in body weight are likely to be due to changes in intake, but there is no clear evidence of a physiological process at work. Studies in parabiotic rats (which share a common blood supply) have shown that when one member of a pair was made obese, its partner lost a large proportion of its body fat (53). In subsequent studies, when overfeeding was stopped, both partners returned to control body composition (54). The authors attribute these changes to mobilization of a putative lipostatic factor, brought about by expansion of the adipose tissue mass. The recent identification of the genetic system encoding and possibly regulating the secretion and actions of a protein "leptin" has again increased interest in a specific feedback from adipose tissue stores that affects appetite. Studies in the *ob/ob* and *db/db* mice are based on the idea that the *ob* gene expresses a protein (leptin) that is believed to be released by adipose tissue to influence certain appetite-controlling pathways in the brain (55). Recently research activity has intensified in trying to understand the role of lipostatic factors regulating the adipose tissue mass with the unraveling of the leptin system that is currently underway in rodents, and to a growing extent in humans (55). It is also of interest that leptin occurs at much higher levels in the plasma of obese subjects (56). The same is true for insulin (57,58). Since the high level of plasma insulin in obese subjects is due to insulin resistance, the concept of leptin resistance in obese subjects has been developed (59). Furthermore, it appears that high-fat diets (60), especially diets high in saturates (61), induce insulin resistance in rodents, and possibly humans (62). High-fat diets also appear to induce leptin resistance in rats (59). Clearly, by the time obesity has developed both the leptin system and enteroinsular axis appear to have been perturbed.

There is clear evidence that chronic administration of leptin has marked effects in decreasing food intake and adiposity of both *ob/ob* and wild-type mice (63), but what is its role in the intact animals under ecological conditions? Is there any evidence from human studies that adipose tissue exerts an appetite-inhibiting action? It is becoming increasingly apparent that the leptin system interacts with other systems. For example, leptin may interact with NPY, which has a role in carbohydrate preference and ingestion (64). Indeed, given the evidence suggesting that the CNS monitors both fat and carbohydrate metabolism in an interrelated manner (44), it would be surprising if the leptin system did not interact with other systems believed to have important effects on feeding.

It is also worth bearing in mind that other changes in body composition occur when body fat is deposited. In humans there is usually an expansion of the fat-free mass. Exactly which components of increased body size and composition exert signals to influence subsequent feeding is not clear. For a given level of training, lean body mass appears to be well regulated and it might be expected that changes in lean body mass will elicit corrective responses of the system controlling feeding behavior (65). Work is yet to be done in humans to elucidate how changes in body size and composition influence feeding behavior.

F. Monitoring of Energy and Nutrient Intake by the Nervous System

There is now an extensive and growing array of both central and peripheral hormones, peptides, and other messengers that can be grouped into functional systems related to the regulation of nutrient balance (66). Such a complexity of signaling systems is necessary to interpret the multiple and complex messages that relay information to the brain about the orosensory, gastrointestinal, metabolic, and neuroendocrine consequences of ingesting foods, which themselves have particular characteristics. In addition, the brain cross-references this experience with prior learned experiences of similar or the same foods.

Despite the fact that protein has a pronounced effect on satiety (see below), it is at present unclear which mechanisms are involved and at what levels they operate. The hypothesis that dietary-induced alterations in the plasma ratio of tryptophan and large neutral amino acids influenced brain serotonin synthesis and that this directly led to alterations in selection between protein-rich and carbohydrate-rich foods is now generally accepted as being oversimplified. It appears from neuroanatomical and feeding studies in rodents that the opioid peptides and growth hormone–releasing hormone both stimulate protein intake in rats given access to a choice of pure macronutrients (66).

Greater progress has been made in understanding the neural pathways involved in monitoring of carbohydrate and fat metabolism (and presumably, by proxy, the metabolic availability of these nutrients). The recent work by Ritter's group has provided important new evidence of the connections between peripheral physiology and regions of the brain concerned with feeding. This work is important because there is relatively little direct evidence of links between the peripheral physiology of the CNS and feeding

behavior. Their neuroanatomical work suggests that both fat and carbohydrate oxidation are separately monitored by the CNS and that these signals are integrated within the brain to monitor overall fuel status (44). Ritter and Calingasan have used the antimetabolic drugs mercaptoactetate (which causes lipoprivation by blocking mitochondrial acyl-CoA-dehydrogenases and so reduces beta oxidation of fatty acids) and 2-DG as tools to produce lipoprivic and glucoprivic signals. Using surgical and chemical lesions together with neurochemical approaches, they have provided important evidence that the response to lipoprivic signals is likely to be dependent on vagal sensory neurones. In other words, they have provided evidence that fatty acid oxidation is monitored in the periphery and these signal are relayed to specific areas of the brain, which they have identified through a combination of lesion and behavioral studies, together with work using markers of neuronal activity in specific regions of the brain. These areas of the brain are also activated by 2-DG-induced glucoprivic feeding. However, glucoprivic feeding appears to be partially mediated by receptor populations that are different from those mediating lipoprivic feeding, since glucoprivic feeding is not dependent on vagal sensory neurons (i.e., not influenced by vagotomy or capsaicin treatment, which damages vagal sensory neurons) and can be stimulated by activation of metabolic receptors actually within the brain, which exist in addition to those monitoring lipoprivic feeding. This is supported by work using another antimetabolite, 2,5-anhydro-D-mannitol, which, unlike 2-DG, does not cross the blood-brain barrier and so only inhibits glucose oxidation in the periphery. 2-DG inhibits glucose oxidation in both the brain and the periphery. The glucoprivic feeding response to 2,5-anhydro-D-mannitol is also characterized by activation of the same immunochemical markers (Fos-like activity) in the same regions of the brain that respond to lipoprivic feeding, the area postrema and nucleus of the solitary tract (the AP/NST). This area receives central vagal sensory terminals. Lesioning of AP/NST that destroys the sensory but not motor nucleus abolishes MA but not 2-DG-induced feeding. Total subdiaphragmatic vagotomy abolishes the feeding response to low (but not high) doses of 2,5-AM. It has been suggested from these lines of evidence that fatty acid oxidation is monitored in the periphery, while glucose oxidation is monitored both in the center and in the periphery. The authors observe that simultaneous activation of these distinct systems appears to produce an integrated feeding response that takes into account the metabolic availability of both carbohydrates and fatty acids (44). This is important since the physiological and behavioral responses of the appetite regulatory system need to be able to take account of both changing metabolic requirements and fluctuations in the environmental supply of metabolic fuels.

Thus the A/P and NST appear important for glucoprivic and lipoprivic feeding. These areas of the brain are linked to the paraventricular nucleus (PVN) and the lateral hypothalamus (LH). Langhans has suggested that a relay from the AP/NST to the PVN/LH via the parabrachial nucleus seems to be required to feed peripherally generated signals to the PVN/LH (67). Both the ventromedial hypothalamus (VMH) and the LH possess glucosensitive neurons. This is important because it is already known that a number of neurochemicals act on the hypothalamic system to influence feeding. These include the stimulation of carbohydrate intake in rodents given access to pure sources of macronutrients by norepinephrine, by γ-aminobutyric acid, and by neuropeptide Y (66). Fat intake appears to be increased by galanin, the opioid peptides, and the mineralocorticoid aldosterone. These substances are also believed to act within the medial hypothalamus (66). Thus the several pathways by which information relating to the metabolic availability of fat and carbohydrate is monitored and integrated are beginning to be delineated. Figure 5 is an adaptation of Langhans' integration of these various lines of evidence (67). The neuronal pathways that relay central and peripheral information regard-

ing fuel status are interlinked with receptor populations for a number of neurochemicals that are themselves related to metabolic fuel status and other aspects of physiological functioning. Now that these central monitoring mechanisms are being mapped, a key challenge will be to understand their quantitative importance in feeding behavior and the nature of their functional responses to changes in energy and nutrient balance in intact animals, responding to physiological changes such as growth and development or pregnancy and lactation.

Regarding disturbances of this system in the development of obesity, Bray (68) has suggested that obesity is associated with imbalances in the autonomic nervous system in concert with the pituitary adrenal axis. Specifically, he has suggested that obesity is associated with a relative or absolute reduction in the activity of the thermogenic component of the sympathetic nervous system, attended or maintained by normal or increased circulating corticosteroids. This concept has considerable utility in unifying a number of observations. First, insulin-resistant obese subjects have been found to show a blunted postprandial thermogenesis. This may well be due to a blunted postprandial glucose oxidation curve, which is, in part, sympathetically mediated. Raben has shown that there is a strong correlation between postprandial glucose disposal

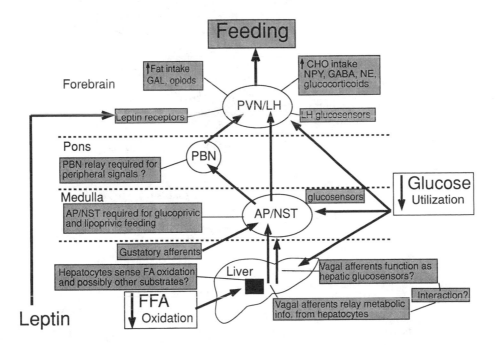

Figure 5 Current understanding of the way in which the central nervous system monitors and integrates physiological and gustatory signals that are associated with the metabolic availability of fat and carbohydrate. Fat appears to be monitored primarily in the periphery; carbohydrate in both the CNS and periphery. These signals are integrated in the area postrema and nucleus of the solitary tract, which itself is linked to the hypothalamic feeding areas of the forebrain. (Adapted from Ref. 67.)

and satiety (20). Second, as a general principle it appears that thermogenic agents appear to exert suppressive effects on appetite, which are possibly mediated through the activity of the SNS (69). This may also be true for the hierarchical effects that dietary macronutrients exert on satiety (see below). Third, there are a number of intermediary messengers in the form of peptides, which are integrated into the functioning of the autonomic nervous system and whose actions are consistent with the hypothesis that food intake and sympathetic activity exhibit reciprocal effects (70). Furthermore, there is evidence that some of these intermediary messengers, e.g., neuropeptide Y, exhibit an altered distribution or functioning in obesity.

To explore the system determining human feeding behavior it is appropriate to consider how central features and components of that system change under different environmental conditions. The most central feature of feeding behavior is food. Food varies in orosensory qualities and in composition. Until recently the orosensory qualities of foods acted as reliable cues that gave accurate information about the nutrient content of food and the physiological consequences of ingesting it. A growing number of advances in food technology have changed this relationship between the sensorial attributes of the diet and its nutrient composition. Figure 6 summarizes the main ways in which food can affect the feeding system.

V. DIET COMPOSITION AND FEEDING BEHAVIOR

Given the current prevalence of obesity on a worldwide scale and the role of overconsumption in generating a positive energy balance that is converted into weight gain, it is important to consider the composition of foods that form the basis of overconsumptiom. In turn, this introduces the key concept of diet composition and feeding behavior. How do the relative amounts of the energy-yielding macronutrients influence the control of food intake? There is a good deal of variation in the experimental results from research on this issue and findings have purported to show inter alia that all macronutrients have equal power to suppress subsequent energy intake, protein exerts a greater suppressive effect on subsequent energy intake than carbohydrate or fat, carbohydrate and fat have similar effects on caloric suppression, fat generates strong signals that suppress appetite, and fat is the least effective of the macronutrients at suppressing appetite.

A. Macronutrients, Satiation, and PI Satiety

1. Protein

Protein appears to be the macronutrient that suppresses energy intake to a greater extent than any of the other macronutrients. Careful retrospective analysis of food records (71) indicates that protein exerts postingestive action over and above the contribution from energy per se. In a recent study by Bingham et al. (72), the food and energy intakes of 160 postmenopausal women living at home in the Cambridge area were measured on four consecutive days in each of the four seasons. This approach produced 16 days of weighed intakes per subject kept over 1 year. The proportion of energy intake from protein correlated negatively with total energy intake ($r = -0.45$), carbohydrate did not correlate at all with total energy intake ($r = 0.0$), and fat correlated positively with total energy intake ($r = 0.18$).

Protein also exerts a large influence on satiety in the laboratory. Some studies using pure macronutrient loads delivered to the stomach or solutions quickly swallowed by subjects wearing noseclips (73,74) have found that all macronutrients have equal satiating power. It is intriguing in this regard that sensory cues (especially taste) may be important in clearly identifying the effects of nutrient ingestion. Miller and Teates (75) found that male Sprague-Dawley rats were able to select from nutritionally different diets in a way that stabilized the protein energy ratio at 0.14. However, when rats were subjected to impairment of oral somatosensory input, they were unable to maintain a stable selection pattern. The authors hypothesized that selection between protein and carbohydrate (or energy) at least "involves an associative learning process in which somatosensory inputs affect feeding activity and/or the properties of the food link dietary choice behavior to later metabolic consequences."

It also appears that there may be a critical threshold in the amount of protein required to suppress subsequent energy intake since studies that have found little effect of protein relative to other macronutrient preloads have only used small amounts of energy as protein in the preload (73,76). Hill and Blundell (77) found that a high-protein (HP) meal (31% of 2.1 MJ) produced a greater sensation of fullness and a decreased desire to eat, relative to a high-carbohydrate (HC) meal (52%) of the same energy content. Hill and Blundell (78) also found that both obese and normal-weight subjects reduced their subsequent meal intakes by 19 and 22%, respectively, after a HP (54% of 2 MJ) meal compared to a HC meal (63% of 2 MJ). Barkeling et al. (79) gave 20 normal-weight women a high-protein (43% of 2.6 MJ) or a high-carbohydrate (69% of 2.6 MJ) lunch and measured the energy intake at

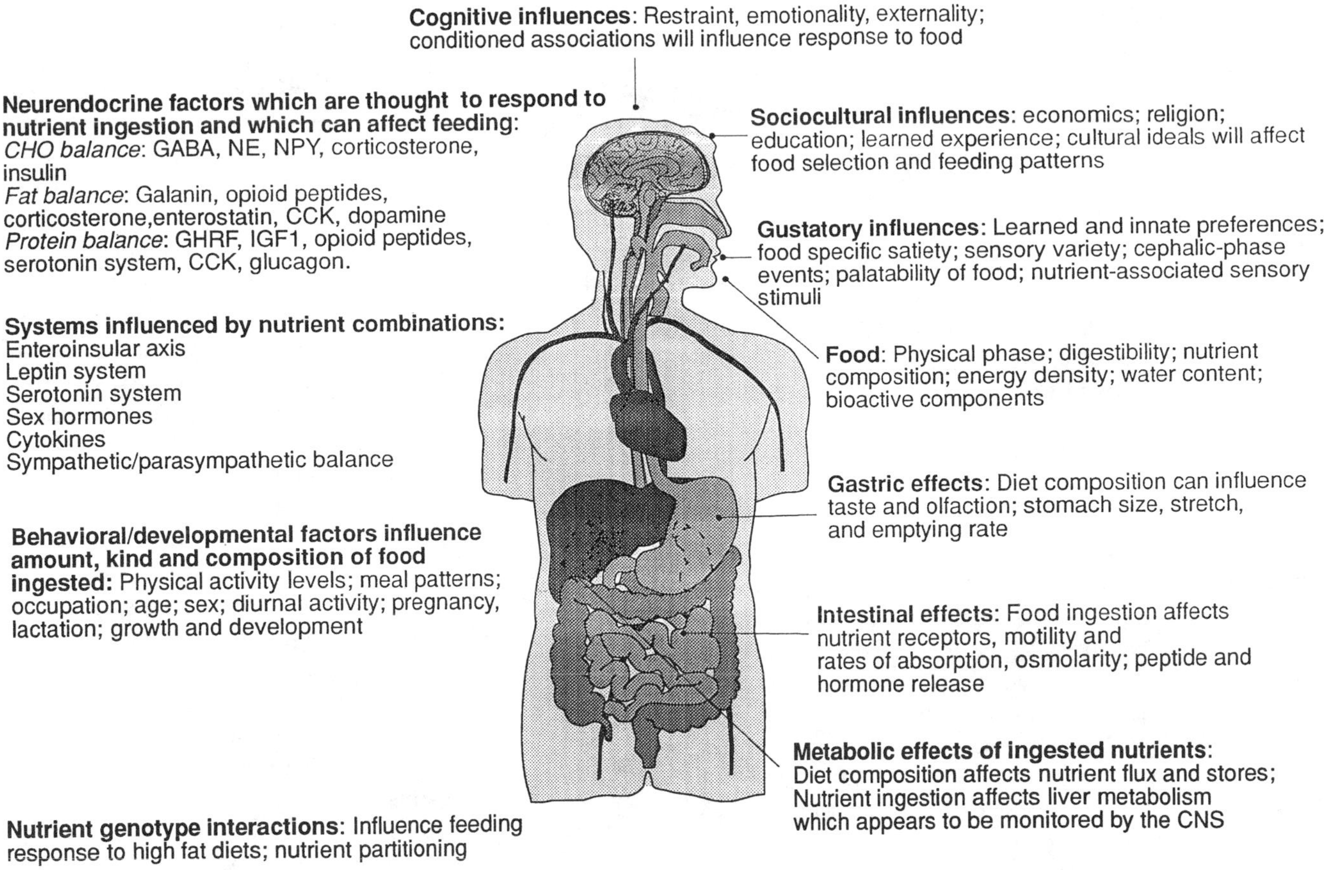

Cognitive influences: Restraint, emotionality, externality; conditioned associations will influence response to food

Neurendocrine factors which are thought to respond to nutrient ingestion and which can affect feeding:
CHO balance: GABA, NE, NPY, corticosterone, insulin
Fat balance: Galanin, opioid peptides, corticosterone,enterostatin, CCK, dopamine
Protein balance: GHRF, IGF1, opioid peptides, serotonin system, CCK, glucagon.

Systems influenced by nutrient combinations:
Enteroinsular axis
Leptin system
Serotonin system
Sex hormones
Cytokines
Sympathetic/parasympathetic balance

Behavioral/developmental factors influence amount, kind and composition of food ingested: Physical activity levels; meal patterns; occupation; age; sex; diurnal activity; pregnancy, lactation; growth and development

Nutrient genotype interactions: Influence feeding response to high fat diets; nutrient partitioning

Sociocultural influences: economics; religion; education; learned experience; cultural ideals will affect food selection and feeding patterns

Gustatory influences: Learned and innate preferences; food specific satiety; sensory variety; cephalic-phase events; palatability of food; nutrient-associated sensory stimuli

Food: Physical phase; digestibility; nutrient composition; energy density; water content; bioactive components

Gastric effects: Diet composition can influence taste and olfaction; stomach size, stretch, and emptying rate

Intestinal effects: Food ingestion affects nutrient receptors, motility and rates of absorption, osmolarity; peptide and hormone release

Metabolic effects of ingested nutrients:
Diet composition affects nutrient flux and stores; Nutrient ingestion affects liver metabolism which appears to be monitored by the CNS

Figure 6 Primary ways in which food and nutrient ingestion influences the main compartments of the human appetite system. Food influences this system through multiple feedbacks at multiple levels, which can be traced through the processes of food location, ingestion, digestion, absorption, and metabolism. Satiety is therefore maintained by a functional sequence or cascade of sequential physiological events that reinforce each other. Removing parts of a food or nutrient's effects on this sequence will therefore diminish its impact on satiety.

a subsequent evening meal. They found that energy intake was depressed by 12% after consumption of the HP meal. Booth et al. (80) also found that a HP meal reduced the intake of a subsequent test meal by 26% relative to a virtually protein-free meal in normal-weight individuals. Thus protein appears to be particularly satiating when given at moderate and large amounts.

This apparent appetite-restraining effect of protein has not yet been given a strong theoretical basis, and there has been little recent investigation of the "protein stat." It is pertinent to note that essential amino acids when ingested in excess of requirements form a physiological stress that must be disposed of by oxidation. It is known that animals will alter feeding behavior to alleviate a physiological stress (81). Pigs, in particular, appear capable of learning to select a protein:energy ratio in the diet that is optimal for growth (82,83), as can rats (75). There is also evidence

that the kind of amino acids ingested may influence satiety. Imbalances in single essential amino acids can greatly affect the feeding behavior of rats (84). The protein:energy ratio of foods may be important in influencing feeding. Malnourished children find it difficult to tolerate nutritional supplements whose protein:energy ratio is too high. Millward has hypothesized that lean tissue deposition may be an important factor driving appetite during catchup growth in children (65). Since several aspects of amino acid status can be influenced in disease, the influence of factors affecting protein and amino acid balance on feeding behavior in the clinical setting may be considerable. At present, we do not know the form or detail of the mechanisms.

2. Carbohydrates

Carbohydrates appear to be efficient inhibitors of appetite in the short term. The potency of ingested carbohydrate is complemented by work showing that 2-deoxy-D-glucose actually increases hunger when given to human subjects (85). The effectiveness of carbohydrate includes the effects of sugars, longer-chain oligosaccharides such as maltodextrin and polysaccharides. Interestingly, the effect of PI satiety is influenced by the structure of starch as indicated by the difference between high-amylose and amylopectin foods (86). One interesting issue is the relationship between the PI satiety effect of carbohydrates and their action on plasma profiles of glucose and insulin. Is the PI satiety effect related to the AUC for insulin, as suggested by some studies (87)? Is the absorption and metabolism of carbohydrate important for the maintenance of satiety in the intermeal interval (18,20–23)?

The notion of satiety and plasma profiles prompts a consideration of the effects of dietary fiber or resistant starch. The evidence is not clear (88). The effects of fiber on the expression of appetite (amount of energy consumed) may depend on whether intrameal or postmeal effects are studied. The time-energy displacement idea has clearly shown the restraining effect on consumption of low-energy-dense foods (89), an action mediated via control of satiation and hence meal size (energy). This phenomenon has been used to limit weight gain in farm animals that do not have access to other foods (26). The PI effects of fiber depend on the amount and type delivered in experimental meals and are likely to be influenced by the proportions of soluble and insoluble fiber, which will have different effects on gastrointestinal processing. It is becoming increasingly apparent that fermentable carbohydrates produce significant quantities of short-chain fatty acids. The absorption and metabolism of acetate, propionate, and butyrate may themselves exert influences on satiety.

3. Fat and Carbohydrate

Perhaps the most controversial area of research on macronutrients involves comparisons of fat and carbohydrate. Carbohydrate has been suggested by several theorists as the central macronutrient influencing feeding behavior by acting as a major lever in a negative feedback loop (18,90–92) or by influencing nutrient selection between proteins and carbohydrates (93). These same models view fat as a poorly regulated macronutrient. The outcome of experiments is critically dependent on the methodology employed. There are signs that general agreement is beginning to emerge. Numerous laboratory studies have now shown that when humans or animals are allowed to feed

ad libitum on high-fat (HF) energy-dense diets, the subjects consume similar amounts (weight) of food but more energy (which is usually accompanied by weight gain) than when they feed ad libitum on lower-fat, less energy-dense diets (6,7,9). The ingestion of systematically manipulated HF, energy-dense diets does not appear to elicit compensatory feeding responses.

Interestingly, if single midday meals are covertly manipulated, by increasing or decreasing their energy density using fat or carbohydrate, under conditions where subjects feed on a range of familiar food items, compensation appears to be more precise (94,95). When experiments are conducted over similar time frames but the diet is systematically manipulated (i.e., subjects cannot select food items of differing composition), compensation for the fat content of the diet is again poor (96). These observations further suggest that both learning and preabsorptive and absorptive-phase factors play a major role in meal-to-meal compensation. Furthermore, a number of prospective observational epidemiological studies show that fat consumption is a risk factor for subsequent weight gain (97). It should be noted that the stimulatory effect of fatty foods on energy intake is due not only to the high energy density but also to the facilitatory action of fat in the mouth. For some time, it has been known that subjects exposed to HF foods tend to overconsume energy but do not much alter the actual amount of food they eat (8); this phenomenon has been termed by Bundell "passive overconsumption." This is important because there is little or no evidence that the PI actions of fat exert positive feedback on food intake (i.e., that fat increases the amount of food eaten). Parenthetically, it should be noted that the use of the term "passive overconsumption" only means that there is no conscious intention to overconsume. There are, however, mediating mechanisms that do account for the excess energy intake. These include the potent orosensory qualities of HF foods, the facilitatory effect of fat in the mouth, and the contribution of fat to a higher dietary energy density.

Fewer studies have compared isoenergetically dense loads of fat and carbohydrate. Recent work by Rolls et al. (98) has suggested that in the very short term preloads of carbohydrate have a greater capacity to suppress energy intake at a test-meal 30 min after the presentation of a preload than do isoenergetically dense loads of fat. Although other work (99) has found no difference in the satiating efficiency of graded HF- and HC-rich loads of energy, Van Stratum et al. (10) found that isoenergetically dense HF and HC diets produced similar energy intakes over 2 weeks in 22 Trappist nuns. This finding has recently been confirmed in men (11). These data again suggest that carbohydrate status per se is not perhaps the major pivotal factor that exerts powerful negative feedback onto subsequent intake.

4. The Fat Paradox

The apparently ambivalent effects of fat have generated a phenomenon referred to as the fat paradox. On the one hand, a fat such as corn oil, infused into the jejunum, has been shown to slow gastric emptying, increase feelings of fullness, and reduce food intake in a test meal. Infusions into the ileum bring about similar effects and also reduce feelings of hunger (100). On the other hand, similar infusions made intravenously exerted no effect on gastric emptying or measures of appetite. Lipid infusions at around 80% of resting energy requirements, over 3 days, produce only partial compensation (43%) of energy intake (101). Similar experiments have been carried out in rats where intraduodenal infusions inhibited food intake whereas intravenous infusions did not (102). These findings imply that, after the ingestion of fat, potent fat-induced satiety signals are generated by preabsorptive rather than postabsorptive physiological responses. In addition, a number of studies—of short- and medium-term duration—have demonstrated the existence of high intakes of energy with HF foods (e.g., diets (7–9,96,104). These studies have demonstrated that HF foods constitute a sufficient, but not a necessary, condition for passive overconsumption (also referred to as HF hyperphagia). This form of hyperphagia should not be possible if fat generates potent satiety signals that impede further eating. How can these two features be reconciled?

There are now some data to indicate that fat-induced satiety signals are not incompatible with the phenomenon of HF hyperphagia. In certain studies in which subjects have been exposed to ranges of HF and HC foods, the fat foods give rise to a markedly high consumption of energy associated with a lower weight of food eaten (103,104). The function of a satiety signal should be to reduce the amount of food that people put into the mouth or alter the kind of food they select. This appears to occur with HF foods (in normal-weight subjects) indicating the operation of an inhibitory influence over eating. However, in the face of the high energy density and possible oral facilitation of fatty foods, this inhibition is either too weak or too slow-acting to prevent the intake of a significant amount of energy. Furthermore, during intestinal infusion studies lipid usually enters the small intestine at a much faster rate than the rate at which the load would empty from the stomach. This interpretation means that in considering the action of dietary fat on appetite control it is necessary to distinguish between fat per se and fat as a contributor to the high energy density of foods. These deductions also suggest behavioral, nutritional, and pharmacological strategies for reducing fat (energy) intake.

5. Carbohydrates and Overeating

While considering the issue of overeating and weight gain, it is worth mentioning that fat is not the only nutrient that can give rise to overconsumption. There is evidence that HC diets can also generate a high energy intake, as for example in the Guru Walla phenomenon, which leads to weight gain (52). We have recently shown that six men overate and gained weight on HC energy-dense diets compared to less-energy-dense diets of the same nutrient ratios and similar sensory characteristics (105). It would be expected that HF diets would be more efficient at inducing weight gain, since excess carbohydrate is less efficiently stored than similar energetic excesses of fat (106), but the phenomenon of weight gain with HC diets must be explained. Does this mean that the metabolism of carbohydrate does not generate a potent physiological response that serves as an inhibitory signal for the control of appetite? Or does it mean that when cognitive cues are disguised, the physiological satiety produced by postabsorptive handling of carbohydrates can be easily overridden? There is no theoretical reason why it is not possible to overeat on HC diets. Clearly the nutrient balance status of any macronutrient is unlikely to exert a rigid leverage on feeding behavior, except in extreme states of balance. The key issue is whether it is probable that HC, energy-dense diets will produce excess energy intakes in real life. Furthermore, the form in which carbohydrates are ingested may be important. Is it less easy to detect a more readily absorbed continuous administration of a nutrient (e.g., in a drink) than a bolus (e.g., as a meal) (107)?

Under both free-living and laboratory conditions, where fat contributes disproportionately to energy density, the available data suggest that there is a hierarchy in the satiating efficiency (i.e., the ability for each MJ of each macronutrient ingested to suppress subsequent energy intake) of the dietary macronutrients such that protein suppresses subsequent energy intakes (per unit of energy ingested) to a greater extent than carbohydrate, which suppresses subsequent energy intake to a greater extent than dietary fat (108). Carbohydrate appears to sit in the middle of this hierarchy. The extent to which the macronutrients differentially affect satiation or PI satiety is yet to be determined. Under more artificial conditions when HF and HC foods are made isoenergetically dense, this differential influence that carbohydrate and fat exert on motivation to eat or actual feeding appears less clear-cut. Under these conditions fat and carbohydrate have similar effects on total energy intake.

This hierarchy is apparent in humans (101) and rats (50) when macronutrients are given as parenteral infusions, suggesting part of these effects are postabsorptive. Alcohol, on the other hand, appears to simply bypass the appetite regulatory system, both in free-living people (109) and in the laboratory (110). More recent evidence suggests that alcohol can actually stimulate energy intake (111). Given its pharmacological properties, it is not surprising that alcohol is not regulated in a manner similar to other macronutrients. At isoenergetic doses in the diet, carbohydrate appears to exert a more acute, immediate effect on subjective hunger while fat exerts a more delayed effect (112). This is consistent with (but not exclusively determined by) their respective rates of absorption and metabolism.

6. Micronutrients

There is currently very little data on the effect of micronutrients on feeding behavior and body weight under normal feeding conditions. There is evidence that rodents will learn to select a diet whose ingestion will alleviate a micronutrient deficiency (81). It may also be supposed that the administration of a micronutrient that will, for instance, improve a deficiency-related defect in nutrient metabolism will improve appetite for that nutrient, and perhaps appetite in general.

B. Issues Concerning Satiety Signals

The pattern of food intake and the physiological events that occur at the end of a meal indicate an important role for preabsorptive signals in terminating eating and in determining the episodic nature of eating. What role is played by postabsorptive processes? The energy (fuel) balance approach to appetite control is based on the idea that the metabolic fate of nutrients in the body exerts important influences over behavior (92). Some hypotheses, such as the idea linking food selection to serotoninergic activity (93), are based exclusively on the understanding that nutrient-induced metabolic activity exerts a directional influence on food consumption. However, some recent studies have indicated that large differences in the oxidation patterns of nutrients (fat and carbohydrate) can occur (after dietary manipulations) that do not appear to exert any influence over the quantitative aspect of food intake (114,115), at least for the following 24 hr. The same group has provided evidence that nutrient metabolism does exert potential influences on energy intake when these relationships are examined over a number of days (9). Logic demands that the requirement for nutrients by the body will exert an influence over the form of behavior

that provides these nutrients, but what is the evidence for this, what is the nature of the mechanism involved, and what are the physiological limits within which the mechanism operates?

Animal studies have suggested that the rate of oxidation of fat and carbohydrate exerts an inhibitory effect on appetite (116–120). Specific proposals have been made by Langhans and Scharrer (116) regarding the increase in intracellular metabolism in hepatocytes. Some of this evidence is indirect. The blockade of glucose oxidation by 2-DG or 2,5-AM (45) or fat oxidation by methylpalmoxirate or 2-mercaptoacetate leads to an increase in food intake in animals (45,116–121). These phenomena have been termed glucoprivic and lipoprivic forms of feeding. These effects are strong phenomena in animals [and, for 2-DG, in humans (85)] and form the basis for useful experimental models; their respective pathways through the brain can be traced by lesioning or biochemical procedures. This work by Ritter's group is extremely important since it indicates the neurochemical processing of metabolic activity (44).

Does this pharmacological blockade of nutrient oxidation indicate the existence of a naturally functioning physiological process? Is the stimulation of eating that occurs following a block of oxidation mirrored by an inhibition of eating when fuel utilization is high? Considering carbohydrate metabolism, experimental results of Raben indicate an extremely high correlation ($r = 0.9$) between hunger and PI measures of carbohydrate oxidation, AUC plasma glucose, insulin, and norepinephrine (20). Campfield and Smith (21) have found that a 6–12% preprandial drop in blood glucose is a robust predictor of meal initiation in animals (21) and humans (22). Stubbs et al. (9) have also found a statistically significant negative relationships between protein and carbohydrate stores and oxidation and the subsequent day's food intake, in normal men living in a calorimeter for 7 days at a time. The same relationships were significant for fat oxidation but not stores. Stubbs et al. (9) have interpreted these data as suggesting that the regulation of nutrient stores by increases in oxidation may partly underlie the greater capacity of protein and carbohydrate to suppress subsequent intake.

The key question here is whether or not the different profiles of nutrient oxidation arising from variations in the diet composition exert an influence over eating behavior. From a biological perspective, an animal could deal with extreme forms of diet composition through metabolic adaptation—with no consequences for behavior. There may be no obligatory requirement to adjust behavior, unless the process of metabolic adaptation incurs a physiological stress. It therefore seems important to establish the conditions under which nutrient-induced metabolic activity exerts either a quantitative or directional influence over eating behavior and whether it is possible to condition these effects. It seems reasonable to hypothesize that under conditions where prior learning cues are removed and extremes of metabolic adaptation are reached, feeding behavior will be altered. Feeding behavior may subsequently be altered before such extremes are reached if the metabolic change is a cue for learning.

In addition it is possible that metabolic (postabsorptive) events achieve biological relevance only if they are accompanied (preceded) by preabsorptive signals. This would indicate that appetite control is achieved jointly by physiological responses generated at different stages in the handling of nutrients following ingestion. The organism presumably recognizes these physiological changes as sequential cues that, by reinforcing each other, cumulatively constitute the "satiety cascade" (122). Removing individual cues from the sequence may well weaken the overall impact of a food or nutrient on satiation or PI satiety.

C. Specific Macronutrient Selection in Humans?

It is clear that human beings display preferences for, and selection of, different types of foods. These foods vary in taste, texture, density, and nutrient composition together with a host of cognitively mediated attributes. Under extreme physiological circumstances, animals and presumably humans can display a strong preference for a dietary component that is in deficit. The literature on salt appetite and on preferences of vitamin-deficient animals for foods that alleviate the deficiency are examples of this (see Ref. 81 for an introductory discussion of these phenomena). Nutrient deficits are not a necessary condition of a physiologically induced preference or aversion. To what extent can humans display a preference or aversion toward a particular macronutrient? What is the mechanism that could mediate this form of behavior? It is likely that a nutrient-based preference could develop through a process of learning. This would need a clearly defined unconditioned signal (arising from the physiological system)—a detection mechanism—linked to a particular sensory/or environmental cue. For instance, rats learn to prefer flavors that are associated with fructose infusions into the portal vein (43,123). These phenomena are most likely to be best observed under conditions where a learned change in feeding behavior will alleviate some physiological stress. The metabolic handling of protein loads constitutes a greater physiological stress than the oxidation/storage of fat or carbohydrate. Under experimental conditions, a number of animal species adopt selection strategies to optimize the protein:energy ratio of their diet and avoid an intake of excess protein (26,82,83). It is worth considering

whether there is any other unconditioned physiological signal that could serve as the source of food-selecting behavior directed to a particular macronutrient under more naturalistic conditions. For instance, athletes tend to consume greater amounts of carbohydrates than the general population. Is any of this selection driven by physiological changes induced by exercise per se? The organoleptic properties of the diet may influence nutrient selection for nonphysiological reasons. It is also important to bear in mind that selection of foods can be influenced by a number of nonphysiological and non-sensory-associated factors. Examining the relative and quantitative importance of physiological versus nonphysiological determinants remains an important area for future investigation.

Of special current interest is the existence of specific fat-seeking or fat-avoiding behavior. Is it possible to manipulate the system nutritionally, physiologically, or pharmacologically to induce individuals to avoid sources of dietary fat? Do we possess a sufficiently sensitive methodology to detect selective preferences for macronutrients? Animal studies suggest that a number of chemical manipulations, including galanin and enterostatin, can selectively alter eating behavior from high- or low-fat diets (66,67). Can this type of behavior be demonstrated in humans? Interestingly, a few studies indicate that short- or medium-term (3 months) manipulation with a serotoninergic drug can apparently selectively alter human fat consumption (124). There is evidence that serotonin activity in the brain is associated with the activity of both CCK and enterostatin, which are peripheral peptides, released in response to fat ingestion (124). Does this form part of a functional loop to enable humans to exercise control over fat consumption, or is it a biological accident that can be exploited for therapeutic purposes?

D. Macronutrients, Appetite, and Obesity

1. Food and Macronutrient Intake in the Etiology of Obesity

Considerable attention has recently focused on the issue of how the macronutrient composition of the diet can influence the current epidemic of obesity in Western society (2). Ingestion of dietary fat does appear to be a risk factor for subsequent weight gain (97), although it is possible to become obese on a HC diet (52). Drenowski (125) and Mela and Sacchetti (126) have produced data that suggest that fatter people prefer fattier foods. There is not a great deal of evidence that preference per se will influence quantitative intake (i.e., how much food is eaten) to an extent that will influence body weight. It is, however, likely that preference influences qualitative food intake, i.e., what foods are eaten. This is important because the phenomenon of passive overconsumption of energy on HF diets is not an issue of quantitative increases in food intake but of qualitative selection of HF, energy-dense foods. It has also been suggested that a genetic predisposition to store rather than oxidize fat may predispose certain individuals to rapid weight gain when they are exposed to a HF diet. Lissner and Heitmann (97) have recently examined prospective data on fat intake and subsequent weight gain and have found that in women, those who exhibited a genetic susceptibility to weight gain showed the greatest tendency to gain weight when exposed to a HF diet. In the 1950s Jean Mayer highlighted the need to distinguish between the dynamic period of rapid weight gain and the stable plateau that body weight appears to reach in obesity. This may well be important since it appears from laboratory experiments that satiation, PI satiety, and hunger are influenced by food intake in obese subjects in a similar way as in lean people (77). Spitzer and Rodin (3) also note that the majority of studies on eating behavior in normal-weight and overweight individuals conducted between 1969 and 1981 were "impressive in their demonstration of the lack of clear overweight-normal weight differences in eating behavior." The situation has not changed much today. They did, however, note that in short-term studies palatability appeared to be the most consistent variable in producing overweight-normal differences in amount of food eaten.

Furthermore, the physiological features and psychological profiles that characterize the obese and may be involved in the maintenance of the obese state may not necessarily be the same features that led to obesity in the first place (18). Understanding the factors that produce sustained increases in energy intake over expenditure and the time course over which this occurs is crucial for understanding the etiology of obesity. It is also worth mentioning that obesity is a generic category which, like skin color, identifies an obvious recognizable feature of individuals, but explains little of the behavior of those individuals. There are likely to be a number of different factors that individually or together influence body weight. For instance, it is well known that not all obese subjects are restrained eaters. Similarly not all obese subjects are insulin-resistant. Since it is presently difficult to categorize which "type" of obesity a person belongs to or indeed how many "types" there are, it is equally difficult to identify the factors bringing about these characteristics.

There has been an ongoing debate over the last few decades on the extent to which changes in energy expenditure or energy intake are the primary factors involved in the etiology of obesity. Prentice et al. (127) argue that the obese have higher absolute energy requirements than do the lean, because of the greater mass of metabolically active tissue. This is true under standardized conditions; however, decreases in physical activity without attendant changes in energy intake will also precipitate a positive energy balance. A recent review of the doubly labeled water literature suggests that the obese do not have a lower energy expenditure due to physical activity, indeed their energy expenditure is higher than that of the control population (128). This higher total daily energy expenditure in the obese is likely to be due to both the increased energy cost of physical activity in the obese and the highly sedentary nature of the general population with whom they are compared. Thus changing patterns of physical activity are important life-style factors that can influence the predisposition to weight gain. At present, the exact nature of the relationship between feeding behavior, nutrient intake, and physical activity patterns is not clear.

Studies of dietary compliance (129–131) suggest that people tend to underreport their intakes of energy during diet survey studies (132,133,134). The obese, however, appear to systematically underreport their intakes of energy relative to expenditure of energy, to a greater degree than do the lean (131,132). These findings certainly contradict the notion that the obese actually require less energy or the same energy to maintain a stable body weight as do the lean. Indeed the findings of significant underreporting of food intake in the obese, together with absolutely higher energy requirements (at least when comparing sedentary lean and overweight individuals), tend to support the contention that the obese are actually consuming less than their usual intakes of energy under the conditions of the studies concerned (3,133,135). In support of the above assertions it seems appropriate to cite diet survey studies that suggest a positive correlation between energy intake and body mass index (wt/ht^2). In these studies the increased energy derived from fat appears to correlate with body mass index (1,136), and particularly with percent body fat (136–141). Likewise, several studies demonstrate a relationship between reduced dietary fat intake and reduced body fatness (142,143) or weight (8,13). These data also suggest a role for the macronutrient composition of the diet in the etiology of obesity. There are, however, a number of studies that do not show a correlation between energy intake and body mass index (144). There are a number of reasons for this. Physical activity, degree of underreporting, differences in metabolic body size, and other factors may all obscure such a relationship. The two factors most regularly cited as risk behaviors for weight gain are high levels of fat intake and low levels of physical activity (145).

The development of obesity is primarily due to an excessive intake of energy relative to that required to stay in energy balance. Since the flexibility of resting metabolism in humans is very limited, it is likely that the development of obesity involves a real hyperphagia, which may be abetted by decreases in physical activity. On experimental overfeeding at least, the interindividual variability in weight gain is very large (146,147). There may therefore be a genetic component associated with nutrient partitioning subsequent to that hyperphagia, which predisposes some people to deposit more fat relative to lean tissue (148–150).

It is therefore likely that nutrient and energy intake is somehow altered during the development of obesity and that regulation may again be reestablished at a higher level of body weight once stable obesity is established (18,92).

Since the majority of weight loss treatments are characterized by initial success and subsequent rebound in weight gain, it is likely that physiological and/or cognitive mechanisms come into play that increase energy intake. Identifying the mechanisms involved in the near-inevitable weight gain subsequent to initial weight loss may provide valuable information pertinent to the development of strategies to improve long-term weight loss.

VI. PALATABILITY AND SENSORY FACTORS

A. Palatability and Food Intake

In considering the capacity for energy intake to rise above energy expenditure, the weakness of inhibitory factors has to be set against the potency of facilitatory processes. The palatability of food is clearly one feature that could exert a positive influence over behavior. The logical status of palatability is that of a construct (it is not an objective feature such as protein content or blood glucose) (151,152). Palatability can be influenced by a number of factors including environmental cues and the physiological state of the organism. However, palatability can be operationally defined according to the amount of food consumed, although some authors feel that this is inappropriate for animal studies (26). The independent index of palatability is usually considered to be the subjective appreciation of pleasantness. This subjective sensation is quantified by expressing it on an objective scale according to standard psychophysical procedures (153). This sensation is often taken to reflect the hedonic dimension of food. The nature of the relationship between palatability, food consumption, and energy balance has never been systematically determined although palatability does influence the cumulative intake curve, and palatability has been invoked as a mediating principle to account for the prolongation of ingestion from a variety of foods due to sensory-specific satiety operating in short-term studies.

It may be hypothesized that palatability would exert a powerful effect on intrameal satiety (while food was being consumed), but is there an enduring legacy that influences PI satiety? And what is the effect of the expectation of getting pleasure from food on the initiation and maintenance of eating? Although almost everyone would agree that palatability exerts a powerful influence on eating behavior, there is no systematic body of data to explain the strength or the limits of the effect (154).

B. Sweetness, Sucrose, and Sweeteners

The effect of these three factors on appetite is steeped in controversy and conflict. Part of this is undoubtedly due to the interference of commercial agencies (such as the sugar lobby and high-intensity-sweeteners industry) in the scientific process. For this reason the designation of the role of sweetness on the control of food intake is confounded by the market prospects of the agents providing the sweetness. Sweetness is one of the most powerful and easily recognized taste sensations. Sweetness is clearly a potent psychobiological phenomenon. Foods are made sweet to increase their attractiveness (raise palatability) and, in turn, to increase consumption (by the eater and purchaser). The most economical account of sweetness is that, like the more general attribute of palatability, it facilitates food intake. This should apply independent of the energy or macronutrient profile associated with the sweetness. However, the effects of the associated energy and nutrients should be considered when assessing the overall action of sweetness in foods.

Some attempts have been made to experimentally uncouple sweetness and energy so as to evaluate the relative contribution of each factor to the control of appetite (155–157). According to the foregoing argument, it may be supposed that sweetness would facilitate while energy would inhibit. After some lively debate, it now seems to be agreed that the consumption of sugars (sweetness plus energy) does lead to energy compensation (a subsequent suppression of intake by an amount roughly equivalent to the amount provided by the sugars), as described by Black and Anderson (158). Different sugars (mono- or disaccharides) may exert somewhat different effects. Since industrial manufacturers largely agree that it is the addition of sweetness to foods that is believed to enhance consumption (a stimulatory effect), it is difficult to argue that it is the sweetness per se that causes the compensation.

From this it follows that high-intensity sweeteners and sucrose should produce different effects on food intake by virtue of their distinctive physiological effects. The suppressive effect of sugar is presumably due to carbohydrate metabolism (see earlier discussion). However, sucrose-like high-intensity sweeteners will also confer a facilitatory action on appetite via sweetness per se. This means that the effects of sweetness will be manifest when present in combination with other nutrients. For example, what would be the effect of HF foods whose palatability has been raised further by the addition of sweetness? Would the effect be detected on satiation or PI satiety?

One implication of this concerns the interpretation of recent analyses of the relationship between obesity and sugar and fat consumption. Using a large data base, it has been shown that the consumption of fat is positively related to body mass index while an inverse relationship is seen for sucrose (159). Initially, these data suggest that sucrose intake is unrelated to obesity. Indeed, it could be argued from these relationships that consuming sucrose either prevents obesity or is the cure for obesity. However, at present the analysis does not indicate how the overall profile of nutrient intake relates to the selection of particular food groups or to actual eating behavior. Furthermore, in that particular analysis both fat and sucrose intake correlated positively with energy intake. Several scenarios could be envisaged. One of these would involve a subgroup of the sample that is overweight, or gaining weight, and whose sugar intake is low but the sugar is consumed along with fat. Other sweetening agents may also be involved. Some proposals concerning the effects of sweet and fat foods have been made (160). This issue is part of a larger problem involving sensory and nutrient interactions in foods and their capacity to stimulate or inhibit food intake.

C. Fat and Fat Mimetics

Currently a number of low-calorie or acaloric fat mimetics are under development. These compounds are poorly absorbed across the gastrointestinal wall and are not metabolized by the colonic microflora. The most extensively studied of these are the olestras, which are a group of compounds that possess a sucrose (rather than glycerol) backbone with more than three fatty acid side chains. Earlier work on the effects of fat mimetics on energy intake in lean men (161,162) and children (163) suggested that energy intake was compensated for when fat in specific items of the diet was covertly replaced by olestra. These studies were relatively short-term and subjects were able to freely select from a variety of familiar food items

throughout the rest of the day, after ingestion of full-fat or olestra-containing breakfasts. Other work by Porikos (164) has shown that compensation was less complete. More recent studies have suggested that under certain conditions, olestra may lead to sustained reductions in energy intakes. Work by Cotton et al. (165) has shown that substituting 55 g of dietary fat with olestra on one day led to poor compensation of energy intake on the subsequent day. Work at the Pennington Research Center has demonstrated that sustained reductions in ad libitum energy intakes are possible using olestra under conditions where the diet has been systematically altered (166,167). Finally, work by Miller et al. (168) suggests that subjects do not compensate well for the reduction in energy and fat intake brought about by the consumption of olestra-based snacks, although compensation is more accurate when subjects are informed of the dietary manipulation. These studies have produced results that are virtually identical to those in which the energy density of the diet is covertly manipulated with dietary fat. This is not surprising since olestra is performing the same function. The olestras therefore act as a useful tool to dissociate the sensory from the nutritional effects of consuming dietary fat. At present there is no evidence that diets containing the sensory characteristic of fats but not the energy density (i.e., foods in which dietary fat has been substituted by olestra) promote overconsumption of energy. However, in the majority of these studies the full-fat, energy-dense food is compared to the fat-substituted food. These comparisons have not therefore been made at the same level of dietary energy density. This is similar to comparing the effects of fat and carbohydrate by using low-fat, less-energy-dense diets versus high-fat, more-energy-dense diets. Furthermore, it is worth asking whether mimicking the sensory properties of fats and sugars actually maintains sensory preference for these nutrients. The fat mimetics show great potential as a tool for assisting in reduction of fat intake in consumers at large and perhaps, if used responsibly, in weight-reducing programs. However, if their use becomes increasingly prevalent, in time their influence on other aspects of eating behavior and physiological functioning should not be ignored.

D. Variety

It has been suggested from a number of short-term studies that have been conducted (169,170–172), together with the cafeteria-diet model, that sensory variety of foods promotes overconsumption of energy. Furthermore, in rats Le Magnen has shown that simply increasing sensory variety can lead to excess energy intake and weight gain, provided the variety is constantly rotated. Increases and decreases in sensory variety that were stable over time had a much less pronounced effect (27). It has also been hypothesized that this effect may be pronounced in people who are more susceptible to environmental cues (173). Unfortunately, to our knowledge, there have been no studies conducted where the effects of increasing or decreasing the sensory variety of a nutritionally controlled diet have been examined on the energy intake of human subjects over a period of several days or more. Increasing the variety of sandwiches served at a single meal may influence energy intake during that meal, but what happens at the next meal? Thus outcomes that appear to be anecdotally obvious need to be confirmed by careful experimental design and studies that examine feeding patterns over several days. At present there is, to our knowledge, no evidence that sensory variety per se leads to large perturbations of energy balance. The mechanism of sensory-specific satiety may well function to maximize the variety of items consumed and hence increase the probability of satisfying nutritional requirements. How important this is in relation to other time and cost-benefit considerations in the feeding strategy of a human or an animal is yet to be determined.

There is therefore a good deal of work to do in considering the relative contribution of sensory versus nutritional determinants of feeding behavior and energy balance. This area of research is of growing importance since the sensory qualities of the diet no longer necessarily provide reliable information regarding its nutritional content. Some individuals may be more disposed to cues such as palatability or olfactory cues associated with certain foods than to internal (physiological) cues. Disturbed sensory functioning is a major factor involved in the loss of appetite due to pathologies or side effects of the drugs used to treat certain illnesses (36).

E. Meal Patterns

Mela and Rodgers (174) have reviewed the role that snack foods and eating patterns might play in the genesis of obesity. They note that early animal data indicate that the consumption of less frequent, larger meals should be more likely to lead to weight gain and fat deposition than the same amount of energy ingested in smaller, more frequent bouts of eating. However, recent work in humans has found that changes in feeding frequency at controlled levels of energy intake had no significant effects on total energy expenditure (175,176). However, a pattern of fewer, larger meals led to greater periodicity in nutrient oxidation/storage patterns, particularly in the ratio of car-

bohydrate to fat oxidized, relative to a feeding pattern of more frequent, smaller meals at the same daily energy intake (175). If factors such as blood glucose dynamics exert important influences on feeding behavior, then feeding frequency may indirectly influence human appetite. When the food intake of animals is limited to only one or two meals per day, but they can feed ad libitum, the gastrointestinal tract becomes enlarged and glucose and amino acids are apparently more rapidly absorbed into the bloodstream (81). Rates of glycogenesis and lipogenesis may also be increased under these conditions, shifting the nutrient oxidation-storage equilibrium in the direction of storage. It has been hypothesized that factors favoring nutrient stores decrease the metabolic availability of nutrients and so decrease postabsorptive satiety (117). Epidemiological data in humans are beginning to emerge that also suggest that energy taken in as numerous small meals appears to correlate with lower body mass index (144). This may be due to factors other than appetite regulation. Furthermore, the animal feeding under these conditions has less chance to compensate for excess energy intakes because it has to "anticipate" an appropriate energy intake in just a few large eating bouts rather than making many small adjustments through snacks. Appetite regulation is such that there would be a tendency to over- rather than underestimate appropriate energy intakes. It is of interest that meal feeding in humans appears to be strongly conditioned, as indicated by the fact that the greatest predictor of hunger and meal initiation in ad libitum feeding humans is usually time of day. Rats typically adjust energy intakes by altering the number of meals they eat, whereas humans tend to adjust meal size. However, if rats are exposed to a human-type meal-feeding pattern, they will adjust energy intakes by altering meal size (177). Since it is likely that gastrointestinal and metabolic satiety signals interact to reinforce each other, the time of the day at which feeding occurs may have implications for body weight regulation. It may be hypothesized that foods eaten late at night are less well detected since the opportunity for metabolic reinforcement of gastrointestinal satiety signals would tend to be bypassed.

The timing and rate of nutrient ingestion and its effects on satiety are likely to be important in the clinical setting. For instance, will the nasogastric administration of a person's energy requirements as tube feeds continuously over 24 h have the same effect on appetite as cyclic administration throughout the day? If the feed were given throughout the night, would subjects feel uncomfortably hungry throughout the day? These issues also have implications for the management of patients on home parenteral nutrition (Elia, M. personal communication). The whole issue of timing and composition of feed administration in the clinical management of patients receiving nutritional support is yet to be investigated in more detail.

The data from humans concerning meal patterns, appetite, and energy balance are difficult to interpret. Unfortunately, this literature contains many methodological problems such as differences in the exact definition of a meal as opposed to a snack. Altered meal patterns, because they may limit the capacity of people to compensate energy intake, may well interact with diet composition to affect appetite and energy balance. Dietary macronutrients appear to exert differential effects on pre- and postabsorptive satiety signals, and the influence of specific nutrients may vary over different time courses.

VII. CONCLUSION

At the time of writing we have attempted to represent the current state of research findings in relation to diet and food intake in humans. We have aimed to point the reader in the direction of some major unresolved issues that still surround the study of human feeding. We have also discussed the apparent resolution of a number of other issues and have commented on the limitations of some of these conclusions. This is important since many research papers still cite "facts" about feeding for which there is still relatively little evidence. It is likely that by the end of the decade a number of issues will be resolved (e.g., the role of dietary fat in producing hyperphagia). Other issues, for instance the neurendocrine and physiological responses to nutrient ingestion, become more complex as they are uncovered. An increasing number of effectors and subsystems are being identified and are known to operate at several levels ranging from the molecular to the whole-body. Over the last few decades greater progress has been made in understanding the nature of the appetite system (through whole-body studies) and in identifying its components (through molecular and biochemical studies, often in animal models) that in understanding how these components operate and interact. We still do not have a synthetic theory of feeding behavior as exists, for example, for biological evolution.

We have emphasized the multifactorial nature of the feeding system and the necessity of a multidisciplinary approach to its study. Owing to the current state of knowledge and the complex nature of the appetite system, we feel that it is not only pertinent, but crucial, to refer the experimental exploration of the systems involved in human feeding to the functioning of real people in the real world. In other words, it is important to maintain the balance between whole-body and invasive, mechanistic studies in linking putative hunger, appetite, and satiety signals to the behaviors they are believed to influence. Given the current emphasis on directing research toward promoting greater human health and well-being, animal and molecular models of compartments of the appetite system provide invaluable information if related to parallel (but less invasive) protocols in humans.

As the food we eat is changed and transformed by food producers and manufacturers for a variety of reasons, understanding the role of the diet in feeding behavior and energy balance is more important than ever. Structured research strategies that seek to understand the mechanisms underlying quantitative and qualitative feeding behavior, within the context of energy and nutrient balance, may help us keep pace with the rapidly changing nature and effects of the diet that we eat.

ACKNOWLEDGMENTS

We are grateful to Alex Johnstone and Joanne Stubbs for assistance in preparation of the manuscript.

REFERENCES

1. Factors influencing body weight (sect 3.4.3) In: Diet nutrition and the prevention of chronic disease. A report of a WHO study group. Geneva: World Health Organization, 1990.
2. Danforth E. Diet and obesity. Am J Clin Nutr 1985; 41: 1132–1145.
3. Spitzer L, Rodin J. Human eating behavior: a critical review of studies in normal weight and overweight individuals. Appetite 1981; 2:293–329.
4. Mattes RD. Gustation as a determinant of ingestion: methodological issues. Am J Clin Nutr 1985; 41:672–683.
5. Hill AJ, Rogers PJ, Blundell JE. Techniques for the experimental measurement of human eating behavior and food intake: a practical guide. Int J Obes 1995; 19(6):361–375.
6. Shepherd R. Sensory influences on salt, sugar and fat intake. Nutr Res Rev 1988; 1:125–144.
7. Duncan KH, Bacon JA, Weinsier RL. The effects of high and low energy density diets on satiety, energy intake, and eating time of obese and non obese subjects. Am J Clin Nutr 1983; 37:763–767.
8. Lissner L, Levitsky DA, Strupp BJ, Kalkwarf HJ, Roe DA. Dietary fat and the regulation of energy intake in human subjects. Am J Clin Nutr 1987; 46:886–892.
9. Stubbs RJ, Harbron CG, Murgatroyd PR, Prentice AM. Covert manipulation of dietary fat and energy density: effect on substrate flux and food intake in men feeding ad libitum. Am J Clin Nutr 1995; 62 2:316–330.

10. Van Stratum P, Lussenburg RN, van Wezel LA, Vergroesen AJ, Cremer HD. The effect of dietary carbohydrate: fat ratio on energy intake by adult women. Am J Clin Nutr 1978; 31:206–212.

11. Stubbs RJ, Harbron CG, Prentice AM. The effect of covertly manipulating the dietary fat to carbohydrate ratio of isoenergetically dense diets on ad libitum food intake in free-living humans. Int J Obes 1996; 20:651–660.

12. Brunswik E. The Conceptual Framework of Psychology. Chicago: University of Chicago Press 1995:102.

13. Kendall A, Levitsky DA, Strupp BJ, Lissner L. Weight-loss on a low fat diet: consequence of the impression of the control of food intake in humans. Am J Clin Nutr 1991; 53:1124–1129.

14. Van Itallie TB, Vanderweele DA. The phenomenon of satiety. In: Björntorp P, Cairella M, Howard AN, eds. Recent Advances in Obesity Research III. London: Libby, 1981: 278–289.

15. Blundell JE. Hunger, appetite and satiety-constructs in search of identities. In: Turner M, eds. Nutrition and Lifestyles. London: Applied Science Publishers, 1979:21–42.

16. Gibbs J, Young R, Smith GP. Cholecystokinin elicits satiety in rats with open gastric fistulas. Nature 1973; 245: 323–325.

17. West DB, Greenwood MRC, Marshall KA. Lithium chloride, cholecystokinin, and meal patterns: evidence that cholecystokinin suppresses meal size in rats without causing malaise. Appetite 1987; 8:221–227.

18. Mayer J. The regulation of energy intake and the body weight. Ann NY Acad Sci 1955; 63:15–43.

19. Pharmacological treatment of obesity: Satellite Symposium to the 6th International Congress on Obesity. In: Bray GA, Inoue S, eds. Am J Clin Nutr 1992; 55 (Suppl 1) .

20. Raben A. Appetite and carbohydrate metabolism. PhD thesis, Royal Veterinary and Agricultural University, Copenhagen, 1995.

21. Campfield LA, Smith FJ. Transient declines in blood glucose signal meal initiation. Int J Obes 1990; 14(Suppl 3): 15–33.

22. Campfield LA, Smith FJ, Rosenbaum M, Geary N. Human hunger: is there a role for blood glucose dynamics? Appetite 1992; 18:244 (letter).

23. Campfield LA, Smith FJ. Functional coupling between transient declines in blood glucose and feeding behavior: temporal relationships. Brain Res Bull 1986; 174: 427–433.

24. Carpenter RG, Grossman SP. Plasma fat metabolites and hunger. Physiol Behav 1982; 30:57–63.

25. Rich AJ, Chambers P, Johnston IDA. Are ketones an appetite suppressant? Journal of Enteral and Parenteral Nutrition 1988; 13:7S.

26. Forbes JM. Voluntary food intake and diet selection in farm animals. 1995 CAB International, Oxon UK.

27. Le Magnen J. Neurobiology of Feeding and Nutrition. San Diego, CA: Academic Press, 1992.

28. Franke LW. The ability of rats to discriminate between diet of various degrees of toxicity. Science 1936; 83:130–135.

29. Kalat JW, Rozin P. Role of interference in taste aversion learning. J Comp Physiol Psychol 1971; 77:53–58.

30. Bernstein IL. Development of food aversion during illness. Proc Nutr Soc 1994; 53:131–137.

31. Rozin P, Kalat JW. Specific hungers and poison avoidance as adaptive specialisations of learning. Psychol Rev 1971; 78:459–486.

32. Rozin P, Rodgers WH. Novel diet preferences in vitamin deficient rats and rats recovering from vitamin deficiencies. J Comp Physiol Psychol 1967; 63:421–428.

33. Booth DA, Lee M, Macleavey C. Acquired sensory control of satiation in man. Br J Psychol 1976; 67:137–47.

34. Booth DA, Mather D, Fuller J. Starch content of associatively conditioned human appetite and satiation, indexed by intake and eating pleasantness of starch-paired flavours. Appetite 1982; 3:163–184.

35. Mook DG. Oral factors in appetite and satiety. Ann NY Acad Sci. 1989; 575:265–280.

36. Mattes RD. Sensory influences on food intake and utilisation in humans. Hum Nutr Appl Nutr 1987; 41A: 77–95.

37. Sawchenko PE, Friedman MI. Sensory functions of the liver. Am J Physiol 1979; 236:R5-R20.

38. Meiselman HL. Determining consumer preference in institutional food service. In: Food Service Systems. New York: Academic Press, 1979:127–153.

39. Dalton S, Linke RA, Simko MD. Reasons related to consistency between intended and actual food choice, including accuracy of and satisfaction with perceived body size. In: Abstr., 67th Annual meeting of the American Dietetic Association, Washingon, DC, 1984:73–74.

40. Cannon WB, Washburn AL. An explanation of hunger. Am J Phys 1912; 29:441–454.

41. Keys A, Brozeck J, Mickelsen O, Longstreet-Taylor H. The Biology of Human Starvation. Minneapolis, MN: University of Minnesota Press, 1950.

42. Medical Research Council Special report series No. 275, (1951) HMSO.

43. Tordoff MG, Ulrich PM, Sandler F. Flavour preferences and fructose: evidence that the liver detects the unconditioned stimulus for calorie based learning. Appetite 1990; 14:29–44.

44. Ritter S, Calingasan NY. Neural substrates for metabolic controls of feeding. In: Fernstrom JD, Miller GD, eds. Appetite and Body Weight Regulation: Sugar, Fat and Macronutrient Substitutes. Boca Raton, FL: CRC Press, 1994.

45. Friedman MI, Rawson NE. Fuel metabolism and appetite control. In: Fernstrom JD, Miller GD, eds. Appetite and Body Weight Regulation: Sugar, Fat and Macronutrient Substitutes. Boca Raton, FL: CRC Press, 1994.

46. Forbes JM. Metabolic aspects of the regulation of voluntary food intake and appetite. Nutr Res Rev 1988; 1: 145–148.

47. Janowitz HD, Grossman MI. Some factors affecting the food intake of normal dogs and dogs with esophagostomy and gastric fistulas. Am J Physiol 1949; 159:143–148.

48. Young RC, Gibbs CJ, Antin J, Holt J, Smith GP. Absence of satiety during sham feeding in the rat. J Comp Physiol Psychol 1974; 87:795–800.

49. Mook DG, Culberson GR, Gelbart RJ, McDonald K. Oropharangeal control of ingestion in rats: Acquisition of sham drinking patterns. Behav Neurosci 1983; 97: 574–584.

50. Walls EK, Koopmans HS. Differential effects of intravenous glucose, amino acids and lipid on daily food intake in rats. Am J Physiol 1992; 262:R225–R234.

51. Norgan NC, Durnin VGA. The effect of 6 weeks of overfeeding on the body weight, body composition and energy metabolism of young men. Am J Clin Nutr 1980; 33:978–988.

52. Pasquet P, Apfelbaum M. Recovery of initial body weight and composition after long-term massive overfeeding in men. Am J Clin Nutr 1994; 60:861–863.

53. Harris RBS, Martin RJ. Specific depletion of body fat in parabiotic partners of tube fed obese rats. Am J Physiol 1984; 247:R380–R386.

54. Harris RBS, Martin RJ. Site of action of putative lipostatic factor: food intake and peripheral pentose shunt pathway. Am J Physiol 1990; 259:R45–R52.

55. Zhang Y, Proenca, Maffei M, Barone M, Leopold L, Friedman JM. Positional cloning of the mouse obese gene and its human homologue. Nature 1994; 372:425–431.

56. Considine RV, Sinha MK, Heiman ML, Kriauciunas A, Stephens TW, Nyce MR, Ohannesian JP, Macro CC, McKee LJ, Bauer TL, Caro JF. Serum immunoreactive-leptin concentrations in normal weight and obese humans. N Engl J Med 1996; 334:292–295.

57. Karam JH, Grodsky GM, Forsham PH. Excessive insulin response to glucose in obese subjects as measured by immunochemical assay. Diabetes 1963; 12:197–204.

58. Bogardus C, Lillioja S, Mott M, Hollenbeck C, and Reaven G. Relationship between degree of obesity and in vivo insulin action man. Am J Physiol 1985; 248:E286–E291.

59. Frederich RC, Hamman A, Anderson S, Lollman B, Lowell BB, Flier JS. Leptin levels reflect body lipid content in mice: evidence for diet induced resistance to leptin action. Nature Med 1995; 1:1311–1314.

60. Storlien LH, James DE, Burleigh KM, Chisholm DJ, Kraegen EW. Fat feeding causes widespread in vivo insulin resistance, decreased energy expenditure and obesity in rats. Am J Physiol 1986; 251:E576–E583.

61. Storlien LH, Jenkins AB, Chisholm DJ, Pascoe WS, Khouri S, Kraegen EW. Influence of dietary fat composition on development of insulin resistance in rats. Diabetes 1991; 40:280–289.

62. Borkman M, Storlien LH, Pan DA, Jenkins AB, Chisholm DJ, Campbell LV. The relationship between insulin sensitivity and the fatty-acid composition of skeletal muscle phospholipids. N Engl J Med 1993; 328:238–44.

63. Halaas JL, Galiwala KS, Maffei M, Cohen SL, Chait BT, Rabinowitz D, Lallone RL, Burley SK, Friedman JM. Weight-reducing effects of the plasma protein encoded by the obese gene. Science 1995; 269:543–546.

64. Stephens TW, Basinski M, Bristow PK, Bue-Valleskey JM, Burgett SG, Craft L, Hale J, Hoffman J, Hsiung HM, Hriauciunas A, MacKellar W, Rosteck PR, Schoner B, Smith D, Tinsley FC, Zhang XY, Heiman M. The role of neuropeptide Y in the antiobesity action of the obese gene product. Nature 1995; 377:530–532.

65. Millward JD. A protein-stat mechanism for regulation of growth and maintenance of the lean body mass. Nutr Res Rev 1995; 8:93–120.

66. Lebowitz SF. Neurochemical-neurendocrine systems in the brain controlling macronutrient intake and metabolism. Trends Neurosci 1992; 15:491–497.

67. Langhans W. Metabolic and glucostatic control of feeding. Proc Nutr Soc 1996; 55:497–515.

68. Bray GA. Obesity—a state of reduced sympathetic activity and normal or high adrenal activity (the autonomic and adrenal hypothesis revisited). Int J Obes 1990; 14(Suppl 3):77–90.

69. Astrup A, Toubro S, Christensen NJ and Quaade F. Pharmacology of thermogenic drugs. Am J Clin Nutr 1992; 55:246S–248S.

70. Bray GA. Peptides affect the intake of specific nutrients and the sympathetic nervous system. Am J Clin Nutr 1992; 55:265S–271S.

71. DeCastro JM. Macronutrient relationships with meal patterns and mood in the spontaneous feeding behavior of humans. Physiol Behav 1987; 39:561–569.

72. Bingham SA, Gill C, Welch A, Day K, Cassidy A, Khaw KT, Sneyd MJ, Key TJA, Roe L, Day NE. Comparison of dietary assessment methods in nutritional epidemiology: weighed records v. 24 h recalls, food-frequency questionnaires and estimated-diet records. Br J Nutr 1994; 72: 619–643.

73. Geliebter AA. Effects of equicaloric loads of protein, fat, and carbohydrate on food intake in the rat and man. Physiol Behav 1979; 22:2647–273.

74. de Graaf C, Schrevrs A, Blauw YH. 1993. Short term effects of different amounts of sweet and non-sweet carbohydrates on satiety and energy intake. Physiol Behav 1993; 54:833–843.

75. Miller MG, Teates JF. Acquisition of dietary self-selection in rats with normal and impaired oral sensation. Physiol Behav 1985; 34:401–408.

76. de Graaf C, Hulshof T, Westrate JA, Jas P. Short-term effects of different amounts of protein, fat and carbohydrates on satiety. Am J Clin Nutr 1992; 55:33–38.

77. Hill AJ, Blundell JE. Comparison of the action of macronutrients on the expression of appetite in lean and obese humans. Ann NY Acad Sci 1990; 597:529–531.

78. Hill AJ, Blundell JE. Macronutrients and satiety: the effects of a high-protein or high-carbohydrate meal on subjective

motivation to eat and food preferences. Nutr Behav 1986; 3:133–144.

79. Barkeling B, Rossner S, Bjorvell H. Efficiency of a high-protein meal (meat) and a high carbohydrate meal (vegetarian) on satiety measured by automated computerised monitoring of subsequent food intake, motivation to eat and food preferences. Int J Obes 1990; 14:743–51.

80. Booth DA, Chase A, Campbell AT. Relative effectiveness of protein in the late stages of appetite suppression in man. Physiol Behav 1970; 5:1299–1302.

81. Lyle LD. Control of eating behavior. In: Wurtman RJ, Wurtman JJ, eds. Nutrition and the Brain. New York: Raven Press, 1977.

82. Kyriazakis I, Emmans GC, Whittemore CT. Diet selection in pigs: choices made by growing pigs given foods of different protein concentrations. Anim Product 1990; 50: 189–199.

83. Kyriazakis I, Emmans GC. Selection of a diet by growing pigs given choices between foods differing in contents protein and rapeseed meal. Appetite 1992; 19:121–132.

84. Fromentin G, Nicolaidis S. Rebalancing essential amino acid intake by self-selection in the rat. Br J Nutr 1996; 75:669–682.

85. Thompson DA, Campbell RG. Hunger in humans induced by 2-deoxy-D-glucose: glucoprivic control of taste preference and food intake. Science 1977; 198:1065–68.

86. Van Amelsvoort JMM, Weststrate JA. Amylose-amylopectin ration in a meal affects post male volunteers. Am J Clin Nutr 1992; 55:712–718.

87. Holt S, Brand J, Soveny C, Hansky J. Relationship of satiety to postprandial glycemic, insulin and cholecystokinin responses. Appetite 1992; 18:129–141.

88. Burley VJ, Blundell JE. Dietary fibre and the pattern of energy intake. In: Krichevsky D, Bonfield C, eds. Dietary Fibre in Health and Disease. Chicago: University of Chicago Press, 1995; 102:243–256.

89. Weinsier RC, Johnston MH, Doleys DM, Bacon JA. Dietary management of obesity: evaluation of the time-energy displacement diet in terms of its efficacy and nutritional adequacy for long term weight control. Br J Nutr 1982; 47:367–479.

90. Russek M. An hypothesis on the participation of hepatic glucoreceptors in the control of food intake. Nature 1963; 197:79–80.

91. Russek M. Current status of the hepatostatic theory of food intake control. Appetite 1981; 2:137–143.

92. Flatt JP. The difference in storage capacities for carbohydrate and for fat, and its implications for the regulation of body weight. Ann NY Acad Sci 1987; 499:104–123.

93. Fernstrom JD. Food induced changes in brain serotonin synthesis is there a relationship to appetite for specific macronutrients? Appetite 1987; 81:63–82.

94. Foltin RW, Fischman MW, Moran TH, Rolls BJ, Kelly TH. Caloric compensation for lunches varying in fat and carbohydrate contents by humans in a residential laboratory. Am J Clin Nutr 1990; 52:969–980.

95. Foltin RW, Rolls BJ, Moran TH, Kelly TH, McNelis AL, Fischman MW. Caloric, but not macronutrient compensation by humans for required eating occasions with meals and snacks varying in fat and carbohydrate. Am J Clin Nutr 1992; 55:331–342.

96. Lawton CL, Burley VJ, Wales JK, Blundell JE. Dietary fat and appetite control in obese subjects: weak effects on satiation and satiety. Int J Obes 1993; 17:409–416.

97. Lissner L, Heitmann BL. Dietary fat and obesity: evidence from epidemiology. Eur J Clin Nutr 1995; 49:79–90.

98. Rolls BJ, Kim-Harris S, Fischman MW, Foltin RW, Moran TH, Stoner SA. Satiety after preloads with different amounts of fat and carbohydrate: implications for obesity. Am J Clin Nutr 1994; 60:476–87.

99. Rolls BJ, Kim S, McNelis AL, Fischman MW, Foltin RW, Moran TH. Time course of effects of preloads high in fat or carbohydrate on food intake and hunger ratings in humans. Am J Physiol 1991; 260:R756–R763.

100. Welch IML, Sepple CP, Read NW. Comparisons of the effects of satiety and eating behavior of infusions of lipid into the different regions of the small intestine. Gut 1988; 29:306–311.

101. Gil K, Skeie B, Kvetan V, Askanazi J, Friedman MI. Parenteral nutrition and oral intake: effect of glucose and fat infusion. Journal of Enteral and Parenteral Nutrition 1991; 15:426–432.

102. Greenberg D, Becker DC, Gibbs J, Smith GP. Infusions of lipid into the duodenum elecit satiety in rats while similar infusions into the vena cava do not. Appetite 1989; 12: 213 (abstract).

103. Green S, Burley VJ, Blundell JE. Effect of fat-containing and sucrose-containing foods on the size of eating episodes and energy intake in lean males: potential for causing overconsumption. Eur J Clin Nutr 1994; 48:547–555.

104. Tremblay A, Lavallee N, Almeras N, Allard L, Despres JP, Bouchard C. Nutritional determinants of the increase in energy intake associated with a high-fat diet. Am J Clin Nutr 1992; 53:134–137.

105. O'Reilly LM, Stubbs RJ, Johnstone AM, Mara OM, Robertson KA. Covert manipulation of the energy density of mixed diets: effects on ad libitum food intake in "free-living" humans. Proc Nutr Soc (in press).

106. Horton TJ, Drougas H, Brachey A, Reed GW, Peters JC, Hill JO. Fat and carbohydrate overfeeding in humans: differing effects on energy storage. Am J Clin Nutr 1995; 62: 19–29.

107. Ramirez I. When does sucrose increase appetite and obesity? Appetite 1987; 9:1–19.

108. Stubbs RJ. Macronutrient effects on appetite. Int J Obes 1995; 19(Suppl 5):S11–S19.

109. DeCastro JM, Orozco S. Moderate alcohol intake and spontaneous eating patterns of humans: evidence of unregulated supplementation. Am J Clin Nutr 1991; 52: 246–253.

110. Tremblay A, Wouters E, Wenker M, St-Pierre S, Bouchard C, Depres JP. Alcohol and a high-fat diet: a combination

favouring overfeeding. Am J Clin Nutr 1995; 62: 639–644.

111. Mattes RD. Dietary compensation by humans for supplemental energy provided as ethanol or carbohydrate in fluids. Physiol Behav 1996; 59:179–187.

112. Johnstone AM, Harbron CG, Stubbs RJ. Macronutrients, appetite and day-to-day food intake in humans. Eur J Clin Nutr 1996; 50:418–430.

113. Kennedy GC. The role of depot fat in the hypothalamic control of food intake in the rat. Proc R Soc (B) 1953; 140:578–592.

114. Shetty PS, Prentice AM, Goldberg GR, Murgatroyd PR, McKenna APM, Stubbs RJ, Volschenk PA. Alterations in fuel selection and voluntary food intake in response to iso-energetic manipulation of glycogen stores in man. Am J Clin Nutr 1994; 60:534–43.

115. Stubbs RJ, Goldberg GR, Murgatroyd PR, Prentice AM. Carbohydrate balance and day-to-day food intake in man. Am J Clin Nutr 1993; 57:897–903.

116. Langhans W, Scharrer E. The metabolic control of food intake. World Rev Nutr Diet 1992; 70:1–68.

117. Friedman MI, Stricker EM. The physiological psychology of hunger: A physiological perspective. Psychol Rev 1976; 83:409–431.

118. Friedman MI, Tordoff MG. Fatty acid oxidation and glucose utilisation interact to control food intake in rats. Am J Physiol 1986; 251:R840–R845.

119. Friedman MI. Body fat and the metabolic control of food intake. Int J Obes 1990; 16(Suppl 3):53–63.

120. Friedman MI, Ramirez I, Bowden CR, Tordoff MG. Fuel partitioning and food intake: role for mitochondrial fatty acid transport. Am J Physiol 1990; 258:R216–R221.

121. Friedman MI, Ramirez I. Relationship of fat metabolism to food intake. Am J Clin Nutr 1985; 42:1093–1098.

122. Blundell JE. The psychobiological approach to appetite and weight control. In: Brownell KD, Fairburn CG eds. Eating Disorders and Obesity: A Comprehensive Handbook. New York: Guildford Press, 1995.

123. Tordoff MG, Freidman MI. Hepatic portal infusions decrease food intake and increase food preference. Am J Physiol 1986; 251:R192–R196.

124. Blundell JE, Lawton CL, Halford JCG. Serotonin, eating behavior and fat intake. Obes Res 1995; 3:S471–S476.

125. Drenowski A. Energy intake and sensory properties of food. Am J Clin Nutr 1995; 62:1081S–5S.

126. Mela DJ, Sacchett DA. Sensory preferences for fats: Relationship with diet and body composition. Am J Clin Nutr 1991; 53:908–915.

127. Prentice AM, Black AE, Murgatroyd PR, Goldberg GR, Coward WA. Metabolism or appetite: questions of energy balance with particular reference to obesity. J Hum Nutr Diet 1989; 2:95–104.

128. Prentice AM, Black AE, Coward WA, Cole TJ. Energy expenditure in overweight and obese adults in affluent societies: an analysis of 319 doubly-labelled water measurements. Eur J Clin Nutr 1996; 50(2):93–97.

129. Bingham SA, Cummings JH. Urine nitrogen as an independent validatory measure of dietary intake: a study of nitrogen balance in individuals consuming their normal diet. Am J Clin Nutr 1985; 42:1276–1289.

130. Bingham SA. The dietary assessment of individuals; methods, accuracy, new techniques and recommendations. Nutr Abstr Rev 1987; 57:705–742.

131. Bingham SA, Welch A, Cassidy A, Runswick S. The use of 24 h urine nitrogen to detect bias in the reported habitual food intake of individuals assessed form weighed dietary records. Proc Nutr Soc 1989.

132. Black AE, Goldberg GR, Jebb SA, Livingstone MBE, Cole TJ, Prentice AM. Critical evaluation of energy intake data using fundamental principles of energy physiology. 2. Evaluating the results of published surveys. Eur J Clin Nutr 1991; 45:583–599.

133. Bandini LG, Schoeller DA, Cyr HN, Dietz WH. Validity of reported energy intake in obese and non-obese adolescents. Am J Clin Nutr 1990; 52:421–425.

134. Goldberg GR, Black A, Jebb SA, Cole TJ, Murgatroyd PR, Coward WA, Prentice AM. Critical evaluation of energy intake using fundamental principles of energy physiology. 1. Derivation of cut-off limits to identify under recording. Eur J Clin Nutr 1991; 45:569–581.

135. Durrant ML, Royston JP, Wloch RT, Garrow JS. The effect of covert energy density of preloads on subsequent ad libitum energy intake in lean and obese subjects. Hum Nutr Clin Nutr 1982; 36C:297–306.

136. Miller WC, Linderman AK, Wallace J and Niederpruem M. (1990) Diet composition, energy intake and exercise in relation to body fat in men and women. Am J Clin Nutr 52:426–430.

137. Dreon DM, Frey-Hewitt B, Ellseworth N, Williams PT, Terry RB, Wood PD. Dietary fat: carbohydrate ratio and obesity in middle-aged men. Am J Clin Nutr 1988; 4: 995–1000.

138. Romieu I, Willet WC, Stampfer MJ, Colditz GA, Sampson L, Rosner B, Hennekends CH, Speizer FE. Energy intake and other determinants of relative weight. Am J Clin Nutr 1988; 47:406–12.

139. Tremblay A, Plourde G, Despres JP, Bouchard C. Impact of dietary fat content and fat oxidation on energy intake in humans. Am J Clin Nutr 1989; 49:799–805.

140. George V, Tremblay A, Despres JP, Le Blanc C, Bouchard C. Effects of dietary fat content on total and regional adiposity in man and women. Int J Obes 1990; 14: 1085–1091.

141. Tucker LA, Kano MJ. Dietary fat and body fat: a multivariate study of 205 females. Am J Clin Nutr 1992; 56: 616–612.

142. Prewitt TE, Schmeisser D, Bowen PE, Aye P, Dolecek TA, Langenberg P, Cole T, Brace L. Changes in body weight, body composition and energy intake in women fed high and low-fat diets. Am J Clin Nutr 1991; 54:304–310.

143. Sheppard L, Lianne AR, Kristal AR, Krushi LH. Weight loss in women participating in a randomised trial of low fat diets. Am J Clin Nutr 1991; 54:821–828.

144. Gibney MJ. Epidemiology of obesity in relation to nutrient intake. Int J Obes 1995; 19:S1–S4.

145. Department of Health. Obesity, Reversing the increasing problem of obesity in England. Report from the Nutrition and Physical Activity Task Forces, Department of Health, London, 1995.

146. Forbes GB, Kreipe RE, Lipinski B. Body composition and the energy cost of weight gain. Hum Nutr Clin Nutr 1982; 36C:487–488.

147. Forbes GB, Brown MR, Weller SE, Lipinski BA. Deliberate overfeeding in women and men energy cost and composition of the weight gain. Br J Nutr 1985; 56:1–9.

148. Poehlman ET, Tremblay A, Depres JP, Fontaine E, Perusse L, Theriault G, Bouchard C. Genotype controlled changes in body composition and fat morphology following overfeeding in twins. Am J Clin Nutr 1986; 43:723–731.

149. Bouchard C, Tremblay A, Depres A, Poehlman JP, Theriault G, Nadeau A, Lupien P, Moorjani S, Dussalt J. Sensitivity to overfeeding: the Quebec experiment with identical twins. Prog Food Nutr Sci 1988; 12:45–72.

150. Bouchard C, Tremblay A, Depres A, Nadeau A, Lupien P, Theriault G, Dussalt J, Moorjani S, Pinault S, Fournier G. The response to long term overfeeding in twins. N Engl J Med 1990; 322:1477–1482.

151. Ramirez I. What do we mean when we say palatable food? Appetite 1990; 14:159–161.

152. Rogers PJ. Why a palatability construct is needed. Appetite 1990; 14:167–170.

153. Hill AJ, Blundell JE. Nutrients and behavior: research strategies for the investigation of taste characteristics food preferences, hunger sensations and eating patterns in man. J Psychol Res 1982; 17:203–212.

154. Ramirez I, Tordoff M, Friedman MI. Dietary hyperphagia and obesity: what causes them? Physiol Behav 1989; 45:163–168.

155. Rogers PJ, Carlyle J, Hill AJ, Blundell JE. Uncoupling sweet taste and calories: comparison of the effects of glucose and three intense sweeteners on hunger and food intake. Physiol Behav 1988; 43:547–552.

156. Rogers PJ, Blundell JE. Separating the actions of sweetness and calories: Effects of saccharin and carbohydrates on hunger and food intake in human subjects. Physiol Behav 1989; 45:1093–1099.

157. Rogers PJ, Burley VJ, Alikhanizadeh LA, Blundell JE. Postingestive inhibition of food intake by aspartame: importance of interval between aspartame administration and subsequent eating. Physiol Behav 1995; 57:489–493.

158. Black RM, Anderson GH. Sweeteners, food intake and selection. In: Fernstrom JD, Miller GD, eds. Appetite and body weight regulation: sugar, fat and macronutrient substitutes. Boca Raton, FL: CRC Press, 1994.

159. Bolton-Smith C, Woodward M. Dietary composition and fat to sugar ratios in relation to obesity. Int J Obes 1994; 18:820–828.

160. Heaton KW, Emmet PW. Extrinsic sugars and the consumption of fat. Am J Clin Nutr 1994; 59(Suppl):774S.

161. Burley VJ, Blundell JE. Evaluation of the action of a nonabsorbable fat on appetite and energy intake in lean, healthy males. In: Aillaud G, ed. Obesity in Europe 91. London: John Libbey, 1991: 63–65.

162. Rolls BJ, Pirraglia PA, Jones MB, Peters JC. Effects of olestra, a noncaloric fat substitute, on daily energy and fat intakes in lean men. Am J Clin Nutr 1992; 56:84–92.

163. Birch LL, Johnson SL, Jones MJ, Peters JC. Effects of a nonenergy fat substitute on children's energy and macronutrient intake. Am J Clin Nutr 1993; 58:326–33.

164. Porikos KA. Study on the effects of olestra on energy intake in 5 obese men. Study sponsored by Proctor and Gamble. Personal communication.

165. Cotton JR, Burley VJ, Blundell JE. Effect on appetite of replacing natural fat with sucrose polyester in meals or snacks across one whole day. Int J Obes 1993; 17(Suppl 2):47.

166. Bray GA, Sparti A, Windhauser MM, York D. Effect of two weeks fat replacement by olestra on food intake and energy metabolism. Annual Meeting of the Federation of American Societies of Experimental Biology, 1995.

167. Sparti A, Windhauser MM, Lovejoy J, Bray G. Subjects eat for carbohydrate not calories after dietary fat replacement with olestra. Annual Meeting of the American Society of Clinical Nutrition, May 1995.

168. Miller DL, Hammer VA, Shide DJ, Peters JC, Rolls BJ. Consumption of fat-free potato chips by obese and restrained males and females. Annual Meeting of the Federation of American Societies of Experimental Biology, April 1995.

169. Rolls B, Rowe E, Rolls E. Appetite and obesity: influences of sensory stimuli and external cues. In: Turner M. Ed. Nutrition and Lifestyles. London: Applied Science Publishers, 1979.

170. Rolls BJ, Rolls E, Rowe EA, Kingston B, Megson A, Gunary R. Variety in a meal enhances food intake in man. Physiol Behav 1981; 26:215–221.

171. Rolls BJ, Rolls ET, Rowe EA. The influence of variety on human food selection and intake. In: Eliot Stellar AVI, ed. The Psychobiology of Human Food Selection. Westport, Connecticut, 1982.

172. Spiegel TA, Stellar E. Effects of variety on food intake of underweight, normal weight and overweight women. Appetite 1990; 15:47–61.

173. Rodin J. Current status of the internal-external hypothesis for obesity: what went wrong. Am Psychol 1981; 36:361–372.

174. Mela D, Rodgers P. 'Snack foods,' overeating and obesity: relationships with food composition, palatability and eating behavior. Br Food J 1993; 95:13–16.

175. Verboecket van der Venne WPHG, Westerterp KR. Influence of the feeding frequency on nutrient utilisation in man: consequences for energy metabolism. Eur J Clin Nutr 1991; 45:161–169.

176. Verboecket van der Venne WPHG, Westerterp KR. Frequency of feeding, weight reduction and energy metabolism. Int J Obes 1993; 17:31–36.

177. DeCastro JM. The meal pattern of rats shifts from postprandial regulation to preprandial regulation when only five meals per day are scheduled. Physiol Behav 1988; 43: 739–746.

14

Experimental Studies on the Control of Food Intake

Henry S. Koopmans
University of Calgary, Calgary, Alberta, Canada

I. INTRODUCTION

The amount of food eaten is a major contributor to the control of body weight and to the development of obesity. It is now well established that daily food intake is internally controlled. Several studies have shown that signals arising in the mouth, throat, and esophagus play only a minor role in controlling food intake. Gastric distension and chemoreception are generally conceded to be the major inhibitors of food intake during a meal. The importance of intestinal signals is still in some dispute. The infusion of large amounts of food into the intestine can diminish feeding or sham-feeding behavior. However, the physiological delivery of a relatively small amount of food into the upper jejunum of crossed-intestines rats has no effect on short-term food intake despite the absorption of nutrients through the intestinal segment.

A large number of studies have examined the role of gastrointestinal and pancreatic hormones on the inhibition of food intake. CCK, bombesin, glucagon, and amyloid peptide have been shown to inhibit food intake when injected into the peritoneal cavity or into the bloodstream. Insulin has been shown to both increase and inhibit food intake. In contrast, a study using cross-circulated rats whose blood was fully mixed every minute showed that the combination of all absorbed nutrients and hormones present in the bloodstream after a meal had no effect on short-term food intake.

Stimulation of the ileum, cecum, or colon has been shown to cause a large loss of weight in animals with jejunoileal bypass or ileal transposition, but it is uncertain whether these signals remain in the physiological range and act in a normal way to inhibit food intake. Studies with parabiotic rats that have their lower guts either unstimulated or doubly stimulated with exogenous food show no specific effect of stimulation of the lower gut on the control of daily food intake. The liver has long been thought to be a regulator of food intake and several studies using portal infusions of glucose have produced reductions in food intake. However, complete liver denervations and portacaval shunts that divert mesenteric blood away from the liver into the systemic blood have no effect on meal patterns or daily food intake.

The most reliable way to cause a large reduction of daily food intake is to infuse nutrients, such as glucose, amino acids, or lipids, directly into the major veins. These infused nutrients, which bypass the gut, can reduce daily food intake by 50–100% of the calories infused. These results, which have been found in all studies, show that the presence of nutrients in the blood and/or their metabolism or storage in tissues is the major controller of daily food intake. Although infused nutrients appear to be the major regulators of daily intake, it is not yet known how or where their presence in the blood or body is sensed. Several investigators believe that metabolic activity controls food intake because the injection of blockers of both glucose and lipid metabolism causes dose-dependent increases in food intake. However, it is possible that these metabolic blockers activate an escape pathway that provides absorbed food to resolve difficulties in metabolism and that the underlying metabolic activities are not part of the normal mechanism that controls food intake.

Another possible source of signals that inhibit food intake is the storage tissues. Most of the research has focused on possible signals from body fat. The surgical removal of some of the fat pads from rats leads to an eventual return to normal fat pad size but does not cause a change in food intake except under special conditions. Recent work on the obese mouse (*ob/ob*) has shown that there is a protein, called leptin, that is present only in adipose tissue and that is released into the bloodstream. Injection of the ob protein into *ob/ob* mice inhibits food intake, increases metabolism, and reduces body weight, but it has no effect in *db/db* mice, which are known to lack a functional ob protein receptor. The ob protein provides a new and interesting way in which energy balance and body weight may be regulated. However, the ready availability of food in developed countries, the increased fat content in the diet, and the reduced amount of exercise also contribute to the development of obesity.

II. INTERNAL SIGNALS CONTROL FOOD INTAKE

The amount of food eaten is an essential component of the control of body weight. Food provides the chemical energy that is required for metabolism and for the storage of nutrients for later use. If the amount of ingested food is inadequate for the body's needs, the animal will burn its endogenous stores of fat and protein and will lose weight. If food is eaten in excess of needs, some of that food will be stored in fat, muscle, and liver for later use. Thus, the proper control of food intake is essential for maintaining a healthy body composition and avoiding obesity.

There is little doubt that daily food intake is controlled by internal signals. If rats are force-fed for a period of time until they become obese, the rats will reduce their food intake, when allowed to do so, and will bring their body weight back down to normal levels (1). Conversely, when the rats' food intake is restricted for a period of time so that they lose weight and become thin, they will increase their food intake, when they are allowed to do so, and will again bring their body weight up to normal levels. Although this study clearly shows that there are internal mechanisms that adjust daily food intake following changes in body weight, it does not show how the task is accomplished. During force feeding and starvation there are changes in the degree of stimulation of the gastrointestinal tract, in the internal metabolic pathways of the liver and other organs, and in the storage of nutrient in muscle and fat. When force feeding or starvation stops, any or all of these changes could be responsible for generating an internal signal that brings cumulative food intake and body weight back to normal levels.

Since food intake is a behavior, it must be mediated by the brain. Although many regions of the brain are involved in the control of daily intake, several important studies have shown that two major regions, the ventromedial hypothalamus and the lateral hypothalamus, are critically involved in the control of daily food intake and body weight (2). If lesions are made in the ventromedial hypothalamus or in the paraventricular nucleus, an animal will begin to eat soon after coming out of the anesthesia, will gorge itself for several hours, and will continue overeating for weeks or months until a new level of body weight has been achieved. Thereafter, food intake is stabilized and the new level of body weight will be defended (3). As with normal rats, if these lesioned, obese rats are overfed and forced to reach a new level of body weight, they will voluntarily reduce their daily food intake and bring body weight back to their previous obese levels (see Fig. 1). If they are starved, they will subsequently increase their food intake until they again reach their previous level of obesity. These obese rats are no longer as accurate in their control of food intake: they become finicky; that is, they respond to improved food quality by overeating and to food adulteration by undereating. Thus, they are more likely to change their body weight in response to changes in the characteristics of their diet than are normal rats. They are also less willing to work for food: if they are required to press a lever several times to get access to food, they will eat less and lose some of their body weight.

Lesions to the lateral hypothalamus cause animals to eat less and lose weight. If the lesions are large, the rats have to be nursed back to health by feeding or intubing liquid diets (4). If the lesions are relatively small, the rats reduce their food intake for a period of time until they have arrived at a lower body weight, and then, they eat to maintain that weight. Lesions that limit or inhibit food intake are difficult to interpret since the absence of a behavior can have several causes. The lesion may have damaged a regulatory center and reset body weight at a new lower level. Alternatively, the lesion may have destroyed the motor capabilities that underlie feeding or a sensory quality that made feeding attractive. The possibility that a motor or sensory deficit may result from a lesion can be explored by depriving the rat of food and lowering its body weight before the lesion is performed (5; see Fig. 2). Rats that are starved before the lesion increase their food intake after the brain surgery, showing that the lesion did not affect the ability to eat or the attractiveness of food. These deprived rats ate more than normal after the surgery

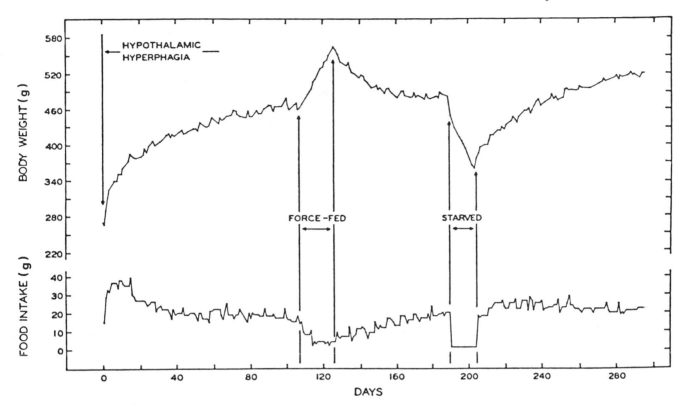

Figure 1 Body weight and food intake of rats given ventromedial hypothalamic lesions, allowed to reach a new level of body weight, and then force-fed or starved. After being force-fed or starved, the rats alter their food intake and bring their body weight back to their new obese level. (From Ref. 3, reprinted with permission.)

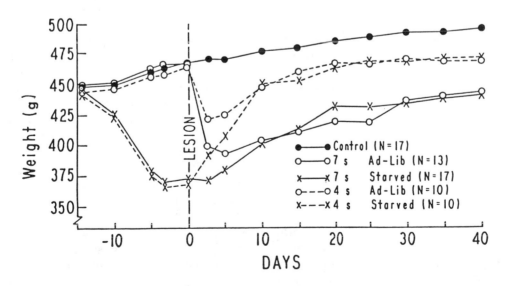

Figure 2 Body weight of rats that were free-fed or starved before being given two different sizes of lesions in the lateral hypothalamus. The rats reach a level of body weight related to the size of the lesion and the starved rats increase their food intake after the lesion. (From Ref. 5, reprinted with permission.)

and stabilized their body weight at the same lower level as nondeprived rats that have had the same sized lesion. These studies demonstrate that the lesion acts by changing the set point for body weight. The combination of the results from VMH and LH lesions shows that there are regions of the brain that respond to internal signals in a way that controls daily food intake. Again, the relationship of these brain regions to peripheral signals generated in the gut, through metabolism, or in storage organs has not been clarified by these studies. The overfeeding or underfeeding of the rats has affected all of the body's organs and all of the processes involved in digesting, absorbing, transporting, metabolizing, and storing food.

Internal regulation of food intake is also demonstrated in nature (6). Rodents that hibernate gain weight during the summer and autumn and then gradually lose weight during the winter as their body temperature drops to just above freezing. Bears also gain weight in the autumn and then retire to their dens where they lower body temperature by a few degrees and slowly lose weight. Birds gain weight twice a year before their annual migrations and arrive at their destinations with little body fat. Deer and walruses gain weight before mating season and then make no effort to eat and lose weight throughout their courtship period. Some birds and mammals reduce their intake during periods when they are incubating eggs or looking after young. Thus, the signals that control daily intake and the deposition of fat are under internal control and vary with external conditions. However, none of these natural experiments demonstrate which internal changes are involved in causing the readily observed changes in food intake and body weight. These internal signals have been shown to be regulatory because birds incubating eggs eat very little of the food that is readily available and they continue to lose weight until the season is at an end (7).

Other types of external challenges have been shown to cause large changes in daily food intake to prevent loss of body weight. When there is a large need for calories, daily food intake can be doubled. Lactating mammals more than double their food intake to provide milk for their young (8). Rats exposed to the cold show large increases in food intake to provide the heat needed to maintain body temperature (9,10).

Internal regulation of food intake can also be demonstrated in pairs of parabiotic rats in which a 30-cm segment of one rat's upper small intestine is disconnected from its own digestive tract and sewn into the intestine of its partner (see Fig. 3). This surgery requires three transections of the small intestines in two rats, but none of the major nerves or blood vessels are cut. As a result of this surgery, one rat in the pair continually loses some of its ingested food into the crossed intestinal segment and

into the bloodstream of its partner. The partner, on the other hand, has its digestive tract shortened by connecting its upper duodenum to its lower jejunum. All of the food eaten by the partner is retained in its own gut and is absorbed into its own bloodstream. One consequence of this surgery is that the rat that loses food into its partner's small intestine and bloodstream exhibits a large (50%) increase in daily food intake, while its partner reduces its daily food intake by about the same amount (11; see Fig. 4). The pair as a whole continues to eat the same total quantity of food and to gain weight at the same rate as controls. The three-fold difference in daily food intake between the two rats in a crossed-intestines pair is sustained for the rest of these animal's lives. This study clearly shows that daily food intake is internally regulated. The rats show large and sustained changes in daily food intake due to a relatively minor surgery. The surgery involves only three transections and reconnections of the small intestines, which in themselves would not cause a sustained change in food intake (12). The altered feeding results from the rerouting of food through the gut and the altered stimulation of the rats' internal organs.

III.   TYPES OF INTERNAL SIGNALS

The most convenient way to describe the possible internal signals that are involved in the control of food intake is to trace the route that the food moves through the body from the moment when it first touches the tongue until it is reduced through metabolism to the waste products of water and carbon dioxide or is stored in tissues for later use. When an animal becomes hungry, it begins to search for food and often uses strategies that minimize its cost in obtaining the food (13,14). Once food is encountered, it is explored through smell and taste. Once identified, the sensory qualities of the food can be compared to previous experiences and an estimate can be made of its satiating properties (15). If the food is found to be acceptable, it is ingested and comes into contact with the mucosa of the tongue where it stimulates taste receptors. At the same time, volatile substances in the food excite odor receptors in the nose. When the food is swallowed, it passes from the mouth through the throat and esophagus into the stomach and can stimulate various stretch and chemoreceptors in these organs. These neural messages may provide part of a short-term signal for the control of intake during a meal. Some of the food in the stomach passes rapidly as a small bolus into the upper small intestine (16). The presence of food in the intestine inhibits and controls stomach emptying (16,17). Within a few minutes after the beginning of a meal, glucose derived from labo-

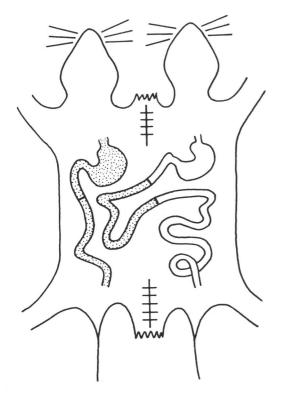

Figure 3 Diagram of a one-way crossed-intestines rat. The stippled gut belongs to the rat on the left. The right rat is continually losing food into the intestine and bloodstream of its partner. No major nerves or blood vessels are cut. (From Ref. 11, reprinted with permission.)

ratory chow is absorbed from the gut and is present in the bloodstream (18, see Fig. 5). This leads to a shift in the release of gut hormones and, once the important pancreatic hormone, insulin, has been released (19), to the transport of some of the absorbed nutrient into tissues. Since most of these changes occur within the first few minutes after feeding and since animals usually require 5–30 min to complete a meal, a large number of internal changes provide possible short-term satiety signals. Our major task is to determine which of these signals are involved in causing the termination of a meal. After a meal ends, the ingested nutrients are transferred slowly from the gut to the bloodstream and, then, to the tissues where they enter various metabolic pathways and provide energy for the cells. Changes in the rate of nutrient transfer may provide signals that terminate one meal or initiate another and may control the subsequent meal patterns throughout the day. Excess nutrients are stored mainly in liver, muscle, and fat and these tissues may provide possible long-term signals that control daily food intake and energy balance.

In short, there are three main types of internal signals that may be involved in the control of food intake. Signals will arise quickly from the gastrointestinal tract due to the stimulation of the mucosa with food and the absorption of nutrients across the gastrointestinal wall. These signals could be involved in the termination of a single meal. Both short-term and medium-term signals can arise from the presence of absorbed nutrients in the bloodstream and their deposition into tissues where they can be used for metabolism or for storage of excess food. Long-term signals that are involved in controlling food intake over several days are more likely to arise from shifts in metabolism and from the storage organs. The relative importance of all of these types of signals for the control of meal and daily food intake is still in considerable dispute. There are a wide range of theories with some supporting evidence for each possibility, but there are few definitive explanations for the underlying control mechanisms.

A. Signals Arising in the Gastrointestinal Tract—Taste and Smell

The nose and mouth are the first organs to come into contact with food. The neural messages generated by the smell and taste of food are sent to the olfactory bulb or to the brainstem and are relayed up to higher centers of the brain. Taste and smell are usually thought to provide chemical messages for the decision about whether and how much to ingest, but they can become rewards in themselves and lead to overeating and obesity. While stimuli from the gut and from other internal organs may be involved in the control of feeding behavior, there is definitely a cognitive component. Animals need to decide when and where to feed and to remember past encounters with food. The particular flavors and textures can then be used to guide feeding behavior. Collier and his collaborators have been the major contributors to laboratory studies that examine the decisions that are made about the cost requirements of finding food and ingesting it. They have shown that increasing the cost of obtaining food by increasing the number of lever presses needed to gain access to a food source leads to a decision to reduce the number of meals each day (20; see Fig. 6). While meal number goes down, the size of the average meal increases so that total daily food intake is held fairly constant (20,21). If the tasks become very complex or require too much effort, the animal may choose to eat somewhat less than its normal daily portion and, thereby, trade off the amount of effort in obtaining food against its level of body weight. Daily food intake may decrease to 80–90% of its previous level. Collier has argued that there is too much emphasis upon a depletion-repletion model of the control

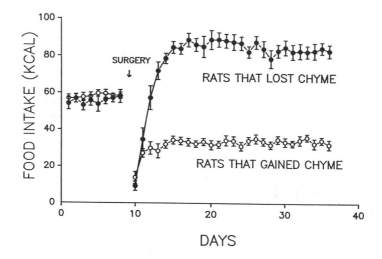

Figure 4 Daily food intake of one-way crossed-intestines rats. The surgery was done on day 9. The rat on the right in Figure 3 that lost food or chyme into the partner's crossed intestinal segment showed a large increase in daily food intake while its partner reduced its daily intake. These large changes in daily food intake are sustained for the rest of the animals' lives.

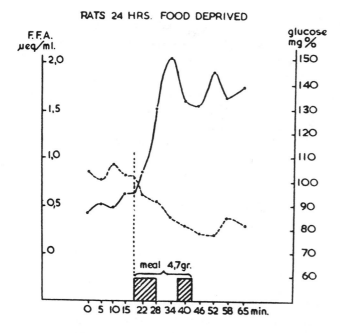

Figure 5 Changes in plasma glucose and free fatty acid levels occur within minutes of the initiation of a laboratory chow meal in 24-hr-food-deprived rats. These changes begin well before the meal has come to an end. (From Ref. 18, reprinted with permission.)

of food intake (22). He notes that changes in external requirements cause large changes in meal patterns, but not in daily intake. He questions whether there are fixed internal signals controlling meal intake and believes that the choice of meal size has a large cognitive component. The counter-argument is that a hungry animal with free access to food will eat more food when it is removed at the same time from the esophagus, stomach, or intestine (11,23). Some internal signals from the gastrointestinal tract or elsewhere in the body must be involved in terminating a meal. Thus, the amount eaten may depend on cognitive estimates of the food's caloric value and availability as well as on tentative signals generated in the gastrointestinal tract or beyond. The cognitive component would be influenced by subsequent confirming or disconfirming signals generated by the metabolism and storage of postabsorptive nutrients.

B. Esophageal and Gastric Fistuli

Once a decision has been made to swallow food, it passes down through the throat and esophagus to the stomach. The early physiologists Bernard and Pavlov did experiments using an esophageal fistula that allowed food that was eaten to pass out of the body before it could reach the stomach. They were trying to determine whether internal signals led to the termination of feeding behavior. They discovered that dogs and horses with esophageal fistuli greatly overate (24). These experiments have been replicated in more recent times and have been given clearer definition. Hull et al. (25) did an experiment on a

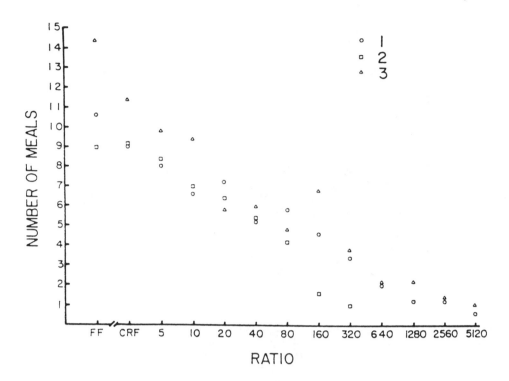

Figure 6 Number of daily meals taken by each of three rats (1, 2, 3) when they are free-feeding (FF) or when they have to press one (CRF) or more times to gain access to food. As the lever-pressing requirement increases, the rats take fewer but larger meals. They maintain their normal level of daily food intake until they reach the highest levels of bar pressing, when they reduce daily intake a little. (From Ref. 20, reprinted with permission.)

single dog and showed that on the first and second sham-feeding session, the dog greatly overate. Their 10-kg dog ate nearly its body weight in food before pausing for 5 min. This group also showed that the dog was gradually able to realize that it was sham feeding during the experimental test and, by the eighth day, the dog refused to eat in the experimental cage. However, when returned to its home cage and offered food, the dog sham-fed, showing that there was a cognitive component in the dog's previous cessation of sham-feeding behavior. This result of excessive feeding after an esophageal fistuli was confirmed by Janowitz and Grossman, who found that dogs sham-fed 4–5 times their normal intake (26).

The sham-feeding paradigm has also been demonstrated in rats. Mook created an esophageal fistula in rats and fed them glucose, sucrose, and saline solutions (27). He found that when the nutrients were prevented from reaching the stomach, intake was greatly increased in a 1-hr test. In addition, the rats showed a preference for higher concentrations of the ingested solution. After creating a gastric fistula in rats, Smith et al. (28) found that the rats continued feeding for more than 2 hr. A rat with a gastric fistula will eat at a normal rate for 15–20 min, but will continue to feed over the next 100 min at a rate that is about half its previous rate (see Fig. 7). The fact that the well-trained rat continues to feed suggests that distension or chemical cues arising in the stomach, in the small intestine, or beyond are important for the inhibition of intake during a single meal. The decrease in the rate of food intake after 20 min shows that mucosal stimulation inhibits the rat's avidity for food or that the animal tires of the motor movements involved in feeding.

There are advantages and disadvantages of the use of either esophageal or gastric fistuli. With an esophageal fistula, the esophagus is transected, usually in the neck, and both ends of the esophagus are externalized or, alternatively, the end leading to the stomach is closed and a gastric tube is inserted. Thus, the food eaten by the animal as well as its salivary secretions pass entirely out of the animal and do not reach the stomach or intestine. Sufficient food and water can be given to the animal by putting the food into the externalized lower esophagus or through the gastric tube. The major advantage of the esophageal fistula is that one can be certain that only the mucosa of the mouth, throat, and upper esophagus is stimulated by food: none of the food can stimulate the wall of the stom-

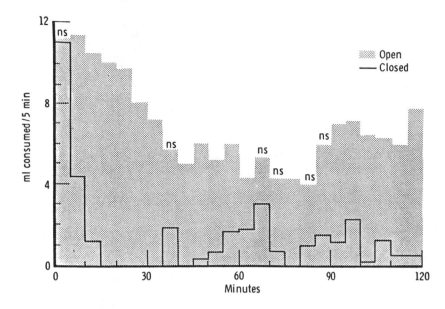

Figure 7 Food intake of rats that have a gastric fistula that is either open or closed. When the fistula is closed, a 17-hr-deprived rat will complete its meal in 15 min and then take a few small meals in the next 2 hr. When the fistula is open and the food drains out of the body, the rat will continue to feed throughout the 2-hr period. (From Ref. 28, reprinted with permission.)

ach or pass into the intestine and be digested and absorbed. The main drawbacks of the esophageal fistula preparation are that the feeding procedure is often quite messy, the animal must be fed by tube, and the fluid and electrolyte content of the saliva must be appropriately replaced. If replacement is inadequate, then subsequent intake may be affected by deficits that the animal can not correct for itself. The gastric fistula does not suffer from these difficulties because most of the time the fistula is closed and food moves through the digestive tract in its normal fashion. Only at the time of the experiment is the fistula opened, the stomach flushed, and the experiment begun. If the animal is fed a liquid diet, most of the food will drain out of the gastric cannula, preventing the distension of the stomach and the associated neural or hormonal signals. However, two studies have shown that some of the nutrient ingested is emptied through the pylorus into the intestine and is absorbed into the bloodstream (29,30). Thus, the weakness of the gastric fistula is that the stomach and the rest of the gut will receive some stimulation of the mucosa by food, which makes the results more difficult to interpret. Of course, the bulk of the food has been lost through the fistula and the intensity of downstream signals is greatly reduced. The use of both the esophageal and the gastric fistula leads to considerable overfeeding, called sham feeding. The sham-feeding animal receives taste stimuli but little or no postingestive

stimuli. Sham feeding will continue well beyond the usual time when feeding ceases in an intact animal.

All of the experiments agree that signals arising from stimulation of the mucosal lining of the mouth, throat, and esophagus with food are not enough to stop feeding behavior. Some additional signals must arise at the level of the stomach or the small intestine to inhibit intake during a single meal. These results are entirely consistent with the results from the crossed-intestines rats mentioned above (11). After the intestinal surgery (see Fig. 3), these rats exhibit a threefold difference in daily food intake. Since all of the food necessarily passes through the mouth, throat, and esophagus, these upper-gut organs are stimulated 3 times as much in one rat as in its partner. If stimulation of these organs were the main signals controlling daily food intake, then the large differences in food intake would not have been seen in these rats. The large, long-term differences in food intake of these crossed-intestines rats show that these mucosal signals play only a minor regulatory role in the control of daily food intake.

C. Signals Arising in the Stomach

The stomach has been thought to be a storage site for food and an inhibitor of food intake since the ancient Greeks understood the anatomy of the gastrointestinal tract (31). In humans and large animals, the bulk of the meal eaten over a relatively short period of time remains in the stomach for more than an hour. After a short period of adjustment following a meal, the rate of gastric emptying becomes steady and a fixed number of calories is delivered to the small intestine per unit time (16,32,33). Because the bulk of the ingested food stays in the stomach after a meal, gastric distension is one obvious mechanism for the short-term inhibition of food intake. An assessment of the total amount of food eaten during a meal would appear to depend to a large extent on two types of signals: (1) the degree of distension of the stomach and (2) the activation of chemoreceptors in the gastric or intestinal wall.

Distension cannot be the only signal involved in the regulation of food intake. Animals will increase their food intake when nonnutritive diluents are added to the diet. Adolph found that rats will adjust their food intake to compensate when the amount of dilution was not too large (34). At higher concentrations of diluents, the rats compromised by reducing intake. Janowitz and Grossman showed a less complete and gradual adjustment to the addition of diluents in the food of dogs and cats (35). A recent study using a liquid fiber that gels in the stomach found diminished reports of hunger in human subjects, but food intake was only slightly reduced and then only after a delay of several hours (36). Thus, gastric distension by itself, without activation of chemoreceptors, is not a major regulator of food intake. Determination of the nutritive characteristics of the food is also essential.

Davis and Campbell (23) did studies that focused on the role of the stomach in the inhibition of food intake. They placed a tube in the stomach of 4-hr food-deprived rats fed a liquid milk or elemental diet and then withdrew the food during the time when the rats were feeding or at various times after the meal was complete. They found that on the first day of continual withdrawal of diet and sham feeding, the rats nearly doubled their 30-min intake. Some food must have remained in the stomach to allow continued removal of the liquid diet by suction and some may have emptied into the duodenum. On subsequent days, their intake increased even further until the rats ate 4–5 times their usual amount of liquid food in a 30-min period. In a second experiment, the rats ate about 17 ml of an attractive liquid diet, sweetened condensed milk. When 8–10 ml of their stomach contents were withdrawn at 10, 30, or 50 min after the meal, the rats responded by eating a nearly equivalent amount of food, which showed that the rats noticed the withdrawal of food and compensated for it by eating more. There are two difficulties with this experiment. Even though the rats were deprived for only 4 hr, they ate 17 ml of this attractive,

high-energy diet, which should either match or exceed stomach capacity. Perhaps the animals were eating to reach full distension and they were not concerned about the number of calories ingested. Furthermore, some of the ingested food would have moved into the duodenum, making it impossible to conclude that the signals that inhibited food intake arose solely in the stomach. There may have been an added intestinal component. Nevertheless these experiments did point to gastric distension as having an important role in the inhibition of a single meal.

Deutsch et al. (37) extended and clarified these studies through the use of a pyloric cuff, which was intended to prevent the food from leaving the stomach. In addition, they added a gastric tube that could drain stomach contents so that the level of gastric pressure would not exceed the normal level after a meal. They fed 12-hr-deprived rats a milk meal while measuring gastric pressure with a water manometer. The rats drank 13.6 ml with the pyloric cuff open and 11.5 ml with the cuff closed. These values were not significantly different and showed that the rats stopped feeding on the basis of gastric distension and chemoreception and did not appear to require stimulation of the duodenum with food. However, the rats drank to stomach capacity, which was demonstrated in overflow experiments to be about 13.6 ml. Thus, it was not clear whether the intake was regulatory for calories eaten or was inhibited by the limits of gastric distension. In a subsequent study, Deutsch and Gonzalez showed rats could eat smaller meals of a liquid diet without noticing the surreptitious delivery of saline into the stomach (38). This study showed that the calories present in the stomach were sensed by the animal. Deutsch (39) claimed that there were nutrient receptors embedded in the wall of the stomach that would become exposed to the lumenal contents as the gastric volume increased. The combination of gastric distension and the caloric concentration, as determined by exposure to the "nutrient receptors," would provide information to the brain to inhibit feeding behavior. One difficulty with the Deutsch theory is that it pays little attention to the anatomy of the stomach when describing the hypothetical nutrient receptors. Neural receptors are not likely to be present in the lumen of the stomach or in the lumen of the gastric glands or pits. First, the gastric contents are highly corrosive and nerve terminals would be readily destroyed. Moreover, there is a constant turnover of mucosal cells throughout the digestive tract and these rapidly dividing cells migrate continuously along the basement membrane. They would override nerve terminals that might be aimed toward the lumen. Furthermore, there have been no descriptions of nerve terminals beyond the lamina propria, the support tissue for the gastric mucosa. Thus, nerves would be able to sense the presence of food in the gastric lumen only if the food was absorbed into the wall of the stomach. Relatively little nutrient is absorbed through the gastric mucosa (40).

Recently, Kaplan et al. (41,42) have challenged the interpretation of the pyloric cuff experiments. They confirm that rats eat the same amount of food whether a pyloric cuff is open or closed, which is the fundamental observation in previous studies (29,37,43). However, they have shown that during the first meal of a food-deprived rat there is a rapid emptying of the stomach that may be as much as 25–40% of the meal (44). When they measure the amount of nutrient in the stomach after a meal with the cuff either open or closed, they find that the gastric contents were 30% greater in the rat with the cuff closed. They conclude that although the rats with a closed cuff eat the same amount of food as rats with an open cuff, they require a larger gastric distension signal to terminate a meal. In short, they believe that the amount of food in the gastrointestinal tract, not just the amount of food in the stomach, controls food intake.

The role of the stomach in the inhibition of food intake has to be affected by the rate of stomach emptying. As food empties, there is less food in the stomach and less gastric distension. McHugh and Moran have a series of experiments on gastric emptying (45–47). They have found that saline empties rapidly in an exponential way from the stomach. On the other hand, nutrients empty rapidly from the stomach for the first 4–5 min, but, thereafter, the presence of nutrient in the small intestine slows down the emptying rate to a steady state until the meal is gone. A fixed number of calories empty from the stomach per unit time regardless of the composition of the food placed in the stomach (32,45). They argue that the intestine inhibits stomach emptying and that distension of the stomach inhibits food intake. Both stomach and intestinal signals are important.

Although there is general agreement that the stomach provides part of the signal that inhibits food intake during a single meal, we still do not know the nature of the signal or how it is transmitted to the brain. Nerves are the most likely route of transmission. The information about the degree of gastric distension or the presence of nutrients in the gastrointestinal walls could be transmitted to the brain through either nerves or hormones. Paintal (48) and Iggo (49) have shown that there are vagal stretch receptors in the stomach. These nerves increase their discharge rate as a linear function of the degree of gastric distension (see Fig. 8). Deutsch has argued that vagotomy eliminates the satiety signals that results from gastric distension after a very large meal, but that gastric nutrient content of the stomach can still be sensed (50,51). A study in which the

stomach and upper intestine was transplanted from one inbred rat into another suggests that an unidentified gastric hormone may inhibit food intake (52). It is unlikely that changes in intragastric pressure are major determinants of the satiety since the relaxation reflex prevents an increase in pressure beyond a fixed level (53,54). Since there is relatively little absorption of food from the stomach (40), a gastric signal is unlikely to be an absorbed nutrient.

There are at least two limitations to a gastric theory of the control of food intake. It is well known that most animals have a circadian rhythm of food intake with meals occurring at times that are appropriate for the animals' nocturnal or diurnal orientation. Rats eat heavily during the early dark phase (55). As implied above, if food empties from the stomach at a fixed caloric rate, then intense eating during the early part of the dark phase should greatly distend the stomach. New meals would have to be initiated while the stomach remains relatively full. Toward the end of the dark phase and throughout the light phase, the rat eats little. At the later part of the light phase, the stomach should be relatively empty, but few meals are initiated. Thus, the degree of gastric distension necessary to provide an inhibitory signal for feeding behavior would have to vary throughout the day. Most of the experiments on stomach emptying have been done on deprived rats, dogs, pigs, or monkeys at a fixed time of day. This procedure would tend to show that food intake is inhibited by gastric distension while studies done over 24 hr must show that the degree of gastric distension varies greatly over the day.

Another limitation of a gastric theory can be seen from the results of the one-way crossed-intestines study that has been previously described (see Fig. 3). Following the surgery, one rat in the pair eats three times as much as its partner and this change persists for the rest of the animals' lives. This means that three times the amount of food passes through the stomach of the rat that eats more. If the stretch or nutrient receptors in the mucosa or in the muscular wall of the stomach were sensing the total caloric value of the food passing through the stomach and using this information to control daily food intake, then the food intake of these rats would lose weight while its partner would gain weight. Since daily food intake did change dramatically, the stomach must not have a way of sensing the total amount of food passing through it. However, gastric distension could retain its importance in the control of food intake if there were changes in the rate of stomach emptying in these rats. If, for example, there were a threefold difference in the rate of gastric emptying for the two rats in a pair, then the degree of distension and chemical stimulation of the two rats' stomachs might re-

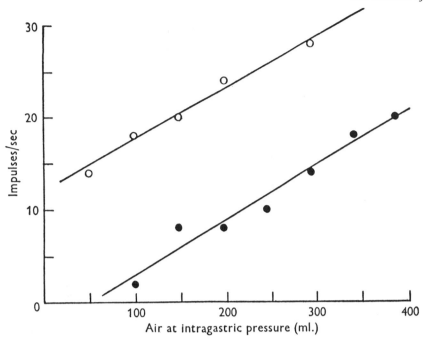

Figure 8 Rate at which single fibers isolated from the vagus nerve of a cat fire as the amount of air in an intragastric balloon is increased to the designated volume. (From Ref. 48, reprinted with permission.)

main the same. Preliminary data suggest that there are large changes in the rate of gastric emptying in these rats and, thus, gastric signals may still be partially responsible for the control of daily intake in these rats.

The results of the crossed-intestines study show that the ultimate control of daily food intake must occur at the level of the small intestine or beyond. It is yet not clear whether intestinal or metabolic signals influence food intake by controlling stomach emptying or by some other response to the absorbed food. Neural or hormonal signals generated in the small intestine may act directly on the brain to inhibit food intake or they may act indirectly on food intake by changing the rate of gastric emptying. Intestinal satiety signals would be generated as the food is absorbed through the mucosa or as absorbed nutrients or released hormones came into contact with the nerves in the wall of the small intestine.

D. Signals Arising in the Intestine

The studies cited above indicate that gastric distension is an important short-term signal that inhibits food intake. However, it is possible that other signals are involved in the termination of a meal. Messages arising in the intestine or in other organs may also be involved in generating satiety signals. Some early studies have shown that the intestine can be a source of signals for the inhibition of

food intake (56,57). These investigators found that the delivery of hyperosmotic nutritive and nonnutritive solutions to the duodenum reduced meal size in the rat. One interpretation of the results of these early infusion experiments is that the intestine is a source of satiety signals during a meal. Another interpretation is that the infusions cause some discomfort or intensify signals in an abnormal way.

Many of the recent studies of intestinal satiety have used the paradigm of the sham-feeding rat. A gastric fistula is implanted into the animal and it is opened during the feeding test. At various times before or after feeding, an infusion of glucose or some other nutrient is made into the duodenum. One rat study found that infusing 2.25 kcal of an elemental liquid diet over 6 min into the duodenum reduced sham feeding most effectively when the infusion began 12 min after the rat began eating (58). This delay may correspond to the time when a rat normally begins to end a feeding bout. Oddly enough, the same infusion of the diet 6–12 min into the duodenum before the rat began sham feeding had no effect on its feeding behavior. This result suggests that the intestinal signal is quite transient and that oral and intestinal signals must occur at the same time for feeding to be inhibited.

Most of the intestinal satiety studies have been done in rats and monkeys. In one rat study, Liebling et al infused a liquid diet with a caloric value of .375 kcal/ml directly into the duodenum. They found a small reduction in sham feeding when 3 ml was infused over 3 min and a larger reduction when 6 ml was infused over 6 min (59). This rate of infusion exceeds the normal rate of delivery (see below). In a similar study in rhesus monkeys, 20, 40, and 60 ml of a liquid diet containing 1 kcal/ml was delivered into the duodenum at a rate of 5 or 7.5 ml/min (60). The 20-ml infusion produced a small, significant inhibition of sham feeding, which increased with increasing dose. In most of these sham-feeding studies, feeding continues throughout the test period in part because gastric distension is not available as a signal to inhibit food intake.

Most of these studies suggest that there is an intestinal signal that inhibits food intake. Such a satiety signal could be transmitted to the brain through the peripheral nerves. Several investigators have recorded from the vagus and from mesenteric nerves. They have found that there is an increased firing rate when glucose or amino acids are placed in the lumen of the intestine (61–64). Other studies have shown that vagotomy prevents the reduced food intake caused by intestinal infusions (57,65). In recent years, Yox et al. have continued the exploration of the way in which intestinal satiety is communicated to the brain. The infusion of 10 cc of maltose or oleic acid at a rate of 0.13 kcal/min reduced food intake while octanoic acid and casein hydrolysate had minimal effects. The effects of maltose and oleic acid on sham feeding can be blocked by capsaicin treatment or by vagotomy (66,67), which again shows that the intestinal signal travels through the vagal afferents to diminish food intake.

In a very interesting study, McHugh and Moran (68) allowed monkeys to drink 150 ml of a 1 kcal/ml glucose solution and found that 21.6 ml passed into the duodenum in 5 min. Then, they infused the 21.6 ml into the intestine of fasted monkeys over 3–5 min and observed their feeding behavior for the next 4 hr. The monkeys with glucose infused directly into their intestine showed a substantially reduced food intake during the first hour compared to monkeys that had delivered the same amount of glucose into their own intestine through normal gastric emptying. Only after 3–4 hr did their food intake return to the same levels as the controls. Thus, the delivery of an appropriate amount of glucose directly into the intestine, but in a less than physiological way, caused a large suppression of food intake. The authors conclude that an intestinal infusion, without the stimuli associated with the taste and swallowing of food and without gastric distension, may have reduced food intake in an abnormal way. They question whether the infusion of nutrients into the intestine produces a normal satiety. If the delivery of food to the intestine makes the animal feel discomfort or malaise, then the reduction of food intake cannot be accu-

rately ascribed to internal mechanisms that normally produce satiety.

What would be a physiological mode and rate of delivery of food into the small intestine? It is obvious that food normally arrives in the intestine after it has been mixed with saliva and processed in the stomach by acid and digestive enzymes. The release of food from the stomach is periodic and results from a pressure differential between the gastric antrum and the duodenal bulb (54). Small spurts of food are delivered into the upper duodenum at the end of the gastric contractions. This food is, then, distributed along the upper small intestine by repeated constrictions of the intestinal circular muscle, which mixes the chyme rapidly with bicarbonate and digestive enzymes secreted from the pancreas and with bile secreted from the liver and gall bladder. Thus, under normal physiological conditions, the food is already partially processed before it reaches the duodenum and, then, it is immediately mixed with intestinal contents. The food must arrive at the duodenal bulb in a predigested state for delivery to be considered normal. Complex foods, such as plant or animal tissues, would be most changed by the digestive process while simplified foods, such as pure sugar or amino acid solutions, would change little. These later, simple foods are most often used in experiments but they rarely occur in nature and are even limited in the kitchen cupboard. Most importantly, the food must be delivered at a rate that is within the normal physiological range. That rate can be estimated by examining the total food intake of a rat or any other animal during a 24-hr period. Adult rats eat between 60 and 100 kcal/day depending on the strain and the physical conditions of the experiment. If this amount of food were delivered to the duodenum at a constant rate throughout the day then 0.04–0.07 kcal would arrive per minute. Since rats eat more heavily in the dark phase, the delivery of food might increase during the night. If the stomach-emptying rate were to double, then 0.14 kcal could be delivered per minute, or only 1.4 kcal during the 10 min that it normally takes a rat to feed. Deliveries of liquid food to the small intestine at a much higher rate are common in the feeding-behavior literature.

An important test of the value of an experiment is whether the delivery of food to the intestine has approximated physiological conditions. Many studies in the literature deliver food at a rate that goes beyond normal physiological limits and the infused food has not been processed by the digestive tract. The study that comes closest to using physiological procedures to assess the importance of intestinal satiety has been done with crossed-intestines rats (69). These rats are parabiotic pairs that have a further surgery in which a 30-cm segment of lower duodenum or upper jejunum is isolated from the intestine of each rat in the pair and then sewn into the intestine of its partner (see Fig. 9). After the surgery, the food eaten by each rat in the pair arrives in the rat's own stomach, travels through a 5-cm segment of upper duodenum that includes the common bile and pancreatic duct, and then passes into the 30-cm crossed segment. Thus, the food has been mixed with saliva and gastric secretions before entering the small intestine and then it is mixed with pancreatic and hepatic secretions before it crosses into the intestines of its partner. Some of this food is digested and absorbed in the partner's upper small intestine and then the remaining food passes back into the lower jejunum of the rat that fed and travels down along the rest of the length of that rat's small intestine and lower gut. The surgery is symmetrical, so that each rat loses some of the food that it eats into the upper small intestine of its part-

ner. The short-term experiment is done by feeding one rat in the pair 10 or 30 min before the partner and then measuring the partner's intake after the crossed segment has been stimulated by food. A rat will normally complete its first meal after a 7-hr fast in 6–8 min. The results of several experiments show that the food intake of both rats is not affected by having a delay of 10 or 30 min. The feeding rat does not overeat even though its own lower duodenum and upper jejunum does not come into contact with food. The unfed partner does not reduce its food intake when allowed to eat even though ingested food of the other rat can be definitively shown to be present in the crossed segment and absorbed into the bloodstream within minutes after feeding. Thus, a 30-cm segment of the small intestine does not alter food intake during a meal after a 7-hr fast especially when the food has be processed by the gut in a highly physiological way.

The major limitation of the crossed intestines experiment is that the 30-cm crossed segment is only part of the normal length of the rat's small intestine, which has a total length of 100–110 cm. Of course, the upper third of the small intestine receives the ingested food more rapidly and is a major site for the absorption of nutrient (70). Nevertheless, it could be argued that it is necessary to stimulate a longer length of intestine to show "intestinal satiety." On the other hand, the experiment is exceptional in its physiological delivery of food into this critical upper intestinal segment. The food has been processed through the mouth, stomach, and upper duodenum and has been mixed with digestive enzymes and salivary, gastric, pancreatic, and intestinal secretions. Experiments have shown that the rate of gastric emptying was slightly higher during the first 10 min after a meal in the crossed-intestines rats compared to control parabiotic pairs (69). Thus, the feeding of one rat in the pair should have delivered slightly more food than is normal to the crossed segment of the partner. Still there was no effect on the partner's food intake when measured at 10 or 30 min. Measurements were made of the absorption of radioactive glucose and amino acids that were present in the diet and it was found that at 10 min there was significantly more radiolabel in the bloodstream of the unfed and hungry rat than in the bloodstream of the fed and satiated rat (69). The conclusion from this experiment is that the combined signals arising in the 30-cm crossed-intestinal segment, including neural, hormonal, and metabolic signals, were insufficient to inhibit short-term food intake. Since the upper small intestine is a major site for the absorption of ingested food, these results suggest that the upper intestine may not generate signals that inhibit food intake. If intestinal signals are normally involved in the control of food intake during a meal, then it is also puzzling that a free-feeding

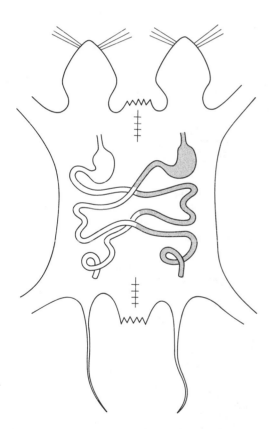

Figure 9 Diagram of two-way crossed-intestines rats. A 30-cm segment of lower duodenum and upper jejunum is isolated from the gastrointestinal (GI) tract of each rat and is connected to the intestine of its partner. The preparation is symmetrical. Each rat loses food into the upper small intestine of its partner and some of that food returns to its own lower jejunum. The stippled GI tract belongs to the rat on the right.

crossed-intestines rat that lacks signals arising in its own 30-cm crossed intestinal segment does not overeat since "satiety" signals are missing in this animal.

The reader might be confused by the seemingly contradictory conclusions drawn between the results from the above study (69; see Fig. 9) and from the one-way crossed-intestines experiment (11; see Fig. 3) in which there was a large change in the daily food intake of both of the parabiotic rats when one rat lost food continually into the crossed segment of its partner. It is important to note that the study described in this section used a symmetrical surgical preparation and was designed to investigate changes in short-term food intake, while the second study (see Fig. 3) was designed to investigate changes in daily food intake due to the continuous loss of calories from one rat to the other. The seeming contradiction about the role of the intestine in the control of short- and long-term intake can be readily investigated in the left rat of the one-way crossed-intestines model (Fig. 3). By feeding the rat on the right 30 min before or after its partner, the rat on the left, which receives nutrients into its 30-cm crossed intestinal segment, can either have its crossed segment stimulated by predigested food when it begins to feed or the intestinal segment can remain empty during feeding. If the signals in the crossed intestinal segment were to inhibit food intake during a meal, then the rat on the left, which has its crossed segment stimulated with food, should eat less while the same rat with an empty crossed segment should eat more. In fact, these rats eat the same amount of food in these two conditions (11). Thus, we can conclude that even in this one-way crossed-intestines preparation where the rats have dramatically changed their daily food intakes, there is no effect of the physiological stimulation of the 30-cm crossed intestinal segment on short-term food intake. Indeed, the two crossed-intestines experiments are consistent in providing data from which one can draw the conclusion that the physiological stimulation of the crossed segment does not alter short-term food intake. An important conclusion from the one-way crossed-intestines experiment is that the short-term and the long-term controls of food intake are clearly different. In the same animals that show large and sustained changes in daily food intake, there is no effect of intestinal stimulation on short-term intake. That is, the same surgery that alters daily food intake in a dramatic way has no effect on short-term food intake after a 7-hr fast. The results from this model show that there are two separate mechanisms for the control of short-term or meal intake and for the control of daily food intake. Although the role of the intestine in the control of short-term food intake is still controversial, the stimulation of the same segment of the small intestine by nutrients with the sub-sequent absorption and metabolism of food has a major effect on the control of daily food intake.

In summary, several experiments have shown that infusion of nutrients into the small intestine can inhibit food intake during a single meal. This inhibition is blocked by vagotomy. When nutrients are infused into the duodenum of rhesus monkeys at the same rate that it is normally released from the stomach, there is an inhibition of food intake that is greater than when the same amount of food is delivered to the intestine by gastric emptying. In addition, when nutrients are delivered to a limited segment of the upper small intestine in a physiological way, there appears to be no effect on short-term food intake. On the other hand, studies that deliver food directly to the intestine usually do so at a nonphysiological rate and in a nonphysiological form. Thus, the presence of a short-term "intestinal satiety" signal during normal feeding has not been adequately demonstrated. The results of the one-way crossed-intestine studies show that there are signals arising at the level of the intestine or resulting from the absorption of food that have no effect on short-term food intake but that do control daily food intake in a very large and significant way. The relative role of the gut in the control of daily intake can be assessed by observing the effect of the infusion of intravenous nutrients that bypass the gut. These studies will be assessed later.

E. The Effect of Gastrointestinal and Pancreatic Hormones on Food Intake

The issue of whether the stomach and small intestine are sources of short-term satiety signals also has direct implications for the role of gastrointestinal hormones in the control of food intake. If an organ generates signals that induce satiety, then its hormones may also provide part of the that signal.

During a normal meal, the ingested food is delivered to the stomach, which allows some food to pass rapidly into the duodenum until intestinal mechanisms inhibit gastric emptying (16). Thus, soon after the beginning of a meal, the mucosal surface of the gut from mouth to mid-ileum has been partially stimulated with nutrients. As previously mentioned, plasma glucose and fatty acid levels change within minutes after the beginning of a meal of laboratory chow (18). Plasma insulin levels also increase rapidly: in part due to cephalic insulin release (71) and in part due to the sustained absorption of glucose and the release of hormones such as GIP and GLI (72). Thus, food has been digested and absorbed and gut hormones have been released long before the end of a meal. This fact leaves the possibility that hormones released by the small intestine during the absorption of food or from the pancreas after nutrients have appeared in the bloodstream could be involved in the termination of a meal.

The gut is the largest endocrine organ in the body (73). After a meal, a large number of gastrointestinal hormones are released, including gastrin, somatostatin, secretin, cholescystokinin, gastric inhibitory polypeptide (GIP), neurotensin, GLI-1, and PYY (74). Any of these hormones, especially those arising in the stomach or upper small intestine, would be considered prime candidates as possible gastrointestinal satiety signals. In addition, pancreatic hormones released by the combination of gut hormones and nutrients may provide additional satiety signals.

The first gut hormones to be examined for a role in the control of food intake during a meal were secretin and cholecystokinin (CCK). Glick et al. (75) injected secretin and CCK separately or together into the peritoneal cavity or into the aorta of rats and found that neither hormone produced a significant reduction of food intake. There was a tendency for the ip injection of CCK to reduce food intake, but the result with multiple tests on six rats was not significant at $p = 0.05$. Koopmans et al. (76) injected cholecystokinin into the peritoneal cavity of mice and found that the mice reduced both their food and water intake, suggesting that their dose of CCK was not specific and may have been causing malaise in the animals. Thereafter, Gibbs et al. (77,78) injected CCK and its octapeptide into the peritoneal cavity of rats and found a dose-dependent reduction of food intake for both forms of CCK. Secretin alone or in conjunction with CCK had no effect on food intake. They injected an intermediate dose of CCK, 20 U/kg ip, and found no effect on water intake. To test the possibility of malaise resulting from the CCK injection, they used a relatively weak test. A one-bottle conditioned aversion paradigm was used with the attractive tastant saccharin paired with the injection of CCK. They found that a high dose of CCK, 40 U/kg, failed to generate a conditioned taste aversion in these rats although lithium chloride, a nauseating poison, was very effective. Deutsch and Hardy (79) challenged these results by doing a more sensitive two-bottle conditioned aversion test with different neutral flavors associated with CCK and vehicle administration. They found that intake of the flavored water associated with the 40 U/kg CCK injection was reduced from 9.4 ml to 3.3 ml for the flavor paired with CCK injection. Thus, at the highest dose, they found a mild conditioned taste aversion, which can be interpreted as due to either malaise or the aversive side of excessive satiety.

The importance of CCK as a satiety signal remains controversial. CCK injected into the peritoneal cavity causes an inhibition of gastric motility and an excitation of duodenal phasic activity (80). A meal usually generates an increase in gastric motility and an inhibition of duodenal activity. Thus, exogenous CCK could be causing unusual gut motility patterns that are communicated by nerves to the brain to inhibit food intake. It is now well established that exogenous CCK requires an intact vagus nerve to cause an inhibition of food intake (81–83). There is also evidence that doses of CCK that inhibit food intake produce plasma levels that are an order of magnitude higher than normal postprandial CCK levels (84). Moreover, iv infusion of a monoclonal antibody to CCK blocked CCK-stimulated pancreatic enzyme secretion, but had no stimulatory effect on food intake (85).

One of the most convincing pieces of evidence that endogenous CCK acts to reduce food intake is that specific CCK antagonists cause an increase in food intake (86–88). Since these antagonists cause an increase in feeding behavior, it is unlikely that the change can be due to some nonspecific cause. There are two known types of CCK receptors: CCK-A receptors, which are present in the pancreas, gall bladder, pyloric sphincter, afferent vagal fibers (89,90) and in specific brain regions, including the area postrema, the nucleus tractus solitarius, and the hypothalamus, and CCK-B receptors, which are distributed widely in the brain and in the stomach (91). Specific blockade of type A receptors, but not of type B receptors, attenuates the inhibition of food intake caused by CCK (92,93). However, these antagonists cross the blood-brain barrier, are distributed throughout the body, and could have their effects either in the periphery or in the brain. Since CCK-A receptors are found in both the brain and the periphery, it is not yet clear where the antagonists act (94). It is possible that CCK-A antagonists act in the brain to increase food intake and not in the periphery.

The ability of the upper-gut peptides gastrin, secretin, and GIP to reduce food intake has been tested using a sham-feeding paradigm on rats with open gastric fistuli (94). It was found that even at relatively high doses, none of these peptides had an inhibitory effect on feeding behavior. However, CCK and CCK octapeptide were effective in inhibiting sham feeding.

Another peptide that has been reported to reduce food intake is bombesin. Its intraperitoneal delivery induced a dose-dependent reduction of food intake (95,96; see Fig. 10). Bombesin is isolated from amphibian skin and has some sequence homology with the mammalian neurotransmitter gastrin-releasing polypeptide (GRP). It normally does not circulate, but its injection into the bloodstream causes the release of several pancreatic and gut hormones (97). Injection of bombesin into the lateral ventricle produced an increase in grooming and resting at a dose below that needed to inhibit food intake. In addition, intraventricular injection was more effective than ip injec-

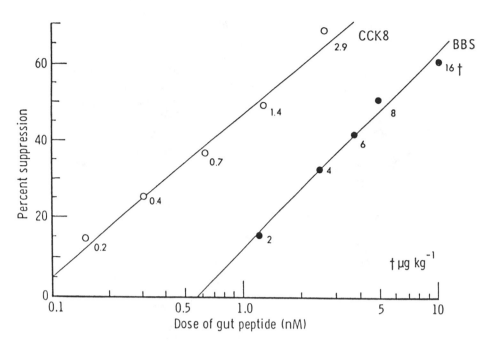

Figure 10   Percent suppression of food intake during the first 15 min of food presentation as increasing amounts of the gut peptides, cholecystokinin octapeptide (CCK8) and bombesin (BBS), are injected into the peritoneal cavity of rats. (From Ref. 96, modified and reprinted with permission.)

tion in inhibiting food intake (98). There is controversy about the way in which bombesin inhibits food intake. One study disconnected all the nerves to the gut by doing a vagotomy and spinal cord transection. They found that complete denervation but not vagotomy alone, inhibited bombesin's effect on food intake (99). However, the rats were 18-hr food-deprived and ate more than normal stomach capacity. This study suggests that bombesin acts peripherally to inhibit food intake. On the other hand, other studies suggest that bombesin may act on the central nervous system. Bombesin-like peptides are present in the paraventricular nucleus, drop during feeding behavior, and rise after the meal is finished (100). In addition, the reduction of food intake induced by peripheral bombesin can be blocked by the intraventricular injection of a bombesin receptor antagonist (101). A bombesin antagonist administered at high doses had no effect on food intake but was able to block bombesin-induced satiety (102). It appears to act independently of CCK.

The pancreatic hormone, glucagon, has long been known to suppress food intake in humans and rodents (103,104). This suppression can be blocked by vagotomy (105) and, more specifically, by hepatic vagotomy (106). The most convincing piece of evidence that glucagon was acting as a satiety agent was that the injection of glucagon antibodies caused an increase in food intake (107,108).

Glucagon reduces food intake when it is infused into the portal vein (104) and is less effective when it is infused into the vena cava (109). All of these results suggest that glucagon acts on the liver to inhibit food intake and that the information about the presence of glucagon is sent to the brain through the hepatic vagal nerve.

Another pancreatic hormone, insulin, has long been thought to be involved in the control of food intake. Insulin rises after a meal and gradually declines as carbohydrate absorption diminishes (19). The "glucostatic" theory originated by Jean Mayer in the 1950s asserted that rats became satiated when there was an arteriovenous (A-V) difference in blood glucose levels indicating the uptake of glucose by peripheral tissues and that they became hungry when the A-V difference disappeared (110). Since insulin is the main hormone that moves glucose out of the bloodstream into cells and, thereby, causes an A-V difference, the theory was essentially an insulin theory of the termination of food intake. Woods and Porte (111) extended this theory to claim that the average plasma insulin level feeds back on the brain to inhibit food intake. Investigators had noted that blood insulin levels tended to increase with increasing obesity, demonstrating the phenomenon of insulin resistance (112,113). Woods and Porte postulated that these elevated blood insulin levels provide a feedback signal that informs the brain about the amount of adipose tissue and, if adipose tissue is excessive, inhibits food intake. One difficulty with this theory is that obese individuals tend to eat more, rather than less, than their lean counterparts (114). The Woods and Porte theory is supported by a number of studies that have shown that insulin delivered intracranially causes a reduction of food intake and a loss of body weight (115,116). However, the critical question is whether peripheral insulin crosses over into the brain to inhibit food intake. It has been shown in dogs that peripheral insulin crosses slowly into the brain and appears in the cerebral spinal fluid (117). Does this insulin alter food intake? There is conflicting evidence. VanderWeele et al. (118) infused 1, 2, and 6 U of insulin in the peritoneal cavity by osmotic minipump into rats and found a small reduction of daily food intake that was not dose-dependent. In diabetic animals that had been allowed to become hyperphagic, increasing doses of insulin reduced daily food intake, but they did not bring food intake back to normal levels (119). In a recent rat study, very low doses of insulin, either 1 or 2 mU, were infused into the hepatic portal vein during each voluntary meal throughout the daylight hours (120). Meal size decreased in a dose-dependent manner while there was no change in the number of meals. Daily intake was not measured. In contrast, Willing et al. (121,122) infused 2–4 U of insulin per day into the vena cava of rats that had been made diabetic just before infusion. The rats' food intake increased with increasing dose until it reached 30–40% above baseline levels (see Fig. 11). During this time, urinary glucose was gradually reduced to zero, showing that the insulin was effective in moving glucose into cells. Overfeeding occurred before glucose had been cleared from the urine and while blood glucose levels were greatly elevated. The same increases in intake were observed whether insulin was infused into the vena cava or into the portal vein. To test whether insulin might cross the blood-brain barrier to affect food intake, Walls and Koopmans (123) continuously infused insulin into the carotid artery leading to the brain. Since blood flow to the brain is less than 3% of cardiac output, blood insulin levels would be greatly elevated while passing through the brain. They found that carotid insulin was no more effective in altering food intake than vena cava insulin, and in both cases, food intake was significantly increased.

When human studies are examined, insulin infusion during a meal either produced no effect or caused an increase in food intake. Woo et al. (124) infused both insulin and glucose to mimic their postprandial levels before the meal began. They found no change in meal size even with substantially elevated insulin levels. Rodin et al. (125) infused insulin while maintaining plasma glucose

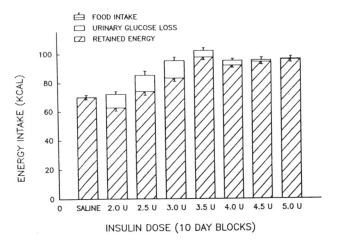

Figure 11 Daily food intake of rats made diabetic after the baseline infusion of saline and, thereafter, infused intravenously with increasing daily doses of insulin. The open bars indicate the amount of glucose lost in the urine of these rats. Daily food intake increases at the lower doses of insulin even though there is an elevated blood glucose and substantial lose of glucose through the urine.

levels. They recorded increased hunger ratings with a high insulin infusion and a substantially increased meal at the end of the infusion. Holt and Miller (126) tested different types of rice meals and found that those meals that allowed rapid absorption of glucose and high plasma insulin levels produced higher hunger ratings and increased food intake at the end of the 2-hr session. In short, human studies have tended to find that insulin increases rather than inhibits food intake.

A third pancreatic hormone, amylin, has recently been shown to inhibit food intake in mice and rats (127,128). Amylin is cosecreted with insulin from the pancreatic beta-cell. It reduces basal and glucose-stimulated insulin secretion (129) and is normally released after a meal. Amylin also decreases food intake when injected intraventricularly (130). Subdiaphragmatic vagotomy does not block its effect (131).

All of these studies show that hormones may play a role in the inhibition of food intake. Another way of testing the role of hormones in the control of food intake is to cross the circulation of two rats in a parabiotic pair. This can be done by connecting the abdominal aorta of each rat with the ascending vena cava of its partner (see Fig. 12). After this surgery, the blood of the two rats is completely mixed every minute (132). The role of blood factors in the control of feeding behavior can be tested by feeding one of the rats in a pair 10 or 30 min before its partner after a 7-hr deprivation. Rats deprived for 7 hr will normally stop eating after 6–8 min based on their own internal satiety signals. The rat fed first will have all of its released hormones and absorbed nutrients diluted into twice its normal amount of blood and removed by twice the amount of tissue. This should lower the plasma levels of all the hormones released by the meal and of all the absorbed nutrients. If these humoral factors are important in the control of meal intake, the rat fed first should eat a larger-than-normal meal to bring these humoral signals up to some specified level. On the other hand, its partner fed 10 or 30 min later will already have elevated hormones and nutrients present in its blood. If these humoral signals are important in the termination of a meal, these rats should eat a smaller meal. The results of this experiment showed that the rats ate the same size meal regardless of whether they ate first and had a low plasma level of hormones or nutrients or ate second when they were already stimulated by these humoral signals. The natural conclusion from this study is that the combination of released hormones and absorbed nutrients is not an important signal in the termination of a meal when these substances flow through the systemic circulation from one rat to the other. Hormones and nutrients may have an effect on food intake by stimulating the liver since all gut hormones released and all water-soluble nutrients absorbed by the intestine must pass through the liver before entering the general circulation. Thus, released hormones could act on the nerves in the wall of the gut or on nerves terminating in the portal vein and liver. However, once these humoral substances pass into the vena cava leading to the heart, they are already being diluted by the blood of the partner arriving into the vena cava. Thus, this study limits the possible signals derived from a meal to neural signals generated in the gastrointestinal tract and the liver. These neural signals may be generated by the local presence of hormones.

The results of the cross-circulation studies do challenge many of the theories that argue that nutrients or hormones present in the blood are involved in the control of meal intake. In fact, the results of the study show that the combination of all hormones normally released after a meal and all of the nutrients absorbed from the gut do not appear to inhibit food intake. Theorists with a different point of view may argue that results from parabiotic rats are not typical of normal, single animals. While it is true that these rats are restrained in their movement by the presence of the partner, the parabiotic surgery is relatively minor and there is no interference with any of the rat's internal organs other than end-to-side connections of grafts to their major blood vessels. No drugs or exogenous hormones have to be given to these animals at the time of testing: there are no concerns about dose, site of action,

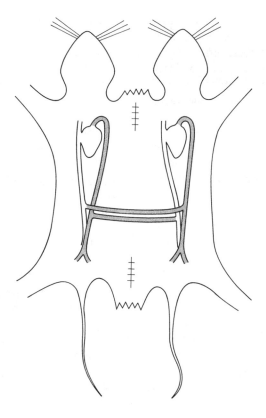

Figure 12 Diagram of conscious rats with continuous cross-circulation of the blood between the two rats. Grafts from other inbred rats are used to connect the descending aorta of one rat to the ascending vena cava of its partner. Thirty percent of cardiac output crosses in each 15 sec circulation time and the blood is completely mixed every minute. The stippled vessels are those that carry only arterial blood.

type of injection, or possible malaise. The only change is that about 30% of their cardiac output flows into their partner during each 15 sec circulation time and, of course, 30% is continuously replaced by blood returning from the partner. In short, the cross-circulated rats are normal parabiotic rats that live for more than a year without special attention. This surgical preparation has the advantage of testing not just the role of one nutrient or hormone at a time, but of testing the role of all of the hormones released from the gut into the bloodstream after a meal and all of the absorbed nutrients simultaneously. Since these hormones are released in a physiological way and the nutrients are absorbed by normal processes, the blood levels should never exceed normal concentrations. Although these rats have some restricted movement, their daily food intake is normal and they do provide an important test of the role of gut hormones and absorbed nutrients on the termination of a meal.

One difficulty in interpreting the cross-circulation study is that these results seem to imply that nerves provide the only signals that inhibit food intake during a single meal. In many ways, an important role for nerves in the termination of a meal is a reasonable hypothesis. The bulk of the food eaten during a meal remains in the stomach and only empties slowly into the intestine. The combination of gastric chemo- and distension receptors would be needed to inform the brain about the amount of food stored in the stomach. Since the stomach of a free-feeding rat is rarely empty, new food eaten can only be recognized by increased gastric distension or some change in the chemical characteristics of the food in the stomach. Thus, the expected internal changes suggest that neural messages are involved in the termination of food intake. On the other hand, there are many studies in which vagotomies have been done with no major long-term effect on food intake. Animals with vagotomies usually lose some weight and have changes in stomach emptying depending on the diet (133,134). However, their food intake does stabilize. If the vagus nerve is not essential for production of a satiety signal and humoral signals play no role in the control of intake, then how does the animal know when to stop feeding? Are the splanchnic nerves essential? Or can the animal shift its attention from one type of signal to another when the internal signals do not produce the expected changes that normally follow feeding?

Very few investigators have attempted a complete gut denervation which requires extensive surgery. There are three reports that claim that all nerves to the gastrointestinal tract have been severed. Grossman et al. (135) did a three-stage operation over several months on dogs that had complete section of the vagus and sympathetic nerves. After recovery, food intake was measured and they found that denervated dogs ate the same size meals as intact dogs. When the dogs were given insulin injections, food intake for both dogs increased by the same amount. Harris et al. (136) followed the same surgical procedure and confirmed that there were no lasting results of nerve section on feeding behavior and found that amphetamine caused a similar decrease in food intake in denervated and intact dogs. Both of these studies showed that the recovered dogs ate normally and that they responded to substances that alter food intake in the same way as normal dogs. However, neither group of experimenters reported a postmortem confirmation that the surgery was complete and that there was no nerve regeneration. More recently, Stuckey et al. (99) performed a two-stage operation on rats doing dorsal rhizotomy and cord section first, allowing the rats to recover for 2–3 weeks, doing some behavioral tests, and, thereafter, doing bilateral vagotomy with another week for recovery. The main objective of this study was to determine how bombesin affected food intake, so no data on meal pattern or daily intake were presented, although the authors state that grossly normal feeding behavior was maintained. It is mentioned that the animals initially lost weight and then maintained it at a reduced level. At postmortem, nerve section was confirmed with the aid of a dissecting microscope, but no functional tests of complete denervation were done. These studies show that it is possible for dogs and rats to feed in a grossly normal way several weeks or months after complete denervation surgery. The surgeries are very difficult and require considerable recovery time.

At present, the conflicting results from the cross-circulation and denervation studies suggest that animals may be able to shift their attention from one signal to another. The cross-circulation studies do not interfere with any of the possible communicating signals within the body because no major nerves are severed and blood flows throughout the bodies of both rats. However, there is about a week of recovery from the time of surgery until the behavioral testing begins. During this time, the rats could learn to ignore changes in blood levels of hormones or nutrients and rely only on intact neural messages to inhibit food intake. In contrast, the denervation studies interfere with one of the major signal systems in the body, but the animals survive and recover after several weeks or months. With major gut denervation, they are able to feed in a fairly normal way. Perhaps during this long adjustment period, they learn to pay attention to mouth and throat signals or to the changes in the blood levels of hormones and nutrients. A possible shift over time to different internal signals seems to be the only way to reconcile the two sets of studies. Further investigation is needed to obtain a clear understanding of the nature of the signals that inhibit food intake after a meal.

F. Signals Arising in the Lower Gut

Jejunoileal bypass surgery has been one of the most successful treatments for causing weight loss in morbidly obese patients. In this surgery, the upper jejunum is connected to the lower ileum so that the food bypasses 80–90% of the length of the small intestine and, as a result, the ingested food is not fully digested and absorbed. Following this surgery, these obese patients lose a substantial amount of weight and manage to keep the weight off (137). The theory behind the surgery was that, by shortening the length of the small intestine, one would reduce the absorptive area of the gut and would prevent the absorption of food. The patients could eat as much as they wanted, but much of the food would pass right through the digestive tract and would fail to be absorbed.

Consequently, patients who were unable to control their food intake would still lose weight. In fact, one consequence of the surgery was that the patients chose to eat less, which contributed to the substantial weight loss (138). This effect has also been observed in rats (139). In fact, the weight loss was largely caused by reduced food intake and not by malabsorption. Part of the reason for this reduction of intake may have been the discomforting lower-gut symptoms. The patients had a lot of diarrhea, bloating, and flatulence and were continually going to the bathroom to eliminate the discomfort. Thus, there may have been aversive conditioning that led to the reduction of food intake.

Another way to test the importance of the lower small intestine in the inhibition of food intake is to move the lower small intestine to the upper regions of the gut without causing any change in the length of the small intestine. In one experiment, a 10- or 20-cm segment of lower ileum was isolated from the lower small intestine and was reconnected to the midduodenum or upper jejunum (140). These rats with ileal transposition showed a decrease in food intake that led to a substantial loss of weight. The ileal transposition surgery was more effective in obese than in lean rats, although the effect was significant in both. These data suggest that overstimulation of the ileum might lead to a reduction of food intake by intensification of lower-gut signals.

The ileal transposition studies showed that malabsorption and its associated discomfort were not essential components of the reduction of food intake that followed jejunoileal bypass (11,140). Increased lower-gut stimulation was sufficient to cause a large reduction of food intake. However, these studies failed to prove that the intensification of ileal signals was reducing food intake through a normal physiological mechanism. It was still possible that the intensified signals were causing a reduction of intake by making the animal uncomfortable, that is, by generating physiological signals that were outside their usual range. One suggestion that the level of stimulation was abnormal was the large number of morphological changes that resulted from the intensified ileal stimulation. There was a 50% increase in the wet weight of the stomach, pancreas and remaining jejunoileum, as well as a fivefold increase of the transposed ileal segment (141,142). These changes in organ size could be interpreted as a hard-wired attempt by the body to reduce ileal stimulation. In a normal rat, similar changes would increase the holding capacity of the stomach, provide more digestive enzymes for the processing of food in the upper small intestine, and increase the absorptive surface of the gut. In addition, ileal stimulation would reduce intestinal transit, leading to less

stimulation of the lower gut (143,144). Reduced food intake could be interpreted as another way in which the organism could prevent food from reaching the lower small intestine (142). However, all of these signals might still be outside the usual physiological range: the intense stimulation of the transposed ileal segment could be making the animal sick. After all, almost all of the ingested food had to pass through this ileal segment before it could be absorbed, which was far from the normal level of stimulation by about 3–5% of the ingested and digestible food. Was there a way to reduce the stimulation of this ileal segment and bring it closer to the normal physiological range?

The degree of the stimulation of the lower gut could be altered by using surgery on another type of parabiotic rat pair. In this surgical preparation, the small intestine of one rat in the pair was transected at the jejunoileal junction, or about halfway down the length of the small intestine. The upper jejunal end of this rat's small intestine was connected end-to-side to the partner's small intestine at the same level (see Fig. 13). The lower ileal end was simply closed so that no more ingested food could enter into its lumen. The result of this surgery was that one rat in the pair (the rat on the right) no longer had its ileum, cecum, and colon stimulated by exogenous food, while its partner had its lower gut doubly stimulated. Instead of a 20–30-fold increase in the amount of ileal stimulation that might be expected in the ileal transposition rats, these rats had their full lower gut either unstimulated or doubly stimulated by chyme that had been appropriately processed for the level of intestinal stimulation (145). Of course, in this preparation, there was also a continual loss of food from the intestine of one rat into the intestine of its partner. The rat that lost food into its partner and that had its lower gut unstimulated increased its daily food intake by 30–40% while its partner that had its lower gut doubly stimulated reduced its own intake by about the same amount. On the surface, this result suggests that food intake is controlled by the lower small intestine, but the results need to be interpreted carefully. Is the change in daily food intake due to the loss of food from one rat to the other or due to the change in lower-gut stimulation? To answer this question, one needs to look at the changes in body weight that occur over an extended period. When the rats were sacrificed 24 days later, it was found that the two rats did not differ significantly in body weight or in the size of their retroperitoneal fat pads. Therefore, the adjustments of daily food intake were appropriate for the amount of food lost from one rat into the intestine of its partner. This result showed that doubling or reducing to nil the exogenous stimulation of the lower gut had no

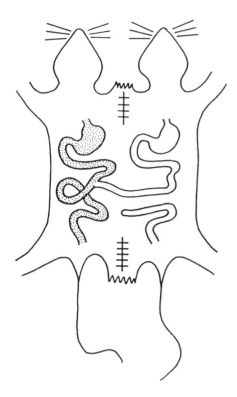

Figure 13 Diagram of rats with doubly stimulated lower guts. The rat on the right has its small intestine transected at the junction between jejunum and ileum. The jejunum is connected end-to-side to the partner's intestine at the jejunoileal junction. The stippled GI tract belongs to the rat on the left. After the surgery, the rat on the left has its lower gut doubly stimulated with chyme while the right rat has no further food enter into its ileum, cecum or colon. (From Ref. 145, reprinted with permission.)

specific effect on the daily food intake of the rats. The changes that were observed could be attributed to the loss of chyme from one rat to the other. The major controller of food intake was the amount of absorbed food and not the stimulation of the lower gut. From these results, one can conclude that the lower gut has no special role in the control of food intake.

G. Signals Arising in the Liver

The liver originates as an outgrowth of gut tissue and plays a significant role in the secretion of bile and the absorption of fat. One of its major functions within the body is the control of the metabolism of glucose, amino acids, and fat. Therefore, the role of the liver in the control of food intake could be seen from the perspective of a gut

organ coming in early contact with food or as a mediator and regulator of metabolism. It is appropriate to review its role in the control of food intake in a section that moves from gut signals to metabolic signals.

The liver is the only organ, other than the gut, that comes into direct contact with a substantial amount of the ingested food. All of the absorbed water-soluble nutrients, including sugars and amino acids, pass through the liver on their way into the general circulation. The liver removes many of these nutrients during the absorptive phase and works to control their levels in the bloodstream. Thus, the liver would be in a position to assess or monitor the total amount of carbohydrate and protein entering from outside, which could be 60–90% of ingested calories. However, the liver does not come into direct contact with all of the absorbed fat since ingested long-chain fat does not enter the portal vein, but instead passes into the intestinal lymphatics, travels through the thoracic duct, and enters the blood at the level of the large veins leading into the heart (146). Thus, the absorbed fat bypasses the liver before it enters the bloodstream. Some of the absorbed fat will go directly to muscle and adipose tissue for use or for storage and would never pass through the liver, making it impossible for the liver to determine the total amount of absorbed fat by direct contact. Of course, the liver could have some indirect way, based on some change in external signals or in the use of a specific metabolic pathway, to evaluate the total amount of external fat entering into the body during the day.

Russek was the first person to propose that the liver was a major organ involved in the regulation of food intake (147). He suggested that hepatic nerves respond to changes in the metabolic activity and the associated membrane hyperpolarization of the hepatocytes. He argued that these changes were communicated to the brain through the hepatic vagus nerve. Niijima has shown that the nerves in the hepatic branches of the vagus decrease their firing rate in an inverse relationship to the glucose concentration in the portal vein (148). Novin and his collaborators infused isotonic glucose into the portal vein of free-feeding rabbits and found that it had little effect on meal intake, but when the glucose was infused into the portal vein in 17-hr-deprived animals, it did reduce food intake over a period of 3 hr (149,150). In contrast, infusion of glucose into the duodenum reduced food intake in free-feeding rabbits but had little effect in deprived rabbits. These data are a little confusing because glucose infused into the duodenum should be very rapidly absorbed into the portal vein and, thus, ought to act in a similar way as direct portal vein infusion. Like portal infusion, duodenal infusion should have reduced the food intake of the deprived rabbits, unless a duodenal signal somehow blocks a later hepatic signal.

The role of the liver in the control of food intake has been more recently investigated by Tordoff and associates. They infused glucose into the portal vein and found that it was more effective than equiosmolar concentrations of NaCl only at the lowest concentration of 0.3 M (151,152). As the dose doubled and quadrupled, the 2-hr food intake of the rats infused with salt continued to decrease, while those infused with glucose remained at the same level (see Fig. 14). In comparison, infusion of the same amount of glucose into the jugular vein had relatively little effect on 2-hr food intake. They also found that the rats with portal glucose infusion had lower plasma glucose levels and increased hepatic glycogen compared to jugularly infused rats. This result is consistent with the fact that the infused portal glucose was altering hepatic metabolism and was being stored as glycogen. One puzzling aspect of these data was that increasing the dose of glucose caused no

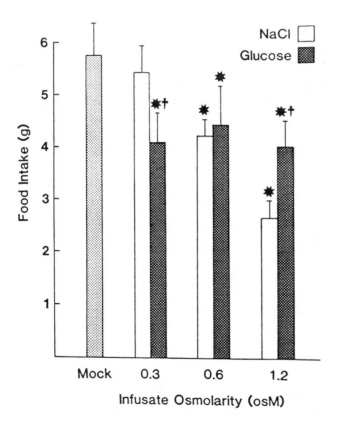

Figure 14 Food intake of rats infused with increasing concentrations of glucose and sodium chloride into the portal vein. *Food intake is significantly different from the control mock infusion. †The two treatments at a single dose differ significantly. There is no dose dependence of glucose infused into the portal vein. (From Ref. 152, reprinted with permission.)

greater reduction of food intake even though the highest dose was the equivalent of 104 kcal/day, or more than a rat would normally eat. The hepatic sensor did not seem to be measuring the amount of water-soluble nutrient passing through the liver during this short time frame. It registered the presence of glucose, but not the amount.

A more recent study has measured daily food intake over a 17-hr period when only 10 or 20 kcal of glucose or amino acids (0.57 or 1.15 kcal/hr) was infused into the portal or the jugular vein. It was found that using these slow infusions of relatively small amounts of glucose produced a significant 5- or 10-kcal reduction of food intake but there was no difference in intake between the portal or vena cava infusions (153). This result suggests that, for integration over the full day, the liver is not the major sensor for the presence of glucose in the blood.

One way to assess the role of the liver in the control of food intake is to allow a substantial amount of water-soluble nutrient to pass through the hepatic sinusoids and see whether it has a direct effect on food intake during a single meal. This objective can be achieved by using the two-way crossed-intestines rat, a symmetrical preparation in which a 30-cm segment of each rat's intestine is connected to the intestine of its partner (see Fig. 9). This preparation was described above, but can be briefly described again. Following this surgery, either rat in the pair has its ingested food move into its own stomach, pass through its upper duodenum, and then travel into the crossed segment of its partner's intestine at a level just below the bile duct (145). Some of each rat's ingested food will be digested in the partner's upper small intestine and absorbed into the partner's bloodstream, and some will continue to travel down the digestive tract back into the gut of the feeding rat. Water-soluble nutrients will be absorbed from the crossed intestinal segment and be delivered to the portal vein of the partner. The effect of these water-soluble nutrients on the hepatic control of food intake can be assessed in these rats by feeding only one rat of a pair after a 7-hr fast. The rat fed first has a lower delivery of absorbed nutrient into its own bloodstream and less stimulation of the liver by food during the 10 min following a meal because its own crossed 30-cm segment of the upper intestine remains unstimulated by food, yet its food intake does not increase, but remains at control levels. The partner rat fed 10 or 30 min later has already had its liver stimulated by the absorbed food, but this rat eats the same amount as its partner's fed earlier or as control rats without their intestines crossed. In fact, when the absorption of glucose-³H or of amino acids-³H was measured in rat pairs where one of the rats was fed the radioactive meal, it was found to be significantly higher at 10 min in the rat that had not yet fed and was hungry than in the feeding partner that had completed its meal and was satiated. These results suggest that the passage of water-soluble nutrients through the liver in a physiologically controlled way does not inhibit food intake during a meal. The liver does not appear to monitor the amount of absorbed nutrient passing through its sinusoids and use this information to alter meal intake.

An alternate way of testing the capacity of the liver to measure the amount of absorbed nutrient passing through its sinusoids and, with this information, alter food intake is to divert the blood coming from the gut into the systemic circulation before it reaches the liver. This can be done by use of a portacaval shunt. In this surgery, the portal vein is clamped and tied just below the liver. The vein is transected on the gut side of the tie and the loose end is connected end-to-side to the ascending vena cava. As a result of this surgery, all of the blood leaving the gut passes directly into the systemic circulation and does not go through the liver on its first pass into the body. The liver is supported only by blood arriving through the hepatic artery, and over the next 10 days it is diminished by 30% in wet weight (154). If the liver were monitoring the total amount of water-soluble nutrient that was entering through the gut and using this information to control food intake, one would predict that the shunted rat would overeat on its first meal after the surgery and would continue to overeat until hepatic signals were adjusted for the reduced caloric load passing through the hepatic artery. In fact, it was found that the shunted rats ate 3.6 ± 0.7 kcal on their first meal compared to 6.2 ± 1.6 kcal for the controls ($p = .18$). These results did not change in subsequent meals. During the first night, the portacaval shunted rats ate an average meal size of 5.1 ± 2.4 kcal while the controls ate 5.5 ± 1.9 kcal ($p = .90$). The shunted rats also ate 7.4 ± 1.7 meals while the controls ate 8.1 ± 2.2 meals ($p = .80$). During the next 8 days of recovery, the shunted rats tended to eat less than controls and they lost somewhat more weight (see Figs. 15 and 16). These results show that the shunted rats ate less food than controls even though their livers were deprived of contact with some of the absorbed nutrient. Some of the absorbed food would pass from gut to muscle or adipose tissue without ever coming into contact with the liver.

An increase in food intake by shunted rats would be predicted by a theory that argues that the liver measures or monitors the total amount of exogenous water-soluble food arriving from the gut and sends a message that controls food intake. To make sure that we were testing rats at their best performance, measurements were also made of meal patterns during the last 6 days of the study when the rat's daily food intake and rate of body weight gain

had stabilized for both the shunted and control rats (154). The rat's first meal after a 7-hr fast was 10.7 ± 1.4 kcal in shunted rats and 10.8 ± 1.2 kcal in controls ($p = .98$). On their average meal over the day, the shunted rats ate 5.1 ± 0.5 kcal while control rats ate 5.9 ± 0.8 kcal ($p = .26$). The number of meals were 15.8 ± 1.6 versus 14.7 ± 1.0, respectively ($p = .70$). Clearly, the food intake of the shunted rats was not larger than and, in fact, was not significantly different from that of controls. This results suggests that the liver does not use information that it may obtain about the amount of absorbed food to control food intake. Russek has argued that the diversion of the blood away from the liver through the use of a portacaval shunt does not change the stimulation of the liver by absorbed food: within one circulation time, he argues, the absorbed nutrients have passed into the hepatic artery and elevated plasma levels (155). However, in shunted rats, a substantial amount of the absorbed nutrient will never pass through the liver. Some portion of the absorbed glucose and amino acids will go directly from the systemic circulation to muscle, fat, and other tissues and will be taken up by these tissues before it can ever reach the liver. Thus, the liver fails to have contact with the full amount of water-soluble nutrient absorbed from the intestine in these portacaval-shunted rats and, therefore, should not be able to assess its total nutrient content.

These last two studies show that the liver does not determine the amount of absorbed nutrient and pass this information to the brain to control food intake. In the first study, there was a physiological delivery of a substantial amount of nutrient from the upper small intestine into the portal vein leading directly to the liver. This delivery over a period of 10, 30, or 60 min did not reduce food intake and, in fact, had no effect on the size of the first meal after a 7-hr fast. In the second study, the diversion of the nutrient-containing portal blood away from the liver did not cause an increase in the first meal after the surgery or in the meals throughout the first day or in the meals taken throughout a 6-day period when daily food intake and body weight gain had stabilized 10 days after the surgery. Thus, both studies show that the liver does not monitor the amount of absorbed food and convey that information to the brain to alter food intake.

Although the liver does not appear to sense the total amount of nutrient absorbed from the gut, it could be involved in relaying information to the brain about metabolic changes taking place in the body, such as the type of nutrient being used for fuel or the fasting-refeeding state, and this information may influence and alter food intake. If the liver were involved in the control of food intake, it would need to send messages to the brain to produce a change. These messages would have to be sent

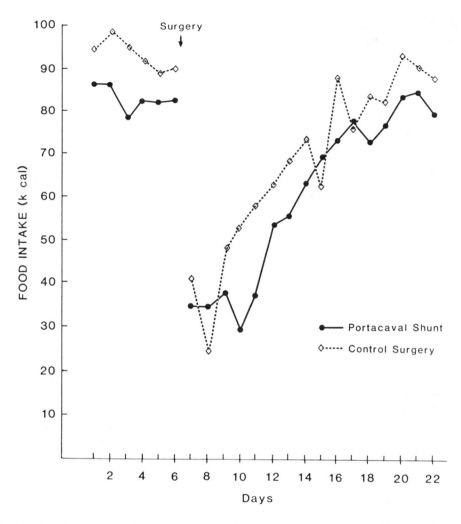

Figure 15 Daily food intake of rats provided with a portacaval shunt or given sham surgery. Measurements of meal patterns were made on the first day after surgery and during the last 6 days when the rats had returned to baseline intake.

by nerves or through the bloodstream. A partial denervation, hepatic vagotomy, has been done in free-feeding rats and produced mixed results. Friedman and Sawchenko (156) found a shift in the day/night rhythm with increased feeding during the day and reduced feeding at night. There was a small change in daily intake but only in male rats. On the other hand, Del Prete and Scharrer (157,158) have shown that hepatic vagotomy caused no change in day/night feeding but the pattern of daytime feeding was altered. These are relatively minor effects of partial denervation of the liver. When a total hepatic denervation is done, the changes in meal pattern completely disappear (159–162). A recent liver transplant study showed a small decrease in daily intake in liver-denervated and transplanted rats, especially in the night (160). Thus,

hepatic denervations appear to have little effect on spontaneous food intake and the hepatic nerves are not much involved in the control of meal patterns. On the other hand, hepatic vagotomies have been shown to affect food intake when it is altered by external treatments, such as infusion of total parenteral nutrition (163) or of glucagon (106). Thus, hepatic nerves may play a role in unusual, external challenges, but they appear not to have much of a role in the normal control of food intake. The other possible way in which the liver could inform the brain about peripheral changes in metabolism is by the release of some humoral factor. The type and quantity of food eaten have an effect on the release of somatomedins or insulin-like growth factors that alter metabolism and enhance growth (164). A specific inhibitor of food intake

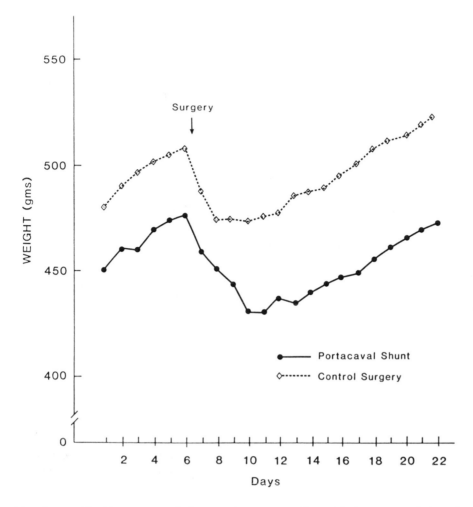

Figure 16 Body weight of rats with either portacaval shunt or sham surgery. Rats with the portacaval shunt lose more weight after surgery but their subsequent weight gain is comparable to that of controls.

secreted from the liver has not been identified, but remains a possibility.

H. Metabolic Signals

Although the liver does not seem to monitor the amount of water-soluble nutrient entering into the bloodstream from the gut, it still responds to changes in the plasma levels of glucose, amino acids, and fats by removing or releasing these nutrients to maintain their blood levels within a well-defined range. That the liver can release glucose in the blood has been known since the days of Claude Bernard. In fact, the liver and various regulatory hormones are very effective in maintaining plasma glucose levels: they are able to substantially limit the surge in plasma glucose that follows a CHO meal and to maintain

plasma glucose levels even under conditions involving extensive exercise when glucose is rapidly being used by the muscles (165). Thus, the liver could acquire some information about the flow of energy through the body without having to monitor the total amount of absorbed nutrient.

It is possible that the liver or some other tissue in the body monitors the plasma levels of the macronutrients and sends this information to the brain to alter food intake. Indeed, there are many theories that claim that plasma nutrient levels are important in the control of food intake. The early version of the "glucostatic" theory stated that elevated plasma levels of glucose inhibit food intake (166). When it was noted that diabetic rats had very high plasma glucose levels and, nevertheless, were hyperphagic, the theory was altered to claim that the use of glucose by the tissues, which produced an arteriovenous

(A-V) difference in plasma glucose, controlled daily food intake (167,168). Because increased levels of plasma insulin are needed to generate an A-V difference in peripheral plasma glucose, the glucostatic theory is closely associated with a theory that insulin inhibits food intake. One argument against the glucostatic theory is that a meal of meat, which contains mostly protein and fat, is highly satiating, suggesting that regulation of glucose transport into cells cannot be the only mechanism involved in control of meal intake. In an alternate approach, the "aminostatic" theory states that increased levels of plasma amino acids are associated with decreased appetite in humans (169). Amino acid levels were found to vary inversely with ratings of hunger. A major argument against the aminostatic theory is that increased protein content of the diet leads to substantially lower levels of plasma amino acids but no major increase in food intake (170,171). Thus, amino acid levels themselves are unlikely to control food intake. The final classic theory, the "lipostatic" theory, states that the amount of body fat controls daily food intake; this will be discussed in greater detail below (172).

One way of testing whether metabolic signals control food intake is to infuse nutrients directly into the bloodstream and to determine whether the infusion reduces daily food intake. Such an infusion bypasses the gut and tests its relevance for the reduction of daily food intake. All relevant studies have shown that the infusion of nutrients into the bloodstream produces a substantial reduction of daily food intake (173–176). These studies show that the presence of these nutrients in the bloodstream or the metabolic consequences of their uptake into the body's tissues generate a signal that feeds back to the brain to inhibit feeding behavior. Each of these nutrients has its own specific effect upon daily food intake (177; see Fig. 17). If 34 kcal of glucose is infused slowly and continuously over a 17-hr feeding period, the rats show a reduction of intake that is equivalent to 55% of the calories infused. When the infusion stops, the rats return in one day to their previous baseline levels of intake. In contrast, infusion of 10 or 20 kcal of an amino acid mixture causes a complete reduction of intake relative to the number of calories infused. Daily food intake is decreased during the first day of infusion and returns within a day to normal at the end of the infusion. Finally, infusion of 20 or 40 kcal of iv lipid provokes a gradual reduction of food intake that stabilizes at a lower level after 4–6 days. The compensation for calories infused averaged only 42% of the calories infused, showing that fat was the least effective in reducing voluntary food intake. When the infusion ceased, daily food intake increased very slowly over several days, showing that the pattern of response to fat infusion was very different from the patterns resulting from

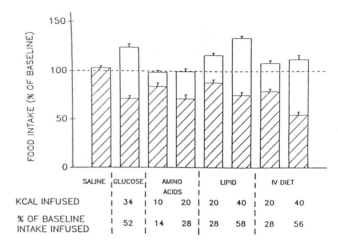

Figure 17 Average daily food and energy intake of rats infused intravenously with saline, glucose, amino acids, lipids, and an iv diet that had the same composition as the oral diet. Slashed bars are the voluntary daily food intake; open bars are the total number of calories infused. The total height of the bar is the total amount of calories ingested and infused. Rats show a 50% compensation for glucose and lipid, nearly complete compensation for amino acids, and 75–80% compensation for the iv diet. (From Ref. 177, reprinted with permission.)

the infusion of water-soluble nutrients. Since the infusion of each of these macronutrients separately might lead to a less-than-complete compensation because of a change in the relative amounts of the macronutrients available to the tissues, we also included an infusion condition in which all of the nutrients were infused in the same proportion as the nutrients in the diet. Infusion of 20 and 40 kcal of iv diet produced reductions of daily food intake that were about 77% of the calories infused. Thus, there was a better adjustment for all three nutrients than for the sum of the nutrients infused separately (177,178). The body was responding partly to the macronutrient composition of the infusate. In addition, the infusion of all three nutrients did not produce full compensation, showing that either signals originating in the gut or signals associated with the circadian pattern of food delivery were important in providing the full signal for the inhibition of food intake.

All of the infusion studies show that the presence of the infused nutrients in the blood or their metabolism and storage in the tissues provides the major signal that controls daily food intake. These infusions of nutrients cause a reduction in food intake without there being a concomitant change in metabolic rate. When glucose is infused into the vena cava, the rats show an immediate reduction of daily food intake, but metabolic rate remains the same (179). There is, of course, a shift in RQ, which reflects the increase in the amount of glucose that is being burned by the tissues. There is also a small increase in metabolic rate on the fourth day of glucose infusion when there has been a sustained increase in carbohydrate calories delivered to the body, but the increase in metabolic rate was only 5% of baseline levels. On the other hand, when fat is infused in the form of an intravenous intralipid, there were gradual changes in food intake but no change in metabolic rate before, during, or after the infusion. Even if infusion of nutrients does not change metabolic rate, it leads to the deposit of excess calories in body fat (180).

Since the infusion of nutrients into the bloodstream is a very effective way of reducing daily food intake, there must be one or several sites within the body where the infused food is translated into a signal that is sent to the brain to alter food intake. One of the most likely sites for the measurement of plasma levels of nutrients would be the brain itself. Several studies have shown that there are neurons in the ventromedial and lateral hypothalamus that are responsive to glucose and amino acids as well as insulin and other hormones (181). These neurons could be assessing the plasma levels of these nutrients and using this information to initiate and control the feeding behavior of the animal.

Another way to assess the effects of nutrients on the control of daily food intake is to draw nutrients that have already been absorbed out of the bloodstream. This can be done with the cross-circulated rats that were described above (see Fig. 12). One rat in a cross-circulated pair can be deprived of food for 4 days while the food intake of its partner is observed. If nutrients are important in the control of daily food intake, the feeding rat that loses half of its ingested food into its partner should increase its daily food intake. We observed that the rats did not significantly change their food intake for 2 days and, thereafter, increased food intake on the 3rd and 4th day by about 30–40%, which was not compensatory for the amount of food lost (132). As a Result, the rats lost weight. When food was again available to both rats, the long-term-feeding rats reduced their intake to baseline levels on the first day. This result suggests that, in cross-circulated rats, a decrease in the blood level of nutrients and the amount of nutrient transferred into tissue is not noticed by the mechanism that controls daily intake for 2 days. This result challenges the hypothesis that metabolism controls daily intake. However, it is in conflict with the results from studies using direct nutrient infusion where water-soluble nutrients reduce daily food intake within the first day of infusion (177,178). It is possible that nutrients are more effective in causing a reduction in food intake than in causing food intake to increase. In any case, the cross-circulation studies show that food absorbed

from the gut has little effect on meal intake and that daily food intake increases only slowly when plasma metabolites are lost into the bloodstream of the partner.

Another way to approach the search for a metabolic signal that controls food intake is to block various metabolic pathways and see whether the blockade causes a change in food intake. Since metabolism is very central to the survival of the organism, one has to be careful to select agents that do not make the animal sick or uncomfortable. Indeed, the most convincing metabolic blockers should cause an increase in food intake, showing that the agent works specifically on feeding behavior and that the animal is healthy enough to respond to the internal stimulus. A series of studies using metabolic blocking agents have suggested that there are metabolic signals that can alter food intake.

The first metabolic blocker that was shown to cause an increase in food intake was 2-deoxy-glucose (2-DG), which is taken up by cells and interferes with glucose utilization (182). 2-DG causes an increase in food intake, activates the sympathoadrenal system, and substantially increases plasma glucose, FFA, epinephrine, and glucagon levels (183–185). Small amounts of 2-DG injected into the brain stimulate food intake (186). There are conflicting data about whether 2-DG acts on the liver to reduce food intake. Some studies claim that hepatic branch vagotomy attenuates the effect of peripherally injected 2-DG (187) while others claim that it enhances the feeding response (188). Still others find no effect of hepatic vagotomy (189,190) or total hepatic denervation (191) on 2-DG-induced feeding.

Another blocker, 2,5-anhydro-d-mannitol (2,5-AM), also interferes with glucose metabolism and increases food intake in a dose-dependent manner (192). 2,5-AM inhibits glycogenolysis and gluconeogenesis (193). It also produces a small decrease in plasma glucose and a significant increase in plasma fatty acids, glycerol, and ketone bodies (194). It is as effective in reducing food intake in diabetic as in normal rats, suggesting that elevated blood glucose and low blood insulin levels are not detrimental to its effect. Low doses of 2,5-AM probably act in the liver. When infused intraportally, it has a faster and larger effect on food intake than when infused intravenously. The effects of small doses of 2,5-AM are eliminated by hepatic vagotomy although higher doses are still effective in increasing food intake. 2,5-AM also affects metabolism: it causes an increase in metabolic rate during the first hour after injection but has no long-lasting effect on whole-body energy expenditure. It does lower RQ with a decrease in carbohydrate metabolism and an increase in fatty acid oxidation (195). 2,5-AM lowers hepatic ATP, which may provide a signal that increases food intake (196).

However, infusion of 100% TPN reduces food intake by 85%, but there are no associated changes in hepatic ATP or ATP to Pi ratio. Thus this ratio does not seem to control food intake during intravenous infusions of nutrients (197). On the 5th day of this study, voluntary daily food intake increases considerably but there are no still changes in hepatic ATP.

There are also a couple of inhibitors of fatty acid metabolism that cause an increase in food intake. Mercaptoacetate (MA) causes an increase in food intake during the day in rats fed a high-fat diet but not a low-fat diet (198). MA impairs mitochondrial beta-oxidation of fatty acids (199) and causes elevation of plasma free fatty acids, no change in plasma glucose, and a reduction of the ketone 3-hydroxybutyrate (198). The effects of mercaptoacetate can be blocked by subdiaphragmatic vagotomy and by destruction of vagal afferents by capsaicin (189), suggesting that the effects of MA are transmitted through the vagus nerve. MA activates the sympathetic nervous system and increases plasma levels of norepinephrine, fatty acids, and glucose (185).

Another fatty acid oxidation inhibitor, methyl palmoxirate (MP), also causes an increase in food intake (200). MP lowers fatty acid oxidation by inhibiting carnitine palmitoyltransferase I, which transports long-chain fatty acids into mitochrondria (201). It elevates plasma free fatty acids and glycerol while lowering ketone bodies (202). MP also interacts with 2-DG, which blocks glucose utilization to cause an increase in food intake at doses that are not effective on their own (see Fig. 18). MP causes an increase in food intake when the rats are fed a high-fat diet rich in long-chain fats but not when they are fed a high-fat diet rich in medium-chain fats (203). Neither MP nor 2-DG alone or together were able to cause an increase in food intake in Syrian hamsters (204).

The fact that these metabolic blockers are effective in increasing food intake does not necessarily imply that the metabolites with which they interfere are normally involved in the control of meal size, meal patterns, or daily food intake. Metabolic blockers do act in a specific way to elevate food intake, but they also put unusual stress on the animal and elevate stress hormones (185). It is possible that these metabolic blockers could be activating an escape pathway that is present only for unusual circumstances when it is necessary to boost plasma metabolite levels. Food intake may be initiated as a last resort whenever metabolites fall to very low levels at a regulating site. After all, when other sources of fuel fail, feeding will provide some nutrient that can be rapidly absorbed (18) and can contribute to maintaining an adequate metabolic rate. However, sudden reductions in the availability of metabolic fuels are not common in animals and most meals

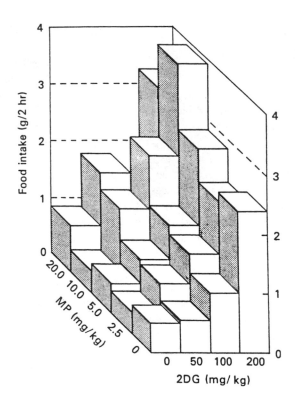

Figure 18 Two-hour food intake of rats injected with the combination of 2-deoxy-d-glucose (2-DG), an antimetabolite for glucose, and methyl palmoxirate (MP), an inhibitor of fatty acid oxidation. The drugs given together have a much larger effect on increasing food intake. (From Ref. 202, reprinted with permission.)

are eaten in a relatively relaxed state without metabolic stress. The increase of food intake provoked by metabolic blockers may provide more of an escape from a severe metabolic deficit than a regular mechanism for the control of food intake.

I. Storage Signals

Early studies by a number of investigators have shown that body weight is regulated. If an animal is force-fed to obesity, it will, when given free access to food, reduce its food intake and return its body weight back toward normal levels (1). In contrast, when an animal is starved or its food intake is restricted, it will slowly lose weight, but when it is given food ad lib again, it will increase its daily food intake and decrease its energy expenditure to bring its body weight back up toward normal levels (205). Since the major change in these animals is the amount of stored fat, several investigators have believed that there is some internal mechanism that measures the amount of body fat and that adjusts food intake and energy expenditure to bring body fat back to its usual level. Unfortunately, these studies only show the presence of internal regulation: they do not show where or how a corrective signal is generated and transmitted. Indeed, as mentioned in the Introduction, the overfeeding or underfeeding of an animal causes changes in the stimulation of the gastrointestinal tract, in the metabolic pathways that are used as well as in the storage of nutrients in tissue. The response to any of these changes could be responsible for bringing food intake and body weight back to normal levels.

The idea that body fat could control food intake was first proposed by Kennedy as a result of his hypothalamic lesion studies. The lipostatic theory states that the amount of body fat controls daily food intake in some way (172). However, the theory does not specify the nature of the signal system that brings body weight back to normal. It could be a metabolite, such as fatty acid or glycerol, or a hormone released by adipose tissue or a chalone, defined as a negative humoral feedback signal controlling tissue size. A number of theorists have tested the role of glycerol by injecting it subcutaneously (sc) or intracerebrally (ic). Glycerol has received considerable attention because it is released by adipose tissue during lipolysis in an amount that is directly proportional to the amount of body fat and to adipocyte size (206,207). When injected sc or ic, it causes a reduction of food intake and a decrease in body weight (208). Glycerol has been fed to rats and causes a somewhat more than compensatory reduction of food intake (209,210), but high levels of glycerol in the diet are highly unusual and adaptation to a new diet would necessarily take time. Only one study has infused glycerol into the bloodstream to try to mimic plasma levels and investigate its effect on daily intake. Glick found in 1980 that a 1-day intra-arterial infusion of glycerol caused a reduction of daily intake that was 3 times the amount of calories infused (209). If his results are accurate, they argue for a role for glycerol in the control of daily intake. These results, however, have not been replicated.

One way to study the role of body fat in the control of food intake is to remove some of the fat in one group of rats and see whether these rats adjust their food intake and energy expenditure to bring body fat back to normal levels. Two studies have found that lean rats that have the inguinal and epididymal fat pads removed will bring their total amount of body fat back to control levels in 3–6 weeks (211,212). Only one of these studies measured food intake under relatively specialized conditions in which Osborne-Mendel rats were fed a high-fat diet that tended to make the rats obese. It was found that after about 20 days of rapid weight gain, the lipectomized rats began to reduce their daily food intake relative to controls

(211). This decrease may have resulted from a decreased capacity for storage. Indeed, these high-fat-fed, lipectomized rats had less body fat at postmortem, but their fat cells were the same size as those of normal controls on the high-fat diet. This study suggests that the changes in food intake resulted from the lack of capacity to store the excess ingested food and not from some regulation of food intake by body fat. Another study did lipectomy of inguinal, retroperitoneal, and epididymal fat pads or sham surgery in ground squirrels just before they began the increase in body weight prior to hibernation (213). The authors found that 4 months later there was no difference in body composition and no significant change in cumulative food intake in the lipectomized squirrels relative to sham controls. Indeed, the lipectomized ground squirrels ate slightly less food and gained slightly more than their sham controls, but neither result was significant. Again, this study shows clear regulation of body fat but no necessary connection between changes in body fat and changes in food intake.

Greenwood (214) has argued that the enzyme that moves fat into tissues, lipoprotein lipase (LPL), acts as a gatekeeper, directing ingested fat into adipose tissue and away from other tissues. She claims that the level of adipose tissue LPL activity could alter feeding behavior in both rodents and humans by sequestering some of the ingested fat away from organs that sense the amount of ingested food. One piece of supportive evidence is that there are elevated LPL levels in young fatty (fa/fa) rats before they become hyperphagic and hyperinsulinemic (215). Furthermore, obese women have been found to have 3.5 times the level of adipose tissue LPL than age-matched lean women (216). Even after the loss of 13 kg, or about half of their excess weight, the obese women's level of LPL in adipose tissue was still 3 times higher than that of their lean counterparts, suggesting that elevated LPL might move some of the ingested fat into adipose tissue and, thereby, maintain their obesity. The idea that the fat component of ingested food might be moved into adipose tissue has become a central component of another theory of the metabolic control of food intake (217,218). Friedman claims that the oxidation of metabolic fuels in the liver generates a signal that controls feeding behavior. If ingested food bypasses these oxidative pathways, which he believes take place in the liver, then this food will not be noticed by the regulating system. He believes that changes in the intramitochrondial oxidation of metabolic fuels govern feeding behavior. If fuel is partitioned so that more fuel moves into adipose tissue, less fuel will be available for oxidation and, thus, the excess fat moved into adipose tissue will not be noticed by the system that regulates food intake. One problem with this oxidation theory is that the intravenous infusion of either glucose or fat into rats produces large changes in daily food intake but no measurable changes in the overall metabolic rate (179). Either the metabolic control of food intake is so tight that food intake changes while metabolism does not or food intake is not controlled by metabolism, but is controlled instead by the amount of circulating nutrients.

Another way to gain insight into the control of the amount of body fat is to investigate the characteristics of genetically obese mice and rats. There are several strains of obese mice, including ob/ob, db/db, agouti, and yellow, as well as two strains of obese rats, fatty (fafa) and corpulent. All of these strains appear to depend on the presence of a recessive gene that leads to obesity. The ob/ob and db/db mice have many characteristics in common: hyperphagia, hyperglycemia, hyperinsulinemia, and marked obesity. Ob/ob mice are infertile and have difficulty maintaining body temperature under cold stress (219). The first attempt to understand the function of the protein product of the ob gene was done in parabiotic mice. Coleman connected ob/ob, db/db, and normal mice together to see whether the slow exchange of blood through the parabiotic union would lead to changes in food intake and body weight (220). Parabiotic connections of two normal, two ob/ob, or two db/db mice produced pairs that grew well and exhibited no changes in intake. In contrast, when db/db mice were connected to either normal or ob/ob mice, these latter mice reduced their food intake, had reduced plasma insulin and glucose levels, and continually lost weight. Some of these normal or ob/ob partners eventually became so thin that they, apparently, died from starvation. Coleman hypothesized that the db/db mice produced a blood-borne satiety factor that the db/db mice could not sense, but which inhibited the food intake of their partners and led to their slow emaciation. In addition, Coleman found that when normal mice were parabiosed with ob/ob mice, the ob/ob mice reduced their food intake and rate of growth, suggesting that normal mice also produced a satiety factor that was lacking in ob/ob mice. In short, ob/ob mice failed to produce an effective blood-borne satiety factor and db/db mice failed to sense its presence. Coleman thought that the genetic defect in db/db mice might be caused by a deficient sensor in the hypothalamus.

Recent investigations have used molecular biology techniques to explore the character of the ob gene. These interesting studies have shown that the ob gene codes for an mRNA that is present only in adipose tissue and this mRNA translates into a protein that is released into the bloodstream. Several studies have shown that when this protein, called leptin, has been injected ip into mice, there is a large reduction in food intake and body weight (see Fig. 19). These reductions are most striking in ob/ob mice that do not make a functional protein themselves, but they also occur in normal mice (221). Ob/ob mice normally have a lower body temperature and lower metabolic rate, but injection of leptin brings these values back up to normal levels, showing that leptin is working on both food intake and energy expenditure to bring body weight back to normal. Leptin also lowers serum insulin and glucose, but these effects may be the result of the reduced food intake. As predicted from the parabiotic experiments of Coleman, the injection of leptin into db/db mice had no effect on food intake, showing that the db/db mice do not have a functional receptor for leptin and are, thus, not affected by the elevated blood leptin levels presumed to be present because of their obesity (222). Recent work has shown that there is a splicing error in the processing of the leptin receptor in db/db mice (223). Leptin receptors have been isolated from the choroid plexus and from the hypothalamus. Leptin is released by adipocytes and appears to act on the brain, probably the hypothalamus. Injection of one-third of the intravenous dose of leptin into the ventricles of ob/ob mice produced similar reductions in food intake, suggesting that a brain region was sensing the presence of leptin (224).

Not long after the announcement of an ob gene protein, researchers measured the expression of the ob gene mRNA in the adipose tissue of obese and normal human subjects and found that it was elevated in the obese (225,226). According to Coleman's theory, this result can occur if the ob gene protein is defective or if there is no functional receptor for leptin. The studies did show the expression of an mRNA for production of a leptin-like protein in obese human subjects. More recently, measurements of immunoreactive leptin have been made in the blood of normal and obese humans (227). These investigators found a significant fourfold increase in the serum levels of leptin-like molecules in obese individuals compared to normal-weight subjects and there was a strong positive correlation between serum concentrations of a leptin-like molecule and the percentage of body fat ($r = .85$). It is not clear whether these leptin-like molecules are restraining food intake in these obese patients or are deformed and ineffective. When seven of these patients were given a low-calorie diet (800 kcal/day), there was a drop in both serum leptin-like material and in the expression of ob mRNA in their adipose tissue. Both of these changes rebounded, in part, when the patients were put on a weight maintenance diet.

The physiological triggers of leptin release have to date only been explored by changes in the expression of the ob gene in the adipose tissues of mice and rats. Fasting led to a substantial fall in the ob mRNA in the epididymal

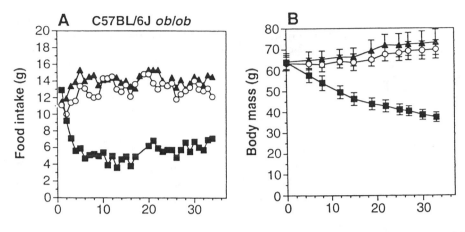

Figure 19   Food intake and body weight of ob/ob mice given a daily ip injection of ob protein for 34 days. ■, rats receiving 5 μg /g/day of ob protein; ○ and ▲, rats receiving vehicle or no treatment. Similar treatment of db/db mice produced no effect. (From Ref. 222, reprinted with permission.)

fat pad of ob/ob mice and refeeding brought it toward normal levels (228). This result was confirmed in Sprague-Dawley rats and was shown to have a circadian rhythm, with the ob gene expression doubling during the 12 hr of dark when the rats were fed (229). Fasting prevented this cyclic fluctuation. A single large injection of insulin (1 IU) into fasted rats led to an increase in ob mRNA expression to the levels of fed controls. Thus, insulin may play some role in ob gene expression and leptin release. Injection of hydrocortisone also led to an increase in ob mRNA and a corresponding decrease in food intake and body weight (230). Although these studies are based only on gene expression and not on blood leptin levels, they suggest that release of leptin may be controlled by hormones as well as by absorbed food.

The leptin results have provided some validation for the "lipostatic" hypothesis (172) with the identification of a possible blood factor released by adipose tissue. This blood factor limits excess body weight by decreasing food intake and increasing energy expenditure. These results are based on the injection of ob protein in a few rodent species and they seem to conflict with the data that show elevated leptin-like material in the blood of obese human subjects who normally eat more and exercise less than their lean counterparts. Whether blood levels of ob protein are involved in the day-to-day control of food intake and energy expenditure still needs further exploration.

IV. RELATIONSHIP OF FOOD INTAKE AND OBESITY

Obesity occurs when food intake exceeds energy expenditure for an extended period (231). One cause of obesity is the ready availability of a large variety of food. The positive taste characteristics of the food seem to override the internal signals that normally inhibit food intake. Rats are known to become obese when given an attractive supermarket diet (232,233). Diets that are high in both fat and carbohydrate have been shown to cause overfeeding and weight gain (234,235).

Mixed meals that have a high fat content tend to cause overeating (234,235). They also prevent the oxidation of the fat component of the diet. Fat oxidation is inhibited by carbohydrate-containing meals because the absorbed glucose releases insulin, which, at low levels, inhibits fatty acid release (236). Insulin also activates lipoprotein lipase, which moves some of the fat into adipose tissue for storage rather than allowing the fat to be transferred to tissues for oxidation (237). In addition, ingested fat is stored at a lower energy cost than fat synthesized from carbohydrate and protein. The cost of storing fat in adipose tissue is only 3% of the ingested calories while the cost of converting carbohydrate into fat requires 23% of the calories consumed (238). When mice are given an increased percentage of their diet as fat, their body fat content increases and a larger percent of the mice have more than 30% of their body composition as fat (239). When human subjects have fat removed from their diet, they lose weight (240). These studies suggest that fat calories are less effective in inhibiting food intake than are carbohydrate or protein calories. This was confirmed in a study in which glucose and lipids were infused intragastrically or intravenously in rats (177,241). The lipid infusion was much less effective in the inhibition of daily food intake. One way to counteract a high-fat content of the diet is to burn fat calories by exercising (242).

The increased proportion of people in North America who have become obese in the last decade (243) shows that the recent increases in the percentage of body fat are not due to our genes but to our behavior and life-style. These observations suggest that the ready accessibility and the pleasant taste of the wide variety of foods currently available in developed countries and their relatively high fat content play a large role in the development of obesity. In addition, the decrease in exercise resulting from desk jobs and television viewing contributes to the reduced calorie output and to the storage of excess energy. A similar phenomenon is seen in laboratory rats that are fed a supermarket diet in a small cage that restricts activity (232). To gain weight, humans and rats must overeat and must override the internal signals that are normally involved in the control of food intake.

ACKNOWLEDGMENTS

The work was supported by grants from MRC and NIH.

REFERENCES

1. Cohn C, Joseph D. Influence of body weight and body fat on appetite of normal lean and obese rats. Yale J Biol Med 1962; 34:598–607.
2. Anand BK, Brobeck JR. Hypothalamic control of food intake in rats and cats. Yale J Biol Med 1951; 24:123–46.
3. Hoebel BG, Teitelbaum P, Weight regulation in normal and hypothalamic hyperphagic rats. J Comp Physiol Psych 1966; 61:189–93.
4. Teitelbaum P, Epstein AN. The lateral hypothalamic syndrome. Psychol Rev 1962; 69:74–90.
5. Keesey RE, Boyle PC, Kemnitz JW, Mitchel JS. (1976) The role of the lateral hypothalamus in determining the body weight set point. In: Novin, D, Wyrwicka W, Bray G, eds. Hunger: Basic Mechanisms and Clinical Implications. New York: Raven Press, 1976:243–255.
6. Mrosovsky N, Sherry DF. Animal anorexias. Science 1980; 207:837–842.
7. Sherry DF, Mrosovsky N, Hogan JA. Weight-loss and anorexia during incubation in birds. J Comp Physiol 1980; 94:89–94.
8. Wade GN, Schneider JE. Metabolic fuels and reproduction in female mammals. Neurosci Biobehav Rev 1992; 16: 235–272.
9. Brobeck, J.R. Food intake as a mechanism of temperature regulation. Yale J Biol Med 1947; 20:545–552.
10. Cottle GN, Carlson LD. Adaptive changes in rats exposed to cold. Am J Physiol 1954; 178:305–308.
11. Koopmans HS. Internal signals cause large changes in food intake in crossed-intestines rats. Brain Res Bull 1985; 14:595–603.
12. Koopmans HS, Sclafani A, Fichtner C, Aravich P. The effects of ileal transposition on food intake and body weight loss in VMH obese rats. Am J Clin Nutr 1982; 35: 284–293.
13. Collier GH. Satiety: an ecological perspective. Brain Res Bull 1985; 14:693–700.
14. Johnson DF, Ackroff K, Peters J, Collier GH. Changes in the rat's meal patterns as a function of the caloric density of the diet. Physiol Behav 1986; 36:929–936.
15. Booth DA. Conditioned satiety in the rat. J Comp Physiol Psych 1972; 81:457–471.
16. McHugh PR. The control of gastric emptying. J Auton Nerv Syst 1983; 9:221–231.
17. Lin HC, Doty JE, Reedy TJ, Meyer TH. Inhibition of gastric emptying by sodium oleate depends on the length of the intestine exposed to acid. Amer J Physiol 1990; 259: G1025–1030.
18. Steffens AB. Blood glucose and FFA levels in relation to the meal pattern in the normal and the ventromedial hypothalamic lesioned rat. Physiol Behav 1969; 4:215–225.
19. Steffens AB. Plasma insulin content in relation to blood glucose level and meal pattern in the normal and hypothalamic hyperphagic rat. Physiol Behav 1970; 5: 147–151.
20. Collier G, Hirsch E, Hamlin PH. The ecological determinants of reinforcement in the rat. Physiol Behav 1972; 9: 705–716.
21. Kanarek RB. Availability and caloric density of the diet as determinants of meal patterns in cats. Physiol Behav 1975; 15:611–618.
22. Collier G. The dialogue between the house economist and the resident physiologist. Nutr Behav 1986; 3:9–26.
23. Davis JD, Campbell CS. Peripheral control of meal size in the rat: effect of sham feeding on meal size and drinking rate. J Comp Physiol Psych 1973; 83:379–387.
24. Rosenzweig MR. The mechanisms of hunger and thirst. In: Postman L, ed. Psychology in the Making. New York: Knopf, 1962:73–143.
25. Hull CL, Livingston JR, Rouse RO, Barker AN. Time, sham, and esophageal feeding as reinforcements. J Comp Physiol Psych 1951; 44:236–245.
26. Janowitz HD, Grossman MI. Some factors affecting the food intake of normal dogs and dogs with esophageostomy and gastric fistulae. Am J Physiol 1949; 159: 143–148.
27. Mook DG. Oral factors in appetite and satiety. Ann NY Acad Sci 1989; 575:265–278.
28. Smith GP, Gibbs J, Young RC. Cholecystokinin and intestinal satiety in the rat. Fed Proc 1974; 33:1146–1149.
29. Scalfani A, Nissenbaum JW. Is gastric sham feeding really sham feeding? Am J Physiol 1985; 248:R387–390.
30. Grill HJ, Berridge KC, Ganster DJ. Oral glucose is the prime elicitor of preabsorptive insulin secretion. Am J Physiol 1984; 246:R88–95.

31. Plato. The Timeaus of Plato. New York: Arno Press, 1973: 271.

32. Hunt JN, Stubbs DF. The volume and energy content of meals as determinants of gastric emptying. J. Physiol (Lond) 1975; 245:209–255.

33. Hunt JN. A possible relation between the regulation of gastric emptying and food intake. Am J Physiol 1980; 239:G1–G4.

34. Adolph BK. Urges to eat and drink in rats. Am J Physiol 1947; 151:110–125.

35. Janowitz HD, Grossman MI. Effects of variations in the nutritive density on intake of food in dogs and cats. Am J Physiol 1949; 258:184–193.

36. Tomlin J. The effect of the gel forming liquid fibre on feeding behavior in man. Br J Nutr 1995; 74:427–436.

37. Deutsch JA, Young WG, Kalogeris TJ. The stomach signals satiety. Science 1978; 201:165–167.

38. Deutsch JA, Gonzalez MF. Gastric nutrient content signals satiety. Behav Neural Biol 1980; 30:113–116.

39. Deutsch JA. Dietary control and the stomach. Prog Neurobiol 1983; 20:313–332.

40. Karel L. Gastric absorption. Physiol Rev 1948; 28: 433–450.

41. Kaplan JM, Siemers W, Grill HJ. Ingestion, gastric fill and gastric emptying before and after withdrawal of gastric contents. Am J Physiol 1994; 267:R1257–1265.

42. Selley RJ, Kaplan JM, Grill HJ. Effect of occluding the pylorus on intraoral intake: a test of the gastric hypothesis of meal termination. Physiol Behav 1995; 58:245–249.

43. Kraly FS, Smith GP. Combined pregastric and gastric stimulation by food is sufficient for normal meal size. Physiol Behav 1978; 21:405–408.

44. Kaplan JM, Spector AC, Grill HJ. Dynamics of gastric emptying during and after stomach fill in the rat. Am J Physiol 1992; 263:R813–820.

45. McHugh PR, Moran TH. Calories and gastric emptying: a regulatory capacity with implications for feeding. Am J Physiol 1979; 236:R254–260.

46. McHugh PR, Moran TH. Accuracy of the regulation of caloric ingestion in the rhesus monkey. Am J Physiol 1978; 235:R29–34.

47. McHugh PR, Moran TH, Wirth JB. Postpyloric regulation of gastric emptying in rhesus monkeys. Am J Physiol 1982; 243:R408–415.

48. Paintal AS. A study of gastric stretch receptors. Their role in the peripheral mechanism of satiation of hunger and thirst. J Physiol (Lond) 1954; 126:255–270.

49. Iggo A. Tension receptors in the stomach and urinary bladder. J Physiol (Lond) 1955; 128:593–607.

50. Gonzalez MF, Deutsch JA. Vagotomy abolishes cues of satiety produced by gastric distension. Science 1981; 212: 1283–1284.

51. Kraly FS, Gibbs J. Vagotomy fails to block the satiating effect of food in the stomach. Physiol Behav 1990; 24: 1007–1010.

52. Koopmans HS. A stomach hormone that inhibits food intake. J Auton Nerv Syst 1983; 6:157–171.

53. Abrahamsson H, Jansson G. Elicitation of reflex vagal relaxation of the stomach from pharynx and esophagus in the cat. Acta Physiol Scand 1969; 28:267–273.

54. Mayer EA. The physiology of gastric storage and emptying. In: Johnson ER, Alpers DH, Christensen J, Jacobson ED, Walsh JH. Physiology of the Gastrointestinal Tract. New York: Raven Press, 1994:929–976.

55. Kersten A. Strubbe JH, Spiteri N. Meal patterning of rats with changes in day length and food availability. Physiol Behav 1980; 25:953–958.

56. Ehman GK, Albert DJ, Jamieson JL. Injections into the duodenum and induction of satiety in the rat. Can J Psych 1971; 25:147–166.

57. Snowdon CT. Production of satiety with small intraduodenal infusions in the rat. J Comp Physiol Psych 1975; 88:231–238.

58. Antin J, Gibbs J, Smith GP. Intestinal satiety requires pregastric food stimulation. Physiol Behav 1977; 18: 421–425.

59. Liebling DS, Eisner JD, Gibbs J, Smith GP. Intestinal satiety in rats. J Comp Physiol Psych 1975; 89:955–965.

60. Gibbs J, Madison SP, Rolls ET. Satiety role for the small intestine examined in sham-feeding Rhesus monkeys. J Comp Physiol Psych 1981; 95:1003–1015.

61. Sharma KN, Nasset ES. Electrical activity in the mesenteric nerves after perfusion of gut lumen. Am J Physiol 1962; 202:725–730.

62. Mei N. Vagal glucoreceptors in the small intestine of the cat. J Physiol (Lond) 1978; 282:485–506.

63. Jeanningros R. Vagal unitary responses to intestinal amino acid infusions in anesthetized cat: a putative signal for protein satiety. Physiol Behav 1982; 28:9–21.

64. Mei N. Intestinal chemosensitivity. Physiol Rev 1985; 65: 211–237.

65. Novin D. The integration of visceral information in the control of feeding. J. Auton Nerv Syst 1983; 9:233–246.

66. Yox DP, Ritter RC. Capsaicin attenuates suppression of sham feeding induced by intestinal nutrients. Am J Physiol 1988; 255:R569–574.

67. Yox DP, Stokesbury PH, Ritter RC. Vagotomy attenuates suppression of sham feeding induced by intestinal nutrients. Am J Physiol 1991; 260:R503–508.

68. McHugh PR, Moran TH. The inhibition of feeding produced by direct intraintestinal infusion of glucose: Is this satiety? Brain Res Bull 1986; 17:415–418.

69. Koopmans HS. The intestinal control of food intake. In: Bray, G, ed. Recent Advances in Obesity Research II. London: Newman Publishers, 1978:33–43.

70. Davenport HW. Physiology of the Digestive Tract. Chicago: Yearbook Meical Publishers, 1971:183–210.

71. Louis-Sylvestre J. Preabsorptive insulin release and hypoglycemia in rats. Am J Physiol 1976; 230:56–60.

72. Walsh JH. Gastrointestinal hormones. In: Johnson LR, Albers DH, Christenson J, Jacobson ED, Walsh JH, eds. Physiology of the Gastrointestinal Tract. New York: Raven Press, 1994:1–128.

73. Grossman MI. Trends in gut hormone research. In: Thompson JC, ed. Gastrointestinal Hormones. Austin: University of Texas Press, 1975:3–10.

74. Go VLW, Michner S, Roddy D, Koch M. Clinical relevance of regulatory gastrointestinal peptides. Clin Biochem 1984; 17:82–88.

75. Glick Z, Thomas DW, Mayer J. Absence of effect of injections of the intestinal hormones secretin and cholecystokinin-pancreozymin upon feeding behavior. Physiol Behav 1971; 6:5–8.

76. Koopmans HS, Deutsch JA, Branson PJ. The effect of cholecystokinin pancreozymin on hunger and thirst in mice. Behav Biol 1972; 7:441–444.

77. Gibbs J, Young RC, Smith GP. Cholecystokinin decreases food intake in rats. J Comp Physiol Psych 1973; 84:488–495.

78. Smith GP, Gibbs J, Young RC. Cholecystokinin and intestinal satiety in the rat. Fed Proc 1974; 33:1146–1149.

79. Deutsch JA, Hardy WT. Cholecystokinin produces bait shyness in rats. Nature 1977; 266:196.

80. Shillabeer G, Davison JS. Endogenous and exogenus cholecystokinin may reduce food intake by different mechanisms. Am J Physiol 1987; 253:R379–382.

81. Smith GP, Jerome C, Chusin BJ, Eterno R, Simansky KJ. Abdominal vagotomy blocks the satiety effect of cholecystokinin in the rat. Science 1981; 213:1036–1037.

82. Lorenz DN, Goldman SA. Vagal mediation of the cholecystokinin satiety effect in rats. Physiol Behav 1982; 29:599–604.

83. Reidelberger RD. Abdominal vagal mediation of the satiety effects of exogenous and endogenous cholecystokinin in rats. Am J Physiol 1992; 263:R1354–1358.

84. Reidelberger RD, Kalogeris TJ, Soloman TE. Plasma CCK levels after food intake and infusion of CCK analogs that inhibit feeding in dogs. Am J physiol 1989; 256:R1148–1154.

85. Reidelberger RD, Varga G, Rosenquiest GL, Liehr RM, Wong H, Walsch JH. Comparative effects of CCK monoclonal antibody on food intake and pancreatic exocrine secretion in rats. Int J Obesity 1991; 15:12.

86. Hewson G, Leighton RG, Hughes J. The cholescystokinin receptor antagonist L364,718 increases food intake in the rat by attenuation of the action of endogenous cholecystokinin. Br J Pharm 1988; 93:79–84.

87. Dourish CT, Rycroft W, Iverson SD. Postponment of satiety by blockade of brain cholecystokinin (CCK-B) receptors. Science 1989; 245:1509–1511.

88. Reidelberg RD, O'Rourke MF. Potent cholecystokinin antagonist L364,718 stimulates food intake in rats. Am J Physiol 1989; 257:R1512–1518.

89. Davison JS, Clarke GD. Mechanical properties and sensitivity to CCK of vagal gastric slowly adapting mechanoreceptors. Am J Physiol 1988; 255:G55–60.

90. Schwartz GJ, McHugh PR, Moran TH. Integration of vagal afferent responses to gastric loads and cholecystokinin in rats. Am J Physiol 1991; 261:R64–69.

91. Reidelberger, RD. Choescystokinin and control of food intake. J Nutr 1994; 124:1327S–1333S.

92. Corwin RL, Gibbs J, Smith GP. Increased food intake after type A but not type B cholecystokinin receptor blockade. Physiol Behav 1991; 50:255–258.

93. Moran TH, Ameglio PJ, Schwartz GJ, Mchugh PR. Blockade of type A, not type B, CCK receptors attenttuates satiety actions of exogenous and endogenus CCK. Am J Physiol 1992; 262:R46–R50.

94. Lorenz DN, Kreielsheimer G, Smith GP. Effect of cholecystokinin, gastrin, secretin and GIP on sham feeding in the rat. Physiol Behav 1979; 23:1065–1072.

95. Gibbs J, Fauser DJ, Rose EA, Rolls BJ, Rolls ET, Maddison SP. Bombesin suppresses feeding in rats. Nature 1979; 282:208–210.

96. Gibbs J, Kulkosky PJ, Smith GP. Effects of peripheral and central bombesin on feeding behavior in rats. Peptides 1981; 2(S2):179–183.

97. Ghatei MA, Jung RT, Stevenson JC, Hillyard CJ, Adrian TE, Lee YC, Christofides ND, Sarson DL, Mashiter K, MacIntyre I, Bloom SR. Bombesin: action on gut hormones and calcium in man. J Clin Endocr Metab 1982; 54:980–985.

98. Gibbs J, Kulkosky PJ, Smith GP. Effects of peripheral and central bombesin on feeding behavior of rats. Peptides 1981; 2(S2):179–183.

99. Stuckey JA, Gibbs J, Smith GP. Neural disconnection of gut from brain blocks bombesin-induced satiety. Peptides 1985; 6:1249–1252.

100. Plamondon H, Merali Z. Push-pull perfusion reveals meal-dependent changes in the release of bombesin-like peptides in the rat paraventricular nucleus. Brain Res 1994; 668:54–61.

101. Motamedi F, Rashidy-Pour A, Zarrindast MR, Bavadi M. Bombesin-induced anorexia requires central bombesin receptor activation: independence from interaction with central catecholinergic systems. Psychopharmacology 1993; 110:193–197.

102. Laferrere B, Leroy F, Bonhomme G, Le Gall A, Basdevat A, Guy-Gand B. Effects of bombesin, of a new bombesin agonist (BIM187) and a new antagonist (BIM189) on food intake in rats, in relation to cholecystokinin. Eur J Pharm 1992; 215:23–28.

103. Stunkard AJ, Van Itallie TB, Reis BB. The mechanism of satiety: effect of glucagon on gastric hunger contractions in man. Proc Soc Exp Biol Med 1955; 89:258–261.

104. Martin JR, Novin D. Decreased feeding in rats following hepatic-portal infusions of glucagon. Physiol Behav 1977; 19:461–466.

105. Martin JR, Novin D, Vander Weele DA. Loss of glucagon suppression of feeding after vagotomy in rats. Am J Physiol 1978; 234:E314–318.

106. Geary N, Smith GP. Selective hepatic branch vagotomy blocks pancreatic glucagon's satiety effect. Physiol Behav 1983; 31:391–394.

107. Langhans W, Ziegler U, Scharrer E, Geary N. Stimulation of feeding in rats by intraperitoneal injection of antibodies to glucagon. Science 1982; 218:894–896.

108. Le Sauter J, Noh U, Geary N. Hepatic portal infusion of glucagon antibodies increases meal size in rats. Am J Physiol 1991; 261:R162–165.

109. Geary N, Le Sauter J, Noh U. Glucagon acts in the liver to control spontaneous meal size in rats. Am J Physiol 1993; 264:R116–122.

110. Mayer J. Regulation of energy intake and body weight: the glucostatic theory and the lipostatic hypothesis. Ann NY Acad Sci 1955; 63:15–42.

111. Woods SC, Porte D. Insulin and the set point regulation of body weight. In Novin D, Wyrwicka W, Bray GA, ed. Hunger: Basic Mechanisms and Clinical Implications. New York: Raven Press, 1976:273–280.

112. Bagdade JD, Bierman EI, Porte DJ. The significance of basal insulin levels in the evaluation of the insulin response to glucose in diabetic and nondiabetic subjects. J Clin Invest 1967; 46:1549–1557.

113. Polonsky KS, Given BD, VanCauter E. Twenty-four hour profiles and pulsatile patterns of insulin secretion in normal and obese subjects. J Clin Invest 1988; 81:442–448.

114. Porikos KP, Pi-Sunyer FX. Regulation of food intake in human obesity: studies with caloric dilution and exercise. Clin Endocrin Metab 1984; 13:547–561.

115. Woods SC, Lotter EC, McKay LD, Porte D. Chronic intracerebroventricular infusion of insulin reduces food intake and body weight in baboons. Nature 1979; 282:503–505.

116. Brief DJ, Davis JD. Reduction of food intake and body weight by chronic intraventricular insulin infusion. Brain Res Bull 1984; 12:571–575.

117. Schwartz MW, Bergman RN, Kahn SE, Taborsky J, Fisher LD, Sipols AJ, Woods SC, Steil GM, Porte, D. Evidence for entry of plasma insulin into cerebrospinal fluid through an intermediate compartment in dogs. J Clin Invest 1991; 88:1272–1281.

118. VanderWeele DA, Pi-Sunyer FX, Novin D, Bush MJ. Chronic insulin infusion suppresses food ingestion and body weight gain in rats. Brain Res Bull 1980; 5(S4):7–11.

119. VanderWeele DA. Insulin and satiety from feeding in pancreatic normal and diabetic rats. Physiol Behav 1993; 54:477–485.

120. VanderWeele DA. Insulin is a prandial satiety hormone. Physiol Behav 1994; 56:619–622.

121. Willing AE, Walls EK, Koopmans HS. Insulin administration leads to increased food intake in diabetic rats eating high and low fat diets. Physiol Behav 1994; 56:983–991.

122. Willing AE, Koopmans HS, Walls EK. Hepatic portal and vena cava insulin infusions lead to increased food intake in diabetic rats. Physiol Behav 1994; 56:993–1001.

123. Walls EK, Koopmans, HS. Increased food intake following carotid and systemic insulin infusions. Int J Obes 1992; 16:153–160.

124. Woo R, Kissileff HR, Pi-Sunyer FX. Elevated postprandial insulin levels do not induce satiety in normal-weight humans. Am J physiol 1984; 247:R745–749.

125. Rodin J, Wack J, Ferrannini E, DeFronzo RA. Effect of insulin and glucose on feeding behavior. Metabolism 1985; 34:826–831.

126. Holt SH, Miller JB. Increased insulin responses to ingested foods are associated with lessened satiety. Appetite 1995; 24:43–54.

127. Morley JE, Flood JF. Amylin decreases food intake in mice. Peptides 1991; 12:865–869.

128. Chance WT, Balasubramaniam S, Stallion A, Fischer JE. Anorexia following the systemic injection of amylin. Brain Res 1993; 607:185–188.

129. Ohsawa H, Kanatsuka A, Yamaguchi T, Makino H, Yoshida S. Islet amylin polypeptide inhibits glucose-stimulated insulin secretion from isolated rat pancreatic islets. Biochem Biophys Res Commun 1989; 160:961–967.

130. Chance WT, Balasubramaniam S, Zhang FS, Wimalawamsa SJ, Fischer JE. Anorexia following intrahypothalamic administration of amylin. Brain Res 1991; 352–354.

131. Lutz TA, Del Prete E, Scharrer E. Subdiaphramatic vagotomy does not influence the anoretic effect of amylin. Peptides 1995; 16:457–462.

132. Koopmans HS, Wang DM, Koslowsky I, Kloiber R. The effect of cross-circulation on food intake. Obes Res 1994; 3:331S.

133. Mordes JP, Herrera G, Silen W. Decreased weight gain and food intake in vagotomized rats. Soc Exp Biol Med 1977; 156:257–272.

134. Louis-Sylvestre J. Feeding and metabolic patterns in rats with truncular vagotomy or with transplanted B-cells. Am J Physiol 1978; 235:E119–125.

135. Grossman MI, Cummins GM, Ivy AC. The effect of insulin on food intake after vagotomy and sympathectomy. Am J Physiol 1947; 149:100–102.

136. Harris SC, Ivy AC, Searle LM. Mechanisms of amphetamine-induced loss of weight; consideration of hunger and appetite. JAMA 1947; 134:1468–1475.

137. Robinson RG, Folstein MF, McHugh PR. Reduced calorie intake following small bowel bypass surgery: a systematic study of the possible causes. Psych Med 1979; 9:37–53.

138. Pilkington TRE, Gazet JC, Ang L, Kalucy RS, Crisp AH, Day S. Explanations for weight loss after jejunoileal bypass in gross obesity. Br Med J 1976; 1:1504–1505.

139. Sclafani A, Koopmans HS, Vasselli JR, Reichmann M. Effects of intestinal bypass surgery on appetite, food intake and body weight in obese and lean rats. Am J Physiol 1978; 234:E389–398.

140. Atkinson RL, Brent EL, Wagner BS, Whipple JH. Energy balance and regulation of body weight after intestinal bypass in rats. Am J Physiol 1983; 243:R658–663.

141. Koopmans HS, Ferri GL, Sarson DL, Polak J, Bloom SR. The effects of ileal transposition and jejunoileal bypass on food intake, body weight, gastrointestinal hormone levels and tissue adaptation. Physiol Behav 1984; 33:601–609.

142. Koopmans HS. An integrated organismic response to lower gut stimulation. Scand J Gastroenterol 1983; 18(S82):143–153.

143. Read NW, Kinsman R. Effect of infusion of nutrient solutions into the ileum on gastrointestinal transit and plasma levels of neurotension and enteroglucagon in man. Gastroenterology 1984; 86:274–280.

144. Soper NJ, Chapman NJ, Kelly KA, Brown ML, Phillips SF, Go VL. The "ileal brake" after ileal pouch-anal anastomosis. Gastroenterology 1990; 98:111–116.

145. Koopmans HS. Endogenous gut signals and metabolites control daily food intake. Int J Obes 1990; 14(S3): 93–102.

146. Tso P. Intestinal lipid absorption. In: Johnson ER, Alpers DH, Christensen J, Jacobson ED, Walsh JH, eds. Physiology of the Gastrointestinal Tract. New York: Raven Press 1994:1867–1908.

147. Russek M. A hypothesis on the participation of hepatic glucoreceptors in the control of food intake. Nature (Lond). 1963; 200:176.

148. Niijima A. Glucose-sensitive afferent nerve fibers in the hepatic branch of the vagus nerve in the guinea-pig. J Physiol 1982; 332:315–323.

149. Novin D, Sanderson JD, Vander Weele DA. The effect of isotonic glucose on eating as a function of feeding condition and infusion site. Physiol Behav 1974; 13:3–7.

150. Novin D. (1976) Visceral mechanisms in the control of food intake. In: Novin D, Wyrwicka W, Bray G, eds. Hunger: Basic Mechanisms and Clinical Implications. New York: Raven Press, 1976:357–367.

151. Tordoff MG, Friedman MI. Hepatic-portal glucose infusions decrease food intake and increase food preference. Am J Physiol 1986; 251:R192–195.

152. Tordoff MG, Tluczek JP, Friedman, MI. Effect of portal glucose concentration on food intake and metabolism. Am J Physiol 1989; 257:R1474–1480.

153. Willing AE, Koopmans HS. Hepatic portal and vena cava glucose and amino acid infusions decrease daily food intake in rats. Neurosci Abstr 1994; 20:1226.

154. Koopmans HS. Hepatic control of food intake. Appetite 1984; 5:127–131.

155. Russek Reply to Koopman's Hepatic control of food intake. Appetite 1984; 5:133–135.

156. Friedman MI, Sawchenko PE. Evidence for hepatic involvement in control of ad libitum food intake in rats. Am J Physiol 1984; 247:R106–113.

157. Del Prete E, Scharrer E. Influence of age and hepatic branch vagotomy on the night/day distribution of food intake in rats. Zeit Ernahr 1993; 32:316–320.

158. Del Prete E, Scharrer E. Circadian effects of hepatic branch vagotomy on the feeding response to 2-deoxy-D-glucose in rats. J Auton Nerv Syst 1994; 6:27–36.

159. Bellinger LL, Mendel VE, Williams FE, Castonquay TW. The effect liver denervation on meal patterns, body weight and body composition of rats. Physiol Behav 1984; 33: 661–667.

160. Bellinger LL, Williams FE. Meal patterns and plasma liver enzymes and metabolites after total liver denervations. Physiol Behav 1995; 58:625–628.

161. Louis-Sylvestre J, Servant JM, Molimard R, Le Magnen J. Effect of liver denervation on feeding pattern of rats. Am J Physiol 1980; 239:R66–70.

162. Louis-Sylvestre J, Larue-Achagiotis C, Michel A, Houssin D. Feeding pattern in liver transplanted rats. Physiol Behav 1990; 48:321–326.

163. Beverly JL, Yang ZJ, Meguid MM. Hepatic vagotomy effects on metabolic challenges during parenteral nutrition in rats. Am J Physiol 1994; 266:R646–649.

164. Phillips LS. Nutritional regulation of somatomedin activity and growth. In: Giordano G, Van Wyk JJ, Minuto F, eds. Somatomedins and Growth. London: Academic Press, 1979:311–323.

165. Sigal RJ, Purdon C, Bilinski D, Vranik M, Marliss E. Glucoregulation during and after intense exercise: effects of beta-blockade. J Clin Endocrinol Metab 1994; 78: 359–366.

166. Mayer J, Bates MW. Blood glucose and food intake in normal and hypophysectomized, alloxan-treated rats. Am J Physiol 1952; 168:812–819.

167. Mayer J. Regulation of energy intake and body weight: the glucostatic theory and the lipostatic hypothesis. Ann NY Acad Sci 1955; 63:15–42.

168. Van Itallie TB. The glucostatic theory 1953–1988: roots and branches. Int J Obes 1990; 14(S3):1–10.

169. Mellinkof SM, Frankland M, Boyle M, Griepel M. Relation between serum amino acid concentration and fluctuations in appetite. J Appl Psych 1956; 8:535–538.

170. Peters JC, Harper AE. Adaptation of rats to diets containing different levels of protein: effects on food intake, plasma and brain amino acid concentrations and brain neurotransmitter metabolism. J Nutr 1985; 115:382–398.

171. Moundras C, Remesy C, Demigne C. Dietary protein paradox: decrease of amino acid availability induced by high-protein diets. Am J Physiol 1993; 264:G1057–1065.

172. Kennedy GC. The role of depot fat in the hypothalamic control of food intake in the rat. Proc Roy Soc B 1952; 140:578–592.

173. Nicolaidis S, Rowland N. Metering of intravenous versus oral nutrients and the regulation of energy balance. Am J Physiol 1976; 231:661–668.

174. Woods SC, Stein LJ, McKay LD, Porte D. Suppression of food intake by intravenous nutrients and insulin in the baboon. Am J Physiol 1984; 247:R393–401.

175. Walls EK, Koopmans HS. Effect of intravenous nutrient infusions on food intake in rats. Physiol Behav 1989; 45: 1223–1226.

176. Meguid MM, Chen TY, Yang ZJ, Campos ACL, Hitch DC, Gleason JR. Effects of continuous graded total parenteral nutrition on feeding indexes and metabolic concomitants in rats. Am J Physiol 1991; E126–140.

177. Walls EK, Koopmans HS. Differential effects of intravenous glucose, amino acids and lipid on daily food intake in rats. Am J Physiol 1992; 262:R225–234.

178. Beverly JL, Yang ZJ, Meguid MM. Factors influencing compensatory feeding during parenteral nutrition in rats. Am J Physiol 1994; 266:R1928–1932.

179. Walls EK, Koopmans HS. Influence of intravenous nutrients on food intake and energy expenditure. Neurosci Abstr 1992; 18:1233.

180. Meguid RA, Beverly JL, Meguid MM. Surfeit calories during parenteral nutrition influences food intake and carcass adiposity in rats. Physiol Behav 1995; 57:265–269.

181. Oomura Y. (1976) Significance of glucose, insulin and free fatty acid on the hypothalamic feeding and satiety neurons. In: Novin D, Wyrwicka W, Bray G, eds. Hunger: Basic Mechanisms and Clinical Implications. New York: Raven Press, 1976:145–157.

182. Smith GP, Epstein AN. Increased feeding in response to decreased glucose utilization in the rat and monkey. Am J Physiol 1969; 217:1083–1087.

183. Yamamoto H, Nagai K, Nakagawa H. Time-dependent involvement of autonomic nervous system in hyperglycemia due to 2-deoxy-D-glucose. Am J Physiol 1988; 255:E928–933.

184. Matsunaga H, Igucho A, Yatomi A, Uemura K, Muira H, Gotoh M, Mano T, Sakamoto S. The relative importance of nervous system and hormones to the 2-deoxy d-glucose-induced hyperglycemia in fed rats. Endocrinology 1989; 124:1259–1264.

185. Scheurink A, Ritter S. Sympathoadrenal responses to glucoprivation and lipoprivation in rats. Physiol Behav 1993; 53:995–1000.

186. Miselis RR, Epstein AN. Feeding induced by intracerebroventricular 2-deoxy-D-glucose in the rat. Am J Physiol 1975; 229:1438–1447.

187. Del Prete E, Scharrer E, Hepatic branch vagotomy attenuates the feeding response to 2-deoxy-D-glucose. Exp Physiol 1990; 75:259–261.

188. Scharrer E, Del Prete E, Giger R. Hepatic branch vagotomy enhances glucoprivic feeding in food-deprived old rats. Physiol Behav 1993; 54:259–264.

189. Ritter S, Taylor JS. Vagal sensory neurons are required for lipoprivic but not glucoprivic feeding in rats. Am J Physiol 1990; 258:R1395–1401.

190. Tordoff MG, Hopfenbeck, Novin D. Hepatic vagotomy (partial hepatic denervation) does not alter ingestive responses to metabolic challenges. Physiol Behav 1982; 28: 417–424.

191. Bellinger CL, Williams FE. Liver denervation does not modify feeding responses to metabolic challenges or hypertonic NaCl induced water consumption. Physiol Behav 1983; 30:463–470.

192. Tordoff MG, Rafka R, DiNovi MJ, Friedman MI. 2,5-anhydro-D-mannitol: a fructose analogue that increases food intake in rats. Am J Physiol 1988; 254:R150–153.

193. Hanson RL, Ho RS, Wisenberg JJ, Simpson R, Younathan ES, Blair JB. Inhibition of gluconeogenesis and glycogenolysis by 2,5-anhydro-D-mannitol. J Biochem 1984; 259: 218–233.

194. Tordoff MG, Rawson NE, Friedman MI. 2,5-anhydro-D-mannitol acts in liver to initiate feeding. Am J Physiol 1991; 261:R283–R288.

195. Park CR, Seeley RJ, Bentham L, Friedman MI, Woods SC. Whole body energy expenditure and fuel oxidation after 2,5-anhydro-D-mannitol administration. Am J Physiol 1995; 268:R299–302.

196. Rawson NE, Blum H, Osbakken MD, Friedman MI. Hepatic phosplate trapping decreased ATP and increased feeding after 2,5-anhydro-D-mannitol. Am J Physiol 1994; 266:R112–R117.

197. Bodoky G, Yang ZJ, Mequid MM, Laviano A, Szeverenyi N. Effects of fasting, intermittent feeding or continuous parenteral nutrition of rat liver and brain energy metabolism as assessed by ^{31}P-NMR. Physiol Behav 1995; 58: 521–527.

198. Scharrer E, Langhans W. Control of food intake by fatty acid oxidation. Am J Physiol 1986; 250:R1003–1006.

199. Bauche F, Sabourault D, Giudicelli Y, Nordmann J, Nordmann R. Inhibition in vitro of acyl-CoA-dehydrogenases by 2-mercaptoacetate in rat liver mitochondria. Biochem J 1983; 215:457–464.

200. Friedman MI, Tordoff MG, Ramirez I. Integrated metabolic control of food intake. Brain Res Bull 1986; 17: 855–859.

201. Tutwiler GF, Ho W, Mohrbacher RJ. 2-Tetradeclycidic acid. Meth Enzymol 1981; 2:533–551.

202. Friedman MI, Tordoff MG. Fatty acid oxidation and glucose utilization interact to control food intake in rats. Am J Physiol 1986; 251:R840–845.

203. Friedman MI, Ramirez I, Bowden CR, Tordoff MG. Fuel partitioning and food intake: role of mitochondrial fatty acid transport. Am J Physiol 1990; W258:R216–221.

204. Lazzarini SJ, Schneider JF, Wade GN. Inhibition of fatty acid oxidation and glucose metabolism does not alter food intake or hunger motivation in Syrian hamsters. Physiol Behav 1988; 44:209–213.

205. Levitsky D, Faust I, Glassman M. The ingestion of food and the recovery of body weight following fasting in the naive rat. Physiol Behav 1976; 17:575–580.

206. Björntorp P, Bergman H, Varnas-Kas E, Lindholm B. Lipid mobilization in relation to body composition in man. Metabolism 1969; 18:112–117.

207. Goldrick RB, McLoughlin GM. Lippolysis and lipogenesis from glucose in human fat cells of different sizes. J Clin Invest 1970; 49:1213–1223.

208. Wirtschafter D, Davis JD. Body weight: reduction by long-term glycerol treatment. Science 1977; 198:1271–1273.

209. Glick Z. Food intake of rats administered with glycerol. Physiol Behav 1980; 25:621–626.

210. Grinker J, Strohmayer AJ, Horowitz J, Hirsch J, Leibel RL. The effect of the metabolite glycerol on food intake and body weight in rats. Brain Res Bull 1980; 5(S4):29–35.

211. Faust IM, Johnson PR, Hirsch J. Surgical removal of adipose tissue alters feeding behavior and the development of obesity in rats. Science 1977; 197:393–396.

212. Larson KA, Anderson DB. The effects of lipectomy on remaining adipose tissue depots in the Sprague-Dawley rat. Growth 1978; 42:469–477.

213. Dark J, Forger NG, Stern JS, Zucker I. Recovery of lipid mass after removal of adipose tissue in ground squirrels. Am J Physiol 1985; 249:R73–78.

214. Greenwood MRC. The relationship of enzyme activity to feeding behavior in rats: lipoprotein lipase as the metabolic gatekeeper. Int J Obes 1985; 9(S1):67–70.

215. Gruen R, Hietanen E, Greenwood MRC. Increased adipose tissue lipoprotein lipase activity during development of the genetically obese rat (fafa). Metabolism 1978; 27:1955–1965.

216. Yost TJ, Eckel RH. Fat calories may be preferentially stored in reduced-obese women: a permissive pathway for resumption of the obese state. J Clin Endocrinol Metab 1988; 67:259–264.

217. Friedman MI, Ramirez I, Bowden CR, Tordoff MG. Fuel partitioning and food intake: role for mitochrondial fatty acid transport. Am J Physiol 1990; 258:R216–221.

218. Friedman MI. Body fat and the metabolic control of food intake. Int J Obes 1990; 14(S3):53–67.

219. Vinter J, Hull D, Batt RA, Tyler DD. The effect of limited feeding on thermogenesis and thermoregulation in genetically obese (ob/ob) mice during cold exposure. Int J Obes 1988; 12:111–117.

220. Coleman DL. Effects of parabiosis of obese with diabetes and normal mice. Diabetologia 1973; 9:294–298.

221. Pellymounter MA, Cullen MJ, Baker MB, Hecht R, Winters D, Boone T, Collins F. Effects of the obese gene product on body weight regulation in ob/ob mice. Science 1995; 269:540–543.

222. Hallas JL, Gajiwala KS, Maffei M, Cohen SL, Chait BT, Rabinowitz D, Lallone RL, Burley SK, Friedman JM. Weight-reducing effects of the plasma protein encoded by the obese gene. Science 1995; 269:543–546.

223. Lee G-H, Proence R, Montez JM, Carroll KM, Darvishzadeh JG, Lee JI, Friedman JM. Abnormal splicing of the leptin receptor in diabetic mice. Nature 1996; 379:632–636.

224. Campfield LA, Smith FJ, Guisez Y, Devos R, Burn P. Recombinant mouse OB protein: evidence for a peripheral signal linking adiposity and central neural networks. Science 1995; 269:546–549.

225. Lonnqvist F, Arner P, Nordfors L, Schalling M. Overexpression of the obese (ob) gene in adipose tissue of human obese subjects. Nature Medicine 1995; 1:950–953.

226. Hamilton BS, Paglia D, Kwan AYM, Dietel M. Increased obese mRNA expression in omental fat cells from massively obese humans. Nature Med 1995; 1:953–956.

227. Considine RV, Sinha MK, Heiman ML, Kriauciunas A, Stephens TW, Nyce MR, Ohannesian JP, Marco CC, McKee LJ, Bauer TL, Caro JF. Serum immunoreactive-leptin concentrations in normal-weight and obese humans. N Engl J Med 1996; 334:292–295.

228. Trayhurn P, Duncan JS, Thomas MEA, Rayner DV. Expression of the ob (obesity) gene in adipose tissue in mice. Int J Obes 1995; 19(S2):34.

229. Saladin R, De Vos P, Guerre-Millo M, Leturque A, Girard J, Steals B, Auwerx J. Transient increase in obese gene expression after food intake or insulin administration. Nature 1995; 377:527–529.

230. De Vos P, Saladin R, Auwerx J, Steals B. Induction of ob gene expression by corticosteroids is accompanied by body weight loss and reduced food intake. J Biol Chem 1995; 270:15958–15961.

231. Flatt JP. Body composition, respiratory quotient and weight maintenance. Am J Clin Nutr 1995; 62:1107S–1117S.

232. Sclafani A, Springer D. Dietary obesity in adult rats: similarities to hypothalamic and human obesity syndromes. Physiol Behav 1976; 17:461–471.

233. Rolls BJ, Van Duijvenvoorde PM, Rowe EA. Variety in the diet enhances intake in a meal and contributes to the development of obesity in the rat. Physiol Behav 1983; 31:21–27.

234. Lucas F, Sclafani A. Hyperphagia in rats produced by a mixture of fat and sugar. Physiol Behav 1990; 47:51–55.

235. Ramirez I, Friedman MI. Dietary hypophagia in rats: role of fat, carbohydrate and energy content. Physiol Behav 1990; 47:1157–163.

236. Umpleby AM, Sonksen, PH. The chalonic action of insulin in man. In: Garrow JS, Halliday D, eds. Substrate and Energy Metabolism. London: Libbey, 1985:169–178.

237. Eckel RH. Lipoprotein lipase: a multifunctional enzyme relevant to common metabolic diseases. N Engl J Med 1989; 320:1060–1068.

238. Flatt JP. Energetics of intermediary metabolism. In: Garrow JS, Halliday D, eds. Substrate and Energy Metabolism in Man. London: Libbey, 1985:58.

239. Salmon DM, Flatt JP. Effect of dietary fat on the incidence of obesity among ad libitum fed mice. Int J Obes 1985; 9:443–449.

240. Kendall A, Levitsky DA, Strupp BJ, Lissner L. Weight loss on a low-fat diet: consequence of the imprecision of the control of food intake in humans. Am J Clin Nutr 1991; 53:1124–1129.

241. Burggraf KK, Willing AE, Koopmans HS. The effects of glucose or lipid infused intravenously or intragstrically on voluntary food intake in the rat. Physiol Behav (in press).

242. Hill JO, Melby C, Johnson SL, Peters JC. Physical activity and energy requirements. Am J Clin Nutr 1995; 62: 1059S–1066S.

243. Pi-Sunyer FX. The fattening of America. JAMA 272: 238–239, 1994.

15

Behavioral Neuroscience of Obesity

Sarah F. Leibowitz
The Rockefeller University, New York, New York

Bartley G. Hoebel
Princeton University, Princeton, New Jersey

I. INTRODUCTION

An animal's brain monitors energy in the environment and within the body and then adjusts eating behavior, energy utilization, and fat stores to maintain a balance. This chapter will discuss how the brain performs this life-giving task. The brain integrates energy-related sensory information, collected from the eyes, ears, nose, tongue, gastrointestinal tract, liver, pancreas, and blood, through receptors specialized to detect nutrient-rich molecules. The hypothalamus is one of the areas that uses this information to adjust physiological functions for storing or utilizing energy at appropriate times. The hypothalamus also contributes to the control of food intake by interacting with mechanisms for voluntary behavior that are essential for obtaining food. This physiological and behavioral control involves connections to the pituitary for endocrine regulation, connections to the hindbrain that subserve essential feeding reflexes, and circuits extending to forebrain systems for choosing, instigating, and reinforcing voluntary behavior. These circuits allow the brain to adjust its physiology and behavior to meet the economic demands of the ecological niche in which the animal lives. We have chosen the hypothalamus as a "base of operations" from which to survey the neuroscience of food intake and obesity.

A. Chapter Outline

This chapter has five parts. (1) It describes most of the known neurochemical systems for controlling eating and body weight (biogenic amines, peptides, proteins, acetylcholine, and amino acids); (2) it relates the hypothalamic components of these systems to endocrine signals that modulate their activity; (3) it relates the hypothalamus to brain circuits for voluntary behavior; (4) it describes disturbances in these neurochemical systems in animal models of obesity or diabetes; and (5) it interprets this evidence in relation to clinical problems and potential therapeutics.

Early investigations of neurochemical mechanisms underlying obesity focused on the monamine neurotransmitters, norepinephrine (NE), dopamine (DA), and serotonin (5-HT), that alter the sensitivity of various brain circuits to biological rhythms and energy homeostasis. Then, peptides were discovered that modulate nutrient balance. These include neuropeptide Y (NPY) and galanin (GAL), which function in the brain to stimulate eating behavior and enhance body weight. These are in contrast to numerous peptides that inhibit feeding. For example, cholecystokinin (CCK), enterostatin (ENT), and glucagon-like peptide 1 (GLP-1) are manufactured in the periphery but also possibly in the brain where they act on specific receptors. Corticotropin-releasing hormone (CRH), oxytocin (OT), and neurotensin (NT) are synthesized in local hypothalamic neurons. Most recently, the protein leptin, produced in adipose tissue, has been isolated and found to act on brain receptors to inhibit feeding and reduce body weight. Many other neurotransmitters and neuromodulators are involved in basic sensorimotor processes, perception, learning, and memory. However, it is the particular monoamines and peptides such as these that are coded for energy-related processes that have served as model systems for unlocking the secrets of the brain for body weight control.

Recent research links these neurochemical systems to powerful endocrine influences. Hormones with metabolic actions in the periphery are controlled and released by signals from the brain; however, they also feed back to have potent effects on the activity of the central systems. These hormones, including the adrenal steroid, corticosterone (CORT), and the pancreatic hormone, insulin, fluctuate markedly in relation to physiological states and biological rhythms. Their interaction with brain neurotransmitters and neuromodulators is critical in determining specific states of nutrient balance and weight gain.

Eating behavior varies enormously depending on the availability of food. People in the frozen north may hunt for days and then eat huge meals and store the excess calories as fat in the manner of many carnivores. The same people in a temperate climate may nibble throughout the day in the manner of a grazing herbivore. To adjust to these extremes, the person's brain encodes and remembers stimuli that represent places, tastes, and nutritious aftereffects of eating. Conditioned stimuli then serve to prime appropriate behavior in the future. Thus, the hypothalamus is part of a massive neural system devoted to encoding, remembering, and choosing stimuli that give rise to instrumental responses for obtaining food before it is actually needed.

Animal models of overeating and obesity include genetically inbred strains, with spontaneous or experimentally induced gene mutations, and outbred strains, with distinct phenotypes but no identified genetic variation. Studies with these rodent stains involve measurements of endogenous neurochemicals and of responses to injected compounds. These investigations have yielded new information on possible interactions between genes and environment and how disturbances in these brain systems may contribute to the development or maintenance of obesity.

The brain has a central role in integrating these different functions. Therefore, it is clinically important to explore these neurochemical and neuroendocrine processes with regard to both the body's energy stores and the ani-

mal's behavior. Characterization of the systems will eventually allow one to link specific gene products, receptor subtypes, neuronal cell groups, and brain pathways to a precise physiological or behavioral trait related to nutrient balance. This information pertaining to normal conditions is essential for understanding disturbances that underlie obesity. It lays the groundwork for identifying pharmacological, nutritional, and behaviorial strategies that are effective in the treatment of this disorder.

B. Brain Areas

In studying brain neurochemicals, it is essential to identify the precise areas and cell groups of the brain that are critical for their effects on body weight regulation and eating behavior. Recent studies of the hypothalamus in laboratory rats reveal specific nuclei or regions that have a direct role in maintaining energy or nutrient balance (Fig. 1). These include the paraventricular nucleus (PVN), ventromedial hypothalamus (VMH), and dorsomedial nucleus (DMN), which control both nutrient intake and metabolism. The medial preoptic area (MPO) just anterior to the PVN is involved in reproductive physiology, which shifts with metabolic fuels and body weight, notably at puberty and during pregnancy. The arcuate nucleus (ARC) and median eminence (ME) in the basomedial hypothalamus control anterior pituitary hormone secretion in relation to nutrient balance. The suprachiasmatic nucleus (SCN) is the master controller of circadian rhythms for both physiological and behavioral processes.

Along with these medial hypothalamic (MH) nuclei there is the lateral hypothalamus (LH), which is like a city train station with a welter of nerve fibers passing through, local circuitry and sensory cell groups (Fig. 1). The complexity of the LH is reflected in the scientific history of this region, which Stellar characterized as a "feeding center" (1). The LH contains glucose-sensitive cells, feeding-related neurons with monoamine and peptide receptors, nerve fibers involved in feeding reward, and fibers of passage subserving motive functions. The perifornical region within the LH (pfLH) may be specialized for potentiating feeding reflexes and reinforcing voluntary motor functions of ingestive behavior. As portrayed in Figure 1 and discussed in the section on DA, some LH fibers support stimulation-induced eating and reinforce self-stimulation. They are shown to be part of a reinforcement circuit from the pfLH to brainstem nuclei, such as the parabrachial nucleus (PBN) and nucleus of the solitary tract (NTS). These nuclei integrate descending information with primary taste input and ascending autonomic signals from the gut. Part of the ascending brainstem output goes to cortical sensory areas, and part goes to as-

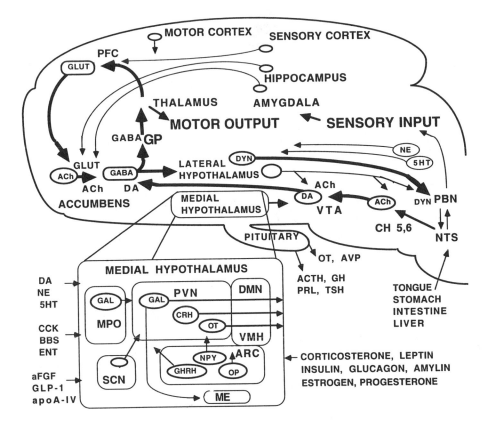

Figure 1 Schematic side view of the brain with emphasis on the medial hypothalamic area (expanded box) and two neural loops (bold arrows). The expanded view of the medial hypothalamus indicates some of the local feeding and satiety neurons and their inputs. For example, galanin cells in the medial preoptic area (MPO) are shown projecting to the paraventricular nucleus (PVN), and these PVN neurons project to the median eminence (ME). The gonadal steroids, estrogen and progesterone, stimulate galanin (GAL) mRNA in the MPO and PVN and thereby affect GAL levels in the ME at puberty when fat ingestion and body fat rise markedly. The NPY neurocircuit projects from neurons in the arcuate (ARC) to terminals in the PVN. This circuit monitors and controls carbohydrate intake and metabolism. Growth hormone–releasing hormone (GHRH) neurons in the ARC project to the MPO and suprachiasmatic nucleus (SCN) and are involved in protein ingestion. Two peptides synthesized in the PVN, corticotrophin-releasing hormone (CRH) and oxytocin (OT), have inhibitory effects on feeding and body weight through projections descending to the hindbrain. The opioids (OP) that are synthesized in the ARC project to multiple brain areas and control both reward and feeding processes. The ventromedial hypothalamus and dorsomedial nucleus are also likely contributors to these neurochemical systems. The circulating hormones corticosterone, leptin, insulin, amylin, glucagon, and the gonadal steroids directly influence the activity of these hypothalamic peptide circuits. Other peptides, cholecystokinin (CCK), bombesin (BBS), enterostatin (ENT), apolipoprotein A-IV (apo A-IV), glucagon-like protein 1 (GLP-1), and acidic fibroblast growth factor (aFGF) also impact on these hypothalamic systems. The biogenic amines dopamine (DA), serotonin (5HT), and norepinephrine (NE) are synthesized in brainstem neurons and innervate the hypothalamic nuclei. Some hormones, such as OT, arginine vasopressin (AVP), growth hormone (GH), adreno-corticotropic hormone (ACTH), and prolactin (PRL), are stored and released in the pituitary; these also modulate eating behavior and body weight. The medial hypothalamus is part of a much larger feeding circuit. Starting in the lower right corner, signals from the tongue and gut enter the brainstem to activate hindbrain structures, the nucleus tractus solitarius (NTS) and parabrachial nucleus (PBN), which ascend to the forebrain. The hypothalamus also senses chemosensory information and sends it to the brainstem. The NTS output goes to the sensory cortex and to the amygdala and hippocampus. Here chemosensory information is combined with other sense modalities (sights, sounds, locations, and codes for safe nutrition vs. toxic foods). The arrows from the hippocampus (place memory), amygdala (emotion memory), and prefrontal cortex (complex choice memory) sweep into the nucleus accumbens (NAc) on glutamate (GLUT) neurons. The NAc is basically a highly encephalinized sensorimotor interface in the cognitive/limbic loop drawn in bold lines from prefrontal cortex (PFC) to the NAc then globus pallidus (GP) and back to the PFC with commands branching off to motor output circuits. The short acetylcholine (ACh) neurons in the NAc may act as gates that are modulated by DA from the ventral tegmental area (VTA) along with NE, 5HT, and OP discussed in the text. The medial and lateral hypothalamus help control the NAc via the loop shown, from the hypothalamus to the VTA and brainstem including a dynorphin (DYN) link, then to cholinergic (CH) cell groups 5 and 6, to the VTA, and to the NAc where DA can be released. By this route, feeding signals can influence DA/ACh balance in the NAc to reinforce or inhibit instrumental behavior for food.

cending acetylcholine (Ach) neurons (J. Connell and B. G. Hoebel, unpublished observations) that connect to mid-brain dopaminergic fibers in the ventral tegmental area (VTA). These DA fibers ascend back through the LH on their way forward to the entirelimbic system including the nucleus accumbens (NAc). The NAc is one of the limbic areas projecting to the LH, thus forming the loop shown in Figure 1.

The prefontal cortex (PFC) takes cortical sensory taste information, transforms it to reflect sensory specific satiety (2) and likely sends it in part to the NAc. The NAc also receives multimodal sensory information from the amygdala and hippocampus, reflecting good and bad experiences with tastes, smells, sights, sounds, and important places in the environment. The NAc output courses its way to motor command systems. Part goes via the globus pallidus (GP), and part descends through the LH to the VTA (not shown). The GP instructs the motor system and feeds back in the loop shown going to the PFC (Fig. 1). The NAc lies at the intersection of these two loops. It serves as a sensorimotor interface that is gated in part by the hypothalamus. These circuits are described in greater detail in Section VII.

C. Sympathetic/Parasympathetic Nervous Systems

The LH and MH have autonomic effects that are in some ways opposite. Lesions in the LH, depending on the exact location, can cause the well-known syndrome of aphagia, sensory neglect, and motor impairment (3,4) and can disinhibit sympathetic signs such as peripheral NE release. Conversely, electrical stimulation of the LH can promote eating, self-stimulation, and parasympathetic functions in peripheral tissues as evidenced by increased cholinergic tone (5–8).

In the MH, electrical stimulation inhibits eating and is aversive. It increases sympathetic neural output to brown adipose tissue (BAT) and stimulates glucose uptake in skeletal muscles (8). Lesions of the MH, including the PVN, cause overeating and an elevated plateau for body weight maintenance (9,10). Ventromedial hypothalamic damage may also destroy neurons necessary for inhibition of peripheral insulin secretion (11). This leads to hyperinsulinemia that is proportional to the elevated level of body weight (12). These lesions unsettle the autonomic nervous system by creating an animal with excessive parasympathetic tone (6).

A similar state of parasympathetic dominance occurs in animals that are genetically obese (13) and in obese men (14). They deposit excess fat with or without overeating, although they do generally overeat, and this hyperphagia further exacerbates their obesity. Spontaneous food intake

is inversely correlated with sympathetic activity (15,16). Paradoxically, low sympathetic tone can be found in both underweight and overweight animals. One possible explanation is that the "overweight" animals may actually be "underweight" in relation to their weight plateau. This is the familiar description of the VMH-lesioned animals, which in their dynamic phase are overeaters and gain weight but are actually underweight relative to their own eventual weight level (9). Thus, as suggested by Bray, low sympathetic activity reflects not only high food intake but also the tendency or "potential" to eat. Perhaps any animal that is under its preferred weight level for a given diet can have a large feeding potential coupled with low sympathetic activity. This could include food-deprived animals, VMH-lesioned animals in the dynamic phase, genetically obese animals, or dietary obese animals that are denied their palatable diet.

The sympathetic nervous system is implicitly defined as primarily an energy output system; the parasympathetic system is considered on the input side of the equation. Energy output on a given food ration can be divided into the thermic effect of food (body heat production), physical exercise, and metabolic rate, all of which affect body weight. A person or animal that is eating normally but gaining weight might have low levels of any of these three output pathways. Described next are a few correlates of these autonomic functions that have been linked to neuropharmacology.

The thermic effect of food refers to the amount of heat produced (thermogenesis) above and beyond basal metabolic rate (17). This measure changes with the animal's weight and is closely related to body fat. When a normal animal or person gains weight by overeating and depositing fat, the thermic effect of a meal increases. This allows the subject to adapt to the extra fat by squandering heat and curtailing further weight gain. During the dynamic phase of overeating after VMH lesions, the thermic effect of food remains low while the animal gains weight rapidly. This low heat production may signal an impaired sympathetic state that occurs in cases of impending obesity (16). High body temperature not only gets rid of unneeded calories; it also inhibits food intake via a histaminergic system in the hypothalamus (18). A hot rat usually eats less (19), and histamine and its receptors may play a role. Thus histamine provides a new pharamacological avenue to control appetite.

Physical activity accounts for a considerable amount of energy expenditure. Hyperactivity contributes to weight loss, whereas a sedentary life can lead to obesity. Food-restricted rats conserve energy by becoming less active and more reactive (20). With the availability of a running wheel, underweight rats may display hyperactivity that exacerbates their weight loss (21). When food is restricted to about 80% of normal body weight, rats exhibit marked changes in the brain, such as a decline in basal levels of DA in the NAc (22,23) leading them to engage in behaviors that release DA (see below). Low basal DA is also observed in the NAc of genetically obese Zucker rates (24). Both the underweight and obese rats can be hypoactive.

The third factor on the output side is basal metabolic rate. By using a computerized metabolism cage that corrects for temperature and activity, Nicolaidis and Even (25) discovered a decline in background metabolism just before a meal. Campfield and Smith (26) show that blood glucose also falls before meals, and as the body's metabolism changes and glucose levels start to rise, the animal initiates a meal. Under controlled conditions, the nadir in blood glucose level is so reliable as a predictor of a meal that one must assume the brain can respond to glucose dynamics or, more likely, to the chemical factors that reverse the decline in glucose. This is a revival of Mayer's glucostatic theory (27). However, Friedman et al. (28) point out that the liver plays a powerful role in responding to fat as well as glucose and creates "metabolic sensations" via vagal signals that are transformed into brain perceptions. Through measurements of the immediate early gene product, c-fos, as an indication of cellular activity, Calingasan and Ritter (29) confirm that the hypothalamus is one of several brain areas that changes its activity in response to decreased utilization of either glucose or fat. Nicolaidis and Even (25) encompass both glucostasis and lipostasis in the suggestion that fuels for the brain are monitored in the hypothalamus as a microcosmic representation of the whole body. Bernadis and Bellinger review the idea that the LH senses its own intermediary metabolism (30).

In summary, a simplified heuristic for remembering hypothalamic functions is to imagine the LH region as a source of output signals that instruct the animal to eat and release insulin. As a meal progresses, MH cell groups send out satiety signals that generally inhibit these parasympathetic functions. Neurochemical inputs that dampen this satiety function (causing disinhibition) can lead to overeating and weight gain until a new higher weight plateau is reached. This complimentary LH versus MH excitatory/inhibitory schema, based on Stellar's original concept (1), is useful for understanding historical developments and formulating general hypotheses. Modern advances in behavioral neuroscience are starting to reveal the complexity and elegance of hypothalamic circuits with multiple transmitters, each with multiple receptors and dynamic properties for controlling specific macronutrients and learned voluntary behaviors.

D. Neuroendocrine Systems

An important function of the hypothalamus is to control hormone secretion from the anterior and posterior pituitary that, in turn, influences hormone synthesis in target organs. Hypothalamic neurosecretory cells produce peptides that are delivered to the portal blood vessels and are transported to the anterior pituitary. These brain peptides include CRH, luteinizing hormone-releasing hormone (LHRH), and thyrotropin-releasing hormone (TRH). The respective pituitary hormones they regulate are adrenocorticotropic hormone (ACTH), luteinizing hormone (LH), and thyroid-stimulating hormone (TSH). These trophic hormones then impact on target glands to stimulate the production, respectively, of the adrenal steroid, corticosterone (CORT); the gonadal steriods, estradiol (E_2) and progesterone (P); and the thyroid hormone, thyroxine. In addition, there are other hypothalamic neurons that synthesize the peptides arginine vasopression (AVP) and OT and send axons to the posterior pituitary where they end in close proximity to the vascular bed of the gland, store, and release their neurosecretory products directly into the blood stream. Each of these hormones, controlled by the hypothalamus and releaseed by the pituitary, has potent metabolic actions in peripheral tissues that affect body fat. In addition, they impact on the brain to produce complex behavioral and physiological responses related to the intake and metabolism of nutrients. As described below, this process is mediated through feedback actions of these hormones on the brain neurochemicals involved in energy balance.

II. BIOGENIC AMINES IN THE CONTROL OF EATING BEHAVIOR AND METABOLISM

Through pharmacological and biochemical studies, specific neurotransmitters and peptides have been identified within the hypothalamic areas and implicated in physiological and behavioral processes that impact on body weight. It is now clear that there is great redundancy involving multiple neurochemicals and their actions, both stimulatory and inhibitory, on eating and metabolism. These systems are activated under diverse physiological states and environmental conditions that affect an organism during its lifetime. This section reviews the evidence implicating biogenic amines in these processes. This is followed by subsequent sections on the peptides, amino acids, and steroids.

A. Norepinephrine

There is support for a strong circadian rhythm of hypothalamic NE and its receptors, suggesting that it plays an important role in the animal's overall state of arousal. Measurements of NE release, receptor activity, and neuronal firing demonstrate a peak at the onset of the natural feeding cycle (31,32). The more excited the animal becomes, the faster noradrenergic neurons fire (33). While this suggests a general role for NE in brain arousal, NE additionally modulates specific types of motivation such as food consumption (Fig. 1).

Hypothalamic injections of NE can have very specific behavioral effefcts (34–36). When injected into the PVN, it enhances lab chow intake, and when a choice of macronutrients is allowed, NE causes a preferential increase in the ingestion of carbohydrate, compared to fat or protein. NE increases body weight after chronic injection in the VMH, and also in the PVN when the animal can express hyperphagia for carbohydrate (10). This catecholamine induces feeding via α_2-noradrenergic receptors concentrated in the PVN. Local administration of antagonists of α_2-receptors reduces feeding. The strongest effect of NE can be seen at the onset of the natural feeding cycle. This shows that physiological rhythms are critical in understanding its function. The same is true of peptides, notably NPY, with which NE coexists, as discussed below.

The arousal effect of NE is consistent with its close interaction with the adrenal steroid, CORT (36,37). Blood levels of this glucocorticoid rise just prior to the active cycle when it has an important role in arousal. It also activates the NE system in the PVN by potentiating α_2-receptor binding and increasing the NE-induced feeding response. The rise in circulating CORT coincides with a natural rise in extracellular NE in the PVN at the onset of the active period (32,38) in association with an increase in appetite for carbohydrate (39). As indicated below, CORT also fosters a rise in blood glucose at the same time that it stimulates carbohydrate intake (37).

As a consequence of this relationship with CORT and perhaps other feeding-stimulatory neurochemicals reviewed below, NE injections in the MH region have effects that are similar to those produced by lesions in this region, including increased food intake, parasympathetic activity, and body weight. Therefore, it appears that NE inhibits, and MH lesions destroy, various satiety signals (40) and sympathetic functions (15). Figure 1 sketches the PVN-MH "satiety" function as part of a descending system, although this is an oversimplification. Not shown is the in-

hibition of the satiety function by the ascending dorsal noradrenergic bundle, which may be a source of the NE that acts at α_2-receptor sites to disinhibit eating (40).

In contrast to NE's feeding-stimulatory action on α_2-noradrenergic receptors, the α_1-receptor subtype in the PVN mediates feeding suppression (35,41). Injections of α_1-agonists reduce food consumption, while specific α_1-antagonists stimulate feeding. A notable example of a drug acting on these receptors is the popular over-the-counter agent phenylpropanolamine. It is effective in the short term in reducing body weight (42) and inhibits feeding by acting on α_1-receptors in the PVN (43). The density of both α_1- and α_2-receptors can vary with body weight (44), which provides support for their role in weight regulation.

Radiolabeled anorectic drugs can be used to mark sites in the brain where they bind (45). Amphetamine (AMPH) and mazindol bind particularly well in the PVN and VMH. Their binding here is reduced by food deprivation in association with a decline in blood glucose. This phenomenon is similar to a glucose-dependant decline reported for α_2-receptor binding in the PVN (46). Based on this, Angel (45) hypothesized that anorectic drug binding inhibits α_2-receptors, thereby reducing carbohydrate intake. Amphetamine is also effective in the LH via other monoamine receptors, as discusssed next.

While the focus of these studies has been on NE's action at α-noradrenergic receptors in the PVN, there is evidence that the LH responds differently. In the perifornical region of the LH, NE or epinephrine suppresses feeding behavior via β-adrenergic receptors (47,48). Destruction of a subset of noradrenergic and adrenergic neurons in the ventral midbrain bundle that projects in part to the hypothalamus causes hyperphagia and body weight gain (42,49). Thus, adrenergic inputs can have different effects on feeding depending on the site of innervation and the receptors that predominate. As a general rule, α_2-receptors foster feeding, while α_1- and β-adrenergic receptors reduce feeding. This pattern of control in the brain may have its counterpart in the periphery where the net lipolytic effect of catecholamines is dependent on a similar functional balance between α_2- and β-adrenergic receptors in fat cells (50).

B. Serotonin

As with NE, circadian changes in the firing rate of serotonergic neurons suggest that they also play an important role in the animal's overall state of arousal. An animal's level of excitement rises as 5-HT neurons fire faster (33). Serotonergic activation is most evident at the onset of the natural feeding cycle. Injection studies show that 5-HT at this time suppresses carbohydrate intake by an action on

MH nuclei including the PVN and VMH (Fig. 1) (51, 52). Microdialysis studies show a significant increase in 5-HT release during the meal (53). Extracellular 5-HT may also increase before the animal starts to eat in reaction to the sight and smell of food (54, 55). Additional 5-HT is released as the animal consumes the food, but it declines to baseline levels over the next 30 min. This time course is consistent with an anticipatory and short postingestive satiety effect for 5-HT rather than a long-lasting action. Perhaps 5-HT potentiates systems for satiety that require postingestive signals in order to become active.

Biogenic amines often have effects that depend on other local neurochemical signals. Hypothalamic 5-HT may act in synergy with other peptides that produce satiety (56), acting when appropriate postingestive signals are present to release cofactors, such as CCK, in the hypothalamus. This peptide may come from serotonergic neurons as a cotransmitter and have longer-lasting effects on feeding than the monoamine alone. CCK may also be released in the hypothalamus in response to vagal inputs that are relayed from the stomach to the hypothalamus (49). The proposal that 5-HT and CCK work together is further supported by the finding that 5-HT receptor blockers antagonize CCK's anorectic effect (57, 58).

The compound, *d*-fenfluramine (Isomeride or Redux), is an anorectic drug that is a 5-HT reuptake blocker at low doses and a releaser of 5-HT at higher doses (59–61). Consistent with results obtained with 5-HT, the feeding-suppressive effect of *d*-fenfluramine is attenuated by various 5-HT receptor antagonists (62–65). Thus, the actions of 5-HT as well as *d*-fenfluramine, or its active metabolite norfenfluramine, may involve specific 5-HT receptors that provide some degree of behavioral specificity. *d*-Fenfluramine additionally increases background metabolism by enhancing utilization of the body's fuels (25). This increased metabolism contributes to weight loss and possibly also to the decrease in food intake.

Serotonin may act, in part, via an inhibitory action on the α_2-noradrenergic system of the MH (35,65). Serotonin and *d*-fenfluramine reduce the hyperphagic actions of NE in the PVN, especially carbohydrate intake. This may explain why *d*-fenfluramine is sold primarily to treat carbohydrate craving and related obesity (66). The interaction between NE and 5-HT may also be a mechanism through which this drug indirectly inhibits the self-stimulation system related to feeding reinforcement (67), thereby contributing to its appetite-reducing property (68).

It is clear that there are other sites, besides the MH, where 5-HT acts in the control of feeding behavior and metabolism. For example, diets with an amino acid imbalance cause primary anorexia and conditioned taste aversion. This effect, which is blocked by 5-HT antagonists, is mediated in part through actions in the piriform cortex (69). Serotonin also contributes to postingestive onset of satiety through brainstem structures (70) as well as its potent actions in the periphery (71).

C. Dopamine

Dopamine and AMPH-related compounds have long been known to suppress feeding through their action in the hypothalamus. However, the full story of DA's actions in the brain is only beginning to unfold. In the hypothalamus, DA has effects in the LH and MH. It also has powerful actions related to feeding behavior in other brain regions, notably the NAc where it is a behavior reinforcer (Fig. 1).

1. Dopamine in the Hypothalamus

Hypothalamic DA contributes to AMPH-induced anorexia (72–74). This is of renewed interest due to the recent upsurge in the use of the dopaminergic and noradrenergic drug, phentermine (75), in combination with *d,l*-fenfluramine, for treatment of obesity (76,77). A variety of catecholaminergic effects may occur in the hypothalamus depending on the site of intervention and the experimental technique used. Hypothalamic DA is released, in part, from an incertohypothalamic cell group, from MH neurons intimately involved in the control of pituitary functions (78), and from DA cell groups (A8, A9, A10) that ascend from the midbrain. Injections of DA in the LH suppress food intake, an action blocked specifically by DA receptor antagonists (72,73). Anorectic doses of AMPH injected in the LH increase extracellular DA, although NE and 5-HT are also increased (79). All three monoamines may suppress feeding and mediate the actions of AMPH under different conditions (40,48,54, 74,80).

As further evidence of a DA satiety function in the LH, some compounds that block DA receptors stimulate eating behavior. This was demonstrated with the nonspecific receptor antagonist chlorpromazine and with the specific D_2-receptor antagonist sulpiride (40,81). Chronic peripheral injections of sulpiride cause hyperphagia and obesity in rats, analogous to the effect sometimes seen in schizophrenic patients undergoing antipsychotic treatment with D_2-antagonists (73,81). This effect may be due, in part, to dopaminergic control of pituitary functions controlling E_2 release (82), or to disinhibition of a behavior reinforcement system that leads to overeating. Sulpiride in the LH has locomotor and reward effects like self-stimulation of the LH (81). Thus, DA can act at hypothalamic D_2-receptors to inhibit instrumental responses, including responses involved in eating.

Using microdialysis to measure extracellular DA, Orosco and Nicolaidis (83) correlated DA release in the MH with eating behavior. Meguid et al. (84) propose that taste and smell may enhance the release of hypothalamic DA at the start of a meal, to organize autonomic reflexes for receiving food. Then, postingestive signals from the liver may subsequently inhibit DA release in both the MH and LH. Diabetic rats that are hyperphagic show enhanced DA turnover in the VMH (85). Thus, DA release may influence eating as well as satiety, depending on the overall state of the systems and their multiple receptor subtypes.

Recording studies in monkeys have found taste-responsive cells in the hypothalamus that are sensitive to DA (86). Some of these cells are tuned to features of the animal's external environment. Other cells that are glucose-sensitive are for monitoring the internal state.

Cells in the hypothalamus, some of which are responsive to DA, influence feeding via an output that connects to the mesolimbic DA system, which passes back through the hypothalamus on its way to the NAc (Fig. 1). As a clear demonstration of this, a DA antagonist injected in the LH causes the release of DA in the NAc (81,87). In the PVN, the feeding-stimulatory peptide GAL also increases NAc DA, as described in Section III. Thus, DA or GAL in the hypothalamus can control the accumbens DA system in an antagonistic fashion and thereby influence eating behavior.

2. Dopamine as a Behavior Reinforcer in the Mesolimbic System

Neurons projecting from the VTA to the NAc can reinforce behavior and are sometimes involved in motivation (87–89). This seems to be based on a dual role in instrumental and classical conditioning. Dopamine is released in the NAc by behavior such as self-stimulation, psychostimulant self-administration, and eating (90–94). Self-stimulation or stimulation-induced feeding in the LH releases DA in the NAc, with or without food present (95). When food-deprived rats eat a meal, DA release in the NAc may be especially salient because the baseline level is low (22,23,96). In addition, DA can be released in the NAc by classically conditioned stimuli, as discussed below.

An increase in extracellular DA in the NAc can be a positive reinforcer. This is shown in rats with NAc cannules for self-injection of AMPH or DA directly into that region (97,98). When rats self-administer cocaine intravenously, they respond in a manner that raises extracellular DA whenever it falls to a low level (99). Neurochemicals are reinforcers if they stimulate DA cells in the VTA,

prime examples being opiates and neurotensin (100,101). This means that the mesolimbic DA system activates a reinforcement process (by definition, a reinforcer increases instrumental responding). Therefore, DA is probably a reinforcer when released by self-stimulation, drugs, or natural behavior such as eating, mating, aggression, and associated stimuli. It appears from a teleological point of view that animals perform voluntary behavior to get the effects of DA release in the NAc and perhaps in other forebrain sites such as the PFC (102).

Dopamine in the NAc is also involved in reinforcing behavior to escape an aversive stimulus. Extracellular DA increases during MH stimulation-escape behavior but not during the same stimulation when it is inescapable (87). Thus, DA may be a negative reinforcer for active escape as well as a positive reinforcer for active approach in feeding situations.

3. Taste Reactions and Dopamine

Dopamine antagonists administered systemically or directly into the NAc block locomotion, instrumental behavior, and sucrose intake (103). Results with the DA antagonist raclopride are particularly interesting. An animal drinking sucrose, with a fistula so it never gets full, acts as if the sucrose has been diluted when treated with this DA blocker. The avidity for sweet taste diminishes when raclopride is given systemically or locally in the NAc (104). Reinforcement may involve both D_1- and D_2-receptors. The literature on this is not clear due to the discovery of new receptor subtypes, the nonspecificity of some pharmaceutical agents, multiple facets of reinforcement, and multiple actions in many brain regions such as the hypothalamus and NAc (105).

A definitive role for mesolimbic DA has been demonstrated by neural recordings from DA cells in the VTA of awake monkeys. Some of the neurons that project to the NAc increase their firing rate during eating (106). As the monkey gains practice at the feeding task, neural activity precedes food presentation. It coincides instead with discriminative stimuli that are a sign of forthcoming food. Thus, with experience, DA release becomes allied with conditioned stimuli and perhaps with secondary reinforcers. This suggests that mesolimbic DA in primates is involved in learning what, where, and when to eat, more than in the act of eating.

4. Body Weight and Dopamine

Microdialysis shows that basal extracellular DA may be as low as half normal in rats at 80% of free-feeding body weight (22,23). Given the demonstration that rats respond for cocaine when accumbens DA decreases to a certain level (99), it is quite possible that animals also respond for food when DA reaches a low level. Drug self-administration, self-stimulation, and eating are all potentiated by food deprivation (107–109), and they all can increase extracellular DA in the NAc. It is therefore likely that animals or people with diminished amounts of DA, for any reason, may have a tendency to take foods or drugs that restore DA.

Although DA depletion in the nigrostriatal pathway causes aphagia and weight loss (110), rats can still eat when DA is depleted in the NAc. For example, Sodersten et al. (111) used 6-hydroxydopamine to deplete accumbens DA to 16% of normal and found that rats can still swallow a normal amount of sucrose when delivered directly into the mouth. Dopamine-depleted animals eat normally when the food is easy to get, but they opt not to perform difficult tasks (112). Rats that bar-press for cocaine and food pellets in alternation stop responding for the dopaminergic drug when DA is depleted, but they still bar-press for food (113). Apparently, accumbens DA serves partly as a priming signal that activates the systems needed for difficult tasks, for learning or switching behavior (114, 115). For simple tasks, other areas such as the striatum, hypothalamus, midbrain, and brainstem may be sufficient. A decerebrate rate, with no forebrain at all, can still swallow food put in its mouth and reject it when full. Thus, the caudal brainstem participates strongly in neural control of feeding (116).

5. Classical Conditioning of Neurotransmitter Release

Dopamine released by a conditioned stimulus, such as a taste, a place, or even an advertisement, may prime instrumental behavior leading to more DA release. When DA is low, as during food restriction, a conditioned stimulus is needed to release the initial DA and start the behavior. Dopamine release in the NAc can be conditioned with food flavors. A flavor associated with intragastric feeding becomes a preferred flavor (117) that releases DA in the NAc (55). Conversely, a flavor that reminds the animal of lithium-induced nausea causes extracellular DA to decrease (118). Thus, conditioned DA release in the NAc probably plays an important role in the animal's decision to approach or avoid food.

There are several components to behavior reinforcement. These include the facets people think of as motivation, drive, wanting or willingness to work, plus the hedonic aspect involved in liking and pleasure and other related concepts such as incentive and satisfaction. Researchers are currently engaged in the fascinating enterprise of dissecting out the roles of DA, as well as opioid

peptides and other neurotransmitters, in these aspects of the total reinforcement process (88,89,102,119–121).

D. Histamine

Histamine, which is synthesized from histidine, is well known for its role in regulating body temperature and stimulating drinking (122,123). Neuronal histamine, in addition, is involved in the regulation of feeding, mastication, and circadian rhythms (123–126). Peripheral histidine injections that increase brain histamine levels cause a concomitant decrease in food intake. Peripheral or ventricular administration of drugs that block histamine receptors enhance feeding. In the hypothalamus, food-deprived rats show increased levels of endogenous histamine, and obese rats exhibit reduced levels (127,128). Pharmacological activation of hypothalamic histamine suppresses feeding through the H_1-receptor subtype. Sites of action include the PVN and VMH, areas richest in histamine and H_1-receptors. Iontophoretic application of H_1-antagonists suppresses neuronal activity in these areas.

Sakata et al. (123) propose a role for hypothalamic histamine in the homeostatic control of energy stores. Fasting and 2-deoxy-D-glucose as well as insulin-induced hypoglycemia all stimulate the turnover of histamine. The essential stimulant is a reduction in glucose utilization and a consequent histamine-dependent decrease in brain glycogen to maintain brain glucose availability. A further role for histamine may be reflected in the impact of high ambient temperatures, which elevate hypothalamic histamine and suppress food intake (129). Histamine injected into the preoptic area reduces body temperature (130). This process of histaminergic thermoregulation raises the possibility that this biogenic amine is also involved in changes of ingestive behavior and body temperature induced by interleukin-1β, which is released in response to infection, injury, and inflammation (129). Ventricular injection of the cytokine suppresses food intake and induces thermogenesis (131,132). These responses, which are accompanied by a rise in histamine turnover, are attenuated by depletion of neuronal histamine in the hypothalamus (133).

III. PEPTIDES THAT INCREASE EATING AND BODY WEIGHT

In studies over the past decade, attention has focused on the peptides that alter eating and body weight with greater potency and longer duration of action relative to the biogenic amines. This section will describe findings obtained with peptides that have stimulatory actions on eating behavior. The following section will examine a larger number of peptides, as well as a few proteins, that function in an inhibitory fashion. These peptides may act in both the periphery and brain, either as neurotransmitters or as paracrine (local acting) and endocrine (long distance) hormones. In some cases, these peptides produce similar effects peripherally and centrally to provide an integrative functional output. In a model case, brain angiotensin neurons are part of a circuit that raises blood pressure in different ways, including stimulation of salt intake and drinking behavior (134,135). Conversely, there is a peptide, atrial naturetic factor, that performs a variety of functions to decrease fluid intake and lower blood pressure (136). The coordinated brain/body functioning of coded peptides gives rise to the integrative peptide theory, which has been a useful heuristic in the study of peptides that increase or decrease eating and body weight (49,137–139).

A. Neuropeptide Y

Evidence indicates that NPY controls the body's nutrient stores through complex behavioral and metabolic actions. It functions via a local hypothalamic circuit as well as through its actions on peripheral organs, including adipose tissue. It controls the secretion of many hormones and is distinguished by its responsiveness to the feedback actions of these hormones and to environmental stimuli that influence hormonal secretion. Neuropeptide Y exhibits temporal patterns of endogenous activity in relation to natural physiological states or stages that, in turn, are accompanied by specific changes in circulating hormones, eating behavior, and nutrient metabolism.

The available evidence links the NPY system to states of carbohydrate ingestion and utilization that shift substrates toward fat synthesis (140–142). The neurocircuit underlying this neurochemical action involves a dense NPY projection that originates in neurons of the ARC and terminates in the medial portion of the PVN (Fig. 1). This projection functions in close association with two circulating hormones involved in glucose homeostatis, namely, CORT and insulin.

I. Effects of NPY and Its Antagonists

The impact of hypothalamic NPY injections on behavioral, physiological, and endocrine responses supports its proposed role in maintaining carbohydrate balance through processes of both ingestion and metabolism. These actions of exogenous NPY, summarized in greater detail in recent reviews (140–145), are most strongly seen in the area of

the PVN where NPY-containing terminals are dense. They include a stimulatory effect both on food intake, especially carbohydrate, and on the utilization of carbohydrate to support fat synthesis. Repeated NPY injections increase body weight (146). The endocrine effects of NPY include enhanced release of CORT, which favors the availability and utilization of glucose. This allows NPY to integrate feeding with the hypothalamopituitary-adrenal (HPA) axis, which serves an important function in nutrient balance (described below). In addition, NPY stimulates the secretion of AVP, and it has an indirect stimulatory effect on insulin secretion to control blood levels of glucose under dynamic conditions. These multiple actions of NPY are accompanied by a reduction in energy expenditure, through an inhibition of sympathetic nervous system activity, and by a diversion of excess energy toward fat synthesis and storage. It may act peripherally to suppress lipolysis in adipose tissue or inhibit gastric acid secretion (147,148).

Do these effects of injected NPY reflect the functions of the endogenous peptide? In support of this possibility, a number of studies have reported feeding suppression with hypothalamic injections of NPY antisera and receptor antagonists (149,150). The available NPY antagonists lack specificity, however, and only with the recent cloning of a potential NPY "feeding" Y_5-receptor (151) can more specific compounds be obtained. Another approach has been to utilize specific antisense oligodeoxynucleotides (ODNs) to NPY mRNA (152). When administered directly into the region of the NPY-synthesizing cell groups of the ARC, the antisense ODNs, but not sense ODNs, cause a reduction in carbohydrates as well as fat ingestion and a decrease in insulin secretion. These effects are associated with a decline in NPY levels of the ARC but not other areas. The importance of this neuropeptide for long-term body weight regulation is suggested by the effectiveness of antisense ODNs to NPY mRNA in attenuating weight gain over a 5-day period of daily injections.

2. Regulatory Feedback Properties of Hypothalamic NPY

A variety of physiological and endocrine signals feed back to regulate NPY gene trancription or translation, as well as peptide synthesis, transport, release, and receptor activity, generally in the ARC-PVN neuronal projection. In these areas, the adrenal steroid CORT acts through glucocorticoid type II receptors with a potent stimulatory effect on NPY gene expression, synthesis, and receptor activity (37,153–158). The behavioral action of NPY is similarly enhanced by CORT, as well as antagonized by a glucocorticoid receptor antagonist. A different pattern becomes evident with the gonadal steriods, E_2 and P. While E_2 inhibits NPY gene expression in the ARC and then NPY release in the PVN, possibly contributing to the steroid's anorectic action, the administration of P has a stimulatory effect on NPY in E_2-primed animals (159–163).

Other hormones or physiological states related to carbohydrate or fat metabolism also impact on the NPY neurocircuit (164–167). Insulin exerts an inhibitory effect on peptide gene expression, producing its strongest effect in NPY neurons of the ARC. This effect on a feeding-stimulatory peptide, whether direct or indirect, may mediate the satiety-producing effects attributed to insulin after its release by a meal (168). Caloric deprivation and antagonists of carbohydrate and fat metabolism also influence NPY's function. Peptide synthesis and gene expression are greatly enhanced by total food restriction (169–173) or by the specific metabolic inhibitor 2-deoxy-D-glucose, which blocks carbohydrate utilization (174). In contrast, an inhibitor of fat oxidation, which favors carbohydrate utilization, has little impact on NPY synthesis. These metabolic inhibitors have distinct behavioral and endocrine effects consistent with these differential peptide changes in the hypothalamus (174,175). Blockade of glucose utlization enhances both NPY in the ARC and circulating CORT levels and stimulates eating, preferentially carbohydrate intake.

The cellular mechanisms involved in these interactions remain to be characterized. Specific regulatory properties of NPY involving second-messenger pathways are suggested by the enhanced production of NPY in response to increased levels of cyclic adenosine 3′,5′-monophosphate (cAMP) (176–180). This potent effect on NPY can be observed through in vivo as well as in vitro manipulations.

3. Physiological States

NPY may function in different physiological states or conditions and in different individuals or subpopulations with distinct patterns of weight regulation. This is supported by studies in rats exhibiting natural variations in their eating patterns, nutrient preferences, and body weight. These investigations argue for clear site specificity, as well as peptide and hormone specificity, in the relationships between the hypothalamic neurochemicals and specific behavioral or physiological traits (181,182). A strong positive correlation is revealed between NPY levels in the ARC or PVN and the animal's daily intake of carbohydrate, as opposed to fat or protein (182).

There are dynamic shifts in NPY gene expression or production in association with natural biological rhythms. Across the diurnal cycle, for example, there are distinct patterns of nutrient intake, circulating hormones, and hypothalamic peptides (37,39,158,183–185). At the start of the active feeding period, a natural rise occurs in NPY gene expression and NPY level in the ARC and PVN. This rise is positively correlated with high levels of CORT and with spontaneous ingestion of carbohydrate but not fat. Peak NPY is also linked to an increase in gluconeogenesis and glycogenolysis, followed by increased utlization of carbohydrate.

Across the 4-day female cycle, interesting relationships between gonadal steroids and hypothalamic peptides become apparent. The peak levels of NPY are seen during proestrus, in the MPO, PVN, and ARC, which may result from the rise in circulating E_2 and P (163,186,187). During development, NPY rises dramatically from birth to maturity (188–191). A pattern of high circulating CORT levels and NPY production in the ARC is characteristic of prepubertal animals, when carbohydrate is the preferred nutrient particulary in female rats (191–195).

4. NPY-Monoamine Interactions

In stimulating feeding at the onset of the active cycle, NPY may interact synergistically with NE and antagonistically with 5-HT (196,197). These monoaminergic neuromodulators and NPY coexist in brainstem neurons that innervate the hypothalamus. The feeding response elicited by NPY is similar to that induced by NE and is reduced by 5-HT. It can be attenuated pharamacologically by fenfluramine. Such neurochemical interactions are necessary to coordinate behavioral patterns as complex as eating initiation and satiety with rhythms, arousal, and stressful events.

B. Galanin

Galanin (GAL), similar to NPY, stimulates feeding and alters metabolism through local hypothalamic circuits. These two peptides systems, however, are anatomically as well as functionally distinct (140). The GAL system, in contrast to NPY, is associated with patterns of fat consumption and signals of fat oxidation. Specific interactions between circulating steroids and this hypothalamic peptide system involve the gonadal steroids, E_2 and P, which affect the GAL projection differently from their effect on the NPY system. Anatomically, the GAL system that is related to eating behavior and metabolism involves a population of neurons in the anterior portion of the PVN and another in the MPO (Fig. 1). These neurons project locally within the PVN, which contains an high concentration of GAL receptors, as well as ventrally to the ME to control pituitary hormone secretion (198).

1. Effects of GAL and Its Antagonists

The behavioral and endocrine actions of GAL in the PVN are very different from those of NPY (140,196,199–201). They include an increase in fat ingestion in addition to carbohydrate intake; this occurs in the same animals that respond to NPY with a specific increase in carbohydrate intake. Repeated injections of antisense ODNs to GAL mRNA into the PVN produce a strong and selective reduction in fat ingestion, accompanied by a decline in PVN GAL levels and weight gain and an increase in circulating insulin. The GAL antagonist M40 blocks GAL-elicited feeding and reduces spontaneous feeding (202,203).

GAL reduces energy expenditure and inhibits sympathetic nervous system activity (204,205). Unlike NPY, it has little effect specifically on carbohydrate or fat utilization, which may offer some explanation for why repeated injections of GAL have little impact on body weight (146,206). The endocrine effects attributed to GAL are, in some cases, diametrically opposite to those of NPY (37,207,208). They include an inhibition of CORT and insulin release, effects that occur both centrally through the PVN and peripherally in the adrenals or pancreas, respectively. GAL also reduces the release of AVP. The gastrointestinal effects of GAL, in contrast to NPY's, involve an increase in gastric acid secretion.

2. Regulatory Feedback Properties of Hypothalamic GAL

In addition to the differential actions of hypothalamic injections of GAL and NPY, these peptide systems exhibit different responsiveness to physiological and endocrine feedback signals. The adrenal steroid, CORT, which stimulates NPY in the ARC, has little impact or transiently inhibits GAL gene expression in PVN neurons and has no effect on GAL's feeding behavioral action in this nucleus (37,209,210). Estradiol alone or in combination with P has a potent stimulatory effect on GAL in the PVN, MPO, and ME (198,211–213). Insulin exerts an inhibitory effect on GAL gene expression and synthesis in the PVN (214). This effect may involve direct actions on brain receptors, as suggested by in vitro studies showing a dramatic decline in GAL immunoreactivity in primary hypothalamic cell cultures (165). This may be related to insulin's satiety-producing effects released by a meal (168).

The hypothalamic GAL system is less responsive than NPY to total food restriction (215). However, GAL but not NPY responds markedly to a specific inhibitor of fat oxidation (216). Pharmacological blockade of fat oxidation reduces fat ingestion, and this behavioral effect is accompanied by a decrease in GAL production in the PVN. With this reduced inability to ingest and metabolize fat, the an-

imals exhibit a compensatory increase in protein intake. The finding that GAL and NPY respond differently to an inhibitor of glucose oxidation or manipulations of cAMP (175,180) provides further evidence that the cellular mechanisms controlling the production of these two peptides are different.

3. Physiological States

These differences between NPY and GAL, in their physiological actions and regulatory signals, suggest that they may function through distinct mechanisms and in different physiological states or conditions. In particular, GAL gene expression and peptide production in the PVN are positively linked to the behavioral response of fat ingestion and also to weight gain (217). This enhanced GAL activity in high-fat-eating rats may be related to the fact that fat consumption and PVN levels of GAL are inversely related to circulating insulin (217). GAL gene expression, along with circulating hormones, shifts markedly in association with natural biological rhythms but differently from NPY (140). The PVN GAL neurons show peak levels during the middle of the feeding cycle, when circulating insulin and CORT levels are naturally declining and spontaneous fat ingestion rises. Across the estrous cycle, peak GAL levels occur during proestrus in the MPO, PVN, and ME (186,198,212,218). This rise in GAL may result from the rise in circulating E_2 and P and may be causally related to the increased nutrient intake, preferentially fat ingestion, that occurs during this stage of the female cycle (Leibowitz SF and Alexander JT, unpublished data).

4. Early Development

Marked shifts in GAL are also detected in periods of development from birth to maturity (188,219,220). Whereas NPY rises significantly around weaning and again at puberty, a particularly sharp rise in GAL levels is evident after puberty. This increase in peptide, detected in the MPO, PVN, and ME, is most dramatic in females and is very likely in response to a surge in gonadal steroids (188,219,220). These neurochemical-neuroendocrine changes may be associated with the sharp rise in fat ingestion and body fat and the decline in insulin sensitivity that is characteristic of this developmental stage (192,221).

5. GAL-Monoamine Interactions

GAL may interact with the biogenic amines in the control of food intake and metabolism. It acts in a synergistic and dependent manner with NE, such that the peptide's stimulatory effect on feeding is blocked by α_2-noradrenergic receptor antagonists or NE synthesis inhibitors (200). In contrast, DA and GAL appear to act in an antagonistic fashion. Dopamine and AMPH, which releases DA, preferentially reduce fat ingestion, and GAL inhibits the production of hypothalamic DA (222).

C. Opioid Peptides

Food palatability depends in part on brain opioids. Therefore, opioid systems may be important in binge eating and diet-induced obesity. As reviewed by Gosnell and Levine (223), systemic morphine increases food ingestion, and the opioid receptor antagonist naloxone reduce intake of palatable food. When macronutrient diets are available, opioid agonists preferentially enhance ingestion of fat-rich diets (224). Patterns of ingesting sweet solutions under the influence of morphine or naloxone suggest that opioids inhibit aversive components of overeating and thereby increase the amount of food ingested (103,225,226). Opioids released in the nervous system by eating palatable food can cause analgesia in rats and humans (227–229). Therefore, some people may eat to suppress pain.

1. Opioid Subsystems

It has been difficult using systemic injections to unravel the roles of various mu, kappa, and delta systems and their multiple receptors. Progress is being made, as summarized in recent reviews (223,230–232). The opioid peptides, dynorphin, β-endorphin, and enkephalin, act primarily via kappa, mu, and delta receptors, respectively (223,233–236). When labeling the brain for opioid peptides and their receptors, the regions involved with taste, autonomic control, feeding, and reward stand out. Bodnar et al. (237) suggest that mu_1-receptors affect body weight and alter physiological responses of the glucostatic and lipostatic systems, whereas some of the kappa-receptor systems can stimulate food palatability.

Early work with local brain injections in the PVN-MH region showed that endorphin, dynorphin, or an enkephalin analog all induce feeding (238,239). Carr (233) reviews evidence that points to a specific opioid pathway involved in feeding and its reinforcement. The threshold for feeding induced by LH stimulation is raised by specific antibodies against dynorphin-A (240). Naloxone also raises the threshold for stimulation-induced eating, and this effect of naloxone, unlike the classic anorexic action of AMPH and phenylpropanolamine, is potentiated by eating. A site where naloxone exerts its anorectic effect via kappa- or mu-receptors lies in the PBN, a brainstem region that relays taste and vagal information to and from

the forebrain. Thus, an identified dynorphin path from LH to PBN may potentiate eating for taste (233,241, 242). In addition, the stimulation of food intake and decrease in sympathetic activity when NPY is injected into the PVN is blocked by naloxone in the NTS. Thus, NPY-induced feeding depends in part on opioids in the NTS (223,243).

2. Opioid Reward

The next question is whether this or a similar pathway is involved in self-stimulation and feeding reinforcement. In support of this proposal, electrodes in the LH that induce feeding also support self-stimulation (244). Moreover, opiate antagonists sometimes decrease self-stimulation (245) as well as stimulation-induced eating. The self-stimulation rate at eating sites in the LH is inhibited by a meal and generally reflects loss of appetite, as long as a control is used for motor effects on bar-press rate (244–247). In a majority of such studies, food deprivation increases LH self-stimulation rate or lowers the threshold (107,233). This effect is reversed by ventricular infusion of naltrexone (233). Therefore, the opioid potentiation by the behavior reinforcement system that is defined by LH self-stimulation in the pfLH is similar to the system for stimulation-induced eating.

The parallels between LH stimulus-induced eating and deprivation-induced effects on self-stimulation led Carr to the hypothesis that a natural incentive mechanism for eating and reward is stimulated by palatable tastes via an opioid system and that both are sensitized by the metabolic needs imposed by weight loss (233). This appetite enhancement mechanism that is reflected in LH self-stimulation seems to involve several limbic regions including the dynorphin pathway that starts in the pfLH and projects to the PBN (241). This may be part of the feeding-reward system that is modulated by food intake, food deprivation, and insulin, as described by Hernandez and Hoebel (246). It is potentiated by dynorphin release and sensitized by an opioid process in response to weight loss or diabetes in the studies of Carr (233). Therefore, dynorphin can be envisioned in Figure 1 as part of the feeding and reinforcement system drawn from the LH to the PBN. From a clinical point of view, it is conceivable that this is part of the metabolism-modulated taste-appetite system that drives bingeing behavior.

Other brain regions for opiate-induced feeding also exist, notably the VTA, NAc, and amygdala (223). In the VTA, morphine has a potent feeding effect that is mimicked by dynorphin (248). Opiates are behavior reinforcers in the VTA as shown by morphine self-injection, conditioned place preference, and potentiation of self-stimulation (93,245,249–251). These effects may be due to opioid suppression of an inhibitory effect produced by the amino acid gamma-amino butyric acid (GABA) on the mesolimbic DA system. In the NAc, rats self-inject morphine or enkephalin (252,253).

3. Inhibition of Opioid Reward

Kappa-agonists have both stimulatory and inhibitory effects on feeding in different parts of the brain. As reviewed above, food deprivation potentiates behavior in part by releasing dynorphin A in the PBN (233). On the other hand, kappa-agonists in the VTA or NAc inhibit the mesolimbic DA system (254) and may play a role in stopping food intake or generating aversion. Thus, there seems to be more than one kappa-opioid system involved in the circuitry for eating (255). Enterostatin, a peptide released by a fatty meal, may suppress food intake by inhibiting a kappa-opioid system (256) that may also be linked to GAL. Logically, enterostatin may inhibit the LH-PBN dynorphin pathway of the feeding-reinforcement system, but this is yet to be demonstrated.

D. Growth Hormone–Releasing Hormone

Evidence suggests a stimulatory role for growth hormone-releasing hormone (GHRH) in feeding behavior (Fig. 1) (257–260). Central injections of GHRH enhance food intake in rats and sheep. The hypothalamic region most responsive to this peptide effect is the area of MPO and SCN, which has a high concentration of GHRH-containing terminals. This feeding-stimulatory action is centrally mediated and independent of the growth hormone–promoting properties of GHRH that involve projections from the ARC to the ME and anterior pituitary.

From injection studies at different times of the circadian cycle, it seems that endogenous GHRH may contribute to the burst of feeding exhibited at the start of the active cycle (258–260). This proposal receives support from experiments with antiserum raised against GHRH, which suppresses natural feeding. Injections of GHRH stimulate intake specifically of protein, having little effect on carbohydrate or fat intake, while an antiserum against GHRH preferentially inhibits protein consumption at the onset of the natural feeding cycle. This may reflect a role of endogenous GHRH, in the MPO/SCN area, in stimulating both growth and the ingestion of the essential nutrients needed for growth.

There is evidence that a growth hormone-releasing peptide (GHRP), acting within the brain, mimics an unidentified native GH-releasing, hormone-amplifying hormone. Ventricular administration of low doses of a newly developed GHRP, KP-102, stimulates feeding in rats (261).

This compound has no effect after systemic administration. It amplifies the feeding-stimulatory effectv of GHRH through a specific receptor for GHRPs possibly in the hypothalamus.

There is likely to be considerable interaction between the different neurochemical systems of the brain controlling eating and body weight. The GHRH system is closely associated with, and may depend on, the opioid system in the PVN. Opiate agonists stimulate the ingestion of protein as well as fat, while the action of GHRH is antagonized by PVN injections of opioid receptor antagonists (257).

E. Melanin-Concentrating Hormone

The novel peptide melanin-concentrating hormone (MCH) has recently been studied in terms of its role in food intake and body weight regulation. A proposed function of MCH in feeding was initially based on both anatomical evidence, showing MCH perikarya restricted largely to the LH area (262), and biochemical results, revealing increased MCH message or synthesis in these neurons at the onset of the natural feeding cycle (263) and after obesity-producing VMH lesions (264). In terms of its regulation, the mRNA expression of MCH neurons in the LH is enhanced by food deprivation, an effect reversed by refeeding (265). It is increased by insulin and by blockade of glucose oxidation. These manipulations activate the sympathoadrenal response, suggesting that MCH affects feeding indirectly by means of a metabolic (lipolytic) action that modulates the response of LH neurons to glucose and free fatty acids (265).

The possible importance of MCH in energy balance is further suggested by a study with a new technique, mRNA differential display with polymerase chain reaction, which is used to identify novel mRNA's differentially expressed in the brain (266). In this report, an mRNA for MCH was overexpressed in genetically obese *ob/ob* mice, compared to their lean littermates. While further investigations are needed to determine whether MCH has a role in the development or maintenance of the genetic obesity, this study demonstrates initial success in the use of this novel technique for revealing genes activated in relation to body weight.

The specific function of MCH remains to be defined. Pharmacological studies have demonstrated both stimulation and suppression of feeding with central injections of this cyclic peptide. At a high does of 5 μg, MCH enhanced feeding (267). In another study (265), lower doses in the cerebral ventricles (100 ng) or LH (1 ng) produced a long-lasting reduction in food intake.

F. Prolactin

Prolactin (PRL) is a peptide hormone that is elevated during lactation, a physiological culmination of the reproductive cycle in female mammals (268). This hormone is synthesized in the anterior pituitary gland but is also expressed, albeit in low concentrations, by cells in the brain, notably the medial basal hypothalamus (269). As the mammary tissue develops the capacity for milk production, there occurs an increase in demand for nutrients, leading the lactating female to look to both metabolic and behavioral adaptations to meet these demands (268). These adaptations include hyperphagia, conservation of energy by reduced activity, decreased rates of nonshivering thermogenesis, lipid synthesis, triglycerol turnover, and more efficient use of nutrients through a change in insulin responsiveness.

Injection studies reveal multiple behavioral as well as physiological actions of PRL related to reproduction. In addition to its well-known actions of enhancing milk production and stimulating growth, PRL acts on behavioral systems. It increases grooming, facilitates sexual receptivity, and promotes maternal behavior (270).

Prolactin also stimulates eating behavior in mammals and in birds. Lactation in rodents is characterized by marked hyperphagia. Prolactin levels and hyperphagia are directly proportional to litter size, suggesting a causal relationship (268,271,272). Systemic administration of PRL in female rats produces an increase in food intake. Interestingly, a protein-rich diet is preferred after PRL injections as well as during lactation (268,271,273). Prolactin is effective when administered into the brain where it functions independently of ovarian hormones (274). Sites of action include nuclei of the medial hypothalamus where PRL receptors are concentrated (270,275). A feedback loop may involve the eating-stimulatory peptide GAL, which is synthesized in PVN neurons and stimulates the release of PRL from the pituitary (276). A hypothalamic β-endorphin-containing circuit may also play a role (277). The possibility that PRL controls fat synthesis is suggested by the finding that inhibition of PRL secretion, by the DA agonist bromocriptine, decreases fat stores and blocks lipogenic responsiveness to insulin in the absence of any changes in food intake (278).

IV. PEPTIDES THAT REDUCE EATING AND BODY WEIGHT

Many peptides have been discovered that have inhibitory effects on feeding and weight gain (Fig. 1). An important question addressed in the investigation of these substances is whether their behavioral or physiological effects are both specific and meaningful in the overall control of energy balance. Discussed below are most of the peptides that have sufficient evidence to support their role in the control of feeding and metabolism. In some cases, these substances are synthesized in peripheral organs and send signals to the brain via the circulation, vagus nerve, or sympathetic afferents. Other peptides are synthesized in the brain to act through local neurocircuits.

A. Insulin

Insulin secretion from the pancreatic β-cells varies in proportion to body adiposity (166,168,279,280). To control body weight, insulin is believed to enter the brain, where it acts as a humoral feedback regulator of food intake and energy balance. Insulin injections into the brain reduce food intake, meal size, and weight gain and stimulate the sympathetic nervous system. One site of action is the hypothalamus, where insulin receptors and intracellular signaling molecules, e.g., insulin receptor substrate-1, are concentrated and where insulin-specific antibodies have opposite effects to insulin itself.

This metabolic hormone enters the brain via a saturable, receptor-mediated transport mechanism (281). It may act, in part, through its effects on the production of brain neurochemicals (166,168,214,282). For example, insulin inhibits gene expression of peptides, such as NPY and GAL, that enhance food ingestion and exert anabolic effects. The insulin-like growth factor, IGF-2, which has anorectic actions, also reduces NPY release in vitro (283). Conversely, insulin stimulates the activity of peptides, such as CCK and CRH, that have satiety or catabolic actions (described below). Thus, overall insulin secretion may link short-term changes in energy intake and expenditure with long-term body weight regulation (168).

B. Leptin (OB Protein)

The experimental study of obesity has been greatly faciliated by the characterization of several single-gene mutations in rodents. One of these is the obese *ob/ob* mouse, which inherits early-onset obesity as a recessive trait. The *ob* gene has recently been cloned and its gene product, leptin, identified and found to be produced exclusively in fat cells (284). Its production is increased by insulin and glucocorticoids, and the protein is secreted into the circulation and enters the brain through a saturable process (285–287).

The receptor upon which leptin acts has also been cloned (288). Defects in this receptor produce the syndrome of the mutant diabetic *db/db* mouse. This structure belongs to the class I cytokine receptor family, and one of the binding proteins may be the extracellular domain analogous to the growth hormone–binding protein, another member of the cytokine family. Leptin produces its biological effects by acting on this extracellular domain of the receptor.

Peripheral or central injection of leptin reduces food intake, insulin secretion, and body weight (287). The satiety effects of leptin reside in the N-terminal region of the peptide sequence (269). Leptin also increases energy expenditure and normalizes blood glucose concentrations in obese mice (289).

With regard to the mechanism of leptin's actions in the brain, it has been demonstrated that this peptide reduces NPY gene expression in the ARC (290), but it has no impact on GAL (291). While hypothalamic NPY may have some role in leptin's actions, the normal or enhanced responsiveness of NPY knockout mice to leptin injection argues against an essential role for NPY (292). The importance of the glucocorticoids and their receptors is demonstrated by the finding that adrenalectomy, similar to leptin itself, attenuates the obesity of *ob/ob* mice (16).

The role of leptin in body weight regulation is under intensive study (287). In both animals and humans, circulating leptin concentrations reflect the amount of adipose tissue in the body, as indicated by a strong positive correlation between these variables. This rise in leptin with obesity may indicate the presence of "leptin resistance" resulting possibly from a reduction of leptin tranport into the brain (293). A rhythmicity of *ob* mRNA levels can be seen across the circadian cycle in relation to food intake, with lowest levels during the inactive period and highest levels 8 hr after the onset of feeding. This rhythm, together with the finding that a large change in circulating leptin can occur under different conditions involving little change in body weight, supports the suggestion that this peptide is related to other factors besides adipose tissue size.

There is evidence that leptin may impact on neuroendocrine systems involved in reproduction and in conserving energy during periods of food deprivation. Fasting markedly reduces circulating leptin and produces endocrine responses including a reduction in gonadal and thyroid hormones and an increase in adrenal hormones (294). These adaptive responses to starvation are prevented by exogenous leptin in the absence of any change in body weight, blood glucose, or ketones. A related finding is that leptin restores fertility in female *ob/ob* mice independent of any effect on body weight (295). This may reflect the close relationship between fat accumulation at puberty and activation of the hypothalamic-pituitary-gonadal axis, with leptin informing the brain of the adequacy of fat stores needed for reproduction.

C. Amylin

Amylin is a 37-amino-acid peptide with extensive sequence overlap with calcitonin gene–related peptide (296). It is coreleased with insulin from pancreatic β-cells in response to a variety of stimuli. These include meal ingestion and elevated blood concentrations of glucose, arginine, and β-hydroxybutyrate.

Amylin has multiple biological actions related to glucose (296,297). Although it is coreleased with insulin, it inhibits insulin secretion and counteracts insulin's metabolic actions. In vivo studies indicate that amylin alone stimulates glycogenolysis, decreases glucose uptake, enhances blood glucose and lactate levels, and induces insulin resistance. These effects, however, generally occur at supraphysiological concentrations. In addition to altering glucose homeostasis, both peripheral and central injections of amylin reduce food intake in rodents (297). Unlike the satiety actions of CCK, this effect of amylin is not altered by abdominal vagotomy, nor is it mediated by a change in gastric emptying. Precise meal pattern analyses reveal a specific action of amylin on the satiety processes at the end of a meal, rather than on feeding rate or on the size and duration of subsequent meals (298).

The possibility that amylin acts centrally remains to be demonstrated. Amylin itself is found in the brain, possibly derived from the circulation (299), and high levels of amylin-binding sites are detected in the hypothalamus (300). Systemic administration of amylin affects neurochemical activity in the brain, causing a rise in hypothalamic concentrations of 5-HT and reduced forebrain DA metabolism (301). These neurochemical changes may contribute to the feeding suppression induced by amylin.

Amylin function is disturbed in both type I insulin-dependent and type II insulin-independent diabetic conditions (296). This peptide is the predominant component of the amyloid deposits in the pancreatic islets of type II diabetic patients. These excess peptide concentrations may contribute to the disordered glucose homeostasis, e.g., glucose intolerance and insulin resistance, suggesting that amylin antagonists may be potential therapeutic agents in these patients. Type I diabetes, however, is associated with decreased production of amylin and decreased release after a meal. In this condition of insulin insufficiency, intravenous infusion of an amylin analog may help to reduce postprandial hyperglycemia.

D. Apolipoprotein A-IV

Apolipoprotein A-IV (apo A-IV) is produced by the small intestine and released into the blood in response to a lipid meal (302–304). After administration of this protein, either systemically or directly into the brain, a significant suppression of feeding can be seen. It is proposed that apo A-IV may be a circulating satiety signal produced specifically by a high-fat meal.

E. Glucagon

Glucagon is released from the pancreas during a meal (305,306). Pharmacological studies indicate that glucagon reduces the size of spontaneous meals, whereas glucagon antibodies increase meal size. The mechanism for glucagon's action may involve signals within the liver, as well as the hepatic branch of the abdominal vagus. The possibility that glucagon acts via stimulation of hepatic glucose production or fatty acid oxidation remains to be firmly established. The finding that this pancreatic peptide interacts synergistically with other gut-brain peptides, such as CCK, suggests that it may contribute in a complex manner to the array of peripheral signals controlling meal size.

F. Glucagon-like Peptide 1

The peptide hormone glucagon-like peptide 1 (GLP–1), results from post-translational processing of proglucagon in the L-cells of the intestinal mucosa. It is secreted in response to the ingestion of mixed meals. This peptide is important for control of blood glucose concentrations (307). It potently stimulates glucose-induced insulin secretion and inhibits glucagon secretion, thereby decreasing hepatic glucose production. Recent evidence indicates that GLP-1 and its specific receptors are present in the hypothalamus (308).

Central administration of GLP-1 potently inhibits feeding, while a GLP-1 antagonist stimulates feeding and enhances the feeding response induced by NPY, suggesting a physiological role (309). A possible site of action is the PVN where the peptide's receptors are concentrated and the immediate early gene, c-*fos*, is stimulated by GLP-1 (309,310). This and other evidence has led to the hypothesis that GLP-1 is a natural mediator of satiety, possibly responding to the postmeal rise in circulating glucose levels. This is suported by studies showing acute onset of anorexia in animals receiving transplantable glucagonoma tumor lines that have high levels of proglucagon mRNA and produce highly elevated plasma levels of GLP-1 and glucagon (311).

G. Cholecystokinin

As an integrative peptide for satiety, CCK has parallel functions in the gut and certain brain regions, such as the PVN-MH (138,312–315). This peptide also has roles in the mesolimbic DA system that provide a challenge to any simple overall explanation of function (58).

1. Peripheral Cholecystokinin

Although CCK-8 is the active peptide that is typically studied in paracrine and neurotransmitter research, CCK-33 is more effective in the periphery due to its endocrine actions at distant sites including the liver (316). This peptide can stimulate the release of OT, which in rats is involved in nausea (see below) (317,318). However, CCK satiety without nausea has also been demonstrated (58,312,319,320). As further evidence for CCK satiety, CCK antagonists can increase food intake when given peripherally or locally in regions such as the PVN-MH (321).

Functioning as a paracrine hormone, CCK is released from secretory cells and nerve fibers in the upper intestine where it works locally to stimulate pancreatic secretion and gallbladder contraction. The peptide also inhibits gastric emptying by constricting the pyloric sphincter (315). Receptors for CCK involved in feeding suppression exist, for example, in the pyloric sphincter, the sensory vagus nerve where they are transported to vagal nerve terminals, and the PBN and PVN. These sites may all be part of a CCK pathway involved in control of feeding. The sequence of events after a meal to promote satiety may include the release of peripheral CCK, which acts on vagal nerve endings in the gut, followed by signals to the hindbrain and hypothalamus through central CCK neurons.

2. Brain Cholecystokinin

To suppress feeding, CCK in the PVN may act by counteracting α_2-NE-induced feeding, synergizing with 5-HT and interacting with E_2 during the estrous period (57,322). The hypothalamic output under the influence of CCK is presumably biased to adjust the hindbrain centers to stop feeding reflexes. The PVN projects back to the vagal motor nucleus where there are cells excited by CCK. Sodersten et al. (111) hypothesize that this involves a hindbrain DA-CCK interaction. The vagal output, in turn, projects back to the gastrointestinal tract. Technical approaches used to demonstrate this circuit include CCK suppression of sham eating, sphincter extirpation, selective vagotomy, CCK receptor binding, local CCK brain injections, receptor antagonists, Fos immunoreactivity and electrophysiological recording (314,315,323–327). Thus, CCK acts in both the body and the brain and sends neural information from one to the other but does not seem to cross the blood-brain barrier. The primary receptor for CCK satiety is the CCK_A subtype, which has the same sequence and overall function in the brain and body (315).

Cholecystokinin can inhibit the learning of food incentives (328). Rats perform fewer responses for food if they have prior experience performing the response under the influence of CCK injections. Apparently, CCK can devalue the incentive properties of food in hungry animals, and this is manifest later when the animals work for less of that food. Similarly, CCK is more effective at suppressing the intake of a flavored solution if the flavor, rather than being neutral, is linked to a caloric reward, ethanol (329). Given that a flavor paired with calories can release DA in the NAc (330), CCK through the circuitry of Figure 1 may inform the brain of "nutritive expectations," as referred to by Fedorchak and Bolles (329). The hypothalamus could be one region where CCK can inhibit conditioned mesolimbic DA release.

Some of the mesolimbic DA neurons contain CCK as a cotransmitter. Thus, CCK is a neurotransmitter in some DA projection sites such as the NAc (331). The NAc has intrinsic CCK neurons as well. Heidbreder, De Witte, and their colleagues (332) have studied the effects of satiety peptides on dopaminergic reinforcement processes as reflected in hypothalamic self-stimulation. Ventricular injection of CCK-8 decreases self-stimulation, as one might predict for a satiety factor when self-stimulation is related to appetite. The same doses of CCK, however, increase self-stimulation rate when injected into the posterior, medial NAc where CCK is a DA cotransmitter (332). One may speculate that CCK potentiates some of the reinforcing effects of DA when the two are released together in the NAc. Thus, CCK in the posterior, medial shell of the NAc is probably involved in locomotion and some aspects of the primary or secondary reinforcement of eating.

H. Bombesin

Soon after bombesin (BBS) was found in the mammalian gut, Gibbs et al. (333) discovered that it had satiety properties. McCoy and Avery (334) conclude that BBS-like peptides fit most of the criteria for an integrative peptide with parallel functions in the body and brain. Peripheral BBS shortens meals and lengthens the time to the next meal, without behavioral or subjective signs of illness (335). However, the story is not simple. There exist several BBS-like peptides, such as gastrin-releasing peptide and forms of neuromedin, which may act within the brain or body (336). Peripherally administered BBS can stimulate

the release of gastrin, CCK, insulin, and other gut peptides that contribute to satiety. When given chronically on an appropriate schedule, BBS can cause weight loss (337).

I. Enterostatin

Enterostatin (ENT) is a satiety peptide derived from pancreatic procolipase by the enzymatic action of trypsin in response to food in the gut, particularly the presence of fat. When given peripherally or into the cerebroventricle, ENT selectively inhibits voluntary intake of fat as opposed to carbohydrate (338,339). Peripheral responses to ENT are dependent upon hepatic vagal afferents to the brain. Systemically administered ENT activates neurons in the PVN, while PVN injections of this peptide significantly reduce food intake, demonstrating a function that parallels its actions in the gut (340).

An ENT circuit in the brain may cause satiety by inhibiting an opioid system that promotes fat ingestion (256). Enterostatin antagonizes kappa-agonists that stimulate fat intake, and a kappa-agonist (U50488) at low doses can interfere with the suppression of fat intake normally caused by ENT. Both ENT and kappa-antagonists suppress an animal's choice of fatty food. Thus, York and Lin (340) propose the existence of a kappa-opioid system in the PVN that controls appetite for fat and is inhibited by ENT. They also demonstrate that ENT inhibits the consumption of a fat-rich diet induced by GAL while having no effect on NPY-elicited feeding (341). This GAL-ENT-kappa system may control the DA/ACh balance in the NAc (see below) for the promotion and inhibition of instrumental responses for fatty food.

J. Corticotropin-Releasing Hormone

A well-known role of CRH is to control the HPA axis, exerting powerful regulatory effects on ACTH, β-endorphin, and glucocorticoid release. In addition, however, this peptide has been implicated in the mediation of the integrated physiological and behavioral responses to stress. These responses are largely independent of the activation of the HPA axis, suggesting a direct action of CRH on brain receptors.

Included in the CRH-induced responses are changes in eating behavior and metabolism involving a constellation of effects favoring a state of negative energy balance (342–346). The specific effects observed with CRH injections into the MH or PVN include a marked suppression of food intake. This is coupled with stimulation of sympathetic outflow that increases lipolysis and energy expenditure and raises blood glucose while inhibiting any increase in insulin secretion. Chronic central CRH administration causes a sustained reduction in food intake and body weight in lean and obese animals. Urocortin, a neuropeptide related to CRH, is considerably more potent than CRH in suppressing feeding and more selective in binding to the CRH_2 receptor, which may mediate the anorectic response (347).

A role of endogenous CRH or urocortin in energy balance is suggested by the evidence that antagonists of CRH receptors or manipulations that reduce CRH biosynthesis potentiate feeding (348). In states of glucocorticoid insufficiency induced by adrenalectomy, CRH expression in the PVN is enhanced. This neurochemical event is associated with a decline in body weight, impaired recovery of weight loss due to food deprivation, and prevention of experimental induced obesity (344). Circulating glucocorticoids normally released by CRH may provide the feedback signal for inhibition of CRH and regulation of adipose tissue.

These effects of CRH may be mediated, in part, by inhibition of endogenous NPY, which normally potentiates eating and weight gain (345,348,349). Administration of CRH reduces NPY-elicited feeding and decreases NPY gene expression in lean and obese rats. Moreover, adrenalectomy, which enhances CRH expression in the PVN, reduces NPY mRNA in the ARC. Thus, conditions associated with changes in eating behavior and body weight have opposite effects on CRH and NPY.

The actions of CRH on metabolism and energy balance may also involve alterations in immune signals, particularly cytokines (346). This is reflected in the stimulatory effect of cytokines such as interleukin-1 on the release of CRH and in the essential role of CRH in the hypophagic effect of interleukin-1 and its impact on fever, thermogenesis, and ACTH release. The possibility of bidirectional communication is suggested by the influence of CRH on immune and inflammatory responses. Thus, the role of this peptide in energy balance must be evaluated in a broad context, as an integrator of the physiological responses to stress in relation to immunity and infection.

K. Oxytocin and Vasopressin

An oxytocinergic pathway for the inhibition of feeding has been suggested (317). Stricker and Verbalis (317) summarize the ingestive effects of pituitary oxytocin (OT) in rats as inhibiting food intake under conditions other than normal satiety, e.g., in states of nausea or dehydration. Central OT injections reduce food intake as well as sodium appetite (350–352), while the OT receptor antagonists stimulate feeding (353). Arginine vasopressin re-

places OT for these functions in primates and, like OT, inhibits feeding in rats (354,355).

Evidence suggests the involvement of other neuromodulators in OT's action. A role for 5-HT is indicated by the stimulatory effect of this monoamine on the release of OT. *d*-Fenfluramine increases pituitary OT release via the PVN and inhibits it via the DMN (356), suggesting a possible function of OT in the action of this anorectic compound. The peptide CRH also stimulates OT, which may be one factor underlying its feeding-suppressive effect (357). Conversely, brain GAL, which stimulates feeding, plays a role in inhibiting pituitary OT release (358).

L. Neurotensin

Neurotensin (NT) increases in the plasma of humans after eating a meal, and the increase is significantly larger if the meal is hot and palatable rather than cold and poorly accepted (359). When NT is injected peripherally in rats, there is no compelling evidence that it causes satiety by itself (360); however, inhibition of feeding and grooming behaviors are reported with large doses (361). Peripheral neurotensin may act physiologically in synergy with other satiety peptides normally released at the same time.

Neurotensin injected in the PVN-MH region decreases food intake provided the active portion of the peptide chain is used (31,360). This peptide interacts closely with the monoamines. Neurotensin modulates hypothalamic NE release (362), and in the mesolimbic system, NT is colocalized with DA in neurons that project from the VTA to the NAc. Neurotensin iontophoresed into the VTA increases DA cell firing rate. These clues led to the demonstration that rats self-inject NT into the VTA (363). Repeated NT injections in the VTA sensitize animals to the hyperactivity produced by subsequent injections, due to increased responsiveness of DA neurons (364). In the posterior, medial NAc where NT is coreleased with DA, injections of NT are like CCK in potentiating self-stimulation (365). On the other hand, NT in parts of the NAc can prevent dopaminergic effects and thus alter motivation. The modulation of motivation by glucocorticoids acting on peptidergic expression in the NAc is reviewed by Angulo and McEwen (366).

M. Calcitonin

In addition to calcitonin, the calcitonin family of peptides includes calcitonin gene-related peptide (CGRP), adrenomedullin, and islet amyloid polypeptide. These peptides are each found to reduce food intake when centrally injected (367–371). The hypothalamus is a main target site for calcitonin-induced anorexia and contains high concentrations of calcitonin receptors. As indicated above, CGRP is structurally similar to a diabetes-associated hormone, amylin, and these peptides have similar biological effects including feeding suppression. In obese women, plasma CGRP concentrations are found to be high (372). While high-carbohydrate meals fail to affect circulating CGRP, high-fat meals cause a significant rise in CGRP levels, suggesting a possible link to dietary obesity.

N. Melanocyte-Stimulating Hormone

Melanocyte-stimulating hormone (MSH) is produced during the processing of pro-opiomelanocortin, with desacetyl-MSH (d-MSH) normally acetylated on the N terminus to produce α-MSH. In relation to obesity, the yellow (agouti) obese mouse shows an increased ratio of d-MSH to α-MSH in the pituitary (267). Pharmacological studies in this genetic mouse strain reveal a feeding-inhibitory effect after central injection of α-MSH, in contrast to a stimulatory effect with peripheral injection of d-MSH (267). The hyperphagia, reduced sympathetic tone, and enhanced metabolic efficiency of the agouti mouse may be attributed to overexpression of the agouti gene product in the brain where it modulates MSH and antagonizes the melanocortin receptor (MC4-R) in the hypothalamus (373).

O. Acidic Fibroblast Growth Factor

Acidic fibroblast growth factor (aFGF) is one of several growth factor peptides that do more than promote mitosis and tissue repair (374). It facilitates learning and memory and, in addition, inhibits eating behavior, according to extensive work by Oomura and his colleagues (375). Proof of a role in satiety comes from an increase in nighttime eating in rats given aFGF antibodies. The peptide is found in both the body and brain where it is synthesized and released from storage sites in ependymal cells of the gut and ventricular walls. When aFGF is released into the CSF by a meal, it permeates the hypothalamic structures and inhibits the same glucose-sensitive cells in the LH that are inhibited by glucose itself. Oomura has hypothesized that blood glucose both stimulates insulin release from the pancreas and releases aFGF from the ventricular lining, with both cooperating in the inhibition of eating via hypothalamic mechanisms.

P. Cyclo(His-Pro)

Cyclo(His-Pro) is derived from TRH. This dipeptide at high doses reduces food intake and causes a reduction in body weight (376). Levels of cyclo(His-Pro) are increased in the LH of obese Zucker rats, and these elevated levels are reduced by dehydroepiandrosterone, which itself reduces feeding and weight gain (377).

Q. Cytokines

Certain cytokines and related chemokines suppress feeding when injected systematically or into the brain. They are released in response to infection, inflammation, and trauma as part of host defense, causing anorexia and specific actions on the immune system. Plata-Salaman and associates (378–381) review the anorexigenic cytokines and chemokines including interferon-gamma, tumor necrosis factor-α, interleukin-1β (IL-Iβ), and interleukin-8, plus anorectic products they activate such as β$_2$-microglobulin. Both β$_2$-microglobulin and IL-1β, acting in the VMH, significantly reduce food intake and meal size, and IL-1β decreases weight gain. These effects can be dissociated from the fever induced by the cytokines. Treatment with IL-1β increases CRH immunoreactivity in the PVN, a possible mediator of the cytokine effects (382). Histamine may play a role in the suppression of food intake by IL-Iβ that stimulates hypothalamic histamine turnover rate and histamine-N-methyltransferase activity (383).

V. ACETYLCHOLINE AND AMINO ACIDS IN FEEDING-RELATED CIRCUITS

It has long been known that nicotine in cigarettes suppresses appetite, and smoking cessation leads to increased body weight. Thus ACh, which acts on nicotine receptors, is particularly relevant to the discussion of obesity. Amino acids are also very important in several contexts. In addition to their direct actions, new evidence suggests that the brain can detect an amino acid imbalance in the diet and thereby affect food choice.

A. Acetylcholine

Acetylcholine has several roles at nicotinic as well as muscarinic receptors in the circuits that control eating. This neurotransmitter acts not only in the hypothalamus; it acts in the VTA where cholinergic cells project onto DA cells (Fig. 1) and in the NAc where ACh interneurons control behavior output. In the LH, the muscarinic agonist carbachol potentiates eating and drinking (347,384–386). In the midbrain VTA, nicotine stimulates dopaminergic cell bodies to release DA in the NAc (387). Nicotine infused into the NAc similarly releases DA (388,389). Thus, cigarettes have a double dopaminergic action by activating the mesolimbic DA projection at both its origin and terminals.

Acetylcholine interneurons in the NAc may contribute to the inhibition of eating behavior. Most, if not all, of the ACh in the NAc comes from interneurons that play a special role in gating motivated behavior output. As a working hypothesis, it is suggested that these ACh interneurons act as gates that control instrumental behavior for reinforcers such as food (390). Just as striatal DA/ACh balance is a factor in Parkinson's disease and Huntington's chorea, accumbens DA/ACh balance may be a factor in disorders of motivated behavior, such as anorexia and binge eating. To test this idea, Mark et al. (390) measured ACh during a meal and found the highest levels to coincide with slowing and stopping of eating. Neostigmine infused intio the NAc to elevate endogenous ACh can stop an ongoing meal. Along with the evidence below, this suggests that accumbens ACh is involved in a "no-go" command that counters the DA "go" signal.

A conditioned taste aversion releases ACh in the NAc when the taste stops the animal from eating a flavor associated with nausea. Thus, the conditioned stimulus raises extracellular ACh at the same time it lowers the release of DA (391). This may contribute to inhibition of behavior output such as eating. This DA/ACh imbalance, with low DA and high ACh release, is very different from what occurs with a normal satiating meal that can raise first extracellular DA and then ACh at the same time (390). This leads to the hypothesis that ACh in the posterior, medial NAc through unidentified receptors can contribute to stopping eating behavior.

B. Amino Acids

The metabolism of energy in the brain is coupled to the formation of several amino acids, including GABA, which serve neurotransmitter roles. This may confer on them a special role in brain mechanisms for eating and body weight regulation. Obese Zucker rats have disturbances in brain GABA that may contribute to their overeating (392). They are refractory to the anorectic effects of the GABA-transaminase inhibitor EOS, which elevates GABA levels in the brain.

The role of GABA in feeding varies in different brain areas. The PVN is the most sensitive site to the feeding-stimulatory effects induced by injections of GABA agonists and the feeding-inhibitory effect of a GABA antagonist (393–395). In the VMH, mixed results with injections of GABA agonists have been obtained (393–396). Panksepp and Meeker (396) have suggested the existence of a metabolically distinct GABA-ergic system that exerts inhibi-

tory control over feeding. This is based on the finding that levels of endogenous GABA are high in the VMH during the light phase when natural feeding is low (397), and conditions associated with decreased feeding cause enhanced levels of VMH GABA (398). The release of GABA is triggered in part by nutrients arriving in the gut.

As indicated in Figure 1, complex sensory inputs to the NAc arrive on glutamate pathways from the PFC, amygdala, and hippocampus. Output signals leave the NAc on GABA pathways of the extrapyramidal motor system to the VTA, GP, and LH. Glutamate projections to the NAc shell stimulate an output pathway that inhibits feeding via GABA neurons to the LH (399). On the other hand, there are glutamate inputs to the LH that stimulate feeding (400–402). In the NTS, glutamate has been implicated in the suppression of feeding by CCK and by glucose-induced satiety (403). A benzodiazepine-GABA system is involved in responses to palatable tastes (404).

VI. STEROID HORMONES AFFECTING FEEDING AND WEIGHT REGULATION

This section reviews evidence supporting a role, either direct or indirect, for the adrenal and gonadal steroids in energy and nutrient balance.

A. Adrenal Steroids

There is a vast literature on the adrenal steroids and their role in controlling feeding and body weight. This literature, which has been extensively reviewed (37,405–408), has led to the conclusion that at normal physiological levels, the steroids corticosterone (CORT) and aldosterone (ALDO) have specific functions in maintaining carbohydrate and fat stores across the daily light/dark cycle. This process is accomplished through behavioral and metabolic actions, which involve the mediation of both the type I and type II steroid receptors. These receptors exist in the brain and act, in part, through their permissive interactions with neurochemical systems that modulate nutrient balance. Under conditions of obesity and repeated stress, the adrenal steroids are elevated, resulting in chronic disturbances in the steroid-neurochemical interactions. In the absence of these steroids, such as after adrenalectomy, all forms of obesity are attenuated (408).

1. Type I and Type II Receptors

Studies of the natural light/dark cycle in normal-weight animals have led to the proposal of distinct functions performed by the different steroid receptors (37). The type I receptor is activated under conditions of low basal levels of circulating CORT (0.5–2.0 μg/dl). It functions tonically throughout the daily cycle to sustain feeding, particulary fat intake, and enhance fat deposition. Fat intake occurs at a fairly constant level across the feeding cycle in almost every meal, although it rises toward the second half of the active phase. This stable behavioral pattern provides a continuous supply of a high-caloric nutrient, which can be readily stored in the stomach or adipose tissue for short- or long-term use, respectively. This tonic control of fat intake, possibly mediated through hypothalamic type I receptors, may be likened to their function in the basal forebrain for maintaining salt balance (409) and in the lower brainstem for continuous monitoring of blood pressure (410).

The type II receptor, in contrast, is activated under conditions of somewhat higher or moderate levels of CORT. It may function phasically during the early hours of the active cycle when CORT normally rises to levels of 3–10 μg/dl but also during periods of stress when even higher levels are achieved (37). A primary function of the type II receptor at the onset of the feeding cycle is to replenish and defend the body's carbohydrate stores through both ingestion and storage. This immediate defense is required to prevent the hypoglycemia that may develop after periods of little eating and continued breakdown of carbohydrate stores. This provides adequate supplies to the brain to stablize neuronal processes (411,412). This phasic, anabolic effect of moderate levels of CORT may be contrasted with the type II receptor actions of higher CORT levels, such as after acute stress or limited food supplies. In addition to stimulating nutrient ingestion, unusually high CORT concentrations actually have catabolic actions on the body's fat and protein stores to provide additional substrates for maintaining normal carbohydrate balance. Under stable conditions, however, the type II receptor subtype is very likely inactive at other times of the circadian cycle or in physiological states when glycogen stores are plentiful, cellular glucose uptake is normal, and circulating CORT levels are low.

Thus, in maintaining the body's nutrient stores from one day to the next, these two receptor subtypes work toward a common goal. Through ingestion and metabolism, they provide the nutrients essential for maintaining the body's carbohydrate and fat stores under different environmental conditions. As circulating CORT levels rise, the priorities of nutrient partitioning favor the actions of type II receptors that restore carbohydrate through behavioral and metabolic processes. Thus, at any moment across the light/dark cycle, but particularly during the initial phase of the feeding cycle, there exists an inverse relation between the carbohydrate and fat content of a meal (39). The differential functions of the receptor subtypes, however, are most evident under conditions of abnormally high CORT levels, when Type II receptor activation exerts catabolic effects on certain tissues to shift essential nutrients toward carbohydrate replenishment and storage.

2. Corticosterone-Peptide Interactions

Receptors mediating these actions of the adrenal steroids across the circadian cycle are located in the brain (37). They are particularly responsive in the hypothalamic PVN, which plays a primary role in controlling CORT release as well as nutrient balance. Neurons in the ARC are similarly responsive to CORT. In maintaining carbohydrate stores, the type II receptors act in part through central neurochemical systems that synthesize NPY in the ARC and the catecholamine NE in the brainstem. As described above, this steroid enhances gene expression, transport, and receptor activity, ultimately potentiating the action of NPY and NE released in the medial PVN. Circulating CORT very likely determines the circadian rhythm of endogenous NPY and noradrenergic activity detected in the hypothalamus.

Natural rhythms of circulating steroids and their receptor subtypes are critical in maintaining normal control of physiological processes (413,414). These rhythms allow for necessary shifts in phases of priming, activation, and rest. Without these rhythms, a chronic state of activation, which constitutes a stress to the organism, will eventually result in pathology. In the control of nutrient balance, the dual-control receptor systems involving type I and type II receptors provide a mechanism that responds to large shifts in circulating CORT and assist in coordinating metabolic processes appropriate for specific circadian periods or environmental challenges. The loss of these rhythms in states of obesity (see below) has clear negative consequences on cellular and physiological functions.

3. Corticosterone-Insulin Interaction

In evaluating the anabolic and catabolic effects of CORT, it is important to consider its actions in relation to the primary metabolic hormone, insulin (37,405). Corticosterone and insulin are well known for their antagonistic actions, particularly in their effects on glucose uptake and metabolism. This antagonism is also evident in their behavioral actions whereby insulin that is released in proportion to the body's fat mass (see above) reduces food intake and attenuates the steroid's stimulatory action on feeding. This interaction between CORT and insulin may occur within the brain as well as in peripheral tissues, possibly involving differential effects on brain neurochemicals such as NPY.

It is now clear, however, that the effects of these hormones may differ in different tissues and physiological or pathological states. For example, an actual synergism in their action is seen in the liver where CORT and insulin both increase glycogen synthesis and lipogenesis, and at the onset of the natural feeding cycle when both hormones normally peak for efficient postprandial storage of the ingested carbohydrates. However, in states of obesity, the antagonism between these hormones becomes exaggerated when circulating CORT levels are abnormally and chronically high. There occurs a compensatory rise in insulin secretion along with increased insulin resistance. The resulting chronic hyperinsulinemia and hypercortisolemia increase hepatic lipogenesis while reducing gluconeogenesis and produce catabolic effects within muscle where CORT's actions outweigh those of insulin. Under these conditions, it is inevitable that brain neurochemistry controlled by these hormones is in a greatly disturbed state.

B. Gonadal Steroids

Reproductive physiology and behavior depend on the availability of oxidizable metabolic fuels. Energetic factors that affect reproduction, such as food availability, ambient temperature, exercise, storage, and mobilization of fatty acids, all affect the availability of metabolic fuels (268,415). These changes in metabolic fuels influence reproduction through actions at multiple sites. These include key sites in the brain and involve alterations in the activity of gonadotropin-releasing hormone neurons and E_2-binding effector neurons. The ovarian steroids E_2 and P play a major role in this process, producing changes in nutrient ingestion, partitioning, and utilization of fuels.

Estradiol is associated with a reduction in eating behavior, adiposity, and body weight in adults (268). Ovariectomy produces the opposite effect such that animals gain weight in an E_2-reversible manner. As described above, these effects of E_2 may be mediated through its influence on hypothalamic peptide systems, such as NPY, CRH, and CCK (161,416–418). For example, E_2 replacement after ovariectomy (OVX) reduces NPY gene expression in the ARC and NPY release in the PVN, which is likely to result in a decline in food intake and loss of body weight. The reverse pattern is seen with steroid effects on CRH and CCK. Estradiol stimulates the production or function of these peptides in the PVN, which normally act to inhibit feeding and decrease weight gain. This combination of hypothalamic events, enhanced catabolic signaling combined with impaired compensatory activation of

anabolic pathways, leads to body weight loss during chronic high levels of E_2 in adults.

In understanding the role of gonadal steroids in feeding and metabolism, one must additionally consider the impact of P, which has diverse actions in relation to E_2 that may involve an early enhancing effect followed by an inhibition. Thus, while E_2 inhibits NPY, P actually stimulates this peptide's production in E_2-primed animals (419), suggesting an antagonism between the two steroids. In contrast, GAL is activated by E_2, alone but to a greater extent with P (213,420). This resulting pattern, of increased NPY and GAL production under the influence of both steroids together, may explain the finding of increased caloric or particularly fat intake and body weight that occurs in females at puberty when the gonadal steroids and peptides rise to peak levels (140,188,192). Thus, the role of P contrasts with that of E_2; it builds energy stores through behavioral as well as metabolic actions, in contrast to the anorexic and lipolytic actions of E_2 (268,415,421). The precise steroid-neurochemical interactions underlying these actions remain to be characterized.

VII. BRAIN AND BEHAVIOR: REINFORCEMENT SYSTEMS AND OVEREATING

Motivation to eat is a major factor in the development and maintenance of obesity. Neural mechanisms have evolved to anticipate the animal's energy needs and avoid past mistakes. The brain learns and remembers a myriad of responses for finding, storing, and rationing food supplies. The animal is both consciously and unconsciously aware of fuel sources within its ecological niche and its own body. It uses innate reflexes plus classical and instrumental conditioning to get food, to know how hard to work for it, and to know how much to eat. Responses that engage the environment are particularly clever when they involve motivation and learning of complex and arbitrary motor sequences that must be chained together from the animal's repertoire of simpler responses. To survey the chemical neuroanatomy of classical and instrumental conditioning of feeding behavior in a few pages is to leave out most of the available information. Nonetheless, some basic principles can be drawn from the above discussion during a brief tour of the feeding-reinforcement circuit as we now know it (49,102).

An overview of Figure 1 indicates that sensory signals from vision, audition, somesthesis, and the chemosenses are entered separately or as multimodal signals into the inputs of two major circuits or loops. One loop from PFC to NAc (the vertical oval) uses sensory information to generate motor output patterns. Thus, the NAc is often referred to as a sensorimotor interface (422). The other loop from the LH to the NAc (the horizontal oval) reinforces output from the sensorimotor interface.

A.   Sensory Input

Chemosensory imputs for taste, olfaction, metabolism, and fuel storage are fed into the NTS, PBN (423,424), hypothalamus, and amygdala. Glucoreceptors are widespread in a network throughout much of the brain (425). The prime example of chemosensory processing is the taste signal that has been traced from the tongue to NTS, where some of it combines with hepatic vagal inputs representing glucose and amino acids in the liver (426). This signal travels on to the PBN, thalamus (directly to the hypothalamus in rodents), and then taste sensory cortex, where cells respond to stimuli on the tongue. Recording studies in monkeys follow this trace from the classic taste cortex to the orbital PFC, where cells respond to the same tastes as a function of appetite and satiety. As a monkey eats a flavorful food and gradually becomes satiated, the PFC cells gradually stop responding to the flavor. This effect is specific for the flavor of a particular food (427). The animal, like the cells in its PFC, no longer responds to one food when satiated but still responds to another. This phenomenon is known as sensory-specific satiety.

B.   Behavior Generator System

As shown in Figure 1, complex sensory information enters the NAc on the glutamate neurons, is gated by ACh neurons, and leaves the NAc on GABA neurons of the motor system. The PFC is involved in making choices, including choices of foods. It projects strongly via glutamate neurons to the NAc and other parts of the striatum. The NAc has various rostral-caudal and shell-core inputs and outputs with functionally distinct neuronal ensembles (428,429). Acetylcholine interneurons in the NAc may act as gates that stop instrumental motor output (390,391). These gating neurons are modulated by DA and other transmitters, such as 5-HT (430) and certain opioids (431). Such influences may thereby disinhibit instrumental motor output. The output from the NAc goes primarily to the ventral GP, then to the thalamus, and out to motor systems (432,433). The information also loops back from the thalamus to the PFC and back to the NAc (30,434), as shown in Figure 1.

C.   Behavior Reinforcement and Inhibition Systems

The hypothalamus is part of a system that evaluates the sensory outcome of behavior and then reinforces behavior. Its functions are important for maintaining a normal body weight. As indicated in the lower part of Figure 1, insulin-sensitive cells in the ARC and cells for circadian rhythm in the SCN influence feeding-related cells in the PVN. Figure 1 further suggests that the pfLH feeding-reinforcement path descends (90,242,435) and connects to the VTA, PBN, and NTS. Recording studies show that pfLH stimulation, which is capable of inducing eating and brain-stimulation reward, has effects on NTS cells that mimic the effects of palatable tastes on the tongue (436). This descending system may connect to the ascending ACh path that stimulates the VTA cells of the mesolimbic DA system (437). The VTA projects to forebrain limbic structures, including the NAc, amygdala, hippocampus, and PFC, that have inputs back to the LH (399,438). Overall, these projections can be viewed as a behavior reinforcement circuit that increases the rate or force of ongoing behavior and recruits responses to associated signals. This is a major portion of the system for reinforcing eating. Thus, it may play a role in overeating, and binge eating in particular.

1.   Mesolimbic Control of Reinforcement

In the NAc, DA helps to reinforce behavior in a variety of ways (88,439,440). The time course of DA release in the NAc fails to fit a simple notion of a feeding reward. In microdialysis experiments, DA release can occur during eating, and DA often remains elevated for up to an hour after the meal is over (95,441). The synaptic overflow of DA into the extracellular space revealed by microdialysis is functional DA. It can have synaptic actions on dopaminergic receptors and at uptake sites some distance from the release site in the manner of "volume transmission" (442). Sometimes DA is released in anticipation of eating, as reflected in a conditioned rise in extracellular DA before a meal (330,443). This agrees with recording studies in monkeys showing that "naïve" DA cells in the VTA fire during eating, but later "learn" to fire during the presentation of discriminative stimuli that signal forthcoming food (106). Therefore, these cells can release DA in response to conditioned discriminative stimuli that predict food.

2.   Hypothalamic Control of Reinforcement

It has been shown for 30 years that the hypothalamus influences complex responses for food. Only now is the mechanism becoming clear. The above discussion depicts a pathway from the LH to the NAc by which the hypothalamus influences operant eating responses. As evidence for this idea, GAL injections into the PVN cause a significant increase in DA release in the NAc (444). This occurs in the absence of food and only in animals that in a separate test with food present exhibit a GAL induced-feeding response. Thus, it is feeding behavior that is likely to be reinforced by the DA-activated circuit in the NAc. Eating or associated stimuli can release more DA, which further reinforces the behavior. This positive feedback may contribute to bingeing on the kinds of foods, rich in fat and carbohydrate, that are enhanced by GAL (140). Hypothalamic injection of GAL not only releases DA that may accelerate eating; it also decreases extracellular ACh in the NAc, thereby disinhibiting eating (444).

Hypothalamic injection of the D_2 antagonist sulpiride is another way to induce eating (445). When injected in the LH, sulpiride causes the release of DA in the NAc in the absence of food, much like GAL. In this case, we have direct evidence of the reinforcing effect, as rats self-inject sulpiride into their own hypothalamus (81). Perhaps any hypothalamic manipulation that releases accumbens DA can motivate the animal to repeat its behavior. This may contribute to obsessive-compulsive behavior when there is no natural satiety factor sufficient to stop it. In the case of eating a meal, a rise in ACh release in the NAc very likely contributes to the stopping or switching of behaviors.

VIII. BRAIN AND PHYSIOLOGY: ANIMAL MODELS OF OBESITY AND DIABETES

In the above sections, studies of different brain neurochemicals have been reviewed. The evidence obtained has suggested potential candidates in the natural control of feeding behavior, metabolism, and food reinforcement. Given the complex set of processes required to control the multiple components of nutrient and energy balance, considerable redundancy and interaction between systems is required to perform the task. The discussion of these systems has so far focused on their potential roles under natural conditions.

This section considers animal models of obesity. The models, of both mice and rats, include genetically inbred strains with spontaneously inherited defects, transgenic or knockout animals with experimentally induced genetic defects, and outbred strains with distinct phenotypes but unknown genetic or environmental influences. This sec-

tion addresses two specific questions. First, are neurochemical systems in the brain disturbed in animals with a differential propensity toward obesity, and, second, do these systems in fact contribute to the development or maintenance of specific symptoms? Helpful in answering these questions are studies that examine young animals prior to their development of obesity.

A. Genetic Rodent Strains

The genetic types of obesity are those that are polygenic or are transmitted by a single recessive or dominant gene, namely, the obese (*ob/ob*), diabetes (*db/db*), fat, tubby, yellow (A^y), and adipose mice and the Zucker fatty (*fa/fa*) rat. The polygenic are the KK, NZO, and C3H. Studies of the biogenic amines in these strains demonstrate a variety of disturbances (446–450). In the obese mice (*ob/ob*) or rats (*fa/fa*), these include higher levels of medial hypothalamic NE, reduced NE turnover, increased α_2-receptor binding, and greater responsiveness to the feeding-stimulatory effect of NE or the α_2-agonist clonidine. While they show greater responsiveness to the feeding-suppressive effects of a β_3-agonist, they exhibit reduced activity of the β_2-adrenergic receptors that decrease feeding (450). The serotonergic system is also depressed in its activity in obese subjects. This is revealed by measurements of the 5-HT metabolite, 5-hydroxy-3-indole acetic acid (5-HIAA), and by their decreased responsiveness to 5-HT administration (446–449,451,452). With regard to histamine, which inhibits food intake, Zucker fatty rats have lower levels of this biogenic amine in the hypothalamus and are unresponsive to the feeding-stimulatory actions of histamine receptor antagonists (453,545). Moreover, GABA transmission may be disturbed as Zucker fatty rats are refractory to the anorectic effects of an inhibitor of GABA transaminase that produces GABA (392).

The genetically obese mice or rats also show distinct changes in their endogenous peptides and their responsiveness to peptide injections. Measurements of peptide levels or gene expression reveal increased hypothalamic activity in peptide systems, including NPY and GAL, that potentiate feeding and body weight gain (173,455–458) and reduce peptide levels of CRH and NT that inhibit feeding (456,459–461). Expression of the CRF_2 receptor transcript is reduced in the VMH of obese Zucker rats (462). This contrasts with a normal expression or production of many other peptides in the brain of the genetically obese strains (456). In injection studies, obese Zucker rats exhibit enhanced responsiveness to a kappa-agonist (463) and to NPY (456,464) but reduced responsiveness to CCK (465). In the genetically obese yellow mouse, there is a reduction of α-MSH and an increase in d-MSH (466); elevated d-MSH levels have been associated with increased food intake and body weight (267).

In light of evidence described earlier, it is reasonable to propose that these changes in endogenous peptide activity or sensitivity to injected peptides are attributable, in part, to specific disturbances in circulating hormones or nutrients characteristic of these genetic strains. These include a decline in insulin sensitivity or secretion, a rise in circulating CORT, and increased ingestion of total calories or specific macronutrients. For example, since gene expression of the feeding-stimulatory peptides, NPY and GAL, are normally suppressed by insulin (166,214), the enhanced activity of these brain systems seen in obese animals may reflect reduced sensitivity to this hormone. In fact, insulin uptake in the brain is decreased in obese Zucker rats (467–469), thereby precluding its normal inhibitory feedback action.

The question is, are these disturbances in brain neurochemicals causally related to specific traits of obesity or diabetes? There is evidence that, in some cases, they are involved in producing as well as maintaining the disorder. Chronic NPY administration causes severe overeating and increased body fat, accompanied by hyperinsulinemia, insulin resistance, and high circulating CORT (140,470,471). Moreover, repeated administration of antisense ODNs to GAL or NPY mRNA in the PVN or ARC, respectively, reduces eating and body weight (152,217). A causal relationship is further supported by evidence indicating increased hypothalamic NPY activity at an early age in genetically obese rats (458,472–474) and a close association between increased NPY or GAL release and the hyperphagia seen in diabetic rats (167,475,476). The dramatic increase in GAL and NPY at puberty, in association with a sharp rise in body fat and weight gain (140), suggests a particular involvement of these peptides in pubertal-onset obesity and a susceptibility to endocrine and behavioral disturbances at this developmental state.

B. Transgenic and Gene Knockout Animals

By overexpressing or knocking out a gene for a specific neurochemical or receptor in the brain, investigators have gained further knowledge as to their causal relationship to obesity. Most notable are mouse strains with disturbed expression of the 5-HT$_{2C}$ receptors or the type II glucocorticoid receptors, which in both cases exhibit increased weight gain or food intake (477,478). The transgenic mouse with an impaired corticosteroid receptor function, by partial knockout of gene expression with type II glucocorticoid receptor antisense RNA, displays a characteristic phenotype of a hyperactive HPA axis, reduced energy expenditure, and adult onset of marked obesity. In light of the above evidence on NPY, with chronic stimulation or blockade, it is perhaps surprising that a knockout mouse for this peptide exhibits normal patterns of food intake and body weight control (292). Apparently they compensate for loss of NPY. These animals show enhanced responsiveness to the anorectic effects of leptin (292), which had been proposed to act in part through inhibition of the NPY system.

C. Outbred Rodent Strains

Genetically heterogeneous strains of rats show a range of eating and body weight patterns that lead them to be obesity resistant (OR) versus prone (OP) to overeating and obesity. For example, when Sprague-Dawley rats are allowed to choose their food from pure macronutrient diets, 30% naturally consume high amounts of fat and gain weight while another 50% consume a high-carbohydrate diet and stay lean (39). Additionally, when rats are fed a single high-fat/high carbohydrate diet, some develop diet-induced obesity while others are resistant (44,479,480). In general, these OP rats have a natural preference for fat while OR rats prefer carbohydrate (338).

In the OP rats compared to the OR rats, alterations in brain neurochemistry are evident. For example, Levin et al. (481,482) show that the OP rats have higher levels of circulating NE, reflecting a decline in NE turnover and sympathetic activity, and an altered ratio of α_2/α_1 noradrenergic receptors in the hypothalamus (44). Rats that choose a high amount of fat in their diet and gain more weight show enhanced gene expression and levels of GAL in the PVN (217). Further, OP rats exhibit greater responsiveness to treatment of ENT, which decreases food intake and body weight gain on a high-fat diet (338,483). They are also more responsive to the stimulatory effects of central administration of GAL but not NPY (484). In each case, these differences in the neurochemical activity and sensitivity may be associated with, and possibly causally related to, the distinct traits of OP and OR rats.

IX. CLINICAL PHARMACOLOGY AND THERAPEUTICS

One main goal of research in this area is to understand basic neural, genetic, physiological, and environmental processes that interact in the control of ingestive behavior. As illustrated in this chapter, multidisciplinary approaches for investigating the brain allow in-depth analyses of specific physiological states and stages, as well as different animal populations. Using similar strategies, models of obesity may then be examined to understand pathological states and causes of obesity. Investigation of the multiple traits of obesity should help in the discovery of strategies to treat and prevent this disorder.

A detailed examination of possible pharmacological and dietary manipulations that may alleviate symptoms of obesity is beyond the scope of this chapter and is covered elsewhere in this book. Specific therapeutic strategies are also discussed in detail elsewhere. Treatments include pharamaceutical agents to stimulate or block specific receptors. They may ultimately involve antisense RNAs to countermand specific protein production and compounds that target specific candidate genes through gene transfer, to correct a gene defect or enhance a normal gene product.

A. Therapeutic Strategies

The foregoing discussions of neurochemical systems suggest basic strategies for developing successful therapeutic measures. The unmistakable impression one gets from the discussion and from Figure 1 is that multiple systems in the brain are involved in the control of nutrient balance and body weight. Thus, there are many possible points of intervention. Because of the redundancy, however, effective treatment may require drugs that influence multiple circuits or target a final common path involved in a particular trait or type of obesity.

Timing will be crucial in designing pharmacological treatments for obesity. As described above, receptor activity and sensitivity shift throughout the day, throughout the estrous cycle, and with age. Individual or group variability, associated with differences in brain neurochemistry or drug responsiveness, also needs to be considered in molding treatments to specific behavioral or metabolic traits. Gender differences are illustrated by the greater sensitivity of the female rat to the anorexic effect of d-fenfluramine and the hypothermic effect of the 5-HT agonist 8-OH-DPAT (485,486). This is consistent with clinical evidence showing that dieting alters the responsiveness of women but not men to the 5-HT precursor tryptophan (487).

The treatment of obesity can be a lifelong process. Serotonergic drugs may maintain their effectiveness for a relatively long period. Specific peptide antagonists may also have long-term efficacy, as suggested by animal studies. Efficacy in humans, however, remains to be demonstrated. Early intervention and possible prevention need to be the focus of any treatment plan. Studies of developmental stages provide clues that may maximize the benefits of dietary or pharmacological interventions. Even in the uterus, a fetus is programmed by its environment and can be born with an avidity for salt or food that depends on the mother's ingestive behavior or hormones (488,489).

Analyses of early predictors to identify individuals at risk will help in devising innovative strategies for preventing the development of eating and body weight disorders.

B. Biogenic Amines

What role might the biogenic amines have in human overeating and obesity? As suggested in the section on DA, it is logical to hypothesize that the overeating component of bulimia is related to instrumental behavior that releases DA in the NAc and its associated systems (490). In underweight rats, extracellular DA in the NAc is low after food deprivation while tissue levels are high, suggesting subnormal amounts of DA release (491,492). This finding is intriguing since the mesolimbic DA system that projects to the NAc is known for its powerful role in arousal, feeding reinforcement (49,89,106,493,494), psychostimulant reward (247), locomotion (93), and incentive motivation (495). As a rule, anything that stimulates the mesolimbic DA system may engender both behavior reinforcement (i.e., behavior repetition/acceleration) and forward locomotion (42,245). Thus, animals may try to maintain a high level of DA release. When they are below their preferred body weight and basal DA is low, exaggerated behaviors, including stimulus-reactive locomotion, increased meal frequency, and drug abuse, may be required to raise extracellular DA to optimal levels. This hypothesis is supported by the finding that a meal or single injection of morphine or AMPH in underweight subjects fails to increase extracellular DA to the high levels of normal controls (492). This may relate to the fact that underweight animals eat more meals and more readily self-administer drugs of abuse (109). The same tendency has been observed in dieting college women (496).

In clinical studies, disturbances in the activity of monoamine systems in patients with eating or body weight disorders have been detected. For example, obese or bulimic patients exhibit a deficiency of brain 5-HT activity and decreased postsynaptic serotonergic receptor responsiveness (497,498). Disturbances in catecholamine function include higher circulating levels of epinephrine and NE in obese subjects (499). Obese humans also show reduced lipolytic NE sensitivity as well as decreased number of α_2-adrenoreceptors (500). Then, responsiveness to L-DOPA-induced growth hormone (GH) release is diminished in obese humans (501). Genetic studies have associated the A1 allele of the D_2 receptor with obesity and carbohydrate perference in obese patients (502).

The pharmacological agents currently available for the treatment of obesity impact on the biogenic amines or their receptors. These agents, which very likely act in part through the monamine receptor systems identified in the hypothalamus and NAc, include appetite suppressants, which influence NE (e.g., phenylpropanolamine), 5-HT (e.g., d-fenfluramine), and multiple monamines, including DA (e.g., AMPH and phentermine). To take advantage of these different systems, Weintraub (76) started a new trend by combining appetite suppressants to get a larger effect while canceling out certain side effects. Thus, dopaminergic drugs are finding new use in the treatment of obesity and overeating. Amphetamine-like side effects are avoided by combining the dopaminergic drug with one that is serotonergic. Stunkard, Berkowitz, and their colleagues (503) report that d-fenfluramine given to obese women for 18 weeks reduces hunger, food craving, and general preoccupation with food, resulting in increased adherenence to dietary guidelines. While the exact neurochemical basis of Fen-Phen action is not known, the appetite-suppressant effects of the biogenic amines in the hypothalamus are likely to be involved. The overall effect of dFen-Phen on the balance of DA and ACh in the NAc is similar to that of a meal, with both DA and ACh being released in the absence of eating (P. Rada and B.G. Hoebel, unpublished results).

C. Peptide Systems

In humans, there is preliminary evidence linking brain peptide function to the pathophysiology of clinical eating disorders. For example, in bulimic patients, disturbances have been detected in CSF content of peptide YY (PYY), a pancreatic polypeptide closely related to NPY that also stimulates eating. A dramatic increase in CSF PYY in bulimics who have abstained from bingeing has led to the proposal that these patients, when initiating a binge, may be responding to heightened levels of PYY (504). There is further evidence that obesity in humans may reflect disturbances in NPY and the HPA axis (498,500,505). In obese humans, a positive association is apparent between CSF levels of this peptide and of CRH, which controls the release of cortisol (506). Further, a sequence variation at the NPY peptide and NPY Y_1 receptor gene in humans is associated with an increase in appetite for carbohydrate and protein in women and men, respectively (507). Pancreatic polypeptide in the blood, which is associated with decreased appetite, rises in response to a meal; however, levels of this peptide are considerably reduced in obese compared to lean subjects (508).

Several lines of evidence implicate the peptide CRH in food-associated symptoms of various neuropsychiatric disorders (344). For example, patients with Cushing's disease, who exhibit hyperphagia, lethargy, and obesity, show a marked decrease in CRH secretion into the CSF. They also have a decreased sensitivity to the feedback actions of circulating cortisol, perhaps due to long-standing hypercortisolism. The opposite pattern is seen in patients with anorexia nervosa. These subjects have increased levels of CRH in the CSF and a blunted ACTH response to CRH. While these neurochemical changes may be related to patterns of eating and body weight, issues of cause and effect as well as specificity of CRH's actions relative to energy balance need further investigation.

In human's, the *ob* gene is expressed exclusively in adipose tissues and it codes for a protein that is 85% homologous to mouse leptin (509,510). To date, no deleterious mutations and only one single-base polymorphism have been detected in the human *ob* gene (511). Possible linkage of extreme obesity to markers flanking the human *ob* gene, however, has recently been suggested (512,513). Clinical trails currently underway should soon reveal the efficacy of leptin in controlling eating and body weight in humans.

Given the evidence that some monamines act in synergy with postingestive peptides to produce satiety, it is likely that drug combinations that include one or more monoamine agonists combined with a peptide-related drug will be more effective. These combinations may give more powerful and selective effects with particularly low doses of any one component. With the recent cloning of the NPY Y_5 "feeding" receptor (151), it is likely that a number of compounds will be synthesized to antagonize this receptor and specifically alter eating behavior and energy metabolism. A GAL receptor has also been cloned, although it is not yet known whether it is specific to GAL's feeding effect (514). Agents that reduce circulating glucose levels or enhance sensitivity to insulin may be of additional value in the treatment of obesity and type II diabetes (515). Besides its anorectic actions, GLP-1 improves pancreatic β-cell and α-cell sensitivity to glucose and stimulates insulin secretion, thereby normalizing basal glucose levels (516,517). Compounds of this nature may be useful under conditions when full insulin replacement therapy is not feasible.

D. Steroid Hormones

A compound that blocks the type II glucocorticoid receptors, RU486, is found to reduce body weight in obese animals (518,519). Tests in humans are currently underway to determine its efficacy over the long term. This may open the door to low-dose combinations of multiple drugs, such as a monamine agonist, peptide-related compound, and glucocorticoid antagonist, to delicately adjust multiple systems rather than using a single strong treatment of just one system component. The latter may be more appropriate for treatment of patients with a single identifiable problem.

ACKNOWLEDGMENTS

Some of the research described in this review has been supported by U.S. Public Health Service Grants MH 43422 (SFL) and MH 30697 (BGH). We thank Mr. Jordan Dourmashkin and Ms. Hi Joon Yu for their assistance in the preparation of this chapter.

REFERENCES

1. Teitelbaum P, Stricker EM. Compound complementarities in the study of motivated behavior. Psychol Rev 1994; 101:312–317.
2. Rolls ET. Neuronal activity related to the control of feeding. In: Ritter RC, Ritter S, Barnes CD, eds. Feeding Behavior Neural and Humoral Controls. Orlando, FL: Academic Press, 1986: 163–190.
3. Lenard L, Jando G, Karadi Z, Hajnal A, Sandor P. Lateral hypothalamic feeding mechanisms: iontophoretic effects of kainic acid, ibotenic acid and 6-hydroxydopamine. Brain Res Bull 1988; 20:847–856.
4. Steffens AB, Strubbe JH, Balkan B, Scheurink JW. Neuroendocrine mechanisms involved in regulation of body weight, food intake and metabolism. Neurosci Biobehav Rev 1990; 14:305–313 (review).
5. Bernardis LL, Bellinger LL. The lateral hypothalamic area revisited: neuroanatomy, body weight regulation, neuroendocrinology and metabolism. Neurosci Biobehav Rev 1993; 17:141–193.
6. Powley TL, Opsahl CA. Autonomic components of the hypothalamic feeding syndromes. In: Novin D, Wyrwicka W, Bray GA, eds. Hunger: Basic Mechanisms and Clinical Implications. New York: Raven Press, 1976: 313–326.
7. Steffens AB, Strubbe JH, Scheurink AJ, Balkan B. Neuroendocrine activity during food intake modulates secretion of the endocrine pancreas and contributes to the regulation of body weight. In: Friedman MI, Tordoff MG, Kare MR, eds. Chemical Senses: Appetite and Nutrition. New York: Marcel Dekkar, 1991: 405–425.
8. Shimazu T. Central nervous system regulation of energy expenditure in brown adipose tissue and skeletal muscle. In: Angel A, Anderson H, Bouchard C, Lace D, Leiter L, Mendelson R, eds. Progress in Obesity Research, 7th ed. London: John Libbey, 1996: 193–199.
9. Hoebel BG, Teitelbaum P. Weight regulation in normal and hypothalamic hyperphagic rats. Comp Physiol Psychol 1996; 61:189–193.
10. Leibowitz SF, Roossin P, Rosenn M. Chronic norepinephrine injection into the hypothalamic paraventricular nucleus produces hyperphagia and increased body weight in the rat. Pharmacol Biochem Behav 1984; 21:801–808.
11. Inoue S. Animal models of obesity: Hypothalamic lesion. In: Bjorntop P, Brodoff BN, eds. Obesity. Philadelphia: JB Lippincott, 1992: 266–277.
12. Woods SC, Lotter EC, McKay LD, Porte D. J. Chronic intracerebroventricular infusion of insulin reduces food intake and body weight of baboons. Nature 1979; 282: 503–505.
13. York DA, Marchington D, Holt SJ, Allars J. Regulation of sympathetic activity in lean and obese Zucker (*fa/fa*) rats. Am J Physiol 1985; 249:E299-305.
14. Peterson HR, Rothschild M, Weinberg CR, Fell RD, McLeish KR, Pfeifer, et al. Body fat and the activity of the autonomic nervous system. N Engl Med 1988; 318: 1077–1083.
15. Bray GA. Hypothalamic and genetic obesity: An appraisal of the autonomic hypothesis and the endocrine hypothesis. In: Sullivan AC, Garattini S, eds. Novel Approaches and Drugs for Obesity. London: John Libbey, 1985: 119–137.
16. Bray GA. Food intake, sympathetic activity and adrenal steroids. Brain Res Bull 1993; 32: 537–541.
17. Jequier E. Energy regulation and thermogenesis in humans. In: Bray GA, Spiegelman BM, eds. Obesity: Towards a Molecular Approach. New York: Wiley-Liss, 1990: 95–106.
18. Sakata T, Ookuma K, Fujimoto K, Fukagawa K, Yoshimatsu H. Histaminergic control of energy balance in rats. Brain Res Bull 1991; 27:371–375.
19. Brobeck JR. Food and temperature. Recent Progr Horm Res 1960; 16:439–459.
20. Campbell BA, Misanin JR. Basic drives. Annu Rev Psychol 1960; 20:57–84.
21. Aravich PF, Doerries, LE, Stanley E, Metcalf A, Lauterio TJ. Glucoprivic feeding and activity-based anorexia in the rat. In: Schneider LH, Cooper SJ, Halmi KA, eds. The Psychology of Human Eating Disorders. New York: New York Academy of Sciences, 1989: 490–492.
22. Pothos EN, Creese I, Hoebel BG. Restricted eating with weight loss selectively decreases extracellular dopamine in the nucleus accumbens and alters dopamine response to amphetamine, morphine and food intake. Neurosci 1995; 15:6640–6650.
23. Pothos EN, Hernandez L, Hoebel BG. Chronic food deprivation decreases extracellular dopamine in the nucleus accumbens: implications for a possible neurochemical link between weight loss and drug abuse. Obes Res 1995; 3 Suppl 4:525S-529S.
24. Shimizu H, Simomura Y, Takahashi M, Uehara Y, Fukatsu A, Sato N. Altered ambulatory activity and related brain monomaine metabolism in genetically obese Zucker rats. Exp Clin Endocrinol 1991; 97:39–44.
25. Nicolaidis S, Even P. Metabolic rate and feeding behavior. Ann NY Acad Sci 1989; 575:86–104 (review).
26. Campfield LA, Smith FJ. Systemic factors in the control of food intake: evidence for patterns as signals. In:

Stricker EM, ed. Handbook of Behavioral Neurobiology. New York: Plenum Press, 1990:183–206.

27. Mayer J. Glucostatic mechanism of regulation of food intake. N Engl J Med 1953; 249:13–16.

28. Friedman MI, Rawson NE, Tordoff MG. Control of food intake. In: Bray GA, Ryan DH, eds. Molecular and Genetic Aspects of Obesity. Baton Rouge: LSU Press, 1996: 318–339.

29. Calingasan NY, Ritter S. Hypothalamic paraventricular nucleus lesions do not abolish glucoprivic or lipoprivic feeding. Brain Res 1992; 595:25–31.

30. Bernardis LL, Bellinger LL. The lateral hypothalamic area revisited: ingestive behavior. Neurosci Biohehav Rev 1996; 20:189–287.

31. Stanley BG, Leibowitz SF, Eppel N, St.-Pierre S, Hoebel BG. Suppression of norepinephrine-elicited feeding by neurotensin: evidence for behavioral anatomical and pharmacological specificity. Brain Res 1985; 343: 297–304.

32. Paez X, Stanley BG, Leibowitz SF. Microdialysis analysis of norepinephrine levels in the paraventricular nucleus in association with food intake at dark onset. Brain Res 1993; 606:167–170.

33. Jacobs BL. Brain monoaminergic unit activity in behaving animals. In: Epstein AN, Morrison AR, eds. Progress in Psychobiology and Physiological Psychology. New York: Academic Press, 1987:171–206.

34. Leibowitz SF, Weiss GF, Yee F, Tretter JB. Noradrenergic innervation of the paraventricular nucleus: specific role in control of carbohydrate ingestion. Brain Res Bulletin 1985; 14:561–567.

35. Currie PJ. Medial hypothalamic a_2-adrenergic and serotonergic effects on ingestive behavior. In: Cooper SJ, Clifton PG, eds. Dopamine Receptor Subtypes and Ingestive Behaviour. London: Academic Press, 1996:285–300.

36. Leibowitz SF. Neurochemical-neuroendocrine systems in the brain controlling macronutrient intake and metabolism. Trends Neurosci 1992; 15:491–497 (review).

37. Tempel, DL, Leibowitz SF. Adrenal steroid receptors: interactions with brain neuropeptide systems in relation to nutrient intake and metabolism. Neuroendocrinol 1994; 6:479–501 (review).

38. Stanley BG, Schwartz DH, Hernandez L, Hoebel BG, Leibowtiz SF. Patterns of extracellular norepinephrine in the paraventricular hypothalamus: relationship to circadian rhythm and deprivation-induced eating behavior. Life Sci 1989; 45:275–282.

39. Shor-Posner G, Ian C, Brennan G, Cohn T, Moy H, Ning A, et al. Self-selecting albino rats exhibit differential preferences for pure macronutrient diets: characterization of three subpopulations. Physiol Behav 1991; 50: 1187–1195.

40. Hoebel BG, Leibowitz SF. Brain monoamines in the modulation of self-stimulation feeding, and body weight. In: Weiner H, Hofer MA, Stunkard AJ, eds. Brain, Behavior and Bodily Disease. New York: Raven Press, 1981.

41. Morien, A, McMahon L, Wellman PJ. Effects on food and water intake of the alpha 1-adrenoceptor agonists amidephrine and SK&F-89748. Life Sci 1993; 53:169–174.

42. Hoebel BG. Brain neurotransmitters in food and drug reward. Am J Clin Nutr 1985; 42:1133–1150 (review).

43. Wellman PJ, Davies BT. Reversal of phenylpropanolamine anorexia in rats by the alpha-1 receptor antagonist benoxathian. Pharmacol Biochem Behav 1991; 38:905–908.

44. Wilmot CA, Sullivan AC, Levin BE. Effects of diet and obesity on brain alpha 1- and alpha 2-noradrenergic receptors in the rat. Brain Res 1988; 453:157–166.

45. Angel I. Central receptors and recognition sites mediating the effects of monamines and anorectic drugs on feeding behavior. Clin Neuropharmacol 1990; 13:361–391.

46. Jhanwar-Uniyal M, Papamichael MJ, Leibowitz SF. Glucose-dependent changes in alpha 2-noradrenergic receptors in hypothalamic nuclei. Physiol Behav 1988; 44: 611–617.

47. Leibowitz SF. Reciprocal hunger-regulating circuits involving alpha- and beta-adrenergic receptors located, respectively, in the ventromedial and lateral hypothalamus. Proc Nat Acad Sci USA 1970; 67:1063–1070.

48. Margules DL. Beta-adrenergic receptors in the hypothalamus for learned and unlearned taste aversions. Comp Physiol Psychol 1970; 73:13–21.

49. Hoebel BG. Neuroscience and motivation: pathways and peptides that define motivation. In: Atkinson RC, Herrnstein RJ, Lindzey G, Luce RD, eds. Steven's Handbook of Experimental Psychology, 2nd ed. New York: Wiley, 1988: 547–625.

50. Lafontan M, Berlan M. Fat cell adrenergic receptors and the control of white and brown fat cell function. J Lipid 1993; 34:1057–1091 (review).

51. Leibowitz SF, Weiss GF, Shor-Posner G. Hypothalamic serotonin: pharmacological, biochemical, and behavioral analyses of its feeding-suppressive action. Clin Neuropharmacol 1988; 11(Suppl 1):S51–71.

52. Leibowitz SF. Hypothalamic serotonin in relation to appetite for macronutrients and eating disorders. In: Vanhoutte PM, ed. Serotonin. Amsterdam, The Netherlands: Kluwer Academic Publishers, 1993:383–391.

53. Schwartz DH, McClane S, Hernandez L, Hoebel BG. Feeding increases extracellular serotonin in the lateral hypothalamus of the rat as measured bh microdialysis. Brain Res 1989; 479:349–354.

54. Schwartz DH, Hernandez L, Hoebel BG. Serotonin release in lateral and medial hypothalamus during feeding and its anticipation. Brain Res Bull 1990; 25:797–802.

55. Mark GP, Schwartz DH, Hernandez L, West HL, Hoebel BG. Application of microdialysis to the study of motivation and conditioning: measurements of dopamine and serotonin in freely-behaving rats. In: Robinson TE, Justice JB, eds. Microdialysis in the Neurosciences. Amsterdam: Elsevier Science Publishing, 1991: 369–385.

56. Cooper SJ, Dourish CT, Barber DJ. Reversal of the anorectic effect of (+)-fenfluramine in the rat by selective

cholecystokinin receptor antagonist MK-329. Br Pharmacol 1990; 99:65–70.

57. Smith GP, Gibbs J. Satiating effect of cholecystokinin. Annals of the NY Acad Sci 1994; 713:236–241 (review).

58. Crawley JN, Corwin RL. Biological actions of cholecystokinin. Peptides 1994; 15:731–755.

59. Campbell DB. Dexfenfluramine: an overview of its mechanisms of action. Rev Contemp Pharmacother 1991; 2: 93–113.

60. Rowland NE, Carlton J. Tolerance to the effects of *d*-fenfluramine in rats, hamsters and mice. In: Ferrari E, Brambilla F, eds. Disorders of Eating Behavior: A Psychoneuroendocrine Approach. Oxford: Perfamon, 1986: 367–374.

61. Samanin R, Garattini S. The neuropharmacology of obesity: experimental studies. Rev Contemp Pharmacother 1991; 2:53–59.

62. Lawton CL, Blundell JE. 5-HT and carbohydrate suppression: effects of 5-HT antagoinists on the action of *d*-fenfluramine and DOI. Pharmacol Biochem Behavio 1993; 46:349–360.

63. Gibson EL, Kennedy AJ, Curzon G. *d*-Fenfluramine- and *d*-norfenfluramine-induced hypophagia: differential mechanisms and involvement of postsynaptic 5-HT receptors. Eur J Pharmacol 1993; 242:83–90.

64. Grignaschi G, Sironi F, Samanin R. The 5-HT1B receptor mediates the effect of *d*-fenfluramine of eating caused by intra-hypothalamic injection of neuropeptide Y. Eur J Pharmacol 1995; 274:221–224.

65. Leibowitz SF, Weiss GF, Suh JS. Medial hypothalamic nuclei mediate serotonin's inhibitory effect on feeding behavior. Pharmacol Biochem Behav 1990; 37:735–742.

66. Wurtman RJ, Wurtman JJ. Carbohydrate craving, obesity and brain serotonin. Appetite 1986; 7(Suppl.):99–103.

67. McClelland RC, Sarfaty T, Hernandez L, Hoebel BG. The appetite suppressant, *d*-fenfluramine, decreases self-stimulation at a feeding site in the lateral hypothalamus. Pharmacol Biochem Behav 1989; 32:411–414.

68. Blundell JE, Rogers PJ. Hunger, hedonics and the control of satiation and satiety. In: Friedman MI, Tordoff MG, Kare MR, eds. Chemical Senses: Appetite and Nutrition. New York: Marcel Dekker, 1991:127–148.

69. Hammer VA, Gietzen DW, Beverly JL, Rogers QR. Serotonin receptor antagonists block anorectic responses to amino acid imbalance. Am J Physiol 1990; 259: R627–R636.

70. Li BH, Spector AC, Rowland NE. Reversal of dexfenfluramine-induced anorexia and c-Fos/c-Jun expression by lesion in the lateral parabrachial nucleus. Brain Res 1994; 640:255–267.

71. Simansky KJ, Jakubow J, Sisk FC, Vaidya AH, Eberle-Wang K. Peripheral serotonin is an incomplete signal for eliciting satiety in sham-feeding rats. Pharmacol Biochem Behav 1992; 43:847–854.

72. Leibowitz SF, Brown LL. Histochemical and pharmacological analysis of catecholaminergic projections to the perifornical hypothalamus in relation to feeding inhibition. Brain Res 1980; 201:315–345.

73. Leibowitz SF, Rossakis C. Pharmacological characterization of perifornical hypothalamic dopamine receptors mediating feeding inhibition in the rat. Brain Res 1979; 172: 115–130.

74. Leibowitz SF. Midbrain-hypothalamic catecholamine projection systems mediating feeding stimulation and inhibition in the rat. Usdin E, Kopin IJ, Barchas J, eds. Catecholamines: Basic and Clinical Frontiers. New York: Pergamon Press, 1979:1675–1677.

75. Garattini S, Borroni E, Mennini T, Samanin R. Differences and similarities amoung anorectic agents. In: Garattini S, Samanin R, eds. Central Mechanisms of Anorectic Drugs. New York: Raven Press, 1978:127–143.

76. Weintraub M. Long-term weight control study: conclusions. Clin Pharmacol Ther 1992; 51:642–646.

77. Hitzig P. Combined dopamine and serotonin agonists: a synergistic approach to alcoholism and other addictive behaviors. Maryland Med J 1993; 42:153–156.

78. Moore KE, Demarest KT, Lookingland KJ. Stress, prolactin and hypothalamic dopaminergic neurons. Neuropharmacology 1987; 26:801–808 (review).

79. Parada M, Hernandez L, Schwartz D, Hoebel BG. Hypothalamic infusion of amphetamine increases extracellular serotonin, dopamine and norepinephrine. Physiol Behav 1988; 44:607–610.

80. Wellman PJ. A review of the physiological bases of the anorexic action of phenylpropanolamine (*d*,1-norephedrine). Neurosci Biobehav Rev 1990; 14:339–355 (review).

81. Parada MA, Puig de Parada M, Hoebel BG. Rats self-inject a dopamine antagonist in the lateral hypothalamus where it acts to increase extracellular dopamine in the nucleus accumbens. Pharamcol Biochem Behav 1995; 52: 179–187.

82. Parada MA, Hernandez L, Paez X, Baptista T, Puig de Parada M, et al. Mechanism of the body weight increase induced by systemic sulpiride. Pharamcol Biochem Behav 1989; 33:45–50.

83. Orosco M, Nicolaidis S. Spontaneous feeding-related monoaminergic changes in the rostromedial hypothalamus revealed by microdialysis. Physiol Behav 1992; 52: 1015–1019.

84. Meguid MM, Yang Z-J, Bellinger LL, Gleason JR, Koseki M, Laviano A, et al. Innervated liver plays an inhibitory role in regulation of food intake. Surgery 1996; 119: 202–207.

85. Shimizu H. Alteration in hypothalamic monoamine metabolism of freely moving diabetic rat. Neurosci Lett 1991; 131:225–227.

86. Karadi Z, Oomura Y, Nishino H, Scott TR, Lenard L, Aou S. Responses of lateral hypothalamic glucose-sensitive and glucose-insensitive neurons to chemical stimuli in behaving rhesus monkeys. Neurophysiol 1992; 67:389–400.

87. Hoebel BG, Rada PV, Mark GP, Parada M, Puig de Parada M, Pothos E, et al. Hypothalamic control of accumbens dopamine: A system for feeding reinforcement. In: Bray GA, Ryan D, eds. Molecular and Genetic Aspects of Obesity. Baton Rouge: LSU Press, 1995.

88. Berridge KC. Food reward: Brain substrates of wanting and liking. Neurosci Biobehav Rev 1996; 20:125.

89. Salamone JD, Cousins MS, McCullough LD, Carriero DL, Berkowitz RJ. Nucleus accumbens dopamine release increases during instrumental level pressing for food but not free food consumption. Pharmacol Biochem Behav 1994; 49:25–31.

90. Wise RA. Common neural basis of brain stimulation reward, drug reward, and food reward. In: Hoebel BG, Novin D, eds. The Neural Basis of Feeding and Reward. Brunswick, ME: Haer Institute, 1982:445–454.

91. Fibiger HC, Phillips AG. Reward, motivation, cognition: Psychobiology of mesotelencephalic dopamine system. In: Mountcastle VB, ed. Handbook of Physiology, Section 1: The Nervous System. Bethesda, MD: American Physiological Society, 1986:647–675.

92. Hoebel BG, Hernandez L, Mark GP, Schwartz DH, Pothos E, Steckel JM, et al. Brain microdialysis as a molecular approach to obesity: Serotonin, dopamine, cyclic-AMP. In: Bray G. Ricquier D, Spiegleman B, eds. Obesity: Towards a Molecular Approach. New York: Alan R Liss, 1990: 45–61.

93. Koob GF, Goeders NE. Neuroanatomical substrates of drug self-administration. In: Liebman JM, Cooper SJ, eds. The Neuropharmacological Basis of Reward. New York: Oxford University Press, 1989:214–263.

94. Kornetsky C, Porrino LJ. Brain mechanisms of drug-inducted reinforcement. In: O'Brien CP, Jaffee JH, eds. Addictive States. Association for Research in Nervous and Mental Diseases. New York: Raven Press, 1992:59–77.

95. Hernandez L, Hoebel BG. Feeding and hypothalamic stimulation increase dopamine turnover in the accumbens. Physiol Behav 1988; 44:599–606.

96. Wilson C, Nomikos GG, Collu M, Fibiger HC. Dopaminergic correlates of motivated behavior: importance of drive. J Neurosci 1995; 15:5169–5178.

97. Hoebel BG, Monaco AP, Hernandez L, Aulisi EF, Stanley BG, Lenard L. Self-injection of amphetamine directly into the brain. Psychopharmacology 1983; 81:158–163.

98. Guerin B, Goeders NE, Dworkin SI, Smith JE. Intracranial self-administration of dopamine into the nucleus accumbens. Soc Neurosci Abstr 1984; 10:1072.

99. Wise RA, Newton P, Leeb K, Burnette B, Pocock D, Justice JB Jr. Fluctuations in nucleus accumbens dopamine concentration during intravenous cocaine self-administration in rats. Psychopharmacology 1995; 120:10–20.

100. Bozarth MA. The mesolimbic dopamine system as a model reward system. In: Wellner P, Scheel-Kruger J, eds. The Mesolimbic Dopamine System: From Motivation to Action. New York: Wiley, 1991:301–333.

101. Glimcher PW, Giovino AA, Hoebel BG. Neurotensin self-finjection in the ventral tegmental area. Brain Res 1987; 403:147–150.

102. Kalivas PW, Barnes CD. Limbic Motor Circuits and Neuropsychiatry. Boca Raton, FL: CRC Press, 1993.

103. Sclafani A, Aravich PF, Xenakis S. Dopaminergic and endorphinergic mediation of a sweet reward. In: Hoebel BG, Novin D, eds. The Neural Basis of Feeding and Reward. Brunswick, ME: Haer Inst, 1982:507–515.

104. Smith GP. Dopamine and food reward. In: Fluharty S, Morrison AM, eds. Progress in Psychobiology and Physiological Psychology. New York: Academic Press, 1995: 83–144.

105. Terry P. Dopamine receptor subtypes and ingestive behaviour. In: Cooper SJ, Clifton PG, eds. Drug Receptor Subtypes and Ingestive Behaviour. London: Academic Press, 1996:223–266.

106. Schultz W, Apicella, P, Ljungberg T. Responses of monkey dopamine neurons to reward and conditioned stimuli during successive steps of learning a delayed response task. J Neurosi 1993; 13:900–913.

107. McClelland RC, Hoebel BG. d-Fenfluramine and self-stimulation: loss of fenfluramine effect on underweight rats. Brain Res Bull 1991; 27:341–345.

108. Carr KD, Papadouka V. The role of multiple opioid receptors in the potentiation of reward by food restriction. Brain Res 1994; 639:253–260.

109. Carroll ME, France CP, Meisch RA. Food deprivation increases oral and intravenous drug intake in rats. Science 1979; 205:319–321.

110. Stricker EM, Zigmond MJ. Recovery of function after damage to central catecholamine-containing neurons: a meurochemical model for the lateral hypothalamic syndrome. In: Sprague JM, Epstein AN, eds. Progress in Psychobiology and Physiological Psychology. New York: Academic Press, 1978:121–188.

111. Sodersten P, Bednar I, Qureshi GA, Carrer H, Qian M, Mamoun H, et al. Cholecystokinin-dopamine interactions in satiety. In: Cooper SJ, Clifton PG, eds. Drug Receptor Subtypes and Ingesdtive Behaviour. London: Academic Press, 1996:19–38.

112. Cousins MS, Salamone JD. Nucleus accumbens dopamine depletions in rats affect relative response allocation in a novel cost/benefit procedure. Pharmacol Biochem Behav 1994; 49:85–91.

113. Koob GF, Robledo P, Markou A, Caine SB. The mesocorticolimbic circuit in drug dependence and reward — a role for the extended amygdala? In: Kalivas PW, Barnes CD, eds. Limbic Motor Circuits and Neuropsychiatry. Boca Raton, FL: CRC Press, 1996:289–310.

114. Kelley AE, Delfs JM. Dopamine and conditioned reinforcement. Psychopharmacology 1991; 103:187–196.

115. Weiss FMT, Lorang MT, Bloom FE, Koob GF. Oral alcohol self-administration stimulates dopamine release in the rat nucleus accumbens: Genetic and motivational determinants. J Pharmacol Exp Ther 1993; 267:250–258.

116. Grill HJ, Kaplan JM. Caudal brainstem participates in the distributed neural control of feeding. In: Stricker EM, ed. Handbook of Behavioral Neurobiology. New York: Plenum Press, 1990:125–149.

117. Sclafani A. Nutritionally based learned flavor preferences in rats. In: Capaldi ED, Powley TL, eds. Taste, Experience and Feeding. Washington, DC: American Psychological Association, 1990:139–156.

118. Mark GP, Blander DS, Hoebel BG. A conditioned stimulus decreases extracellular dopamine in the nucleus accumbens after the development of a learned taste aversion. Brain Res 1991; 551:308–310.

119. The Neuropharmacological Basis of Reward. New York: Oxford University Press, 1989.

120. The Mesolimbic Dopamine System: From Motivation to Action. New York: Wiley, 1991.

121. Horvitz JC, Richardson WB, Ettenberg A. Dopamine receptor blockade and reductions in thirst produce differential effects on drinking behavior. Pharamcol Biochem Behav 1993; 45:725–728.

122. Leibowitz SF. Histamine: modification of behavioral and physiological components of body fluid homeostasis. In: Yellin TO, ed. Histamine Receptors. New York: SP Medical and Scientific Books, 1977:219–253.

123. Sakata T, Kurokawa M, Oohara A, Yoshimatsu H. A physiological role of brain histamine during energy deficiency. Brain Res Bull 1994; 35:135–139.

124. Sheiner JB, Morris P, Anderson GH. Food intake suppression by histidine. Pharmacol Biochem Behav 1985; 23: 721–726.

125. Ookuma K, Yoshimatsu H, Sakata T, Fujimoto K. Hypothalamic sites of neuronal histamine action on food intake by rats. Brain Res 1989; 490:268–275.

126. Ookuma K, Sakata T, Fukagawa K, Yoshimatsu H, Kurokawa M, Machidori, et al. Neuronal histamine in the hypothalamus suppresses food intake in rats. Brain Res 1993; 628:235–242.

127. Yoshimatsu H, Machidori H, Doi T, Kurokawa M, Ookuma K, Kang M, et al. Abnormalities in obese Zuckers: defective control of histaminergic functions. Physiol Behav 1993; 54:487–491.

128. Machidori H, Sakata T, Yoshimatsu H, Ookuma K, Fujimoto K, Kurokawa, et al. Zucker obses rats: defect in brain histamine control of feeding. Brain Res 1992; 590: 180–186.

129. Sakata T. Histamine receptor and its regulation of energy metabolism. Obes Res 1995; 3:541s–548s.

130. Brezenoff HE, Lomax P. Temperature changes following microinjection of histamine into the thermoregulatory centers of the rat. Experientia 1970; 26:51–52.

131. Hashimoto M. Characterization and mechanism of fever induction by interleukin-1 beta. Pflugers Arch Eur Physiol 1991; 419:616–621.

132. Plata-Salaman CR, Oomura Y, Kai Y. Tumor necrosis factor and interleukin-1 beta: suppression of food intake by direct action in the central nervous system. Brain Res 1988; 448:106–114.

133. Kang M, Yoshimatsu H, Oogawa R, et al. Hypothalamic neuronal histamine modulates physiological responses induced by interleukin-1 beta. Am J Physiol 1995; 269: R1308–R1313.

134. Lind RW, Swanson LW, Ganten D. Angiotensin II immunoreactive pathways in the central nervous system of the rat: evidence for a projection from the subfornical organ to the paraventricular nucleur of the hypothalamus. Clin Exp Hypertension — Part A, Theory Prac 1984; 6: 1915–1920.

135. Eng R, Miselis RR. Polydipsia and abolition of angiotensin-induced drinking after transections of subfornical organ efferent projections in the rat. Brain Res 1981; 225: 200–206.

136. Schulkin J, Fluharty SJ. Neuroendocrinology of sodium hunger: Angiotensin, corticosteriods, and atrial natriuretic hormone. In: Schulkin J, ed. Hormonally Induced Changes in the Mind and Brain. San Diego: Academic Press, 1993:13–50.

137. Epstein AN. The physiology of thirst. In: Pfaff DW, ed. The Physiological Mechanisms of Motivation. New York: Springer-Verlag, 1982:164–214.

138. Hoebel BG. Integrative peptides. Brain Res Bull 1985; 14: 525–528.

139. Pert CB, Ruff MR, Weber RJ, Herkenham M. Neuropeptides and their receptors: a psychosomatic network. J Immunol 1985; 135:820s–826s.

140. Leibowitz SF. Brain peptides and obesity: pharmacologic treatment. Obes Res 1995; 3:573s–589s.

141. Dryden S, Frankish H, Wang Q, Williams G. Neuropeptide Y and energy balance: one way ahead for the treatment of obesity? Eur J Clin Invest 1994; 24:293–308 (review).

142. Billington CJ, Briggs JE, Harker S, Grace M, Levine AS. Neuropeptide Y in hypothalamic paraventricular nucleus: a center coordinating energy metabolism. Am J Physiol 1994; 266:R1765–70.

143. Dumont Y, Martel JC, Fournier, A, St-Pierre S, Quirion R. Neuropeptide Y and neuropeptide Y receptor subtypes in brain and peripheral tissues. Prog Neurobiol 1992; 38: 125–167 (review).

144. Dube MG, Sahu A, Kalra PS, Kalra SP. Neuropeptide Y release is elevated from the microdissected paraventricular nucleus of food-deprived rats: an in vitro study. Endocrinology 1992; 131:684–688.

145. Stanley BG. Neuropeptide Y in multiple hypothalamic sites controls eating behavior, endocrine, and autonomic systems for body energy balance. In: Colmers WF, Wahlestedt C, eds. The Biology of Neuropeptide Y and Related Peptides. Totowa, NJ: Humana Press, 1993:457–509.

146. Stanley BG, Kyrlouli SE, Lampert S, Leibowitz SF. Neuropeptide Y chronically injected into the hypothalamus: a powerful neurochemical inducer of hyperphagia and obesity. 1986; 7:1189–1192.

147. Humphreys GA, Davison JS, Veale WL. Injection of neuropeptide Y into the paraventricular nucleus of the hypothalamus inhibits gastric acid secretion in the rat. Brain Res 1988; 456:241–248.

148. Valet P, Berlan M, Beauville M, Crampes F, Montastruc JL, Lafontan M. Neuropeptide Y and peptide YY inhibit lipolysis in human and dog fat cells through a pertussis toxin-sensitive G protein. J Clin Invest 1990; 85: 291–295.

149. Stanley BG, Magdalin W, Seirafi A, Nguyen MM, Leibowitz SF. Evidence for neuropeptide Y mediation of eating produced by food deprivation and for a variant of the Y1 receptor mediating this peptide's effect. Peptides 1992; 13:581–587.

150. Leibowitz SF, Xuereb M, Kim T. Blockade of natural and neuropeptide Y-induced carbohydrate feeding by a receptor antagonist PYX-2. NeuroReport 1992, 3:1023–1026.

151. Gerald C, Walker MW, Criscolone L, Gustafson EL, Batzi-Hartmann C, Smith KE, et al. A receptor subtype involved in neuropeptide-Y-induced food intake. Nature 1996; 382:156.

152. Akabayashi A, Wahlestedt C, Alexander JT, Leibowtiz SF. Specific inhibition of endogenous neuropeptide Y synthesis in arcuate nucleus by antisense oligonucleotides suppresses feeding behavior and insulin secretion. Brain Res Mol Brain Res 1994; 21:55–61.

153. Corder R, Pralong F, Turnill D, Saudan P, Muller AF, Gaillard RC. Dexamethasone treatment increases neuropeptide Y levels in rat hypothalamic neurones. Life Sci 1988; 43:1879–1886.

154. Dean RG, White BD. Neuropeptide Y expression in rat brain: effects of adrenalectomy. Neurosci Lett 1990; 114: 339–344.

155. Larsen PJ, Jessop DS, Chowdrey HS, Lightman SL, Mikkelsen JD. Chronic administration of glucocorticoids directly upregulates prepro-neuropeptide Y and Y1-receptor mRNA levels in the arcuate nucleus of the rat. Neuroendocrinol 1994; 6:153–159.

156. Ponsalle, P, Srivastava L, Unt R, White JD. Glucocorticoids are required for food-deprivation induced increases in hypothalamic neuropeptide-Y expression. J Neuroendocrinol 1992; 4:585–591.

157. White BD, Dean RG, Edwards GL, Martin RJ. Type II corticosteriod receptor stimulation increases NPY gene expression in basomedial hypothalamus of rats. Am J Physiolo 1994; 266:R1523–9.

158. Akabayashi A, Watanabe Y, Wahlestedt C, McEwen BS, Paez X, Leibowitz SF. Hypothalmic neuropeptide Y, its gene expression and receptor activity: relation to circulating corticosterone in adrenalectomized rats. Brain Res 1994; 665:201–212.

159. McCarthy HD, Crowder RE, Dryden S, Williams G. Megestro acetate stimulates food and water intake in the rat: effects on regional hypothalmic neuropeptide Y concentrations. Eur Pharmacol 1994; 265:99–102.

160. Urban JH, Bauer-Dantoin AC, Levine JE. Effects of steroid replacement on neuropeptide-Y (NPY) gene expression in the arcuate nucleus (ARC) of ovariectomized (OVX) rats. Soc Neurosci Abst 1992; 18:110 (abstract).

161. Bonavera JJ, Dube MG, Kalra PS, Kalra SP. Anorectic effects of estrogen may be mediated by decreased neuropeptide-Y release in the hypothalamic paraventricular nucleus. Endocrinology 1994; 134:2367–2370.

162. Brann DW, McDonald JK, Putnam CD, Mahesh VB. Regulation of hypothalamic gonadotropin-releasing hormone and neuropeptide Y concentrations by progesterone and corticosteroids in immature rats: correlation with luteinizing hormone and follicle-stimulating hormone release. Neuroendocrinology 1991; 54:425–432.

163. Kalra SP, Crowley WR. Neuropeptide Y: a novel neuroendocrine peptide in the control of pituitary hormone secretion, and its relation to luteinizing hormone. Frontiers Neuroendocrinol 1992; 13:1–46 (review).

164. Silva I, Wang J, Felber M, Akabayashi A, Leibowitz SF. Impact of insulin on neuropeptide-Y (NPY) in the hypothalamic arcuate and paraventricular nuclei in vivo and in vitro. Soc Neurosci Abst 1995; 21:1392 (abstract).

165. Wang J, Andrews D, Liu H, Leibowitz SF. Insulin inhibits galanin in the hypothalamic paraventricular nucleus: in vivo and in vitro studies. Neurosci Abstr 1995; 21:1392 (abstract).

166. Schwartz MW, Sipols A, J., Marks JL, Sanacora G, White JD, Scheurink A, et al. Inhibition by hypothalamic neuropeptide Y gene expression by insulin. Endocrinology 1992; 130:3608–3616.

167. Sahu A, Sninsky CA, Phelps CP, Dube MG, Kalra PS, Kalra SP. Neuropeptide Y release from the paraventricular nucleus increases in association with hyperphagia in streptozotocin-induced diabetic rats. Endocrinology 1992; 131:2979–2985.

168. Kaiyala KJ, Woods SC, Schwartz MW. New model for the regulation of energy balance and adiposity by the central nervous system. Am J Clin Nutr 1995; 62:1123S–1134S (review).

169. Beck B, Jhanwar-Uniyal M, Burlet A, Chapleur-Chateau M, Leibowtiz SF, Burlet C. Rapid and localized alterations of neuropeptide Y in discrete hypothalamic nuclei with feeding status. Brain Res 1990; 528:245–249.

170. Sahu A, Kalra PS, Kalra SP. Food deprivation in ingestion induce reciprocal changes in neuropeptide Y concentrations in the paraventricular nucleus. Peptides 1988; 9: 83–86.

171. Calza L, Giardino L, Battistini N, Zanni M, Galetti S, Protopapa F, et al. Increase of neuropeptide Y-like immunoreactivity in the paraventricular nucleus of fasting rats. Neurosci Lett 1989; 104:99–104.

172. Sanacora G, Kershaw M, Finkelstein JA, White JD. Increased hypothalamic content of preproneuropeptide Y messenger ribonucleic acid in genetically obese Zucker rats and its regulation by food deprivation. Endocrinology 1990; 127:730–737.

173. Jhanwar-Uniyal M, Chua SC, Jr. Critical effects of aging and nutritional state on hypothalamic neuropeptide Y and galanin gene expression in lean and genetically obese Zucker rats. Brain Res 1993; 3:195–202.

174. Kanarek RB, Marks-Kaufman R, Ruthazer R, Gualtieri L. Increased carbohydrate consumption by rats as a function of 2-deoxy-D-glucose administration. Pharmacol Biochem Behav 1983; 18:47–50.

175. Akabayashi A, Zaia CTBV, Silva I, Chae HJ, Leibowitz SF. Neuropeptide Y in the arcuate nucleus is modulated by alterations in glucose utilization. Brain Res 1993; 621: 343–348.

176. Barnea A, Cho G, Hajibeigi A, Aguila MC, Magni P. Dexamethasone-induced accumulation of neuropeptide-Y by aggregating fetal brain cells in culture: a process dependent on the developmental age of aggregates. Endocrinology 1991; 129:931–938.

177. Lerchen RA, Yum DY, Krajcik R, Minth-Worby CA. Transcriptional vs. posttranscriptional control of neuropeptide Y gene expression. Endocrinology 1995; 136:833–841.

178. Sabol SL, Higuchi H. Transcriptional regulation of the neuropeptide Y gene by nerve growth factor: antagonism by glucocorticoids and potentiation by adenosine 3',5'-monophosphate and phorbol ester. Mol Endocrinol 1990; 4:384–392.

179. Higuchi H, Yang HY, Sabol SL. Rat neuropeptide Y precursor gene expression. mRNA structure, tissue distribution, and regulation by glucocorticoids, cyclic AMP, and phorbol ester. J Biol Chem 1988; 263:6288–6295.

180. Akabayashi A, Zaia CT, Gabriel SM, Silva I, Cheung WK, Leibowitz SF. Intracerebroventricular injection of dibutyryl cyclic adenosine 3',5'-monophosphate increases hypothalamic levels of neuropeptide. Brain Res 1994; 660: 323–328.

181. Beck B, Stricker-Krongrad A, Burlet A, Nicolas JP, Burlet C. Specific hypothalamic neuropeptide Y variation with diet parameters in rats with food choice. NeuroReport 1992; 3:571–574.

182. Jhanwar-Uniyal M, Beck B, Jhanwar YS, Burlet C, Leibowitz SF. Neuropeptide Y projection from arcuate nucleus to parvocellular division of paraventricular nucleus: specific relation to the ingestion of carbohydrate. Brain Res 1993; 631:97–106.

183. Larue-Achagiotis C, Martin C, Verger P, Louis-Sylvestre J. Dietary self-selection vs. complete diet: body weight gain and meal pattern in rats. Physiol Behav 1992; 51: 995–999.

184. Miller GD, Hrupka BJ, Gietzen DW, Rogers QR, Stern JS. Rats on a macronutrient self-selection diet eat most meals from a single food cup. Appetite 1994; 23:67–78.

185. Jhanwar-Uniyal M, Beck B, Burlet C, Leibowitz SF. Diurnal rhythm of neuropeptide Y-like immunoreactivity in the suprachiasmatic, arcuate and paraventricular nuclei and other hypothalamic sites. Brain Res 1990; 536:331–334.

186. Alexander JT, Akabayashi A, Gabriel AM, Baskin LE, Owen CJ, Leibowtiz SF. Galanin and neuropeptide-Y immunoreactivity in hypothalamic nuclei in relation to the estrous cycle. Soc Neurosci Abstr 1995; 21:1888 (abstract).

187. Bauer-Dantoin AC, Urban JH, Levine JE. Neuropeptide Y gene expression in the arcuate nucleus is increased during preovulatory luteinizing hormone surges. Endocrinology 1992; 131:2953–2958.

188. Alexander JT, Akabayashi A, Gabriel SM, Thomas BE, Leibowitz SF. Galanin and neuropeptide Y immunoreactivity in brain nuclei of female and male rats in relation to puberty. Soc Neurosci Abstr 1994; 20:99 (abstract).

189. Allen JM, McGregor GP, Woodhams PL, Polak JM, Bloom SR. Ontogeny of a novel peptide, neuropeptide Y (NPY) in rat brain. Brain Res 1984; 303:197–200.

190. Kagotani Y, Hashimoto T, Tsuruo Y, Kawano H, Daikoku S, Chihara K. Development of tne neuronal system containing neuropeptide Y in the rat hypothalamus. Int J Dev Neurosci 1989; 7:359–374.

191. Sutton SW, Mitsugi N, Plotsky PM, Sarkar DK. Neuropeptide Y (NPY): a possible role in the initiation of puberty. Endocrinology 1988; 123:2152–2154.

192. Leibowitz SF, Lucas DJ, Leibowitz KL, Jhanwar YS. Developmental patterns of macronutrient intake in female and male rats from weaning to maturity. Physiol Behav 1991; 50:1167–1174.

193. Lesniewska B, Miskowiak B, Nowak M, Malendowicz LK. Sex differences in adrenocortical structure and function. XXVII. The effect of ether stress on ACTH and corticosterone in intact, gonadectomized, and testosterone- or estradiol-replaced rats. Res Exp Med 1990; 190:95–103.

194. Patchev VK, Hayashi S, Orikasa C, Almeida OF. Implications of estrogen-dependent brain organization for gender differences in hypothalamo-pituitary-adrenal regulation. FASEB J 1995; 9:419–423.

195. Sapolsky RM, Meaney MJ. Maturation of the adrenocortical stress response: neuroendocrine control mechanisms and the stress hyporesponsive period. Brain Res 1986; 396:64–76 (review).

196. Tempel DL, Leibowitz SF. Diurnal variations in the feeding responses to norepinephrine, neuropeptide Y and galanin in the PVN. Brain Res Bull 1990; 25:821–825.

197. Dryden S, McCarthy HD, Malabu UH, Ware M, Williams G. Increased neuropeptide Y concentrations in specific hypothalamic nuclei of the rat following treatment with methysergide: evidence that NPY may mediate serotonin's effects on food intake. Peptides 1993; 14:791–796.

198. Merchenthaler I, Lopez FJ, Negro-Vilar A. Anatomy and physiology of central galanin-containing pathways. Prog Neurobiol 1993; 40:711–769 (review).

199. Chae HJ, Hoebel BG, Tempel DL, Paredes M, Leibowitz SF. Neuropeptide-Y, galanin and opiate agonists have differential effects on nutrient ingestion. Soc Neurosci Abstr 1995; 21:Abstract.

200. Kyrkouli SE, Stanley BG, Hutchinson R, Seirafi RD, Leibowitz SF. Peptide-amine interactions in the hypothalamic paraventricular nucleus: analysis of galanin and neuro-

peptide Y in relation to feeding. Brain Res 1990; 521: 185–191.

201. Tempel DL, Leibowitz KJ, Leibowitz SF. Effects of PVN galanin on macronutrient selection. Peptides 1988; 9: 309–314.

202. Leibowitz SF, Kim T. Impact of a galanin antagonist on exogenous galanin and natural patterns of fat ingestion. Brain Res 1992; 599:148–152.

203. Corwin RL, Robinson JK, Crawley JN. Galanin antagonists block galanin-induced feeding in the hypothalamus and amygdala of the rat. Eur J Neurosci 1993; 5:1528–1533.

204 Mendendez JA, Atrens DM, Leibowitz SF. Metabolic effects of galanin injections into the paraventricular nucleus of the hypothalamus. Peptides 1992; 13:323–327.

205. Nagase H, Bray GA, York DA. Effect of galanin and enterostatin on sympathetic nerve activity to interscapular brown adipose tissue. Brain Res 1996; 709:44–50.

206. Smith BK, York DA, Bray GA. Chronic cerebroventricular galanin does not induce sustained hyperphagia or obesity. Peptides 1994; 15:1267–1272.

207. Koenig JI, Hooi SC, Maiter DM. On the interaction of galanin within the hypothalamo-pituitary axis of the rat. In: Hokfelt T, Bartfai T, Jacobowtiz T, Ottson DT, eds. Galanin: A New Multifunctional Peptide in the Neuroendocrine System. New York: Macmillan, 1991:331–342.

208. Kondo K, Murase T, Otake K, Ito M, Oiso Y. Centrally administered galanin inhibits osmotically stimulated arginine vasopressin release in conscious rats. Neurosci Lett 1991; 128:245–248.

209. Hedlund PB, Koenig JI, Fuxe K. Adrenalectomy alters discrete galanin mRNA levels in the hypothalamus and mesencephalon of the rat. Neurosci Lett 1994; 170:77–82.

210. Akabayashi A., Watanabe Y, Gabriel SM, Chae HJ, Leibowitz SF. Hypothalamic galanin-like immunoreactivity and its gene expression in relation to circulating corticosterone. Mol Brain Res 1994; 25:305–312.

211. Bloch GJ, Eckersell C, Mills R. Distribution of galaninimmunoreactive cells within sexually dimorphic components of the medial preoptic area of the male and female rat. Brain Res 1993; 620:259–268.

212. Brann DW, Chorich LP, Mahesh VB. Effect of progesterone on galanin mRNA levels in the hypothalamus and the pituitary: correlation with the gonadotropin surge. Neuroendorcrinology 1993; 58:531–538.

213. Gabriel SM, Washton DL, Roncancio JR. Modulation of hypothalamic galanin gene expression by estrogen in peripubertal rats. Peptides 1992; 13:801–806.

214. Tang C, Akabayashi A, Manitiu A, Leibowitz SF. Insulin modulates galanin gene expression in the hypothalamic paraventricular nucleus. J Neuroendorcrinol 1996; In press.

215. Beck B, Burlet A, Nicolas JP, Burlet C. Galanin in the hypothalamus of fed and fasted lean and obese Zucker rats. Brain Res 1993; 623:124–130.

216. Manitiu A, Nascimento J, Akabayashi A, Leibowitz SF. Inhibition of fatty acid oxidation via injection of mercap-

toacetate. Internation Behav Neurosci Abstr 1994; 3:67 (abstract).

217. Akabayashi A, Koenig JI, Watanabe Y, Alexander JT, Leibowitz SF. Galanin-containing neurons in the paraventricular nucleus: a neurochemical marker for fat ingestion and body weight gain. Proc Nat Acad Sci USA 1994; 91: 10375–10379.

218. Marks DL, Smith MS, Vrontakis M, Clifton DK, Steiner RA. Regulation of galanin gene expression in gonadotropin-releasing hormone neurons during the estrous cycle of the rat. Endocrinology 1993; 132:1836–1844.

219. Gabriel SM, Kaplan LM, Martin JB, Koenig JI. Tissuespecific sex differences in galanin-like immunoreactivity and galanin mRNA during development in the rat. Peptides 1989; 10:369–374.

220. Rossmanith WG, Marks DL, Clifton DK, Steiner RA. Induction of galanin gene expression in gonadotropinreleasing hormone neurons with puberty in the rat. Endorcrinology 1994; 135:1401–1408.

221. Arslanian SA, Kalhan SC. Correlations between fatty acid and glucose metabolism. Potential explanation of insulin resistance of puberty. Diabetes 1994; 43:908–914.

222. Nordstrom O, Melander T, Hokfelt T, Bartfai T, Goldstein M. Evidence for an inhibitory effect of the peptide galanin on dopamine release from the rat median eminence. Neurosci Lett 1987; 73:21–26.

223. Gosnell BA, Levine AS. Stimulation of ingestive behavior by preferential and selective opiod agonists. In: Cooper SJ, Clifton PG, eds. Drug Receptor Subtypes and Ingestive Behavior. London: Academic Press, 1996: 147–166.

224. Leibowitz SF. Opioid, a-noradrenergic and adrenocorticotropin systems of hypothalamic paraventricular nucleus. In: Weiner H, Baum A, eds. Perspective in Behavioral Medicine, Eating Regulation and Discontrol. Hillsdale, NJ: Lawrence Erlbaum Associates, 1987: 113–136.

225. Siviy SM, Calcagnetti DJ, Reid LD. A temporal analysis of naloxone's suppressant effect on drinking. Pharmacol Biochem Behav 1982; 16:173–175.

226. Rudski JM, Billington CJ, Levine AS. Naxolone's effects on operant responding depend upon level of deprivation. Pharmacol Biochem Behav 1994; 49:377–383.

227. Cooper SJ. Sweetness, reward and analgesia. Trends Pharmacol Sci 1984; 322–323.

228. Kanarek RB, White ES, Biegen MT, Marks-Kaufman. R. Dietary influences on morphine-induced analgesia in rats. Pharmacol Biochem Behav 1991; 38:681–684.

229. Blass EM, Hoffmeyer LB. Sucrose as an analgesic for newborn infants. Pediatrics 1991; 87:215–218.

230. Bodnar RJ. Opioid receptor subtype antagonists and ingestion. In: Cooper SJ, Clifton PG, eds. Drug Receptor Subtypes and Ingestive Behaviour. San Diego, CA: Acadmic Press, 1996:127–166.

231. Nencini P. Sensitization to the ingestive effects of opioids. In: Cooper SJ, Clifton PG, eds. Drug Receptor Subtypes

and Ingestive Behaviour. San Diego, CA: Academic Press, 1996:193–218.

232. Vaccarino FJ. Dopamine-opioid mechanisms in ingestion. In: Cooper SJ, Clifton PG, eds. Drug Receptor Subtypes and Ingestive Behaviour. San Diego, CA: Academic Press, 1996:219–232.

233. Carr KD. Opioid receptor subtypes and stimulation-induced feeding. In: Cooper SJ, Clifton PG, eds. Drug Receptor Subtypes and Ingestive Behavior. San Diego CA: Academic Press, 1996:167–192.

234. Reid LD. Endogenous opioid peptides and regulation of drinking and feeding. Am J Clin Nutr 1985; 42: 1099–1132 (review).

235. Morley JE, Levine AS, Gosnell BA, Kneip J, Grace M. The kappa opioid receptor, ingestive behaviors and the obese mouse (*ob/ob*). Physiol Behav 1983; 31:603–606.

236. Cooper SJ. Evidence for opioid involement in controls of drinking and water balance. In: Rodgers RJ, Cooper SJ, eds. Endorphins, Opiates and Behavioural Processes. New York: Wiley, 1988:187–216.

237. Bodnar RJ, Beczkowska IW, Koch JE. Opioid receptor subtypes differentially alter palatable fluid intake in rats. Appetite 1993; 21:165.

238. Leibowitz SF, Hor L. Endorphinergic and alpha-noradrenergic systems in the paraventricular nucleus: effects on eating behavior. Peptides 1982; 3:421–428.

239. McLean S, Hoebel BG. Feeding induced by opiates injected into the paraventricular hypothalamus. Peptides 1983; 4:287–292.

240. Carr KD, Bak TH, Simon EJ, Portoghese PS. Effects of the selective kappa opioid antagonist, nor-binaltorphimine, on electrically-elicited feeding in the rat. Life Sci 1989; 45:1787–1792.

241. Zardetto-Smith AM, Moga MM, Magnuson DJ, Gray TS. Lateral hypothalamic dynorphinergic efferents to the amygdala and brainstem in the rat. Peptides 1988; 9: 1121–1127.

242. Carr KD, Aleman DO, Bak TH, Simon EJ. Effects of parabrachial opioid antagonism on stimulation-induced feeding. Brain Res 1991; 545:283–286.

243. Levine AS, Grace M, Billington CJ. The effect of centrally administered naloxone on deprivation and drug-induced feeding. Pharmacol Biochem Behav 1990; 36:409–412.

244. Hoebel BG. Brain-stimulation reward and aversion in relation to behavior. In: Wauquier A, Rolls ET, eds. Brain-Stimulation Reward. Amsterdam: Elsevier/North-Holland, 1976:335–372.

245. Wise RA. Opiate reward: sites and substrates. Neurosci Biohehav Rev 1989; 13:129–133 (review).

246. Hernandez L, Hoebel BG. Hypothalamic reward and aversion: A link between metabolism and behavior. In: Veal WL, Lederis K, eds. Current Studies of Hypothalamic Function, Vol. 2, Metabolism and Behavior. Basel: Karger, 1978:72–92.

247. Wise RA. The brain and reward. In: Leibman JM, Cooper SJ, eds. The Neuropharmacological Basis of reward. New York: Oxford University Press, 1989:377–424.

248. Hamilton ME, Bozarth MA. Feeding elicited by dynorphin (1–13) microinjections into the ventral tegmental area in rats. Life Sci 1988; 43:941–946.

249. De Witte P, Heidbreder C, Roques BP. Kelatorphan, a potent enkephalinases inhibitor, and opioid receptor agaonists DAGO and DTLET, differentially modulate self-stimulation behaviour depending on the site of administration. Neuropharmacology 1989; 28:667–676.

250. Glimcher PG, Giovino AA, Margolin DH, Hoebel BG. Endogenous opiate reward induced by an enkephalinase inhibitor, thiorphan, injected into the ventral midbrain. Behav Neurosci 1984; 98:262–268.

251. Carr GD, Fibiger HC, Phillips GD. Conditioned place preference as a measure of drug reward. In: Liebman JM, Cooper SJ, eds. The Neuropharmacological Basis of Reward. New York: Oxford University Press, 1989:264–319.

252. Goeders NE, Lane TD, Smith JE. Self-administration of methionine enkephalin into the nucleus accumbens. Pharmacol Biochem Behav 1984; 20:451–455.

253. Olds ME. Reinforcing effects of morphine in the nucleus accumbens. Brain Res 1982; 237:429–440.

254. Shippenberg TS, Bals-Kubik R. Involvement of the mesolimbic dopamine system in mediating the aversive effects of opioid antagonists in the rat. Behav Pharmacology 1995; 6:99–106.

255. Cooper SJ. Interactions between endogenous opioids and dopamine: Implications for reward and aversion. In: Willner P, Scheel-Kruger J. eds. The Mesolimbic Dopamine System: From Motivation to Action. New York: Wiley, 1991:331–366.

256. Lin L, Okada S, York DA, Bray GA. Structural requirements for the biological activity of enterostatin. Peptides 1994; 15:849–854.

257. Dickson PR, Vaccarino FJ. GRF-induced feeding; evidence from protein selectivity and opiate involvement. Peptides 1994; 15:1343–1352.

257. Dickson PR, Feifel D, Vaccarino FJ. Blockade of endogenous GRF at dark onset selectively suppresses protein intake. Peptides 1995; 16:7–9.

259. Vaccarino FJ, Feifel D, Rivier J, Vale W. Antagonism of central growth hormone-releasing factor activity selectively attenuates dark-onset feeding in rats. J Neurosci 1991; 11:3924–3927.

260. Vaccarino FJ, Hayward M. Microinjections of growth hormone-releasing factor into the medial preoptic area/suprachiasmatic nucleus region of the hypothalamus stimulate food intake in rats. Regul Peptides 1988; 21:21–28.

261. Okada K, Ishi S, Minami S, Sugihara H, Shibasaki T, Wakabayashi I. Intracerebroventricular administration of the growth hormone releasing peptide KP-102 increases food intake in free-feeding rats. Endrocrinology 1996; 137: 5155.

262. Bittencourt JC, Presse F, Arias C, Peto C, Vaughan J, Nahon JL, et al. The melanin-concentrating hormone system of the rat brain: an immuno- and hybridization histochemical characterization. J Neurol 1992; 319:218–245.

263. Presse F, Nahon JL. Differential regulation of melanin-concentrating hormone gene expression in distinct hypothalamic areas under osmotic stimulation in rat. Neuroscience 1993; 55:709–720.

264. Deray A, Griffond B, Colard C, Jacquemard C, Bugnon C, Fellmann D. Activation of the rat melanin-concentrating hormone neurons by ventromedial hypothalamic lesions. Neuropeptides 1994; 27:185–194.

265. Presse F, Sorokovsky I, Max JP, Nicolaidis S, Nahon JL. Melanin-concentrating hormone is a potent anorectic peptide regulated by food-deprivation and glucopenia in the rat. Neuroscience 1996; 71:735–745.

266. Qu Z, Ling PR, Tahan SR, Sierra P, Onderdonk AB, Bistrian BR. Protein and lipid refeeding changes protein metabolism and colonic but not small intestinal morphology in protein-depleted rats. J Nutr 1996; 126:906–912.

267. Shimizu H, Shargill NS, Bray GA, Yen TT, Gesellchen PD. Effects of MSH on food intake, body weight and coat color of the yellow obese mouse. Life Sci 1989; 45:543–552.

268. Wade GN, Schneider JE. Metabolic fuels and reproduction in female mammals. Neurosci Biobehav Rev 1992; 16:235–272 (review).

269. Dutt A, Kaplitt MG, Kow LM, Pfaff DW. Prolactin, central nervous system and behavior: a critical review. Neuroendocrinology 1994; 59:413–419 (review).

270. Crumeyrolle-Arias M, Latouche J, Jammes H, Djiane J, Kelly PA, Reymond MJ, et al. Prolactin receptors in the rat hypothalamus: autoradiographic localization and characterization. Neuroendocrinology 1993; 57:457–466.

271. Dial J, Avery DD. The effects of pregnancy and lactation on dietary self-selection in the rat. Physiol Behav 1991; 49:811–813.

272. Noel MB, Woodside B. Effects of systemic and central prolactin injections on food intake, weight gain, and estrous cyclicity in female rats. Physiol Behav 1993; 54:151–154.

273. Heil SH, Cramer CP. Prolactin injections result in dose-dependent protein consumption in rats. Int Soc Dev Psychobiol 1993; (abstract).

274. Sauve D, Woodside B. The effect of central administration of prolactin on food intake in virgin female rats is dose-dependent, occurs in the absence of ovarian hormones and the latency to onset varies with feeding regimen. Brain Res 1996; 729:75–81.

275. Hnasko RM, Buntin JD. Functional mapping of neural sites mediating prolactin-induced hyperphagia in doves. Brain Res 1993; 623:257–266.

276. Koshiyama H, Kato Y, Inoue T, Murakami Y, Ishikawa Y, Yanaihara N, et al. Central galanin stimulates pituitary prolactin secretion in rats: possible involvement of hypothalamic vasoactive intestinal polypeptide. Neurosci Lett 1987; 75:49–54.

277. Horvath TL, Kalra SP, Naftolin F, Leranth C. Morphological evidence for a galanin-opiate interaction in the rat mediobasal hypothalamus. J Neuroendocrinol 1995; 7:579–588.

278. Cincotta AH, Meier AH. Reduction of body fat stores by inhibition of prolactin secretion. Experientia 1987; 43:416–417.

279. McGowan MK, Andrews KM, Kelly J, Grossman SP. Effects of chronic intrahypothalamic infusion of insulin on food intake and diurnal meal patterning in the rat. Behav Neurosci 1990; 104:373–385.

280. VanderWeele DA. Insulin is a prandial satiety hormone. Physiol Behav 1994; 56:619–622.

281. Baura GD, Foster DM, Porte D, Jr., Kahn SE, Bergman RN, Cobelli C, et al. Saturable transport of insulin from plasma into the central nervous system of dogs in vivo. A mechanism for regulated insulin delivery to the brain. J Clin Invest 1993; 92:1824–1830.

282. Schwartz MW, Figlewic DP, Baskin DG, Woods SC, Porte D, Jr. Insulin in the brain: a hormonal regulator of energy balance. Endoc Rev 1992; 13:387–414 (review).

283. Sahu A, Dube MG, Phelps CP, Sninsky CA, Kalra PS, Kalra SP. Insulin and insulin-like growth factor II suppress neuropeptide Y release from the nerve terminals in the paraventricular nucleus: a putative hypothalamic site for energy homeostasis. Endocrinology 1995; 136:5718–5724.

284. Zhang Y, Procena R, Maffei M, Barone M, Leopold L., Friedman JM. Positional cloning of the mouse obese gene and its human homologue [published erratum appears in Nature 1995 Mar 30; 374(6521):479] [see comments]. Nature 1994; 372:425–432.

285. Banks WA, Kastin AJ, Huang W, Jaspan JB, Maness LM. Leptin enters the brain by a saturable system independent of insulin. Peptides 1996; 17:305–311.

286. Woods SC, Chavez M, Park CR, Reidy C, Kaiyala K, Richardson RD, et al. The evaluation of insulin as a metabolic signal influencing behavior via the brain. Neurosci Biobehav Rev 1996; 20:139–144 (review).

287. Caro JF, Sinha MK, Kolaczynski JW, Zhang PL, Considine RV. Leptin: the tale of an obesity gene. Diabetes 1996; 45:1455.

288. Tartaglia LA, Dembski M, Weng X, Deng N, Culpepper J, Devos R, et al. Identification and expression cloning of a leptin receptor, OB-R. Cell 1995; 83:1263–1271.

289. Campfield LA, Smith FJ, Guisez Y, Devos R, Burn P. Recombinant mouse OB protein: evidence for a peripheral signal linking adiposity and central netural networks [see comments]. Science 1995; 269:546–549.

290. Stephens TW, Basinski M, Bristow PK, Bue-Valleskey JM, Burgett SG, Craft L, et al. The role of neuropeptide-Y in the antiobesity action of the obese gene product. Nature 1996; 377:530–532.

291. Leibowitz SF, Wang J. Circulating leptin: specific effects on brain peptides involved in eating and body weight regulation. Obes Res 1996; 4:1S Abstract.

292. Erickson JC, Cleff KE, Palmiter RD. Sensitivity to leptin and susceptibility to seizures of mice lacking neuropeptide-Y. Nature 1996; 381:415–418.

293. Kolaczynski JW, Nyce MR, Considine RV, Boden G, Nolan JJ, Henry R, et al. Acute and chronic effects of insulin on leptin production in humans: studies in vivo and in vitro. Diabetes 1996; 45:699–701.

294. Ahima RS, Prabakaran D, Mantzoros C, Qu D, Lowell B, Maratos-Flier E, et al. Role of leptin in the neuroendocrine response to fasting. Nature 1996; 382:250–252.

295. Barash IA, Cheung CC, Weigle DS, Ren H, Kabigting EB, Kuijper JL, et al. Leptin is a metabolic signal to the reproductive system. Endocrinology 1996; 137–3144.

296. Cooper GJ. Amylin compared with calcitonin gene-related peptide: structure, biology, and relevance to metabolic disease. Endocr Rev 1994; 15:163–201 (review).

297. Edwards BJ, Morley JE. Amylin. Life Sci 1992; 51: 1899–1912 (review).

298. Lutz TA, Geary N, Szabady MM, Del Prete E, Scharrer E. Amylin decreases meal size in rats. Physiol Behav 1995; 58:1197–1202.

299. Banks WA, Kastin AJ, Maness LM, Huang W, Jaspan JB. Permeability of the blood-brain barrier to amylin. Life Sci 1995; 57:1993–2001.

300. Sexton PM, Paxinos G, Kenney MA, Wookey PJ, Beaumont K. In vitro autoradiographic localization of amylin binding sites in rat brain. Neuroscience 1994; 62: 553–567.

301. Chance WT, Balasubramaniam A, Stallion A, Fischer JE. Anorexia following the systemic injection of amylin. Brain Res 1993; 607:185–188.

302. Hayashi H, Nutting DF, Fujimoto K, Cardelli JA, Black D, Tso P. Transport of lipid and apolipoproteins A-I and A-IV in intestinal injuries lymph of the rat. J Lipid Res 1990; 31:1613–1625.

303. Fujimoto K, Fukagawa K, Sakata T, Tso P. Suppression of food intake by apolipoprotein A-IV is mediated through the central nervous system in rats. J Clin Invest 1993; 91: 1830–1833.

304. Okumura T, Fukagawa K, Tso P, Taylor IL, Pappas TN. Mechanism of action of intracisternal apolipoprotein A-IV in inhibiting gastric acid secretion in rats. Gastroenterology 1995; 109:1583–1588.

305. Geary N. Pancreatic glucagon signals postprandial satiety. Neurosci Biobehav Rev 1990; 14:323–338 (review).

306. Geary N, Le Sauter J, Noh U. Glucagon acts in the liver to control spontaneous meal size in rats. Am J Physiol 1993; 264:R116–22.

307. Kreymann B, Williams G, Ghatei MA, Bloom SR. Glucagon-like peptide-1 7–36: a physiological incretin in man. Lancet 1987; 2:1300–1304.

308. Kreymann B, Ghatei MA, Burnet P, Williams G, Kanse S, Diani AR, et al. Characterization of glucagon-like peptide-1-(7–36)amide in the hypothalamus. Brain Res 1989; 502:325–331.

309. Turton MD, O'Shea D, Gunn I, Beak SA, Edwards CM, Meeran K, et al. A role for glucagon-like peptide-1 in the central regulation of feeding. Nature 1996; 379:69–72.

310. Shughrue PJ, Lane MV, Merchenthaler I. Glucagon-like peptide-1 receptor (GLP1-R) mRNA in the rat hypothalamous. Endocrinology 1996; 137:5159.

311. Madsen OD, Karlsen C, Blume N, Jensen HI, Larsson LI, Holst JJ. Transplantable glucagonomas derived from pluripotent rat islet tumor tissue cause severe anorexia and adipsia. Scand J Clin Lab Invest 1995; 220(Suppl.): 27–35.

312. Gibbs J, Smith GP. Gut peptides and feeding behavior: The model of cholecystokinin. In: Ritter RC, Ritter S, Barnes CD, eds. Feeding Behavior Neural and Humoral Controls. Orlando, FL: Acadmic Press, 1986:329–352.

313. Galef J, B.G., Beck M. Diet selection and poison avoidance by mammals individually and in social groups. In: Stricker EM, ed. Handbook of Behavioral Neurobiology, Vol 10. New York: Plenum Press, 1990:329–349.

314. Schwartz DH, Dorfman DB, Hernandez L, Hoebel BG. Cholecystokinin: 1. CCK antagonists in the PVN induce feeding, 2. Effects of CCK in the nucleus accumbens on extracellular dopamine turnover. In: Wang RY, Schoenfeld R, eds. Neurology and Neurobiology: Cholecystokinin Antagonists. New York: Alan R Liss, 1988:285–305.

315. Moran TH. Receptor subtype and affinity state underlying the satiety actions of cholecystokinin (CCK). In: Cooper SJ, Clifton PG, eds. Drug Receptor Subtypes and Ingestive Behaviour. London: Academic Press, 1996:1–18.

316. Smith GP, Dorre D, Melville L. CCK-33 inhibits food intake after intraportal and intravenous administration. Soc Neurosci Abstr 1996; 22:17 (abstract).

317. Verbalis JG, McCann MJ, McHale CM, Stricker EM. Oxytocin secretion in response to cholecystokinin and food: differentiation of nausea from satiety. Science 1986; 232: 1417–1419.

318. Deutsch JA, Hardy WT. Cholecystokinin produces bait shyness in rats. Nature 1977; 266:196.

319. Mueller K, Hsaie S. Specificity of cholecystokinin satiety effect: Reduction of food but not water intake. Pharmacol Biochem Behav 1977; 6:643–646.

320. Flood JF, Silver AJ, Morley JE. Do peptide-induced changes in feeding occur because of damages in motivation to eat? Peptides 1990; 11:265–270.

321. Dourish CT. Behavioral analysis of the role of CCK-A and CCK-B receptors in the control of feeding in rodents. In: Dourish CT, Cooper SJ, Inverson SD, Inverson LL, eds. Multiple Cholecystokinin Receptors in the CNS. Oxford: Oxford University Press, 1992:234–253.

322. Geary N, Trace D, McEwen B, Smith GP. Cyclic estradiol replacement increases the satiety effect of CCK-8 in ovariectomized rats. Physiol Behav 1994; 56:281–289.

323. Corp ES, McQuade J, Moran TH, Smith GP. Characterization of type A and type B CCK receptor binding sites in rat vagus nerve. Brain Res 1993; 623:161–166.

324. Crawley JN. Cholecystokinin modulates dopamine mediated behaviors: Differential actions in medial posterior versus anterior nucleus accumbens. Annal NY Acad Sci 1994; 713:138–142.

325. Gibbs J, Smith GP, Greenberg D. Cholecystokinin: A neuroendocrine key to feeding behavior. In: Schulkin J, ed. Hormonally Induced Changes in Mind and Brain. Orlando, FL: Academic Press, 1993:51–69.

326. Li B-H, Rowland NE. Effects of vagotomy on cholecystokinin-and dexfenfluramine-induced fos-like immunoreactivity in the rat brain. Brain Res Bull 1995; 37: 589–593.

327. Salaman CR, Fukada A, Oomura Y, Minami T. Effects of sulphated cholecystokinin octapeptide (CCK-8) on the dorsal motor nucleus of the vagus. Brain Res Bull 1988; 21:839–842.

328. Balleine B, Davies A, Dickinson A. Cholecystokinin attenuates incentive learning in rats. Behav Neurosci 1995: 109:312–319.

329. Fedorchak PM, Bolles RC. Nutritive expectancies mediate cholecystokinin's suppression-of-intake effect. Behav Neurosci 1988; 102:451–455.

330. Mark GP, Smith SE, Rada PV, Hoebel BG. An appetitively conditioned taste elicits a preferential increase in mesolimbic dopamine release. Pharmacol Biochem Behav 1994; 48:651–660.

331. Hokfelt T, Skirboll L, Rehfeld JF, Goldstein M, Markay K, Dann O. A subpopulation of mesencephalic dopamine neurons projecting to limbic areas contains a cholecystokinin-like peptide: evidence from immunohistochemistry combined with retrograde tracing. Neuroscience 1980; 5:2093–2124.

332. Heidbreder C, Gewiss M, De Mott B, Mertens I, De Witte P. Balance of glutamate and dopamine in the nucleus accumbens modulates self-stimulation behavior after injection of cholecystikinin and neurotenson in the rat brain. Peptides 1992; 13:441–449.

333. Gibbs J, Fauser DJ, Row EA, Rolls BJ, Rolls ET, Maddison SP. Bombesin suppresses feeding in rats. Nature 1979; 282:208–210.

334. McCoy JG, Avery DD. Bombesin: potential integrative peptide for feeding and satiety. Peptides 1990; 11: 595–607.

335. Kulkosky PJ, Gray L, Gibbs J, Smith GP. Feeding and selection of saccharin after injections of bombesin, LiCl, and NaCl. Peptides 1981; 2:61–64.

336. Lee MC, Schiffman SS, Pappas TN. Role of neuropeptides in the regulation of feeding behavior: A review of cholecystokinin, bombesin, neuropeptide Y, and galanin. Neurosci Biobehav Rev 1994; 18:313–323.

337. West DB, Williams RH, Bragert DJ, Woods SC. Bombesin reduces food intake of normal and hypothalamically obese rats and lowers body weight when given chronically. Peptides 1982; 3:61–67.

338. Okada S, York DA, Bray GA, Mei J, Erlanson-Albertsson C. Differential inhibition of fat intake in two strains of rat by the peptide enterostatin. Am J Physiol 1992; 262: R1111–R1116.

339. Lin L, McClanahan S, York DA, Bray GA. The peptide enterostatin may produce early satiety. Physiol Behav 1993; 53:789–794.

340. York DA, Lin L. Enterostatin: A peptide regulator of fat ingestion. In: Bray GA, Ryan DH, eds. Molecular and Genetic Aspects of Obesity. Baton Rouge: Louisiana State Unversity Press, 1996:281–297.

341. Lin L, Gehlert DR, York DA, Bray GA. Effect of enterostatin on the feeding response to galanin and NPY. Obes Res 1993; 1:186–192.

342. Arase K, York DA, Shimizu H, Shargill N, Bray GA. Effects of corticotropin-releasing factor on food intake and brown adipose tissue thermogenesis in rats. Am J Physiol 1988; 225:255–259.

343. Egawa M, Yoshimatsu H, Bray GA. Effect of corticotropin releasing hormone and neuropeptide Y on electrophysiology activity of sympathetic nerves to interscapular brown adipose tissue. Neuroscience 1990; 34:771–775.

344. Glowa JR, Barrett JE, Russell J, Gold PW. Effects of corticotropin releasing hormone on appetitive behaviors. Peptides 1992; 13:609–621 (review).

345. Menzaghi F, Heinrichs SC, Pich EM, Tilders FJ, Koob GF. Functional impairment of hypothalamic corticotropin-releasing factor neurons with immunotargeted toxins enhances food intake induced by neuropeptide Y. Brain Res 1993; 618:76–82.

346. Rothwell NJ. Central effects of CRF on metabolism and energy balance. Neurosci Biobehav Rev 1990; 14: 263–271 (review).

347. Spina M, Merlo-Pich E, Chan RKW, Basso Am, Rivier J Vale W, et al. Appetite-suppressing effects of urocortin, a CRF-related neuropeptide. Science 1996; 273:1561.

348. Heinrichs SC, Menzaghi F, Pich EM, Hauger RL, Koob GF. Corticotropin-releasing factor in the paraventricular nucleus modulates feeding induced by neuropeptide Y. Brain Res 1993; 611:18–24.

349. Bchini-Hooft van Huijsduijnen OB, Rohner-Jeanrenaud F, Jeanrenaud B. Hypothalamic neuropeptide Y messenger ribonucleic acid levels in pre-obese and genetically obese (fa/fa) rats; potential regulation thereof by corticotropin-releasing factor. J Neuroendocrinol 1993; 5:381–386.

350. Olson BR, Drutarosky MD, Chow MS, Hruby VJ, Stricker EM, Verbalis JG. Oxytocin and an oxytocin agonist administered centrally decreased food intake in rats. Peptides 1991; 12:113–118.

351. Verbalis JG, Blackburn RE, Olson BR, Stricker EM. Central oxytocin inhibition of food and salt ingestion: a mechanism for intake regulation of solute homeostasis. Regul Peptides 1993; 45:149–154 (review).

352. Blackburn RE, Samson WK, Fulton RJ, Stricker EM, Verbalis JG. Central oxytocin inhibition of salt appetite in rats: evidence for differential sensing of plasma sodium and osmolality. Proc Nat Acad Sci USA 1993; 90: 10380–10384.

353. Olson BR, Drutarosky MD, Stricker EM, Verbalis JG. Brain oxytocin receptor antagonism blunts the effects of anorexigenic treatments in rats: evidence for central oxytocin inhibition of food intake. Endocrinology 1991; 129: 785–791.

354. Langhans W, Delprete E, Scharrer E. Mechanisms of vasopressin's anorectic effect. Physiol Behav 1991; 49: 169–176.

355. Reghunandanan V, Badgaiyan RD, Marya RK, Maini BK. Suprachiasmatic injection of a vasopressin antagonist modifies the circadian rhythm of food intake. Behav Neur Biol 1987; 48:344–351.

356. Van De Kar LD, Rittenhouse PA, Li Q, Levy AD, Brownfield MS. Hypothalamic paraventricular, but not supraoptic neurons, mediate the serotonergic stimulation of oxytocin secretion. Brain Res Bull 1995; 36:45–50.

357. Olson BR, Drutarosky MD, Stricker EM, Verbalis JG. Brain oxytocin receptors mediate corticotropin-releasing hormone-induced anorexia. Am J Physiol 1991; 260: R448–52.

358. Bjorkstrand E, Hulting A-L, Meister B, Uvnas-Moberg K. Effect of galanin on plasma levels of oxytocin and cholecystokinin. NeuroReport 1993; 4:10–12.

359. Melchior JC, Rigaud D, Chayvialle JA, Colas-Linhart N. Palatability of a meal influences release of beta-endorphin, and of potential regulators of food intake in healthy human subjects. Appetite 1994; 22:233–244.

360. Stanley BG, Hoebel BG, Leibowitz SF. Neurotensin: effects of hypothalamic and intravenous injections on eating and drinking in rats. Peptides 1983; 4:493–500.

361. Sandoval SL, Kulkosky PJ. Effectsd of peripheral neurotensin on behavior of the rat. Pharmacol Biochem Behav 1992; 41:385–390.

362. Lee TF, Rezvani AH, Hepler JR, Myers RD. Neurotensin releases norepinephrine differentially from perfused hypothalamus of sated and fasted rat. Am J Physiol 1987; 252:E102–9.

363. Glimcher PG, Giovino AA, Hoebel BG. Neurotensin self-injection in the ventral tegmental area. Brain Res 1987; 403:147–150.

364. Kalivas PW, Taylor S. Behavioral and neurochemical effect of daily injection will neurotensin into the ventral tegmental area. Brain Res 1985; 358:70–76.

365. Rompre P-P, Gratton A. Mesencephalic microinjections of neurotension-(1–13) and its C-terminal fragment, neurotensin-(8–13), potentiate brain stimulation reward. Brain Res 1993; 616:154–162.

366. Angulo J., A., McEwen BS. Molecular aspects of neuropeptide regulation and function in the corpus striatum and nucleus accumbens. Brain Res Rev 1994; 19:1–28.

367. Chait A, Suaudeau C, De Beaurepaire R. Extensive brain mapping of calcitonin-induced anorexia. Brain Res Bull 1995; 36:467–472.

368. Krahn DD, Gosnell BA, Levine AS, Morley JE. Effects of calcitonin gene-related peptide on food intake. Peptides 1984; 5:861–864.

369. Chance WT, Balasubramaniam A, Zhand FS, Wimalawansa SJ, Fischer JE. Anorexia following the intrahypothalamic administration of amylin. Brain Res 1991; 539: 352–354.

370. Freed WJ, Perlow MJ, Wyatt RJ. Calcitonin: inhibitory effect on eating in rats. Science 1979; 206:850–852.

371. Taylor GM, Meeran K, O'Shea D, Smith DM, Ghatei MA, Bloom SR. Adrenomedullin inhibits feeding in the rat by a mechanism involving calcitonin gene–related peptide receptors. Endocrinology 1996; 137:3260.

372. Zelissen PM, Koppeschaar HP, Lips CJ, Hackeng WH. Calcitonin gene-related peptide in human obesity. Peptides 1991; 12:861–863.

373. Lu D, Willard D, Patel IR, Kadwell S, Overton L, Kost T, et al. Agouti protein is an antagonist of the melanocyte-stimulating-hormone receptor. Nature 1994; 371: 799–802.

374. Hanai K, Oomura Y, Kai Y, Nishikawa K, Shimizu N, Morita H, et al. Central action of acidic fibroblast growth factor in feeding regulation. Am J Physiol 1989; 256: R217–23.

375. Oomura Y, Sasaki K, Li AJ. Memory facilitation reduced by food intake. Physiol Behav 1993; 54:493–498.

376. Prasad C. Neurobiology of cyclo(His-Pro). Ann NY Acad Sci 1989; 553:232–251 (review).

377. Prasad C, Mizuma H, Brock JW, Porter JR, Svec F, Hilton C. A paradoxical elevation of brain cyclo(His-Pro) levels in hyperphagic obese Zucker rats. Brain Res 1995; 699: 149–153.

378. Plata-Salaman CR, Sonti G, Borkoski JP, Wilson C, Ffrench-Mullen JMH. Anorexia induced by chronic central administration of cytokines at estimated pathophysiological concentrations. Physiol Behav 1996; 59: 867–871.

379. Plata-Salaman CR. Interferons and central regulation of feeding. Am J Physiol 1992; 263:R1222–7.

380. Plata-Salaman CR, Borkoski JP. Chemokines/intercrines and central regulation of feeding. Am J Physiol 1994; 266: R1711–R1715.

381. Plata-Salaman CR, Sonti G, Borkoski JP. Modulation of feeding by beta 2-microglobulin, a marker of immune activation. Am J Physiol 1995; 268:R1513–R1519.

382. Rivest S, Rivest C. Stress and interleukin-1 beta-induced activation of c-fos, NGFI-B and CRF gene expression in the hypothalamic PVN: comparison between Spraque Dawley, Fisher-344 and Lewis rats. J Neuroendocrinol 1994; 6:101–117.

383. Kang M, Yoshimatsu H, Chiba S, Kurokawa M, Ogawa R, Tamari Y, et al. Hypothalamic neuronal histamine modulates physiological responses injduced by interleukin-1 beta. Am J Physiol 1995; 269:R1308–R1313.

384. Chance WT, Lints CE. Eating following cholinergic simulation of the hypothalamus. Physiol Psych 1977; 5: 440–444.

385. Fukuda M, Ono T, Nakamura K, Tamura R. Dopamine and ACh involvement in plastic learning by hypothalamic neurons in rats. Brain Res Bull 1990; 25:109–114.

386. Singer G, Kelly J. Cholinergic and adrenergic interaction in the hypothalamic control of drinking and eating behavior. Physiol Behav 1972; 8:885–890.

387. Museo E, Wise RA. Place preference conditioning with ventral tegmental injections of cytisine. Life Sci 1994; 55:1179–1186.

388. Mifsud J-C, Hernandez L, Hoebel BG. Nicotine infused into the nucleus accumbens increases synaptic dopamine as measured by in vivo microdialysis. Brain Res 1989; 478:365–367.

389. Nisell M, Nomikos GG, Svensson TH. Infusion of nicotine in the ventral tegmental area or the nucleus accumbens of the rat differentially affects accumbal dopamine release. Pharmacol Toxicol 1994; 75:348–352.

390. Mark GP, Rada P, Pothos E, Hoebel BG. Effects of feeding and drinking on acetylcholine release in the nucleus accumbens, striatum, and hippocampus of freely behaving rats. J Neurochem 1992; 58:2269–2274.

391. Mark GP, Weinberg JB, Rada PV, Hoebel BG. Extracellular acetylcholine is increased in the nucleus accumbens following the presentation of an aversively conditioned taste stimulus. Brain Res 1995; 688:184–188.

392. Coscina DV, Castonguay TW, Stern JS. Effects of increasing brain GABA on the meal patterns of genetically obese vs. lean Zucker rats. Int J Obe Relat Metab Disord 1992; 16:425–433.

393. Tsujii S, Bray GA. GABA-related feeding control in genetically obese rats. Brain Res 1991; 540:48–54.

394. Kelly J, Rothstein J, Grossman SP. GABA and hypothalamic feeding systems. I. Topographic analysis of the effects of microinjections of muscimol. Physiol Behav 1979; 23:1123–1124.

395. Kelly J, Grossman SP. GABA and hypothalamic feeding systems. II. A comparison of GABA, glycine and acetylcholine agonists and their antagonists. Pharmacol Biochem Behav 1979; 11:647–652.

396. Panksepp J, Meeker RB. The role of GABA in the ventromedial hypothalamic regulation of good intake. Brain Res Bull 1980; 5:453–460.

397. Cattabeni F, Maggi A, Monduzzi M, De Angelis L, Racagni G. GABA: circadian fluctuations in rat hypothalamus. J Neurochem 1978; 31:565–567.

398. Meeker RB, Myers RD. GABA and glutamine: possible metabolic intermediaries involved in the hypothalamic regulation of food intake. Brain Res Bull 1980; 5:253–259.

399. Maldonado-Irizarry CS, Swanson CJ, Kelley AE. Glutamate receptors in the nucleus accumbens shell control feeding behavior via the lateral hypothalamus. J Neurosci 1995; 15:6779–6788.

400. Stanley BG. Glutamate and its Receptors in Lateral Hypothalamic Stimulation of Eating. In: Cooper SJ, Clifton PG, eds. Dopamine Receptor Subtypes and Ingestive Behaviour. London: Academic Press, 1996:301–322.

401. Stanley BG, Willett VL, ed, Donias HW, Ha LH, Spears LC. The lateral hypothalamus: a primary site mediating excitatory amino acid-eliciting eating. Brain Res 1993; 630:41–49.

402. Stanley BG, Ha LH, Spears LC, De MG, 2d. Lateral hypothalamic injection of glutamate, kainic acid, D,L-alpha-amino-3-hydroxy-5-methyl-isoxazole propionic acid or N-methyl-D-aspartic acid rapidly elicit intense transient eating in rats. Brain Res 1993; 613:88–95.

403. Bednar I, Qian M, Qureshi GA, Kallstrom L, Johnson AE, Carrer H, et al. Glutamate inhibits ingestive behaviour. J Neuroendocrinol 1994; 6:403–408.

404. Berridge KC, Pecina S. Benzodiazepines, appetite, and taste palatability. Neurosci Biobehav Rev 1995; 19:121–131 (review).

405. Dallman MF, Strack AM, Akana SF, Bradbury MJ, Hanson ES, Schribner KA, et al. Feast and famine: critical role of glucocorticoids with insulin in daily energy flow. Frontiers Neuroendocrinol 1993; 14:303–347 (review).

406. Devenport L, Knehans A, Sundstrom A, Thomas T. Corticosterone's dual metabolic actions. Life Sci 1989; 45:1389–1396.

407. King BM. Glucocorticoids and hypothalamic obesity. Neurosci Biobehav Rev 1988; 12:29–37 (review).

408. Gray GA, Fisler JS, York DA. Neuroendocrine control of the development of obesity: understanding gained from studies of animal models. Frontiers Neuroendocrinol 1996; 11:128–181.

409. Epstein AN. Neurohormonal control of salt intake in the rat. Brain Res Bull 1991; 27:315–320 (review).

410. Gomez-Sanchez EP, Fort C, Thwaites D. Central mineralocorticoid receptor antagonism blocks hypertension in Dahl S/JR rats. Am J Physiol 1992; 262:E96–9.

411. Virgin CE, Jr., Ha TP, Packan DR, Tombaugh GC, Yang SH, Horner HC, et al. Glucocorticoids inhibit glucose transport and glutamte uptake in hippocampal astrocytes: implications for glucocorticoid neurotoxicity. J Neurochem 1991; 57:1422–1428.

412. Sapolsky RM, Krey LC, McEwen BS. The neuroendocrinology of stress and aging: the glucocorticoid cascade hypothesis. Endocr Rev 1986; 7:284–301 (review).

413. McEwen BS. Non-genomic and genomic effects of steroids on neural activity. Trends Pharmacol Sci 1991; 12:141–147 (review).

414. Born J, DeKloet ER, Wenz H, Kern W, Fehm HL. Gluco- and antimineralocorticoid effects on human sleep: a role of central corticosteroid receptors. Am J Physiol 1991; 260:E183–8.

415. Wade GN, Schneider JE, Li H. Control of fertility by metabolic cues. Am Physiol 1996; 270:1–20.

416. Baskin DG, Norwood BJ, Schwartz MW, Koerker DJ. Estradiol inhibits the increase of hypothalamic neuropeptide Y messenger ribonucleic acid expression induced by

weight loss in ovariectomized rats. Endocrinology 1995; 136:5547–5554.

417. Swanson LW, Simmons DM. Differential steroid hormone and neural influences on peptide and mRNA levels in CRH cells of the paraventricular nucleus: a hybridization histochemical study in the rat. J Comp Neurol 1989; 285: 413–435.

418. Butera PC, Xiong M, Davis RJ, Platania SP. Central implants of dilute estradiol enhance the satiety effect of CCK-8. Behav Neurosci 1996; 110:823–830.

419. Laferrere B, Wurtman RJ. Effect of *d*-fenfluramine on the serotonin release in brain of anasthetized rats. Brain Res 1989; 504:258–263.

420. Merchenthaler I, Lennard DE, Lopez FJ, Negro-Vilar A. Neonatal imprinting predetermines the sexually dimorphic, estrogen-dependent expression of galanin in luteinizing hormone-releasing hormone neurons. Proc Nat Acad Sci USA 1993; 90:10479–10483.

421. Puerta M, Venero C, Castro C, Ablenda M. Progesterone does not alter sympathetic activity in tissues involved in energy balance. Eur J Endocrinol 1996; 134:508–512.

422. Mogenson GJ, Brudzynski SM, Wu M, Yang CR, Yim CY. From motivation to action: a review of dopaminergic regulation of limbic −> nucleus accumbens −> ventral palladium > pedunculopontine nucleus circuitries involved in limbic-motor integration. In: Kalivas PW, Barnes CD, eds. Limbic Motor Circuits and Neuropsychiatry: Boca Raton, FL: CRC Press, 1993:193–236.

423. Spector AC. Gustatory function in the parabrachial nuclei: Implications from lesion studies in rats. Rev Neurosci 1995; 6:143–175.

424. Travers SP, Norgren R. Organization of orosensory reponses to the nucleus of the solitary tract of the rat. J Neurophysiol 1995; 73:2144–2162.

425. Lennard DE, Eckert WA, Merchanthaler I. Corticotropin-releasing hormone neuronsa in the paraventricular nucleus project to the external zone of the median eminence: a study combining retrograde labeling with immunocytochemistry. J Neuroendocrinol 1993; 5: 175–181.

426. Niijima A, Meguid MM. An electrophysical study on amino acid sensors in the hepato-portal system in the rat. Obes Res 1995; 3:741S–745S.

427. Rolls ET. The Neurophysiology of Feeding. In: Sullivan AC, Garattini S, eds. Noval Approaches and Drugs for Obesity. London: John Libbey, 1985:139–150.

428. Meredith GE, Blanf B, Groenewegen HJ. The distribution and compartamental organization of the cholinergic neurons in nucleus accumbens. Neuroscience 1989; 31: 327–345.

429. Pennartz CMA, Groenewegen HJ, Lopes da Silva F, H. The nucleus accumbens as a complex of functionally distinct neuronal ensembles: An integration of behavioral, electrophysiological and anatomical data. Prog Neurobiol 1994; 42:719–761.

430. Rada PV, Mark GP, Hoebel BG. In vivo modulation of acetylcholine in the nucleus accumbens of freely moving rats. I. Inhibition by serotonin. Brain Res 1993; 619: 98–104.

431. Stoof JC, Drukarch B, De Boer P, Westerink BHC, Groenewegen HJ. Regulation of the activity of striatal cholinergic neurons by dopamine. Neuroscience 1992; 47: 755–770.

432. Koob GF, Swerdlow NR. The functional output of the mesolimbic dopamine system. In: Kaklivas PW, ed. The Mesocorticolimbic Dopamine System. New York: New York Academy of Sciences, 1988:216–217.

433. Olive MF, Bertolucci M, Evans CJ, Maidment NT. Microdialysis reveals a morphine-induced increase in pallidal opioid peptide release. NeuroReport 1995; 6:1093–1096.

434. Parent A, Hazrati L-N. Functional anatomy of the basal ganglia. I. The cortico-basal ganglia-thalamo-cortical loop. Brain Res Rev 1995; 20:91–127.

435. Shizgal P, Kiss I, Bielajew C. Psychophysical and electrophysiological studies of the substrate for brain stimulatkion reward. In: Hoebel BG, Novin D, eds. The Neural Basis of Feeding and Reward. Brunswick, ME: Haer Institute, 1982:419–430.

436. Hernandez L, Murzi E, Schwartz DH, Hoebel BG. Neuroelectrophysiological and neurochemical approach to a hierarchical feeding organization. In: Björntorp P, Brodoff B, eds. Obesity. Philadelphia: JB Lippincott, 1992: 171–183.

437. Yeomans JS, Mathur A, Tampakeras M. Rewarding brain stimulation: Role of tegmental cholinergic neurons that activate dopamine neurons. Behav Neurosci 1993; 107: 1077–1087.

438. Heimer L, Alheid GF. Piecing together the puzzle of basal forebrain anatomy. In: Napier TC, ed. The Basal Forebrain. New York: Plenum Press, 1991:1–42.

439. Salamone JD. Behavioral pharmacology of dopamine systems: a new synthesis. In: Willner P, Scheel-Kruger J, eds. The Mesolimbic Dopamine System: From Motivation to Action. New York: Wiley, 1991:599–613.

440. Wise RA, Spindler J, de Wit H, Gerber GJ. Neuroleptic-induced "anhedonia" in rats: pimozide blocks the reward quality of food. Science 1978; 201:262–264.

441. Radhakishun FS, van Ree JM, Westerink BH. Scheduled eating increases dopamine release in the nucleus accumbens of food-deprived rats as assessed with on-line brain dialysis. Neurosci Lett 1988; 58:351–356.

442. Agnati, LF, Bjelke B, Fuxe K. Volume transmission in the brain. Am Sci 1992; 80:362–373.

443. Blackburn JR, Phillips AG, Jakubovic A, Fibiger HC. Dopamine and preparatory behavior. II. A neurochemical analysis. Behav Neurosci 1989; 103:15–23.

444. Hoebel BG, Rada P, Mark GP, Hernandez L. The power of integrative peptides to reinforce behavior by releasing dopamine. In: Strand FL, Beckwith BE, Chronwell B, Sandman CA, eds. Models of Neuropeptide Action. New York: New York Academy of Sciences, 1994:36–41.

445. Parada MA, Hernandez L, De Parada MP, Paez X, Hoebel BG. Dopamine in the lateral hypothalamus may be involved in the inhibition of locomotion related to food and water seeking. Brain Res Bull 1990; 25:961–968.

446. Currie PJ, Wilson LM. Central injection of 5-hydroxytryptamine reduces food intake in obese and lean mice. NeuroReport 1992, 3:59–61.

447. Currie PJ, Wilson LM. Yohimbine attenuates clonidine-induced feeding and macronutrient selection in genetically obese (ob/ob) mice. Pharmacol Biochem Behav 1992; 43:1039–1046.

448. Currie PJ. Differential effects of NE, CLON, and 5-HT on feeding and macronutrient selection in genetically obese (ob/ob) and lean mice. Brain Res Bull 1993; 32:133–142.

449. Routh VH, Murakami DM, Stern JS, Fuller CA, Horwitz BA. Neuronal activity in hypothalamic nuclei of obese and lean Zucker rats. Int J Obes 1990; 14:879–891.

450. Tsujii S, Bray GA. Food intake of lean and obese Zucker rats following ventricular infusions of adrenergic agonists. Brain Res 1992; 587:226–232.

451. Shimizu H, Uehara Y, Negishi M, Shimomura Y, Takahashi M, Fukatsu A, et al. Altered monoamine metabolism in the hypothalamus of the genetically obese yellow (Ay/a) mouse. Exp Clin Endocrinol 1992; 99:45–48.

452. Garthwaite TL, Kalkhoff RK, Guansing AR, Hagen TC, Menahan LA. Plasma free tryptophan, brain serotonin, and an endocrine profile of the genetically obese hypergycemic mouse at 4–5 months of age. Endocrinology 1979; 105:1178–1182.

453. Yoshimatsu H, Sakata T, Machidori H, Fujimoto K, Yamatodani A, Wada H. Ginsenoside Rg1 prevents histaminergic modulation of rat adaptive behavior from elevation of ambient temperature. Physiol Behav 1993; 53:1–4.

454. Machidori H, Sakata T, Yoshimatsu H, Ookuma K, Fujimoto K, Kurokawa M, et al. Zucker obese rats: defect in brain histamine control of feeding. Brain Res 1992; 590: 180–186.

455. Schwartz MW, Baskin DG, Bukowski TR, Kuijper JL, Foster D, Lasser G, et al. Specificity of leptin action on elevated blood glucose levels and hypothalamic neuropeptide Y gene expression in ob/ob mice. Diabetes 1996; 45: 531–535.

456. Wilding JP, Gilbey SG, Bailey CJ, Batt RA, Williams G, Ghatei MA, et al. Increased neuropeptide-Y messenger ribonucleic acid (mRNA) and decreased neurotensin mRNA in the hypothalamus of the obese (ob/ob) mouse. Endocrinology 1993; 132:1939–1944.

457. Beck B, Stricker-Krongrad A, Nicolas JP, Burlet C. Chronic and continuous intracerebroventricular infusion of neuropeptide Y in Long-Evans rats mimics the feeding behaviour of obese Zucker rats. Int J Obes Relat Metab Disord 1992; 16:295–302.

458. Beck B, Burlet A, Bazin R, Nicolas JP, Brulet C. Elevated neuropeptide Y in the arcuate nucleus of young obese Zucker rats may contribute to the development of their overeating. J Nutr 1993; 123:1168–1172.

459. Beck B, Burlet A, Bazin R, Nicolas JP, Burlet C. Early modification of neuropeptide Y but not of neurotensin in the suprachiasmatic nucleus of the obese Zucker rat. Neurosci Lett 1992; 136:185–188.

460. Beck B, Nicolas JP, Burlet C. Neurotensin decreases with fasting in the ventromedian nucleus of obese Zucker rats. Metabolism 1995; 44:972–975.

461. Nakaishi S, Nakai Y, Fukata J, Naito Y, Usui T, Fukushima M, et al. Immunoreactive corticotropin-releasing hormone levels in discrete hypothalamic nuclei of genetically obese Zucker rats. Neurosci Lett 1993; 159:29–31.

462. Richard D, Rivest R, Naimi N, Timofeeva E, Rivest S. Expression of corticotropin-releasing factor and its receptors in the brain of lean and obese Zucker rats. Endocrinology 1996; 137:4786.

463. Ferguson-Segall M, Flynn JJ, Walker J, Margules DL. Increased immunoreactive dynorphin and leu-enkephalin in posterior pituitary of obese mice (ob/ob) and supersensitivity to drugs that act at kappa receptors. Life Sci 1982; 31:2233–2236.

464. Stricker-Krongrad. A, Max JP, Musse N, Nicolas JP, Burlet C, Beck B. Increased threshold concentrations of neuropeptide Y for a stimulatory effect on food intake in obese Zucker rats — changes in the microstructure of the feeding behavior. Brain Res 1994; 660:162–166.

465. McLaughlin CL, Baile CA. Cholecystokinin, amphetamine and diazepam and feeding in lean and obese Zucker rats. Pharmacol Biochem Behav 1979; 10:87–93.

466. Shimizu H, Bray GA, Retzius T, York DA. Acetylation to d-MSH in pituitary may be an important factor in the development of obesity in yellow mice. Clin Res 1986; 36:193a.

467. Baskin DG, Stein LJ, Ikeda H, Woods SC, Figlewicz DP, Porte D, Jr., et al. Genetically obese Zucker rats have abnormally low brain insulin content. Life Sci 1985; 36: 627–633.

468. Figlewicz DP, Ikeda H, Hunt TR, Stein LJ, Doras DM, Woods SC, et al. Brain insulin binding is decreased in Wistar Kyoto rats carrying the 'fa' gene. Peptides 1986; 7: 61–65.

469. Stein LJ, Doras DM, Baskin DG, Figlewicz DP, Porte D, Jr., Woods SC. Reduced effect of experimental peripheral hyperinsulinemia to elevate cerebrospinal fluid insulin concentrations of obese Zucker rats. Endocrinology 1987; 121:1611–1615.

470. Zarjevski N, Cusin I, Vettor R, Rohner-Jeanrenaud F, Jeanrenaud B. Intracerebroventricular administration of neuropeptide Y to normal rats has divergent effects on glucose utlization by adipose tissue and skeletal muscle. Diabetes 1994; 43:764–769.

471. Zarjevski N, Cusin I. Vettor R, Rohner-Jeanrenaud F, Jeanrenaud B. Chronic intracerebroventricular neuropeptide-Y administration to normal rats mimics hormonal and metabolic changes of obesity. Endocrinology 1993; 133: 1753–1758.

472. Chua S, LaChaussee JL. Molecular patholgenesis of obesity in the fatty rat. Appetite 1993; 21:303.

473. Chung WK, Truett GE, Smoller, JW, Hirsch J, Liebel RL. Increased hypothalamic preproneuropeptide Y mRNA in six to nine day old fatty (*fa/fa*) rats. Soc Neurosci Abst 1992; 18:A1785 Abstract.

474. Sanacora G, Finkelstein JA, White JD. Developmental aspect of differences in hypothalamic preproneuropeptide Y messenger ribonucleic acid content in lean and genetically obese Zucker rats. J Neurosci 1992; 4:353–357.

475. McKibbin PE, McCarthy HD, Shaw P, Williams G. Insulin deficiency is a specific stimulus to hypothalamic neuropeptide Y: a comparison of the effects of insulin replacement and food restriction in streptozocin-diabetic rats. Peptides 1992; 13:721–727.

476. Williams G, Steel JH, Cardoso H, Ghatei MA, Lee YC, Gill JS, et al. Increased hypothalamic neutopeptide Y concentrations in diabetic rat. Diabetes 1988; 37:763–772.

477. Tecott LH, Sun LM, Akana SF, Strack AM, Lowenstein DH, Dallman MF, et al. Eating disorder and epilepsy in mice lacking 5-HT2c serotonin receptors. Nature 1995; 374:542–546.

478. Richard D, Chapdelaine S, Deshaies Y, Pepin MC, Barden N. Energy balance and lipid metabolism in transgenic mice bearing an antisense GCR gene construct. Am J Physiol 1993; 265:R146–50.

479. Levin BE. Increased brain 3H-paraminoclonidine (alpha 2-adrenoceptor) binding associated with perpetuation of diet-induced obesity in rats. Int J Obes 1990; 14:689–700.

480. Levin BE, Triscari J, Sullivan AC. The effect of diet and chronic obesity on brain catecholamine turnover in the rat. Pharmacol Biochem Behav 1986; 24:299–304.

481. Levin BE, Planas B. Defective glucoregulation of brain alpha 2-adrenoceptors in obesity-prone rats. Am J Physiol 1993; 264(Pt 2):R305–11.

482. Levin BE. Reduced norepinephrine turnover in organs and brains of obesity-prone rats. Am J Physiol 1995; 268:R389–94.

483. Okada S, Lin L, York DA, Bray GA. Chronic effects of intracerebral ventricular enterostatin in Osborne-Mendel rats fed a high-fat diet. Physiol Behav 1993; 54:325–329.

484. Lin L, York DA, Bray GA. Comparison of Osborne-Mendel and S5B/PL strains of rat: central effects of galanin, NPY, β-casomorphin and CRH on intake of high-fat and low-fat diets. Obes Res 1996; 4:117–124.

485. Rowland NE, Carlton J. Effects of fenfluramine on food intake, body weight, gastric emptying and brain monamines in Syrian hamsters. Brain Res Bull 1986; 17:575–581.

486. Uphouse L, Salamanca S, Caldarola-Pastuszka M. Gender and estrous cycle differences in the response to the 5-HT1A agonist 8-OH-DPAT. Pharmacol Biochem Behav 1991; 40:901–906.

487. Goodwin GM, Fairburn CG, Cowen PJ. Dieting changes serotonergic function in women, not men: implications for the aetiology of anorexia nervosa? Psychol Med 1987; 17:839–842.

488. Jones AP, Dayries M. Maternal hormone manipulations and the development of obesity in rats. Physiol Behav 1990; 47:1107–1110.

489. Epstein AN. Prospectus: Thirst and salt appetite. In: Sticker EM, ed. Handbook of Behavioral Neurobiology: Neurobiology of Food and Fluid Intake, 10th ed. New York: Plenum Press, 1990:489–512.

490. Hoebel BG, Hernandez L, Mark GP, Pothos E. Microdialysis in the study of psychostimulants and the neural substrate for reinforcement: Focus on dopamine and serotonin. In: Frascella J, Brown R, eds. Neurobiological Approaches to Brain-Behavior Interaction, NIDA Research Monograph. Rockville, MD: DHHS publication, 1992: 1–34.

491. Hoebel BG, Hernandez L. Microdialysis studies of psychostimulants. National Institute on Drug Abuse Research Monograph Series 1990; 95:343–344.

492. Pothos, E, Hernandez L, Auerbach SB, Creese I, Hoebel BG. Changes in body weight can alter the mesolimbic dopamine system and its response to food and drugs. Neuropsychopharmacology 1993; 9:30–31S.

493. Hoebel BG, Hernandez L, Schwartz DH, Mark GP, Hunter GA. Microdiaysis studies of brain norepinephrine, serotonin and dopamine release during ingestive behavior. In: Schneider L, Cooper SJ, Halmi KA, eds. The Psychobiology of Human Eating Disorders. New York: New York Academy of Sciences, 1989:171–193.

494. Schneider LH. Orosensory self-stimulation by sucrose involves brain dopaminergic mechanisms. In: Schneider LH, Cooper SJ, Halmi KA, eds. The Psychobiology of Human Eating Disorders. New York: New York Academy of Sciences, 1989:307–320.

495. Robinson TE, Berridge KC. The neural basis of drug craving: an incentive sensitization theory of addiction. Brain Res Rev 1993; 18:247–291 (review).

496. Krahn DD, Kurth C, Demitrack M, Drewnowski A. The relationship of dieting severity and bulimic behaviors to alcohol and other drug use in young women. J Substance Abuse 1992; 4:341–353.

497. Jimerson DC, Lesem MD, Kaye WH, Brewerton TD. Low serotonin and dopamine metabolite concentrations in cerebrospinal fluid from bulimic patients with frequent binge episodes. Arch Gen Psychiatry 1992; 49:132–138.

498. Strombom U, Krotkiewski M, Blennow K, Mansson J, Ekman R, Björntorp P. The concentrations of monamine metabolites and neuropeptides in the cerebrospinal fluid of obese woman with different body fat distribution. Int J Obes 1996; 20:361–368.

499. Weidmann P, de Courten M, Boehlen L, Shaw S. The pathogenesis of hypertension in obese subjects. Drugs 1993; 46(Suppl 2):197–208 (review).

500. Reynisdottir S, Wahrenberg H, Carlstrom K, Rossner S, Arner P. Catecholamine resistance in fat cells of woman

with upper-body due to obesity decreased expression of beta 2-adrenoceptors. Diabetologia 1994; 37:428–435.

501. Lee EJ, Kim KR, Lee KM, Lim SK, Lee HC, Lee JH, et al. Reduced growth hormone response to L-dopa and pyridostigmine in obesity. Int J Obes Relat Metab Disord 1994; 18:465–468.

502. Noble EP, Noble RE, Ritchie T, Syndulko K, Bohlman MC, Noble LA, et al. D2 dopamine receptor gene and obesity. Int J Eat Disord 1994; 15:205–217.

503. Stunkard AJ, Berkowitz RJ, Tanrikut C, Reiss E, Young L. d-Fenfluramine treatment of binge eating disorder. Obes Res 1996; 3:341s (abstract).

504. Kaye WH, Berrettini W, Gwirtsman H, George DT. Altered cerebrospinal fluid neuropeptide Y and peptide YY immunoreactivity in anorexia and bulimia nervosa. Arch Gen Psychiatry 1990; 47:548–556.

505. Kramlik SK, Altemus M, Castonguay TW. The effects of the acute administration of RU 486 on dietary fat preference in fasted lean and obese men. Physiol Behav 1993; 54:717–724.

506. Brunani A, Invitti C, Dubini A, Piccoletti R, Bendinelli P, Maroni P, et al. Cerebrospinal fluid and plasma concentrations of SRIH, beta-endorphin, CRH, NPY and GHRH in obese and normal weight subjects. Int J Obes Relat Metab Disord 1995; 19:17–21.

507. Cote G, Tremblay A, Dionne DT, Bouchard C. DNA sequence variation at the NPY and NPY Y1 receptor loci and human food intake. Obes Res 1995; 3:354s (abstract).

508. Lieverse RJ, Masclee AA, Jansen JB, Lamers CB. Plasma cholecystokinin and pancreatic polypeptide secretion in response to bombesin, meal ingestion and modified sham feeding in lean and obese persons. Int J Obes Relat Metab Disord 1994; 18:123–127.

509. Considine RV, Considine EL, Williams CJ, Nyce MR, Magosin SA, Bauer L, et al. Evidence against either a premature stop codon or the absence of obese gene mRNA in human obesity. J Clin Invest 1995; 95:2986–2988.

510. Masuzaki H, Ogawa Y, Isse N, Satoh N, Okazaki T, Shigemoto M, et al. Human obese gene expression. Adipocyte-specific expression and regional differences in the adipose tissue. Diabetes 1995; 44:855–858.

511. Considine RV, Considine EL, Williams CJ, Nyce MR, Zhang P, Opentanova, et al. Mutation screening and identification of a sequence variation in the human ob gene coding region. Biochem Biophy Res Commun 1996; 220:735–739.

512. Clement K, Garner C, Hager J, Philippi A, LeDuc C, Carey A, et al. Indication for linkage of the human OB gene region with extreme obesity. Diabetes 1996; 45:687–690.

513. Reed DR, Ding Y, Xu W, Cather C, Green ED, Price RA. Extreme obesity may be linked to markers flanking the human OB gene. Diabetes 1996; 45:691–694.

514. Parker EM, Izzarelli DG, Nowak HP, Mahle CD, Iben LG, Wang J, et al. Cloning and characterization of the rat GALR1 galanin receptor from Rin14B insulinoma cells. Brain Res Mol Brain Res 1995; 34:179–189.

515. Crepaldi G, Del Prato S. What therapy do our NIDDM patients need? Insulin releasers. Diabetes Res Clin Pract 1995; 28(Suppl.):S159–65 (review).

516. D'Alessio DA, Prigeon RL, Ensinck JW. Enteral enhancement of glucose disposition by both insulin-dependent and insulin-independent processes. A physiological role of glucagon-like peptide I. Diabetes 1995; 44:1143–1437.

517. Otonkoski T., Hayek. A Constitution of a biphasic insulin response to glucose in human fetal pancreatic beta-cells with glucagon-like peptide 1. J Clin Endocrinol Metab 1995; 80:3779–3783.

518. Trocki O, Baer DJ, Castonguay TW. Comparison of effects of adrenalectomy and RU-486 in rats given a choice of maintenance diet and fat supplement. Am J Physiol 1995; 269(Pt 2):R-708–19.

519. Langley SC, York DA. Effects of antiglucocorticoid RU 486 on development of obesity in obese fa/fa Zucker rats. Am J Physiol 1990; 259(Pt 2):R539–R544.

16

Development of White Adipose Tissue

Gérard Ailhaud
University of Nice-Sophia Antipolis, Nice, France

Hans Hauner
Heinrich-Heine-University Dusseldorf, Dusseldorf, Germany

I. INTRODUCTION

In contrast to the development of brown adipose tissue (BAT), which takes place mainly before birth, the development of white adipose tissue (WAT) represents a continuous process throughout life, and the acquisition of fat cells appears to be an irreversible process. At the cellular level, this phenomenon raises the question of the characteristics of the cells constituting the adipose tissue organ. This leads in turn to the question of the nature of the factors that regulate the formation of new fat cells from dormant adipose precursor cells. Once adipose tissue is formed, adipocytes represent between one-third and two-thirds of the total number of cells. The remaining cells are blood cells, endothelial cells, pericytes, adipose precursor cells of varying degree of differentiation, and, most likely, fibroblasts (1). The existence of very small fat cells in addition to mature adipocytes has also been documented (2). Figure 1 summarizes the various cell types present in this tissue, based on ultrastructural studies in vivo and biological studies in vitro. The population of adipose precursor cells corresponds presumably to those cells previously defined in developing and adult rodents as "interstitial cells," "non-lipid-filled mesenchymal cells," or "other mesenchymal cells," which includes both "undifferentiated" and "poorly differentiated" mesenchymal cells (3). At present, it cannot be assessed to which extent various morphological descriptions represent only different stages of the cell lineage leading to the characteristic adipocyte phenotype. From the biological perspective, hundreds of different cell types present in the whole body arise from a single fertilized egg. With development, stem cells become increasingly committed to specific lineages. In that respect, the establishment of embryonic stem (ES) cell lines has opened new experimental approaches as ES cells are able to generate various lineages under appropriate culture conditions, including the adipose lineage (4). The latter originates from mesenchymal multipotent stem cells that develop into unipotent adipoblasts by largely unknown mechanisms. Commitment of adipoblasts gives rise in vitro to preadipose cells (usually termed preadipocytes), i.e., cells that have expressed early markers but not yet late markers and that have not yet accumulated triacylglycerol stores. It remains unclear whether adipoblasts, which are formed during embryonic development, are still present postnatally or whether only preadipocytes are present in vivo. Clearly, in vitro studies with ES cells should provide clues to answer these critical questions and to characterize the key molecular events of adipoblast formation. In vitro, preadipose cells undergo terminal differentiation to immature adipose cells containing small lipid droplets and then to mature fat cells (usually termed adipocytes) filled with large droplets (Fig. 1). It is likely, but not proven, that the maturation process, i.e., the last step in terminal differentiation, occurs as completely in vitro as it does in vivo.

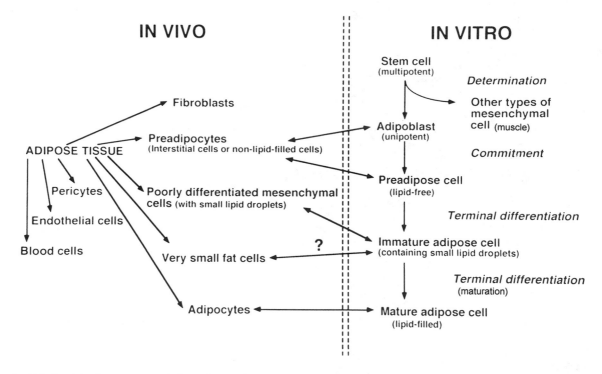

Figure 1   Relationships between morphological types in vivo and stages of cell differentiation in vitro. The adipocyte fraction corresponds to adipocytes and some very small fat cells. The stromal-vascular fraction corresponds to a mixture of the other cell types.

II. REGULATION OF ADIPOSE TISSUE MASS IN VIVO

A. Phylogeny and Ontogeny of Adipose Tissue

Among invertebrates, adipose tissue represents an important organ in insects whereas its quantitative importance decreases in arachnids, crustaceans, and molluscs in which liver appears as a new organ. Among vertebrates, adipose tissue develops extensively in homeotherms, although its proportion of body weight can vary greatly between species (up to 40% of body weight in cetaceans) or within a species as it is the case in migrating birds and hibernating mammals.

The development of WAT shows wide differences between species. It cannot be detected macroscopically during embryonic life and at birth in most rodents (mouse, rat), whereas it is present at birth in the guinea pig, rabbit, pig, and human. Studies of embryonic development in pig (5) and human (6) have emphasized the tight coordination of angiogenesis in time and space with the formation of fat cell clusters.

Histologically, WAT appears well vascularized, each adipocyte being actually in contact with a single capillary. Thus blood supply is adequate to support the active entry and release of metabolites as well as the secretion of various peptide and nonpeptide molecules. The innervation of WAT was known to be perivascular only. In rat, the sole innervation is postganglionic sympathetic and noradrenergic (7). However, sympathetic innervation of WAT has been reported (8), albeit less extensively than that of BAT where sympathetic adrenergic neurons are innervating directly brown adipocytes.

The characterization of specific growth factors able to trigger and modulate the development of capillaries and fat cell clusters is still in its infancy. Ubiquitous angiogenesis factors have been described, some of which [the transforming growth factor-β (TGF-β) and prostaglandin E_2 (PGE$_2$)] being synthesized and secreted by adipocytes (3). 1-Butyrylglycerol is solely secreted by adipocytes and appears to act as a potent angiogenesis factor only in this tissue (9). In addition, endothelial cells as well as fibroblasts and other cells of mesenchymal origin, including preadipocytes and adipocytes, secrete insulin-like growth factor-I (IGF-I) and IGF-binding protein(s). This suggests the involvement of IGF-I in the hyperplastic development of adipose tissue during embryogenesis.

B. Adipose Tissue Development in Early Life

Most studies on the early development of adipose tissue are exclusively based on morphological methods due to the lack of appropriate cell culture models. The "primitive fat organ" of Wassermann develops in the embryo from poorly defined predetermined "anlagen" long before a visible fat deposition takes place. At this early stage, cells that later will develop into adipocytes are morphologically undistinguishable from other cell types of the connective tissue (10). Only later does fat deposition allow the retrospective identification of these cells as designated preadipocytes. Light microscopy studies in human fetuses suggest that the first traces of a fat organ are detectable between the 14th and 16th week of prenatal life. Aggregation of mesenchymal cells in close association with the formation of blood vessels was described as the first indication of adipogenesis in humans (10,11). The first primitive organ structures to be identified at sites where fat accumulates characteristically are fat lobules, long before typical vacuolated fat cells are distinguishable. After the 23rd week of gestation, the number of fat lobules remains constant, while in the subsequent weeks the size of the lobules is continuously growing (11). At the sites of early fat development, the multilocular aspect of adipocytes predominates and probably reflects the early developmental stage (6). This is interesting, since the morphological development in vitro resembles the developmental steps in vivo. Preadipose cells either from clonal cell lines or from primary cultures usually exhibit a multilocular appearance, not only during early, but also during late, stages of in vitro differentiation when the characteristic markers of mature fat cells are fully expressed.

Brown and white adipocytes cannot be discriminated during prenatal development by conventional light microscopy studies. The available data do not provide any evidence of significant site- or sex-related differences in early development, supporting the concept that the marked regional differences in adipose tissue distribution in males and females fully develop later in life, presumably under the control of sex hormones. Although some microscopic studies postulate that the second trimester may be a critical period for the development of obesity in later life, the descriptive nature of these data does not allow any firm conclusion in this respect.

At the beginning of the third trimester, adipocytes are found in the principal fat depot areas but are still rather small (6). At birth, body fat accounts for approximately 16% of body weight as assessed by whole-body counting of ^{40}K. Analysis of biopsy samples of adipose tissue revealed that the increase in body fat during the first year of life from about 0.7 to 2.8 kg is entirely due to an increase in fat cell size, while fat cell number remains unchanged (12). Other studies on this issue gave controversial results, particularly with regard to the development of fat cell number during the first year of life. Such differences may be largely explained by variations in methodology and the general difficulties in assessing total-body fat cell number. In addition, most studies were cross-sectional, which makes interpretation of results more difficult. Longitudinal studies showed a continuous increase in fat cell weight between 1 and 12 months of age (13). It has also been pointed out that in fetal life and early infancy adipose tissue is composed of different cell populations: lipid-containing cells but also many cells that are essentially lipid-free and are not readily recognized as adipocytes. Small cells in the early stages of fat accumulation may make an important contribution to the adipose cell mass at this age. Therefore, it is tempting to assume that a gradual accumulation of body fat after birth is mainly reflected by increasing fat cell size (14).

C. Physiology of Adipose Tissue Cellularity in Humans

Apart from species differences, the development of adipose tissue varies according to sex and age. Moreover, the ability of rodents and humans to increase the number of adipocytes, depending on the nature of the diet and the localization of the adipose depot, has long been known (15). The formation of new fat cells following the proliferation of "dedifferentiated" cells during refeeding after a prolonged period of food deprivation, as well as the proliferation of mature adipocytes, still remain controversial events, which, if existing, should be of low magnitude.

Many studies during the last 25 years have been dealing with changes of adipose tissue cellularity throughout life. Based on such observations, a hypothesis was early established that postulated the existence of sensitive periods in adipose tissue development during childhood. Two peaks for accelerated adipose tissue growth were reported: one after birth and another between 9 and 13 years (16). Later studies using different techniques support this hypothesis. When thymidine kinase activity was measured as an index of cellular proliferation, Baum and co-workers found that adipose tissue enzyme activity was highest in infants during the first year after birth. A second, but much smaller, peak in enzyme activity was found in the preadolescent years (17). There is only one study in which cell proliferation and differentiation was measured in cultured stromal cells isolated from adipose tissue samples of children at different ages. Despite some limitations, the results of this study also suggest that the capacity for cell proliferation and differentiation in adipose tissue is highest during the first year of life and less pronounced in the years before puberty (18). Irrespective of this debate on the existence of sensitive periods in adipose tissue growth, Knittle and co-workers demonstrated in a large cohort of children that, starting by age of 2, children show a small, but continuous increase in both cell size and number during childhood even over a 4-year observation period (19).

The rate of cell proliferation in adipose tissue slows down during adolescence and, at weight stability, fat cell number seems to remain fairly constant in adult life. An expansion of adipose tissue mass is believed to be largely due to an enlargement of existing fat cells; only in severe obesity total fat cell number can increase up to threefold (20). However, aging animals are able to increase the fat cell number in most of their adipose depots in response to a high-carbohydrate or a high-fat diet (15) whereas a recent in vitro study showed that adult humans are able to form new adipocytes at any age; even adipose tissue samples obtained from individuals above the age of 60 contain a significant proportion of cells that can undergo differentiation (21). In contrast to established preadipocyte clonal lines from rodents, most stromal cells from human adipose tissue seem to be already in a late stage of development. They obviously do not require postconfluent cell division to enter the terminal differentiation program (22). The morphological appearance of the stromal cell fraction isolated from human adipose tissue is rather homogeneous (Fig. 2). The majority of cells exhibit tiny lipid droplets arranged around the nucleus, which can easily be detected by Oil Red O staining or electron microscopy.

D. Hormonal Effects on Adipose Tissue Growth

Lessons learned from defined endocrinological disorders indicate that hormones can affect both the adipose tissue mass and its distribution pattern. The various hormones reported to be related with dynamic changes of the adipose tissue so far are summarized in Table 1. The role of some hormones that may be of particular physiological importance is described next in more detail.

1. Thyroid Hormones

Hypothyroidism in rats induces a transient hypoplasia, whereas hyperthyroidism induces a transitory hyperplasia of retroperitoneal and epididymal fat tissues (23), which is in favor of an accelerating effect of tri-iodothyronine (T_3) on the precocious formation of (mature) fat cells. Interestingly, in hypophysectomized pig fetuses, but not in intact fetuses, thyroxine (T_4) profoundly enhances adipose

tissue development by hyperplasia and hypertrophy, which points to a role of T_4 as an adipogenic agent, at least in early developmental stages, and suggests that growth hormone (GH) antagonizes the adipogenic potential of thyroid hormones (24).

2. Insulin

Insulin is an anabolic hormone that potently supports lipid storage in adipose tissue, but it is also a powerful growth-promoting factor. Insulin favors lipid accumulation not only via stimulation of glucose uptake and increased lipoprotein lipase (LPL) activity but also by inhibition of catecholamine-induced lipolysis. The lipogenic effect of insulin is already evident in fetal life, since hyperinsulinemia in the fetal circulation of mothers with gestational diabetes frequently results in macrosomia. In streptozotocin-diabetic rats, insulin stimulates the in vivo cell proliferation in white adipose tissue. This growth-stimulating effect was observed in interstitial cells rather than in other cell types including lipid-containing cells (25). In cell culture experiments insulin was found to be a positive modulator of adipose differentiation in cells of the Ob17 preadipose clonal line (26) as well as in rat and human adipocyte precursor cells in primary culture (21,27). In contrast, the growth-promoting effect of supraphysiological insulin concentrations may be exerted via the IGF-I receptor. An interesting phenomenon in this context is insulin-induced lipohypertrophy of diabetic subjects. This clinical observation is frequently made, when insulin is repeatedly injected at the same site, and can reach striking extensions, particularly in young women. Analysis of adipose tissue cellularity revealed that fat cell size is only moderately increased in lipohypertrophic areas as compared to unaffected sites, strongly suggesting that additional fat cells are locally recruited (Hauner and co-workers, unpublished data).

3. Growth Hormone

It has long been known that GH deficiency is associated with an increased body fat mass. Children with GH deficiency have enlarged fat cells but a reduced number compared to healthy children (28). Treatment with GH normalizes these disturbances of adipose tissue cellularity (28,29). The increased body fat mass in GH-deficient subjects is mainly localized in the abdominal region, and administration of GH results in preferential reduction of fat cell size in the abdomen (29). Studies using computerized tomography (CT) suggest that the visceral depots are particularly sensitive to the effect of GH. A 6-month treatment with recombinant GH of patients with adult-onset GH deficiency resulted in a 4.7-kg reduction of adipose

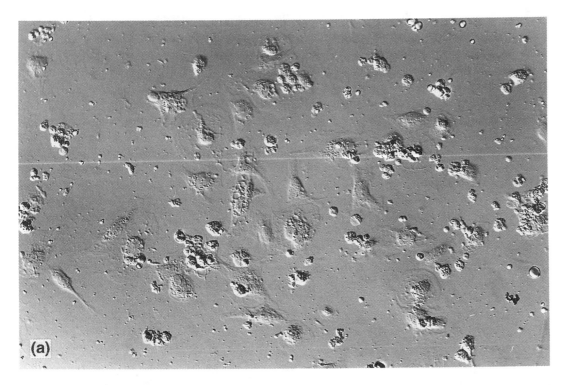

Figure 2 Human adipose precursor cells before and after terminal differentiation. Human adipose precursor cells were maintained in differentiation medium (21) for 12 hr (a), 4 days (b), and 15 days (c). Micrographs were taken with interference contrast. Magnification ×250.

tissue mass. Subcutaneous adipose tissue decreased by an average of 13%, whereas visceral adipose tissue was reduced by 30% (30). In contrast, in patients with acromegaly a reduced fat mass was observed that returns to normal after treatment of the hormone excess by octreotide or pituitary surgery. Interestingly, resting energy expenditure was increased in acromegaly and related to the concentrations of insulin-like growth factor-I indicating that GH is a regulator not only of body composition but also of energy metabolism (31).

The mechanisms for the slimming effects of GH are only partially understood. Chronic administration of GH to GH-deficient children was found to induce a significant reduction in basal lipogenesis and a decreased antilipolytic action of insulin leading to a significant reduction of adipocyte size, but only in the abdominal depot (29). In cultured human adipose tissue pieces, GH counteracted the stimulatory effect of glucocorticoids on LPL activity without affecting LPL mRNA levels (32). (LPL activity is well known to be the gatekeeper for the uptake of triglycerides from the circulation into adipose tissue, which is quantitatively the most important mechanism for lipid storage.) On the other hand, recent data suggest that GH has an intrinsic lipolytic activity, which can be demonstrated in fat cells from GH-deficient adults and is even enhanced after long-term GH administration (33). As many biological actions of GH are mediated via the induction of IGF-I synthesis, attention has been paid to the question of whether the metabolic effects of GH on adipose tissue are exerted by IGF-I. Studies in porcine preadipocyte cultures have shown that GH is able to increase IGF-I mRNA at least twofold. Since the increase in local IGF-I production was associated with a decrease in adipocyte development, the authors concluded that local IGF-I may contribute to suppression of the adipocyte phenotype (34). In contrast, IGF-I increased adipose conversion in rabbit adipocyte precursors. The stromal-vascular cells from the perirenal adipose tissue were found to secrete large amounts of IGF-I and IGF-binding proteins (35). Similar results have been obtained in cultured human preadipocytes. Upon stimulation by GH, stromal cells respond with an increased synthesis and release of IGF-I, which is followed by increased DNA synthesis as assessed by tritiated thymidine incorporation. It was also demonstrated that adipose cells have specific GH receptors and that the hormone exerts a variety of direct metabolic effects such as inhibition of glu-

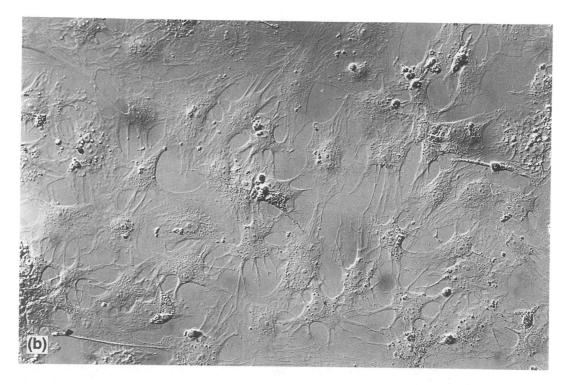

Figure 2   *(Continued)*.

cose uptake and stimulation of lipolysis, which may cause a net loss of stored lipids (36).

4.   Glucocorticoids

Clinical observations suggest that patients suffering from glucocorticoid excess develop an increased adipose tissue mass with a characteristic preferential accumulation of fat in the trunk and neck region. In a recent study using CT, surgical treatment of women with Cushing's disease was associated with a significant reduction of all adipose tissue depots except for leg adipose tissue. However, visceral, head, and neck adipose tissue depots were more markedly reduced than other depots (37). Studies of adipose tissue cellularity in Cushing's syndrome have shown that this expansion is primarily due to enlarged abdominal fat cells (38). This effect can be at least partly explained by the finding that fat cells from the abdominal depot exhibit more cytoplasmic glucocorticoid receptors and higher receptor mRNA compared with adipocytes from other regions (39). In Cushing's syndrome fat cell hypertrophy in the abdomen appears to be due to elevated adipocyte LPL activity and also to low lipolytic activity (38). The role of glucocorticoids and the importance of the hypothalamic-pituitary-adrenal axis in the excessive de-

velopment of adipose tissue have been documented in two models of transgenic mice. In a first model (40), a reduction of the glucocorticoid receptor in the brain and also in liver and kidneys was obtained with an antisense mRNA, whereas in a second model (41), overexpression of corticotropin-releasing factor (CRF) was achieved. In both cases, the observed increase in corticotropin and corticosterone levels was accompanied by increase in adipose tissue mass, with the development of Cushing's syndrome in CRF-overexpressing mice. Finally, glucocorticoids are known to be potent promoters of the adipose differentiation process, a mechanism that may also contribute to adipose tissue expansion during glucocorticoid excess (21).

5.   Sex Steroids

The role of sex steroids in the hyperplastic development of adipose tissue has not yet been well documented. Direct effects of sex steroids have been postulated for decades, but information on their molecular receptors in adipocytes of animals and humans remain scanty. Androgen receptors and estrogen receptors have been characterized in rat adipocytes (42,43) whereas estrogen receptor mRNA has been detected in human adipocytes (44). In primates, a

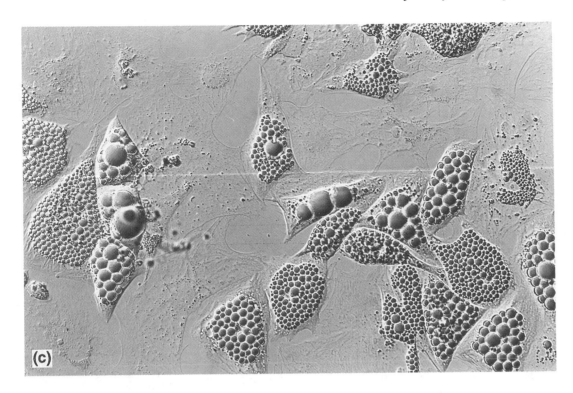

Figure 2 (*Continued*).

large proportion of androgens in men (40%) and a preponderance of estrogens in women (75% before menopause, ~100% after menopause) are synthesized in peripheral tissues (including adipose tissue) from adrenal precursor steroids, suggesting an intracrine effect of sex steroids in adipocytes (45,46).

Studies by magnetic resonance imaging (MRI) indicate that puberty in girls is associated with the preferential accumulation of adipose tissue in the gluteal and femoral region (47), suggesting that the divergence of sex steroid metabolism and serum levels among boys and girls may be responsible for the development of sex-specific fat distribution patterns at this age (48). In middle-aged women, decreased estrogen production during menopause may cause a shift in fat distribution toward a more abdominal pattern. Estrogen replacement therapy appears to result in a reduced amount of trunk adipose tissue as determined by dual energy X-ray absorptiometry (49).

In men, low testosterone levels are associated with enlarged visceral adipose tissue depots (50). When middle-aged, abdominally obese men are treated with testosterone, a small decrease in visceral fat mass in conjunction with an improvement of insulin resistance and associated metabolic disturbances is observed (51). A possible expla-

Table 1 Effect of Selected Hormones, Cytokines, and Growth Factors on Adipose Tissue Cellularity from In Vivo and In Vitro Studies

Factor	Fat cell size	Fat cell number	Fat mass
Insulin			
Excess	↑	(↑)	↑
Cortisol			
Excess	↑	(↑)	↑
Growth hormone			
Excess	↓	↑	↓
Deficiency	↑	↓	↑
Testosterone			
Deficiency	↑	n.d.	↑
Tri-iodothyronine			
Excess	↓	↑	Normal
Deficiency	Normal	↓	↓
TNF-α	↓	n.d.	↓
EGF	↓	↓	↓

n.d. = not determined.

nation for this observation is that androgens are positive effectors of lipolysis in concert with GH, thereby decreasing the size of the abdominal fat cells, but may not be directly involved in the regulation of fat cell formation (50). Another interesting finding is that alcoholic men have more adipose tissue localized in intra- and retroperitoneal depots than abstinent men, also possibly due to a lower androgen activity (52).

6. Nutrients

Quite recently, fatty acids (FA) have been shown in vitro to trigger terminal differentiation of preadipose into adipose cells (see below). In vivo, the effects of increased FA uptake on adipose tissue development have been remarkably illustrated in transgenic mice overexpressing human LPL in skeletal and cardiac muscle. Increased FA entry in both tissues is associated with weight loss due to some loss of muscle mass and, quite strikingly, to the virtually complete disappearance of adipose tissue (53). In vivo also, the nature of FA present in triacylglycerol molecules is of importance in adipose tissue development as feeding rats a diet rich in saturated fat leads to a threefold increase in the number of adipocytes in the retroperitoneal depot compared to the number of adipocytes in animals fed a diet rich in polyunsaturated fat, which indicates that saturated FA are more potent than unsaturated FA in promoting mitotic clonal expression and/or terminal differentiation of preadipose cells (54).

In addition to hormones, normal glucose homeostasis appears to be essential for adipose tissue development. Transgenic mice overexpressing the glucose transporter GLUT4 selectively in adipose tissue have enhanced glucose disposal in vivo and develop increased adiposity due to adipocyte hyperplasia (55). In contrast, mice deficient in GLUT4 by disrupting the gene exhibit growth retardation accompanied by a severe reduction in adipose depots despite a nearly normal glycemia (56). The possibility to reduce WAT development by enhancing nonshivering thermogenesis has been impressively illustrated by constructing transgenic mice in which the uncoupling protein (UCP) gene was driven the by fat-specific adipocyte FABP promoter. The expression of UCP in both BAT *and* WAT promoted a marked reduction in body weight and WAT mass (57).

E. Lipectomy

Surgical removal of adipose tissue and careful observation of its regeneration is another appropriate approach to study the regulation of adipose tissue growth and body weight in vivo. To date, many studies have been performed to investigate the effect of lipectomy on adipose tissue regeneration in a variety of species and depots and under various conditions (58). However, the results of

these studies were inconclusive, since the response to lipectomy was found to depend on various factors such as species, region of excision, time after operation, extent of removal, and type of diet. Nevertheless, in most animal studies a clear tendency for regeneration of the lost tissue was apparent at least in the perirenal and subcutaneous fat depots, but restoration at the site of excision was not always complete. In both rat and rabbit, the regenerative response was highest in the perirenal fat depot (59,60). In contrast, surgical removal of the epididymal fat pads did not lead to regeneration. These data are to some extent compatible with in vitro findings indicating that adipocyte precursor cells from the perirenal region have a higher capacity for proliferation and differentiation (27,61). Morphological studies in rats showed that adipose tissue regeneration in the inguinal site occurs in close association with revascularization and blood supply. Immediately after lipectomy, thymidine kinase activities are elevated at the sites of removal but slowly drop in the subsequent course to a level that is still above normal. Both total fat cell number and average fat cell size continuously increase during this process until the original tissue size is restored. Thus, the regeneration of adipose tissue resembles the processes that occur in developing adipose tissue and involves the new formation of fat cells from preadipocytes (62).

Two other aspects are of potential importance. One question is whether adipose tissue regrowth after lipectomy can also occur at other sites, thereby replacing the lost tissue mass. Faust and co-workers reported a compensatory fat deposition in nonexcised tissues after removal of epididymal and inguinal fat pads in rats (59). In another study, subcutaneous and bilateral epididymal lipectomy in castrated male rats resulted in compensatory increases of mesenteric and perirenal fat depots due to an increase in fat cell size compared to sham-operated rats (63). If this latter observation holds true in humans, surgical removal of significant amounts of subcutaneous adipose tissue could cause a redistribution of lipid stores to visceral sites, thereby favoring undesirable metabolic effects (48,64).

It is largely unknown whether the site-specific differences in regenerative capacity are due to inherent characteristics of the local tissue or to differences in the local environment. Circumstantial observations in humans are apparently in favor of the former possibility: skin transplantation from the abdomen to the forearm or to the back of the hand can lead to local hypertrophy of the transplant in case of body weight gain. However, the cellular composition of the subcutis may vary markedly depending on the anatomical location, and some particular skin areas may lack preadipose cells, which normally excludes the development of fat cells. Surprisingly, systematic studies on adipose tissue regrowth are missing in humans despite of the widespread application of suction lipectomy and dermolipectomy for cosmetic reasons, particularly in women. Much work needs to be done to ascertain to which degree and under which conditions adipose tissue regrowth can occur in humans.

F. Regional Differences in Adipose Tissue Growth

Many studies in animals and humans indicate that various aspects of adipocyte growth and function depend on the anatomical origin of the cells (48,64). The available methodology may not always allow an accurate assessment of differences, particularly if they are only modest. Regional differences may concern not only the metabolism of adipocytes but also the capacity to form new adipocytes.

Many cell culture studies were dealing with possible regional differences in adipose tissue growth. In rats, it has been repeatedly demonstrated that perirenal preadipose cells replicate more extensively under cell culture conditions than epididymal cells (61). In addition, perirenal cells differentiated more readily by morphological and biochemical criteria (27,61). In vitro differentiation of epididymal preadipocytes was also less pronounced than that of inguinal subcutaneous preadipocytes (65). These results are in good agreement with those obtained in adipose tissue cellularity studies (66). Available data also suggest that the composition of the preadipocyte precursor pool differs from region to region (61,67). Djian and co-workers reported that the adipocyte precursor populations derived from rat perirenal and epididymal fat are composed of cell clones that vary in capacity for replication and differentiation. Since these differences between rat perirenal and epididymal depots were still detectable during secondary culture, the authors assumed that this variation among fat depots may have an intrinsic basis (61). Possible explanations for this variability may include differences among fat depots in the distribution of hormone receptors such as glucocorticoid and adrenergic receptors that are involved in adipose tissue metabolism and growth (48,64).

Apart from receptor distribution, it is also likely that regional differences in adipose tissue growth may result from differences in the local environment of the cells. Innervation and blood flow are two major determinants of the local milieu. Comparative studies have noticed that mesenteric fat cells receive more blood than subcutaneous cells (68). In accordance with this finding, the stromal-vascular cell fraction of omental adipose tissue contains a high proportion of endothelial cells, while the same fraction obtained from subcutaneous adipose tissue is almost free of endothelial cells (21). It is obvious that a better blood supply may provide greater levels of humoral factors that are involved in the regulation of adipose tissue growth and also more substrates for lipid accumulation. In an elegant approach, Cousin and co-workers have recently demonstrated that a local sympathetic denervation of white adipose tissue in rats induces preadipocyte proliferation without affecting metabolic function. The surgical denervation also resulted in an accelerated recruitment of precursors as assessed by increased expression of an early marker of adipose differentiation (69). In agreement with these results, exposure to norepinephrine of rat adipocyte precursor cells in primary culture was found to suppress proliferation (70).

Only sparse data are available on site-specific differences in adipose tissue cellularity and growth in humans. They indicate that intra-abdominal fat cells are smaller than subcutaneous cells, while published results on variations in fat cell size among subcutaneous depots are inconclusive or found to be influenced by many factors such as age, hormonal status, diet, and others. A comparison of adipose tissue cellularity between young and middle-aged women revealed that the latter had more body fat than the former. This difference was exclusively explained by larger fat cells in all depots, while the younger women had a significantly higher total fat cell number. The age-related increase in fat cell size was particularly pronounced in the abdominal depot. The authors concluded from their studies that abdominal fat cells are more sensitive to nutritional and/or hormonal factors than those from other regions (71).

Very limited information is available on regional differences of adipose tissue development in humans. Pettersson and co-workers compared the capacity for adipose differentiation in stromal cells from omental and subcutaneous adipose tissue samples. They reported that more omental than subcutaneous cells were converted into adipocytes in an enriched viscous suspension medium (72). However, in this system high serum concentrations were used, which are now known to strongly inhibit adipose differentiation in human cells due to a high mitogenic and antiadipogenic activity. In a recent study, the capacity for adipose differentiation was compared in cultured stromal cells from the abdominal and femoral adipose tissue obtained from obese women by needle biopsy. Under serum-free, hormone-supplemented culture conditions, glycerol-3-phosphate dehydrogenase (GPDH) activities used as an index of adipose differentiation was on average significantly higher in the cells from the abdominal region, while other parameters such as number of stromal cells per gram adipose tissue were not significantly different (73). These findings could help to explain why changes in depot size are greater in the abdominal region as compared to other regions.

III. DEVELOPMENTAL ISSUES IN THE LEAN AND OBESE STATE

A. Adipose Tissue Cellularity in Obesity

An excessive amount of body fat can result from enlarged fat cells or an increase in fat cell number or a combination of both. In humans, the study of Salans and co-workers emphasized that childhood-onset obesity is characterized by a combination of fat cell hyperplasia and hypertrophy, in contrast to adulthood-onset where fat cell hypertrophy is predominant (16). Indeed, studies in lean and obese children suggest that obese children exhibit more rapid and earlier elevations in both cell number and cell size during childhood and adolescence (19). In contrast, studies in adults indicated that obese subjects have larger adipose cells than lean subjects but no significant increase in fat cell number (16). However, further studies revealed that development of hyperplasia can also occur in adult life. During excessive weight gain as seen in severely obese adults, both fat cell size and number increase independent of the time of onset of obesity (20). It was concluded from such studies in humans and animals that an increase in the number of mature fat cells does not occur until existing cells reach a critical cell size (20,74). Since fat cell size is varying in different adipose tissue depots, it was speculated that this phenomenon is regulated at the local level (13,74; see below). In addition, there is now convincing evidence that new adipocytes can be recruited throughout the whole lifetime (21).

The few studies comparing adipose tissue growth in lean and obese humans do not allow any firm conclusions concerning main characteristics of fat cell proliferation and differentiation. Pettersson and co-workers reported that the replication rates of cultured stromal-vascular cells isolated from adipose tissue of lean and obese subjects were similar. In addition, no difference in the capacity for differentiation was observed between cells from nonobese and obese individuals regardless of tissue site, arguing against a genetic predisposition at the cellular level (72). On the other hand, Roncari and co-workers reported an exaggerated replication and differentiation of cultured adipocyte precursor cells from massively obese subjects as compared to lean controls, which may indicate that in this particular subgroup an intrinsic defect could be responsible for fat cell hyperplasia and facilitate the development of massive obesity in humans (75). Up to now, these data await confirmation from other groups.

Apart from these limited data in humans, many in vitro studies have been performed in animal models of obesity to determine if there are significant differences in the capacities and mechanisms to form new adipocytes between obese and lean animals and, in particular, to look for intrinsic differences in genetic obesity. Most studies have been carried out in Zucker rats. Compared with lean rats, a decreased as well as an increased adipogenic capacity of preadipocytes derived from obese Zucker rats has been reported. However, under strictly controlled serum-free culture conditions, the only difference between lean and obese animals was that adipose conversion in cells from older obese rats was lower than from lean controls (76). It may be speculated that due to a higher adipogenic activity, preadipose cells in advanced stages of development are recruited more extensively and rapidly in obese as compared to lean animals. Thus, the conclusion is that the metabolic consequences induced by the *fa* gene and leading to obesity cause secondary changes in the cellular composition of the stromal cell fraction. Other studies on this issue did not describe consistent differences in the capacity for preadipocyte proliferation and differentiation between obese and lean animals, arguing against an intrinsic basis for the above-mentioned differences in adipose tissue cellularity.

B. Modulation of Adipose Tissue Cellularity by Diet and Weight Change

The relationship between nutrition and adipose tissue cellularity is the crucial clue for the understanding of adipose tissue expansion. It was found, as a conclusion from many studies, that early nutrition can potently affect fat cell number in adult life. On the other hand, early undernutrition in the rat can partly impede the formation of fat cells. In the adult rat, feeding a high-fat diet can also increase fat cell number (74), while energy restriction is only associated with a decrease in fat cell size but not in number, indicating that dietary manipulation in adulthood cannot reduce fat cell number (66). This has been elaborated in experiments where rats were overnourished for a long period of time, which resulted in both an increase in fat cell size and number. Discontinuation of the experimental diet was followed by a decline in average fat cell size until it reached the levels of normal control rats. However, fat cell number remained at the high level achieved during overfeeding (66).

It is uncertain whether extreme dietary restrictions can affect fat cell number. In a study of severe long-term food deprivation causing up to 99% reduction in white adipose tissue mass, there was no evidence that fat cells were lost.

After refeeding, no change in fat cell number was observed despite marked changes in endothelial and nonadipocyte mesenchymal cell number in adipose tissue (77). These data are not consistent with the results of some older studies that showed a decrease in fat cell number after long-term weight reduction (78). In a more recent study, induction of diabetes in rats by streptozotocin resulted not only in a marked reduction of fat cell size, but also in a decrease in white adipose tissue cellularity as assessed by quantitative cellular analysis. Interestingly, the tiny adipocytes were characterized by the presence of multilocular triglyceride droplets (79). It is also interesting to know whether fat cell hyperplasia found in the obese state can decline during prolonged maintenance of reduced weight. Again, in most studies, the number of fat cells was not normalized in either form of obesity even after extended periods of weight reduction. Obviously, an established fat cell hyperplasia cannot be reversed by extreme nutritional intervention including prolonged maximal starvation (77,78).

It is tempting to assume that some of the contradictory findings are due to limitations of the applied methods. For various reasons, the classic methodological approaches for the determination of adipose tissue cellularity are inaccurate and do not allow a reliable identification of the cell populations present in adipose tissue. This makes it extremely difficult to distinguish early preadipocytes as well as tiny fat cells from other cell types in adipose tissue.

In humans, short-term studies have also demonstrated that moderate weight changes are only associated with changes in fat cell weight but not in fat cell number (80,81). To date, there is only one study that investigated the long-term effects of weight change on adipose tissue cellularity. The authors reported that prolonged reduction of body weight in adult women over 6–9 years reduced the number of monolocular adipocytes (13). Other evidence for a possible reduction of fat cell number by weight loss comes from a study of morbidly obese subjects undergoing gastric surgery. After a mean weight loss of 30–40 kg fat cell size was markedly decreased in all adipose tissue depots. In addition, the calculated fat cell number was significantly reduced (82). Irrespective of methodological limitations, these reports raise the possibility that at least some adipocytes can completely lose their lipids and regain a state of lipid depletion. This remains an important issue, since it was repeatedly hypothesized that persistence of hypercellularity may contribute to the difficulties encountered by postobese subjects to maintain a reduced body weight.

Adipose tissue growth seems to depend not only on total caloric intake but also on the composition of the diet.

Older animal studies have already suggested that dietary fat can induce hyperplastic adipose tissue growth independent of body weight gain (83,84). This effect was also observed when strictly isocaloric diets were fed (85). Saturated fatty acids proved to be more effective in promoting adipose tissue expansion in Sprague-Dawley rats than polyunsaturated fatty acids (54). This presumptive relationship between fat intake and adipose tissue growth may be substantiated by recent in vitro data demonstrating that exogenous triglycerides can promote adipose differentiation. This new findings may provide a better insight at the cellular level as to why a fat-rich diet favors adipose tissue expansion in humans (86).

IV. STUDIES OF ADIPOSE TISSUE DEVELOPMENT IN VITRO

Cell culture techniques have the advantage that the effects of single factors can be studied under strictly defined conditions. This methodology is an ideal tool to unravel mechanisms of hormone action or cell development. However, in vivo the physiological function of a specific cell type or organ strongly depends on its communication with the environment. As part of a complex, highly integrated organism, the adipose tissue depots are interacting with surrounding but also with distant tissues by various forms of communication. To fully understand and corroborate the physiological importance of in vitro findings in any tissue it is essential to perform additional in vivo studies that consider the cross-talk among the various tissues. This point has been remarkably illustrated in the last couple of years with the cloning of the *ob* gene and the various roles played by leptin.

A. Clonal Cell Lines and Cell Strains

Cells of clonal lines fall into three categories: (1) totipotent embryonic stem cells giving rise to embryoid bodies able to generate cells of all lineages (ES cells), (2) multipotent stem cells can follow myogenic, chondrogenic, or adipogenic pathways, and (3) cells that have already undergone determination to the adipose lineage, termed preadipocyte clonal lines (Table 2).

The process of adipose cell differentiation has been primarily investigated in cells of preadipocyte clonal lines such as 3T3-L1, 3T3-F442A, Ob17, 1246, 3T3-T, and ST13, which are all aneuploid. Some investigators have turned to the study of adipose precursor cells derived from the stromal-vascular fraction of adipose tissues from various species, including the human; these cells are dip-

Table 2 Clonal Cell Lines and Cell Strains

Cell lines	Species	Origin	Ref.	Category
ES	Mouse embryo	Blastocytes	4	I
1246	Embryocarcinoma cells injected into C3H mouse	Clonal line T-984	87	II
C1	Embryonal carcinoma cells transfected with recombinant plasmid PK4	Clonal line 1003-PK4	88	II
RCJ3.1	Fetal rat	Calvaria	89	II
TAI	Mouse embryo	5-azacytidine-treated 10T1/2 fibroblasts	90	II
30A5	Mouse embryo	5-azacytidine-treated 10T1/2 fibroblasts	90	II
azaCyd CHEF-18	Hamster embryo	5-azacytidine-treated CHEF-18 fibroblasts	87	II
BSM2	Young mouse	Bone marrow	91	III
+/+2.4	Adult mouse	Bone marrow	92	III
3T3-L1	Swiss mouse embryo	Variant embryo fibroblast	87	III
3T3-F442A	Swiss mouse embryo	Variant embryo fibroblast	87	III
A31T	Balb mouse embryo	Variant embryo fibroblast	87	III
Ob17	C57 BL/6J ob/ob adult mouse	Epididymal fat pad	87	III
HGFu	C57 BL/6J +/? adult mouse	Epididymal fat pad	87	III
ST13	DDN mouse	Mammary carcinoma	87	III
MC3T3-G2/PA6	Newborn mouse	Calvaria	87	III
MS3-2A	Adult mouse	Bone marrow stroma	87	III
BFC-1	C57 BL/6J adult mouse	SV fraction of BAT	87	III

Cell strains	Species	Origin	Ref.	
	Mouse	SV cells of epididymal fat pad	87	III
	Rat	SV cells of epididymal, perirenal, subcutaneous and inguinal fat pad	87	III
	Hamster	SV cells of perirenal and subcutaneous fat tissue	87	III
	Pig	SV cells of perirenal and subcutaneous fat tissue	87	III
	Rabbit	SV cells of perirenal fat tissue	87	III
	Bovine	SV cells of subcutaneous adipose tissue	87	III
	Ovine	SV cells of perirenal and subcutaneous adipose tissue	87	III
	Human	SV cells of subcutaneous and omental adipose tissue	87	III
	Mouse	Bone marrow	87	III
	Rat	Bone marrow	87	III
	Human	Bone marrow	87	III

Category I corresponds to totipotent cells, category II to multipotent cells, and category III to unipotent cells.

loid but have a limited life span. When transplanted into animals, cells from both sources develop into mature fat cells. In vitro they differentiate, in the presence of an appropriate hormonal milieu, to yield cells that have most, if not all, the morphological, ultrastructural and biochemical characteristics of adipocytes, including hormonal responses. Adipose precursor cells resemble fibroblasts while growing at low density, but at growth arrest induced by various means (serum or calcium deprivation, thymidine block, or merely by confluence), the differentiation process takes place and culminates in a large triacylglycerol accumulation.

The process of adipose cell differentiation, which can be analyzed in vitro with preadipocyte clonal lines, corresponds to the phenotypic changes: adipoblast → preadipose cell (usually termed preadipocyte) → immature adipose cell → mature adipose cell (usually termed adipocyte) (Fig. 3). The differentiation process of adipose precursor cells isolated from fat tissue and present in the stromal-vascular fraction corresponds primarily to the sequence preadipose cell (preadipocyte) → immature adipose cell → mature adipose cell (adipocyte), although the presence of adipoblasts cannot be excluded. This conclusion is based on the fact that mouse, rat, and human stromal-vascular cells contain the bulk of A2COL6/pOb24 mRNA and express LPL and IGF-I mRNAs, i.e., have already expressed early markers (stage 3 of Fig. 3). Morphologically, after reaching confluence, fibroblast-like cells become round, enlarge, and accumulate triacylglycerol droplets in their cytoplasm. The main events, based on numerous studies by various investigators, are summarized in Figure 3. Preadipocyte factor 1 (Pref-1) is a transmembrane protein present in, but not unique to, adipoblasts and preadipocytes, which decreases to nondetectable levels during terminal differentiation. Constitutive expression of Pref-1 in 3T3-L1 cells inhibits differentiation, suggesting that Pref-1 maintains preadipocytes in the nonterminally differentiated state (93). Growth arrest at the G_1/S stage of the cell cycle, rather than contact among arrested cells, is necessary to trigger the formation of preadipocytes from adipoblasts. This commitment is associated with the emergence of potential regulatory genes and proteins such as A2COL6/pOb24, AP27, FSP27, ADRP, LPL, and PPARδ, as well as the emergence of a selective uptake of long-chain fatty acids by means of a fatty acid translocase (FAT). The regulation of expression of these early genes takes place primarily at a transcriptional level and appears to be independent of various hormones, which, in contrast, are required for terminal differentiation. DNA synthesis precedes the expression of late and very late genes, which is associated with a limited growth resumption of these committed, early marker-expressing cells followed by the induction of the CCAAT/enhancer-binding protein α (C/EBPα) and the enzymatic machinery required for fatty acid synthesis and esterification. Cell division of preadipose cells appears to be essential for terminal differentiation (defined by the emergence of GPDH activity), at least in rodent cells, provided cells are exposed to the appropriate hormonal milieu (see below). The observations made in vitro are in agreement with those made in vivo in rodents, which showed: (1) after pulse labeling with [³H]thymidine, the labeling indices of cells from the subcutaneous adipose tissue were highest in partially differentiated cells (esterase positive, e.g., presumably LPL-

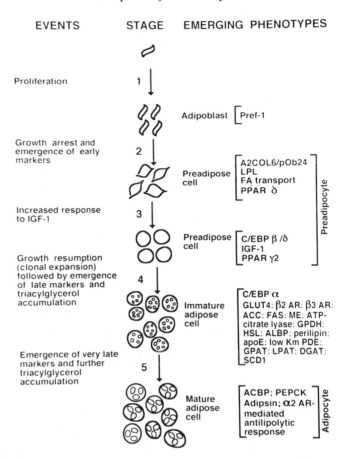

Figure 3 Multiple stages of adipose cell differentiation. The scheme is based on data obtained with cells of preadipoyte clonal lines and adipose precursor cells. Pref-1, preadipocyte factor 1; A2COL6/pOb24, α2-chain collagen VI; LPL, lipoprotein lipase; FA transport, fatty acid transport; PPAR, peroxisome proliferator-activated receptor; C/EBP, CCAAT/enhancer-binding protein; IGF-I, insulin-like growth factor I; GLUT-4, insulin-sensitive glucose transporter 4; β2-AR, β2-adrenoreceptor; β3-AR, β3-adrenoreceptor; α2-AR, α2-adrenoreceptor; ACC, acetyl-CoA carboxylase; FAS, fatty acid synthetase; ME, malic enzyme; GPDH, glycerol-3-phosphate dehydrogenase; ALBP, adipocyte lipid-binding protein (aP2); HSL, hormone-sensitive lipase; apoE, apolipoprotein E; low-K_m PDE, low-K_m phosphodiesterase; GPAT, glycerophosphate actyltransferase; LPAT, lysophosphatidate acyltransferase; DGAT, diglyceride acyltransferase; SCD-1, stearoylCoA desaturase 1; ACBP, acyl CoA–binding protein; PEPCK, phosphoenolpyruvate carboxykinase.

positive) containing no lipid droplets (94) and (2) only cells that had replicated their DNA were able to express GPDH activity and to accumulate triacylglycerol (95).

However, there is also evidence that cultured human adipocyte precursor cells can develop into adipocytes without cell division, indicating that these cells have already undergone critical mitosis in vivo and may be in a late stage of the developmental program (22).

B. Adipogenic Factors and Second-Messenger Pathways

Adipogenic factors or external inducers are required to trigger the terminal differentiation of preadipose into adipose cells whereas antiadipogenic factors are able to counteract their effects. The responsiveness of preadipose cells to external signals that induce/repress differentiation may vary for various reasons: (1) differences in the stage of adipose lineage at which clonal cell lines have been established (e.g., category I, II, or III, see Table 2 for details) and (2) differences in the stage—early, intermediate, or late—at which cells are exposed to various agents; in that respect the effects of hormones on differentiating cells should be distinguished from their effects in fully differentiated cells. To add further complication, the (fetal) bovine serum used in many experiments contains positive and negative effectors, the relative proportions of which cannot be controlled. This has led many investigators to use serum-free medium, particularly in the case of preadipose cell strains (Table 2). In some instances, the fact that one signal can substitute for an inducer from a separate signal transduction pathway indicates a redundancy of certain signaling systems in adipocyte differentiation.

From a general point of view, the distinction between obligatory and modulating hormones is not as clear-cut as originally thought. Moreover, since rodent preadipose cells undergo mitoses during terminal differentiation, a clear distinction between mitogenic and adipogenic factors is difficult to make. In that respect, besides their well-known role in the control of lipolysis, a new role of catecholamines as mitogens has been proposed but remains controversial since the proliferation of white preadipocytes (96) and that of brown preadipocytes (97) have been reported either to be stimulated via α_2-adrenoreceptor- and β-adrenoreceptor-mediated agents, respectively, or to be inhibited in the case of white preadipocytes (70). The contribution of catecholamines to hyperplasia of fat deposits remains an intriguing possibility and requires further physiological studies. Despite these limitations, a limited panoply of factors appears to be required for the terminal differentiation of preadipose into adipose cells from clonal lines, excluding the requirement for a single adipogenic hormone. IGF-I, glucocorticoids, and cAMP-elevating agents are well-established inducers. T_3 and retinoids appear also to be required. In addition, long-chain fatty acids (FA) act directly or indirectly as positive modulators of terminal differentiation whereas angiotensin II (A-II) ap-

pears implicated in a paracrine/autocrine mechanism. This panoply of factors is even more limited with respect to adipose precursor cells from adipose tissue as stimulation by glucocorticoids (or prostacyclin), IGF-I, and insulin is sufficient to trigger terminal differentiation (3).

1. IGF-I and Insulin

IGF-I and insulin at nonphysiologically high concentrations behave as mitogens that bind to IGF-I receptor present at high levels in preadipose cells. GH, which stimulates differentiation of 3T3 and Ob17 preadipocytes, appears to function (via an autocrine/paracrine mechanism) by activating expression and secretion of IGF-I. IGF-I receptor is a ligand-dependent tyrosine kinase, which acts by initiating a tyrosine kinase-mediated pathway implicating Ras and Raf-I as signal mediators (98). Tyrosine kinase–mediated pathways appear crucial as MAP kinase was shown to be essential for differentiation of 3T3-L1 preadipose cells probably by means of growth stimulation in response to serum or insulin at high concentrations (99). When present within a physiological range of concentrations, insulin is not a mitogen and appears as a mere modulator of the expression of genes and corresponding enzymes involved in triacylglycerol accumulation in differentiated cells (26).

2. Glucocorticoids and cAMP-Elevating Agents

Glucocorticoids, including the synthetic glucocorticoid dexamethasone, stimulate terminal differentiation of preadipose cells from different clonal lines and that of preadipose cells from various cell strains, including human. Glucocorticoids act, at least in part, by increasing arachidonic acid availability and prostacyclin production, which then acts as an autocrine/paracrine adipogenic hormone. Prostacyclin can substitute for glucocorticoids and induces a rise in cAMP and Ca^{2+} intracellular levels, both signals triggering the terminal differentiation of Ob1771 preadipose cells as well as modulating positively that of rat and human preadipocytes (3). In contrast to Ob1771 cells, both glucocorticoids and cAMP-elevating agents are required for terminal differentiation of 3T3-L1 preadipose cells (98).

3. Tri-iodothyronine and Retinoids

T_3 also appears to be implicated in the terminal differentiation of preadipose cells. A dramatic decrease in the adipogenic activity of the serum-free medium could be observed in the absence of T_3 accompanied by an increase of the mitogenic potency. Thus, T_3 at physiological concentrations ($EC_{50} \sim 0.1$ nM) appears to modulate both proliferation and differentiation (100). The all-*trans* retinoic acid appears at physiological concentrations to be a potent stimulatory hormone of the terminal differentiation of preadipose Ob17 cells and that of rat preadipocytes, and it can substitute for T_3. T_3 receptors and retinoic acid receptor-α (RARα) are implicated in the responses of Ob1771 preadipose cells to T_3 and retinoids, respectively (101).

4. Fatty Acids (FA)

Both long-chain FA (saturated, unsaturated, and nonmetabolizable) and peroxisome proliferators (agents that increase peroxisome proliferation) are able to activate terminal differentiation in synergy with the other adipogenic factors (86). The mechanisms by which these effectors are active have recently been thoroughly studied. The cloning and properties of three members of the peroxisome proliferator-activated receptor (PPAR) gene family, which are members of the steroid/thyroid hormone receptor family, have improved our understanding of these points (see below).

5. Angiotensin II

A-II is likely to arise from angiotensinogen present in adipocytes as adipose tissue is the most important extrahepatic source and as angiotensinogen accumulates in late differentiated adipose cells (102). When preadipose and adipose cells are cocultured and exposed to A-II, A-II binds to specific receptors in adipocytes, which respond by a specific increase in prostacyclin production (103). Since prostacyclin acts in preadipocytes only (see above), this leads to the formation of new fat cells. This autocrine/paracrine mechanism may be operating in vivo, as A-II triggers adipose tissue prostacyclin production (104) and as the renin-angiotensin system may play a role in adipose tissue development (105,106).

C. Antiadipogenic Factors

Various factors that inhibit or abolish differentiation of adipose precursor cells have been reported (3), including platelet-derived growth factor (PDGF) and TGF-β. The most intriguing results are those obtained in preadipose cells with TGF-β since, except for pig preadipocytes (107), terminal differentiation appears irreversibly blocked after its removal, in contrast to various other factors where partial or complete recovery of the differentiated phenotype is observed (3). The situation remains unclear with regard to fibroblast growth factor (FGF) and epidermal growth factor (EGF), which have been claimed to be inhibitory or to be without effect, depending on the origin of target cells. In vivo, subcutaneous administration of EGF to newborn rats results in a large decrease of the weight of inguinal fat pads, which suggests the delayed formation of adipocytes from preadipocytes (108). The effects of tumor necrosis factor-α (TNF-α) are multiple, since it inhibits the expression of several differentiation-specific genes and induces a phenotypic "dedifferentiation" on a long-term basis. The TNF-signaling pathway involves a regulatory role of c-*myc* that is distinct from its role in cell proliferation (109). Dehydroepiandrosterone and some structural analogs, as well as many fat-soluble vitamins, are known to abolish terminal differentiation of 3T3-L1 preadipose cells (3). Retinoids have been reported also to inhibit differentiation, but the supraphysiological concentrations used in those studies raise serious doubt about their physiological relevance. In summary, no specific antiadipogenic factor has been yet reported, but, considering the diversity of the adipogenic factors so far described, such a finding appears a remote possibility.

V. MOLECULAR MECHANISMS OF ADIPOSE CELL DIFFERENTIATION

The differentiation process is characterized by a coordinate increase in the expression of most adipocyte proteins and a decrease in the expression of preadipocyte proteins. In most cases, alteration of the transcriptional rate of the corresponding genes accounts for almost all the changes. Thus extensive studies have been carried out to identify *cis*-acting promoter elements of the target genes and cognate *trans*-acting factors that control their transcription. "Master regulators" of adipocyte gene transcription have been described in the last few years. A combination of positive-acting factors from the C/EBP family and PPAR family as well as negative-acting factors [C/EBPα undifferentiated protein (CUP), C/EBP homologous protein-10 (CHOP-10)] are implicated, the time course of appearance allowing the orderly progression of the differentiation program (98).

A. *Trans*-Acting Factors

C/EBPα, the first identified member of this family shown to bind to CCAAT sequence (termed C/EBP binding site), emerges when clonal expression ceases and terminal differentiation begins, whereas other members of this family, C/EBPβ and δ, are present in growing adipoblasts and are expressed transiently in preadipose cells. The emergence of C/EBPα is rapid as autoactivation of the C/EBPα gene occurs through its C/EBP binding site. C/EBPα behaves as a "master regulator" as (1) it binds specifically to C/

EBP sites within the promoters of three adipocyte genes (ALBP, SCD1, GLUT4) that are coordinately expressed during terminal differentiation, (2) constitutive expression of anti-sense C/EBPα RNA prevents terminal differentiation, (3) ectopic expression in fibroblastic cells induces differentiation to adipose cells, and (4) C/EBPα gene inactivation by homologous recombination leads to mice unable to develop the first adipose depot that appears in the scapular region of control animals (98). Although C/EBPα has critical functions in terminally differentiated adipose cells, its role is not unique to adipose tissue as it is also expressed in other lipid-synthesizing tissues such as BAT, liver, and intestine. Among other positive-acting factors, mPPARγ_2, a member of the PPAR family (110), appears quite specific as it is predominantly expressed in mouse WAT and BAT (111). mPPARδ (also called FAAR or mNUC1; 112,113), the mouse homolog of the human NUC1, emerging earlier than mPPARγ_2 during differentiation, is expressed in mice in a variety of lipogenic tissues (WAT, BAT, intestine) and a few nonlipogenic tissues (skeletal muscle, heart). Forced expression of C/EBPα (98), PPARγ_2 (114), and mPPARδ (112) in fibroblasts is sufficient to activate the transcription of various lipid-related genes encoding for late markers of adipose differentiation and to induce terminal differentiation provided appropriate activators are present in the cell environment. Moreover, forced expression of both C/EBPα and PPARγ_2 in fibroblasts brings synergy and leads to maximal adipocyte differentiation (114). PPAR isoforms bind to members of the retinoic X receptor (RXR) family as heterodimers and are activated by a broad diversity of molecules, including natural compounds, such as fatty acids, prostaglandins, or leukotrienes, and synthetic molecules, such as nonmetabolizable fatty acids, fibrates, or thiazolidinediones. Prostaglandin D$_2$ metabolites such as prostaglandin J$_2$ and derivatives may be the actual physiological ligands of PPARγ_2 (115–117) whereas long-chain saturated and unsaturated fatty acids, which act as potent activators of PPARδ, are postulated but not proven to be also ligands (112). A better knowledge of the natural ligands of the various PPARs and insights into the biosynthesis of certain prostaglandins from arachidonic acid in adipose cells may provide an important clue for the link existing between the FA composition of food and fat cell formation in animals and humans.

B. Trans-Differentiation

The multipotentiality of progenitor mesodermal cells from certain clonal lines has been illustrated in vitro by the concomitant differentiation of cells into myotubes, chondrocytes, and adipocytes. Exogenous regulatory factors appear to play a crucial role in the determination into a specific differentiation lineage. Exposure to fatty acids or thiazolidinediones of C2C12N myoblasts expressing m-PPARδ and of muscle satellite cells (118), as well as exposure of G8 myoblasts overexpressing both PPARγ_2 and C/EBPα (119), prevents the formation of myotubes and leads to the expression of a typical adipose differentiation program, indicating that these adipogenic inducers specifically convert the differentiation pathway of myoblasts into that of adipoblasts.

These in vitro findings raise the possibility that such an event takes place in vivo, particularly in some pathological states characterized by lipid accumulation in muscle cells or in obesity when numerous fat cells pervade muscle tissue. It could be speculated that, in the obese state, hyperlipidemia increases the flux of FA acting as PPAR activators that enter muscle cells, leading in turn to increased susceptibility to convert myoblasts to adipose cells.

REFERENCES

1. Johnson PR, Greenwood MRC. Adipose tissue. In: Weiss L, ed. Cell and Tissue Biology—A Textbook of Histology. Baltimore: Urban & Schwarzenberg, 1988:191–209.
2. Julien P, Despres JP, Angel A. Scanning electron microscopy of very small fat cells and mature fat cells in human obesity. J Lipid Res 1989; 30:293–299.
3. Ailhaud G, Grimaldi P, Négrel R. Cellular and molecular aspects of adipose tissue development. Annu Rev Nutr 1992; 12:207–233.
4. Keller GM. In vitro differentiation of embryonic stem cells. Curr Opin Cell Biol 1995; 7:862–869.
5. Hausman GJ. Identification of adipose tissue primordia in perirenal tissues of pig fetuses: utility of phosphatase histochemistry. Acta Anat 1987; 128:236–242.
6. Poissonnet CM, Burdi AR, Garn SM. The chronology of adipose tissue appearance and disturbance in human fetus. Early Hum Dev 1984; 10:1–11.
7. Ballantyne B, Raftery AT. The intrinsic autonomic innervation of white adipose tissue. Cytobios 1974; 10: 187–197.
8. Fredholm BB. In: Cryer A, Van RLR, eds. New Perspectives in Adipose Tissue: Structure, Function and Development. London: Butterworths, 1985:45–64.
9. Dobson DE, Kambe A, Block E, Dion T, Lu H, Castellot JJ Jr, Spiegelman BM. 1-butyrylglycerol: a novel angiogenesis factor secreted by differentiating adipocytes. Cell 1990; 61:223–230.
10. Wassermann F. The development of adipose tissue. In: Renold AE, Cahill GF, eds. Handbook of Physiology. Section 5: Adipose Tissue. Washington, DC: American Physiological Society, 1965:87–100.

11. Poissonnet CM, Burdi AR, Bookstein FL. Growth and development of human adipose tissue during early gestation. Early Hum Dev 1983; 8:1–11.

12. Häger A, Sjöström L, Arvidsson B, Björntorp P, Smith U. Body fat and adipose tissue cellularity in infants: a longitudinal study. Metabolism 1977; 26:607–614.

13. Sjöström L, William-Olsson T. Prospective studies on adipose tissue development in man. Int J Obes 1981; 5: 597–604.

14. Boulton TJC, Dunlop M, Court JM. The growth and development of fat cells in infancy. Pediatr Res 1978; 12: 908–911.

15. Faust IM, Miller WH Jr. Hyperplastic growth of adipose tissue in obesity. In: Angel A, Hollenberg CM, Roncari DAK, eds. The Adipocyte and Obesity: Cellular and Molecular Mechanisms. New York: Raven Press, 1983:41–51.

16. Salans LB, Cushman SW, Weismann RE. Studies of human adipose tissue. Adipose cell size and number in nonobese and obese patients. J Clin Invest 1973; 52:929–941.

17. Baum D, Beck RQ, Hammer LD, Brasel JA, Greenwood MRC. Adipose tissue thymidine kinase activity in man. Pediatr Res 1986; 20:118–121.

18. Hauner H, Wabitsch M, Pfeiffer EF. Proliferation and differentiation of adipose tissue derived stromal-vascular cells from children of different ages. In: Björntorp P, Rössner S, eds. Obesity in Europe 88: Proceedings of the 1st European Congress on Obesity. London-Paris: Libbey, 1989:195–200.

19. Knittle JL, Timmers K, Ginsberg-Fellner F, Brown RE, Katz DP. The growth of adipose tissue in children and adolescents. Cross-sectional and longitudinal studies of adipose cell number and size. J Clin Invest 1979; 63:239–246.

20. Hirsch J, Batchelor B. Adipose tissue cellularity in human obesity. Clin Endocrinol Metab 1976; 5:299–311.

21. Hauner H, Entenmann G, Wabitsch M, Gaillard D, Ailhaud G, Négrel R, Pfeiffer E. Promoting effect of glucocorticoids on the differentiation of human adipocytes precursor cells cultured in a chemically defined serum. J Clin Invest 1989; 84:1663–1670.

22. Entenmann G, Hauner H. Relationship between replication and differentiation in cultured human adipocyte precursor cells. Am J Physiol 1996; 270:C1011–C1016.

23. Levacher C, Sztalryd C, Kinebanyan MF, Picon L. Effects of thyroid hormones on adipose tissue development in Sherman and Zucker rats. Am J Physiol 1984; 246: C50–C56.

24. Hausman GJ. The influence of thyroxine on the differentiation of adipose tissue and skin during fetal development. Pediatr Res 1992; 32:1255–1261.

25. Géloen A, Collet AJ, Guay G, Bukowiecki LJ. Insulin stimulates in vivo cell proliferation in white adipose tissue. Am J Physiol 1989; 256:C190–C196.

26. Amri E-Z, Grimaldi P, Négrel R, Ailhaud G. Adipose conversion of Ob17 cells. Insulin acts solely as a modulator in the expression of the differentiation program. Exp Cell Res 1984; 152:368–377.

27. Wiederer O, Löffler G. Hormonal regulation of the differentiation of rat adipocyte precursor cells in primary culture. J Lipid Res 1987; 28:649–658.

28. Bonnet F, Lodeweyckx MV, Eeckels R, Malvaux P. Subcutaneous adipose tissue and lipids in blood in growth hormone deficiency before and after treatment with human growth hormone. Pediatr Res 1974; 8:800–5.

29. Rosenbaum M, Gertner JM, Leibel RL. Effects of systemic growth hormone (GH) administration on regional adipose tissue distribution and metabolism in GH-deficient children. J Clin Endocrinol Metab 1989; 69:1274–81.

30. Bengtsson B-A, Eden S, Lönn L, Kvist H, Stokland A, Lindstedt G, Bosaeus I, Tölli J, Sjöström L, Isaksson OGP. Treatment of adults with growth hormone (GH) deficiency with recombinant human GH. J Clin Endocrinol Metab 1993; 76:309–17.

31. O'Sullivan AJ, Kelly JJ, Hoffman DM, Freund J, Ho KKY. Body composition and energy expenditure in acromegaly. J Clin Endocrinol Metab 1994; 78:381–386.

32. Ottosson M, Vikman-Adolfsson K, Enerbäck S, Elander A, Björntorp P, Eden S. Growth hormone inhibits lipoprotein lipase activity in human adipose tissue. J Clin Endocrinol Metab 1995; 80:936–941.

33. Harant I, Beauville M, Crampes F, Rivière D, Tauber M-T, Tauber J-P, Garrigues M. Response of fat cells to growth hormone (GH): effect of long term treatment with recombinant human GH in GH-deficient adults. J Clin Endocrinol Metab 1994: 78:1392–1995.

34. Gaskins HR, Kim J-W, Wright JT, Rund LA, Hausman GJ. Regulation of insulin-like growth factor-I ribonucleic acid expression, polypeptide secretion, and binding protein activity by growth hormone in porcine preadipocyte cultures. Endocrinology 1990; 126:622–630.

35. Nougues J, Reyne Y, Barenton B, Chery T, Darandel V, Soriano J. Differentiation of adipocyte precursors in a serum-free medium is influenced by glucocorticoids and endogenously produced insulin-like growth factor-I. Int J Obes 1993; 17:159–167.

36. Wabitsch M, Braun S, Hauner H, Heinze E, Ilondo M, Shymko R, De Meyts P, Teller W. Mitogenic and antiadipogenic properties of human growth hormone in human adipocyte precursor cells in primary culture. Pediatr Res 1996; 40:450–456.

37. Lönn L, Kvist H, Ernest I, Sjöström L. Changes in body composition and adipose tissue distribution after treatment of women with Cushing's syndrome. Metabolism 1994; 43:1517–1522.

38. Rebuffé-Scrive M, Krotkiewski M, Elfverson J, Björntorp P. Muscle and adipose tissue morphology and metabolism in Cushing's syndrome. J Clin Endocrinol Metab 1988; 67:1122–1128.

39. Rebuffé-Scrive M, Brönnegard M, Nilsson A, Eldh J, Gustafsson J-A, Björntorp P. Steroid hormone receptors in human adipose tissues. J Clin Endocrinol Metab 1990; 71: 1215–1219.

40. Pepin MC, Pothier F, Barden N. Impaired type II glucocorticoid-receptor function in mice bearing antisense RNA transgene. Nature 1992; 355:725–728.

41. Stenzel-Poore MP, Cameron VA, Vaughan J, Sawchenko PE, Vale W. Development of Cushing's syndrome in corticotropin-releasing factor transgenic mice. Endocrinology 1992; 130:3378–3386.

42. Xu X, De Pergola G, Björntorp P. The effects of androgens on the regulation of lipolysis in adipose precursor cells. Endocrinology 1990; 126:1229–1234.

43. Pedersen SB, Börglum JD, Eriksen EF, Richelsen B. Nuclear estradiol binding in rat adipocytes. Regional variations and regulatory influences of hormones. Biochim Biophys Acta 1991; 1093:80–86.

44. Mizutani T, Nishikawa Y, Adachi H, Enomoto T, Ikegami H, Kurachi H, Nomura T, Miyake A. Identification of estrogen receptor in human adipose tissue and adipocytes. J Clin Endocrinol Metab 1994; 78:950–954.

45. Labrie F. At the cutting edge: intracrinology. Mol Cell Endocrinol 1991; 78:C113–C118.

46. Labrie F, Simard J, Luu-The V, Trudel C, Martel C, Labrie C, Zhao HF, Rheaume E, Couet J, Breton N. Expression of 3β-hydroxysteroid dehydrogenase/Δ4–Δ5 isomerase (3β-HSD) and 17β-hydroxysteroid dehydrogenase (17β-HSD) in adipose tissue. Int J Obes 1991; 15:91–99.

47. de Ridder CM, de Boer RW, Seidell JC, Nieuwenhoff CM, Jeneson JAL, Bakker CJG, Zonderland ML, Erich WBM. Body fat distribution in pubertal girls quantified by magnetic resonance imaging. Int J Obes 1992; 16:443–449.

48. Kissebah AH, Krakower GR. Regional adiposity and morbidity. Physiol Rev 1994; 74:761–811.

49. Haarbo J, Marslew U, Gotfredsen A, Christiansen C. Postmenopausal hormone replacement therapy prevents central distribution of body fat after menopause. Metabolism 1991; 40:1323–1326.

50. Björntorp P. The regulation of adipose tissue distribution in humans. Int J Obes 1996; 20:291–302.

51. Marin P, Holmäng S, Jönsson L, Sjöström L, Kvist H, Holm G, Lindstedt G, Björntorp. The effects of testosterone treatment on body composition and metabolism in middle-aged obese men. Int J Obes 1992; 16:991–997.

52. Kvist H, Hallgren P, Jönsson L, Pettersson P, Sjöberg C, Sjöström L, Björntorp P. Distribution of adipose tissue and muscle mass in alcoholic men. Metabolism 1993; 42:569–573.

53. Levak-Frank S, Radner H, Walsh AM, Stollberger R, Knipping G, Hoefler G, Sattler W, Breslow JL, Zechner R. Muscle-specific overexpression of lipoprotein lipase causes a severe myopathy characterized by proliferation of mitochondria and peroxisomes in transgenic mice. J Clin Invest 1995; 96:976–986.

54. Shillaber G, Lau DC. Regulation of new fat cell formation in rats: the role of dietary fats. J Lipid Res 1994; 35:592–600.

55. Shepherd PR, Gnudi L, Tozzo E, Yang H, Leach F, Kahn BB. Adipose cell hyperplasia and enhanced glucose disposal in transgenic mice overexpressing GLUT4 selectively in adipose tissue. J Biol Chem 1993; 268:22243–22246.

56. Katz EB, Stenbit AE, Hatton K, DePinho R, Charron MJ. Cardiac and adipose tissue abnormalities but not diabetes in mice deficient in GLUT4. Nature 1995; 377:151–155.

57. Kopecky J, Clarke G, Enerbäck S, Spiegelman B, Kozak LP. Expression of the mitochondrial uncoupling protein gene from the aP2 gene promoter prevents genetic obesity. J Clin Invest 1995; 96:2914–2923.

58. Faust IM, Kral J. Growth of adipose tissue following lipectomy. In: Cryer A, Van RLR, eds. New Perspectives in Adipose Tissue: Structure, Function and Development. London: Butterworths, 1987:319–332.

59. Faust IM, Johnson PR, Hirsch J. Adipose tissue regeneration following lipectomy. Science 1977; 197:391–393.

60. Reyne Y, Nougues J, Vezinhet A. Adipose tissue regeneration in 6-month-old and adult rabbits following lipectomy. Proc Soc Exp Biol Med 1983; 174:258–264.

61. Djian P, Roncari DAK, Hollenberg CH. Influence of anatomic site and age on the replication and differentiation in rat adipocyte precursors in culture. J Clin Invest 1983; 72:1200–1208.

62. Roth J, Greenwood MRC, Johnson PR. The regenerating fascial sheath in lipectomized Osborne-Mendel rats: morphological and biochemical indices of adipocyte differentiation and proliferation. Int J Obes 1981; 5:131–143.

63. Larson KA, Anderson DB. The effects of lipectomy on remaining adipose tissue depots in the Sprague-Dawley rat. Growth 1978; 42:469–477.

64. Leibel RL, Edens NK, Fried SK. Physiological basis for the control of body fat distribution in humans. Annu Rev Nutr 1989; 9:417–443.

65. Grégoire F, Todoroff G, Hauser N, Remacle C. The stroma-vascular fraction of rat inguinal and epididymal adipose tissue and the adipoconversion of fat cell precursors in primary culture. Biol Cell 1990; 69:215–222.

66. Faust IM. Nutrition and the fat cell. Int J Obes 1980; 4:314–321.

67. Wang H, Kirkland JL, Hollenberg CH. Varying capacities for replication of rat adipocyte precursor clones and adipose tissue growth. J Clin Invest 1989; 83:1741–1746.

68. Crandall DL, Goldstein BM, Huggins F, Cervoni P. Adipocyte blood flow: influence of age, anatomic location, and dietary manipulation. Am J Physiol 1984; 247:R46–R51.

69. Cousin B, Casteilla L, Lafontan M, Ambid L, Langin D, Berthault M-F, Pénicaud L. Local sympathetic denervation of white adipose tissue in rats induces preadipocyte proliferation without noticeable changes in metabolism. Endocrinology 1993; 133:2255–2262.

70. Jones DD, Ramsay TG, Hausman GJ, Martin RJ. Norepinephrine inhibits rat pre-adipocyte proliferation. Int J Obes 1992; 16:349–354.

71. Krotiewski M, Sjöström L, Björntrop P, Smith U. Regional adipose tissue cellularity in relation to metabolism in

young and middle-aged women. Metabolism 1975; 24: 703–710.

72. Pettersson P, Van RLR, Karlsson M, Björntorp P, Adipocyte precursor cells in obese and nonobese humans. Metabolism 1985; 34:808–812.

73. Hauner H, Entenmann G. Regional variation of adipose differentiation in cultured stromal-vascular cells from the abdominal and femoral adipose tissue of obese women. Int J Obes 1991; 15:121–126.

74. Faust IM, Johnson PR, Stern JS, Hirsch J. Diet-induced adipocyte number increase in adult rats: a new model of obesity. Am J Physiol 1978; 235:E279–E286.

75. Roncari DAK, Lau DCW, Kindler S. Exaggerated replication in culture of adipocyte precursors from massively obese persons. Metabolism 1981; 30:425–427.

76. Grégoire FM, Johnson PR, Greenwood MRC. Comparison of the adipoconversion of preadipocytes derived from lean and obese Zucker rats in serum-free cultures. Int J Obes 1995; 19:664–670.

77. Miller WH, Faust IM, Goldberger AC, Hirsch J. Effects of severe long-term food deprivation and refeeding on adipose tissue cells in the rat. Am J Physiol 1983; 245: E74–E80.

78. Hausberger FX. Effect of dietary and endocrine factors on adipose tissue growth. In: Renold AE, Cahill GF, eds. Handbook of Physiology. Section 5: Adipose Tissue. Washington, DC: American Physiological Society, 1965: 519–528.

79. Géloen A, Roy PE, Bukowiecki LJ. Regression of white adipose tissue in diabetic rats. Am J Physiol 1989; 257: E547–E553.

80. Björntorp P, Carlgren G, Isaksson B, Krotkiewski M, Larsson B, Sjöström L. Effect of an energy-reduced dietary regimen in relation to adipose tissue cellularity in obese women. Am J Clin Nutr 1975; 28:445–452.

81. Knittle JL, Ginsberg-Fellner F. Effect of weight reduction on in vitro adipose tissue lipolysis and cellularity in obese adolescents and adults. Diabetes 1972; 21:754–761.

82. Näslund I, Hallgren P, Sjöström L. Fat cell weight and number before and after gastric surgery for morbid obesity in women. Int J Obes 1988; 12:191–197.

83. Lemonnier D. Effect of age, sex, and site on the cellularity of the adipose tissue in mice and rats rendered obese by a high-fat diet. J Clin Invest 1972; 51:2907–2915.

84. Herberg L, Döppen W, Major E, Gries FA. Dietary-induced hypertrophic-hyperplastic obesity in mice. J Lipid Res 1975; 15:580–585.

85. Oscai LB, Brown MM, Miller WC. Effect of dietary fat on food intake, growth and body composition in rats. Growth 1984; 48:415–424.

86. Amri E, Ailhaud G, Grimaldi PA. Fatty acids as signal transducing molecules: involvement in the differentiation of preadipose to adipose cells. J Lipid Res 1994; 35: 930–937.

87. Ailhaud G, Amri E, Bertrand B, Barcellini-Couget S, Bardon S, Catalioto RM, Dani C, Deslex S, Djian P, Doglio A, Pradines-Figuères A, Forest C, Gaillard D, Grimaldi P, Négrel R, Vannier C. Cellular and molecular aspects of adipose tissue growth. In: Bray G, Ricquier D, Spiegelman B, eds. Obesity: Towards a Molecular Approach. New York: Alan R Liss, 1990:844–856.

88. Poliard A, Nifuji A, Lamblin D, Plee E, Forest C, Kellermann O. Controlled conversion of an immortalized mesodermal progenitor cell towards osteogenic, chondrogenic or adipogenic pathways. J Cell Biol 1995; 130: 1461–1472.

89. Grigoriadis AE, Heersche JNM, Aubin JE. Differentiation of muscle, fat, cartilage, and bone from progenitor cells present in a bone-derived clonal cell population: effect of dexamethasone. J Cell Biol 1988; 106:2139–2151.

90. Konieczny SF, Emerson CP. 5-Azacytidine induction of stable mesodermal stem cell lineages from 10T1/2 cells: evidence for regulatory genes controlling determination. Cell 1984; 38:791–800.

91. Pietrangeli CE, Hayashi SI, Kinead PW. Stromal cell lines which support lymphocyte growth: characterization, sensitivity to radiation and responsiveness to growth factors. Eur J Immunol 1988; 18:863–872.

92. Anklesaria P, Klassen P, Sakakeeny MA, Fitzgerald TJ, Harrison D, Rybak ME, Greenberger JS. Biological characterization of cloned permanent stromal cell lines from anemic S1/S1d mice and +/+ littermates. Exp Hermatol 1987; 15:636–644.

93. Smas CM, Sul HS. Pref-1, a protein containing EGF-life repeats, inhibits adipocyte differentiation. Cell 1993; 73: 725–734.

94. Pilgrim C. DNA synthesis and differentiation in developing white adipose tissue. Dev Biol 1971; 26:69–76.

95. Cook JR, Kozak LP. sn-glycerol-3-phosphate dehydrogenase gene expression during mouse adipocyte development in vivo. Dev Biol 1982; 92:440–448.

96. Bouloumié A, Planat V, Devedjian JC, Valet P, Saulnier-Blache JS, Record M, Lafontan M. α2-Adrenergic stimulation promotes preadipocyte proliferation. Involvement of mitogen-activated protein kinases. J Biol Chem 1994; 269:30254–30259.

97. Nedergaard J, Herron D, Jacobsson A, Rehnmark S, Cannon B. Norepinephrine as a morphogen?: its unique interaction with brown adipose tissue. Int J Deve Biol 1995; 39:827–837.

98. MacDougald OA, Lane D. Transcriptional regulation of gene expression during adipocyte differentiation. Annu Rev Biochem 1995; 64:345–373.

99. Sale EM, Atkinson PG, Sale GJ. Requirement of MAP kinase for differentiation of fibroblasts to adipocytes, for insulin activation of p90 S6 kinase and for insulin or serum stimulation of DNA synthesis. EMBO J 1995; 14: 674–684.

100. Darimont C, Gaillard D, Ailaud G, Négrel R. Terminal differentiation of mouse preadipocyte cells: adipogenic and antimitogenic role of tri-iodothyronine. Mol Cell Endocrinol 1993; 98:67–73.

101. Safonova I, Darimont C, Amri E, Grimaldi P, Ailhaud G, Reichart U, Shroot B. Retinoids are positive effectors of adipose cell differentiation. Mol Cell Endocrinol 1994; 104:201–211.

102. Saye JA, Lynch KR, Peach MJ. Changes in angiotensinogen messenger RNA in differentiating 3T3-F442A adipocytes. Hypertension 1990; 15:867–871.

103. Darimont C, Vassaux G, Ailhaud G, Négrel R. Differentiation of preadipose cells: paracrine role of prostacyclin upon stimulation of adipose cells by angiotensin II. Endocrinology 1994; 135:2030–2036.

104. Darimont C, Vassaux G, Gaillard D, Ailhaud G, Négrel R. In situ microdialysis of prostaglandins in adipose tissue: stimulation of prostacyclin release by angiotensin II. Int J Obes 1994; 18:783–788.

105. Lazard D, Briend-Sutren MM, Villageois P, Mattei MG, Strosberg AD, Nahmias C. Molecular characterization and chromosome localization of a human angiotensin II AT2 receptor gene highly expressed in fetal tissues. Receptors Channels 1994; 2:271–280.

106. Harp JB, DiGirolamo M. Components of the renin-angiotensin system in adipose tissue: changes with maturation and adipose mass enlargement. J Gerontol. 1995; 50A:B270–B276.

107. Richardson RL, Hausman GJ, Gaskins HR. Effect of transforming growth factor-beta on insulin-like growth factor 1- and dexamethasone-induced proliferation and differentiation in primary cultures of pig preadiopocytes. Acta Anat 1992; 145:321–326.

108. Serrero G, Mills D. Physiological role of epidermal growth factor on adipose tissue development in vivo. Proc Natl Acad Sci USA 1991; 88:3912–3916.

109. Ninomiya-Tsuji J, Torti FM, Ringold GM. Tumor necrosis factor-induced c-myc expression in the absence of mitogenesis is associated with inhibition of adipocyte differentiation. Proc Natl Acad Sci USA 1993; 90:9611–9615.

110. Schoonjans K, Staels B, Auwerx J. Role of the peroxisome proliferator activated receptor (PPAR) in mediating the effects of fibrates and fatty acids on gene expression. J Lipid Res 1996; 37:907–925.

111. Tontonoz P, Hu E, Graves RA, Budavari AI, Spiegelman BM. mPPARγ_2: tissue-specific regulator of an adipocyte enhancer. Genes Dev 1994; 8:1224–1234.

112. Amri E, Bonino F, Ailhaud G, Abumrad NA, Grimaldi PA. Cloning of a protein that mediates transcriptional effects of fatty acids in preadipocytes. Homology to peroxisome proliferator-activated receptors. J Biol Chem 1995; 270: 2367–2371.

113. Kliewer SA, Forman BM, Blumberg B, Ong ES, Borgmeyer U, Mangelsdorf DJ, Umesono K, Evans RM. Differential expression and activation of a family of murine peroxisome proliferator-activated receptors. Proc Natl Acad Sci USA 1994; 91:7355–7359.

114. Tontonoz P, Hu E, Spiegelman BM. Stimulation of adipogenesis in fibroblasts by PPARγ_2, a lipid-activated transcription factor. Cell 1994; 79:1147–1156.

115. Kliewer SA, Lenhard JM, Willson TM, Patel I, Morris DC, Lehmann JM. A prostaglandin J_2 metabolite binds peroxisome proliferator-activated receptor γ and promotes adipocyte differentiation. Cell 1995; 83:813–819.

116. Forman BM, Tontonoz P, Chen J, Brun RP, Spiegelman BM, Evans RM. 15-Deoxy-$\Delta^{12,14}$-prostaglandin J_2 is a ligand for the adipocyte determination factor PPARγ. Cell 1995; 83:803–812.

117. Yu K, Bayona W, Kallen CB, Harding HP, Ravera, McMahon G, Brown M, Lazar MA. Differential activation of peroxisome proliferator-activated receptors by eicosanoids. J Biol Chem 1995; 270:23975–23983.

118. Teboul L, Gaillard D, Staccini L, Inadera H, Amri EZ, Grimaldi P. Thiazolidinediones and fatty acids convert myogenic cells into adipose-like cells. J Biol Chem 1995; 270:28183–28187.

119. Hu E, Tontonoz P, Spiegelman BM. Transdifferentiation of myoblasts by the adipogenic transcription factors PPARγ and C/EBPα. Proc Natl Acad Sci USA 1995; 92: 9856–9860.

17

Adipose Tissue as a Storage Organ

Peter Arner
Karolinska Institute and Huddinge Hospital, Huddinge, Sweden

Robert H. Eckel
University of Colorado Health Sciences Center, Denver, Colorado

I. INTRODUCTION

Adipose tissue is the body's largest energy reservoir. Energy is stored in fat cells as triacylglycerols (TG). The major source for adipocyte TG is circulating chylomicrons and very-low-density lipoproteins (VLDL) in which TG is hydrolyzed by lipoprotein lipase (LPL) located on the capillary walls of adipose tissue so that free fatty acids (FFA) and monoacylglycerol are formed. FFA are probably taken up by the fat cell through active transport; a specific FFA-transporting protein has been described (2). Once taken up by the fat cells, FFA are esterified to TG. The circulating albumin-bound FFA can also be taken up by the fat cells and be esterified to TG. During lipolysis, intracellular TG undergo hydrolysis through the action of another lipase, which is located inside the fat cell—hormone-sensitive lipase (HSL)—so that glycerol and FFA are formed. These products leave the fat cells and are transported by the bloodstream to other tissues (mainly liver for glycerol and liver plus muscle for FFA).

Some of the FFA that are formed during lipolysis do not, however, leave the fat cell. Instead they are reesterified to intracellular TG. They glycerol formed during lipolysis is not reutilized to a major extent because fat cells contain only minimal amounts of the enzyme glycerol kinase. In a normal weight man, about 100–300 g of TG is hydrolyzed and synthesized each 24 hr in the total fat depot (15). It is possible that slight alterations in this high turnover rate can be important for the development of obesity. This chapter reviews quantitative and regulatory aspects of lipid storage and mobilization in human adipose tissue. It is estimated that several thousand articles have been published relating in one way or another to adipose tissue metabolism. In light of space limitations, we will as often as possible cite reviews that cover a large number of major publications in the area.

II. LIPOGENESIS

The term "lipogenesis" has been used loosely and can indicate the incorporation of any TG precursor into complex lipids, e.g., TG, or, more specifically, the generation of acyl carbons from adipocyte-derived precursors, i.e., glucose. To distinguish these definitions in adipose tissue, examples of each are appropriate. When the incorporation of glucose into TG is measured, most of the glucose carbon in TG resides in the glycerol backbone, not acyl side chains. However, when ^3H_2O or ^{14}C acetate is employed, the isotopes are almost exclusively positioned in fatty acids. This latter scenario could also be entitled de novo lipogenesis. From this point, lipogenesis will represent this more conservative definition.

In humans, lipogenesis rarely occurs (48,66). The storage of fatty acids in the adipose organ is almost entirely dependent on the uptake of fatty acids released from circulating triglyceride-rich lipoproteins by LPL (46,52,116).

However, because patients with LPL deficiency do accumulate adipose tissue TG (20), other mechanisms including lipogenesis must be considered. The key enzymes that enhance lipogenesis include fatty acid synthase and acetyl CoA carboxylase. Although these enzymes are regulated by both glucose and insulin (42), even when glucose transport in adipose tissue is enhanced 10-fold, i.e., in transgenic mice with adipose tissue–specific overexpression of GLUT-4, a very small amount of the total glucose metabolized (1%) enters triglyceride fatty acids (115). Yet, in the absence of LPL, lipogenic enzyme induction must be greater and contribute to the maintenance of adipose tissue TG stores.

Alternative pathways by which adipose tissue TG stores are maintained have been insufficiently examined. One pathway is the adipsin/acylation stimulating protein system (ASP) described by Cianflone et al. (25). ASP is a plasma protein identical to the third component of complement known as C3adesArg. Adipocytes have the capability of synthesizing and secreting all three proteins necessary to form C3a, including adipsin (complement factor D), factor B, and C3 (23). Once generated, ASP can increase TG synthesis in fibroblasts, and in cultured human adipocytes as well (24). The most substantial effect of ASP appears to be an increase in the activity of diacylglycerol acyltransferase, which generates diglyceride from phosphatidate (121). Yet, the importance of ASP to TG synthesis in human physiology remains untested. Moreover, the availability of fatty acids must still be met by lipogenesis or uptake from the circulation.

Other possible mechanisms for the uptake of fatty acids from the circulation in the absence of LPL include albumin-bound FFA and/or the VLDL receptor. At present, the relative contribution of albumin-bound FFA in meeting adipocyte TG stores remains unclear. The VLDL receptor has a similar distribution as LPL but its function is unknown (27). Evidence to support a minimal role of this protein in physiology is the absence of a phenotype in transgenic mice with knockouts in the VLDL receptor (Hobbs, H., personal communication). In addition, in transgenic mice that lack LPL in adipose tissue but express it in skeletal muscle, the fatty acid composition of adipose tissue TG fatty acids is altered to indicate enhanced lipogenesis rather than uptake from the circulation (palmitate > linoleic acid) (Zechner, R., personal communication).

In summary, in the presence of LPL, fatty acids are generated from the hydrolysis of TG-rich lipoprotein TGs by LPL; when LPL is absent, the data support enhanced lipogenesis as the mechanism for their deposition.

III. LIPOLYSIS

A. Control of Hormone-Sensitive Lipase

During intracellular lipolysis, TG are broken down in a stepwise fashion via diacylglycerol (DG) and monoacylglycerol (MG) to form 3 moles of FFA and 1 mole of glycerol per mole of completely hydrolyzed TG. Under most conditions, TG are completely hydrolyzed, although up to 10% can be partly hydrolyzed to MG and DG in human fat cells (10). If no reesterification occurs, the molar ratio of FFA versus glycerol is 3:1. This ratio decreases when reesterification occurs. In addition, some FFA can be trapped in the intracellular water space of fat cells. Although the latter FFA pool can vary considerably during lipolysis (6), the changes are very small in comparison to the changes in FFA that are attributed to lipolysis and reesterification. The rate-limiting step for lipolysis is HSL. This enzyme catalyzes the hydrolysis of TG to DG and DG to MG. Finally, MG are hydrolyzed by a monoacylglycerol lipase. The latter enzyme is in abundance and is not regulated by hormones. On the other hand, HSL is subject to intense regulation.

HSL is activated by phosphorylation. The phosphorylation is regulated by the classic cyclic AMP pathway (Fig. 1). Hormones and other substances regulate the formation and breakdown of cyclic AMP. Cyclic AMP activates protein kinase A, which in turn stimulates the phosphorylation of HSL (111). Lipolysis is stimulated by hormones acting on cell-surface receptors coupled to adenylyl cyclase via so-called Gs proteins (30). This activates the cyclase, which stimulates the formation of cyclic AMP from ATP.

Lipolysis can be inhibited by cell surface receptors in two different ways. Some hormones and parahormones are coupled to adenylyl cyclase via so-called Gi proteins. This inhibits adenylyl cyclase so that less cyclic AMP is produced, leading to a decreased activation of protein kinase A and thereby decreased phosphorylation of HSL (30). Other hormones act through receptors that are linked to phosphadityl inositol kinase 3 (PIK-3). The most extensively investigated of the latter type of receptors is the insulin receptor (62,81,92). When insulin binds to its receptor, the receptor is activated by phosphorylation on tyrosine residues, which causes tyrosine phosphorylation on intracellular substrates such as insulin receptor substrate I (IRS-1). These tyrosine-phosphorylated substrates bind to a 85-kDa subunit of PIK-3 and thereby activate the catalytic subunit of the enzyme. Through yet undefined mechanisms, the signaling through PIK-3 activates an isoenzyme in the phophodiesterase family phosphodiesterase III (PDE III). The latter enzyme catalyses the break-

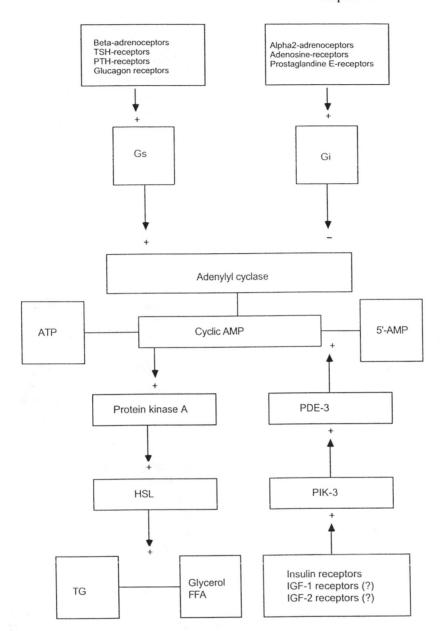

Figure 1 Receptor-mediated lipolysis in human fat cells. Gs, Gi = stimulatory or inhibitory GTP sensitive coupling protein; PDE = 3 = phosphodiesterase of type III; PIK-3 = phosphatidylinositol-3-kinase; HSL = hormone-sensitive lipase; TG = triacylglycerol; FFA = free fatty acid; IGF = insulin-like growth factor; + = stimulation; − = inhibition.

down of cyclic AMP to inactive 5'AMP, causing a decrease in the cyclic AMP level so that protein kinase A is inactivated and HSL is less phosphorylated causing less TG to be hydrolyzed. HSL is also dephosphorylated by phosphatases that are less well characterized.

A number of hormones and parahormones inhibit lipolysis in fat cells of most species. Insulin and, probably, insulin-like growth factor I (IGF-1) and II (IGF-2) inhibit

lipolysis through the PIK-3/PDE III pathway. Prostaglandins of the E type, adenosine, and neuropeptide Y act through Gi-coupled receptors. A number of hormones have pronounced lipolytic effects in adipocytes of laboratory animals, acting through Gs receptors. These include, for example vasopressin, secretin, glucagon, parathyroid hormone, TSH, and ACTH. In humans, however, these hormones are usually either ineffective or weak (glucagon, TSH, parathyroid hormone). The major lipolytic hormones in humans (and in most other species) are the catecholamines. Unlike all other hormones, they have a dual effect on lipolysis, which is stimulation through the Gs-coupled β-1-, β-2- and β-3-adrenoceptors and inhibition via Gs-coupled α-2 adrenoreceptors (61). There are marked species differences in the expression and function of these adrenoceptor subtypes. For example, in rodents β-3-receptors play a dominant role whereas in humans β-2 and α-2-adrenoceptors dominate (41,45). Thus, in humans the lipolytic effect of catecholamines is dependent on the balance between α- and β-adrenoceptors. Usually the lipolytic β-effect predominates.

B. Nonhormonal Control of HSL

When isolated fat cells or pieces of adipose tissue are incubated in vitro in the absence of hormones or other regulatory substances, there is a spontaneous release of glycerol and FFA into the incubation medium. It is also possible to enhance glycerol and FFA production in the absence of hormones by physical manipulation of fat cells (82). This nonhormonal process is usually referred to as basal lipolysis. The rate of basal lipolysis varies considerably between species but is high in human adipose tissue (0.5–1.5 μmol/g tissue pieces/hr). The mechanisms for maintenance of basal lipolysis are unknown, but a number of factors might be involved.

It is possible that adenylyl cyclase, which is the only known endogenous stimulator of cyclic AMP production, has a spontaneous activity. This could be because some Gs receptors are coupled to adenylyl cyclase even in the absence of hormone binding. It has been demonstrated that β-adrenoceptors can be coupled to and activate adenylyl cyclase in the absence of a receptor agonist (22). It could also be that HSL has a basal activity causing nonhormonal maintenance of the lipolysis rate. HSL has two phosphorylation sites; only one of these is subjected to hormonal regulation. The other site might be involved in maintenance of basal lipolysis.

Another possibility is that physical interactions occur between the fat droplet and HSL. It has been demonstrated in rat fat cells that the enzyme is translocated from the cytosol to the fat droplet following catecholamine stimulation (40). This translocation is believed to be important for lipolysis activation and seems to involve a docking protein called perilipin (47). However, some of the protein is attached to the lipid droplet even in the absence of hormones; this might maintain a spontaneous hydrolysis of TG in the fat droplet that is near the enzyme protein. It has been suggested that phosphatidylcholine at the surface of the lipid droplet modifies the activity of adjacent HSL molecules, thereby regulating lipolysis (82).

An interesting feature of basal lipolysis is its strong relationship with the fat cell size, in particular in human fat cell cells (15). Large fat cells, usually present in adipose tissue of obese subjects, have a much higher rate of lipolysis than small ones, which usually are obtained from nonobese subjects. Body-weight reduction is accompanied by a reduction in fat cell size and a concomitant decrease in the basal rate of lipolysis.

When humans are investigated in vivo after an overnight fast, a significant rate of lipolysis is observed (28). In vivo administration of high doses of insulin cannot decrease the rate of lipolysis in situ to zero (28). Local administration of β- plus α-adrenergic receptor antagonists in concentrations sufficient to obtain total adrenergic blockade does not abolish the resting lipolysis rate in situ when measured after an overnight fast with microdialysis (3). Taken together these data suggest that there is a nonhormonal regulation of the adipose tissue lipolysis also in vivo—at least in humans.

A potential regulator of basal lipolysis could be local adenosine production, as reviewed in Ref. 7. Adenosine has potent antilipolytic effects in human fat cells, and interstitial adenosine concentrations sufficiently high to cause an antilipolytic effect have been demonstrated in vivo in human adipose tissue (71). However, the physiological role of adenosine for human lipolysis is yet unclear. Furthermore, adenosine leaks out of human adipocytes only when they are artificially damaged (55).

IV. LIPOPROTEIN LIPASE

LPL is a secretory glycoprotein synthesized in a number of tissues including adipose tissue where it plays an important role in the provision of fatty acids for their uptake and storage as TG (33). Expression of LPL in adipose tissue occurs as an early marker of differentiation after preadipocytes are committed to differentiate into adipocytes (117). Following transcription and translation, LPL is progressively glycosylated and trimmed in the endoplasmic reticulum and Golgi apparatus where activation also occurs (107). LPL is then packaged into secretory vesicles from which secretion occurs. After secretion, the active lipase is transported to the capillary endothelium where it is bound to glycosaminoglycans and made available for the hydrolysis of circulating triglyceride-rich lipoproteins (chylomicrons and VLDL) (Fig. 2). Following activation by apolipoprotein CII and hydrolysis, the resultant lipolysis products, in particular FFA, can displace LPL from

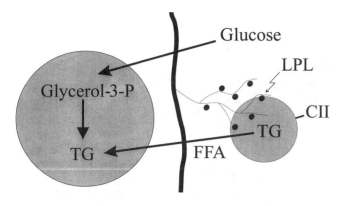

Figure 2 Transport of triglyceride lipoprotein triglyceride fatty acids (FFA) in adipose tissue. Lipoprotein lipase (LPL) is activated by apolipoprotein CII on chylomicrons and very-low-density lipoproteins. Triglycerides (TG) is formed from glucose-derived glycerol 3-P and FFA.

the endothelium where the enzyme can bind to lipoproteins and be transported back to the liver. In the liver, or perhaps other tissues, LPL bound to lipoproteins may facilitate the uptake of lipoproteins by cell surface receptors, i.e., the LDL receptor or the LDL receptor-related protein (LRP) (109).

A. Role and Regulation of LPL in Adipose Tissue:

As already mentioned above, LPL is important in the provision of fatty acids for TG storage in adipose tissue (32). Only in the absence of the enzyme do other pathways, i.e., lipogenesis, become relevant. LPL also has other roles. These include phospholipase and cholesteryl ester lipase activities that are minimal and of uncertain importance physiologically. In addition, the provision of fat-soluble vitamin esters and their uptake by adipose tissue may be facilitated by LPL (16).

Because LPL is made in a number of other tissues of the body, adipose tissue competes for lipoprotein TG fatty acids with other tissues to maintain its fatty acid availability and accumulation. It is therefore not surprising to discover that the regulation of LPL in adipose tissue is often divergent from that in skeletal muscle, another major organ wherein fatty acid uptake is important to the physiological role of the tissue.

1. Gender

Most studies have demonstrated higher levels of adipose tissue LPL in women than men (32). And, in women, adipose tissue LPL is higher in the femoral/gluteal subcutaneous region than in the abdominal wall (9,94,123).

At present, limited data exist to demonstrate different lipase activities in visceral versus subcutaneous adipose tissue (44,96).

2. Feeding

The ingestion of a meal increases adipose tissue LPL. This increase has been demonstrated in biopsies of adipose tissue (32), and in plasma effluents from adipose tissue (29). In general, when meals are high in carbohydrate the increase in adipose tissue LPL is higher than when the fat content is high (91). A similar effect of carbohydrate versus fat is seen after weeks of feeding (114); however, this difference is less well substantiated. The carbohydrate dependency of this response implicates a role for insulin in the regulation of the adipose tissue enzyme.

3. Insulin

As demonstrated by the euglycemic clamp technique (101), and human subcutaneous adipose tissue cultures (44), adipose tissue LPL is increased by insulin. Of interest, near-maximal stimulation is seen at serum insulin concentrations that are within the physiological range for humans (~35 µU/ml) (32). And, this regulation by insulin is similar between femoral/gluteal adipose tissue and the abdominal wall (124). In human omental adipose tissue organ cultures (44) or cultured isolated adipocytes (57), this effect of insulin is less apparent. In fact, in omental adipose tissue culture this stimulatory effect of insulin requires the presence of dexamethasone (44), while in cultured human adipocytes the concentration of insulin needed is quite high, suggesting that the IGF-1 receptor may be mediating the response (57). A partial explanation for these differences is the source of adipose tissue utilized for in vitro versus in vivo studies. In vitro studies typically use visceral adipose tissue whereas measurements of LPL that are carried out as part of the euglycemic clamp have employed subcutaneous adipose tissue. It is well appreciated that visceral adipose tissue is less responsive to insulin than subcutaneous adipose tissue.

4. Catecholamines

In tissue culture or in animals, catecholamines typically decrease adipose tissue LPL (31,32,84,93). Moreover, this effect may occur at the level of LPL gene transcription (84,93). However, only recently has the lack of a similar effect of isoproterenol infusions on adipose tissue LPL in humans been documented (35). This is particularly curious because LPL activity and mRNA in vastus lateralis muscle are increased by isoproterenol (35). The differences in response between humans and animals are particularly interesting when one considers that catecholamines stimulate lipolysis in animals and humans. An explanation for these differences remains to be provided.

5. Exercise/Training

Following exercise in humans, adipose tissue LPL is increased (79,102). This change presumably relates to the amount of TG depletion that occurred during the previous exercise period. In trained individuals, LPL in adipose tissue is lower or unchanged (63,104,108) while LPL in skeletal muscle is higher (104,108). When detrained, subjects experience an increase in the adipose tissue and decrease in the skeletal muscle enzyme (108). This may reflect degrees of catecholaminergic tone in tissues that relate to training/detraining. A seasonal component, related or unrelated to training, has also been suggested (88).

6. Growth Hormone

Growth hormone is lipolytic, and therefore it is not surprising that acromegaly (106) or growth hormone infusions (85) decrease adipose tissue LPL in humans. Of interest, however, IGF-1 increases LPL in cultured isolated human adipocytes (57). In vivo, however, despite the regulatory relationship between growth hormone and IGF-1, the role of growth hormone at the adipose tissue level appears to dominate.

7. Tumor Necrosis Factor-α (TNF-α)

The discovery of TNF-α (cachectin) related to the ability of the cytokine to inhibit LPL in cultured 3T3-L1 cells (56). This effect is now known to occur, at least in part, at the level of LPL gene transcription (78,127). However, only recently has adipose tissue been identified as a source of TNF-α, and has it been recognized that local production of the cytokine can contribute to insulin resistance in tissues (49). Moreover, when adipose tissue LPL was related to adipose tissue TNF-α mRNA, an inverse relationship was found (59). However, despite reciprocal changes in adipose tissue LPL and TNF-α mRNA with weight reduction, there was no relationship between the magnitude of change of these two variables (59). The physiological and pathophysiological role of TNF-α in adipose tissue in vivo remains to be determined.

8. Steroids

The effect of steroids on adipose tissue LPL is dependent on the type of steroid. When used in adipose tissue organ cultures in vitro, glucocorticoids increase LPL by either decreasing the degradation of the active lipase (4), and/or increasing its synthesis (86). Women with Cushing's syndrome have increases in abdominal subcutaneous adipose tissue LPL (95). Of interest, the number of glucocorticoid receptors in visceral adipose tissue is four times that in the subcutaneous region (87).

Estrogens and estrogen levels appear to be associated with a decrease in LPL activity in gluteal subcutaneous adipose tissue (51). This effect is of interest when one considers the important role of estrogens in controlling the distribution of subcutaneous adipose tissue. The recent identification of estrogen receptors in human adopose tissue (77) renders this effect open to more intense investigation. The effect of androgens on adipose tissue LPL also appears region-dependent. Men treated with testosterone, but not dihydrotesterone, had decreases in adipose tissue LPL in the abdominal but not the femoral adipose tissue depot (73,97). Because the change in LPL following testosterone, administration related to the change in incorporation of radioactive trioleate into adipose tissue, a more rapid turnover of TG in the abdominal than femoral region was suggested. Because testosterone but not dihydrotestosterone altered the lipase, aromitization of testosterone to estradiol may be important in generation of this effect. Recent unpublished data also suggest such an effect (Iverius, P., personal communication).

V.   ADIPOSE TISSUE METABOLISM IN LEAN AND OBESE PERSONS

A.   Lipolysis

Most studies on TG turnover in fat cells in the obese state have focused on lipolysis. It is well established that the circulating FFA levels are increased in obese subjects. Furthermore, isotopic turnover studies performed after an overnight fast show an increase in the overall rate of lipolysis in vivo in obesity. However, when the rate is related to the total fat mass, obese subjects have normal or even decreased rates of lipolysis after an overnight fast (28). The latter is in consonance with recent direct in vivo studies of lipolysis after an overnight fast in subcutaneous adipose tissue. With the aid of microdialysis it was observed that, under these conditions, the rate of lipolysis per tissue weight was normal in the obese state (53). Thus, increased overall rates of "basal" lipolysis in vivo causing elevated circulating FFA level in the obese might just be a mass effect due to the enlargement of the body fat. The basal rate of lipolysis in vitro is also increased in adipose tissue of obese subjects, which probably reflects the enlargement of fat cell size in obesity. When, however, the increase in fat cell size is accounted for, the differences in basal rate of lipolysis in vitro between lean and obese subjects disappear (5).

It is frequently observed that the hormonal regulation of lipolysis—in particular the action of catecholamines—is impaired in obesity. A number of in vivo studies have shown blunted catecholamine-induced lipolysis in obese subjects (28). The same is true for in vitro studies when the subcutaneous adipose tissue has been investigated. This depot constitutes about 80% of the total fat mass. The molecular mechanisms behind in vitro lipolytic catecholamine resistance are partly elucidated. In simple obesity it seems to be caused by decreased expression and function of β-$_2$-adrenoceptors and increased function of α-$_2$-adrenoceptors (75,99). When obesity is accompanied by insulin resistance, the lipolytic catecholamine resistance in subcutaneous fat cells is further enhanced owing to an additional defect in the ability of cyclic AMP to activate lipolysis (98). The human data with catecholamines are in close harmony with those obtained using animal models. Thus, catecholamine-induced lipolysis in dogs and rodents is decreased in obesity (61).

It is less clear to what extent insulin action on lipolysis is altered in obesity. This might be due to difficulties in obtaining reproducible experimental conditions when inhibition of lipolysis is measured. For lipolysis in vitro, insulin, adenosine, and prostaglandins have complex interactions with catecholamines. The rate of lipolysis is critically dependent on the prevailing concentration of insulin and catecholamine at the adipocyte level. Usually, antilipolysis in vitro is determined in the absence of catecholamines or in the presence of a fixed concentration of catecholamines. It is probably necessary to use a number of combinations of catecholamine-insulin concentrations to get a clear picture of antilipolysis. Consequently, increased, decreased, or normal antilipolytic actions of insulin have been demonstrated in fat cells obtained from obese subjects (5). Also, in vivo data on antilipolysis are conflicting, showing normal or decreased antilipolytic action of insulin in the obese state (5,28). This is in marked contrast to the findings with insulin action on glucose transport in fat cells or glucose uptake by adipose tissue, invariably showing insulin resistance in obese subjects (21). Preservation or only partial reduction of the antilipolytic effect of insulin could be of importance for maintenance or acceleration of obesity in overweight subjects who are resistant to other actions of insulin such as those on glucose metabolism and LPL (see below) as discussed in detail (Ref. 5). Other antilipolytic mechanisms may also be involved in obesity, e.g., decreased antilipolytic actions

of prostaglandins and adenosine observed in subcutaneous fat cells of obese subjects (7). The latter data should, however, be interpreted with caution because the complex interactions between adenosine and prostaglandins, on the one hand, and catecholamines, on the other hand, were not evaluated.

Whether adipocyte reesterification is altered in obesity is unknown at present. This process is difficult to study in small biopsy samples and has not been examined in detail in humans so far.

B. Lipogenesis

Limited reports exist to demonstrate that glucose incorporation into acylglycerides is increased in human adipose tissue from obese subjects. The capacity of fat cells to synthesize lipids is enhanced in vitro in obesity, which as least in part can be explained by the increase in fat cell size. However, Edens et al. (39) demonstrated lower rates of ^{14}C glucose incorporation into acylglyceride in intraabdominal than subcutaneous adipose tissue, but comparison to lean subjects was not reported. They went on to suggest that this process may help to limit adipocyte size within the visceral depot. The mechanisms behind this increase are unknown. In human adipose tissue, Belfiore et al. (12) reported that the activity of ATP citrate lyase, but not that of malate dehydrogenase, was increased in obese compared to normal weight controls. This discrepancy in relative enzyme activities suggests that the change in lipogenesis is at most of moderate degree, affecting the most rate-limiting step, ATP citrate lyase (the enzyme responsible for the generation of acetyl CoA from citrate in the cytosol). Of potential interest is the recent discovery that TG synthesis in fat cells can be stimulated by ASP. This protein is increased in adipose tissue of obese subjects (110).

C. Lipoprotein Lipase

The literature is more than sufficient to document that activities of adipose tissue LPL are increased in obese subjects (32). In general, the quantity of heparin-releasable adipose tissue LPL relates to BMI and adipocyte size. Here, the manner in which the data are presented is important. If LPL activity is expressed per gram of adipose tissue, increases may not be seen. However, when LPL activity is expressed per adipocyte, increases are typical. A defense of the latter relates to the adipocyte as the source of the lipase. Despite the increases in adipose tissue LPL activity, steady-state levels of LPL mRNA are not increased (83). These differences suggest that the differences in activity between normal weight and obese subjects can be explained by posttranslational differences in processing of the enzyme.

The regulation of adipose tissue by insulin and meals in obese subjects, however, parallels the insulin resistance seen for other actions of insulin. Using the euglycemic clamp technique, near-maximal adipose tissue LPL responses are seen in normal-weight subjects at steady-state insulin concentrations of ~35 μU/ml whereas in obese subjects, the insulin dose-response curve is shifted to the right, with concentrations of ~100 μU/ml required for maximal responsiveness (32). In general, there is a relationship between the responsiveness of the adipose tissue enzyme and the amount of glucose required to maintain euglycemia (38), supporting the lipase response as being another manifestation of insulin resistance. A similar lack of adipose tissue LPL responsiveness to a high-carbohydrate meal has also been demonstrated (36). Overall, this deficiency of LPL responsiveness to meals and insulin may be an adaptive mechanism in the attempt to limit additional TG deposition (34). Currently being examined is whether or not relative insulin sensitivity in normal-weight and obese subjects predicts weight (and adipose mass) stability versus increases in body fat.

VI. ADIPOSE TISSUE METABOLISM AS A CAUSE OR CONSEQUENCE OF OBESITY

A. Lipolysis

It is necessary for our understanding of the pathogenesis of obesity to find out whether metabolic abnormalities observed in adipose tissue of obese subjects are primary or secondary phenomenon. One way to address this uncertainty is to study obese subjects before and after weight reduction, when the body weight is at a new steady state.

Relatively few studies have been published on weight-reduced obese subjects. A reduction of body weight to a level still considered as overweight is accompanied by a decreased basal rate of lipolysis and improved catecholamine-induced lipolysis in vitro (5). These data suggest that the abnormalities in basal and catecholamine-induced lipolysis at least in part are secondary phenomena. Further indirect support for this assumption are the studies in *ob/ob* mice. Fat cells from these mice are catecholamine-resistant due to alteration in G-protein-mediated signaling pathways (11). However, the monogenic defect causing obesity in these mice is caused by alterations of a specific protein that is not a part of G-protein signaling (128).

Much less is known about primary or secondary defects in insulin action. Antilipolysis appears not to be

studied in this respect yet. Insulin-induced glucose metabolism of human adipocytes is not changed when obese subjects are investigated before and after weight reduction (126). An intriguing possibility is that the insulin resistance of adipose tissue is caused by other fat-specific factors that regulate adipocyte insulin action. Again, studies in rodents and humans suggest that adipocytes produce TNF-α, which interferes with the insulin receptor signaling causing inhibited insulin action (50). The production of this cytokine is increased in fat cells of obese rodents (50) and adipose tissue from obese humans (49,59). In rodents, increased TNF-α causes a further inhibition of insulin action (50). Thus, in obesity the insulin resistance of adipose tissue (and maybe of other tissues as well) could be caused by local production of fat specific factors such as TNF-α.

In theory, primary defects in reesterification might be present in adipose tissue of certain individuals. Approximately 50% of newly hydrolyzed FFA are reesterified in subcutaneous adipose tissue of obese weight-stable individuals; during weight reduction this proportion drops to 10% (65). The role of reesterification for obesity cannot, however, be determined until further studies on normal-weight and postobese weight-stable subjects are performed.

B. Lipogenesis

Few data address the impact of weight reduction on glucose incorporation into acylglycerides in adipose tissue from human subjects. Moreover, the reports that exist are conflicting. In one study, the incorporation of acetate into total lipids was decreased by 40%, but measurements were taken 5 days into a fast (89). In a classic study by Bray (19), two small groups of severely obese subjects were studied, one male and during weight maintenance, the second female and during weight regain after marked weight reduction. When compared to the first group, women undergoing active weight regain had increases in basal lipogenesis, and for "nibblers" increases in insulin-stimulated lipogenesis. Of interest, even in the weight gain environment, <5% of glucose carbon was directed to acylglycerides. Overall, these studies are insufficient to make any conclusions on the role of increased lipogenesis in the production of obesity or weight regain following weight reduction.

C. Lipoprotein Lipase

Much more data are available to support a role of adipose tissue LPL overexpression in the recidivism of the obese state. Schwartz and Brunzell (103) were the first to report increases in adipose tissue LPL activity in fasted weight-maintaining reduced-obese subjects. In a more recent report by Kern et al. (58), this increase in adipose tissue LPL activity was paralleled by increases in LPL mass and mRNA. It is important to stress weight maintenance because measurements of adipose tissue LPL in hypocaloric subjects are decreased rather than increased or unchanged (32).

In several studies, adipose tissue LPL was not increased following isocaloric maintenance of the reduced obese state, but the responsiveness of the enzyme to insulin (36) (Fig. 3) or high-fat meals (122) was sufficiently altered to predict an adipose tissue environment capable of enhanced lipid uptake and storage. The concomitant decreases in skeletal muscle LPL would further favor such a partitioning (37). A plethora of rodent data supports this pathophysiology (13,26). Still unclear, however, is whether or not alterations in the expression of adipose tissue or skeletal muscle LPL and the responsiveness of the enzyme to nutrients predict the development of obesity. It also remains controversial as to whether the reduced obese state reflects the metabolic environment that predicts obesity in the never obese.

Recently, evidence suggests that the LPL gene may predict responses to overfeeding, acute exercise, or exercise training. RFLPs at the BamHI and PvuII sites related to the response of adipose tissue LPL to chronic perturbations (18). In twin studies, not only was the level of subcutaneous adipose tissue LPL measured in suprailiac biopsies characterized by a significant heritable level (90), but the response to short-term overfeeding (17) and an acute and strenuous bout of exercise was greater in monozygotic than dizygotic twin pairs (102). Moreover, in separate studies, the HindIII RFLP for the LPL gene has been associated with hypertriglyceridemia in subjects with visceral obesity (119). Finally, following suction lipectomy, the amount of LPL activity in a nonlipectomized adipose tissue control site predicted whether or not adipose tissue expansion would occur in the control site up to 18 months after liposuction (125). Overall, these data support the importance of LPL in regulating the adipose tissue mass and, potentially, the related metabolic sequelae of obesity in humans.

Because of the limited data on the effect of body weight reduction on metabolism in adipose tissue of reduced obese subjects, it is hard to draw any firm conclusions about the primary and secondary metabolic changes. More investigations are needed, such as family studies, longitudinal studies, and investigations on obese subjects after complete normalization of body weight.

Obesity is age-dependent, most subjects increasing their fat stores when they become older. Basal and cate-

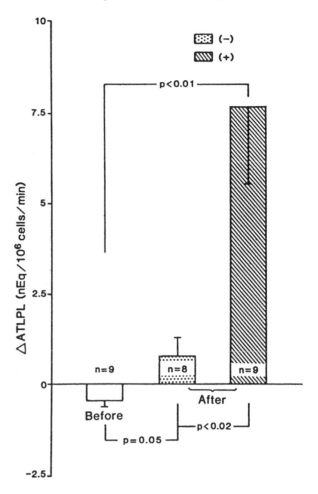

Figure 3 Adipose tissue lipoprotein lipase (ATLPL) responsiveness to insulin: effect of weight reduction plus or minus stabilization. The change (Δ) in gluteal ATLPL after 6 hr of insulin infusion (40 mU m^{-2} min) and maintenance of fasting euglycemia with a variable glucose infusion is shown before weight loss (open bar), immediately after weight loss (stippled bar), and after weight loss with 3 months of isocaloric stabilization (hatched bar). Paired analysis of ATLPL immediately after weight loss with initial ATLPL and that obtained after weight loss plus 3 months of isocaloric weight stabilization was carried out in eight of nine subjects. Comparisons of ATLPL before and after weight loss plus stabilization were performed in all nine subjects.

cholamine-induced lipolysis in vivo and in vitro are decreased in normal-weight old versus young subjects (69). An age-dependent inhibition of HSL function may cause this change (69). In addition, insulin-induced antilipolysis and glucose metabolism (100) and LPL (118) are lower in adipose tissue of elderly as compared to young nonobese subjects. Thus, some of the changes observed in the action of catecholamines and insulin on adipose tissue of elderly obese subjects may only reflect the physiologies of normal aging.

VII. ADIPOSE TISSUE METABOLISM AND FAT TOPOGRAPHY

A. Lipolysis

It is well known that body fat distribution differs between normal-weight men and women favoring a peripheral distribution in women and a central one in men. Also, in obesity the distribution of body fat is subject to variation. Some subjects have central (abdominal) obesity while others have a peripheral type of obesity. The latter form is common among women and the former among men. A number of epidemiological studies suggest that abdominal but not peripheral obesity has strong associations with metabolic and cardiovascular complications (60). The enlargement of the inner visceral fat depot appears to be the major factor contributing to increased metabolic cardiovascular morbidity in abdominal obese subjects (1,60,67). It has been speculated that visceral fat is dangerous because portal FFA derived from the enlarged visceral fat mass can cause a number of metabolic disturbances in the liver (Table 1) leading to hypertriglyceridemia, hyperinsulinemia, insulin resistance, and hyperglycemia/glucose intolerance (14,43). These are typical features for the metabolic (insulin resistance) syndrome, a cornerstone of which is abdominal obesity. However, it is possible that changes in metabolism of adipose tissue in combination with enlargement of certain fat depots play a role in the metabolic complications of abdominal obesity.

The abnormalities in lipolysis regulation discussed previously are more readily observed in abdominal obesity than in other forms of obesity (1,60). Thus, greater resistance to the lipolytic effect of catecholamines and the antilipolytic effect of insulin is found in subjects with ab-

Table 1 Possible Consequences for the Liver of Elevated Portal Free Fatty Acids

Event	Mechanism
Hyperglycemia	Increased stimulation of gluconeogenesis by fatty acids
Hyperinsulinemia	Decreased insulin degradation
Insulin resistance	Inhibited insulin receptor binding and intracellular signaling
Hypertriglyceridemia	Stimulated lipoprotein production because of increased availability of substrate

dominal as compared to peripheral obesity (28). It is possible that this link between abnormal in vivo regulation of lipolysis and upper body obesity is caused by regional variations in lipolysis regulation.

Site differences in lipolysis regulation are frequently demonstrated in vitro and in vivo even in normal-weight subjects (64). Lipolysis is less marked in the gluteal/femoral as compared to abdominal subcutaneous adipose tissue. Catecholamines are less lipolytic in the former than the latter region, owing to increased α_2-adrenoceptor function and decreased β-adrenoceptor expression in the gluteal/femoral fat cells (64). The site differences are more marked in women than in men, which may explain why women have more fat in the peripheral sites than men. There are also regional differences in both visceral and subcutaneous adipose tissue in normal-weight subjects (8). They also occur in adipose tissue of laboratory animals. In humans, lipolysis is more marked in the former region owing to increased lipolytic activity of catecholamines and decreased antilipolytic activity of insulin, prostaglandins, and adenosine in the former region. The mechanisms behind these regional differences are known in some detail (Table 2) and are localized at the level of expression and function of agonist receptors.

In upper-body obesity the regional variations in lipolysis between visceral and subcutaneous fat cells are further increased (Fig. 4). Catecholamine resistance is observed in subcutaneous abdominal fat cells, which seems to be caused by multiple changes in the lipolysis cascade, i.e., decreased β_2-adrenoceptor expression, increased function of α_2-adrenoceptors, and decreased function of HSL (75,98,99). In visceral fat, on the other hand, catecholamine action is increased owing to an increased β_3-receptor function and decreased α_2-adrenoceptor function (70). These findings taken together suggest that catecholamine-induced lipolysis is decreased in subcutaneous fat but increased in visceral fat following catecholamine stimulation. This would cause a marked increased in portal FFA in relation to peripheral venous FFA and could thus be a mechanism responsible for the hepatic insulin resistance in abdominal obesity. It should, however, be borne in mind that this speculation is based entirely on in vitro observations. Unfortunately, for ethical reasons it is not possible to directly study portal FFA flux in vivo in humans. Furthermore, it is not clear if the regional variations in antilipolytic hormones/parahormones in normal-weight subjects are further changed in abdominal obesity. The regional differences in the antilipolytic effect of insulin have not been examined so far. However, this hormone caused a much more marked inhibition of lipolysis in subcutaneous as compared to visceral adipocytes of massively obese women (76).

Table 2 Mechanisms for Regional Variations in Lipolysis Between Visceral and Subcutaneous Adipocytes

Hormone/parahormone	Action on lipolysis in the visceral region	Mechanism
Catecholamines	Increased	1. Increased expression/function of beta$_1$-, beta$_2$-, and beta$_3$-adrenoceptors 2. Decreased expression of alpha$_2$-adrenoceptors
Insulin	Decreased	1. Decreased receptor affinity 2. Decreased postreceptor signaling
Adenosine	Decreased	Decreased receptor expression
Prostaglandin-E	Decreased	Decreased receptor expression

B. Lipogenesis

At present, few studies of the comparative rates of lipogenesis or lipogenic enzyme activities between adipose tissue depots have been published. In the study of Edens et al. (39), intra-abdominal adipose tissue from both severely obese men and women accumulated 50% less ^{14}C-glucose into ^{14}C-acylglyceride than subcutaneous adipose tissue. Similar data were reported by Maslowska et al. (74).

C. Lipoprotein Lipase

In normal-weight subjects, gender-based differences in adipose tissue LPL have been found between adipose tissue

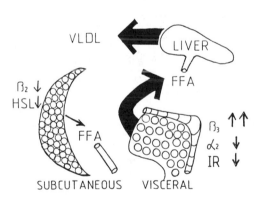

Figure 4 Altered adipocyte lipolysis in upper-body obesity. Catecholamine-induced lipolysis is blunted in subcutaneous fat cells owing to decreased β$_2$-adrenoceptor expression and impaired function of hormone-sensitive lipase (HSL) but improved in visceral fat cells due to increased function of β$_3$-adrenoceptors and decreased function of α$_2$-adrenoceptor and insulin receptors. This causes a relative redistribution of mobilization of free fatty acids (FFA) favoring direct delivery to the liver by the portal system. As a consequence liver function is altered leading among other things to increased production of very low density lipoproteins (VLDL).

regions. In men, adipose tissue LPL activity is higher in the abdominal wall than in the gluteal/femoral region (9); in women, the opposite is found (9,94,12). In general, these differences relate to rates of uptake of orally administered FA (73). In subcutaneous sites of normal weight women, however, the regulation of adipose tissue LPL by insulin is similar between depots (123). In obese women (63,123) and men (73), fasting adipose tissue LPL activities were not different between the abdominal wall and gluteal regions, and the regulation of the enzyme by insulin (123) and exercise (63) was also similar.

Again, when studied ex vivo in organ culture, the insulin stimulatory effect on LPL was less in omental than in subcutaneous adipose tissue pieces (44). Dexamethasone, however, increased the activity and mRNA in omental, but not subcutaneous pieces. When added together, the effect of insulin and dexamethasone was greater in omental than subcutaneous adipose tissue. How these effects relate to in vivo expression and regulation of the enzyme and lipid balance in adipose tissue regions remains untested.

VIII. GENETIC AND MOLECULAR BIOLOGY ADVANCES

With the recent advances in molecular biology technology it is possible to study the function of regulatory proteins by reconstitution experiments in dividing cell lines and transgenic or knockout experiments in living animals. In addition, techniques are available to specifically inhibit regulatory genes in nondividing cells. These techniques have recently been introduced in the investigations on the regulation of fat cell metabolism. For example, transgenic approaches have been used to selectively overexpress the glucose transporter protein GLUT4 in adipocytes (105) and to disrupt the adipocyte β$_3$-adrenoceptor gene in mice (112). Moderate degrees of obesity are seen in these two transgenic models. Overexpression of HSL in a preadipocyte cell line prevents differentiated adipocytes from taking on the appearance of fat cells, i.e., accumulating TG (113). The value of adipose tissue-specific overexpression of HSL in transgenic animals or following gene therapy is under study by several groups, but at present an associated phenotype in these animals has yet to be reported. The further study of the many factors that either enhance, e.g., insulin, IGF-1, FA and other peroxisomal enhancers, glucocorticoids, thiazolidinediones, and TGF-β, or prevent, e.g., prostaglandins, cytokines, and endothelin-1, adipocyte differentiation may yield important and new strategies to limit the adipose tissue mass in children and/or more severe obesity in adults (117). In addition, better understanding of the process of differentiation, including adipose tissue-specific enhancers and the transcription factors that orchestrate preadipocyte differentiation, should be similarly productive.

An alternative approach is to study how tissue-specific expression of genes that relate to the adipose mass are regulated, and how over- or underexpression of these genes in adipose tissue or alternative tissues controls fuel partitioning and phenotype. Here, strain differences may be important. An example is the overexpression of LPL in skeletal muscle, which in C57B1/CBA mice produces leanness and even death when the overexpression is zealous (68). However, in FVB mice only moderate leanness with moderate overexpression and even obesity in high overexpressors results (54). Although these differences are likely strain-related, they do indicate that in at least FVB mice compensatory mechanisms exist to prevent adipose tissue loss when lipoprotein lipid fuels are diverted away from the adipose organ. Another example of a gene that is important to lipid metabolism and has tissue-specific regulation is acetyl CoA carboxylase. This gene has two promoters (PI and PII), which are differentially regulated in the liver and adipose tissue. Under normal conditions, only PI is operational in adipose tissue and PII in liver (72). In Wistar rats, starvation leads to a marked decrease in gene expression from both promoters, whereas high-fat diets induce the activity of both PI and PII in the liver, but only PI in adipose tissue. In Zucker obese rats, the major increase in lipogenesis is from the liver with the overexpression of the carboxylase coming from the PI promoter. By selectively altering the expression of the PI promoter, a strategy could be developed that not only limits the small amount of additional TG fatty acids in adipose tissue, but more important, decreases the substrate delivery to adipose tissue from hepatically produced VLDL. The ultimate impact on the phenotype has yet to be examined.

Another area of potential importance for our understanding of adipose tissue metabolism is the search for natural gene mutations. Using modern molecular genetic methods it is now possible to screen for point mutations and other mutations in so-called candidate genes or to scan the whole genome looking for mutations in genes with yet unknown function. For adipose tissue specific genes, candidate gene mutations have so far only been observed in or near the β_3-adrenoceptor, TNF-α and LPL. A missence mutation in codon 64 of the gene for the β_3-adrenergic receptor that leads to the replacement of tryptophan by arginine in the receptor protein has been published. However, the frequency of the mutation is not increased in obese subjects but is associated with an increased capacity to gain weight in severely obese subjects (27) and/or an earlier onset of non-insulin-dependent diabetes mellitus (120). As already mentioned, an LPL gene HindIII polymorphism is described that associates with dyslipidemia in upper-body-obese subjects (119). A linkage between obesity and polymorphisms near TNF-α is observed in Pima Indians (80). The possible importance of these genetic variations for adipose tissue function remains, however, to be established; at present, no direct studies on fat cells having the altered genotype have been published.

IX. SUMMARY

TG, which are stored in adipocytes in adipose tissue, are the body's major source of energy. The turnover of TG in fat cells is rapid and mainly regulated by two lipases. LPL, which is located on the capillary walls of adipose tissue, controls the uptake of circulating TG by adipocytes whereas the intracellularly located hormone sensitive lipase (HSL) controls the hydrolysis (lipolysis) of adipocyte TG. Among hormones, only insulin and catecholamines have pronounced metabolic effects on human adipose tissue metabolism. Insulin stimulates LPL and inhibits HLS; the opposite is true for catecholamines. In addition, a paracine regulation of these enzymes occurs, involving adenosine, prostaglandin E, TNF-α, and acylation-stimulating protein. There are regional variations in adiopcyte turnover of TG favoring lipid mobilization in the visceral fat depots and lipid storage in the peripheral subcutaneous sites. These site variations can at least in part be explained by regional variations in the action of hormones and parahormones. The hormonal regulation of adipocyte turnover of TG is altered in obesity; this is most marked in upper-body obesity. There is resistance to insulin stimulation of LPL; however, LPL activity in fasted obese subjects is increased and remains so following weight reduction. Whether the antilipolytic effect of insulin is altered or not is unclear at present. Catecholamine-induced lipolysis is enhanced in visceral fat but decreased in subcutaneous fat. The latter may cause a redistribution of lipid mobilization in upper-body obesity favoring release of lipids to the portal system, which exclusively drains the visceral fat depot. A high flux of portal lipids can disturb liver function and in part cause several of the metabolic complications to upper-body obesity. Overall, despite the remarkable knowledge that exists about adipose tissue as a storage organ, the molecular age has produced the need for a more in-depth and basic understanding that will explain why energy storage differs so widely.

REFERENCES

1. Abate N, Garg A. Heterogeneity in adipose tissue metabolism: causes, implications and management of regional adiposity. Prog Lipid Res 1995; 34:53–70.
2. Abumrad NA, Melki, SA, Harmon CM. Transport of fatty acid in isolated rat adipocyte and in differentiating preadipose cells. Biochem Soc Trans 1991; 18:1130–1132.
3. Andersson K, Arner P. Cholinoceptor-mediated effects on glycerol output from human adipose tissue using in situ microdialysis. Br J Pharmacol 1995; 115:1155–1162.
4. Appel B, Fried SK. Effects of insulin and dexamethasone on lipoprotein lipase in human adipose tissue. Am J Physiol 1992; 262:E695–E699.
5. Arner P. Control of lipolysis and its relevance to development of obesity in man. Diabetes Metab Rev 1988; 4: 507–515.
6. Arner P. Metabolism of fatty acids: An overview. In: Bray GA, Ricquier D, Spiegelman BM, eds. Obesity: Towards a Molecular Approach. New York: Wiley-Liss, 1990: 159–172.
7. Arner P. Adenosine, prostaglandins and phosphodiesterase as targets for obesity pharmacotherapy. Int J Obes 1993; 17:S57–S59.
8. Aner P. Differences in lipolysis between human subcutaneous and omental adipose tissues. Ann Med 1995; 27: 435–438.
9. Arner P, Lithell H, Wahrenberg H, Bronnegard M. Expression of lipoprotein lipase in different human subcutaneous adipose tissue regions. J Lipid Res 1991; 32: 423–429.
10. Arner P, Östman J. Mono- and diacylglycerol in human adipose tissue. Biochim Biophys Acta 1974; 369: 209–221.
11. Begin-Heick N. Quantification of the α and β subunits of the tranducing elements (G_s and G_i) of adenylate cyclase in adipocyte membranes from lean and obese (*ob/ob*) mice. Biochem J 1990; 268:83–89.
12. Belfiore F, Borzi V, Napoli E, Rabuazzo AM. Enzymes related to lipogenesis in the adipose tissue of obese subjects. Metabolism 1976; 25:483–493.
13. Bessesen DH, Robertson AD, Eckel RH. Weight reduction increases adipose but decreases cardiac LPL in reduced-obese Zucker rats. Am J Physiol 1991; 261:E246–E251.
14. Björntorp P. Fatty acids, hyperinsulinemia and insulin resistance: which comes first? Curr Opin Lipidol 1994; 5: 166–174.
15. Björntorp P, Östman J. Human adipose tissue dynamics and regulation. Adv Metab Disord 1971; 5:277–327.
16. Blaner WS, Obunike JC, Kurlandsky SB, al-Haideri M, Piantedosi R, Deckelbaum RJ, Goldberg IJ. Lipoprotein lipase hydrolysis of retinyl ester. Possible implications for retinoid uptake by cells. J Biol Chem 1994; 269: 16559–16565.
17. Bouchard C. Inheritance of human fat distribution and adipose tissue metabolism. In: Vague J, Björntorp P, Guy-Grand B, Rebuffe-Scrive M, Vague P, eds. Metabolic Complications of Human Obesities. Amsterdam: Elsevier, 1985.
18. Bouchard C, Despres JP, Mauriege P, Marcotte M, Chagnon M, Dionne FT, Belanger A. The genes in the constellation of determinants of regional fat distribution. Int J Obes 1991; 15:9–18.
19. Bray GA. Lipogenesis in human adipose tissue: Some effects of nibbling and gorging. J Clin Invest 1972; 51: 537–548.
20. Brun LD, Gagne C, Julien P, Tremblay A, Moorjani S, Bouchard C, Lupien PJ. Familial lipoprotein lipase-activity deficiency: study of total body fatness and subcutaneous fat tissue distribution. Metabolism 1989; 38:1005–1009.
21. Caro JF, Dohm LG, Pories WJ, Sinha MK. Cellular alterations in liver, skeletal muscle and adipose tissue responsible for insulin resistance in obesity and type II diabetes. Diabetes Metab Rev 1989; 5:665–689.
22. Chidiac P, Hebert TE, Valiquette M, Dennis M, Bouvier M. Inverse agonist activity of β-adrenergic antagonists. Pharmacol Exp Ther 1993; 45:490–499.
23. Choy LN, Rosen BS, Spiegelman BM. Adipsin and an endogenous pathway of complement from adipose cells. J Biol Chem 1992; 267:12736–12741.
24. Cianflone K, Roncari DAK, Maslowska M, Baldo A, Forden J, Sniderman AD. Adipsin/acylation stimulating protein system in human adipocytes: regulation of triacylglycerol synthesis. Biochemistry 1994; 33:9489–9495.
25. Cianflone K, Sniderman A, Walsh M, Vu H, Gagnon J, Rodriguez M. Purification and characterization of acylation stimulating protein. J Biol Chem 1989; 264:426–430.
26. Cleary M, Vasselli J, Greenwood M. Development of obesity in Zucker obese (fa/fa) rat in absence of hyperphagia. Am J Physiol 1980; 238:E284–E292.
27. Clement K, Vaisse C, Manning BJ, Basevant A, Guy-Grand B, Rutz J, Silver KD, Shuldiner AR, Froguel P, Strosberg AD. Genetic variation in the β_3-adrenergic receptor and an increased capacity to gain weight in patients with morbid obesity. N Engl J Med 1995; 333:352–354.
28. Coppack SW, Jensen MD, Miles JM. In vivo regulation of lipolysis in humans. J Lipid Res 1994; 35:177–193.

29. Coppack SW, Yost TJ, Fisher RM, Eckel RH, Miles JM. Periprandial systemic and regional lipase activity. Am J Physiol 1996; 270:E718–E722.

30. Davies JI, Souness JE. The mechanisms of hormone and drug action on fatty acid release from adipose tissue. Rev Pure Appl Pharmacol 1981; 2:1–112.

31. Deshaies Y, Geloen A, Paulin A, Marette A, Bukowiecki LJ. Tissue-specific alterations in lipoprotein lipase activity in the rat after chronic infusion of isoproterenol. Horm Metab Res 1993; 25:13–16.

32. Eckel RH. Adipose tissue lipoprotein lipase. In: Borensztajn J, ed. Lipoprotein Lipase. Chicago: Evener, 1987: 79–132.

33. Eckel RH. Lipoprotein lipase. A multifunctional enzyme relevant to common metabolic diseases. N Engl J Med 1989; 320:1060–1068.

34. Eckel RH. Insulin resistance: an adaptation for weight maintenance. Lancet 1992; 340:1452–1453.

35. Eckel RH, Jensen DR, Schlaepfer IR, Yost TJ. Tissue-specific regulation of lipoprotein lipase by isoproterenol in normal weight humans. Am J Physiol 1996; 271: R1280–R1286.

36. Eckel RH, Yost TJ. Weight reduction increases adipose tissue lipoprotein lipase responsiveness in obese women. J Clin Invest 1987; 80:992–997.

37. Eckel RH, Yost TJ, Jensen DR. Sustained weight reduction in moderately obese women results in decreased activity of skeletal muscle lipoprotein lipase. Eur J Clin Invest 1995; 25:396–402.

38. Eckel RH, Yost TJ, Jensen DR. Alterations in lipoprotein lipase in insulin resistance. Int J Obes 1995; 19:S16–S21.

39. Edens NK, Fried SK, Kral JG, Hirsh J, Leibel RL. In vitro lipid synthesis in human adipose tissue from three abdominal sites. Am J Physiol 1993; 265:E374–E379.

40. Egan JJ, Greenberg AS, Chang M, Wek SA, Moos MC, Londos C. Mechanism of hormone stimulated lipolysis in adipocytes: Translocation of hormone sensitive lipase to the lipid storage droplet. Proc Natl Acad Sci USA 1992; 89:8537–8541.

41. Enocksson S, Shimizu M, Lönnqvist F, Nordenstrom J, Arner P. Demonstration of an in vivo functional b$_3$-adrenoceptor in man. J Clin Invest 1995; 95:2239–2245.

42. Foufelle F, Gouhot B, Pegorier JP, Perderau D, Girard J, Ferre P. Glucose stimulation of lipogenic enzyme gene expression in cultured white adipose tissue. A role for glucose 6-phosphate. J Biol Chem 1992; 267:20543–20546.

43. Frayn KN, Williams CM, Arner P. Are increased plasma non-esterified fatty acid concentrations a risk marker for coronary heart disease and other chronic diseases? 1996; 90:243–253.

44. Fried SK, Russell CD, Grauso NL, Brolin RE. Lipoprotein lipase regulation by insulin and glucocoroticoid in subcutaneous and omental adipose tissues of obese women and men. J Clin Invest 1993; 92:2191–2198.

45. Galitzky J, Lafontan M, Nordenström J, Arner P. Role of vascular alpha-2 adrenoceptors in regulating lipid mobi-

lization from human adipose tissue. J Clin Invest 1993; 91:1997–2003.

46. Galton DJ. Lipogenesis in human adipose tissue. J Lipid Res 1968; 9:19–26.

47. Greenberg AS, Egan JJ, Wek SA, Moos MCJ, London C, Kimmel AR. Isolation of cDNAs for perilipins A and B: Sequence and expression of lipid droplet-associated proteins of adipocytes. Proc Natl Acad Sci USA 1993; 90: 12035–12039.

48. Hellerstein MK, Christiansen M, Kaempfer S, Kletke S, Wu K, Reid JS, Mulligan K, Hellerstein NS, Schakleton CHL. Measurement of de novo lipogenesis in humans using stable isotopes. J Clin Invest 1991; 87:1841–1852.

49. Hotamisligil GK, Arner P, Caro JF, Atkinson RL, Spiegelman BM. Increased adipose tissue expression of tumor necrosis factor-α in human obesity and insulin resistance. J Clin Invest 1995; 95:2409–2415.

50. Hotamisligil GK, Spiegelman BM. Tumor necrosis factor a: a key component of the obesity-diabetes link. Diabetes 1994; 43:1271–1278.

51. Iverius PH, Brunzell JD. Relationship between lipoprotein lipase activity and plasma sex steroid level in obese women. J Clin Invest 1988; 82:1106–1112.

52. Jacobsen BK, Trygg K, Hjermann I, Thomassen MS, Real C, Norum KR. Acyl patterns of adipose tissue triglycerides, plasma fatty acids, and diet of a group of men participating in a primary coronary prevention program (the Oslo Study). Am J Clin Nutr 1983; 38:906–913.

53. Jansson PA, Larsson A, Smith U, Lönnroth P. Glycerol production in subcutaneous adipose tissue in lean and obese humans. J Clin Invest 1992; 89:1610–1617.

54. Jensen DR, Morin CL, Schlaepfer IR, Pennington DS, Marcell T, Gutierrez-Hartmann A, Eckel RH. Transgenic mice with overexpression of skeletal muscle lipoprotein lipase: divergent effects of differential overexpression on body lipid. Obes Res 1995; 3:361s.

55. Kather H. Purine accumulation in human fat cell suspensions. J Biol Chem 1988; 263:8803–8809.

56. Kawakami M, Pekala PH, Lane MD, Cerami A. Lipoprotein lipase suppression in 3T3-L1 cells by an endotoxin-induced mediator from exudate cells. Proc Natl Acad Sci USA 1982; 79:912–916.

57. Kern PA, Marshall S, Eckel RH. Regulation of lipoprotein lipase in primary cultures of isolated human adipocytes. J Clin Invest 1985; 75:199–208.

58. Kern PA, Ong JM, Saffari B, Carty J. The effects of weight loss on the activity and expression of adipose-tissue lipoprotein lipase in very obese humans. N Engl J Med 1990; 322:1053–1059.

59. Kern PA, Saghizadeh M, Ong JM, Bosch RJ, Deem R, Simsolo RB. The expression of tumor necrosis factor in human adipose tissue. Regulation by obesity, weight loss, and relationship to lipoprotein lipase. J Clin Invest 1995; 95:2111–2119.

60. Kissebah AH, Krakower GR. Regional adiposity and morbidity. Am Physiol Soc 1994; 74:761–811.

61. Lafontan M, Berlan M. Fat cell adrenergic receptors and the control of white and brown fat cell function. J Lipid Res 1993; 34:1057–1091.

62. Lam K, Carpenters CL, Ruderman NB, Friel JC, Kelly KL. The phosphatidylinositol 3-kinase serine kinase phosphorylates IRS-1. J Biol Chem 1994; 269:20648–20652.

63. Lamarche B, Despres JP, Moorjani S, Nadeau A, Lupien PJ, Tremblay A, Theriault G, Bouchard C. Evidence for a role of insulin in the regulation of abdominal adipose tissue lipoprotein lipase response to exercise training in obese women. Int J Obes Relat Metab Disord 1993; 17: 255–261.

64. Leibel RL, Edens NK, Fried SK. Physiologic basis for the control of body fat distribution in humans. Annu Rev Nutr 1989; 9:417–443.

65. Leibel RL, Hirsch J, Berry EM, Gruen RK. Alterations in adipocyte free fatty acid re-esterification associated with obesity and weight reduction in man. Am J Clin Nutr 1985; 42:198–206.

66. Leitch CA, Jones PJH. Measurement of human lipogenesis using deuterium incorporation. J Lipid Res 1993; 34: 157–163.

67. Lemieux S, Despres JP. Metabolic complications of visceral obesity: Contribution to the etiology of type 2 diabetes and implications for prevention and treatment. Diabetes Metab 1994; 20:375–393.

68. Levak-Frank S, Radner H, Walsh AM, Stollberger R, Knipping G, Hoefler G, Sattler W, Breslow JL, Zechner R. Muscle-specific overexpression of lipoprotein lipase causes a severe myopathy characterized by proliferation of mitochondria and peroxisomes in transgenic mice. J Clin Invest 1995; 96:1–11.

69. Lönnqvist F, Nyberg B, Wahrenberg H, Arner P. Catecholamine-induced lipolysis in adipose tissue of the elderly. J Clin Invest 1990; 85:1614–1621.

70. Lönnqvist F, Thorne A, Nilsell K, Hoffstedt J, Arner P. A pathogenic role of visceral fat β_3-adrenoceptors in obesity. J Clin Invest 1995; 95:1109–1116.

71. Lönnroth P, Jansson PA, Fredholm BB, Smith U. Microdialysis of intercellular adenosine concentration in subcutaneous tissue in humans. Am Physiol. Soc 1989; 256: E250–E255.

72. Lopez-Cassilas F, Ponce-Castaneda MV, Kim KH. In vivo regulation of the activity of the two promoters of the rat acetyl coenzyme-A carboxylase gene. Endocrinology 1991; 129:1049–1058.

73. Mårin P, Oden B, Björntorp P. Assimilation and mobilization of triglycerides in subcutaneous abdominal and femoral adipose tissue in vivo in men: effects of androgens. J Clin Endocrinol Metab 1995; 80:239–243.

74. Maslowska MH, Sniderman AD, McLean LD, Cianflone K. Regional differences in triacylglycerol synthesis in adipose tissue and in cultured preadiopocytes. J Lipid Res 1993; 34:219–228.

75. Mauriege P, Despres JP, Prud'homme D, Pouliot MC, Marcotte M, Tremblay A, Bouchard C. Regional variation in adipose tissue lipoysis in lean and obese men. J Lipid Res 1991; 32:1625–1633.

76. Mauriege P, Marette A, Atgie C, Bouchard C, Theriault G, Bukowiecki LK, Marceau P, Biron S, Nadeau A, Despres JP. Regional variation in adipose tissue metabolism of severely obese premenopausal women. J Lipid Res 1995; 36:672–684.

77. Mizutani T, Nishikawa Y, Adachi H, Enomoto T, Ikegami H, Kurachi H, Nomura T, Miyake A. Identification of estrogen receptor in human adipose tissue and adipocytes. J Clin Endocrinol Metab 1994; 78:950–954.

78. Morin CL, Shclaepfer IR, Eckel RH. Tumor necrosis factor-a eliminates binding of NF-Y and an octamer-binding protein to the lipoprotein lipase promoter in 3T3-L1 adipocytes. J Clin Invest 1995; 95:1684–1689.

79. Nikkila EA. Role of lipoprotein lipase in metabolic adaptation to exercise and training. In: Borensztajn J, Lipoprotein Lipase, ed. Chicago: Evener Publishers, 1987: 187–199.

80. Norman RA, Bogardus C, Ravussin E. Linkage between obesity and a marker near the numor necrosis factor-alpha locus in Pima Indians. J Clin Invest 1995; 96:158–162.

81. Okada T, Kawano Y, Sakakibara T, Hazeki O, Ui M. Essential role of phosphatidylinositol 3-kinase in insulin-induced glucose transport and antilipolysis in rat adipocytes. J Biol Chem 1994; 269:3568–3573.

82. Okuda H, Morimoto C, Tsujita T. Role of endogenous lipid droplets in lipolysis in rat adipocytes. J Lipid Res 1994; 35:36–44.

83. Ong JM, Kern PA. Effect of feeding and obesity on lipoprotein lipase activity, immunoreactive protein, and messenger RNA levels in human adipose tissue. J Clin Invest 1989; 84:305–311, 1989.

84. Ong JM, Saffari B, Simsolo RB, Kern PA. Epinephrine inhibits lipoprotein lipase gene expression in rat adipocytes through multiple steps in posttranscriptional processing. Mol Endocrinol 1992; 6:61–69.

85. Ottosson M, Vikman-Adolfsson K, Enerback S, Elander A, Björntorp P, Eden S. Growth hormone inhibits lipoprotein lipase activity in human adipose tissue. J Clin Endocrinol Metab 1995; 80:936–941.

86. Ottosson M, Vikman-Adolfsson K, Enerback S, Olivecrona G, Björntorp P. The effects of cortisol on the regulation of lipoprotein lipase activity in human adipose tissue. J Clin Endocrinol Metab 1994; 79:820–825.

87. Pedersen SB, Jonler M, Richelsen B. Characterization of regional and gender differences in glucocoricoid receptors and lipoprotein lipase activity in human adipose tissue. J Clin Endocrinol Metab 1994; 78:1354–1359.

88. Persson B. Seasonal variation of lipoprotein lipase activity in human subcutaneous adipose tissue. Clin Sci Mol Med 1974; 47:631–634.

89. Petrasek R, Rath R, Masek J. Influence of a five-day fast on the incorporation of acetae-1-C-14 into total lipids and CO_2 in subcutaneous adipose tissue of obese women. Physiol Bohemoslov 1975; 24:335–337.

90. Poehlman ET, Despres JP, Marcotte M, Tremblay A, Theriault G, Bouchard C. Genotype dependency of adaptation in adipose tissue metabolism after short-term overfeeding. Am J Physiol 1986; 250:E480–E485.

91. Pykalisto OJ, Smith PH, Brunzell JD. Determinants of human adipose tissue lipoprotein lipase. Effect of diabetes and obesity on basal- and diet-induced activity. J Clin Invest 1975; 56:1108–1117.

92. Rahn T, Ridderstrale M, Tornqvist H, Manganiello V, Fredrikson G, Belfreage P, Degerman E. Essential role of phospatidylinositiol 3-kinase in insulin-induced activation and phosphorylation of the cGMP-inhibited cAMP phosphodiesterase in rat adipocytes. FEBS Lett 1994; 350:314–318.

93. Raynolds MV, Awald PD, Gordon DF, Gutierrez-Hartmann A, Rule DC, Wood WM, Eckel RH. Lipoprotein lipase gene expression in rat adipocytes is regulated by isoproterenol and insulin through different mechanisms. Mol Endocrinol 1990; 4:1416–1422.

94. Rebuffe-Scrive M, Enk L, Crona N, Lönnroth P, Abrahamsson L, Smith U, Björntorp P. Fat cell metabolism in different regions in women. J Clin Invest 1985; 75:1973–1976.

95. Rebuffe-Scrive M, Krotkiewski M, Elfverson J, Björntorp P. Muscle and adipose tissue morphology and metabolism in Cushing's syndrome. J Clin Endocrinol Metab 1988; 67:1122–1128.

96. Rebuffe-Scrive, Lönnroth P, Mårin P, Wesslau C, Björntorp P. Regional adipose tissue metabolism in men and postmenopausal women. Int J Obes 1987; 11:347–355.

97. Rebuffe-Scrive M, Mårin P, Björntorp P. Effect of testosterone on abdominal adipose tissue in men. Int J Obes 1991; 15:791–795.

98. Reynisdottir S, Ellerfeldt K, Wahrenberg H, Lithell H, Arner P. Multiple lipolysis defects in the insulin resistance (metabolic) syndrome. J Clin Invest 1994; 93:2590–2599.

99. Reynisdottir S, Wahrenberg H, Carlström K, Rössner S, Arner P. Catecholamine resistance in fat cells of women with upper-body obesity due to decreased expression of beta2-adrenoceptors. Diabetologia 1994; 37:428–435.

100. Rowe JW, Minaker KL, Pallotta JA, Flier JS. Characterization of the insulin resistance of aging. J Clin Invest 1983; 71:1581–1587.

101. Sadur CN, Eckel RH. Insulin stimulation of adipose tissue lipoprotein lipase. Use of the euglycemic clamp technique. J Clin Invest 1982; 69:1119–1125.

102. Savard R, Bouchard C. Genetic effects in the response of adipose tissue lipoprotein lipase activity to prolonged exercise. A twin study. Int J Obes 1990; 14:771–777.

103. Schwartz RS, Brunzell JD. Increase of adipose tissue lipoprotein lipase activity with weight loss. J Clin Invest 1981; 67:1425–1430.

104. Seip RL, Angelopoulos TJ, Semenkovich CF. Exercise induces human lipoprotein lipase gene expression in skeletal muscle but not adipose tissue. Am J Physiol 1995; 268:E229–E236.

105. Shepherd PR, Gnudi L, Tozzo E, Yang H, Leach F, Kahn BB. Adipose cell hyperplasia and enhanced glucose disposal in transgenic mice overexpressing GLUT4 selectively in adipose tissue. J Biol Chem 1993; 268:22243–22246.

106. Simsolo RB, Ezzat S, Ong JM, Saghizadeh M, Kern PA. Effects of acromegaly treatment and growth hormone on adipose tissue lipoprotein lipase. J Clin Endocrinol Metab 1995; 80:3233–3238.

107. Simsolo RB, Ong JM, Kern PA. Characterization of lipoprotein lipase activity, secretion, and degradation at different sites of post-translational processing in primary cultures of rat adipocytes. J Lipid Res 1992; 33:1777–1784.

108. Simsolo RB, Ong JM, Kern PA. The regulation of adipose tissue and muscle lipoprotein lipase in runners by detraining. J Clin Invest 1993; 92:2124–2130.

109. Skottova N, Savonen R, Lookene A, Hultin M, Olivecrona G. Lipoprotein lipase enhances removal of chylomicrons and chylomicron remnants by perfused rat liver. J Lipid Res 1995; 36:1334–1344.

110. Sniderman A, Cianflone K, Eckel RH. Levels of acylation stimulating protein in obese women before and after moderate weight loss. Int J Obes 1991; 15:327–332.

111. Strålfors P, Olsson H, Belfrage P. Hormone-sensitive lipase. In: Boyer PD, Krebs EG, eds. The Enzymes. New York: Academic Press, 1987:147–177.

112. Susulic VS, Frederich RC, Lawitts J, Tozzo E, Kahn BB, Harper M, Himms-Hagen J, Flier JS, Lowell BB. Targeted disruption of the β_3-adrenergic receptor gene. J Biol Chem 1995; 270:29483–29492.

113. Sztalryd C, Komaromy MC, Kraemer FB. Overexpression of hormone-sensitive lipase prevents triglyceride accumulation in adipocytes. J Clin Invest 1995; 95:2652–2661.

114. Taskinen MR, Nikkila EA, Ollus O. Serum lipids and lipoproteins in insulin-dependent diabetic subjects during high-carbohydrate, high fiber diet. Diabetes Care 1983; 6:224–230.

115. Tozzo E, Shepherd PR, Gnudi L, Kahn BB. Transgenic Glut-4 overexpression in fat enhances glucose metabolism: preferential effect on fatty acid synthesis. Am J Physiol 1995; 31:E956–E964.

116. van Staveren W, Deurenberg P, Katan MB, Burema J, de Groot L, Hoffmans D. Validity of the fatty acid composition of subcutaneous fat tissue microbiopsies as estimate of the long-term average fatty acid composition of the diet of separate individuals. Am J Epidemiol 1986; 123:455–463.

117. Vasseur-Cognet M, Lane MD. *Trans*-acting factors involved in adipogenic differentiation. Curr Opin Genet Dev 1993; 3:238–245.

118. Vessby B, Lithell H, Boberg J, Hellsing K, Werner I. Gemfibrozil as a lipid lowering compound in hyperlipoproteinaemia. A placebo-controlled cross-over trial. Proc R Soc Med 1976; 69(Suppl 2):32–37.

119. Voh MC, Lamarche B, Moorjani S, Prud'homme D, Nadeau A, Bouchard C, Lupien PJ, Depres JP. The lipoprotein lipase HindIII polymorphism modulates plasma triglyceride levels in visceral obesity. Arterioscler Thromb 1995; 15:714–720.

120. Walston J, Silver K, Bogardus C, Knowler WC, Celi FS, Austin S, Manning B, Stosberg AD, Stern MP, Raben N, Sorkin JD, Roth J, Shuldiner AR. Time of onset of non-insulin-dependent diabetes mellitus and genetic variation in the β_3-adrenergic-receptor gene. N Engl J Med 1995; 333:343–347.

121. Yasruel Z, Cianflone K, Sniderman AD, Rosenbloom M, Walsh M, Rodriguez MA. Effect of acylation protein on the triacylgylcerol synthetic pathway of human adipose tissue. Lipids 1991; 26:495–499.

122. Yost TJ, Eckel RH. Fat calories may be preferentially stored in reduced-obese women: a permissive pathway for resumption of the obese state. J Clin Endocrinol Metab 1988; 67:259–264.

123. Yost TJ, Ecekl RH. Regional similarities in the metabolic regulation of adipose tissue lipoprotein lipase. Metabolism 1992; 41:33–36.

124. Yost TJ, Jensen DR, Eckel RH. Tissue-specific lipoprotein lipase: Relationships to body composition and body fat distribution in normal weight humans. Obes Res 1993; 1:1–4.

125. Yost TJ, Rodgers CM, Eckel RH. Suction lipectomy: outcome relates to region-specific lipoprotein lipase activity and interval weight change. Plast Reconstr Surg 1993; 92: 1101–1108.

126. Zawadki JK, Bogardus C, Foley JE. Insulin action in obese non-insulin-dependent diabetics and in their isolated adipocytes before and after weight loss. Diabetes 1987; 36: 227–336.

127. Zechner R, Newman TC, Sherry B, Cerami A, Breslow JL. Recombinant human cachectin/tumor necrosis factor but not interleukin-1 alpha downregulates lipoprotein lipase gene expression at the transcriptional level in mouse 3T3-L1 adipocytes. Mol Cell Biol 1988; 8:2394–2401.

128. Zhang Y, Proenca R, Maffei M, Barone M, Leopold L, Friedman JM. Positional cloning of the mouse obese gene and its human homologue. Nature 1994; 372:425–431.

18

Diverse Roles of Adipose Tissue in the Regulation of Systemic Metabolism and Energy Balance

Susan K. Fried and Colleen D. Russell
Rutgers University, New Brunswick, New Jersey

I. INTRODUCTION

Prior to the 1950s, the main functions of adipose tissue were considered to be insulation against heat loss and protection of internal organs against traumatic injury (1). With the availability of radiolabeled substrates, it was rapidly realized that adipose tissue was not an inert reservoir for excess ingested energy (1). Rather, it was established that adipocyte triglyceride stores are continuously turning over at a rate that is tightly controlled by hormones. The physiological, cellular, and molecular mechanisms regulating the primary function of the adipocyte, to store excess ingested energy as triacylglycerol and to release fatty acids to meet the energy needs of other tissues, have been rapidly unfolding in the past several decades. Research of the past decade has uncovered many novel metabolic functions of adipose tissue, apart from its central role in triglyceride metabolism. There is also increasing evidence that in addition to the classical actions of insulin and counterregulatory hormones on adipocyte metabolism, the adipocyte plays an active role in modulating its own metabolism, and hence its size, via autocrine and paracrine mechanisms that may function as "adipostats" (2,3).

In addition to releasing free fatty acids and glycerol that serve as substrates for energy metabolism in other tissues, the adipocyte may contribute substantially to whole-body lactate and amino acid production (4,5). Although the adipocyte has not yet been shown to be the equal of the hepatocyte in terms of the sheer number of its metabolic roles or secretory products, the diversity of fat cell functions is nonetheless impressive (3,6). Like the hepatocyte, the adipocyte synthesizes and secretes proteins that participate in lipid transport [cholesterol ester transfer protein (CETP), retinol-binding protein (RBP)] or metabolism [acylation-stimulating protein (ASP)] (4,7). These proteins may have local influences within adipose tissue and may also be secreted and function systemically.

Adipose tissue also participates in a variety of endocrine systems. Newly discovered roles of the adipocyte/adipose tissue include the following: (1) adipocyte production of the cytokine tumor necrosis factor (TNF) may play an etiological role in the development of adipocyte (as well as systemic) insulin resistance in obesity, (2) the local production of angiotensinogen may play a role in the development of obesity-induced hypertension, (3) synthesis of estrogens by adipose tissue may mediate effects of obesity on the risk for osteoporosis and cancer. Thus, an expansion of the adipose mass (cell size and number) has pleiotropic effects on endocrine and metabolic events at the whole-body level that may contribute to the pathogenesis of metabolic complications of obesity.

Most recently, the cloning of the *ob* gene and the discovery that it is expressed exclusively in the adipocyte establishes, for the first time, a true endocrine function of the adipocyte (8). The *ob* gene product (named leptin) is secreted from the adipocyte and is found in serum. When administered to mice, leptin has potent effects on the central regulation of both feeding and energy expenditure

(9–12). Thus, leptin appears to be the long-sought-after "feedback signal" that links the status of fat stores to the regulation of food intake and body weight. It remains to be established whether leptin is the only hormone of this type secreted by the adipocyte. Nevertheless, available evidence points to the importance of integrated paracrine (including TNF) and endocrine (leptin) mechanisms that function to limit the expansion of fat stores.

This chapter will review the literature on the regulation of recently identified metabolic and endocrine functions of adipose tissue and discuss implications for the regulation of metabolism and the development of obesity and its metabolic complications. Because detailed reviews of several specific topics of this field were recently published (3,4,6,7,13), our main goal is to provide an integrative overview of newly identified functions of the adipocyte and adipose tissue.

II. ADIPOCYTE METABOLIC PRODUCTS

A. Lactate

Most in vitro studies of adipocyte glucose metabolism assess only the conversion of glucose into CO_2 and triacylglycerol, fatty acids, and glyceride glycerol. While valid for the adipocytes of young rats (where the sum of these products accounts for ~90% of the glucose utilized), this method underestimates adipocyte glucose metabolic rates in other models (4,14). In large adipocytes from older rats and human adipocytes, glucose conversion to lactate (and pyruvate) can account for only 40–80% of adipocyte glucose metabolism (14,15). Glycogen is a minor product (4).

Microdialysis and arteriovenous (A-V) difference studies of abdominal subcutaneous human adipose tissue demonstrate a net production of lactate in both the postprandial state and after a load of glucose (16–18). A-V difference studies of Frayn et al. show that that only 13–15% of the glucose taken up by adipose tissue is converted to lactate after glucose or meal ingestion but the value rises to 30–35% after an overnight fast (16,17). The increase in relative rates of lactate production with starvation in human adipose tissue is similar to results observed in vitro in isolated adipocytes from fed versus starved rats (4,19).

The rate of adipocyte lactate production is sensitive to in vitro incubation conditions. When adipocytes are incubated at low fat cell concentrations, lactate production accounts for an increased proportion of glucose metabolism (30% compared to 15% of the total glucose metabolized in the presence of insulin) (20). The mechanisms influencing the production of lactate by adipocytes under there conditions are not known, but adenosine has been

ruled out as a mediator (20). It is therefore possible that alterations in adipose tissue blood flow or paracrine/autocrine factors could influence adipocyte lactate production in vivo. The net output of lactate from adipose tissue may also depend on its rate of utilization via the glyceroneogenic pathway (particularly under conditions of low blood flow) (21).

It has been proposed that adipose tissue could contribute substantially to whole-body lactate production, and in particular may serve as a significant source of gluconeogenic substrate (4). However, it is difficult to quantify the contribution of adipose tissue to whole-body lactate turnover (22). Data from microdialysis studies combined with measurements of adipose tissue blood flow show that apparent lactate release from adipose tissue in the fasting state is similar per kilogram of adipose tissue in lean and obese subjects (implying greater production per cell in the obese) (23). Glucose ingestion appears to increase adipose tissue lactate production, but only in lean subjects (23). It is estimated that total daily body lactate appearance is ~1350 mmol/day. In the postabsorptive state, adipose tissue produces ~10 μmol/kg/min of lactate, or 144 mmol/10 kg/day, which accounts for approximately 10% of the total, assuming that all adipose depots produce lactate at a similar rate (23). If in humans, as in rats, visceral (mesenteric) adipose tissue produces more lactate, measurement of the contribution of only subcutaneous adipose tissue may yield a minimal estimate (4). Additionally, the contribution of lactate to whole-body production may be higher in obesity because the absolute number and size of adipocytes are increased.

B. Amino Acids

Few investigators have addressed the role of adipose tissue in amino acid metabolism. Studies in vitro show that adipose tissue can take up branched-chain amino acids and glutamate and product glutamine (5,24). Glutamine is of particular interest because it functions to transport carbon and nitrogen between different tissues. Analysis of whole-body studies of glutamine turnover reveals that skeletal muscle, lung, and hepatic production cannot account for whole-body utilization of glutamine, leading to the proposal that adipose tissue may be a site of glutamine production (5). Microdialysis studies of rat inguinal fat pad by Kowalski and Watford demonstrate a net output of glutamine in the fasted state (5). Using an A-V difference method, Frayn and colleagues have demonstrated a net glutamine and alanine output, as well as glutamate uptake by human subcutaneous adipose tissue (24). A recent microdialysis study of human adipose tissue revealed a net output of a number of amino acids (25). Clearly, adipose tissue should not be discounted in studies assessing whole-body amino acid metabolism. It will be of great interest to determine whether adipose glutamine production increases during different conditions when whole-body glutamine utilization is known to be increased (pregnancy, stress, infection) (5).

III. ROLE OF THE ADIPOCYTE SECRETORY PRODUCTS IN LIPID TRANSPORT AND METABOLISM

A. Cholesterol Ester Transfer Protein (CETP)

CETP stimulates the transfer of cholesterol ester from HDL into VLDL and triglycerides from VLDL into HDL. CETP levels are inversely correlated with plasma high-density lipoprotein (HDL) levels (26). Though low HDL levels are strongly statistically linked to coronary heart disease risk, the relationship of CETP to the development of atherogenesis is complex and depends on the level of triglyceridemia (27). Studies in Tall's laboratory demonstrate that adipose tissue is a major source of CETP in hamsters and that adipocytes synthesize and secrete this protein. Adipose tissue CETP mRNA levels were found to be regulated by the level of cholesterol in the diet and by fasting (whereas CETP expression in other tissues was unaffected) (28). Like this rodent model, expression of CETP in human adipose tissue is also very high and responds to dietary cholesterol (29,30). Furthermore, plasma HDL levels are more highly correlated (inversely) with adipose tissue CETP mRNA levels than plasma CETP levels, suggesting that CETP is locally active in HDL metabolism within adipose tissue (26,30). CETP is hypothesized to help recycle cholesterol deposited in adipose tissue. After esterification by lecithin cholesterol acyltransferase, cholesterol derived from adipocytes is transfered to chylomicron remnants and then delivered to the liver (26,28). There may be important interactions of CETP with lipoprotein lipase (LPL), another secretory product of the adipocyte, in the regulation of lipid transport (26). Lipolysis of triglyceride-rich lipoproteins by LPL leads to the buildup of fatty acids on the surface of lipoprotein particles, increasing binding of CETP and transfer activity (26).

The mobilization of adipocyte cholesterol may also involve interaction of CETP and apolipoprotein E (Apo E), which is also synthesized by adipose tissue. In human adipose tissue, Apo E mRNA levels are high and Apo E is synthesized, but no Apo E secretion (into serum-free medium) can be detected (31). Surprisingly, Apo E is predominantly expressed in stromal-vascular cells rather than adipocytes, at least in rat adipose tissue (32). Additional work is needed to assess whether Apo E is secreted from adipocytes or stromal cells in the presence of an acceptor such as HDL and functions extracellularly, or whether it mainly functions intracellularly.

CETP is hypothesized to play a role in lowering HDL levels in obesity. In obese subjects, low HDL levels are associated with increased plasma CETP activity and mass, independent of postheparin plasma lipoprotein lipase and hepatic lipase activities (33,34). CETP levels are correlated positively with total fat mass and negatively with the ratio of visceral to subcutaneous fat mass, but are not independently related to visceral fat mass (34). Thus, subcutaneous fat may express higher levels of CETP and so may be of particular importance in regulating plasma CETP levels. The quantitative contribution of adipose tissue production to plasma CETP in obesity is not yet established. Research is also needed to clarify the hormonal and substrate regulators of adipose tissue CETP synthesis and secretion.

B. The Adipocyte and Retinoid Metabolism

A chance observation by Makover and colleagues (35) led to the discovery that adipose tissue was among the peripheral tissues that express retinol binding protein (RBP), a plasma protein that delivers retinol to tissue and whose expression was previously thought to be restricted to the liver. Studies in Blaner's laboratory later demonstrated that RBP mRNA is expressed almost exclusively in adipocytes rather than stromal-vascular cells (32). On a per cell basis, RBP expression in adipocytes is approximately 25% of hepatocyte levels (32). Expression of RBP mRNA is similar in the six major adipose depots in the rat and all show significant stores of retinal and retinyl esters (15–20% of total-body stores) (32). Importantly, isolated adipocytes synthesize RBP and secrete it into the culture medium (32). The importance of adipocyte RBP in the mobilization of adipose tissue retinoid stores during weight loss or dietary deficiency and the mechanisms regulating adipose RBP expression remain to be established.

IV. ENDOCRINE FUNCTIONS OF ADIPOSE TISSUE

A. Implications for Systemic and Local Adipocyte Metabolism

1. Angiotensinogen

Angiotensinogen is a precursor of angiotensin II which has potent vasoconstrictor effects (36). Angiotensinogen is expressed abundantly in liver and in a number of peripheral tissues, including adipose tissue (37,38). Rat adipocytes synthesize and secrete this protein, and the levels of angiotensinogen mRNA are comparable to those in liver

(37). Angiotensinogen gene expression is highly differentiation-dependent in cultured murine adipocytes (39). Adipose tissue possesses the enzymatic machinery to convert angiotensinogen into angiotensin II. This active form (angiotensin II) may also influence adipocyte differentiation by interactions with adipocyte angiotensin receptors (40), inducing adipose cells to produce prostacyclin (41–43).

In rodents, the level of angiotensinogen expression is increased in obesity and, in contrast to expression in liver, is regulated by nutritional status (44). Fasting decreases and refeeding increases mRNA levels above control (fed) levels (44). These alterations in angiotensinogen gene expression are paralleled by changes in angiotensinogen secretion from isolated adipocytes (44) Frederich et al. hypothesized that alterations in adipose tissue angiotensinogen expression may explain the hypotensive effects of caloric restriction and the hypertension associated with obesity (44). It was also hypothesized that angiotensinogen plays a role in local adipose tissue blood flow and, hence, rates of fatty acid reesterification (44). Thus, by affecting both substrate availability and preadipocyte differentiation, angiotensinogen factors in the regulation of adipose size in response to nutritional signals.

2. Estrogens

The presence of estrogens in the plasma of postmenopausal women led to the discovery that adipose tissue was an active extraglandular producer of certain steroid hormones (45–47). Circulating C19 precursors of adrenal origin (mainly and androstenedione) are converted to estrone and estradiol via adipose tissue P450 aromatase. In vitro experiments suggest that the bulk of adipose aromatase activity resides in the stromal-vascular cells (48,49). Production of estrogens by adipose tissue is positively correlated with age and body weight/fat mass (50–52). Because aromatase activity itself does not appear to increase with obesity, it has been hypothesized that the increased fat mass and adrenal output (androgen precursors) may incur a "passive" increase in estrogen production by adipose tissue (50). Levels of aromatase activity are fairly consistent among the major adipose depots, although that of the buttocks may be slightly higher (53). In vitro studies of adipose stromal cells indicate that aromatase expression can be increased by glucocorticoids (54) and cAMP analogs (55). The significance of these findings with respect to adipose tissue estrogen production in vivo requires further investigation.

Adipose tissue is the principal source of estrogens in postmenopausal women (45,51). The major estrogen formed here, estrone, is less potent than estradiol, but estrone concentrations may be increased severalfold in morbidly obese postmenopausal women (45,52). Local estrone production in breast adipose tissue has been linked to breast cancer incidence (56,57). Aromatase expression has been found to be highest in the quadrant of breast adipose tissue containing a tumor, although it is not completely clear whether an increased local concentration of estrogens is an initiating event or a simply a consequence of the cancer (56,58). Obesity-related increases in adipose estrogen production have also been associated with endometrial cancer (59), yet potentially have a beneficial effect on osteoporosis through estrogen actions on bone (59). Estrogens also have complex effects on food intake and energy metabolism (60). Clearly, many questions about the regulation and consequences of adipose tissue estrogen production remain to be answered.

B. Leptin: Endocrine Signal from the Adipocyte to the Brain

The notion that the body fat content is regulated by "some aspect of the synthesis or transport of fat," known as the "lipostatic hypothesis," dates to the classic paper of Kennedy in 1953 (61). Though it is generally agreed that body weight is regulated, the idea that total body fat content per se (or adipocyte size) is a regulated entity is still debated (62,63). There was, however, evidence for a blood-borne signal that was produced in obese animals and regulated food intake. As demonstrated by Hervey, parabiosis of an obese animal (secondary to hyperphagia produced by lesions of the ventromedial hypothalmus (VMH) or stimulation of the lateral hypothalmus) could reduce food intake and markedly deplete body fat in the control lean partner (64,65). Similarly, subsequent studies showed that overfeeding elicits a blood-borne factor that decreases food intake and may have metabolic effects on adipocyte lipogenesis (62,66). Parabiosis studies of genetically obese mice by Coleman established that a blood-borne signal produced in obese (*db*/db) animals [with mutations at the *db* (diabetes) locus] inhibited food intake in lean animals. In contrast, parabiosis of an obese (*ob*/*ob*) mouse to lean littermates has no effect on the lean partner and moderates the obesity of the *ob*/*ob* mouse. These results led Coleman to hypothesize that the *ob*/*ob* mouse lacks the ability to produce a satiety factor and the *db*/*db* mutant is unable to detect it (62,67).

Considerable effort using traditional physiological and biochemical methods did not lead to the identification of this "satiety" factor, nor even insight into its tissue source. The search for a neural, metabolic, or hormonal link that could relay information about the size of fat stores to brain appears to have culminated in the discovery of the adipocyte hormone "leptin" in the laboratory of Friedman.

Zhang et al. (8) used a reverse genetics approach involving genetic and physical mapping techniques, to clone the *ob* gene (leptin) and its human homologe in 1994. The gene for leptin was expressed exclusively in adipocytes (8). The coding sequence of the leptin gene is highly conserved among species; the human and mouse leptin cDNA sequences show high similarity the 3′ and 5′ untranslated regions of leptin mRNA, however, show only 30% homology between mice and human sequences. The rat homolog of leptin has also been cloned (68,69). The rat and mouse amino acid sequences are 84% identical. The 4.5-kb human *ob* mRNA encodes an 18-kDa protein including a signal sequence of 2KD that is cleaved in the presence of microsomes. The 16-kDa fragment is translocated into the microsomal lumen, consistent with the behavior of a secreted protein (8). The circulating form of leptin is also 16K, as assessed by Western analysis, suggesting that leptin is not posttranslationally processed (9). Different mutations in leptin were identified in two *ob/ob* mouse strains. The original strain (C57/BL6 *ob/ob*) overexpresses leptin mRNA in adipose tissue with a nonsense mutation that produces a premature stop codon, and the other strain shows no leptin mRNA expression, presumably owing to a mutation in the gene's promoter region (8). No mutations of the *ob* gene have yet been identified in the small number of human patients examined so far (70). However, linkage of extreme obesity (BMI > 45–50) to polymorphisms in the ob locus have been detected by sib-pair analysis in families in Philadelphia (71) and Paris (72).

The genomic organization of the mouse (73) and human (74,75) *ob* gene has been described. A 763-bp mouse *ob* gene promoter drove expression only in transfected primary rat adipose cells. The minimal promoter (-161) contained Sp1 and CCAAT/enhancer binding protein (C/EBP) motifs. Cotransfection with C/EBPα, a transcription factor known to be important in regulating adipocyte differentiation, markedly stimulated *ob* gene transcription (73). A 300-bp fragment of the human *ob* 5′-flanking region was even more active than a 3-kb sequence in driving expression of a reporter gene in 3T3-F44A adipocytes, suggesting a role for remote inhibitory elements (74). A number of putative binding sites for transcription factors, including an Sp-1 site, cAMP response element, CCAAT/enhancer binding protein, and glucocorticoid response elements, were present in the human *ob* promoter. Several repetitive sequences that may influence *ob* transcription were also noted (74).

Several groups have now reported that intraperitoneal administration of recombinant leptin to *ob/ob* mice or their lean littermates leads to a marked reduction in food intake and body weight (9–12). Administration of leptin also decreases food intake and body weight of lean and dietary-induced obese mice (9–11), though the effects are of smaller magnitude than in *ob/ob* mice. As predicted, leptin has no effect on food intake in *db/db* mutants that appear to have a defective leptin receptor (11,76–78). Recombinant leptin also exhibits metabolic effects, decreasing plasma insulin, glucose, and cortisol and raising body temperature, energy expenditure, and motor activity in *ob/ob* mice to normal levels in lean controls (11,79). However, no detectable increase in energy expenditure resulted from leptin administration to lean mice (11). As demonstrated by pair-feeding experiments, decreased food intake does not completely account for the fat-depleting effects of leptin administration in lean or *ob/ob* mice (80). The effects of leptin on body weight are fully reversible; food intake returns to baseline upon cessation of treatment. Impressively, effects of administration of leptin into the lateral ventricles of the cerebrum (i.c.v.) are particularly dramatic. After a lag time of 30 min, the mice given leptin i.c.v. consumed no food for 6.5 hr (10). Thus leptin has a longer duration of action then neuropeptides that regulate feeding (10). As a secreted adipocyte protein influencing the neural control of feeding and metabolism (10), leptin therefore fits the standard criteria of a true hormone.

Serum levels of leptin are elevated 2–20-fold in several models of obesity, including mice with MSG-induced hypothalamic obesity or VMH-lesioned rats (81,82), transgenic mice lacking brown adipose (UCP-DTA) (83), and genetic obesities in rodents (*db/db* mice, Zucker fatty rats, fat, tub, A^y (9,71,82–85). The magnitude of the differences between lean and obese strains is roughly proportionate to the degree of obesity. Leptin mRNA levels are not increased prior to the development of obesity in Zucker fatty rats (86). As expected, immunoreactive leptin protein is not present in the serum of *ob/ob* mice (83). Acquired obesity due to high-fat feeding is also associated with an increase in leptin expression (85,87–89). Increased leptin mRNA levels are observed with high-fat feeding, which result solely from adipocyte hypertrophy, consistent with the idea that leptin reflects fat cell size (85). The increase is leptin expression is proportional to the level of fatness determined by body composition analysis in mice fed low- and high-fat diets (89). Because caloric intake of the high-fat diet was not decreased in the face of elevated leptin levels, it was suggested that the diet altered the set point for body weight by altering sensitivity to leptin (89).

The relative abundance of leptin mRNA varies severalfold across different fat depots (90,91). There are also variations in responsiveness to overfeeding or insulin infusion among depots (90,91). Thus, some adipose tissue depots may provide stronger leptin signals than others, suggesting that the expansion of some adipose tissue depots may have weaker impacts on food intake and energy expenditure.

Leptin expression is also elevated in the adipose tissue (70,92,93) and serum (70,84,94) of obese humans, as reported by several laboratories. Adipose tissue leptin mRNA levels are increased approximately twofold and serum leptin levels are increased up to 10-fold in obese compared to lean subjects (70,92,93). The range of serum leptin concentrations at a given level of body fat is high, approximately 10-fold (84,94). Serum leptin levels are correlated with serum insulin levels, but the tightest correlate is percentage body fat (94). Plasma leptin levels decline upon weight loss (84,94). Leptin levels in patients with NIDDM are somewhat lower than those in equally obese nondiabetics, but higher than in lean persons (95). No gender differences in leptin levels have been noted in humans matched for body fat (94). However, several groups have reported that the levels and degree of variability of serum leptin levels are greater in women than men (84,94). Leptin mRNA levels determined by in situ hybridization were higher in adipose tissue of women than men (93), suggesting gender differences in leptin production. Interestingly, it was also noted that female mice also showed higher leptin expression than males at equal levels of body fatness (89). Consistent with this possibility, in rat adipocytes, estrogen caused a twofold increase in leptin mRNA levels (96).

Several recent reports show that leptin mRNA expression varies with nutritional status in a manner compatible with its putative role as a feedback regulator of appetite and energy expenditure. Starving rats for 1–3 days markedly decreases (and refeeding increases) adipocyte leptin mRNA levels in lean mice or rats (88,97–99). In contrast, starvation had little impact on leptin mRNA levels in *ob/ob* mice (97) or Zucker fatty rats (86). It has been speculated that the continued elevation of leptin mRNA in starvation in obese animals was due to persistent hyperinsulinemia. Consistent with this hypothesis, induction of hyperinsulinemia increased leptin mRNA levels in normal lean rats (86,91). Furthermore, treatment of *fa/fa* rats or *db/db* mice with the insulin-sensitizing drug thiazolidinedione, which lowered plasma insulin levels, also decreased leptin mRNA levels and circulating leptin levels (100). As discussed below, the relative importance of insulin and other hormones and metabolism in regulating leptin productions remains to be established.

Chronic nutritional manipulations that influence the level of adiposity also affect leptin expression. Semistarvation for 10 days also decreased leptin expression in normal animals (99). Obesity produced by tube-feeding rats twice their normal intake until they are 130% overweight led to a further increase in leptin mRNA levels (90). However, the acute effect of a meal-feeding pattern of food intake incurred during control tube feeding also increased leptin mRNA levels two- to threefold in 2 days in the absence of excess calorie intake or weight gain. The question of whether leptin expression is influenced by level of fatness or food intake per se has also been addressed by treating obese high-fat fed mice with a β_3-adrenergic drug that normalized the level of adiposity. Despite continued hyperphagia, levels of leptin mRNA were equal to values in leans. Thus, available evidence indicates that level of adiposity does affect leptin expression but that acute variations in nutritional status can also influence leptin expression.

In rats, serum leptin levels exhibit a diurnal variation. Increased serum leptin during the dark phase is associated with food intake. In contrast, in humans there is no correlation between serum leptin levels and insulin or glucose levels in response to meals during the day (95). Suprisingly, leptin levels in lean, obese, and non-insulin-dependent diabetic subjects increase during sleep, leading to the speculation that leptin suppresses appetite during the night (95).

Leptin mRNA levels are increased at a late stage of differentiation of cultured adipocyte cell lines (82,98,101). Similarly, leptin expression appears to be a feature only of fully differentiated rodent or human adipocytes. It is absent from the stromal-vascular fraction, which contains preadipocytes (102,103).

The role of specific hormones in modulating leptin expression in differentiated fat cells has been addressed by several groups, with somewhat conflicting results. Insulin was found to cause a modest increase (104) or no change (96) in leptin mRNA levels in primary cultures of rat adipocytes. In ob17 adipocytes (101), but not 3T3-L1 adipocytes (98), insulin increased leptin mRNA levels approximately twofold. It was concluded that insulin increased leptin at the transcriptional level because actinomycin D blocked the effect. Additionally, although leptin mRNA showed a rapid turnover (half-life of approximately 2 hr) in ob17 adipocytes, it was the same in the presence of absence of insulin (101).

In contrast to the ability of insulin administration to cause a prompt increase in leptin expression in rodents (86,91,104), several groups have failed to detect an effect of standard hyperinsulinemic-euglycemic clamps on leptin levels in lean, obese, or NIDDM patients (105,106). However, a rise in serum leptin levels after 72 hr of sustained hyperinsulinemia was recently reported (105). Consistent with this finding, in one report, isolated human adipocytes cultured with insulin for 72 hr showed a transient increase in leptin mRNA levels at 48 hr and an increase in secreted leptin at 72 hr (105).

Administration of pharmacological doses of the glucocorticoid dexamethasone to rats increases leptin mRNA levels. It was postulated that the ensuing rise in leptin explained the decreased food intake (107,108). Dexamethasone also caused a rapid increase in leptin mRNA levels in isolated rat adipocytes (96). The effect was detectable within 1 hr and reached a maximum (four- to eightfold increase) after 7 hr (96). The increase in leptin mRNA level was partially blocked by inhibition of protein synthesis, suggesting that dexamethasone may influence the expression of proteins that affect the rate of transcription or stability of leptin mRNA levels (96).

Agents that increase cyclic AMP decrease leptin expression in vivo and in vitro (85,101,108). Thus, adrenergic agonists that increase lipolysis and deplete fat stores also signal an increase in food intake.

A role for leptin in the pathogenesis of anorexia during infection has also been postulated. Administration of endotoxin and cytokines (TNF-α, IL-1) to hamsters increased leptin mRNA levels and circulating leptin protein (109).

Leptin mRNA may also be expressed in brown adipose tissue, although contamination by white adipocytes has not definitively been ruled out. In brown adipose tissue, leptin mRNA appears to be regulated by fasting in a parallel manner to white adipose tissue (99). Cold exposure markedly decreased brown, but not white, adipose tissue leptin mRNA levels, while β_3-adrenergic agonist decreased expression in both tissues (99). These data are consistent with a recent finding that agents that increase cAMP decrease leptin expression in isolated adipocytes (108).

Additional studies are needed (and sure to be rapidly forthcoming) to evaluate the hormonal and substrate factors that regulate the expression of leptin mRNA, synthesis and secretion in adipocytes. The intriguing possibility that increased cell size (swelling) per se could influence leptin gene expression has been suggested (92). It will also be important to assess whether the alterations in serum leptin levels are mainly a function of the number of adipocytes, their size, or both. Consistent with the notion that adipocyte size regulates leptin expression, preliminary evidence shows a higher expression of leptin mRNA in large versus small human adipocytes (92).

The recent identification, cloning, and mapping of brain receptors for leptin (OB-R) 76,77,110) to the *db* locus provide a molecular explanation for the similar phenotypes of *ob/ob* and *db/db* mice. *db/db* mice produce an abnormally spliced OB-R that lacks the intracellular domain thought to be important in signal transduction (77,78). A soluble form of the leptin receptor is also ex-

pressed in adipose and several other tissues (78). In addition to being expressed in the hypothalmus, the OB-R is present in peripheral tissues, including adipose tissue, suggesting that leptin may also have autocrine functions as well (78). Though administration of leptin in vivo decreases leptin mRNA levels in adipose tissue, in vitro addition of leptin to isolated fat cells does not down-regulate leptin expression (108).

V. AUTOCRINE AND PARACRINE MECHANISMS REGULATING ADIPOSITY

A. Evidence that Fat Cell Size is Regulated

The question of whether total body fat stores, fat cell number, or fat cell size is regulated has been addressed by assessing the response to surgical excision of adipose tissue (lipectomy, LPX). The literature is controversial with respect to whether regrowth of excised adipose tissues occurs and whether total body lipid stores are defended by compensatory enlargement of remaining depots (111). The depot excised (subcutaneous vs. gonadal), species, diet, age, hormonal status, and strain all influence the results (111–115). No regrowth of epididymal fat depots after lipectomy has been reported (111). Regeneration of subcutaneous fat depots reproducibly occurs after long periods of follow-up or when high-fat diets are fed (for a review see Ref. 111). Regrowth is more robust in hibernating species that seasonally adjust their body fat stores (112,116,117). Nevertheless, the LPX model has been useful for generating hypotheses about the role of fat cell size in regulating food intake.

Removing fat cells from an animal might logically be expected to increase food intake by decreasing leptin output, but this remains to be directly examined. An early report by Leibelt et al. showed hyperphagia in gold thioglucose obese mice in response to removal of epididymal fat pads (118). However, no increase in food intake has been noted in subsequent studies in nonobese animals (62,112,113,115). Lack of regrowth and lack of compensatory growth of other depots in genetically lean animals was observed by Kral (115) and by Faust et al. (114). Both investigators concluded that fat cell size may be regulated. Faust et al. provided evidence that feeding behavior was linked to adipocyte size in lipectomized rats fed a high-fat diet (113). After surgical removal of 25% of the adipocytes in rats, there was no immediate effect of lipectomy on food intake or body weight, and no difference in total-body fat stores after 19 weeks on a low-fat "chow" diet. When LPX and control groups were exposed to a high-fat diet, a similar degree of hyperphagia initially occurred in both groups. However, after a few weeks, the LPX group began to eat less than the control group and, accordingly, accumulated less total body fat. These data were interpreted as evidence that adipocyte hypertrophy "may not be a completely passive occurrence." Faust et al. went on to speculate that "it is likely that adipocyte resistance to enlargement was responsible for restraining the development of obesity" in lipectomized rats. In other words, LPX rats have fewer total fat cells to store lipid in and so reach maximum fat cell size more rapidly than controls. This attainment of maximum fat cell size incurs a down-regulation of food intake, presumably via some negative feedback mechanism.

While leptin was probably one signal that was restraining food intake in this experimental paradigm, there are most likely others, including the paracrine effects of adipocyte production of TNF and perhaps other cytokines that have a direct effect on adipocyte metabolism, limiting the capacity to store triglycerides (see below). Despite having a malfunctioning leptin pathway, Zucker *fa/fa* rats (like *db/db* mice) are able to regulate their body weight and appear to modulate their food intake in response to changes in fat cell size (119). Thus, there are likely to be multiple mechanisms restraining the expansion of adipose stores in response to a change in diet or other environmental challenges. Figure 1 illustrates potential feedback mechanisms by which adipocyte size may influence adipocyte metabolism and food intake.

B. Adipocyte TNF-α as a "Feedback" Regulator of Adipocyte Metabolism and Fat Cell Size

Hotamisligil et al. first reported that mRNA for the cytokine TNF-α was overexpressed in the adipose tissue of obese Zucker (*fa/fa*) rats and other genetic models of obesity (*db/db*, *tub/tub*, *ob/ob*), but not in acquired obesity models (MSG-induced) (120). There was no detectable expression of other cytokines in adipose tissue. Moreover, adipose tissue fragments from the obese animals secreted more TNF-α than that from lean controls (120). This result was unexpected because TNF-α overproduction by immune cells, in response to infection or neoplasia, had been thought to be a cause of cachexia, which entails a loss of fat stores (121). This "wasting syndrome" could be induced by the exogenous administration or production of human TNF-α in mouse models (121). Metabolic alterations associated with TNF-α overproduction include hypertriglyceridemia, increased lipolysis, decreased adipose tissue lipoprotein lipase activity and lipogenic gene expression, and insulin resistance in vivo. Furthermore, relatively high doses of hTNF-α induce a "dedifferentia-

tion" or lipid depletion of mouse adipocyte cell lines in vitro, including the down-regulation of a number of adipose-specific genes (122,123). These cachectic effects of TNF-α are seemingly incompatible with the enlarged adipose mass characteristic of obesity. However, in contrast to the effects of high doses of human TNF-α, which causes dedifferentiation, prolonged exposure of cultured mouse 3T3-F442A adipocytes to low doses of murine TNF-α causes a specific down-regulation of the expression of the mRNAs for the insulin-sensitive glucose transporter (GLUT4) and adipsin genes (120,123). In addition, low doses of murine TNF-α inhibit insulin receptor tyrosine kinase activity (98). Differential effects of murine and human TNF-α may be a consequence of the fact that hTNF-α interacts with only one of the two TNF-α receptors (the 55 kDa but not the 75 kDa) that affect different signaling pathways (13,121).

The fact that TNF-α is overexpressed in adipocytes of several obese-diabetic rodent models and appears to cause adipocyte insulin resistance led to the proposal that TNF-α could act as an "adipostat" or feedback regulator of adipocyte size (2). Serum levels of TNF-α, usually undetectable in lean rats, are elevated in Zucker fatty rats, though at still quite low levels, suggesting that adipose tissue production of TNF-α could affect systemic metabolism. To assess the potential importance of TNF-α in the insulin resistance of the Zucker fatty rat, Hotamisligil et al. infused soluble TNF-α receptor-IgG fusion protein to neutralize the effects of endogenous TNF-α (120,124). They observed a marked improvement in whole-body insulin sensitivity as assessed by a hyperinsulinemic-euglycemic clamp. This was due to an improvement in peripheral, but not hepatic, insulin action. Additional studies revealed that in vivo neutralization of TNF-α normalizes muscle and fat insulin receptor autophosphorylation and insulin receptor substrate-1 (IRS-1) phosphorylation (124). On the whole-body level, infusion of the soluble TNF-α receptor-IgG fusion protein decreases plasma glucose, plasma insulin, and free fatty acid levels (124). It has been suggested that the decline in FFA in this model was due to a enhancement of insulin's antilipolytic effect, though this has not yet been directly demonstrated (124). These data suggest that TNF-α plays an etiological role in the peripheral insulin resistance observed in obese diabetic animals.

Using a highly sensitive polymerase chain reaction assay, TNF-α expression was also detected in rat and human skeletal muscle and shown to be increased in insulin-resistant states in human subjects (125). Increased TNF-α production by macrophages from *ob/ob* and *db/db* mice has also been demonstrated (126). Thus, the relative con-

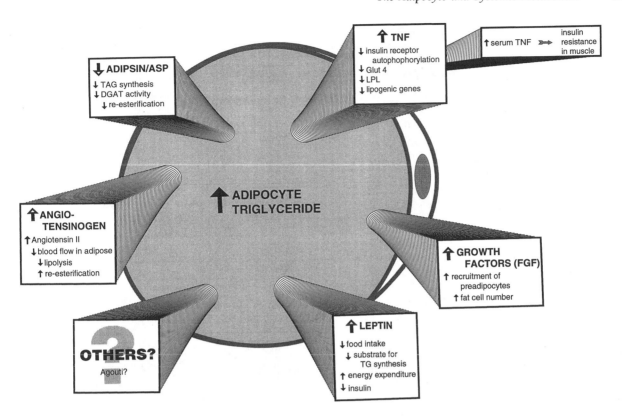

Figure 1 Feedback regulation of adiposity. The adipocyte produces a number of endocrine and paracrine factors that may serve as feedback signals to regulate fat cell size. These may serve as "adipostats" that slow further expansion of fat cell size and normally help maintain body fat levels within narrow limits. Regulatory failures that lead to sustained increases in fat cell size may also stimulate the recruitment of preadipocytes, which would lead to hyperplastic obesity. TAG, triacylglycerol; ASP, acylation-stimulating factor; TNF, tumor necrosis factor-α; FGF, fibroblast growth factor.

tribution of local and systemic production of TNF-α to muscle insulin resistance requires further investigation. It is not clear that adipose tissue is acting as an endocrine organ with regard to TNF-α.

It is noteworthy that the metabolic alterations characteristic of enlarged adipocytes from spontaneously obese, aging rats (decreased fatty acid synthesis, decreased insulin effect on glucose transport, increased lactate production) (4,127,128) are nearly identical to those produced by TNF-α, suggesting a causative role. These changes in adipocyte metabolism would normally serve to limit the expansion of fat cell size by decreasing rates of triacylglyceride synthesis. Consistent with the hypothesis that TNF-α protects against excess expansion of the adipose mass, a preliminary report found increased adiposity in mice in which the TNF-α receptor was knocked out (129). It remains to be determined whether specifically knocking out expression of adipocyte TNF-α or its receptor will influence the development of obesity or obesity-related insulin resistance. Additional studies are also needed to assess developmental aspects of adipose tissue TNF-α expression relative to the onset of tissue insulin resistance. The molecular mechanisms regulating adipose tissue TNF-α expression in response to nutritional or hormonal signals also remain to be elucidated.

The exciting observation that TNF-α may play a role in the development of insulin resistance in obese rodent models has been followed up with two recent studies of obese, nondiabetic humans. Adipose tissue TNF-α mRNA levels are elevated several fold in obese compared to lean subjects. In agreement with the initial studies on rodent adipose tissue, Kern et al. (130) found that TNF-α was expressed almost exclusively in human adipocytes, not in stromal cells or contaminating macrophages present in adipose tissue. Moreover, they found that adipose tissue TNF-α levels were proportional to body mass index or percent body fat, except in morbidly obese subjects (BMI > 45). The lack of elevated TNF-α expression in adipose tissue of severely obese subjects is hypothesized to be due to a regulatory failure, contributing to the high level of obesity. Both groups found that adipose tissue fragments from obese subjects also secrete more TNF-α, though plasma levels are undetectable (83,130).

Levels of TNF-α expression in adipose tissue tightly correlated with the level of hyperinsulinemia, a marker of insulin resistance in the obese normoglycemic subjects they studied (131). Both Kern et al. (130) and Hotamisligil et al. (131) find that TNF-α expression is decreased after weight reduction and stabilization at the lower body weight. The decline in TNF-α is associated with an increase in the expression of lipoprotein lipase (LPL) activity (130). Because TNF-α is known to decrease human adipose tissue LPL activity and LPL mRNA (132), it is tempting to speculate on a causal role for TNF-α in restraining the activity of human adipose tissue LPL in obesity and in increasing its activity after weight loss (83,133). In keeping with this idea, TNF-α has been shown to decrease GLUT4 levels and increase lipolysis (120,133), both characteristics of enlarged adipocytes from obese subjects. Taken together, these results support the hypothesis that TNF-α may have a role in the development of adipocyte insulin resistance in human obesity, and in limiting increases in adipocyte size. However, because serum levels of TNF-α are not elevated in obese humans, effects of adipose-derived TNF-α on muscle insulin resistance are tentative. It is possible that by regulating triglyceride uptake and efflux from adipose tissue (i.e., availability of fatty acid substrate for muscle), TNF-α could indirectly influence muscle insulin resistance. TNF-α increases lipolysis in humans in vivo (134) and in primary cultures of newly differentiated human preadipocytes (133). An effect of TNF-α in vitro in isolated adipocytes has not yet been demonstrated. Thus, while a paracrine role for TNF-α in adipose tissue metabolism in human obesity is supported by available evidence, it is not clear whether adipose production of this cytokine plays a direct role in the insulin resistance of muscle or in influencing the development of NIDDM in obese subjects. Interestingly, in Pima Indians, a population with a high prevalence of obesity and NIDDM, a linkage between obesity/body fat percent and a polymorphism in the TNF-α locus has recently been reported (135).

C. Adipsin, the Alternative Pathway of Complement and Acylation Stimulating Protein

Adipsin is a serine protease that is secreted by adipocytes. It was originally identified and cloned by Spiegelman and colleagues as a highly differentiation-dependent gene in 3T3-L1 adipocytes (136,137). Adipsin expression is markedly down-regulated in rodent obesities, and this is probably a consequence of elevated levels of insulin and glucocorticoids present in the obese state (138–140).

Sequence comparison revealed that mouse adipsin showed a high degree of similarity with human complement D (123), the initial and rate-determining enzyme in the alternative pathway of complement; adipsin is the murine version of this protein. Likewise, human adipsin is identical to complement D (141). Choy et al. (142) demonstrated that mouse adipose tissue synthesizes all of the proteins of the alternative complement pathway [factors C3, D (adipsin), and B]. The proximal (nonlytic) portion of the pathway is operative in adipose tissue. When adipose tissue fragments are incubated in vitro, this proteolytic cascade results in the generation of biologically active C3a (an anaphylatoxin), Ba and Bb, and other proteolytic fragments (142). The activity of the alternative complement pathway in cultured adipocyte cell lines and other tissues requires stimulation by cytokines. However, the proximal pathway is fully active in adipose tissue fragments even without stimulation by cytokines, possibly as a result of endogenous cytokine production. Additional research is needed to determine the primary functions(s) of the alternative complement pathway and how its activity in adipose tissue is controlled. A possible pathophysiological role for this pathway is suggested from the fact that partial acquired lipodystrophy is associated with constitutive activation of the alternative complement pathway (6,142).

It was originally speculated that the presence of the alternative pathway of complement in adipose tissue suggested a role in immunity, adipogenesis, or energy balance (6). An alternative hypothesis has been put forth by Sniderman and Cianflone (7,143). This group purified a 14-kD a serum protein that stimulated triacylglycerol synthesis in fibroblasts and adipocytes and hence was named acylating stimulating protein (ASP) (144,145). The serum concentration of this protein increased after a meal containing fat (146). Baldo et al. (143) demonstrated that ASP results from the cleavage of the terminal arginine residue from C3a by plasma carboxypeptidases. Because C3a is the end product of the alternative complement pathway, of which adipsin (complement D) is a main component, Sniderman and colleagues propose that the pathway be called the "adipsin-ASP pathway" (7).

ASP stimulates triglyceride synthesis to a greater extent than insulin, and furthermore, the ASP effect is additive with that of insulin (147,148). ASP stimulates the activity of diacylglycerol acyltransferase, the final enzyme in the triglyceride synthetic pathway (148) and is therefore hypothesized to also play a role in the regulation of reesterification. Consistent with an direct intracellular function of ASP, this protein also stimulates triglyceride synthesis when added to microsomes prepared from human adipose tissue (148).

More recent studies by Cianflone et al. demonstrate that human adipocytes also express mRNAs for adipsin, C3, and factor B, as well as produce factor C3a (147,149). They also showed that C3a generated in vitro has similar activity to ASP purified from plasma in stimulating triglyceride synthesis in differentiating human preadipocytes and fibroblasts (147). Human preadipocytes and fibroblasts secrete small amounts of ASP, which can increase eightfold upon differentiation of human preadipocytes in culture (147,149). Thus, a paracrine role of ASP in regulating human adipose tissue metabolism seems likely.

The fact that ASP is more potent than insulin in stimulating triacylglycerol synthesis in human adipose tissue supports a role for this protein in determining the rate at which fatty acids (derived from circulating triacylglycerols hydrolyzed by LPL) are esterified and stored in human adipose tissue. However, in contrast to results in rodent models, serum levels of adipsin tend to be increased in obese human subjects while adipsin secretion per fat cell is normal (150,151). However, considering that adipsin production is not increased in proportion to the increased adipocyte size, which is a contrast to many other adipocyte proteins, the relatively lower production of ASP could play a role in limiting the rate of triglyceride synthesis as fat cells enlarge. Consistent with this hypothesis, in vivo studies show that the esterification of triglyceride-fatty acids released by lipoprotein lipase is less efficient in obese than lean subjects (152–154). Further investigation will clarify whether the major role of ASP is in regulating local triacylglyceride uptake by fat cells and whether adipose tissue contributes to the pool of serum ASP and thus to systemic triglyceride clearance. The relationship of the activity of the adipsin-ASP pathway to the regulation of adipocyte size as well as the mechanisms of action of ASP must also be resolved.

D. Adipocyte Secretory Products and the Regulation of Adipocyte Number

As discussed in detail in another chapter, adipocytes secrete a number of hormones that exert paracrine effects on preadipocyte growth and differentiation. These include fibroblast growth factors (FGFs) and insulin-like growth factor I, as well as angiotensin II. Thus, local influences on the regulation of adipocyte number can potentially ac-

commodate failures in the feedback regulation of adipocyte size.

VI. OTHER ADIPOCYTE SECRETORY PRODUCTS WITH POSSIBLE METABOLIC ROLES

A. Acrp30: Adipocyte Complement-Related Protein of 30 kDa

Another novel secretory product expressed exclusively by adipocytes, Acrp30, has recently been discovered by screening a subtraction cDNA library of mRNAs induced during differentiation of 3T3-L1 adipocytes (155). Acrp30 shows similarity to complement factor C1q and a hibernation-specific protein isolated from the plasma of Siberian chipmunks. Western analysis showed that Acrp30 is a relatively abundant serum protein. The function of this protein is still unknown, but like adipsin, its secretion is modulated by insulin, suggesting that its expression may be regulated by nutritional status. Spiegelman's group also reported cloning of this protein, dubbing it "AdipoQ" and noting that its expression is markedly reduced in the adipose tissue of obese mice and humans (156).

B. Agouti

The *agouti* gene encodes a secreted protein that acts in a paracrine manner to antagonize the melanocyte-stimulating hormone receptor and thereby regulates mouse coat color. It is normally expressed only in skin of mice. Dominant mutations in the *agouti* locus cause agouti to be expressed in all tissues, producing a syndrome consisting of yellow fur, obesity, hyperinsulinemia, and insulin resistance (157). Ectopic expression of agouti in transgenic mice reproduces this syndrome (158). In contrast to mice, the human agouti gene is normally expressed in adipose tissue and testis (159) among other tissues (159), suggesting a role for this protein in regulating adipose tissue function. Agouti may produce insulin resistance by elevating the concentration of intracellular free calcium (160).

VII. SUMMARY AND CONCLUSIONS

We have reviewed the evidence that adipose tissue can regulate its own function (adipocyte metabolism, cell size and number) through the production of autocrine, paracrine, and endocrine signals. By regulating food intake, the adipocyte literally controls the flow of substrate available for storage of triglyceride. The efficiency of deposition is also affected by local regulation of blood flow (via adipocyte production of angiotensinogen), local production of TNF-α, which influences insulin signaling and lipogenic gene expression, and local production of ASP-adipsin, which may regulate intracellular triglyceride synthesis. There are undoubtedly many other mechanisms yet to be uncovered that regulate the level of energy stores by modulating the deposition and mobilization of adipose triglyceride pools. As discussed by Ailhaud, mechanisms also exist that allow mature adipocytes to signal the expansion of their size via recruitment of preadipocytes, subsequently causing development of hyperplastic obesity.

It is possible to conceive of the adipocyte as existing to meet the energy and substrate demands of other tissues in the body by producing lactate and glutamine, as well as fatty acids and glycerol. It is clear that future studies of systemic amino acid and glucose/lactate metabolism must take into account the contribution of adipose tissue. Growing evidence also indicates that the adipocyte is not a simple passive reservoir for lipid-soluble compounds, but also is involved in the regulated production of proteins involved in whole-body and local metabolism of lipids (fat-soluble vitamins, cholesterol) including CETP and RBP. Adipose tissue may have previously gotten short shrift as a dynamic metabolic organ, but as the pace at which novel genes can be identified quickens, new roles for adipose tissue are rapidly being exposed.

The era when "fat" was considered a metabolically inactive tissue of limited interest has surely ended. As pointed out by Frayn and colleagues (161), although adipose tissue consumes little oxygen relative to other tissues, "white adipose tissue is an exceptionally efficient participant in the regulation of fuel selection in the body as a whole." It is also important to realize that adipose tissue is not simply a recipient of hormonal and substrate commands from the rest of the body. Instead, depending on its triglyceride inventory, adipose tissue may actively increase or decrease food intake and energy expenditure.

REFERENCES

1. Wertheimer HE. Introduction—a perspective. In: Renold AE, Cahill GF, eds. Handbook of Physiology. Washington, DC: American Physiological Society, 1965:5–12.
2. Spiegelman BM, Hotamisligil GS. Through thick and thin: wasting, obesity and TNF-α. Cell 1993; 73:625–627.
3. Flier JS. The adipocyte: storage depot or node on the energy information superhighway? Cell 1995; 80:15–8.
4. DiGirolamo M, Newby FD, Lovejoy J. Lactate production in adipose tissue: a regulated function with extra-adipose implications. FASEB J 1992; 6:2405–2412.
5. Kowalski TJ, Watford M. Production of glutamine and utilization of glutamate by rat subcutaneous adipose tissue in vivo. Am J Physiol 1994; 266:E151–154.
6. Spiegelman BM, Choy L, Hotamisligil GS, Graves RA, Tontonoz P. Regulation of adipocyte gene expression in differentiation and syndromes of obesity/diabetes. J Biol Chem 1993; 268:6823–6826.
7. Sniderman AD, Cianflone K. The adipsin-ASP pathway and regulation of adipocyte function. Ann Intern Med 1994; 26:389–393.
8. Zhang Y, Proenca R, Maffei M, Barone M, Leopold L, Friedman JM. Positional cloning of the mouse obese gene and its human homologue. Nature 1994; 372:425–432.
9. Halaas JL, Gajiwala KS, Maffei M, et al. Weight-reducing effects of the plasma protein encoded by the *obese* gene. Science 1995; 269:543–545.
10. Campfield LA, Smith FJ, Guisez Y, Devos R, Burn P. Recombinant mouse OB protein: evidence for a peripheral signal linking adiposity and central neural networks. Science 1995; 269:546–549.
11. Pellymounter MA, Cullen MJ, Baker MB, et al. Effects of the *obese* gene product on body weight regulation in *ob/ob* mice. Science 1995; 269:540–549.
12. Weigle DS, Bukowske TR, Foster DC, et al. Recombinant ob protein reduces feeding and body weight in the *ob/ob* mouse. J Clin Invest 1995; 96:2065–2070.
13. Hotamisligil GS, Spiegelman BM. Tumor necrosis factor α: a key component of the obesity-diabetes link. Diabetes 1994; 43:1271–1278.
14. Marin P, Rebuffe-Scrive M, Smith U, Björntorp P. Glucose uptake in human adipose tissue. Metabolism 1987; 36:1154–1160.
15. Crandall D, Fried SK, Francendese AA, Nickel M, Digirolamo M. Lactate release from isolated rat adipocytes: influence of cell size, glucose concentration, insulin and epinephrine. Horm Metab Res 1983; 15:326–329.
16. Coppack SW, Frayn KN, Humphreys SM, Whyte PL, Hockaday TDR. Arteriovenous differences across human adipose and forearm tissues after overnight fast. Metabolism 1990; 39:384–390.
17. Frayn KN, Coppack SW, Humphreys SM, Whyte PI. Metabolic characteristics of human adipose tissue in vivo. Clin Sci 1989; 76:509–516.
18. Hagstrom E, Arner P, Ungerstaedt U, Bolinder J. Subcutaneous adipose tissue: a source of lactate production after glucose ingestion in humans. Am J Physiol 1990; 258:E888–893.
19. Newby DF, Wilson LK, Thacker SV, DiGirolamo M. Adipocyte lactate production remains elevated during refeeding after fasting. Am J Physiol 1990; 259:E865–871.
20. DiGirolamo M, Thacker SV, Fried SK. Effects of cell density on in vitro glucose metabolism by isolated adipocytes. Am J Physiol 1993; 264:E361–366.
21. Francendese AA, DiGirolamo M. Alternative substrates for triacylglycerol synthesis in isolated adipocytes of different size from the rat. Biochem J 1981; 194:377–384.

22. Watford M, Fried SK. Adipose tissue metabolism can now be directly studied in vivo. TIBS 1991; 16:201–202.

23. Jansson P-A, Larsson A, Smith U, Lonnroth P. Lactate release from the subcutaneous tissue in lean and obese men. J Clin Invest 1994; 93:240–246.

24. Frayn KN, Khan K, Coppack SW, Elia M. Amino acid metabolism in human subcutaneous adipose tissue in vivo. Clin Sci 1991; 80:471–474.

25. Maggs DG, Jacob R, Rife F, et al. Interstitial fluid concentrations of glycerol, glucose, and amino acids in human quadricep muscle and adipose tissue. J Clin Invest 1995; 96:370–377.

26. Tall AR. Plasma cholesteryl ester transfer protein. J Lipid Res 1993; 34:1255–1274.

27. Hayek T, Masucci-Magoulas L, Jiang X, et al. Decreased early atherosclerotic lesions in hypertriglyceridemic mice expression cholesteryl ester transfer protein transgene. J Clin Invest 1995; 96:2071–2074.

28. Jiang XC, Moulin P, Quinet E, et al. Mammalian adipose tissue and muscle are major sources of lipid transfer protein mRNA. J Biol Chem 1991; 266:4631–4639.

29. Martin LJ, Connelly PW, Nancoo D, et al. Cholesteryl ester transfer protein and high density lipoprotein responses to cholesterol feeding in men: relationship to apolipoprotein E genotype. J Lipid Res 1993; 34:437–446.

30. Quinet EM, Huerta P, Nancoo D, Tall AR, Marcel YL, McPherson R. Adipose tissue cholesteryl ester transfer protein mRNA in response to probucol treatment: cholesterol and species dependence. J Lipid Res 1993; 34:845–852.

31. Zechner R, Moser R, Newman TC, Fried SK, Breslow JL. Apolipoprotein E gene expression in mouse 3T3-L1 adipocytes and human adipose tissue and its regulation by differentiation and lipid content. J Biol Chem 1991; 266:10583–10588.

32. Tsutsumi C, Okuno M, Tannous L, et al. Retinoids and retinoid-binding protein expression in rat adipocytes. J Biol Chem 1992; 267:1805–1810.

33. Dullaart RPF, Sluiter WJ, Dikkeschei LD, Hoogenberg K, Van Tol A. Effect of adiposity on plasma lipid transfer protein activities: a possible link between insulin resistance and high density lipoprotein metabolism. Eur J Clin Invest 1994; 24:188–194.

34. Arai T, Yamashsita S, Hirano K, et al. Increased plasma cholesteryl ester transfer protein in obese subjects. A possible mechanism for the reduction of serum HDL cholesterol levels in obesity. Arterioscler Thromb 1994; 14:1129–1136.

35. Makover A, Soprano A, Wyatt ML, Goodman DS. Localization of retinol-binding protein messenger RNA in the rat kidney and in perinephric fat tissue. J Lipid Res 1989; 30:171–180.

36. Crandall DL, Herzlinger HE, Saunders BD, Kral JG. Developmental aspects of the adipose tissue renin-angiotensin system: therapeutic implications. Drug Dev Res 1994; 32:117–125.

37. Cassis LA, Saye J, Peach MJ. Location and regulation of rat angiotensinogen mesenger RNA. Hypertension 1988; 11:591–596.

38. Campbell DJ. Circulating and tissue angiotensin systems. J Clin Invest 1987; 79:1–6.

39. Saye JA, Cassis LA, Sturgill TW, Lynch KR, Peach MJ. angiotensionogen gene expression in 3T3-L1 adipocytes. Am J Physiol 1989; 256:C448–451.

40. Crandall DL, Herzlinger HE, Saunders BD, Armellino DC, Kral JG. Distribution of angiotensin II receptors in rat and human adipocytes. J Lipid Res 1994; 35:1378–1385.

41. Darimont C, Vassaux G, Ailhaud G, Negrel R. Differentiation of preadipose cells: Paracrine role of prostacyclin upon stimulation of adipose cells by angiotensin-II. Endocrinology 1994; 135:2030–2036.

42. Jonsson JR, Game PA, Head RJ, Frewin DB. The expression and localisation of the angiotensin-converting enzyme mRNA in human adipose tissue. Blood Pressure 1994; 3:72–75.

43. Darimont C, Vassaux G, Gaillard D, Ailhaud G, Negrel R. In situ microdialysis of prostaglandins in adipose tissue: stimulation of prostacyclin release by angiotensin II. Int J Obes 1994; 18:783–788.

44. Frederich, Jr., Kahn BB, Peach MJ, Flier JS. Tissue-specific nutritional regulation of angiotensinogen in adipose tissue. Hypertension 1992; 19:339–344.

45. Grodin IM, Siiteri PK, McDonald PC. Source of estrogens production in postmenopausal women. J Clin Endocrinol Metab 1973; 36:207–214.

46. Schindler AE, Ebert A, Friedrich E. Conversion of androstenedione to estrone by human fat tissue. J Clin Endocrinol Metab 1972; 35:627–630.

47. Deslypere JP, Verdonck L, Vermeulen A. Fat tissue: A steroid reservoir and site of steroid metabolism. J Clin Endocrinol Metab 1985; 61:564–570.

48. Ackerman GE, Smith ME, Mendelson CR, MacDonald PC, Simpson ER. Aromatization of androstenedione by human adipose tissue stromal cells in monolayer culture. J Clin Endocrinol Metab 1981; 53:412–417.

49. Price T, Aitken J, Head J, Mahendroo MS, Means GD, Simpson ER. Determination of aromatase cytochrome P450 messenger RNA in human breast tissues by competitive polymerase chain reaction (PCR) amplification. J Clin Encrinol Metab 1992; 74:1247–1252.

50. Cleland WH, Mendelson CR, Simpson ER. Effects of aging and obesity on aromatase activity of human adipose cells. J Clin Endocrinol Metab 1985; 60:174–177.

51. Hemsell DL, Grodin JM, Breuner PF, Sitteri PK, MacDonald PC. Plasma precursors of estrogens II. Correlation of the extent of conversion of plasma androstenedione to estrone with age. J Clin Endocrinol Metab 1974; 38:476–479.

52. Edman CD, MacDonald PC. Effect of obesity on conversion of plasma androstenedione to estrone in ovulatory and anovulatory young women. Am J Obstet Gynecol 1978; 130:456–461.

53. Bulun SE, Simpson ER. Competitive RT-PCR analysis indicates levels of aromatase cytochrome P450 transcripts in adipose tissue of buttocks, thighs and abdomen of women increase with age. J Clin Endocrinol Metab 1994; 78:798–803.

54. Simpson ER, Ackeman GE, Smith ME, Mendelson CR. Estrogen formation in stromal cells of adipose tissue of women: induction by glucocorticosteroids. Proc Natl Acad Sci USA 1981; 78:5690–5694.

55. Mendelson CR, Cleland WH, Smith ME, Simpson ER. Regulation of aromatase activity of stromal cells derived from human adipose tissue. Endocrinology 1982; 111: 1077–1085.

56. O'Neill JS, Elton RA, Miller WR. Aromatase activity in adipose tissue from breast quadrants: a link with tumor site. Br J Med 1988; 296:741–743.

57. Miller WR, O'Neill J. The importance of local synthesis of estrogen within the breast. Steroids 1987; 50:537–548.

58. Bulun SE, Mahendroo MS, Simpson ER. Aromatase gene expression in adipose tissue: relationship to breast cancer. J Steroid Biochem 1994; 49:4–6.

59. MacDonald PC, Edman CD, Porter JC, Sitteri PK. Effect of obesity on conversion of plasma androstenedione to estrone in postmenopausal women with and without endometrial concer. Am J Obstet Gynecol 1978; 130: 448–455.

60. Reid IR, Ames R, Evans MC, et al. Determinants of total body and regional bone mineral bone density in normal postmenopausal women—a key role for fat mass. J Clin Endocrinol Metab 1992; 75:45–51.

61. Kennedy GC. Role of depot fat in hypothalamic control of food intake in rat. Proc R Soc Lond B 1953; 140: 578–592.

62. Harris RBS. Role of set-point theory in regulation of body weight. FASEB J 1990; 4:3310–3318.

63. Weigle DS. Appetite and the regulation of body composition. FASEB J 1994; 8:302–310.

64. Hervey GR. The effects of lesions in the hypothalmus in parabiotic rats. J Physiol Lond 1959; 145:336–352.

65. Martin RJ, White BD, Hulsey MG. The regulation of body weight. Sci Am 1991; 79:528–541.

66. Harris RBS, Martin RJ. Specific depletion of body fat in parabiotic partners of tube-fed obese rats. Am J Physiol 1984; 247:R380–386.

67. Coleman DL. Obese and diabetes: two mutant genes causing diabetes-obesity syndromes in mice. Diabetologia 1978; 14:141–148.

68. Ogawa Y, Masuzaki H, Isse N, et al. Molecular cloning of rat obese cDNA augmented gene expression in genetically obese Zucker fatty (fa/fa) rats. J Clin Invest 1995; 96: 1647–1652.

69. Murakami T, Shima K. Cloning of rat obese cDNA and its expression in obese rats. Biochem Biophys Res Commun 1995; 209:944–952.

70. Considine RV, Considine EL, Williams CJ, et al. Evidence against either a premature stop codon or the absence of obese gene mRNA in human obesity. J Clin Invest 1995; 95:2986–2988.

71. Reed DR, Ding Y, Xu D, Cather C, Green ED, Price RA. Extreme obesity may be linked to markers flanking the human OB gene. Diabetes 1996; 45:691–694.

72. Clement K, Garner C, Hager J, et al. Indication for linkage of the human OB gene region with extreme obesity. Diabetes 1996; 45:687–690.

73. He Y, Chen H, Quon M, Reitman M. The mouse obese gene. Genomic organization, promoter activity and activation by CCAAT/enhancer-binding protein a. J Biol Chem 1995; 270:28887–28891.

74. Gong D, Bi S, Pratley RE, Weintraub BD. Genomic structure and promoter analysis of the human obese gene. J Biol Chem 1996; 271:3971–3974.

75. Isse N, Ogawa Y, Tamura N, et al. Structural organization and chromosomal assignment of the human obese gene. J Biol Chem 1995; 270:27728–27733.

76. Chua SC, Chung WK, Wu-Peng S, et al. Genotypes of mouse diabetes and rat fatty due to mutations in the OB (leptin) receptor. Science 1996; 271:994–996.

77. Chen H, Chariat O, Tartaglia LA, et al. Evidence that the diabetes gene encodes the leptin receptor: identification of a mutation in the leptin receptor gene in db/db mice. Cell 1996; 84:491–495.

78. Lee G, Proenca R, Montez JM, et al. Abnormal splicing of the leptin receptor in diabetic mice. Nature 1996; 379: 632–635.

79. Stephens TW, Basinski M, Bristow PK, et al. The role of neuropeptide Y in the antiobesity action of the obese gene product. Nature 1995; 377:530–532.

80. Levin N, Nelson C, Gurney A, Vandlen R, De Sauvage R. Decreased food intake does not completely account for adiposity reduction after ob protein infusion. Proc Natl Acad Sci USA 1996; 93:1726–1730.

81. Funahashi T, Shimomura I, Hiraoka H, et al. Enhanced expression of rat obese (ob) gene in adipose tissues of ventromedial hypothalamus (VMH)-lesioned rats. Biochem Biophys Res Commun 1995; 211:469–475.

82. Maffei M, Fei H, Lee G, et al. Increased expression in adipocytes of ob RNA in mice with lesions of the hypothalamus and with mutation at the db locus. Proc Natl Acad Sci USA 1995; 92:6957–6960.

83. Frederich RC, Lollmann B, Hamann A, et al. Expression of ob mRNA and its encoded protein in rodents. Impact of nutrition and obesity. J Clin Invest 1995; 96: 1658–1663.

84. Maffei M, Halaas J, Ravussin E, et al. Leptin levels in human and rodent: measurement of plasma leptin and ob RNA in obese and weight-reduced subjects. Nature Med 1995; 1:1155–1161.

85. Collins S, Surwit RS. Pharmacologic maniulation of ob expression in a dietary model of obesity. J Biol Chem 1996; 271:9437–9440.

86. Cusin I, Dainsbury A, Doyle P, Rohner-Jeanrenaud F, Jeanrenaud B. A relationship leading to clues to the understanding of obesity. Diabetes 1995; 44:1467–1470.

87. Masuzaki H, Ogawa Y, Hosaoda K, Kawada T, Fushiki T, Nakao T. Augmented expression of the obese gene in the adipose tissue from rats fed high-fat diet. Biochem Biophys Res Commun 1995; 216:355–358.

88. Mizuno TM, Bergen H, Funabashi T, et al. Obese gene expression: reduction by fasting and stimulation by insulin and glucose in mice, and persistent elevation in acquired (diet-induced) and genetic (yellow agouti) obesity. Proc Natl Acad Sci USA 1996; 93:3434–3438.

89. Frederich RC, Hamann A, Anderson S, Lollmann B, Lowell BB, Flier JS. Leptin levels reflect body lipid content in mice: Evidence for diet-induced resistance to leptin action. Nature Med 1995; 1:1311–1314.

90. Harris RBS, Ramsay TG, Smith SR, Bruch RC. Early and late stimulation of ob mRNA expression in meal-fed and overfed rats. J Clin Invest 1996; 97:2020–2026.

91. Zheng D, Jones JP, Usala SJ, Dohm GL. Differential expression of ob mRNA in rat adipose tissues in response to insulin. Biochem Biophys Res Commun 1996; 218: 434–437.

92. Hamilton BS, Paglia D, Kwan AYM, Dietel M. Increased *obese* mRNA expression in omental fat cells massively obese humans. Nature Med 1995; 1:953–956.

93. Lonnqvist F, Arner P, Nordfors L, Schalling M. Overexpression of the obese (*ob*) gene in adipose tissue of human obese subjects. Nature Med 1995; 1:950–953.

94. Considine RV, Sinha MK, Heiman ML, et al. Serum immunoreactive-leptin concentrations in normal-weight and obese humans. N Engl J Med 1996; 334:292–295.

95. Sinha MK, Ohannesian JP, Heiman ML, et al. Nocturnal rise of leptin in lean, obese, and non-insulin dependent diabetes mellitus subjects. J Clin Invest 1996;97: 1334–1347.

96. Murakami T, Iida M, Shima K. Dexamethasone regulates obese expression in isolated rat adipocytes. Biochem Biophys Res Commun 1995; 214:1260–1267.

97. Trayhurn P, Moira EA, Duncan JS, Rayner DV. Effects of fasting and refeeding on *ob* gene expression in white adipose tissue of lean and obese (*ob/ob*) mice. FEBS Lett. 1995; 368:488–490.

98. Macdougald OA, Hwang CS, Fan H, Lane MD. Regulated expression of the obese gene product (leptin) in white adipose tissue and 3T3-L1 adipocytes. Proc Natl Acad Sci USA 1995; 92:9034–9037.

99. Moinat M, Deng C, Muzzin P, et al. Modulation of obese gene expression in rat brown and white adipose tissues. FEBS Lett 1995; 373:131–134.

100. Zhang B, Graziano MP, Doebber TW, et al. Downregulation of the expression of the obese gene by an antidiabetic thiazolidinedione in Zucker diabetic fatty rats and *db/db* mice. J Biol Chem 1996; 271:9455–9459.

101. Leroy P, Dessolin S, Villageois P, et al. Expression of *ob* gene in adipose cells. J Biol Chem 1996; 271:2365–2368.

102. Hauner H, Entenmann G, Wabitsch M, Gaillard D, Ailhaud G. Promoting effect of glucocorticoids on the differentiation of human adipocyte precursor cells cultured in a chemically defined medium. J Clin Invest 1989; 84: 1663–1670.

103. Masuzaki H, Ogawa Y, Isse N, et al. Human obese gene expression. Adipocyte-specific expression and regional differences in the adipose tissue. Diabetes 1996; 44: 855–858.

104. Saladin R, De Vos P, Guerre-Millo M, et al. Transient increase in obese gene expression after food intake or insulin administration. Nature 1995; 377:527–529.

105. Kolaczynski JW, Nyce MR, Considine RB, et al. Acute and chronic effect of insulin on leptin production in humans. Studies in vitvo and in vitro. Diabetes 1996; 45:699–701.

106. Dagogo-Jack S, Fanelli C, Paramore D, Brotheres J, Landt M. Plasma leptin and insulin relationships in obese and nonobese humans. Diabetes 1996; 45:695–698.

107. De Vos P, Saladin R, Auwerx J, Staels B. Induction of ob gene expression by corticosteroids is accompanied by body weight loss and reduced food intake. J Biol Chem 1995; 270:15958–15961.

108. Slieker LJ, Sloop KW, Surface PL, et al. Regulation of expression of ob mRNA and protein by glucocorticoids and cAMP. J Biol Chem 1996; 271:5301–5304.

109. Grunfeld C, Zhao C, Fuller J, et al. Endotoxin and cytokines induce expression of leptin, the *ob* gene product, in hamsters. A role for leptin in the anorexia of infection. J Clin Invest 1996;97:2152–2157.

110. Tartaglia LA, Dembski M, Weng X, et al. Identification and expression cloning of a leptin receptor, OB-R. Cell 1995; 83:1263–1271.

111. Faust IM, Kral JG. Growth of adipose tissue following lipectomy. In: Cryer A, Van RLR, eds. New Perspectives in Adipose Tissue: Structure, Function and Development. London: Butterworths, 1985:319–332.

112. Hamilton JM, Wade GN. Lipectomy does not impair fattenting induced by short photoperiods or high fat diets in female syrian hamsters. Physiol Behav 1988; 43:85–92.

113. Faust IM, Johnson P, Hirsch J. Surgical removal of adipose tissue alters feeding behavior and the development of obesity in rats. Science 1977; 197:393–396.

114. Faust IM, Johnson PR, Hirsch J. Noncompensation of adipose mass in partially lipectomized mice and rats. Am J Physiol 1976; 231:538–544.

115. Kral J. Surgical reduction of adipose tissue in the male Sprague-Dawley rat. Am J Physiol 1996; 231:1090–1096.

116. Mauer MM, Bartness TJ. Body fat regulation after partial lipectomy in Siberian hamsters is photoperiod dependent and fat pad specific. Am J Physiol 1994; 266:R870–878.

117. Mauer MM, Bartness TJ. A role for testosterone in the maintenance of sesonally appropriate body mass but not in lipectomy-induced body fat compensation in Siberian hamsters. Obes Res 1995; 3:31–41.

118. Leibelt RA, Ichinoe S, Nicholson N. Regulatory influences of adipose tissue on food intake and body weight. Ann NY Acad Sci 1965; 131:559–582.

119. Vasselli JR, Fiene JA, Maggio CA. Relationship of adipocyte size to hyperphagia in developing male obese Zucker rats. Am J Physiol 1992; 262:1233–1238.

120. Hotamisligil GS, Shargill NS, Spiegelman BM. Adipose expression of tumor necrosis factor-α: direct role of obesity-linked insulin resistance. Science 1993; 259:87–91.

121. Tracey KJ, Cerami A. Tumor necrosis factor, other cytokines and disease. Annu Rev Cell Biol 1993; 9:317–343.

122. Petruschke T, Hauner H. Tumor necrosis factor-a prevents the differentiation of human adipocyte precursor cells and causes delipidation of newly developed fat cells. J Clin Endocrinol Metab 1993; 76:742–747.

123. Torti FM, Dieckmann B, Beutler B, Cerami A, Ringold GM. A macrophage factor inhibits adipocyte gene expression: an in vitro model of cachexia. Science 1985; 229:867–869.

124. Hotamisligil GS, Budavari A, Murray D, Spiegelman BM. Reduced tyrosine kinase activity of the insulin receptor in obesity-diabetes central role of tumor necrosis factor-α. J Clin Invest 1994; 94:1543–1549.

125. Saghizadeh M, Ong JM, Garvey WT, Henry RR, Kern PA. The expression of TNFα by human muscle. Relationship to insulin resistance. J Clin Invest 1996; 97:1111–1116.

126. Yamakawa T, Tanaka S, Yamakawa Y, et al. Augmented production of tumor necrosis factor-α in obese mice. Clin Immunol Immunopathol 1995; 75:51–56.

127. DiGirolamo M, Howe D, Esposito J, Thurman L, Owens JS. Metabolic patterns and insulin responsiveness of enlarging fat cells. J Lipid Res 1974; 15:332–338.

128. Zentella A, Manogue K, Cerami A. Cachectin/TNF-mediated lactate production in cultured myocytes is linked to activation of a futile substrate cycle. J Biol Chem 1993; 264:13369–13372.

129. Oster MH, Levin N, Moore M, Cronin MJ. TNF receptor-II (R2) knock-out mice develop diet induced obesity. FASEB J 1995; 9:A186 (Abstract).

130. Kern PA, Saghizadeh M, Ong JM, Bosch RJ, Deem R, Simsolo RB. The expression of tumor necrosis factor in human adipose tissue. Regulation by obesity, weight loss, and relationship to lipoprotein lipase. J Clin Invest 1995; 95:2111–2119.

131. Hotamisligil GS, Arner P, Caro JF, Atkinson RL, Spiegelman BM. Increased adipose tissue expression of tumor necrosis factor-α in human obesity and insulin resistance. J Clin Invest 1995; 95:2409–2415.

132. Fried SK, Zechner R. Effects of cachectin/tumor necrosis factor on human adipose tissue lipoprotein lipase activity, mRNA levels, and biosynthesis. J Lipid Res 1989; 30:1917–1923.

133. Hauner H, Petruschke T, Russ M, Rohrig K, Eckel J. Effects of tumour necrosis factor alpha (TNFα) on glucose transport and lipid metabolism of newly-differentiated human fat cell culture. Diabetologia 1995; 38:764–771.

134. Starnes F, Warren RS, Jeevanandam M, et al. Tumor necrosis factor and the acute metabolic response to tissue injury in man. J Clin Invest 1988; 82:1321–1325.

135. Norman RA, Bogardus C, Ravussin E. Linkage between obesity and a marker near the tumor necrosis factor-α locus in Pima Indians. J Clin Invest 1995; 96:158–162.

136. Cook KS, Min HY, Johnson D, et al. Adipsin: A circulating serine protease homolog secreted by adipose tissue and sciatic nerve. Science 1987; 237:402–404.

137. Cook KS, Groves DL, Min HY, Spiegelman BM. A developmentally regulated mRNA from 3T3 adipocytes encodes a novel serine protease homologue. Proc Natl Acad Sci USA 1986; 82:6480–6484.

138. Spiegelman BM, Lowell B, Napolitano A, et al. Adrenal glucocorticoids regulate adipsin gene expression in genetically obese mice. J Biol Chem 1989; 264:1811–1815.

139. Lowell BD, Flier JS. Differentiation dependent biphasic regulation of adipsin gene expresion by insulin and insulin-like growth factor-1 in 3T3-F442A adipocytes. Endocrinology 1990; 127:2898–2906.

140. Flier J., Cook KS, Usher P, Spiegelman BM. Severly impaired adipsin expression in genetic and acquired obesity. Science 1987; 237:405–408.

141. White RT, Damm D, Hancock N, et al. Human adipsin is identical to complement factor D and is expressed at high levels in adipose tissue. J Biol Chem 1992; 267:9210–9213.

142. Choy L., Rosen B, Spiegelman BM. Adipsin and an endogenous pathway of complement from adipose cells. J Biol Chem 1992; 12736–12740.

143. Baldo A, Sniderman AD, St-Luce S, et al. The adipsin-acylation stimulating protein system and regulation of intracellular triglyceride synthesis. J Clin Invest 1993; 92:1543–1547.

144. Germinario R, Sniderman AD, Manuel S, Lefebvre SP, Baldo A, Cianflone K. Coordinate regulation of triacylglycerol synthesis and glucose transport by acylation-stimulating protein. Metabolism 1993; 42:574–580.

145. Cianflone K, Sniderman AD, Walsh MJ, Vu J, Gagnon J, Rodriguez MA. Purification and characterization of acylation stimulating protein. J Biol Chem 1989; 264:426–430.

146. Cianflone K, Vu H, Walsh M. Sniderman AD. The metabolic response of ASP to an oral fat load. J Lipid Res 1989; 30:1727–1733.

147. Cianflone K, Roncari DAK, Maslowska M, Baldo A, Forden J, Sniderman AD. Adipsin/acylation stimulating protein system in human adipocytes: Regulation of triacylglycerol synthesis. Biochemistry 1994; 33:9489–9495.

148. Yasruel Z, Cianflone K, Sniderman AD, Rosenbloom M, Walsh M, Rodriquez MA. Effect of acylation simulating protein on the triacylglycerol synthetic pathway of human adipose tissue. Lipids 1991; 26:495–499.

149. Cianflone K, Maslowska M. Differentiation-induced production of ASP in human adipocytes. Eur J Clin Invest 1995;25:817–825.

150. Napolitano A, Lowell BB, Damm D, et al. Concentrations of adipsin in blood and rates of adipsin secretion by adipose tissue in humans with normal, elevated and diminished adipose tissue mass. Int J Obes 1994; 18:213–218.

151. Sniderman AD, Cianflone K, Eckel RH. Levels of acylation stimulating protein in obese women before and after moderate weight loss. Int J Obes 1991; 15:333–336.

152. Frayn KN, Shadid S, Hamlani R, et al. Regulation of fatty acid movement in human adipose tissue in the postabsorptive-to-postprandial transition. Am J Physiol 1994; 266:E3083–317.

153. Coppack SW, Evans RD, Fisher RM, et al. Adipose tissue metabolism in obesity: lipase action in vivo before and after a mixed meal. Metabolism 1992; 41:264–272.

154. Potts JL, Coppack SW, Fisher RM, Humphreys SM, Gibbons GF, Frayn KN. Impaired postprandial clearance of triacylglycerol-rich lipoproteins in adipose tissue in obese subjects. Am J Physiol 1995; 31:E5885–594.

155. Scherer PE, Williams S, Fogliano M, Baldini G, Lodish HF. A novel serum protein similar to C1q, produced exclusively in adipocytes. J Biol Chem 1996; 270: 26746–26749.

156. Hu E, Liang P, Spiegelman BM. AdipoQ is a novel adipose-specific gene dysregulated in obesity. J Biol Chem 1996; 271:10697–10703.

157. Manne J, Argeson AC, Siracusa LD. Mechanisms for the pleiotropic effects of the agouti gene. Proc Natl Acad Sci USA 1995; 92:4721–4724.

158. Klebig ML, Wilkinson JE, Geisler JG, Woychik RP. Ectopic expression of the agouti gene in transgenic mice causes obesity, features of type II diabetes and yellow fur. Proc Natl Acad Sci USA 1996; 92:4728–4732.

159. Wilson BD, Ollmann MM, Kang L, Stoffel M, Bell GI, Barsh GS. Structure and function of ASP, the human homolog of the mouse agouti protein Hum Mol Genet 1996; 4:223–230.

160. Zemel Mb, Kim JH, Woychik RP, et al. Agouti regulation of intracellular calcium: role in the insulin resistance of viable yellow mice. Proc Natl Acad Sci USA 1995; 92: 4733–4737.

161. Frayn KN, Humphreys SM, Coppack SW. Fuel selection in white adipose tissue. Proc Nutr Soc 1995; 54:177–189.

19

Brown Adipose Tissue

Jean Himms-Hagen
University of Ottawa, Ottawa, Ontario, Canada

Daniel Ricquier
National Center of Scientific Research, Meudon, France

I. INTRODUCTION

A. Definition of Brown Adipose Tissue

For many years biological and medical scientists have recognized the existence of deposits of a distinct brown-colored fatty tissue located at various sites in the bodies of a variety of mammals. Macroscopically similar to white adipose tissue (WAT), this tissue has been simply referred to as brown adipose tissue (BAT). The unilocular lipid-storing cells of WAT have been referred to as white adipocytes, whereas the multilocular lipid storing cells of BAT have been referred to as brown adipocytes. Intensive studies carried out during the past three decades, principally on laboratory rodents, have now furnished substantial information about internal metabolic processes of BAT* and some understanding of one physiological role of BAT within the mammalian organism, thermogenesis. These studies have revealed the presence within brown adipocytes of abundant mitochondria (which give them their brown color) and a unique mitochondrial protein not found in any other tissue. Because it enables the oxidation of substrates to proceed without the phosphorylation of ADP, this protein has become known as uncoupling protein (UCP). It has an important role in the thermogenic

---

*For further, more detailed information on this topic the reader is referred to books (1,2) and recent reviews (3–9).

capacity of BAT. Because it is readily identified in histological preparations, it can serve as a marker enabling the precise identification of mature brown adipocytes. This technique has now revealed that brown adipocytes are not limited to the discrete tissue masses hitherto recognized as BAT but are more widely distributed throughout the mammalian body.

BAT has traditionally been regarded as occurring in discrete depots, in interscapular, subscapular-intramuscular, axillary, intercostal, perirenal, and periaortic regions. The distribution is similar in rodents and in newborn human infants (Fig. 1). The distribution differs from that of WAT depots, which are in periovarian, mesenteric, epididymal or parametrial, retroperitoneal, inguinal, and other subcutaneous regions.

BAT contains several different cell types. Most abundant are mature multilocular brown adipocytes and endothelial cells associated with the vasculature. However, mature multilocular brown adipocytes, which express mRNA for UCP and contain abundant mitochondria and appreciable amounts of UCP, can also under certain circumstances be distributed within what have traditionally been regarded as WAT depots. They become more visible and acquire abundant mitochondria when the tissues have been subjected to chronic stimulation (see below). Thus, adipocytes with potential thermogenic properties are more generally distributed than previously thought. The physiological significance of the existence of these cells is as

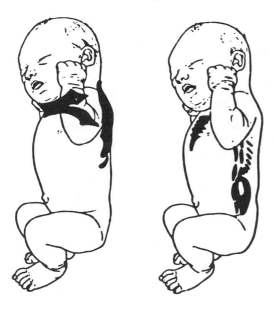

Figure 1 Distribution of depots of BAT in a newborn infant. (Left) Superficial intramuscular depots; (right) deeper depots in the thorax and abdomen. (From Dawkins MJR, Hull D. The production of heat by fat. Copyright © August 1965 by Scientific American Inc. All rights reserved.)

yet not clear. Their existence should not be ignored in considering some of the newer endocrine functions of adipose tissue.

Because brown adipocytes can occur in both "brown" and "white" adipose tissue depots, it is necessary to define our nomenclature for these cells. The terms "convertible adipose tissue" (10) and "masked brown adipocytes" (11) have been proposed. Here we use the term "dormant" brown adipocyte to mean a cell that does not express appreciable amounts of mRNA for UCP under resting conditions but does have the potential to do so when intensively stimulated by norepinephrine or by a β_3-adrenoceptor (AR) agonist. These cells are assumed to be present in WAT depots, mixed in among the mature white adipocytes. The nature of their innervation, if any, is unknown. They can be "awakened" when appropriately stimulated and then take on the appearance, characteristic gene expression, and large thermogenic capacity of mature brown adipocytes. Moreover, just as "white" adipose tissue depots can contain dormant or awakened brown adipocytes, so can "brown" adipose tissue depots contain mature unilocular white adipocytes, adjacent to the mature brown adipocytes (see below). Thus, adipose tissues at different locations and at different times span a spectrum, from typical BAT, in which most cells are innervated, mul-

tilocular mature brown adipocytes that express UCP, to typical WAT, in which the most visible cells by routine histology are noninnervated, unilocular mature white adipocytes that do not express UCP, even when stimulated by a β_3-AR agonist. The physiological significance of such plasticity of adipose tissues is not clear. Whether adult humans, often considered to possess little or no active BAT, have dormant brown adipocytes in their WAT depots is unknown, but human infants have been demonstrated to have uncoupling protein not only in BAT depots but also in a WAT depot (retroperitoneal) (12). The targeting by drugs for the treatment of obesity of this plasticity of adipose tissues is worth exploration.

B. Function of BAT and Its Control by the Sympathetic Nervous System

Interscapular BAT of the rat has been the most intensively studied BAT depot. Within this depot, the brown adipocytes receive a direct sympathetic innervation and their thermogenic function is controlled directly by norepinephrine acting upon adrenergic receptors (ARs). The production of heat by the brown adipocytes of this and other innervated BAT depots is important for thermoregulation, i.e., the maintenance of thermal balance, and is referred to as nonshivering thermogenesis to distinguish it from heat generated in muscles by shivering. It is evoked in mammals housed at temperatures below thermoneutrality and is controlled by norepinephrine secreted from the sympathetic nerves in the BAT. Newborn human infants, born with abundant BAT deposits (Fig. 1), can almost double their oxygen consumption when exposed to mild cold, an increase that occurs primarily in their BAT (13). The thermogenic capacity of the brown adipocyte, as reflected in the concentration of UCP in its mitochondria, matches closely the needs for thermoregulation. Thus, this concentration is extremely low in adult rats and mice living at thermoneutrality, rising manyfold at colder temperatures (14). At the usual temperatures at which rats and mice are housed, the concentration of UCP in their brown adipocyte mitochondria is already much higher than that at thermoneutrality. The thermogenic activity and capacity of BAT necessarily reflect the environmental temperature at which the animal has been living.

Thermogenic activity and capacity of BAT also reflect the nutritional status of the animal. Thus, both are reduced in the fasting state, increased in the fed state, and further increased when animals overeat a varied and palatable diet. Diet-induced thermogenesis refers to a sympathetic-mediated increase in energy expenditure for thermogenesis in BAT induced by this last type of diet.

Thermogenesis by the brown adipocyte is not continuous but occurs in episodes (15). It is hypothesized to serve not only to maintain body temperature but also to integrate feeding episodes with the animal's thermoregulatory needs, providing both initiation and termination signals for a single meal (16) (see below).

C. Abundance of Mitochondria and Unique Expression of UCP in BAT

The more intensively a brown adipocyte is stimulated by norepinephrine, the more abundant become its mitochondria and its total content of UCP. This is true of all species studied. In some species there is also a simultaneous and marked selective increase in synthesis of UCP, so the concentration of this protein in the mitochondria increases (rat, mouse, guinea pig), but this increase is absent or less marked in other species (Siberian and Syrian hamsters, Richardson's ground squirrel) (8). Conversely, a brown adipocyte that receives but little stimulation expresses very little UCP and contains very few mitochondria. The capacity to express UCP when stimulated is unique to the brown adipocyte, indeed defines a cell as a brown adipocyte (see below).

D. Subtypes of Adrenergic Receptors in BAT

Mature brown adipocytes in rats, mice, and newborn human infants contain β_3-ARs. These receptors are also present on the dormant brown adipocytes present in retroperitoneal WAT, at least in rats. The β_3-AR is, however, a late marker of the differentiated state and is absent from the precursor interstitial cells in the BAT. These precursor cells contain β_1-ARs and proliferate and differentiate in response to an action of norepinephrine on these receptors. Thus, stimulation by the endogenous neurotransmitter, norepinephrine, brings about hyperplasia of the BAT. Selective β_3-AR agonists are unable to recruit new cells within an adipose depot, although they can bring about marked mitochondrial proliferation within brown adipocytes already present (17).

α_1-ARs are also present in brown adipocytes. They interact synergistically with β_3-ARs to stimulate the activity of adenylate cyclase (18,19), to bring about induction of adenylate cyclase type III (19), and to induce c-*fos* expression (20). In rats, they participate synergistically in the action of norepinephrine to increase thyroxine 5′-deiodinase activity, hence in the selective increase in UCP synthesis brought about by the facilitative action of T_3 on the cAMP-mediated induction of UCP synthesis (21–24). In mice, β_3-ARs alone are able to mediate this effect (25).

In some species, α_2-ARs play an important inhibitory role in brown adipocyte responsiveness to norepinephrine but in most they do not.

E. BAT Function is Insulin-Dependent

Insulin has a direct action on brown adipocytes to increase glucose uptake via translocation of GLUT 4 (26,27). The sensitivity of BAT to this action of insulin is enhanced when thermogenesis is stimulated, as in a cold-exposed rat (28). In contrast, BAT usually develops resistance to insulin early in the development of obesity in animal models. Insulin also plays a vital role in maintaining the thermogenic capacity of BAT, influencing the synthesis of UCP and of GLUT 4 (29,30). However, insulin deficiency results in a low sympathetic activity (7), and there is a complex interaction between insulin and the sympathetic innervation in the control of BAT (31). Norepinephrine also has a direct effect on brown adipocytes to increase glucose entry but this does not require the translocation of glucose transporters to the plasma membrane (26,32,33).

F. BAT is Usually Atrophied in Animal Models of Obesity

BAT of obese animals is generally in a relatively atrophied state, usually secondary to a low activity of its sympathetic innervation. It has a very low content of UCP and a low capacity for thermogenesis (see Refs. 3,4). The concept that a deficit in energy expenditure due to lack of BAT thermogenesis might contribute to the development of obesity (34) has formed the basis of many studies of BAT in obese animals performed by many different researchers. However, in none was it possible to quantitate the contribution of the deficit to the obesity. Although the deficit usually preceded the development of hyperphagia, the hyperphagia that eventually occurred in most of these animal models of obesity obviously contributed to the obesity as much as, if not more than, the high metabolic efficiency due to the deficit in BAT thermogenesis.

Evidence for a causal relationship of lack of BAT thermogenesis to development of obesity has now been provided by the development of obesity in transgenic mice with genetic ablation of brown adipocytes (35). In these mice, brown adipocytes die when they are stimulated to express UCP because of the simultaneous expression of a transgene in which a toxigene is linked to the promoter of the UCP gene. That raising these mice at thermoneutrality to obviate the deficit in energy expenditure due to lack of BAT thermogenesis prevents both the obesity and the hyperphagia (36) provides evidence both for the important role for BAT thermogenesis in energy balance in animals living at temperatures below thermoneutrality and for a role of BAT thermogenesis in restraining food intake.

G. β_3-Adrenoceptors in Brown Adipocytes as a Target for Antiobesity Drugs

The development of selective β_3-AR agonists targeted to these receptors in brown and white adipocytes has been the subject of much research over the last 20 years. The first compounds developed were not completely devoid of any action on β_1- or β_2-ARs and, when tested in humans, induced side effects, such as increased heart rate and tremor. Much more highly selective products have now been developed. However, although they work well in rats and mice, as expected from their being targeted to rodent β_3-ARs, their efficacy in humans remains uncertain both because of the different pharmacology of the human β_3-AR and because of the unknown distribution and abundance of brown adipocytes, whether dormant or not, in human adipose tissues. The concept that a single compound could at the same time mobilize triacylglycerol stores from white adipocytes and promote their combustion in brown adipocytes remains, however, sufficiently attractive that further research on the development of such compounds for use in humans will undoubtedly continue.

II. MORPHOLOGY AND INNERVATION

A. Morphology, Origin, and Location of Brown Adipocytes

In the typical BAT depot, mature multilocular brown adipocytes and endothelial cells associated with the vasculature are the predominant cell types and are equally abundant. Of lesser abundance are the interstitial cells; these are precursor cells that can be induced to proliferate and differentiate into new mature brown adipocytes when the BAT is subjected to chronic stimulation by norepinephrine. Protoadipocytes and preadipocytes, stages in the differentiation of new mature cells, are usually detectable only when hyperplasia is being induced by chronic stimulation (37–39). A few mature white adipocytes are usually also present (40,41).

A typical mature, thermogenically competent brown adipocyte is characterized by the presence of multiple triacylglycerol droplets of various sizes and of abundant large mitochondria. These mitochondria contain closely packed cristae that are characterized by the presence of UCP. Such cells are present not only in typical BAT depots but also in typical white adipose tissue depots when these have been subjected to chronic stimulation by cold expo-

sure or by treatment with a β_3-AR agonist (see below). The origin of the mature brown adipocytes that appear in white adipose tissue depots subjected to chronic β_3-AR stimulation is not clear. It is unlikely that proliferation of precursors occurs in these depots because such precursors do not possess β_3-ARs. Described as dormant brown adipocytes, they are presumably very small cells with no morphological resemblance to brown adipocytes until their β_3-ARs are stimulated, upon which mitochondrial proliferation and expression of UCP give them the morphology of mature brown adipocytes. They are possibly a vestige of the brown adipocytes that were present in the depot at an early stage of development. However, different WAT depots contain different proportions of mature white adipocytes and dormant brown adipocytes. Not only can the latter be awakened when suitably stimulated, they can even acquire the innervation characteristic of mature brown adipocytes (42).

B. Vasculature of BAT and Blood Flow

The bilaterally symmetrical interscapular BAT of the rat has symmetrical thoracodorsal arterial and venous blood vessels supplying each side. In addition, a single centrally placed vein, Sulzer's vein, provides the major venous drainage. Arteriovenous anastomoses provide a means for control of entry of blood into the capillary bed that supplies the parenchymal cells of the BAT (43). Their closure shunts blood into the capillary bed whereas their opening shunts the blood directly into the venous drainage and away from the capillary bed, thus depriving the parenchymal cells of oxygen and inhibiting thermogenesis. Blood flow through BAT can increase up to 200-fold during the transition from the resting state to the thermogenically active state (15,44–46). The physiological significance of this arrangement is discussed further below.

C. Innervation of BAT

The most frequently studied BAT depot, in the interscapular location in the rat and mouse, has each of its two sides innervated by five to seven intercostal nerves as well as by paravascular nerves that run along the symmetrical arteries and veins. Most investigators find no cross-innervation between the two sides (47,48). The major nerves are extremely heterogeneous with most of the fibers traversing the BAT and proceeding on to the skin of the back. Parenchymal cells are innervated by abundant noradrenergic sympathetic nerves and also by less abundant capsaicin-sensitive, CGRP-containing sensory nerves. The vasculature has a complex innervation, with endings containing norepinephrine alone, or norepinephrine plus

NPY, or substance P, or CGRP. Arteriovenous anastomoses are innervated by nerves containing norepinephrine, CGRP, or substance P (43,49). Human BAT resembles rat BAT in its innervation and neurotransmitters (50,51).

Study of the central brain regions involved in control of BAT thermogenesis and growth has involved placement of lesions, or electrical or chemical stimulation of discrete brain areas (7). A generalization made on the basis of such studies has been that the lateral hypothalamus generally exerts an inhibitory influence on BAT whereas the ventromedial hypothalamus exerts an excitatory influence (7). Recent evidence has provided a new insight into the control of BAT by the hypothalamus. Electrical stimulation of the ventromedial hypothalamus induces a decrease in BAT temperature for as long as the stimulation is applied and a large increase in BAT temperature once the stimulation is stopped (52,53). Both effects require an intact innervation, and the reduction in temperature is mediated via the lateral hypothalamus. Control of reduction in temperature is suggested to be via opening of arteriovenous anastomoses via release of neuropeptides whereas the increase in temperature involves both the closing of the arteriovenous anastomoses, shunting the blood to the capillary bed, and the direct action of norepinephrine on the parenchymal cells. It is suggested that norepinephrine from sympathetic nerves closes the arteriovenous anastomoses via an action on α_1-ARs, directing blood to the capillary bed, where it acts on β_3-ARs on brown adipocytes to increase thermogenesis. This suggestion would explain the observed synergism between α_1- and β-adrenergic agonists to increase BAT blood flow in vivo (46). Selective β_3-adrenergic agonists are less effective than norepinephrine in increasing blood flow through BAT (54), probably because they lack the ability to act on the α_1-ARs to close the arteriovenous anastomoses.

The turning up and turning down of the temperature of BAT by the hypothalamus allows fine control of the temperature of the BAT, particularly important during feeding episodes (see below).

III. DEVELOPMENT AND OCCURRENCE

A. Fetal Development

BAT is present in the newborn or young of most species that require nonshivering thermogenesis to compensate for heat loss when they leave the maternal nest. The precise time at which brown fat develops during the perinatal period varies between species, obviously related to differences in the degree of maturity at birth. In most species, BAT differentiates during fetal life, but it may have reached its full development already at birth, as in the case of

guinea pigs, or only during the days following birth, as in rats, or even later at several weeks, in Syrian hamsters (55,56).

During the last week of fetal development, rapid growth of BAT in mouse and rat is accompanied by morphological differentiation of adipocytes, increase in number and complexity of mitochondria, and pronounced changes in mitochondrial enzymes such as cytochrome c oxidase and F1-ATPase; the UCP appears for the first time 2 days before birth and rapidly increases in the next few days (57–60). In bovine fetus, low levels of UCP and of UCP mRNA are present in perirenal adipose tissue at the beginning of the third trimester of gestation; the levels then increase until birth (61). UCP is present in adipose tissue of fetal rhesus monkeys delivered by cesarean section on day 135 of gestation (82% of term) (62) and in interscapular and perirenal adipose tissues of fetal reindeer 2 weeks before birth (63).

In the human fetus, all developing adipose tissue has the brownish-orange color that is considered typical for the perirenal and interscapular fat in rodents and accounts for about 1% of body weight (64). Using the histological criteria of multilocularity, brown adipocytes are present in human embryos at the 20th week of gestation (65,66). Characteristic BAT (67) and UCP is present in premature infants at 25–27 weeks of gestation (65,68,69) and doubles between the 25th and the 32nd week (69).

B. Occurrence in Different Species

1. BAT in Small Mammals

BAT is present during the whole life span in insect eaters (hedgehog, mole, shrew), hibernators (hamster, squirrel, marmot, doormouse, spermophile, bats) or nonhibernating rodents (mouse, rat), and carnivores (polecat, marten, badger). The presence of BAT in small mammals and its importance, either at birth in lagomorphs (rabbit) and hystricomorphs (guinea pig), or during the first weeks of life or cold exposure in rat and mouse, or at arousal from hibernation, have been recognized for a long time (see Ref. 1). It represents 1% of body weight in adult rat and 5% in newborn rabbit and newborn guinea pig (64).

2. BAT in Large Mammals (Except Humans)

BAT is present in newborn lambs (70,71), cattle (71), goats (72,73), dogs (74,75), reindeer (63), and young monkeys (macaque, rhesus, chimpanzee, baboon, and marmoset) (76,77). BAT does not occur in prototherian mammals (monotremes) or in metatherian mammals (marsupials) (78). Although there is some histological evidence for the presence of small amounts of BAT in pigs, a sensitive immunoreactive system is unable to detect UCP in adipose tissue of pigs at the age of 4 days or several weeks (79). In fact, although the UCP gene is present in domestic and wild pigs, no expression of the UCP mRNA can be detected (D. Ricquier, unpublished data).

3. BAT in Humans

Six major depots constituting 90% of the total brown fat have been identified in the infant: these depots are in cervical, axillary, perirenal, periadrenal, and pericardiac regions and in the posterior part of the abdominal cavity; the remaining 10% is found in other sites: along thoracic aorta, intercostal arteries, abdominal aorta, saphenous veins, and in omentum (Fig. 1) (68,80).

With increasing age, BAT accumulates lipid, and increasing proportions of the cell population become unilocular, so ultimately it may be indistinguishable from white fat on histological grounds. Although it is mainly unilocular, adult fat occurring at sites that contained BAT in the fetus and infant can be considered as inactive BAT. Clusters of typical BAT-type multilocular cells have been found in adults, at all the sites in which it occurs in infancy. It is more readily identified in younger subjects and those exposed to cold environments, but it has been found in subjects of all ages (65,68,81–83). BAT may also exist in humans as a tumor termed hibernoma (84–86).

BAT of newborn infants has a thermogenic function similar to that in animals (87). Indeed, the BAT of a newborn infant can double the resting metabolic rate on exposure to mild cold (26°C) (13). There is some evidence for more active BAT in infants kept at 22–27°C than 34°C, and in undersized infants who have greatest problems with temperature maintenance (88). It has been reported that multilocular brown fat is more conspicuous in infants dying with "crib death" (65,88) where there is an increase in circulating catecholamines; crib death certainly has a heterogeneous etiology and it has been proposed that BAT may be contributing to some cases through excessive thermogenesis. Increased BAT activity was also measured in children with malignant disease (89). That volatile anesthetics inhibit thermogenesis in animal brown adipocytes suggests that these agents could contribute to hypothermia in infants during surgery (90,91).

In adult humans the contribution of BAT to any process of temperature control or metabolic regulation remains controversial (68,81). BAT in human adults is, however, of interest because, if present and functionally active, it may have a regulatory role in body weight. In adult humans the distinction between brown and white fat cannot be made macroscopically, and it is impossible to give an estimate of how much brown fat adults retain from neonatal life or to quantitate the contribution of BAT to nonshivering thermogenesis and diet-induced thermogenesis in humans. Some evidence suggests that BAT may retain some thermogenic function. Sleeping energy expenditure is reduced in obese type 2 diabetic women during mild cold exposure (88), suggesting that a defect in thermogenesis similar to that in genetically obese animals may be present. Perirenal fat had reverted to a typical brown fat-type histology in two elderly subjects dying after admission to hospital with hypothermia (92). More abundant multilocular BAT and presence of UCP have been reported in the cervical adipose tissue of outdoor workers and alcoholics, but not in indoor workers (82,83). Such evidence is quite persuasive for a thermogenic function of BAT in humans.

The most useful index of both the identification of brown adipocytes and their thermogenic capacity is their content of UCP. Using specific antiserum against purified human UCP or rat UCP, it has been possible to demonstrate that UCP is present in BAT mitochondria of infants and adults (12,68,81,83,93). UCP is present at low concentrations in BAT of preterm infants and at higher concentrations in infancy (68). The most striking situation in adult life when BAT returns to its "active" histological appearance is in the presence of pheochromocytoma, a catecholamine-secreting tumor of the chromaffin tissue (93–95). UCP and UCP mRNA were also detected in human hibernoma in patients with (84) or without (86) pheochromocytoma. UCP was immunologically detected in subscapular and pericarotid fat from alcohol consumers (83). Cloning of a DNA probe specific for UCP allowed the detection of UCP mRNA in adipose depots of infants and adults (12,84,96). In adults, significant UCP mRNA was present in perirenal adipose tissue from patients with pheochromocytoma and also in perirenal adipose tissue of individuals in pathological situations other than pheochromocytoma (12) and in human hibernoma (84,86).

In conclusion, the role of BAT in diet-induced thermogenesis and body weight regulation remains uncertain because quantitation of BAT and its thermogenic capacity is exceedingly difficult in adults. From the concentrations of UCP in adult adipose tissue in sites of BAT, it would seem, however, that this tissue could not account for more than 1 or 2% of overall energy expenditure.

C. Growth of BAT Induced by Cold Acclimation

The coordinated growth of BAT that occurs during acclimation to cold involves hyperplasia (more mature brown adipocytes) and expansion of the mitochondrial mass, both in the brown adipocytes already present and in the new brown adipocytes. Interstitial precursor cells are stimulated to proliferate. They then differentiate via proto-adipocytes and preadipocytes into mature cells (37,38,97). This proliferation is induced by an action of norepinephrine on a β_1-AR on the precursor cells (98). Chronic treatment of rats with a selective β_3-adrenergic agonist is unable to induce hyperplasia of BAT (99–101). In contrast, the mitochondrial proliferation involves an action of norepinephrine on a β_3-AR on the mature cells; expression of the β_3-AR is a late marker of differentiation (98,99). Chronic stimulation results in induction of synthesis of adenyl cyclase type III (19) such that, despite a down-regulation of β_3-ARs (102), the capacity of the tissue to respond to norepinephrine is preserved. A selective increase in UCP synthesis and insertion into the mitochondria is also induced by norepinephrine and is facilitated by the T_3 produced by the increased activity of thyroxine 5′-deiodinase also brought about by the norepinephrine, an effect that requires an action of the norepinephrine on both β- and α_1-ARs (21–24). All these consequences of cold acclimation require the participation of the nerves that innervate BAT and can be mimicked by chronic administration of norepinephrine (37,59,103–106).

IV. PHYSIOLOGICAL FUNCTIONS AND THEIR CONTROL

A. Role in Thermogenesis During Cold Exposure (Small Mammals and Newborn Infants)

The most obvious and longest-known role for BAT thermogenesis is in the maintenance of homeothermy, that is, in thermoregulation. In mammals, all metabolic processes release heat in all organs of the body (107). However, overall metabolic heat production can be subdivided into two components. First, obligatory thermogenesis is a necessary consequence of the metabolic reactions that are essential for life in the resting state. It occurs continuously in all organs of the body regardless of the temperature to which the animal is exposed and includes the heat necessarily released during the ingestion and processing of the food eaten. Second, facultative thermogenesis is extra heat production that can be fairly rapidly switched on and off over and above obligatory thermogenesis. Facultative thermogenesis includes heat generated specifically for thermoregulatory purposes. There are two main components, cold-induced nonshivering thermogenesis, which occurs in BAT and is sympathetic-mediated, and cold-induced shivering thermogenesis, which occurs in skeletal muscles and is mediated by the motor nerves to the mus-

cles. Facultative thermogenesis also includes heat produced as a by-product of muscle metabolism during voluntary exercise.

For energy balance to be achieved, both obligatory thermogenesis and the additional facultative thermogenesis must be balanced by an equal intake of energy. It must be realized, therefore, that facultative thermogenesis is contributing to overall energy expenditure at all temperatures below thermoneutrality (which is 28–29°C for the rat and 32–36°C for the newborn baby). At mild cold temperatures, this facultative thermogenesis takes the form of BAT thermogenesis, with shivering evoked only at cooler temperatures. Smaller animals have a greater surface area in relation to their metabolic mass and a lesser opportunity for insulation than do larger animals. Smaller animals thus have a greater heat loss per unit metabolic mass than do larger animals and a greater need to increase their heat production in the cold. The use of BAT thermogenesis to combat cold is developed to its greatest extent in smaller mammals that live successfully in a wide variety of habitats, some rather cold. The use of BAT thermogenesis is also common in newborn mammals, even in larger species that lack it when adults, such as humans and many ruminants such as sheep and cows.

The most frequently studied species, the laboratory rat, once its BAT has grown in response to long-term acclimation to cold at 4°C, is able to supplement its resting obligatory heat production by three- to fourfold when exposed to cold or when infused with norepinephrine to switch on BAT thermogenesis (44–46). Most of this extra heat production occurs in its BAT (44–46), a remarkable capacity for metabolism by such a small amount of tissue. The newborn human infant likewise has a remarkable capacity to supplement its obligatory energy expenditure at thermoneutrality (34–35°C) by more than twofold when it is exposed to very mild cold (26–28°C, actually not cold at all for an adult) (13). The newborn infant is unable to shiver and this increase in thermogenesis occurs primarily in BAT (108).

B. Role in Thermogenesis in Hibernators During Arousal from Hibernation

The thermogenic function of BAT was first discovered in studies of hibernating animals; indeed, BAT was known as the "hibernating gland" for many years because of its abundant presence in hibernators. There is no doubt that thermogenesis in BAT plays an important part in the rapid warming up of the body that occurs when a hibernating animal arouses from hibernation to euthermia (109). Shivering thermogenesis in muscle also contributes to this warming up, the relative contributions of nonshivering thermogenesis in BAT and shivering thermogenesis in muscle varying from species to species.

Many hibernating species develop seasonal hyperphagia and obesity in preparation for the energy needs of the hibernating state and arousal (110). They also grow more BAT at the same time. The way in which this is controlled, i.e., growth of BAT without simultaneous activation of thermogenesis, is still not understood for any species studied. It seems not to be mediated by the sympathetic nervous system.

C. Role in Energy Balance

A role for BAT thermogenesis in energy balance was proposed in 1979 on the basis of two lines of evidence. First, defective BAT thermogenic function in an animal model of obesity, the genetically obese *ob/ob* mouse, suggested that a deficit in energy expenditure in BAT might contribute to the development of obesity (3,4,34). Second, stimulated BAT growth and thermogenesis in rats overeating a varied and palatable "cafeteria" diet suggested that enhanced energy expenditure for diet-induced thermogenesis in BAT in normal animals might help to defend against obesity (111,112) (see below). Numerous studies during the intervening years have reinforced these suggestions but have been unable to make any quantitative assessment of the role of BAT thermogenesis in energy balance. The recent finding of early development of obesity in an animal model that virtually lacks functional BAT, the UCP-DTA mouse (35), has provided convincing evidence for an important role for BAT in energy balance. However, these mice also eventually become hyperphagic, which also contributes to their obesity. Since raising these mice at thermoneutrality prevents both the obesity and the hyperphagia (36), the hyperphagia may be secondary to the lack of heat production by the BAT. An additional role for BAT in control of energy balance lies in its participation in thermoregulatory feeding (see below).

D. Role in Control of Thermoregulatory Feeding (Rodents and Newborn Infants)

A recently proposed thermoregulatory feeding hypothesis ascribes to BAT thermogenesis a central role in control of both onset and termination of a feeding episode in rats living in a constant environment with a regular lighting schedule (16). Episodes of greatly increased sympathetic nervous system activity, 8–12/day and mostly during the dark phase when body temperature is high, initiate bouts of BAT thermogenesis, such that temperature of the body starts to rise. The greatly increased utilization of glucose by the stimulated BAT results in a transient dip in blood glucose concentration, known from other evidence to precede and to initiate the onset of a meal. The rat starts to eat while BAT thermogenesis and the increase in body temperature continue. Termination is brought about by the high level of core temperature in response to thermo-regulatory needs. Feeding stops, stimulation of the sympathetic nervous system ceases, BAT thermogenesis is switched off, and body temperature starts to decrease slowly until the next burst of sympathetic activity is initiated, again for thermoregulatory needs. When the precise control of an increase in BAT temperature is lost, as in many animal models of obesity that have atrophied BAT, the termination signal is weakened and meal size increases. Feeding is thus viewed as the outcome of a thermoregulatory event. Rats do not eat to warm up. They start to eat only after they have started to warm up and stop eating once they have warmed up. Feeding can also be initiated by other cues, such as presentation of palatable food. The BAT-generated termination signal, however, is probably also important for meals initiated for reasons of palatability.

The thermoregulatory feeding hypothesis most likely applies to newborn human infants in the first few weeks of life as well (108). These infants possess abundant BAT deposits with a sufficient capacity for thermogenesis to allow them to more than double their energy expenditure when exposed to very mild cold. The cyclic feeding pattern of newborn infants fed on demand during the first few weeks of life follows precisely the pattern outlined above for rats, except that they do not have a circadian rhythm in body temperature and eat meals at fairly frequent intervals through the day and night. The cry with which the infant attracts the mother's attention is part of the arousal initiated by the start of the episode of increased sympathetic activity and BAT thermogenesis, as is the nutritive suckling response and the behavior of the mother. A similar cold-induced vocalization in newborn rats is closely associated with stimulated BAT thermogenesis and respiratory activation (113).

BAT thermogenesis is seen here as an integral part of a physiological feeding control system that links thermal balance with energy balance. The hypothalamus plays an integrating role in both thermal balance and energy balance via its influence on BAT thermogenesis and on routes of blood flow through BAT. The mediation of the sympathetically mediated thermoregulatory feeding control system by β_3-ARs in BAT reveals another important role for the existence of this subtype of β-AR in rats and newborn human infants. The resistance of the β_3-AR to desensitization ensures that loss of receptor function during a feeding episode, such as might occur if it were mediated by β_1- or β_2-ARs, is avoided and precise timing of the meal duration and size can occur.

E. Role in Diet-Induced Thermogenesis

Diet-induced thermogenesis in BAT of rats was originally described as a sympathetically mediated increase in energy expenditure for thermogenesis in BAT, brought about by overeating a varied and palatable diet (111,112). Prolonged overeating of such a diet resulted in growth of BAT, hence increased the capacity for diet-induced thermogenesis. Diet-induced thermogenesis decreases feed efficiency and thus is believed to combat the obesity that would otherwise result from the overeating. A new and complementary view of the physiological significance of diet-induced growth of BAT is provided by the postulated role of BAT in control of episodes of thermoregulatory feeding (see above). The increased capacity for BAT thermogenesis would be expected to allow more rapid warming during a feeding episode, hence more rapid attainment of the termination signal for feeding. This would result in ingestion of smaller meals. Diet-induced thermogenesis in BAT can thus also be viewed as a defense mechanism against hyperphagia, combatting the induction of hyperphagia by the variety and palatability of the foods offered.

Obese animals are generally found to have an impaired capacity for diet-induced growth and thermogenesis in BAT, secondary to the low activity and responsiveness of their sympatheitc nervous system to diet (3–5).

The interpretation of the term "diet-induced thermogenesis" has varied among researchers in this field, some using it to describe any increase in energy expenditure after a meal, including the energy cost of processing the food itself, more properly called the thermic effect of the food (107). Using the definition above, i.e., an increase in energy expenditure for thermogenesis in BAT that is mediated by activation of the sympathetic nervous system, and given the rather small number of thermogenically competent and innervated brown adipocytes in adult humans, it seems likely that the capacity of adult humans for diet-induced thermogenesis in brown adipocytes is rather small.

V. MOLECULAR MECHANISMS AND THEIR CONTROL

A. Differentiation Program of Brown Adipocytes Versus White Adipocytes

Obvious morphological and functional differences demonstrate that white and brown adipocytes are different (Fig. 2). Earlier studies on the ontogenic development of adipose tissue have led to some confusion in the area; during the differentiation of WAT, the adipocytes go through a stage which, at the magnification of light microscopy, has a morphological appearance similar to brown adipocytes. This apparent continuum of morphology from multilocular to unilocular adipocytes led to the suggestion that brown fat is a tissue that is, in fact, identical with embryonic white fat and that persists in a permanently embryonic state. Brown fat is now, however, recognized as a tissue in its own right; it is not an immature form of white fat or a transition form in the genesis of adipose tissue (56,114).

I. Two Types of Adipocyte Exist

It is presently accepted that two types of adipose tissues exist. Certain precursors have the potential to develop only into brown adipocytes, while others develop only into white adipocytes (114). This is illustrated by the fact that when precursor cells are isolated from a characteristic BAT depot, these precursors differentiate in vitro into UCP-containing brown adipocytes (115,116) whereas precursors obtained from a characteristic white-type depot never express UCP upon differentiation (117).

The existence of two types of precursor cells is strongly supported by analysis of the development of white and brown adipose tissues in young Syrian hamsters (118). Adipocyte precursor cells appear in the interscapular region at about 12 days' gestation. Shortly after birth, they accumulate lipid forming a single droplet that increases in size and this adipose depot appears to be WAT at this stage of development. By 3–4 days of age a second cell type appears among the unilocular cells in close association with the circulatory system. These new cells increase in number during development and they look like typical multilocular brown adipocytes, packed with mitochondria. They constitute almost 100% of the tissue mass by 15 days. The adipose depot has the appearance of BAT. UCP appears in interscapular adipose tissue only on the 7–8th day of life in the hamster and its specific content increases 80 times between day 8 and day 17 (118). At birth the histological appearance of inguinal fat is similar to that of interscapular tissue, and unilocular cells develop and mature without appearance of multilocular stages; brown adipocyte precursors and brown adipocytes never appear in inguinal deposits, which retain the appearance of WAT depots. These results indicate that the precursor cells of brown adipocytes are present at birth in the interscapular deposits, and that these cells differ from those of the inguinal region.

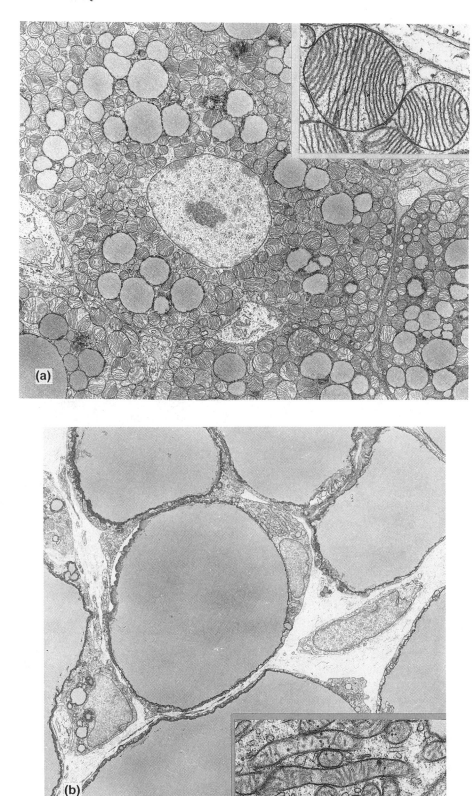

Figure 2   Ultrastructure of brown and white adipocytes of a young rat. (a) Interscapular BAT (×7000; inset ×26,500). (b) Epididymal WAT (×5000, inset ×36,500). Insets show details of the mitochondrial structure of these two types of adipocyte. Note the greater number, size, and density of cristae of mitochondria in brown adipocytes compared with white adipocytes.

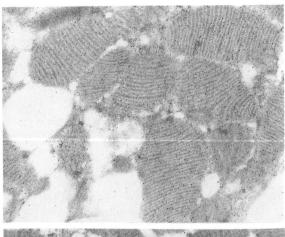

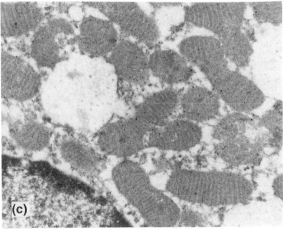

(c)

Figure 2 (*Continued.*) (c) UCP in the cristae of BAT by immunogold labeling (×34,000). Interscapular BAT of young rats maintained either at 4°C (top) or 20°C (bottom) is shown. Note the much greater density of gold particles on the cristae of BAT mitochondria of the cold-acclimated rat, indicative of a greater concentration of UCP in these membranes. (Electron micrographs prepared by Dr. Saverio Cinti.)

2. Adipose Depots Are Heterogeneous

For a long time it has been considered that certain adipose depots are exclusively brown or white. In fact, several reports indicate that many depots generally considered as either brown or white also contain a minority of adipocytes of the other type. Typical brown adipocytes are present in parametrial fatpad of mouse (119) and rat (11). Typical brown adipocytes were characterized in periovarian fat tissue using electron microscopy and detection of UCP mRNA and UCP by immunocytochemistry, immunoelectron microscopy, and Western analysis of isolated mitochondria (11,120). Many UCP-containing adipocytes were also detected in several white-type adipose depots of

baboons (121). In human adults, islets of multilocular adipose cells embedded in white adipose tissue depots have been described (12,51). These observations are in agreement with the detection of UCP (68,83,122) and UCP mRNA (12) in white adipose depots of human adults.

3. Plasticity of Adipose Tissues and Role of Dormant Brown Adipocytes

In large mammals such as sheep, cattle, goats, reindeer, and humans (61,63,65,68,71–73), most of the tissue that is of the brown type in newborns and infants takes on the appearance of the white type with advancing age.

Acclimatization of mice for 1 week at 5°C and then exposure for 1 hour 2–3 times daily at −20°C for 1 week induces appearance of a significant amount of UCP mRNA of UCP in mitochondria in the inguinal fatpad, which is generally considered to be white adipose tissue (10). Such a phenomenon was not observed in other white adipose depots. Morphological and morphometric analysis showed that inguinal adipose tissue appeared as BAT whereas, in control mice, inguinal adipose tissue was UCP-negative and appeared as WAT. Conversely, after readaptation to 28°C, inguinal adipose tissue of cold-stressed mice did not contain UCP and again resembled white adipose tissue. These observations led Lončar (10) to propose the existence of a third type of adipose tissue termed "convertible adipose tissue," suggesting that adipocytes forming this depot, although they appear to be of the white type at room temperature, have the potential to express UCP and develop thermogenic mitochondria under severe cold exposure. Interestingly, Lončar (10) also reported that adipocytes of other adipose depots of the white type maintain their original phenotype during cold stress and are unable to be converted into brown adipocytes; they are genuine white adipocytes.

The spectacular reinduction of typical and functional brown adipocytes in adult patients with pheochromocytoma (93–95), in adult dogs treated with a β_3-AR agonist (75), in WAT depots of rats treated with a β_3-AR agonist (100,101), and in periovarian WAT of cold-exposed or β_3-agonist-treated rats (11,120) could be explained both by recruitment of brown adipocyte precursors and by activation of "dormant" brown adipocytes (see Introduction), i.e., cells that need the appropriate stimulus to express UCP and all features that make brown adipocytes mophologically and functionally distinct from white adipocytes.

In conclusion, the question of what makes adipoblasts that are apparently similar to be engaged in the differentiation program of either white or brown adipocytes has not been solved. We believe there exist two types of adipocytes deriving from distinct precursor cells: (1) white adipocytes, which will never contain thermogenic mitochondria or express UCP, and (2) brown adipocytes, which, according to species, age, and anatomical location, may either maintain a brown adipocyte phenotype or be inactive and dormant and appear under an apparent phenotype of the white type or of a precursor cell; however, under certain conditions (cold exposure, pheochromocytoma, pharmacological treatment), such dormant brown adipocytes recover their brown adipocyte phenotype.

B. High Content of Mitochondria and Its Control

A very large amount of mitochondria is the most obvious and spectacular feature of brown adipocytes (Fig. 2) and it confers on brown adipocytes their very high oxidative capacity. The appearance is quite different from that of the white adipocyte (Fig. 2). Brown adipocyte mitochondria are unique in that they contain UCP in their inner membrane (Fig. 2) and, in contrast to mitochondria of other tissues, they contain relatively little F_0F_1-ATPase and have a relatively low capacity for oxidative phosphorylation (123). White and brown preadipocytes both possess a relatively high number of mitochondria, but upon differentiation the former have lost a high proportion of their mitochondria while the latter have increased and developed their mitochondria. The understanding of the differential mechanism of control of mitochondriogenesis is probably the key to elucidate the molecular mechanisms of white and brown adipocyte specific differentiation.

C. Expression of UCP

UCP occupies a central role in brown fat biology both because it is a marker unique to brown adipocytes and because it confers on mitochondria and brown adipocytes their physiological capacity to dissipate oxidation energy as heat. These features of the UCP have led investigators to try to elucidate the cell-specific control of transcription of the UCP and the mechanism of the uncoupling activity of the protein.

I. UCP Is a Regulated Proton Translocator of the Inner Mitochondrial Membrane

In agreement with early postulates that heat production and uncoupling in brown fat mitochondria result from proton reentry into the matrix (124), purification and reconstitution experiments established that UCP is a membranous proton translocator (6,125). Such experiments, as well as analysis of isolated mitochondria and brown adipocytes, demonstrated that purine nucleotides inhibit

UCP under conditions where heat production is not needed. Upon stimulation of cells by norepinephrine and subsequent lipolysis, free fatty acids directly activate UCP, which provokes heat production (126) (Fig. 3). The exact mechanism of ion transport by UCP is not explained yet. Three models for the role of fatty acids in H^+/OH^- transport have been proposed (9): fatty acids are activators that stimulate the H^+-translocating pathway; fatty acids anions are translocated by UCP; the carboxyl group of fatty acids acts as H^+ acceptor or donor.

The primary structure of the UCP was established both by amino acid sequencing and by cDNA or gene sequencing for several species (6,125,127–133), including humans (96). The first and most striking observation that arose from sequence analysis was that UCP, which was the second mitochondrial carrier to be sequenced, is related to the ADP/ATP carrier and is a member of the mitochondrial transporter family, which also consists of the phosphate carrier, the oxoglutarate/malate carrier, and the citrate carrier; all these carriers probably derive by triplication from a common ancestor (6,125,134).

Predictions of secondary structure of UCP and other mitochondrial transporters suggested the presence of six transmembrane α-helices linked by hydrophilic loops (134). This predicted folding of the UCP in the membrane was confirmed by the localization of epitopes present on one side or the other side of the membrane (135, 136). Using 2-azido-ATP labeling (137) and expression of UCP mutants in yeasts (138), amino acids forming the nucleotide-binding site were identified. Except for the folding of UCP in the membrane and the identification of the amino acids involved in nucleotide binding, limited information on its functional organization is available; in particular, the amino acid residues participating in the activator effect of fatty acids and the proton translocation itself are unknown but they will be probably identified using recombinant expression of mutated UCPs.

2. Control of UCP Expression

Denervation of interscapular brown fat of rats and treatment of animals with catecholamines have demonstrated that norepinephrine released by sympathetic fibers innervating brown adipocytes is the main physiological activator of UCP synthesis (7,80). The development of primary culture system (115,116,139) as well as isolation of immortalized brown adipocyte cell lines (140–143) allowed the demonstration of the direct activation of UCP synthesis by norepinephrine in brown adipocytes.

UCP synthesis is strongly regulated at the transcriptional level (59,115) and mRNA stabilization can also participate in maintaining a high level of UCP mRNA

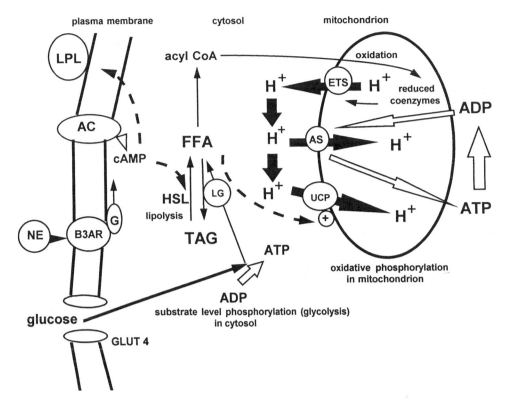

Figure 3 Major metabolic processes in a mature brown adipocyte when thermogenesis is stimulated by norepinephrine released from sympathetic nerves in the BAT. Norepinephrine (NE) released from a nearby sympathetic nerve interacts with a β_3-adrenoceptor (B3AR). Via activation of a G-protein (G), adenylate cyclase is stimulated to make cyclic AMP (cAMP). The concentration of cAMP increases. This stimulates the activity of protein kinase A, which then phosphorylates inactive hormone-sensitive lipase (HSL) to make it active. The increase in hormone-sensitive lipase activity increases the rate of lipolysis and the concentration of fatty acids (FFA) increases. The increase in FFA level has two effects. First, they are the signal for the increased operation of the uncoupling protein (UCP) in the inner mitochondrial membrane, which allows protons to enter the mitochondrion more rapidly, thus dissipating the proton gradient created by the electron transport system (ETS). Second, they are activated to acyl CoA, transported into the mitochondrion via the carnitine shuttle, and serve there as the fuel for thermogenesis. Their oxidation in the fatty acid β-oxidation cycle and the tricarboxylic acid cycle generates reduced coenzymes. The rate of operation of the electron transport system (ETS) increases because it is no longer restrained by the proton gradient against which it pumps protons. The reduced coenzymes are oxidized more rapidly; hence the rate of operation of the two cycles that produce them likewise increases. Synthesis of ATP by the proton-translocating ATP synthetase (AS) slows because the energy of the proton gradient is no longer sufficient to drive it. The overall effect is that oxidation of fatty acids derived from endogenous triacylglycerol stores (TAG) is increased, the energy released appearing as heat. Fatty acids can also be derived from blood-borne lipoproteins (chylomicrons and very low density lipoproteins) by the stimulated BAT because cAMP induces the synthesis of lipoprotein lipase (LPL). The brown adipocyte, operating in this uncoupled mode, might become depleted of its ATP but for the stimulation by norepinephrine also of glucose entry. This effect involves activation of the glucose transporter, GLUT 4, but not its translocation to the plasma membrane. The glucose which enters is metabolized via glycolysis, providing ATP by substrate level phosphorylations. The major product is lactate, which is exported to the blood, conveyed to the liver, and reconverted to glucose by gluconeogenesis. Some of the pyruvate produced in glycolysis is converted to fatty acids via lipogenesis (LG) and these fatty acids are then oxidized or cycled back into triacylglycerol. The brown adipocyte is also able to increase glucose uptake in response to insulin, a response that does involve translocation of GLUT 4 to the plasma membrane (not shown). This occurs after a meal, when the glucose that enters is used for synthesis of triacylglycerols, both fatty acids and the glycerol backbone, to replenish the fat stores in the brown adipocyte.

(144,145). The main effect of norepinephrine on UCP induction results from recruitment of β_1-, β_3-, and, to a lesser extent α_1-adrenoreceptors (9,80). UCP synthesis can be triggered by addition of cAMP to differentiated brown adipocytes (115,116,140). Besides norepinephrine, UCP synthesis requires other hormones such as T3, which amplifies fourfold the transcriptional response of the UCP gene to norepinephrine (139,144,146–148) and insulin (29,31,139) or IGF-1 (148). In lambs, UCP mRNA synthesis in in vitro differentiated brown adipocytes is dependent on glucocorticoids (149) whereas rat UCP gene expression is inhibited by corticosterone (150) although it was reported that addition of dexamethasone to cultured rat brown adipocytes after confluence elevated the mRNA level of UCP (151). Recent studies of rat UCP gene promoter demonstrated that retinoids, alone or in synergy with cAMP, can also activate UCP gene transcription (152,153).

The analysis of molecular events controlling the unique transcription in brown adipocytes and its regulation by hormones has been undertaken. The start site for transcription of the rat and mouse UCP gene and several DNase I-hypersensitive sites have been identified in the 5′-flanking region. Analysis of mouse and rat UCP gene promoter by transfection experiments and transgenic mice revealed both tissue-specific and adrenergic response elements in 3 kb of 5′-flanking DNA (152,153). A 200-bp enhancer element located at −2.3 kb was first identified by Cassard-Doulcier et al. (152) and confirmed by three other studies (23,154,155). Whether this enhancer is involved or not in the specific transcription mechanism is a matter of debate; an alternative hypothesis for the specific transcription of UCP gene in brown adipocytes is based on the possible existence of an inhibitory region downstream of the enhancer (152). In agreement with the well-known functional control of UCP gene transcription, Kozak et al. (154) identified cyclic-AMP-response elements located in the enhancer and in the proximal region of the promoter. The UCP gene enhancer has a complex organization and it contains regulatory elements that can bind both retinoid receptors (155,156) and thyroid hormone receptors (23,156); this enhancer can also bind CCAAT/enhancer binding proteins (157). In addition to these cis elements, in vitro analysis of interactions between DNA and nuclear proteins identified NF1, ets1, and Sp1 as putative trans factors (156). The dissection of the UCP gene will have to be extended to identify the exact transcription factors and molecular mechanisms that control its tissue-specific transcription.

D. The β_3-Adrenoceptor: Species Differences in Expression, Pharmacology, and Control Mechanisms

In the mid-1970s it became apparent that β-ARs of the rat white adipocyte are neither β_1- or β_2-AR but are atypical (158). The main features of atypical β-ARs, now termed β_3-ARs, are that they mediate responses that are insensitive to most standard β-AR antagonists, they have a low affinity for norepinephrine, they can be activated by certain antagonists of β_1- and β_2-ARs such as CGP 12177, and they are activated by novel agonists, BRL37344 and notably CL-316,243 (17,158–165).

1. β_3-Adrenoceptor Structure and Gene

The presence of β_3-AR in brown adipocytes was definitively established by the cloning of β_3-AR gene and cDNA (165–169). The β3AR is present in brown and white adipocytes of most small mammals except the guinea pig (170,171) and is the predominant β-AR in BAT of the rat (172). The presence of β_3-ARs in brown adipocytes of large mammals will be discussed below.

The β_3-AR gene and cDNAs have been cloned for human (166,173–176), mouse (167), rat (168,169), and bovine (177). The rat and mouse β_3-ARs are 80% and 82% identical, respectively, to the human β_3-AR. In fact, the level of homology between the different cloned β_3-ARs is higher (93 or 94%) in regions that are predicted to be transmembranous segments. The β_3-AR differs from both β_1-AR and β_2-AR in having a low sequence homology and a short carboxy-terminal tail. The β_3-AR lacks serine and threonine residues, which are potential phosphorylation sites for the β-AR kinase in the carboxy-terminal tail and a consensus sequence for protein kinase A-mediated phosphorylation, both in the third intracellular loop and in the carboxy-terminal tail; moreover, tyrosine residues possibly involved in agonist-promoted down-regulation are lacking (158,160,161,178,179). At the genomic level, the β_3-AR gene differs from other AR genes in that it contains several exons (161,165,169,175,176,180–182).

2. Physiological Function of β_3-Adrenoceptor in BAT

Many in vivo and in vitro studies have demonstrated that the β_3-AR plays an important role in rodent BAT thermogenesis. β_1-AR stimulation of adenylyl cyclase of rat BAT occurs at low norepinephrine concentration whereas activation of β_3-ARs only occurs at higher concentration of norepinephrine (161,183). Treatment of rats with a β_3AR agonist increases the level of UCP mRNA (59,184). The treatment of adult dogs with a β_3-AR agonist, now known as a partial agonist, induced a spectacular reinduction of BAT (75). The synthesis of DNA in mouse brown fat precursor cells is due to the exclusive stimulation of β_1-AR by norepinephrine; as the brown adipocyte differentiates, it acquires β_3-ARs (185,186). In primary culture, β_3-AR agonists strongly activate UCP synthesis in differentiated brown adipocytes (115,116, 139,187); such an effect apparently results from cAMP induction. The β_3-AR also participates in the control of glucose utilizaton by BAT (188), which is known to be stimulated by norepinephrine (189).

Recently, the exact role of β_3-AR in BAT was reevaluated using CL-316,243, a new, highly selective β_3-AR agonist in rodents (99,100,101). When administered to rats, this compound induced a doubling of BAT protein content without hyperplasia and provoked a marked proliferation of mitochondria, with no change in UCP concentration in mitochondria. Such data point out a particular role of β_3-ARs in mitochondrial proliferation in mature brown adipocytes. Thus, CL-316,243-induced hypertrophy of BAT differed from that induced by chronic stimulation of the tissue by norepinephrine, which also induces hyperplasia and a selective increase in UCP concentration in mitochondria. Selective β_3-AR agonists are unable to recruit new cells in BAT since they lack the β_1-AR-mediated effect of norepinephrine in precursor cells. They can, however, prevent or reverse diet-induced obesity in rats (99), genetic obesity in *fa/fa* rats (100,101) and yellow KK mice (190), and hypothalamic obesity in monosodium glutamate–treated mice (191). In fact, mature brown adipocytes of rodents possess both β_1-ARs and β_3-ARs; at low concentrations, norepinephrine stimulates respiration in brown adipocytes mainly through β_1-ARs; β_3-ARs may represent the physiological receptors for the neurotransmitter secreted from sympathetic nerve endings when its concentration is very high and also as soon as the high-affinity β_1-ARs are desensitized (192,193).

A transgenic mouse that lacks β_3-ARs and has no thermogenic response to a selective β_3-AR agonist does nevertheless have a normal thermogenic response to norepinephrine and normal growth and accumulation of UCP in its BAT in a cold environment (194), as well as a normal increase in thyroxine 5′-deiodinase activity (195). These effects are presumably mediated by the action of norepinephrine on β_1-ARs, which are overexpressed in BAT and substitute for β_3-ARs when these are absent (194).

3. The β_3-Adrenoceptor in Human BAT

β_3-AR mRNA can be detected in human WAT (122,175,196–198) but the existence of a functional β_3-AR in human white fat cells is still a matter of debate

(161–164). However, β_3-AR mRNAs are abundant in UCP-containing perirenal adipose tissue from infant and also from adult patients with pheochromocytoma (122, 175,181) and binding studies using a selective agonist for the β_3-AR (199) indicate the presence of β_3-ARs in infant BAT (200). These data show that human brown adipocytes can transcribe the β_3-AR gene. However, the difficulty in obtaining fresh BAT has not permitted a functional assay of β_3-AR in human BAT. Even if human brown adipocytes have functional β_3-ARs, it remains to be demonstrated whether the low amount of BAT present in human adults can contribute to a physiological response to β_3-AR agonists and whether such compounds will be efficient antiobesity drugs. Humans may well resemble the bovine rather than the rodent in that β_3-ARs and UCP are present in fetal and neonatal life but both disappear with age as BAT is replaced by WAT (201).

4. β_3-Adrenoceptor Regulation

The level of β_3-AR mRNA is lower by 60% and 71%, respectively, in brown and white fat in obese (*fa/fa*) Zucker rats (168). Impaired expression and activity of β_3-AR was also described in obese (*ob/ob*) mice (202). Adrenalectomy of *fa/fa* rats increases the low level of β_3-AR mRNA to normal but is without effect in lean rats, suggesting a suppressive influence of excess glucocorticoids on expression of this gene (203). It might be supposed that amelioration by adrenalectomy of the low sympathetic activity that is known to occur in BAT of obese animals (3,4) brought about this effect. However, excessive sympathetic stimulation, as during cold exposure, down-regulates β_3-ARmRNA in BAT, an effect prevented by denervation (102). Moreover, treatment of cultured brown adipocytes by β-adrenergic agonists or cAMP results in a marked down-regulation of β_3-AR mRNA level within several hours (186). However, other studies of β_3-AR mRNA in animals exposed to cold or injected with norepinephrine or adrenalectomized and studies based on denervation of BAT led to complex results that do not explain the role of the neurotransmitter in β_3-AR mRNA regulation (158,161,204).

Thyroid status influences the level of all three subtypes of β-AR in BAT. In the hypothyroid state, β_1- and β_2-AR mRNAs are reduced, apparently secondary to the increase in sympathetic nervous system activity in the tissue (205). In contrast, β_3-ARmRNA and β_3-AR number are increased in BAT in the hypothyroid state but are decreased in WAT, both changes reversed by thyroid hormone (206).

The structural differences between β_3-AR and other β-ARs mentioned above (the β_3-AR lacks most of the amino acid residues involved in the phosphorylation normally associated with desensitization of β-ARs) suggest that β₃-AR could be coupled to stimulatory G-proteins in a different way from β₁- and β₂-ARs and that the β₃-AR may desensitize less than β₁- and β₂-ARs (158,160,161). In agreement with this hypothesis, analysis of β₃-AR expressed in heterologous systems indicated that the β₃-AR did not display short-term agonist-promoted desensitization (207,208). In addition, long-term norepinephrine infusion in animals induced desensitization of β₁-AR and β₂-AR but not of β₃-AR in white adipocytes (209). However, a physiological desensitization was observed in β₃-adrenergically stimulated hamster brown adipocytes by a group (210) that explained this phenomenon by a significant decrease in the amount of functional G-protein per unit of adenylate cyclase that occurs in the plasma membranes of cold-acclimated animals (211,212).

β₃-ARs play certainly a major role in brown adipocytes, which have a dense noradrenergic innervation. Their biological importance is high in BAT of rodents, hibernators, and probably, newborn human infants. Although their importance in adult humans is not well established, they are receptors of interest to develop selective thermogenic and antiobesity compounds.

E. Expression of Other Factors and Proteins

In addition to UCP and β₃-AR which have been extensively studied, BAT expresses a number of proteins of interest such as type II thyroxine 5'-deiodinase and adipocyte determination and differentiation factor 1 (ADD1). As also shown for WAT, BAT has the capacity to synthesize and sometime secrete many peptide factors, which supports the idea that it possesses functions different from lipid metabolism and thermogenesis (213,214).

1. Thyroxine 5'-Deiodinase

Most metabolic effects of thyroxine are due to triiodothyronine produced by deiodination of thyroxine. Three different thyroxine 5'-deiodinases (types I, II, and III) can convert thyroxine to triiodothyronine. These enzymes differ in the molecular site of their deiodination, substrate specificity, reaction kinetics, inhibitor sensitivity, tissue distribution, and physiological regulation. Rat BAT contains a high activity of type II thyroxine 5'-deiodinase, which is insensitive to propylthiouracil and has a low K_m for T_4; in contrast, rat epididymal fat contains only type I 5'-deiodinase activity (215). Development and maturation of brown adipose tissue in rodents, bovines, ovines, and humans is preceded by 5' deiodinase induction (9). However, in contrast with rodent (215) or human brown fat (216) where the type II 5'-deiodinase predominates, the

main form of thyroxine deiodinase in BAT of fetal calves and in BAT of young goats and newborn lambs is type I (73,217,218).

There are no available structural data on type II 5'-deiodinase. Physiological studies of BAT revealed that this enzyme can be induced by norepinephrine and contribute to UCP synthesis. Norepinephrine injections or acute cold exposure of rats or hamsters provokes a large increase in BAT type II 5'-deiodinase (9,219). Silva and Larsen (220) calculated that activated BAT can be an extrathyroidal source of triiodothyronine. Conversely, the decreased norepinephrine content of BAT from obese animals is accompanied by a decreased type II 5'-deiodinase activity and a lack of cold-induced increase of 5' D-II activity (9,221,222). There are conflicting data concerning the type of AR mediating the induction of BAT type II 5'-deiodinase by norepinephrine. In rats, it is mediated by a synergistic effect of α₁- and β-adrenergic agents and a role for cAMP was reported (24). In mouse brown adipocytes in culture, the main induction pathway of type II 5'-deiodinase involves an increase in cAMP levels resulting from activation of β₃-ARs (25,223).

The importance of T_3 in the activation of UCP gene transcription by norepinephrine has been mentioned above. T_4 deiodination is required for an optimal synthesis of UCP in brown adipose tissue (224–226). The direct role of T_3 in UCP gene transcription was recently confirmed by in vitro analysis of the UCP promoter (156) and the delineation of a T_3-response unit in the rat UCP promoter (23).

2. ADD1

ADD1 is a novel member of the transcription factor family (227). This protein plays a role in the regulation of determination- and differentiation-specific gene expression in adipocytes and its mRNA is expressed predominantly in BAT. The high level of ADD1 expression in BAT could reflect an important role in differentiation of brown adipocytes (227).

3. Secreted Peptide Factors

The recent cloning of the ob gene, defective in the genetically obese ob/ob mouse, had provided evidence for another protein secreted by adipose tissue, the OB protein (228,229). The OB protein, now named leptin, is synthesized and secreted by white adipocytes. Its expression is increased in animal models of obesity (except the ob/ob mouse) (228), as is the level that circulates in blood (230). Expression of the ob gene in BAT is, however, rather weak (230–236) or even not detectable (237,238) unless the animals are obese (230,233,234,238,239). However, sympathetic stimulation by cold exposure and administration of a β_3-AR agonist both reduce the expression of the *ob* gene in BAT (232). It would seem that only when sympathetic nervous system activity is very low, as in the obese animals, is there appreciable expression of leptin in BAT. Treatment of genetically obese *ob/ob* mice with the OB protein reverses their hypothermic state (240) suggesting that, among other things, it increases sympathetic nervous system activity in BAT.

Brown adipocytes synthesize and secrete lipoprotein lipase under the influence of norepinephrine. This enzyme promotes free fatty acid uptake from blood-borne triacylglycerols during cold-induced β-adrenergic activation of BAT (9,241–243).

The adipose tissues are the most important source of angiotensinogen. Brown adipocytes from multiple anatomical sites in the rat express angiotensinogen mRNA and secrete angiotensinogen (244–247). In addition, there is some evidence that angiotensinogen is processed to the angiotensin peptides in rat BAT, and that angiotensin II modulates norepinephrine release when tested in BAT slices (248,249). It was also demonstrated that angiotensin II participates, through interaction with receptors, in the enhanced sympathetic activity of cold-induced thermogenesis of rats (250).

Following the demonstration that adipsin that is expressed in BAT (and in WAT) is in fact the factor D of the alternative pathway of complement activation, Spiegelman and his colleagues identified other factors of this pathway in adipocytes (251).

4. Secreted Lipid Factors

Although it was mainly studied in WAT, brown adipocytes are probably able to secrete prostaglandins and monobutyrin. The former participate in regulation of lipolysis and adipose differentiation; the latter, which results from the acylation of diacylglycerol by butyryl-CoA, stimulates both angiogenesis and vasodilatation of microvascular beds (214,252).

The adipose masses are likely to constitute an important site of extragonadal sex steroid formation. In fact, studies performed in the 1960s have established that rodent BAT contains significant amounts of hydrocortisone, cortisone, corticosterone, 11-deoxycorticosterone, and 17-hydroxycortexone. A more recent study of steroids in BAT of Alp marmot, badger, and rat confirmed and extended the presence of several different steroids (253). In addition to the previously identified steroids mentioned above, androsterone, progesterone, 3α-hydroxy-5α-pregnan-20-one, 3α-hydroxy-5β-pregnan-20-one, 3α,21-dihydroxy-5α-pregnan-20-one, 3α,21-dihydroxy-5β-pregnan-one,

and 3β,21-dihydroxy-5α-pregnan-one were also identified and quantified (253). The physiological role of these different steroids has not been analyzed.

VI. PERSPECTIVE

Concepts of the function of BAT have changed during the last few years and since the publication of the two major books devoted to this tissue (1,2). BAT was originally defined as a heat-producing tissue. It was thought to be important mainly in small mammals living in a cold climate, in hibernators during arousal from hibernation, and in newborn mammals, including human infants, during the neonatal period. BAT was thus of interest mainly to researchers working on thermoregulation. Elucidation of the unique mitochondrial thermogenic process, involving the UCP, brought BAT to the attention of mitochondriologists. BAT then became of interest to a much wider range of research interests when its implication in energy balance and obesity became apparent some 16 years ago. Shortly thereafter, the rapid development of a molecular biological approach to the study of obesity included molecular biology of both brown and white adipocytes. This last approach has now provided new and important information about the potential role of defects in brown adipocytes in the development of obesity and hyperphagia.

The brown adipocyte has proved to be of value in deciding the function of the β_3-AR (17,161–165). This receptor has a lower affinity than β_1- or β_3-ARs for the endogenous neurotransmitter norepinephrine, and the need for its existence is not clear. As far as the brown adipocyte is concerned, the importance lies in the response of this receptor type to the high concentration of norepinephrine released from the nerves, ensuring that only neurally released, but not circulating, norepinephrine stimulates thermogenesis. The β_3-AR is also more resistant to desensitization than the other two types, a desirable property for one that must mediate a chronically stimulated state, as in the animal living in the cold, or the intense stimulation during a feeding episode, as is hypothesized to occur in rats and newborn infants (16,108). While not essential for BAT function, as shown by the fairly normal BAT function in the β_3-AR knockout mouse, the β_3-AR presumably allows optimal functioning of the tissue.

The physiological significance of the association of an isoform of the human β_3-AR with early-onset obesity and NIDDM in four different ethnic populations (254–257) has not been explained in terms of the function of this receptor. However, the β_3-AR is of greatest physiological importance in newborn infants, which possess abundant

BAT that expresses β_3-ARs (122,181,200). One might speculate that, if indeed BAT is involved in control of feeding episodes in newborn infants (108), an altered β_3-AR in the BAT might lead to altered control of feeding patterns very early in life (17).

The more recent concept that mature brown adipocytes can coexist in varying proportions with mature white adipocytes in many adipose tissues and that these proportions can be varied by chronic stimulation of β-ARs has led to the concept of the presence of dormant brown adipocytes in WAT depots, perhaps a vestige of cells present in neonatal life. The normal physiological role of these dormant brown adipocytes is uncertain, but targeting of antiobesity drugs to these cells to increase energy expenditure is an attractive possibility. There is no doubt that adipose tissues are more plastic than originally believed and that future elucidation of their functions will produce further surprises. The adipocyte, whether brown or white, may indeed be "a node on the energy information superhighway" (213).

Finally, it must be emphasized that physiologically the brown adipocyte functions in a milieu that would usually include neurons, both adrenergic and peptidergic and on both adipocytes and blood vessels, a blood supply that is controlled by neurons, and other cell types, including white adipocytes. Both its thermogenic function and its growth are controlled by the hypothalamus via its nerves, primarily in relation to thermoregulatory needs, but these needs are closely associated with control of feeding, both thermoregulatory feeding and that associated with diet-induced thermogenesis. Understanding the physiological function of the brown adipocyte requires not only a knowledge of the nature of its genes, of their control, and of its metabolic processes, but also an understanding of the milieu in which it functions, both in BAT and in WAT.

ADDENDUM

The cloning of mouse and human cDNAs encoding a protein structurally and functionally related to the UCP of BAT was recently reported (Fleury C, Neverova M, Collins S, Raimbault S, Champigny O, Levi-Meyrueis C, Bouillaud F, Seldin MF, Surwit RS, Ricquier D, Warden CH. Uncoupling protein-2: a novel gene linked to obesity and hyperinsulinemia. Nature Genetics, 1997, in press). This novel protein, referred to as UCP2, has 59% amino acid identity to UCP and its predicted secondary structure is very similar to that of UCP. Expression of UCP2 in yeast revealed its likely uncoupling action on respiration. High levels of UCP2 were detected in muscle, white and brown adipose tissues, and in tissues containing numerous macrophages and lymphocytes. The UCP2 gene maps to rodent and human chromosome regions that have been linked to obesity and hyperinsulinemia. Expression is high in white adipose tissue of a strain of mouse resistant to obesity and is further increased by fat feeding. Overall, results suggest that UCP2 might represent a new energy dissipative pathway, important in energy balance, body weight regulation and thermogenic responses to inflammatory stimuli.

ACKNOWLEDGMENTS

We are grateful to Dr. Saverio Cinti, Istituto di Morfologia Umana Normale, Facoltá di Medicina e Chirurgia, Universitá di Ancona, 60131, Ancona, Italy, for preparing the electron micrographs of BAT shown in Figure 2. Work of the authors mentioned in this review has been supported by grants from the Medical Research Council of Canada (JH-H) and Centre de la Recherche Scientifique, Meudon, France (DR).

REFERENCES

1. Lindberg O, ed. Brown Adipose Tissue. New York: Elsevier, 1970.
2. Trayhurn P, Nicholls DG, eds. Brown Adipose Tissue. London: Arnold, 1986.
3. Himms-Hagen J. Brown adipose tissue thermogenesis and obesity. Progr Lipid Res 1989; 28:67–115.
4. Himms-Hagen J. Brown adipose tissue thermogenesis; role in thermoregulation, energy regulation and obesity. In: Schönbaum E, Lomax P, eds. Thermoregulation: Physiology and Biochemistry. New York: Pergamon, 1990: 327–414.
5. Himms-Hagen J. Brown adipose tissue thermogenesis: interdisciplinary studies. FASEB J 1990; 4:2890–2989.
6. Ricquier D, Casteilla L, Bouillaud F. Molecular studies of the uncoupling protein. FASEB J 1991; 5:2237–2242.
7. Himms-Hagen J. Neural control of brown adipose tissue thermogenesis, hypertrophy, and atrophy. Front Neuroendocrinol 1991; 12:38–93.
8. Himms-Hagen J. Neural and hormonal responses to prolonged cold exposure. In: Fregly M, Blatteis, CM, eds. Adaptation to the Environment. New York: Oxford University Press, 1995; 6:439–480.
9. Ricquier D, Cassard-Doulcier A-M. The biochemistry of white and brown adipocytes analysed from a selection of proteins. Eur J Biochem 1993; 218:785–796.
10. Lončar D. Convertible adipose tissue in mice. Cell Tissue Res 1991; 266:149–161.
11. Cousin B, Cinti S, Morroni M, Raimbault S, Ricquier D, Pénicaud L, Casteilla L. Occurrence of brown adipocytes

in rat white adipose tissue: molecular and morphological characterization. J Cell Sci 1992; 103:931–942.

12. Garruti G, Ricquier D. Analysis of uncoupling protein and its mRNA in adipose tissue deposits of adult humans. Int J Obes 1992; 16:383–390.

13. Brück K. Heat production and temperature regulation. In: Stave U, ed. Perinatal Physiology. New York: Plenum Press, 1978:455–498.

14. Himms-Hagen J. Brown adipose tissue and cold-acclimation. In: Trayhurn P, Nicholls DG, eds. Brown Adipose Tissue. London: Arnold, 1986:214–267.

15. Closa D, Gómez-Sierra J-M, Latres E, Alemany M, Remesar X. Short-term oscillations of aortic core temperature and thermogenic organ blood flow in the rat. Exp Physiol 1993; 78:243–253.

16. Himms-Hagen J. Role of brown adipose tissue in control of thermoregulatory feeding in rats: a new hypothesis that links thermostatic and glucostatic hypotheses for control of food intake. Proc Soc Exp Biol Med 1995; 208: 159–169.

17. Himms-Hagen J, Danforth E, Jr. The potential role of beta-3 adrenoreceptor agonists in the treatment of obesity and diabetes. Curr Opin Endocrinol Diabetes. 1996; 3:59–65.

18. Ma SWY, Foster DO. Potentiation of in vivo thermogenesis in rat brown adipose tissue by stimulation of α_1-adrenoceptors is associated with increased release of cyclic AMP. Can J Physiol Pharmacol 1984; 62:943–948.

19. Granneman JG. Expression of adenylyl cyclase subtypes in brown adipose tissue: neural regulation of type III. Endocrinology 1995; 136:2007–2012.

20. Thonberg H, Zhang S-J, Tvrdik P, Jacobsson A, Nedergaard J. Norepinephrine utilizes α_1- and β-adrenoceptors synergistically to maximally induce c-fos expression in brown adipocytes. J Biol Chem 1994; 269:33179–33186.

21. Silva JE. Full expression of uncoupling protein gene requires the concurrence of norepinephrine and triiodothyronine. Mol Endocrinol 1988; 2:706–713.

22. Bianco AC, Kieffer JD, Silva JE. Adenosine 3',5'-monophosphate and thyroid hormone control of uncoupling protein messenger ribonucleic acid in freshly dispersed brown adipocytes. Endocrinology 1992; 130: 2625–2633.

23. Rabelo R, Schifman A, Rubio A, Sheng X, Silva JE. Delineation of thyroid hormone-responsive sequences within a critical enhancer in the rat uncoupling protein gene. Endocrinology 1995; 136:1003–1013.

24. Raasmaja A, Larsen PR. α_1- and β-adrenergic agents cause synergistic stimulation of the iodothyronine deiodinase in rat brown adipocytes. Endocrinology 1989; 125:2502–2509.

25. Pavelka S, Heřmanská J, Baudyšová M, Houštěk J. Adrenergic control of type II iodothyronine 5'-deiodinase activity in cultured mouse brown adipocytes. Biochem J 1993;292:303–308.

26. Marette A, Bukowiecki LJ. Stimulation of glucose transport by insulin and norepinephrine in isolated rat brown adipocytes. Am J Physiol 1989; 257:C714–C721.

27. Slot JW, Geuze HJ, Gigengack S, Lienhard GE, James DE. Immuno-localization of the insulin regulatable glucose transporter in brown adipose tissue of the rat. J Cell Biol 1991; 113:123–135.

28. Vallerand AL, Pérusse F, Bukowiecki LJ. Stimulatory effects of cold exposure and cold acclimation on glucose uptake in rat peripheral tissues. Am J Physiol 1990; 259: R1043–R1049.

29. Géloën A, Trayhurn P. Regulation of the level of uncoupling protein in brown adipose tissue by insulin. Am J Physiol 1990; 258:R418–R424.

30. Burcelin R, Kandé J, Ricquier D, Girard J. Changes in uncoupling protein and GLUT4 glucose transporter expression in interscapular brown adipose tissue of diabetic rats: relative roles of hyperglycaemia and hypoinsulinaemia. Biochem J 1993; 291:109–113.

31. Géloën A, Trayhurn, P. Regulation of the level of uncoupling protein in brown adipose tissue by insulin requires the mediation of the sympathetic nervous system. FEBS Lett 1990; 267:265–267.

32. Nikami H, Shimizu Y, Endoh D, Yano H, Saito M. Cold exposure increases glucose utilization and glucose transporter expression in brown adipose tissue. Biochem Biophys Res Commun 1992; 185:1078–1082.

33. Shimizu Y, Nikami H, Saito M. Sympathetic activation of glucose utilization in brown adipose tissue in rats. J Biochem 1991; 110:688–692.

34. Himms-Hagen J. Obesity may be due to a malfunctioning of brown fat. Can Med Assoc J 1979; 121:1361–1364.

35. Lowell BB, Susulic VS, Hamann A, Lawitts JA, Himms-Hagen J, Boyer BB, Kozak L, Flier JS. Development of morbid obesity in transgenic mice following the genetic ablation of brown adipose tissue. Nature (Lond) 1993; 366:740–742.

36. Melnyk A, Harper M-E, Himms-Hagen J. Raising at thermoneutrality prevents obesity in brown adipose tissue (BAT)-ablated mice. Am J Physiol 1997 (in press).

37. Géloën A, Collet AF, Guay G, Bukowiecki LJ. Beta-adrenergic stimulation of brown adipocyte proliferation. Am J Physiol 1988; 254:C175–C182.

38. Géloën A, Collet AJ, Guay G, Bukowiecki LJ. In vivo differentiation of brown adipocytes in adult mice: an electron microscopic study. Am J Anat 1990; 188:366–372.

39. Goglia F, Géloën A, Lanni A, Minaire Y, Bukowiecki LJ. Morphometric-stereologic analysis of brown adipocyte differentiation in adult mice. Am J Physiol 1992; 262: C1018–C1023.

40. Sbarbati A, Morroni M, Zancanaro C, Cinti S. Rat interscapular brown adipose tissue at different ages: a morphometric study. Int J Obes 1991; 15:581–588.

41. Morroni M, Barbatelli G, Zingaretti MC, Cinti S. Immunohistochemical, ultrastructural and morphometric evi-

dence for brown adipose tissue recruitment due to cold acclimation in old rats. Int J Obes 1995; 19:126–131.

42. Giordano A, Morroni M, Santone G, Marchesi GF, Cinti S. Tyrosine hydroxylase, neuropeptide Y, substance P, calcitonin gene-related peptide and vasoactive intestinal peptide in nerves of rat periovarian adipose tissue: an immunohistochemical and ultrastructural investigation. J Neurocytol 1996; 25:125–136.

43. Nnodim JO, Lever JD. Neural and vascular provisions of rat interscapular brown adipose tissue. Am J Anat 1988; 182:283–293.

44. Foster DO, Frydman ML. Nonshivering thermogenesis in the rat. II. Measurements of blood flow point to brown adipose tissue as the dominant site of the calorigenesis induced by noradrenaline. Can J Physiol Pharmacol 1978; 56:110–122.

45. Foster DO, Frydman ML. Tissue distribution of cold-induced thermogenesis in conscious warm- or cold-acclimated rats reevaluated from changes in tissue blood flow: the dominant role of brown adipose tissue in the replacement of shivering by nonshivering thermogenesis. Can J Physiol Pharmacol 1979; 57:257–270.

46. Foster DO. Quantitative role of brown adipose tissue in thermogenesis. In: Trayhurn P, Nicholls DG, eds. Brown Adipose Tissue. London: Arnold, 1986:31–51.

47. Foster DO, Depocas F, Zaror-Behrens G. Unilaterality of the sympathetic innervation of each pad of rat interscapular brown adipose tissue. Can J Physiol Pharmacol 1982; 60:107–113.

48. Watanabe J, Mishiro K, Amatsu T, Kanamura S. Absence of paravascular nerve projection and cross-innervation in interscapular brown adipose tissues of mice. J Auton Nerv Syst 1994; 49:269–276.

49. Norman D, Mukherjee S, Symons D, Jung RT, Lever JD. Neuropeptides in interscapular and perirenal brown adipose tissue in the rat: a plurality of innervation. J Neurocytol 1988; 17:305–311.

50. Lever JD, Mukherjee S, Norman D, Symons D, Wheeler MH, Connacher A, Jung RT. Catecholaminergic and peptidergic nerves in naturally occurring and pheochromocytoma-associated human brown adipose tissue. Clin Anat 1989; 2:157–166.

51. Lever JD, Jung RT, Nnodim JO, Leslie PJ, Symons D. Demonstration of a catecholaminergic innervation in human perirenal brown adipose tissue at various ages in the adult. Anat Rec 1986; 215:251–255.

52. Woods AJ, Stock MJ. Biphasic brown fat temperature responses to hypothalamic stimulation in rats. Am J Physiol 1994; 266:R328–R337.

53. Woods AJ, Stock MJ. Inhibition of brown fat activity during hypothalamic stimulation in the rat. Am J Physiol 1996; 270:R605–R613.

54. Thurlby PL, Ellis RDM. Differences between the effects of noradrenaline and the β-adrenoceptor agonist BRL 28410 in brown adipose tissue and hind limb of the anesthetized rat. Can J Physiol Pharmacol 1986; 64:1111–1114.

55. Néchad M. Structure and development of brown adipose tissue. In: Trayhurn P, Nicholls DG, eds. Brown Adipose Tissue. London: Arnold, 1986:1–30.

56. Nedergaard J, Connolly E, Cannon B. Brown adipose tissue in the mammalian neonate. In: Trayhurn P, Nicholls DG, eds. Brown Adipose Tissue. London: Arnold, 1986: 152–213.

57. Houštěk J, Kopecký J, Rychter Z, Soukup T. Uncoupling protein in embryonic brown adipose tissue—existence of nonthermogenic and thermogenic mitochondria. Biochim Biophys Acta 1988; 935:19–25.

58. Houštěk J, Kopecký J, Baudysova M, Janikova D, Pavelka S, Klement P. Differentiation of brown adipose tissue and biogenesis of thermogenic mitochondria in situ and in cell culture. Biochim Biophys Acta 1990; 1018:243–247.

59. Ricquier D, Bouillaud F, Toumelin P, Mory G, Bazin R, Arch J, Pénicaud L. Expression of uncoupling protein mRNA in thermogenic or weakly thermogenic brown adipose tissue. Evidence for a rapid β-adrenoceptor-mediated and transcriptionally regulated step during activation of thermogenesis. J Biol Chem 1986; 261: 13905–13910.

60. Obregon M-J, Jacobsson A, Kirchgessner T, Schotz MC, Cannon B, Nedergaard J. Postnatal recruitment of brown adipose tissue is induced by the cold stress experienced by the pups. Biochem J 1989; 259:341–346.

61. Casteilla L, Forest C, Robelin J, Ricquier D, Lombet A, Ailhaud G. Characterization of mitochondrial-uncoupling protein in bovine fetus and newborn calf. Am J Physiol 1987; 252:E627–E636.

62. Strieleman PJ, Gribskov CL, Kemnitz JW, Schalinske KL, Claude P, Parada I, Shrago E, Swick RW. Brown adipose tissue from fetal rhesus monkey (*Macaca mulatta*): morphological and biochemical aspects. Comp Biochem Physiol 1985; 81B:393–399.

63. Soppela P, Nieminin M, Saarela S, Keith JS, Morrison JN, MacFarlane S, Trayhurn P. Brown fat-specific mitochondrial uncoupling protein in adipose tissues of newborn reindeer. Am J Physiol 1991; 260:R1229–R1234.

64. Girardier L. Brown fat: an energy dissipating tissue. In: Mammalian Thermogenesis. Girardier L, Stock MJ, eds. London: Chapman and Hall, 1983:50–98.

65. Lean MEJ, James WPT. Brown adipose tissue in man. In: Trayhurn P, Nicholls DG, eds. Brown Adipose Tissue. London: Arnold, 1986:339–365.

66. Moragas A, Torán N. Prenatal development of brown adipose tissue in man. A morphometric and biomathematical study. Biol Neonate 1983; 43:80–85.

67. Zancanaro C, Carnieli VP, Moretti C, Benati D, Gamba P. An ultrastructural study of brown adipose tissue in preterm human newborns. Tissue Cell 1995; 27:339–348.

68. Lean MEJ, James WPT, Jennings G, Trayhurn P. Brown adipose tissue uncoupling protein content in infants, children and adult humans. Clin Sci 1986; 71:291–297.

69. Houštěk J, Vísek K, Pavelka S, Kopecký J, Krejčová E, Heřmanská J, Čermáková M. Type II iodothyronine 5'-

deiodinase and uncoupling protein in brown adipose tissue of human newborns. J Clin Endocrinol Metab 1993; 77:382–387.

70. Clarke L, Darby CJ, Lomax MA, Symonds ME. Effect of ambient temperature during 1st day of life on thermoregulation in lambs delivered by cesarean section. J Appl Physiol 1994; 76:1481–1488.

71. Casteilla L, Champigny O, Bouillaud F, Robelin J, Ricquier D. Sequential changes in the expression of mitochondrial protein mRNA during the development of brown adipose tissue in bovine and ovine species. Sudden occurrence of uncoupling protein mRNA during embryogenesis and its disappearance after birth. Biochem J 1989; 257:665–671.

72. Trayhurn P, Thomas MEA, Keith JS. Postnatal development of uncoupling protein, uncoupling protein mRNA and GLUT4 in adipose-tissues of goats. Am J Physiol 1993; 265:R676–R682.

73. Nicol F, Lefranc H, Arthur JR, Trayhurn P. Characterization and postnatal development of 5′-deiodinase activity in goat perirenal fat. Am J Physiol 1994; 267:R144–R149.

74. Ashwell M, Stirling D, Freeman S, Holloway BR. Immunological, histological and biochemical assessment of brown adipose tissue activity in neonatal, control and β-stimulant-treated adult dogs. Int J Obes 1987; 11: 357–365.

75. Champigny O, Ricquier D, Blondel O, Mayers RM, Briscoe MG, Holloway BR. β_3-Adrenergic receptor stimulation restores message and expression of brown-fat mitochondrial uncoupling protein in adult dogs. Proc Natl Acad Sci USA 1991; 88:10774–10777.

76. Rothwell MJ, Stock MJ. Biological distribution and significance of brown adipose tissue. Comp Biochem Physiol 1985; 82A:745–751.

77. Rothwell NJ, Stock MJ. Thermogenic capacity and brown adipose tissue activity in the common marmoset. Comp Biochem Physiol 1985; 81A:683–686.

78. Hayward JS, Lisson PA. Evolution of brown fat: its absence in marsupials and monotremes. Can J Zool 1992; 70:171–179.

79. Trayhurn P, Temple NJ, Van Aerde J. Evidence from immunoblotting studies on uncoupling protein that brown adipose tissue is not present in the domestic pig. Can J Physiol Pharmacol 1989; 67:1480–1485.

80. Nedergaard J, Cannon B. Brown adipose tissue: development and function. In: Polin RA, Fox WW, eds. Fetal and Neonatal Physiology, vol 1. Philadelphia: WB Saunders, 1992:314–325.

81. Lean MEJ. Evidence for brown adipose tissue in humans. In: Björntorp P, Brodoff BN, eds. Obesity. Philadelphia: JB Lippincott, 1992:117–129.

82. Huttunen P, Hirvonen J, Kinnula V. The occurrence of brown adipose tissue in outdoor workers. Eur J Appl Physiol 1981; 46:339–345.

83. Kortelainen M-L, Pelletier G, Ricquier D, Bukowiecki LJ. Immunohistochemical detection of human brown adipose tissue uncoupling protein in an autopsy series. J Histochem Cytochem 1993; 41:759–764.

84. Bouillaud F, Villarroya F, Hentz E, Raimbault S, Cassard A-M, Ricquier D. Detection of brown adipose tissue uncoupling protein in adult patients by a human genomic probe. Clin Sci 1988; 75:21–27.

85. Brooks JJ, Perosio PM. Adipose Tissue. In: Sternberg SS, ed. Histology for Pathologists. New York; Raven Press, 1992:33–60.

86. Zancanaro C, Pelosi G, Accordini C, Balercia G, Sbabo L, Cinti S. Immunohistochemical identification of the uncoupling protein in human hibernoma. Biol Cell 1994; 80:75–78.

87. McIntyre J, Hull D, Nedergaard J, Cannon B. Thermoregulation. In: Gluckman PD, Heymann MA, eds. Perinatal and Pediatric Pathophysiology: a clinical perspective. London: Arnold, 1993:357–368.

88. Lean MEJ. Brown adipose tissue and obesity. In: Belfiore F, Jeanrenaud B, Papalia D, eds. Obesity: Basic Concepts and Clinical Aspects. Basel: Karger, 1992:37–49.

89. Bianchi A, Bruce J, Cooper AL, Childs C, Kohli M, Morris ID, Morris-Jones P, Rothwell NJ. Increased brown adipose tissue activity in children with malignant disease. Horm Metabol Res 1989; 21:640–641.

90. Ohlson KBE, Mohell N, Cannon B, Lindahl SGE, Nedergaard J. Thermogenesis in brown adipocytes is inhibited by volatile anesthetic agents. A factor contributing to hypothermia in infants. Anesthesiology 1994; 81:176–183.

91. Dicker A, Ohlson KBE, Johnson L, Cannon B, Lindahl SGE, Nedergaard J. Halothane selectively inhibits nonshivering thermogenesis. Possible implications for thermoregulation during anesthesia of infants. Anesthesiology 1995; 82:491–501.

92. Aherne W, Hull D. Brown adipose tissue and heat production in the newborn infant. J Pathol Bacteriol 1966; 91:223–234.

93. Bouillaud F, Combes-George M, Ricquier D. Mitochondria of human brown adipose tissue contain a 32 000-M$_r$ uncoupling protein. Biosci Rep 1983; 3:775–780.

94. Ricquier D, Néchad M, Mory G. Ultrastructural and biochemical characterization of human brown adipose tissue in pheochromocytoma. J Clin Endocrinol Metab 1982; 54:803–807.

95. Lean MEJ, James WPT, Jennings G, Trayhurn P. Brown adipose tissue in patients with phaeochromocytoma. Int J Obes 1986; 10:219–227.

96. Cassard A-M, Bouillaud F, Mattei M-G, Hentz E, Raimbault S, Thomas M, Ricquier D. Human uncoupling protein gene: structure, comparison with rat gene, and assignment to the long arm of chromosome 4. J Cell Biochem 1990; 43:255–264.

97. Géloën A, Collet AJ, Bukowiecki LJ. Role of sympathetic innervation in brown adipocyte proliferation. Am J Physiol 1992; 263:R1176–R1181.

98. Bronnikov G, Houstek J, Nedergaard J. β-Adrenergic cAMP-mediated stimulation of proliferation of brown fat

cells in primary culture—mediation via β_1—but not via β_3—adrenoceptors. J Biol Chem 1992; 267:2006–2013.

99. Himms-Hagen J, Cui J, Danforth E, Jr, Taatjes DJ, Lang SS, Waters BL, Claus TH. Effect of CL 316,243, a thermogenic β_3-agonist, on energy balance and brown and white adipose tissues in rats. Am J Physiol 1994; 266: R1371–R1382.

100. Himms-Hagen J, Ghorbani M. Reversal of obesity in fa/fa rats by treatment with a β_3-adrenoceptor agonist, CL 316,243: cellularity and biochemical characteristics of white and brown adipose tissues. Obes Res 1995; 3 (Suppl 3):406s.

101. Ghorbani M, Himms-Hagen J. Reversal of obesity in fa/fa rats by treatment with a β_3-adrenoceptor agonist, CL 316,243: appearance of abundant brown adipocytes in retroperitoneal white adipose tissue. Obes Res 1995; 3 (Suppl 3):407s.

102. Granneman JG, Lahners KN. Differential adrenergic regulation of β_1- and β_3-adrenoceptor messenger ribonucleic acids in adipose tissues. Endocrinology 1992; 130:109–114.

103. Ricquier D, Mory G, Bouillaud F, Thibault J, Weissenbach J. Rapid increase of mitochondrial uncoupling protein and its mRNA in stimulated brown adipose tissue. Use of a cDNA probe. FEBS Lett 1984; 178:240–244.

104. Bouillaud F, Ricquier D, Mory G, Thibault J. Increased level of mRNA for the uncoupling protein in brown adipose tissue of rats during thermogenesis induced by cold exposure or norepinephrine infusion. J Biol Chem 1984; 259:11583–11586.

105. Mory G, Bouillaud F, Combes-George M, Ricquier D. Noradrenaline controls the concentration of the uncoupling protein in brown adipose tissue. FEBS Lett 1984; 166: 393–396.

106. Tsuhazaki K, Nikami H, Shimizu Y, Kawada T, Yoshida T, Saito M. Chronic administration of β-adrenergic agonists can mimic the stimulative effect of cold exposure on protein synthesis in rat brown adipose tissue. J Biochem 1995; 117:96–100.

107. Girardier L, Stock MJ. eds. Mammalian Thermogenesis. London: Chapman and Hall, 1983.

108. Himms-Hagen J. Does thermoregulatory feeding occur in newborn infants? A novel view of the role of brown adipose tissue thermogenesis in control of food intake. Obes Res 1995; 3:361–369.

109. Lyman CP, Willis JS, Malan A, Wang LCH, eds. Hibernation and Torpor in Mammals and Birds. New York: Academic Press, 1982.

110. Bauman WA. Hibernation: a model of adaptive hyperlipogenesis and associated metabolic features. In: Björntorp P, Brodoff BN, eds. Obesity. Philadelphia: JB Lippincott, 1992:206–219.

111. Rothwell NJ, Stock MJ. A role for brown adipose tissue in diet-induced thermogenesis. Nature 1979; 281:31–35.

112. Rothwell NJ, Stock MJ. Brown adipose tissue and diet-induced thermogenesis. In: Trayhurn P, Nicholls DG, eds. Brown Adipose Tissue. London: Arnold, 1986:269–298.

113. Blumberg MS, Efimova IV, Alberts JR. Thermogenesis during ultrasonic vocalization by rat pups isolated in a warm environment. Dev Psychobiol 1992; 25:497–510.

114. Cannon B, Nedergaard J. Adipocytes, preadipocytes, and mitochondria from brown adipose tissue. In: Hausman GJ, Martin RJ, eds. Biology of the Adipocyte. New York: Van Nostrand Reinhold, 1987.

115. Rehnmark S, Néchad M, Herron D, Cannon B, Nedergaard J. α- and β-adrenergic induction of the expression of the uncoupling protein thermogenin in brown adipocytes differentiated in culture. J Biol Chem 1990; 265: 16464–16471.

116. Kopecký J, Baudyšová M, Zanotti F, Janíková D, Pavelka S, Houštěk J. Synthesis of mitochondrial uncoupling protein in brown adipocytes differentiated in cell culture. J Biol Chem 1990; 265:22204–22209.

117. Ailhaud G, Grimaldi P, Négrel R. Cellular and molecular aspects of adipose tissue development. Annu Rev Nutr 1992; 12:207–233.

118. Houstek J, Janikova D, Bednar J, Kopecky J, Sebastian J, Soukup T. Postnatal appearance of uncoupling protein and formation of thermogenic mitochondria in hamster brown adipose tissue. Biochim Biophys Acta 1990; 1015: 441–449.

119. Young P, Arch JRS, Ashwell M. Brown adipose tissue in the parametrial fat pad of the mouse. FEBS Lett 1984; 167:10–14.

120. Cousin B, Casteilla L, Dani C, Muzzin P, Revelli JP, Pénicaud L. Adipose tissues from various anatomical sites are characterized by different patterns of gene expression and regulation. Biochem J 1993; 292:873–876.

121. Viguerie-Bascands N, Bousquet-Mélou A, Galitzky J, Ricquier D, Berlan M, Casteilla L. Evidence for numerous brown adipocytes lacking functional β_3-adrenoceptors in fat pads from non-human primates. J Clin Endocrinol Metab 1996; 81:368–375.

122. Krief S, Lönnqvist F, Raimbault S, Baude B, Van Spronsen A, Arner P, Strosberg AD, Ricquier D, Emorine LJ. Tissue distribution of β_3-adrenergic receptor mRNA in man. J Clin Invest 1993; 91:344–349.

123. Houštěk J, Andersson U, Tvrdík P, Nedergaard J, Cannon B. The expression of subunit c correlates with and thus may limit the biosynthesis of the mitochondrial F_0F_1-ATPase in brown adipose tissue. J Biol Chem 1995; 270: 7689–7694.

124. Nicholls DG, Locke RM. Thermogenic mechanisms in brown fat. Physiol Rev 1984; 64:1–64.

125. Klingenberg M. Mechanism and evolution of the uncoupling protein of brown adipose tissue. Trends Biochem Sci 1990; 15:108–112.

126. Nicholls DG, Rial E. Brown fat mitochondria. Trends Biochem Sci 1984; 9:489–491.

127. Aquila H, Link TA, Klingenberg M. The uncoupling protein from brown fat mitochondria is related to the mitochondrial ADP/ATP carrier. Analysis of sequence homologies and of folding of the protein in the membrane. EMBO J 1985; 4:2369–2376.

128. Klaus S, Casteilla L, Bouillaud F, Ricquier D. The uncoupling protein UCP: a membranous mitochondrial ion carrier exclusively expressed in brown adipose tissue. Int J Biochem 1991; 23:791–801.

129. Bouillaud F, Weissenbach J, Ricquier D. Complete cDNA-derived amino acid sequence of rat brown fat uncoupling protein. J Biol Chem 1986; 261:1487–1490.

130. Ridley RG, Patel HV, Gerber GE, Morton RC, Freeman KB. Compete nucleotide sequence and derived amino acid sequence of cDNA encoding the mitochondrial uncoupling protein of rat brown adipose tissue: lack of a mitochondrial targeting presequence. Nucleic Acids Res 1986; 14:4025–4035.

131. Casteilla L, Bouillaud F, Forest C, Ricquier D. Nucleotide sequence of a cDNA encoding bovine brown fat uncoupling protein. Homology with ADP binding site of ADP/ATP carrier. Nucleic Acids Res 1989; 17:2131.

132. Kozak LP, Britton JH, Kozak UC, Wells JM. The mitochondrial uncoupling protein gene. Correlation of exon structure to transmembrane domain. J Biol Chem 1988; 263:12274–12277.

133. Balogh AG, Ridley RG, Patel HV, Freeman KB. Rabbit brown adipose tissue uncoupling protein mRNA: use of only one of two polyadenylation signals in its processing. Biochem Biophys Res Commun 1989; 161:156–161.

134. Walker JE. The mitochondrial transporter family. Curr Opin Struct Biol 1992; 2:519–526.

135. Miroux B, Casteilla L, Klaus S, Raimbault S, Grandin S, Clément JM, Ricquier D, Bouillaud F. Antibodies selected from whole antiserum by fusion proteins as tools for the study of the topology of mitochondrial membrane proteins. J Biol Chem 1992; 267:13603–13609.

136. Miroux B, Frossard V, Raimbault S, Ricquier D, Bouillaud F. The topology of the brown adipose tissue mitochondrial uncoupling protein gene determined with antibodies against its antigenic sites revealed by a library of fusion proteins. EMBO J 1993; 12:3739–3745.

137. Winkler E, Klingenberg M. Photoaffinity labeling of the nucleotide-binding site of the uncoupling protein from hamster brown adipose tissue. Eur J Biochem 1992; 203:295–304.

138. Bouillaud F, Arechaga I, Petit PX, Raimbault S, Levi-Meyrueis C, Casteilla L, Laurent M, Rial E, Ricquier D. A sequence related to a DNA recognition element is essential for the inhibition by nucleotides of proton transport through the mitochondrial uncoupling protein. EMBO J 1994; 12:1990–1997.

139. Klaus S, Cassard-Doulcier A-M, Ricquier D. Development of Phodopus sungorus brown preadipocytes in primary cell culture: effect of an atypical beta-adrenergic agonist, insulin, and triiodothyronin on differentiation, mitochon-drial development, and expression of the uncoupling protein UCP. J Cell Biol 1991; 115:1783–1790.

140. Ross SR, Choy L, Graves RA, Fox N, Solevjeva V, Klaus S, Ricquier D, Spiegelman BM. Hibernoma formation in transgenic mice and isolation of a brown adipocyte cell line expressing the uncoupling protein gene. Proc Natl Acad Sci USA 1992; 89:7561–7565.

141. Klaus S, Choy L, Champigny O, Cassard-Doulcier A-M, Ross S, Spiegelman B, Ricquier D. Characterization of the novel brown adipocyte cell line HIB 1B. Adrenergic pathways involved in regulation of uncoupling protein gene expression. J Cell Sci 1994; 107:313–319.

142. Kozak UC, Kozak LP. Norepinephrine-dependent selection of brown adipocyte cell lines. Endocrinology 1994; 134:906–913.

143. Benito M, Porras A, Santos E. Establishment of permanent brown adipocyte cell lines achieved by transfection with SV40 large T antigen and *ras* genes. Exp Cell Res 1993; 209:248–254.

144. Rehnmark S, Bianco AC, Kieffer JD, Silva JE. Transcriptional and posttranscriptional mechanisms in uncoupling protein mRNA response to cold. Am J Physiol 1992; 262: E58–E67.

145. Picó C, Herron D, Palou A, Jacobsson A, Cannon B, Nedergaard J. Stabilization of the mRNA for the uncoupling protein thermogenin by transcriptional/translational blockade and by noradrenaline in brown adipocytes differentiated in culture: a degradation factor induced by cessation of stimulation? Biochem J 1994; 302:81–86.

146. Bianco AC, Sheng X, Silva JE. Triiodothyronine amplifies norepinephrine stimulation of uncoupling protein gene transcription by a mechanism not requiring protein synthesis. J Biol Chem 1988; 263:18168–18175.

147. Silva JE. Hormonal control of thermogenesis and energy dissipation. Trends Endocrinol Metab 1993; 4:25–32.

148. Guerra C, Porras A, Roncero C, Benito M, Fernandez M. Triiodothyronine induces the expression of the uncoupling protein in long term fetal rat brown adipocyte primary cultures: role of nuclear thyroid hormone receptor expression. Endocrinology 1994; 134:1067–1074.

149. Casteilla L, Nouguès J, Reyne Y, Ricquier D. Differentiation of ovine brown adipocyte precursor cells in a chemically defined serum-free medium. Importance of glucocorticoids and age of animals. Eur J Biochem 1991; 198: 195–199.

150. Moriscot A, Rabelo R, Bianco AC. Corticosterone inhibits uncoupling protein gene expression in brown adipose tissue. Am J Physiol 1993; 265:E81–E87.

151. Shima A, Shinohara Y, Doi K, Terada H. Normal differentiation of rat brown adipocytes in primary culture judged by their expression of uncoupling protein and the physiological isoform of glucose transporter. Biochim Biophys Acta 1994; 1223:1–8.

152. Cassard-Doulcier A-M, Gelly C, Fox N, Schrementi J, Raimbault S, Klaus S, Forest C, Bouillaud F, Ricquier D. Tissue-specific and β-adrenergic gene regulation of the

mitochondrial uncoupling protein gene: control by *cis*-acting elements in the 5′-flanking region. Mol Endocrinol 1993; 7:497–506.

153. Boyer BB, Kozak LP. The mitochondrial uncoupling protein in brown fat: correlation between DNase I hypersensitivity and expression in transgenic mice. Mol Cell Biol 1991; 11:4147–4156.

154. Kozak UC, Kopecky J, Teisinger J, Enerbäck S, Boyer BB, Kozak LP. An upstream enhancer regulating brown-fat-specific expression of the mitochondrial uncoupling protein gene. Mol Cell Biol 1994; 14:59–67.

155. Alvarez R, De Andrés J, Yubero P, Viñas O, Mampel T, Iglesias R, Giralt M, Villarroya F. A novel regulatory pathway of brown fat thermogenesis. Retinoic acid is a transcriptional activator of the mitochondrial uncoupling protein gene. J Biol Chem 1995; 270:5666–5673.

156. Cassard-Doulcier A-M, Larose M, Matamala JC, Champigny O, Bouillaud F, Ricquier D. In vitro interactions between nuclear proteins and uncoupling protein gene promoter reveal several putative transactivating factors including Ets1, retinoid X receptor, thyroid hormone receptor, and a CACCC box-binding protein. J Biol Chem 1994; 269:24335–24342.

157. Yubero P, Viñas O, Iglesias R, Mampel T, Villarroya F, Giralt M. Identification of tissue-specific binding domains in the 5′-proximal regulatory region of the rat mitochondrial brown fat uncoupling protein gene. Biochem Biophys Res Commun 1994; 204:867–873.

158. Arch JRS, Kaumann AJ. β_3- and atypical β-adrenoceptors. Med Res Rev 1993; 13:663–729.

159. Largis EE, Burns MG, Muenkel HA, Dolan JA, Claus TH. Antidiabetic and antiobesity effects of a highly selective β_3-adrenoceptor agonist (CL 316,243). Drug Dev Res 1994; 32:69–76.

160. Lafontan M, Berlan M. Fat cell adrenergic receptors and the control of white and brown fat cells function. J Lipid Res 1993; 34:1057–1091.

161. Lafontan M. Differential recruitment and differential regulation by physiological amines of fat cell β-1, β-2 and β-3 adrenergic receptors expressed in native fat cells and in transfected cells. Cell Signal 1994; 6:363–392.

162. Giacobino J-P. β_3-Adrenoceptor: an update. Eur J Endocrinol 1995; 132:377–385.

163. Lowell BB, Flier JS. The potential significance of $\beta(3)$ adrenergic receptors. J Clin Invest 1995; 95:923–924.

164. Granneman JG. Why do adipocytes make the β_3-adrenergic receptor? Cell Signal 1995; 7:9–15.

165. Strosberg AD, Pietri-Rouxel F. Function and regulation of the β_3-adrenoceptor. Trends Pharmacol Sci 1996; 17:373–381.

166. Emorine LJ, Marullo S, Briend-Sutren M-M, Patey G, Tate K, Delavier-Klutchko C, Strosberg AD. Molecular characterization of the human β_3-adrenergic receptor. Science 1989; 245:1118–1121.

167. Nahmias C, Blin N, Elalouf J-M, Mattei MG, Strosberg AD, Emorine LJ. Molecular characterization of the mouse β_3-adrenergic receptor: relationship with the atypical receptor of adipocytes. EMBO J 1991; 10:3721–3727.

168. Muzzin P, Revelli J-P, Kuhne F, Gocayne JD, McCombie WR, Venter JC, Giacobino J-P, Fraser CM. An adipose tissue-specific β-adrenergic receptor. Molecular cloning and down-regulation in obesity. J Biol Chem 1991; 266:24053–24058.

169. Granneman JG, Lahners KN, Chaudhry A. Molecular cloning and expression of the rat β_3-adrenergic receptor. Mol Pharmacol 1991; 40:895–899.

170. Himms-Hagen J, Triandafillou J, Bégin-Heick N, Ghorbani M, Kates A-L. Apparent lack of β_3-adrenoceptors and of insulin regulation of glucose transport in brown adipose tissue of guinea pigs. Am J Physiol 1995; 268:R98–R104.

171. Carpéné C, Castan I, Collon P, Galitzky J, Moratinos J, Lafontan M. Adrenergic lipolysis in guinea pig is not a β_3-adrenergic response: comparison with human adipocytes. Am J Physiol 1994; 266:R905–R913.

172. Muzzin P, Revelli J-P, Fraser CM, Giacobino J-P. Radioligand binding studies of the atypical β_3-adrenoceptor in rat brown adipose tissue using [^{3}H]CGP 12177. FEBS Lett 1992; 298:162–164.

173. Tate KM, Briend-Sutren M-M, Emorine LJ, Delavier-Klutchko C, Marullo S, Strosberg AD. Expression of three human β-adrenergic receptor subtypes in transfected chinese hamster ovary cells. Eur J Biochem 1991; 196:357–361.

174. Liggett SB, Schwinn DA. Multiple potential regulatory elements in the 5′ flanking region of the β_3-adrenergic receptor. DNA Seq 1991; 2:61–63.

175. Granneman JG, Lahners KN, Chaudhry A. Characterization of the human β_3-adrenergic receptor gene. Mol Pharmacol 1993; 44:264–270.

176. Lelias JM, Kaghad M, Rodriguez M, Chalon P, Bonnin J, Dupre I, Delpech B, Bensaid M, Lefur G, Ferrara P, Caput D. Molecular cloning of a human β_3-adrenergic receptor cDNA. FEBS Lett 1993; 324:127–130.

177. Pietri-Rouxel F, Lenzen G, Kapoor A, Drumare MF, Archimbault P, Strosberg AD, Manning BSJ. Molecular cloning and pharmacological characterization of the bovine β_3-adrenergic receptor. Eur J Biochem 1995; 230:350–358.

178. Emorine LJ, Fève B, Pairault J, Briend-Sutren M-M, Marullo S, Delavier-Klutchko C, Strosberg AD. Structural basis for functional diversity of β_1-, β_2- and β_3-adrenergic receptors. Biochem Pharmacol 1991; 41:853–859.

179. Strosberg AD. Structure/function relationship of proteins belonging to the family of receptors coupled to GTP-binding proteins. Eur J Biochem 1991; 196:1–10.

180. Granneman JG, Lahners KN, Rai DD. Rodent and human β_3-adrenergic receptor genes contain an intron within the protein-coding block. Mol Pharmacol 1992; 42:964–970.

181. Granneman JG, Lahners KN. Analysis of human and rodent β_3-adrenergic receptor messenger ribonucleic acids. Endocrinology 1994; 135:1025–1031.

182. Van Spronsen A, Nahmias C, Krief S, Briend-Sutren M-M, Strosberg AD, Emorine LJ. The promoter and intron-exon structure of the human and mouse β_3-adrenergic-receptor genes. Eur J Biochem 1993; 213: 1117–1124.

183. Galitzky J, Carpéné C, Bousquet-Mélou A, Berlan M, Lafontan M. Differential activation of β_1-, β_2- and β_3-adrenoceptors by catecholamines in white and brown adipocytes. Fundam Clin Pharmacol 1995; 9:324–331.

184. Muzzin P, Revelli J-P, Ricquier D, Meier MK, Assimacopoulos-Jeannet F, Giacobino J-P. The novel thermogenic β-adrenergic agonist Ro 16-8714 increases the interscapular brown-fat β-receptor-adenylate cyclase and the uncoupling-protein mRNA level in obese (*fa/fa*) Zucker rats. Biochem J 1989; 261:721–724.

185. Nedergaard J, Bronnikov G, Golozoubova V, Rehnmark S, Bengtsson T, Thonberg H, Jacobsson A, Cannon B. Brown adipocyte differentiation: an innate switch in adrenergic receptor endowment and in adrenergic response. In: Ditschuneit H, Gries FA, Hauner H, Schusdziarra V, Wechsler JG, eds. Obesity in Europe. London: John Libbey, 1994: 73–80.

186. Klaus S, Muzzin P, Revelli J-P, Cawthorne MA, Giacobino J-P, Ricquier D. Control of β_3-adrenergic receptor gene expression in brown adipocytes in culture. Mol Cell Endocrinol 1995; 109:189–195.

187. Champigny O, Holloway BR, Ricquier D. Regulation of UCP gene expression in brown adipocytes differentiated in primary culture. Effects of a new β-adrenoceptor agonist. Mol Cell Endocrinol 1992; 86:73–82.

188. Liu Y-L, Stock MJ. Acute effects of the β_3-adrenoceptor agonist, BRL 35135, on tissue glucose utilisation. Br J Pharmacol 1995; 114:888–894.

189. Liu X, Pérusse F, Bukowiecki LJ. Chronic norepinephrine infusion stimulates glucose uptake in white and brown adipose tissues. Am J Physiol 1994; 266:R914–R920.

190. Yoshida T, Sakane N, Wakabayashi Y, Umekawa T, Kondo M. Anti-obesity and anti-diabetic effects of CL 316,243, a highly specific β_3-adrenoceptor agonist, in yellow KK mice. Life Sci 1994; 54:491–498.

191. Yoshida T, Sakane N, Wakabayashi Y, Umekawa T, Kondo M. Anti-obesity effect of CL 316,243, a highly specific β_3-adrenoceptor agonist, in mice with monosodium-L-glutamate-induced obesity. Eur J Endocrinol 1994; 131: 97–102.

192. Zhao J, Unelius L, Bengtsson T, Cannon B, Nedergaard J. Coexisting β-adrenoceptor subtypes: significance for thermogenic process in brown fat cells. Am J Physiol 1994; 267:C969–C979.

193. D'Allaire F, Atgié C, Mauriège P, Simard P-M, Bukowiecki LJ. Characterization of β_1- and β_3-adrenoceptors in intact brown adipocytes of the rat. Br J Pharmacol 1995; 114: 275–282.

194. Susulic V, Frederich RC, Lawitts JA, Tozzo E, Kahn BB, Harper M-E, Himms-Hagen J, Flier JS, Lowell BB. Targeted disruption of the β_3-adrenergic receptor gene. J Biol Chem 1995; 270:29483–29492.

195. Harper M-E, Kates A-L, Himms-Hagen J. No response to selective β_3-adrenoceptor (AR) agonist (CL 316,243) but normal responses to non-selective β-AR agonists and cold in β_3-AR knockout mice. Obes Res 1995; 3(Suppl 3): 406s.

196. Lönnqvist F, Krief S, Strosberg AD, Nyberg B, Emorine LJ, Arner P. Evidence for a functional β_3-adrenoceptor in man. Br J Pharmacol 1993; 110:929–936.

197. Revelli J-P, Muzzin P, Paoloni A, Moinat M, Giacobino J-P. Expression of the β_3-adrenergic receptor in human white adipose tissue. J Mol Endocrinol 1993; 10:193–197.

198. Berkowitz DE, Nardone NA, Smiley RM, Price DT, Kreutter DK, Fremeau RT, Schwinn DA. Distribution of β_3-adrenoceptor mRNA in human tissues. Eur J Pharmacol Mol Pharmacol 1995; 289:223–228.

199. Muzzin P, Boss O, Mathis N, Revelli J-P, Giacobino J-P, Willcocks K, Badman GT, Cantello BCC, Hindley RM, Cawthorne MA. Characterization of a new, highly specific, β_3-adrenergic receptor radioligand, [^{3}H]SB 206606. Mol Pharmacol 1994; 46:357–363.

200. Deng C, Paoloni-Giacobino A, Kuehne F, Boss O, Revelli JP, Moinat M, Cawthorne MA et al. Respective degree of expression of β_1-, β_2- and β_3-adrenergic receptors in human brown and white adipose tissues. Br J Pharmacol 1996; 118:929–934.

201. Casteilla L, Muzzin P, Revelli J-P, Ricquier D, Giacobino J-P. Expression of β_3- and β_3-adrenergic-receptor messages and adenylate cyclase β-adrenergic response in bovine perirenal adipose tissue during its transformation from brown into white fat. Biochem J 1994; 297:93–97.

202. Collins S, Daniel KW, Rohlfs EM, Ramkumar V, Taylor IL, Gettys TW. Impaired expression and functional activity of the β_3- and β_1-adrenergic receptors in adipose tissue of congenitally obese (C57BL/6J *ob/ob*) mice. Mol Endocrinol 1994; 8:518–527.

203. Okada S, Onai T, Kilroy G, York DA, Bray GA. Adrenalectomy of the obese Zucker rat: effects on the feeding response to enterostatin and specific mRNA levels. Am J Physiol 1993; 265:R21–R27.

204. Onai T, Kilroy G, York DA, Bray GA. Regulation of beta(3)-adrenergic receptor mRNA by sympathetic nerves and glucocorticoids in BAT of Zucker obese rats. Am J Physiol 1995; 38:R519–R526.

205. Rubio A, Raasmaja A, Maia AL, Kim K-R, Silva JE. Effects of thyroid hormone on norepinephrine signaling in brown adipose tissue. I. β_1- and β_2-adrenergic receptors and cyclic adenosine 3′,5′-monophosphate generation. Endocrinology 1995; 136:3267–3276.

206. Rubio A, Raasmaja A, Silva JE. Effects of thyroid hormone on norepinephrine signaling in brown adipose tissue. II. Differential effects of thyroid hormone on β_3-adrenergic receptors in brown and white adipose tissue. Endocrinology 1995; 136:3277–3284.

207. Nantel F, Bonin H, Emorine LJ, Zilberfarb V, Strosberg AD, Bouvier M, Marullo S. The human β_3-adrenergic receptor gene is resistant to short-term agonist-promoted desensitization. Mol Pharmacol 1993; 43:548–555.

208. Liggett SB, Freedman NJ, Schwinn DA, Lefkowitz, RJ. Structural basis for receptor subtype-specific regulation revealed by a chimeric β_3-/β_2-adrenergic receptor. Proc Natl Acad Sci USA 1993; 90:3665–3669.

209. Carpéné C, Galitzky J, Collon P, Esclapez F, Dauzats M, Lafontan M. Desensitization of beta-1 and beta-2, but not beta-3, adrenoceptor-mediated lipolytic responses of adipocytes after long-term infusion. J Pharmacol Exp Ther 1993; 265:237–247.

210. Unelius L, Bronnikov G, Mohell N, Nedergaard J. Physiological desensitization of β_3-adrenergic responses in brown fat cells: involvement of a post-receptor process. Am J Physiol 1993; 265:C1340–C1348.

211. Svoboda P, Unelius L, Cannon B, Nedergaard J. Attenuation of $G_s\alpha$ coupling efficiency in brown-adipose-tissue plasma membranes from cold-acclimated hamsters. Biochem J 1993; 295:655–661.

212. Chambers J, Park J, Cronk D, Chapman C, Kennedy FR, Wilson S, Milligan G. β_3-Adrenoceptor agonist-induced down-regulation of $G_s\alpha$ and functional desensitization in a Chinese hamster ovary cell line expressing a β_3-adrenoceptor refractory to down-regulation. Biochem J 1994; 303:973–978.

213. Flier JS. The adipocyte: storage depot or node on the energy information superhighway. Cell 1995; 80:15–18.

214. Ailhaud G, Grimaldi P, Négrel R. A molecular view of adipose tissue. Int J Obes 1992; 16(Suppl 2):S17–S21.

215. Leonard JL, Mellen SA, Larsen PR. Thyroxine 5'-deiodinase activity in brown adipose tissue. Endocrinology 1983; 112:1153–1155.

216. Houštěk J, Vízek K, Pavelka S, Kopecký J, Krejčová J, Heřmanská J, Čermánová M. Type II iodothyronine 5'-deiodinase and uncoupling protein in brown adipose tissue of newborns. J Clin Endocrinol Metab 1993; 77: 382–387.

217. Giralt M, Casteilla L, Viñas O, Mampel T, Iglesias R, Robelin J, Villarroya F. Iodothyronine 5'-deiodinase activity as an early event of prenatal brown-fat differentiation in bovine development. Biochem J 1989; 259:555–559.

218. Trayhurn P, Thomas MEA, Duncan JS, Nicol F, Arthur JR. Presence of the brown fat-specific mitochondrial uncoupling protein and iodothyronine 5'-deiodinase in subcutaneous adipose tissue of neonatal lambs. FEBS Lett 1993; 322:76–78.

219. Silva JE, Larsen PR. Adrenergic activation of triiodothyronine production in brown adipose tissue. Nature (Lond) 1983; 305:712–713.

220. Silva JE, Larsen PR. Potential of brown adipose tissue type II thyroxine 5'-deiodinase as a local and systemic source of triiodothyronine in rats. J Clin Invest 1985; 76: 2296–2305.

221. Wu SY, Stern JS, Fisher DA, Glick Z. Cold induced increase in brown fat thyroxine 5' monodeiodinase is attenuated in Zucker obese rat. Am J Physiol 1987; 252: E63–E67.

222. Kates A-L, Himms-Hagen J. Defective regulation of thyroxine 5'-deiodinase in brown adipose tissue of ob/ob mice. Am J Physiol 1990; 258:E7–E15.

223. Houštěk J, Pavelka S, Baudyšová M, Kopecký J. Induction of type II iodothyronine 5'-deiodinase and mitochondrial uncoupling protein in brown adipocytes differentiated in cell culture. FEBS Lett 1990; 274:185–188.

224. Bianco AC, Silva JE. Optimal response of key enzymes and uncoupling protein to cold in brown adipose tissue depends on local T_3 generation. Am J Physiol 1987; 253: E255–E263.

225. Giralt M, Martin I, Iglesias R, Viñas O, Villarroya F, Mampel T. Ontogeny and perinatal modulation of gene expression in rat brown adipose tissue. Unaltered iodothyronine 5'-deiodinase activity is necessary for the response to environmental temperature at birth. Eur J Biochem 1990; 193:297–302.

226. Reiter RJ, Klaus S, Ebbinghaus C, Heldmaier G, Redlin U, Ricquier D, Vaughan MK, Steinlechner S. Inhibition of 5'deiodination of thyroxine suppresses the cold-induced increase in brown adipose tissue messenger ribonucleic acid for mitochondrial uncoupling protein without influencing lipoprotein lipase activity. Endocrinology 1990; 126:2550–2554.

227. Tontonoz P, Kim JB, Graves RA, Spiegelman BM. ADD1: a novel helix-loop-helix transcription associated with adipocyte determination and differentiation. Mol Cell Biochem 1993; 13:4753–4759.

228. Zhang Y, Proenca R, Maffei M, Barone M, Leopold L, Friedman JM. Positional cloning of the mouse obese gene and its human homologue. Nature (Lond) 1994; 372: 425–432.

229. Zhang Y, Proenca R, Maffei M, Barone M, Leopold L, Friedman JM. Positional cloning of the mouse obese gene and its human homologue (correction). Nature 1995; 374:479.

230. Frederich RC, Löllmann B, Hamann A, Napolitano-Rosen A, Kahn BB, Lowell BB, Flier JS. Expression of the ob mRNA and its encoded protein in rodents. Impact of nutrition and obesity. J Clin Invest 1995; 96:1658–1663.

231. Maffei M, Fei H, Lee G-H, Dani C, Leroy P, Zhang Y, Proenca R, Negrel R, Ailhaud G, Friedman JM. Increased expression in adipocytes of ob RNA in mice with lesions of the hypothalamus and with mutations at the db locus. Proc Natl Acad Sci USA 1995; 92:6957–6960.

232. Moinat M, Deng CJ, Muzzin P, Assimacopoulos-Jeannet F, Seydoux J, Dulloo AG, Giacobino JP. Modulation of obese gene expression in rat brown and white adipose tissues. FEBS Lett 1995; 373:131–134.

233. Masuzaki H, Ogawa Y, Shigemoto M, Satoh N, Mori K, Tamura N, Hosoda K, Yoshimasa Y, Jingami H, Nakao K. Adipose tissue-specific expression of the obese (ob) gene

in rats and its marked augmentation in genetically obese-hyperglycemic Wistar fatty rats. Proc Japan Acad Ser B 1995; 71:148–152.

234. Vydelingum S, Shillabeer G, Hatch G, Russell JC, Lau DCW. Overexpression of ob gene in the JCR-LA-corpulent rat. Biochem Biophys Res Commun 1995; 216:148–153.

235. Murakami T, Iida M, Shima K. Dexamethasone regulates *obese* expression in isolated rat adipocytes. Biochem Biophys Res Commun 1995; 214:1260–1267.

236. MacDougald OA, Hwang C-S, Fan H, Lane MD. Regulated expression of the obese gene product (leptin) in white adipose tissue and 3T3-L1 adipocytes. Proc Natl Acad Sci USA 1995; 92:9034–9037.

237. Trayhurn P, Thomas MEA, Duncan JS, Rayner DV. Effects of fasting and refeeding on *ob* gene expression in white adipose tissue of lean and obese (*ob/ob*) mice. FEBS Lett 1995; 368:488–490.

238. Murakami T, Shima K. Cloning of the rat obese cDNA and its expression in obese rats. Biochem Biophys Res Commun 1995; 209:944–952.

239. Ogawa Y, Masuzaki H, Isse N, Okazaki T, Mori K, Shigemoto M, Satoh N, Tamura N, Hosoda K, Yoshimasa Y, Jingami H, Kawada T, Nakao K. Molecular cloning of the *obese* cDNA and augmented gene expression in genetically obese Zucker fatty (*fa/fa*) rats. J Clin Invest 1995; 96:1647–1652.

240. Pelleymounter MA, Cullen MJ, Baker MB, Hecht R, Winters D, Boone T, Collins F. Effect of the *obese* gene product on body weight regulation in ob/ob mice. Science 1995; 269:540–543.

241. Carneheim C, Nedergaard J, Cannon B. β-Adrenergic stimulation of lipoprotein lipase in rat brown adipose tissue during acclimation to cold. Am J Physiol 1984; 246:E327–E333.

242. Mitchell JRD, Jacobsson A, Kirchgessner TG, Schotz MC, Cannon B, Nedergaard J. Regulation of expression of the lipoprotein lipase gene in brown adipose tissue. Am J Physiol 1992; 263:E500–E506.

243. Giralt M, Martin I, Vilaró S, Villarroya F, Mampel T, Iglesias R, Viñas O. Lipoprotein lipase mRNA expression in brown adipose tissue: translational and/or posttranslational events are involved in the modulation of enzyme activity. Biochim Biophys Acta 1990; 1048:270–273.

244. Campbell DJ, Habener JF. Cellular localization of angiotensinogen gene expression in brown adipose tissue and mesentery: quantification of messenger ribonucleic acid abundance using hybrodization in situ. Endocrinology 1987; 121:1616–1626.

245. Cassis LA, Saye J, Peach MJ. Location and regulation of rat angiotensinogen messenger RNA. Hypertension 1988; 11:591–596.

246. Frederich RC, Kahn BB, Peach MJ, Flier JS. Tissue-specific nutritional regulation of angiotensinogen in adipose tissue. Hypertension 1992; 19:339–344.

247. Crandall DL, Herzlinger HE, Saunders BD, Kral JB. Developmental aspects of adipose tissue renin-angiotensin system: therapeutic implications. Drug Dev Res 1994; 32:117–125.

248. Cassis LA, Dwoskin LP. Presynaptic modulation of neurotransmitter release by endogenous angiotensin II in brown adipose tissue. J Neural Transm 1991; (Suppl 34):129–137.

249. Cassis LA, Dwoskin LP. Acute and chronic losartan administration: effect on angiotensin II content and modulation of [³H]norepinephrine release from rat interscap-ular brown adipose tissue. J Neural Transm (Gen Sect) 1994; 98:159–163.

250. Cassis LA. Role of angiotensin II in brown adipose tissue thermogenesis during cold acclimation. Am J Physiol 1993; 265:E860–E865.

251. Spiegelman BM, Choy L, Hotamisligil GS, Graves RA, Tontonoz P. Regulation of adipocyte gene expression in differentiation and syndromes of obesity/diabetes. J Biol Chem 1993; 268:6823–6826.

252. Wilkison WO, Spiegelman BM. Biosynthesis of the vasoactive lipid monobutyrin. Central role of diacylglycerol. J Biol Chem 1993; 268:2844–2849.

253. Wagner H, Nusser D, Sachs M. Steroid profiles of brown adipose tissue. J Steroid Biochem Mol Biol 1991; 39:405–407.

254. Walston J, Silver K, Bogardus C, Knowler WC, Celi FS, Austin S, Manning B, Strosberg AD, Stern MP, Raben N, Sorkin JD, Roth J, Shuldiner AR. Time of onset of non-insulin-dependent diabetes mellitus and genetic variation in the β3-adrenergic-receptor gene. N Engl J Med 1995; 333:342–347.

255. Widén E, Lehto M, Kanninen T, Walston J, Shuldiner AR, Groop LC. Association of a polymorphism in the β3-adrenergic-receptor gene with features of the insulin resistance syndrome in Finns. N Engl J Med 1995; 333:348–351.

256. Clément K, Vaisse C, Manning BStJ, Basdevant A, Guy-Grand B, Ruiz J, Silver KD, Shuldiner AR, Froguel P, Strosberg AD. Genetic variation in the β3-adrenergic receptor and an increased capacity to gain weight in patients with morbid obesity. N Engl J Med 1995; 333:352–354.

257. Kadowaki H, Yasuda K, Iwamoto K, Otabe S, Shimokawa K, Silver K, Walston J, Yoshinaga H, Kosaka K, Yamada N, Saito Y, Hagura R, Akanuma Y, Shuldiner A, Yazaki Y, Kadowaki T. A mutation in the β3-adrenergic receptor gene is associated with obesity and hyperinsulinemia in Japanese subjects. Biochem Biophys Res Commun 1995; 215:555–560.

20

Resting Energy Expenditure, Thermic Effect of Food, and Total Energy Expenditure

Yves Schutz and Eric Jéquier
University of Lausanne, Lausanne, Switzerland

I. METHODS OF MEASURING ENERGY EXPENDITURE IN HUMANS

A. Introduction

Three main methods are used to measure energy expenditure in humans: indirect calorimetry, direct calorimetry, and the doubly labeled water technique. These methods are based on different principles and do not measure the same type of energy.

Indirect calorimetry is the best method to measure resting energy expenditure, the thermic effect of food, and the energy expended for physical activity. It has the advantage of being relatively simple; it can be used either with a ventilated hood system (for a resting subject), or with a respiration chamber, when a 24-hr measurement is needed. A first advantage of indirect calorimetry is the immediate response of oxygen consumption (measured by the method of respiratory gas exchange) in relation with the real oxygen consumption in the tissues and organs within the body. There is no delay in measuring oxygen consumption because the body has negligible O_2 stores. A second advantage of indirect calorimetry in comparison with other methods is the possibility to assess nutrient oxidation rates, when oxygen consumption, CO_2 production, and urinary nitrogen excretion are measured.

Direct calorimetry is the method of choice for studies aiming at assessing thermoregulatory responses. The method consists in measuring heat losses, not heat pro-

duction. In many circumstances, heat losses differ from heat production and there is a change in heat stored. For instance, after a meal, heat production begins to rise 20–30 min after the onset of eating, whereas heat loss increases only later; the consequence of the different time courses of heat production and heat loss is a rise in body temperature.

The method of direct calorimetry consists in the measurement of the heat dissipated by the body by radiation, convection, conduction, and evaporation (1). Under conditions of thermal equilibrium in a subject at rest and in postabsorptive conditions, heat production, measured by indirect calorimetry, is identical to heat dissipation, measured by direct calorimetry (Fig. 1). This is an obvious confirmation of the first law of thermodynamics, which states that the energy released by oxidative processes is ultimately transformed into heat (and external work during exercise). In steady-state conditions, the identity between heat production and heat loss in a resting subject (Fig. 1) corroborates the validity (for the whole body) of the method of indirect calorimetry.

The third method, *the doubly labeled water technique*, is based on the difference in the rates of turnover of ^2H_2O and $H_2\ ^{18}O$ in body water. The subject is given a single oral dose of $^2H_2\ ^{18}O$ to label body water with both isotopes ^2H and ^{18}O. A rapid exchange of ^{18}O occurs between water and carbon dioxide due to the action of carbonic anhydrase. As a result, after equilibrium of $^2H_2\ ^{18}O$ in the water pool and equilibrium of ^{18}O with carbon dioxide,

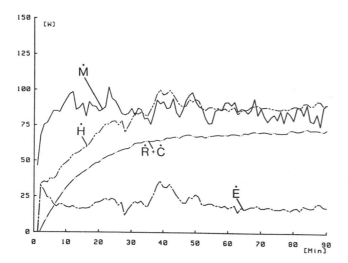

Figure 1   Metabolic rate (Ṁ), total heat losses (Ḣ), radiative and convective heat losses (Ṙ + Ċ), and evaporative heat losses (Ė) in a male subject aged 25 years, exposed at 28°C in a direct calorimeter. Note that after 30 min of temperature equilibration within the calorimeter, the values of M and H are similar, indicating that heat production is identical to heat losses.

^{18}O is lost both as $H_2{}^{18}O$ and as $CO^{18}O$, whereas ^{2}H is lost only as $^{2}H_2O$. The difference in the rate of turnover of $H_2{}^{18}O$ and $^{2}H_2O$ is an estimate of CO_2 production rate. To calculate the subject's energy expenditure, the mean respiratory quotient (RQ) must be known. Energy expenditure is obtained by multiplying $\dot{V}CO_2$ by the energy equivalent of CO_2 production. The latter varies from 21.0 to 27.7 kJ/L CO_2 at respiratory quotients of 1.0 to 0.7, respectively. The disappearance rates of the isotopes can be measured in urine, blood, or saliva, for a period equivalent to two to three biological half-lives. This corresponds to about 14 days in adult subjects. Thus, the method provides a mean value of energy expenditure for a 2-week period. It is not possible to calculate the day-to-day variation in energy expenditure with the doubly labeled water technique.

Several validation studies in both infants and adults have consistently shown a good agreement between the $\dot{V}CO_2$ determined by the doubly labeled water and that assessed by indirect calorimetry. Issues have been raised regarding two-point versus multiple-point isotopic sampling, the extent of the fractionation of the isotopes, the difference between the oxygen and hydrogen dilution space, as well as the inherent precision of the analysis by mass spectrometry (2). Roberts et al. (3) have recently conducted an interlaboratory comparison of the doubly labeled water method using standards containing varying amounts of $^{2}H_2$ and ^{18}O as well as dose specimens. Sur-

prisingly, there was substantial variability between laboratories in the results and some laboratories obtained physiologically impossible energy expenditure (i.e., below the resting value). The type of calculation used had little effect on the accuracy of the technique. As a result, the average coefficient of variation for the doubly labeled water method, which is often claimed to be 5%, was not attained by a few laboratories, mostly due to the quality of the isotopic analysis. The impact of deuterium and ^{18}O pool size determination on the calculation of total energy expenditure constitutes an important issue (4) since hydrogen tracer dilutes into a pool significantly larger than the body water pool due to the presence of labile hydrogen. This justifies the need for a correction factor for the isotope pool size. It seems that the best approach is to use a pool size based on the average of the deuterium and ^{18}O pool space (4).

A recent study by Speakman (5) indicated that the error for $\dot{V}CO_2$ estimated by doubly labeled water was not normally distributed. Depending on the difference in the elimination rate constants of the two labels, the duration of the experiment, and the initial isotopic dose, the precision error (99% confidence interval for mean) using duplicate analysis varied enormously (between 3 and 47%). By increasing the number of replicates from two to five, the error could be substantially reduced. The issue of shifts in baseline abundance of deuterium of ^{18}O tracers is important since it may generate errors in the derivation of CO_2 and H_2O turnover rates and hence calculated energy expenditure. Jones (6) suggested that optimally the subject should first equilibrate with the new water source when a doubly labeled water study is performed. Alternatively, correction for shifting baseline can be made by measuring isotopic abundance changes in a control group of subjects who do not receive the doubly labeled water dose, but ingest the same diet as the experimental group and perform similar activities.

B. Indirect Calorimetry: The Method of Choice to Measure Energy Expenditure and Nutrient Oxidation Rates

1. Measurement of Energy Expenditure

The term "indirect calorimetry" stems from the fact that the heat released by chemical processes within the body can be indirectly calculated from the rate of oxygen consumption ($\dot{V}O_2$). The main reason for the close relation between energy metabolism and $\dot{V}O_2$ is that the oxidative phosphorylation in the respiratory chain is coupled with a continuous synthesis of adenosine triphosphate (ATP). The energy expended within the body to maintain electrochemical gradients, to support biosynthetic processes, and to generate muscular contraction cannot be directly provided by nutrient oxidation. Almost all chemical processes requiring energy depend on ATP hydrolysis. It is the rate of ATP utilization that determines the overall rate of substrate oxidation and therefore $\dot{V}_{O_2}$. With the exception of anaerobic glycolysis, ATP synthesis is coupled with substrate oxidation. Because there is a proportionality between $\dot{V}_{O_2}$ and ATP synthesis, and because each mole of ATP synthesized is accompanied by the production of a given amount of heat, one understands the rationale of using $\dot{V}_{O_2}$ measurement to calculate heat production within the body (7).

The study of the regulation of energy metabolism and nutrient utilization in humans has recently raised great interest thanks to advances in the construction of open-circuit ventilated hood indirect calorimeters and comfortable respiration chambers (8).

With the measurement of $\dot{V}_{O_2}$ (in liters of O_2/min) at STPD conditions (standard temperature (0°C), pressure (760 mmHg), and gas dry), metabolic rate (M), which corresponds to heat production, can be calculated (in kilojoules per minute) as follows:

$$M = 20.3 \times \dot{V}_{O_2} \qquad (1)$$

The number 20.3 is a mean value (in kJ/L) of the energy equivalent for the consumption of 1 L (STPD) oxygen. The value of the energy equivalent of oxygen depends on the composition of the fuel mixture oxidized (Table 1). The error in using Eq. (1) instead of an equation that takes into account the type of fuels oxidized [Eq. (2) and (3), see below] is not greater than ±2%.

The heat released by the oxidation of each of the three macronutrients (carbohydrates, fats, and proteins) can be calculated from three measurements: oxygen consumption ($\dot{V}_{O_2}$), carbon dioxide production ($\dot{V}_{CO_2}$), and urinary nitrogen excretion (N).

Simple equations for computing metabolic rate (or energy expenditure) from these three determinations are written under the form:

$$M = a\,\dot{V}_{O_2} + b\,\dot{V}_{CO_2} - c\,N \qquad (2)$$

The factors a, b, and c depend on the respective constants for the amount of O_2 used and the amount of CO_2 produced during oxidation of the three classes of nutrients (Table 1). An example of such a formula (Brouwer's equation) is given below:

$$M = 16.18\,\dot{V}_{O_2} + 5.02\,\dot{V}_{CO_2} - 5.99\,N \qquad (3)$$

where M is in kilojoules per unit of time, $\dot{V}_{O_2}$ and $\dot{V}_{CO_2}$ are in liters STPD per unit of time, and N is in grams per unit of time. Slightly different factors for the amounts of O_2 used and of CO_2 produced during oxidation of the nutrients are used by other authors, and the values for the factors a, b, and c are modified accordingly. The difference in energy expenditure calculated by the various formulae is not greater than 3%. Detailed information about these calculations is given elsewhere (7–9).

2. Measurement of Nutrient Oxidation Rates

As an example, let us assume that a subject is oxidizing g grams per minute of carbohydrate (as glucose), f grams per minute of fat, and is excreting n grams per minute of urinary nitrogen. The following equations, based on Table 1, describe $\dot{V}_{O_2}$ and $\dot{V}_{CO_2}$:

$$\dot{V}_{O_2} = 0.746\,g + 2.02\,f + 6.31\,n \qquad (4)$$

$$\dot{V}_{CO_2} = 0.746\,g + 1.43\,f + 5.27\,n \qquad (5)$$

Table 1 Oxygen Consumed, CO_2 Produced, and Heat Released from Oxidation of Nutrients

Nutrients	O_2 consumed[a]	CO_2 produced[a]	RQ	kJ/g	kcal/g	kJ/L	kcal/L	kJ/L	kcal/L
Starch	0.829	0.829	1.00	17.6	4.20	21.2	5.06	21.2	5.06
Saccharose	0.786	0.786	1.00	16.6	3.96	21.1	5.04	21.1	5.04
Glucose	0.746	0.746	1.00	15.6	3.74	21.0	5.01	21.0	5.01
Lipid	2.019	1.427	0.71	39.6	9.46	19.6	4.69	27.7	6.63
Protein	1.010	0.844	0.83	19.7	4.70	19.5	4.66	23.3	5.58
Lactic acid	0.746	0.746	1.00	15.1	3.62	20.3	4.85	20.3	4.85

[a]In liters per gram of substrate oxidized.
RQ = respiratory quotient = $\dot{V}_{CO_2}/\dot{V}_{O_2}$.
Source: Data from Livesey G, Elia M. Am J Clin Nutr 1988; 47:608–628.

We can solve Eq. (4) and (5) for the unknown g and f as follows:

$$g = 4.59 \dot{V}_{CO_2} - 3.25 \dot{V}_{O_2} - 3.68\,n \qquad (6)$$

$$f = 1.69 \dot{V}_{O_2} - 1.69 \dot{V}_{CO_2} - 1.72\,n \qquad (7)$$

Because 1 g urinary nitrogen arises from approximately 6.25 g protein, the protein oxidation rate (p in grams per minute) is given by the equation

$$p = 6.25\,n \qquad (8)$$

Other metabolic processes (such as lipogenesis, gluconeogenesis, and ketogenesis) may influence the calculated oxidation rates of nutrients. However, intermediate metabolic processes do not influence the results of Eq. (6) and (7), provided intermediate substrates do not accumulate within the body or are not excreted from the body. When there is accumulation or excretion of an intermediate or end product other than CO_2 and H_2O, this approach to compute the oxidation rates of nutrients is no longer valid, and correction factors must be applied to take into account the changes in the pool size of the intermediates or end products.

II. RESTING AND BASAL METABOLIC RATES (RMR AND BMR)

A. Whole-Body, Organs, and Tissue Metabolic Rates

There is an arbitrary distinction between RMR and BMR in the literature. RMR may be considered equivalent to BMR if the measurements are made in postabsorptive conditions. It seems difficult to partition RMR into various subcomponents since the metabolic rate of individual organs and tissues is difficult to assess in humans under noninvasive experimental conditions. By measuring the arteriovenous difference in concentration of O_2 across an organ or tissue, combined with the assessment of blood flow perfusing this organ or tissue, the $\dot{V}_{O_2}$ of an organ or tissue can be estimated in vivo (based on the reverse Fick equation), but this requires invasive procedure such as arterial and venous catheterization. The error of measurement will largely increase if the rate of blood perfusion of an organ is high as compared to its $\dot{V}_{O_2}$, indicating a low arteriovenous oxygen difference.

Elia (10) has written an excellent review of the contribution of organs and tissue to the metabolic rate. The major part of the whole-body RMR stems from organs with high metabolic activity such as the liver, kidneys, brain, and heart, although these account for a small proportion of the total body weight (5%, Table 2). Per unit organ weight, the kidneys and heart have a metabolic rate more than twice as high as the liver and the brain. In contrast, the metabolic rate of muscle per unit body weight is nearly 35 times lower than that of the heart and kidneys. Since the proportion of muscle to nonmuscle changes with age from birth to adulthood, the RMR per unit body weight is not constant with age (11). The tissue with the lowest metabolic activity per unit body weight is adipose tissue, which accounts for only 4% of the whole-body RMR in nonobese subjects. Calculations show that this value can increase up to 10% or more in obese subjects with large excess body fat (Schutz et al., unpublished). The "residual" metabolic rate (16%) not explained by the tissues and organs mentioned above can be accounted for by skin and intestines (which have a relatively large protein mass and protein turnover), as well as bones and lungs.

B. Body Composition: Effect of Fat-Free Mass and Fat Mass

The excess body weight of the obese is primarily constituted by fat tissue, but also a small component of associated lean tissue. Although the exact nature of extra lean tissue in obesity is largely unknown, it seems logical to expect a greater absolute RMR in obese adults (12) and children (13) characterized by an excess fat mass and a slight increase in fat-free mass. Numerous studies have demonstrated that the major factor explaining the variation in RMR between individuals is fat-free mass (14). Fat-free mass (FFM) is a heterogeneous component that can be partitioned into muscle mass and nonmuscle mass. Unfortunately, there is no simple and accurate way to assess these two subcomponents. Due to the larger variation, between individuals, in fat mass, as compared to FFM, and due to the fact that in grossly obese women fat mass can represent a nonnegligible component of total RMR, the prediction models for RMR that include both FFM and fat mass explain significantly more variance in RMR than FFM alone (14). In addition, age, sex, and family membership are additional factors that should be taken into account.

The effects of gender on resting metabolic rate are explained by differences in body composition. Caution should be used when comparing resting metabolic rate expressed per kilogram FFM in men and women, because the composition of FFM is influenced by gender. The muscle mass of men being larger than that of women, this fact tends to lower the value of RMR per kilogram FFM in men when compared to that of women. This is explained by a greater component of a tissue with a low metabolic rate (resting muscle) in men than in women

Table 2 Contribution of Different Organs and Tissues to Total Body Weight and Basal Metabolic Rate (BMR) in an Average Man of 70 kg with a BMR of 1680 kcal/day (7.03 MJ/day)

	Tissue or organ weight (kg)	Contribution of tissue or organ weight to body weight (%)	Organ metabolic rate per unit weight (kcal/kg/day)	Contribution to BMR (% total)
Liver	1.8	2.6	200	21
Brain	1.4	2.0	240	20
Heart	0.33	0.5	440	9
Kidneys	0.31	0.4	440	8
Muscle	28.0	40.0	13	22
Adipose tissue	15.0	21.4	4.4	4
Δ = miscellaneous tissues (bones, skin, intestines, lungs, etc.)	23.2	33.1	12	16
Total	70.00	100	24 (mean)	100

Source: Ref. 10.

(Table 2). According to recent data (15,16), women have a lower RMR than men (3–10%) even after adjustment for FFM, fat mass, age, and VO_2max. Various mechanisms could explain this observation, such as hormonal status, differences in the composition of the FFM, muscular fiber type composition (17), and Na,K-ATPase activity (18), as well as differences in the activity of the neoglucogenic pathway, differences in the central body temperature, and sympathetic nervous system activity (15).

Physiological variations in sex hormones during the phases of the menstrual cycle in women offer the opportunity to assess, in addition to the change in basal body temperature, the effect of hormonal variation on RMR. Previous studies have indicated an increase in RMR (19) and sleeping metabolic rate (20) in the luteal phase of the menstrual cycle, although recent data in Indian (21) and Dutch (22) women did not show any differences. In a study in which heat production and heat losses were measured by both direct and indirect calorimetry (23), we failed to find any significant differences in RMR (heat production) and heat losses during the luteal phase of the menstrual cycle in young women. By combining indirect calorimetry, direct calorimetry, and thermometry, skin thermal conductance and skin blood flow could be calculated. We observed a decrease in these two latter parameters during the luteal phase that indicates an increase in cutaneous thermal insulation. We concluded that during the luteal phase, the decreased thermal conductance in women exposed to a neutral environment allows the maintenance of a higher internal temperature (23).

Aging leads to a progressive decrease in RMR. Classically, this has been attributed to the reduction in muscle mass accompanying aging (24). A drop in the metabolic activity per unit tissue mass is also likely to occur if the loss of FFM does not fully account for the lower RMR (25). In a recent study, we explored the change in RMR and whole-body protein turnover in healthy elderly and lean Gambian men (26). It was found that adjusted for FFM, the RMR was significantly lower by 13% in elderly as compared to young individuals. This was not explained by a decrease in protein turnover, since the protein turnover adjusted for FFM was not different between the two groups. The extent of the decline in RMR in obese male and female individuals remains to be investigated.

C. Effect of Previous Dietary Intake

Postabsorptive RMR (or BMR) is typically measured 12 hr after the last meal, in order to diminish the effect of "residual" postprandial thermogenesis. Nevertheless, the relative composition of the diet eaten the previous days (i.e., the food quotient, FQ), largely influences the respiratory quotient during postabsorptive RMR (27). Isocaloric substitution of low versus high carbohydrate diets has much more influence on the RQ than on the rate of RMR (28). The extent to which short-term overfeeding will increase both the RQ and the RMR depends on the duration of overfeeding: one single-day surfeit energy intake increases the RQ above the FQ (indicating fat storage), but the rise in RMR is very limited and most of the effect is seen on dietary-induced thermogenesis (29).

D. Hormonal Factors

Many studies have demonstrated that catecholamines increase RMR (30–32). Both β_1 and β_2-adrenoceptors are involved in this sympathetically mediated thermogenesis (33). Subcutaneous or intravenous injections of epinephrine increase the RMR by about 20% with large interstudy variation and in a dose-dependent manner (30). Many different organs are involved in the epinephrine-mediated thermogenesis, but the major part of the effect seems to occur in skeletal muscles and in the heart. The mechanism by which epinephrine exerts its thermogenic action may be via a specific stimulation at the cellular level, extrasubstrate cycling (e.g., Cori cycle), and activation of skeletal muscle and cardiac activities.

It has been known for several decades that administration of thyroid hormones increases the RMR since this test was used, several decades ago, as a diagnostic tool until hormonal concentrations could be determined. The response on the RMR is not immediate and appears after several days of hormonal administration. Hyperthyroid patients have an increased metabolic rate, which is dependent on the T3 blood concentration and may reach up to 180% of the standard reference value (34). There is no general agreement about the mechanism of action of thyroid hormones: they may increase the Na,K-ATPase activity in various tissues and may also lead to a stimulation in the rate of protein turnover.

E. Familial and Genetic Effects

A decade ago, Bogardus et al. (35) observed that part of the unexplained variance in RMR could be accounted for by family membership, indicating that the level of RMR is partially genetically determined. The twins studies of Bouchard et al. (36) have shown that the RMRs of monozygotic twins have more resemblance than that of dizygotic twins after statistical adjustment for differences in body size and body composition. An excellent and recent account of the part played by genetic factors in the etiology of human obesity as well as their metabolic implications has recently been published by Bouchard et al. (37).

III. THERMIC EFFECT OF FOOD IN HUMANS

The energy expenditure increases significantly after a meal, a phenomenon that was first attributed to the intake of protein under the term "specific dynamic action." It was subsequently recognized that not only protein intake, but also carbohydrate and, to a lesser extent, fat intake stimulate energy expenditure. This effect is now called dietary-induced thermogenesis or the thermic effect of food.

The thermic effect of food is mainly due to the energy cost of nutrient absorption, processing, and storage. The total thermic effect of food over 24 hr represents about 10% of the total energy expenditure in sedentary subjects.

A. Techniques for Measurement of the Thermic Effect of Food

The best technique to assess the thermic effect of a meal is to measure the energy expenditure following a meal during 3–5 hr and to compare the values with a control test during the same period of time, after a zero-energy drink is given. Alternatively, one often measures resting energy expenditure in a postabsorptive subject during 1 hr to get a stable baseline. Thereafter, a meal is given to the subject and energy expenditure is continuously measured with a ventilated hood during 3–5 hr. The area under the curve over the baseline (considered a constant reference value) represents the thermic effect of the meal.

B. Effect of Energy Intake and Dietary Composition on the Thermic Effect of Food

The thermic effect of the nutrients mainly depends on the energy costs of processing and/or storing the nutrient. Expressed in percent of the energy content of the nutrient, values of 8, 2, 20–30, and 22% have been reported for glucose, fat, protein, and ethanol, respectively (7,38,39).

Glucose-induced thermogenesis mainly results from the cost of glycogen synthesis and substrate cycling (38). Glucose storage as glycogen requires 2 mol ATP/mol. In comparison with the 38 mol ATP produced on complete oxidation of glucose, the energy cost of glucose storage as glycogen corresponds to 5% (or 2/38) of the energy content of glucose stored. Cycling of glucose to glucose-6-phosphate and back to glucose, to fructose-1,6-diphosphate and back to glucose-6-phosphate, or to lactate and back to glucose is occurring at varying rates, and these are energy-requiring processes that may increase the thermic effect of carbohydrates.

The thermic effect of dietary fat is very small; an increase of 2% of its energy content has been described during infusion of an emulsion of triglyceride (40). This slight increase in energy expenditure is explained by the ATP consumption in the process of free fatty acid reesterification to triglyceride. As a consequence, the dietary energy of fat is used very efficiently.

The thermic effect of proteins is the highest of all nutrients (20–30% of the energy content of proteins). Ingested proteins are degraded in the gut into amino acids. After absorption, amino acids may be deaminated, their amino group transferred to urea, and their carbon skeleton converted to glucose. These biochemical processes require the consumption of energy amounting to ≈25% of the energy content of amino acids. The second pathway of amino acid metabolism is protein synthesis; the energy expended for the synthesis of the peptide bonds also represents $\cong 25\%$ of the energy content of amino acids. Therefore, irrespective of their metabolic pathway, the thermogenesis induced after amino acids absorption represents about 25% of their energy content.

The thermic effect of ethanol amounts to about 22% of its energy content (39). The acute effects of ethanol ingestion include a decrease in the plasma free fatty acids level and a change in the cellular redox state in the liver cells, with an inhibition of lipid oxidation.

C. Effect of Gender and Age on the Thermic Effect of Food

The thermic effect of food is apparently not influenced by gender. More than a decade ago we observed that the thermic effect of an oral load of glucose was negatively correlated with age (41). The effects of age on the thermic effect of food are entirely explained by the decrease in FFM with age (42). Thus, when the thermic effect of food is corrected for the FFM, both young and elderly subjects have similar values (42).

D. Effect of Body Composition and Nutritional Status on the Thermic Effect of Food

The effect of body composition on the thermic effect of food has been well studied. The hypothesis of a "thrifty gene," a genetic propensity to increase the efficiency of energy utilization, has been proposed to explain how humans have survived during periods of famine over the million years of evolution. According to this hypothesis, there has been a strong selective pressure to eliminate individuals with a low metabolic efficiency, whereas those with a "thrifty gene" have had greater chance of survival thanks to a more efficient energy metabolism. When exposed to conditions of plenty, those with a thrifty gene have an increased risk to become obese.

In support of this hypothesis, it has been reported that thermogenesis is decreased in most obese individuals (43). Thermogenesis is the energy expenditure above basal metabolic rate due to food intake, cold exposure, thermogenic agents, and psychological influences. The most important factor that stimulates thermogenesis is food intake (38). However, caffeine (44) and nicotine (45) are thermogenic agents that stimulate energy expenditure. Cold exposure does not play a significant role in stimulating energy expenditure under usual life conditions (46). Humans avoid cold exposure by wearing clothes and maintaining room temperature in the comfort zone.

Dietary thermogenesis includes two components: the "obligatory" costs of digesting, absorbing, processing, and storing the nutrients and a "facultative" component. The facultative component of thermogenesis depends on the sympathetic nervous system (47). Carbohydrate overfeeding induces a sustained rise of urinary norepinephrine (48), and infusions of glucose and insulin increase plasma norepinephrine levels (49). Additional evidence of the activation of the sympathetic nervous system after carbohydrate infusion is the reduction of the glucose-induced thermogenic response by ß-adrenergic blockade with propranolol (50,51).

The possible contribution of a thermogenic defect in the etiology of obesity is controversial. The thermogenic responses to glucose or meal ingestion are either decreased (52–61) or unaltered (62–68) in obese subjects. The thermic effect of infused insulin-glucose was found to be reduced in insulin-resistant and non-insulin-dependent diabetes mellitus (NIDDM) obese patients (69–71). The thermic effect of insulin-glucose was found to be proportional to the rate of glucose storage. This concept is supported by Ravussin et al. (72), who showed a similar thermic effect of glucose in lean and obese subjects when they were infused at the rate of insulin needed to obtain a predetermined glucose uptake. Obese subjects had to be infused with a larger rate of insulin infusion to get the same rate of glucose uptake as that of lean subjects. With a similar rate of glucose uptake, the thermogenic response was the same in lean and in obese subjects. It can be concluded that obese subjects with impaired glucose tolerance and NIDDM obese patients have a decreased rate of glucose storage after a meal (or a glucose load), which is accompanied by a reduced rate of storage of glucose as glycogen in muscles, with an economy of energy expenditure.

It is interesting to evaluate the possible role of a thermogenic defect in the weight gain that occurs in most patients after cessation of hypocaloric therapy. We calculated that a thermogenic defect can account for a maximal energy saving of ≈ 125 kcal/day. Because the increase in body weight is accompanied by a rise in energy expenditure of approximately 25 kcal/day/kg weight gain (8), it can be calculated that a weight gain of 5 kg (i.e., a rise in energy expenditure of ~125 kcal/day) completely offsets the effect of the thermogenic defect (73). Therefore, a thermogenic defect is a factor that contributes to the weight gain after cessation of dietary therapy but it has a modest effect (73). It is likely that an abnormality in the control of food intake plays the most important role in the development of obesity or in relapse of body weight gain after a hypocaloric diet. Obese individuals, even those with a low basal metabolic rate per unit lean body mass, expend more energy than lean sedentary individuals (74). Thus, the important conclusion is that the concept of "small eaters" who remain obese with daily energy intake less than 1800 kcal/day is certainly wrong.

E. Control of the Thermic Effect of Food by the Autonomic Nervous System and by Hormones

The sympathetic nervous system (SNS) plays a role in the control of energy expenditure. As already described, the thermogenic response to food ingestion includes a facultative component that depends on the activity of the SNS (14–18). Recent evidence shows that oral (75) or iv (76) glucose administration stimulates muscle sympathetic nerve activity (NSNA). Increased activity of the SNS may contribute to the thermic effect of food since β-adrenergic blockade with propranolol decreases glucose-induced thermogenesis (50,51). However, the metabolic effects of catecholamines released at sympathetic nerve endings or by the adrenal medulla remain unclear (77).

Since the parasympathetic nervous system is involved in the cephalic phase of insulin secretion at the beginning of a meal (78), a role for this system has also been investigated in the control of the thermic effect of food (79). Cholinergic blockade with atropine decreases the thermic effect of a meal (79). This effect can be explained in part by the fact that atropine slows gastric emptying and reduces intestinal motility. Thus, the thermogenic mechanisms that are dependent on the parasympathetic nervous system may be related to intestinal absorption and the subsequent rate of storage of the absorbed nutrients.

The main hormone involved in the thermic effect of a meal is insulin. There is a reduced thermogenic response to a meal in obese subjects with insulin resistance and in obese NIDDM patients. Thus, either insulin resistance and/or a relative defect in insulin secretion induces a reduced glucose-induced thermogenesis. The latter is due in part to an impaired rate of glucose storage as glycogen in muscles; whether a reduced activation of the SNS plays a role is still unknown.

F. Familial and Genetic Effects on Thermic Effect of Food

Genetic factors may contribute to the interindividual differences observed in the components of energy expenditure. Studies on the genetic effect of energy expenditure associated with the thermic effect of food are limited. Bouchard et al. (36) measured the thermic effect of a 1000-kcal meal during 4 hr in 21 pairs of dizygotic twins and 37 pairs of monozygotic twins, as well as in 31 parent-offspring pairs. The results suggest a genetic effect of $<1/3$

of the total thermic effect of food. Expressed in absolute values, the standard deviation of the thermic effect of food over 4 hr reached about 20 kcal, and the 95% confidence intervals were therefore ± 40 kcal, or $\pm 4\%$ of the energy intake. These data confirm that the variance of the thermic effect of food between individuals represents a relatively small proportion of the total energy turnover. By comparison, the 95% confidence intervals were about ± 250 kcal/day for resting energy expenditure, or about $\pm 10\%$ of total energy expenditure.

IV. COMPONENTS OF TOTAL ENERGY EXPENDITURE IN THE LEAN AND OBESE STATES

A. Absolute Versus Relative Values

It has been customary to distinguish different components of total energy expenditure (TEE): basal metabolic rate, postprandial thermogenesis (or thermic effect of food), and physical activity. This distinction is important since the reasons for an abnormal 24-hr energy expenditure can be ascribed to a combination of abnormal subcomponents. The resting metabolic rate represents the energy expended in resting conditions under fasting state and comfortable environmental conditions; the thermic effect of food represents the net increase in postabsorptive resting metabolic rate in response to the ingestion of a meal or to an increase in total food intake (diet-induced thermogenesis). Extra non-meal-mediated thermogenic stimuli may occur due to cold or heat exposure, as well as psychological factors (emotion or stress), or may result from the administration of hormones and drugs. Physical activity is the most variable (and hence least predictable) component of total energy expenditure. In contrast to the other components, it can be voluntarily modified by the behavior of the subject. In absolute terms, the TEE of the obese has been shown to be greater than that of lean individuals, both in the confinement of a respiration chamber (12,43,80) and in free-living conditions (81). The relative rate of TEE can be expressed as a multiple of some baseline values such as RMR. This approach has been used by the International Expert Committee for calculating the energy requirement by the so-called "factorial" method (82). Since both the RMR and TEE of obese subjects are greater in absolute value, it seems of interest to calculate the ratio between the latter and the former. This provides a rough index of physical activity ("physical activity level"), but the contribution of the thermic effect of foods represents a small confounding factor. Since the energy cost for a given activity is proportional to body weight, in particular for weight-bearing activities, the absolute energy expenditure during weight-bearing activity will be linearly related to body weight (83). A flat (or a negative) relationship between the energy expenditure due to physical activity and the degree of obesity would indicate that the greater absolute cost of physical activity among obese subjects is largely offset by the depressed activity level. A recent study by Rising et al. (84) has shown that obesity was associated with lower levels of physical activity. The key question is to know whether a low level of physical activity is the *consequence* or the *cause* of obesity, or both.

Normalization of total energy expenditure in the obese appears to be difficult since the RMR is proportional to FFM (and fat mass) whereas the energy expenditure–related physical activity is proportional to body weight. Although there is a statistical bias in normalizing the TEE by RMR (85), it nevertheless seems to be a reasonable way (as compared to other alternatives) to express the free-living energy expenditure. The fact that both the absolute RMR and the energy cost for a given activity are greater in the obese explains why the TEE expressed in relative value (TEE/RMR) is not expected to be dramatically different from that observed in a nonobese subject. In this context, it is of interest to review the magnitude of the ratio TEE/RMR in nonobese and obese adult subjects. Table 3 shows an overview of different experimental studies recently published in the literature (86–92). Globally considered, there is no strong evidence that the ratio TEE/RMR is systematically lower in obese individuals than in lean subjects, although the variations among and within studies were substantial (Table 3). This confirms our previous results in the respiration chamber (12).

Compilations of total daily energy expenditure results (using a meta-analysis approach) in individuals of various body weight and gender have been recently made by

Schulz and Schoeller (93) and Carpenter et al. (85). In all these studies, energy expenditure was assessed by the doubly labeled water technique. In the former study (93), it was found that the increase weight of men (but not of women) was associated with a tendency for the TEE/RMR ratio to be lower (93), corroborating the notion that obesity tends to depress physical activity in obese men.

Due to the increase in prevalence and incidence of childhood obesity, it seems also important to study the energy metabolism in children as they grow through puberty in order to initiate early therapeutic intervention and prevent subsequent obesity in adults. Blunted physical activity due to a greater placidity and sedentary life-style are associated with low TEE (94–96). A classic study by Dietz et al. (97) has shown that the amount of time dedicated to watching television was related to the degree of obesity in childhood. The relationship between a low level of physical activity and the accumulation of body fat in children has been the subject of a number of recent studies in both infants and children of Caucasian and Pima Indian origin (94,98,99). The classic study by Roberts et al. (99) has suggested that infants who are overweight at 1 year of age had a low total energy expenditure 9 months earlier (i.e., at 3 months of age) compared with a control group of children. The blunted rate of energy expenditure can be considered as one of the causal factors since at the time the infants were measured (3 months) they were not overweight. Although the total daily energy expenditure in free-living condition in obese children is, expressed in absolute value, either greater than (100) or similar (101) to a matched group of lean children, this does not imply that the obese children have the same level of physical activity since the same type of activity will involve a greater energy cost in obese children. Taken together, these studies suggest that a reduced physical activity–related energy expenditure constitutes an important factor in the etiology of the subsequent excess weight gain. The recent study of Davies and White (102) has shown a negative association between the level of physical activity as determined by the ratio between TEE and resting metabolic rate (physical activity level) and the percentage of body fat in a sample of 77 boys and girls.

B. Effect of Weight Loss on Energy Expenditure

When significant weight loss occurs, energy expenditure decreases, whereas weight gain leads to a rise in energy expenditure (103,104). This will depend on the respective effect of the individual factors influencing the three components of TEE: resting energy expenditure will decrease as a function of the loss of FFM, the absolute thermic effect of food will be lower as a result of the restricted

Table 3 Total Energy Expenditure (TEE) Expressed as a Multiple of Resting Metabolic Rate (RMR) in Obese and Nonobese Subjects

	Authors	Ref.	TEE/RMR
I. Obese individuals			
American women	Lichtman et al. (1992)	86	1.68
American women	Welle et al. (1992)	87	1.73
British women	Livingstone et al. (1990)	88	1.39
Pima Indian	Ravussin et al. (1991)	89	1.56
II. Nonobese individuals			
American men	Goran et al. (1993)	90	1.70
American men	Roberts et al. (1991)	91	1.98
British men	Livingstone et al. (1990)	88	1.88
Dutch men	Westerterp et al. (1991)	92	1.64

dietary intake, and, for a given rate of physical activity, the absolute energy expenditure due to physical activity will drop because of the lower body size. In a prospective study of weight loss and relapse in body weight gain, we found that the rate of TEE and RMR essentially followed the change in body weight and body composition (105). The progressively reduced (or increased) energy expenditure accompanying weight loss (or weight gain) constitutes one of the major factors that explain the decrease in the rate of weight loss (or weight gain) with time (103). Another factor is the change in dietary compliance during dieting, which seems to be an individual characteristic (106).

REFERENCES

1. Jéquier E. Direct and indirect calorimetry in man. In: Garrow JS, Halliday D, eds. Substrate and Energy Metabolism. London: J Libbey, 1985:82–92.
2. Schoeller DA, Taylor PB, Shay K. Analytic requirements for the doubly labeled water method. Obes Res 1995; 3(Suppl 1):15–20.
3. Roberts SB, Dietz W, Sharp T, Dallal GE, Hill JO. Multiple laboratory comparison of the doubly labeled water technique. Obes Res 1995; 3(Suppl 1):3–13.
4. Matthews DE, Gilker CD. Impact of ^{2}H and ^{18}O pool size determinations on the calculation of total energy expenditure. Obes Res 1995; 3(Suppl 1):21–29.
5. Speakman JR. Estimation of precision in DLW studies using the two-point methodology. Obes Res 1995; 3(Suppl 1):31–39.
6. Jones PJH. Correction approaches for doubly labeled water in situations of changing background water abundance. Obes Res 1995; 3(Suppl 1):41–48.
7. Jéquier E, Acheson K, Schutz Y. Assessment of energy expenditure and fuel utilization in man. Annu Rev Nutr 1987; 7:187–208.
8. Jéquier E, Schutz Y. Long-term measurements of energy expenditure in humans using a respiration chamber. Am J Clin Nutr 1983; 38:989–998.
9. Frayn NN. Calculation of substrate oxidation rates in vivo from gaseous exchange. J Appl Physiol 1983; 55:628–634.
10. Elia M. Organ and tissue contribution to metabolic rate. In: Kinney JM, Tucker HN. Energy Metabolism: Tissue Determinants and Cellular Corollaries. New York: Raven Press, 1992:61–79.
11. Weinsier RL, Schutz Y, Bracco D. Reexamination of the relationship of resting metabolic rate to fat-free mass and to the metabolically active components of fat-free mass in humans. Am J Clin Nutr 1992; 55:790–794.
12. Schutz Y, Jéquier E. Energy expenditure. Lancet 1986; 1:101–102 (letter).
13. Maffeis C, Schutz Y, Zoccante L, Pinelli L. Resting metabolic rate in six-to-ten-year-old obese and nonobese children. J Pediatr 1993; 122:556–562.
14. Nelson KM, Weinsier RL, Long CL, Schutz Y. Prediction of resting energy expenditure from fat-free mass and fat mass. Am J Clin Nutr 1992; 56:848–856.
15. Ferraro R, Lillioja S, Fontvielle AM, Rising R, Bogardus C, Ravussin E. Lower sedentary metabolic rate in women compared to men. J Clin Invest 1992; 90:1–5.
16. Arciero PJ, Goran MI, Poehlman ET. Resting metabolic rate is lower in women than in men. J Appl Physiol 1993; 75:2514–2520.
17. Zurlo F, Larson K, Bogardus C, Ravussin E. Skeletal muscle metabolism is a major determinant of resting energy expenditure. J Clin Invest 1990; 86:1423–1427.
18. Poehlman ET, Toth MJ, Webb GD. Erythocyte Na-K pump activity contributes to the age-related decline in resting metabolic rate. J Clin Endocrinol Metab 1993; 76:1054–1057.
19. Solomon SJ, Kurzer MS, Calloway DH. Menstrual cycle and basal metabolic rate in women. Am J Clin Nutr 1982; 36:611–616.
20. Bisdee JT, James WPT, Shaw MA. Changes in energy expenditure during the menstrual cycle. Br J Nutr 1989; 61:187–199.
21. Piers LS, Diggavi SN, Riijskamp J, van Raaif JMA, Shetty PS, Hautvast JGAJ. Resting metabolic rate and thermic effect of a meal in the follicular and luteal phases of the menstrual cycle in well-nourished Indian women. Am J Clin Nutr 1995; 61:296–302.
22. Westsrate JA. Resting metabolic rate and diet-induced thermogenesis: a methodological reappraisal. Am J Clin Nutr 1993; 58:592–601.
23. Frascarolo P, Schutz Y, Jéquier E. Decreased thermal conductance during the luteal phase of the menstrual cycle in women. J Appl Physiol 1990; 69:2029–2033.
24. Shock NW, Yiengst MJ. Age changes in basal respiratory measurements and metabolism in males. J Gerontol 1955; 10:31–40.
25. Poehlman ET, Goran MI, Gardner AW, Ades PA, Arciero PJ, Katzman-Rooks SM, Montgomery SM, Toth MJ, Sutherland PT. Determinants of decline in resting metabolic rate in aging females. Am J Physiol 1993; 264:E450–E455.
26. Benedek C, Berclaz P-Y, Jéquier E, Schutz Y. Resting metabolic rate and protein turnover in apparently healthy elderly Gambian men. Am J Physiol 1995; 268:E1083–E1088.
27. Acheson KJ, Schutz Y, Bessard T, Ravussin E, Jéquier E, Flatt JP. Nutritional influences on lipogenesis and thermogenesis after a carbohydrate meal. Am J Physiol 1984; 246:E62–E70.
28. Schutz Y. Abnormalities of fuel utilization as predisposing to the development of obesity in humans. Obes Res 1995; 3(Suppl 2):173S–178S.

29. Schutz Y. The adjustment of energy expenditure and oxidation to energy intake: the role of carbohydrate and fat balance. Int J Obes 1993; 17(Suppl 3):S23–S27.

30. Sjöström L, Schutz Y, Gudinchet F, Hegnell L, Pittet PG, Jéquier E. Epinephrine sensitivity with respect to metabolic rate and other variables in women. Am J Physiol 1983; 245:E431–E442.

31. Staten MA, Matthews DE, Cryer PE, Bier M. Physiological increments in epinephrine stimulate metabolic rate in humans. Am J Physiol 1987; 253:E322–E330.

32. Mansell PI, Fellows IW, MacDonald IA. Enhanced thermogenic response to epinephrine after 48-h starvation in humans. Am J Physiol 1990; 258:R87–R93.

33. Blaak EE, Saris WHM, Vanbaak MA. Adrenoceptor subtypes mediating catecholamine-induced thermogenesis in man. Int J Obes 1993; 17(Suppl 3):78–81.

34. Randin JP, Schutz Y, Scazziga B, Lemarchand Beraud T, Felber JP, Jéquier E. Unaltered glucose-induced thermogenesis in Graves' disease. Am J Clin Nutr 1986; 43: 738–744.

35. Bogardus C, Lillioja S, Ravussin E, Abbott W, Zawadzki JK, Young A, Knowler WC, Jacobowitz R, Moll PP. Familial dependence of the resting metabolic rate. N Engl J Med 1986; 315:96–100.

36. Bouchard C, Tremblay A, Nadeau A, Després JJ, Thériault G, Boulay MR, Lortie G, Leblanc C, Fournier G. Genetic effect in resting and exercise metabolic rates. Metabolism 1989; 38:364–370.

37. Bouchard C, Dériaz O, Pérusse L, Tremblay A. Genetics of energy expenditure in humans. In: Bouchard C, ed. The Genetics of Obesity. Ann Arbor, MI: CRC Press; 1994: 135–145.

38. Tappy L, Jéquier E. Fructose and dietary thermogenesis. Am J Clin Nutr 1993; 58(suppl.):766S–770S.

39. Suter PM, Jéquier E, Schutz Y. Effect of ethanol on energy expenditure. Am J Physiol 1994; 266:R1204–R1212.

40. Thiébaud D, Acheson K, Schutz Y, Felber JP, Golay A, DeFronzo RA, Jéquier E. Stimulation of thermogenesis in men after combined glucose long-chain triglyceride infusion. Am J Clin Nutr 1983; 37:603–611.

41. Golay A, Schutz Y, Broquet C, Moeri R, Felber JP, Jéquier E. Decreased thermogenic response to an oral glucose load in older subjects. J Am Geriatr Soc 1983; 31: 144–148.

42. Bloesch D, Schutz Y, Breitenstein E, Jéquier E, Felber JP. Thermogenic response to an oral glucose load in man: comparison between young and elderly subjects. J Am Coll Nutr 1988; 7:471–483.

43. Jéquier E, Schutz Y. Energy expenditure in obesity and diabetes. Diabetes Metab Rev 1988; 4:583–593.

44. Bracco D, Ferrara JM, Arnaud MJ, Jéquier E, Schutz Y. Effects of caffeine on energy metabolism, heart rate, and methylxanthine metabolism in lean and obese women. Am J Physiol 1995; 269:E671–E678.

45. Hofstetter A, Schutz Y, Jéquier E, Wahren J. Increased 24-hour energy expenditure in cigarette smokers. N Engl J Med 1986; 314:79–82.

46. Jéquier E, Gygax PH, Pittet PH, Vannotti A. Increased thermal body insulation: relationship to the development of obesity. J Appl Physiol 1974; 36:674–678.

47. Welle S, Lilavivat U, Campbell RG. Thermic effect of feeding in man: increased norepinephrine levels following glucose but not protein or fat consumption. Metabolism 1981; 30:953–958.

48. Schutz Y, Acheson KJ, Jéquier E. Twenty-four-hour energy expenditure and thermogenesis: response to progressive carbohydrate overfeeding in man. Int J Obes 1985; 9: 111–114.

49. Rowe JW, Young JB, Minaker KL, Stevens AL, Pallotta J, Landsberg L. Effect of insulin and glucose infusions on sympathetic nervous system activity in normal man. Diabetes 1981; 30:219–225.

50. Acheson K, Jéquier E, Wahren J. Influence of beta-adrenergic blockade on glucose-induced thermogenesis in man. J Clin Invest 1983; 72:981–986.

51. Acheson K, Ravussin E, Wahren J, Jéquier E. Thermic effect of glucose in man: obligatory and facultative thermogenesis. J Clin Invest 1984; 74:1572–1580.

52. Bessard T, Schutz Y, Jéquier E. Energy expenditure and postprandial thermogenesis in obese women before and after weight loss. Am J Clin Nutr 1983; 38:680–693.

53. Kaplan ML, Leveille GA. Calorigenic response in obese and non-obese women. Am J Clin Nutr 1976; 23: 1108–1113.

54. Pittet P, Chappuis P, Acheson KJ, de Techtermann F, Jéquier E. Thermic effect of glucose in obese subjects studied by direct and indirect calorimetry. Br J Nutr 1976; 35: 281–289.

55. Shetty PS, Jung RT, James WPT, Barrand MA, Callingham BA. Postprandial thermogenesis in obesity. Clin Sci 1981; 60:519–525.

56. Danforth E Jr, Daniels RJ, Katzeff HL, Ravussin E, Garrow JS. Thermogenic responsiveness in Pima Indians. Clin Res 1981; 29:663A.

57. Golay A, Schutz Y, Meyer HU, Thiébaud D, Curchod B, Maeder E, Felber JP, Jéquier E. Glucose-induced thermogenesis in nondiabetic and diabetic obese subjects. Diabetes 1982; 31:1023–1028.

58. Schwartz RS, Ravussin E, Massari M, O'Connell M, Robbins DC. The thermic effect of carbohydrate versus fat feeding in man. Metabolism 1983; 32:581–589.

59. Schutz Y, Bessard T, Jéquier E. Diet induced thermogenesis measured over a whole day in obese and non obese women. Am J Clin Nutr 1984; 40:542–552.

60. Swaminathan R, King RFGJ, Holmfield J, Siwek RA, Baker M, Wales JK. Thermic effect of feeding carbohydrate, fat, protein and mixed meal in lean and obese subjects. Am J Clin Nutr 1985; 42:177–181.

61. Segal KR, Gutin B, Nyman AM, Pi-Sunyer FX. Thermic effect of food at rest, during exercise, and after exercise

in lean and obese men of similar body weight. J Clin Invest 1985; 76:1107–1112.

62. Sharief NN, MacDonald I. Differences in dietary induced thermogenesis with various carbohydrates in normal and overweight men. Am J Clin Nutr 1982; 35:267–272.

63. Welle SL, Campbell RG. Normal thermic effect of glucose in obese women. Am J Clin Nutr 1983; 37:87–92.

64. Felig P, Cunningham J, Levitt M, Hendler R, Nadel E. Energy expenditure in obesity in fasting and postprandial state. Am J Physiol 1983; 244:E45–E51.

65. Segal KR, Gutin B. Thermic effects of food and exercise in lean and obese women. Metabolism 1983; 32:581–589.

66. Blaza S, Garrow JS. Thermogenic response to temperature, exercise and food stimuli in lean and obese women, studied by 24 h direct calorimetry. Br J Nutr 1983; 49:171–180.

67. Anton-Kuchly B, Laval M, Choukroun ML, Manciet G, Roger P, Varene P. Postprandial thermogenesis and hormonal release in lean and obese subjects. J Physiol (Paris) 1985; 80:321–329.

68. Vernet O, Christin L, Schutz Y, Danforth E, Jéquier E. Enteral vs parenteral nutrition: comparison of energy metabolism in lean and moderately obese women. Am J Clin Nutr 1986; 43:194–209.

69. Ravussin E, Bogardus C, Schwartz RS, Robbins DC, Wolfe RR, Horton ES, Danforth E, Sim EAH. Thermic effect of infused glucose and insulin in man: decreased response with increased insulin resistance in obesity and non-insulin-dependent diabetes mellitus. J Clin Invest 1983; 72:893–902.

70. Bogardus C, Lillioja S, Mott D, Zawadski J, Young A, Abbott W. Evidence for reduced thermic effect of insulin and glucose infusions in Pima Indians. J Clin Invest 1985; 75:1264–1269.

71. Golay A, Schutz Y, Felber JP, DeFronzo RA, Jéquier E. Lack of thermogenic response to glucose/insulin infusion in diabetic obese subjects. Int J Obes 1986; 10:107–116.

72. Ravussin E, Acheson KJ, Vernet O, Danforth E Jr, Jéquier E. Evidence that insulin resistance is responsible for the decreased thermic effect of glucose in human obesity. J Clin Invest 1985; 76:1268–1273.

73. Weinsier RL, Bracco D, Schutz Y. Predicted effects of small decreases in energy expenditure on weight gain in adult women. Int J Obes 1993; 17:693–700.

74. Ravussin E, Lillioja S, Knowler WC, Christin L, Freymond D, Abbott WGH, Boyce V, Howard BW, Bogardus C. Reduced rate of energy expenditure as a risk factor for body weight gain. N Engl J Med 1988; 318:467–472.

75. Berne F, Fagius J, Niklasson F. Sympathetic response to oral carbohydrate administration. Evidence from microelectrode nerve recordings. J Clin Invest 1989; 84:1403–1409.

76. Vollenweider P, Tappy L, Randin D, Schneiter Ph, Jéquier E, Nicod P, Scherrer U. Differential effects of hyperinsulinemia and carbohydrate metabolism on sympathetic nerve activity and muscle blood flow in humans. J Clin Invest 1993; 92:147–154.

77. Tappy L, Girardet K, Schwaller N, Vollenweider L, Jéquier E, Nicod P, Scherrer U. Metabolic effects of an increase of sympathetic activity in healthy humans. Int J Obes 1995; 19:419–422.

78. Berthoud H-R, Bereiter DA, Trimble ER, Siegel EG, Jeanrenaud B. Cephalic phase, reflex insulin secretion. Neuroanatomical and physiological characterization. Diabetologia 1981; 20:393–401.

79. Nacht CA, Christin L, Temler E, Chioléro R, Jéquier E, Acheson KJ. Thermic effect of food: possible implication of parasympathetic nervous system. Am J Physiol 1987; 253:E481–E488.

80. Blaza S, Garrow JS. Thermogenic response to temperature, exercise and food stimuli in lean and obese women, studied by 24 h direct calorimetry. Br J Nutr 1983; 49:171–180.

81. Prentice AM, Black AE, Coward WA, Davies HL, Goldberg GR, Murgatroyd PR, Ashford J, Sawyer M, Whitehead RG. High levels of energy expenditure in obese women. Br Med J 1986; 292:983–987.

82. Schutz Y, Jéquier E. Energy needs: assessment and requirements. In: Shils ME, Shike M, eds. Modern Nutrition in Health and Disease. Philadelphia: Lea & Febiger, 1994; 101–111.

83. Schutz Y. Rôle de l'inactivité physique dans l'étiologie de l'obésité. Rev Thér 1989; 5:281–290.

84. Rising R, Harper IT, Fonvielle AM, Ferraro RT, Spraul M, Ravussin E. Determinants of total daily energy expenditure: variability in physical activity. Am J Clin Nutr 1994; 59:800–804.

85. Carpenter WH, Poehlman ET, O'Connell M, Goran MI. Influence of body composition and resting metabolic rate on variation in total energy expenditure: a meta-analysis. Am J Clin Nutr 1995; 61:4–10.

86. Lichtman SW, Pisarska K, Berman ER, Pestone M, Dowling H, Offenbacher E, Weisel H, Heshka S, Matthews DE, Heymsfield SB. Discrepancy between self-reported and actual caloric intake and exercise in obese subjects. N Engl J Med 1992; 327:1893–1898.

87. Welle S, Forbes GB, Statt M, Barnard RR, Amatruda JM. Energy expenditure under free-living conditions in normal weight and overweight women. Am J Clin Nutr 1992; 55:14–21.

88. Livingstone MBE, Prentice AM, Strain JJ, Coward WA, Black AE, Barker ME, McKenna PS, Whitehead RG. Accuracy of weighted dietary records in studies of diet and health. Br Med J 1990; 300:708–712.

89. Ravussin E, Harper I, Rising R, Bogardus C. Energy expenditure by doubly labeled water: validation in lean and obese subjects. Am J Physiol 1991; 261:E402–E409.

90. Goran MI, Beer WH, Poehlman ET, Wolfe RR, Young VR. Variation in total energy expenditure in young, healthy free living men. Metabolism 1993; 42:487–496.

91. Roberts SB, Heyman MB, Evans WJ, Fuss P, Tsay R, Young VR. Dietary energy requirements of young adult men, determined by using doubly labeled water method. Am J Clin Nutr 1991; 54:499–505.

92. Westerterp KR, Meijer GAL, Saris WHM, Soeters PB, Winants Y, Hoor FT. Physical activity and sleeping metabolic rate. Med Sci Sports Exerc 1991; 23:166–170.

93. Schulz LO, Schoeller DA. A compilation of total daily energy expenditures and body weights in healthy adults. Am J Clin Nutr 1994; 60:676–681.

94. Fontvieille AM, Harper TT, Ferraro T, Spraul M, Ravussin E. Daily energy expenditure by five year old children measured by doubly labelled water. J Pediatr 1993; 123: 201–206.

95. Goran MI, Carpenter WH, Poehlman ET. Total energy expenditure in 4 to 6 year old children. Am J Physiol 1993; 264:E706–E711.

96. Davies PSW, Coward WA, Tyler H, White A. Total energy expenditure and energy intake in the pre-school child: a comparison. Br J Nutr 1994; 72:13–20.

97. Dietz WH, Gortmaker SL. Do we fatten our children at the TV set? Television viewing and obesity and adolescents. Pediatrics 1985; 75:807–812.

98. Fontvielle AM, Krisha A, Ravussin E. Decreased physical activity in Pima Indians compared with Caucasian children. Int J Obes 1993; 17:445–452.

99. Roberts SB, Savage J, Coward WA, Chew B, Lucas A. Energy expenditure and intake in infants born to lean and overweight mothers. N Engl J Med 1988; 318: 461–466.

100. Maffeis C, Pinelli L, Zaffanello M, Schena F, Iacumin P, Schutz Y. Daily energy expenditure in free-living conditions in obese and non-obese children: comparison of doubly labelled water ($^2H_2$ ^{18}O) method and heart-rate monitoring. Int J Obes 1995; 19:671–677.

101. DeLany JP, Harsha DW, Kime JC, Kumler J, Melancon L, Bray GA. Energy expenditure in lean and obese prepubertal children. Obes Res 1995; 3(Suppl 1):67–72.

102. Davies PSW, White GA. Physical activity and body fatness in pre-school children. Int J Obes 1995; 19:6–10.

103. Schutz Y. Macronutrients and energy balance in obesity. Metabolism 1995; 44:(Suppl 3) 7–11.

104. Weinsier RL, Nelson KN, Hensrud DD, Darnell BE, Hunter GR, Schutz Y. Metabolic predictors of obesity. Contribution of resting energy expenditure, thermic effect of food, and fuel utilization to four-year weight gain of post-obese and never-obese women. J Clin Invest 1995; 95: 980–985.

105. Froidevaux F, Schutz Y, Christin L, Jéquier E. Energy expenditure in obese women before and during weight loss, after refeeding and in the weight-relapse period. Am J Clin Nutr 1993; 57:35–42.

106. Lyon XH, Di Vetta V, Milon H, Jéquier E, Schutz Y. Compliance to dietary advice directed towards increasing the carbohydrate to fat ratio of the everyday diet. Int J Obes 1995; 19:260–269.

21

Energy Expenditure in Physical Activity

James O. Hill
University of Colorado Health Sciences Center, Denver, Colorado

Wim H. M. Saris
University of Maastricht, Maastricht, The Netherlands

I. ENERGY EXPENDITURE DURING PHYSICAL ACTIVITY

A. Definitions and Assessment Methods

1. Physical Activity, Energy Expenditure, and Physical Fitness

Human beings obey the laws of thermodynamics and must fuel all physical activity by extracting energy from food. There are many ways of measuring and expressing physical activity. Measurements of physical activity are often expressed in terms of energy expenditure. Alternatively, physical activity can be expressed as the amount of work performed (watts); as the time period of activity (hours, minutes); as units of movements (counts); or even as a numerical score derived from responses to a questionnaire. Activity can also be defined as an overt intentional behavior (e.g., the number of social contacts).

The term "energy expenditure" is not synonymous with the term "physical activity." One may expend the same amount of energy in a short burst of strenuous exercise as in a less intense endurance type of activity, yet the physiological effects of these two could differ. For example, high-intensity exercise may lead to a proportionally higher carbohydrate versus fat oxidation than low-intensity exercise and thus may affect substrate balance differently.

It is important to realize that energy expenditure is related to body size, so a small, lean person who is very active may expend a similar number of kilojoules per day as a tall, obese person who is sedentary. Since for the average adult the resting metabolic rate (RMR) is fairly close to 3.5 ml/kg/min of oxygen, or 1 kcal/kg body weight/hr, the energy cost of activities can be expressed as multiples of RMR and called METs (an abbreviation of "metabolic"). The use of METs is a simple approach to estimate energy expenditure, taking body weight into account. Recently, an extensive compendium of MET values of all types of activities was published by Ainsworth et al. (1). MET values provide an indication of intensity of physical activity and, when summed over time, can be used to compare level of physical activity between individuals. The physical activity level (PAL) is another means of providing information about level of physical activity. The PAL is calculated as total daily energy expenditure (TEE) divided by RMR. For sedentary subjects the PAL is around 1.5. This value can increase to around 3.5–4.5 under extreme exercise conditions. Prentice et al. (2) have noted the importance of considering differences in body size when interpreting measurements of physical activity. Caution must be used when making comparisons of energy expended in physical activity between individuals who differ markedly in body size.

The gross energy cost of exercise that can be maintained for more than a few minutes varies roughly between 2.0 METs (leisure walking) and 8.0 METs (running 5 mph). However, to expend more energy (e.g., 18 METs;

running 10 mph) for a longer period of time, the aerobic fitness of an individual has to be far beyond the level that is observed in the general population. An individual who has an aerobic fitness of 35 ml/kg/min, which is the average for a normal-weight 40-year-old woman, is not able to expend more than 7 METs (corresponding to 70% of her VO_2max) for more than 30 min. A deterioration in aerobic fitness can thus reduce the ability to be active.

2.   Assessment Methods

The greatest obstacle in validating field methods of assessing habitual physical activity in humans is the lack of an adequate criterion to which to compare these techniques. La Porte et al. (3) have listed more than 30 techniques that have been used for comparison purposes.

The doubly labeled water (DLW) technique has provided a better standard for assessing energy expended in physical activity (4). This method is now used widely by obesity researchers to assess energy expended in physical activity. This technique allows assessment over relatively long periods of time (10–14 days) in free-living subjects. There is generally good agreement between energy expenditure measured by the DLW technique and measurement by respirometry. Using these data, we can estimate the DLW techniques as having an accuracy of 1–3% with a precision of 2–8%. One disadvantage of the technique is its relatively high cost, usually limiting the number of subjects who can be studied.

For estimation of energy expended in physical activity in larger groups, heart rate recording, combined with accelerometers to measure movements, appears to be the most accurate technique. Use of physical activity questionnaires is less accurate. To date, there have been few studies of comparison of such questionnaires with the DLW method (4).

B.   Components of Energy Expenditure

For measurement purposes, total daily energy expenditure can be divided into components. These usually include sleeping/resting metabolic rate (SMR/RMR), the thermic effect of food (TEF), and the energy expended in physical activity (EE_{ACT}) (5). An individual's overall level of physical activity can have an impact on each component of energy expenditure and can modify the fuel mixture oxidized by the body. The way in which this occurs varies with characteristics of the activity (e.g., intensity, duration) and of the subject performing the activity (e.g., age, gender, training status, body composition, and genetic background).

C.   Determinants of EE_{ACT}

EE_{ACT} represents a significant portion of total daily energy expenditure. The range of EE_{ACT} is wide, from about 15% of total daily energy expenditure in very sedentary individuals to 50% or more of total daily energy expenditure in highly active individuals (6,7). Because this component of energy expenditure is the most variable component of energy expenditure, both within and between subjects (8), its potential role in body weight regulation and in the etiology of obesity deserves close examination. For example, Dauncey (7) estimates that differences in minor activity throughout the day can account for differences of 20% in 24-hr energy expenditure. Such differences, if not compensated for by changes in energy intake, can lead to significant changes in body weight and/or body composition.

The total amount of energy expended during physical activity is determined by the amount of activity performed and the efficiency with which it is performed. The total amount of physical activity performed over a day is the sum of planned exercise, activities associated with daily living (e.g., walking, stair climbing, etc.), and unproductive muscular activities such as fidgeting and shivering. In comparing energy expenditure between individuals, EE_{ACT} is more variable than the other components of energy expenditure. For example, Ravussin et al. (8) measured physical activity by radar in a whole-room calorimeter and found that the energy expended in physical activity varied from 830 to 4180 kJ/day. These large differences in physical activity were seen in subjects confined to a small room with no access to exercise equipment. Differences in amount of physical activity performed may be even greater in a free-living situation.

I.   Amount of Physical Activity Performed

Very limited data are available regarding determinants of participation in physical activity. A major obstacle is the lack of accurate techniques to quantify physical activity. Most available studies rely on self-reports of physical activity participation.

Variation due to Genetic Background. It is likely that genetics play some role in determining the amount of physical activity performed. Data in support of this notion were reviewed by Bouchard et al. (9). Based on twin and family studies, the heritability for physical activity level has been estimated as between 29 and 62%. Analysis of self-reports of physical activity from the Finnish Twin Registry, consisting of 1537 monozygotic and 3057 dizygotic twins, estimated a 62% heritability level for age-adjusted physical activity (10). Analyses of self-reported physical activity from the Quebec Family Study, consisting of 1610 members of 375 families, showed a heritability level of 29% for habitual physical activity (11).

Variation due to Age. Many data sets consistently show a decline in physical activity with aging (12–14), with the decline occurring in both men and women. However, some data suggest that during the period 1986–1990, activity levels increased more in elderly subjects than in young adults (14).

Variation due to Gender. Adult men and women in the United States report similar levels of aerobic and moderate physical activity (14,15). In other countries, such as Canada, England, and Australia, men report 1.5–3 times more aerobic or moderate activity than women (13,16,17). Women in the United States appear to have increased their physical activity more than men during the period 1986–1990 (14,15). In children, a consistent gender difference is found, with boys being more active than girls (18).

Variation due to Body Composition. Substantial data suggest that overweight individuals are less active than their lean counterparts (19–21). This appears to be true across all ages, for both genders, and for all ethnic groups. We cannot, however, conclude on the basis of available evidence that a low level of physical activity contributes to development of obesity. It is equally possible that development of obesity leads to a reduction in physical activity. Reduced activity may partly be balanced by increased energy cost of weight-bearing activities. In fact, moving around with a higher body mass implies a higher energy cost.

Variation due to Education. Groups with more education consistently report more leisure-time physical activity than groups with less education. In the United States, high-education groups are 2–3 times more likely to be active than low-education groups (12,14,15).

Seasonal Variations in Physical Activity. Limited data are available regarding differences in amount of physical activity performed during different seasons. Data from Canada suggest wide differences in time spent in physical activity due to season. Time spent in these activities was twice as high during the summer months compared to the winter months (16).

2. Determinants of the Energy Cost of Physical Activity

The other major determinant of EE_{ACT} is the efficiency with which exercise (i.e., work) is performed. Work efficiency can be defined as the amount of work performed divided by the energy expended in performing the work. Although it is clear that work efficiency is not constant for all human subjects, the extent of individual differences and their importance in body weight regulation is unclear. Several studies have reported differences in work efficiency between groups of subjects, and these will be discussed below.

It is logical that differences in morphology/metabolism of skeletal muscle may play a role in determining work efficiency. Blei et al. (22), using ^{31}P NMR spectroscopy, reported that human muscle varied nearly twofold in both energy cost per twitch (energy cost) and recovery time constants (oxidative capacity) across individuals.

Body Weight/Body Composition. It requires more energy to move a larger body mass, and several investigators (23–25) demonstrated that energy expended in physical activity during weight-bearing physical activity increased with increasing body mass. It is important to take into account the greater cost of physical activity of a larger body mass when assessing differences in physical activity between obese and nonobese subjects. An obese person who is slightly less active than a lean counterpart may expend as much as or more total energy in physical activity.

It is less clear whether work efficiency varies with body composition, independently of body weight. Some studies (26–29) have found no differences in work efficiency between obese and nonobese subjects, while others (30,31) have found a greater work efficiency in the obese. Most studies not finding differences in work efficiency have used cycle ergometers with a moderate workload, while those finding differences have used cycle ergometers with heavy loads or treadmills. Work efficiency may vary with type and intensity of physical activity. There are some data suggesting that oxygen consumption increases more rapidly in obese than lean individuals as workload increases (30). This would be consistent with a greater work efficiency in the obese.

Effects of Changes in Body Weight/Body Composition. Several studies have reported that efficiency of work is reduced following weight reduction. Foster et al. (32) measured the energy cost of walking in 11 obese women before weight loss and at 9 and 22 weeks post weight loss. They determined that the energy cost of walking (after controlling for loss of body weight) decreased substantially by 22 weeks after weight loss. They estimated that with a 20% loss of body weight, subjects would expend about 427 kJ/hr less during walking than before weight loss. Geissler et al. (33) compared energy expenditure during different physical activities and found that energy expenditure was about 15% lower in the postobese compared to controls across different activities. deBoer et al. (34) found that sleeping metabolic rate declined appropriately for the decline in fat-free mass (FFM) when obese subjects lost weight but that total energy expenditure declined more than expected for the change in FFM. Similar results were obtained by Leibel et al. (35), who speculate that an increased work efficiency may be partially responsible for weight regain following weight loss.

Alternatively, Froidevaux et al. (36) measured the energy cost of walking in 10 moderately obese women before and after weight loss and during refeeding. Total energy expended during treadmill walking declined with weight loss but was entirely explained by the decline in body mass. Net efficiency of walking did not change. Poole and Henson also found no change in efficiency of cycling after caloric restriction in moderately obese women (28). Weigle and Brunzell demonstrated that about 50% of the decline in energy expenditure with weight loss was eliminated when they replaced weight lost by energy restriction with external weight worn in a specially constructed vest (37). Thus, although it is clear that total energy expenditure declines with weight loss, the extent to which changes in work efficiency contribute to this decline is controversial.

Role of Skeletal Muscle Metabolism in Determining Work Efficiency. Differences in skeletal muscle morphology/metabolism have been suggested to play a role in differences in work efficiency. Henriksson (38) has suggested that changes in muscle morphology in response to energy restriction lead to changes in the relative proportion of type I versus type II fibers in human subjects. Some studies suggest that type II fibers have a greater fuel economy than type I fibers (39,40). Since type II fibers appear to be better preserved during starvation than type I fibers (38), overall fuel economy and work efficiency may be increased following energy restriction and loss of body mass. However, a recent study on muscle fiber type before and after a 10.8-kg weight loss in obese females did not show any changes in the fiber type distribution (41).

The potential contribution of skeletal muscle differences to differences in work efficiency between weight-stable lean and obese subjects is more controversial. Substantial data suggest that obese subjects oxidize pro-

portionally more carbohydrate and less fat than lean subjects in response to perturbations in energy balance (42–44) and that differences in morphology/metabolism of skeletal muscle and sympathetic nervous system activity (45) may underlie some of the whole-body differences (44,46). However, it is not clear to what extent such differences contribute to differences in work efficiency. Further, such differences may arise from both genetic and environmental causes.

Genetic Contributions to Work Efficiency. Very little information is available to allow estimation of the genetic contribution to differences in efficiency of work. Bouchard et al. (47) assessed the energy cost associated with common body postures (sitting, standing) and low-intensity activities (walking, stair climbing, etc.) in 22 pairs of dizygotic and 31 pairs of monozygotic twins. All subjects were classified as sedentary. A significant genetic effect for energy expenditure was found with low-intensity activities (from 50 to 150 watts) even after correction for differences in body weight. No genetic effect was seen for activities requiring energy expenditure greater than 6 times resting energy expenditure.

Effects of Age on Work Efficiency. Work efficiency may vary with age. For example, Villagra et al. (48) demonstrated that children are about 10% more energy efficient during squatting exercises than adults. There is little information available to evaluate the effects of aging in adults on work efficiency. Skeletal muscle mass is often lost as a subject ages, and if the loss involves a greater proportion of type I versus type II fibers, work efficiency could increase with age.

Effects of Exercise Training on Work Efficiency. If work efficiency varies as a function of exercise training, training-induced effects in skeletal muscle could be important. Alterations in physical activity can alter the fiber-type proportions of skeletal muscle as well as induce significant changes in enzyme activities. Aerobic exercise training results primarily in the transformation of type IIb into type IIa fibers, while transformation of type II fibers into type I fibers is not common unless the exercise training has been extremely intense over a long period. Type I fibers have a greater mitochondrial density, are more oxidative, and are more fatigue-resistant than type IIb fibers. Type IIb fibers are glycolytic in nature with lower mitochondrial content and are more prone to fatigue. Type IIa fibers are intermediate in their mitochondrial content and, in humans, closely resemble type I fibers in oxidative capacity. However, an overlap of oxidative capacity exists between fiber type groups. Type I and type IIa fibers are more energy efficient than type IIb fibers and the proportions of these fiber types will vary according to the type of exercise training performed. It has been shown that even independently of fiber-type alterations, the activities of important enzymes in oxidative and glycolytic pathways can be modified as a result of exercise training and can lead to improvements in metabolic efficiency.

Sharp et al. (49) found that there was not a significant relationship between VO_2max and EE_{ACT} in a group of men and women studied in a whole-room calorimeter. Cross-sectional studies indicate that training may increase the efficiency of the activity when being trained. Elite runners and cyclists have lower energy expenditure at a certain speed when compared to not specifically trained individuals. Differences can account for 15% (running) up to 50% (swimming) (50,51). Children have a higher energy cost calculated per kilogram body weight for the same activity compared to adults.

Effects of Gender on Work Efficiency. There are several reports that female athletes, unlike male athletes, are more energy-efficient than their sedentary counterparts (52–54). There are reports in the literature of increased energy efficiency in female runners (52), dancers (53), and swimmers (54) as compared to sedentary females. Most reports make conclusions regarding energetic efficiency based on indirect rather than direct measurements of energy intake and/or expenditure. For example, Mulligan and Butterfield (52) concluded that female runners had increased energy efficiency since their self-reported energy intake was less than their estimated energy expenditure. In the few studies in which both intake and expenditure were measured directly, no evidence of increased energy efficiency was seen in female runners (55) or cyclists (56). Thus, the question of whether female athletes show a different energy efficiency than sedentary females is controversial. If this proves to be true, the extent to which such differences might be due to differences in work efficiency is unknown.

D. Postexercise Energy Expenditure

Energy expenditure does not return to pre-exercise levels immediately upon cessation of the physical activity, and the period of increased energy expenditure following exercise is called excess postexercise energy expenditure. The factors that determine the extent to which postexercise energy expenditure occurs have not been clearly defined, leaving a controversy regarding the overall importance of postexercise energy expenditure for overall energy balance. A good review of these factors is provided by Bahr (57).

Some have suggested energy expenditure can be elevated as long as 24 hr after a bout of exercise (58), while others have suggested baseline energy expenditure is restored within a few minutes after exercise cessation (59). Further, it appears that the magnitude and duration of the postexercise increase in energy expenditure is related to the intensity and duration of the exercise bout, with longer, more intense exercise likely to produce a more significant postexercise increase in energy expenditure (60). Over a 12-hr period excess postexercise energy expenditure has been found to vary between 24 kcal after 120 min cycling at 100 watt and 157 kcal after cycling 80 min at 70% VO_2max (61). Compared to the energy expenditure during exercise itself, the postexercise increase above RMR is modest and has been found to increase energy expenditure by exercise by another 3–15%.

In a review of this phenomenon, Poehlman et al. (62) concluded that, from a practical point of view, an exercise prescription for the general public of low ($<50\%$ VO_2max) and moderate intensity (50–70% VO_2max) would result in an extra postexercise energy expenditure of only 9 to maximal 30 kcal/bout. It is unlikely that these differences will significantly influence body weight regulation. In this regard, it is questionable whether the moderate exercise usually prescribed for moderately obese humans is sufficient to produce appreciable postexercise increase in energy expenditure.

E. Effects of Increased Physical Activity on Other Components of Energy Expenditure

I. Resting Metabolic Rate (RMR)

Conflicting data have been reported regarding whether changes in physical activity alter RMR independently of changes in FFM. In several cross-sectional investigations, an elevated RMR was seen in endurance-trained individuals compared to sedentary, untrained subjects, independent of differences in body composition (62,63). Arciero et al. (64) recently studied over 500 healthy men and women and reported that peak VO_2 was a significant predictor of RMR, independent of body weight and body composition. Other studies have found highly fit, trained subjects to have RMR values no different from those of sedentary controls (65,66). Sharp et al. (49) used a whole-room calorimeter to perform a cross-sectional study of the relationships among RMR, body composition, and physical fitness. They reported that physical fitness (assessed as maximum oxygen consumption) was unrelated to RMR, TEF, EE_{ACT}, or total daily energy expenditure independently of body composition. The reasons for the discrepant findings are unknown, but may be related to differences between studies in the time interval between the last bout of exercise and measurement of RMR, and to the level of energy intake during the days immediately preceding RMR measurement. Another important factor is the lack of precise methods to measure daily physical activity. In one study using the DLW method, a positive relation between EE_{ACT} and RMR was found ($r^2 = 0.72$) (67). Subjects in this study were not involved in any kind of training, which underlines the importance of the precision of the technique to quantify physical activity in order to detect any relationship. Finally, it is impossible to determine cause-and-effect relationships from cross-sectional analyses.

Several of the studies that first identified higher RMR values in trained athletes allowed 24 hr between the last exercise bout and RMR measurement. Because subjects abstained from exercise for this relatively long period (compared to the usual 10–12-hr fast), an acute effect of exercise on RMR was largely discounted, and investigators suggested the increased RMR values in athletes might be due to adaptations to chronic exercise (68). Several well-conducted studies, which used a longer interval (48–56 hr) between previous exercise and RMR measurement, failed to find elevations of RMR in trained subjects (69,70). Together these studies suggest that any elevation of RMR in trained athletes may reflect the acute perturbations of strenuous exercise, rather than adaptation to training.

Since acute changes in energy intake and energy balance can influence RMR, it is important to separate effects of exercise from effects of alterations in energy intake. Contrary to several of the aforementioned studies, Ballor and Poehlman (71) observed an elevation of RMR in trained women who had abstained from exercise for at least 36 hr. Energy consumption was not controlled during the period of exercise abstention, and if the subjects failed to lower their usual energy intake during this period, they would have been acutely overfed. Overfeeding is associated with a rapid increase in energy expenditure (72,73). In another study (74), RMR was not increased in subjects who underwent an exercise training program for 9 weeks, but the subjects were found to be underfed based on energy expenditure determinations using DLW. Melby et al. (75) have previously observed that RMR decreases in exercising athletes when they move to an energy-deficit state. From earlier studies, it was suggested that the combination of high energy expenditure and energy intake (high energy flux or turnover) could elevate RMR in endurance-trained athletes, even when they are in energy balance (76). Data from Bullough et al. (77) support this hypothesis. RMR in exercise-trained individuals was influenced by the total flux of energy through the body (total

energy expenditure at steady state). Also, in trained versus untrained subjects, RMR was elevated under acute conditions of high exercise energy expenditure and high energy intake, but this elevation was attenuated as the time interval increased from the last exercise bout to the measurement of RMR. These data suggest that RMR may be chronically elevated in individuals who engage in daily high-intensity, prolonged exercise, due to an effect of acute exercise rather than an adaptation to chronic exercise. It should be noted that the amount of exercise performed by nonathletes for the purpose of weight control is typically of much lower intensity and duration and would likely have little, if any, impact on RMR.

2. Thermic Effect of Food

There is no consistent picture of how a change in physical activity effects TEF. Some investigators report an increase in TEF with increased physical fitness level (78), others report the opposite (79,80), and some find no effect (81). Witt et al. (82) have proposed that the magnitude of TEF is influenced by the length of time interval between the last exercise bout and TEF measurement. It is difficult on the basis of the published literature to determine if physical activity has a reproducible effect on this component of energy expenditure. The measurement of TEF itself has a large coefficient of variation (35%), which might explain the observed differences in the published results.

Exercise could acutely affect energy expenditure through its interaction with food. Some data suggest a synergistic relationship between the energy expended in physical activity and that due to TEF (83). Further, Segal et al. (84,85) have suggested that obese humans show a smaller increase in energy expenditure in response to the combined effects of a single meal and exercise than do nonobese humans. However, others using a whole-room calorimeter have concluded that, at least with moderate activity, there is little evidence to support a synergistic relationship between energy expenditure due to TEF and that produced by physical activity over a whole day (86,87). Dauncey (7) reviewed this area and concluded that the majority of research suggests the energy cost of human activity is independent of food intake and that there is not a synergistic relationship between the thermic effect of food and that of exercise.

II. SUBSTRATE OXIDATION DURING PHYSICAL ACTIVITY

Body weight regulation involves balancing total energy intake and expenditure. It also involves maintaining, over some period of time, a balance between intake and oxidation of protein, carbohydrate, and fat. Thus, it is useful to consider factors that influence both the amount and composition of fuel used during physical activity. When assessing factors that influence substrate oxidation, it is important to consider influences both during performance of exercise and during the postexercise recovery period.

Substrate oxidation during exercise is often estimated from the whole-body respiratory quotient (RQ), which provides an indication of the relative proportion of carbohydrate and fat being oxidized. In comparing RQ between exercise condition, it is important to consider total energy expended as well as RQ. Especially at low-intensity exercise, a relatively high proportion of lipids is oxidized, mainly as a result of the preferential oxidation of free fatty acids in the type I fibers. For example, at 20% Vo_2max RQ is about 0.80, meaning that 62% of the local substrate utilization is derived from fat. At 80% Vo_2max more type II fibers are involved and the *R* value is about 0.9, leading to a contribution of fat oxidation of only 21%. It has been argued that low-intensity exercise is optimal for maximizing fat oxidation during exercise. However, more important than the change in *R* value is the increase in energy expenditure turnover at higher exercise intensity levels. Therefore, the optimal level for a maximal fat oxidation during exercise is around 60% Vo_2max. Lower-intensity exercise, while oxidizing proportionally more fat than high-intensity exercise, must be performed for a longer period to oxidize a greater absolute amount of fat.

A. Characteristics of the Physical Activity

While the intensity of the exercise is the major determinant of amount of energy expended in exercise, both the intensity and duration of exercise influence the source of fuel used for exercise (88). At maximal or supramaximal work intensities [$\geq$100% maximal oxygen uptake (Vo_2max)], energy is derived from the anaerobic breakdown of substrates including glycogen (89). This extremely high intensity of work can only be maintained for a very short period (90,91). With submaximal exercise there is a balance between aerobic and anaerobic metabolism (92). The main fuel source during submaximal exercise, performed at high work intensities (>70–75% Vo_2max) is carbohydrate with a much lesser contribution from fat (93). As exercise intensity declines, lipid becomes increasingly important as a fuel source whereas the contribution of carbohydrate declines (94). By contrast, protein oxidation during exercise is small (95). Exercise that is predominantly aerobic can be maintained for long periods, up to many hours in trained individuals (96), with lipid oxidation increasing as time progresses (97,98).

1. Circulating Versus Intramuscular Fuel Sources

Carbohydrate and fat can be derived both from the circulation [free fatty acids (FFAs) and glucose] and within the muscle (intramuscular triglyceride-derived FFAs or IMTGs and glycogen) (98). It is well established that FFAs released from adipose tissue lipolysis are a major source of circulating lipid fuel during exercise (97–99). The contribution of IMTGs as a fuel source during exercise is now increasingly recognized (100–103). This is implied from the observation that IMTG stores decline significantly following prolonged activity (90,101) and from the inability of plasma FFA uptake or turnover to account for all the lipid oxidized during exercise (98,100,104). Circulating triglycerides are considered to be used minimally as an exercise fuel source (105) particularly under fasting conditions (106). The balance between the use of circulating versus intramuscular fuels is also dependent on the duration and intensity of activity.

2. Exercise Duration

Intramuscular fuel sources are the most important during initial exercise, with an increasing contribution from circulating fuels as exercise progresses (97,103,107). During the initial phase of exercise, carbohydrate is mainly supplied from intramuscular glycogen stores (94,98,108). After approximately 30–40 min of exercise, the contribution of blood glucose increases (97) and remains relatively constant (103,109) until the later stages of prolonged exercise, when it declines (108). The blood glucose level is maintained through an increase in hepatic glucose production (94,97,108). Initially, this is mainly due to hepatic glycogenolysis, but with prolonged exercise, gluconeogenesis becomes more important (97,109,110).

The factors that regulate IMTG oxidation and determine the relative contribution of FFA versus IMTG to fat oxidation are not well understood. However, IMTG appear to be utilized more during the initial phase of moderate exercise with an increasing contribution from circulating FFA as time progresses (89,90).

Although the contribution of protein to fuel utilization during exercise is small, <11% of total energy expended (111), this can increase with very prolonged exercise. Protein contributes to energy production directly via oxidation of branched chain amino acids (BCAA) and indirectly through the increased release of the gluconeogenic precursor alanine (95). Protein synthesis in muscle declines whereas proteolysis in other tissues can increase the circulating BCAA (95,112). This increases the amino acid pool available for oxidation. As gluconeogenesis becomes more important during exercise, alanine release also rises (113).

3. Exercise Intensity

The effect of exercise intensity on circulating versus intramuscular fat and carbohydrate utilization is demonstrated in the study of Romijn et al. (103). This study identified a hierarchy for fuel utilization over 30 min of different intensity exercise. At 25% VO_2max, circulating fuels, specifically FFA, were primarily oxidized whereas with 65% VO_2max exercise, energy provision was accounted for equally by circulating and intramuscular fuels, and by lipid and carbohydrate. Both IMTG and glycogen were used in roughly equal proportions. At an intensity of 85% VO_2max, muscle glycogen was primarily utilized, with lesser contributions from circulating blood glucose, FFA, and IMTGs. Oxidation of BCAA increases with higher work intensities (112) but still remains small relative to total oxidation.

4. Aerobic Versus Anaerobic Exercise

The energy expended during aerobic and anaerobic exercise depends on the intensity of each. There is no indication that one is performed with a systematically different work efficiency than the other. The type of exercise, however, can influence substrate oxidation during exercise. Exercise in which anaerobic metabolism predominates, relies more on carbohydrate than does exercise in which aerobic exercise predominates (93). Therefore, proportionally more carbohydrate and less fat will be oxidized when anaerobic versus aerobic metabolism predominates during exercise. However, it appears that the situation is reversed during the postexercise recovery period. During this period, fat oxidation may be higher following anaerobic exercise than following aerobic exercise (114,115). Thus, to determine the total amount of fat and carbohydrate oxidized due to a bout of aerobic versus anaerobic exercise, both the exercise and postexercise recovery period must be considered.

B. Characteristics of the Exercising Individual

Both the amount of energy expended during exercise and the source of fuel for the added energy expenditure are influenced by several characteristics of the exercising individual.

I. Training Status

While increasing physical fitness does not alter the amount of energy expended in physical activity, it does alter the source of fuel for the exercise. The most frequently assessed measure of physical fitness is aerobic fitness as determined by VO_2max. The main effect of increasing VO_2max is to increase fat utilization during exercise performed at the same absolute workload (99,116–118). This is partly due to the lower relative intensity of the exercise. Even so, fat oxidation may be increased at the same relative work intensity in trained versus untrained individuals (107,108). Increased fat oxidation in trained subjects is greatly facilitated by morphological and enzymatic adaptations in skeletal muscle following training (119,120). Increased proportions of oxidative type I fibers and decreased proportions of type IIb fibers (except in sprint athletes) result following exercise training, so skeletal muscle is more adapted to fat oxidation. Similarly, the activity of important enzymes in fat and carbohydrate oxidation is modified. It has been shown that the increased rate of triglyceride–fatty acid cycling in trained subjects at rest is partially responsible for increasing the availability of circulating FFA for oxidation during exercise (121). Exercise training leads to an increased ability to remove FFA from the circulation (107), which will also facilitate an increase in FFA oxidation. In addition, some of the increased fat oxidation in trained individuals may be due to a greater reliance on IMTG as an exercise fuel source. This is suggested by a greater decline in IMTG post exercise following a period of training (116) and an inability of the increased FFA uptake to account for all the increase in total fat oxidation observed during exercise (118,122). This increased lipid oxidation essentially spares both muscle glycogen and blood glucose (116,118,122). Other training adaptations relating to carbohydrate metabolism include a greater capacity for muscle glycogen storage (123) and an increased lactate clearance, which provides more gluconeogenic substrate (124).

2. Gender

Some studies have found that females oxidize proportionally more lipid during exercise of a similar intensity compared to males (125–129). However, this has not always been observed (130–132). Protein oxidation during moderate-intensity exercise appears to be lower in females versus males, although for both genders its overall contribution to total fuel oxidation remains small (128). The stage of menstrual cycle in females may also affect the pattern of fuel oxidation. Although few adequately controlled studies have been performed in this area, there is a suggestion of increased lipid oxidation during exercise performed in the luteal versus follicular phase of the menstrual cycle (133,134). Further work is warranted to more accurately elucidate potential gender-related aspects of exercising fuel metabolism.

3. Age

It has been suggested that the ability to oxidize fat during exercise declines with age (135). If true, this could be due to changes in the morphology and metabolism of skeletal muscles, and/or to availability of lipid substrate during exercise.

4. Body Composition

There is some suggestion that fuel oxidation during exercise is influenced by body composition. Wade et al. (136) proposed that obese subjects used substrates differently from lean subjects during exercise. Obese subjects oxidized less fat during exercise than lean subjects. The authors related the lower fat oxidation to a lower proportion of type I (oxidative) muscle fibers in the obese as compared to lean subjects. Geerling et al. (137) replicated this study and failed to find a difference in RQ during exercise when lean and obese objects performed exercise at equivalent workloads after adjustment for body composition. It remains to be determined whether and how body composition influences substrate oxidation during exercise and whether characteristics of skeletal muscle influence this process.

III. THE ROLE OF PHYSICAL ACTIVITY IN THE ETIOLOGY OF OBESITY

There are clear theoretical reasons why level of physical activity should be important in body weight regulation. As described above, physical activity is a major factor determining total level of energy expenditure. Increases in physical activity will increase total energy expenditure and decreases in physical activity will reduce total energy expenditure. Unless such changes are accompanied by compensatory changes in energy intake, weight loss will result.

Physical activity is also a major determinant of fat balance. Maintaining a high level of physical activity provides a means of consuming a high-fat diet without increasing body fat mass. It is becoming clear that obesity is a result of positive fat balance since protein and carbohydrate balances appear to be well maintained even following challenges to body weight regulation (e.g., diet and exercise alterations). Fat oxidation and intake, however, are not acutely responsive to changes in each other, so following a challenge to body weight regulation, fat balance may only be restored following a change in the body fat mass. When one consumes a diet high in fat, fat balance can be achieved by having a large body fat mass or having a high level of physical activity. Similarly, increasing physical activity without a change in fat intake will increase fat oxidation above fat intake and produce negative fat balance and loss of body fat mass.

A. The Relationship Between Physical Activity and Body Fatness

In this section, evidence for a link between physical activity and the amount and location of body fat will be examined. Particular attention will be given to characteristics of the physical activity that may be important for body weight regulation.

1. Is a Low Level of Physical Activity a Risk Factor for Development of Obesity?

The recent report from NHANES III shows that the prevalence of obesity has increased over the past 8 years from about 25% to 33% in U.S. adults (138). Which environmental condition has led to the dramatic increase in prevalence of obesity in Western society: the abundance of food or the lack of activity? Both conditions have changed drastically over the past century. Unfortunately, population-based records of food intake are not very accurate, and physical activity data are completely lacking. It is interesting to note that national household surveys of different countries show a decrease in energy intake. For example, in Great Britain, energy intake decreased by more than 500 kcal from 1970 to 1990 (139). During the same time, however, body mass index (BMI) and average body weight increased by 1.0 BMI unit and 2.5 kg, respectively. These figures imply that EE declined by even more than 500 kcal. The problem is that we do not have any data to show whether this might be the case, other than anecdotal information on the number of automobiles and occupational mechanization.

Negative relationships between measures of physical activity (usually self-reports) and indices of obesity (usually BMI) are seen in most data sets obtained from the general U.S. population (140,141). The relationship appears to be similar in men and women, and across all ages (142–144). Further, there is evidence for a similar relationship in African-Americans (145), Hispanics (146), and Native Americans (147).

While BMI is a reproducible measure, self-reports of physical activity have been criticized as potentially unreliable. At least two studies using DLW to measure the energy expended in physical activity have shown a significant negative relationship between physical activity and BMI (148,149).

Further, studies in which subjects are followed over time suggest that changes in physical activity are associated with changes in body fatness. This can be illustrated in the three studies summarized in Table 1 (150–152). In each study, physical activity was related to BMI at baseline and 2–10 years later. In all studies, the level of physical activity was negatively related to BMI at baseline, and level of physical activity at follow-up was negatively related to change in BMI from baseline to follow-up. In two of the three studies the level of physical activity at baseline was negatively related to change in BMI from baseline to follow-up. Finally, all studies suggest a negative relationship between change in level of physical activity and change in BMI.

Reduced levels of physical activity with age in the general population may play a role in development of obesity. Reductions in physical activity could alter fiber-type composition toward a greater proportion of glycolytic type IIb fibers, which have a reduced capacity for fat utilization and may predispose to fat accumulation. This could lead to a vicious cycle of reduced physical activity resulting in increased type IIb fiber proportions and a decline in fat oxidation and promotion of obesity. This obesity could then lead to further reduction in physical activity and so promote an even greater proportion of type IIb fibers.

2. Is Body Fatness Linked to Particular Characteristics of Physical Activity?

It is not clear which characteristics of physical activity influence body weight regulation. In most of the studies discussed above, the self-reports of physical activity capture total dose of physical activity. There is scant data about how other characteristics of physical activity, such as type, intensity, duration, and frequency, affect body weight regulation independently of total dose of physical activity.

Both aerobic and resistance exercise have been used successfully in weight reduction programs, and although the latter may preserve or increase fat-free mass, both seem to reduce body fat similarly when total dose of activity is considered (153). Further, a variety of aerobic activities have been successfully used in weight reduction studies (154).

While moderate-intensity exercise uses proportionally more fat than high intensity, there is some suggestion that

exercise of greater intensity is associated with lower BMI than exercise of moderate intensity (155). It should be realized that in many cases, moderate-intensity exercise must be performed for a longer period to produce as much fat oxidation as high-intensity exercise. It is not possible with the available data to conclusively separate effects of intensity from effects of total amount of physical activity.

A great deal of new information suggests that short bouts of activity may be just as effective for body weight regulation as longer bouts. Jakicic et al. (156) demonstrated similar weight loss in overweight subjects given an exercise program consisting of the same dose of activity as either 30-min or 10-min bouts of exercise.

Few data are available regarding how frequency of physical activity impacts upon body weight regulation. Most experts recommend that people exercise 3–5 days/week, and while such recommendations are reasonable, we have no data at present to allow determination of optimum frequency of exercise for body weight regulation.

Finally, many obesity experts are recommending decreases in sedentary activities and increases in life-style activities in addition to increases in planned exercise. Many Americans spend a great deal of time in sedentary activities such as sitting at a desk and watching television. Energy expenditure during such activities is very low. By trying to reduce time spent in sedentary activity (even without specifying a specific alternative), total energy expenditure can be increased. Epstein et al. (157) have shown the effectiveness of such strategy in children. Total energy expenditure can also be greatly increased by increasing life-style activities such as taking the stairs instead of the elevator and parking further away from one's destination.

3. Is Level of Physical Activity Related to Body Fat Distribution?

Only a few studies have examined the relationship between physical activity and body fat distribution (usually assessed as waist-to-hip ratio, WHR). The CARDIA study (145) found a negative relationship between levels of physical activity and WHR in African-American men and women and in Caucasian men. The relationship was not found in Caucasian women. Physical activity was negatively related to WHR and to waist circumference in the European Fat Distribution Study (158). Few studies have examined this relationship and much more information is needed. It may be that visceral adipose tissue is preferentially lost during negative energy balance, regardless of how it is produced. Alternatively, negative energy balance produced by physical activity may lead to preferential re-

Table 1 Are Changes in Physical Activity Associated with Changes in BMI?

	Health Worker Study (French et al.) (2 years)	Healthy Women Study (Owens et al.) (3 years)	NHANES I Follow-Up Study (Williamson et al.) (10 years)
Baseline physical activity negatively related to BMI	Yes	Yes	Yes
Baseline physical activity negatively related to change in BMI	Yes	Yes	No
Follow-up physical activity negatively related to change in BMI	Yes	Yes	Yes
Change in physical activity negatively related to change in BMI	Yes	Yes	Small effect

duction in visceral adipose tissue as compared to negative energy balance produced by energy restriction.

Weight loss produced by physical activity includes substantial reduction of visceral adipose tissue (159). However, it is not clear whether weight loss produced by exercise alone or exercise combined with energy restriction includes a greater proportion of visceral adipose tissue reduction than weight loss produced by energy restriction alone.

It is also unclear whether men and women show a similar reduction in visceral adipose tissue with weight loss and particularly with exercise. Wing and Jeffery (160) assessed WHR in men and women participating in a 6-month behavioral weight loss program. They found a greater reduction in WHR in men versus women at the end of the program and at the 12-month follow-up period. However, at the 18-month follow-up period, the results were reversed, with women showing a greater reduction in WHR than men. Schwartz et al. (161) examined body fat loss due to endurance exercise training in young and elderly men. They found greater loss of visceral adipose tissue in younger versus older men. The way in which physical activity affects loss of visceral adipose may be affected by genetics (162).

B. Do Changes in Physical Activity Lead to Changes in Body Fatness in the Overweight?

In this section, we will consider how increases in physical activity can impact upon overall fatness. In particular, we will consider how physical activity can affect amount of weight loss, composition of weight loss, change in body fat distribution, and maintenance of weight loss.

It is clear that substantial weight loss can be produced by exercise alone. This is illustrated in the study by Lee

et al. (163) where overweight men were drafted into the Singapore army and subjected to 20 weeks of supervised vigorous exercise. The average loss of body weight in this study was 12.5 kg in 20 weeks. Subjects were free to consume as much food as they desired. While the study by Lee et al. (163) represents an extreme physical activity program, it does illustrate that physical activity alone can produce weight loss. Less intense physical activity programs will produce slower weight loss and may require much longer time periods to produce significant changes in body weight. In a 1-year study on sedentary subjects who were trained to run a marathon, a loss of about 2.5 kg fat was found (164). In another 40-week study, where subjects were trained to run a half marathon, a fat loss of 3.8 kg in men was found and a concomitant increase of 1.6 kg fat free mass, while the corresponding changes in women were 2.0 kg and 1.2 kg, respectively (165).

Increases in physical activity will increase energy expenditure. This will produce negative energy balance, negative fat balance, and weight loss unless subjects increase energy intake. While we can accurately estimate the effects of a given increase in physical activity on energy expenditure, we know little about effects of such changes on energy intake. Thus, we still do not have the ability to predict the effects of a given increase in physical activity on weight loss. Another factor that might play a role in the level of energy expenditure is the compensation in daily activities outside the training hours, leading to no extra increase in energy expenditure on a daily basis. In lean and obese women no indication of compensation was observed (166), while in lean males training stimulated physical activity during the nonexercising part of the day (167). In 10-year-old obese boys with a normal daily physical activity level compared to lean counterparts, a training program resulted in a 10% increase of the total energy expenditure (TEE) (168). About 50% of this increased expenditure could be accounted for by the training program. It was concluded that other energy-consuming factors, such as TEF or daily physical activity outside the training hours, must also have increased. These findings are in contrast to a group of elderly subjects, where a significant compensation was found during a training program (169).

C. Physical Activity During Energy Restriction

To prevent negative effects of energy restriction during weight loss on RMR, TEF, and possibly EE_{ACT}, it has been suggested that the addition of an exercise program to the energy restriction diet accelerates fat loss, preserves FFM, and prevents or decelerates the decline in RMR more effectively than a diet alone. Reviews on this subject showed a modest FFM preservation and an additional extra fat mass loss (35,170–172). Most exercise studies do not show an effect on the decline in RMR during the weight loss period. Especially in those studies with a comparison of RMR adjusted for FFM, the evidence for no extra effect, other than a proportional decrease with the changes in body composition, is overwhelming. Most published studies are of short duration and of questionable power to detect the expected additional effect of physical activity on body weight.

The long-term studies of Wood and colleagues (173,174) show that adding physical activity to caloric restriction programs can increase the amount of weight and fat loss. In one study (173), men and women were randomly assigned to a control group, a group receiving food restriction alone (diet only), or a group receiving diet and physical activity (diet and exercise). After 1 year, men in the diet and exercise group lost about 4 kg more of body fat and body weight than subjects in the diet-only group. This suggests that energy intake compensation may have been in the order of 50% of total calories expended in physical activity. For women, the differences were less and were only about 1 kg of total body weight and 1.5 kg of body fat. This could suggest that caloric compensation was greater in women than men.

D. Long-Term Effects of Physical Activity on Weight Maintenance

Many formerly obese subjects claim to need a lifelong diet or extreme levels of exercise to maintain their weight loss. In general, long-term success in weight maintenance in the obese has been rare. This has led to speculations about a postobesity syndrome characterized by a persistently lower level of energy expenditure. A study by Leibel et al.

(35) showed that weight loss resulted in decreased, total, nonresting, and resting energy expenditure levels adjusted for metabolic mass when measured after weight stabilization. These compensatory changes in energy expenditure, which oppose the maintenance of a body weight that is different from the usual weight, were comparable in the obese and nonobese. These results suggest a physiological resistance to changes in body weight, irrespective of the level of body fatness. This raises the question of whether it requires a lower-than-normal food intake for obese individuals to maintain a nonobese weight and whether it is necessary to maintain this low intake indefinitely. One way to escape this vicious cycle is to increase expenditure and lipid oxidation by elevating activity levels. So far, prospective long-term studies are very limited, but the results are encouraging.

Despite the relative small effects of exercise on acute loss of body weight and body fat mass, the benefits of physical activity for body weight and body fat regulation become apparent when long-term maintenance of body weight losses is examined. Substantial data suggest that subjects who exercise are better at maintaining weight losses at periods greater than 1 year following initial weight loss than subjects who do not exercise. A well-controlled study by King et al. (175), on the effect of a minimal intervention strategy on weight maintenance through energy restriction alone or exercise alone over 1 year, clearly showed better results for the exercise group. Dieters showed a more variable pattern of weight gain and weight loss during the maintenance year than did exer-

Table 2 Proposed Mechanisms Linking Exercise with the Success of Weight Maintenance

1. Increased energy expenditure
2. Better aerobic fitness
3. Improvement of body composition
   Fat loss
   Preservation of lean body mass
   Reduction of visceral fat depot
4. Increased capacity for fat mobilization and oxidation
5. Control of food intake
   Short-term reduction of appetite
   Reduction of fat intake
6. Stimulation of thermogenic response
   Resting metabolic rate
   Diet-induced thermogenesis
7. Change in muscle morphology and biochemical capacity
8. Increased insulin sensitivity
9. Improved plasma lipid and lipoprotein profile
10. Reduced blood pressure
11. Positive psychological affects

cisers. This argues favorably for activity as an intervention strategy. Van Dale et al. (176) followed a group of obese women over a period of 18–40 months post treatment. Like other investigators, they observed that body weight maintenance after a diet or diet/exercise treatment was very difficult. In contrast, a better weight maintenance was observed in a smaller number of subjects (13%) who had regular exercise (three times or more per week) after their weight loss period. These subjects maintained most of their weight loss. Perhaps the most interesting observation was the restoration of RMR adjusted for metabolic mass, which contrasted the unsuccessful group, who still had a 10% lower RMR adjusted for metabolic mass. Kayman et al. surveyed a group of subjects 1 year after weight loss and found that 80% of those individuals who had maintained the weight loss reported regular physical activity while only 20% of those who had relapsed reported regular exercise (177). Finally, self-reported data from successful reduced-obese subjects in the National Weight Control Registry indicate expending an average of 2800 kcal/week in physical activity (178).

However, information is lacking on mechanisms, even though it is known that exercise induces a number of favorable physiological alterations affecting body composition, thermogenic response, muscle morphology, blood lipid profile, physiological well-being, self-esteem, and motivation. Therefore, a variety of factors may act together to explain why regular physical activity may contribute to long-term success in the maintenance of weight loss (Table 2).

The current recommendation for physical activity in adults in the United States is 30 min or more of moderate-intensity physical activity on most, preferably all, days of the week (179). This recommendation fulfills the criteria necessary to sustain an active life-style. Thus, increases in physical activity, while of minimal importance in acute weight loss, play a major role in determining the success of long-term weight maintenance.

REFERENCES

1. Ainsworth BE, Haskell WL, Leon AS, et al. Compendium of physical activities. Classification of energy costs of human physical activities. Med Sci Sports Exerc 1993; 25: 71–80.
2. Prentice AM, Goldberg GR, Murgatroyd PR, Cole TJ. Physical activity and obesity: problems in correcting expenditure for body size. Int J Obes 1996; 20:688–691.
3. La Porte RE, Montoye HJ, Caspersen CJ. Assessment of physical activity in epidemiologic research: problems and prospects. Public Health Rep 1985; 100:131–146.
4. Montoye HJ, Kemper HCG, Saris WHM, Washburn RA. Measuring Physical Activity and Energy Expenditure. Champaign, IL: Human Kinetics Publishers, 1996.
5. Hill JO, Pagliassotti MJ, Peters JC. Nongenetic determinants of obesity and fat topography. In: Bouchard C, ed. Genetic Determinants of Obesity, Boca Raton, FL: CRC Press, 1994:35–48.
6. Livingstone MBE, Strain JJ, Prentice AM, Coward WA, Nevin GB, Barker ME, Hickey HJ, McKenna PG, Whitehead RG. Potential contribution of leisure activity to the energy expenditure patterns of sedentary populations. Br J Nutr 1991; 65:145–155.
7. Dauncey MJ. Activity and energy expenditure. Can J Physiol Pharmacol 1990; 68:17–27.
8. Ravussin E, Lillioja S, Anderson TE, Christin L, Bogardus C. Determinants of 24-hour energy expenditure in man: methods and results using a respiratory chamber. J Clin Invest 1986; 78:1568–1578.
9. Bouchard C, Dériaz O, Pérusse L, Tremblay A. Genetics of energy expenditure in humans. In: Bouchard C, ed. The Genetics of Obesity, Boca Raton, FL: CRC Press, 1994: 135–146.
10. Kaprio J, Koskenvuo M, Sarna S. Cigarette smoking, use of alcohol, and leisure-time physical activity among same sexed adult male twins. Prog Clin Biol Res 1981; 69: 37–46.
11. Pérusse L, Tremblay A, Leblanc C, Bouchard C. Genetic and environmental influences on level of habitual physical activity and exercise participation. Am J Epidiol 1989; 129:1012–1022.
12. Stephens T, Caspersen CJ. The demography of physical activity. In: Bouchard C, Shephard RJ, Stephens T, eds. Physical Activity, Fitness, and Health. Champaign, IL: Human Kinetics Publishers, 1994:203–213.
13. Activity and Health Research. Allied Dunbar National Fitness Survey: Main Findings. London: The Sports Council and the Health Education Authority, 1992.
14. Caspersen CJ, Merritt RK. Trends in physical activity patterns among older adults: the behavioral risk factor surveillance system, 1986–1990. Med Sci Sports Exerc 1992: 24:S26.
15. Merritt RK, Caspersen CJ. Trends in physical activity patterns among young adults: the behavioral risk factor surveillance system, 1986–1990. Med Sci Sports Exerc 1992: 24:S26.
16. Stephens T, Craig CL. The Well-Being of Canadians: Highlights of the 1988 Campbell's Survey. Ottawa: Canadian Fitness and Lifestyle Research Institute, 1990.
17. Risk Factor Prevalence Study Management Committee. Risk Factor Prevalence Study: Survey no. 3 1989. Canberra: National Heart Foundation of Australia and Australia Institute of Health, 1990.
18. Saris WHM, Elvers JWH, Van 't Hof M, Binkhorst RA. Changes in physical activity profiles of children aged 6 to 12 years. In: Rutenfranz J, ed. Children and Exercise XII.

Champaign, IL: Human Kinetics Publishers, 1986: 121–130.

19. Matsushima M, Kriska A, Tajima N, LaPorte R. The epidemiology of physical activity and childhood obesity. Diabetes Res Clin Pract 1990; 10(Suppl 1):S95–S102.

20. Pacy PJ, Webster J, Garrow JS. Exercise and obesity. Sports Med 1986; 3:89–113.

21. Thompson JK, Jarvie GJ, Lahey BB, Cureton KJ. Exercise and obesity: etiology, physiology, and intervention. Psych Bull 1982; 91:55–79.

22. Blei ML, Conley KE, Odderson IR, Esselman PC, Kushmerick MJ. Individual variation in contractile cost and recovery in human skeletal muscle. Proc Natl Acad Sci USA 1993; 90:7396–7400.

23. Miller AT, Blyth CS. Influence of body type and body fat content on the metabolic cost of work. J Appl Physiol 1955; 8:139–141.

24. Passmore R. Daily energy expenditure in man. Am J Clin Nutr 1956; 4:692–708.

25. Jéquier E and Schutz Y. The contribution of BMR and physical activity to energy expenditure. In: Cioffi LA, James WPT, Van Itallie TB, eds. The Body Weight Regulatory System: Normal and Disturbed Mechanisms. New York: Raven Press, 1981:89–96.

26. Bray GA, Whipp BJ, Koyal SN, Wasserman K. Some respiratory and metabolic effects of exercise in moderately obese men. Metabolism 1977; 26:403–412.

27. Hanson JS. Exercise responses following production of experimental obesity. J Appl Physiol 1973; 35:587–591.

28. Poole DC, Henson LC. Effect of acute caloric restriction on work efficiency. Am J Clin Nutr 1988; 47:15–18.

29. Whipp BJ, Bray GA, Koyal SN. Exercise energetics in normal man following acute weight gain. Am J Clin Nutr 1973; 26:1284–1286.

30. Dempsey JA, Reddan W, Balke B, Rankin J. Work capacity determinants and physiologic cost of weight-supported work in obesity. J Appl Physiol 1966; 21:1815–1820.

31. Maloiy GMO, Heglund NC, Prager LM, Cavagna CA, Taylor CR. Energetic cost of carrying loads: have African women discovered an economic way? Nature 1986; 319: 668–669.

32. Foster GD, Wadden TA, Kendrick ZV, Letizia KA, Lander DP, Conill AM. The energy cost of walking before and after significant weight loss. Med Sci Sports Exerc 1995; 27:888–894.

33. Geissler CA, Miller DS, Shah M. The daily metabolic rate of the post-obese and the lean. Am J Clin Nutr 1987; 45: 914–920.

34. deBoer JO, van ES AJH, Roovers LCA, van Raaij JM, Hautvast JG. Adaptation of energy metabolism of overweight women in low-energy intake, studied with whole-body calorimeters. Am J Clin Nutr 1986; 44:585–595.

35. Leibel RL, Rosenbaum M, Hirsch J. Changes in energy expenditure resulting from altered body weight. N Engl J Med 1995; 332:621–628.

36. Froidevaux F, Schutz Y, Christin L, Jéquier E. Energy expenditure in obese women before and during weight loss, after refeeding, and in the weight-relapse period. Am J Clin Nutr 1993; 57:35–42.

37. Weigle DS, Brunzell JD. Assessment of energy expenditure in ambulatory reduced-obese subjects by the techniques of weight stabilization and exogenous weight replacement. Int J Obes 1990; 14(Suppl 1):69–81.

38. Henriksson J. The possible role of skeletal muscle in the adaptation to periods of energy deficiency. Eur J Clin Nutr 1990; 44(Suppl 1):55–64.

39. Wendt IR, Gibbs CL. Energy production of rat extensor digitorum longus muscle. Am J Physiol 1973; 224: 1081–1086.

40. Crow M, Kushmerick MJ. Chemical energetics of slow and fat-twitch muscles of the mouse. J Gen Physiol 1982; 79:147–166.

41. Saris WHM, Kempen KPG, Van Baak MA. Muscle fiber type, body fatness and substrate oxidation during exercise in obese females. Int J Obes 1994: 18(Suppl 2):96.

42. Thomas CD, Peters JC, Reed GW, Abumrad NN, Sun M, Hill JO. Nutrient balance and energy expenditure during ad libitum feeding of high-fat and high-carbohydrate diets in humans. Am J Clin Nutr 1992; 55:934–942.

43. Zurlo F, Lillioja S, Esposito-Del Puente A, Nyomba BL, Raz I, Saad MF, Swinburn BA, Knowler WC, Bogardus C, Ravussin E. Low ratio of fat to carbohydrate oxidation as predictor of weight gain: study of 24-h RQ. Am J Physiol 1990; 259:E650–E657.

44. Zurlo F, Nemeth PM, Choksi RM, Sesodia S, Ravussin E. Whole-body energy metabolism and skeletal muscle biochemical characteristics. Metabolism 1994; 43:481–486.

45. Blaak EE, Van Baak MA, Kemerink GJ, Pakbiers MTW, Herdendal GAR, Saris WHM. β-Adrenergic stimulation of energy expenditure and forearm skeletal muscle metabolism in lean and obese men. Am J Physiol 1994; 267: E316–E322.

46. Chang S, Graham B, Yakubu F, Lin D, Peters JC, Hill JO. Metabolic differences between obesity-prone and obesity-resistant rats. Am J Physiol 1990; 259:R1103–R1110.

47. Bouchard C, Tremblay A, Nadeau A, Després JP, Thériault G, Boulay MR, Lortie G, Leblanc C, Fournier G. Genetic effect in resting and exercise metabolic rates. Metabolism 1989; 38:364–370.

48. Villagra F, Cooke CB, McDonagh MJN. Metabolic cost and efficiency in two forms of squatting exercise in children and adults. Eur J Appl Physiol 1993; 67:549–553.

49. Sharp TA, Reed GW, Sun M, Abumrad NN, Hill JO. Relationship between aerobic fitness level and daily energy expenditure in weight-stable humans. Am J Physiol 1992; 263:E121–E128.

50. Costill DL. Inside Running: Basic of Sport Physiology. Indianapolis: Benchmark Press, 1986.

51. Holmer I. Physiology of swimming man. Acta Physiol Scand 1974; (Suppl 407).

52. Mulligan K, Butterfield GE. Discrepancies between energy intake and expenditure in physically active women. Br J Nutr 1990; 64:23–36.

53. Dahlstrom M, Jansson E, Nordevang E, Kaijser L. Discrepancy between estimated energy intake and requirements in female dancers. Clin Physiol 1990; 10:11–25.

54. Jones PL, Leitch CA. Validation of doubly labeled water for measurement of caloric expenditure in collegiate swimmers. J Appl Physiol 1993; 74:2909–2914.

55. Schulz LO, Alger S, Harper I, Wilmore JH, Ravussin E. Energy expenditure of elite female runners measured by respiratory chamber and doubly labeled water. J Appl Physiol 1992; 72:23–28.

56. Horton TJ, Drougas HJ, Sharp TA, Martinez LR, Reed GW, Hill JO. Energy balance in endurance-trained female cyclists and untrained controls. J Appl Physiol 1994; 76:1937–1945.

57. Bahr R. Excess post exercise oxygen consumption—magnitude, mechanisms, and practical implications. Acta Physiol Scand 1992; 144(Suppl 605):1–70.

58. Bielinski R, Schutz Y, Jequier E. Energy metabolism during the postexercise recovery in man. Am J Clin Nutr 1985; 42:69–82.

59. Freedman-Akabas, S, Colt E, Kissileff HR, Pi-Sunyer FX. Lack of sustained increase in V_{O_2} following exercise in fit and unfit subjects. Am J Clin Nutr 1985; 41:545–549.

60. Brehm BA, Gutin B. Recovery energy expenditure for steady state exercise in runners and nonexercisers. Med Sci Sports Exerc 1986; 18:205–210.

61. Saris WHM, Van Baak MA. Consequences of exercise on energy expenditure. In: Hill AP, Wahlqvist ML, eds. Exercise and Obesity. London: Smith Gordon, 1994:85–101.

62. Poehlman ET. A review: Exercise and its influence on resting energy metabolism in man. Med Sci Sports Exerc 1989; 21:515–525.

63. Poehlman ET, McAuliffe TL, Van Houten DR, Danforth E Jr. Influence of age and endurance training on metabolic rate and hormones in healthy men. Am J Physiol 1990; 259:E66–E72.

64. Arciero P, Goran MI, Poehlman ET. Resting metabolic rate is lower in women than in men. J Appl Physiol 1993; 75:2514–2520.

65. Broeder CE, Burrhus KA, Svanevik LS, Wilmore JH. The effects of aerobic fitness on resting metabolic rate. Am J Clin Nutr 1992; 55:795–801.

66. Lundholm K, Holm G, Lindmark L, Larsson B, Sjostrom L, Björntorp P. Thermogenic effect of food in physically well-trained elderly men. Eur J Appl Physiol 1986; 55:486–492.

67. Westerterp KR, Meyer GAL, Saris WHM, Soeters PB, Winants Y, Ten Hoor F. Physical activity and sleeping metabolic rate. Med Sci Sport Exerc 1991; 23:166–170.

68. Poehlman ET, Melby CL, Badylak SF. Resting metabolic rate and postprandial thermogenesis in highly trained and untrained males. Am Clin Nutr 1988; 47:793–798.

69. Herring JL, Mole PA, Meredith CN, Stern JS. Effect of suspending exercise training on resting metabolic rate in women. Med Sci Sports Exerc 1992; 24:59–65.

70. Schulz LO, Nyomba BL, Alger S, Anderson TE, Ravussin E. Effect of endurance training on sedentary energy expenditure measured in a respiratory chamber. Am J Physiol 1991; 260:E257–261.

71. Ballor DL, Poehlman ET: Restng metabolic rate and coronary heart disease risk factors in aerobically and resistance-trained women. Am J Clin Nutr 1992; 56:968–974.

72. Acheson KJ, Schutz Y, Bessard T, Anantharaman K, Flatt JP, Jequier E. Glycogen storage capacity and de novo lipogenesis during massive carbohydrate overfeeding in man. Am J Clin Nutr 1988; 48:240–247.

73. Horton TJ, Drougas H, Brachey A, Reed GW, Peters JC, Hill JO. Fat and carbohydrate overfeeding in humans: different effects on energy storage. Am J Clin Nutr 1995; 62:19–29.

74. Bingham SA, Goldberg GR, Coward WA, Prentice AM, Cummings JH. The effect of exercise and improved physical fitness on basal metabolic rate. Br J Nutr 1989; 61:155–173.

75. Melby CL, Schmidt WD, Corrigan D. Resting metabolic rate in weight-cycling collegiate wrestlers compared with physically active, noncycling control subjects. Am J Clin Nutr 1990; 52:409–414.

76. Poehlman ET, Melby CL, Badylak SF, Calles J. Aerobic fitness and resting energy expenditure in young adult males. Metabolism 1989; 38:85–90.

77. Bullough RC, Melby CL, Harris MA, Gillette CG. Interaction of acute changes in exercise energy expenditure and energy intake on resting metabolic rate. Am J Clin Nutr 1995; 61:473–481.

78. Hill JO, Heymsfield SB, McManus CB III, DiGirolamo M. Meal size and thermic response to food in male subjects as a function of maximum aerobic capacity. Metabolism 1984; 33:743–749.

79. Gilbert JA, Misner JE, Boileau RA, Ji L, Slaughter MH. Lower thermic effect of a meal post-exercise in aerobically trained and resistance-trained subjects. Med Sci Sports Exerc 1991; 23:825–830.

80. LeBlanc J, Diamond P, Cote J, Labrie A. Hormonal factors in reduced postprandial heat production of exercise-trained subjects. J Appl Physiol 1984; 56:772–776.

81. Owen OE, Kavle E, Owen RS, Polansky M, Caprio S, Mozzoli MA, Kendrick ZV, Bushman MC, Boden GA. Reappraisal of caloric requirements in healthy women. Am J Clin Nutr 1986; 44:1–19.

82. Witt KA, Snook JT, O'Dorisio TM, Zivony D, Malarkey WB. Exercise training and dietary carbohydrate: effects on selected hormones and the thermic effect of feeding. Int J Sport Nutr 1993; 4:272–289.

83. Miller DS, Mumford P, Stock M. Gluttony. 2. Thermogenesis in overeating man. Am J Clin Nutr 1967; 20:1223–1229.

84. Segal KR, Gutin B, Albu J, Pi-Sunyer, F.X. Thermic effect of food and exercise in lean and obese men of similar lean body mass. Am J Physiol 1987; 252:E110–E117.

85. Segal KR, Pi-Sunyer FX. Exercise and obesity. Med Clin North Am 1989; 73:217–236.

86. Dalosso HM, James WPT. Whole-body calorimetry studies in adult men. 2. The interaction of exercise and overfeeding on the thermic effect of a meal. Br J Nutr 1984; 52:65–72.

87. Dauncy MJ, Bingham SA. Dependence of 24 h energy expenditure in man on the composition of the nutrient intake. Br J Nutr 1983; 50:1–13.

88. Gollnick PD. Metabolism of substrates: energy substrate metabolism during exercise as modified by training. Fed Proc 1985; 44:353–357.

89. Cerretelli P. Energy sources for muscular exercise. Int J Sports Med 1992; 13:S106–S109.

90. Karlsson J. Lactate in working muscles after prolonged exercise. Acta Physiol Scand 1971; 82:123–130.

91. Symons DJ, Jacobs I. High intensity exercise performance is not impaired by low intramuscular glycogen. Med Sci Sports Ex 1989; 21:550–557.

92. Sahlin K. Muscle glucose metabolism during exercise. Ann Med 1990; 22:85–89.

93. Brooks GA, Mercier J. Balance of carbohydrate and lipid utilization during exercise: the "crossover" concept. J Appl Physiol 1994; 76:2253–2261.

94. Wahren J. Glucose turnover during exercise in man. Ann NY Acad Sci 1977; 301:45–55.

95. Hood DA, Terjung RL. Amino acid metabolism during exercise and following endurance training. Sports Med 1990; 9:23–35.

96. Stein TP, Hoyt RW, O'Toole M, Leskiw MJ, Schluter MD, Wolfe RR, Hiller WDB. Protein and energy metabolism during prolonged exercise in trained athletes. Int J Sports Med 1989; 10:311–316.

97. Ahlborg G, Felig P, Hagenfeldt, Hendler R, Wahren J. Substrate turnover during prolonged exercise in man. Splachnic and leg metabolism of glucose, free-fatty acids, and amino acids. J Clin Invest 1974; 53:1080–1090.

98. Essen B, Hagenfeldt L, Kaijser L. Utilization of blood-borne and intramuscular substrates during continuous and intermittent exercise in man. J Physiol 1977; 265:489–506.

99. Kiens B, Essen-Gustavsson B, Christensen NJ, Saltin B. Skeletal muscle substrate utilization during submaximal exercise in man: effect of endurance training. J Physiol 1993; 469:459–478.

100. Havel RJ, Pernow B, Jones NL. Uptake and release of free fatty acids and other metabolites in the legs of exercising men. J Appl Physiol 1967; 23:90–99.

101. Essen B. Intramuscular substrate utilization during prolonged exercise. Ann NY Acad Sci 1977; 301:30–44.

102. Brouns F, Saris WHM, Beckers E, Aldercreutz H, van der Vusse GJ, Keizer HA, Kuipers H, Menheere P, Wagenmakers AJM, ten Hoor F. Metabolic changes induced by sustained exhaustive exercise cycling and diet manipulation. Int J Sports Med 1989; 10:S49–S62.

103. Romijn JA, Coyle EF, Sidossis, LS, Gastaldelli A, Horowitz JF, Endert E, Wolfe RR. Regulation of endogenous fat and carbohydrate metabolism in relation to exercise intensity and duration. Am J Physiol 1993; 265:E380–E391.

104. Jansson E, Kaijser L. Effect of diet on the utilization of blood-borne and intramuscular substrates during exercise in man. Acta Physiol Scand 1982; 115:19–30.

105. Hargreaves M, Kiens B, Richter EA. Effect of increased free fatty acid concentrations on muscle metabolism in exercising men. J Appl Physiol 1991; 70:194–201.

106. Griffiths AJ, Humphreys SM, Clark MOL, Frayn KN. Forearm substrate utilization during exercise after a meal containing both fat and carbohydrate. Clin Sci 1994; 86:169–175.

107. Turcotte LP, Richter EA, Kiens B. Increased plasma FFA uptake and oxidation during prolonged exercise in trained vs. untrained humans. Am J Physiol 1992; 262:E791–E799.

108. Bergstrom J, Hultman E. A study of the glycogen metabolism during exercise in man. Scand J Clin Lab Invest 1967; 19:218–228.

109. Bosch AN, Dennis SC, Noakes TD. Influence of carbohydrate ingestion on fuel substrate turnover and oxidation during prolonged exercise. J Appl Physiol 1994; 76:2364–2372.

110. Ahlborg G, Juhlin-Dannfelt A. Effect of β-receptor blockade on splachnic and muscle metabolism during prolonged exercise in men. J Appl Physiol 1994; 76:1037–1042.

111. Friedman JE, Lemon PWR. Effect of chronic endurance exercise on retention of dietary protein. Int J Sports Med 1989; 10:118–123.

112. Millward DJ, Bowtell JL, Pacy P, Rennie MJ. Physical activity, protein metabolism and protein requirements. Proc Nutr Soc 1994; 53:223–240.

113. Felig P, Wahren J. Amino acid metabolism in exercising man. J Clin Invest 1971; 50:2703–2714.

114. Melby CL, Scholl C, Edwards G, Bullough R. Effect of acute resistance exercise on postexercise energy expenditure and resting metabolic rate. J Appl Physiol 1993; 75:1847–1853.

115. Maehlum S, Grandmontagne M, Newsholme EA, Sejersted, OM. Magnitude and duration of excess postexercise oxygen consumption in healthy young subjects. Metabolism 1986 35:425–429.

116. Hurley BF, Nemeth PM, Martin WH, Hagberg JM, Dalsky GP, Holloszy JO. Muscle triglyceride utilization during exercise: training effect. J Appl Physiol 1986; 60:562–567.

117. Coggan AR, Kohrt WM, Spina RJ, Bier DM, Holloszy JO. Endurance training decreases plasma glucose turnover and oxidation during moderate exercise in men. J Appl Physiol 1990; 68:990–996.

118. Martin WH, Dalsky GP, Hurley BF, Matthews DE, Bier DM, Hagberg JM, Rogers MA, King DS, Holloszy JO. Ef-

fect of endurance training on plasma free fatty acid turnover and oxidation during exercise. Am J Physiol 1993; 265:E708–E714.

119. Holloszy JO, Coyle EF. Adaptations of skeletal muscle to endurance exercise and their metabolic consequences. J Appl Physiol 1984; 56:831–838.

120. Hoppeler H. Exercise-induced ultrastructural changes in skeletal muscle. Int J Sports Med 1986; 7:187–204.

121. Romijn JA, Klein S, Coyle EF, Sidossis LS, Wolfe RR. Strenuous endurance training increases lipolysis and triglyceride-fatty acid cycling at rest. J Appl Physiol 1993; 75:108–113.

122. Jansson E, Kaijser L. Substrate utilization and enzymes in skeletal muscle of extremely endurance-trained men. J Appl Physiol 1987; 62:999–1005.

123. Saltin G. Metabolic fundamentals in exercise. Med Sci Sports Exerc 1973; 5:137–146.

124. Donovan CM, Brooks GA. Endurance training affects lactate clearance not lactate production. Am J Physiol 1983; 244:E83–E92.

125. Blatchford FK, Knowlton RG, Schneider DA. Plasma FFA responses to prolonged walking in untrained men and women. Eur J Appl Physiol 1985; 53:343–347.

126. Froberg K, Pedersen PK. Sex differences in endurance capacity and metabolic response to prolonged heavy exercise. Eur J Appl Physiol 1984; 52:446–450.

127. Tarnopolsky LJ, MacDougall JD, Atkinson SA, Tarnopolsky MA, Sutton JR. Gender differences in substrate for endurance exercise. J Appl Physiol 1990; 308;302–308.

128. Phillips SM, Atkinson SA, Tarnopolsky MA, MacDougall JD. Gender differences in leucine kinetics and nitrogen balance in endurance athletes. J Appl Physiol 1993; 75: 2134–2141.

129. Tarnopolsky MA, Atkinson SA, Phillips SM, MacDougall JD. Carbohydrate loading and metabolism during exercise in men and women. J Appl Physiol 1995; 78:1360–1368.

130. Costill DL, Fink WJ, Getchell LH, Ivy JL, Witzmann FA. Lipid metabolism in skeletal muscle of endurance-trained males and females. J Appl Physiol 1979; 47:787–791.

131. Powers SK, Riley W, Howley ET. Comparison of fat metabolism between trained men and women during prolonged aerobic work. Res Q Exerc Sport 1980; 51: 427–431.

132. Brewer J, Williams C, Patton A. The influence of high carbohydrate diets on endurance running performance. Eur J Appl Physiol 1988; 57:698–706.

133. Nicklas BJ, Hackney AC, Sharp RL. The menstrual cycle and exercise: performance, muscle glycogen, and substrate responses. Int J Sports Med 1989; 10:264–269.

134. Hackney AC, McCracken-Compton MA, Ainsworth B. Substrate responses to submaximal exercise in the mid-follicular and midluteal phases of the menstrual cycle. Int J Sport Nur 1994; 4:299–308.

135. Calles-Escandón J, Arciero PJ, Gardner AW, Bauman C, Poehlman ET. Basal fat oxidation decreases with aging in women. J Appl Physiol 1995; 78:266–271.

136. Wade AJ, Marbut MM, Round JM, Muscle fibre type and aetiology of obesity. Lancet 1990; 335:805–808.

137. Geerling BJ, Alles MS, Murgatroyd PR, Goldberg GR, Harding M, Prentice AM. Fatness in relation to substrate oxidation during exercise. Int J Obes 1994; 18:453–459.

138. Pi-Sunyer FX. Medical hazards of obesity. Ann Intern Med 1993; 119:655–660.

139. MAFF household food consumption and energy expenditure (annual reports). London: AMSO, 1940–1994.

140. Hill JO. Physical activity, body weight and body fat distribution. In: Leon A, ed. Physical Activity and Cardiovascular Health. (in press).

141. Kuczmarski RJ, Flegal KM, Campbell SM, et al. Increasing prevalence of overweight among US adults. JAMA 1994; 272:205–211.

142. Eck LH, Hackett-Renner C, Klesges LM. Impact of diabetic status, dietary intake, physical activity, and smoking status on body mass index in NHANES II. Am J Clin Nutr 1992; 56:329–333.

143. Reaven PD, Barrett-Connor E, Edelstein S. Relation between leisure-time physical activity and blood pressure in older women. Circulation 1991; 83:559–565.

144. Obarzanek E, Schreiber GB, Crawford PB, et al. Energy intake and physical activity in relation to indexes of body fat: the National Heart, Lung, and Blood Institute Growth and Health Study. Am J Clin Nutr 1994; 60:15–22.

145. Slattery ML, McDonald A, Bild DE, et al. Associations of body fat and its distribution with dietary intake, physical activity, alcohol, and smoking in blacks and whites. Am J Clin Nutr 1992; 55:943–949.

146. Mayer EJ, Burchfiel CM, Eckel RH, et al. The role of insulin and body fat in associations of physical activity with lipids and lipoproteins in a biethnic population: the San Luis Valley Diabetes Study. Arterioscler Thromb 1991; 11: 973–984.

147. Fontvieille AM, Kriska A, Ravussin E. Decreased physical activity in Pima Indian compared with Caucasian children. Int J Obes 1993; 17:445–452.

148. Davies, PSW, Gregory J, White A. Physical activity and body fatness in pre-school children. Int J Obes 1995; 19: 6–10.

149. Schulz LO, Schoeller DA. A compilation of total daily energy expenditures and body weights in healthy adults. Am J Clin Nutr 1994; 60:676–681.

150. Williamson DF, Madans J, Anda RF, et al. Recreational physical activity and ten-year weight change in a US national cohort. Int J Obes 1993; 17:279–286.

151. Owens JF, Matthews KA, Wing RR, et al. Can physical activity mitigate the effects of aging in middle-aged women. Circulation 1992; 85:1265–1270.

152. French SA, Jeffery RW, Forster JL, et al. Predictors of weight change over two years among a population of working adults: the Healthy Worker Project. Int J Obes 1994; 18:145–154.

153. Ballor DL, Keesey RE. A meta-analysis of the factors affecting exercise-induced changes in body mass, fat mass

and fat-free mass in males and females. Int J Obes 1991; 15:717–726.

154. Ballor DL, Poehlman ET. Exercise-training enhances fat-free mass preservation during diet-induced weight loss: a meta-analytical finding. Int J Obes 1994; 18:35–40.

155. Tremblay A, Després J-P, Leblanc C, et al. Effect of intensity of physical activity on body fatness and fat distribution. Am J Clin Nutr 1990; 51:153–157.

156. Jakicic JM, Wing RR, Butler et al. Prescribing exercise in multiple short bouts versus one continuous bout: effects on adherence, cardiorespiratory fitness, and weight loss in overweight women. Int J Obes 1995; 19:893–901.

157. Epstein LH, Valoski AM, Vara LS et al. Effects of decreasing sedentary behavior and increasing activity on weight change in obese children. Health Psych 1995; 14:109–115.

158. Seidell JC, Cigolini M, Deslypere J-P, et al. Body fat distribution in relation to serum lipids and blood pressure in 38-year-old European men: the European Fat Distribution Study. Atherosclerosis 1991; 86:251–260.

159. Després JP, Pouliot MC, Moorjani S, et al. Loss of abdominal fat and metabolic response to exercise in obese women. Am J Physiol 1991; 261:E159–E167.

160. Wing RR, Jeffery RW. Effect of modest weight loss on changes in cardiovascular risk factors: Are there differences between men and women or between weight loss and maintenance. Int J Obes 1995; 19:67–73.

161. Schwartz RS, Shuman WP, Larson V, et al. The effect of intensive endurance exercise training on body fat distribution in young and older men. Metabolism 1991; 40:545–551.

162. Bouchard C, Tremblay A, Després JP, et al. The response to exercise with constant energy intake in identical twins. Obes Res 1994; 2:400–411.

163. Lee L, Kumar S, Chin Leong L. The impact of five-month basic military training on the body weight and body fat of 197 moderately to severely obese Singaporean males aged 17 to 19 years. Int J Obes 1994; 18:105–109.

164. Janssen GME, Graef CJJ, Saris WHM. Food intake and body composition in novice athletes during a trained period to run a marathon. Int J Sport Med 1989; 10(Suppl 1):S17–S21.

165. Westerterp KR, Meyer GAL, Janssen GME, Saris WHM, Ten Hoor F. Long-term effect of physical activity on energy balance and body composition. Br J Nutr 1992; 68:21–30.

166. Van Dale D, Saris WHM, Schoffelen PFM, Ten Hoor F. Effect of adding exercise to energy restriction, 24 h energy expenditure, resting metabolic rate and daily physical activity. Eur J Clin Nutr 1989; 43:441–451.

167. Meyer GAL, Janssen GME, Westerterp KR, Verhoeven F, Saris WHM, Ten Hoor F. The effect of a 5 month training programme on physical activity. Evidence for a sex difference in the metabolic response to exercise. Eur J Appl Physiol 1991; 62:11–17.

168. Blaak EE, Westerterp KR, Bar-Or O, Saris WHM. Effect of training on total energy expenditure and spontaneous activity in obese boys. Am J Clin Nutr 1992; 55:777–782.

169. Goran MI, Poehlman ET. Endurance training does not enhance total energy expenditure in healthy elderly persons. Am J Physiol 1992; 263:E950–E957.

170. Saris WHM. The role of exercise in the dietary treatment of obesity. Int J Obes 1993; 17(Suppl 1):S17–S21.

171. Prentice AM, Goldberg GR, Jebb SA, Black AE, Murgatroyd PR. Physiological response to slimming. Proc Nutr Soc 1991; 50:441–458.

172. Donnelly JE, Pronk NP, Jacobsen DJ, et al. Effects of a very-low calorie diet and physical-training regimens on body composition and resting metabolic rate in obese females. Am J Clin Nutr 1991; 54:56–61.

173. Wood PD, Stefanick ML, Williams PT, et al. The effects on plasma lipoproteins of a prudent weight-reducing diet, with or without exercise, in overweight men and women. N Engl J Med 1991; 325:461–466.

174. Stefanic ML. Exercise and weight control. Exerc Sport Sci Rev 1993; 21:363–396.

175. King AC, Frey-Hewitt B, Dreon D, Wood P. Diet versus exercise in weight maintenance: the effects of minimal intervention strategies on long term outcomes in men. Arch Intern Med 1989; 149:2741–2746.

176. Van Dale D, Saris WHM, Ten Hoor F. Weight maintenance and resting metabolic rate 18–40 months after a diet-exercise treatment. Int J Obes 1990; 14:347–359.

177. Kayman S, Bruvold W, Stern JS. Maintenance and relapse after weight loss in women: behavioral aspects. Am J Clin Nutr 1990; 52:800–807.

178. Klem ML, Wing RR, McGuire MT, et al. A descriptive study of individuals successful at long-term weight maintenance of substantial weight loss. Am J Clin Nutr (in press).

179. Pate RR, Pratt M, Blair SN et al. Physical activity and public health. JAMA 1995; 273:402–407.

22

Endocrine Determinants of Obesity

Peter G. Kopelman
St. Bartholomew's and The Royal London School of Medicine and Dentistry at Queen Mary and Westfield College, London, England

I. INTRODUCTION

Obesity results from a fundamental disorder of energy balance with energy stores in the body (largely fat tissue) being too large either because energy intake is too high or because expenditure has been too low. The development of obesity involves a complex interaction between genetic and environmental factors, which, in turn, alter metabolic and endocrine function. Obesity may be characterized by alterations in endocrine function, although such changes are largely a consequence of increasing body fatness. The cellular mechanisms involved in these changes and their relationship to the metabolic aberrations associated with the distribution of adipose tissue are now better understood, and it has become clear that such metabolic alterations may be closely involved with the development of important complications of obesity—ischemic heart disease, cerebrovascular events, and diabetes mellitus. This chapter will review the alterations in endocrine function found in obesity—insulin secretion, adrenocortical function, sex steroid secretion and binding, and growth hormone release—and will discuss the evidence that such changes may play a role in either the determination of corpulence or the perpetuation of the obese state. A possible common etiological pathway between obesity and the polycystic ovary syndrome will be considered and evidence for a genetic basis to altered endocrine function reviewed.

II. INSULIN SECRETION IN OBESITY

Obesity is characterized by an elevated fasting plasma insulin and an exaggerated insulin response to an oral glucose load (1). However, obesity and body fat distribution influence glucose metabolism through independent but additive mechanisms. Kissebah and colleagues (2) have demonstrated that increasing upper body obesity, as measured by the ratio of waist to hip circumference (WHR), is accompanied by a progressive increase in the glucose and insulin response to an oral glucose challenge. The in vivo insulin sensitivity in individuals was assessed further by determining the steady-state plasma glucose (SSPG) and insulin (SSPI) attained during a simultaneous intravenous infusion of somatostatin, insulin, and dextrose. Since endogenous insulin production was suppressed by somatostatin and the SSPI was comparable in each situation, SSPG directly measured the subjects' ability to dispose of an intravenous glucose load under the same insulin stimulus. SSPG can be taken as an index of insulin resistance. The results showed a positive correlation between WHR, as a measure of increasing upper body obesity, and SSPG. After adjustment for the effects of overall fatness (% ideal body weight), WHR remained independently correlated with SSPG, suggesting that the location of body fat is an independent factor influencing the degree of insulin sensitivity and, in turn, metabolic profile.

Measurement of portal plasma insulin levels (as an index of insulin secretion) shows similar levels in upper body and lower body obesity, but hepatic insulin extraction, both basally and during stimulation by intravenous or oral glucose, is reduced in upper body obesity (3). As a consequence, posthepatic insulin delivery is increased in upper body obesity, leading to more marked peripheral insulin concentrations. In other words, an increase in relative body weight is associated with a moderate decline in hepatic and peripheral insulin sensitivity, whereas upper body obesity is characterized by greater decreases in hepatic and peripheral insulin sensitivity as well as a marked reduction in the maximal stimulation of peripheral glucose utilization. Studies of insulin sensitivity and responsiveness of skeletal muscle and the relationship to overall glucose disposal in premenopausal women, with varying body fat distribution, have revealed a significant decline as WHR increases (4). Insulin-stimulated activity of the glucose-6-phosphate independent form of glycogen synthase (GSI) was measured in quadricep muscle biopsies taken during a somatostatin-insulin-dextrose infusion. Despite comparable degrees of SSPI in all women, significant reductions in % GSI were seen as the degree of upper body fatness increased and this was accompanied by decreased efficiency in insulin-stimulated glucose disposal (reflected by increasing SSPG at similar SSPI levels). Furthermore, a significant trend was reported for a decreased number of cellular insulin receptors associated with increasing WHR, which was associated in some subjects with reduced glucose disposal during supramaximal insulin stimulation. Such findings suggest a defect at both the level of the insulin receptor and in postreceptor events.

The possibility that insulin resistance in obesity is due to either a decreased number of insulin-sensitive glucose transporters (GLUT) or an inability to stimulate recruitment of transporters from microsomes to the plasma membrane has been investigated in obese humans. Garvey and colleagues (5) measured GLUT 4 expression in adipocytes—GLUT 4 is the transporter that mediates the bulk of insulin-stimulated transport activity. They found that obesity led to a depletion of intracellular GLUT 4 transporters with fewer carriers being available for insulin-mediated recruitment to the cell surface. Furthermore, the cellular content of GLUT 4 was determined by the GLUT 4 mRNA over a wide range of body weight. In non-insulin-dependent diabetic patients (NIDDM) profound insulin resistance was caused by a more severe depletion of GLUT 4 mRNA compared to simple obesity, and transporter loss involved both plasma membrane and intracellular compartments (5). In both groups of patients, pretranslational suppression of GLUT 4 transporters entirely accounted for impaired cellular insulin responsiveness in adipose tissue. In contrast, no significant differences were

seen in skeletal muscle GLUT 4 content and GLUT 4 mRNA activity was similar to that seen control subjects (6). These studies demonstrated that GLUT 4 gene expression in the muscles studied is not affected by insulin-resistant states. Other mechanisms that potentially could impair glucose transport activity in skeletal muscle include decreased functional activity of the transporters or an impairment of insulin-stimulated translocation of intracellular GLUT 4 to the cell surface. It has been demonstrated that chronic exposure to high concentrations of glucose and insulin reduces the subsequent ability of insulin to maximally stimulate glucose transport by inhibiting transporter translocation (7). The in vivo efficacy of skeletal muscle glucose uptake has been shown to be inversely proportional to the glycosylated hemoglobin value in NIDDM subjects (8). Thus hyperglycemia and/or hyperinsulinemia could induce at least a component of insulin resistance in muscle via such mechanisms. A possible hypothesis for the pathogenesis of diabetes associated with obesity is that insulin resistance in adipocytes occurs as the initial lesion and impaired glucose tolerance leads to postprandial hyperglycemia and hyperinsulinemia. These factors result in a cascade of events including insulin resistance in muscle (from a defect in transporter translocation) and eventual secretory exhaustion of pancreatic β cells.

An additional factor contributing to the insulin insensitivity of obesity may be the excessive plasma levels of free fatty acids derived from portal adipose tissue (9). Enlarged abdominal adipocytes show an enhance sensitivity to lipolytic stimuli and increased FFA production. This results in relative insulin resistance to the antilipolytic action of insulin in abdominal obesity and may contribute to systemic insulin resistance, particularly in liver and muscle (10).

III. ADRENOCORTICAL FUNCTION IN OBESITY

Obese subjects have a normal circulating plasma cortisol concentration with a normal circadian rhythm and normal urinary free cortisol but an accelerated degradation of cortisol, which is compensated by an increased cortisol production rate (11,12). It is considered that the increase in metabolic clearance of cortisol is secondary to a decrease in cortisol-binding globulin plasma concentrations. Slavnov and Epshein (13) have reported a moderate elevation in plasma corticotropin (ACTH) levels in obesity, which may explain the increased cortisol production. The increased peripheral clearance rate of cortisol is probably mediated by binding to the glucocorticoid receptor that is present in glucocorticoid-responding tissue (14). An increased peripheral density of this receptor will be followed by an increased metabolic clearance rate. Enlarged visceral adipocytes, as found in abdominal obesity, could be the site where this occurs because such tissue appears to have a higher density of glucocorticoid receptors than other adipose tissue (15). This may be one explanation for the functional hypercortisolism associated with abdominal obesity in subjects who are only moderately overweight. Cortisol inhibits the antilipolytic effect of insulin in human adipocytes, and this may be particularly pronounced in visceral abdominal fat containing a high density of the glucocorticoid receptor (16). The localization of fat is crucial for the insulin-stimulated expression of LPL activity mediated by the glucocorticoid receptor (17).

The increased peripheral clearance and the obesity-associated acceleration in overall adrenocortical function also leads to an increase in adrenal androgen production. Urinary 17-ketosteroids (17-KS), which measure various androgen metabolites including etiocholananolone, androsterone, dehydroepiandrosterone (DHEA), and its sulfate conjugate (DHEAS), are elevated in obese subjects (18). The changes in adrenal androgen production may simply occur in compensation for an increasing metabolic clearance but there is additional evidence to suggest alterations in adrenocortical dynamics. Kurtz and colleagues (19) noted an increased turnover of DHEA in obese women. These authors demonstrated a significant correlation between upper body obesity (WHR) and the metabolic clearance of DHEA and androstenedione, which suggests that the androgenic effects of DHEA may have a role in fat distribution. In premenopausal women serum DHEA concentration correlates positively with trunk fat and negatively with leg fat accumulation whereas no such effect is seen in men (20,21). A shift in fat accumulation in women toward abdominal obesity may be an androgenic effect of DHEA. In healthy postmenopausal women, androgen levels are inversely related to fasting plasma glucose levels and are predictive of central obesity 10–15 years later (22). Brody et al. (23) have reported a positive correlation between body weight and changes in DHEA and the DHEA/17-hydroxyprogesterone ratio after exogenous administration of ACTH. This is suggestive of hyperresponsiveness of adrenal androgens in obesity. Weaver and colleagues (24) have also provided evidence for increased ACTH release in obesity by reporting an association between the ACTH response to insulin-induced hypoglycemia and increasing body weight. Moreover, alteration in adrenocortical production of adrenal androgens probably reflects the influence of other factors including adrenal androgens themselves. In vitro studies have suggested a lesser degree of inhibition of human 17-

hydroxylase activity by DHEA as compared to the inhibition of human 17,20-desmolase activity (25). The increased adipose tissue breakdown and the higher urinary excretion of DHEA in such circumstances could lead to decreased intra-adrenal concentrations of the steroid. As a consequence, the inhibition of 17,20-desmolase will be further diminished and a selective increase in the production of DHEA and its metabolites will occur.

DHEA may therefore contribute to the establishment of a vicious cycle of events—the greater androgenic action of DHEA contributing to abdominal fat cell accumulation with resulting hyperglycaemia and hyperinsulinemia. The latter depresses the SHBG concentration, which results in an increase in free testosterone levels and increased visceral fat accumulation.

IV. CUSHING'S SYNDROME AND OBESITY

There are many clinical similarities between subjects with upper body obesity and the increased adiposity found in patients with Cushing's syndrome. Cushing's syndrome may be characterized by insulin resistance, impaired glucose tolerance, hypertension, hyperlipidemia, centrally localized adipose tissue, and muscle weakness (26). In addition, decreased plasma SHBG concentrations and increased free testosterone levels are features of Cushing's syndrome. An overlap between upper body obesity (UBO) and Cushing's syndrome is found not only with regional fat distribution but also with alterations in muscle type. UBO shows a relative decrease in type 1 to type IIb muscle fibers as found in Cushing's syndrome (26). Furthermore, women with UBO and women with Cushing's syndrome do not show the typical female increase in fat size and LPL activity in femoral adipocytes as compared to abdominal adipocytes. Instead, LPL activity in enlarged abdominal fat cells is increased 2–3 times that seen in normal-weight women. It is likely that this results from a combined action of increased cortisol and insulin at the receptor level: human adipose tissue exposed in vitro for prolonged periods to high concentrations of cortisol shows an increase in LPL activity but only in the presence of insulin (16). These findings suggest cortisol has a preferential effect on abdominal adipose tissue because no clear difference from normal is found in adipose tissue taken from the femoral region. This could reflect the increased numbers of glucocorticoid receptors found in abdominal adipocytes (15). The diminished lipolysis in Cushing's syndrome results in a decreased capacity of abdominal fat cells to activate fat mobilization, which, in turn, contributes to the enlargement of abdominal adipocytes. Thus, upper body adiposity in Cushing's syndrome may be due to a combination of increased LPL activity and decreased lipolytic activity—it is likely that elevated cortisol concentrations are involved in the former but the mechanisms for the latter are uncertain. Undoubtedly, direct effects of cortisol on cellular insulin sensitivity are an important contributor to peripheral insulin resistance.

Rebuffe-Scrive and colleagues (26) have shown that muscle tissue from the vastus lateralis in women with Cushing's syndrome contains a normal amount of glycogen but very low glycogen synthase activity, the likely consequence of diminished insulin sensitivity. Fiber composition in such women (and in women with UBO who were not cushingoid) was characterized by a relative abundance of type IIb and a scarcity of type 1 muscle fibers compared to women with gynaeoid (lower body) obesity. Moreover, a correlation was seen between the proportion of type 1 muscle fibers and insulin sensitivity and between type IIb fibers and insulin resistance: type 1 fibers show higher insulin sensitivity and bind insulin more efficiently. The metabolic environment has a direct effect on muscle fiber sensitivity because subjects with rheumatoid arthritis treated chronically with high doses of prednisolone have a lower proportion of type 1 and a higher proportion of type IIb fibers than similar patients who have not been treated with steroids (27). Thus the altered distribution of muscle fiber type in Cushing's syndrome results from excessive endogenous glucocorticoid activity. In women with abdominal obesity without Cushing's syndrome, alterations in muscle fiber type may reflect similar hormonal changes combined with a genetic predisposition.

V. REGIONAL DISTRIBUTION OF BODY FAT

Fat topography can be defined at two levels: first, by individual differences in adipose tissue cell characteristics and, second, by the anatomical distribution of body fat (28,29). Excess fat may be primarily stored either in the abdominal region (upper body fat) or in the gluteal-femoral region (lower body fat). The factors responsible for fat localization in the upper or lower parts of the body and the association of regional adiposity with morbidity are unknown but the differences in the control of adipose tissue lipolysis may play a role.

Differences are found in rates of lipolysis in adipose tissue fragments obtained from different anatomical sites. Human adipose tissue is richly endowed with a and B adrenoreceptors—binding of agonists to B receptors enhances lipolysis whereas agonists that bind to a2 receptors

inhibit lipolysis. In both men and women, the lipolytic response to noradrenaline (a2 and B) is more marked in abdominal than gluteal or femoral tissues (29). Furthermore, detailed analysis in men and women suggests that the usual pattern of male fat distribution (greater abdominal fat accumulation) reflects greater a2 activity in the abdominal tissue of men (30). There is considerable evidence that lipoprotein lipase (LPL) plays a controlling rate in the regional distribution of fat. There are significant gender and regional differences in LPL activity that largely parallel variations for fat size. Premenopausal women have higher LPL activities in gluteal and femoral regions than men but the differences disappear after the menopause (31). In addition, women have quantitatively more LPL in gluteal and femoral tissue, which contains larger fat cells, than they do in abdominal adipose tissue. In contrast, men show minimal regional variations in LPL activity or fat cell size. These differences in fat distribution between men and women may explain the tendency for premenopausal women to deposit fat preferentially in lower body fat depots.

The biochemical mechanisms regulating adipose tissue LPL activity are not completely understood. A regional difference is seen in the response of adipose tissue to catecholamine-induced lipolysis, which is probably localized at the adrenoreceptor level: stimulation of the protein kinase complex, the most distal part of the activating chain, abolishes the lipolytic difference between site and gender (32). Insulin is permissive for LPL synthesis and glucocorticoids enhance the activity of LPL when added with insulin in vitro (16). Sex steroids have been implicated in the regional distribution of body fat and gender differences are seen in LPL activity particularly during pregnancy and lactation (33). Regional variation in receptors for glucocorticoids or sex steroids could play a role in determining regional differences in adipose tissue. The reverse situation may also be true—adipose tissue having an effect on the production of sex hormones.

VI. SEX STEROID SECRETION IN OBESITY

Significant associations are seen in reproductive endocrinology between excess body fat and ovulatory dysfunction, hyperandrogenism, and hormone-sensitive carcinomas (34). The topography of fat distribution is correlated with these changes (35). The differences in fat distribution relate to the difference in androgenicity and to the variations in insulin action seen between upper body and lower body obesities. However, obesity influences the menstrual cycle independent of fat distribution (36). Menarche frequently occurs at a younger age in obese girls and menstrual abnormalities are common in adulthood (37). Weight loss has a salutary effect on ovulatory function with the return of menses in previously amenorrheic obese women (38). Obese women may be characterized by distinct alterations in circulating sex hormone levels (36). Androstenedione and testosterone concentrations are commonly elevated whereas sex hormone–binding globulin (SHBG) is reduced. The plasma ratio of estrone to estradiol is also increased in obesity. Interestingly, a similar pattern of changes of sex steroid concentrations and binding are found in women with the polycystic ovary syndrome (39).

Evans and colleagues (35) have shown body weight and WHR are inversely correlated with SHBG levels and directly correlated to free testosterone concentrations. Others have described a higher production rate from the adrenal cortex and ovaries and increased metabolic clearance of testosterone and dihydrotestosterone (DHT) (36). The clearance of testosterone increases as SHBG decreases, the consequence of an increased fraction of unbound testosterone available for hepatic extraction and clearance (37). Such a mechanism may protect some obese subjects from the development of frank hirsutism. Fat tissue is able to sequester various steroids, including androgens, probably as a result of their lipid solubility. Most sex steroids appear to be preferentially concentrated within adipocytes rather than in the plasma (38). As a result, the overall steroid pool in severely obese subjects is far greater than that of normal-weight individuals—the volume of fat in obese subjects is much larger than the intravascular space and tissue steroid concentration is 2–13 times higher than in plasma. Fat may serve not only as a reservoir but also as a site for steroid metabolism. Androgens can be irreversibly aromatized to estrogens or reversibly converted to other androgens (39).

There are two possible explanations for this obesity-related increase in androgen production rate. The first possibility is a hypothalamic-pituitary-gonadal and adrenal compensation for the higher MCR, in effect a "servo-control" mechanism (19). Alternatively, the increase in ovarian and adrenal production is stimulated by other factors such as insulin with a consequent reduction in hepatic production of SHBG and an increase in metabolic clearance rate (MCR) of bound steroids (40). Independently increased androgen levels may stimulate upper body fat deposition with an additional increase in the steroidal MCR through adipose tissue sequestration and androgen metabolism (38).

VII. ESTROGEN METABOLISM IN OBESITY

Excess body fat leads to alterations in estrogen metabolism that affect the hypothalmic-pituitary-ovarian axis and may lead to ovarian dysfunction (41). The production of estrogen and its precursors, including androstenedione and testosterone, decreases with age and particularly with the menopause. In premenopausal women, mean 24-hr plasma estrone and estradiol levels do not differ between obese and normal-weight women (42). However, obese women demonstrate lower circulating SHBG levels and thereby an increased fraction of circulating estradiol. In postmenopausal obese women, serum levels of estrone and estradiol are correlated with the degree of obesity and fat mass (43). SHBG levels are lower in these older obese women, suggesting elevated estradiol concentrations. Davidson and colleagues (44) have shown that estrone and estradiol levels decline earlier in obese women compared to normal-weight controls—age must be taken into account when comparing groups of postmenopausal women.

Aromatization of androstenedione to estrone has been demonstrated in vivo in adipose tissue from premenopausal and postmenopausal women and is closely related to body weight (45). Aromatase activity is detected primarily in the stroma of adipose tissue and not in intact adipocytes (46). Peripheral aromatization increases with age and is 2–4 times higher in postmenopausal women (47). Androstenedione is the major substrate for peripheral estrogen formation. In contrast, only a small amount of testosterone is converted to estradiol although this may be of greater clinical significance. Longcope and colleagues (48) have reported significant associations between body weight and conversion of testosterone to estradiol.

The interconversion of estrone to estradiol has been observed in vivo and in vitro in adipose tissue with a greater conversion being found in omental fat than subcutaneous fat (49,50). Adipose tissue 17-β-hydroxysteroid dehydrogenase activity, measured by the conversion of estrone to estradiol, is higher in premenopausal than in postmenopausal women and all women have a higher activity compared to men (50). Estrogens should not be considered passive by-products of obesity because they have been shown in vitro to promote adipose tissue proliferation by inducing replication and proliferation of adipocyte precursors (51).

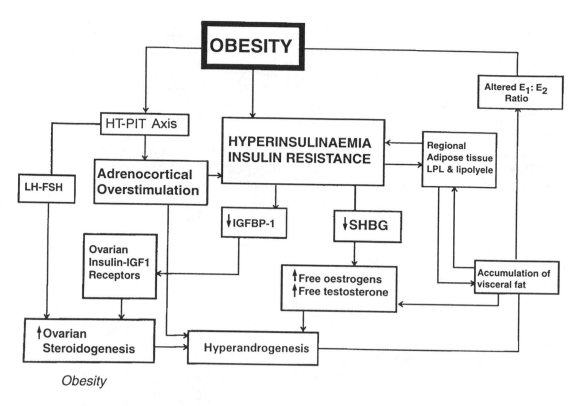

Obesity

Figure 1 Scheme of events seen in association with the development of obesity emphasizing a relationship between alterations in endocrine function and abdominal (or visceral) accumulation of body fat. IGFBP-1, insulin-like growth factor–binding protein; SHBG, sex hormone–binding globulin.

VIII. SEX HORMONE BINDING GLOBULIN IN OBESITY

SHBG is a circulating globulin produced by the liver that binds in high affinity but low capacity to many of the circulating sex hormones (52). Alterations in SHBG levels have a profound impact on the metabolism and action of bound steroids. A decrease in SHBG concentration is associated with an increase in metabolic clearance and free fraction of testosterone and estradiol. Furthermore, blood conversion rates of testosterone and androstenedione are positively correlated with the free fraction of testosterone but independent of total serum testosterone. The low affinity of SHBG for estradiol relative to testosterone results in an estrogen amplification effect on sensitive tissues (particularly the liver) with decreasing SHBG plasma levels (52). The mechanism by which obesity decreases the production of SHBG is unclear. It is possible that obesity-related hyperandrogenism leads to an initial reduction in SHBG levels, a greater metabolic clearance of testosterone and estradiol, and a new sex hormone equilibrium (41). Kirschner and colleagues (53) have investigated androgen

and estrogen production in women and related this to body fat topography. UBO is characterized by higher total serum testosterone concentrations with increased production rates, increased estradiol levels, and reduced SHBG concentrations in comparison to lower body obesity. Evans et al. (35) have previously reported a linear correlation between SHBG levels and WHR. It is of interest that Kirschner et al. also found lower peripheral aromatization of androstenedione to estrone in UBO compared to comparable women whose obesity was distributed in the femoral-gluteal regions.

The hypothesis that insulin may regulate the hepatic production of SHBG is supported by the finding of a direct inhibitory action of insulin on SHBG secretion by cultured human hepatoma cells (54). Peiris and colleagues (55) have shown UBO to be associated with increased pancreatic insulin production and decreased hepatic insulin clearance. Thus, increasing splanchnic insulin concentrations may account for decreased hepatic SHBG production in this type of obesity. These authors also showed the severity of the peripheral insulin resistance to be positively correlated with the magnitude of free

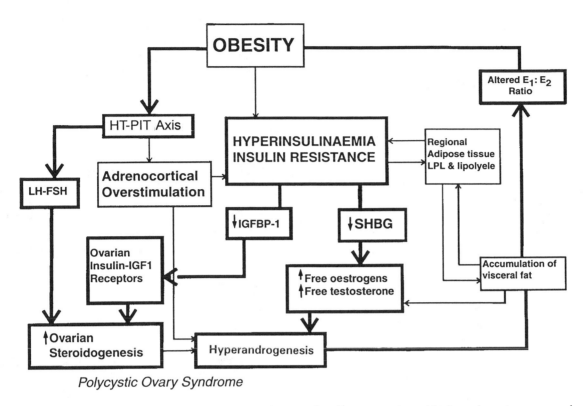

Figure 2 Scheme illustrating the alterations in endocrine function found in association with the polycystic ovary syndrome. The pathways of likely primary importance are highlighted by bold arrows and boxes—note the overlap with the changes seen with obesity per se.

testosterone—the greater the free testosterone level, the greater the degree of insulin resistance. The changes in circulating androgens do not appear to influence plasma insulin levels but, conversely, increasing plasma insulin may increase androgen secretion by a number of mechanisms, including direct stimulation of androgen production by the ovary (40). Recent evidence suggests that both insulin and insulin-like growth factor 1 (IGF-1) may be important regulators of ovarian thecal and stromal androgen production with an interaction at the receptor level on the ovarian stroma of these two hormones (56).

IX. GROWTH HORMONE SECRETION IN OBESITY

Growth hormone (GH) is an important regulator of body mass throughout life: subcutaneous fat is markedly increased in GH-deficient children as well as in GH-deficient adults (57). Interestingly, in these subjects fat deposition occurs predominantly on the trunk. Moreover, hypopituitary patients have abnormally high amounts of intra-abdominal fat, which may be decreased by 30% after 6

months of treatment with growth hormone (58). Such evidence suggests that relative GH deficiency or insensitivity could play a role in the perpetuation of the obesity.

An impaired GH response to insulin-induced hypoglycemia is found in association with obesity but this seems likely to be a consequence rather than a cause of extreme obesity (59). Sims and colleagues (60) have confirmed that weight gain decreases the GH response to all types of provocative stimuli whereas the GH response to hypoglycemia significantly increases in obese subjects following weight loss. An input of food in excess of energy expenditure appears to be important because impaired GH responsiveness is not a characteristic of subjects who are overweight as the result of increased musculature induced by vigorous exercise (61). In this situation, energy expenditure is balanced by an increase in appropriate protein and energy intake whereas 10 days of overfeeding with carbohydrate can produce impaired GH responsiveness without an increase in body weight (62). The explanation for the decreased output of GH in obesity has not been fully elucidated. It has been suggested that the altered GH secretion results from alterations in IGF-1 and its binding proteins (63). Synthesis of IGF-1 is stimulated by insulin, and the hyperinsulinemia of obesity could directly enhance IGF-1 production and suppress the production of GH from the pituitary by a negative feedback mechanism. A negative feedback effect of IGF-1 has been demonstrated in pituitary cells in culture (64). However, several authors have reported that IGF-1 circulating levels in obese adults are normal (65). By contrast, IGF-binding proteins 1 and 3 (IGFBP-1, IGFBP-3) are both reduced in obesity with decreased plasma concentrations of IGFBP-1 being inversely related to fasting plasma insulin and WHR (66,67). A reduced level of IGFBP-1 suggests enhanced biological activity of IGF-I, which, in turn, may feed back on the hypothalamic-pituitary axis to suppress GH release. It is of interest that IGF-1, GH, and insulin have all been shown to promote the conversion of preadipocytes to adipocytes and may, therefore, play a role in upper body fat deposition (68). Moreover, substantial weight reduction will reverse the documented alterations in insulin, GH, IGF-1, and its binding proteins (69).

X. POLYCYSTIC OVARY SYNDROME AND OBESITY

The polycystic ovary syndrome (PCOS) is the most common endocrine disorder of reproduction (70). Moderate obesity is frequently found in association with the syndrome and this has led to speculation that obesity and PCOS may be causally related. Such speculation was originally underlined by Stein and Leventhal's description of the syndrome but subsequent studies have emphasized the diversity of the clinical features that may be associated with the classic ovarian morphology (71,72). The ovaries in PCOS show thickened cortices with subcapsular follicles of which an increased number are atretic. In addition, there is hyperplasia of the theca cells and immature granulosa cells of the follicles, which are unable to convert thecal androgens into estrogens by aromatization. The ovarian stroma, which is formed largely from atretic follicles, is androgen-producing and usually hyperplastic in PCOS. Many of these features are seen in ovaries from obese women with normal menstrual function, but in this circumstance the ovary is not enlarged (73). A similar ovarian morphology is also reported in women with Cushing's disease and congenital adrenal hyperplasia, syndromes that are associated with hyperandrogenism (70). What are the common features of PCOS and obesity and how is it possible to distinguish PCOS from obesity?

PCOS is characterized by increased plasma androstenedione, increased testosterone, and a reversed estradiol: estrone ratio. Furthermore, SHBG is reduced in women with PCOS with a similar relationship to body fat distribution as found in obesity (35,74). In PCOS (in contrast to obesity) the ovaries appear to be the major source of androgens with the production being dependent on LH; adrenal androgen production is ACTH-dependent (70). Testosterone is formed in peripheral tissues by conversion from androstenedione, DHEA, and DHEAS, while estrone is both secreted by the ovaries and derived from extragonadal aromatization. In both PCOS and obesity, aromatization rates of androstenedione to estrone by adipose tissue are positively correlated with body weight (75). In contrast to obesity, PCOS is characterized by alterations in gonadotropin release. An increased secretion of LH relative to FSH is seen in PCOS with the elevated LH levels resulting from an increased amplitude of LH pulses (76). It appears that the increased LH pulse reflects an increased pituitary sensitivity to gonadotropin-releasing hormone (GnRH) (72,76).

Women with PCOS show hyperinsulinemia and insulin resistance (77). Although the degree of hyperinsulinemia is proportional to body weight, normal-weight women with PCOS also show insulin resistance. Investigations confirm a situation in PCOS identical with obesity—increasing upper body fatness is associated with increasing peripheral insulin resistance and decreasing hepatic extraction (40). It is possible that androgens may directly diminish insulin action because significant positive correlations are seen between androgen and insulin levels in PCOS (77). However, suppression of gonadal steroid production by 12 weeks of treatment with a long-acting analog of GnRH did not significantly alter plasma insulin levels, hepatic glucose production, or peripheral glucose disposal (78).

The primary etiological event in PCOS is unknown. One suggestion is that increased LH pulses relative to FHS result in arrested folliculogenesis and increased ovarian estrogen production. This is secondary to LH-dependent thecal androgen secretion and insufficient granulosa cell estrogen production (because of relative FSH deficiency). Increased LH release produces thecal and stromal hyperplasia and anovulation results from the disordered gonadotropin release. This results in the formation of subcapsular follicular cysts: androgens directly cause thickening of the ovarian cortex and increased rates of follicular atresia. The androgens also feed back on the hypothalamic-pituitary axis by their peripheral conversion to estrogens. This tonic estrogen feedback, predominantly by estradiol, leads to greater sensitivity to GnRH and increased LH pulses with a vicious cycle of events being created. However, there are several mechanisms by which obesity per se is independently involved in the development of chronic hyperandrogenic anovulation (79), and a better understanding of these may provide clues to the role of fatness in the pathogenesis of PCOS.

Alterations in the peripheral metabolism of sex steroids in obesity, which result in increased extraglandular aromatization of androstenedione to estrogen and decreased SHBG, will affect the hypothalamic-pituitary regulation through feedback mechanisms. Other factors are also involved because decreased SHBG and increased androgen production occur in obese women both with and without reproductive dysfunction (36). Hyperinsulinemia may independently alter gonadotropin secretion and ovarian steroidogenesis to produce PCOS (56). A correlation has been shown between hyperinsulinemia and hyperandrogenism in women with PCOS; obese women with PCOS are significantly more hyperinsulinemic than nonobese women with PCOS (80). Nestler and colleagues (81) have observed a corresponding fall in plasma insulin and testosterone concentrations in obese women with PCOS given diazoxide without any apparent effect on pulsatile gonadotropin secretion or the response to GnRH stimulation. These effects, which were not seen in normal-weight women, underline the influence of obesity as a predisposing factor and suggest a different sensitivity of steroidogenesis in the face of hyperinsulinemia. An additional mechanism by which insulin may influence androgen secretion is represented by its action on IGF-BP1, which can be synthesized in ovarian cells and is regulated by insulin (82,83). Lean women with PCOS demonstrate a positive correlation between hyperinsulinemia and IGF-1 concentrations and a negative association with IGFBP-1, a pattern identical to that seen in obesity (77). Since IGF-BP1 acts as an inhibitor of IGF-1 production, its decrease in hyperinsulinemic states may favor an increase in androgen production by increasing ovarian concentrations of IGF-1 (84). IGF-1 is a potent amplifier of LH-induced androgen synthesis (85). Thus, an interaction between insulin and growth factors at the receptor level may lead to alterations in ovarian stimulation. Whatever the precise mechanisms, obesity is an undoubted compounding factor—weight reduction in women with PCOS generally improves the hormonal abnormalities and restores ovulation (86).

In summary, obesity is common in PCOS but is not directly associated with discernible changes in gonadotropin release. The finding that weight reduction improves menstrual function in some obese women with PCOS is strong evidence that obesity contributes to the hormonal abnormalities found in PCOS. A plausible explanation for the association is that the gonadotropin abnormalities of PCOS, insulin resistance, and some marker(s) for obesity represent genetic defects at a different, but anatomically close, locus, which overlap to result in a heterogeneous disorder.

XI. GENETIC DETERMINANTS OF OBESITY

There is increasing evidence to suggest a genetic basis to extreme obesity. Studies of adopted children and twins provide considerable information as to whether childhood environment or genetic inheritance is predominant in determining fatness (87,88). Such studies have also demonstrated a genetic basis to the distribution of fat tissue (89). Nevertheless, these studies simply measure hereditability (the genetic influence) found among persons living in a particular range of environmental conditions. The important implication is that environmental factors augmented by hereditary tendencies are crucial and potentially reversible—a point to emphasize when possible primary abnormalities of endocrine function are considered in obesity. However, common human metabolic disorders can rarely be reduced to simple Mendelian phenotypes—they are complex multifactorial traits evolving under the influence of numerous affectors, including social, physiological, metabolic, and molecular factors. Segregation of the genes is not easily detected in familial or pedigree studies, and whatever the influence of the gene(s) on the etiology, it is generally attenuated or exacerbated by nongenetic factors. An understanding of the genetic basis of such traits requires an appropriate conceptual framework, adequate phenotype measurements, proper samples of unrelated persons and nuclear families or extended pedigrees, and extensive candidate gene typing and other molecular markers (90).

The susceptibility gene concept is of importance for the various phenotypes that may be relevant to the endocrine determinants of obesity. A susceptibility gene is defined as one that increases the susceptibility or risk of a disease but is not necessary for disease expression. An allele at a susceptibility gene may make it more likely that the carrier will become affected but the presence of that allele is not sufficient by itself to explain the occurrence of the disease. It merely lowers the threshold for the person to develop the disease. To further complicate the genetic circumstance, clinical manifestations are also modulated by a variety of gene-environment interactions. These effects result from an individual's "sensitivity" to environmental exposures or life-style differences, e.g., alcohol intake, cigarette smoking, exercise, and so forth. This explains why trends from genetic epidemiological studies of the heritability level that examine segregation of major genes and gene-nutrition or gene-physical activity interaction effects have shown only moderate heritability. Interestingly, the highest heritability coefficients seem to be for various indicators of android and gyneoid fat distribution, for plasma DHEA and DHEAS, and for plasma cortisol concentrations (90).

To simplify the task, animal models of obesity have been widely studied. A relationship has been described in laboratory-bred, genetically obese rodents between hyperinsulinemia and altered hypothalamic-pituitary function that is present before the onset of obesity (91). In these animals the hypothalamus appears to play an important role in the maintenance of a normal blood glucose by integrating the afferent signal, i.e., circulating blood glucose concentrations, with the central regulation of autonomic activity to the pancreas. Rodent models of obesity, whether produced by lesions of the ventromedial nucleus or homozygous *ob* and *fa* genes, are all characterized by hyperinsulinemia and insulin resistance. Recently the characteristics of an obesity gene in the *ob/ob* mouse have been detailed and a human homolog found (92): in this animal the complexity of the trait has been reduced to a single gene disorder resulting in a dichotomous phenotype with the affected animals reaching 3 times the normal body weight. The investigators identified a 650,000-base-pair region on chromosome 6 as containing *ob*, which narrowed the search to 0.02% of the genome. Six genes were isolated in sequence with one being found to be exclusively expressed in adipose tissue in normal mice, rendering it a likely candidate gene. Sequence data suggested that this gene encodes a secreted protein. When its structure was compared in normal and obese mice, a premature stop codon was found in the latter animals that resulted in the translocation of a truncated protein, and expression of this mutated gene was found to be 20 times greater than in the control animals. When the human genome was screened, an *ob* homolog that was 84% identical with the mouse *ob* gene was found, which establishes *ob* as a highly preserved, biologically important gene. These findings invite the hypothesis that the *ob* gene product is a soluble factor synthesized and secreted by adipose tissue that signals satiety presumably by interacting with specific receptors in the hypothalamus. The nature of human obesity as a complex trait predicts that the effect of *ob*, if any, will be less spectacular in humans than in the mouse model, except possibly in selected pedigrees. Additional genes will have to be found to explain all of the trait's genetic variance.

The study of candidate genes in population association studies in humans has revealed associations between obesity, body fat distribution, or hyperinsulinemia with the genes for insulin, apolipoprotein D, and the glucocorticoid receptor. Interestingly, all these associations are also found with diabetes, suggesting an important genetic overlap between the two disorders.

A. Insulin Gene

The INS gene has been cloned and localized to the short arm of chromosome 11 (11p15.5) (93). It is closely linked with a hypervariable region (HVR) of DNA, characterized by variation in the number of tandem repeats 14 base pairs in length (94). There exist distinct classes of alleles depending on the number of repeats—class 1 alleles are 0–600 bp, class 2 are 600–1200 bp, and class 3 are greater than 1200 bp in length. Associations exist between non-insulin-dependent diabetes and the class 3 allele: an association between the HVR and NIDDM has been reported in South Indians in whom the main determinant of diabetes is UBO (95,96). An investigation of British Caucasian extremely obese women with normal glucose tolerance has shown a positive association between the class 3 allele and fasting hyperinsulinemia and with various indices of insulin secretion and resistance (97). As this region lies 5′ to the INS gene, it has been postulated that the HVR is in linkage disequilibrium with mutations in the regulatory sequences important for transcriptional activity of the gene or, alternatively, that the HVR has a direct effect on gene regulation.

B. Glucocorticoid Receptor

The glucocorticoid receptor is widely distributed and expressed in many tissues and has been extensively investigated as a model for transcriptional regulation. The chronic effect of glucocorticoids is exerted by the regulation of gene expression by means of transcriptional enhancement that contains glucocorticoid response elements (GREs) near hormone-responsive promoters. GREs are active only on binding of the receptor-steroid complex. The glucocorticoid receptor consists of three structural domains: the hormone-binding, the DNA-binding, and the modulatory region or N-terminal domain (98,99). These regions are essential for the receptor to act as a transcription factor effecting gene expression of the target genes. Mutations or polymorphisms in these domains could therefore lead to the altered expression of genes involved in glucose and insulin homeostasis. An association has been found between hyperinsulinemia and the 4.5-kb Bcl I restriction fragment length polymorphism (RFLP) of the GCR gene in extremely obese women (100). Furthermore, a linkage of obesity with the Bcl I RFLP and two microstatellites in the same chromosomal region of the GCR gene has been reported in obese sib pairs (101). Such findings provide strong presumptive evidence that mutations in the GCR gene may play a role in obesity and hyperinsulinemia.

C. Apolipoprotein D

An association has been described between the apolipoprotein D (Apo D) gene and NIDDM (102). More recently, the application of a Taq 1 restriction enzyme digestion has revealed an association between the 2.2-kb allele of the Apo D gene with obesity and hyperinsulinemia—no association was seen with the 2.7-kb allele (103). This suggests an association the Apo D polymorphism itself and obesity or linkage disequilibrium between the Apo D gene and another gene in close proximity (e.g., the GLUT 2 locus). Preliminary studies of GLUT 2 polymorphism have failed to show any association with obesity.

The results from these investigations support the hypothesis of a genetic basis to the metabolic and endocrine alterations associated with obesity. They indicate a likely complex genetic background to human obesity and the potential dangers of extrapolating findings from laboratory-bred rodents to the human situation. However, the findings to date must remain speculative until larger numbers of subjects have been investigated.

XII. CONCLUSIONS

Rodent models of obesity, whether produced by lesions of the ventromedial nucleus or by homozygous *ob* and *fa* genes, are all characterized by hyperinsulinemia and insulin resistance. In young preobese *fa/fa* Zucker rats, hypersecretion of insulin is completely abolished by acute cholinergic blockade, which indicates a parasympathetic origin of the hypersecretion and suggesting an early defect mediated by the vagus nerve (104). In adult *fa/fa* rats (and the obesity models), hyperinsulinemia is associated with increased lipogenesis and decreased glucose uptake in muscle and this appears to be the explanation for the development of insulin resistance (105). In addition, such animals have an abnormal regulation of corticosterone with 24-hr urinary excretion rates being twice as great in the obese *fa/fa* rat compared to lean littermates. Moreover, the obese animals show increased concentrations of CRF in the median eminence of the hypothalamus and a corresponding increase in pituitary ACTH secretion (106). Thus the initial abnormalities of endocrine function in the

rodent models of obesity appear to originate in the central nervous system. This central abnormality results in dysregulation of autonomic function and hyperinsulinemia and alterations in adrenocortical activity leading to hypercortisolism. The peripheral tissue changes seen in these circumstances are the consequence rather than a cause, although they undoubtedly add to the obese situation. The heterogeneity of human obesity makes direct comparison with laboratory-bred rodents unwise; however, there are striking similarities between endocrine determinants of rodent and human obesity.

Human obesity is characterized by hyperinsulinemia, which, in turn, is correlated with the degree of fatness. The distribution of fat tissue is important in determining the degree of hyperinsulinemia with the highest plasma insulin concentrations generally being associated with UBO. Furthermore, characteristic changes in adrenocortical activity are recognized in human obesity with increased turnover of cortisol and increased secretion of androgens. The increased production of androgens further enhances UBO: an increasing volume of body fat alters the peripheral metabolism of sex hormones and increases insulin resistance. Increasing insulin secretion suppresses hepatic formation of SHBG and IGFBP-1, which, in turn, influences sex steroid and IGF-1 cellular action. A proposed scheme of alterations found in obesity is shown in Figure 1.

The polycystic syndrome differs from obesity by virtue of alterations in hypothalamic-pituitary-gonadal function. Obesity is not a prerequisite for the development of the syndrome although it is a frequent accompaniment. Hyperinsulinemia is present in most patients with PCOS, and it is possible to propose a similar sequence of events to those seen in obesity that link alterations in sex steroid secretion and peripheral metabolism with changes in ovarian function. Once again, the situation is accentuated by weight gain, particularly in the upper body segments (Fig. 2).

Our understanding of the endocrine mechanisms involved in the determination and perpetuation of obesity has increased substantially during the past 10 years as better methods have become available to investigate cellular events. The role of subtle endocrine changes in influencing adipose tissue deposition and metabolism is now better appreciated and this has resulted in several plausible hypotheses about the origins of obesity. The study of biochemical markers of the metabolic changes described in this chapter as candidate genes for obesity will undoubtedly lead to an even better understanding. It is likely that an exciting new phase of obesity research has begun.

REFERENCES

1. Kolterman OG, Insel J, Sackow M, Olefsky M. Mechanisms of insulin resistance in human obesity. J Clin Invest 1980; 65:1272–1284.
2. Kissebah AH, Vydelingum N, Murray R. Relation of body fat distribution to metabolic complications of obesity. J Clin Invest 1982; 54:254–260.
3. Peiris AN, Mueller RA, Smith GA. Splanchnic insulin metabolism in obesity: influence of body fat distribution. J Clin Invest 1986; 78:1648–1657.
4. Evans DJ, Murray R, Kissebah AH. Relationship between skeletal muscle insulin resistance, insulin-mediated glucose disposal and insulin binding effects of obesity and body fat topography. J Clin Invest 1984; 74:1515–1525.
5. Garvey WT, Maianu L, Huecksteadt TP, et al. Pretranslational suppression of a glucose transporter protein causes cellular insulin resistance in non-insulin dependent diabetes and obesity. J Clin Invest 1991; 87:1072–1081.
6. Garvey WT, Maianu L, Hancock JA, Golichowski AM, Baron A. Gene expression of GLUT 4 in skeletal muscle from insulin-resistant patients with obesity, IGT, GDM and NIDDM. Diabetes 1992; 41:465–475.
7. Garvey WT, Olesfky JM, Matthaei S, Marshall S. Glucose and insulin coregulate the glucose transport system in primary cultured adipocytes: a new mechanism of insulin resistance. J Biol Chem 1987; 262:189–197.
8. Baron A, Laakso M, Brechtel G, Edelman SV. Reduced capacity and affinity of skeletal muscle for insulin-mediated glucose uptake in non-insulin dependent diabetic subjects. J Clin Invest 1991; 87:1186–94.
9. Bolinder J, Kager L, Ostman J, Arner P. Differences at the receptor and post-receptor levels between human omental and subcutaneous tissue in the action of insulin on lipolysis. Diabetes 1983; 32:117–122.
10. Krotkiewski M, Björntorp P. Muscle tissue in obesity with different distribution of adipose tissue, effects of physical training. Int J Obes 1986; 10:331–341.
11. Migeon CJ, Green OC, Eckert JP. Study of adrenocortical function in obesity. Metabolism 1963; 12:718–730.
12. Galvao-Tales A, Graves L, Burke CW, et al. Free cortisol in obesity: effect of fasting. Acta Endocrinol 1976; 81:321–329.
13. Slavnov VN, Epshein EV. Somatotrophic, thyrotrophic and adrenotrophic functions of the anterior pituitary in obesity. Endocrinologie 1977; 15:213–218.
14. Rebuffe-Scrive M, Bronnegard M, Nilsso A, et al. Steroid hormone receptors in human adipose tissues. J Clin Endocrinol Metab 1990; 71:1215–1219.
15. Bronnegard M, Arner P, Hellstrom L, et al. Glucocorticoid receptor messenger ribonucleic acid in different regions of human adipose tissue. Endocrinology 1990; 127:1689–1696.
16. Cigolini M, Smith U. Human adipose tissue in culture. VIII. Studies on the insulin-antagonistic effect of glucocorticoids. Metabolism 1979; 28:502–510.
17. Smith U, Hammerstein J, Björntorp P, Kral JG. Regional differences and effect of weight reduction on human fat metabolism. Eur J Clin Invest 1979; 16:302–309.
18. Simkin V. Urinary 17-ketosteroid and 17-ketogenic steroid excretion in obese patients. N Engl J Med 1961; 264:974–977.
19. Kurtz BR, Givens JR, Kominder S, et al. Maintenance of normal circulating levels of Δ-androstenedione and dehydroepiandrosterone in simple obesity despite increased metabolic clearance rates: evidence for a servo-controlled mechanism. J Clin Endocrinol Metab. 1987; 64:1261–1267.
20. Williams DP, Boyden TW, Pamenter RW, et al. Relationship of body fat percentage and fat distribution with dehydroepiandrosterone sulphate in premenopausal females. J Clin Endocrinol Metab 1993; 77:80–85.
21. Usiskin KS, Butterworth S, Clore JN, et al. Lack of effect of dehydroepiandrosterone sulphate in obese men. Int J Obes 1990; 14:457–463.
22. Khaw K-T, Barret-Connor E. Fasting plasma glucose levels and endogenous androgens in non-diabetic postmenopausal women. Clin Sci 1191; 80:199–203.
23. Brody S, Carlstrom K, Lagrelius A, et al. Adrenal steroids in post-menopausal women: relation to obesity and bone mineral content. Maturitas 1987; 9:25–32.
24. Weaver JU, Kopelman PG, McLoughlin L, et al. Hyperactivity of the hypothalamo-pituitary-adrenal axis in obesity: a study of ACTH, AVP, β-lipoprotein and cortisol responses to insulin-induced hypoglycaemia. Clin Endocrinol 1993; 39:345–350.
25. Couch RM, Muller J, Winter JSD. Regulation of the activities of 17-hydroxylase and 17,20 desmolase in the human adrenal cortex: genetic analysis and inhibition by endogenous steroids. J Clin Endocrinol Metab 1986; 63:613–618.
26. Rebuffe-Scrive M, Krotkiewski M, Elfverson J, Björntorp P. Muscle and adipose tissue morphology and metabolism in Cushing's syndrome. J Clin Endocrinol Metab 1988; 67:1122–1128.
27. Danneskiold-Samsoe B, Grimby G. The influence of prednisolone on the muscle morphology and muscle enzymes in patients with rheumatoid arthritis. Clin Sci 1986; 71:692–701.
28. Bouchard C, Bray GA, Hubbard V. Basic and clinical aspects of regional fat distribution. Am J Clin Nutr 1990; 52:946–950.
29. Krotkiewski M, Björntorp P, Sjostrom L, Smith U. Impact of obesity on metabolism in men and women: importance of regional adipose tissue distribution. J Clin Invest 1983; 72:1150–1162.
30. La Fontan M, Dang-Tran L, Berlan M. Alpha-adrenergic antilipolytic effect of adrenaline in human fat cells of the thigh: comparison with adrenal responsiveness of different fat deposits. Eur J Clin Invest 1975; 9:261–266.
31. Rebuffe-Scrive M, Björntorp P. Regional adipose tissue metabolism in man. In: Vague J, Björntorp P, Guy-Grand

B, eds. Metabolic Complications of Human Obesities. Amsterdam: Excerpta Medica, 1985:149–159.

32. Wahrenberg H, Lonnqvist F, Arner P. Mechanisms underlying regional differences in lipolysis in human adipose tissue. J Clin Invest 1989; 84:458–467.

33. Rebuffe-Scrive M, Enk L, Crona N, et al. Fat cell metabolism in different regions in women. Effects of menstrual cycle, pregnancy and lactation. J Clin Invest 1985; 75:1973–1976.

34. Kirschner MA, Schneider G, Ertel NH, Worton E. Obesity, androgens, oestrogens and cancer risk. Cancer Res 1982; 42:3281–3285.

35. Evans DJ, Hoffman RG, Kalkhoff R, Kissebah AH. Relationship of androgenic activity of body fat topography, fat cell morphology and metabolic aberrations premenopausal women. J Clin Endocrinol Metab 1983; 57:304–310.

36. Samojlik E, Kirschner MA, Silber D, et al. Elevated production in metabolic clearance rates of androgens in morbidly obese women. J Clin Endocrinol Metas 1984; 59:949–954.

37. Vermulen A, Ando S. Metabolic clearance rate and interconversion of androgens and the influence of free androgen fractions. J Clin Endocrinol Metas 1979; 48:320–326.

38. Feher T, Brodrogi L. A comparative study of steroid concentrations in human adipose tissue and peripheral circulation. Clin Chim Acta 1982; 126:135–141.

39. Longcope C, Karot, Horton R. Conversion of blood androgens to estrogens in normal adult men and women. J Clin Invest 1969; 48:2191–2201.

40. Barbieri RL, Hornstein MD. Hyperinsulinaemia and ovarian hyperandrogenism: cause and effect. Endocrinol Metab Clin North Am 1988; 17:685–703.

41. Aziz R. Reproductive endocrinologic alterations in female asymptomatic obesity. Fertil Steril 1989; 52:703–725.

42. Zhang Y-W, Stern B, Rebar RW. Endocrine comparison of obese menstruating and amenorrhoeic women. J Clin Endocrinol Metab 1984; 58:1077–1083.

43. Meldrum DR, Davidson BJ, Tatryn IV, Judd HL. Changes in circulating steroids with aging in post-menopausal women. Obstet Gynaecol 1981; 57:624–628.

44. Davidson BJ, Gambone JC, Lagasse LV, et al. Free oestradiol in postmenopausal women with and without endometrial cancer. J Clin Endocrinol Metab 1981; 52:404–408.

45. Schinder AE, Ebert A, Friedrich E. Conversion of androstenedione to oestrone by human fat tissue. J Clin Endocrinol Metab 1972; 35:627–630.

46. Ackerman GE, Smith AE, Mendelson CR, et al. Aromatization of androstenedione by human adipose tissues-tromal cells in monolayer culture. J Clin Endocrinol Metab 1981; 53:412–417.

47. Hemsell DL, Grodin JM, Brenner PF, et al. Plasma precursors of oestrogen. II. Correlation of the extent of conversion of plasma androstenedione to oestrone with age. J Clin Endocrinol Metab 1974; 38:476–479.

48. Longcope C, Baker R, Johnston CC Jr. Androgen and oestrogen metabolism: relationship to obesity. Metabolism 1986; 35:235–237.

49. Longcope C, Layne DS, Tait JF. Metabolic clearance rates and interconversions of oestrone and 17-β-oestradiol in normal males and females. J Clin Invest 1986; 47:93–106.

50. Deslypere JP, Verdonek L, Vermuulen A. Fat tissue: a steroid reservoir and site of steroid metabolism. J Clin Endocrinol Metab 1987; 61:564–570.

51. Roncari DAK, Van RLR. Promotion of human adipocyte precursor replication in 17-β-oestradiol in culture. J Clin Invest 1977; 62:502–508.

52. Anderson DC. Sex hormone binding globulin. Clin Endocrinol 1974; 3:69–96.

53. Kirschner MA, Samojlik M, Drejka M, et al. Androgen-oestrogen metabolism in women with upper body obesity versus lower body obesity. J Clin Endocrinol Metab 1990; 70:473–479.

54. Plymate SR, Matej LA, Jones RA, Friedl KE. Inhibition of sex hormone binding globulin production in human hepatoma (hep G2) cell line by insulin and prolactin. J Clin Endocrinol Metab 1988; 67:460–464.

55. Peiris AN, Mueller RA, Strieve MF, et al. Relationship of androgenic activity to splanchnic insulin metabolism and peripheral glucose utilisation in premenopausal women. J Clin Endocrinol Metab 1987; 64:162–169.

56. Barbieri RL, Makris A, Randall RW, et al. Insulin stimulates androgen accumulation in incubations of ovarian stroma obtained from women with hyperandrogenism. J Clin Endocrinol Metab 1986; 62:904–910.

57. Tanner JM, Whitehouse RH. The effect of human growth hormone on subcutaneous fat thickness in hyposomatrophic and hypopituitary dwarfs. J Endocrinol 1967; 39:263–275.

58. Bengtsson BA, Eden S, Lonn L, et al. Treatment of adults with growth hormone deficiency with recombinant human GH. J Clin Endocrinol Metab 1994; 78:960–967.

59. Kopelman PG. Neuroendocrine function in obesity. Clin Endocrinol 1988; 28:675–689.

60. Sims EAH, Danforth EH, Horton ES, et al. Endocrine and metabolic effects of experimental obesity in man. Recent Prog Hormone Res 1973; 29:457–487.

61. Kalkhoff R, Ferrow C. Metabolic differences between obese overweight and muscular overweight men. N Engl J Med 1971; 284:1236–1239.

62. Merimee TJ, Fineberg SE. Dietary regulation of human growth hormone secretion. Metabolism 1973; 22:1491–1497.

63. Glass AR, Burman KD, Dahms WT, Boehm TM. Endocrine function in human obesity. Metabolism 1981; 30:89–104.

64. Glass AR. Endocrine aspects of obesity. Med Clin North Am 1989; 73:139–160.

65. Rasmussen MH, Juul A, Kjems LL, et al. Lack of stimulation of 24 hour growth hormone release by hypocaloric

diets in obesity. J Clin Endocrinol Metab 1995; 80: 796–801.

66. Weaver JU, Kopelman PG, Holly JMP, et al. Decreased sex hormone binding globulin (SHBG) and insulin-like growth factor binding protein (IGFBP-1) in extreme obesity. Clin Endocrinol 1990; 32:641–646.

67. Bang P, Brismar K, Rosenfeld RG, Hall K. Fasting affects serum insulin-like growth factors (IGFs) and IGF-binding proteins differently in patients with non-insulin-dependent diabetes versus healthy non-obese and obese subjects. J Endocrinol Metab 1994; 78:960–967.

68. Ailhaud G, Grimaldi P, Negrel R. A molecular view of adipose tissue. Int J Obes 1992; 16(Suppl 2):517–521.

69. Rasmussen MH, Hvidberg A, Juul A, et al. Massive weight loss restores 24 hour growth hormone release profiles and seurm insulin-like growth factor 1 levels in obese subjects. J Clin Endocrinol Metab 1995; 80:1407–1415.

70. Dunaif A. Polycystic ovary syndrome and obesity. In: Björntorp P, Brodoff BN, eds. Obesity. Philadelphia: JP Lippincott, 1992:594–605.

71. Stein IF, Leventhal ML. Amenorrhoea associated with bilateral polycystic ovaries. Am J Obest Gynecol 1935; 29: 181–191.

72. Conway GS, Honour JW, Jacobs HS. Heterogeneity of the polycystic ovary syndrome: clinical, endocrine and ultrasound features in 556 patients. Clin Endocrinol 1989; 30: 459–470.

73. Fisher ER, Gregonon R, Stephen T, et al. Ovarian changes in women with morbid obesity. Obstet Gynaecol 1974; 44:839–844.

74. Hausner H, Ditschieneit HM, Pal SB, et al. Fat distribution, endocrine and metabolic profile in obese women with and without hirsutism. Metabolism 1988; 37:281–286.

75. Edman CD, MacDonald PC. Effect of obesity on conversion of plasma and androstenedione to oestrone in ovulatory and anovulatory young women. Am J Obstet Gynecol 1978; 130:456–461.

76. Yen SSC, Chaney C, Judd HL. Functional aberrations of the hypothalamic-pituitary system in polycystic ovary syndrome: a consideration of the pathogenesis. In: James VHT, Serio M, Giusti, eds. The Endocrine Function of the Human Ovary. Proceedings of the Serono Symposium. London: Academic Press, 1976:373–385.

77. Conway GS, Jacobs HS, Holly JMP, Wass JAH. Effects of luteinising hormone, insulin, insulin-like growth factor small binding protein-1 in the polycystic ovary syndrome. Clin Endocrinol 1990; 33:593–603.

78. Geffner ME, Kaplan SA, Bersch N, et al. Persistance of insulin resistance in polycystic ovary disease after inhibition of ovarian steroid secretion. Fertil Steril 1986; 45: 327–333.

79. Kiddy DS, Sharp PS, Scanlon MF, et al. Differences in clinical and endocrine features between obese and non-obese subjects with polycystic ovary syndrome: an anal-ysis of 263 consecutive cases. Clin Endocrinol 1990; 32: 213–220.

80. Franks S, Kiddy D, Sharp P, et al. Obesity and polycystic ovary syndrome. Ann NY Acad Sci 1991; 626:201–206.

81. Nestler JE, Barlascini CO, Matt DW, et al. Suppression of serum insulin by diazoxide reduces serum testosterone levels in obese women with PCOS. J Clin Endocrinol Metab 1989; 68:1027–1032.

82. Suikkar A-M, Koivisto VA, Rutanen E-M, et al. Insulin regulates the serum levels of low molecular weight insulin-like growth factor binding protein. J Endocrinol Metab 1988; 66:266–272.

83. Koistinen R, Suikkari A-M, Tiifinen A, Kountula K. Human granulosa cells contain insulin-like growth factor binding protein (IGF-BP1) mRNA. Clin Endocrinol 1990; 32:635–640.

84. Holly JMP. The physiological role of IGFBP-1. Acta Endocrinol 1991; 124:55–62.

85. Erikson GF, Magoffin DA, Dyer CA, Hofeditz C. The ovarian androgen producing cells: a review of structure function/relationships. Endocr Rev 1985; 6:371–399.

86. Kiddy DS, Hamilton-Fairley D, Bush A, et al. Improvement in endocrine and ovarian function during dietary treatment of obese women with polycystic ovary syndrome. Clin Endocrinol 1992; 36:105–111.

87. Sorenson TIA, Price RA, Stunkard AJ, Schulsinger F. Genetics of obesity in adult adoptees and their biological siblings. Br Med J 1989; 298:87–90.

88. Bouchard C, Tremblay A, Despres J-P, et al. The response to longterm overfeeding in identical twins. N Engl J Med 1990; 322:1477–1482.

89. Bouchard C, Despres J-P, Mauriege P. Genetic and non-genetic determinants of regional fat distribution. Endocr Rev 1993; 14:72–93.

90. Bouchard C. Genetics and the metabolic syndrome. Int J Obes 1995; 19(Suppl 1):S52–S59.

91. Jeanrenaud B. A hypothesis on the aetiology of obesity: dysfunction of the central nervous system as a primary cause. Diabetologia 1985; 28:502–513.

92. Zhang Y, Proenca R, Maffei M, et al. Positional cloning of the mouse obese gene and its human homologue. Nature 1995; 372:425–432.

93. Bell GI, Picket RL, Rutter WJ, et al. Sequence of the human insulin gene. Nature 1980; 284:26–32.

94. Bell GI, Karam JH, Rutter WJ, et al. Polymorphic cDNA region adjacent to 5′ end of the human insulin gene. Proc Natl Acad Science USA 1981; 78:5759–5763.

95. Permutt MA, Elbein SC. Insulin gene in diabetes analysis through RFLP. Diabetes Care 1990; 13:364–375.

96. Ramachandran A, Snehalatha C, Dharmaraj D, et al. Preview of glucose intolerance in Asian Indians: urban-rural differenes and significance of upper body adiposity. Diabetes Care 1991; 15:1348–1355.

97. Weaver JU, Kopelman PG, Hitman GA. Central obesity and hyperinsulinaemia in women associated with poly-

morphism in the 5′ flanking region of the human insulin gene. Eur J Clin Invest 1992; 22:265–270.

98. Hollenberg SM, Weinberger C, Ong ES, et al. Primary structure and expression of a functional human glucocorticoid receptor cDNA. Nature 1985; 318:635–641.

99. Encio IJ, Detera-Wadleigh SD. The genomic structure of the human glucocorticoid receptor. J Biol Chem 1990; 266:7182–7188.

100. Weaver JU, Hitman GA, Kopelman PG. An association between Bc11 restriction fragment length polymorphism of the glucocorticoid receptor locus and hyperinsulinaemia in obese women. J Mol Endocrinol 1992; 9:295–300.

101. Clement K, Phillipi A, Pividal R, et al. Linkage analysis of glucocorticoid receptor gene in 85 multiplex families with morbid obesity. In J Obes 1994; 18(Suppl 2):O39.

102. Baker WA, Hitman GA, Ilawrami K, et al. Apolipoprotein D gene polymorphism: a new genetic marker for type 2 diabetic subjects from Naurua and South India. Diabetic Med 1994; 11:947–952.

103. Vijayaraghavan S, Hitman GA, Kopelman PG. Apolipoprotein-D polymorphism: a genetic marker for obesity and hyperinsulinaemia. J Clin Endocrinol Metab 1994; 79:568–570.

104. Rohner-Jeanrenaud F, Bobbioni E, Ionescu E, et al. Central nervous system regulation of insulin secretion. In: Shabo AJ, ed. Advances in Metabolic Disorders, vol 10. New York, Academic Press, 1993:193–220.

105. Penicaud L, Rohner-Jeanrenaud F, Jeanrenaud B. In vivo metabolic changes as studied longitudinally after ventromedial hypothalamic lesions. Am J Physiol 1986; 250: E662–E668.

106. Cunningham JJ, Calles-Escandon J, Garrido F, et al. Hypercorticosteronuria and diminished pituitary responsiveness to corticotrophin-releasing factor in obese Zucker rats. Endocrinology 1986; 118:998–1001.

23

Sympathoadrenal System and Metabolism

Arne Astrup
Royal Veterinary and Agricultural University, Frederiksberg, Denmark

Ian Andrew MacDonald
University of Nottingham Medical School, Nottingham, England

I. ANATOMY AND PHYSIOLOGY OF SYMPATHOADRENAL SYSTEM

The autonomic nervous system consists of sympathetic and parasympathetic nerves that arise from characteristic levels of the spinal cord. In each case, a preganglionic neuron exits in the spinal cord, with the parasympathetic ganglia being in or close to the target organ or tissue, while the sympathetic ganglia are generally close to the spinal cord (mainly in the sympathetic trunk). Thus, the parasympathetic nerves are characterized by long preganglionic and short postganglionic neurons, whereas the sympathetic nerves have short preganglionic and long postganglionic neurons. A further anatomical distinction between the two branches of the autonomic nervous system is that the parasympathetic preganglionic nerves originate in either the mesencephalon, pons, medulla oblongata, or the sacral region of the spinal cord, whereas the sympathetic preganglionic nerves arise from the thoracic and lumbar regions of the spinal cord (Fig. 1). It is clear from Figure 1 that the majority of organs and tissues are innervated by both sympathetic and parasympathetic nerves. Major exceptions are the blood vessels, sweat gland, and adipose tissue, which have only a sympathetic nerve supply. The adrenal medulla is also unique, in that it is effectively a sympathetic ganglion, but instead of having postganglionic fibers it releases hormones directly into the bloodstream. There are many situations in which sympathetic nervous activation and adrenal medullary secretion are dissociated, and it is probably appropriate to consider them separately in most cases. Thus, the term "sympathoadrenal system" is more appropriate for this discussion.

A major structural difference between sympathetic and parasympathetic postganglionic nerves is the ways in which they innervate the target issues. The parasympathetic nerves generally branch, with a nerve terminal being in close opposition to the target cell. By contrast, the sympathetic nerves have a series of varicosities along their length, so each nerve releases neurotransmitters from a number of sites.

The nerves illustrated in Figure 1 represent the efferent part of the autonomic nervous system. In many cases, activation of these nerves occurs as part of a reflex mechanism, with many of the afferent signals traveling to the brain in afferent nerve fibers that travel in the sympathetic and parasympathetic nerve trunks. In most cases, the integration of these afferent signals occurs in the hypothalamus, which is also affected by inputs from higher brain centers. Thus, the hypothalamus can be viewed as the major regulator of autonomic activity, and this is undoubtedly of major importance in the control of metabolism.

In most cases, in tissues with both sympathetic and parasympathetic innervation, the effects of stimulation of these nerves are opposite. This is better viewed as part of a reciprocal control system rather than being antagonistic,

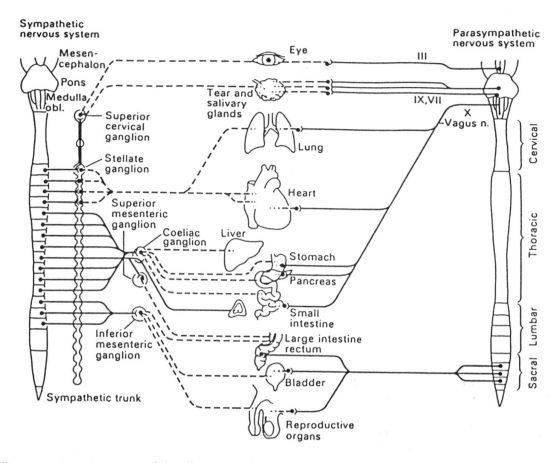

Figure 1 Diagrammatic representation of the efferent part of the autonomic nervous system. Sympathetic innervation of the blood vessels, sweat, and piloerector muscles is not shown. (Reproduced with permission from Brain RL. Clinical Neurology, 6th ed, revised by Bannister, R. Oxford: Oxford University Press, 1985: 124.)

as it is clear that the autonomic nervous system provides a high level of control of physiological systems. The main exceptions are the salivary glands, where both types of autonomic nerves increase salivary secretion, although the composition of the fluid produced differs for the two nerve types. The main aspects of autonomic function that are of specific interest in relation to metabolism and obesity concern the regulation of the cardiovascular system, gastrointestinal function, pancreatic hormone secretion, and adipose tissue lipolysis. The last two aspects are considered in more detail below, but these effects are likely to occupy a lower priority in terms of the maintenance of homeostasis to the cardiovascular and gastrointestinal effects of the autonomic nervous system.

It is clear that the single most important role of the autonomic system is the maintenance of an adequate blood pressure to sustain vital organ function. This is achieved by sympathetic and parasympathetic control of cardiac output (i.e., heart rate and force of contraction)

and sympathetic control of the blood vessels. In most vascular beds, stimulation of the sympathetic nerves produces vasoconstriction, reducing tissue blood flow and potentially raising blood pressure. In some tissues (e.g., adipose tissue, skeletal muscle, and some skin areas), sympathetic activation can also produce vasodilatation and an increase in blood flow. However, in most tissues blood flow increases because of the effects of local metabolites, or due to a reduction in sympathetic vasoconstrictor activity. The different effects of sympathetic nerves on blood vessels are due to the release of different neurotransmitters, or activation of different receptor subtypes. Any nonspecific stimulation of antagonism of the sympathetic nervous system directed at producing metabolic effects will also have significant cardiovascular effects that could be undesirable.

In relation to gastrointestinal function, sympathetic activation has a general inhibitory effect, reducing intestinal motility and gastric emptying. This is in marked contrast to its general stimulatory effect on many other physiological processes. In most physiological situations, the sympathetic nervous system is activated in a discrete manner, with stimulation of some tissues and no effect on others. This is exemplified by the study of Muntzel et al., who showed that administration of insulin directly into the brain of rats activated sympathetic outflow to the hindlimbs (mainly skeletal muscle) but not to the adrenal glands or kidneys (1). It is only in extreme circumstances, e.g., profound hypotension or activation of the "fight and flight" response, that there is generalized sympathetic activation.

In metabolic situations such as overfeeding, fasting, or hypoglycemia in rats, there is selective activation or inhibition of sympathetic activity in some organs, with no change in others (2). Thus, any consideration of the role of altered sympathetic nervous system activity or adrenal medullary secretion in the development, maintenance, or treatment of obesity must recognize the selectivity of the effects on physiological regulation.

II. NEUROTRANSMITTERS AND RECEPTORS IN THE AUTONOMIC NERVOUS SYSTEM

The central nervous system control of the autonomic nervous system involves a large number of different neurotransmitters and neuromodulators (reviewed in Ref. 3). These neuromodulators are normally peptide molecules and are released with the classical neurotransmitters, having a variety of effects altering the response to the neurotransmitter. The detail of such central control of autonomic efferent activity is beyond the scope of this chapter. However, alteration of this central control, either by direct effects on the neurotransmitter or due to alterations in the neuromodulators, will affect autonomic efferent nerve activity.

A. Peripheral Neurotransmitters

The principal neurotransmitter in the autonomic ganglia (both sympathetic and parasympathetic) is acetylcholine, but a number of neuropeptides are also present and may serve a neuromodulatory role (4). The main difference between sympathetic and parasympathetic nerves is in the postganglionic neurotransmitters. Parasympathetic nerves almost exclusively release acetylcholine (and some peptides) from the nerve terminal to have effects on the target issues. By contrast, sympathetic nerves release norepinephrine or acetylcholine, together with a number of neuropeptides.

The original simplistic view that norepinephrine and acetylcholine were the only neurotransmitters released by the postganglionic autonomic nerve fibers have been shown to be inappropriate. It is now apparent that in the intestine and urinary bladder (and probably in many other tissues) there are some autonomic nerves that can produce functional responses even when norepinephrine and acetylcholine effects are blocked. This nonadrenergic, noncholinergic neurotransmission was originally thought by Burnstock (5) to involve ATP as the neurotransmitter (i.e., purinergic neurons), but it is now clear that a number of substances, such as peptides (NPY, CGRP), amines (5HT and dopamine), and even nitric oxide (6), may be important neurotransmitters. However, definitive roles for these substances have not yet been established, so it is unclear what contribution they might make to the sympathetic nervous system control of metabolism.

B. Autonomic Receptors

Because of the uncertainty about the actual roles of nonadrenergic, noncholinergic neurotransmissions, this section will focus on the receptors for acetylcholine and catecholamines (norepinephrine/epinephrine). The autonomic ganglia have the nicotinic class of cholinergic receptors on the postganglionic nerves. Thus, acetylcholine released from the preganglionic nerve binds to these nicotinic receptors to initiate the action potentials in the postganglionic nerves. Although the postganglionic parasympathetic nerves also release acetylcholine, the receptors on the target cells are of the muscarinic cholinergic type. Thus, while both ganglia and end-organ receptors in the parasympathetic system are stimulated by acetylcholine, they are antagonized by different drugs. The autonomic ganglia are blocked by high doses of drugs such as curare, while the muscarinic receptors in the target tissues are blocked only by drugs such as atropine (Fig. 2).

The sympathetic postganglionic neurons are more complex, in that in some tissues the neurotransmitter is acetylcholine acting on muscarinic receptors (e.g., sweat glands), while in most tissues norepinephrine is released to act upon a variety of types of adrenoceptor. The main grouping of adrenoceptors is into α and β types, with at least two types of α-adrenoceptor and three types of β-adrenoceptor. α-Adrenoceptors are particularly common in blood vessels, and their stimulation by norepinephrine leads to vasoconstriction. By contrast, stimulation of β-adrenoceptors usually causes dilatation of vascular or bronchial smooth muscle. A major distinction between α- and β-adrenoceptors is in their second-messenger mechanisms. The importance of second messengers as mediators of cell responses was first identified for

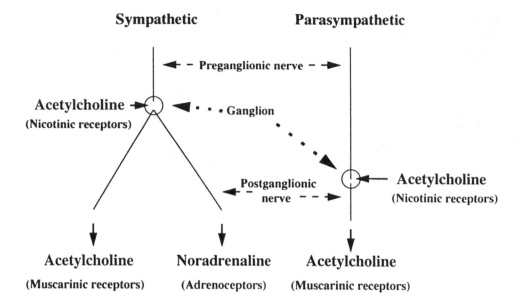

Figure 2   Diagrammatic representation of the autonomic neurotransmitters at the ganglia and neuroeffector junctions.

β-adrenoceptors in liver, where the liberation of cyclic AMP due to the activation of adenylate cyclase produces the metabolic response. It is now clear that cyclic AMP generation is a key feature of most, if not all, β-adrenoceptor-mediated responses, although the detailed mechanisms are rather complex and vary between tissues and receptor types, involving G-proteins and other membrane components. α-Adrenoceptor activation leads to the production of different second messengers, in particular through activation of phosphatidylinositol and diacylglycerol production, and causes an increase in intracellular calcium and often a decrease in cyclic AMP.

Norepinephrine and epinephrine have fairly similar potencies for α- and β-adrenoceptors, so the actual effects of sympathetic activation or increased plasma epinephrine will vary between different tissues depending on the relative proportions of the different receptors and which ones are being activated. For example, skeletal muscle blood vessels have both α- and β-adrenoceptors, with most of the α-receptors being close to the sympathetic nerves, and most of the β-receptors on the endothelial surface of the blood vessels. Thus, sympathetic activation usually (but not always) produces predominantly α₁-adrenoceptor stimulation and vasoconstriction, whereas a physiological increase in plasma epinephrine activates β₂-adrenoceptors and produces vasodilation.

It was originally thought that the different types of adrenoceptors were restricted to specific tissue types or locations within tissues, but it is now clear that this is not the case, and most tissues will have a mixture of receptors.

III. METHODS FOR ASSESSING SYMPATHETIC ACTIVITY

A number of techniques are routinely used to assess the activity of the sympathetic nervous system, but none of them is able to provide reliable information under all experimental conditions. When assessing sympathetic activity, three important components must be recognized: the neural reflex arc, end-organ responsiveness, and the existence of any compensatory systems (7). The following sections consider the ways in which sympathetic nerve activity can be assessed, but it is clear that, when possible, one should use more than one of these techniques to obtain a more reliable assessment, and also that functional correlates of these indices of sympathetic activity should also be determined.

A.   Efferent Neural Activity

1.   Microneurography

The activity of the efferent sympathetic nerves can be determined either by direct nerve recording (microneurography) or indirectly from spectral analysis of the variability of heart rate or blood pressure. The use of the technique of microneurography to assess sympathetic nerve firing rates was pioneered by Wallin and colleagues (8) and it has since been used by many investigators in a variety of situations. The technique involves the insertion of a fine, tungsten microelectrode into a nerve, and so is restricted to peripheral nerves such as the peroneal nerve in the leg. Thus, the technique can only provide information on the activity of sympathetic nerves supplying the skin and skeletal muscle, and while measurements are being made, the subject must rest quietly, remaining still, to avoid breaking the electrode. Despite these limitations, the technique has been used in a number of situations to identify sympathetic efferent contributions to cardiovascular control. For example, skeletal muscle sympathetic activity and blood pressure show a good correlation (8) and skin sympathetic activity correlates well with finger vasoconstriction when the whole body is cooled (9). It is clear from these early studies, and subsequent work, that muscle sympathetic nerve activity is mainly related to the control of blood pressure, and that an increase in nerve firing rate is usually associated with vasoconstriction in skeletal muscle. However, this is not always the case, as during hypoglycemia (10) or hyperinsulinemic euglycemia (11) there is an increase in muscle blood flow despite increased muscle sympathetic nerve activity (12, 13). Furthermore, muscle sympathetic activity increases after food intake (14) but this is sometimes associated with muscle vasodilation (15).

Thus, assessing peripheral sympathetic nerve firing rate in humans provides an index of the activity of the sympathetic innervation of skeletal muscle, but in some circumstances this may not reflect overall sympathetic activity in the whole body. An example of this is the proposal that sympathetic activity may be altered in obesity (see below). From the measurement of plasma or urinary catecholamines in obese and nonobese subjects, reported in the literature, there is no clear consensus as to whether the obese have altered sympathetic activity. However, the few studies that report measurements of muscle sympathetic nerve activity in lean and obese subjects consistently report increased activity in the obese. Thus, depending on how sympathetic activity is assessed, one would conclude the obese are either the same as, or different from, the lean (16).

2. Heart Rate Variability

An alternative way of assessing sympathetic activity involves measuring the variations in heart rate, or systolic blood pressure, that occur in the frequency domain. This technique requires several minutes of continuous data collection from subjects in a steady state (usually resting quietly) and involves the application of spectral analysis techniques to identify the dominant frequencies that underlie the variability in the physiological variable. The majority of studies using this approach have been based on recording heart rate (actually the intervals between successive R waves in the electrocardiogram) and provide infor-

mation on both sympathetic and parasympathetic influences (e.g., 17). The major limitation of this technique is that it does not provide a clear index of cardiac sympathetic activity, but rather that the low (approx. 0.15 Hz) and high (approx. 0.30 Hz) frequency peaks are related to combined sympathetic/parasympathetic and just parasympathetic influences, respectively. The high-frequency (parasympathetic) component is predominantly determined by the respiratory frequency, whereas the low frequency is more related to baroreflex control of the heart. If one wishes to use this technique to assess cardiac sympathetic activity, it is important to control the respiratory component, and to be aware that measurements should be made in a steady state, as alterations in plasma catecholamines can affect heart rate.

B. Neurotransmitter Release

No reliable techniques are available for the assessment of acetylcholine release in vivo, as the neurotransmitter is hydrolyzed too rapidly in the synaptic cleft. It is also difficult to quantify norepinephrine release from sympathetic neurons, because this neurotransmitter can undergo a number of different metabolic fates (Fig. 3): reuptake into the neuron, metabolism in the sympathetic cleft, uptake into surrounding tissues, or spillover into the plasma. The fact that some of the released norepinephrine appears in the plasma provides the basis of measuring plasma catecholamines to obtain an index of sympathetic activity. More useful quantitative assessments of sympathetic activ-

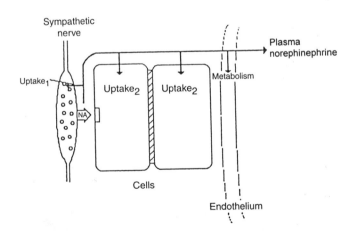

Figure 3 Routes of norepinephrine uptake and spillover into plasma after release from sympathetic nerves (varicosities). (Reproduced from Macdonald IA. How do we study autonomic activity in humans? Fundam Clin Pharmacol 1995; 9:443–449, with permission.)

ity can be obtained from measurements of norepinephrine spillover into the plasma, or of urinary norepinephrine excretion.

C. Norepinephrine Spillover into Plasma

The rate of norepinephrine spillover can be quantified using radioactive tracer techniques and has been applied in a variety of different metabolic and cardiovascular states (18). The fundamental assumption underlying the use of this technique to assess neurotransmitter release is that there is a constant relationship between release, synaptic metabolism, neuronal reuptake, tissue uptake, and spillover into the plasma. Such an assumption would be difficult to evaluate experimentally, but one should be aware that drugs that alter neuronal reuptake would invalidate it. The main practical problem with using this technique to assess sympathetic activity is whether a regional or a whole-body assessment is needed. For example, forearm venous blood samples will be affected by norepinephrine uptake from arterial blood into forearm tissue, and local release. This can provide a good index of local sympathetic activity but is inappropriate for assessing the whole body. A more reliable index of whole-body sympathetic activity is provided if spillover measurements use either systemic arterial or pulmonary arterial blood samples. Additional, useful information can be obtained if venous blood samples are taken from vascular beds such as heart, kidney, and splanchnic bed (19) but the techniques are rather invasive and may be inappropriate for many subject groups.

D. Plasma Catecholamines

Measurement of plasma norepinephrine concentration per se provides limited information on sympathetic activity. This is because norepinephrine in the plasma arises from both spillover from sympathetic nerves and release from the adrenal medulla. Thus, alteration in plasma norepinephrine could be the result of changes in adrenal medullary activity. However, in most situations alterations in sympathetic nerve activity are responsible for changes in plasma norepinephrine, although the site of blood sampling can affect the magnitude of any changes observed. In most cases it is more appropriate to use arterial (reviewed in Ref. 20) or arterialized-venous (21) blood samples if plasma norepinephrine is to be used to assess whole-body sympathetic activity. This is because forearm venous plasma norepinephrine concentrations are determined by the balance between uptake of norepinephrine into forearm tissue from arterial blood and spillover from sympathetic nerves into the venous blood. Thus, altera-

tions in forearm sympathetic activity and blood flow will have a substantial effect on any index of sympathetic activity that is derived.

In principle, the use of plasma epinephrine concentrations or measurement of adrenal spillover into plasma to assess adrenal medullary activity would be less prone to the errors described above for norepinephrine. In most circumstances, this is true provided arterial or arterialized-venous samples are used. However, for useful comparison to be made between subjects, or within subjects over time, it is essential that the kinetics relating epinephrine release to its clearance and metabolism are comparable. For example, the nonselective β-adrenoceptor antagonist propranolol reduces the clearance of catecholamines from the plasma, resulting in higher plasma epinephrine concentrations for a given rate of release or infusion (22).

Some studies have used measurements of platelet catecholamines to provide a longer-term index of the level of sympathetic nervous, or adrenal medullary, activity (23). The attraction of this approach is that while the half-life for plasma catecholamines is short (1–1.5 min) that for platelet catecholamines is substantially longer. Thus, fewer samples would be needed to obtain an overall assessment and short-term disturbances are unlikely to have a major effect if platelet catecholamines are used. However, this approach is not widespread and has not been fully validated or compared extensively with the other techniques.

E. Urinary Catecholamines

The urinary excretion of catecholamines provides a longer-term index of the plasma concentrations that existed during the period of urine formation (24). The main drawbacks of this approach are that alterations in catecholamine metabolism will change the relationship between the excretion of the free amines, conjugated amines, and other metabolites, and the accuracy and completeness of the urine collection could vary between subjects. Thus, in principle, more useful information on sympathoadrenal activity could be gained from measurements of urinary rather than plasma catecholamines, but errors can occur in some circumstances.

F. Other Indices

The peptide cotransmitters that are released with norepinephrine may also spill over into the plasma, but little is known of the kinetics of this process or its comparability to norepinephrine spillover. Thus, plasma NPY concentration can be measured and changes observed in situations in which norepinephrine also changes (25). However, it is also apparent that the disappearance kinetics for NPY are very different for norepinephrine, thus limiting the usefulness of plasma NPY as an index of sympathetic activity.

G. Summary

A variety of techniques exist to assess sympathetic activity, but all are of limited value alone, and much more useful information would be obtained from combining several methods. An example of this is the study of response to food ingestion by Cox et al. (19). They measured muscle sympathetic nerve activity and regional and whole-body norepinephrine spillover and showed substantial variation in different parts of the body. The drawback of this approach is the invasive nature of the techniques. However, wherever possible at least two techniques should be used when comparing groups of subjects.

IV. AUTONOMIC CONTROL OF METABOLISM

In considering the autonomic control of metabolism, it is worth distinguishing between effects of the sympathetic and parasympathetic innervation of organ and tissues and the hormonal actions of the adrenal medullary catecholamines. Furthermore, the autonomic control of metabolism can be either due to direct effects of metabolic processes or an indirect consequence of changes in regulatory hormones (such as insulin). It is quite clear that the autonomic control of metabolism can occur as part of a discrete regulatory system, with simultaneous activation of some parts of the autonomic nervous system and suppression of other parts. In addition, metabolic effects of autonomic activation can be considered in two categories: as part of a normally regulated physiological process (e.g., the response to starvation) or secondary to the autonomic response to a "stressful" stimulus. For example, the glucose intolerance and fat mobilization produced by sympathoadrenal activation during stress may confer survival value, but the benefits of such a response are not always clear. More importantly, the metabolic consequences of such responses to stress may contribute to the etiology of type II diabetes and obesity and are considered in more detail later.

A. The Parasympathetic Nervous System

The main parasympathetic effects on metabolism are a consequence of the vagal control of insulin secretion from the pancreas. The main role of the parasympathetic innervation of the pancreas appears to be to control the pulsatile release of insulin that occurs during the fasting period and to mediate the early insulin response to feeding. The latter is particularly evident during the dephalic and gastric phases of food ingestion and probably primes the liver for glycogen synthesis in advance of direct effects of absorbed glucose on the pancreas. The major autonomic effects on metabolism are due to sympathoadrenal influences on carbohydrate and fat metabolism and on overall energy expenditure.

B. Sympathoadrenal Effects on Carbohydrate Metabolism (Fig. 4)

Activation of the sympathoadrenal system leads to a prompt and sustained rise in blood glucose. The main effects of plasma epinephrine (i.e., adrenal medullary activation) are a transient increase in hepatic glucose production (by both glycogenolysis and gluconeogenesis) and more sustained reduction in skeletal muscle glucose uptake. The direct effects of epinephrine on carbohydrate metabolism are mediated mainly by β-adrenoceptors (26) but there may also be some stimulation of hepatic α-adrenoceptors (27). Probably of greater importance are the indirect effects of plasma epinephrine and of the SNS on the pancreas. Under normal circumstances, both plasma epinephrine and the sympathetic nerves reduce insulin secretion from the pancreatic β-cells, via stimulation of α_2-adrenoceptors (28). In addition, they can increase glucagon release from the α-cells by stimulation of β-adrenoceptors.

In addition to the effects of plasma epinephrine on liver glucose output and pancreatic insulin secretion, it is also capable of stimulating glycogenolysis in muscle. The absence of glucose-6-phosphatase in muscle means that the glycogenolysis leads to increased lactate production, with the lactate then available (via transport in the blood) for hepatic gluconeogenesis.

C. Sympathoadrenal Control of Lipid Metabolism

As with the effects of carbohydrate metabolism, the sympathoadrenal system has major effects on lipid metabolism via the inhibition of insulin release from the pancreas. Under normal circumstances, insulin increases triacylglycerol accumulation in adipose tissue by the combined effects of stimulating lipoprotein lipase and inhibiting hormone-sensitive lipase activities. Reducing insulin release will thus decrease triacylglycerol clearance from plasma and increase lipolysis in adipose tissue. A reduction in plasma insulin is probably the main mediator of the lipolytic response in the first few hours of starvation.

In addition to these indirect effects on lipid metabolism, both plasma epinephrine and the sympathetic nerves

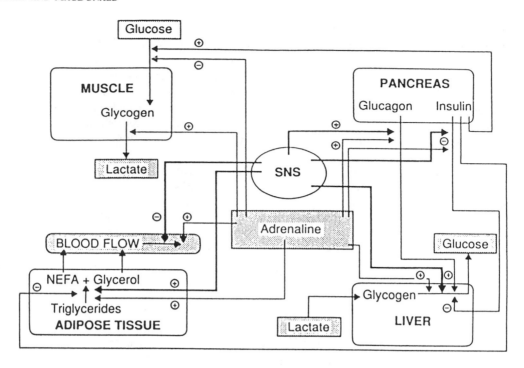

Figure 4 Summary of the metabolic effects of the sympathetic nervous system (SNS) and plasma epinephrine. Shaded boxes represent the plasma compartment, thick lines are sympathic nerves, other lines represent exchange through the bloodstream. (Reproduced with permission from Webber J, Macdonald IA. Metabolic actions of catecholamines in man. In: Bouloux, ed. Catelochamines — Baillere-Tindalls Clinics in Endocrinology and Metabolism. (1993: 393–413.)

have direct effects on adipose tissue lipolysis. The main effect of catecholamines (especially plasma epinephrine) is to stimulate lipolysis via the activation of β-adrenoceptors. Epinephrine also increases adipose tissue blood flow (via activation of vascular β-adrenoceptors), whereas sympathetic activation may initially cause vasoconstriction via α-adrenoceptor stimulation (29). The adipocytes may also have α_2-adrenoceptors, which have antilipolytic effects that appear to dominate in some situations, e.g., in subcutaneous tissue removed from obese subjects (30). Due to the stimulation of lipolysis and increasing circulating levels of free fatty acids, increased sympathetic activity is generally associated with decreased glucose oxidation and increased fat oxidation. The increased fat oxidation can take place without a concurrent increase in plasma FFA levels, which suggests that stimulation of lipolysis in intramuscular triglyceride stores can occur (31).

D. Sympathoadrenal Control of Energy Expenditure

Total energy expenditure can be broken down into three major components: resting metabolic rate (RMR), the thermic effect of food, and the energy cost of physical activity.

All three components are influenced by the sympathoadrenal system. They can be quantified by indirect calorimetry in combination with the doubly labeled water technique.

I. Resting Metabolic Rate

RMR accounts for 60–80% of daily energy expenditure and varies greatly between individuals. Most of the variation between subjects can be accounted for by differences in size of fat-free mass (FFM) and fat mass. However, after adjustment for differences in body composition, RMR still differs markedly between subjects. RMR has a genetic component, which is expressed mainly, but not entirely, through the genetic influence on FFM and fat mass. A number of studies of different designs, and using various techniques to assess sympathetic activity, have shown that differences in sympathetic activity in Caucasians can account for some of the variability in RMR unexplained by body composition (Table 1). The stimulatory sympathetic effect on RMR is mediated through stimulation of β-adrenoceptors in the target tissues, because the β-adrenergic antagonist propranolol reduces RMR (32). The magnitude of the reduction in RMR caused by propranolol

Table 1 Correlation Between Different Indices of Sympathetic Nervous System (SNS) Activity and Resting Metabolic Rate (RMR) Adjusted for Body Size and Composition in Caucasians and Pima Indians

SNS assessment	Caucasians	Pima Indians
β-Blockade	$r = -0.57$ ($p < 0.001$)	NS
Urinary norepinephrine excretion	$r = 0.78$ ($p < 0.0001$)	NS
Muscle SNS activity	$r = 0.51$ ($p < 0.05$)	NS
Plasma norepinephrine	$r = 0.35$ ($p < 0.003$)	—

Pima Indians have low levels of SNS, and unlike in Caucasians, RMR does not correlate with SNS activity.
Source: Refs. 32, 33, 35.

was highest in subjects with the greatest positive deviations (i.e., RMR greater than predicted from body size and composition), suggesting that differences between individuals in sympathetic activation of β-adrenoceptors contribute to variations in RMR. Further evidence is provided by cross-sectional studies showing that RMR adjusted for body size and composition is positively correlated to urinary norepinephrine excretion (32), muscle sympathetic tone measured by microneurography (33), plasma norepinephrine spillover rate (34), and plasma norepinephrine concentration (35). The sympathetically mediated component of RMR may have a genetic basis as pairs of monozygotic twins have a higher resemblance with regard to muscle sympathetic nervous activity than pairs of unrelated individuals matched for gender and age (36). However, shared environmental influences such as physical fitness and diet composition might be alternative explanations for this finding.

2. Thermic Effect of Food

The sympathoadrenal system plays an important role in the regulation of postprandial energy and substrate metabolism. The thermic effect of nutrients can be partitioned into an obligatory and a facultative thermogenesis (37), where the facultative component appears to be mediated by the sympathoadrenal system because it can be abolished by β-adrenergic antagonists. Ingestion of food, and of carbohydrate-rich meals in particular, results in a biphasic activation of the sympathoadrenal system. One component is an insulin-mediated activation of the sympathetic nervous system. This activation is partly a hemodynamic reflex, but it may cause a weak thermogenic effect in skeletal muscle, white adipose tissue, liver, heart, and other tissues. The second thermogenic component occurs later when blood glucose starts to decline, which elicits an increased epinephrine release from the adrenal medulla, sufficient to exceed the threshold of a thermogenic

effect. The administration of central or peripheral inhibitors of the sympathoadrenal system reduces the thermic effect of meals by 30–40% depending on experimental circumstances (37,38). The quantitative contribution of the sympathoadrenal system to meal-induced thermogenesis is highly dependent on the composition of the meal, particularly the carbohydrate and fructose content.

Both oral and intravenous glucose administration are accompanied by a thermogenic effect and by stimulation of muscle sympathetic nerve activity (39,40). About 25% of the meal-induced facultative thermogenesis can be estimated to take place in skeletal muscle (41). The activation of the sympathetic nervous system by carbohydrate has been attributed to a central action of insulin on hypothalamic areas, but the sympathetic nervous system is also activated by fructose (42), which does not increase plasma insulin. It is likely that an insulin-independent splanchnic vasodilatation triggers a sympathetic reflex of hemodynamic nature. Insulin also seems to cause splanchnic and skeletal muscle vasodilatation, which is counteracted by increased SNS activity (7).

3. 24-Hour Energy Expenditure

Measurements of 24-hr EE integrate RMR, thermic effect of food, and the energy expended on physical activity. RMR is the most important component, and differences between subjects in RMR can explain more than 70% of the variation in the size of total free-living EE (43). As physiological differences in sympathetic activity are responsible for differences in the individual's level of RMR, for the thermic effect of food, and probably also for spontaneous physical activity (44), 24-hr EE adjusted for body size and composition correlates positively with indices of sympathetic activity (32,35). The contribution of the sympathoadrenal system to 24-hr EE in nontrained subjects probably accounts for 300–400 kJ/day, although studies using pharmacological inhibition of β-adrenoceptors have provided slightly lower reductions (200–300 kJ/day) (45,46). The estimates achieved by administration of competitive β-adrenergic antagonists such as propranolol should, however, be interpreted with caution because they are inhibitors, not blockers. Moreover, they also inhibit the clearance of catecholamines from the circulation and produce higher plasma levels of norepinephrine and epinephrine, which may attenuate the β-receptor inhibition. After differences in body size and composition, spontaneous physical activity, and thyroid hormone status have been taken into account, the difference in 24-hr EE between normal subjects with low and high sympathetic activity is ~750 kJ/day (35), which probably provides a more realistic estimate of the physiological range.

Environmental changes, such as a low ambient temperature (47), physical fitness (48), and high dietary carbohydrate content (49), may further increase sympathetic activity and the sympathetically mediated thermogenesis. Differences in diet composition may be responsible for a more chronic influence on 24-hr EE, at least in a subgroup of susceptible individuals. The dietary carbohydrate content is positively related to indices of sympathetic activity and energy expenditure (34), and isocaloric increases in dietary carbohydrate content increase plasma noradrenaline concentrations and plasma T_3 levels more than diets lower in carbohydrate (49,50) and produce a slightly higher 24-hr energy expenditure in formerly obese subjects (49). The effects may be confined to simple carbohydrates, e.g., sucrose (51).

4. Receptor Subtype Mediation

When the sympathoadrenal system is stimulated, all types of adrenoceptors are activated, but thermogenesis is primarily mediated by β_1- and β_2-adrenoceptors. The existence of biologically active β_3-adrenoceptors in human cells has been controversial. Nevertheless, the isolation of a gene coding for the human β_3-adrenoceptor (52), the demonstration of the expression of β_3-adrenoceptor mRNA in human fat cells, and recent *in vivo* data (53) support the existence of functional β_3-adrenoceptors in humans. Some studies have suggested that a significant proportion of the thermogenic response induced by catecholamines and sympathomimetics such as ephedrine is due to β_3-adrenoceptor activation (54,55), and that a mutation in the β_3-receptor gene may play a role in the development of some types of obesity (56).

V. THE EFFECT OF ENERGY IMBALANCE AND PHYSICAL ACTIVITY ON SYMPATHOADRENAL ACTIVITY

A. Under- and Overnutrition

Changed energy expenditure is a fundamental response of the human body to overnutrition and undernutrition in an attempt to maintain a constant lean body mass, and the SNS is an important regulator of the metabolic processes controlling fuel and energy fluxes (57,58).

Acute energy restriction leads to a reduction of the sympathoadrenal drive, resulting in a reduced energy expenditure. Overfeeding increases SNS activity, expending some of the surplus energy by accelerating metabolism. Response to energy restriction also results in modulation of the adrenergic receptor number and sensitivity.

Young and Landsberg (59) were the first to show a close link between SNS activity and fasting, using the norepinephrine turnover technique in rats. They demonstrated a significant decrease in norepinephrine turnover in the cardiac tissue of 48-hr starved rats, which was completely reversed by 1 day of overfeeding. Energy restriction in humans also leads to a decrease in circulating levels of norepinephrine and to lower urinary excretion of norepinephrine and its metabolites (60–62). The adaptive response of the SNS to energy restriction and energy overfeeding in normal-weight subjects was elegantly shown by measurements of norepinephrine turnover during undereating for 10 days (VLED, 2 MJ/day), a weight maintenance diet and a hyperenergetic diet (+4.2 MJ/m²), respectively (63). Norepinephrine turnover rate increased significantly with increasing energy intake and was a more sensitive index than plasma norepinephrine levels, which rose only insignificantly. In conclusion: in normal-weight subjects sympathetic activity changes in response to short-term changes in energy intake. There are marked differences between individuals, which may partly explain the differences in susceptibility to gain fat during overfeeding (64). The carbohydrate content of the iso- and hyperenergetic diet also influences sympathetic activity and energy expenditure. Overfeeding by carbohydrate produces higher sympathetic activity and thermogenic responses than does fat overfeeding (65). Sucrose seems to be a more potent stimulator of sympathetic activity than complex carbohydrates (51).

B. Physical Activity and Training

The sympathetic nervous system activity increase is part of the response to the altered substrate demand during acute and prolonged physical exercise (training) and may cause an increase in RMR and fat oxidation. During weight loss, induced by either dietary energy restriction or an exercise training program, norepinephrine turnover was found to decrease by 20% in the diet group, but remained unchanged in the exercise group (66). It has been shown that administration of propranolol, a nonselective β-antagonist, to trained and sedentary males results in a decrease in RMR and fat oxidation in the trained subjects, whereas no change occurs in the sedentary group (48).

Hence the reduction in sympathetic activity caused by energy restriction is counteracted by a training program. Endurance training is accompanied both by a higher sympathetic drive and by enhanced β-adrenoceptor sensitivity, which favors a higher RMR and an increased utilization of fatty acids relative to carbohydrate as fuel.

VI. THE INVOLVEMENT OF THE SYMPATHOADRENAL SYSTEM IN THE ETIOLOGY OF OBESITY

Animal models indicate that reduced sympathetic nervous activity may have an etiological role in the development of most obesities (67). In humans a low sympathetic activity is a risk factor for weight gain, and in obese subjects it is associated with a poorer diet-induced weight loss. The mechanisms linking a low sympathetic activity to fat gain and resistance to slimming are probably a combination of the sympathetic influence on RMR, spontaneous physical activity, the response of energy expenditure to overfeeding, and an impaired suppression of hunger, which may, in part, be mediated through impaired fat utilization.

A. Animal Models of Obesity

The observation that most animal models of obesity are associated with a low sympathetic activity is the basis for the hypothesis that a low sympathetic activity is central for the efferent mediation of the positive energy balance (67). Bray proposed the "**M**ost **O**besities k**N**own **A**re **L**ow **I**n **S**ympathetic **A**ctivity" (MONA LISA) hypothesis (Fig. 5) (68). Genetic influences on the development of experimental obesity involve the failure to activate the sympathetic nervous system appropriately in response to nutrient intake, which seems to require normal or increased levels of circulating corticosteroids (68). One of the most extensively studied models is the VMH hypothalamic-lesioned animal, where the low sympathetic activity has been demonstrated indirectly by measurements of impaired fat mobilization, i.e., reduced fatty acid concentrations during various lipolytic stimuli, and directly by elec-

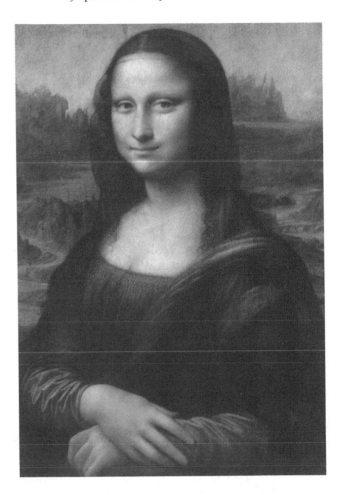

Figure 5 What has Mona Lisa to do with sympathetic activity and obesity? The MONA LISA hypothesis stands for **M**ost **O**besities k**N**own **A**re **L**ow **I**n **S**ympathetic **A**tivity (68).

trical measurements of efferent nerve activity in sympathetic fibers supplying brown adipose tissue and pancreas (69). The low sympathetic activity may lead to lower thermogenesis and stimulation of subsequent food intake, and consequently to a positive energy balance and obesity. An enhanced food intake may be the predominant mechanism leading to the positive fat balance. Sakaguchi et al. found an inverse relationship between sympathetic activity and food intake where the highest levels of food intake were associated with the lowest levels of sympathetic activity and *vice versa* (70). It has been proposed that postprandial heat production may serve as an indirect satiety signal to terminate eating (68). In obese animals the impairment of the sympathetic activation following meals may decrease their postprandial heat production and thus indirectly increase food intake. A second mechanism may be a decreased activation of β₃-adrenoceptors, which normally leads to inhibition of feeding. A third link between sympathetic activity and food intake may work through substrate utilization and the glycogenostatic appetite mechanism (71). Though the mechanisms linking a low sympathetic activity to appetite control are less well understood, a number of observations support their existence in humans (Fig. 6). Furthermore, in concert with the impact of a low sympathetic activity on various components of energy expenditure, the quantitative importance for energy balance is substantial.

B. Sympathoadrenal Activity in Obesity

One of the major problems in assessing the role of sympathetic activity for the development of obesity is the limitation of examining obese subjects, because any abnormality of the SNS may be secondary to the obese state rather than being causal. There is evidence that factors that are dissociated from each other, such as a positive energy balance, body weight gain, and enlarged body fat stores, may stimulate sympathetic activity, probably as a counterregulatory mechanism aimed at limiting weight gain. If a low sympathetic activity plays a causal factor in obesity, it may be apparent in the preobese state, but may not be detected in subjects moving along an ascending weight curve or once the obese state is reached.

Nevertheless, there have been a large number of studies comparing SNS activity, based on plasma or urinary catecholamine measurements, in lean and obese individuals. Young and Macdonald reviewed the relevant literature on data published from 1980 to 1995. This period was chosen because of the possibility of unreliable catecholamine assays prior to 1980 (73). Only studies involving normotensive and nondiabetic subjects were included. Table 2 shows the updated collated results on norepinephrine and epinephrine in obese and lean subjects (16). It is clear that there is no consensus as to whether the obese have a lower sympathetic activity than the lean when plasma or urine norepinephrine is used as the index of sympathetic activity. In ~30% of the studies, however, the obese groups had lower norepinephrine levels than the lean groups, which opens the possibility that subgroups of obese may have lower sympathetic activity. In contrast, the majority of studies indicate that obese subjects tend to have lower epinephrine levels, a finding that certainly needs further consideration. Some of the other tests of sympathetic and autonomic functions suggest that increasing fatness is inversely related to autonomic activity (74). A rather different conclusion may be drawn from the studies using direct muscle sympathetic nerve activity (MSNA) measurement. In the four studies of Caucasian subjects in which MSNA was related to body fatness, a consistent

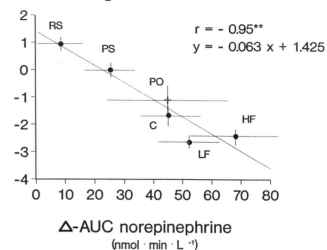

Figure 6 Correlation between mean change in postprandial hunger rating (visual analog scales) and plasma norepinephrine response (Δ-AUC). Data are group means ± SEM from different meal test studies. RS, resistant starch meal; PS, pregelatinized starch meal; PO, postobese group, high-fat meal; C, control group, high-fat meal; LF, low-fiber meal; HF, high-fiber meal. The regression line is given. (Reproduced with permission from Ref. 72.)

positive relationship was found (33,40,75,76), though much variation in MSNA for a given body fat mass still exists. Thus, even when MSNA is used as an index, there will be some obese individuals with a reduced sympathetic activity, but it may be more easily detected in preobese and postobese individuals, where it is not confounded by the effect of enlarged body fat stores and antecedent positive energy balance, factors that may stimulate sympathetic activity.

For Pima Indians, an ethnic group with a very high prevalence of obesity, the situation is different. In this group there is no relationship between β-adrenoceptor inhibition and energy expenditure (32). Pima Indians have lower sympathetic activity than weight-matched Caucasians, and they do not exhibit the relationship between urinary noradrenaline excretion and energy expenditure, and between MSNA and energy expenditure, found in Caucasians. Nor does their MSNA increase with increasing body fat content (33,76). Most important, it has recently been shown in a prospective study that urinary norepinephrine excretion, adjusted for body size, correlated negatively with weight gain observed during a 3-year follow-up ($r = -0.30$) (77).

These results demonstrate that Pima Indians have lower sympathetic activity than Caucasians, which may partly

Table 2 Indices of Sympathetic Nervous System and Adrenal Medullary Activity in Lean and Obese

	Obese < lean	Obese = lean	Obese > lean
Sympathetic nervous system	14	21	11
Adrenal medulla	12	21	1

Plasma or urine norepinephrine was used to assess sympathetic nervous system activity, epinephrine value to assess adrenal medullary secretion.
Source: Reproduced with permission from Ref. 16.

contribute to their lower RMR for a given body size and composition. The finding that their sympathetic activity does not correlate with body fatness suggests that they are unable to increase their sympathetic activity as a counter-regulatory mechanism to avoid body weight gain. The finding that a low sympathetic activity in Pima Indians is a predictor of subsequent weight gain further stresses its etiological importance.

C. β-Adrenergic Sensitivity in Obesity

The transmission of the sympathetic signaling to the target tissues requires an intact number and sensitivity of β-adrenoceptors. Blaak et al. (78) found an impaired thermogenic response to stepwise infusion of the β-adrenoceptors agonist isoprenaline in obese subjects compared with normal-weight subjects. Weight reduction improved, but did not normalize, the response (78). Mutations in the genes coding for the β-adrenoceptors may be partly responsible for this phenomenon. A missense mutation in the $β_3$-adrenoceptors genes has been reported to be associated with a marginally lower metabolic rate (79). The prevalence of this mutation is higher in Pima Indians than in Caucasians, and this mutation may be a factor responsible for a lower metabolic rate, impaired thermogenic responses to sympathetic stimulation (54), and a lower fat oxidation.

D. Abnormalities in Sympathetic Responsiveness to Under- and Overfeeding in Obesity

While the sympathetic activity recorded in obese subjects under more or less well-characterized static phases is difficult to interpret, a more informative approach is to study the sympathetic reactivity to changes in energy balance, i.e., under- and overfeeding. Young and Landsberg demonstrated a decrease in sympathetic activity of 48-hr starved rates (59). They found a decrease in norepinephrine turnover in cardiac tissue during starvation, which was completely reversed by 1 day of refeeding. Human

studies using various techniques have confirmed this reduction of sympathetic activity during energy restriction and have suggested that it may be at least partly responsible for the decrease in RMR that accompanies energy restriction and fasting (60–62). Few studies have examined the adaptive response of the SNS to energy restriction and energy surplus.

1. Sympathetic Response to Food Intake

It has been suggested that the facultative component of meal-induced thermogenesis mediated by the sympathoadrenal system is reduced in obese subjects, and that it could play a causal role in the development and maintenance of obesity. The finding that the thermic effect of food remained reduced after a major weight loss and that the sympathetic response to carbohydrate also remained smaller in the reduced-obese than in a nonobese control group supports this suggestion (80). However, in more carefully controlled studies in which postobese individuals were entirely weight normalized and weight stable before examination, the thermic effect of food did not differ between postobese subjects and controls (81). Furthermore, in a prospective study a low thermic effect of food was not found to be associated with subsequent weight gain (82). There is therefore no evidence to support a causal role in obesity of a low postprandial sympathetic activity.

2. Response to Overfeeding

Underfeeding leading to a 10% decrease in body weight is accompanied by a reduction in total energy expenditure and RMR (83). Likewise, maintenance of a body weight at a level 10% above initial weight is associated with a compensatory increase in energy expenditure. These compensatory changes in energy expenditure cannot be accounted for by changes in body size and composition (83) and may be partly attributed to regulatory changes in sympathoadrenal activity.

O'Dea et al. assessed sympathetic activity by the norepinephrine turnover technique during 10 days of underfeeding (2 MJ/day), a weight maintenance diet, and a hyperenergetic diet ($+4.2$ MJ/m^2 surface area) in normal-weight subjects (63). The results can be compared with those reported in a subsequent paper in which obese subjects underwent the same protocol (84). The results are presented in Table 3 (58). In the normal-weight subjects norepinephrine turnover rate increased during overfeeding, despite an insignificant increase in plasma norepinephrine levels. By contrast, norepinephrine turnover rate failed to increase in response to overfeeding in the obese subjects (84). The absence of any reduction in norepinephrine turnover with undereating and the blunted increase with overfeeding indicate that sympathetic responsiveness to changes in energy status is impaired in obese individuals. In line with these results, Vollenweider et al. found that basal MSNA was substantially higher in obese than in lean subjects (40), but the MSNA increase found in the lean subjects during a hyperinsulinemic euglycemic clamp was almost absent in a group of obese subjects. It is possible that the obese subjects had already taken advantage of the stimulating effect of hyperinsulinemia on MSNA, and that a subsequent increase in insulin levels did not further increase muscle sympathetic firing rate. These studies conducted in obese individuals do not elucidate whether the lack of sympathetic responsiveness to hyperinsulinemia, as induced by overfeeding, precedes or is consequent to the obese state. A small study of responses to a hyperinsulinemic euglycemic clamp in postobese subjects and matched controls failed to detect any differences in the increase in plasma norepinephrine levels (85). Measurement of norepinephrine turnover or MSNA could perhaps have revealed an impaired increase among the postobese subjects. More studies are clearly needed to clarify this question.

In the Quebec overfeeding study, where 12 pairs of monozygotic twins were overfed 4.2 mJ/day for 100 days, Bouchard et al. demonstrated that weight gain varied from 4.3 to 13.3 kg, but within each pair fat gain was very similar (64). It was estimated that in the pair who gained the least weight about 60% of the extra energy must have

been dissipated. Unfortunately, no data on changes in sympathetic activity were reported in the study, but it is tempting to speculate that genetically determined differences in sympathetic responsiveness may partly explain the observed between-pairs differences in weight gain.

3. Sympathoadrenal Activity in Postobese Subjects

Due to the confounding effects of excessive fat depots on sympathetic activity and energy expenditure, formerly obese subjects, who have remained weight stable close to ideal body weight for extended periods, have become subject to studies of responsiveness to various stimulations of the sympathoadrenal system.

When sympathetic activity, assessed by plasma norepinephrine concentrations, has been studied following medium- and high-fat diets, sympathetic activity has been found normal in postobese subjects (46,47,49–51,55). Postobese subjects also have a normal sympathetic and thermogenic response to moderate cold exposure (47) and to β-adrenergic inhibition (46). The sympathetic response to meals has been found reduced (80,86) or normal (81), and a difference between postobese subjects and controls may be due to poor matching of groups for body composition and aerobic capacity (87) and to lack of control of antecedent energy balance and diet composition. By contrast, there is a more sustained effect of dietary macronutrient composition on sympathetic activity and energy expenditure. The basal sympathetic activity varies with the antecedent dietary carbohydrate content, which seems to possess a stimulatory effect on sympathetic activity in postobese subjects, which is much more pronounced than in never-obese subjects, where the effect may be hardly detectable. This should be taken into consideration when studying sympathetic activity and energy expenditure in postobese subjects. Lean and James (50) reported that reducing the dietary fat/carbohydrate ratio increased 24-hr energy expenditure of postobese subjects above that of a matched control group, whereas a diet providing a high fat/carbohydrate ratio suppressed energy expenditure be-

Table 3 Norepinephrine Turnover During Undereating, Weight Maintenance, and Overeating in Normal-Weight and Obese Subjects

	Hypoenergetic (2 MJ/day)		Isoenergetic		Hyperenergetic ($+4.2$ MJ/m^2/day)	
	Lean	Obese	Lean	Obese	Lean	Obese
Plasma norepinephrine, pg/ml	154	138	173	157	192	136
Norepinephrine appearance rate, μg/min/m^2	0.21	0.18	0.26	0.16	0.38	0.19

Source: Composed of data from two separately published studies (63,83) using the same protocol and methodology, and collected by Saris (58). Reproduced with permission from Ref. 58.

low the levels of the control group. The high-fat/low-carbohydrate diet may contribute to promoting weight gain in the postobese by reducing energy expenditure, and this mechanism is in line with the general concept that obesity develops as an interaction between susceptible genes and certain environmental factors. Due to the genetic heterogeneity of obesity, however, many of the results produced by studies comprising smaller groups of postobese individuals can only be suggestive and studies with different carbohydrate contents should be addressed separately. Two compilations of data in postobese subjects excluded studies in which the subjects consumed low-fat/high-carbohydrate diets. The largest study on 28 postobese subjects and 28 matched controls found RMR, adjusted for differences in body size and composition, was 8% lower among the postobese (88). A meta-analysis on RMR in postobese subjects has confirmed that RMR for a given body composition is 4–5% lower in the postobese than in controls (89). An impaired thermogenic sensitivity to β-adrenergic stimulation has also been reported in postobese subjects (78,86,90). It is possible that a lower plasma T_3 concentration may be contributing to a lower β-adrenergic sensitivity and responsiveness (91), which in turn may be responsible for the lower RMR and thermogenic responses of the postobese (88).

After consumption of a high-carbohydrate/medium-fat diet, 24-hr energy expenditure, heart rate, and plasma norepinephrine concentrations were higher in postobese women than in tightly matched controls (92). In a subsequent study comparing three isoenergetic diets with either low, medium, or high carbohydrate contents, it was found that plasma norepinephrine concentration was 50% higher on the high-carbohydrate than on the low-carbohydrate diet in both postobese subjects and never-obese controls, but 24-hr energy expenditure was increased only in the postobese, i.e., 4% above the control group (49). The similar plasma norepinephrine levels suggested that an increased β-adrenergic sensitivity of the postobese subjects was responsible.

A recent, strictly controlled 5-day calorimetry study showed that the T_3 and T_3/T_4 ratio of postobese subject decreased markedly when the diet was switched from a diet with a low to a high ratio of fat/carbohydrate, whereas no change was found among the controls (93).

Obese subjects tend to have lower epinephrine levels (see above), which also have been reported in postobese individuals (94). It may be speculated whether a lower circulating epinephrine level may contribute to a low RMR, fat oxidation, and changed fat partitioning.

In conclusion, there is evidence that postobese subjects consuming medium- and high-fat diets have lower RMR than tightly matched controls. Withdrawal of the stimu-

latory impact of dietary carbohydrate on sympathetic tone and on thyroid hormone levels by high-fat diets in postobese subjects may be responsible for their lower energy expenditure. It is possible that the lower T_3 levels found in the postobese than in controls on high-fat diets may cause a decreased β-adrenergic sensitivity. Sympathetic activity and energy expenditure in postobese subjects can be increased to normal or even supranormal levels by low-fat/high-carbohydrate diets.

4. Sympathetic Activity as a Predictor of Weight Loss in Obesity

As already mentioned, a low sympathetic activity is a risk factor for, or a predictor of, subsequent weight gain in Pima Indians. Similar studies have so far not been reported in Caucasians. Two studies, however, have reported that a low sympathetic activity in obese patients undergoing a dietary weight loss program is associated with a smaller weight loss (95,96). Astrup et al. studied prognostic metabolic markers for long-term weight loss in obese women undergoing 36 weeks of dietary treatment (4.2 mJ/day) (95). They found that postprandial plasma norepinephrine was positively associated with the maximum attained weight loss (average 16.2 kg, $r = 0.30$) after controlling for pretreatment 24-hr energy expenditure, fat oxidation, and plasma dihydrotestosterone. Patients who were less successful, i.e., the lower 50 percentile of attained weight loss at week 36, tended to have lower pretreatment plasma norepinephrine. The importance of basal sympathetic tone for weight loss prognosis has been confirmed in a study in which 63 obese patients underwent an 8-week VLED (2.8 MJ/day) (96). Both pretreatment levels of norepinephrine and epinephrine levels were independently associated with a decrease in body fat (%). Successful patients, i.e., the upper 50 percentile of decrease in body fat, had higher pretreatment plasma norepinephrine levels than those in the lower 50 percentile. These studies show that plasma norepinephrine is a predictor of body weight and fat loss during low-energy diets in obese subjects. They do not clarify whether plasma norepinephrine is the mediating factor or a just a marker. Taken together with the well-established role of the sympathetic nervous system for regulation of energy balance, however, a causal role can be considered probable. Whether the sympathetic tone influences appetite and food intake or acts predominantly on energy expenditure is not clear. That the relationship between baseline plasma norepinephrine existed even after controlling for baseline 24-hr energy expenditure and fat oxidation (97) suggests that the effect is exerted through the intake side of the energy balance equation.

VII. PHARMACOLOGICAL AGENTS INTERACTING WITH THE SYMPATHOADRENAL SYSTEM

A. Compounds Promoting Obesity

Pharmacological agents interfering with the sympathoadrenal system may influence energy intake, nutrient partitioning, and energy expenditure, and chronic treatment may have an important impact on body composition and size. Central and peripheral inhibitors of the sympathetic nervous system tend to promote fat and weight gain and to reduce lean body mass and usually occur as side effects to compounds used in the treatment of hypertension and ischemic heart disease.

I. β-Adrenergic Antagonists

Treatment of hypertension, angina pectoris, various arrhythmias, and liver disease by β-adrenergic antagonists clearly demonstrates a weight gain as compared to treatment with diuretics or placebo (98,99). The lack of body composition measurements makes it difficult to assess to what extent the observed weight gains can be attributed to fat gain. In patients with chronic liver disease, treatment by propranolol induced a weight gain of 1.8 kg/6 months, 3.9 kg/9 months, and 5.7 kg/year, which was entirely due to fat gain (100). In a randomized trial of propranolol versus placebo in patients after a myocardial infarction, the mean weight gain above placebo was 1.4 kg after 2 and 3 years of follow-up. This weight gain could not be accounted for by group differences in physical activity, fluid retention, or use of diuretics (101). The average weight gain reported during propranolol use seems to be higher than those in patients treated by selective β_1-adrenergic inhibitors, such as atenolol and oxprenolol (102).

Though the mean weight gain does not seem to be clinically important, the proportion of patients experiencing a substantial weight gain or increase in visceral fat may be more significant. It is also likely that treatment with β-blockers may increase the incidence of insulin resistance and type 2 diabetes (103). The weight and fat gain observed during pharmacological inhibition of β-adrenoceptors should not readily be translated into the physiological importance of the sympathoadrenal system for body weight regulation. Inhibition of β-receptors, rather than blockade, is achieved by the use of therapeutic doses of the pharmacological agents. Moreover, agents such as propranolol reduce the clearance of endogenous catecholamines and raise plasma levels of norepinephrine and epinephrine, which may attenuate the pharmacological inhibition. Furthermore, propranolol may act as an

agonist on the human β_3-adrenoceptor (104,105). This stimulation may counteract the positive energy balance caused by β_{1+2} antagonism. In conclusion, evidence exists to support the hypothesis that body weight and fat gain occur during therapeutic use of β-adrenergic antagonists, and that this may have clinical importance in some patients.

2. Other Compounds

A number of drugs promoting weight gain and obesity may exert some inhibitory effect on the sympathoadrenal system. Examples are tricyclic antidepressant drugs, which cause a reduction in RMR, and the thermic effect of food (106). Whether these findings involve inhibition of the sympathoadrenal system remains to be determined. Sodium valproate, a widely used antiepileptic drug, causes weight gain in more than 50% of the treated patients (107) and has been shown to suppress fasting and postprandial plasma levels of norepinephrine and epinephrine (108).

B. Pharmacotherapy of Obesity

A number of sympathomimetic compounds with anorectic or thermogenic effects are either currently in use or are presently being introduced as adjuvants to dietary treatment of obesity. Although the impact of some of the compounds (amphetamine, phentermine, ephedrine, diethylpropion, sibutramine) is considered to consist of a central anorectic effect and a peripheral thermogenic effect, the latter is conceivably mediated through a central activation of the sympathetic nervous system. Some of the sympathomimetic agents act predominantly by causing release of endogenous norepinephrine, but they may also possess direct β-adrenergic and α-adrenergic properties (97). How the central inhibition of food intake is mediated is unclear. Increased tone of the noradrenergic neurons in the hypothalamus increases appetite, and this effect is mediated by α_2-adrenoceptors localized to the paraventricular nucleus (109). The anorectic effects of sympathomimetics have been considered to be mediated through dopaminergic receptors (109), but this monoamine system cannot be responsible for the effect because the weight loss produced by chronic treatment with ephedrine is abolished in hypertensive patients treated with the β-adrenergic antagonist propranolol, but preserved in patients treated with diuretics (97). Consequently, both the appetite suppression and the thermogenic effect of sympathomimetics are mediated by β-adrenoceptors.

Increased energy expenditure can be achieved by stimulation of all three β-adrenoceptors, and during chronic treatment by an ephedrine/caffeine combination the thermogenic effect may amount to a 5–10% increase in 24-hr energy expenditure, which produces a 15 g/day increase in fat oxidation (110). Agents with predominant β_2-agonistic properties (clenbuterol, cimaterol) are also thermogenic and have been used to manipulate growth and body composition, enhancing the deposition of body protein and reducing fat stores, thereby being termed repartitioning compounds (111). Similar effects can also be induced during chronic treatment in humans (45,110).

Selective β_3-adrenergic agonists may cause weight loss in rodents without hemodynamic and CNS side effects. Therefore, a number of β_3-agonists have been tested in humans, but the outcome has generally been disappointing (112–114). Reasons for the failure of some β_3-agonists in humans have included a poor pharmacokinetic profile and a failure of prodrugs to be metabolized to selective β_3-agonists (113). Most β_3-agonists have been selected based on screening in rodents, and the human and the rat β_3-receptor differ pharmacologically, so those compounds that have been evaluated in humans have much lower efficacy at the human than the rat receptor. Even modest effects on 24-hr energy expenditure, however, may cause fat loss in the long-term treatment. Obese patients treated for 2 weeks with a selective β_3-agonist, ZD 2079, increased daily energy expenditure by 230 kJ/day as compared with placebo (115), but the true potential of β_3-adrenoceptor agonists in treatment of obesity can only be evaluated when compounds with good selectivity and efficacy at the human β_3-receptor have been identified.

In the evaluation of drugs for treating obesity, secondary end-points as risk factors should also be considered (116,117). In this context there is a tendency for hemodynamic and metabolic side effects, predominantly due to β_{1+2}-receptor stimulation, to subside because tolerance develops as a matter of down-regulation of receptors. β-Adrenoceptor agonists may also possess beneficial effects on insulin sensitivity (113) and blood lipids (118).

REFERENCES

1. Muntzel MS, Morgan DA, Mark AL, Johnson AK. Intracerebroventricular insulin produced non-uniform regional increases in sympathetic nerve activity. Am J Physiol 1994; 267:R1350–R1355.

2. Landsberg L, Young JB. The influence of diet on the sympathetic nervous system. Neuroendocr Perspect 1985; 4: 191–218.

3. Bennaroch EE. Central neurotransmitters and neuromodulators in cardiovascular regulatio. In: Bannister R, Mathias CJ, eds. Autonomic Failure, 3rd ed. Oxford: Oxford University Press, 1992:36–53.

4. Matthews MR. Autonomic ganglia in multiple system atrophy and pure autonomic failure. In: Bannister R, Mathias CJ, eds. Autonomic Failure, 3rd ed. Oxford: Oxford University Press, 1992:593–621.

5. Burnstock G. Purinergic nerves. Pharmacol Rev 1972; 24: 509–581.

6. Bredt DS, Hwang PM, Snyder SH. Localisation of nitric oxide synthase indicating a neural role for nitric oxide. Nature 1990; 347:768-770.

7. Mathias CJ, Bannister R. Investigation of autonomic disorders. In: Bannister R, Mathias CJ, eds. Autonomic Failure: A Textbook of Disorders of the Autonomic Nervous System, 3rd ed. Oxford: Oxford University Press, 1992: 255–290.

8. Wallin BG, Sundlöf G, Lindblad LE. Baroreflex mechanisms controlling sympathetic outflow to the muscles in man. In: Sleight P, ed. Arterial Baroreceptors and Hypertension. Oxford: Oxford University Press, 1980:101–108.

9. Bini G, Hagbarth KE, Hynninen P, Wallin BG. Thermoregulatory and rhythm-generating mechanisms governing the sudomotor and vasoconstrictor outflow in human cutaneous nerves. J Physiol 1980; 306:537–552.

10. Macdonald IA, Bennett T, Gal, EAM, Green JH, Walford S. The effect of propranolol or metroprolol on thermoregulation during insulin-induced hypoglycaemia in man. Clin Sci 1982; 63:301–310.

11. Scott AR, Bennett T, Macdonald IA. Effects of hyperinsulinaemia on the cardiovascular response to graded hypovolaemia in normal and diabetic subjects. Clin Sci 1988; 75:85–92.

12. Fagius J, Niklasson F, Berne C. Sympathetic outflow in human muscle nerves increases during hypoglycaemia. Diabetes 1986; 35:1124–1129.

13. Berne C, Fagius J, Pollare T, Hjemdahl P. The sympathetic response to euglycaemic hyperinsulinaemia. Diabetologia 1992; 35:873–879.

14. Fagius J, Berne C. Increase in muscle nerve sympathetic activity in humans after food intake. Clin Sci 1994; 86: 159–167.

15. Mansell PI, Macdonald IA. The effects of underfeeding on the physiological responses to food ingestion in normal weight women. Br J Nutr 1988; 60:39–48.

16. Macdonald IA. Advances in our understanding of the role of the sympathetic nervous system in obesity. Int J Obes 1995; 19 (Suppl 7):52–57.

17. Malliani A, Payani M, Lombardi F, Cerutti S. Cardiovascular neural regulation explored in the frequency domain. Circulation 1991; 84:482–492.

18. Esler M, Jennings G, Lambert G, Meredith I, Horne M, Eisenhofer. Overflow of catecholamine neurotransmitter to the circulation: source, fate and function. Physiol Rev 1990; 70:963–985.

19. Cox HS, Kaye DM, Thompson JM, Turner AG, Jennings GL, Itsiopoulos C, Esler MD. Regional sympathetic nervous activation after a large meal in humans. Clin Sci 1995; 89:145–154.

20. Hjemdahl P. Plasma catecholamines — analytical challenges and physiological limitations. Bailliere's Clin Endocrinol Metab 1993; 7:307–353.

21. Liu D, Andreasson K, Lins PE, Adamson U, Macdonald IA. Adrenaline and noradrenaline response to insulin-induced hypoglycaemia in men: should the hormone levels be measured in arterialized venous blood? Acta Endocrinol 1993; 128:95–98.

22. Cryer PE, Rizza RA, Haymond MW, Gerich JE. Epinephrine and norepinephrine are cleared through beta-adrenergic, but not alpha-adrenergic, mechanisms in man. Metabolism 1980; 29:1114–1118.

23. Chamberlain KG, Pestel RG, Best JD. Platelet catecholamine contents and cumulative indexes of sympathoadrenal activity. Am J Physiol 1990; 259:E141–E147.

24. Kopp U, Bradley T, Hjemdahl P. Renal venous outflow and urinary excretion of norepinephrine, epinephrine and dopamine during graded renal nerve stimulation. Am J Physiol 1983; 244:E52–E60.

25. Lundberg JM, Martinsson A, Hemsen A, Theodorsson-Norheim E, Svedenhag J, Ekblom J, Hjemdahl P. Co-release of neuropeptide Y and catecholamines during physical exercise in man. Biochem Biophys Res Commun 1985; 133:30–36.

26. Sacca L, Vigorito C, Cicala M, Ungaro B, Sherwin RS. Mechanisms of epinephrine-induced glucose intolerance in normal humans: role of the splanchnic bed. J Clin Invest 1982; 69:284–293.

27. Rosen SG, Clutter WE, Shah SD, Miller JP, Bier DM, Cryer PE. Direct α-adrenergic stimulation of hepatic glucose production in human subjects. Am J Physiol 1983; 245:E616–E626.

28. Ruffolo RR, Nichols AJ, Hieble JP. Metabolic regulation by α_1 and α_2-adrenoceptors. Life Sci 1991; 49:171–183.

29. Hjemdahl P, Linde B. The influence of circulatory NE and Epi on adipose tissue vascular resistance and lipolysis in humans. Am J Physiol 1983; 245:H447–H452.

30. Richelsen B, Pedersen S B, Møller-Pedersen T, Bak JF. Regional differences in triglyceride breakdown in human adipose tissue: effects of catecholamines, insulin and prostaglandin E_2. Metabolism 1991; 40:990–996.

31. Tappy L, Girardet K, Schwallewr N, Vollenweider L, Jéquier E, Nicod P, Scherrer U. Metabolic effects of an increase of sympathetic activity in healthy humans. Int J Obes 1995; 19:419–422.

32. Saad MF, Alger SA, Zurlo F, Young JB, Bogardus C, Ravussin E. Ethnic differences in sympathetic nervous system-mediated energy expenditure. Am J Physiol 1991; 261:E789–E794.

33. Spraul M, Ravussin E, Fontvieille AM, Rising R, Larson DE, Anderson EA. Reduced sympathetic nervous activity. A potential mechanism predisposing to body weight gain. J Clin Invest 1993; 92:1730–1735.

34. Toth MJ, Poehlman ET. Sympathetic nervous system activity and resting metabolic rate in vegetarians. Metabolism 1994; 43:621–625.

35. Toubro S, Sørensen TIA, Rønn B, Christensen NJ, Astrup A. Twenty-four-hour energy expenditure: the role of body composition, thyroid status, sympathetic activity, and family membership. J Clin Endocrinol Metab 1996; 81:2670–2674.

36. Wallin B, Kunimoto M, Sellgren J. Possible genetic influence on the strength of human muscle nerve symjpathetic activity at rest. Hypertension 1993; 22:282–284.

37. Acheson KJ, Jéquier E, Wahren J. Influence of β-adrenergic blockade on glucose-induced thermogenesis in man. J Clin Invest 1983; 72:893–902.

38. Astrup A, Christensen NJ, Simonsen L, Bülow J. Effects of nutrient intake on sympathoadrenal activity and thermogenic mechanisms. J Neurosci Methods 1990; 34:187–192.

40. Berne C, Fagius J, Niklasson F. Sympathetic response to oral carbohydrate administration. Evidence from microelectrode nerve recording. J Clin Invest 1989; 84:1403-1409.

40. Vollenweider P, Randin D, Tappy L, Jéquier E, Nicod P, Scherrer U. Impaired insulin-induced sympathetic neural activation and vasodilation in skeletal muscle in obese humans. J Clin Invest 1994; 93:2365–2371.

41. Astrup A, Simonsen L, Bülow J, Madsen J, Christensen NJ. Epinephrine mediates facultative carbohydrate-induced thermogenesis in human skeletal muscle. Am J Physiol 1989; 257:E430–E345.

42. Tappy L, Randin JP, Felber JP, Chiolero R, Simonsen DC, Jéquier E, DeFronzo R. Comparison of thermogenic effect of fructose and glucose in normal humans. Am J Physiol 1986; 250:E718–E724.

43. Westerterp KR, Meyer GAL, Saris WHM. Physical activity and sleeping metabolic rate. Med Sci Sports Exerc 1991; 23:166–170.

44. Christin L, O'Connell M, Bogardus C, Danforth E Jr, Ravussin E. Norepinephrine turnover and energy expenditure in Pima Indian and white men. Metabolism 1993; 4:723–729.

45. Acheson KJ, Ravussin E, Schoeller DA, Christin L, Bourquin L, Baertschi P, Danforth E, Jéquier E. Two-week stimulation or blockade of the sympathetic nervous system in man: influence on body weight, body composition, and twenty four-hour energy expenditure. Metabolism 1988; 37:91–98.

46. Buemann B, Astrup A, Madsen J, Christensen NJ. A 24-h energy expenditure study on reduced-obese and non-obese women: effect of β-blockade. Am J Clin Nutr 1992; 56:662–670.

47. Buemann B, Astrup A, Christensen NJ, Madsen J. Effect of moderate cold exposure on 24-h energy expenditure: similar response in post obese and nonobese women. Am J Physiol 1992; 263:E1040–E1045.

48. Tremblay A, Coveney JP, Després JP, Nadeau A, Prud'homme D. Increased resting metabolic rate and lipid oxidation in exercise-trained individuals: evidence for a

role of beta adrenergic stimulation. Can J Physiol Pharmacol 1992; 70:1342–1347.

49. Astrup A, Buemann B, Christensen NJ, Toubro S. Failure to increase lipid oxidation in response to increasing dietary fat content in formerly obese women. Am J Physiol 1994; 266:E592–E599.

50. Lean MEJ, James WPT. Metabolic effects of isoenergetic nutrient exchange over 24 hours in relation to obesity in women. Int J Obes 1988; 12:15–27.

51. Raben A, Anderson K, Karberg MA, Holst JJ, Astrup A. Modified potato starches: beneficial impact on glucose metabolism and appetite sensations. Am J Clin Nutr In press.

52. Emorine LJ, Marullo S, Briend-Sutren M-M, Patey G, Tate K, Delavier-Klutchko C, Strosberg AD. Molecular characterization of the human β_3-adrenergic receptor. Science 1989; 245:1118–1121.

53. Newnham DM, Ingram CG, Mackie A, Lipworth BJ. β-adrenoceptor subtypes mediating the airways response to BRL 35135 in man. Br J Clin Pharmacol 1993; 36:565–571.

54. Liu Y-L, Toubro S, Astrup A, Stock MJ. Contribution of β_3-adrenoceptor activation to ephedrine-induced thermogenesis in humans. Int J Obes 1995; 19:678–685.

55. Toubro S, Astrup A. The selective β_3-agonist ZD2079 stimulates 24-h energy expenditure through increased fidgetting. A 14 day, randomized placebo-controlled study in obese subjects. Int J Obes 1995; 19/2:O70.

56. Clément K, Vaisse C, Manning BSJ, Silver KD, Basdevant A, Guy-Grand B, Shuldiner AR, Froguel Ph, Strosberg AD. Genetic variation in the β_3-adrenergic receptor and an increased capacity to gain weight in patients with morbid obesity. N Engl J Med 1995; 333:352–354.

57. Macdonald IA, Webber J. Feeding, fasting and starvation: factors affecting fuel utilization. Proc Nutr Soc 1995; 54:267–274.

58. Saris WHM. Effects of energy restriction and exercise on the sympathetic nervous system. Int J Obes 1995; 19(Suppl 7):17–23.

59. Young JB, Landsberg L. Suppression of sympathetic nervous system during fasting. Science 1977; 196:1473–1475.

60. Shetty PS, Jung RT, James WPT. Effect of catecholamine replacement with levodopa on the metabolic response to semi-starvation. Lancet 1979; 1:77–79.

61. Bessard T, Schulz Y, Jequir E. Energy expenditure and post-prandial thermogenesis in obese women before and after weight loss. Am J Clin Nutr 1983; 38:680–693.

62. Jung RI, Shetty PS, James WPT. The effect of refeeding after semi-starvation on catecholamine and thyroid metabolism. Int J Obes 1980; 4:95–100.

63. O'Dea K, Ester MD, Leonars P, Stockigt JR, Nestel P. Noradrenaline turnover during under and overeating in normal weight subjects. Metabolism 1982; 31:896–899.

64. Bouchard C, Tremblay A, Després JP, Nadeau A, Lupien PJ, Thériault G, Dussault J, Moorjani S, Pinault S, Four-

nier G. The response to long-term overfeeding in identical twins. N Engl J Med 1990; 322:1477–1482.

65. Horton TJ, Drougas H, Brachey A, Reed GW, Peters JC, Hill JO. Fat and carbohydrate overfeeding in humans: different effects on energy storage. Am J Clin Nutr 1995; 62:19–29.

66. Schwartz RS, Jaeger LF, Weight RC, Lakshminaratan S. The effect of diet or exercise on plasma norepinephrine kinetics in moderate obese young men. Int J Obes 1990; 14:1–11.

67. Bray GA, York DA, Fisler JS. Experimental obesity: a homeostatic failure due to defective nutrient stimulation of the sympathetic nervous system. Vitam Horm 1989; 45:1–125.

68. Bray GA. The MONA LISA Hypothesis. Most obesities known are low in sympathetic activity. In: Oomura Y, Tarui S, Inoue S, Shimazu T, eds. Progress in Obesity Research. London: John Libbey, 1990:61–66.

69. Sakaguchi T, Bray GA, Eddlestone G. Sympathetic activity following paraventricular or ventromedial hypothalamic lesions in rats. Brain Res Bull 1988; 20:461–465.

70. Sakaguchi T, Takahashi M, Bray GA. Diurnal changes in sympathetic activity: relation to food intake and to insulin injected into the ventromedial or suprachiasmatic nucleus. J Clin Invest 1988; 82:2812–2816.

71. Astrup A, Flatt JP. Metabolic determinants of body weight regulation. In: Bouchard C, Bray G, eds. Regulation of Body Weight: Biological and Behavioural Mechanisms. Life Sciences Research report 57. Chichester: Wiley, 1996:193–210.

72. Raben A, Holst JJ, Christensen NJ, Astrup A. Determinants of postprandial appetite sensations: macronutrient intake and glucose metabolism. Int J Obes 1996; 20:161–169.

73. Young JB, Macdonald IA. Sympathoadrenal activity in human obesity: heterogeneity of findings since 1980. Int J Obes 1992; 16:959–967.

74. Peterson HR, Rothschild M, Weinberg CR, Fell RD, McLeish KR, Pfeifer MA. Body fat and the activity of the autonomic nervous system. N Engl J Med 1988; 318:1077–1088.

75. Scherrer U, Randin D, Tappy L, Vollenweider P, Jéquier E, Nicod P. Body fat and sympathetic nerve activity in healthy subjects. Circulation 1994; 89:2634–2640.

76. Spraul M, Anderson EA, Bogardus C, Ravussin E. Muscle sympathetic nerve activity in response to glucose ingestion. Impact of plasma insulin and body fat. Diabetes 1994; 43:191–196.

77. Tataranni PA, Young JB, Ravussin E. A low sympathetic nervous system activity is associated with body weight gain in Pima Indians. Int J Obes 1996; 20(Suppl 4):63.

78. Blaak EE, Van Blaak MA, Kester ADM, Saris WHM. β-adrenergically mediated thermogenic and heart rate responses: Effect of obesity and weight loss. Metabolism 1995; 44:520–524.

79. Walston J, Silver K, Bogardus C, Knowler WC, Celi FS, Austin S, Manning B, Strosberg AD, Stern MP, Raben N, Sorkin JD, Roth J, Shuldiner AR. A missense mutation in the β_3-adrenergic receptor gene in Pima Indians and other populations with obesity and diabetes mellitus. N Engl J Med 1995; 333:343–347.

80. Astrup A, Andersen T, Christensen NJ, Bülow J, Madsen J, Berum L, Quaade F. Impaired glucose-induced thermogenesis and arterial norepinephrine response persist after weight reduction in obese humans. Am J Clin Nutr 1990; 51:331–337.

81. Raben A, Andersen HB, Christensen NJ, Madsen J, Holst JJ, Astrup A. Evidence for an abnormal postprandial response to a high-fat meal in women predisposed to obesity. Am J Physiol 1994; 267:E549–E559.

82. Tataranni PA, Larson DE, Snitker S, Ravussin E. Thermal effect of food in humans: methods and results from use of a respiratory chamber. Am J Clin Nutr 1995; 61: 1013–1019.

83. Leibel RL, Rosenbaum M, Hirsch J. Changes in energy expenditure resulting from altered body weight. N Engl J Med 1995; 332:621–628.

84. Bazelmans J, Nestel PJ, O'Dea K, Ester MD. Blunted norepinephrine responsiveness to changing energy status in obese subjects. Metabolism 1982; 31:896–899.

85. Toubro S, Western P, Bülow J, Macdonald I, Raben A, Christensen NJ, Madsen J, Astrup A. Insulin sensitivity in post-obese women. Clin Sci 1994; 84:407–413.

86. Dulloo AG, Miller DS. The thermogenic properties of ephedrine/methylxanthine mixtures: human studies. Int J Obes 1986; 10:467–481.

87. Eckel RH, Ailhaud G, Astrup A, Flatt JP, Hauner H, Levine AS, Prentice AM, Ricquier D, Steffens AB, Woods SC. What are the metabolic and physiological mechanisms associated with the regulation of body weight? In: Bouchard C, Bray GA, eds. Regulation of Body Weight: Biological and Behavioral Mechanisms. Chichester: Wiley, 1996: 225–238.

88. Astrup A, Buemann B, Toubro S, Ranneries C, Raben A. Low resting metabolic rate in subjects predisposed to obesity: a role for thyroid status. Am J Clin Nutr 1996; 63: 879–883.

89. van de Werken K, Toubro S, Buemann B, Raben A, Astrup A. Meta-analysis on resting energy expenditure in postobese versus controls: a preliminary report. Int J Obes 1996; 20(Suppl 4):29.

90. Jung RT, Shetty PS, James WPT, Barrand MA, Callingham BA. Reduced thermogenesis in obesity. Nature 1979; 279: 322–323.

91. Bilezikian JP, Loeb JN. The influence of hyperthyroidism and hypothyroidism on α- and β-adrenergic receptor systems and adrenergic responsiveness. Endocr Rev 1983; 4: 378–388.

92. Astrup A, Buemann B, Christensen NJ, Madsen J. 24-hour energy expenditure and sympathetic activity in postobese women consuming a high-carbohydrate diet. Am J Physiol 1992; E281–E288.

93. Buemann B, Toubro S, Astrup A. Lower plasma T_3 level in postobese women after 3 days on a high fat diet. Int J Obes 1996; 20(Suppl 4):28.

94. Andersen HB, Raben A, Astrup A, Christensen NJ. Plasma adrenaline concentration is lower in post-obese than in never-obese women in the basal state, in response to sham-feeding and after food intake. Clin Sci 1994; 87: 69–74.

95. Astrup A, Buemann B, Gluud C, Bennett P, Tjur T, Christensen NJ. Prognostic markers for diet-induced weight loss in obese women. Int J Obes 1995; 19:275–278.

96. Kempen KPG, Saris WHM, Blaak EE, Stegen JCHC, Keseter ADM. Predictors of fat loss during very-low calorie diet in obese females. Metabolism (submitted).

97. Astrup A. The sympathetic nervous system as a target for intervention in obesity. Int J Obes 1995; 19(Suppl 7): S24–S28.

98. Bengtsson C. Comparison between alprenolol and chlorthalidone as antihypertensive agents. Acta Med Scand 1972; 191:433–439.

99. Gonasun LM, Langrall H. Adverse reactions to pindolol administration. Am Heart J 1982; 104:482–486.

100. Hayes PC, Stewart WW, Bouchier IAD. Influence of propranolol on weight and salt and water homeostasis in chronic liver disease. Lancet 1984; 2:1064–1068.

101. Rössner S, Taylor CL, Byington RP, Furberg CD. Long term propranolol treatment and changes in body weight after myocardial infarction. Br Med J 1990; 300:902–903.

102. Bai TR, Webb D, Hamilton M. Treatment of hypertension with beta-adrenoceptor blocking drugs. J Royal Coll Phys 1982; 16:239–241.

103. Skarfors ET, Lithell HO, Selinus I, Aberg H. Do antihypertensive drugs precipitate diabetes in predisposed men? Br Med J 1989; 298:1147–1151.

104. Blin N, Nahmias C, Drumare MF, Strosberg AD. The β_3-adrenergic receptor: a single subtype responsible for atypical β-mediated effects. Br J Pharmacol 1994; 112: 911–919.

105. Strosberg AD. Adrenergic, dopaminergic and histaminergic drugs. Structure, function and regulation of the three β-adrenergic receptors. Obes Res 1995; 3(Suppl 4): 501S–505S.

106. Fernstrom MH. Drugs that cause weight gain. Obes Res 1995; 3(Suppl 4):435S–439S.

107. Dinesen H, Gram L, Andersen T. Weight gain during treatment with valproate. Acta Neurol Scand 1984; 70: 65–69.

108. Breum L, Astrup A, Gram, Andersen T, Stokholm K, Christensen NJ, Werdelin L, Madsen J. Metabolic changes during treatment with valproate in humans: implication for untoward weight gain. Metabolism 1992; 41: 666–670.

109. Liebowitz SF. Neurochemical control of macronutrient intake. In: Oomura Y, Tarui S, Inoue S, Shimazu T, eds.

Progress in Obesity Research. London: John Libbey, 1990: 13–18.

110. Astrup A, Buemann B, Christensen NJ, Toubro S, Thorbek G, Victor OJ, Quaade F. The effect of ephedrine/caffeine mixture on energy expenditure and body composition in obese women. Metabolism 1992; 41:686–688.

111. Stock MJ. New approaches to the control of obesity in animals and their clinical potential. In: Somogyi JC, Hejda S, eds. Nutrition in the Prevention of Disease. Basel, Switzerland: Karger, 1989:32–37.

112. Astrup A, Toubro S, Christensen NJ, Quaade F. Pharmacology of thermogenic drugs. Am J Clin Nutr 1992; 55: 246S–248S.

113. Arch JRS, Wilson S. Prospects for β_3-adrenoceptor agonists in the treatment ofg obesity and diabetes. Int J Obes 1996; 20:191–199.

114. Yen TT. β-agonists as antiobesity, antidiabetic and nutrient partitioning agents. Obes Res 1995; 3(Suppl 4): 531S–536S.

115. Toubro S, Astrup A. The selective β_3-agonist ZD2079 stimulates 24-h energy expenditure through increasing fidgetting. A 14 day, randomised placebo-controlled study in obese subjects. Int J Obes 1995; 19/2.O70.

116. Bray GA. Pharmacologic treatment of obesity: symposium overview. Obes Res 1995; 3(Suppl 4):415S.

117. Astrup A, Breum L, Toubro S. Pharmacological and clinical studies of ephedrine and other thermogenic agonists. Obes Res 1995; 3(Suppl 4):537S-540S.

118. Buemann B, Marckmann, Christensen NJ, Astrup A. The effect of ephedrine plus caffeine on plasma lipids and lipoproteins during a 4.2 mJ/day diet. Int J Obes 1994; 18: 329–332.

24

Energy Expenditure and Substrate Oxidation

Jean-Pierre Flatt
University of Massachusetts Medical School, Worcester, Massachusetts

Angelo Tremblay
Laval University, Ste.-Foy, Quebec, Canada

I. FACTORS DETERMINING TOTAL SUBSTRATE OXIDATION

The rate of substrate oxidation varies considerably during the day, being dictated by the body's need to regenerate the ATP used in carrying out its metabolic functions, in digesting and storing nutrients, and in moving and performing physical tasks. The amount of heat generated is generally sufficient to allow maintenance of body temperature by regulation of heat dissipation, aided when necessary by measures seeking to maintain comfort through appropriate clothing and control of environmental temperatures. Situations where substrate oxidation is activated for the sake of thermogenesis are avoided as much as possible.

The energy expended in the resting state depends primarily on the size of the lean body mass, plus the metabolic costs for processing ingested nutrients. The energy expended for specific physical activities is highly reproducible and in many cases roughly proportional to body weight (1). Overall energy expenditure for weight-maintaining adults is thus determined primarily by body size and by the intensity and duration of the physical activities undertaken. In sedentary individuals total daily energy expenditure (TEE) varies typically between 1.4 and 1.7 times the rate of resting energy expenditure (REE) extrapolated to 24 hr.

A. Efficiency of Oxidative Phosphorylation and P:O Ratio

It is difficult to assess the efficiency of oxidative phosphorylation and the P:O ratio in intact cells, because the ATP turnover due to the cell's metabolic activities is not readily measurable. Pahud et al. (2) were nevertheless able to assess the efficiency of oxidative phosphorylation in humans by combining direct and indirect calorimetry measurements in young men pedaling on a bicycle ergometer at different levels of work output. During sustained aerobic work, the mechanical work performed was equivalent to 27% of the energy contained in the increment in substrate oxidation elicited by pedaling. During the first minutes of pedaling against a suddenly increased resistance, the mechanical work produced (measured electrically with the bicycle ergometer) plus the energy appearing in the form of heat (measured by direct calorimetry and from the increase in the subjects' body temperature) exceeded the energy liberated by substrate oxidation (determined by indirect calorimetry). This implies that preformed high-energy bonds (ATP and creatine phosphate) were utilized to accomplish part of the mechanical work during this phase of the test. The characteristics of this latter process allowed them to determine that the *coupling coefficient*, which describes the efficiency with which chemical energy can be converted into work in muscles, is 41%. The difference in the two observed efficiencies is due to the fact that a fraction only of the energy liberated by the oxidation of metabolic fuels is recovered in the form of ATP. The ratio 27%/41% = 0.66 thus provides an estimate of the efficiency with which the energy liberated by substrate oxidation is recovered in the form of ATP in human muscles.

During the complete oxidation of 1 mol of glucose, approximately 689 (ΔG, kcal/mol) × 0.66 = 450 kcal of free energy is therefore recovered in the form of high-energy bonds. Since the ΔG for ATP hydrolysis in muscle is about −14.3 kcal/mol and oxidative phosphorylation operates at near-equilibrium conditions, one would expect 450/14.3 = 31.5 mol ATP to be formed, which corresponds to a P:O ratio of 31.3/12 = 2.6 (3). This is in reasonably good agreement with other evaluations of the P:O ratio in intact cells (3). In reality, such experiments provide evaluations of the increments in ATP generation divided by the increments in oxygen consumption, i.e., "ΔP:ΔO ratios." These are higher than the P:O ratio prevailing in resting cells, in which this ratio is lower due to a certain rate of proton leakage through the mitochondrial membrane (4). While ATP turnover based on estimates of the ΔP:ΔO ratio will thus be overestimated, this uncertainty is not of great importance when increments in ATP turnover are to be assessed. Considering the number of assumptions and sources of possible errors inherent in these estimates, a value of 2.6 still seems to be consistent with the "traditional" values of three and two high-energy bonds regenerated per mitochondrial NADH per $FADH_2$ or cytoplasmic NADH reoxidized, respectively. To maintain consistency with common practices, these values were used in computing the amounts of ATP yielded by the oxidation of metabolic fuels (Table 1) (5,6) and in the assessment of the metabolic costs of processes based on their ATP-related stoichiometries (Fig. 1) (5).

Except for some reactions catalyzed by peroxidases, and for diverse hydroxylations catalyzed by oxygenases (where the ultimate reaction with oxygen is often catalyzed by the cytoplasmic cytochrome P450), reaction with oxygen is mediated only by cytochrome oxidase, the ultimate enzyme in the mitochondrial respiratory chain. This explains why substrate oxidation in vivo is closely controlled by the rate of ADP formation (i.e., the rate of ATP utilization) under most circumstances, except in brown adipose tissue (BAT). BAT mitochondria contain a unique *uncoupling protein* (UP). In the presence of fatty acids produced by catecholamine-stimulated lipolysis (7) this protein creates a proton-conducting pathway that allows NADH reoxidation to occur at rates much higher than those determined when proton reentry is coupled to ATP regeneration. This permits rapid substrate oxidation

and heat production, important for the maintenance of body temperature in small animals exposed to cold, as well as in raising body temperature during arousal from hibernation. Activation of this proton conductance pathway during overfeeding can play an important role in enhancing energy dissipation, thereby limiting fat accumulation during overfeeding in small animals (8,9). This mechanism for energy dissipation does not appear to operate to a significant extent in humans, however (7).

B. Costs Associated with ATP Generation

The number of moles of ATP formed per mole of glucose, fatty acid, and amino acid oxidized is shown in Table 1, as well as the number of ATP required to initiate their degradation (negative numbers), and in the case of amino acid oxidation to carry out gluconeogenesis and ureagenesis. To evaluate the costs of ATP expenditures associated with these and other metabolic processes, the amount of substrate that needs to be oxidized to regenerate a given amount of ATP must be assessed. Such evaluations depend therefore not only on the P:O ratio, but also on the amounts of ATP expended for the transport, activation, and handling of the metabolic fuels whose oxidation provides the energy for ATP regeneration.

I. Substrate Handling and Storage Costs

In the case of glucose, 38 ATPs are produced during the oxidation of one glucose molecule, but two are used for its activation to glucose-6-P and fructose-di-P, so that the ATP yield is 36/38 = 95%. If one allows for the fact that some 15–25% of the glucose released by the liver is recycled via the *Cori cycle* and the *glucose-alanine cycle* (at a net cost of 4 ATP/glucose recycled), only some 90% of the ATP generated by oxidation of glucose derived from liver glycogen are available to replace ATPs used in peripheral tissues. Significant portions of the carbohydrates supplied by the diet are initially stored in the form of muscle glycogen (10), so a substantial part of the glucose released by the liver is in fact regenerated from lactate released by breakdown of muscle glycogen. The cost of gluconeogenesis would then consume additional ATP. Assuming that this applies to half of the glucose released by the liver, the net ATP yield during glycogen oxidation is reduced to about 82% (Fig. 1). The heat of combustion (ΔH) for glucose is 670 kcal/mol (11). (Note that the ΔH for glucose oxidation is very similar to the ΔG for this process, i.e., −689 kcal/mol, which is generally the case when complete oxidations of biological substrates are considered.) The ΔH for fructose-1, 6-di P oxidation may be

Table 1 Stoichiometry of Substrate Oxidation and High-Energy Bond Production

Substrate	RQ (kcal/L O₂)	Products
$C_6H_{12}O_6$ + 6 O_2 *Glucose*	RQ = 1.00 (4.99 kcal/L 02) →	6 CO_2 + 6 H_2O + 670 kcal[a] [+38 − 2 = + 36 ~][b]
$C_6H_{1(5}$ + 6 O_2 *Glucosyl-*	RQ = 1.00 (5.05 kcal/L 02) →	6 CO_2 + 6 H_2O + 678 kcal[a] [+38 − 1 = + 37 ~]
[c]4.5 $C_6H_{12}O_6$ + 4 O_2 *Glucose*	RQ = 2.75 (7.06 kcal/L 02) →	$C_{16}H_{32}O_2$ + 11 CO_2 + 11 H_2O + 630 kcal *Palmitate* [+ 40 − 34 = 6 ~]
$C_{16}H_{32}O_2$ + 23 O_2 *Palmitate*	RQ = .696 (4.68 kcal/L 02) →	16 CO_2 + 16 H_2O + 2398 kcal [+ 131 − 2 = + 129 ~]
$C_{57}H_{107}O_6$[d] + 78 O_2 *Triglyceride*	RQ = 71[d] (4.69 kcal/L 02)[d] →	57 CO_2 + 52 H_2O + 8139 kcal [+ 459 − 7 = + 452 ~]
$C_{4.6}H_{8.4}O_{1.8}N_{1.25}$[f] + 1.5$O_2$ + 0.2 H_2O *Protein*	(RQ = 0.40) (liver) →	0.6 Urea + 0.6 CO_2 + 0.35 Gluc + 0.3 KB [+8.2 − 4.6 = + 3.6 ~]
.35 Gluc + .3 KB + 3.3 O_2	(RQ = 1.0) (periphery) →	3.3 CO_2 + 3.1 H_2O [+ 20.6 − 1 = + 19.6 ~]
$C_{4.6}H_{8.4}O_{1.8}N_{1.25}$ + 4.8 O_2 *Protein*	RQ = .835[e] (4.66 kcal/L O_2)[e] →	0.6 Urea + 4.0 CO_2 + 2.9 H_2O + 520 kcal [+ 28.8 − 5.6 = + 23.2 ~][g]

[a] See Ref. 11.

[b] The number of high-energy bonds (~) produced, minus those utilized, as well as the overall ~ yield is shown in square brackets.

[c] Based on stoichiometry reported for lipogenesis in rat adipose tissue (6).

[d] Palmityl-stearyl-oleyl triglyceride, which is representative of the usual fatty acid pattern in human adipose fat.

[e] Coefficients given by Livesey and Elia (13).

[f] Approximate composition of a protein mixture containing 1000 mmol of amino-acyl residues in 110 g, to have 16% of its weight as N and 50% as C, to be oxidized with an RQ of 0.835 and to generate 3.6 g glucose per g of N.

[g] ATP stoichiometry is based on McGilvery (14).

Source: Adapted from Ref. 5.

estimated at 685 kcal/mol. The release of 685 kcal, then reflects the turnover of 38 mol of ATP or 685/38 = 18 kcal/mol ATP when glucose is the metabolic fuel oxidized. However, since 18% of the ATP generated merely replaces the ATP spent for substrate handling, an amount of glucose containing 18/0.82 = 22 kcal must be oxidized to replace 1 mol of ATP consumed by a given metabolic process. To evaluate the energy expended in regenerating ATP by oxidation of fat, one has to consider that some of the free fatty acids produced by triglyceride hydrolysis in adipose tissue are reesterified before leaving adipose tissue, at a cost of 7 ATP/triglyceride reconstituted. Some of the free fatty acids (FFA) released into the circulation are removed and reesterified by the liver, to be reexported in the form of lipoproteins, requiring twice 2.33 ATP/FFA (Fig. 1) (5). The extent to which the lipolytic rate exceeds

the rate of fatty acid oxidation appears to be rather variable (12). If one assumes that lipolysis proceeds at twice the rate of fat oxidation and that half of the fatty acids that escape oxidation are reesterified in adipose tissue while the other half are returned to adipose tissue via lipoproteins secreted by the liver, 3.5 ATP are expended per mole of fatty acid oxidized. Oleate is the most common fatty acid in human triglycerides. During its oxidation 146 ATP/mol are generated, while 2 ATP are expended for its activation to oleyl-CoA. The ATP yield for fat oxidation is thus approximately 140.5/146 = 96%. In view of the large amount of ATP generated per mole of fatty acid oxidized, some variations in the relative rate of FFA reesterification will not greatly modify this yield. The ΔH for oleate oxidation is 2657 kcal/mol (11), and that for oleyl-CoA can be estimated at 2670 kcal/mol, so 2670/146 =

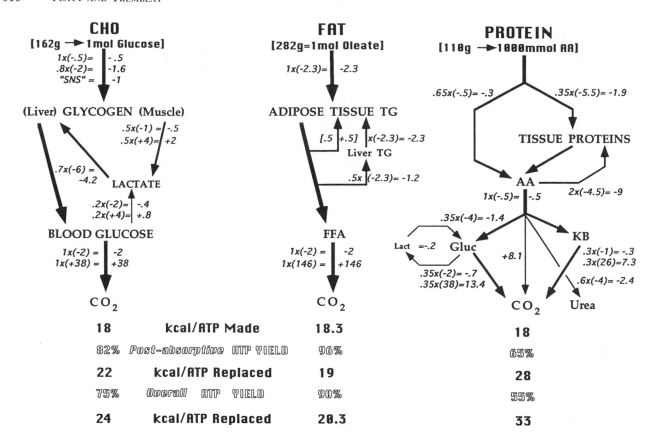

Figure 1 ATP yields during oxidation of carbohydrate, fat, and protein. Figures in brackets show moles of substrate flowing through various metabolic pathways, and in parentheses, the moles of ATP produced and expended per mole of substrate metabolized, assuming a P:O ratio of 3 for the reoxidation of mitochondrial NADH. (Reproduced with permission from Ref. 5.)

18.3 kcal are released per mole of ATP turned over. The energy expenditure per mole of ATP utilized and replaced by fatty acid oxidation thus comes to 18.3/0.96 = 19 kcal/mol ATP (as compared to 22 kcal/mol ATP during glycogen oxidation (Fig. 1).

By taking into account the known heats of combustion and the amino acid content of various proteins, Livesey and Elia concluded that the RQ during protein oxidation is 0.835, and that 4.7 kcal is released per gram of protein metabolized to CO_2, water, and urea, rather than 0.80 and 4.32, respectively, as originally proposed by Loewy (13). In the course of their oxidation, 110 g × 4.70 kcal/g = 517 kcal and 28.8 mol of ATP are generated (14), or 517/28.8 = 18 kcal/mol ATP. (With Loewy's coefficients, the corresponding value is 16.5 kcal/mol ATP generated, which is not consistent with the values of 18.0–18.3 kcal/mol ATP generated during carbohydrate and fat oxidation.) Since the costs of gluconeogenesis and ureagenesis consume 5.5 mol ATP per 1000 mmol of mixed AA oxidized, or about 20% of the amount generated (Table

1), the oxidation of 18/0.8. = 22.5 kcal of protein is required to generate 1 mol of ATP. Only some of the amino acids produced by protein breakdown are oxidized (possibly about 1/3) (15), so oxidation of amino acids derived from endogenous protein turnover is always accompanied by protein resynthesis, a process requiring about 5 ATP/amino acid reincorporated into protein (i.e., 4 for the synthesis of the peptide bond plus an estimated one additional mole for amino acid transport, mRNA synthesis, etc.). This would consume 10 ATP in addition to the 5.5 utilized for glucose and urea synthesis per mole of amino acid oxidized. The net ATP yield associated with the oxidation of amino acids derived from the turnover of endogenous proteins would accordingly be in the order of (28.8 − 15.5)/28.8 = 45%. Thus, in situations where amino acids contribute 15% or 20% of the fuel mix oxidized, if this is considered to imply commensurate differences in protein turnover rates, one would expect a 3% difference in metabolic rates. Part of the variability in basal metabolic rates is indeed explained by differences in protein turnover (16). Furthermore, it is well known that elevations in urinary nitrogen excretion and in resting metabolic rates run a parallel course following trauma or during sepsis (17).

The ATP yielded by different nutrients is further decreased when one takes into account the costs incurred for their initial transport and storage after ingestion. Assuming that in addition to the two ATPs used for the synthesis of glycogen, .5 ATP are expended for active transport and intestinal enzyme synthesis and motility, this would entail an energy expenditure equivalent to 2.5 × (22.5 kcal per mol ATP replaced at a postprandial RQ of .89) = 56 kcal, or 56/670 = 8% for the storage of dietary carbohydrate as glycogen. The fact that some of the ingested glucose is used without prior conversion into glycogen (assumed to be 20% in Fig. 1) is approximately offset by the stimulation of the sympathetic nervous system induced by carbohydrate intake (18). In studies in which the amount of glycogen synthesis could be calculated from indirect calorimetry data, the energy expended for glucose storage was evaluated at 4–6% of the glucose energy infused, accounting for about 2/3 of the observed increase in energy expenditure above the fasting rate, the remainder being attributable primarily to increased catecholamine secretion (18). When the catecholamine effect is curtailed by administration of adrenergic blocking agents, the thermic effect observed is consistent with the predicted metabolic expense for glucose storage. Taking into account the energy dissipated during the postprandial phase, the net ATP yield from dietary carbohydrate comes to about .92 × 82% (the net ATP yield for glycogen oxidation) = 75%. In the case of fat, the predictable cost for the initial deposition of dietary fat comes to about 3% of the energy provided by dietary fat, though addition of fat generally appears to raise postprandial energy expenditure by 5–10% of the energy provided by the added fat (19). The net ATP yield from dietary fat would thus be reduced to .93 × 96% (the yield from endogenous fat), or about 90%. These considerations suggest that the oxidation of 18/0.75 = 24 kcal of dietary carbohydrate or the oxidation of 18.3/0.90 = 20.3 kcal of dietary fat is needed to replace 1 mol of ATP, or that some 15–20% more energy may be required to sustain metabolism with dietary carbohydrate than with dietary fat, even in the absence of lipogenesis.

2. Diet Composition and Energy Expenditure

In animal studies, Donato and Hegsted (20) reported that 35% of the energy consumed in excess of maintenance requirements were retained when the excess was provided in the form of fat, as compared to 28% when the excess

was carbohydrate. In mice whose 24-hr energy expenditure was measured individually for many consecutive days, the use of carbohydrate as a fuel, as compared to fat, was accompanied by 9–12% higher rates of energy expenditure (5). Hurni et al. (21) found sleeping metabolic rates, BMRs, and 24-hr energy expenditure to be 5–8% higher in a group of volunteers when they were consuming a high-carbohydrate diet (80% of energy as CHO, 5% as fat), as compared to a mixed diet (55% CHO and 30% fat). On the other hand, Abbott et al. (22) could find no difference in 24-hr expenditure among obese Pima Indians adapted to diets providing 42% fat and 43% carbohydrate, or 20% fat and 65% carbohydrate. However, in many studies in which total daily energy expenditure was measured while the proportions of CHO and fat in the diet differed substantially, slightly higher energy expenditures on high-carbohydrate than on high-fat diets have been observed, though the differences were not statistically significant (23–25). Since a 15% difference in net ATP yields, applied to the proportion of carbohydrate exchanged for fat, would only lead to a relatively minor difference in overall expenditure, this effect remains uncertain.

The increase in resting energy expenditure, i.e., the thermic effect of food (TEF) elicited by protein consumption, varies between 20 and 30% (26,27). The ATP required to absorb and transport dietary amino acids into cells and then to convert them into protein may be estimated at about 5.5 mol of ATP per mole of mixed amino acids. If the amino acids are oxidized instead, the ATP expenditure for transport, urgeagenesis, and gluconeogenesis also comes to about 5.5 mol of ATP (14,28). The TEF of protein is therefore essentially the same when either (or any combination) of these two processes is involved, i.e., (5.5 × 22.5 kcal/ATP replaced)/(110 g × 4.70 kcal/g) = 25% (29). However, depending on the proportion of amino acids initially converted into protein, subsequent costs for protein turnover will vary, until an amount of amino acids equivalent to that initially incorporated into protein has in turn been degraded and converted into glucose and urea. Protein intake can thus be expected to influence energy expenditure beyond the postprandial phase. For instance, in patients receiving fixed amounts of energy by intravenous infusion, but in whom 0.31 g of dextrose/kg body weight/day was replaced by an equicaloric amount of amino acids (to provide 364 instead of 180 mg of amino acid nitrogen/kg body weight/day), an increase in energy expenditure of 2.2 kcal/kg/day was observed (30). This is equivalent to 40% of the energy content of the additional dose of amino acids. Considering that the amino acids were provided intravenously, and that there was a concomitant decrease in metabolic costs for handling glucose, one would expect dietary protein to raise the metabolic rate by an amount approaching half of its energy content.

Based on the "best guesses" described above, the ATP expended for substrate handling (transport, storage, recycling, and activation) dissipates about 10%, 25%, or 45% of the ATP produced in the metabolic degradation of dietary fat, carbohydrate, or protein, respectively. The *net ATP yields* are thus estimated to decline from 90% with fat, to 75% with carbohydrate, and 55% with protein. On this basis, a change in protein intake from 75 g to 100 g/day would be expected to increase energy expenditure by about 50 kcal/day. Depending on the composition of the diet consumed and the time elapsed after food intake, the cost for replacing 1 mol of ATP would be expected to vary between 20 and 22 kcal. This is some 10–20% more than the 18 kcal released per mole of ATP turned over.

3. Cost for Glucose Conversion to Fat

Several reactions in the fatty acid synthesizing pathway require ATP, so conversion of glucose into fat requires a substantial energy investment. If the costs for prior conversion of glucose into glycogen, as well as for the transport of fatty acid synthesized in the liver to adipose tissue, are also included, the cost for conversion of dietary carbohydrate into fat may be assessed at some 25% (6,31). In subjects consuming a Western diet, fatty acid synthesis from glucose appears to be of minor quantitative significance (32), as even the ingestion of an unusually large carbohydrate load of 500 g is accommodated by expansion of the glycogen reserves, without increases in body fat (33). Contrary to still commonly held expectations, dissipation of dietary energy by conversion of glucose into fat is therefore not a reason why high-carbohydrate diets are less conducive to obesity than high-fat diets.

4. Costs for Maintaining Energy Reserves

The costs for nutrient storage include not only the ATP expenditure required for their initial incorporation into the body's stores, but also those involved in maintaining and moving the tissues that contain these reserves. The resting metabolic rate increases by about 7–10 kcal/day/kg of additional body weight in adult women and men (34). Due to the cost of moving the additional weight, this causes a greater increase in energy expenditure, however, ranging from 10–15 in sedentary to 20–30 kcal/day/kg of additional body weight in moderately to very active individuals. Typically it takes about 1 year for these costs to be equal to the initial energy investment. The degree of physical activity is thus another factor affecting the cost of energy storage, even though it does not imply any

change in the efficiency with which metabolic processes or ATP turnover occurs. Furthermore, the self-correcting effect that changes in body weight exert in compensating for deviations from the energy balance are greater in physically active and in "fidgety" subjects (35) than in sedentary individuals, a phenomenon that totally escapes detection when resting metabolic rates are compared.

5. Futile Cycles

Interconversion of intracellular substrates can cause ATP dissipation if they involve ATP-consuming reactions (e.g., fructose-1,6-diphosphate hydrolysis by fructose diphosphatase and resynthesis by phosphofructokinase). Such *substrate cycles* that cause no net change in the organism but dissipate ATP have sometimes been referred to as *futile cycles*. Elaborate mechanisms have evolved to regulate the activity of enzymes involved in catalyzing opposite transformation to prevent high rates of wasteful substrate interconversions. Complete suppression of these interconversions is not always achieved, however, as it may not be compatible with the quick responses needed to allow for rapid changes in ATP production when needed (36). Other intracellular substrate cycles include interconversions of glucose and glucose-6-P, or synthesis and breakdown of phosphoenolpyruvate by enzymes involved in the gluconeogenic pathway. When fatty acids are produced by triglyceride hydrolysis in adipose tissue, some are reesterified on the spot. In spite of this, FFA are released from adipose tissue in amounts greater than used for energy production; the excess is reesterified in the liver, to be reexported to adipose tissue in the form of lipoproteins (12). This also causes ATP dissipation without net change in the system, but the fact that lipolysis proceeds at higher than minimal rates helps to ensure an adequate supply of circulating FFA and promotes fat oxidation, since it is enhanced by high circulating FFA levels (37). It has been difficult to design tracer studies capable of providing accurate estimates of some of these substrate cycling rates, but the available information suggests that they account for only a few percent of total energy expenditure (38). The increase in peripheral substrate mobilization caused by higher catecholamine levels during overfeeding and the increased release of various mobilizing hormones during periods of stress cause an increase in substrate traffic, which may account for about one-fourth of the rise in resting metabolic rates under these conditions (39).

There has also been interest in examining the possibility that transfer of reducing equivalents from mitochondrial to cytoplasmic NADH, through a set of reactions involving glycerol-3-phosphate dehydrogenase (GPDH), may alter metabolic efficiency, since only two, instead of three, high-energy bonds can be generated from cytoplasmic NADH (40). Overexpression of GPDH in transgenic mice considerably reduces their body fat content (41), but the extent to which this enzyme affects the turnover of reducing-equivalent is unknown. Its influence would be reflected in the resting metabolic rates, as are the effects of futile cycles.

The activity of substrate cycles tends to be enhanced by thyroid hormones (42) and their potential role in energy dissipation has therefore been of some interest. However, their impact on energy expenditure is far less than that of the ATP-dependent sodium extrusion constantly carried out by the cell membranes' sodium-potassium ATPase, which may account for some 20% of basal energy expenditure, though data to establish this with some certainty are not available (43). Proton leakage through the mitochondrial membrane also demands a certain rate of substrate oxidation at rest to maintain a proton gradient sufficient to drive ATP resynthesis, which in isolated hepatocytes was found to account for 20% of resting energy expenditure (4). Even though these two phenomena do not result in changes in the system, one cannot really consider them to be "futile", since they are essential in maintaining membrane potentials and cell integrity. Increases in sodium-potassium ATPase activity induced by thyroxine suggests that enhanced Na^+ pumping may account for increases in energy expenditure caused by elevation of thyroxine levels, though a high number of ATPase molecules does not by itself cause or prove that Na^+ fluxes are increased. Thyroid status also appears to affect the rate of proton leakage through the mitochondrial membrane (44).

C. Metabolic Efficiency

When compared to daily energy turnover, the amount of energy retained during growth and during the development of obesity is rather small, amounting to a difference of only a few percent between intake and expenditure. Because a positive energy balance can, in principle, be attributed to excessive intake or to reduced expenditure, there has been considerable interest in the possible significance of even small differences in *metabolic efficiency* for the development or the prevention of obesity.

Metabolic efficiency can be defined in many ways. The most readily applied approach is to relate physical work output to energy expenditure. During low-intensity exertion, the efficiency of the process appears to be low because most of the energy expended serves to regenerate the ATP dissipated for maintenance metabolism. The intensity of the workload, relative to resting energy expenditure, is thus the major variable determining the apparent

overall metabolic efficiency. To obtain a better measure of metabolic efficiency, it is important to relate the amount of work produced to the change in metabolic rate that it causes. Typical values for the *net efficiency* of aerobic work range from 25 to 27% in humans and animals (2,26). Relating energy deposited in the carcass to total amount of food energy consumed is an important practical consideration in judging *feed efficiency* in the production of meat. As in the case of increasing workloads, overall or *gross nutrient efficiency* rises markedly as the amount of excess energy consumed becomes larger relative to maintenance energy expenditure (Fig. 2). In a situation characterized by rather small changes in body size over time, gross nutrient efficiency is close to zero, which in terms of characterizing potential metabolic differences between lean and obese is essentially meaningless. In trying to assess the efficiency with which food energy is processed, it is therefore important to assess energy retention relative to the amount consumed in excess of maintenance requirements. The accuracy of such an approach is limited,

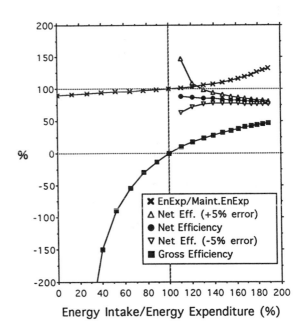

Figure 2 Effect of level of energy intake on "gross" and "net" nutrient efficiencies. Energy expenditure (x) is considered to increase during overfeeding (dissipating 20% of the energy consumed above maintenance requirements) and to decline during underfeeding (attenuating the energy deficit by 5%). "Gross Efficiency" is the % of energy retained relative to energy consumed (■). It is determined primarily by the level of energy intake. "Net Efficiency" (●) is the fraction of energy consumed above maintenance levels that is retained. It is greatly affected by minor errors, i.e., a 5% overestimate (Δ) or a 5% underestimate (∇), particularly in the range of modest excess intakes.

particularly in humans, because the maintenance energy requirements accounts for a rather large fraction of the energy consumed, and because these requirements keep changing as body weight and physical activities vary during the weeks needed to produce measurable changes in body composition. Thus even small errors in estimating maintenance requirements have a considerable impact on the net efficiency value obtained (Fig. 2), and the reliability of such evaluations in characterizing potential differences in metabolic efficiencies is questionable.

Differences in ATP dissipation through ion pumping, futile cycles, and protein turnover are all included in the measured resting metabolic rates. These are closely correlated with the size of the fat-free mass and the fat mass, and resting energy expenditures are thus higher in obese compared to lean subjects of the same heights (45), but a certain degree of variability among individuals remains. The importance often attributed to such differences appears to be founded on the presumption that changes in energy expenditure will not be offset by changes in energy intake. Under conditions where energy intake could be "clamped" at some particular level, a 5% difference in resting energy expenditure would be offset by a difference in body weight of 5–8 kg in a sedentary individual, or less in a physically active individual. When access to food is not restricted, energy balance is determined overwhelmingly by the factors influencing food intake, and by the adjustments in food intake that serve to compensate for recent substrate imbalances, rather than by the overall rate of energy turnover (46). Pregnancy, for instance, leads to the deposition of a few kilograms of additional fat in spite of an increase in resting energy expenditure (47). Arguments about the possible role of minor differences in resting metabolic rates in promoting or preventing obesity and in playing a role in body weight maintenance are therefore hollow, if they are not linked to considerations of the factors controlling energy intake; if they fail to do so, they may end up creating a conceptual trap.

D.   Cold Exposure

Exposure to low environmental temperatures raises energy expenditure and can modify the composition of the fuel mix oxidized. Thus the RQ of ad libitum–fed rats was 0.92 at thermal neutrality, 0.87 during acute cold exposure (acclimation to 25°C and test at 15°C), and 0.77 at chronic cold (acclimation and test at 15°C) (48). This is consistent with other data showing a preferential contribution of lipid to nonshivering thermogenesis in cold-exposed animals (49,50).

The impact of cold exposure has also been studied in humans. Acute exposure to a temperature of 5°C causes resting O_2 consumption to nearly double after 2 hr (51). Under these conditions, changes in the respiratory exchange ratio over the 2 hr of cold exposure were not significant at rest and during exercise. Spending a day in a respiratory chamber at 16°C was perceived to be uncomfortably cool and rectal temperatures in the morning were 0.11°C lower than when the ambient temperature was 24°C. Yet this elicited only a 2% increase in 24-hr energy expenditure, covered by increased glucose oxidation (52). When one considers that individuals generally adjust clothing when exposed to cold, the changes in resting energy expenditure induced by a cold environment are not likely to be substantial. Since a wide range of cold exposures can be survived, the use of glucose obviously can adjust itself to carbohydrate intake, regardless of the stimuli that may cause changes in the RQ at the onset of cold exposure. However, one may keep in mind some incidental observations, whose validity remains to be established. For instance, cold exposure may elicit vigorous movements reflecting efforts to restore blood flow and to raise body temperature, or on the contrary, it may inhibit motion. There also seems to be a prevailing perception of increased hunger when exposed to cold, and of a tendency to gain fat during the cold season.

II.   MEASUREMENT OF SUBSTRATE OXIDATION AND ENERGY EXPENDITURE

Changes in the body's substrate content due to metabolism can be calculated from CO_2 production, O_2 consumption, and urinary nitrogen excretion data. This experimental approach has provided a wealth of data on human energy expenditure (26,27,53,54). The results of this "indirect calorimetry" are consistent with data obtained by direct measurement of heat production, i.e., "direct calorimetry," but the former has the advantage of providing information on the relative amounts of carbohydrate, fat, and protein used. Attention must be given to careful calibrations, to permit accurate determinations of the respiratory quotient, and hence of the relative proportions of carbohydrate and fat oxidized. When combined with precise assessment of the amounts of nutrients consumed, indirect calorimetry allows establishment of substrate or nutrient balances over periods of one or several days, which are far too small to be established by body composition measurements. During recent years, indirect calorimetry has been complemented by the application of the doubly labeled water (DLW) technique, which has allowed determination of energy expenditure (but not substrate balances) in free-living subjects (45).

A. 24-hr Energy Expenditure by Indirect Calorimetry Using Metabolic Chambers

Modern gas analyzers and on-line data processing have stimulated the construction of respiratory chambers in which subjects can be studied over 24-hr periods or for several consecutive days with reasonable comfort, though in a confined environment in which sedentary behavior can be modified by prescribed amounts of exercise on a treadmill or equivalent device (53). Reproducible measurements of daily energy expenditure can be achieved that are accurate within a few percent. Under the best conditions, errors in carbohydrate and fat balances can be reduced to ± 20 and ± 10 g/day, respectively (55). Numerous studies have been performed to quantify daily energy expenditure and substrate balances, notably to compare differences in energy expenditure in lean and obese subjects and the effects of overfeeding. It was found, among other things, that a high 24-hr RQ is a risk factor for long-term body weight gain (56,57). Twenty-four-hour indirect calorimetry also provides a means to study the adjustment of the fuel mix oxidized to changes in the diet's composition (24,25,58). Other important results relate to the role of sympathetic nervous system activity on daily macronutrient utilization (59) and to the measurement of net lipogenesis induced by deliberate and sustained overconsumption of carbohydrates (31).

B. 24-hr Energy Expenditure Based on Heart Rate Measurements

Continuous heart rate monitoring offers a possibility to measure energy expenditure around the clock, but it requires that the relationship between heart rate and oxygen consumption be established individually. The approach has been validated by concomitant indirect calorimetry and doubly labeled water (DLW) measurements (60,61). This "heart rate O_2 method" has been successfully used in trained and untrained individuals to measure daily energy expenditure and compensations in nonprescribed daily activities (62).

C. Energy Turnover in Free-Living Subjects

The lack of means to assess energy expenditure and substrate oxidation under free-living conditions has long been a major barrier for obesity research. This problem was finally resolved thanks to a method conceived by Lifson et al. in the 1950s (63) to assess energy expenditure in small animals. It is based on the administration of an initial dose of $^2H_2^{18}O$. The difference in the rate of ^{18}O elimination, which is lost in water and CO_2, relative to the rate of deuterium (^2H) elimination, lost as water only, allows assessment of the CO_2 production rate, which correlates closely with oxygen consumption and energy expenditure (64). It took nearly three decades before the first paper describing the application of this DLW technique in humans was published (65). A number of methodological problems and potential pitfalls were encountered, leading on occasion to physiologically impossible results. Comparison of results obtained by several groups of investigators have confirmed the validity of the method, and the conditions and calculations for its successful applications have been defined with increasing detail (66).

Measurements of energy turnover by the DLW method in sedentary subjects led to downward revisions of common assumptions about minimum maintenance requirements (67). Other studies (68) led to a reduction of the additional energy allowances during pregnancy from 500 to 300 kcal/day (47). The long-held belief about the low maintenance energy requirements in overweight "small eaters" was shown to be attributable to underreporting of habitual food intake (45,69,70). It also became possible to assess energy expenditure under conditions of extreme physical demand, demonstrating energy turnovers reaching 5000–8000 kcal/day in bicycle racers (71). Roberts et al. found energy expenditure to be lower in babies born to obese parents compared to those born to lean parents (72). According to Goran and Poehlman, the technique can be used to evaluate compensations in energy expenditure in response to exercise training (73).

D. Diet-Induced Thermogenesis

Diet-induced thermogenesis (DIT) includes all increases in resting energy expenditure induced by food consumption, which comprise the thermic effect of food (TEF) as well as increases in energy expenditure between meals that may be induced by food consumption, in particular by excessive food consumption. In humans, most of these increments in resting energy expenditure are explained by "obligatory" factors such as digestion, metabolism, and storage of macronutrients including the cost for the synthesis of the constituents of newly formed tissues, and the physiological processes that are essential for their maintenance. "Nonobligatory" or "facultative" components contributing to DIT are catecholamine-mediated increases in energy expenditure elicited by carbohydrate consumption during the TEF and the stimulation of substrate oxidation in brown adipose tissue (BAT) through activation of a protein-conducting pathway elicited by sympathetic nervous system innervation, which has the effect of uncoupling substrate oxidation from oxidation phosphorylation (7,8). The quantitative importance of facultative thermogenesis can be substantial in animals, and suppression of BAT thermogenesis greatly enhances the development of obesity in animals (9).

Investigations into the physiological role of BAT in humans have not yielded comparable results. Although the presence of BAT has been demonstrated in humans (74), experimental evidence suggests that skeletal muscle is the main site of cold-influenced thermogenesis (75). A number of overfeeding studies have been performed to evaluate the potential role of DIT in human studies in which energy expenditure was directly measured either by indirect calorimetry or by the DLW method, but dissipation of excess dietary energy through *Luxuskonsumption* (a term sometimes used to describe elevated DIT during overfeeding) could not be detected. Most of the increases in 24-hr energy expenditure that were found during overfeeding could be explained by the cost of substrate handling, tissue accretion, and maintenance of an enlarged body (76–79).

E.   Physical Activity

The metabolic changes observed during and for many hours after exercise can substantially modify macronutrient utilization and energy expenditure. As depicted in Figure 3, RQ increases during exercise, indicating that carbohydrate is the main substrate contributing to the increase in energy production. Figure 3 also illustrates that the RQ during exercise is influenced by numerous factors such as the intensity and duration of exercise. It is well established that RQ is increased to a greater extent by high than low to moderate intensity exercise (80) and that the RQ progressively declines when exercise duration is increased. Exercise RQ also tends to be lower in trained than in nontrained individuals (81).

Resting RQ can be reduced for 15–20 hr after prolonged vigorous exercise (82,83). However, no data are currently available to establish how long and how much the resting RQ is decreased after exercise. Since high-intensity exertion is as effective in inducing fat loss as aerobic work (84), one can infer that high-intensity exercise must have a substantial effect in enhancing postexercise lipid oxidation. This may be due to the glycogen depletion it induces, but another important observation is that high-intensity training increases the potential of skeletal muscle to oxidize lipid to a greater extent than aerobic exercise of moderate intensity, at least as judged by the rise in muscle β-hydroxyacyl-CoA degydrogenase (HADH) activity (84).

Since exercise permits weight maintenance at lower degrees of adiposity, it substitutes for an expansion of the fat mass in bringing about rates of fat oxidation commensurate with fat intake. The overall effect of exercise is therefore to increase fat oxidation more than glucose oxidation (85). Human subjects who are high fat oxidizers during exercise consumed less food when they subsequently could eat at will, and they were more likely to be in negative energy and lipid balance compared to low fat oxidizers (86,87). Of particular interest is the hypothesis that exercise is likely to induce greater fat losses in obese individuals who have a high capacity to oxidize fat during and after exercise. The potential link between exercise-induced changes in substrate oxidation and postexercise energy intake and balance needs to be investigated.

F.   Variability of Daily Energy Expenditures, Intakes, and Balances

Daily energy expenditures of subjects confined to a respiratory chambers are substantially lower than in free-living subjects (88,89), and the spontaneous variations in physical activity associated with free-living conditions cannot manifest themselves. On the other hand, DLW measurements that provide assessment of overall energy expenditure over periods of 7–10 days do not resolve variations in energy expenditure from day to day. Future methodological developments may permit us to assess substrate oxidation under free-living conditions, a potential suggested by recent animal studies (90). These variations must be evaluated on the basis of estimates calculated from activity logs. Much more data are available on daily food intakes. Bingham et al. (91) found the coefficients of variation for daily food intake to vary greatly among individuals, with an average value of ±22%. It seems to be generally held that variations in food intake

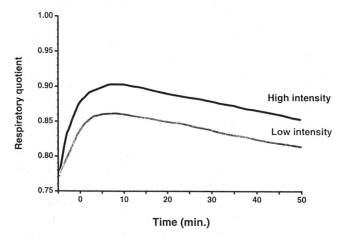

Figure 3   Variations in respiratory quotient during low- and high-intensity exercise. (Adapted from Ref. 80.)

are substantially greater than variations in energy expenditure. Deviations from the energy balance are thus probably comparable in size to the variability in intakes. The extent of daily variations in food intake, energy expenditure, and the size of daily deviations from energy balance could potentially influence body weight maintenance, inasmuch as changes in food intake in response to positive or negative energy balances may not occur with the same accuracy (92).

III. FACTORS DETERMINING SUBSTRATE OXIDATION RATES

Overall energy expenditure is determined by an individual's size and physical activity and is only modestly affected by nutrient intake. Amino acid oxidation rates vary only moderately, increasing somewhat after protein ingestion (15) and during vigorous exertion (93), but declining when protein intakes are reduced. By contrast, the organism has considerable freedom in modifying the relative contributions made by glucose and FFA to the fuel mix oxidized. Such great flexibility in fuel utilization is made possible by the ability of most cells to interchangeably use metabolic intermediates derived from carbohydrates, fats, and proteins to regenerate ATP. It allows adaptation to food supplies varying widely in their macronutrient distribution (provided proteins provide at least some 10%, and essential fatty acids at least 1% of total energy) (47).

A. Substrate Oxidation by Different Tissues

The contribution made by various tissues to the body's oxygen consumption, or in effect to overall energy turnover, is described in Table 2 (14), but their contribution to overall fuel utilization depends on their metabolic functions (94). The central nervous system's (CNS) rate of energy expenditure is particularly high for its size (2% of body weight), as it accounts for nearly 20% of resting energy expenditure in adults (95). Since it cannot use FFA, it is critically dependent on an adequate supply of glucose (about 80 mg/min). However, after adaptation to starvation, ketone bodies can provide about two-thirds of the brain's energy needs (96). Red blood cells also depend on glucose, as they lack mitochondria and must generate ATP by substrate-level phosphorylation during glucose degradation to lactate. They use about 1 g of glucose per hour (95,97), but this has very little impact on the body's fuel economy, since 98% is converted to lactate (97), which can be reconverted into glucose by the liver.

About one-quarter of resting energy expenditure occurs in the splanchnic bed (98). It has become evident that the gut derives a substantial part of its energy by partial degradation of glutamine, its glucogenic moiety reaching the liver (28). Conversion of the glucogenic moieties of the amino acids is a feature of amino acid degradation even under fed conditions (28). One can therefore presume that conversion of pyruvate to acetyl-CoA in the liver is effectively inhibited during most of the day, a conclusion that is consistent with the lack of hepatic fatty acid synthesis under habitual living conditions (32).

The heart accounts for some 10% of resting energy expenditure. Its constant and critical requirement for fuel is aptly matched by its ability to utilize all types of substrates that may be available, including notably some of the lactate produced by working skeletal muscles. Although skeletal muscles make up three-quarters of the body cell mass (BCM), the muscle accounts for only 20–30% of energy expenditure at rest (95). During exertion, substrate oxidation in the muscle mass can increase 20-fold (Table 2) (14), with the increase being even greater in particular muscle groups. In the postabsorptive state, fatty acids are the main oxidized fuel in muscle (94,99), whereas during exertion, great demands are initially placed on the muscles' own glycogen reserve, with a subsequent shift toward increasingly greater use of fatty acids, mobilized from muscle fat stores as well as from adipose tissue (Fig. 3). Since muscle is ready to oxidize fatty acids as well as glucose (37,100), exercise enhances the body's ability to adjust the use of glucose and fatty acids to the dietary supply (Fig. 4). This may explain why fat oxidation can more readily keep up with fat intake in physically active adults and in most children and adolescents as they are naturally more active than adults.

B. Glucose Turnover and Glucose Oxidation

Some of the glucose utilized by various tissues is converted to lactate (*Cori cycle*) or to alanine (*glucose-alanine*

Table 2 Relative Oxygen Consumption of Different Tissues[a]

	At rest	Light work	Heavy work
Brain	0.20	0.20	0.20
Abdominal organs	0.25	0.24	0.24
Kidneys	0.07	0.06	0.07
Skin	0.02	0.06	0.08
Heart	0.11	0.23	0.40
Skeletal muscles	0.30	2.05	6.95
Other	0.05	0.06	0.06
Total	1.00	3.00	8.00

[a]Whole body at rest = 1.00; actual value near 3.8 ml O_2 min^{-1} kg^{-1}.
Source: Adapted from Ref. 14.

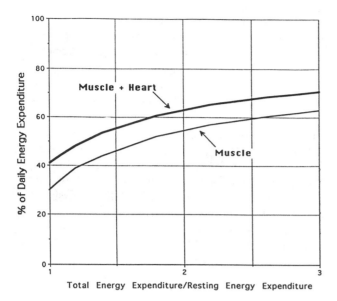

Figure 4 Impact of physical activity (described as the ratio of total to resting energy expenditure) on the contribution of skeletal and heart muscle metabolism to total energy turnover. (Calculated from the information provided in Table 2, assuming that half of the exercise-induced increase in energy expenditure is due to work of light and half to work of heavy intensity.)

cycle), which are readily reconverted into glucose by the liver. Glucose turnover is thus substantially greater than the rate of glucose oxidation. Carbohydrate oxidation determined by indirect calorimetry describes the change in the body's carbohydrate content. The energy content of glycogen (4.18 kcal/g) and of glucose (3.7 kcal/g) differ by 10% (because 1 mol of water is removed when glucose is incorporated into the glycogen or starch). It is thus important to be consistent and to specify which of the two is being considered. During the degradation of amino acid mixtures, 55–60 g of glucose is generated by gluconeogenesis from 100 g of protein, even in the fed state when plenty of glucose is available (28). In indirect calorimetry calculations, the oxidation of the glucose formed by gluconeogenesis from amino acids is included in the coefficients describing CO_2 production and oxygen consumption from protein. Glucose oxidation determined with the help of tracers is thus measurably greater than "carbohydrate disappearance" established by indirect calorimetry. Similarly, the glycerol liberated during the oxidation of triglycerides (about 10 g/100 g of triglycerides, or 5% of the triglyceride energy) is converted into glucose before being oxidized, the CO_2 produced and the oxygen consumed being again included in the coefficients for fat oxidation. This is why the RQ for triglyceride oxidation is slightly higher (by about 0.007) than that for fatty acid oxidation (13).

C. Starvation Ketosis

The body's glycogen reserves are limited to a few hundred grams (101) and during periods of starvation or marked carbohydrate deprivation they can provide enough glucose to the brain for only a few days (96,102). Survival during starvation is made possible by the induction of ketogenesis in the liver, when insulin levels become very low and FFA levels concomitantly rise (103). Acetoacetate plus β-hydroxy-butyrate production reaches 100–120 g/day by the third day of total starvation. Circulating ketone body levels rise only progressively, as some are used by skeletal muscle during the initial days of starvation, since muscle is ready to use ketone bodies whenever they are produced, for example during prolonged physical effort. When starvation ketosis is fully developed, ketone body levels reach a plateau of 5–6 mM. At this level, they provide about two-thirds of the brain's fuel needs, but 5–15 g of β-hydroxy-butyrate and acetoacetate is lost in the urine per day. The urinary loss of limited amounts of these anions can be offset by excretion of N in the form of ammonium instead of urea, as this provides the cations needed, thereby preventing the development of metabolic acidosis (96). In the total absence of insulin, ketone levels rise to far higher levels, in part because the overabundance of circulating fuels decreases peripheral ketone body utilization. Urinary losses then become far greater, leading to metabolic acidosis.

D. Regulation of Substrate Oxidation

In view of the critical need to maintain high ATP levels, of the functional importance of proteins, and of the need to ensure a sufficient supply of glucose for the brain, the main goals for metabolic fuel regulation are to assure the distribution of substrates in amounts sufficient to support oxidative phosphorylation at the required rates, to maintain homeostasis, and to bring about the use of metabolic fuels in such proportions as to minimize changes in protein content and to maintain glycogen levels within a desirable range. This is detrimental to the body's ability to regulate the fat balance (104), which is not a problem in the short term, since such gains or losses of fat are very small in comparison to the body's large fat stores (50,000–200,000 kcal in adults and even more in obese subjects). However, if the fat balance is not accurately regulated, neither is the overall energy balance.

1. Hormonal Regulation of Substrate Availability

The composition of the fuel mix oxidized is mainly controlled by adjustment of circulating substrate and hormone levels. These levels are markedly influenced by nutrient intake. The impact of changes in substrate levels on their rates of utilization during the postprandial phase is enhanced by the release of insulin, which promotes transport and storage of glucose, amino acids, and fats, while inhibiting the release of glucose from the liver and of fatty acids from adipose tissue. The decline in circulating FFA levels brought about by the antilipolytic action of insulin complemented by the direct and indirect effects of insulin in activating pyruvate dehydrogenase (PDH) (105) leads to an increase in glucose oxidation and to a commensurate decrease in fatty acid oxidation. The decline in insulin secretion when glucose absorption from the gut is completed, complemented by the release of catecholamines and glucagon, activates the mobilization of the body's glycogen and fat reserves to assure an adequate supply of glucose and of FFA in the circulation (106,107). These effects are greatly enhanced when the demand for metabolic fuels is magnified by physical efforts.

2. Body Composition and Fuel Composition

Between meals and efforts, the composition of the fuel mix oxidized is influenced by the size of the body's protein pools, the degree of repletion of its glycogen reserves, and the size and distribution of the adipose tissue depots. This is the simple consequence of the fact that the influence of hormones on substrate fluxes is determined by the intensity of the endocrine signals *multiplied* by the size of the targets they influence, and that hormone secretion is itself influenced by prevailing substrate levels.

The gains or losses that occur when the oxidation of glucose, FFA, and amino acids do not match their intakes lead to changes in body composition, until the impact of these changes on the composition of the fuel mixture oxidized complements the body's endocrine and enzymatic regulatory phenomena in such a way that the fuel mix oxidized matches, on average, the macronutrient distribution in the diet (108). As evidenced by the stability of body composition commonly observed, the effect of these changes in bringing about the adjustment of fuel composition to nutrient intake is universal and remarkably effective, but the body composition for which this adjustment is achieved can vary greatly between individuals, depending on interactions between inherited and circumstantial factors (107).

3. Adjustment of Amino Acid Oxidation to Protein Intake

The ability to quantify changes in the body's protein content by monitoring the nitrogen (N) balance has led to the early recognition of the organism's tendency to maintain a stable protein content, or to allow for an appropriate rate of protein accretion during growth or recovery from disease or undernutrition. This occurs regardless of differences in the carbohydrate-to-fat ratio of the diet. Detailed metabolic studies during starvation have revealed how the organism is able to minimize protein losses during food deprivation (96). Its regulatory features also enable it to avoid needless and costly buildup of its protein content when high-protein diets are consumed, but the mechanisms accounting for this are not well understood. Daily protein intakes, generally between 50 and 100 g in adults, are small compared to the body's total protein content, of which about half (some 6 kg) is intracellular and engaged in active turnover. When changing from situations of high to low protein intake, or vice versa, a few days are required before N balance is again achieved. The small gains or losses of proteins that are thereby incurred appear to be prerequisites for the reestablishment of N balance, demonstrating that relatively minor changes in protein content play a significant role in the adjustment of amino acid oxidation rates to protein intake. Small gains or losses of protein thus appear able to influence amino acid oxidation and to bring about the corrective responses needed to compensate for the small deviations from even N balance that occur from day to day.

4. Adjustment of Glucose Oxidation to Carbohydrate Intake—Influence of Glycogen Stores

The body's glycogen stores (200–500 g in adults) (101) are not much larger than the amount of carbohydrate usually consumed in 1 day. In view of the importance of the hepatic glycogen stores in maintaining stable blood glucose levels and of muscle glycogen availability in permitting appropriate muscular responses to sudden demands, biological evolution was compelled to develop regulatory mechanisms (including endocrine signals) that give high priority to the adjustment of carbohydrate oxidation to carbohydrate availability (108,109). Glucose oxidation thus declines rapidly when ingestion of food fails to replenish the glycogen reserves in a timely fashion. On the other hand, the body's metabolism quickly shifts to the predominant use of glucose after carbohydrate ingestion. This manifests itself by a prompt postprandial rise in the respiratory quotient (RQ) to an extent and for periods determined by the amounts and the types of carbohydrates consumed. This response is important since inappropriate curtailment of fat oxidation when carbohydrates provide the bulk of food energy would lead to a negative fat balance or require substantial de novo fat synthesis (at substantial metabolic cost) during part of the day. After large carbohydrate intakes, high rates of carbohydrate oxidation persist for many hours, allowing dissipation of the built-up glycogen reserves (33). If massive consumption of carbohydrates is deliberately kept up for several days, glycogen stores become saturated and further accumulation is prevented by conversion of glucose into fat, which may drive the overall RQ to values greater than 1.0 (31). However, the regulation of appetite is such that glycogen levels are spontaneously maintained far below the range at which de novo lipogenesis is induced, and loss of carbohydrate by conversion into fat is quantitatively insignificant (less than 5 g/day) in adults consuming mixed diets (32).

The degree of repletion of the body's glycogen stores thus greatly influences the contribution made by glucose to the fuel mix oxidized. Gains or losses of glycogen are therefore effective in bringing about changes in glucose oxidation when the influx of carbohydrate varies (24,110) or when physical exertion has caused unusual glycogen depletion. As in the case of protein, this is in part a simple mass effect, since insulin is less effective in curtailing glucose release from the liver when the hepatic glycogen reserves have been built up (111).

5. Adjustment of Fat Oxidation to Fat Intake—Influence of Adipose Tissue Mass and Distribution

As a consequence of the fact that amino acid and glucose oxidation rates adjust themselves to the amounts of protein and carbohydrate consumed, fat oxidation is determined primarily by the gap between total energy expenditure and the amounts of energy ingested in the form of carbohydrates and proteins (46). Fat oxidation rates are thus set primarily by parameters unrelated to the body's fat economy, rather than by the amounts of fat consumed. Furthermore, short-term gains or losses of fat are so small in comparison to the body's large fat stores that they are unlikely to elicit changes in food intake or in fat oxidation. Given the lack of direct regulatory mechanisms serving to adjust fat oxidation to fat intake (112), one may wonder why body fat content should nevertheless tend to remain fairly constant, even when diets differing widely in fat content are consumed.

Various factors contribute to this adjustment. For instance, if fat replaces carbohydrate in meals, the postprandial inhibition of fat oxidation is lessened, since the postprandial rise in RQ is related primarily to the amount of carbohydrate consumed. The presence of fat in a meal delays its absorption and this will also attenuate the postprandial rise in the RQ. When meals containing very large amounts of fat are consumed (e.g., 80 g), some of the fatty acids liberated from chylomicrons by lipoprotein lipase escape capture by adipose cells and enter the pool of circulating FFA, promoting fat oxidation, though only modestly (e.g., 10 g in 6 hr) (113). Finally, glycogen levels may tend to be maintained in a lower range when the proportion of carbohydrate in the diet is reduced, resulting in lower insulin levels and hence higher rates of FFA release and oxidation between meals (24). However, this cannot be expected to produce an exact compensation, since FFA levels and oxidation rates are controlled by insulin, whose secretion is determined primarily by the need to maintain appropriate blood glucose levels.

While short-term errors in the fat balance are too small to affect the size of the body's fat stores, circulating FFA levels, fat oxidation, or food intake, the cumulative effects of repeated imbalances between fat intake and fat oxidation can in time lead to substantial changes in the size of the adipose tissue mass. Expansion of the fat mass leads to higher FFA levels and turnover (114). The role that changes in the adipose tissue mass plays in the establishment of the steady state of weight maintenance can be inferred by considering the changes in substrate balances induced by a period of food restriction. After a few days on reduced intake and during the first days of the subsequent period of weight regain, further losses or gains of protein and glycogen are minimal and account for only a minor part of the energy imbalance. Due to the contribution made by endogenous fat to the fuel mix oxidized during caloric deprivation, the average RQ is lower than usual during the period of weight loss. During weight regain, on the other hand, the 24-h RQ is greater than usual, reflecting the oxidation of a fuel mix containing a higher proportion of glucose than the diet, as part of the fat consumed is stored. At some point, the situation is encountered for which the two conditions necessary for weight maintenance are again satisfied; i.e., food intake is commensurate with energy expenditure and the average RQ matches the diet's *food quotient* (FQ), which describes the ratio of CO_2 produced to O_2 consumed during the biological oxidation of a representative sample of the diet (29,108). What one would like to know in this regard is whether this should be attributed to the increase in energy expenditure associated with weight gain, or whether some other phenomenon is involved.

This issue could be precisely examined in mice (Fig. 5) (107). The unusually elevated rate of food consumption following a period of food restriction abated when the fat mass had regained its initial size. The balance between energy expenditure and food intake was not achieved by an increase in energy expenditure due to weight gain, but by a decrease in food consumption, as the degree of adiposity was approached, for which the RQ became again equal to the FQ. Enlargement of the fat depots thus promotes fat oxidation, just as filled glycogen stores promote glucose oxidation (25,111), but the increase in fat oxidation brought about by expansion of the adipose tissue mass is "chronic" rather than related to recent food consumption. This chronic effect can be enhanced by a type of insulin resistance typically induced by excessive fat accumulation, whose effect is to promote fatty acid, but to inhibit glucose oxidation (46,57,115). The influence of the adipose tissue mass on the composition of the fuel mix oxidized explains why the particular body composition will in time be reached (or approached) for which the fat oxidation is commensurate with fat intake.

6. Alcohol Intake and Oxidation

Alcohol is not generally considered to contribute greatly to dietary energy intake, but alcohol sales data indicate that alcohol provides about 5% of overall energy intake in the United States. In the Quebec Family Study, alcohol energy represented 17% and 11% of daily energy intake of adult males and females, respectively, in the upper quartile for the alcohol intake (116).

Many epidemiological studies have investigated the association between alcohol consumption and the intake of macronutrients. Some reported a negative association between alcohol and carbohydrate intake (116,117); others found reduced protein, fat, and carbohydrate intake in moderate alcohol drinkers (118). However, other studies showed that energy and macronutrient intakes were not altered by alcohol intake, suggesting that alcohol energy often represents just an additional source of dietary energy (119–123). Studies on the impact of alcohol intake on energy expenditure show that the thermic effect of alcohol is slightly higher than that of carbohydrate, but lower than that of protein (124). Alcohol drives its oxidation, regardless of the level of other fuels, but only up to a rate that covers a minor fraction of total energy turnover. The maximal rate of alcohol oxidation varies among individuals, being generally higher in men than in women and enhanced in habitual alcohol consumers (125). In examining the impact of alcohol oxidation on the use of other fuels, one sees that its main effect is to reduce fat oxidation (123,126). The inhibitory effect of alcohol on fat oxidation means that alcohol intake is equivalent to fat intake in influencing the fat and energy balances. Alcohol consumption was indeed found to raise total energy intake,

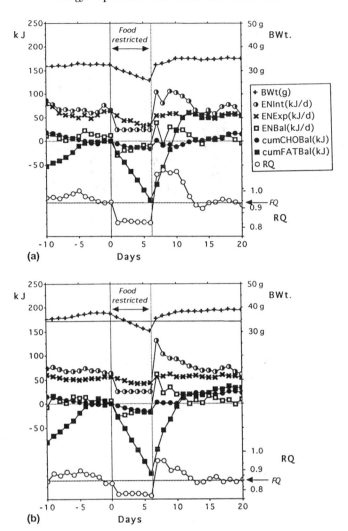

Figure 5 Effect of temporary food restriction on body fat and glycogen content in mice. Shown are average body weights, cumulative carbohydrate and fat balances, and daily energy expenditures, intakes and balances in two groups of five female CD1 mice, during a 6-day period of food restriction to 40% of average ad libitum intake, and during the preceding and following days of ad libitum intake. One group was maintained on a diet containing 13% (a), the other on a diet containing 41% (b) of dietary energy as fat, 19% as casein and the balance as cornstarch plus sucrose (1:1). (Reproduced with permission from Ref. 107.)

particularly when a high-fat diet was consumed (Fig. 6) (116), in a manner that could not be explained by the high-energy density of the items consumed (127). Inactive individuals reporting a high fat and alcohol intake are characterized by increased subcutaneous adiposity, particularly in the trunk area (116).

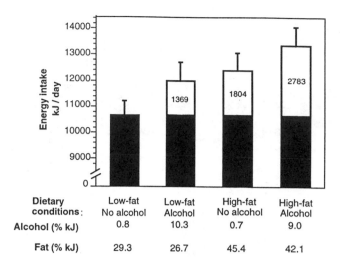

Figure 6   Effect of dietary fat content and alcohol on daily energy intake (means ± SE). (Adapted from Ref. 116.)

IV.   SUBSTRATE BALANCES AND WEIGHT MAINTENANCE

When the steady state of weight maintenance has become established, the concept of *nutrient partitioning* is rather meaningless, since over a period of a few days all the nutrients consumed are oxidized, whereas preferential retention of one type of nutrient varies from day to day, to compensate for short-term deviations from equilibrated substrate balances. It is the nature of these compensatory responses that needs to be examined to understand what brings about body weight stability.

A.   Fuel Composition and Energy Balance

Because of the organism's tendency to adjust glucose oxidation to carbohydrate intake and to maintain stable glycogen stores, the fuel mix oxidized on days during which excess food is consumed is enriched in carbohydrate. This manifests itself by an elevated 24-hr RQ that reveals that fat oxidation is inhibited on such days, in spite of increased intake (108). Excess energy will therefore be retained primarily in the form of fat. When food consumption is insufficient to cover energy expenditure, the substrates obtained from food have to be supplemented by drawing on the body's energy reserves, primarily from endogenous fat, to prevent excessive glycogen losses. The addition of endogenous fat to the fuel mix oxidized causes the 24-hr RQ to be lower than on days during which energy balance is achieved. There is thus a strong positive correlation between the RQ and the energy balance

(108,128,129). Fig. 7 (left panel) shows that the relationship between energy balance and RQ depends on the carbohydrate content of the diet. Full lines show the correlations for diets providing 25, 40, or 55% of dietary energy as fat, assuming that carbohydrate balance is exactly preserved. The slope of these correlations is attenuated when part of the imbalance in the energy balance is absorbed by gains or losses of glycogen, as shown by the dotted lines, based on the assumption that 20% of the energy imbalance is absorbed by changes in the glycogen stores.

B.   RQ/FQ Concept and Energy Balance

To avoid ambiguity about the implications that a particular RQ value may have in judging whether the fuel mix oxidized contains more or less fat than the diet, it is convenient to compare the RQ to the FQ. The relationship between RQ and energy balance can be normalized by considering the RQ/FQ ratio in relation to the ratio of energy intake divided by energy expenditure (Fig. 7, right panel). The fact that the slopes of the lines are slightly different for different diets does not negate the fact that RQ/FQ ratios greater than 1.0 imply positive energy balances, whereas RQ/FQ ratios less than 1.0 indicate negative energy balances. Weight maintenance, which depends on protein, carbohydrate, and fat balances being all close to zero, corresponds to the situation where the respiratory quotient is equal, on average, to the diets' FQ (108).

The need to satisfy the RQ = FQ condition creates constraints in the system, as it shows that a balance must be reached between the influences that the body's glycogen stores and the size of the adipose tissue exert on the relative proportions of glucose and FFA being oxidized (107,108). This creates a reason for a particular degree of fatness to become established as long as an individual's diet and life-style, as well as habitual glycogen levels, are constant (cf. Fig. 5). It is therefore not necessary to postulate the existence of some mysterious set-point to explain body weight stability.

C.   Importance of Food Intake Regulation and Variations in Energy Expenditure in Bringing About Weight Maintenance

Numerous factors capable of influencing food intake have been recognized and studied, but their relative importance and contribution to weight maintenance has been difficult to establish in humans, in whom nonphysiological factors contribute to stabilize or to alter food consumption. Whatever may be involved, it is evident at least that the

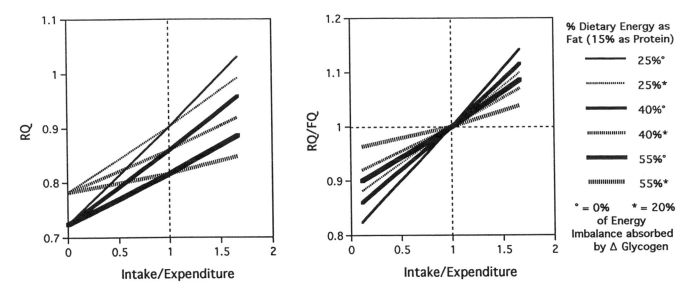

Figure 7 Relationships between the RQ, the RQ/FQ ratio, and energy balance, assuming that carbohydrate balances are equilibrated, or that 20% of the energy imbalances are absorbed by gains or losses of glycogen (dotted lines). (Reproduced with permission from Ref. 129.)

spontaneous drive to eat provides for carbohydrate intakes sufficient to maintain glycogen levels adequate to prevent hypoglycemia and to carry out habitual workloads, and that food intake is spontaneously restrained to keep glycogen levels well below the range for which appreciable rates of de novo lipogenesis would be induced, even when there is free access to a large variety of appetizing foods (31,33). *Diurnal regulation* of food intake effectively serves to avoid overloading of the digestive system, but does not prevent substantial day-to-day deviations from energy and substrate balances nor the existence of individual weekly patterns of food intake (130). Yet individuals reach a plateau at which their body fat content remains nearly constant over prolonged periods. Since changes in energy expenditure can only modestly attenuate the impact of deficient or excessive food consumption, it is changes in food intake that must reverse such deviations. Weight stability is therefore achieved thanks to corrective changes in food consumption that compensate for the deviations from energy balance that occur from day to day in free-living individuals.

D. Factors Influencing Body Composition for Which Substrate Oxidation Matches Nutrient Intake

1. Dietary Fat Content

One of the most significant changes in dietary habits during this century has been a marked increase in the fat content of the diet, which is generally believed to have contributed significantly to the increased incidence of obesity in affluent societies (86,131–133), although other factors (107), notably a reduced level of physical activity, are also important (134). The overfeeding associated with the consumption of mixed diets providing substantial amounts of fat can be attributed in part to the high energy density of high-fat foods (135), to the inability of fat intake to promote fat oxidation (112,136), and to *passive overconsumption* due to the failure of dietary lipid to promote an adequate level of satiety, as suggested by the fact that fat preloads suppress subsequent energy intake less than carbohydrate preloads (137,138). Animal studies show that the steady state of weight maintenance under ad libitum feeding conditions becomes established for higher body fat contents as the fat content of the diet increases, presumably because expansion of the fat mass is required to raise fat oxidation (107,108), supporting the concept that obesity represents an adaptation to high-fat diets (139). A certain predilection for fat in the foods consumed has often been noted in overweight subjects, and epidemiological data show correlations between dietary fat consumption and adiposity (86,131–133).

2. Physical Activity

Vigorous physical activity is known to influence body weight and fat stores and it has been repeatedly observed that obese individuals tend to be less physically active than lean subjects. The Canada Fitness Survey demonstrated that individuals reporting regular practice of vigorous activities were leaner than those not performing such activities (140). In addition, obese individuals who had managed to lose weight and maintained an exercise routine regained less weight than those who did not (141). The negative association between activity level and body fatness was recently described by Rising et al., using the ratio of TEE/REE as an index of physical activity (142).

Intervention studies in which exercise was prescribed show that the weight loss achieved depends on the amount of exercise performed (143). Exercise is most susceptible to induce a negative energy balance in subjects with a high capacity to oxidize fat (87) and when postexercise consumption of high-fat food is avoided (144,145). When the effect of a high-intensity intermittent training program was compared to that of an aerobic training program of moderate intensity (which raised energy expenditure more than twice as much), the former was found to cause a ninefold greater subcutaneous fat loss when expressed per MJ expended in training. In addition, the high-intensity program induced a greater increase in the potential of skeletal muscle to oxidize fatty acids, as judged by muscle β-hydroxy-acylCoA dehydrogenase activity (84).

When fat loss becomes sufficient to decrease fat mobilization and oxidation (85,146), the ability of exercise to induce negative fat and energy balances declines. The effect of exercise in promoting fat oxidation is therefore offset and a new steady state at a lower degree of adiposity is approached.

3. Hormones

Hormones can influence substrate oxidation by altering overall energy expenditure and the relative proportions of amino acids, glucose, and fatty acids being oxidized. The impact on body weight most clearly attributable to hormone-induced changes in energy expenditure occurs in cases of frank hypothyroidism or hyperthyroidism, whereas the effect of other hormones on adiposity is elicited primarily through their influence on the control of food intake and/or substrate metabolism.

In the case of amino acids and glucose, the effect of altered hormone levels or of altered responsiveness to their action can be offset by changes in the size of the protein and amino acid pools, and in glycogen stores and blood glucose levels, without affecting body composition in a readily detectable manner. Hormones that reduce fat oxidation, by inhibiting fat mobilization or by enhancing glucose oxidation, tend to raise the amount of body fat

needed for fat oxidation to become commensurate with fat intake, and this can lead to changes in body composition and body weight that are very much perceived and quantifiable. Insulin is the main hormone curtailing fat oxidation, whereas growth hormone and catecholamines have the opposite effect. An important site for the expression of the antagonistic effects of these hormones is on the regulation of pyruvate dehydrogenase (PDH), the enzyme catalyzing the irreversible step in the oxidation of carbohydrate. Thus, insulin promotes the activation of PDH, whereas increases in FFA and acetyl-CoA levels, elicited by catecholamines and growth hormone or by expansion of the adipose tissue mass, inhibit PDH (105). Interestingly, insulin and FFA levels are both elevated in obesity. The balance between the effects of elevated insulin and FFA levels on PDH activity would appear to have some importance, since body weight gain over several years tends to be less in obese subjects exhibiting insulin resistance (115).

The effect of β-adrenergic agonists tends to be more pronounced on lipid oxidation than on thermogenesis, whereas administration of β-blockers such as propranolol over a 2-week period resulted in a decrease in daily lipid oxidation that was three times greater than the decrease in energy expenditure, while carbohydrate oxidation was increased (59). Acute stimulation of sympathetic activity by exposing the lower body to negative pressure was found to induce a substantial increase in lipid oxidation, whereas energy expenditure was not altered (147). According to the RQ/FQ concept (108,129), a decrease in the use of fat relative to glucose is likely to increase food consumption, and a high RQ has indeed been a predictor for weight gain (56,57).

The situation is in reality much more complex than it appears by considering only the effects of hormones on peripheral fuel metabolism, notably because the neurosystems involved in the regulation of food intake are also influenced by insulin (148). Furthermore, hyperinsulinemia increases plasma noradrenaline (149) and muscle sympathetic nerve activity (150,151). Increases in sympathetic activity decrease energy intake and stimulate thermogenesis (7,8,152). However, since muscle sympathetic nerve activity represents only one component of sympathetic nervous system activity, it is not yet possible to generalize from this peripheral effect. In addition, high insulin levels in the CNS inhibit food intake (153), in part by inhibiting the fasting-related increase in the synthesis and release of neuropeptide Y (154), a peptide known to increase energy intake and to reduce thermogenesis (155). The hyperinsulinemia brought about by enlargement of the fat stores thus tends to restrain further weight gain through central effects as well (148). Conversely, the normalization of insulinemia achieved by weight reduction (156,157) may explain increasing resistance to further weight loss. Glucocorticoid hormones promote fat deposition, and they are in fact essential for the development of obesity in many genetically obese animals (158). As in the case of insulin, their action appears to be mediated by the CNS as well as by peripheral effects (152). Growth hormone exerts the opposite leverage, as, among other effects, it promotes fat oxidation relative to glucose oxidation (159). The balance of these various endocrine effects ultimately has to be judged by the impact they have on the size of the fat mass for which weight maintenance tends to occur.

4. Drugs

Considerable efforts have been made to develop drugs that induce body weight loss, either by increasing energy expenditure or by curbing food intake. At present, most of the commonly used weight-reducing drugs act through their anorectic effects. When food intake is not restricted, the effectiveness of thermogenic stimuli for weight reduction depends on food intake not increasing enough to compensate for the increase in energy expenditure. The phenomena regulating food intake thus remain an essential component in any rationale by which the impact of increases in energy expenditure in eliciting weight reduction is to be explained, and the ultimate issue in explaining the weight-reducing influences of drugs (as well as of exercise) is why food intake regulation did not elicit an increase in food intake commensurate with the increase in energy expenditure. Since the RQs must on average be below the FQ to achieve weight reduction (46), weight-reducing drugs can be selected for their ability to help in achieving this condition, rather than merely for increasing energy expenditure.

E. Daily Substrate Oxidation Patterns in Lean and Obese Individuals

Fat oxidation after an overnight fast is higher in obese than in lean subjects, in part due to higher BMR and in part to lower RQs (146). The negative correlation between RQ and adiposity reflects the influence of the adipose tissue mass in raising FFA levels and in promoting fat relative to glucose oxidation. However, one should also allow for the fact that obese subjects often tend to consume diets with a higher fat content (86,131,132) which could contribute to their relatively low postabsorptive RQ. Whatever the case may be, the average 24-hr RQ is equal to the

diet's FQ in weight-stable subjects be they lean or obese. If one assumes that the lower postabsorptive RQ observed in obese individuals is not imputable to a difference in the macronutrient composition of their diet, one has to expect that the RQ will be higher in obese than in normal subjects during some periods of the day. This issue remains to be explored.

F. Substrate Oxidation and Predisposition to Obesity

Most individuals reach a state of approximate weight maintenance in which the average composition of the fuels they oxidize matches the nutrient distribution in their diets. A rate of fat accumulation resulting in a gain of 1 kg of adipose tissue in a year represents a retention of only about 1% of the energy consumed, making it difficult to detect differences in fuel oxidation under normal conditions. Nevertheless, under rigorously standardized conditions, it was found that subjects tending to have high 24-hr RQs, i.e., those tending to burn more glucose but less fat, were at a higher risk of gaining weight during subsequent years (56,57). The view that burning as much fat as consumed is an important factor in promoting obesity is further supported by the fact that adjustment of fat oxidation to increased fat intake occurs more slowly in obese than in lean subjects (23), placing them at greater risk for weight gain. Furthermore, it was found that a low skeletal muscle oxidative capacity is associated with increased adiposity (160) and that skeletal muscle fatty acid utilization was reduced in women displaying visceral obesity (161).

Since adjustment of fuel oxidation to intake is achieved pretty much equally well in lean and in obese subjects, once their fat mass has reached the size needed for fat oxidation to be commensurate with fat intake, it is necessary to compare postobese individuals to lean controls to identify possible difference in metabolic regulation. Such studies show daily fat oxidation measured by indirect calorimetry to be lower in the postobese subjects (52,162,163). Furthermore fat oxidation rises more slowly in postobese subjects than in lean individuals in response to an increase in dietary fat content (164,165). It thus appears that individuals predisposed to obesity are characterized by a reduced fat oxidation when they are tested in a postobese state. In ex-obese long-distant runners tested after a 39.5-kg weight loss, epinephrine stimulated adipose tissue lipolysis much less than in runners who had never experienced problems with body weight control (166).

G. Interactions Between Genetic and Environmental Factors

The powerful role of inheritance on obesity has long been recognized (167). However, the great increase in the prevalence of obesity in industrialized countries (168), in populations whose gene pool has been relatively constant, shows that environmental factors also assume considerable importance. These facts can be reconciled by recognizing that some genotypes are more affected than others when exposed to environmental factors that influence substrate oxidation and balances. The genotype-environment interactions have been investigated by subjecting monozygotic twins to standardized nutritional and exercise conditions and by comparing within-pair to between-pair responses. Such studies show that heredity is a significant determinant of changes in body weight, energy expenditure, and body fatness induced by training (169,170) or overfeeding (171–173). The observation of Heitman et al. that weight gain was greatest in subjects predisposed to obesity (because at least one of their parents was overweight) and who were consuming diets with a relatively high fat content (174) supports the view that genetic traits may increase the risk of developing obesity by affecting the regulation of glucose versus fat oxidation.

V. CONCLUSIONS

When access to foods is unrestricted, stability of body weight is achieved in spite of differences in energy expenditure, whether these be due to differences in resting metabolic rates, in metabolic efficiency, or in physical activity. Since energy expenditure is not markedly affected by variations in food intake in humans, maintenance of energy balance is overwhelmingly determined by the factors controlling food intake. Adjustment of the composition of the substrate mix oxidized to the macronutrient distribution in the diet plays a crucial role in enabling regulation of food intake to occur in a manner tending to bring about short-term corrections in food consumption that sustain long-term weight stability. In individuals in whom fat oxidation tends to be low relative to glucose oxidation, substantial expansion of the adipose tissue is often necessary before this weight-maintaining situation is reached.

ACKNOWLEDGMENTS

This publication was made possible in part by Grant DK 33214 from the National Institute of Health. Its contents are solely the responsibility of the author and do not necessarily represent the official views of the National Institute of Health. Thanks are also expressed to Dr. Natalie Alméras for her collaboration.

REFERENCES

1. Astrand P-O, Rodahl K. Textbook of Work Physiology, 2nd ed. New York: Mc-Graw Hill, 1977.
2. Pahud P, Ravussin E, Jéquier E. Energy expended during oxygen deficit period of submaximal exercise in man. J Appl Physiol 1980; 48:770–775.
3. Flatt JP, Pahud P, Ravussin E, et al. An estimate of the P:O ratio in man. T I B S 1984; 9:251–255.
4. Brand MD, Couture P, Else PL, et al. Evolution of energy metabolism. Proton permeability of the inner membrane of liver mitochondria is greater in a mammal than in a reptile. Biochem J 1991; 275:81–86.
5. Flatt J. Energy costs of ATP synthesis. In: Kinney JH, Tucker H, ed. Energy Metabolism: Tissue Determinants and Cellular Corollaries. New York: Raven Press, 1992: 319–342.
6. Flatt JP. Conversion of carbohydrate to fat in adipose tissue: an energy-yielding and, therefore, self-limiting process. J Lipid Res 1970; 11:131–143.
7. Himms-Hagen J. Thermogenesis in brown adipose tissue as an energy buffer: implications for obesity. Engl J Med 1984; 311:1549–1558.
8. Rothwell NJ, Stock MJ. Regulation of energy balance. Annu Rev Nutr 1981; 1:235–56.
9. Lowell BB, S-Susulic V, Hamann A, et al. Development of obesity in transgenic mice after genetic ablation of brown adipose tissue. Nature 1993; 366:740–742.
10. DeFronzo RA, Ferrannini E. Regulation of hepatic glucose metabolism in humans. Diabetes/Metab Rev 1987; 3: 415–459.
11. Weast RC. Handbook of Chemistry and Physics, 57th ed. Cleveland, Ohio: CRC Press, 1976.
12. Elia M, Zed C, Neale G, et al. The energy cost of triglyceride-fatty acid recycling in non-obese subjects after an overnight fast and four days of starvation. Metabolism 1987; 36:251–255.
13. Livesey G, Elia M. Estimation of energy expenditure, net carbohydrate utilization, and net fat oxidation and synthesis by indirect calorimetry: evaluation of errors with special reference to the detailed composition of fuels. Am J Clin Nutr 1988; 47:608–623.
14. McGilvery RW, Goldstein G. Biochemistry. A Functional Approach. Philadelphia: WB Saunders, 1979.
15. Garlick PJ, Clugston GA, Swick RW, et al. Diurnal pattern of protein and energy metabolism in man. Am J Clin Nutr 1980; 33:1983–1986.
16. Welle S, Nair KS. Relationship of resting metabolic rate to body composition and protein turnover. Am J Physiol 1990; 258:E990–E998.
17. Kinney JM, Elwyn DH. Protein metabolism and injury. Annu Rev Nutr 1983; 3:433–466.

18. Acheson KJ, Ravussin E, Wahren J, et al. Thermic effect of glucose in man, obligatory and facultative thermogenesis. J Clin Invest 1984; 74:1572–1580.

19. Dallosso HM, James WPT. Whole-body calorimetry studies in adult men. 1. The effect of fat over-feeding on 24 h energy expenditure. Bf J Nutr 1984; 52:49–64.

20. Donato KA, Hegsted DM. Efficiency of utilization of various energy sources for growth. Proc Natl Acad Sci USA 1985; 82:4866–4870.

21. Hurni M, Burnand B, Pittet PH, et al. Metabolic effects of a mixed and a high-carbohydrate low-fat diet in man, measured over 24 h in a respiration chamber. Br J Nutr 1982; 47:33–43.

22. Abbhott WGH, Howard BV, Ruotolo G, et al. Energy expenditure in humans: effects of dietary fat and carbohydrate. Am J Physiol 1990; 258:E347–E351.

23. Thomas CD, Peters JC, Reed GW, et al. Nutrient balance and energy expenditure during ad libitum feeding of high fat and high carbohydrate diets in humans. Am J Clin Nutr 1992; 55:934–942.

24. Shetty PS, Prentice AM, Goldberg GR, et al. Alterations in fuel selection and voluntary food intake in response to isoenergetic manipulation of glycogen stores in humans. Am J Clin Nutr 1994; 60:534–543.

25. Stubbs RJ, Harbron CG, Murgatroyd PR, et al. Covert manipulation of dietary fat and energy density: effect on substrate flux and food intake in men eating ad libitum. Am J Clin Nutr 1995; 62:316–329.

26. Kleiber M. The Fire of Life and Introduction to Animal Energetics. New York: Robert E. Krieger Publishing Company, 1975.

27. Lusk G. The Elements of the Science of Nutrition, 4th ed. Philadelphia: WB Saunders, 1928.

28. Jungas RL, Halperin ML, Brosnan JT. Quantitative analysis of amino acid oxidation and related gluconeogenesis in humans. Physiol Rev 1992; 72:419–448.

29. Flatt JP. The biochemistry of energy expenditure. Rec Adv Obes Res 1978; 2:211–228.

30. Shaw SN, Elwyn DH, Askanazi J, et al. Effects of increasing nitrogen intake on nitrogen balance and energy expenditure in nutritionally depleted adult patients receiving parenteral nutrition. Am J Clin Nutr 1983; 37:930–940.

31. Acheson KJ, Schutz Y, Bessard T, et al. Glycogen storage capacity and de novo lipogenesis during massive carbohydrate overfeeding in man. Am J Clin Nutr 1988; 48:240–247.

32. Hellerstein MK, Christiansen M, Kaempfer S, et al. Measurement of de novo hepatic lipogenesis in humans using stable isotopes. J Clin Invest 1991; 87:1841–1852.

33. Acheson KJ, Schutz Y, Bessard T, et al. Nutritional influences on lipogenesis and thermogenesis after a carbohydrate meal. Am J Physiol 1984; 246:E62–E70.

34. Owen OE, Holup JL, D'Alessio DA, et al. A reappraisal of the caloric requirements of men. Am J Clin Nutr 1987; 46:875–885.

35. Ravussin E, Lillioja S, Anderson TE, et al. Determinants of 24-h energy expenditure in man. J Clin Invest 1986; 78:1568–1578.

36. Newsholme EA, Leech AR. Biochemistry for the Medical Sciences. Chichester: Wiley, 1983.

37. Randle PJ, Hales CN, Garland PB, et al. The glucose fatty-acid cycle: its role in insulin sensitivity and the metabolic disturbances of diabetes mellitus. Lancet 1963; 1:785–789.

38. Wolfe RR. The role of triglyceride–fatty acid cycling and glucose cycling in thermogenesis and amplification of net substrate flux in human subjects. In: Müller MJ, Danforth E, Burger AG, eds. Hormones and Nutrition in Obesity and Cachexia. New York: Springer, 1990.

39. Wolfe RR, Herndon DN, Jahoor F, et al. Effect of severe burn injury on substrate cycling by glucose and fatty acids. N Engl J Med 1987; 317:403–408.

40. Lardy H, Su CY, Kneer N, et al. Dehydroepiandrosterone induces enzymes that permit thermogenesis and decrease metabolic efficiency. In: Lardy H, Stratman F, eds. Hormones, Thermogenesis, and Obesity. New York: Elsevier, 1989:415–426.

41. Kozak LP, Kozak UC, Clarke GT. Abnormal brown and white fat development in transgenic mice overexpressing glycerol 3-phosphate dehydrogenase. Genes Dev 1991; 5:2256–2264.

42. Shulman GI, Ladenson PW, Wolfe MH, et al. Substrate cycling between gluconeogenesis and glycolysis in euthyroid, hypothyroid, and hyperthyroid in man. J Clin Invest 1985; 76:757–764.

43. Clausen T, Van Hardeveld C, Everts ME. Significance of cation transport in control on energy metabolism and thermogenesis. Physiol Rev 1991; 71:733–774.

44. Brand MD, Steverding D, Kadenbach B, et al. The mechanism of the increase in mitochondrial proton permeability induced by thyroid hormones. Eur J Biochem 1992; 206:775–781.

45. Schoeller DA, Field CR. Human energy metabolism: What we have learned from the doubly labeled water method. Annu Rev Nutr 1991; 11:355–373.

46. Flatt JP. Importance of nutrient balance in body weight regulation. Diabetes/Metab Rev 1988; 4:571–581.

47. Recommended Dietary Allowances, 10 ed. Washington, DC: National Academy Press, 1989.

48. Refinetti R. Effect of ambient temperature on respiratory quotient of lean and obese Zucker rats. Am J Physiol 1989; 256:R236–R239.

49. Pagé E, Chénier L. Effects of diets and cold environment on the respiratory quotient of the white rat. Rev Can Biol 1953; 12:530–541.

50. Wilson S, Thurlby PL, Arch J RS. Substrate supply for thermogenesis induced by the β-adrenoceptor agonist BRL 26830A. Can J Physiol Pharm 1987; 65:113–119.

51. Graham TE, Sathasivam P, MacNaughton KW. Influence of cold, exercise, and caffeine on catecholamine and metabolism in men. J Appl Physiol 1991; 70:2052–2058.

52. Buemann B, Astrup A, Christensen N, et al. Effect of moderate cold exposure on 24 h energy expenditure: similar response in postobese and nonobese women. Am J Physiol 1992; 263:E1040–E1045.

53. Jéquier E, Acheson K, Schutz Y. Assessment of energy expenditure and fuel utilization in man. Annu Rev Nutr 1987; 7:187–208.

54. McLean JA, GT. Animal and Human Calorimetry. Cambridge: Cambridge University Press, 1987.

55. Murgatroyd PR, Shetty PS, Prentice AM. Techniques fopr the measurement of human energy expenditure: a practical guide. Int J Obes 1993; 17:549–568.

56. Zurlo F, Lillioja S, Esposito-Del Puente A, et al. Low ratio of fat to carbohydrate oxidation as predictor of weight gain: study of 24h RQ. Am J Physiol 1990; 259:E650–E657.

57. Seidell JC, Muller DC, Sorkin JD, et al. Fasting respiratory exchange ratio and resting metabolic rate as predictors of weight gain: the Baltimore Longitudinal Study on Aging. Int J Obese 1992; 16:667–674.

58. Hill JO, Peters JC, Reed GW, et al. Nutrient balance in humans: effects of diet composition. Am J Clin Nutr 1991; 54:10–17.

59. Acheson KJ, Ravussin E, Schoeller DA, et al. Two-week stimulation or blockade of the sympathetic nervous system in man: influence on body weight, body composition, and twenty four-hour energy expenditure. Metabolism 1988; 37:91–98.

60. Spurr GB, Prentice A, Murgatroyd P, et al. Energy expenditure from minute-by-minute heart-rate recording: comparison to indirect calorimetry. Am J Clin Nutr 1988; 48:552–559.

61. Livingstone MBE, Prentice AM, Coward WA, et al. Simultaneous free-living energy expenditure by the doubly labeled water method and the heart-rate monitoring. Am J Clin Nutr 1990; 52:59–65.

62. Alméras N, Mimeault N, Serresse O, et al. Non-exercise daily energy expenditure and physical activity pattern in male endurance athletes. Eur J Appl Physiol 1991; 63:184–187.

63. Lifson N, Gordon GB, McClintock R. Measurement of total carbon dioxide production by means of $D_2{}^{18}O$. J Appl Physiol 1955; 7:704–710.

64. Elia M. Energy equivalents of CO_2 and their importance in assessing energy expenditure when using tracer techniques. Am J Physiol 1991; 260:E75–E88.

65. Schoeller DA, Van Santen E. Measurement of energy expenditure in humans by doubly labeled water method. J Appl Physiol 1982; 53:955–959.

66. Roberts SB, Dietz W, Sharp T, et al. Multiple laboratory comparison of the doubly labeled water technique. Obes Res 1995; 3:S3–S13.

67. Prentice AM, Coward WA, Davies HL, et al. Unexpectedly low levels of energy expenditure in healthy women. Lancet 1985; 1:1419–1422.

68. Heini A, Schutz Y, Diaz E, et al. Free-living energy expenditure measured by two independent techniques in pregnant and nonpregnant Cambian women. Am J Physiol 1991; 261:E9–E17.

69. Tremblay A, Seale J, Alméras N, et al. Energy requirements of a postobese man reporting a low intake at weight maintenance. Am J Clin Nutr 1991; 54:1–3.

70-. Prentice AM, Black AE, Coward WA, et al. Energy expenditure in overweight and obese adults in affluent societies: an analysis of 319 doubly-labelled water measurements. Eur J Clin Nutr 1996; 50:93–97.

71. Westerterp KR, Saris WHM, van Es M, et al. Use of the doubly labelled water technique in humans during heavy sustained exercise. J Appl Physiol 1986; 61:2162–2167.

72. Roberts SB, Savage J, Coward WA, et al. Energy expenditure and intake in infants born to lean and overweight mothers. Engl J Med 1988; 318:461–466.

73. Goran MI, Poehlman ET. Endurance training does not enhance total energy expenditure in healthy elderly persons. Am J Physiol 1992; 263:E950–E957.

74. Heaton JM. The distribution of brown adipose tissue in the human. Journal of anatomy 1972; 112:35–39.

75. Astrup A, Bülow J, Madsen J, et al. Contribution of brown adipose tissue and skletal muscle to thermogenesis induced by ephedrine in man. Am J Physiol 1985; 248:E507–E515.

76. Norgan NG, Durnin JVGA. The effect of 6 weeks of overfeeding on the body weight, body composition, and energy metabolism of young men. Am J Clin Nutr 1980; 33:978–988.

77. Ravussin E, Schutz Y, Acheson KJ, et al. Short-term mixed-diet overfeeding in man:no evidence for "luxus-konsumption." Am J Physiol 1985; 249:E470–477.

78. Diaz EO, Prentice AM, Goldberg GR, et al. Metabolic response to experimental overfeeding in lean and overweight healthy volunteers. Am J Clin Nutr 1992; 56:641–655.

79. Tremblay A, Coveney S. Després JP, et al. Increased resting metabolic rate and lipid oxidation in exercise-trained individuals: evidence for a role of β-adrenergic stimulation. Can J Physiol 1992; 70:1342–1347.

80. Wasserman K, Hansen EJ, Sue DY, et al. Principles of Exercise Testing and Interpretation. Philadelphia: Lea & Fabiger, 1987:274.

81. Coggan AR, Kohrt MW, Spina RJ, et al. Endurance training decreases plasma glucose turnover and oxidation during moderate-intensity exercise in men. J Appl Physiol 1990; 68:990–996.

82. Tremblay A, Fontaine E, Nadeau A. Contribution of postexercise increment in glucose storage to variations in glucose-induced thermogenesis in endurance athletes. Can J Physiol Pharm 1985; 63:1165–1169.

83. Bielinski R, Schutz Y, Jéquier E. Energy metabolism during the post-exercise recovery in man. Am J Clin Nutr 1985; 42:69–82.

84. Tremblay A, Simoneau J, Bouchard C. Impact of exercise intensity on body fatness and skeletal muscle metabolism. Metabolism 1994; 43:814–818.

85. Flatt JP. Integration of the overall effects of exercise. Int J Obes 1995; 19:S31–S40.

86. Tremblay A, Plourde G, Després JP, et al. Impact of dietary fat content and fat oxidation on energy intake in humans. Am J Clin Nutr 1989; 49:799–805.

87. Alméras N, Lavallée N, Després J-P, et al. Exercise and energy intake: Effect of substrate oxidation. Physiol Behav 1995; 57:995–1000.

88. Ravussin E, Lillioja S, Knowler WC, et al. Reduced rate of energy expenditure as a risk factor for body-weight gain. N Engl J Med 1988; 318:467–472.

89. Stubbs JR, Rit P, Coward WA, et al. Covert manipulation of the ratio of dietary fat to carbohydrate and energy density: effect on food intake and energy balance in free-living men eating ad libitum. Am J Clin Nutr 1995; 62: 330–337.

90. Speakman JR, Racey PA. The equilibrium concentration of oxygen-18 in body water: implications for the accuracy of the doubly-labelled water technique and a potential new method of measuring RQ in free-living animals. J Theor Biol 1987; 127:79–95.

91. Bingham SA, Gill C, Welch A, et al. Comparison of dietary assessment methods in nutritional epidemiology: weighed records v. 24h recalls, food-frequency questionnaires and estimated-diet records. Br J Nutr 1994; 72:619–643.

92. Ramirez I, Tordoff MG, Friedman MI. Dietary hyperphagia and obesity: what causes them? Physiol Behav 1989; 45:163–168.

93. Romijn JA, Coyle EF, Sidossis LS, et al. Regulation of endogenous fat and carbohydrate metabolism in relation to exercise intensity and duration. Am J Physiol 1993; 265: E380–E391.

94. Elia M. General integration and regulation of metabolism at the organ level. Proc Nutr Soc 1995; 54:213–232.

95. Geigy Scientific Tables, 7th ed. Ardsley, NY: Geigy Pharmaceuticals, 1970.

96. Cahill GF. Starvation in man. N Engl J Med 1970; 282(12):668–675.

97. Murphy JR. Erythrocyte metabolism. II. Glucose metabolism and pathways. J Lab Clin Med 1960; 55:286–302.

98. Müller MJ. Hepatic fuel selection. Proc Nutr Soc 1995; 54:139–150.

99. Coppack SW, Frayn KN, Humphreys SM, et al. Arteriovenous differences across human adipose and forearm tissues after overnight fast. Metabolism 1990; 39(4): 384–390.

100. Nuutila P, Koivisto VA, Knuuti J, et al. Glucose-free fatty acid cycle operates in human heart and skeletal muscle in vivo. J Clin Invest 1992; 89:1767–1744.

101. Björntorp, P, Sjöström L. Carbohydrate storage in man: speculations and some quantitative considerations. Metabolism 1978; 27:1853–1865.

102. Klein S, Wolfe RR. Carbohydrate restriction regulates the adaptive response to fasting. Am J Physiol 1992; 262: 631–636.

103. Keller U, Lustenberger J, Müller-Brand J, et al. Human ketone body production and utilization studied using tracer techniques: regulation by free fatty acids, insulin, catecholamines, and thyroid hormones. Diabetes/Metab Rev 1989; 5:285–298.

104. Abbott WGH, Howard BV, Christin L, et al. Short-term energy balance: relationship with protein, carbohydrate, and fat balances. Am J Physiol 1988; 255:E332–E337.

105. Randle PJ, Priestman DA, Mistry SC, et al. Glucose fatty acid interactions and the regulation of glucose disposal. J Cell Biochem 1994; 55S:1–11.

106. Cahill GF Jr. Physiology of insulin in man. Diabetes 1971; 20:785–799.

107. Flatt JP. McCollum Award Lecture, 1995: Diet, lifestyle and weight maintenance. Am J Clin Nutr 1995; 62: 820–836.

108. Flatt JP. Dietary fat, carbohydrate balance, and weight maintenance: effects of exercise. Am J Clin Nutr 1987; 45:296–306.

109. Mayer J, Thomas DW. Regulation of food intake and obesity. Science 1967; 156:328–337.

110. Stubbs RJ, Murgatroyd PR, Goldberg GR, et al. Carbohydrate balance and the regulation of day-to-day food intake in humans. Am J Clin Nutr 1993; 57:897–903.

111. Clore JN, Helm ST, Blackard WG. Loss of hepatic autoregulation after carbohydrate overfeeding in normal man. J Clin Invest 1995; 96:1967–1972.

112. Flatt JP, Ravussin E, Acheson KJ, et al. Effects of dietary fat on postprandial substrate oxidation and on carbohydrate and fat balances. J Clin Invest 1985; 76:1019–1024.

113. Griffiths AJ, Humphreys SM, Clark ML, et al. Immediate metabolic availability of dietary fat in combination with carbohydrate. Am J Clin Nutr 1994; 59:53–59.

114. Björntorp P, Bergman H, Varnauskas E, et al. Lipid mobilization in relation to body composition in man. Metabolism 1969; 18:840–851.

115. Swinburn BA, Nyomba BL, Saad MF, et al. Insulin resistance associated with lower rates of weight gain in Pima Indians. J Clin Invest 1991; 88:168–173.

116. Tremblay A, Wouters E, Wenker M, et al. Alcohol and a high-fat diet: a combination favoring overfeeding. Am J Clin Nutr 1995; 62:639–644.

117. Colditz GA, Giovannucci E, Rimm ER, et al. Alcohol intake in relation to diet and obesity in women and men. Am J Clin Nutr 1991; 54:49–55.

118. Jones BR, Barrett-Connor E, Criqui MH, et al. A community study of calorie and nutrient intake in drinkers and nondrinkers of alcohol, Am J Clin Nutr 1982; 35: 135–139.

119. Bebb HT, Houser HB, Witschi JC, et al. Calorie and nutrient contribution of alcoholic beverages to the usual diets of 155 adults. Am J Clin Nutr 1971; 24:1042–1052.

120. Gruchow HW, Sobocinski KA, Barboriak JJ, et al. Alcohol consumption, nutrient intake and relative body weight among US adults. Am J Coll Nutr 1985; 42:289–295.

121. de Castro JM, Orozco S. Moderate alcohol intake and spontaneous eating patterns of humans: evidence of unregulated supplementation. Am J Clin Nutr 1990; 52: 246–253.

122. Veenstra J, Schenkel JAA, van Erp-Baart AMJ, et al. Alcohol consumption in relation to food intake and smoking habits in the Dutch National Food Consumption Survey. Eur J Clin Nutr 1993; 47:482–489.

123. Prentice AM. Alcohol and obesity. Int J Obes 1995; 19: S44–S50.

124. Suter PM, Jéquier E, Schutz Y. Effect of ethanol on energy expenditure. ASm J Physiol 1994; 266:R1204–R1212.

125. Lieber CS. Herman Award Lecture, 1993: A personal perspective on alcohol, nutrition, and liver. Am J Clin Nutr 1993; 58:430–442.

126. Suter PM, Schutz Y, Jéquier E. The effect of ethanol on fat storage in healthy subjects. N Engl J Med 1992; 326: 983–987.

127. Tremblay A, St-Pierre S. The hyperphagic effect of high-fat and alcohol persists after control for energy density. Am J Clin Nutr 1996; 63:479–482.

128. Jéquier E. Calorie balance versus nutrient balance. In: Kinney JH, Tucker H, eds. Energy Metabolism: Tissue Determinants and Cellular Corollaries. New York: Raven Press, 1992: 123–134.

129. Flatt JP. The RQ/FQ concept and weight maintenance. In: Angel A, Anderson H, Bouchard C, et al. eds. Recent Advances in Obesity Research. London: Libby, 1986; 49–66.

130. Tarasuk V, Beaton GH. The nature and individuality of within subject variation in energy intake. Am J Clin Nutr 1991; 54:464–470.

131. Dreon DM, Frey-Hewitt B, Ellsworth N, et al. Dietary fat: carbohydrate ratio and obesity in middle aged men. Am J Clin Nutr 1988; 47:995–1000.

132. Romieu I, Willett WC, Stampfer MJ, et al. Energy intake and other determinants of relative weight. Am J Clin Nutr 1988; 47:406–412.

133. Lissner L, Heitmann BL. Dietary fat and obesity: evidence from epidemiology. Eur J Clin Nutr 1995; 49:79–90.

134. Prentice AM, Jebb SA. Obesity in Britain: gluttony or sloth? Br Med J 1995; 311:437–439.

135. Porikos KP, Booth G, Van Italie TB. Effect of covert nutritive dilution on the spontaneous food intake of obese individuals: a pilot study. Am J Clin Nutr 1977; 30: 1638–1644.

136. Schutz Y, Flatt JP, Jéquier E. Failure of dietary fat intake to promote fat oxidation: A factor favoring the development of obesity. Am J Clin Nutr 1989; 50:307–314.

137. Rolls BJ, Kim-Harris S, Fischman MW, et al. Satiety after preloads with different amounts of fat and carbohydrate: imploications for obesity. Am J Clin Nutr 1994; 60: 476–487.

138. Blundell JE, Cotton JR, Delargy H, et al. The fat paradox: fat-induced satiety signals versus high fat overconsumption. Int J Obes 1995; 19:832–835.

139. Astrup A, Buemann B, Western P, et al. Obesity as an adaptation to a high fat diet: evidence from as cross-sectional study. Am Clin Nutr 1994; 59:350–355.

140. Tremblay A, Després J, Leblanc C, et al. Effect of intensity of physical activity on body fatness and fat distribution. Am J Clin Nutr 1990; 51:153–157.

141. Ewbank PP, Darga LL, Lucas CP, Physical activity as a predictor of weight maintenance in previously obese subjects. Obes Res 1995; 3:257–264.

142. Rising R, Harper IT, Fontvielle AM, et al. Determinants of total daily energy expenditure: variability in physical activity. Am J Clin Nutr 1994; 59:800–804.

143. Ballor DL, Keesey RE, A meta-analysis of the factors affecting exercise-induced changes in body mass, fat mass, and fat-free mass in males and females. Int J Obes 1991; 15:717–726.

144. Tremblay A, Alméras N, Boer J, et al. Diet composition and postexercise energy balance. Am J Clin Nutr 1994; 59:975–979.

145. King NA, Blundell JE. High-fat foods overcome the energy expenditure induced by high-intensity cycling or running. Eur J Clin Nutr 1995; 49:114–123.

146. Schutz Y, Tremblay A, Weinsier RL, et al. Role of fat oxidation in the long term stabilization of body weight in obese women. Am J Clin Nutr 1992; 55:670–674.

147. Tappy L, Girardet K, Shwaller N, et al. Metabolic effects of an increase of sympathetic activity in healthy humans. Int J Obes 1995; 19:419–422.

148. Woods SC, Figlewicz Latteman DP, Schwartz MW, et al. A re-assessment of the regulation of adiposity and appetite by the brain insulin system. Int J Obes 1990; 14:69–76.

149. Rowe JW, Young JB, Minaker KL, et al. Effect of insulin and glucose infusions on sympathetic nervous system activity in normal man. Diabetes 1981; 30:219–225.

150. Berne C, Fagius J, Pollare T, et al. The sympathetic response to euglycaemic hyperinsulinemia. Diabetologia 1992; 35:873–879.

151. Vollenweider P, Randin D, Tappy L, et al. Impaired insulin-induced sympathetic neural activation and vasodilation in skeletal muscle in obese humans. J Clin Invest 1994; 93:2365–2371.

152. Bray GA. Obesity—A state of reduced sympathetic activity and normal or high adrenal activity: the autonomic and adrenal hypothesis revisited. Int J Obes 1990; 14: 77–92.

153. Kalyala KJ, Woods SC, Schwartz MW. New model for the regulation of energy balance and adiposity by the central nervous system. Am J Clin Nutr 1995; 62:1123S–1134S.

154. Schwartz MJ, Marks J, Sipols AJ, et al. Central insulin administration reduces neuropeptide Y mRNA expression in the arcuate nucleus of food-deprived lean (Fa/Fa) but not obese (fa/fa) Zucker rats. Endocrinology 1991; 128: 2645–2647.

155. Williams G, McKibbin PE, McCarthy HD. Hypothalamic regulatory peptides and the regulation of food intake and energy balance: signals or noise? Proc Nutr Soc 1991; 50: 527–544.

156. Tremblay A, Sauvé L, Després JP, et al. Metabolic characteristics of postobese individuals. Int J Obes 1989; 13: 357–366.

157. Tremblay A, Despres JP, Maheux J, et al. Normalization of the metabolic profile in obese women by exercise and a low fat diet. Med Sci Sports Exerc 1991; 23(12): 1326–1331.

158. Saito M, Bray GA. Adrenalectomy and food restriction in the genetically obese (ob/ob) mouse. Am J Physiol 1984; 246:R20–R25.

159. Salomon F, Cuneo RC, Hesp R, et al. The effects of treatment with recombinant human growth hormone on body composition and metabolism in adults with growth hormone deficiency. N Engl J Med 1989; 321:797–803.

160. Simoneau JA, Bouchard C. Skeletal muscle metabolism and body fat content in men and women. Obes Res 1995; 3:23–29.

161. Colberg S, Simoneau J, Theate F, et al. Skeletal muscle utilization of free fatty acids in women with visceral obesity. J Clin Invest 1995; 95:1846–1853.

162. Lean MEJ, James WPT. Metabolic effects of isoenergetic nutrient exchange over 24 hours in relation to obesity in women. Int J Obes 1988; 8:641–648.

163. Buemann B, Astrup A, Madsen J, et al. A 24-h energy expenditure study on reduced-obese and nonobese women: effect of β-blockade. Am J Clin Nutr 1992; 56: 662–670.

164. Astrup A, Buemann B, Christensen NJ, et al. Failure to increase lipid oxidation in response to increasing dietary fat content in formerly obese women. Am J Physiol 1994; 266:E592–E599.

165. Raben A, Anderson HB, Christensen NJ, et al. Evidence for an abnormal postprandial response to a high fat meal in women predisposed to obesity. Am J Physiol 1994; 267:E549–E559.

166. Tremblay A, Després JP, Bouchard C. Adipose tissue characteristics of ex-obese long-distance runners. Int J Obes 1984; 8:641–648.

167. Bouchard C, Perusse L. Heredity and body fat. Annu Rev Nutr 1988; 8:259–277.

168. Kuczmarski RJ, Flegal KM, Campbell SM, et al. Increasing prevalence of overweight among US Adults. JAMA 1994; 272:205–211.

169. Poehlman ET, Tremblay A, Nadeau A, et al. Heredity and changes in hormones and metabolic rates with short-term training. Am J Physiol 1986; 250:E711–E717.

170. Bouchard C, Tremblay A, Després JP, et al. The response to exercise with constant energy intake in identical twins. Obes Res 1994; 2:400–410.

171. Poehlman ET, Tremblay A, Fontaine E, et al. Genotype dependency of dietary induced thermogenesis: its relation with hormonal changes following overfeeding. Metabolism 1986; 35:30–36.

172. Poehlman ET, Tremblay A, Després JP, et al. Genotype-controlled changes in body composition and morphology following overfeeding in twins. Am J Clin Nutr 1986; 43: 723–731.

173. Bouchard C, Tremblay A, Despres JP, et al. The response to long term overfeeding in identical twins. N Engl J Med 1990; 322:1477–1482.

174. Heitman BL, Lissner L, Sørensen TIA, et al. Dietary fat intake and weight gain in women genetically predisposed for obesity. Am J Clin Nutr 1995; 61:1213–1217.

25

Skeletal Muscle and Obesity

Jean-Aimé Simoneau
Laval University, Ste.-Foy, Quebec, Canada

David E. Kelley
University of Pittsburgh School of Medicine, Pittsburgh, Pennsylvania

I. INTRODUCTION

Skeletal muscle has a key role in the consumption of carbohydrate and lipid. Obesity causes insulin resistance of muscle, as has been recognized for several decades. A main characteristic of this is decreased capacity for insulin-stimulated glucose storage, yet it is unclear how this specific metabolic defect could contribute to weight gain and accretion of fat mass. Clearly, insulin resistance contributes to the risk that obese individuals have for developing the metabolic complications of diabetes, hypertension, and cardiovascular disease. Recent data implicate skeletal muscle as a site of inefficient utilization of lipid, findings that link muscle to the development or maintenance of the obese state. The purpose of this chapter is to describe these characteristics and relate them to abnormalities of carbohydrate and fat metabolism by muscle.

II. STRUCTURE AND COMPOSITION OF SKELETAL MUSCLE AND OBESITY

A. Overall Muscle Mass

It is of interest to ask the question as to whether obese individuals, who have an excess of total fat, also possess a greater muscle mass than lean subjects, otherwise paired for age and sex. Some studies report that fat-free mass is significantly higher in obese subjects. In general, obese individuals with a body mass index (BMI) ranging from 35 to 40 kg/m^2 and weighing about 100 kg have approximately 5 kg more fat-free mass than do lean subjects with a BMI of 25 and weighing about 70 kg. Such small difference does not necessarily mean that muscle mass is greater in obese compared to lean persons. Magnetic resonance imaging has been used to assess the distribution of fat and lean tissue in humans. Ross et al. (1) compared total and regional lean tissue distribution in obese men and women with this technology. It was found, not unexpectedly, that obese women have significantly less total lean tissue than obese men. This difference was observed regardless of which body segment (head and arms, abdomen and torso, hip and pelvic region and legs) was evaluated. To our knowledge, there has not been a comparative studies of obese and lean individuals that has used similar technology.

Using another technology, Landin et al. (2) examined the effects of body weight on total-body potassium and fat content in lean and obese middle-aged men and women. Total-body potassium, calculated from the natural isotope ^{40}K determined in a whole-body counter, was higher in obese men and obese women compared to their lean counterparts. These authors reported that higher total-body potassium content in obese subjects is predominantly due to increased skeletal muscle mass.

B. Intramuscular Fat Content

An additional interesting finding of the study of Landin et al. (2) was that obese men had higher skeletal muscle fat content, as determined in muscle biopsies, than did lean men. Muscle fat content was proportional to increased body weight ($r = 0.67$). This relationship was, however, not found in women. These observations suggested that a greater accretion of fat into muscle occurs in obesity. Using computed tomography (CT) of the thigh, Kelley et al. observed similar findings (3). Obese men had a specific increase of thigh muscle possessing lower-than-normal Houndsfield values (ranging from 1 to 35 Houndsfield Units) for computed tomography attenuation. Because adipose tissue has a negative attenuation value on imaging with computed tomography (generally ranging from -200 to -1), these results were suggestive of an increased fat deposition within muscle, a phenomenon previously reported in other types of diseases (4). A more recent study by our laboratories has confirmed this observation in obese women, who also have skeletal muscle characterized by a greater amount of tissue with low attenuation values (5) (Fig. 1). Similar to the study of Landin et al. (2), our study was not able to distinguish the location of fat (intra- vs. extramuscular fat). In skeletal muscle, fat can be found within connective tissue between muscle fibers or fat can be stored directly within muscle cells. How obesity affects these two compartments remains unclear.

Several ultrastructural investigations of human skeletal muscle have shown that lipid droplets can accumulate within muscle cells and that, in general, the total volume occupied by fat accounts for less than 1% of total cell volume. For instance, the volume percentage occupied by lipid in skeletal muscle of women represents values ranging from 0.5% to 0.7% depending on the fiber type investigated (6). To our knowledge, no studies have yet convincingly demonstrated that lipid droplets or fat is stored in large amount within the muscle cell of obese individuals when compared to lean subjects. Fat accretion within the muscle cell may suggest the existence of a metabolic defect that impedes entry of fatty acids into mitochondria and therefore favors fatty acid reesterification and, accordingly, storage of fat into muscle. Fat accretion in muscle (as detected by CT) is negatively related to insulin sensitivity and visceral obesity (5). Interestingly, and consistent with this, a recent study by Pan et al. (7) revealed that triglyceride storage within muscle is negatively related to insulin sensitivity. Muscle triglyceride concentration and waist/thigh ratio (a measure of central adiposity) related independently to, and explained 44% of, the variance in the nonoxidative component of insulin sensitivity determined at physiological levels. Similarly, in a collaborative study between our laboratories (5), low attenuation muscle tissue of the thigh and visceral obesity accounted for about 60% of the variance in leg glucose storage, the latter being a metabolic pathway that is a strong indicator of insulin sensitivity.

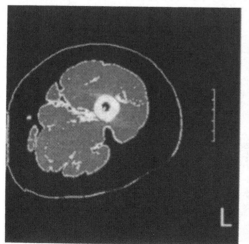 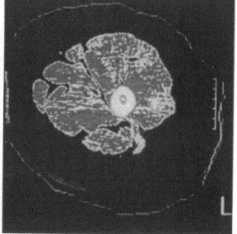

Figure 1   Cross-sectional computed tomography scans of midthigh from two women, with low attenuation muscle highlighted using a region of interest set to attenuation values of 0–35 Hounsfield units. (Left) Left thigh of a lean woman (BMI = 19.2 kg/m²); (right) thigh of an obese woman (BMI = 33.4 kg/m²).

C. Membrane Characteristics of Skeletal Muscle

Another aspect of the altered lipid composition of skeletal muscle in obesity is related to phospholipid composition of mitochondrial and sarcolemmal membranes. There is evidence that muscle membrane fatty acid composition influences overall substrate metabolism and insulin sensitivity (8). Gas liquid chromatography analyses of skeletal muscle biopsies obtained from lean and obese individuals reveal that the percentage of certain long-chain polyunsaturated fatty acids (C20–22) correlates negatively ($r = -0.47; p < 0.01$) with body mass index (9). A proposed mechanism for the effect of altered membrane phospholipid composition upon insulin action and substrate metabolism is altered membrane fluidity, which could affect signal transduction and substrate transport (10). Interestingly, Pehowich (11) has shown that pyruvate oxidation was 28% higher in hypothyroid heart mitochondria from animals fed the omega-3 fatty acid diet compared to those fed the omega-6 fatty acid diet. Although the total phospholipid fatty acid composition was not affected by hypothyroid state, the data suggested that membrane levels of cardiolipin and its omega-3 fatty acid content were able to modulate pyruvate transport in hypothyroid mitochondria. Interestingly, cardiolipin is known to be required for full cytochrome c oxidase activity, the regulatory step of the mitochondrial oxidative phosphorylation. An area for important future research will be whether alterations in the relative distribution of inner-membrane phospholipids can be achieved by dietary manipulation and whether such manipulations can improve metabolic performance of muscle.

D. Muscle Fiber Morphology

Two studies from Krotkiewski et al. (12,13) have reported significant and positive correlations (with an r of about 0.4) between total-body fat and type I or type II muscle fiber areas. These results, indicating larger muscle fibers in obesity, fit nicely with the results described previously indicating elevated fat-free mass in obese subjects. No difference in muscle fiber size was found, however, between obese women exhibiting genoid as compared to androgenic profiles of fat distribution (13). The number of capillaries surrounding muscle fibers may play an important role in substrate utilization, and a reduced capillary density of muscle has been described in obesity. Krotkiewski et al. (12) have reported significant and negative correlations between fasting insulin level (indicative of insulin resistance) and the number of capillaries per area of type I ($r = -0.80$) or type IIA ($r = -0.62$) skeletal muscle

fibers in humans. As recently reviewed by Björntorp (14), if a reduced capillarity of skeletal muscle is a common phenotype of obesity, then a limited transfer of insulin from the capillary binding site to the extravascular space could reduce the rate at which this hormonal signal is perceived by muscle. Binding of insulin is occurring in the capillary endothelium (15) and insulin is transferred through the endothelial cells to reach the insulin receptors located at the surface of the muscle cells. The development of microdialysis techniques may provide unique opportunities to directly sample substrate concentrations of interstitial fluid in vivo. In human peripheral tissues, adipose tissue has been the tissue mostly investigated and measurements in lymph or in extracellular fluid have shown that the transfer of insulin appears to be particularly slow since the extracellular concentrations of insulin never reached those in circulation (16).

E. Muscle Fiber Type Proportion

It is a commonly thought that type I muscle fibers in humans are better endowed for substrate oxidation than type II fibers. Reflecting this concept, it has been proposed that fiber type composition of skeletal muscle in which type II fibers predominate would be a determinant of obesity, owing to the lower substrate oxidation potential of this fiber type. In the testing of this hypothesis, conflicting results have been obtained. Recent studies have reported that individuals with a high percentage of total-body fat exhibit a low percentage of type I fibers in the vastus lateralis muscle (17,18). Among more than 400 individuals, Simoneau and Bouchard have shown that vastus lateralis muscle in about 25% of North American Caucasian men and women contains less than 35% of type I fiber (19). Interestingly, nearly one of three adults in the United States is overweight (20), a prevalence that is about equivalent to the proportion of individuals in the population with a predominance of fast-twitch skeletal muscle characteristics. To date, there are three studies that conclude that variability between subjects in skeletal muscle fiber type proportion is related to differences in body fat content or BMI. Wade et al. (18), on the basis of a rather small group of men ($N = 11$), suggested that at least 40% ($r = -0.65$) of the variability in fatness was related to variation in fiber type I proportion of vastus lateralis muscle and concluded that fatter men exhibited a higher proportion of type II fiber than leaner subjects. Hickey et al. (21) demonstrated a negative correlation ($r = -0.50; p < 0.01$) between percentage of type I fibers in the rectus abdominous muscle and body mass index. A more modest correlation coefficient ($r = -0.32; p < 0.01$) was reported between the fiber type I proportion of vastus lateralis muscle and percent body fat in the study of Lillioja et al. (17) that involved 23 Caucasians and 41 Pima Indian nondiabetic men. On the other hand, Krotkiewski et al. (13) have shown an absence of significant relationship between the proportion of type I fibers and obesity.

It is possible that the significant relationships previously found could have been confounded by physical fitness of the subjects, which was not controlled. Several reports have examined whether there is a relationship between skeletal muscle fiber type distribution and body fat content, among individuals with different levels of physical fitness. From these studies, a significant and negative correlation can be shown between percent of type I fibers in vastus lateralis muscle and total-body fat content. This is one of the reasons why comparisons of muscle characteristics of individuals with similar physical fitness level (e.g., VO$_2$max) but with large variation in body fat content need to be done to determine whether skeletal muscle characteristics can discriminate lean and fat individuals of either sex. A main finding of a recent study from Simoneau and Bouchard (22) is the absence of a relationship between the proportion of type I muscle fibers and the amount of subcutaneous fat within a large sample of women or of men, as well as the lack of difference in the proportion of type I muscle fibers between individuals exhibiting substantial differences in subcutaneous fat content but who were paired on the basis of VO$_2$max expressed per kilogram of body weight (22). Recent collaborative studies between Segal and Simoneau have shown, however, that when lean and obese subjects are paired on the basis of fat-free mass and VO$_2$max (whether expressed per kilogram of weight or kilogram of fat-free mass), vastus lateralis muscle of obese individuals had a small but significantly higher proportion of type IIB fibers than muscle of lean subjects [29% vs. 17%; (23)].

F. Distinction Between Fiber Type Proportion and Metabolic Capacities of Skeletal Muscle

One reason why it has been proposed that fiber type composition of skeletal muscle is important in substrate metabolism is because skeletal muscle composed of a high proportion of type I fibers is insulin-sensitive owing to a greater number of insulin receptors (24). Björntorp (11) recently challenged this concept since he found that skeletal muscle of female rats treated with testosterone exhibited a pronounced change in fiber type composition (increase in type II fibers) while the number of insulin receptors remained unchanged. He also demonstrated that chronic exposure of female rats to hyperinsulinemia was followed by shift in fiber proportion from type I to type II, yet despite this, there was an improvement in insulin sensitivity. These two animal experiments strongly suggest that muscle fiber type composition is not of primary importance in the regulation of insulin sensitivity.

The rationale that fiber type distribution depicts the relative capacity of skeletal muscle for substrate oxidation may not be correct. Although there is no doubt that a large variation exists in the proportion of type I fiber in skeletal muscles among humans (19), the impact of this on substrate oxidation is more controversial. It is not evident that type I fibers of human skeletal muscle are better endowed for substrate oxidation than type II fibers. Previous studies involving microphotometric determinations (25), ultrastructural investigations (26), or microbiochemical activity determinations in dissected single fibers (27) have shown that large variation exists in the metabolic profile within each fiber type (i.e., type I, IIA, and IIB fibers) of human skeletal muscle. Although the studies do report higher average mitochondrial enzyme activities or volume density in type I than in type IIA or type IIB fibers, more than 50% of type I fibers have aerobic-oxidative enzyme activities that are similar to those of type II fibers (25,26). Accordingly, it is important to make a distinction between muscle enzyme capacities for substrate oxidation and muscle fiber type per se. Muscle fiber type is usually established on the basis of histochemical adenosinetriphosphatase (ATPase) staining (Fig. 2). Distinct myosin isoforms exist in skeletal muscle, and the presence of different myosin heavy chains is responsible for the existence of different fiber types when they are stained with the use of the ATPase (28). The specificity of this technique is based on the fact that myofibrillar actomyosin ATPases (mATPase) display distinct stabilities at acid or alkaline pH values (29). Investigation of the functional properties of these different fibers revealed that type IIB fibers exhibit the highest maximum unloaded shortening velocity in comparison to the other fibers (30).

Although the presence of different fiber types may give some pertinent information on the speed of contraction of muscle, it has very low predictive capacity for the glycolytic or aerobic-oxidative metabolic capacities of the same muscle. The metabolic diversity of the muscle fibers is better identified by combining conventional mATPase histochemistry with biochemical analyses of total muscle homogenates or by analyses of single muscle fibers. It has been shown that covariance between fiber type proportion established from mATPase stains and enzyme activity levels of skeletal muscle is low in human (31). Thus, skeletal muscles with given enzyme activity levels may exhibit large differences in fiber type distribution or vice versa.

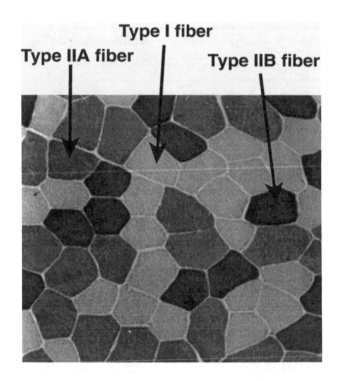

Figure 2 Sections (10 μm thick) of human skeletal muscle were stained for myofibrillar adenosine triphosphatase (mATPase) according to an established technique (19) to determine the proportion of the different fiber types (I, IIA, and IIB).

No difference was found, for instance, in the activity level of succinate dehydrogenase, a regulatory enzyme marker for the Krebs cycle, in samples taken from soleus or vastus lateralis muscles of the same individuals (32) even though these muscle groups exhibit large difference in fiber type I proportion (about 80% for soleus and 50% for vastus lateralis). A vastus lateralis muscle with as little as 15% of type I fibers can possess about the same level of citrate synthase, another enzyme marker for the Krebs cycle, as that of a vastus lateralis muscle with as much as 85% of type I fibers (33) (Fig. 3). These observations indicate that fiber type proportion is a poor marker of the aerobic-oxidative metabolism of skeletal muscle in human.

G. Metabolic Potential of Skeletal Muscle

Rather than solely examining fiber type proportions, another and arguably a better description of the metabolic potential of skeletal muscle is to directly determine muscle enzyme activities. This approach is to select key marker enzymes, chosen because they regulate diverse metabolic pathways and because the particular enzymes catalyze

rate-limiting reactions for each respective pathway of substrate utilization. With this approach, one can obtain an overall metabolic profile of skeletal muscle. The biochemical methodology most commonly used has been to determine maximal activity (V_{max}) of each enzyme chosen for the metabolic profile. The activities of enzymes catalyzing nonequilibrium reactions (i.e., regulatory enzymes) provide a semiquantitative index of both maximal metabolic flux and fuel utilization, while the activities of enzymes catalyzing reactions close to equilibrium provide only qualitative information about the importance of particular metabolic pathways and the principal fuels supporting activity (34). A panel of metabolic markers (Fig. 4) can be assayed according to their role as key regulatory enzymes of glycolysis (PFK, HK), glycogenolysis (PHOS), aerobic oxidative metabolism (CS), oxidative phosphorylation (COX), fatty acid oxidation (CPT, HADH), and anaerobic regeneration of ATP (CK). The rationale for assaying maximal activity of regulatory enzymes has previously been carefully and thoroughly justified (35) and is based on conventional Michaelis-Menten kinetics. Importantly, and what is most pertinent to a consideration of substrate metabolism in obesity, is that the influence of maximal enzyme activity may be greatest at substrate concentrations below the K_m of the enzyme (35), and these are the conditions that prevail during daily living. In collaborative studies between the authors' laboratories, a strong relationship among insulin resistance, obesity, and perturbations of oxidative and glycolytic capacities was found and

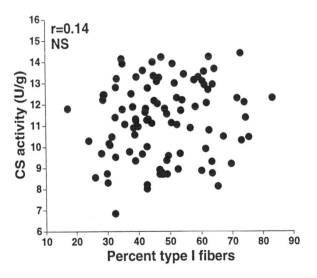

Figure 3 Relationship between proportion of type I fibers and citrate synthase (CS) activity in human vastus lateralis muscle (Unpublished results from Thériault, Thériault, and Simoneau).

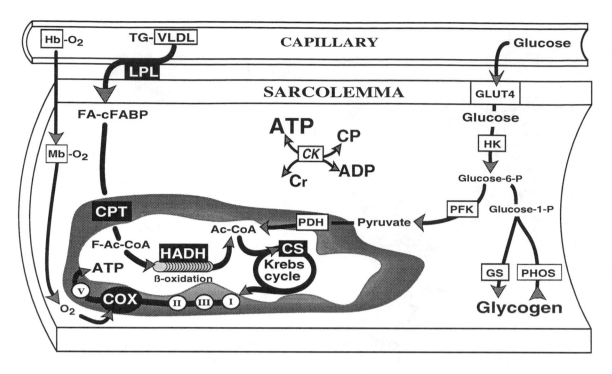

Figure 4 Schematic view of different metabolic markers of skeletal muscle. LPL, lipoprotein lipase; cFABP, cytosolic fatty acid binding protein; CPT, carnitine palmitoyl transferase; HADH, beta-hydroxyacyl CoA dehydrogenase; CS, citrate synthase; COX, cytochrome c oxidase; HK, hexokinase; PFK, phosphofructokinase; PDH, pyruvate dehydrogenase; GS, glycogen synthase; PHOS, glycogen phosphorylase.

these findings will be the topic of the rest of this chapter after a review of the relationship between obesity and insulin resistance.

III. INSULIN RESISTANCE, SUBSTRATE METABOLISM BY SKELETAL MUSCLE, AND OBESITY

A. Insulin Resistance

Obesity causes insulin resistance (36). The link between excess weight and insulin resistance has been recognized for many years, yet despite continued investigation the precise etiology of insulin resistance in obesity remains uncertain. Because insulin has many effects and regulates protein, lipid, and carbohydrate metabolism, the term "insulin resistance" can have many connotations and definitions. In this chapter, insulin resistance will be used to refer to a reduced stimulation of glucose utilization. Reduced utilization of glucose by skeletal muscle largely accounts for systemic insulin resistance (37). Insulin resistance can be discerned in a number of ways, including an abnormally high level of circulating insulin in the face of

normal fasting levels of glucose. This is a reasonable index of insulin resistance in obesity (38,39). Even more typical of the insulin resistance of obesity is an exaggerated insulin response to glucose ingestion, most particularly if found in the setting of normal glucose tolerance (40,41). More precise quantification of insulin sensitivity (and hence resistance) has been achieved with methods such as the euglycemic, insulin infusion, the so-called "glucose clamp" (42). Other techniques, such as intravenous glucose tolerance with mathematical modeling of the glucose and insulin curves, the so-called "minimal model," have also proven to be of great value in the quantification of insulin resistance (43). With these techniques, and most particularly with the glucose clamp method, it can be clearly demonstrated that obesity causes insulin resistance.

Among overweight individuals, the severity of insulin resistance is correlated with the degree of obesity, though in a nonlinear manner (44). In males, beyond a body fat content of approximately 30% the impairment of insulin sensitivity is not further aggravated by greater adiposity. In men, and to an even more pronounced extent in women, the relationship between obesity and insulin resistance is influenced by body fat distribution and is greater in proportion to upper body fat distribution (45). The issue of body fat distribution as it relates to insulin resistance is a particularly interesting topic and can be extended beyond consideration of upper versus lower body fat distribution. As cited previously, fat deposition within muscle is a powerful marker of insulin resistance (5), and this component of fat distribution contributes to insulin resistance independently from overall adiposity. The negative effects of obesity to cause insulin resistance can be modulated by physical activity and training, such that insulin resistance tends to be less severe among obese individuals with higher indices of aerobic power (46). Also, brief periods of physical training, perhaps even a single session of vigorous exercise, can temporarily improve insulin sensitivity in obese subjects (47), similar to the acute effects of exercise on insulin sensitivity in lean individuals.

B. Substrate Metabolism by Skeletal Muscle

During insulin-stimulated conditions, glucose that is taken up by skeletal muscle can be either stored as glycogen or undergo glycolysis and be either oxidized or released from muscle as lactate, the latter pool exchanging freely with alanine (34). Therefore, rate of glucose utilization per se does not reveal the nature of the metabolic defect associated with insulin resistance in obesity, at least with regard to whether glucose oxidation or storage is predominantly affected. One method commonly used to make this assessment is indirect calorimetry, with estimation of the rates of glucose oxidation from values for systemic gas exchange (48,49). When indirect calorimetry is performed in conjunction with the insulin infusion method, the rates of glucose utilization (determined from rates of exogenous glucose infusion required to maintain euglycemia) can be partitioned into oxidative and nonoxidative glucose metabolism, with the latter predominantly reflecting glycogen storage though this does include lactate formation as well (50). Often, infusions of glucose isotopes are used with these methods to refine determination of systemic glucose utilization and to assess insulin regulation of hepatic (endogenous) glucose production (51).

The insulin resistance of obesity seems to affect the pathway of glucose storage more severely than that of glucose oxidation (52–54). In comparison with lean individuals, obese subjects generally have either normal rates of insulin-stimulated glucose oxidation or relatively modest reductions in this pathway. Recognition of this metabolic pattern in the insulin resistance of obesity has spurred a thorough examination of the insulin regulation of the glycogen synthesis pathway, with particular focus on the enzyme glycogen synthase, which is generally regarded as a rate-limiting step in glycogen synthesis (34). Insulin stimulates the activity of glycogen synthase, reversible dephosphorylation of this enzyme, and obesity is associated with insulin resistance in the stimulation of glycogen synthase (52,54). Insulin-stimulated glycogen synthase activity is correlated with rates of insulin-stimulated nonoxidative glucose metabolism (52,55). These findings indicate the key role of glycogen formation in the pathophysiology of the insulin resistance in obesity.

Impaired insulin stimulation of glycogen synthase activity is an important defect, but clearly it is not the only impairment within the cellular cascade of insulin action. Classic investigations into the nature of the cellular defect of insulin action in obesity centered upon downregulation of insulin receptors and insulin bindings (56). These studies gave way to the concept that "postreceptor" defects were a principal cause of insulin resistance. The exact sequence of insulin signaling and "second-messenger" systems remains elusive but considerable progress has been made in recent years (57). It is becoming apparent that the insulin resistance of obesity involves initial steps in insulin signaling (58–62). Decreased content and tyrosine phosphorylation of the insulin beta-receptor subunit, decreased content and tyrosine phosporylation of IRS-1 and decreased content of the p85 subunit of PI 3-kinase, and decreased PI 3-kinase activity associated with IRS-1 were also observed in the skeletal muscle from obese individuals. Each of these is a step of insulin signaling in human skeletal muscle that is necessary for normal stimulation of glucose uptake.

The defect of insulin-stimulated glucose storage is not inconsistent with a primary defect of insulin-stimulated glucose transport into muscle, which, in muscle, is mediated by a tissue-specific isoform of the glucose transport (Glut 4) family (63). Dohm et al. (64) have demonstrated that insulin-stimulated glucose transport is markedly impaired in skeletal muscle of morbidly obese individuals, and that this defect can be greatly improved with weight loss (65). However, content of Glut 4 is not different in obese compared to lean individuals (66), though exercise training does increase muscle content of Glut 4 in obese individuals and this is associated with improved insulin sensitivity (67). The finding that Glut 4 content is essentially normal in obesity raises the possibility that functional defects of glucose transport may be related to the process of insulin-stimulated Glut 4 translocation (68). Recent studies from our laboratories further implicate a defect of glucose transport in the insulin resistance of obesity. Using positron emission tomography to image skeletal muscle uptake of the glucose analog [18]fluoro-deoxy-glucose (FDG), we have found that obese individuals have a marked defect in insulin stimulation of glucose transport (69).

C.   Hemodynamic Factors and Insulin Action

It is likely that the list of cellular defects of insulin action that are associated with obesity will continue to lengthen in the future, but some recent studies have also increased awareness of the potential importance of hemodynamic factors in the pathogenesis of insulin resistance in obesity. Baron et al. (70,71) have shown that obesity is associated with impaired insulin stimulation of blood flow to skeletal muscle. Since insulin stimulation of blood flow contributes to improve substrate and hormone availability, attenuation of this hemodynamic response is likely to contribute to insulin resistance of glucose uptake. Another aspect of the relationship between blood flow and insulin sensitivity involves delivery of insulin across capillary endothelium. Interstitial concentrations of insulin within muscle, as revealed by measurement of insulin concentration in lymph, correlate more strongly with rates of glucose utilization than do arterial concentrations of insulin (72). The time course by which insulin activates glucose utilization within skeletal muscle lags behind the time course of arterial insulin concentrations. There is, however, remarkably close correspondence between the temporal appearance of insulin within lymph and the activation of glucose utilization within skeletal muscle, findings that clearly demonstrate that "prereceptor" events, related to insulin delivery across the capillary endothelium, have an important role in defining the kinetics of insulin action in humans. These concepts are pertinent to insulin resistance in obesity. Not only do obese individuals have less sensitivity to insulin at steady-state conditions, but the onset of insulin activation of glucose utilization is delayed in obese compared to nonobese individuals (73). The discrepancy between obese and lean individuals in the time required for insulin to achieve steady-state stimulation of glucose utilization is greatest at insulin concentrations within the low physiological range. For all of these reasons, it is likely that this aspect of insulin resistance has the greatest physiological significance during prandial conditions of daily living (74). Delays in insulin delivery and activation of glucose utilization could be factors in altered insulin action during postprandial metabolism given the intrinsically non-steady-state conditions of insulin concentration and the relatively brief intervals of peak insulin concentrations during postprandial metabolism. It seems logical to postulate that some of the morphological alterations of skeletal muscle that are associated with obesity, most specifically a reduced capillary density,

contribute to the delayed activation of glucose utilization by insulin.

IV.   GLUCOSE AND FATTY ACID SUBSTRATE COMPETITION IN MUSCLE: THE ROLE IN INSULIN RESISTANCE OF OBESITY AND THE RELATIONSHIP OF SUBSTRATE METABOLISM WITH OXIDATIVE AND GLYCOLYTIC CAPACITIES OF MUSCLE

A.   Glucose and Fatty Acid Substrate Competition

An area of long-standing interest and potential importance in the pathogenesis of insulin resistance in obesity is glucose and fatty acid substrate competition. Glucose and fatty acid substrate competition is commonly referred to as the "Randle cycle," in reference to the hypothesis that fatty acid oxidation by muscle, driven by a concentration-dependent uptake of plasma free fatty acids (FFA), inhibits glucose oxidation and glycolysis, with consequent inhibition of glucose uptake (75–77). Because adipose tissue is increased in obesity and insulin suppression of lipolysis is often impaired (78,79), the metabolic milieu seems appropriate for glucose/FFA substrate competition to contribute to insulin resistance in obese individuals. Skepticism persists regarding the role of substrate competition as a mechanism of insulin resistance in obesity (49,80,81). As previously described, the metabolic profile of insulin-resistant glucose metabolism in skeletal muscle of obese individuals is characterized by a substantial impairment in glycogen synthesis with lesser defects of glucose oxidation or glycolysis, which is different from that predicted by the Randle cycle. However, interest has been renewed in the potential role of substrate competition in obesity (82), spurred in part by several recent clinical investigations (83–85) that have challenged the tenets of the hypothesis as originally proposed by Randle. In fact, some recent studies suggest that part of the expression of insulin resistance of skeletal muscle in obesity is an impaired capacity for utilization of plasma FFA.

B.   Lipid and Carbohydrate Utilization by Skeletal Muscle

Skeletal muscle has the capacity to utilize lipid or carbohydrate for energy production. During postabsorptive conditions, skeletal muscle predominantly relies on lipid oxidation as reflected in a respiratory quotient across the forearm in lean individuals of approximately 0.71–0.82

(86–88). There is also a high rate of extraction of plasma FFA by skeletal muscle during fasting conditions, of approximately 40% (87), and oxidation of plasma FFA taken up by muscle accounted for nearly 80% of resting oxygen consumption by muscle. Insulin suppresses lipolysis and stimulated glucose uptake, oxidation, and storage in skeletal muscle, thereby transiently shifting the predominant substrate utilized for energy production (89). Studies by Kelley et al. (83) have been among the investigations that have reexamined glucose/FFA substrate competition and its effects on skeletal muscle glucose metabolism. In lean healthy volunteers, "clamping" plasma FFA at postabsorptive levels, by giving an infusion of lipid emulsion along with insulin and glucose infusions, induced skeletal muscle insulin resistance by the 4th hour of infusion (83). Regional indirect calorimetry, net balance of lactate across the leg, and glucose uptake were measured to determine the metabolic pattern of the insulin resistance induced by FFA. When FFA were maintained at fasting concentrations during insulin-stimulated conditions, the rate of glucose utilization was reduced. A large fraction of the reduction in rates of glucose utilization was due to reduced glucose storage in muscle. There was some impairment of glucose oxidation, though of lesser amplitude than the defect in glucose storage. However, there was no apparent reduction in overall rates of glycolysis (i.e., glucose oxidation + lactate release), since rates of lactate release from muscle increased in proportion to the defect of glucose oxidation (83).

Maintaining FFA at postabsorptive levels during insulin infusion also impeded insulin stimulation of key enzymes of glucose oxidation and storage. In vastus lateralis muscle, insulin activation of pyruvate dehydrogenase (PDH) and glycogen synthase (GS) was reduced during FFA replacement compared to control studies of insulin alone. The enzyme data and the data on glucose metabolism are quite consistent with studies reported by Boden and his colleagues (84,85), in which it was also found that FFA impaired insulin stimulation of glucose storage and glycogen synthase activity in skeletal muscle but had little effect on insulin-stimulated rates of glycolysis despite inhibition of glucose oxidation. In those studies, FFA did not influence citrate concentrations in skeletal muscle, as might have been expected from the original hypothesis of Randle et al. (75,77). A key point emphasized by Boden et al. (84,85) is that there is an apparent lag of several hours before elevated levels of FFA impair insulin stimulation of glucose storage, while the inhibition of glucose oxidation is manifested promptly. This latter factor may be one explanation as to why the effects of FFA on inhibition of glucose storage have not been appreciated in

earlier studies, which generally were limited to a duration of approximately 2 hr. Therefore, the pattern of insulin resistance induced by FFA bears strong similarity to that observed in obesity and NIDDM (90). Data on FFA uptake by muscle have not been widely examined. Recently, in a collaborative effort between our laboratories, we undertook studies to address the issue of skeletal muscle utilization of FFA in obese individuals and the relationship of this to insulin resistance of obesity (91).

Among lean and obese healthy young women (range of BMI from 19 to 39 kg/m^2), there was a wide range of insulin sensitivity, as assessed by insulin-stimulated glucose uptake across the leg, during euglycemic insulin infusions. Rates of insulin-stimulated glucose storage were negatively correlated with visceral obesity ($r = -0.59$, $p < 0.01$), which, among several components of obesity (e.g., total fat mass, subcutaneous abdominal fat, thigh fat, and BMI), was the strongest marker of insulin resistance of skeletal muscle. One exception was that fat content in muscle, determined noninvasively by a CT technique, was equal to visceral fat in predicting insulin resistance of muscle. However, during steady-state insulin-stimulated conditions, rates of FFA uptake and lipid oxidation across the leg had relatively little variation between subjects, and therefore it seems unlikely that insulin resistance of obesity is primarily caused by increased uptake of plasma FFA.

C. FFA Utilization by Skeletal Muscle in Obesity

Another key goal of this study was to examine the effects of obesity on FFA utilization by skeletal muscle during postabsorptive (fasting) conditions. Visceral obesity was negatively correlated with basal rates of FFA utilization by muscle ($r = -0.60$, $p < 0.01$; Fig.5), despite the fact that women with increased visceral fat had neither lower plasma FFA nor lower rates for systemic appearance of FFA. Our interpretation of these data is that muscle in women with visceral obesity has a reduced capacity for utilizing plasma FFA and analysis of skeletal muscle enzyme capacities supports this concept. Activity of muscle carnitine palmitoyl transferase (CPT) was negatively correlated with visceral fat ($r = -0.76$, $p < 0.05$), and rates of FFA uptake were correlated with CPT activity. The CPT complex mediates transport of long-chain acyl CoA esters across the mitochondrial membrane, via a carnitine shuttle, and is regarded as a rate-limiting step in the oxidation of long-chain FFA. The findings that basal rates of FFA utilization by muscle are lower in obesity may be important for the pathogenesis of this disorder of fuel balance. This study by our laboratories is not the first to suggest

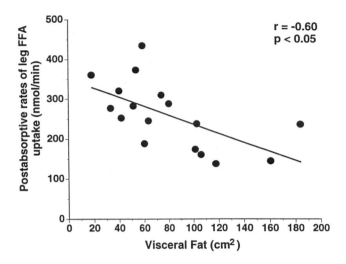

Figure 5 Relationship between postabsorptive rates of leg FFA uptake and visceral fat in human (Reproduced from Ref. 91 by copyright permission of the American Society for Clinical Investigation).

this concept. Ravussin and his colleagues have reported several studies that indicate that a metabolic component of the risk for weight gain is an impaired capacity for oxidation of fat calories (92,93). Their data indicate that, even after adjustment for factors such as energy balance, adiposity, and sex, a high 24-hr respiratory quotient predicted weight gain over subsequent years (92). Subjects with a high respiratory quotient (0.877) were 2.5 times more likely to gain 5 kg or more body weight than those with a low respiratory quotient (0.822) (94,95). Interestingly, inverse relationships between 24-hr respiratory quotient and the activity levels of skeletal muscle HADH (96) and lipoprotein lipase (93) were found, which suggest strongly that muscle is an important tissue contributing to impaired lipid oxidation. Other investigators have found that visceral obesity is negatively correlated with muscle LPL activity (97). Therefore, an important area for clinical investigation and basic research is whether the capacity of muscle for lipid utilization is impaired in obesity and whether there is compensation of this defect once obesity state is attained.

In this collaborative study between our laboratories (91), we also found that visceral obesity was linked to the activity levels of several marker enzymes of oxidative and glycolytic capacities. Citrate synthase (CS), an enzyme of the TCA cycle activity and a strong marker of oxidative capacity, was negatively correlated with visceral obesity ($r = -0.51$, $p < 0.05$). Conversely, CS activity was positively correlated with rates of lipid oxidation across the

leg during fasting conditions and positively correlated with rates of glucose uptake during insulin-stimulated conditions. These data indicate that oxidative capacity, as exemplified by CS activity, influences both postabsorptive utilization of FFA and insulin sensitivity. Conversely, glycolytic potential of muscle, as reflected by activity of phosphofructokinase (PFK), a regulatory enzyme in the glycolytic pathway, is increased in individuals with visceral obesity. In particular, the ratio of PFK/CS activity was a strong marker of insulin resistance (Fig. 6). Also, creatine kinase (CK), a cytosolic enzyme that catalyzes a key step in anaerobic regeneration of ATP, was increased in proportion to obesity and insulin resistance. Taken together, this pattern of enzyme activity indicates that insulin-resistant muscle is disposed toward anaerobic and glycolytic generation of energy. Our interpretation of the enzyme and metabolic data is that substrate metabolism by skeletal muscle in obesity is perturbed during both basal and insulin-stimulated conditions. During basal conditions this is manifest as a reduced capacity in obese individuals for the utilization of plasma FFA by muscle. During insulin-stimulated conditions, the primary defect that is manifest in obesity is within glucose transport and glucose storage pathways. The data suggest that these defects occur together, as suggested by the correlation between fasting rates of lipid oxidation in muscle and insulin-stimulated rates of glucose storage in muscle ($r = 0.61$, $p < 0.05$). In a multiple regression model, basal rates of lipid oxidation across the leg and visceral obesity accounted for nearly 60% of the variance in insulin resistance (91).

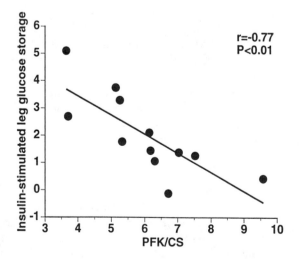

Figure 6 Relationship between insulin-stimulated leg glucose storage and the phosphofructokinase (PFK) to citrate synthase ratio of skeletal muscle in human [Drawn from the results published by Simoneau et al. (5)].

Thus, capacity of muscle to utilize fat during basal conditions and insulin sensitivity for glucose utilization seem to be interrelated metabolic capacities of skeletal muscle, and oxidative capacity may be an important link between insulin sensitivity and capacity for lipid oxidation. As mentioned above, women with visceral obesity had lower activity of citrate synthase in muscle and this enzyme is a key enzymatic marker of muscle mitochondrial content and of overall aerobic-oxidative potential of muscle (98). This enzyme catalyzes formation of citrate from acetyl CoA, the latter representing the biochemical convergence of FFA and glucose metabolism within the mitochondria (34).

If this hypothesis is correct, a reduced oxidative capacity of skeletal muscle might predispose toward obesity by reducing oxidation of fat calories, thereby increasing storage of fat as adipose tissue. Also, FFA taken up by muscle but not oxidized might contribute to triglyceride accumulation within skeletal muscle. Animal studies indicate that accumulation of triglycerides within muscle is a powerful marker of the emergence of insulin resistance in muscle (99). In collaborative studies between the authors' laboratories (5), fat content of muscle, as assessed by CT, was strongly correlated with the oxidative capacity of muscle. Lower density of muscle was negatively correlated with citrate synthase activity and positively correlated with glycolytic capacity and strongly correlated with the ratio of PFK to CS (Fig. 7). Our interpretation is that accumulation of fat within muscle, as revealed by low density on CT imaging, occurs in the presence of an impaired

capacity for oxidation of fat calories and this accumulation of intramuscular fat potentiates insulin resistance in obesity.

Obesity may also predispose to the operation of a "reverse Randle cycle", a term used to denote that increased glucose availability may inhibit utilization of lipid by skeletal muscle. Clinical investigations have demonstrated that in lean individuals, hyperglycemia stimulates systemic glucose oxidation independent of insulin (55) and that this response occurs in skeletal muscle in conjunction with glycemic stimulation of pyruvate dehydrogenase in muscle (100). Recent findings led Sidossis and Wolfe (101) to conclude that, contrary to the prediction of the glucose–fatty acid cycle theory, the intracellular availability of glucose (rather than FFA) determines the nature of substrate oxidation in human subjects. In recent additional studies, it has been found that skeletal muscle glucose oxidation in obese subjects is stimulated by hyperglycemia to an even greater extent than in lean individuals (102). In the studies of Mandarino et al. (102), somatostatin was infused to suppress endogenous insulin secretion and basal amounts of insulin were given as replacement, along with glucagon. During these conditions, skeletal muscle in obese subjects derived nearly 80% of energy production from glucose oxidation during hyperglycemic conditions compared to 40% in muscle of lean individuals (102). Thus, under matched conditions of glucose and FFA availability, skeletal muscle in obese individuals seems more responsive than muscle of lean individuals to the effect of glucose to stimulate glucose oxidation and inhibit lipid oxidation.

In summary, there has been a long-standing interest in the potential role that glucose/FFA substrate competition may have in the pathogenesis of insulin resistance in obesity. A number of recent investigations indicate that skeletal muscle in individuals with obesity has a diminished capacity for utilization of FFA. This impairment may be important to the pathogenesis of obesity and insulin resistance. However, these studies indicate that insulin resistance in obesity does not seem to be caused by increased uptake and oxidation of plasma FFA. Instead, a decreased oxidative capacity of skeletal muscle appears to be related to the expression of insulin resistance in obesity and obesity is associated with a diminished rate of FFA utilization by muscle.

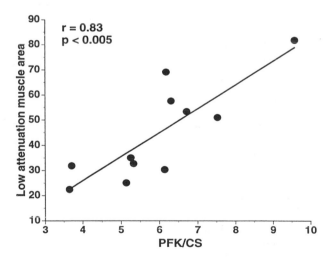

Figure 7 Relationship between low attenuation muscle area determined by CT scans of the thigh and the phosphofructokinase (PFK) to citrate synthase ratio of skeletal muscle in human [Drawn from the results published by Simoneau et al. (5)].

V. SUMMARY AND CONCLUSIONS

In summary, the composition and biochemistry of skeletal muscle is altered in obese as compared to nonobese individuals. The nature of these alterations suggests that they may contribute substantially to the development and maintenance of the obese state. Such a key role is certainly consistent with the capacity that skeletal muscle has to utilize both carbohydrate and lipid fuels and with the major role that skeletal muscle can have in overall fuel balance. A key structural abnormality of skeletal muscle in obesity is increased content of fat, though the precise characterization of how much is within muscle fibrils is as yet uncertain. Accretion of fat within muscle tissues appears to strongly correlate with insulin resistance. This fat accretion within muscle of obese individuals may not be simply a passive process, paralleling fat storage in other tissues. Instead, and of particular metabolic interest, is the emerging concept that biochemical characteristics of skeletal muscle in obese individuals dispose to fat accumulation in muscle. These biochemical characteristics of muscle in obese individuals have long been recognized to include insulin resistance in pathways of glucose metabolism and more recent studies indicate as well a reduced capacity for the utilization of fat calories. The task at present is to more precisely define the nature of the defects within the pathways of fat metabolism, to discern the contribution of environmental and genetic influences, and, finally, to utilize these insights to develop effective treatment strategies. An effort to modify skeletal muscle of obese individuals so that its capacity for substrate utilization, and in particular fat oxidation, is improved should be among the goals of treatment for obesity. Whether capacity for fat oxidation by muscle can be enhanced by pharmacological treatment is largely unknown, and though it is clear that nutritional and exercise interventions can improve insulin sensitivity of skeletal muscle in obese individuals, much remains to be learned about optimal behavioral methods to attain this goal.

ACKNOWLEDGMENTS

The authors would like to acknowledge the sources of financial support for their collaborative studies from the University of Pittsburgh General Clinical Research Center (#5MO1RR00056), the University of Pittsburgh Obesity and Nutrition Research Center (1P30DK46204), the National Institute of Health (1R01 DK49200-01), a Veterans Affairs Merit Award (DEK), a University Research Fellow of the Fonds de la Recherche en Santé du Québec (JAS), and the National Sciences and Engineering Research Council of Canada.

REFERENCES

1. Ross R, Shaw KD, Rissanen J, Martel Y, Guise Jd, Avruch L. Sex differences in lean and adipose tissue distribution by magnetic resonance imaging: anthropometric relationships. Am J Clin Nutr 1994; 59:1277–1285.
2. Landin K, Lindgärde F, Saltin B, Wilhelmsen L. Decreased skeletal muscle potassium in obesity. Acta Med Scand 1988; 223:507–513.
3. Kelley DE, Slasky S, Janosky J. Skeletal muscle density: effects of obesity and non-insulin dependent diabetes mellitus. Am J Clin Nutr 1991; 54:509–515.
4. Bulcke J, Crolla D, Termotte JL, Baert A, Palmer Y, Bergh Rvd. Computed tomography of muscle. Muscle Nerve 1981; 4:67–72.
5. Simoneau J-A, Colberg SR, Thaete FL, Kelley DE. Skeletal muscle glycolytic and oxidative enzyme capacities are determinants of insulin sensitivity and muscle composition in obese women. FASEB J 1995; 9:273–278.
6. Wang N, Hikida RS, Staron RS, Simoneau J-A. Muscle fiber types of women after resistance training—quantitative ultrastructure and enzyme activity. Pflügers Arch 1993; 424:494–502.
7. Pan DA, Milner MR, Lillioja S, Storlien LH. Muscle lipid composition is related to body fatness and insulin action in humans. Int J Obes 1995; 19:213 (abstract).
8. Pan DA, Lillioja S, Milner MR, et al. Skeletal muscle membrane lipid composition is related to adiposity and insulin action. J Clin Invest 1995; 96:2802–2808.
9. Storlien LH, Pan DA, Milner MR, Lillioja S. Skeletal muscle membrane lipid composition is related to adiposity in man. Obes Res 1993; 1(Suppl 2):77S.
10. Pan DA, Hulbert AJ, Storlien LH. Dietary fats, membrane phospholipids and obesity. J Nutr 1994; 124:1555–1565.
11. Pehowich DJ. Hypothyroid state and membrane fatty acid composition influence cardiac mitochondrial pyruvate oxidation. Biochim Biophys Acta 1995; 1235:231–238.
12. Krotkiewski M, Bylund-Fallenius A-C, Holm J, Björntorp P, Grimby G, Mandroukas K. Relationship between muscle morphology and metabolism in obese women: the effects of long-term physical training. Eur J Clin Invest 1983; 13:5–12.
13. Krotkiewski M, Seidell JC, Björntorp P. Glucose tolerance and hyperinsulinaemia in obese women: role of adipose tissue distribution, muscle fibre characteristics and androgens. J Intern Med 1990; 228:385–392.
14. Björntorp P. Insulin resistance: the consequence of a neuroendocrine disturbance? Int J Obes 1995; 19:(Suppl 1):S6–S10.
15. Rasio E. The capillary barrier to circulating insulin. Diabetes Care 1982; 5:158–161.
16. Jansson P-AT, Forvelin JP, vonSehenk HP, Smith UP, Lönnroth PN. Measurements by microdyalysis of the insulin concentration in subcutaneous interstitial fluid-importance of the endothelial barrier for insulin. Diabetes 1993; 42:1469–1473.

17. Lillioja S, Young A, Cutler C, et al. Skeletal muscle capillary density and fiber type are possible determinants of in vivo insulin resistance in man. J Clin Invest 1987; 80: 415–424.

18. Wade AJ, Marbut MM, Round JM. Muscle fibre type and aetiology of obesity. Lancet 1990; 335:805–808.

19. Simoneau J-A, Bouchard C. Human variation in skeletal muscle fiber-type proportion and enzyme activities. Am J Physiol 1989; 257:E567–E572.

20. Williamson DF. Descriptive epidemiology of body weight and weight change in U.S. adults. Ann Intern Med 1993; 119:646–649.

21. Hickey MS, Carey JO, Azevedo JL, et al. Skeletal muscle fiber composition is related to adiposity and in vitro glucose transport rate in humans. Am J Physiol 1995; 268: E453–E457.

22. Simoneau J-A, Bouchard C. Skeletal muscle metabolism and body fat content in men and women. Obes Res 1995; 3:23–29.

23. Segal K, Chatr-Aryamontri B, Rosenbaum M, Simoneau J-A. Effects of hypertension and obesity on postprandial thermogenesis in men. Am J Clin Nutr 1995; 61:895.

24. Kraegen EW, James DE, Jenkins AB, Chisholm DJ. Dose-response curves for in vivo insulin sensitivity in individual tissues in rat. Am J Physiol 1985; 11:E353–E362.

25. Reichmann H, Pette D. A comparative microphotometric study of succinate dehydrogenase activity levels in type I, IIA and IIB fibres of mammalian and human muscles. Histochemistry 1982; 74:27–41.

26. Hoppeler H. The range of mitochondrial adaptation in muscle fibers. In: Pette D, ed. The Dynamic State of Muscle Fibers. New York: Walter de Gruyter, 1990:567–586.

27. Lowry CV, Kimmey JS, Felder S. Enzyme patterns in single human muscle fibers. J Biol Chem 1978; 253: 8269–8277.

28. Staron RS, Johnson P. Myosin polymorphism and differential expression in adult human skeletal muscle. Comp Biochem Physiol 1993; 106B:463–475.

29. Pette D, Staron RS. Cellular and molecular diversities of mammalian skeletal muscle fibers. Rev Physiol Biochem Pharmacol 1990; 116:1–76.

30. Sweeney HL, Kushmerick MJ, Mabuchi K, Gergely J, Sréter FA. Velocity of shortening and myosin isozymes in two types of rabbit fast-twitch muscle fibers. Am J Physiol 1986; 251:C431–C434.

31. Simoneau J-A, Lortie G, Boulay MR, Thibault M-C, Thériault G, Bouchard C. Skeletal muscle histochemical and biochemical characteristics in sedentary male and female subjects. Can J Physiol Pharmacol 1985; 63:30–35.

32. Gollnick PD, Sjödin B, Karlsson K, Jansson E, Saltin B. Human soleus muscle: a comparison of fiber composition and enzyme activities with other leg muscles. Pflügers Arch 1974; 348:247–255.

33. Simoneau J-A. Le muscle squelettique et les désordres fonctionnels et métaboliques chez l'humain. Sci Sport 1991; 6:105–111.

34. Newsholme EA, Leech AR. Biochemistry for the Medical Sciences. Chicester: Wiley, 1983.

35. Gollnick PD, Saltin B. Significance of skeletal muscle oxidative enzyme enhancement with endurance training. Clin Physiol 1982; 2:1–12.

36. Olefsky JM. Decreased insulin binding to adipocytes and monocytes from obese subjects. J Clin Invest 1976; 57: 1165–1172.

37. DeFronzo RA, Gunnarsson R, Björkman O, Olsson M, Wahren J. Effects of insulin on peripheral and splanchnic glucose metabolism in noninsulin-dependent (Type II) diabetes mellitus. J Clin Invest 1985; 76:149–155.

38. Laakso M. How good a marker is insulin level for insulin resistance? Am J Epidemiol 1993; 137(9):959–965.

39. Olefsky J, Farquhar JW, Reaven G. Relationship between fasting plasma insulin level and resistance to insulin-mediated glucose uptake in normal and diabetic subjects. Diabetes 1973; 22(7):507–513.

40. Polonsky KS, Given DB, Hirsch L, et al. Quantitative study of insulin secretion and clearance in normal and obese subjects. J Clin Invest 1988; 81:435–441.

41. Polonsky KS, Given BD, Cauter EV. Twenty-four-hour profiles and pulsatile patterns of insulin secretion in normal and obese subjects. J Clin Invest 1988; 81:442–448.

42. DeFronzo RA, Tobin JD, Andres R. Glucose clamp technique: a method of quantifying insulin secretion and resistance. Am J Physiol 1979; 237:E214–E223.

43. Bergman RN, Finegood DT, Ader M. Assessment of insulin sensitivity in vivo. Endocr Rev 1985; 6:45–86.

44. Bogardus C, Lillioja S, Mott D, Hollenbeck C, Reaven G. Relationship between degree of obesity and in vivo insulin action in man. Am J Physiol 1985; 248:E286–E291.

45. Evans DJ, Murray M, Kissebah AH. Relationship between skeletal muscle insulin resistance, insulin-mediated glucose disposal, and insulin binding: effects of obesity and body fat topography. J Clin Invest 1984; 74:1515–1525.

46. Yki-Järvinen H, Koivisto VA. Effects of body composition on insulin sensitivity. Diabetes 1983; 32:765–969.

47. Devlin JT, Horton SE. Effects of prior high-intensity exercise on glucose metabolism in normal and insulin-resistant men. Diabetes 1985; 34:973–979.

48. Felber JP, Meyer HU, Curchod B, et al. Glucose storage and oxidation in different degrees of human obesity measured by continuous indirect calorimetry. Diabetologia 1981; 20:39–44.

49. Lillioja S, Bogardus C, Mott D, Kennedy A, Knowler W, Howard B. Relationship between insulin-mediated glucose disposal and lipid metabolism in man. J Clin Invest 1985; 75:1106–1115.

50. Thiebaud D, Jacot E, DeFronzo RA, Maeder E, Jéquier E, Felber JP. The effect of graded doses of insulin on total glucose uptake, glucose oxidation, and glucose storage in man. Diabetes 1982; 31:957–963.

51. Gerich JE, Rizza RA, Mandarino LJ. Assessment of insulin action in humans with observations on the insulin resis-

tance in noninsulin-dependent diabetes mellitus. I. Excerpta Med 1982; 35:74–96.

52. Bogardus C, Lillioja S, Stone K, Mott D. Correlation between muscle glycogen synthase activity and in vivo insulin action in man. J Clin Invest 1984; 73:1185–1190.

53. Felber JP, Golay A, Felley C, Jéquier E. Regulation of glucose storage in obesity and diabetes: metabolic aspects. Diabetes Metab Rev 1988; 4(7):691–700.

54. Yki-Järvinen H, Mott D, Young AA, Stone K, Bogardus C. Regulation of glycogen synthase and phosphorylase activities by glucose and insulin in human skeletal muscle. J Clin Invest 1987; 80:95–100.

55. Yki-Järvinen H, Bogardus C, Howard B. Hyperglycemia stimulates glucose oxidation in humans. Am J Physiol 1987; 253:E376–E382.

56. Kolterman O, Gray R, Griffin J, et al. Receptor and post-receptor defects contribute to insulin resistance in non-insulin-dependent diabetes mellitus. J Clin Invest 1981; 68:957–969.

57. Cheatham B, Kahn CR. Insulin action and the insulin signaling network. Endocr Rev 1995; 16:117–141.

58. Goodyear LJ, Giorgino F, Sherman LA, Carey J, Smith RJ, Dohm GL. Insulin receptor phosphorylation, insulin receptor substrate-1 phosphorylation, and phosphatidylinositol 3-kinase activity are decreased in intact skeletal muscle strips from obese subjects. J Clin Invest 1995; 95: 2195–2204.

59. Caro JF, Sinha MDK, Raju SM, et al. Insulin receptor kinase in human skeletal muscle from obese subjects with and without noninsulin dependent diabetes. J Clin Invest 1987; 79:1330–1337.

60. Ahmad F, Considine RV, Goldstein BJ. Increased abundance of the receptor-type protein-tyrosine phosphatase LAR accounts for the elevated insulin receptor dephosphorylating activity in adipose tissue of obese human subjects. J Clin Invest 1995; 6:2806–2812.

61. Clausen JO, Hansen T, Bjorbaek C, et al. Insulin resistance: interactions between obesity and a common variant of insulin receptor substrate-1. Lancet 1995; 346: 397–402.

62. Kusari J, Kenner KA, Suh KI, Hill DE, Henry RR. Skeletal muscle protein tyrosine phosphatase activity and tyrosine phosphatase IB protein content are associated with insulin action and resistance. J Clin Invest 1994; 93:1156–1162.

63. Stephens JM, Pilch PF. The metabolic regulation and vesicular transport of GLUT 4, the major insulin-responsive glucose transporter. Endocr Rev 1995; 16:529–546.

64. Dohm GL, Tapscott EB, Pories WJ, et al. An in vitro human muscle preparation suitable for metabolic studies. J Clin Invest 1988; 82:486–494.

65. Friedman JE, Dohm L, Leggett-Frazier N, et al. Restoration of insulin responsiveness in skeletal muscle of morbidly obese patients after weight loss. J Clin Invest 1992; 89:701–705.

66. Garvey WT, Maianu L, Hancock JA, Golichowski AM, Baron A. Gene expression of GLUT4 in skeletal muscle from insulin-resistant patients with obesity, IGT, GDM, and NIDDM. Diabetes 1992; 41:465–475.

67. Houmard JA, Shinebarger MH, Dolan PL, et al. Exercise training increases GLUT-4 protein concentration in previously sedentary middle-aged men. Am J Physiol 1993; 264:E896–E901.

68. Kahn BB. Facilitative glucose transporters: Regulatory mechanisms and dysregulation in diabetes. J Clin Invest 1992; 89:1367–1374.

69. Kelley DE, Mintun MA, Watkins SC, et al. The effect of NIDDM and obesity on glucose transport and phosphorylation in skeletal muscle. J Clin Invest 1996; 97: 2705–2713.

70. Laakso M, Edelman SV, Brechtel G, Baron AD. Decreased effect of insulin to stimulate skeletal muscle blood flow in obese man. J Clin Invest 1990; 85:1844–1852.

71. Baron AD. Cardiovascular actions of insulin in humans. Implications for insulin sensitivity and vascular tone. Ballieres Clin Endocrinol Metab 1993; 7:961–987.

72. Castillo C, Bogardus C, Bergman R, Thuillez P, Lillioja S. Interstitial insulin concentrations determine glucose uptake rates but not insulin resistance in lean and obese men. J Clin Invest 1994; 93:10–16.

73. Prager R, Wallace P, Olefsky JM. In vivo kinetics of insulin action on peripheral glucose disposal and hepatic glucose output in normal and obese subjects. J Clin Invest 1986; 78:472–481.

74. Baron AD, Laakso M, Brechtel G, Hoit B, Watt C, Edelman SV. Reduced postprandial skeletal muscle blood flow contributes to glucose intolerance in human obesity. J Clin Endocrinol Metab 1990; 70:1525–1533.

75. Randle PJ, Newsholme EA, Garland PB. Regulation of glucose uptake by muscle. Biochemistry 1964; 93:652–665.

76. Randle PJ. Fuel selection in animals. Biochem Soc Trans 1986; 14:799–806.

77. Randle PJ, Garlan PB, Hales CN, Newsholme EA. The glucose-fatty acid cycle. Its role in insulin sensitivity and the metabolic disturbances of diabetes mellitus. Lancet 1963; 1:785–789.

78. Jensen M, Haymond M, Rizza R, Cryer P, Miles J. Influence of body fat distribution of free fatty acid metabolism in obesity. J Clin Invest 1989; 83:1168–1173.

79. Reynisdottir S, Ellerfeldt K, Wahrenberg H, Lithell H, Arner P. Multiple lipolysis defects in the insulin resistance (metabolic) syndrome. J Clin Invest 1994; 93:2590–2599.

80. Felber JP, Ferrannini E, Golay A, et al. Role of lipid oxidation in the pathogenesis of insulin resistance of obesity and type II diabetes. Diabetes 1987; 36:1341–1350.

81. Saloranta C, Koivisto V, Widen E, et al. Contribution of muscle and liver to glucose-fatty acid cycle in human. Am J Physiol 1993; 264:E599–E605.

82. McGarry JD. What if Minkowski had been ageusic? An alternative angle on diabetes. Science 1992; 258:766–770.

83. Kelley DE, Mokan M, Simoneau J-A, Mandarino LJ. Interaction between glucose and free fatty acid metabolism in human skeletal muscle. J Clin Invest 1993; 92:91–98.

84. Boden G, Jadali F, White J, et al. Effects of fat on insulin-stimulated carbohydrate metabolism in normal men. J Clin Invest 1991; 88:960–966.

85. Boden G, Chen X, Ruiz J, White J, Rossetti L. Mechanisms of fatty acid–induced inhibition of glucose uptake. J Clin Invest 1994; 93:2438–2446.

86. Andres R, Cader G, Zierler K. The quantitatively minor role of carbohydrate in oxidative metabolism by skeletal muscle in intact man in the basal state. Measurement of oxygen and glucose uptake and carbon dioxide and lactate production in the forearm. J Clin Invest 1956; 35: 671–682.

87. Dagenais G, Tancredi R, Zierler K. Free fatty acid oxidation by forearm muscle at rest, and evidence for an intramuscular lipid pool in the human forearm. J Clin Invest 1976; 58:421–431.

88. Baltzan M, Andres R, Cader G, Zierler K. Heterogeneity of forearm metabolism with special reference to free fatty acids. J Clin Invest 1962; 41:116–125.

89. Kelley DE, Reilly JP, Veneman T, Mandarion LJ. Effects of insulin on skeletal muscle glucose storage, oxidation, and glycolysis in humans. Am J Physiol 1990; 258: E923–E929.

90. Kelley DE, Mokan M, Mandarino LJ. Intracellular defects in glucose metabolism in obese patients with noninsulin-dependent diabetes mellitus. Diabetes 1992; 41:698–706.

91. Colberg SR, Simoneau J-A, Thaete FL, Kelley DE. Skeletal muscle utilization of free fatty acids in women with visceral obesity. J Clin Invest 1995; 95:1846–1853.

92. Zurlo F, Lillioja S, Esposito-DelPuente A, Nyomba BL, Raz I, Ravussin E. Low ratio of fat to carbohydrate oxidation as predictor of weight gain: a study of 24-h RQ. Am J Physiol 1990; 259:E650–E657.

93. Ferraro R, Eckel R, Larson E, et al. Relationship between skeletal muscle lipoprotein lipase activity and 24-hour macronutrient oxidation. J Clin Invest 1993; 92:441–445.

94. Ravussin E, Swinburn BA. Pathophysiology of obesity. Lancet 1992; 340:404–408.

95. Ravussin E. Metabolic differences and the development of obesity. Metabolism 1995; 44:S12–S14.

96. Zurlo F, Nemeth PM, Choksi RM, Sesodia S, Ravussin E. Whole-body energy metabolism and skeletal muscle biochemical characteristics. Metabolism 1994; 43:481–486.

97. Richelsen B, Pedersen S, Moeer-Pedersen T, Schmitz O, Moller N, Borglum J. Lipoprotein lipase activity in muscle tissue influenced by fatness, fat distribution and insulin obese females. Eur J Clin Invest 1993; 23:226–233.

98. Howald H, Pette D, Simoneau J-A, Uber A, Hoppeler H, Cerretelli P. Effects of chronic hypoxia on muscle enzyme activities. Int J Sports Med 1990; 11:S10–S14.

99. Storlien L, Jenkins A, Chisholm D, Pascoe W, Khouri S, Kraegen E. Influence of dietary fat composition on development of insulin resistance in rats: relationship to muscle triglyceride and w-3 fatty acids in muscle phospholipids. Diabetes 1991; 40:280–289.

100. Mandarino L, Consoli A, Jain A, Kelley DE. Differential regulation of intracellular glucose metabolism by glucose and insulin in human muscle. Am J Physiol 1993; 265: E898–E905.

101. Sidossis LS, Wolfe RR. Glucose and insulin-induced inhibition of fatty acid oxidation: the glucose-fatty acid cycle reversed. Am J Physiol 1996; 270:E733–E738.

102. Mandarino LJ, Consoli A, Kelley DE. Effects of obesity and NIDDM on glucose and insulin regulation of substrate oxidation in skeletal muscle. Am J Physiol 1996; 270:E463–E470.

26

Nutrient Partitioning

W. P. T. James
Rowett Research Institute, Aberdeen, Scotland

Peter J. Reeds
USDA/ARS Children's Nutrition Research Center and Baylor College of Medicine, Houston, Texas

I. INTRODUCTION

It has been argued (1) that genetically determined differences in nutrient partitioning, i.e., the channeling of food carbon into either protein or lipid (2), among individuals are of sufficient magnitude to contribute to the development of obesity. In this chapter we will discuss information on the changes in body composition during growth and with the development of obesity, and assess data on the control of body composition. These effects imply changes in the regulation of protein and lipid deposition during normal growth and reproduction and these changes in farm livestock as well as humans will be assessed.

It is important to distinguish between the short-term channeling of carbon to protein or fat synthesis and the net effect of metabolic turnover on the accumulation of body protein or fat. Thus, a high rate of protein synthesis and breakdown may occur in a small mass of tissue that does not expand progressively because overall synthesis and breakdown rates are the same. Nevertheless, the partitioning of energy into protein rather than fat deposition during growth and development alters the whole efficiency of metabolism (Fig. 1). As shown in Figure 1, at the level of interorgan flows of fuel, the distribution of macronutrients, such as carbohydrate or fat, is either channeled to meet the need for ATP production (oxidation and energy expenditure) or the macronutrients are stored as energy. Thus, at many levels of intracellular metabolism

the body makes decisions on the regulated partition of a finite supply of organic nutrients between different pathways. The amino acids are also allocated to the production of different cellular structures, enzymes, and regulatory proteins; this is a form of intracellular partitioning that may have an impact on tissue protein accretion rates. At each regulatory level there are poorly characterized mechanisms that allow the organism to sense the inflow of organic substrates and the degree to which some genetically determined body compositional goal has been achieved, and then to adjust metabolically to achieve this goal. So, from an obesity perspective, the regulatory questions include not only the sensing of energy imbalance but also the body compositional goal. Not only may this compositional goal be genetically programmed, but the sensing mechanism of that appropriate body compositional goal may also be adjusted by the process of gaining both lean and fat tissue. As will be dealt with later, the maintenance of excessive weight, i.e., of both fat and lean tissues, may actually represent a new goal that is once more defended in the face of reduced intakes despite this new goal not being compatible with optimal health.

II. GROWTH AS A NUTRIENT PARTITIONING PHENOMENON

The regulation of nutrient partitioning is difficult to study in humans or animals because it involves monitoring

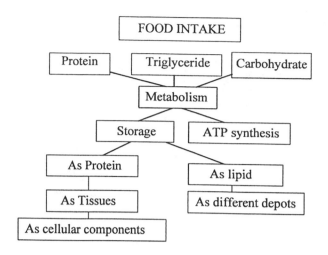

Figure 1 Decisions in nutrient partitioning.

the fluctuating rates of protein and energy metabolism throughout a 24-hr cycle and with remarkable accuracy. This accuracy is needed if the small increment in protein or fat deposition is to be assessed from these measurements. For example, even the accretion of 10 kg of excess fat over a period of a year represents the storage of <10% of total energy intake, so discriminating such a change from the daily fluctuations in nutrient storage is well beyond the accuracy of even the most sophisticated measurements. This means that it is necessary to assess first the impact of diet and other factors on the consequences of the regulatory processes, i.e., by monitoring changes in body composition. Once the factors affecting body composition become clear, it may be possible to assess the processes involved. Since these metabolic studies are much easier to conduct on animals than on humans, the animal literature will be used extensively to test hypotheses emerging from the human data.

In every species studied, postnatal development is characterized by a continuously changing, but closely regulated, ratio between the rates of protein and lipid storage. At any given stage of development, the organism seems to adjust to achieve some preprogrammed body compositional goal, which itself also changes continuously with time. Figure 2 is a composite of human data produced over the years by Fomon et al. (3) and Forbes (4). This shows that, at birth, lean tissues account for about 3 kg and fat for about 0.5 kg in a normal baby. This 15% of body fat increases during the first year of life to 25% in boys and girls, particularly when bottle- rather than breast-fed, but as the lean body mass (LBM) progressively rises, the proportion of fat slowly falls to about 18% in 3–4-year-old children. Dugdale and Payne (5) have esti-

mated that during the first 5 years boys and girls show a smooth increase in the ratio of total calories deposited as protein rather than fat (the p ratio) from about 0.2 at birth to 1.0 at the age of 3 in boys before it then drops to a nadir at 7 years of age. Girls have a similar rise and fall, but this is delayed by 1–2 years and the fall is less steep but then slowly declines to about 0.1 by 16 years of age. Careful body compositional studies show boys not only with a greater LBM for their age than girls, a feature evident from birth up to 5 years of age, but also with a reducing proportion of fat from 5 to 10 years of age (6). Thus, boys tend to enter their pubertal spurt with, on average, about 12% fat and show a further acute rise in the p ratio to 1.0 by the age of 12–13 before it declines to about 0.3 at 16 years of age. Girls' body fat has already increased to 15–20% as they enter puberty and their p ratio shows no pubertal spurt at all. These figures are based on American studies in the early postwar period when very few children were obese.

These differences in the p ratio mean that once puberty is established, the difference between boys and girls in their body composition becomes very marked, with boys rapidly increasing their LBM to a peak of about 350 g/cm height at 19 years accompanied by a change in body fat content, which, after an initial rise of 12–18% in early puberty, falls sharply from the age of about 13 years to a

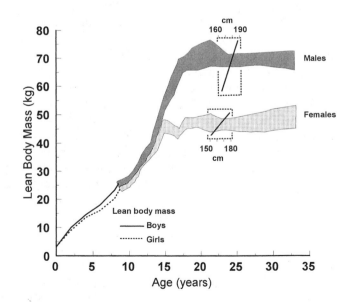

Figure 2 Changes in lean body mass with age. Collated and integrated data redrawn from Forbes (8) and Fomon (3). The adult relationship of lean body mass to height in both men and women is shown as an insert. The shaded area denotes the expected 95% confidence limits.

level of 10% by the late teens. The LBM of girls, however, increases to its peak of only about 250 g/cm height at 15 years, but body fat rises to about 25% of total body weight. These differences in LBM signify not only differences in bone mass, but a major difference in muscle mass. Thus, Cheek (7) has calculated that with the onset of puberty the small (5–10%) preexisting difference in the muscle mass of boys during childhood changes so that during puberty muscle mass increases from about 10 kg at the age of 10 years in boys to about 26 kg in 18-year-olds. This compares with a rise in muscle mass to 20 kg in late-teenage girls. Forbes (8) showed that the slope of the regression of LBM against height in 22–25-year-old men is much steeper (690 g/cm) than for women (290 g/cm), this slope not only reflecting the importance of the larger bone mass in men but particularly the greater muscle mass of males throughout life.

These carefully documented changes during growth and puberty are affected by dietary inadequacy, infection, and other diseases, but at any age before maturity there is a hierarchy of priorities in terms of growth and these priority tissues and functions are protected when there are inappropriate intakes (9). Thus there are fundamental differences in the susceptibility of protein rather than fat deposition to changes in intake. Whereas the rate of protein deposition is ultimately dependent on an adequate supply and balance of the essential amino acids, lipid accumulation can derive from any organic substrate that is metabolized to acetyl CoA. Furthermore, whereas there is an upper limit on the capacity of the body to deposit protein, which appears to be genetically controlled, the capacity to synthesize and deposit lipid seems to be unlimited. To illustrate this point, Figure 3 summarizes data on the influence of feed intake on the relative rates of protein and lipid deposition of growing pigs (10). As intake increases, protein deposition also increases linearly at first and then plateaus to a maximum. This plateau can, however, be changed to only a modest extent by further increases in intake. In contrast, lipid deposition increases linearly across all intakes. This phenomenon can also be observed in recent data on the growth and body composition of human-milk and formula-fed infants (Table 1; Motil et al., personal communication), who, despite 21% and 66% differences in energy and protein intake, show identical lean body masses but different body fat masses. Figure 3 also illustrates another phenomenon characteristic of the growing mammal. If the intake of young animals is restricted to a level that allows only energy equilibrium, they can still gain protein despite being in a state of negative fat balance. In other words, the growing animal protects protein deposition at the expense, if necessary, of fat deposition. A similar feature is seen in growing chil-

dren, who may increase their height and lean body mass while actually losing weight.

Similar phenomena are also evident in the distribution of protein among different organs. In all species so far studied, the relative rates of organ growth show a characteristic allometric relationship with one another. Thus, in neonates, the organs involved in digestion, absorption, and early metabolism (i.e., the intestinal tract, pancreas, and liver) grow particularly rapidly, while there is a close and linear relationship between the rate of muscle protein deposition and the rate of weight gain (Fig. 4).

A. Underfeeding in Children and Young Animals

The phenomenon of "protected" protein deposition under conditions of inadequate nutrition is also seen in the allocation of amino acids to new protein deposition among the different organs of the body (11–13). Thus, an inadequate protein intake substantially reduces the growth of skeletal muscle and the skin, but has a relatively small effect on the rate of protein deposition in bone and, of critical importance to the energetics of the organism, in the gastrointestinal tract. Few studies have been conducted on prolonged over- or underfeeding under highly controlled conditions in children, but a few conclusions can be drawn from monitoring the net effect of nutrient partitioning on body compositional changes. Children, when underfed, compensate by becoming less active and, as food becomes more restricted, growth stops. Although there is a tendency, based on animal studies, to consider the cost of growth to be a large proportion of the energy needed by a growing child, in practice the cost of growth of a baby is modest after the first 3 months of life and amounts to about 2% of the energy used by a 1-year-old child. Nor is energy provision the key to longitudinal growth. This was shown in early feeding studies this century and, more recently, it has been shown that longitudinal growth is particularly responsive to the intake of animal protein (14, 15). In states of severe underfeeding leading to marasmus, there is a particular loss of both body fat and muscle with eventually selective loss of the noncollagen protein content of the body (16). More modest underfeeding may also have lifelong effects, with Shetty suggesting, from his studies on the body composition of Indian adults, that their relatively small muscle mass reflects the long-term impact of marginal protein and energy intakes during childhood (17).

B. Responses to Overfeeding in Children

Children who become obese in general tend to be taller, so some nutrient partitioning effect must have been in-

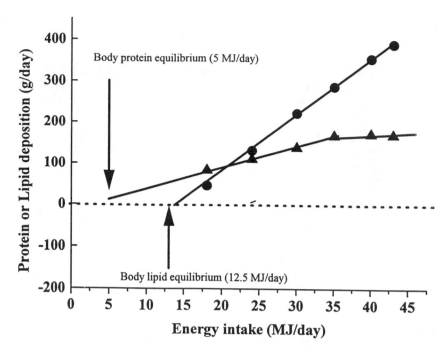

Figure 3 Relationship growth between feed intake and protein and lipid deposition in growing pigs. (From Bikker, et al., 1995.)

duced, but it is unknown whether this increase in stature reflects the modest response in longitudinal bone growth to a marked excess intake of protein and energy or whether there is also a genetic interaction with genetically prone obese children more likely to show accelerated longitudinal growth when consuming excessive amounts of food. What is clear is that the lean tissue mass increases in overweight children and that this increase seems proportionately as great as in adult life (8).

III. NUTRIENT PARTITIONING IN THE ADULT

A. Influence of Gender and Reproduction

It is at the pubertal stage of development that marked gender differences in size, growth rate, and body composition become most evident (18). The mature females of most mammalian species are smaller, have lower muscle mass per unit skeleton, and a higher contribution of fat to body mass. It is reasonable to assume that these inherent differences in the body composition of adult males and females reflect the influence of the sex steroids. Manipulation of steroid endocrine status by ablating the appropriate secretory organs or by exogenous hormonal manipulation alters the relative rates of body protein and lipid deposition in adults (see below).

Maturity is characterized by the virtual suppression of long-term protein deposition, while at the same time the organism retains the ability to deposit fat. The specific rate of protein deposition in grams per day falls abruptly with sexual development, and even in those species (such as the rat, mouse, and pig) in which the epiphyses fail to close, the subsequent rate of protein deposition in the adult is much lower. The genetic-environmental interactions on the processes controlling tissue deposition, which during growth lead to a targeted adult weight of lean tissue, are not normally seen as continuing to have an impact in adult life. Yet when adults or mature animals are semistarved, protein-depleted, or put through a phase of infective or traumatic stress with the loss of lean tissue, there is clear evidence that regulatory processes are reactivated to restore the body protein mass to its former state. This occurs in animals on protein and energy intakes which, in a nondepleted animal, would simply maintain body protein balance. Thus, metabolic pathways are induced that conserve amino acids and enhance protein deposition until the previous protein mass is more or less restored. The nature of these pathways remains obscure.

In the female, pregnancy and lactation temporarily alter the protein and lipid relationships in a marked and closely regulated fashion (19). In many respects pregnancy, and especially lactation, can be regarded as a restoration of growth, inasmuch as the mature female, who would not

Table 1 Protein and Energy Intake and the Accretion of Lean Body and Fat Mass by Breast- and Formula-Fed Infants over the First 3 Months of Life

| Group | Average daily intake | | Accretion | |
	Protein (g/kg)	Energy (kJ/kg)	Lean body mass (kg)	Fat mass (kg)
Breast-fed	1.48	391	1.05 ± 0.99	0.79 ± 0.22
Formula-fed	2.45	472	1.05 ± 0.10	1.02 ± 0.30

Source: Data of Motil (personal communication) reanalyzed with permission.

normally carry out a long-term net deposition of protein, resumes the ability to deposit protein, but does so in very specific components of the body. In fact, it could be argued that the changes in glucose homeostasis that are the natural accompaniment of pregnancy (20,21) reflect the operation of regulatory mechanisms that ensure an adequate supply of nutrients to the fetus. As a consequence, the ability of maternal tissues to sequester organic nutrients is temporarily inhibited.

Lactation is also a period during which there is a fundamental resetting of metabolic regulation, so that the *net* production of protein, lipid, and carbohydrate in the mammary secretions can be maintained and protected. Although voluntary appetite increases during lactation, it is clear that, in a way that is analogous to the achievement of a growth target, the lactating female possesses mechanisms that ensure the production of milk in adequate quantities and composition. Milk composition, in terms of the relative quantities of protein, lipid, and carbohydrate, is highly characteristic of a species, but within a species there is a remarkably small interindividual variation in gross milk composition provided nutrition is ad-

equate. Thus the lactating mammal, under conditions of inadequate nutrition, mobilizes body protein and fat in amounts that are appropriate to ensure the nutritional adequacy of milk (Table 2) (22). These observations are, of course, reminiscent of the protective phenomena in growing individuals and might reflect the operation of similar regulatory mechanisms.

These observations on growth and responsiveness to dietary or physiological stresses have three implications: first, that the magnitude of the lean body mass is genetically determined; second, that there are mechanisms that allow the adult to sense differences between the actual and the programmed lean body mass; third, that repletion can occur via an increase in the nutritional efficiency of protein storage. Such regulatory mechanisms can also be observed at the level of specific organs because alterations in functional demand will reactivate the growth of specific organs. Thus, the skeletal muscles of adults will readily hypertrophy under the normal conditions of resistance training provided the exercise includes eccentric movement, i.e., involving a lengthening of the muscle under tension; this has a specific effect in inducing the muscle damage that seems necessary for muscle hypertrophy (23), and both the liver and kidney will increase in mass following subtotal hepatectomy or unilateral nephrectomy (24), (25). The fact that these tissue growth phenomena can also occur with no change in the arterial supply of substrates implies that the reactivation of the growth mechanism is manifest in the ability of the cells to extract more amino acids at the same circulating concentration.

B. Nutrient Partitioning on Underfeeding

The classic semistarvation studies conducted on young adult volunteers by Keys and his colleagues (26), together with several other studies collated by Forbes (8), and extended by Ferro-Luzzi et al. (27), demonstrate that, provided energy intakes are >1100 kcal/day, there is a smooth curvilinear relationship between the level of body

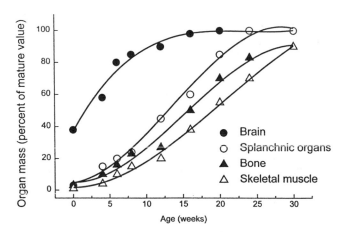

Figure 4 Organ mass growth changes during growth in the pig.

Table 2 Effect of Protein Intake on the Milk Protein Output and Maternal Protein and Lipid Balance in Lactating Cattle

Protein (g)	Milk protein output (g)	Body balance	
		Protein (g)	Lipid (g)
820	390	−130	−80
980	470	−90	−270
1120	515	−6	−285
1308	550	+42	−225

Source: Recalculated from Whitelaw et al. (22).

fat at the onset of semistarvation and the proportion of lean tissue lost. Thus, at a high body fat mass, e.g., 50 kg, about 20% of the tissue lost is LBM; at 20 kg body fat about 30% of the loss is lean tissue, but by the time body fat mass has fallen to 10 kg, half the tissue being lost is lean. Forbes and Ferro-Luzzi have translated these data into tissue changes in relation to BMI (Fig. 5). When energy intakes fall below 1100 kcal/day, the proportion of lean tissue lost rises progressively as food intake falls (8) unless special measures are taken to maintain or even increase the protein intake, as in protein-sparing modified fasts. This form of nutrient partitioning seems to reflect the potential for adults with large adipose tissue mass to fuel tissue metabolism preferentially by free fatty acids released from adipose tissue and which, through the Randle cycle, will tend to suppress its glucose utilization and therefore any need for amino acid-derived glucose production. Any greater tendency to ketosis when free fatty acids are in abundant supply will also reduce glucose

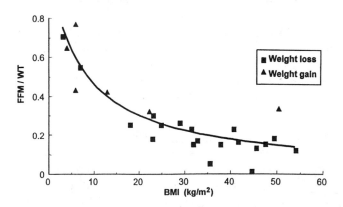

Figure 5 The relationship between adult body mass index and the proportion of fat free mass lost or gained during weight change. Redrawn from Ferro-Luzzi (27).

needs. The ratio of protein/total energy loss, or an analogous ratio of lean tissue/fat tissue loss, has been calculated by Dugdale and Payne (5) from Keys' semistarvation studies (26) and used as a biological feature of the individual's responsiveness to energy imbalance. They subsequently showed (28) that the *p* ratio for individuals, although very different, did show only small changes on prolonged fasting. However, recent recalculations by Dulloo et al. (29), although showing a significant correlation ($r = 0.34$) between the individual *p* ratio of the Minnesota volunteers on semistarvation and when they were refed, did demonstrate a consistent difference in the *p* ratio on underfeeding and overfeeding. This therefore demonstrates that individuals can be ranked in terms of their *p* ratio but that the ratios can be shifted by nutritional means (see below).

I. Sex Differences in Response to Underfeeding

Given their greater body fat, women would be expected to respond to semistarvation with a smaller proportional loss of lean tissue and therefore of urinary N than men. Widdowson (30) noted that females resist starvation better than males, lose a smaller proportion of body protein, and, in humans as well as animals, have less chance of dying under the stress of undernutrition. Thus, 60% of those affected by undernutrition in postwar Germany were male and, experimentally, when 10-day-old pigs were subjected to severe and prolonged undernutrition allowing growth only to 5–6 kg at 1 year of age, 87% of the female pigs remained alive whereas only 22% of the males survived.

These, and other studies, have been reviewed by Hoyenga and Hoyenga (31), who proposed that under evolutionary selective pressure mammalian females had evolved better survival mechanisms. Widdowson's experiment on young pigs with nearly identical body fat contents suggests that the sex differences are intrinsic and not simply a reflection, as in older animals, of the greater survival of the fatter female animals.

Human studies show that female volunteers, on fasting, lose less N than men (32), and the sex differences in urinary nitrogen losses are also seen in obese men and women (33). The greater proportionate loss of fat than lean tissue may also be inferred from cross-sectional studies on very underweight men and women studied in nine national surveys in Asia, Africa, and the Pacific where data are available that allow estimates of both the muscle and fat areas of the arm. In women with a BMI <20 the decline in the arm muscle area is very modest as BMI falls from 18 to 15 because there is a selective loss from their greater fat mass, but in men, as the residual body fat diminishes, muscle tissue is being lost more readily (34). Again, this may simply, reflect the impact of greater energy reserves in the body fat of women.

Mechanistically it seems clear that insulin levels fall further in women than in men during fasting and women have a more rapid rise in both free fatty acids and ketone concentrations; these changes have been linked to a more rapid rise in plasma glucagon levels in women (35). Whether these responses can be considered intrinsic to the sex differences is unclear; comparisons of the insulin and glucagon reactions to fasting in lean and obese adults are hampered by the coexisting insulin resistance in the obese, so it is unclear what the effect of excess body fat per se has on plasma glucagon, and whether women show greater responses than men at equivalent levels of body fat remains uncertain. It is noteworthy, however, that in Figure 5 Forbes (8) and Ferro-Luzzi et al. (27) have combined a whole range of studies on men and women and neither author has suggested an intrinsic difference in the partitioning of lean/fat loss during fasting between men and women of equivalent BMI, with women having more fat. Most of Forbes' data relate to women, but Ferro-Luzzi et al. (27) have now reanalyzed all the available data on the impact of seasonal stress of food inadequacy on the weight loss of men and women living in the Third World. The fall in fat free mass is limited to <2%; the men, however, show a greater weight loss at each level of BMI consistent with their higher proportionate loss of fat-free mass.

C. Nutrient Partitioning in Overfeeding

In adults, overfeeding leads to an increase in lean tissue deposition, but the fraction of weight gain as lean tissue steadily declines as the overfeeding continues. These data are shown in Figure 5. Normal-weight adults fed 80,000 kcal excess deposit about 35% of the weight gain as lean tissue. In Forbes' (8) analyses of women with anorexia nervosa, with a normal body weight and with different grades of obesity, the gradient of LBM deposited is marked at low levels of body fat, but the gradient becomes progressively less steep once body fat exceeds 40 kg (Fig. 6). Dulloo (36) has noted that, after the male Minnesota volunteers were refed back to their prestarvation weight, they had a smaller LBM and a greater fat mass than before the experiment began. Those given food ad libitum continued to overeat and put on excess fat until the LBM had recovered. Dulloo (36) therefore suggests that the hyperphagia may be a response to the incompletely restored LBM, a feature suggested many years ago when Ashworth was studying the extraordinary responses in food intake of recovering malnourished babies. These babies eat vo-

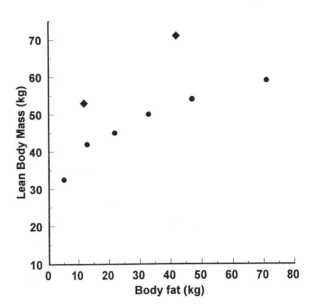

Figure 6 The relationship between lean body mass and total body fat in adult men and women. Redrawn from Forbes (8) with his data for women (●). Superimposed are data for men (◆) based on K⁴⁰ studies with K⁴² standardization as described by James et al. (43).

raciously to increase their growth to 15 times the normal rate until they achieve the appropriate weight for their height at which point most children overnight shut off their appetite (37,38). Later studies in malnourished children suggested that the failure to truly regain lean tissue could relate to inappropriate micronutrient supply, particularly of trace elements such as zinc (39). Thus, as with some malnourished children, the Minnesota men may have been rehabilitated on a relatively poor-quality diet.

1. The Significance of Nutrient Partitioning in Relation to Energy Metabolism and Obesity

Payne and Dugdale (40) first proposed that incremental gains in tissue protein and fat could be simulated on a computer and that the gain in tissue mass led to an increase in energy expenditure that limited further weight gain. They proposed, on the basis of their recalculation of the Keys' semistarvation study, that each individual had a p value that reflected the fraction of energy that was lost or laid down as protein rather than fat and that those with high p values deposited more lean tissue at greater energetic cost and with a greater maintenance cost. These costs limited further weight gain and represented a buffer against weight change such that the normal slow fluctuations in body weight over years could best be explained by a shift in the balance between input and output but without the need to invoke any very fine tuning of appetite and food intake to explain the limited weight changes. Thus, random fluctuations in intake could be accommodated by the buffering effects of nutrient deposition and the costs of storage, with the individual propensity to weight gain being dependent on the constitutive p value for that individual. Their impressive computer simulations allowed them to mimic the subsequent responses to deliberate overfeeding or semistarvation studies conducted by Garrow and Stalley (41).

Payne and Dugdale's computer simulations have been taken further by Schutz and his colleagues (42), who have used recent studies on whole-body calorimetry and body compositional changes on overfeeding to simulate the slow progressive rise in body weight when physical activity falls or intake rises. A plateau weight is eventually reached, but this may take 5–10 years to achieve. The extent of the weight gain depends, as predicted by Payne and Dugdale, on both the fraction of energy laid down as protein, i.e. as LBM rather than fat, and on the extent of energy imbalance. The lower the p ratio, the greater the final weight gain and the longer it takes to achieve a plateau weight.

The implications of these findings can now be related to the body compositional analyses considered earlier. There seem to be three fundamental issues governing the p value: first, interindividual differences, which may well be genetically determined; second, a sex-dependent difference in p values with males having higher p values than females; third, superimposed on the individual setting of the p ratio are the steady adaptive effects relating to the magnitude of the reduced or excess weight perhaps related to the body fat content and whether underfeeding or overfeeding is underway. Whereas it was possible earlier to explain the reduced protein loss and nitrogen excretion when fasting obese rather than lean individuals on the basis of the substrate-induced selective oxidation of fatty acids and the impact of glucagon and insulin responses, the converse limitation in protein accumulation on overfeeding is not readily explained as a fatty acid-related phenomena induced by fat storage.

It seems more likely, from animal studies, that there is usually a genetically set limit to protein stores that can be raised by overfeeding, but only to a modest degree. Overfeeding is likely to lead to increases in gastrointestinal mass and gut protein turnover and to increased hepatic protein enzyme mass and activity as the excess food is processed, and some further increases in cytoplasmic proteins of adipose tissue will result as the tissue expands to accommodate the excess energy deposited as lipid. Furthermore, the increase in body weight will induce an in-creased muscle mass as hypertrophy in response to the physical need to move a greater body weight around as part of normal daily activity. These changes can, however, be expected to be modest.

2. Sex Differences in the Response to Overfeeding

Given the marked sex differences in response to underfeeding and the individual setting of the p ratio, one might expect to find clear evidence that men have a higher p ratio than women on overfeeding, if only because of their lower initial body fat. Men, with their greater musculature, are able to attain even greater muscle mass than women after physical training, so it seems reasonable to expect men to have a higher p ratio on overfeeding. Forbes (8) concluded that the data on men were too limited to allow such a conclusion, but if our original male data on LBM (43) are superimposed on Forbes' data on women (Fig. 6), then not only do normal weight men already have, as expected, a greater LBM at a fat mass of 15 kg, but the increment in LBM at the fat mass of 45 kg in the obese men is about twice that observed in the women. This provides preliminary evidence to suggest that at an equivalent fat mass men have a higher p ratio than women both on semistarvation and on overfeeding.

This difference between men and women may, in part, explain the almost universal finding that women have a higher prevalence of obesity than men despite being weight conscious and attempting repeatedly to slim. Because women have a more restricted limit to their gain in lean tissues, particularly as it relates to muscle mass, an equivalent 100-kcal excess in women will lead to proportionately less lean tissue and more fat being deposited. This, in turn, means that more energy has to be stored for longer and a greater weight gain will occur until finally the energy cost of physical movement plus the impact of the markedly expanded adipose tissue allows them to achieve a new state of energy balance, having stored much more energy than men under similar circumstances.

IV. EXPERIMENTAL MANIPULATION OF NUTRIENT PARTITIONING: THE ANIMAL HUSBANDRY EXPERIENCE

Over the last 20 years those concerned with commercial animal production have responded to economic and consumer pressures by producing animals that use their diets efficiently and produce "leaner" carcasses. The strategies used have been dietary manipulation, conventional breeding, and the use of exogenous growth-promoting substances.

Genetic selection has produced such fast-growing animals, e.g., chickens and pigs, that the physiological limits in terms of long-term adult health and reproductive capacity are now being compromised. Genetic selection, by producing larger adult animals, has not altered body composition much and the lean cuts of meat simply reflect a composition appropriate for age but a larger mass at a younger age. Thus, the genotype control of the relative rates of protein and lipid gain is little changed and the dominant link is between an increase in appetite, growth rates, and final body size.

It is important to distinguish between a change in energy balance affecting fat deposition alone and an increase in protein deposition which, by entraining increases in energy metabolism, leads to a reduction in fat accretion. In the latter case, there is no intrinsic change in the processes of metabolic efficiency but it does reflect a "true" influence on nutrient partitioning, i.e., the distribution of the deposition of excess carbon.

There is a large literature on the selection of pigs for various growth traits, but a high proportion of this literature concentrates on weight gain and its nutritional efficiency rather than on nutrient partitioning. Nevertheless, high ratios of weight gain to feed intake often imply weight deposited with high protein:lipid ratios, and a high ratio of carcass to total preslaughter weight often indicates a high muscle:viscera ratio.

Over the period 1940–1987, numerous reports on changing weight gain and feed efficiency in pigs of broadly similar genetic background (Large White and Landrace) show that between 8 and 26 weeks of age pigs grow from 25 to 95 kg, but the amount of feed needed has fallen, muscle accretion has been enhanced, and fat deposition lowered remarkably (Fig. 7) (44). Thus, the ratio of muscle mass:bone length has increased by almost 50% and there has been a fundamental resetting of the relationship between muscle and fat deposition. Thus the *p* ratio, considered earlier in human studies, has risen because the animal uses its dietary protein more efficiently for muscle protein deposition and uses its dietary carbon less efficiently for the deposition of fat. These changes are almost the mirror image of changes in the chemical composition of the body and the organ composition of body protein in genetically obese rodents (45). Yet birth weight and growth in the first 6 weeks of the pig's life has barely changed and voluntary intake and skeletal and visceral organ size are little different.

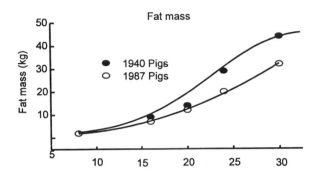

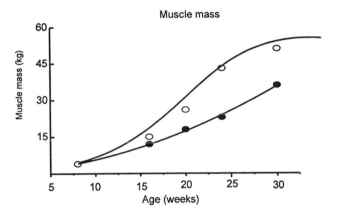

Figure 7 Changes in body composition of pigs following 50 years of selection.

A. Impact of Growth Promoters

I. Growth Hormone (Somatotropin)

It has been suggested for many years that growth hormone (GH), secreted from the anterior pituitary, plays a key role in the regulation of body weight gain in general and bone growth in particular (46), features confirmed with transgenic animals that overexpress the natural hormone (47) or overexpress mutated forms of growth hormone with greater or lesser effectiveness (48). The partitioning of nutrients between protein and lipid deposition is also altered. Thus, animals with mutations involved in the somatotrophic axis and little dwarf mice (49) are not only smaller than their heterozygous littermates, but are also relatively obese, in some examples substantially obese. Correction of the defect by administration of GH, and recently via virtually directed hepatic expression of GH, not only restores linear growth to normal, but also normalizes the relative rates of protein and lipid deposition (50).

These studies indicate the physiological role of GH. The exogenous administration of large amounts of recombinant growth hormone to both animals (51) and humans

(46) stimulates growth and protein deposition while at the same time reducing fat accretion. This is also of great interest to agricultural and medical scientists wishing to manipulate growth and body composition in farm livestock and in catabolic patients (52). Three studies on the effects of exogenous growth hormone on the growth and body composition of commercial strains of pigs (53–55) illustrate the increase in protein-partitioning and protein-depositing capacity of the animal when growth hormone (admittedly in very large doses) was used.

Untreated animals (Figs. 8a and 8b) receiving low-protein diets became relatively obese and an increase in dietary protein, but not energy, intake altered the composition, but not the rate, of weight gain. When animals received a diet containing less than 13% crude protein,

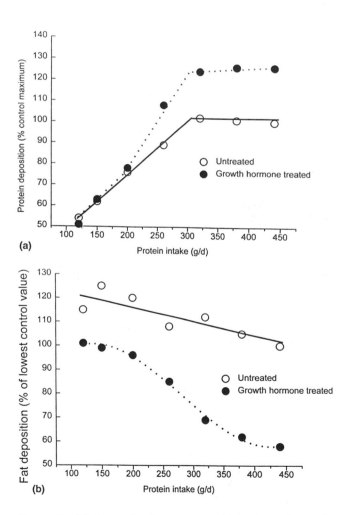

(a)

(b)

Figure 8 (a) Interaction between protein intake and growth hormone effect on protein deposition in pigs. (b) Interaction between protein intake and growth hormone effort on lipid deposition in pigs.

GH had no discernible effect either on nitrogen balance or on protein accretion. Yet lipid deposition was lowered even at low protein intake. As protein supply improved, GH induced a greater increase in protein deposition and markedly reduced fat storage. Finally, Figure 8a shows that the efficiency of protein utilization changes as protein supply rises. Between 120 g and 190 g protein (equivalent to 13–18% of energy as protein) growth hormone induced a substantial increase in the partial efficiency of dietary protein use, but above 18% dietary protein the GH-treated animals continued to deposit more protein, and hence a higher proportion of their protein intake. Above 320 g/day the slopes of the lines relating protein intake to protein deposition were identical, and close to zero in both groups of animals. Growth hormone had apparently increased both the capacity of the animal to deposit protein and the efficiency of protein deposition. The general effect, therefore, was for GH to bring about a true nutrient partitioning effect by altering, to borrow pharmacological terms, the sensitivity and responsiveness of protein and lipid deposition to dietary protein intake. In association with these changes, substantial reduction in lipid deposition is apparent at the lower protein intakes (Fig. 8b). There is then an accentuated decline in fat storage on GH treatment as the higher protein intake allows preferential deposition of protein.

The effect of GH on the growth allometry of different organs seems unremarkable, as judged by the studies on GH-overexpressing transgenic mice: the absolute rate of whole-body protein deposition was increased with little or no effect on the distribution of body protein. So, the animals were larger but of normal proportions. When, however, exogenous growth hormone is given after the period of postnatal development, the tissues are not exposed continuously to high levels of endogenous growth and the growth of the viscera is selectively enhanced. The protein mass within the gastrointestinal tract seems to be particularly responsive, perhaps because of the effects of IGF-1 secretion induced by GH in the liver. IGF-1 administration is particularly effective in stimulating the growth of the gastrointestinal tract, the spleen, and the kidneys (56,57). Despite the obvious effects of growth hormone on muscle protein synthesis in GH-deficient mutants (58), the effects of growth hormone on skeletal muscle growth seems to depend (see below) on the distinct GH effects on long-bone growth.

The persistently high levels of GH also induce diverse effects on carbohydrate, lipid, and protein metabolism through insulin secretion. A hyperinsulinemic state suggestive of insulin resistance affects predominantly adipocyte metabolism (59). Insulin may, however, mediate some of the effects of GH, which may amplify tissue insulin sensitivity and thereby increase the efficiency of protein utilization. Finally, in ruminants with GH as an important regulator of lactation, GH both stimulates the mobilization of body lipid during peak lactation and supports the production of milk protein and lipid (60). These wide-ranging effects of GH are not confined to farm livestock; GH induces protein deposition in adult humans, particularly if they have suffered some trauma (52). Given that the traumatic state is often associated with insulin resistance of protein metabolism, this again suggests that GH has selective effects on insulin-regulated protein turnover.

These wide-ranging effects involving pharmacological or transgenic manipulation of circulating growth hormone levels can now be put into physiological context by relating the data to elegant analyses of the condition of African Pygmies, who have a unique genetic variation in the GH-IGF-I axis. The defect involves a resistance to the action of GH originally considered consistent with a reduction in the number of GH receptors controlling the expression of IGF-I (61). Thus, the circulating levels of IGF-I are slightly reduced (by 18%) during childhood but the expected fourfold surge in IGF-I during adolescence is limited to only a 50% increase. The prepubertal growth rate of these children is not the smallest, ranking 18th of 38 ethnic groups (62), but there is a complete failure of the pubertal spurt. IGF-II levels are normal, as are the surges in testosterone in boys and estradiol in girls during puberty (61). The circulating GH-binding protein, now recognized as the GH receptor dissociated from the membrane, is present at half the normal concentration consistent with a receptor deficiency, but Merimee *et al.* (63) have identified a variant allele in the GH receptor that could explain the poor responsiveness to the normal circulating levels of GH. Infusion studies with GH demonstrated resistance to lipolysis in these Pygmies, a feature distinct from the action of IGF-I, so the clinical picture is consistent with that of pure GH receptor resistance.

Any attempt to relate the animal data on nutrient partitioning to the body composition and responsiveness of these African Pygmies is difficult because the Pygmies operate within an environment where the energy and protein intake is limited. Thus, any propensity to obesity is difficult to discern and the impact of GH on nutrient partitioning may be marginal, as in animals at low protein and energy intakes (Fig. 8). Yet, the recognized greater musculature of the male adult Pygmies is consistent with the effects of the normal levels of sex steroids and implies that the bone elongation and thinning in puberty is GH-dependent but that much of the muscle mass per unit length is testosterone-dependent (see below). Nevertheless, in GH-deficient Swedish children given either daily injections or continuous infusions of GH there was, in the short term, a decrease in body fat and an increase in LBM estimated from body impedance measurements (64). This effect would be consistent with the animal data suggesting an interaction between GH and a plentiful intake of protein, which may, in humans as well as ruminants, affect both IGF-I and binding protein levels through an insulin-mediated mechanism (64).

2. β-Adrenergic Agonists

In the early 1980s it became clear from studies both in rodents and subsequently in farm livestock that some specific β_2-adrenergic agonists have the ability not only to reduce fat accretion, but to induce fat loss while markedly increasing protein deposition. Clenbuterol (65) and cimeterol both have a specific effect on skeletal muscle accretion, which, in treated animals, resists muscle catabolism induced by lactation, denervation, and trauma (66). These effects suggest an important and specific role for the sympathetic nervous system and the β_2-receptor in regulating muscle protein deposition. However, the pharmacology of these agents is particularly complex (67) and may be mediated by the β_3 or "atypical" adrenergic receptor. Blockade of the α-adrenergic receptor induces a similar muscle growth response as that induced by the β_2-adrenergic agonist (68). A transient hyperinsulinemia also occurs, but the insulin resistance seems confined to carbohydrate and lipid metabolism. The drug's impact depends on the level of protein intake (67), but because it does not increase appetite its effect is to increase the efficiency of muscle protein deposition.

In contrast to GH, the β-adrenergic agonists also exert a weak thermogenic effect, thus in part accounting for body fat loss. The parallels and contrasts between β-adrenergic and GH effects on nutrient partitioning are therefore illuminating. Growth hormone slows lipid deposition, stimulates protein deposition, particularly in the viscera, and has little effect on overall energy expenditure. The β-adrenergic agonists induce fat loss, exert a muscle-specific effect, and are weakly thermogenic. On the other hand, both agents apparently increase the nutritional efficiency of protein deposition, cause insulin resistance, and apparently switch the animal toward a more lipid-based use of energy.

3. Steroids

In considering the role of steroid hormones in the regulation of nutrient partitioning and, by implication, their potential use in the amelioration of pathological changes in nutrient partitioning, it is important to separate the glucocorticoids from those hormones normally associated with sexual maturation. First, despite the critical role of leptin and its receptor (see below), there is abundant evidence that aberrations in glucocorticoid function are an important contributor to establishment of the phenotype of a variety of genetically obese rodents (69). Second, the effects of glucocorticoids on protein mass vary markedly between different organs. Both naturally occurring and synthetic glucocorticoids are potent suppressors of muscle, skeletal, and skin protein deposition, but enhance the mass of nonexportable hepatic proteins. Third, unlike growth hormone and the β_2-adrenergic agonists, the insulin resistance associated with persistently elevated glucocorticoid levels is not confined to its effects on carbohydrate and lipid metabolism but includes changes in the regulation of protein metabolism. Thus, glucocorticoid blocks the effect of insulin on tissue protein synthesis and simultaneously activates hepatic amino acid catabolism.

4. Sex Steroids and Body Composition

It has long been known in agricultural practice that castration of the male leads to a marked reduction in the rate of muscle accretion, and until recently, the practice was to first castrate the animal to induce docility but then to inject androgenic-type anabolic steroids to enhance the deposition of muscle protein. The castration did not reduce the pubertal spurt relating to the GH-IGF-I axis, but simply the partition of energy between protein deposition in the longer muscle of the adult animal and fat stores. Thus, there was a reduction in deposited fat as well as an increase in muscle protein. Nevertheless, there is an interaction between the sex hormones and the GH-IGF-I axis because animals either surgically castrated or immunocastrated by immunization with a conjugate of gonadotropin-hormone-releasing-hormone (GnRH) show a fall in serum IGF-I levels compared with uncastrated males (70). Thus, there may be a growth factor interaction leading to changes in muscle mass with the interpulse interval in GH secretion being less in prepubertal female than male sheep but not in rats or humans (71). The sheep data are complicated by the effect of testosterone in promoting increases in food intake, which then has the effect of increasing GH and/or IGF-I levels. When nonpharmacological doses of testosterone are given to castrated animals under conditions where food intake is controlled (72), protein accretion occurs without discernible changes in plasma GH. This protein accretion is probably achieved by a reduction in protein breakdown rates with lower amino acid catabolism rather than by increased rates of protein synthesis that were measured directly (73). Consistent with this is the fall in urinary 3-methylhistidine derived from myofibrillar protein breakdown in both castrated and adrenalectomized male rats (74).

The surge in testosterone in pubertal boys seems responsible for the increase in muscle mass and LBM (Fig. 2). When testosterone is injected into normal male volunteers, there is a clear increase in LBM together with an increase in muscle mass, as judged by changes in creatinine excretion (75). The impact of estrogens on protein metabolism is less evident than their role in altering body fat accumulation and distribution (76).

V. LEPTIN

Current understanding of leptin and its role in energy balance is dealt with elsewhere in this volume. Of relevance, however, is the overall effect of leptin on body composition. Within 6 months of leptin's discovery, three groups (77–79) independently showed that injection of recombinant leptin into *ob/ob* mice in addition to lowering their food intake, body weight, and fat mass, also normalized their insulin concentrations and blood glucose as well as increasing their energy expenditure toward that of their lean littermates.

It is not clear, however, whether leptin also interacts with the distribution of carbon storage between protein and fat. In two of the early papers on the effects of leptin injection, LBM was apparently unaffected by leptin injection at doses that profoundly affected food intake and body fat mass. This suggests that leptin may allow the animal to preserve tissue protein. However, the methods used to determine LBM in these studies included the skeleton in the lean, and it is noticeable that leptin injection lowered body water thereby suggesting a possible lowering of body protein content. Given that leptin's protein structure is reminiscent of that of the lymphokines (80), a feature shared with both prolactin and GH, leptin may have some analogous effects, e.g., on immune function and nutrient partitioning. The question remains whether leptin is "merely" involved in linking body fat mass, energy expenditure, and appetite or whether it exerts further direct peripheral effects on protein metabolism.

VI. ENERGETICS AND MEASURING THE REGULATION OF NUTRIENT PARTITIONING

It is clear from the foregoing that the deposition of dietary carbon can only occur when sufficient carbon is available for storage. This seemingly obvious point needs to encompass the incremental storage of more lipid or protein after each meal than is lost in the intervening periods of fasting. Long-term deposition is, in a very good sense, the summation of many episodes of short-term storage and loss.

Thus, it is clear that the mechanisms regulating nutrient partitioning should operate as part of the fast/fed cycle.

The fundamental physiological viability of the body depends on protecting the ability to sustain ATP synthesis; this must always remain the highest regulatory priority for free-living organisms and animals. Thus, carbon storage only occurs when the physiological demands for ATP have been satisfied. Many different organic substrates can provide the energy for ATP synthesis, but there are dietary substrates that are preferentially oxidized and possibly genetic differences in the "preferred" contributions of carbohydrate, protein, and fat to oxidative metabolism. Indeed, this concept lies at the heart of the food quotient/respiratory quotient (FQ/RQ) hypothesis of Flatt (81). Thus, altering energy expenditure at a constant energy intake can, in theory, alter the protein and lipid contributions of carbon to oxidative metabolism. Because of the necessity for maintaining ATP synthesis, altering one storage pathway automatically changes the contribution of the precursors for this pathway to the central oxidative pathways of metabolism. Thus, the oxidation of some other organic macronutrient changes to maintain ATP synthesis. One example of this metabolic integration is the response to stimulating protein deposition under conditions in which energy intake is constant by restoring to amino acid balance an originally inappropriate amino acid intake in a growing animal (82). To cope with the subsequent surge in protein synthesis there is an automatic demand that the oxidation of either dietary fat or carbohydrate increases with a restriction on their own deposition during growth. As protein deposition occurs, the amount of energy needed to fuel this process is greater than the amount of energy used in storing fat of an equivalent energy content. Maintaining that stored energy at its new level also involves the use of greater energy because the energy cost of continuous protein turnover substantially exceeds the cost of sustaining fat stores (83).

Therefore, when interpreting the results of an experiment in which some genetic, physiological, or pharmacological factor has altered the contributions of protein and lipid accretion to overall energy storage at the mechanistic level, it is important to distinguish between (1) a simple redistribution of the substrates for ATP synthesis, (2) a change in energy balance, merely as a result of the different energetic efficiencies of protein and lipid accretion, and (3) specific and direct interactions of the regulatory factor with the metabolic processes that lead to protein and fat accretion.

The logic of the work on body compositional change is that the effects of those hormonal or other factors that control protein synthesis and/or breakdown can be observed by monitoring short-term changes in protein synthesis and breakdown either on a whole-body basis or in terms of individual organs.

In the last 25 years there have been major advances in our ability to measure protein synthesis and breakdown on a whole-body basis, but as yet it remains unclear whether the p ratio of lean/fat tissue deposition is reflected as proposed by Dugdale and Payne in the diurnal cycling of protein synthesis and breakdown. The proposal itself was generated at the London School of Hygiene in the early 1970s at a time when Waterlow, Garlick, Millward, and ourselves were developing a variety of techniques for monitoring both protein synthesis and breakdown in humans and animals during fasting and feeding. We demonstrated early, with a ^{14}C tyrosine technique, that protein intake and changes in total food intake altered both protein synthesis and breakdown, with the muscle and viscera showing very different responses (84). We then proposed that the C^1 labeling of L-leucine was a more appropriate technique (85), and Clugston and Garlick (86) then made a special study of obese and lean individuals to test the Dugdale/Payne hypothesis. They used a 24-hr constant infusion of $[1-^{14}C]$ leucine with a 12-hr feeding followed by a 12-hr fasting cycle. They concluded that, although there was a surge in estimated protein synthesis on feeding, the ratio of energy derived from protein and utilized by the obese during fasting was $13.9 \pm 1.1\%$ in the obese, a value similar to the $16.2 \pm 1.5\%$ in the lean. These studies, with hindsight, must be considered with caution because only obese women were studied and compared with two lean women and three lean men on intakes which, in energy terms, were matched to the resting metabolic rate but where protein intakes were held constant regardless of the individual's LBM. The studies were also conducted before Garlick had developed his phenylalanine technique for short-term muscle synthesis measurements in humans, before the keto acid was used as a more appropriate measure of intracellular labeling of leucine, and before it was possible to monitor short-term changes in the synthesis of hepatic export protein, in the entry of nitrogenous compounds into the urea cycle, and avoid the problems of label recycling. Thus, we should reserve judgment on whether it is possible to measure acutely the flow of carbon into and from protein and lipid during a diurnal cycle and relate these to the long-term changes in the partition coefficient demonstrable from the body compositional changes set out in this chapter.

VII. CONCLUSIONS

Changes in nutrient partitioning are fundamental to the development of obesity, with a multiplicity of hormones being potentially involved. Over the last 20 years the data on body compositional changes on overfeeding and underfeeding have led to plausible explanations for the steady accumulation of body fat and the achievement of a new stage of energy balance in the obese. The suggestion that the preferential channeling of carbon into protein deposition can affect both the rate and extent of weight gain now needs to be linked to carefully controlled isotopic studies that assess whether the body compositional changes reflect the diurnal surge of amino acids into protein. The energetics of maintaining an enhanced protein mass will also be affected by whether the protein mass is maintained by increasing synthetic rates or by reducing protein breakdown rates since the two processes have very different energetics. Much of the detail of the control of nutrient partitioning have very different energetics. Much of the detail of the control of nutrient partitioning will have to be worked out in animal studies, but novel isotopomer techniques (87) are now becoming available for monitoring the flux of carbon through different pathways, so an analysis of the basis of nutrient partitioning may now be possible.

ACKNOWLEDGMENTS

This work is a publication of the USDA/ARS Children's Nutrition Research Center, Department of Pediatrics, Baylor College of Medicine and Texas Children's Hospital, Houston, TX. Funding has been provided in part from the USDA/ARS under Cooperative Agreement No. 58-6258-6100. Mention of trade names, commercial products, or organizations does not imply endorsement by the U.S. Government. We are grateful to the Scottish Office Agriculture, Environment, and Fisheries Department for supporting this work.

REFERENCES

1. Bouchard C. The genetics of body fat content. In: Angel A, Anderson H, Bouchard C, Lau D, Leiter L, Mendelson R, eds. Progress in Obesity Research. London: John Libbey, 1996:733–742.
2. Bouchard C, Tremblay A, Depres JP, et al. The response to long-term overfeeding in identical twins. N Engl J Med 1990; 322:1477–1482.
3. Fomon SJ, Haschke F, Ziegler EE, Nelson SE. Body composition of reference children from birth to age 10 years. Am J Clin Nutr 1982; 35:1169–1175.
4. Forbes GB. Body composition in adolescence. In: Falkner F, Tanner J, eds. Human Growth: An Advanced Treatise, Vol II. New York: Plenum Press, 1978:239–272.
5. Dugdale AE, Payne PR. Pattern of lean and fat deposition in adults. Nature 1977; 206:349–351.
6. Novak LP. Age and sex differences in body density and creatinine excretion of high school children. Ann NY Acad Sci 1963; 110:545–577.
7. Cheek DB. Body composition, hormones, nutrition and adolescent growth. In: Graumbach MM, Grave GD, Mayer FE, eds. Control of Onset of Puberty. New York: Wiley, 1974: 426–447.
8. Forbes GB. Human Body Composition: Growth, Aging, Nutrition, and Activity. New York: Springer-Verlag, 1987.
9. Hammond J. Physiological limits to intensive production in animals. Br Agric Bull 1952; 4:222–224.
10. Bikker P, Karabinas V, Verstegen MW, Campbell RG. Protein and lipid accretion in body components of growing gilts (20 to 45 kilograms) as affected by energy intake. J. Anim Sci 1995; 73:2355–2363.
11. Seve B, Reeds PJ, Fuller MF, Cadenhead A, Hay SM. Protein synthesis and retention in some tissues of the young pig as influenced by dietary protein intake after early weaning. Reprod Nutr Develop 1986; 26:849–861.
12. Fiorotto ML, Burrin DG, Perez M, Reeds PJ. Intake and use of milk nutrients by rat pups suckled in small, medium or large litters. Am J Physiol 1991; 260:R1104–R1113.
13. Ebner S, Schoknecht P, Reeds PJ, Burrin DG. Growth and metabolism of gastrointestinal and skeletal muscle tissue in protein-malnourished neonatal pigs. Am J Physiol 1994; 266:R1736–R1743.
14. Proos LA, Hofvander Y, Tuvemo T. Menarcheal age and growth pattern of Indian girls adopted in Sweden. II. Catch-up growth and final height. Indian J Pediatr 1991; 58:105–114.
15. Lampl M, Johnson FE, Malcolm LA. The effects of protein supplementation on the growth and skeletal maturation of New Guinean school children. Ann Hum Biol 1978; 5: 219–227.
16. James WPT. Research in malnutrition and its application to parenteral feeding. In: Johnston IDA, ed. Advances in Parenteral Nutrition. Lancaster: MTP Press, 1978:521–531.
17. Shetty PS. Chronic undernutrition and metabolic adaptation. Proc Nutr Soc 1993; 52:267–284.
18. Faulkner F, Tanner JM, eds. Human Growth: A Comprehensive Treatise. New York: Plenum Press, 1985.
19. Hytten FE, Chamberlain GVP. Clinical Physiology of Obstetrics. Oxford: Blackwell Scientific Publications, 1980.
20. Catalano PM, Tyzbir ED, Wolfe RR, Calles J, Roman NM, Amini SB, Sims EA. Carbohydrate metabolism during pregnancy in control subjects and women with gestational diabetes. Am J Physiol 1993; 264:E60–E67.
21. Catalano PM, Drago NM, Amini SB. Maternal carbohydrate metabolism and its relationship to fetal growth and body composition. Am J Obstet Gynecol 1995; 172:1464–1470.

22. Whitelaw FG, Milne JS, Orskov ER, Smith JS. The nitrogen and energy metabolism of lactating cows given abomasal infusions of casein. Br J Nutr 1986; 55:537–556.

23. Gregory PW, Low RB, Stirewalt WS. Changes in skeletal-muscle myosin isozymes with hypertrophy and exercise. Biochem J 1986; 238:55–61.

24. Kujubu DA, Norman JT, Herschman HR, Fine LG. Primary response gene expression in renal hypertrophy and hyperplasia: evidence for different growth initiation processes. Am J Physiol 1991; 260:F823–F827.

25. Michalopoulos GK. Liver regeneration: molecular mechanisms of growth control. FASEB J 1990; 4:176–187.

26. Keys A, Anderson JT, Brozek J, Henschel A, Mickelsen O, Taylor HL. The Biology of Human Starvation. Minneapolis: University of Minnestoa Press, 1950.

27. Ferro-Luzzi A, Branca F, Pastore G. Body mass index defines the risk of seasonal energy stress in the Third World. Eur J Clin Nutr 1994; 48(Suppl 3):S165–S178.

28. Henry CJK, Rivers JPW, Payne PR. Protein-energy metabolism in starvation reconsidered. Eur J Clin Nutr 1988; 42:543–549.

29. Dulloo AG, Jacquet J, Girardier L. Autoregulation of body composition during weight recovery in humans: the Minnesota Experiment revisited. Int J Obes 1996; 20:393–405.

30. Widdowson EM. The responses of the sexes to nutritional stress. Proc Nutr Soc 1976; 35:175–180.

31. Hoyenga KB, Hoyenga KT. Gender and energy balance: sex differences in adaptations for feast and famine. Physiol Behav 1982; 28:545–563.

32. Broom J, Fleck A, Davidson DF, Rosenberg C, Durnin JVGA. Biochemical adaptations in early starvation: observations on sex differences. Proc Nutr Soc 1978; 37:91A.

33. Elia M. Effect of starvation and very low calorie diets on protein-energy interrelationships in lean and obese subjects. In: Scrimshaw NS, Schürch B, eds. Protein-Energy Interactions. Lausanne: IDECG c/o Nestlé Foundation, 1991:249–284.

34. Ferro-Luzzi A, James WPT. Adult malnutrition: simple assessment techniques for use in emergencies. Br J Nutr 1996; 75:3–10.

35. Merimee TJ, Misbin RI, Pulkkinen AJ. Sex variations in free fatty acids and ketones during fasting: evidence for a role of glucagon. J. Clin Endocrinol Metab 1978; 46:414–419.

36. Dulloo AG. Human pattern of food intake and fuel-partitioning during weight recovery after starvation: a theory of autoregulation of body composition. Proc Nutr Soc, 1997; 56:(in press).

37. Ashworth A. Ad lib feeding during recovery from malnutrition. Br J Nutr 1974; 31:109–112.

38. James WPT. Appetite control and other mechanisms of weight homeostasis. In: Blaxter Sir Kenneth, Waterlow JC, eds. Nutritional Adaptation in Man. London: John Libbey, 1985:141–154.

39. Golden BE, Golden MN. Effect of zinc on lean tissue synthesis during recovery from malnutrition. Eur J Clin Nutr 1992; 46:697–706.

40. Payne PR, Dugdale AE. Mechanisms for the control of body weight. Lancet 1977; 1:583–586.

41. Garrow JS, Stalley S. Is there a "set-point" for human body-weight? Proc Nutr Soc 1975; 34:84A.

42. Weinsier RL, Bracco D, Schutz Y. Predicted effects of small decreases in energy expenditure on weight gain in adult women. Int J Obes 1993; 17:693–700.

43. James WPT, Bailes J, Davies HL, Dauncey MJ. Elevated metabolic rates in obesity. Lancet 1978; 1:1122–1125.

44. Reeds PJ, Burrin DG, David TA, Fiorotto ML, Mersmann HJ, Pond WG. Growth regulation with particular reference to the pig. In: Hollis GR, ed. Growth of the Pig. Wallingford: CAB International, 1993:1–32.

45. Reeds PJ, Haggarty P, Fletcher JM, Wahle KWJ. Tissue and whole-body protein synthesis in immature Zucker rats and their relationship to protein deposition. Biochem J 1982; 204:393–398.

46. Isaksson O, Binder C, Hall K, et al, eds. Growth Hormone—Basic and Clinical Aspects. Amsterdam: Elsevier Science, 1987.

47. Palmiter RD, Brinster RL, Hammer RE, Trumbauer ME, Rosenfeld MG, Birnberg NC, Evans RM. Dramatic growth of mice that develop from eggs microinjected with metallothionine-growth hormone fusion genes. Nature (Lond) 1982; 300:611–615.

48. Knapp JR, Chen WY, Turner ND, Byers FM, Kopchick JJ. Growth patterns and body composition of transgenic mice expressing mutated bovine somatotropin genes. J Anim Sci 1994; 72:2812–2819.

49. Donahue LR, Beamer WG. Growth hormone deficiency in "little" mice results in aberrant body composition, reduced insulin-like growth factor-I and insulin-like growth factor-binding protein-3 (IGFBP-3), but does not affect IGFBP-2, -1 or -4. J Endocrinol 1993; 136:91–104.

50. Hahn T, Copeland KE, Woo S. Adeno-viral mediated hepatic growth hormone expression normalizes growth and protein deposition in lit mice. Endocrinology 1997; 138: (in press).

51. Boyd RD, Bauman DE. Mechanisms of action for somatotropin in growth. In: Campion DR, Hausman GJ, Martin RJ, eds. Current Concepts of Animal Growth Regulation. New York: Plenum Press, 1989:257–293.

52. Nguyen TT, Gilpin DA, Meyer NA, Herndon DN Current treatment of severely burned patients. Ann Surg 1996; 223(1):14–25.

53. Campbell RG, Johnson RJ, King RH, Taverner MR, Meisinger DJ. Interaction between dietary protein content and exogenous porcine growth hormone on protein and lipid accretion rates in pigs. J Anim Sci 1990; 68:3217–3225.

54. Caperna TJ, Steele NC, Komarek DR, McMurtry JP, Rosebrough RW, Solomon MB, Mitchell AD. Influence of dietary protein and recombinant porcine somatotropin administration in young pigs: growth, body composition and hormone status. J Anim Sci 1990; 68:4243–4252.

55. Krick BJ, Boyd RD, Roneker KR, Beerman DH, Bauman DE, Ross DA, Meisinger DJ. Porcine somatotropin affects

the dietary lysine requirement and net lysine utilization for growing pigs. J. Nutr 1993; 123:1913–1922.

56. Lo HC, Hinton PS, Peterson CA, Ney DM. Simultaneous treatment with IGF-I and GH additively increases anabolism in parenterally fed rats. Am J Physiol 1995; 269: E368–E376.

57. Read LC, Tomas FM, Howarth GS et al. Insulin-like growth factor-I and its N-terminal modified analogues induce marked gut growth in dexamethasone-treated rats. J Endocrinol 1992; 133:421–431.

58. Pell JM, Bates PC. Differential actions of growth hormone and insulin-like growth factor-I on tissue protein metabolism in dwarf mice. Endocrinology 1992; 130:1942–1950.

59. Wray-Cahen D, Bell AW, Boyd RD et al. Nutrient uptake by the hindlimb of growing pigs treated with porcine somatotropin and insulin. J Nutr 1995; 125:125–135.

60. Lanna DP, Houseknecht KL, Harris DM, Bauman DE. Effect of somatotropin treatment on lipogenesis, lipolysis, and related cellular mechanisms in adipose tissue of lactating cows. J Dairy Sci 1995; 78:1703–1712.

61. Merimee TJ. Growth hormone and IGF abnormalities of the African Pigmy. In: LeRoith D, Raizada MK, eds. Molecular and Cellular Biology of Insulin-like Growth Factors and Their Receptors. New York: Plenum Press, 1989: 73–80.

62. Meredith HV. Research between 1960 and 1970 on the standing height of young children in different parts of the world. Adv Child Dev Behav 1978; 12:1–59.

63. Merimee TJ, Hewlett BS, Wood W, Bowcock AM, Cavalli-Sforza LL. The growth hormone receptor gene in the African Pigmy. Trans Assoc Am Phys 1989; 102:163–169.

64. Johansson J-O, Oscarsson J, Bjarnason R, Bengtsson B-Å. Two weeks of daily injections and continuous infusion of recombinant human growth hormone (GH) in GH-deficient adults. 1. Effects on insulin-like growth factor-I (IGF-I), GH and IGF binding proteins, and glucose homeostasis. Metabolism 1996; 45:362–369.

65. Reeds PJ, Hay SM, Dorward P, Palmer RM. The effect of Clenbuterol on protein deposition in the rat. Lack of effect on muscle protein biosynthesis. Br J Nutr 1986; 56: 249–258.

66. Maltin CA, Reeds PJ, Delday MI, Hay SM, Smith FG, Lobley GE. Inhibition and reversal of denervation-induced atrophy by the beta-agonist growth promoter, Clenbuterol. Biosci Rep 1986; 6:811–818.

67. Reeds PJ, Mersmann HJ. Protein and energy requirements of animals treated with β-adrenergic agonists. A discussion. J Anim Sci 1991; 69:1532–1550.

68. Lindsay DB, Hunter RA, Sillence MN. The use of non-peptide hormones and analogues to manipulate animal performance. In: Buttery PJ, Boorman KN, Lindsay DB, eds. The Control of Fat and Lean Deposition. Oxford: Butterworths-Heinemann, 1922:277–298.

69. Bray GA. Obesity—a disease of nutrient or energy balance. Nutr Rev 1987; 45:33–43.

70. Lobley GE, Connell A, Morris B et al. The effect of active immunization against gonadotropin-hormone-releasing-hormone on growth performance and sample joint composition of bulls. Anim Prod 1992; 55:193–202.

71. Gatford KL, Fletcher TP, Clarke IJ et al. Sexual dimorphism of circulating somatotropin, insulin-like growth factors I and II, insulin-like growth factor binding proteins, and insulin relationships to growth rate and carcass characteristics in growing lambs. J Anim Sci 1996; 74:1314–1325.

72. Lobley GE, Connell A, Buchan V, Skene PA, Fletcher JM. Administration of testosterone to wether lambs: effects on protein and energy metabolism and growth hormone status. J. Endocrinol 1987; 115:429–445.

73. Lobley GE, Connell A, Milne E, et al. Muscle protein synthesis in response to testosterone administration in wether lambs. Br J Nutr 1990; 64:691–704.

74. Santidrian S, Moreyra M, Munro HN, Young VR. Effect of testosterone on the rate of myofibrillar protein breakdown in castrated and adrenalectomized male rats measured by the urinary excretion of 3-methylhistidine. Metabolism 1982; 31:1200–1205.

75. Forbes GB, Porta CR, Herr BE, Griggs RC. Sequence of changes in body composition induced by testosterone and reversal of changes after drug is stopped. JAMA 1992; 267(3):397–399.

76. Forbes GB. Body size and composition of perimenarchal girls. Am J Dis Child 1992; 146:63–66.

77. Pelleymounter MA, Cullen MJ, Baker MB, Hecht R, Winters D, Boone T, Collins F. Effects of the obese gene product on body weight regulation in ob/ob mice. Science 1995; 269: 540–543.

78. Halaas JL, Gajiwala KS, Maffei M, Cohen SL, Chait BT, Rabinowitz D, Lallone RL, Burley SK, Freidman JM. Weight-reducing effects of the plasma protein encoded by the obese gene. Science 1995; 269:543–546.

79. Campfield LA, Smith FJ, Guisez Y, Devos R, Burn P. Recombinant mouse OB protein: evidence for a peripheral signal linking adiposity and central neural networks. Science 1995; 269:546–549.

80. Madej T, Boguski MS, Bryant SH. Threading analysis suggests that the obese gene product may be a helical cytokine. FEBS lett 1995; 373:13–18.

81. Flatt JP. The RQ/FQ concept and weight maintenance. In: Angel A, Anderson H, Bouchard C, Lau D, Leiter L, Mendelson R, eds. Progress in Obesity Research. London: John Libbey, 1996:749–766.

82. Fuller MF, Cadenhead A, Mollison G, Seve B. Effects of the amount and quality of dietary protein on nitrogen metabolism and heat production in growing pigs. Br J Nutr 1987; 58:277–285.

83. Pullar JD, Webster AJF. The energy cost of fat and protein deposition in the rat. Br J Nutr 1977; 37:355–363.

84. Garlick PJ, Millward DJ, James WPT, Waterlow JC. The effect of protein deprivation and starvation on the rate of protein synthesis in tissues of the rat. Biochim Biophys Acta 1975; 414:71–84.

85. James WPT, Sender PM, Garlick PJ, Waterlow JC. The choice of label and measurement technique in tracer studies of body protein metabolism in man. IAEA Symposium on Dynamic Aspects of Isotope Technique in Man. 1974: 461–472.

86. Clugston GA, Garlick PJ. The response of protein and energy metabolism to food intake in lean and obese man. Hum Nutr Clin Nutr 1982; 36C:57–70.

87. Berthold HK, Wykes L, Jahoor F, Klein PD, Reeds PJ. The use of uniformly labeled substrates and mass isotopomer analysis to study intermediary metabolism. Proc Nutr Soc 1994; 53:345–354.

27

Etiology of the Metabolic Syndrome

Per Björntorp
Sahlgren's Hospital, University of Gothenburg, Gothenburg, Sweden

I. HISTORICAL BACKGROUND

It has long been realized that certain metabolic symptoms often occur together, and that these symptoms predict the development of disease. The oldest examples are probably that elevated serum cholesterol precedes cardiovascular disease (CVD) and occurs most frequently in subject with hypertension. Insulin resistance clearly precedes non-insulin-dependent diabetes mellitus (NIDDM) and is also a risk factor for CVD. Clinicians know from experience that, for example, NIDDM and CVD often occur in the same patient, who may display several metabolic abnormalities. Thus, the combination of metabolic disturbances, as well as hypertension, and certain diseases is nothing new for clinicians, and as early as the 1920s (1), there were reports suggesting that such clusters of phenomena may constitute "syndromes."

Recently it has been suggested that a number of metabolic risk factors and the diseases they predict should be collected under a common name constituting a syndrome of metabolic abnormalities. Different names have been suggested. Although several clinicians and researchers had seen such a syndrome previously, it was probably Reaven (2) who first articulated these thoughts and called this cluster of phenomena syndrome X. This syndrome was described as a combination of insulin resistance, dyslipidemia, and hypertension, risk factors for NIDDM and CVD. Other authors have suggested terms such as the plurimetabolic syndrome (3), the "deadly quartet" (4), and

added other metabolic aberrations to the cluster, most notably abdominal obesity, which is part of the deadly quartet (4). This seems highly pertinent because abdominal obesity is probably one of the most frequent components of the syndrome, as will be reviewed below. The term I use for the condition in this review is simply the metabolic syndrome (MS). The advantage of this term is that it is descriptive, covering the essence of the syndrome, namely that it is expressed as multiple metabolic abnormalities, which have in common that they are predictors, "risk factors," for the development of CVD, NIDDM, and stroke. Because of its apparent multiple associations with poor life-style factors, frequently following urbanization, it has been suggested that this is a "civilization syndrome" (5). It is anticipated that once the basic etiology of the syndrome has been revealed, there will be a more appropriate name, which is not only descriptive.

II. DEFINITION

There is no consensus about which factors should be included under the MS. Most authors include a core of phenomena consisting of insulin resistance, dyslipidemia (elevated very-low-density lipoproteins, combined with low concentrations of high-density lipoproteins), and hypertension. Reaven does not include obesity in his original description of syndrome X(2), and it is true that insulin resistance might occur without obesity. On the other hand, the most prevalent associate to insulin resistance is no doubt obesity, particularly when localized to central regions (6). In addition, quantitative analyses of the frequency of clustering of the different components of the MS in epidemiological studies suggest that abdominal body fat distribution, as indicated by an elevated waist/hip circumference ratio (WHR), is found as frequently in the syndrome as insulin resistance. In fact, the WHR shows this association independently of obesity, as indicated by the body mass index (BMI) (7), suggesting that the central distribution of body fat is more important than total fat mass. It seems likely that visceral fat mass is the adipose tissue compartment contributing most strongly to this statistical association (6,8–18).

Other factors, such as hyperuricemia, physical inactivity, hyperandrogenicity in women, growth hormone deficiency, and smoking tobacco, might be considered to be part of MS. There is considerable statistical and mechanistic support for such contentions (5), but there is currently no consensus as to the definition of the factors that should be included.

III. THE EVIDENCE FOR A METABOLIC SYNDROME

The question then is, why has the idea now begun to be considered seriously that the clustering of the metabolic symptoms and diseases mentioned in the previous section might indeed constitute a syndrome, when clinical experience and previous reports have long since indicated this possibility. Collecting clinical observations into a "syndrome" often means that certain signs are occurring together, but that the underlying cause is not apparent. The observation that clinical phenomena cluster in a syndrome often precedes the establishment of an etiological diagnosis, which is usually necessary to lead research into etiological directions.

Epidemiological evidence points in the direction of the presence of a MS. It is long since well established that certain metabolic factors indicate risk for specific diseases. For example, dyslipidemia is known to be associated with CVD. This was first observed in retrospective studies. However, when modern epidemiological research started, it became apparent that CVD, NIDDM, and stroke were preceded by several risk factors. In addition, metabolic risk factors were found to be largely similar for these diseases. A core of factors, constituting insulin resistance, dyslipidemia, hypertension, and abdominal obesity, or, more specifically, a larger-than-normal proportion of body fat localized to central regions, was found to be a predictor for all these diseases. However, the power of each risk factor seemed to have a certain profile in relation to the diseases. Lipids were associated with particularly closely with CVD, insulin resistance with NIDDM, and hypertension with stroke. This probably means that there are some risk factors that are more closely coupled than others with the triggering mechanisms for a specific disease. Nevertheless, there are also statistical connections between the mentioned diseases and other less specific metabolic risk factors. For example, hypertension is a risk factor for NIDDM (19,20), but it is difficult to imagine a pathogenetic mechanism where elevated blood pressure would cause NIDDM. This is probably only a statistical association. But the mere fact that the metabolic factors, including blood pressure elevation, often occur together is a statistical argument for MS.

Another question is how often the full-blown syndrome is found in an individual. Clinical, anecdotal observations suggest that a middle-aged man with hypertension, insulin resistance, abdominal obesity, and dyslipidemia is seen very frequently. However, when this question is analyzed in individuals on a population basis, the results become somewhat different from clinical experience. In a recent epidemiological study of women, hypertriglyceridemia, elevated insulin, and high blood pressure were defined as values that were more than two standard deviations above the mean values in that population. One of these factors was frequently found elevated in association with elevated WHR. However, when two or more abnormalities were included in the calculations, the prevalence of such individuals decreased sharply, and the full-blown syndrome, including all factors, was seldom seen (7). A similar analysis in men, starting with blood pressure as the selection variable, showed essentially the same results (21). This has also been reported recently in children (22). In conclusion, on a population basis individuals with the complete MS are not frequently found. However, particularly insulin resistance and abdominal obesity are tightly coupled statistically (6), and often followed by dyslipidemia and hypertension.

In summary, metabolic factors, including hypertension and abdominal distribution of body fat, indicating elevated risk to develop NIDDM, CVD, and stroke, are frequently seen in clusters. Statistical evidence suggests that this might constitute a syndrome, although all the components of the syndrome are not often seen in the same individual in epidemiological studies.

A stronger argument for the collection of these statistical data into a syndrome would be if the etiological background factor(s) could be revealed. If this were possible, then what is now called a syndrome might be turned into a clinical entity, a defined disease, or group of closely related diseases. Are there possibilities for mechanistic links between the descriptive and statistical associations?

Reaven (2) has built his synthesis of syndrome X on such evidence, which is, to a large extent, a product of his own excellent work through the years. Reaven suggests that insulin resistance is the key factor to a chain of subsequent events leading to the development of the syndrome. Insulin resistance is now largely accepted as an established precursor condition to NIDDM. The mechanism is believed to be an exhaustion of insulin production, resulting in NIDDM. Furthermore, Reaven was the first to show that hyperinsulinemia, a consequence of insulin resistance, regulates the production of atherogenic lipoproteins in the liver (23), another pathogenetic link between the cluster of risk factors and, particularly, CVD. Reaven has also provided evidence for the possibility that insulin resistance may be a causal factor for the development of hypertension (2,24), which has also been suggested by other researchers (25,26). However, this is still the weakest link in this potential pathogenic chain of events. Although the statistical coupling is well established, the current state of information does not allow conclusions about the etiological mechanisms (27). Nevertheless, the available evidence is sufficiently convincing to suggest that insulin resistance may produce most of the components of the MS through mechanisms that are conceptually reasonable.

The accumulation of visceral fat is probably as common as insulin resistance in the MS and is closely associated with insulin resistance in statistical analyses (6,7). Evidence for placing visceral fat depots at the etiological center of the different components of the MS has been presented (28). The trigger mechanisms may be the release of free fatty acids (FFA) from the visceral fat depots into the portal vein, which subsequently affect hepatic mechanisms leading to dyslipidemia, hyperglycemia, and hyperinsulinemia, which are all parts of MS (28). Taken together, both insulin resistance with hyperinsulinemia and visceral fat accumulation might provide reasonable explanatory mechanisms for the rest of the MS.

There are, however, components of the MS that do not fit particularly well into these schemes. Insulin resistance, as the primary cause of the MS, is closely coupled statistically to visceral obesity (6). There is, however, no directly apparent mechanistic hypothesis to explain how visceral accumulation of storage fat can follow from insulin resistance. It is somewhat easier to see a pathway through which insulin resistance might follow from visceral fat accumulation. Visceral depots are particularly sensitive to stimuli that mobilize FFA (28). FFA are, in turn, powerful inducers of both hepatic and muscular insulin resistance (29,30). The question, then, is whether the quantity of FFA mobilized from visceral depots is sufficient to induce systemic insulin resistance. Unfortunately, quantitative measurements are hampered by the difficulties of measuring FFA flux directly in the portal vein of humans. Estimations from lipolysis rates in vitro, visceral fat mass, and hepatic clearance of FFA suggest that portal and systemic FFA concentrations will be sufficient to induce both hepatic and muscular insulin resistance (28). Radioisotope dilution measurements of portal FFA flux in the hepatic veins (31) do not provide evidence for such a contention, however. Unfortunately, none of these methods provide conclusive results for measurements of portal FFA flux. Measurements of the effects of portal FFA, which are not possible in humans, can be performed in rats, however. Such evidence suggests that FFA produce a decreased hepatic clearance of insulin providing a basis for peripheral hyperinsulinemia, but this is only found in young and not in older rats (32), and the applicability to human beings is uncertain.

Recent studies in human beings have, however, provided useful information. The triglyceride content of the liver can be estimated by the degree of attenuation in computerized tomography (CT) scans, low attenuation indicating high triglyceride content. Such measurements show inverse relationships to visceral fat mass. Although circumstantial, this evidence suggests that hepatic triglyceride content may follow from visceral fat accumulation, presumably via large FFA fluxes. This in turn was associated with insulin resistance and hyperinsulinemia (33, 34). Previous studies have shown directly that hepatic triglyceride content is directly proportional to peripheral insulin concentration in humans (35), similar to observations in rats, with a lower hepatic clearance of insulin (32). Furthermore, hepatic clearance of insulin in humans is inversely related to the WHR (36). These data are compatible with a decreased hepatic clearance of insulin via inhibition by portal FFA or hepatic triglyceride, leading to peripheral hyperinsulinemia.

Insulin resistance and visceral fat accumulation may provide reasonable explanations for the genesis of several, but not all, of the other symptoms of the MS. Both are statistically strongly interrelated. The combination of insulin resistance and visceral fat accumulation may well amplify various other components of the MS along the lines outlined above. An alternate explanation might be that both these cardinal symptoms of the MS are parallel phenomena, caused by another, independent yet common factor. Such a possibility will be discussed later.

In summary, there are currently mechanistic pathways to link several of the statistically defined clusters of abnormalities in the MS starting out either from insulin resistance or from visceral fat accumulation. This strengthens the contention of the presence of a MS. However, neither insulin resistance nor visceral fat accumulation can explain all of the abnormalities in the MS, particularly not those of endocrine nature as will be described below. Therefore, it seems likely that another, overriding cause may be the basic abnormality.

In conclusion, it is suggested that the MS is currently a statistical reality that is useful to stimulate research efforts into potential etiological mechanisms.

IV. DIAGNOSIS AND PREVALENCE

How should the MS be diagnosed? This obviously depends on its definition. If one accepts that the symptoms and diseases mentioned in previous sections are components of the MS, then the presence of one of them would be a sign of the syndrome, excluding of course specific diseases, such as, for example, lipoprotein lipase deficiency, causing hypertriglyceridemia, or renal artery occlusion, causing hypertension. The first suggestion for diagnosis is then that any expression of the components of the syndrome would provide evidence for its presence.

A more conservative viewpoint is the following. Since both insulin resistance and visceral accumulation of body fat are prevalent components of the MS and have reasonable pathogenic associations with several other parts of the syndrome (see above), it seems reasonable to suggest that both these factors are minimum requirements for establishing the diagnosis.

This definition has been applied in this review in population studies where the WHR has often been used as a criterion for the MS and where strong statistical interrelationships have been demonstrated between the WHR and particularly insulin. Elevated triglycerides and blood pressure are often accompanying abnormalities. The diagnosis of the MS then rests primarily on the combination of elevated WHR (central obesity) and insulin resistance in these studies.

The prevalence of the MS is of course directly dependent on its definition. It is abundantly clear, however, that insulin resistance, dyslipidemia, hypertension, and elevated WHR are very prevalent components. Exact figures can only be obtained from epidemiological studies, but then difficulties are encountered in setting borderlines for these abnormalities. It seems, however, reasonably safe to state that one or more of the components of the MS are found by middle age in a large fraction or urbanized populations.

If we accept insulin resistance as a diagnostic criterion, the prevalence of this phenomenon has been estimated to be in the order of 25% in westernized populations (37), but is probably much higher in certain other populations, such as the Pima Indians, Australian aborigines, and pop-

ulations in certain Pacific Islands (for review, see Ref. 38). The prevalence also most likely varies with age and perhaps with gender, but no data are available.

The prevalence of an enlarged proportion of body fat as visceral fat seems to follow in parallel with the prevalence of insulin resistance. In the absence of defined borderlines it is difficult to state absolute figures. However, in the fifth quintile of the WHR a high prevalence of metabolic abnormalities and increased risk for CVD are common, and NIDDM is clearly elevated in westernized middle-aged populations (for review, see Ref. 5). This suggests that about 20% of such populations have too much central obesity.

V. TECHNIQUES FOR EVALUATION

The next question is how insulin resistance and visceral body fat accumulation can be measured. This depends on the situation. The gold standard for measurement of systemic insulin resistance is generally considered to be the euglycemic, hyperinsulinemic clamp (40,41). The gold standard for determining visceral fat mass is CT scans or magnetic resonance imaging (MRI) scans (42). Both can only be performed in research laboratories with considerable technical and economical resources. Therefore, in clinical or epidemiological settings we need alternatives.

The area of insulin resistance measurements has recently been thoroughly reviewed (39). As far as measurement of visceral fat mass is concerned, substitutes of CT scan determination have different degrees of accuracy. Epidemiologically, the WHR, or related measurements, have been employed in estimations of risk for CVD, NIDDM, stroke, overall mortality, or in relationship to metabolic components or hypertension, showing rather strong predictive power (43–52). This is, however, a fairly poor measurement of visceral fat mass (53). Abdominal sagittal diameter seems to be a better estimate (53), but has so far only occasionally been used in prospective epidemiological studies (54). For obvious reasons, CT scan measurements are difficult to perform for such surveys, because of the complexity and expense of this technique. There is as yet only one perspective study with CT scan, showing a stronger relationship with visceral fat than with other body fat compartments for the development of NIDDM (51). These few studies suggest that visceral fat accumulation, measured either directly (51) or by substitutes (54), is closely connected with the development of disease. The documentation of the value of WHR or related measurements is, however, more extensive (43–52), including several population-based prospective studies. The relationship between the WHR and the components of the MS, as well as the predictive risk of disease, is usually linear, allowing better possibilities for delineation of a desirable WHR than, for example, a desirable BMI. The WHR is, however, a rather poor measurement of visceral fat mass (53). The question then arises, does the WHR measure additional components carrying information pertinent to the MS?

VI. THE WAIST/HIP CIRCUMFERENCE RATIO

What does the WHR measure? This requires a consideration of the different components of this rather complex ratio. First, if we look a the waist circumference, this consists of the subcutaneous fat layer, muscles, visceral organs, and the intestinal content at the level of measurement. Nevertheless, waist circumference gives a reasonably good estimate of visceral fat content, not least in young men (15,53).

The hip circumference contains mainly the skeletal frame and muscles in the gluteal region. This means that a large group of muscles is included in this measurement. The mass and function of muscles are of major importance for systemic insulin sensitivity (55). Since insulin resistance is a statistical companion to an elevated WHR, it is conceivable that a large WHR, depending on gluteal or generalized muscle atrophy, might be an indicator of muscular insulin resistance. This assumption is supported by the findings of endocrine perturbations in the MS. As will be reviewed in more detail below, recent findings indicate that cortisol secretion is elevated and sex steroids and growth hormone secretion are inhibited. All these hormones exert profound effects on muscle mass and structure and on insulin sensitivity, and it may well be that the hip circumference carries information about such perturbations.

This has never been directly tested, but some observations deserve mention in this connection. First, the muscular atrophy of Cushing's syndrome is in line with this concept. Furthermore, alcoholics are known to have elevated cortisol secretion and decreased sex steroid hormones (56). They also have a profound increase in the WHR, depending on both enlargement of visceral fat mass and a relative atrophy of gluteal muscle mass (57). The hypogonadism of men with the MS (58–60) would be expected to be followed by relative muscle atrophy. Upon treatment of such men with testosterone muscle mass, structure and insulin sensitivity are restored toward normal (61–63). Analogous observations have been made for growth hormone (64), another hormone that is deficient in the MS (65).

One may speculate that the hormonal changes of muscle mass, structure, and function may well vary in different muscular regions, similar to adipose tissue. Muscle tissue is not a homogeneous entity. Among animals there is often a clear specialization of muscles into athletic, sprint-type muscles and muscles used for endurance activity. The former are characterized by white, type II, slow-twitch fibers with mainly glycolytic metabolism and a low density of insulin receptors. The latter muscles are dominated by so-called type I fibers, which appear red because of a high concentration of myoglobin. Such muscles are highly insulin-sensitive because of a high density of insulin receptors (66,67). Human beings do not have such a clear specialization of muscles, although there is some regional variation (68). Muscle atrophy follows several endocrine diseases and mainly affects large central muscles in diabetes. Furthermore, the hormones with aberrant secretion in the MS clearly affect not only muscle mass, but also fiber composition and insulin sensitivity with regional differences (Section IX, B). It is not too far-fetched to imagine that the endocrine abnormalities in the MS not only affect muscle mass in general, but also show a regional specificity. Very little is known about this interesting possibility.

It is thus conceivable that the hip circumference actually provides information on the status of hormones that regulate muscle mass, as well as their structure and insulin sensitivity. The endocrine disturbances of the MS may also cause the redistribution of depot fat to visceral adipose tissue (Section IX, A). Therefore, there is an intriguing possibility that the WHR is an indicator of the both cardinal symptoms of the MS, namely insulin resistance and visceral fat accumulation. This might explain the close association between the WHR and insulin resistance and the unique power of the WHR to predict disease.

VII. THE ROLE OF OBESITY

At this point it is pertinent to discuss whether obesity is necessary for the expression of the MS. Obesity is defined as an increased mass of total adipose tissue triglycerides. By this definition, obesity is not necessarily associated with enlargement of the visceral fat depots. For example, consider the average middle-aged man in the Gothenburg study of "men born [in] 1913." He is about 175 cm tall and his body weight is about 75 kg, of which about 15 kg is total body fat (69). His visceral fat mass might be approximately 5 kg (53). Suppose this man doubles his visceral fat mass, from 5 to 10 kg; then his total body fat would be 20 kg, and his BMI would have changed from

24.6 to 26.1. A doubling of his visceral fat mass then results in a small change in the BMI, a measurement of overweight. In other words, visceral fat mass can vary dramatically within a narrow change of total body fat or BMI. Furthermore, his metabolic risk factors would, from a statistical viewpoint, be expected to rise considerably, much more than would be expected from the small elevation of BMI.

From an epidemiological point of view, the WHR has a stronger predictive power than the BMI for stroke, NIDDM, and, particularly CVD, where the Gothenburg studies actually tend to show a negative relationship with BMI to the risk of developing CVD (70). Actually, the WHR relationship to CVD, to NIDDM, to stroke, and to overall mortality is independent of BMI (43,70,71). But, as discussed above, it seems likely that the WHR contains information other than visceral fat mass. Visceral fat mass has been evaluated prospectively in first-generation Japanese-Americans and found to be superior to other body fat compartments as a predictor of NIDDM (51), and the sagittal abdominal diameter, a surrogate measurement of visceral fat mass, has been suggested to be a stronger predictor than BMI for CVD (54). It is clear that, as an epidemiological predictor for prevalent disease, measurements or approximations of visceral fat mass are superior to total body fat measurements.

This also seems clear when comparing the statistical associations between the components of the MS, blood glucose, insulin, triglycerides, and blood pressure, on the one hand, and the BMI or WHR on a population basis, on the other hand. Within each quintile of the BMI, the WHR was associated with one or more of these risk factors, suggesting a relationship to the WHR, independent of BMI (7).

In case-control studies, where visceral fat mass has been measured by CT scan, it is also clear that the correlations between insulin resistance, dyslipidemia, glucose intolerance, and hypertension, on the other hand, and body fat compartments, on the other, are strongest for visceral fat mass (6,8–18). In addition, the endocrine abnormalities associated with the MS, when measured in relation to body fat compartments, have shown stronger correlations to visceral than to total or subcutaneous body fat (63,65).

Information from CT scan studies has suggested that abdominal subcutaneous fat might provide additional information (72). In addition, a recent study has suggested that the subcutaneous fat depot of the neck is almost as strongly related to the metabolic risk factor pattern of the MS as is visceral fat mass (73). In addition to visceral fat enlargement, this "buffalo hump" is the typical fat accu-mulation pattern seen with hypercortisolism and Cushing's syndrome. As will be reviewed in a following section, the MS is most likely characterized by a hypersensitive hypothalamopituitary-adrenal (HPA) axis, with elevated cortisol secretion, providing a clue to the origin of the specific body fat distribution of the MS.

These data clearly indicate that central, visceral fat mass displays stronger associations to the MS than total body fat does. In fact, some of the observations are compatible with no significant, additional role of total body fat. This can probably not be generalized, however. For example, in the prospective studies of NIDDM in both the TOPS study (74) and the Gothenburg study (46), the BMI seems to add risk in excess to that of the WHR itself. Whether this is due to a larger absolute amount of visceral fat with elevated BMI or statistical risk added by other fat depots is not known.

In summary, visceral fat seems to be the body fat compartment that shows the strongest statistical associations to the metabolic abnormalities of the MS, as well as to its accompanying diseases in prospective studies. Observations suggest that total body fat may contribute additional risk under certain conditions, while sometimes even a protective effect seems to be apparent. The important message from this analysis is that the MS may occur without obesity in conventional terms. Interestingly, this is in concert with Reaven's view, not including obesity in syndrome X (2). The distribution of body fat, whether in abundance or not, seems to be the most important factor.

VIII. ENDOCRINE PERTURBATIONS

Several endocrine abnormalities, in addition to hyperinsulinemia, have now been described in the MS. These comprise both steroid and peptide hormones. The central disturbance is probably an overproduction of cortisol. This was described by early investigators in the field as elevated urinary output of both 17-keto and 17-ketogenic steroids in women with android obesity (75). Cortisol secretion is a much-studied problem in obesity in general, where an increased production combined with an elevated turnover seems to result in normal or even low plasma cortisol levels (for review, see Ref. 76). Recent studies have now shown that output of free cortisol is indeed elevated in proportion to the WHR or the abdominal sagittal diameter. This is, however, apparently not a very robust phenomenon and seems to require measurements under "field conditions" (77). The reason for this is probably that the HPA axis is abnormally sensitive to stimuli and the oversecretion of cortisol is seen only upon stimulation. This statement is based on the following observations.

Stimulatory tests of the entire HPA axis have been performed, showing exaggerated responses. ACTH administration is followed by increased cortisol production (77–79). This might be interpreted to mean that the adrenals are hypersensitive to ACTH stimuli and/or hypertrophied, which may in turn be a consequence of the hyperactivity over the HPA axis. At the level of the pituitary, corticotropin-releasing hormone (CRH) stimulation is followed by a rather dramatic increase in ACTH, cortisol, and β-endorphin concentrations in the circulation (79, 80). Furthermore, CRH and arginine vasopressin administration is similarly followed by increased ACTH and cortisol secretion (81). These results probably mean that the CRH receptors in the pituitary are hyperresponsive or hypersensitive to stimuli either directly to CRH or via the amplifying effects of arginine vasopressin (81). Finally, physical and mental laboratory stress tests are followed by increased cortisol secretion (77,82), showing a hypersensitive response, to physiological central stimuli of the HPA axis.

The total picture then indicates a hyperresponsiveness or hypersensitivity to stimuli at all levels of the HPA axis from the central nervous system to the adrenals, where our original findings (77) have been confirmed and expanded independently by several laboratories. It should be noted, however, that these studies have mainly been performed in women. The question then is why the HPA axis is hyperactive. There are two principal possibilities. By repeated challenges the HPA axis becomes hyperreactive, perhaps by modification of regulatory central adrenergic neurons (83). This is often followed by elevated nadir levels of cortisol in the afternoon, but not necessarily by an elevated peak morning concentration. Indeed, morning serum cortisol levels seem to be low. With a total increase of urinary cortisol output (77), this might mean that the afternoon concentration is elevated. Full diurnal concentration curves are currently being measured.

The HPA axis is regulated by a feedback control, mediated via glucocorticoid receptors in the central nervous system, particularly in the hippocampus (85). When these receptors are occupied by cortisol, the CRH production will be inhibited. Upon repeated or chronic overstimulation of the HPA axis, the glucocorticoid receptors are down-regulated or even irreversibly destroyed, which is then seen as a hyperresponsiveness of the HPA axis. This can be examined by the dexamethasone inhibition test. Such tests with the conventional 1-mg dose do not show any abnormalities (77). We have, however, recently found that the inhibition is less than normal, inversely related to the WHR, at lower doses of dexamethasone (84). This finding then shows a diminished feedback control of the HPA axis and suggests a mild down-regulation of central glucocorticoid receptors.

High androgen concentrations in women are another endocrine abnormality comprised of overproduction of both testosterone (T) and androstenedione (for review, see Ref. 18), both of which become abnormally elevated upon ACTH stimulation (78), suggesting that these hormones have adrenal origin. The increase in androgens may, therefore, actually be a consequence of the hyperactivity of the HPA axis.

Sex-specific steroid hormones seem to be low in both men and women with the MS. Several laboratories have now shown that T values in men are decreased (58–60, 86). A recent study of the men born in 1913 in Gothenburg, who were then 67 years of age, has evaluated the relative hypogonadism. Low values of free T and sex hormone–binding globulin (SHBG) were found to be tightly coupled to the WHR, insulin resistance, and NIDDM and were also risk factors for development of NIDDM, prospectively. Luteinizing hormone (LH), however, did not show such correlations. The relation of insulin resistance with low free T seemed to be independent of LH concentrations, indicating that gonadal as well as pituitary hypogonadism may be responsible (87).

Single determinations of 17-β estradiol in women have not revealed abnormalities (18), but this needs to be evaluated more carefully over the menstrual cycle. Menstruation is frequently irregular or absent (74), resulting in low progesterone production, suggesting abnormalities in the pituitary-gonadal axis in women.

Insulin-like growth factor I (IGF-I) is inversely correlated with visceral fat content, and not related to total or subcutaneous fat mass, measured by CT scan. There were also negative correlations of IGF-I with insulin resistance (65). IGF-I can be stimulated by growth hormone (GH) secretion and is therefore a surrogate measurement of GH secretion (88). Direct measurements of diurnal GH secretion show that GH secretion is diminished in the MS (89, and T. Ljung et al., unpublished).

Taken together, the endocrine abnormalities of the MS comprise an increased sensitivity of the HPA axis with elevated secretions of ACTH and cortisol. In addition, hyperandrogenicity is a characteristic of women with the syndrome, probably another consequence of the hyperactive HPA axis. Other abnormalities are decreased gender-specific sex steroid hormone secretions, probably mainly due to a diminished activity of the pituitary-gonadal axis, as well as a low GH secretion. Interestingly, these latter abnormalities may also well be derived from the increased activity of the HPA axis. It is well established that an increased CRH production secondarily decreases the production of gonadotropin-releasing hormone, as well as growth hormone–releasing hormone. The latter is also inhibited by cortisol (90). There is thus a realistic possibility that the hypersensitivity of the HPA axis is the primary factor that secondarily inhibits the pituitary-gonadal as well as the GH axes. This then obviously places hyperactivity of the HPA axis in the center of the etiology of the other endocrine and neuroendocrine abnormalities. This is summarized in Figure 1.

Activity of the central sympathetic nervous system should also be considered in relation to the HPA axis, because the CRH-producing center is closely connected with the central regulation of the sympathetic nervous system (90). Some observations have been made pertinent to this question. Upon stress tests in the laboratory, central regulation of hemodynamics appear abnormal in the MS. Instead of the normal increase of blood pressure and heart rate with a concomitant decreased peripheral resistance, a depressive reaction, including an increased peripheral resistance, seems to occur (91). The elevated blood pressure in the MS may have a similar origin. Abnormal circulatory reactions to stress have also recently been reported in obese women (81). We have recently noted that this might be particularly pronounced in men with MS (T. Ljung et al., unpublished). This area needs much more work. The

thyroid axis has not been sufficiently studied in the syndrome.

IX. CONSEQUENCES OF THE ENDOCRINE ABNORMALITIES

A. Body Fat Distribution

The hormones involved in the endocrine abnormalities of the MS have profound effects on adipose tissue metabolism and show regional specificity. This will be briefly reviewed, with emphasis on the effects on human adipose tissue, because of the marked species differences in adipose tissue metabolism. A detailed review has been published recently (91a). First, the cellular and molecular mechanisms will be reviewed, followed by physiological, clinical, and interventional observations.

Cortisol is a powerful inducer of lipoprotein lipase (LPL) activity, in the presence of insulin. This is due to a combined effect on gene transcription and a stabilization of the enzyme, with no apparent effects on translation (92). In the presence of GH a marked inhibition is seen, apparently a posttranscriptional effect (93). The cortisol effect is mediated via a specific glucocorticoid receptor in adipose tissue (94). Cortisol, in the presence of insulin, does not activate the lipolytic machinery in human adipose tissue; in fact, there is even some inhibition. However, when GH is added, a marked stimulation of lipolysis occurs (95). In summary, cortisol in the presence of insulin is clearly a hormone that causes triglyceride accumulation in adipocytes. GH counteracts these activities. Hypercortisolemia and hyperinsulinemia as well as low GH secretion are characteristics of the MS, therefore providing a milieu for lipid accumulation.

Other hormones than GH that show low concentrations in the MS, the sex steroid hormones, also exert profound effects on adipose tissue metabolism. T inhibits the activities of LPL as well as glycerophosphate dehydrogenase, another triglyceride accumulating enzyme (96). Since in vivo T and GH act in the presence of cortisol, it is important that the cortisol effects on LPL are inhibited by T (M. Ottosson et al., unpublished). GH is also a powerful inhibitor of cortisol-induced LPL activity by a posttranslational effect (93). Regarding lipid mobilization, both T an GH, particularly in combination, display profound stimulatory effects at several levels on lipolysis. These include expression of β-adrenergic receptors, adenyl cyclase activity, and protein kinase A and/or hormone sensitive lipase activity, while the G-proteins do not seem to be involved. Most of these effects appear to be expressed at the level

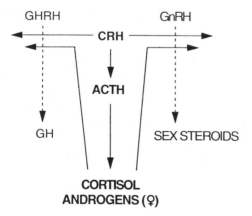

Figure 1 Overview of endocrine abnormalities in the metabolic syndrome: Elevated sensitivity of the hypothalamopituitary-adrenal axis is followed by elevated secretion of corticotropin-releasing hormone (CRH), adrenocorticotropin (ACTH), cortisol, and, in women, adrenal androgens. Secondarily growth hormone-releasing hormone (GHRH) and gonadotropin-releasing hormone (GnRH) are inhibited, followed by low growth hormone (GH) and sex steroid hormone secretions.

of gene transcription (97–100). The effects of T are probably mediated via a specific androgen receptor, which seems to be positively autoregulated by its ligand (100,101).

Both T and GH are lower than normal in men with the MS. Clearly then, when the hormones are deficient, the lipid-mobilizing effects as well as the antagonizing effects on triglyceride assimilation exerted by these hormones will be diminished. The net effect will then be to promote lipid accumulation.

To conform with the findings described above, the elevated T levels in women with the MS would be expected to diminish fat stores. Studies suggest, however, that T exerts different effects on male and female adipose tissue. In oophorectomized rats, estrogen restores full lipolytic potential, while T does not (102).

A specific androgen receptor is present in both male and female adipose tissue and shows the same affinity to androgen ligands. Estrogens negatively influence the expression of the androgen receptor (M. Li and P. Björntorp, unpublished), perhaps protecting from androgen effects. Taken together, it seems then that in females lipolysis needs estrogens for full effects, while androgens exert incomplete stimulation. Furthermore, estrogens seem to protect from the effects of T by down-regulating the androgen receptor density. This might be interpreted to mean that, in females, T does not exert its full lipolytic effect, particularly in the presence of estrogens, which may actually diminish androgen-receptor-mediated T effects. Low GH concentration would also decrease lipolytic effects, even in the presence of T.

This interpretation of androgen effects in adipose tissue from females is, however, an attempt to integrate the currently available information, which is clearly incomplete and rests mainly on results of studies in rats. The data suggest, however, that androgen effects on female adipose tissue are not necessarily those seen in male adipose tissue. The hyperandrogenicity of women with MS might not be sufficient to prevent lipid accumulation in the presence of the powerful effects of cortisol and insulin, which promote lipid accumulation. Recent studies in transsexual women treated with androgens provide indirect evidence for this contention (103). Visceral fat accumulation occurs in such women, but apparently only after oophorectomy, suggesting that the ovaries might protect from central accumulation of body fat. Clearly, however, this important problem requires further studies in human adipose tissue.

The mechanisms for the effects of estrogens and progestogens on human adipose tissue are enigmatic. Direct effects of these hormones cannot be demonstrated in vitro in a sensitive tissue culture system where other steroid hormones, such as cortisol and T, display marked effects (M. Ottosson, unpublished observations). This may be due to the apparent lack of specific receptors for these hormones in human adipose tissue. Neither ligand-binding techniques nor immunoassays of receptor protein show any receptors (104). Furthermore, significant amounts of mRNA cannot be demonstrated by the solution hybridization technique or PCR (105). Nevertheless, the female sex steroid hormones most likely exert effects on human adipose tissue, because both body fat distribution and metabolism change with menopause and can be restored upon hormonal substitution therapy (106). In the absence of direct effects and specific receptors, one can only speculate on the mechanism(s) of action. Maybe these hormones modify the signals induced by other steroid hormone receptors. Progestogens compete for the glucocorticoid receptor at physiological concentrations (107,108) and estrogen probably down-regulates the androgen receptor density, as noted above. Furthermore, it is also possible that female sex steroid hormones may modify the effects of peptide hormones such as GH and insulin, either by direct actions in adipose tissue or by changing the secretion of these hormones (109). This is an important area for further research.

Taken together (see Fig. 2), cortisol and insulin, which are present in excess in the MS, exert powerful effects leading to accumulation of triglyceride both by expressing LPL and by inhibiting lipid mobilization in the adipocyte. In men T and GH, which are deficient, have opposite effects, inhibiting triglyceride accumulation and efficiently promoting lipid mobilization. It is thus apparent that the endocrine perturbations in the MS would be expected to promote lipid accumulation.

The typical specific localization of these effect to visceral depots may be a consequence of several circumstances. First, this depot normally has a higher cellular display per unit mass because of smaller fat cells (110), and therefore more active cytoplasmic mass with hormonal receptors and enzymes involved in adipocyte metabolism. Furthermore, there is abundant blood flow (111) and a denser innervation (112) than in other adipose tissues. These characteristics by themselves would be expected to be associated with more pronounced changes of metabolism after endocrine abnormalities, because this will be a highly reactive adipose tissue region. Furthermore, there is direct evidence for a higher density of the GR in each adipocyte in this depot, measured with ligand-binding technique (107), steady-state mRNA levels (104), and as protein mass (113). Evidence from studies in the male rat shows a higher density of the androgen receptor in intra-abdominal than in subcutaneous adipocytes

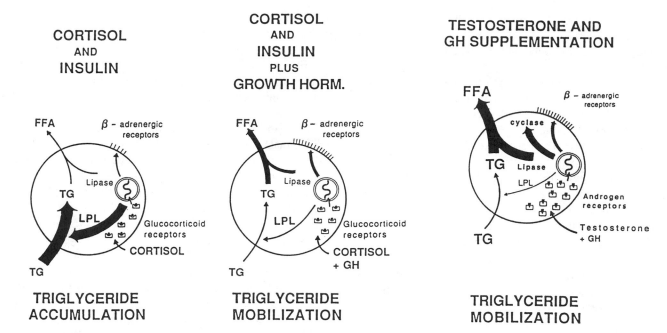

CORTISOL
AND
INSULIN

CORTISOL
AND
INSULIN
PLUS
GROWTH HORM.

TESTOSTERONE AND
GH SUPPLEMENTATION

TRIGLYCERIDE
ACCUMULATION

TRIGLYCERIDE
MOBILIZATION

TRIGLYCERIDE
MOBILIZATION

Figure 2 Schematic overview of the effects on adipose tissue metabolism of hormonal abnormalities involved in the metabolic syndrome. Cortisol, via glucocorticoid receptors, and insulin (left) lead to expression of lipoprotein lipase (LPL). Growth hormone (GH) inhibits LPL and stimulates lipolysis (middle), amplified by testosterone (right), which also increases the density of the androgen receptor. TG, triglycerides; FFA, free fatty acids. For other details, see text.

(101). Indirect evidence in humans also suggests a higher density of the androgen receptor because visceral adipose tissue from young men with higher T values shows more pronounced T-specific effects than visceral adipose tissue from elderly men with lower T secretion (114). All these characteristics of the visceral fat depot would, in concert, make this adipose tissue more sensitive to hormonal responses. Consequently, with combined hormonal perturbations, promoting lipid accumulation, such as in the MS, this would be expected to be most pronounced in visceral fat depots. This is summarized schematically in Figure 3.

These data are mainly deductions from studies using cell culture, where factors in the integrated tissue such as blood flow and innervation are eliminated. Studies on intact subjects can, however, be performed in vivo by administration orally of small amounts of labeled oleic acid mixed with triglycerides (115). The resulting labeled triglycerides are distributed among different adipose tissues and can be measured over time using needle biopsies. Since the label cannot be transformed into carbohydrate, and the label of other lipids in circulation and in adipose tissue presumably is much lower than that in triglycerides, it is possible to compare the uptake of triglyceride in different adipose tissues with time. Early biopsies measure the immediate uptake after lipid ingestion (up to about 4

hr). In later biopsies the uptake after recirculation from other tissues, apparently mainly in muscles, can be estimated (116,117). This occurs for several days and the lipid is thereafter secondarily distributed among adipose tissues as in the first phase. Upon monthly biopsies for several months, the turnover of this lipid can then be measured (116).

Studies in men have shown the following order for uptake of labeled triglyceride: subcutaneous femoral < sub-

VISCERAL   SUBCUTANEOUS

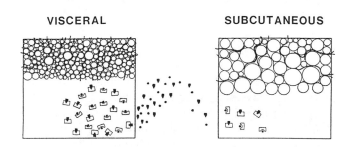

Figure 3 Differences between visceral and subcutaneous adipose tissue. Visceral adipose tissue is characterized by smaller fat cells, more blood flow, and higher density of nerves, as well as glucocorticoid and androgen receptors. Filled circles, cortisol. Arrowheads, testosterone.

cutaneous abdominal < omental = retroperitoneal adipose tissue. The half-life of the label is approximately 8, 6, and 4 months, respectively. The intra-abdominal values have been deduced from comparisons of the uptake figures, assuming similar differences in turnover in a steady state of intra-abdominal fat masses during the observation time. This is a reasonable assumption with a constant body weight in the men examined. These results suggest a high turnover of intra-abdominal adopise tissue (118, 119).

Although this conclusion of a high turnover of visceral fat seems reasonably sound, we have performed additional studies directly on this problem. Since repeated biopsies of visceral fat are not possible in humans, these studies were performed in male rats. Mesenteric adipose tissue showed twice the uptake and turnover in comparison with other adipose tissue regions, which is in good agreement with the observations and assumptions from the human data (120,121).

When slightly hypogonadal men are substituted with T, the in vivo effects of T on fat distribution may be examined. These studies show that uptake or turnover of triglycerides is apparently not affected in femoral adipose tissue. However, in subcutaneous abdominal adipose tissue uptake is inhibited and turnover increased. The most dramatic effect was, however, seen in intra-abdominal fat depots where uptake was only 50% of that in controls, and turnover presumably increased in parallel, using the same deductions used above (118,119). Similar studies in male rats are in agreement, showing that the effects of T are more pronounced on both lipid uptake and turnover in mesenteric adipose tissue (121).

This method has also been utilized in premenopausal women, with glucose as the tracer. The results show a lower uptake and slower turnover in femoral than in abdominal adipose tissues. The half-lives were 18 versus 12 months, respectively (122). Consequently, the sluggishness of metabolism of femoral adipose tissue is found in both men and women. Whether the much longer turnover times in women than men are a gender characteristic cannot be safely concluded, however, because the glucose label in the study of women is mainly incorporated into the glycerol moiety of the triglyceride and may recirculate differently than the oleic acid tracer used in the studies in men.

Results obtained with this method are particularly valuable because they provide integrated information on the regional metabolism of adipose tissue in humans. We have not yet been able to test other hormones with this method. The effects of the female sex steroid hormones might be better understood by such studies, because the mechanisms of action of these hormones are currently un-

clear. The results obtained so far are, however, in excellent agreement with the results from studies using tissue culture, described in the previous section. These detailed cellular studies provide the mechanistic details.

Studies using tissue culture conditions and those done in vivo are also in excellent agreement with physiological, clinical, and intervention data. If we examine the proportion of visceral adipose tissue mass in relation to total body fat mass, it is evident that when the balance between lipid accumulation stimulated by cortisol and insulin is in relative excess compared with the lipid-mobilizing hormones, T in men and GH, visceral fat accumulation is seen (see Fig. 4). Cushing's syndrome, with high cortisol and insulin and low T and GH, is an example. When Cushing's syndrome is successfully treated, body fat distribution is normalized (123). With aging, where cortisol and insulin are normal, but GH is low (124), in men, T is low (125),

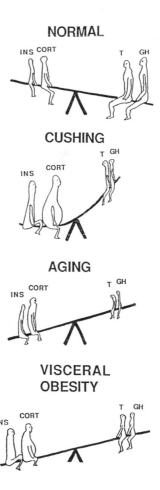

Figure 4 Balance between hormones accumulating (INS, insulin; CORT, cortisol) and mobilizing (T, testosterone; GH, growth hormone) storage fat in/from visceral adipose tissue in different physiological and clinical conditions.

and in women after menopause, estrogen is low, and there is a tendency to visceral fat accumulation (126). Isolated GH deficiency in adults shows a similar picture, which is reversible with GH substitution (64). Finally, when men with the MS, where T is low and there is visceral fat accumulation, are treated with T, visceral fat is diminished (63), and we have recently noticed a marked, specific decrease of visceral fat mass after GH treatment of men with MS (unpublished observations).

Although the mechanism of the effects of progesterone and estrogen is not known, it seems likely that the descriptive effects of estrogens in women are very similar to those of T in men. With menopause, visceral fat accumulates, which can be prevented by replacement therapy with estrogens (127).

In summary, then, the results of molecular, physiological, clinical, and intervention studies are in excellent agreement with the interpretation that the balance between lipid-accumulating and lipid-mobilizing hormones regulates the net mass of visceral fat, which is a particularly flexible tissue with a high turnover rate for triglyceride. The lipid-accumulating hormones are thus cortisol and insulin, antagonized by sex steroids and GH, which also exert permissive effects on lipid mobilization. The elevated cortisol and insulin in the MS would then be expected to be followed by visceral fat accumulation, which would be further exaggerated in men who have low concentrations of T and GH, which prevent visceral fat accumulation. Although information on some remaining details is currently not available, particularly the problem of androgen effects in women, it seems that the body of available information now allows us to conclude that the endocrine abnormalities in the MS are to a large extent responsible for the accumulation of visceral fat typical of that syndrome. This is summarized in Figure 5. In addition, genetic factors are involved, which are reviewed separately in another chapter.

It should also be mentioned that the density of the insulin receptor seems to be lower in adipocytes from visceral fat in comparison with other depots (128). By itself this would be expected to provide diminished insulin effects in this region. This may, however, be compensated for by the marked increase of insulin concentrations found in the MS with its systemic insulin resistance and elevated insulin secretion.

Another potentially interesting feature of visceral body fat in humans is the recently reported presence of the lipolytic β_3-adrenergic receptor (129). This might provide a mechanism for the high lipolytic sensitivity and responsiveness of this adipose tissue (130,131), but is in apparent contradiction with the specific accumulation of body fat in visceral adipose tissue in the MS, unless there is a

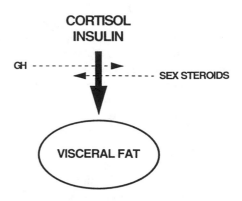

Figure 5 Elevated secretion of cortisol and insulin in combination with low growth hormone (GH) and sex steroid hormones leads to visceral fat accumulation.

low density of the β-adrenergic receptor in the MS. Furthermore, it is not clear whether the steroid hormone abnormalities in the MS may in fact regulate β-adrenergic-receptor density. This area is reviewed in detail in another chapter.

B. Insulin Resistance

The hormones that show abnormal concentrations in the MS also exert profound effects on the regulation of systemic insulin sensitivity. The ability of cortisol to induce insulin resistance is well established. Sex steroid hormones also regulate insulin sensitivity. T seems to optimize the sensitivity of muscles to insulin in men in a rather narrow range of concentrations around those seen in normal, young men (about 15–40 nmol/L). This assumption is based on the following rather consistent evidence. Below the normal range of T concentrations, insulin resistance is found in case-control studies (58) and in epidemiological studies (59,60,86,87). Furthermore, men with NIDDM have low T values, and the degree of insulin resistance appears to be inversely parallel to the T concentrations (132,133). In addition, low T values predict the development of NIDDM in men (87). When men with low T and the MS are given T to approach the normal concentration range, insulin sensitivity is markedly improved, as well as the plasma lipid profile and blood pressure (62, 63). Finally, men taking large doses of anabolic androgens, placing them above the critical concentration limit, become severely insulin resistant (134,135).

There is thus convincing evidence that T concentrations are associated with insulin sensitivity in men. The mechanisms have been studied in a rat model where castration is followed by insulin resistance. Substitution to normal T values restored normal insulin sensitivity, and administration of large doses again induces insulin resistance (136). In both situations of insulin resistance the insulin-sensitive part of the glycogen synthase in muscle is inhibited, and in the hypergonadal state apparently also glucose transport, suggesting the possibility of different mechanisms of action at high and low T concentrations.

In women, too, high concentrations of T are also parallel to insulin resistance in both case-control (18) and epidemiological studies (137,138). Furthermore, hyperandrogenicity is a powerful predictor of NIDDM (137, 138), as well as of development of CVD and hypertension in women (139,140). In addition, women with established NIDDM have high concentration of T in serum, parallel to their insulin resistance (133). Finally, when transsexual women are given T, they become insulin resistant (141).

There are also studies that suggest that hyperinsulinemia, a consequence of insulin resistance, acts as a gonadotropin, stimulating androgen secretion (reviewed in Refs. 142 and 143). Much of this evidence is derived from in vitro experiments. Long-term exposure to hyperinsulinemia did not elevate androgen concentrations in normal women (144). Furthermore, chronic, isolated, insulin exposure in rats is followed by increased rather than decreased insulin sensitivity (145,146). Taken together, it seems that there is now a fairly extensive background of information indicating that hyperandrogenicity in women is followed by insulin resistance.

This is strongly supported by studies in female rats, which become severely insulin resistant upon exposure of moderate doses of T (147,148), and where the detailed mechanisms have been studied. This effect is already present by 48 hr and occurs only at submaximal insulin values during clamp studies, but is normalized at maximal concentrations of insulin (148). Neither FFA, glycerol, nor estrogen levels in plasma are elevated, suggesting that the effect is indeed that of T. At the cellular level in muscle both insulin regulation of glucose transport and glycogen synthase are inhibited. The glucose transporter Glut 4 protein content is decreased, and plasma membrane translocation by insulin is absent. Furthermore, glycogen synthase protein is diminished, but insulin receptor density and tyrosine kinase activity are unaltered (149). There are thus several mechanisms involved at the level of the muscle cell. It is, however, probable that some of these abnormalities are due to the absence of estrogen effects, which seem to have similar consequences (see below) (149). Estrogen and androgens may interact in muscle, by estrogen down-regulating the androgen receptor, as has been observed in adipose tissue (M. Li and P. Björntorp, unpublished). Furthermore, as will be discussed in a later section, hyperandrogenicity in this rat model is followed

by severe restriction of insulin delivery through the capillaries.

It might appear confusing that both too high and too low levels of androgens are followed by insulin resistance, leaving a "window" of normal T values where muscular insulin resistance is optimal. This picture seems consistent in both men and women, with the range of the male window being about between 15 to 40 nmol/L, and the female window having an upper limit of about 3–5 nmol/L of T, and no lower limit. It seems possible that the mechanisms might be different for the induction of insulin resistance above and below the window, being more pronounced for glucose transport above the window, while glycogen synthase is inhibited below it (135,136,147, 148). If this is the case, the window phenomenon would be easier to understand, but conclusive evidence is not currently available.

Oophorectomy in rats is followed by insulin resistance (147,150), and substitution with 17-β estradiol restores this abnormality to normal, while progesterone seems to exert the opposite effect (150). The mechanism for the effect of 17-β estradiol on insulin resistance is probably localized mainly to insulin-stimulated glucose transport (150), affecting both Glut 4 protein mass and translocation mechanisms (149). It seems that this might be the major effect of 17-β estradiol, while the effects of T are an additional perturbation of glycogen synthase function and protein mass. This is supported by the observation that there is a close correlation between whole-body insulin sensitivity, on the one hand, and glycogen synthesis and glycogen synthase protein mass in the muscle on the other (147–149).

Insulin itself seems to regulate insulin sensitivity. Upon exposure to insulin, insulin resistance usually develops (151). Furthermore, blood pressure elevation is considered to be a common correlate (for review, see Ref. 152). This might, however, not necessarily be the effect of insulin itself, because induction of hyperinsulinemia is followed by increased secretion of counterregulatory hormones, as well as elevated activity of the sympathetic nervous system to protect from hypoglycemia. When these counterregulatory events are controlled, and hypoglycemia is prevented by glucose administration, exposure to insulin at physiological blood concentrations has quite different effects. Insulin resistance does not occur, rather increased insulin sensitivity is found. The underlying mechanisms seem to depend on the time of exposure and include effects on both glucose transport and glycogen synthase (145,146). Under these conditions blood pressure elevation is not induced either (153). It therefore seems reasonable to suggest that insulin resistance and hypertension, induced by increased exposure to insulin in the intact organism, are due to the counterregulatory systems, notably for the latter the sympathetic nervous system, as suggested previously (152), and/or increased hormonal secretions from the adrenals. The elevated activity of the HPA axis in the MS, including the adrenals, as well as the suggestive evidence of increased central sympathetic nervous system activity (see above), might therefore be important not only for the induction of insulin resistance, but also for the development of hypertension, which often follows the MS.

GH is conventionally considered to cause insulin resistance. This has, however, mainly been tested with large doses of GH (154). Totally GH-deficient patients are insulin resistant (64). Upon administration of GH to GH-deficient humans, insulin sensitivity is first further decreased, but then returns back to pretreatment conditions (64). The importance of the sex-specific diurnal GH-secretion rhythm (109), as well as potential effects of binding proteins, does not seem to have been taken into account in studies of GH effects. In a recent study we have observed that when GH is administered physiologically in small doses to men with MS and a relative GH deficiency, insulin resistance is indeed improved (unpublished observations).

There is considerable evidence that not only cortisol but also abnormally low GH and T concentration in men and hyperandrogenicity in women, which characterize the MS, are followed by insulin resistance. The role of estrogens, if any, is not known because whether estrogen secretion is abnormal in the MS has not been studied conclusively (see above).

FFA also probably play a major role. The endocrine perturbations of the MS most likely lead to a centralization of body fat in visceral depots. These depots are highly sensitive to lipolytic stimuli and will therefore produce large amounts of FFA, which are powerful inducers of insulin resistance (29). This will most likely affect the liver, which is directly exposed, but these fat depots may also contribute significantly to the elevated FFA concentrations in the systemic circulation (for review, see above). Furthermore, portal FFA may induce not only insulin resistance of the liver, but also overproduction of very-low-density lipoproteins, gluconeogenesis, and cause "leakage" of insulin by the liver by inhibiting hepatic clearance of insulin, as suggested previously (28). These mechanisms may therefore add not only to the hyperinsulinemia, but also to the generation of the other metabolic perturbations of the MS.

It may also be considered that the endocrine perturbations may result in elevated circulating FFA due to direct stimulatory effects on lipolysis regulation and/or inhibition of reesterification of FFA in adipose tissue.

Cortisol is lipolytic in the presence of GH and so is T (see above). In the rat the major role of cortisol on insulin resistance has been demonstrated to be via FFA (155), although other, direct effects have been demonstrated (156). Furthermore, cortisol may well inhibit fatty acid reesterification and thereby contribute to elevated FFA outflux from adipose tissue. Similarly, T in hyperandrogenic women would be expected to contribute to a "permissive" effect on lipolysis, although other direct effects on insulin resistance in muscle have been clearly shown (see above). This field has recently been reviewed (157).

In summary, the endocrine perturbations of the MS may be considered to induce insulin resistance by two principal mechanisms, one directly and another indirectly by inducing FFA mobilization. Together this would provide powerful effects to create insulin resistance. This is summarized in Figure 6.

C. Capillary Turnover

The hormones involved in the MS apparently also exert changes in the turnover of capillary endothelial cells and capillarization. This may be of additional significance for the insulin action on effector cells by regulation of insulin availability. Previous (158) and recent (159,160) studies have shown that insulin probably binds to capillary endothelial cells before it is delivered into the interstitial space where it interacts with the insulin receptor on the muscle cell. This delivery may be rate limiting under certain conditions. Combining the clamp methodology with microdialysis technique, Holmäng et al. (161), in our laboratory, have recently been able to show that insulin concentration in the interstitial space is equal to that in the circulation below about 250 μU/ml, and only about 25% at higher circulating insulin concentrations. This suggests

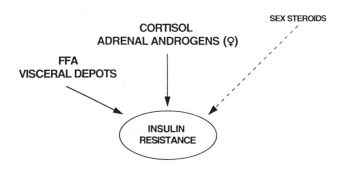

Figure 6 Elevated secretion of adrenal hormones (cortisol and, in women, androgens) in combination with low sex steroids and elevated free fatty acids (FFA) from lipolytically sensitive visceral depots induces insulin resistance.

a saturable transcapillary transport of insulin, with a rate-limiting barrier above about 250 μU/ml.

This is apparently hormonally regulated. Administration of T to female rats shifts the half-maximal transcapillary transport barrier of insulin to the left; in other words, there seems to be a capillary barrier for insulin even at lower plasma concentrations (A. Holmäng and P. Lönnroth, unpublished). This most likely contributes to the marked apparent insulin inefficiency found with hyperandrogenicity in females (147,148) and may depend on a low capillary density and/or diminished utilization of available capillaries (160). The obese Zucker rat seems to lack the barrier (161), but this is apparently not due to the prevailing hyperinsulinemia, because chronic insulin exposure does not seem to have similar effects (145, 146).

Direct measurements of hormonal influences on capillary turnover have been performed recently. Exposure of insulin alone is followed by a dramatic increase (10–20 times) of mitoses in capillary endothelial cells, which is maximal after 2–3 days and then returns to near control values, resulting in a moderate (10–20%) net increase of capillary density measured histochemically. Cortisol exposure in the presence of insulin not only abolishes this insulin effect, but also decreases the number of mitoses below that of controls, with a resulting diminution of capillarization (162). It seems possible that T may exert similar effects (147).

Taken together, these observations have opened up a novel field of regulation of insulin sensitivity in addition to the dilatation of capillaries by insulin, which has been reported to be deficient with insulin resistance (163). Capillaries seem to regulate insulin delivery in a rather complex way, including both availability of binding surface due not only to dilatation (163), but also to turnover of capillaries, as well as changes of the capacity of the transcapillary insulin barrier (160–162).

Since the hormones found to be abnormal in the MS are involved, these capillary regulations are of interest for this syndrome. Decreased capillarization has indeed been found in the MS (164,165). It may be considered that this is another consequence of the endocrine perturbations. For example, cortisol and T excess seems to lead to rarefaction of capillaries even in the presence of hyperinsulinemia (147,148,162). It may also be speculated that these abnormalities include other functional defects than those found in transcapillary insulin transport (160,162 and A. Holmäng and P. Lönnroth, unpublished). Immature, not fully functioning capillary endothelium may also allow protein leakage. Microalbuminuria might be a consequence thereof and has recently been observed in the MS without hypertension and found to be parallel to the prevailing insulin resistance (166). This leads to the intriguing possibility that the microangiopathy of NIDDM, which is often already apparent at the clinical debut of NIDDM, is indeed a consequence of the preceding endocrine perturbations with insulin resistance characteristic of the MS as a prediabetic condition. This area is therefore of considerable interest for further exploration.

D. Myosins

The myosin composition of skeletal muscle is changed in the MS, with a higher-than-normal proportion of white, glycolytic type II fibers at the expense of red, oxidative type I fibers (164,165). Interestingly, a similar change of myosin content can apparently be brought about with elevated levels of cortisol (167) or T (147). Insulin alone seems to exert similar effects (145). It therefore seems possible that insulin regulates the synthesis of type II myosin. It is thus conceivable that the endocrine abnormalities of the MS are also responsible for the abnormal skeletal muscle fiber (myosin) composition, with an abundance of type II fibers (164,165). With this background we speculated that myocardial myosin composition might also be affected. Using the rat model with isolated, chronic hyperinsulinemia (145,146), a marked increase of myocardial mass, with hypertrophied myosin fibers was found. This was associated with decreased cardiac output and elevated peripheral circulatory resistance (153).

These results suggest that hyperinsulinemia, following insulin resistance, may also have central circulatory consequences, where myocardial hypertrophy and poor pump capacity of the heart may be central features. These observations are clearly of interest for the MS, a severely hyperinsulinemic condition. Recent studies have indicated that left ventricular hypertrophy may be found in the MS, correlating with insulin resistance, but being independent of hypertension (168,169). Left ventricular hypertrophy is a malignant condition associated with myocardial malfunction and increased mortality (170). There is thus an intriguing possibility that the MS is associated with malfunction of central hemodynamics, other than those associated with hypertension and ischemic heart disease. This might be due to changes in myocardial myosin synthesis, brought about by the multiple endocrine abnormalities in the MS, including the hyperinsulinemia following insulin resistance.

E. Dementia

Another recent development in this area is more speculative but nevertheless highly interesting (171). The MS has several features of premature aging. The decrease of sex steroid and GH secretion seen in the MS occurs with normal aging (124,125). There is also some evidence for a sensitization of the HPA axis with aging (172), a finding consistent with results of studies in the MS (see above). The metabolic disturbances or the MS are more prevalent in older subjects, and NIDDM, CVD and stroke, predicted by the MS, are more frequent in elderly than in younger persons. Some of the non-Alzheimer dementias, particularly multi-infarction and the noninfarction dementias, are clearly also diseases of aging. The latter is characterized by white matter atrophy of the brain and leakage of albumin into the cerebrospinal fluid, which probably are a consequence of microcirculatory disturbances in the brain (173). The HPA axis of such patients has been found to be hypersensitive as tested with the dexamethasone inhibition test (174). NIDDM, hypertriglyceridemia, and hypertension are prevalent (C.A. Gottfries, personal communication). There are thus several endocrine and metabolic features that occur in common in both noninfarction dementia and the MS, and both show evidence of capillary malfunction (see above). It might be considered that this type of dementia may be another, late manifestation of the tissue-damaging effect of the MS, mediated via capillary malfunction. Preliminary studies suggest that in the Gothenburg study of men born in 1913, the symptoms of the MS precede the development of decreased cognitive function (G. Tibblin, personal communication). This area clearly needs further development.

X. SUMMARY OF THE CONSEQUENCES OF THE ENDOCRINE PERTURBATIONS

As reviewed above, there is considerable evidence ranging from clinical and intervention observations to cellular-molecular studies, suggesting that the combined endocrine perturbation of the MS may actually cause redistribution of body fat to visceral depots. Similarly, there is considerable evidence that insulin resistance may be another consequence. In other words, both of the cardinal symptoms of the MS, insulin resistance and visceral fat accumulation, may indeed be caused by the endocrine abnormalities. In addition, the hyperinsulinemia and insulin resistance, in combination with the perturbation of the counterregulatory hormones, may well also induce hypertension, perhaps via activation of the sympathetic nervous system. Capillary abnormalities, seen in the MS, seem to be inducible by hormonal changes similar to those seen in the MS. This might mean that the microangiopathy of NIDDM originates already during the endocrine and metabolic perturbations of the MS, which pre-

cede NIDDM. Furthermore, there is a possibility that the endocrine abnormalities of the MS might include myocardial hypertrophy with perturbations of central hemodynamic regulation, amplified by activation of the sympathetic nervous system and hypertension. More speculatively, the MS may also be a precursor state to certain forms of dementia (see Fig. 7). Clearly, then, the apparently basic endocrine abnormalities are of considerable interest as potential inducers of a multitude of symptoms and diseases.

XI. THE HYPOTHALAMO-PITUITARY-ADRENAL AXIS

The endocrine abnormalities of the MS consist of a relative hypercortisolemia, hyperandrogenicity in women, low T in men, and low GH secretion. There is also evidence for perturbations along the central sympathetic nervous axis. As reviewed above (see Fig. 1), there is considerable evidence that the hypersensitive HPA axis of the MS may in fact be the primary lesion of the syndrome, because the other endocrine abnormalities may follow as consequences thereof. In concert, the combined endocrine abnormalities then seem to be responsible for visceral fat accumulation and most of the metabolic and circulatory perturbations, as reviewed in preceding sections. Therefore, it is of obvious interest to examine potential background factors to the hypersensitivity of the HPA axis in the MS, because a majority of the multiple abnormalities of the MS seem possible to derive from this perturbation.

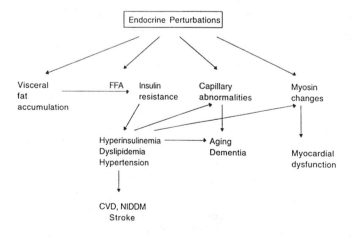

Figure 7 Putative consequences of the endocrine abnormalities in the metabolic syndrome (elevated cortisol, and, in women, androgens, low growth, and sex-specific steroid hormones). FFA, free fatty acids; CVD, cardiovascular disease; NIDDM, non-insulin-dependent diabetes mellitus.

As mentioned above, the HPA axis of the MS shows a hyperactivity after simulations at all levels from central mental or physical stress tests, after CRH and arginine vasopressin stimulation of the CRH receptors in the pituitary and ACTH challenge of the adrenals. There is now also evidence of a deficient feedback inhibition of the HPA axis. (See Fig. 8 for overview.)

What are the conditions that result in this picture? First, various repeated or chronic environmental stressors are followed by an identical condition. This is well known from animal experimentation, and this type of stress response has been characterized as a helplessness, depressive, or defeat reaction (175,176) and is also followed by decreased secretion of sex steroids and GH. The initiating factors may be, for example, toxins, electric shocks, or milder challenges such as changes in social hierarchy (83, 85,175–179). In humans such reactions also occur although the stress reaction after laboratory stress tests is often of a mixed type (77,82,177,180). Elderly athletes, subjecting themselves to frequent stress in the form of exhausting long-distance running, seem to develop a similar chronic stress syndrome with elevated HPA axis activity (181). Other activators of the HPA axis in humans are alcohol abuse, seen in extreme cases as a pseudo-Cushing syndrome (57,182). Furthermore, tobacco smoking, another toxin affecting the central nervous system, shows similar effects (183). Several psychiatric diseases are also associated with hyperactivity of the HPA axis, notably depression (183–185), but also panic and anxiety syndromes (186).

Several of these potential background factors to a hypersensitive HPA axis have been found in the MS. First, in population studies subjects with the MS, defined as an elevated WHR, associated with elevated insulin, report a feeling of perceived stress and poor well-being in general. They are frequently sick and absent from work often with a psychosomatic type of disease such as peptic ulcer. A significantly higher proportion of the men are out of work, either unemployed or because of early retirement. When employed they report problems with adaptation at work and with work management. In men there is a strong relationship to being divorced and living alone, and they have less hobbies during their leisure time, including physical activities. These relationships are independent of BMI, alcohol intake, and smoking (187,188).

There are also socioeconomic observations of interest. The type of work is often physical labor, presumably with relatively low income, and the men have poor housing conditions and belong to a low social class (187,188). In a previous study of the men born in 1913 we found a negative relationship with education (187), which was not found in a recent study of a similar cohort of men born

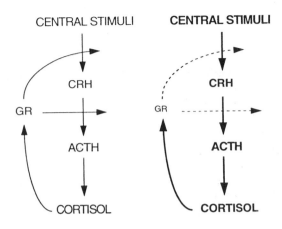

Figure 8 Regulation of corticotropin-releasing hormone (CRH), adrenocorticotropic hormone (ACTH), and cortisol secretion by central stimuli and feedback inhibition by glucocorticoid receptors (GR) in the pituitary and the brain. Left, normal; right, hyperactivity.

in 1944 (188). This might be due to marked changes with social equalization of the education system between these years. Men (187) and women (189) show in essence the same results, except in the employment variables. The women also have more infections.

This problem has recently been studied also by other laboratories. Associations between the WHR with metabolic abnormalities and lower levels of perceived social support has been reported (190). In young black and white adults relationships between the WHR and psychosocial handicaps have been found (191). In Mexican-American men associations between central body fat distribution and job stress have been reported. This relationship is disappearing after adjustment for education, a proxy for social class (192). In Japanese-Americans visceral fat mass was inversely related to educational level, disappearing after statistical adjustment for insulin (193).

These results taken together have been interpreted to mean that these are subjects who show several signs of stress with a depressive type of reaction (reports of perceived stress, absenteeism, psychosomatic disease, infections). The endocrine abnormalities are also typical for such a stress reaction (175,176). Their psychosocial and socioeconomic background, for example with unemployment, poorly paid work, problems at work, and living alone, may well provide a basis for such a reaction.

Various stressors in the environment are perceived differently depending on the personal coping capability (194). The individual personality characteristics are therefore an important component. Such studies have not yet been performed in men, but women show an interesting profile with high ranking in variables suggesting a personality type that might fit with that of women in independent work position (189). We have never found such a professional association (189), but these were women of a generation when the possibility of choosing a profession was comparatively limited. A more recent study has shown that women with a similar personality profile and independent professions often are hyperandrogenic (195), in apparent agreement with our findings (137). The use of strong liquor and smoking tobacco (189) might be consistent with such a personality type. This is a field that urgently needs further exploration.

Previous studies in women (189) and a recent study in men (196) have provided consistent evidence for involvement of psychiatric symptoms. Psychiatric disease in general is more frequent, and there are signs of anxiety and depressive traits as well as frequent sleep problems. It seems likely that the psychological and socioeconomic handicaps reported might provide a background for the development of such symptoms. These observations are of particular interest because of the known relationships to increased activity of the HPA axis, due to a diminished feedback inhibition in conditions with depression and anxiety (184–187).

Smoking tobacco has consistently been reported to be associated with an elevated WHR (189,197–201), also after adjustment for age and obesity (201), including prospective studies (202). Recent studies have also shown that smoking tobacco induces insulin resistance (203, 204). This is the expected outcome because of the known endocrine response to smoking, including cortisol secretion (183).

Alcohol consumption is not that consistently reported to be associated with an elevated WHR, but has been found in both men and women, in some case-control or population studies (189,205–207), but not in all (208, 209). It seems possible that a certain minimal amount of alcohol is needed to express the syndrome. For example, in women the association is most pronounced with intake of strong alcohol beverages (189), and socially integrated alcoholics have a high WHR (210), depending on both increased visceral fat mass and atrophy of gluteofemoral muscles (57). Alcohol concentrations in blood above 1‰, corresponding to a couple of drinks, have been reported to be followed by an elevation of serum cortisol (56).

Cytokines, particularly interleukin-6, have recently been reported to be powerful stimulators of the HPA axis. These are usually produced by inflammatory processes, but tumor necrosis factor α is overproduced in adipose tissue in certain obese rat strains and produces pronounced insulin resistance (211). These are factors of in-

terest that have not yet been examined in relation to the HPA axis and insulin resistance in the MS.

In summary, there are a number of observations suggesting that a depressive type of a stress reaction may be an etiological factor in the MS. There are also observations indicating that several psychosocial and socioeconomic handicaps might provide background factors. Intervention studies are very helpful in determining cause-effect relationships. Such studies are for obvious reasons difficult to perform in human beings, but have been made in non-human primates. Changing social hierarchy among cynomolgus monkeys has been used as a stressor, an apparently mild form of intervention, reminiscent of the psychosocial and socioeconomic handicaps we have found in humans. These monkeys develop a hypersensitive HPA axis due to a decreased feedback control, with a decreased inhibitory effect of dexamethasone at low doses, enlarged adrenals, and menstrual irregularities. Androgens are produced in excess after adrenal challenge. These monkeys then develop a full-blown MS, including insulin resistance, elevated triglycerides, hypertension, decreased glucose tolerance, and coronary atherosclerosis, and they accumulate visceral fat (179,212,213, and C. Shively, personal communication, 1995). Chronic stress and exogenous glucocorticoids have also been reported to induce a selective mass increase of mesenteric adipose tissue in rats (214). These experiments provide strong support to our interpretation that psychosocial and socioeconomic stress is an etiological factor in humans with the MS.

The psychiatric associations with the MS may also be consequences of socioeconomic and psychosocial handicaps and are known to activate the HPA axis, as do smoking tobacco and alcohol excess. We then have a number of factors that are known to sensitize the HPA axis and that are found in the MS. One or more of these factors may be found in a person with the MS, and they may act in concert or individually. It also seems highly likely that the socioeconomic-psychosocial handicaps may induce psychiatric vulnerability and the use of stimulants such as alcohol and smoking. This is a hypothesis we have entertained and tested based on our own data from human studies (5,8,9,215–221), as summarized in Figure 9. A hypothesis involving cortisol as a major factor in the pathogenesis, based mainly on detailed work in animals on metabolic regulations (222,223), is in excellent agreement with our interpretations.

It should be noted, that this hypothesis is not in contradiction to the interpretation that the effects of FFA are the major etiological factor in insulin resistance and the MS, followed by NIDDM (224). Instead, our hypothesis provides an etiological background to the elevated FFA concentrations (see above). Another possibility for the etiology of visceral fat mass increase, insulin resistance, and the other components of the MS is genetic susceptibility. As will be summarized in the final part of this review, as well as in more detail in another chapter, there is currently no conclusive evidence of polymorphisms or deletions of appropriate genes with functional consequences explaining any of the components of the MS. Nevertheless, it is anticipated that genetic susceptibility at different levels will form a basis for disease development under the pressure of environmental factors.

A recent concept, developed by Barker, suggests that several diseases in adult life originate from the intrauterine environment (225). This is suggested to be the case for an elevated WHR, insulin resistance, and the development into NIDDM. Although this finding needs confirmation, it has some interesting bearing on the hypothesis provided above. There is evidence that the HPA axis can be "imprinted" to an increased sensitivity by factors presumably activating the axis in utero (226,227). Undernutrition during critical periods of fetal life, the main basis for the Barker phenomenon, might provide a milieu for such "imprinting" due to the stress of starvation. This then would be compatible with an increased sensitivity of the HPA axis described in the MS in the adult, and therefore in line with the hypothesis described here and previously. This is another area of important research in the efforts to disclose the origin of the MS.

In summary, the hypothesis we have formulated and tested does not seem to be in disagreement with other currently prevailing opinions of the potential etiology of the MS; instead it seems to include several additional factors providing an overriding possibility to understand the factors leading to the MS.

The potential possibility that a hypersensitivity of the HPA axis might provide the missing link between psychosocial-socioeconomic factors and somatic disease makes this field of research particularly exciting. The mechanism for this connection had long been sought. Studies in this field have been particularly difficult because the end-points examined have usually been the diseases, for example CVD. It is interesting that the psychosocial and socioeconomic factors we have described to be associated with the WHR (187–189,196) are those related to CVD (228,229). The long-presumed chain of events leading from psychosocial and socioeconomic factors to disease end-points is of course disturbed by numerous confounders. By examining the proximal, central part of this chain, the HPA axis, possibilities may improve to find noxious environmental factors. For this purpose simpler tests than those now available will have to be developed. We are

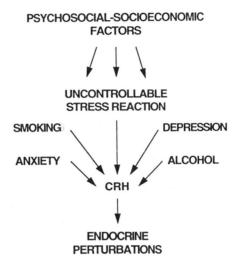

Figure 9 Factors that activate the hypothalamopituitary-adrenal axis via interactions with corticotropin-releasing hormone (CRH) and its releasing factors.

now employing simplified dexamethasone inhibition tests as well as diurnal measurements of cortisol at critical time points, applicable on an outpatient basis. With these methodological simplifications we hope to be able to examine sufficiently large groups to better characterize noxious psychosocial and socioeconomic environmental factors.

Since the MS is a precursor state to CVD and NIDDM (see above) it is of interest to examine the status of the HPA axis in these diseases. Obviously, single serum cortisols are not informative due to the large diurnal variations. Urinary output of cortisol is more reliable, but is also not a robust measurement, depending probably on the challenge of the HPA axis the day of measurement (77).

Some studies have been reported in diabetes. Abnormal dexamethasone inhibition tests were found in diabetic patients (both insulin-dependent and non-insulin-dependent) in relation to diabetic control (230). Diurnal cortisol curves have been reported in NIDDM with good metabolic control and found to be elevated (231), similarly for β-endorphin and ACTH (232). Furthermore, diminished inhibition by dexamethasone of cortisol and ACTH has been reported in diabetes, related to neuropathy (233). Although suggestive, these results do not definitely exclude an effect of glucose homeostasis or depressive traits on the HPA axis.

The effects of "stress" on diabetic control are well established (see, for example, Ref. 234). The potential pathogenic role seems, however, to have been studied mainly in animals (235,236).

These studies are suggestive for a role of an elevated activity of the HPA axis in NIDDM, but interpretations are hampered by confounding factors.

XII. THE CENTRAL NERVOUS SYSTEM

The HPA axis is regulated from several brain centers via serotonergic neurons (237–239). Interestingly, serotonin (5-hydroxytryptamine, 5-HT) receptors are also involved in the psychiatric diseases associated with the MS, as well as with alcohol and smoking (240). Carbohydrate craving, which seems to be an additional characteristic of the MS (241), is also mediated via 5-HT receptors. Consistent with this we have recently found low concentrations of 5-hydroxyindolacetic acid in the cerebrospinal fluid, closely coupled to CRH in women with central obesity and the MS (241). This is an area of interesting further research not least from the aspect of development of novel pharmaceutical treatment. Methods are available for exploring this further including neuropharmacological probing as well as imaging brain techniques where not only brain structures may be examined, but also metabolism and receptor binding of transmitters (242).

XIII. GENETIC ASPECTS

Obviously, genetic factors probably play major roles in the MS. One of the main expressions of the MS, visceral fat accumulation, is strongly determined genetically (243–246). Insulin resistance, the other main characteristic of the MS, has also clearly a genetic component. Large efforts have been made to discover genetic abnormalities in peripheral, insulin-responsive tissues, including studies on the insulin receptor and its signaling system, the glucose transporters, and rate-limiting glycolytic enzymes, so far without convincing results except in rare cases. The glycogen synthase system in muscle has attracted particular attention, but no genetic polymorphisms or deletions of functional importance have so far been found (247). It is anticipated that several genetic defects may occur in the MS, but no certain candidate genes have so far been disclosed. It seems likely that the phylogenetic expression of the MS must first be better defined before such candidate genes can be selected. Currently it seems that genes in the central nervous system might turn out to be particularly interesting. For example, the diurnal cortisol profile is similar in monozygotic twins (248). Genes at this level have not been studied earlier in relation to the MS. This chapter has reviewed the phylogenetic expression of the

MS on the basis of a genetic background. The genetic factors are reviewed in more detail in another chapter.

ACKNOWLEDGMENT

The secretarial assistance of Ms. Raija Saikkonen is gratefully appreciated.

REFERENCES

1. Kylin E. Studien über das Hypertonie-hyperglykämie-hyperurikämi-syndrome. Zentralbl Inn Med 1923; 44: 105–127.
2. Reaven GH. Role of insulin in human disease. Diabetes 1988; 37:1595–1607.
3. Enzi G, Crepaldi G. Subcutaneous and visceral obesity: two distinct clinical entities. Medicographic 1986; 8: 18–21.
4. Kaplan NM. The deadly quartet. Upper-body obesity, glucose intolerance, hypertriglyceridemia and hypertension. Arch Intern Med 1989; 149:1514–1520.
5. Björntorp P. Visceral obesity: a "civilization syndrome." Obes Res 1993; 1:206–222.
6. Kissebah AH, Evans DJ, Peiris A, Wilson CR. Endocrine characteristics in regional obesities: role of sex steroids. In: Vague J, Björntorp P, Guy-Grand B, Rebuffé-Scrive M, Vague P, eds. Metabolic Complications of Human Obesities. Amsterdam: Excerpta Medica, 1985:115–130.
7. Lapidus L, Bengtsson C, Björntorp P. The quantitative relationship between "the metabolic syndrome" and abdominal obesity in women. Obes Res 1994; 2:372–377.
8. Björntorp P. Abdominal obesity and the development of noninsulin dependent diabetes mellitus. Diabetes/Metab Rev 1988; 4:615–622.
9. Björntorp P. The associations between obesity, adipose tissue distribution and disease. Acta Med Scand 1987; 723: 121–134.
10. Sjöström L. Impacts of body weight, body composition and adipose tissue distribution on morbidity and mortality. In: Stunkard AJ, Wadden TA, eds. Obesity: Theory and Therapy, 2nd ed. New York: Raven Press, 1993.
11. Björntorp P, Bengtsson C, Blohmé G, Jonsson A, Sjöström L, Tibblin E, Tibblin G, Wilhelmsen L. Adipose tissue fat cell size and number in relation to metabolism in randomly selected middle-aged men and women. Metabolism 1971; 20:927–932.
12. Després J-P. Obesity and lipid metabolism: relevance of body fat distribution. Curr Opin Lipid 1991; 2:5–15.
13. Després J-P, Moorjani S, Lupien PJ, Tremblay A, Nadeau A, Bouchard C. Genetic aspects of susceptibility of obesity and related dyslipidemia. Mol Cell Biochem 1992; 113: 151–169.
14. Després J-P, Moorjani S, Lupien PJ, Tremblay A, Nadeau A, Bouchard C. Regional distribution of body fat, plasma lipoproteins, and cardiovascular disease. Arteriosclerosis 1990; 10:497–511.

15. Després J-P, Prud'homme D, Pouliot MC, Tremblay A, Bouchard C. Estimation of deep abdominal adipose tissue accumulation from simple anthropometric measurements in men. Am J Clin Nutr 1991; 54:471–477.

16. Hauner H, Ditschuneit HH, Pol SB, Pfeiffer EF. Fettgewebsverteilung und Adipositaskomplikationen bei Übergewichtigen Frauen mit und ohne Hirsutismus. Dtsch Med Wochenschr 1987; 112:709–713.

17. Kissebah AH. Health risks of obesity. Med Clin North Am 1989; 73:111.

18. Kissebah AH, Peiris AN. Biology of regional fat distribution: relationship to non-insulin-dependent diabetes mellitus. Diabetes Metab Rev 1989; R:83–109.

19. Drury PL. Diabetes and arterial hypertension. Diabetologia 1983; 24:1–9.

20. Fuller JH. Epidemiology of hypertension associated with diabetes mellitus. Hypertension 1985; 7(Suppl II):3–78.

21. Eriksson H, Welin L, Wilhelmsen L, Larsson B, Ohlsson LO, Svärdsudd K, Tibblin G. Metabolic disturbances in hypertension: results from the population study Men Born in 1913. J Intern Med 1992; 232:389–395.

22. Guillaume M, Lapidus L, Beckers F, Lambert A, Björntorp P. High prevalence of cardiovascular risk factors in children from the Belgian Luxembourg Province. The Belgian Luxembourg Child Study. Am J Epidemiol 1996; 144:867–880.

23. Reaven GM, Lerner RL, Stern MP, Farquhar JW. Role of insulin in endogenous hypertriglyceridemia. J Clin Invest 1967; 46:1756–1767.

24. Reaven GM, Hoffman BB. A role for insulin in the aetiology and course of hypertension? Lancet 1987; 2:435–436.

25. De Fronzo RA. The effect of insulin on renal sodium metabolism. A review of clinical implications. Diabetologia 1981; 21:165–171.

26. Ferrannini E, Buzzigoli G, Bonadonna R, Giorico MA, Oleggini M, Graziadei L. Insulin resistance in essential hypertension. N Engl J Med 1987; 317:350–357.

27. Izzo J, Swislocki A. Insulin resistance: Is it truly the link? (Workshop III). Am J Med 1991; 90:26S–31S.

28. Björntorp P. "Portal" adipose tissue as a generator of risk factors for cardiovascular disease and diabetes. Arteriosclerosis 1990; 10:493–6.

29. Randle P, Garland P, Hales N, Newsholme E. The glucose-fatty acid cycle: its role in insulin sensitivity and the metabolic disturbances of diabetes mellitus. Lancet 1963; 1:785–789.

30. Ferrannini E, Barrett EJ, Bevilaqua MP, De Fronzo RA. Effects of fatty acids on glucose production and utilization in man. J. Clin Invest 1983; 72:1737–1744.

31. Martin ML, Jensen MD. Effects of body fat distribution on regional lipolysis in obesity. J Clin Invest 1991; 88:609–613.

32. Svedberg J, Strömblad G, Wirth A, Smith U, Björntorp P. Fatty acids in the portal vein of the rat regulate hepatic insulin clearance. J Clin Invest 1991; 88:2054–2058.

33. Goto T, Onumua T, Takebe K, Kral JG. The influence of fatty liver on insulin clearance and insulin resistance in non-diabetic Japanese subjects. Int J Obesity 1995; 19:841–845.

34. Banerji MA, Buckley C, Chaiken RL, Gordon D, Lebovitz HE, Kral JG. Liver fat, serum triglycerides and visceral adipose tissue in insulin-sensitive and insulin-resistant black men with NIDDM. Int J Obes 1995; 19:846–850.

35. Kral JG, Lundholm K, Sjöström L, Björntorp P, Scherstén T. Hepatic lipid metabolism in severe human obesity. Metabolism 1977; 26:1025–1031.

36. Peiris A, Mueller RA, Smith GA, Struve MF, Kissebah AH. Splanchnic insulin metabolism in obesity: influence of body fat distribution. J Clin Invest 1986; 78:1648–1657.

37. Zavaroni J, Bonini L, Fantuzzi A, Dall'aglio E, Passeri M, Reaven GM. Hyperinsulinemia, obesity and syndrome X. J Intern Med 1994; 235:51–56.

38. Zimmet PZ. Kelly West lecture 1991. Challenges in diabetes epidemiology—from West to the rest. Diabetes Care 1992; 15:232–252.

39. Ferrannini E, Cobelli C. The kinetics of insulin in man. II. Role of the liver. Diabetes/Metab Rev 1987; 3:365–397.

40. De Fronzo RA, Tobin JD, Andres R. Glucose clamp technique: a method for quantifying insulin secretion and resistance. Am J Physiol 1979; 237:E214–223.

41. De Fronzo RA. Pathogenesis of type 2 (non-insulin dependent) diabetes mellitus: a balanced overview. Diabetologia 1992; 35:389–397.

42. Sjöström L, Kvist H, Cederblad Å, Tylén U. Determination of total adipose tissue and body fat in women by computed tomography, 40K and tritium. Am J Physiol 1986; 250:E736–745.

43. Lapidus L, Bengtsson C, Larsson B, Pennert K, Rybo E, Sjöström L. Distribution of adipose tissue and risk of cardiovascular disease and death: a 12 year follow up of participants in the population study of women in Gothenburg, Sweden. Br Med J 1984; 288:1257–1261.

44. Larsson B, Svärdsudd K, Wilhelmsen L, Björntorp P, Tibblin G. Abdominal adipose tissue distribution. Obesity and risk of cardiovascular disease and death: 13 year follow up of participants in the Study of Men Born in 1913. Br Med J 1984; 288:1401–1404.

45. Lundgren H, Bergström C, Blohmé G, Lapidus L, Sjöström L. Adiposity and adipose tissue distribution in relation to the incidence of diabetes in women: results from a prospective study in Gothenburg, Sweden. Int J Obes 1989; 13:413–423.

46. Ohlsson L, Larsson B, Svärdsudd K, Welin L, Eriksson H, Wilhelmsen L, Björntorp P, Tibblin G. The influence of body fat distribution on the incidence of diabetes mellitus. Diabetes 1985; 34:1055–1058.

47. Ducimetiere P, Richard J, Cambien F. The pattern of subcutaneous fat distribution in middle-aged men and the risk of coronary heart disease: the Paris Prospective Study. Int J Obes 1986; 10:229–240.

48. Stokes J, Garrison RJ, Kannel WB. The independent contribution of various indices of obesity to the 22-year incidence of coronary heart disease: the Framingham Heart Study. In: Vague J, et al., eds. Metabolic Complications of Human Obesities. New York: Elsevier Science Publishers, 1985:49–57.

49. Donahue R, Abbot P, Bloom R, Reed E, Katsuhiko-Yano DM. Central obesity and coronary heart disease in men. Lancet 1987; 2:821–824.

50. Terry R, Page WF, Haskell WL. Waist/hip ratio, body mass index and premature cardiovascular disease mortality in U.S. Army veterans during a twenty-three year follow up study. Int J Obes 1992; 16:417–423.

51. Bergstrom RW, Newell-Morris LL, Leonetti DL., Shuman WP, Wahl PW, Fujimoto WY. Association of elevated fasting C-peptide level and increased intraabdominal fat distribution with the development of NIDDM in Japanese-American men. Diabetes 1990; 39:104–111.

52. Haffner SM, Stern MP, Mitchell BD, Hazuda HP, Patterson JK. Incidence of type II diabetes in Mexican Americans predicted by fasting insulin and glucose levels, obesity and body fat distribution. Diabetes 1990; 39:283–288.

53. Kvist H, Chowdhury B, Grangård U, Tylén U, Sjöström L. Total and visceral adipose tissue volumes derived from measurements with computed tomography in adult men and women: predictive equations. Am J Clin Nutr 1988; 48:1351–1361.

54. Seidell JC, Andres R, Sorkin JD, Muller DC. The sagittal waist diameter and mortality in men: the Baltimore Longitudinal Study of Aging. Int J Obes 1994; 18:61–67.

55. De Fronzo RA. The triumvirate: β-cell muscle, and liver. A collusion responsible for NIDDM. Diabetes 1988; 37: 667–687.

56. Cicero TJ. Sex differences in the effects of alcohol and other psychoactive drugs on endocrine function. In: Israel Y, Kalant O, Kalant H, eds. Research Advances in Alcohol and Drug Problems. New York: Plenum Press, 1980: 544–593.

57. Kvist H, Hallgren P, Jönsson L, Pettersson P, Sjöberg C, Sjöström L, Björntorp P. Distribution of adipose tissue and muscle mass in alcoholic men. Metabolism 1993; 42: 569–573.

58. Seidell JC, Björntorp P, Sjöström L, Kvist H, Sannerstedt R. Visceral fat accumulation in men is positively associated with insulin glucose and C-peptide levels, but negatively with testosterone levels. Metabolism 1990; 39:897.

59. Khaw KT, Chir MBB, Barrett-Connor E. Lower endogenous androgens predict central adiposity in men. Am J Epidemiol 1992; 2:675–682.

60. Haffner SH, Waldez RA, Stern MP, Katz MS. Obesity, body fat distribution and sex hormones in men. Int J Obes 1993; 17:643–649.

61. Mårin P, Krotkiewski M and Björntorp P. Androgen treatment of middle aged, obese men: effects on metabolism, muscle and adipose tissues. Eur J Med 1992; 1:329–336.

62. Mårin P, Holmäng S, Jönsson L, Sjöström L, Kvist H, Holm G, Lindstedt G, Björntorp P. The effects of testosterone treatment on body composition and metabolism in middle-aged obese men. Int J Obes 1992; 16:991–997.

63. Mårin P, Holmäng S, Gustafsson C, Jönsson L, Kvist H, Elander A, Eldh J, Sjöström L, Holm G, Björntorp P. Androgen treatment of abdominally obese men. Obes Res 1993; 1:245–251.

64. Bengtsson B-Å, Edén S, Lönn L, Kvist H, Stokland A, Lindstedt G, Bosaeus I, Tölli J, Sjöström L, Isaksson OGP. Treatment of adults with growth hormone deficiency with recombinant human growth hormone. J Clin Endocrinol Metab 1993; 76:309–317.

65. Mårin P, Kvist H, Lindstedt G, Sjöström L, Björntorp P. Low concentrations of insulin-like growth factor-I in abdominal obesity. Int J Obes 1993; 17:83–89.

66. Bonen AM, Hagg S, Watson-Wright WM. Insulin binding and glucose uptake differences in rodent skeletal muscles. Diabetes 1980; 30:702–704.

67. Kraeghen EW, James DE, Jenkins AB, Chisholm DJ. Dose-response curves for in vivo insulin sensitivity in individual tissues in rats. Am J Physiol 1985; 11:E353–362.

68. Susheela AK, Walton JN. Note on the distribution of histochemical fibre types in some normal human muscles. A study on autopsy material. J Neurol Sci 1969; 8:201–207.

69. Björntorp P, Berchtold P, Tibblin G. Insulin secretion in relation to adipose tissue in men. Diabetes 1971; 20: 65–70.

70. Larsson B, Svärdsudd K, Welin L, Wilhelmsen L, Björntorp P, Tibblin G. Abdominal adipose tissue distribution, obesity and risk of cardiovascular disease and death: 13 year follow up of participants in the study of men born in 1913. Br Med J 1984; 288:1401–1404.

71. Björntorp P. Abdominal fat distribution and disease: An overview of epidemiological data. Ann Med 1992; 24: 15–18.

72. Bouchard C, Després J-P, Mauriège P. Genetic and non-genetic determinants of regional fat distribution. Endocr Rev 1993; 14:72–93.

73. Sjöström CD, Håkangård CA, Lissner L, Sjöström L. Body compartment and subcutaneous adipose tissue distribution. Risk factor patterns in obese subjects. Obes Res 1995; 3:9–22.

74. Rimm A, Werner L, Bernstein RH, Van Yserloo B. Disease and obesity in 73,532 women. Obes Bariat Med 1972; 1: 77–82.

75. Krotkiewski K, Butruk E, Zembrzuska Z. Les fonctions corticosurrenales dans les divers type morphologiques d'obesité. Diabete 1966; 19:229–233.

76. Strain GW, Zumoff B, Strain JJ. Cortisol production in obesity. Metabolism 1980; 29:980–985.

77. Mårin P, Darin N, Amemeiya T, Andersson B, Jern S, Björntorp P. Cortisol secretion in relation to body fat distribution in obese premenopausal women. Metabolism 1992; 41:882–886.

78. Vague J, Vague P, Boyer J, Cloix M. Anthropometry of obesity, diabetes, adrenal, and beta-cell functions. In: Rodriques RR et al., eds. Exc Med Int Congr 1970; 23: 517–525.

79. Pasquali R, Cantobelli S, Casimirri F, Capelli M, Bortoluzzi L, Flamia R, Labate AMM, Barbara L. The hypothalamic-pituitary-adrenal axis in obese women with different patterns of body fat distribution. J Clin Endocrinol Metab 1993; 77:341–346.

80. Pasquali R, Casimirri F, Cantobelli S, Buratti P, Bortoluzzi L, Capelli M, Labate AMM, Barbara L. β-endorphin response to exogenous corticotrophin-releasing hormone in obese women with different patterns of body fat distribution. Int J Obes 1993; 17:593–596.

81. Pasquali R, Anconetani B, Chattat R, Biscotti M, Spinucci G, Casimirri F, Vicennati V, Carcello A, Labate AMM. The hypothalamic-pituitary-adrenal axis activity and its relationship to the automic nervous system in women with visceral and subcutaneous obesity. Effects of the corticotropin-releasing factor/arginine-vasopressin test and of stress. Metabolism 1996; 45:351–356.

82. Moyer AE, Rodin J, Grilo CH, Cummings N, Larsson LM, Rebuffé-Scrive M. Stress-induced cortisol response and fat distribution in women. Obes Res 1994; 2:255–262.

83. Dallman MF. Stress update. Adaptation of the hypothalamo-pituitary adrenal axis to chronic stress. Trends Endocr Metab 1993; 4:62–69.

84. Ljung T, Andersson B, Björntorp P, Mårin P. Inhibition of cortisol secretion by dexamethasone in relation to body fat distribution, a dose-response study. Obes Res 1996; 4: 277–282.

85. Sapolsky RM, Krey LC, McEwen BS. The neuroendocrinology of stress and aging: The glucocorticoid cascade hypothesis. Endocr Rev 1986; 7:289–301.

86. Nilsson PM, Möller L, Solstad K. Adverse effects of psychosocial stress on gonadal function and insulin levels in middle-aged males. J Intern Med 1995; 237:479–486.

87. Tibblin G, Adlerberth A, Lindstedt G, Björntorp P. The pituitary-gonadal axis and health in elderly men. The Study of Men Born in 1913. Diabetes 1996; 45: 1605–1609.

88. Clemmons DR, Van Wyk JJ. Factors controlling blood concentrations of somatomedin C. J Clin Endocrinol Metab 1984; 13:113–143.

89. Mårin P, Rosmond R, Bengtsson B-Å, Gustafsson C, Holm G, Björntorp P. Growth hormone secretion after testosterone administration to men with visceral obesity. Obes Res 1994; 2:263–270.

90. Chrousos G, Gold P. The concept of stress and stress system disorders. JAMA 1992; 267:1244–1252.

91. Jern S, Bergbrant A, Björntorp P, Hansson L. Relation to central hemodynamics to obesity and body fat distribution. Hypertension 1992; 19:520–527.

91a. Björntorp P. The regulation of adipose tissue distribution in humans. Int J Obes 1996; 20:291–302.

92. Ottosson M, Vikman-Adolfsson K, Enerbäck S, Olivecrona G, Björntorp P. The effects of cortisol on the regulation of lipoprotein lipase activity in human adipose tissue. J Clin Endocrinol Metab 1994; 79:820–825.

93. Ottosson M, Vikman-Adolfsson K, Enerbäck S, Elander A, Björntorp P, Edén S. Growth hormone inhibits lipoprotein lipase activity in human adipose tissue. J Clin Endocrinol Metab 1995; 80:936–941.

94. Ottosson M, Mårin P, Karason K, Elander A and Björntorp P. Blockade of the glucocorticoid receptor with RU 486: effects in vitro and in vivo on human adipose tissue lipoprotein lipase activity. Obes Res 1995; 3:233–240.

95. Ottosson M, Lönnroth P, Björntorp P, Edén S. Differential effects of cortisol and growth hormone on lipolysis in human adipose tissue (submitted for publication).

96. Xu X, De Pergola G, Björntorp P. Steroid hormone effects on adipose tissue growth and metabolism. In: Crepaldi G, Tiengo A, Enzi G, eds. Diabetes, Obesity and Hyperlipidemias IV. Amsterdam: Elsevier, 1990:173–178.

97. Xu X, De Pergola G, Björntorp P. The effects of androgens on the regulation of lipolysis in adipose precursor cells. Endocrinology 1990; 126:1229–1234.

98. Xu X, De Pergola G, Björntorp P. Testosterone increases lipolysis and the number of beta-adrenoceptors in male rat adipocytes. Endocrinology 1991; 128:379–382.

99. Xu X, De Pergola G, Eriksson P, Fu L, Carlsson B, Yang S, Edén S, Björntorp P. Postreceptor events involved in the up-regulation of β-adrenergic receptor mediated lipolysis by testosterone in rat white adipocytes. Endocrinology 1993; 132:1651–1657.

100. De Pergola G, Xu X, Yang S, Giorgino R, Björntorp P. Upregulation of androgen receptor binding in male rat fat pad adipose precursor cells exposed to testosterone: study in a whole cell assay system. J Steroid Biochem Mol 1990; 37:553–558.

101. Sjögren J, Li M, Björntorp P. Androgen hormone binding to adipose tissue in rats. Biochim Biophys Acta 1995; 1244:117–120.

102. De Pergola G, Holmäng A, Svedberg J, Giorgino R, Björntorp P. Testosterone treatment of ovariectomized rats: Effects on lipolysis regulation in adipocytes. Acta Endocrin (Copenh) 1990; 123:61–66.

103. Elbers JMH, Asscheman H, Seidell JC, Gooren LJG. Increased accumulation of visceral fat after long-term androgen administration in women. Int J Obes 1995; 19(Suppl. 2):25 (abstract).

104. Rebuffé-Scrive M, Brönnegård M, Nilsson A, Eldh J, Gustafsson JÅ, Björntorp P. Steroid hormone receptors in human adipose tissues. J Clin Endocrinol Metab 1990; 71: 1215–1219.

105. Brönnegård M, Ottosson M, Böös J, Marcus C, Björntorp P. Lack of evidence for estrogen and progesterone receptor in human adipose tissue. J Steroid Biochem Mol Biol 1994; 51:275–281.

106. Rebuffé-Scrive M, Eldh J, Hafström L-O, Björntorp P. Metabolism of mammary, abdominal and femoral adipocytes

in women before and after menopause. Metabolism 1986; 35:792–797.

107.   Rebuffé-Scrive M, Lundholm K, Björntorp P. Glucocorticoid binding of human adipose tissue. Eur J Clin Invest 1985; 15:267–272.

108.   Xu X, Hoebeke J, Björntorp P. Progestin binds to the glucocorticoid receptor and mediates antiglucocorticoid effect in rat adipose precursor cells. J. Steroid Biochem 1990; 36:465–471.

109.   Edén S, Jansson JO, Oscarsson J. Sexual dimorphism of growth hormone secretion. In: Isaksson O, Binder C, Hall K, Hökfelt B, eds. Growth Hormone: Basic and Clinical Aspects. Amsterdam: Excerpta Medica, 1987:115–129.

110.   Mårin P, Andersson B, Ottosson M, Olbe L, Chowdhury B, Kvist H, Holm G, Sjöström L, Björntorp P. The morphology and metabolism of intraabdominal adipose tissue in men. Metabolism 1992; 41:1242–1248.

111.   West DB, Prinz WA, Greenwood MRC. Regional changes in adipose tissue blood flow and metabolism in rats after a meal. Am J Physiol 1989; 257:R711–716.

112.   Rebuffé-Scrive M. Neuroregulation of adipose tissue: molecular and hormonal mechanisms. Int J Obes 1991; 15:83–86.

113.   Peeke P, Oldfield E, Alexander H, Fraker D, Alexander J, Wells J, Chrousos G. Glucocorticoid receptor expression in patient with Cushing Syndrome. North American Society for the Study of Obesity, Minneapolis, Minnesota, 1993 (abstract).

114.   Rebuffé-Scrive M, Björntorp P. Regional adipose tissue metabolism in man. In: Vague J, et al, eds. Metabolic Complications of Human Obesities. Amsterdam: Elsevier, 1985:149–159.

115.   Björntorp P, Enzi G, Ohlson R, Persson B, Sponbergs P, Smith U. Lipoprotein lipase activity and uptake of exogenous triglycerides in fat cells of different size. Horm Metab Res 1975; 7:230–237.

116.   Mårin P, Rebuffé-Scrive M, Björntorp P. Uptake of triglyceride fatty acids in adipose tissue in vivo in man. Eur J Clin Invest 1990; 20:158–165.

117.   Li M, Björntorp P. Triglyceride uptake in muscles in rats. Obes Res 1995; 3:419–426.

118.   Mårin P, Odén B, Björntorp P. Assimilation and mobilization of triglycerides in subcutaneous abdominal and femoral adipose tissue in vivo in men: effects of androgens. J Clin Endocrinol Metab 1995; 80:239–243.

119.   Mårin P, Lönn L, Andersson B, Odén B, Olbe L, Bengtsson B-Å, Björntorp P. Assimilation of triglycerides in subcutaneous and intraabdominal adipose tissue in vivo in men: effects of testosterone. J Clin Endocrinol Metab 1996; 81:1081–1022.

120.   Li M, Yang S, Björntorp P. Metabolism of different adipose tissue in vivo in the rat. Obes Res 1993; 1:459–468.

121.   Li M, Björntorp P. Effects of testosterone and triglyceride uptake and mobilization in different adipose tissues in male rats in vivo. Obes Res 1995; 3:113–119.

122.   Mårin P, Rebuffé-Scrive M, Smith U, Björntorp P. Glucose uptake in human adipose tissue. Metabolism 1987; 36:1154–1160.

123.   Lönn L, Kvist H, Ernest J, Sjöström L. Changes in body composition and adipose tissue distribution after treatment of women with Cushing's syndrome. Metabolism 1994; 43:1517–1522.

124.   Veldhuis JD. Dynamics of the hypothalamo-pituitary testicular axis. In: Yen SSG, Jaffe RB, eds. Reproductive Endocrinology. Philadelphia: WB Saunders, 1991:409–459.

125.   Vermeulen A. Androgens in the aging male. J Clin Endocrinol Metabol 1991; 73:221–224.

126.   Ashwell M, Cole TJ, Dixon AK. Obesity: New insight into the anthropometric classification of fat distribution shown by computed tomography. Br Med J 1985; 290:1692–1694.

127.   Haarbo J, Marslew U, Gottfredsen A, Christiansen C. Postmenopausal hormone replacement therapy prevents central distribution of body fat after menopause. Metabolism 1991; 40:323–326.

128.   Bolinder J, Kager L, Östman J, Arner P. Differences at the receptor and postreceptor levels between human mental and subcutaneous adipose tissue in the action of insulin on lipolysis. Diabetes 1983; 32:117–123.

129.   Lönnqvist F, Krief S, Strosberg AD, Nyberg B, Emorine LJ, Arner P. Evidence for a functional β3-adrenoceptor in man. Br J Pharmacol 1993; 110:929–936.

130.   Rebuffé-Scrive M, Andersson B, Olbe L, Björntorp P. Metabolism of adipose tissue in intraabdominal depots of non-obese men and women. Metabolism 1989; 38:453–458.

131.   Rebuffé-Scrive M, Anderson B, Olbe L, Björntorp P. Metabolism of adipose tissue in intraabdominal depots in severely obese men and women. Metabolism 1990; 39:1021–1025.

132.   Barrett-Connor E, Khaw KT, Yen SSC. Endogenous sex hormone levels in older adult men with diabetes mellitus. Am J Epidemiol 1990; 132:895–901.

133.   Andersson B, Mårin P, Lissner L, Vermeulen A, Björntorp P. Testosterone concentrations in women and men with NIDDM. Diabetes Care 1994; 17:405–411.

134.   Cohen J, Hickman R. Insulin resistance and diminished glucose tolerance in powerlifters ingesting anabolic steroids. J Clin Endocrinol Metabol 1987; 64:960–971.

135.   Björntorp P. Androgens, the Metabolic Syndrome and non-insulin dependent diabetes mellitus. Ann NY Acad Sci 1993; 676:242–252.

136.   Holmäng A, Björntorp P. The effects of testosterone on insulin sensitivity in male rats. Acta Physiol Scand 1992; 146:505–510.

137.   Lindstedt G, Lundberg PA, Lapidus L, Lundgren H, Bengtsson C, Björntorp P. Low sex-hormone-binding globulin concentration as independent risk factor for development of NIDDM 12-yr follow-up of population study of women in Gothenburg, Sweden. Diabetes 1991; 40:123–128.

138. Haffner SM, Valdez RA, Morales PA, Hazuda HP, Stern MP. Decreased sex hormone-binding globulin predicts non-insulin-dependent diabetes mellitus in women but not in men. J Clin Endocrinol Metab 1993; 77:56–60.

139. Lapidus L, Bengtsson C, Björntorp P, Lissner L, Lindstedt G. Lower sex-hormone-binding globulin concentration is a predictor for cardiovascular mortality in women. A 20-year follow-up of the population study of women in Gothenburg, Sweden (submitted for publication).

140. Lapidus L, Andersson B, Bengtsson C, Björkelund C, Björntorp P, Lissner L, Lundberg PA, Lindstedt G. Sex-hormone-binding globulin concentration and hypertension. Results from the population study of women in Göteborg. J Hypertens 1994; 12(Suppl 3):202 (abstract).

141. Polderman KH, Gooren LJ, Asscherman H, Bakker A, Heine RJ. Induction of insulin resistance by androgens and estrogens. J Clin Endocrinol Metab 1994; 79:265–271.

142. Poretsky L, Kalin ML. The gonadotropic function of insulin. Endocr Rev 1987; 8:132–141.

143. Barbieri RL, Ryan KJ. Hyperandrogenism, insulin resistance, and acanthosis nigricans syndrome: a common endocrinopathy with distinct pathophysiologic features. Am J Obstet Gynecol 1983; 14:90–98.

144. Nestler JE, Clore JN, Strauss III JF, Blackard WG. The effects of hyperinsulinemia on serum testosterone, progesterone, dehydroepiandrosterone sulfate, and cortisol levels in normal women and in a woman with hyperandrogenism, insulin resistance, and acanthosis nigricans. J Clin Endocrinol Metab 1987; 64:180–184.

145. Holmäng A, Brzezinska Z, Björntorp P. Effects of hyperinsulinemia on muscle fiber composition and capillarization in rats. Diabetes 1993; 42:1073–1081.

146. Holmäng A, Jennische E, Björntorp P. The effects of long-term hyperinsulinaemia on insulin sensitivity in rats. Acta Physiol Scand 1995; 153:67–73.

147. Holmäng A, Svedberg J, Jennische E, Björntorp P. Effects of testosterone on muscle insulin sensitivity and morphology in female rats. Am J Physiol 1990; 259: E555–560.

148. Holmäng A, Larsson BM, Brzezinska Z, Björntorp P. Effects of short-term testosterone exposure on insulin sensitivity of muscles in female rats. Am J Physiol 1992; 262: E851–855.

149. Rincon J, Holmäng A, Wahlström E, Lönnroth P, Björntorp P, Zierath JR, Wallberg-Henriksson H. Mechanisms behind insulin resistance in rat skeletal muscle following oophorectomy and additional testosterone treatment. Diabetes 1996; 45:615–621.

150. Kumagai S, Holmäng A, Björntorp P. The effects of oestrogen and progesterone on insulin sensitivity in female rats. Acta Physiol Scand 1993; 149:91–97.

151. Olefsky JM. Lilly Lecture 1980; Insulin resistance and insulin action: an in vitro and in vivo perspective. Diabetes 1981; 30:148–162.

152. Landsberg L. Pathophysiology of obesity-related hypertension: Role of insulin an sympathetic nervous system. J Cardiovasc Pharmacol 1994; 23:S1–8.

153. Holmäng A, Yoshida N, Jennische E, Björntorp P. The effects of hyperinsulinemia on blood pressure regulation, central hemodynamics and myocardial mass in rats. Eur J Clin Invest 1996; 26:973–978.

154. Davidson MB. Effect of growth hormone on carbohydrate and lipid metabolism. Endocr Rev 1987: 115–131.

155. Guillaume-Gentil C, Assimacopoulos-Jeannet F, Jeaurenaud B. Involvement of non-esterified fatty acid oxidation in glucocorticoid-induced peripheral insulin resistance in rats. Diabetologia 1993; 36:899–906.

156. Carter-Su C, Okamoto K. Effect of insulin and glucocorticoids on glucose transporters in rat adipocytes. Am J Physiol 1987; 252:E441–453.

157. Björntorp P. Fatty acids, hyperinsulinemia, and insulin resistance: which comes first? Curr Opin Lipid 1994; 5: 166–174.

158. Rasio E, Mack E, Egdahl R, Herrera M. Passage of insulin across vascular membranes in the dog. Diabetes 1968; 17: 668–672.

159. Yang YJ, Hope JD, Ader M, Bergman RN. Insulin transport across capillaries is rate limiting for insulin action in dogs. J Clin Invest 1989; 84:1620–1628.

160. Holmäng A, Björntorp P, Rippe B. Tissue uptake of insulin and inulin in red and white skeletal muscle in vivo. Am J Physiol 1992; 263 (Heart Circ Physiol 32):H1171–1176.

161. Holmäng A, Björntorp P, Lönnroth P. Interstitial muscle insulin and glucose levels in normal and insulin resistant Zucker rats (submitted for publication).

162. Holmäng A, Jennische E, Björntorp P. Rapid formation of capillary endothelial cells in skeletal muscle after insulin exposure. Diabetologia 1996; 39:206–211.

163. Laakso M, Edelman SV, Brechtel G, Baron AD. Decreased effect of insulin to stimulate skeletal muscle blood flow in obese man. A novel mechanism for insulin resistance. J Clin Invest 1990; 85:1844–1852.

164. Krotkiewski K, Björntorp P. Muscle tissue in obesity with different distribution of adipose tissue. Effects of physical training. Int J Obes 1986; 10:331–341.

165. Lillioja S, Young AA, Culter CL, Joy JL, Abbott WGH, Zawadski JK, Yki-ärvinen H, Christin L, Secomb TW, Bogardus C. Skeletal muscle capillary density and fiber type are possible determinants of in vivo insulin resistance in man. J Clin Invest 1987; 80:415–424.

166. Forsblom C, Ekstrand A, Eriksson J, Groop L. Microalbuminuria in nondiabetic first degree relatives of type 2 diabetic patients. Diabetologia 1992; 32(Suppl 1):A61 (abstract).

167. Rebuffé-Scrive M, Krotkiewski M, Elfverson J, Björntorp P. Muscle and adipose tissue morphology and metabolism in Cushing's syndrome. J Clin Endocrinol Metab 1988; 67:1122–1128.

168. Uusitupa M, Vanninen E. Insulin and left ventricular hypertrophy. J Intern Med 1992; 232:335–339.

169. Lind L, Lithell H, Pollare T. Is it hyperinsulinemia or insulin resistance that is related to hypertension and other metabolic cardiovascular risk factors? J Hypertens 1993; (Suppl 1):S11–16.

170. Messerli MH. Hypertension, left ventricular hypertrophy, ventricular ectopy and sudden death. Am J Hypertens 1993; 6:335–336.

171. Bjöntorp P. Neuroendocrine ageing. J Intern Med 1995; 238:401–404.

172. Heuser IJ, Gotthardt U, Schweiger U, Schmider J, Lammers CH, Dettling M, Holsboer F. Age-associated changes of pituitary-andrenocortical hormone regulation in humans: Importance of gender. Neurobiol Aging 1994; 15: 227–231.

173. Wallin A, Blennow K, Gottfries CG, Karlsson I, Svennerholm L. Blood-brain barrier function in vascular dementia. Acta Neurol Scand 1990; 81:318–322.

174. Balldin J, Gottfries CG, Karlsson I, Lindstedt G, Wålinder J. Dexamethasone suppression test and serum prolactin in dementia disorders. Br J Psychiatry 1983; 143:277–281.

175. Henry JP, Stephens PM. Stress, Health, and the Social Environment. A Sociobiological Approach to Medicine. New York: Springfield, 1977.

176. Mason JW. A review of psychoendocrine research on the pituitary-adrenal cortical system. Psychosom Med 1968; 30:576–607.

177. McEwen BS, Cameron H, Chao HM, Gould E, Magarinos AM, Watanabe Y, Woolley S. Adrenal steroids and plasticity of hippocampal neurons: toward an understanding of underlying cellular and molecular mechanisms. Cell Mol Neurobiol 1993; 13:457–482.

178. Rivier C. Neuroendocrine mechanisms of anterior pituitary regulation in the rat exposed to stress. In: Brown MR, Koob GF, Rivier C, eds. Stress: Neurobiology and Neuroendocrinology. New York; Marcel Dekker, 1991:119–136.

179. Kaplan JR, Adams MR, Koritnik DR, Rose JC, Manuch SB. Adrenal responsiveness and social status in intact and ovariectomized Macaca fascicularis. Am J Primatol 1986; 11:181–193.

180. Frankenhaeuser M. The sympathetic-adrenal and pituitary-adrenal response to challenge: Comparison between the sexes. In: Dembroski TM, Schmidt TH, Blümchen G, eds. Biobehavioral Bases of Coronary Heart Disease. Human Physiology. Basel, Switzerland: Karger, 1983; 2: 91–105.

181. Heuser IJE, Wark HJ, Keul J, Holsboer F. Hypothalamo-pituitary-adrenal axis function in elderly endurance athletes. J Clin Endocrinol Metab 1991; 73:485–488.

182. Smals AG, Kloppenberg PW, Njo T. Alcohol induced Cushingoid syndrome. Br Med J 1976; 2:19–28.

183. Gossain VV, Sherma NK, Srivastava L, Michelakis AM, Rowner CR. Hormonal effects of smoking. II: Effects on plasma cortisol, growth hormone and prolactin. Am J Med Sci 1986; 29:325–327.

184. Carrol BJ. The dexamethasone suppression test for melancholia. Br J Psychiatry 1982; 140:292–304,

185. Sachar EJ. Disrupted 24 hour patterns of cortisol secretion in psychotic depression. Arch Gen Psychiatry 1973; 18: 19–26.

186. Roy-Byrne PP, Unde TW, Post RM, Gallereci W, Chrousos G, Gold PW. The corticotropin-releasing hormone stimulation test in patients with panic disorders. Am J Psychiatry 1986; 143:896–899.

187. Larsson B, Seidell J, Svärdsudd K, Welin L, Tibblin G, Wilhelmsen L, Björntorp P. Obesity, adipose tissue distribution and health in men. The study of men born in 1913. Appetite 1989; 13:37–44.

188. Rosmond R, Lapidus L, Björntorp P. The influence of occupational and social factors on obesity and body fat distribution in middle-aged men. Int J Obes 1995; 20: 599–607.

189. Lapidus L, Bengtsson C, Hällström T, Björntorp P. Obesity, adipose tissue distribution and health in women. Results from a population study in Gothenburg, Sweden. Appetite 1989; 12:25–35.

190. Wing RR, Matthews KA, Kuller LH, Meilahn EN, Plantinga P. Waist to hip ratio in middle-aged women. Associations with behavioral and pyschosocial factors and with changes in cardiovascular risk factors. Arterioscler Thromb 1991; 11:1250–1257.

191. Kaye SA, Folsom AR, Jacobs Jr DR, Hughes GH, Flack JM. Psychosocial correlates of body fat distribution in black and white young adults. Int J Obes 1993; 17: 271–277.

192. Georges E, Wear ML, Mueller WH. Body fat distribution and job stress in Mexican-American men of the Hispanic health and nutrition examination survey. Am J Hum Biol 1992; 4:657–667.

193. Leonetti DL, Bergstrom RW, Shuman WP, Wahl PW, Jenner DA, Harrison GA, Fujimoto WY. Urinary catecholamines, plasma insulin, and environmental factors in relation to body fat distribution. Int J Obes 1991; 15: 345–357.

194. Karasek RA, Russell RS, Theorell T. Physiology of stress and regeneration in job related cardiovascular illness. J Hum Stress 1982; 3:29–42.

195. Purifoy FE, Koopmans LH. Androstenedione, testosterone and free testosterone concentration in women with various occupations. Soc Biol 1979; 26:179–188.

196. Rosmond R, Lapidus L, Mårin P, Björntorp P. Mental distress, obesity and body fat distribution in middle-aged men. Obes Res 1996; 4:245–252.

197. Haffner SM, Stern MP, Hazuda HP, Pugh J, Patterson JK, Malina R. Upper-body and centralized adiposity in Mexican Americans and non-Hispanic whites: relationship to body mass index and other behavioral and demographic variables. Int J Obes 1986; 10:493–502.

198. Barrett-Connor E, Khaw K-T. Cigarette smoking and increased central adiposity. Ann Intern Med 1989; 111: 783–787.

199. Den Tonkelaar I, Seidell JC, Van Noord PAH, Baanders-Van Halewijn EA, Ouwehand IJ. Fat distribution in relation to age, degree of obesity, smoking habits, parity and estrogen use—a cross sectional study in 11,853 Dutch women. Int J Obes 1990; 14:753–761.

200. Seidell JC, Cigolini CM, Deslypere J-P, Charzewska J, Ellsinger B-M, Cruz A. Body fat distribution in relation to physical activity and smoking habits of 38-year-old European men—the European Fat Distribtuion Study. Am J Epidemiol 1991; 133:257–265.

201. Seidell JC. Environmental influences on regional fat distribution. Int J Obes 1991; 15:31–35.

202. Shimokata H, Tobin HJD, Muller DC, Elahi D, Coon PJ, Andres R. Studies in the distribution of body fat. I. Effects of age, sex, and obesity. J Gerontol 1989; 44:M66–73.

203. Facchini FS, Hollenbeck CB, Jeppesen J, Chen YDI, Reaven GM. Insulin resistance and cigarette smoking. Lancet 1992; 339:1128–1130.

204. Smith U. Smoking elicits the insulin resistance syndrome: New aspects of the harmful effect of smoking. J Intern Med 1995; 237:435–447.

205. Troisi RJ, Weiss ST, Segal MR, Cassano PA, Vokonas PS, Landsberg L. The relationship of body fat distribution to blood pressure in normotensive men: the normative aging study. Int J Obes 1990; 14:515–525.

206. Van Barneveld T, Seidell JC, Traag N, Hautvast JGAJ. Fat distribution and γ-glutamyl transferase in relation to serum lipids and blood pressure in 38-year-old Dutch males. Eur J Clin Nutr 1989; 43:809–818.

207. Cigolini M, Targher G, Bergamo Andreis IA, Touoli M, Filippi F, Muggeo M, De Sandre G. Moderate alcohol consumption and its relation to visceral fat and plasma androgens in healthy women. Int J Obes 1996; 20:206–212.

208. Haffner SM, Valdez R, Morales PA, Mitchell BD, Hazuda HP, Stern MP. Greater effect of glycemia on incidence of hypertension in women than in men. Diabetes Care 1992; 15:1277–1284.

209. Selby JV, Newman B, Quesenberry CP Jr, Fabsitz RR, Carmelli D, Meaney FJ, Slemenda C. Genetic and behavioral influences on body fat distribution. Int J Obes 1990; 14:593–602.

210. Pettersson P, Ellsinger BM, Sjöberg C, Björntorp P. Fat distribution and steroid hormones in women with alcohol abuse. J Intern Med 1990; 228:311–316.

211. Matorakis G, Chrousos G, Weber J. Recombinant interleukin 6 activates the hypothalamo-pituitary-adrenal axis in humans. J Clin Endocrinol Metab 1993; 27:1690–1694.

212. Shively C, Clarkson FB, Miller C, Weingand KW. Body fat distribution as a risk factor for coronary artery atherosclerosis in female cynomolgus monkeys. Arteriosclerosis 1987; 7:226–231.

213. Jayo JM, Shively CA, Kaplan JR, Manuck SB. Effects of exercise and stress on body fat distribution in male cynomolgus monkeys. Int J Obes 1993; 17:597–604.

214. Rebuffé-Scrive M, Walsh UA, McEwen BS, Rodin J. Effect of chronic stress and exogenous glucocorticoids on regional fat distribution and metabolism. Physiol Behav 1992 52:583–590.

215. Björntorp P. Classification of obese patients and complications related to the distribution of surplus fat. Am J Clin Nutr 1987; 45:1120–1125.

216. Björntorp P. Possible mechanisms relating fat distribution and metabolism. In: Bouchard C, Johnston F, eds. Fat Distribution During Growth and Later Health Outcomes. New York: Alan R Liss, 1988:175–191.

217. Björntorp P. Obesity and diabetes. In: Alberti KGMM, Kral JP eds. The Diabetes Annual 5. Amsterdam: Elsevier, 1990:373–395.

218. Björntorp P. Visceral fat accumulation: the missing link between psycho-social factors and cardiovascular disease? J Intern Med 1991; 230:195–201.

219. Björntorp P. Obesity, insulin resistance and diabetes. In: Alberti KGMM, Kral LP, eds. The Diabetes Annual 6. Amsterdam: Elsevier, 1991:347–370.

220. Björntorp P. Metabolic implications of body fat distribution. Diabetes Care 1991; 14:1132–1143.

221. Björntorp P. Psychosocial factors and fat distribution. In: Ailhaud G, et al, eds. Obesity in Europe 91. London: John Libbey, 1992:377–387.

222. Brindley DN, Rolland Y. Possible connections between stress, diabetes, obesity, hypertension and altered lipoprotein metabolism that may result in atherosclerosis. Clin Sci 1989; 77:453–461.

223. Rivera MP, Svec F, Is cortisol involved in upper-body obesity? Med Hypoth 1989; 30:95–100.

224. Reaven GM. The fourth Musketeer—from Alexandre Dumas to Claude Bernard. Diabetologia 1995; 38:3–13.

225. Law CM, Barker DJP, Osmond C, Fall S, Simmonds SJ. Early growth and abdominal fatness in adult life. J Epidemiol Commun Health 1992; 46:184–186.

226. Reul JMHM, Stec J, Wiegers JG, Labeur MS, Linthorst ACE, Arzt E, Hosboer F. Prenatal immune challenge alters the hypothalamic-pituitary-adrenal axis in adult rats. J Clin Invest 1994; 93:2600–2607.

227. Joffe JM. Hormonal mediation of the effects of prenatal stress on offspring behavior. In: Gottlieb G, ed. Studies on the Development of Behavior and Nervous System: Early Influences, vol 4. New York: Academic Press, 1978: 108–144.

228. Orth-Gomér K, Johnson JV. Social network interaction and mortality. A six year follow-up study of a random sample of the Swedish population. J Chronic Dis 1987; 40:949–957.

229. Welin L, Tibblin G, Svärdsudd K, Wilhelmsen L. Social influences on mortality in a prospective population study. Lancet 1985; 1:915–918.

230. Hudson JI, Hudson MG, Rotschild AJ, Vignati L, Schatzberg AF, Melby JC. Abnormal results of dexamethasone suppression tests in non-depressed patients with diabetes mellitus. Arch Gen Psychiatry 1984; 41:1086–1089.

231. Cameron OG, Thomas B, Tiongco D, Hariharan M, Gaeden JR. Hypercortisolism in diabetes mellitus. Diabetes Care 1987; 10:662–663.

232. Vermes J, Steinmetz E, Schooal J, Van de Ween EA, Tilders FJH. Increased levels of immunoreactive β-endorphin and corticotropin in non-insulin dependent diabetes mellitus. Lancet 1985; 2:725–726.

233. Tsigos C, Young RJ, White A. Diabetic neuropathy is associated with increased activity of the hypothalamic-pituitary-adrenal axis. J Clin Endocrinol Metab 1993; 76:554–558.

234. Surwit RS, Feinglos NM. The effect of relaxation on glucose tolerance in non-insulin dependent diabetes mellitus. Diabetes Care 1983; 7:203–204.

235. Surwit RS, McCubbin JA, Livingston EG, Feinglos MS. Classically conditioycemia in the obese mouse. Psychosom Med 1985; 47:565–568.

236. Surwit RS, McCubbin JA, Kuhn JA, McGee CM, Gerstenfeld D, Feinglos MN. Alprazolam reduces stress hyperglycemia in ob/ob mice. Psychosom Med 1986; 48:278–282.

237. Sanval-Emeric E. Corticotropin-releasing factor (CRF)—a review. Psychoneuroendocrinology 1986; 11:277–294.

238. Fuller RW. The involvement of serotonin in regulation of pituitary-adrenal function. Frontier Neuroendocrinology 1992; 13:250–270.

239. Chaouloff F. Physiopharmacological interactions between stress hormones and central serotonergic systems. Brain Res Rev 1993; 18:1–32.

240. Eriksson E, Humble M. Serotonin in psychiatric pathophysiology. In: Pohl R, Gershow S, eds. The Basis of Psychiatric Treatment, vol. 3. Basel: Karger, 1990:66–119.

241. Strömbom U, Krotkiewski K, Blennow K, Månsson JE, Ekman R, Björntorp P. The concentrations of monoamine metabolites and neuropeptides in the cerebrospinal fluid of obese women with different body fat distribution. Int J Obes 1996; 20:361–368.

242. Ågren H, Reibring L, Hartvig P, Tedroff J, Bjurling P, Lundqvist H, Långström B. Monoamine metabolism in human prefrontal cortex and basal ganglia. PET studies using $[\beta\text{-}^{11}C]$1-5-hydroxytryptophan and $[\beta\text{-}^{11}C]$L-DOPA in healthy volunteers and patients with unipolar major depression. Depression 1993; 1:71–81.

243. Bouchard C. Genetic factors in the regulation of adipose tissue distribution. Acta Med Scand 1988; 723(Suppl):135–141.

244. Bouchard C, Pérusse L, Leblanc C, Tremblay A, Thériault G. Inheritance of the amount and distribution of human body fat. Int J Obes 1988; 12:205–215.

245. Bouchard C. Genes and body fat. Am J Hum Biol 1993; 5:425–432.

246. Bouchard C, Tremblay A, Després J-P, Nadeau A, Lupien PJ, Thériault G, Dussault J, Moorjani S, Pinault S, Fournier G. The response to long-term overfeeding in identical twins. N Engl J Med 1990; 322:1477–1482.

247. Groop L, Lehto M, Orho M. Non-insulin dependent diabetes mellitus: a genetic and metabolic nightmare. Diab Nutr Metab 1994; 7:253–261.

248. Linkowski P, Van Ouderbergen A, Kerkhofs M, Bosson D, Mendlewicz J, Van Canter E. Twin study of the 24-cortisol profile: evidence for genetic control of the human circardian clock. Am J Physiol 1993; 264:E173–181.

28

Clinical Manifestations of the Metabolic Syndrome

Ahmed H. Kissebah, Glenn R. Krakower, Gabriele E. Sonnenberg, and Magda M. I. Hennes
Medical College of Wisconsin, Milwaukee, Wisconsin

I. INTRODUCTION

Reaven and associates were the earliest to undertake experiments that demonstrated that deterioration in glucose tolerance is a function of the ability of the β cell to compensate for defect(s) in insulin action. Their subsequent studies documented that in insulin-resistant states, resistance to insulin-stimulated glucose uptake is associated with resistance to insulin suppression of plasma FFA concentration. These observations suggested that the relationships between insulin resistance, plasma insulin levels, and glucose intolerance are mediated by changes in ambient plasma FFA concentrations. In his Banting Lecture (1), Reaven summarized this research and provided further evidence to describe how resistance to insulin-stimulated glucose uptake, glucose intolerance, and hyperinsulinemia are fundamental characteristics of some patients with hypertension. Resistance to insulin-stimulated glucose uptake is also associated with increased plasma triglyceride and decreased HDL-cholesterol concentrations, known metabolic precursors of increased risk for coronary artery disease. It has therefore been postulated that a series of related variables, named "syndrome X", tends to occur in the same individuals and may be highly significant in the origins of coronary artery disease. This syndrome includes resistance to insulin-stimulated glucose uptake, glucose intolerance, hyperinsulinemia, increased plasma VLDL-TG, decreased HDL cholesterol, and high blood pressure. Because of the close linkage of these metabolic features with the abdominal body fat distribution pattern and its biological mechanisms, the more collective term "metabolic syndrome" was subsequently introduced.

Obesity is associated with decreased longevity and increased morbidity from a variety of disorders and diseases, including hyperglycemia, hyperlipidemia, hypertension, and cardiovascular disease (2,3). In addition to these associations, obesity is thought to cause or exacerbate a variety of other health problems, including reproductive and sexual dysfunctions, as well as some forms of cancer. A growing body of evidence suggests that fat distribution, specifically the pattern known as abdominal, upper-body, or android obesity, is a major predictor of metabolic health risks independent of the degree of overweight. Thus localization of fat in the abdominal, and specifically the visceral, region has emerged as a significant precursor of hyperinsulinemia, increased plasma triglycerides, decreased HDL levels, elevated blood pressure, as well as increased morbidity and mortality. Even in apparently healthy individuals, this form of obesity and its associated insulin resistance are predictive of glucose intolerance, increased blood pressure, and specific forms of dyslipidemia.

Although awareness of regional fat patterning has been demonstrated from the earliest recorded works of humankind, the abdominal type, or android form, was only first described clinically in 1719 (4). Descriptive accounts continued for nearly 200 years, when measurements and photographs of human obesity biotypes were taken in various pathological states. By the early 1920s relationships between obesity and diabetes were beginning to be observed.

More than 50% of obese persons studied were found to have abnormal glucose tolerance (5,6). Joslin et al. reported in 1936 that over half of the diabetic patients they studied were obese (7). Vague first described the clinical importance of regional adipose tissue distribution as a correlate of obesity complications. While the lower-body, or gynoid, obesity typically seen in women is benign, the upper-body phenotype is commonly associated with such health problems as diabetes, gout, and atherosclerosis in both men and women (8). Unfortunately, the early reports from Vague and others used imprecise methods for assessing body fat, which were generally difficult to reproduce. Nevertheless, the regional distinctions and their relationships to health risks have ultimately been confirmed by newer, more quantitative, and more reproducible technologies developed over the past few years.

Hyperinsulinemia, as first measured by insulin immunoassay, and its relationship to insulin resistance were both demonstrated in early studies of obesity (9). Their relationship to abdominal obesity and its complications only became apparent in latter years, however (10,11). Indeed studies from our laboratory pioneered the scientific basis for this connection and paved the way for studies from others, with the eventual documentation of a strong linkage between the amount of abdominal-visceral fat and disturbances in insulin action and splanchnic dynamics, as well as their connections with the adverse metabolic profiles, morbidities, and other components of the metabolic syndrome.

Visceral obesity, which is associated with alterations in glucose-insulin homeostasis, a characteristic dyslipidemia, and increased blood pressure, has evolved as an important feature of the metabolic syndrome (10,11). Indeed the presence of high levels of visceral fat may represent a prevalent marker of a cluster of metabolic alterations increasing the risk for coronary heart disease (12). Insulin resistance seems to be a central component of the interrelationships between visceral obesity, the plasma lipoprotein-lipid profile, and the risk of NIDDM and coronary heart disease (1). As reviewed recently (3), the cause-effect relationships between visceral fat and the associated metabolic complications are far from clear, but the pathway of potential linkages between abdominal/visceral obesity and the adverse metabolic profile appears to involve complex interactions between genetics, environment, and phenotypic traits.

II. CLINICAL COMPONENTS: CONTRIBUTIONS OF ABDOMINAL OBESITY

The following account will describe characteristic features of the metabolic syndrome and the contributions of abdominal obesity to its expression.

A. Glucose Intolerance and NIDDM

By the early 1980s it was clear that location of fat has prognostic importance in diabetes. The first large-scale epidemiological study to establish a correlation between the frequency of NIDDM as a function of regional fat distribution was performed on a large cohort of Caucasian women from the TOPS (Take Off Pounds Sensibly) membership (Fig. 1A; 13). This study showed that after adjustment for total body fat, women with relatively more fat around the waist, as measured by the waist-to-hip ratio (WHR), had a higher prevalence rate for diabetes. Nonobese women with a lower-body fat distribution profile have a 2.0% prevalence of diabetes, increasing to 6.1% in the moderately obese. In contrast, nonobese women with an upper-body fat distribution profile have a prevalence of diabetes of 5.6%, while in moderately obese women with upper-body obesity, the prevalence of NIDDM increases to 16.5%. Women with an upper-body fat predominance and moderate obesity have a relative risk for diabetes that is 10.3-fold greater than for nonobese women with a lower-body fat distribution. Statistical analysis of the data established that the effects of obesity and body fat distribution on the frequency of diabetes in women are independent from each other and additive. In subsequent analysis of this cohort, relationships between WHR and degree of obesity with NIDDM frequency were analyzed by multiple regression analysis. While both have an important role in determining insulin sensitivity and, in turn, the metabolic profile, other factors such as genetic background are also important. For example, the relative risk of diabetes was found to increase with increasing levels of upper-body obesity at all levels of family history of diabetes, and similarly increases with increasing family history at each level of WHR (Fig. 1B; 14). Thus, in moderately obese women with abdominal fat patterning, the frequency of NIDDM increases from 6.5% in women with no family history to 23.6% in women with a strong family history index of NIDDM, suggesting significant influences of the genetic component(s).

West and Kalbfleisch have summarized many earlier studies that supported the concept that upper-body adipose tissue is associated with greater risk of NIDDM (15). Numerous cross-sectional and prospective studies have

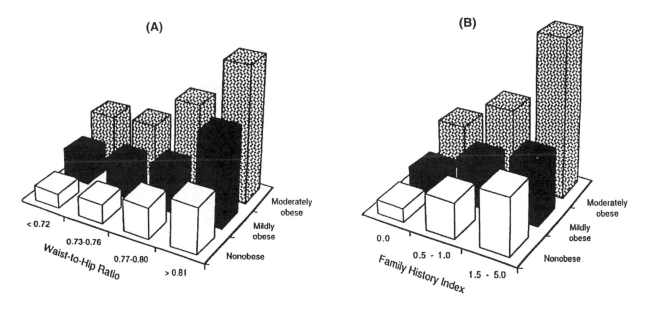

Figure 1 Influence of body fat distribution and heritability on the frequency of NIDDM. (A) Frequency of NIDDM in nonobese and obese women of varying WHR and degree of obesity. (Data from Ref. 13.) (B) Frequency of NIDDM in relation to family history index and degree of overweight in women with WHR 0.75–0.80. (Data from Ref. 14.).

subsequently shown that abdominal, or centralized, body fat distribution is an independent risk factor for NIDDM in several ethnic groups (3).

Our group provided the first scientific documentation of the significant metabolic adversity of abdominal obesity (10). Fasting and postprandial hyperinsulinemia were found to be associated with glucose intolerance in upper-body-obese women, and both metabolic parameters were associated with hypertrophy of adipocytes in the abdominal region. This allowed an important segregation for obese subjects into those with upper-body obesity, with larger fat cells and high glucose and insulin areas, and those with lower-body obesity, with smaller abdominal fat cells and much lower glucose and insulin areas. In subsequent studies, upper-body fat predominance was found to be associated with diminished in vivo insulin sensitivity (16). In healthy, premenopausal women, increasing WHR was accompanied by progressively increasing fasting plasma glucose and insulin levels. Waist-to-thigh ratio was also found to be significantly correlated with insulin action in Pima Indian women, independent of the degree of obesity (17).

Most of the initial studies were performed using WHR as a measure of regional fat distribution. WHR has proven effective in predicting changes in glucose-insulin homeostasis, while being rapid, inexpensive, and applicable to field studies evaluating the role of regional obesity. But the notion that abdominal fat plays a major role in the met-

abolic disorders and increased mortality risk has led to a need for more specific and quantitative methods. One method of choice is computed tomography (CT) scanning, which has been adapted for the direct visualization of abdominal and subcutaneous fat. Studies using the CT techniques have demonstrated the visceral fat mass to be a higher correlate of the fasting and postglucose challenge plasma insulin and lipid levels and blood pressure than total body fat mass (18,19). The CT techniques have also been used to establish correlations of intra-abdominal fat deposition with high plasma glucose responses and glucose intolerance (20,21).

Mechanisms for these changes in glucose tolerance and insulin sensitivity were explored in studies designed to determine the basis for the hyperinsulinemia of abdominal obesity. Increases in insulin production were correlated with the degree of overweight but not with the site of body fat localization or the degree of peripheral insulin insensitivity (22). Pancreatic insulin production is increased threefold in response to a 50–60% reduction in insulin sensitivity, while the same increase in production is induced by a much smaller reduction in peripheral insulin sensitivity in the lower-body-obese women. The limited capacity to mount a commensurate increase in insulin secretion may be due to a secretary defect. Some abdominally obese individuals have also been shown to exhibit lower amplitude and large periodicity variances in the ultradian insulin pulsatilities (23). These may reflect markers of early dysfunction of the β cell.

Abdominally obese subjects, on the other hand, demonstrate a marked decline in hepatic insulin extraction and clearance, which correlates closely with the degree of peripheral insulinemia and insulin insensitivity (22,24,25). Though this reduction may compensate the increased peripheral insulin demand, it could result in diminished hepatic insulin action, which has the potential to impair insulin-mediated suppression of hepatic glucose production. Thus weight gain with lower-body obesity is associated with a milder decline in peripheral insulin sensitivity, which is compensated by increased pancreatic insulin production, while abdominal obesity is characterized by a more severe form of insulin resistance and an additional reduction in hepatic insulin removal, resulting in a much higher degree of peripheral hyperinsulinemia.

The coexistence of hyperinsulinemia and impaired glucose tolerance in abdominal obesity thus suggests that insulin resistance and the accompanying adaptations in splanchnic insulin dynamics are fundamental factors in these associations. Identification of the exact locus of the insulin resistance and the biological pathways in the progression to NIDDM is therefore of great interest.

B. Dyslipidemia and Coronary Heart Disease

Vague and co-workers (26) first observed that atherosclerosis is more closely related to the android, or upper-body obesity than to general obesity. Total plasma cholesterol was also shown to be increased. This relationship was soon confirmed and extended to plasma triglyceride levels. Relationships between body fat distribution and morbidities from cardiovascular disease were first reported in the prospective Gothenburg Study (27). This longitudinal study of 1462 women concluded that WHR is positively correlated with the 12-year incidence of myocardial infarction, angina, stroke, and death independently of age or BMI. Similar relationships between body fat distribution and coronary heart disease, stroke, and mortality have been reported in other prospective studies as well. In a study of 792 men in Gothenburg, Sweden, who were followed up for 13 years, WHR was more strongly associated with stroke, ischemic heart disease, and death than was BMI (28). Using trunk-to-thigh skinfold measurements, an independent association of body fat distribution to CHD was demonstrated among 7746 men in Paris, followed for 6.6 years, while the Honolulu Heart Study of 7692 Japanese men followed for 12 years and then the Framingham Heart Study of men and women followed for 22 years have demonstrated associations between subscapular skinfold measurements and CHD (3,29).

Relationships of upper-body obesity with plasma lipid and lipoprotein concentrations have also been demonstrated (see Refs. 3 and 29 for reviews). This was noted early by our group (10), who showed that abdominally obese women had significantly higher fasting plasma triglyceride levels than lower-body obese, whose triglyceride levels were similar to those of nonobese controls. Adipose tissue distributed centrally in the abdominal region, and particularly visceral rather than subcutaneous fat, is distinctly associated with hyperlipidemia, compared with generalized distributions of body fat. These lipoprotein abnormalities are characterized by elevated VLDL and IDL levels, small, dense LDL with elevated apolipoprotein B levels, and decreased HDL$_{2b}$ levels. In healthy men and women, WHR was found to be positively correlated with decreased HDL cholesterol and increased total cholesterol, LDL cholesterol, and triglyceride levels, independent of BMI. WHR is also significantly correlated with VLDL-TG, and the LDL-apoB/LDL cholesterol ratio. Plasma apoAI is lower and apoB levels are higher in android than in gynoid obesity. Abdominal fat deposition was also associated with an increased concentration of small, dense LDL particles, a condition associated with an increased risk of coronary heart disease (Fig. 2). WHR was positively correlated with small LDL, IDL and VLDL. Overall adiposity was not significantly associated with plasma lipoprotein levels after adjusting for regional adiposity patterns.

Studies in genetic epidemiology have shown that the regional distribution has a significant genetic component. Furthermore, standardized intervention studies in identi-

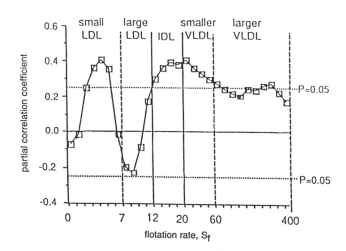

Figure 2 Relationship between fat patterning and lipoprotein size. Pearson correlation coefficients between components of the VLDL-LDL flotation spectrum and WHR, adjusted for skinfold thickness ratios and % body fat. (Adapted from Ref. 186.)

cal twins have shown that some individuals are more susceptible than others to exhibit potentially atherogenic responses under given environmental conditions. Variations in genes relevant to lipid and lipoprotein metabolism may thus alter the relation of abdominal obesity to dyslipoproteinemias, implying that while some individuals with abdominal obesity may be susceptible to develop dyslipoproteinemias, others may be protected from acquiring overt disruptions in lipoprotein metabolism (30). The nature of these genes and their linkage and interaction in the expression of dyslipoproteinemias in abdominal obesity are areas of extensive research interest.

C. Blood Pressure and Hypertension

The link between high blood pressure and obesity was first described by Favier in 1945 (31) and confirmed in later reports (see Ref. 3 for review). Upper-body fat localization and increased visceral fat mass were found to be associated with increased systolic and diastolic blood pressure (10). These associations are independent of the degree of overweight or total-body fat mass (Table 1). Epidemiological studies have shown a strong relationship between blood pressure and mortality and morbidity from coronary artery disease. The positive association of high WHR with elevated blood pressure has been reported in both white and black individuals. A strong relationship between obesity and hypertension is observed in men less than 45 years old (32). Overweight men younger than 45 have not only threefold more hypertension but also fivefold greater prevalence of fasting insulin values greater than 11 μU/ml compared with lean men of similar age (33).

A large body of evidence suggests that hyperinsulinemia and altered insulin sensitivity might be the events that link abdominal or visceral adiposity with hemodynamic changes leading to hypertension (34,35). Impaired glucose tolerance and newly diagnosed diabetes were found to be associated with systolic blood pressure, while an association was found between diabetes and increased blood pressure in both men and women. This association was partially eliminated after adjusting for level of obesity. The Bogalusa Heart Study, which provided evidence that peripheral resistance to insulin activity is related to higher diastolic blood pressure among children, also showed a clear association between insulin concentrations during an oral glucose tolerance test and the central distribution of body fat (36). Modan et al. provided further evidence that insulin resistance and/or hyperinsulinemia may be linked to the increased peripheral vascular resistance of elevated blood pressure (37). It is not understood, however, whether insulin is directly responsible for elevating blood pressure in abdominal obesity, whether hyperinsulinemia and increases in blood pressure occur independently, or whether both result from some other mechanism. Several areas that will be discussed in detail include effects on catecholamine activity, renal sodium and water retention, the renin-angiotensin system, and nitric oxide.

Clear genetic linkages between visceral obesity and hypertension are still unclear. Hypertension results from abnormalities in the vascular, cardiogenic, renal, neurogenic, and endocrine control systems, which normally regulate blood pressure. Familial aggregation, population, and twin studies all point to important genetic influences on the level of blood pressure in childhood and adolescence. A significant portion of the variability in systolic and diastolic blood pressure appears under genetic control. The fact that there are a dozen or more different intermediate phenotypes in hypertension highlights the probable contribution of an overlapping array of a variety of genetic variants to the association between abdominal obesity and the increased blood pressure.

III. BIOLOGY OF REGIONAL ADIPOSITY: RELATIONSHIP TO INSULIN ACTIONS AND SPLANCHNIC DYNAMICS

The primary function of insulin is to accelerate the removal of glucose, fatty acids, and amino acids from the blood. This is accomplished through many different tions, among them accelerating glucose muscle and adipose tissue, altering activities of enzymes metabolizing these substances, and regulating the transcription of selected genes. Insulin resistance, a pathological condition where the biological response to insulin

Table 1 Correlation Coefficients Between Body Fat Topographical Parameters and Mean Blood Pressure

Parameter	r
Body mass index	0.18
Waist-to-hip ratio	0.09
Visceral fat area	0.54*
Subcutaneous fat area	−0.18
Visceral/subcutaneous ratio	0.61*

Changes in mean blood pressure were correlated with indices of body fat in 26 obese, hypertensive Japanese women after weight reduction. *$p < .001$.
Source: Adapted from Ref. 187.

is decreased, is a common feature of the metabolic syndrome associated with upper-body obesity. This section will detail the relationships between this form of obesity with insulin resistance and compensatory changes in splanchnic insulin dynamics.

A. Insulin Resistance

After developing a means to describe changes in the level of blood sugar and how they can be accurately measured, Himsworth noted that a large segment of the diabetic population was insulin insensitive (38). Different amounts of insulin were infused after alimentary hyperglycemia to define the ratio of insulin area to the degree of hyperglycemia, a measure of the degree of insulin insensitivity. He subsequently described how increased secretion of insulin was clinically linked to diabetogenic obesity (39). Relative to insulin-sensitive diabetics, insulin-insensitive diabetics were found to be older and more obese, have hypertension, and exhibit arteriosclerosis.

That insulin resistance can be observed in both lean and obese subjects suggests the presence of heterogeneous factors in the pathophysiology of this condition, among them genetic and environmental influences. This is further complicated by the fact that abdominal obesity, which is strongly associated with insulin resistance, itself has strong genetic and environmental components. Regardless of the origins, the reduced action of insulin observed leads to compensatory hyperinsulinemia, which may further contribute to the insulin-resistant state.

Quantitative measurements of in vivo insulin sensitivity are essential in order to compare the relative importance of insulin resistance to other factors in the pathogenesis of hyperglycemia and direct research into specific cellular defects that contribute to the reduction in insulin action. In addition, an accurate measure of insulin sensitivity should help in assessing the usefulness of therapeutic regimens and possibly predict future metabolic pathologies. Understanding the basis of these technologies and their limitations is therefore essential in the accurate interpretation of data addressing these issues.

I. Methods Evaluating Insulin Resistance

The insulin tolerance test was first used to measure the decline in plasma glucose levels that occurs during the 30–40 min after the intravenous administration of glucose. This simple procedure suffers from the side effects of inducing hypoglycemia and the fact that counterregulatory hormones blunt the fall in plasma glucose concentration, meaning that the fall in this parameter is the result of a complex interplay of multiple hormones rather than

a simple estimate of insulin-stimulated glucose uptake. Himsworth and Kerr avoided the hypoglycemia by combining glucose and insulin challenges (39). Oral glucose is given with intravenous insulin, and the degree to which the plasma glucose response to the oral glucose is blunted over the next hour serves as an estimate of in vivo insulin action.

Reaven and co-workers developed the impedance test (later known as the pancreatic suppression test) to determine in vivo the tissues' insensitivity to insulin-mediated glucose uptake (40). The insulin suppression test is based on the ability of comparable steady-state plasma levels of insulin to promote disposal of a glucose challenge. Steady-state exogenous insulin and glucose are infused while insulin secretion is suppressed. Using this procedure they demonstrated that marked insulin resistance exists in subjects later defined as NIDDM (41). This unique way to quantify in vivo insulin action directly has been limited for several reasons. Since the rate of glucose infusion is fixed, the insulin suppression test cannot be used to test for insulin dose-response profiles. As the impedance test originally described used a combination of norepinephrine and β-adrenergic blockage to suppress insulin secretion, its application to study individuals with hypertension or other cardiovascular morbidities was not recommended. Side effects of this combination in some individuals thus prevented the widespread application of this technique. This method, however, was subsequently modified by Harano et al. (42), who infused somatostatin in place of epinephrine and propanolol to block insulin secretion. Nagulesparan et al. (43) subsequently modified the somatostatin test to adjust insulin dosage by body weight, yielding similar plasma insulin values in all subjects, and the steady-state plasma glucose value at 90 min was used as an index of total body glucose removal. Ratzmann and colleagues (44) used this somatostatin test to confirm some of the earlier results of Reaven's group.

Andres and his group (45) were the first to propose that a dose-response relationship between the concentration of insulin and some index of insulin action could be used to express whole-body insulin action. The glucose clamp procedures were therefore developed to quantify the ability of exogenous insulin to stimulate glucose utilization under steady-state conditions. This procedure has proven useful in identifying physiological abnormalities that predict the development of NIDDM. The hyperglycemic insulin clamp (46), performed by raising the plasma glucose concentration to 125 mg/dl above the basal plasma glucose level and maintaining that concentration, was developed first. The amount of glucose infused from 20 min to 2 hr to maintain this steady-state plasma glucose concentration was used to approximate the amount of glucose utilized. The ratio of this amount of glucose to the mean steady-state plasma insulin concentration thus provided a measure of in vivo insulin action. Since endogenous insulin secretion was not inhibited and could vary among individuals, and since the ratio assumed that the relationship between insulin level and glucose uptake was linear over the range of the endogenous secretion, this methodology has not been considered entirely precise for measurements of insulin action. In addition, estimates of insulin action with this technique have also been criticized, since they are based on the assumption that glucose utilization is independent of variations in plasma glucose level (47).

The euglycemic glucose clamp was subsequently developed. In this procedure, euglycemia during insulin infusion is maintained by the exogenous infusion of glucose, so the amount of glucose needed to maintain euglycemia becomes a direct measure of insulin sensitivity. Insulin is infused at a constant rate to attain a constant and predetermined degree of insulinemia, which is usually attained within 30 min from the start of iv infusion. To prevent a decline in plasma glucose, frequent assays of glucose are made, and glucose is infused to maintain plasma glucose at basal levels. From this, the necessary glucose infusion rate, calculated as the difference of the insulin-induced increment in glucose utilization rate and the endogenous hepatic output, is viewed as a measure of insulin action. With the addition of labeled glucose infusion, hepatic glucose output can be assessed in the nonsteady state, and from this all components of glucose fluxes can be calculated.

These methodologies, with minor adaptations, have proved useful for measuring insulin resistance in a variety of pathological and altered physiological states, but as indicated above, no one procedure will describe insulin resistance in cellular or molecular terms, or in terms of the location of the insulin resistance. One common approach to measuring the rate of glucose production is the isotope dilution method developed by deBodo and colleagues (48). The pool of glucose in the body is labeled using an infusion of tracer-tagged glucose (usually 3-³H-glucose) 90–150 min prior to insulin infusion. At steady-state glycemia, the tracer is diluted only by endogenous glucose production, and glucose production rate then equals glucose utilization rate. Steele (49) developed equations to calculate hepatic glucose output during the insulin clamp procedure, when the total rate of glucose appearance in the extracellular fluid is that resulting from the sum of hepatic glucose output and the exogenous glucose infused. Since Steele extended the primed-constant tracer infusion technique to the non-steady-state situation, isotope dilution techniques have been commonly used. Such

experiments have led investigators to believe that the liver is more sensitive to insulin than extrahepatic tissues, primarily by regulating hepatic glucose production. However, this procedure was found to be inaccurate during all non-steady-state situations tested (50,51), glucose production being underestimated. Data from Norwich suggested that if the plasma specific activity is maintained constant during the non-steady-state experiment, then turnover rates can be accurately determined by the tracer technique (52). This can be done by adding appropriate amounts of tracer to the glucose infusate (Hot-GINF; 53). This has been validated by comparing simultaneous measurements of hepatic arteriovenous balance during euglycemic clamp studies in dogs (54), and the two procedures have recently been compared in human studies under non-steady-state conditions (55,56). The conventional isotope dilution technique overestimated suppression of glucose production and underestimated stimulation of the glucose disappearance rate, however, compared to results obtained with the Hot-GINF procedure.

Another means of estimating substrate oxidation is through the use of indirect calorimetry. The heat production generated by biochemical processes can be assessed from measurements of V_{O_2} and V_{CO_2} in conjunction with the measurement of urinary nitrogen excretion. Energy released from the oxidation of substrates is coupled to high-energy molecule synthesis, whereas the metabolic reactions consuming energy are coupled to ATP hydrolysis, each process ultimately releasing heat. Indirect calorimetry represents a noninvasive technique for the short-term acute studies (57). Indirect calorimetry allows the calculation of overall substrate disappearance rate by the body but does not permit the assessment of the flux of various intermediate metabolic processes. These processes are susceptible to the influence of the respiratory quotient (which leads to over- or underestimation of the true rate of substrate oxidation in various metabolic states). In addition, the calculations involved are not valid when intermediate metabolites accumulate or when end products other than CO_2, water, and urea are released.

Isotopic labeling of substrates provides an independent way of assessing substrate utilization (57). Stable isotopes, used for estimation of the substrate disappearance rate, are able to quantify substrate transformations by using a dilution principle and to estimate the rate of appearance of the tracer irrespective of its origin. In this procedure enriched substrate can be given and its oxidation followed by measuring enrichment of excretion products, such as CO_2 when ¹³C is given (58,59). Stable isotope tracer techniques are safe, allow study of nitrogen-containing substances, and do not disappear by decay, permitting longer-term study or sample storage. In addition, it is possible to study multiple substrates enriched with different stable isotopes administered by different routes, or to combine this technique with radioactive tracers. Unfortunately, the sample preparation is often time-consuming, and quantifying the abundance of stable isotopes requires special equipment and a high degree of technical expertise. Nevertheless, indirect calorimetry and tracer techniques are complementary, and their combination allows the partitioning of postprandial substrate oxidation according to their exogenous and endogenous origins.

As the maintenance of glucose homeostasis depends on the simultaneous occurrence of insulin secretion, stimulation of glucose uptake, and suppression of hepatic glucose production, defects at the level of the β cell, muscle, or liver can thus lead to the development of glucose intolerance or overt diabetes mellitus (60). The introduction of elevated fatty acids to the discussion adds adipose tissue as a fourth site for insulin resistance. Insulin resistance in obesity has been reported to be more marked in peripheral than in hepatic tissues (61). Understanding the primary defects of glucose intolerance and NIDDM requires methodologies that distinguish metabolic events among these tissues. The concept of nutritive versus shunt capillary flow, that only part of the total blood supply is available for interchange of metabolites or hormones, with the rest being shunted through the vascular network with no effective interchange (62), has redirected research efforts in this field. Coupling these techniques with plethysmography (to measure local blood flow) and indirect calorimetry allows calculation of oxidative and nonoxidative glucose metabolism in specific regions, such as forearm muscle (63). These procedures, however, are time-consuming and unsuitable for screening large numbers of individuals. Newer methodologies involving noninvasive procedures, such as functional magnetic resonance imaging and spectroscopy, to measure capillary blood flow and substrate distribution should prove invaluable for studies of the skeletal muscle component of the insulin resistance.

The minimal model approach was developed to permit quantitation of specific parameters to describe the subject's metabolic status (64). Based on frequently sampled intravenous glucose tolerance test data, Bergman and his associates have considered a series of computer models and chose one that adequately describes the data, of sufficient simplicity to allow estimation of the coefficients for one individual from a single test. This approach thus estimates insulin sensitivity using the simplest model of glucose disappearance, where glucose acts to increase its own utilization and retard its endogenous production. This procedure allows analysis of the contributions of both glucose and insulin to glucose tolerance. In the original methodology the insulin sensitivity index is determined from the

3-hr IVGTT, submitting the temporal pattern of glucose and insulin to computer analysis (65). Injecting tolbutamide 20 min after glucose (66) or somatostatin 1 min prior to glucose (67) substantially improves the precision of the estimated insulin sensitivity index. Replacing tolbutamide with insulin permitted study of diabetic individuals and subjects with severe insulin resistance (68,69). It is also possible to calculate the insulin-independent disappearance of glucose using the tolbutamide-modified IVGTT. Because of its simplicity, this methodology has commonly been used to survey large numbers of individuals for insulin resistance in population studies (66).

One important advantage of minimal modeling methodology is its easy adaptation to the study of various metabolic states. It has therefore been adapted for the study of first-phase insulin secretory response by determining plasma C-peptide concentrations and subsequently deconvoluting these into insulin secretion rates. Analysis of plasma fatty acids in these samples should also allow study of suppression of FFA in the poststimulated state. The minimal model approach appears to correlate well with data obtained from clamp procedures.

2. Mechanisms of Insulin Resistance in Abdominal Obesity

The first scientific documentation of the significant role of insulin resistance in mediating the metabolic events of abdominal obesity was presented in 1982 (10), where fasting and postprandial hyperinsulinemia were found to be associated with glucose intolerance in upper-body-obese women. Figure 3 shows glucose and insulin profiles attained during oral glucose stimulation as a function of body fat distribution. In the fasting state, as well as at all time points during the oral glucose challenge, both plasma glucose and insulin excursions are higher in the abdominally obese. As many as two-thirds of all abdominally obese women have demonstrated impaired glucose tolerance or unsuspected diabetic profiles. The coexistence of hyperinsulinemia and high glucose excursions in this group suggests that the abnormalities in glucose tolerance are mediated by diminished insulin sensitivity. Krotkiewski et al. confirmed these findings, reporting similar results among men (11). In subsequent studies upperbody fat predominance was found to be associated with diminished in vivo insulin sensitivity both during oral glucose loading (16) and using the pancreatic suppression test (25). Increasing WHR is accompanied by progressively increasing fasting plasma glucose and insulin levels during oral glucose tolerance test and diminished insulin sensitivity in healthy premenopausal women, as determined using the somatostatin glucose impedance test. Par-

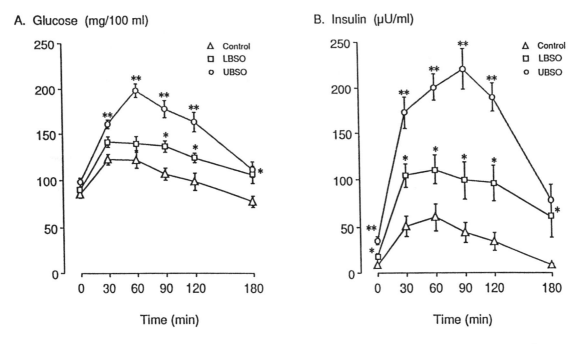

Figure 3 Plasma glucose (A) and insulin (B) responses during oral glucose tolerance testing in nonobese and obese women with either the upper- or lower-body fat distribution. (Data from Ref. 10.)

tial and multiple regression analysis revealed that the effects of body fat topography are independent of and additive to those of obesity. The associations between body fat topography and obesity with parameters of glucose intolerance were analyzed by a multiple regression model with interaction that tested for additivity of WHR and the degree of overweight. Both were found to have independent roles in determining insulin sensitivity and, in turn, the metabolic profile. Subsequent studies using CT techniques demonstrated the visceral fat mass to be a significantly higher correlate of the fasting and postglucose challenge plasma insulin levels than total body fat mass (18,19). This relationship is due primarily to the intra-abdominal fat mass and its linkages to the cumulative insulin response during oral glucose stimulation (Table 2).

The correlations of in vivo insulin sensitivity with glucose and insulin suggest that the glucose intolerance of upper-body obesity is partially due to diminished sensitivity of insulin-mediated glucose disposal. Dose-response studies were performed to further characterize the quantitative and qualitative aspects of these defects. Using the insulin euglycemic clamp technique with the inclusion of 3-³H-glucose infusion to measure the effects of insulin on hepatic glucose production as well as on peripheral glucose utilization, Peiris and co-workers (25) found that basal glucose production among lean and upper- and lower-body-obese individuals is completely suppressed at

an insulin infusion rate of 40 mU/min/m². The dose-response curve for glucose utilization in the lower-body obese is shifted slightly to the right, and maximal glucose utilization is normal. The upper-body obese curve, on the other hand, exhibits a greater rightward shift and a marked reduction in maximal glucose utilization, suggesting that both insulin sensitivity and responsiveness are reduced. This pattern also suggests that the defect in glucose utilization involves a rate-limiting step. The degree of diminished sensitivity and the suppression of maximal responsiveness are similar to what is observed in obese individuals with overt NIDDM. This similarity implies that the defect in glucose utilization in the nondiabetic abdominally obese is of the same severity and is quantitatively and qualitatively similar (at least in kinetic terms) to that seen in diabetics (Fig. 4).

Since skeletal muscle is the major tissue for glucose utilization, and since the insulin resistance appears localized to skeletal muscle (63,70), impaired insulin sensitivity in this tissue could play an important role in the pathogenesis of diminished glucose disposal. Abdominally obese subjects also demonstrate a significant decline in percent glycogen synthase-I (GS-I) response in quadriceps muscle at submaximal plasma insulin levels (71). This decline correlates with the reduction in peripheral glucose utilization. At maximal insulin levels, however, % GS-I response is normal, despite a marked reduction in pe-

Table 2 Standardized Canonical Correlation of the Anthropometric and Metabolic Parameters in Premenopausal Women

Variable	Canonical correlate
Metabolic variable	
Cumulative insulin	—0.74*
Triglyceride	—0.34
Total cholesterol	—0.17
HDL/total cholesterol	—0.12
Systolic blood pressure	—0.18
Diastolic blood pressure	—0.12
Anthropometric variable	
Visceral fat mass	—0.83*
Fat mass	—0.58
Waist/hip ratio	—0.08
Subscapular	—0.67
Subscapular/tricep ratio	—0.02

Canonical correlations comparing sets of anthropometric and metabolic variables in healthy premenopausal women showing a wide range of adiposity and body fat distribution.
*$p < 0.001$.
Source: Data from Ref. 29.

ripheral glucose disposal, suggesting that additional defect(s) that influence other pathways of glucose metabolism are involved. Furthermore, both glucose oxidation and nonoxidative disposal (glycogen synthesis and anaerobic glycolysis) are impaired in abdominal obesity (61). Insulin-activated pyruvate dehydrogenase (% PDH), a rate-limiting enzyme in glucose oxidation, is also impaired. As with GS-I, at maximal insulin level the % PDH response is normal, despite reduced peripheral glucose utilization (Fig. 5). The dissociations suggest that the defect(s) leading to the insulin insensitivity involves an earlier rate-limiting step in glucose metabolism. Abdominal obesity is thus associated with defects in insulin-regulated oxidative and nonoxidative glucose disposal, as well as in insulin suppression of hepatic glucose production.

That insulin-mediated vasodilation is impaired in a number of insulin-resistant states suggests a connection between insulin resistance and hemodynamic mechanisms (72,73). Systemic insulin infusions are accompanied by dose-dependent increases in skeletal muscle blood flow, which are significantly diminished in obese subjects. It has also been claimed that insulin's action to increase skeletal muscle perfusion could account for as much as one-third of its overall effects to stimulate glucose uptake (74,75). In this regard, a defect in this hemodynamic action could result in insulin resistance. On the other hand, our studies, shown in Figure 6, indicate no significant differences in cardiac output and forearm blood flow responses during insulin infusion in both normotensive and hypertensive abdominally obese or lean individuals at euglycemia. These findings, however, do not rule out the notion that the microcirculatory redistribution of blood prefusion to regions of greater capacity to metabolize and store glucose as glycogen might be a new candidate site influencing insulin actions in skeletal muscle.

As shown in Table 3, body fat distribution determined by WHR is negatively correlated with the degree of capillary density in skeletal muscle. In addition, the percentage of type I relative to type IIb fibers is reduced with increasing WHR. Muscle fiber surface areas are all increased with increasing WHR. Furthermore, the degree of capillary rarefaction is correlated with the decline in insulin-mediated peripheral glucose utilization. This reduced capillarization might precede both diminished insulin sensitivity and changes in type I-to-IIb fiber ratio. It is well known that regions with predominantly slow-twitch versus those with fast-twitch fibers display different capillary densities (76), with resulting differences in blood supply. Blood flow through the slow-twitch fibers is approximately threefold greater than in the fast-twitch fibers. Reduced capillary density might thus play some role in initiating changes in muscle fiber activity and eventually in muscle fiber composition. Collectively the above studies indicate that a number of mechanisms, including vascular, neurohumoral, and metabolic components, participate in the etiology of the marked peripheral insulin resistance observed in abdominal obesity.

B. Splanchnic Insulin Dynamics

Splanchnic insulin dynamics represents the sum of events involved in insulin secretion, uptake, and clearance. Insulin is secreted by the pancreas into the portal vein in response to such stimuli as glucose, arginine, and other secretagogues. Insulin travels first to the liver, where 40–60% is removed via saturable, receptor-mediated processes, with much of the rest being removed by the kidneys and skeletal muscle (see Ref. 77 for review). Increased pancreatic insulin secretion in obesity is closely paralleled by the increase in relative body weight but is uninfluenced by the site of body fat predominance (24). Diminished insulin clearance and hepatic insulin extrac-

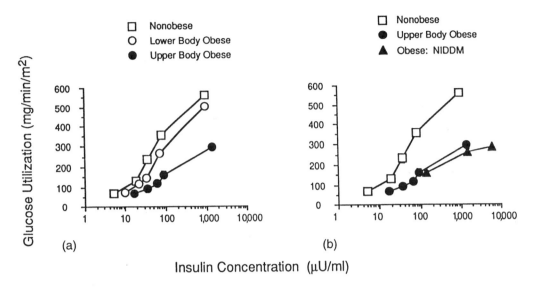

Figure 4 Dose-response effects of insulin on glucose uptake during hyperinsulinemic euglycemic clamps. (a) Glucose utilization as a function of body fat distribution; (b) glucose utilization in nondiabetic abdominally obese and in obese subjects with NIDDM. (Data from Ref. 25.)

tion, on the other hand, are closely aligned with the higher levels of peripheral insulinemia and the greater degree of insulin insensitivity when adiposity is predominantly localized to the abdominal region (78). Together with the increase in pancreatic insulin production, the decrease in insulin extraction attempts to compensate the insulin resistance of abdominal obesity. The following account will describe methods commonly used to evaluate splanchnic insulin dynamics and discuss the role of the pancreas and adaptive mechanisms that influence prevailing plasma insulin levels in abdominal obesity.

I. Methods Evaluating Splanchnic Insulin Dynamics

Traditionally, insulin secretion profiles have been evaluated by measurements of the plasma hormone levels in

the basal state, during oral or iv glucose, standard meal, hyperglycemic clamp, or after administration of specific secretagogues. As pancreatic insulin secretion profiles cannot be evaluated directly because of potential variations in the hepatic extraction of insulin, a number of procedures have evolved whereby plasma C-peptide concentrations are measured instead. This choice is based on the notion that C-peptide is secreted in equimolar amounts to insulin but is not extracted by the liver to a significant extent. As reviewed by Hovorka and Jones (79), C-peptide exhibits linear kinetics over a broad range of plasma concentrations under fasting and fed conditions. As cross-reactivity with proinsulin is generally lower than for insulin, calculations based on plasma C-peptide levels should

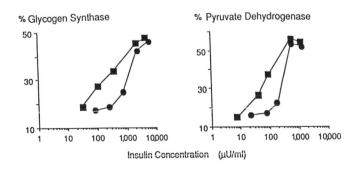

Figure 5 Dose-response effects of insulin on skeletal muscle enzyme activities. The active forms of glycogen synthase and pyruvate dehydrogenase are determined in skeletal muscle biopsies and expressed as percentages of total activities. (■) Nonobese; (●) upper-body obese. (Data from Evans et al., unpublished.)

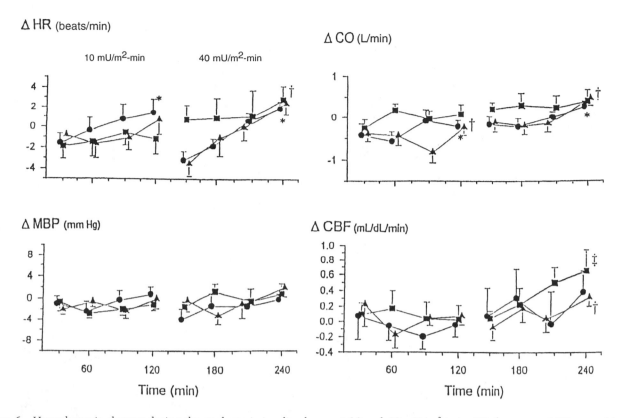

Figure 6 Hemodynamic changes during the euglycemic insulin clamps at 10 and 40 mU/m²/min. HR, heart rate; MBP, mean blood pressure; CO, cardiac output; CBF, calf blood flow. (●) Upper-body obese hypertensives; (■) upper-body obese normotensives; (▲) lean normotensives. Significance is shown versus baseline. (Data from Ref. 73.)

therefore reflect more precise estimates of insulin secretion than those relying on plasma insulin levels.

Waldhausl et al. (80) measured hepatic vein C-peptide concentrations and splanchnic blood flow to calculate the pancreatic insulin production rate in humans. Radziuk had earlier described a mathematical model that was applicable to the calculation of non-steady-state C-peptide secretion rates based on peripheral measurements, fitting the data decay curve to a multi-exponential model (81). It was not certain, however, whether hepatic extraction and MCR of C-peptide could change under physiological circumstances or whether peripheral plasma C-peptide concentrations could mirror insulin secretion at all times. Meistas et al. attempted another measure, using a contin-

Table 3 Relationship of Body Fat Distribution to Muscle Fiber Density and Capillary Density

	Type I (r)	Type IIa (r)	Type IIb (r)
WHR: fiber area	0.46*	0.46*	0.41*
WHR: capillary density	−0.48*	−0.39*	−0.46*
Maximum strength	0.15	0.24	0.24

Samples obtained from skeletal muscle biopsies. Fiber areas and capillary densities determined histographically. Maximum strength determined by ergometry.
*$p < 0.005$.
Source: Data from A. H. Kissebah (unpublished).

uous blood withdrawal system that allows calculation of integrated values for C-peptide and insulin concentrations over a 24-hr period (82). The secretion rate of each peptide was calculated as the product of its pooled 24-hr plasma concentration and metabolic clearance rate. Faber and colleagues proposed that the time course of insulin secretion could further be evaluated by determining plasma C-peptide levels after a bolus injection of C-peptide (83). A multicompartmental model describing the kinetics of C-peptide and insulin was subsequently proposed by Eaton et al. (84). Suppressing endogenous C-peptide secretion with somatostatin, however, allowed estimates of parameters of C-peptide kinetics in each individual (85).

The urinary excretion of C-peptide has also been examined as a possible means of measuring insulin secretion. Kaneko et al. first reported that C-peptide in urine increased in parallel with an oral glucose load (86), and urinary C-peptide excretion would be highly correlated to plasma C-peptide and insulin levels. Due to the possible influence of small changes in GFR, tubular function, and renal plasma flow on C-peptide excretion, however, it was necessary to evaluate the urinary C-peptide concentration in relation to its plasma concentration rather than studying changes in absolute urinary C-peptide excretion values (87).

Polonsky and co-workers (88), as well as our group (24), advanced these earlier attempts and subsequently developed a noninvasive means of evaluating insulin secretion dynamics. The insulin secretion rate is calculated by deconvoluting the plasma C-peptide concentrations using the kinetic coefficients of C-peptide turnover measured in the same individual. The kinetic coefficient parameters are derived from the plasma disappearance curve following either the stimulation of endogenous secretion or the injection of an exogenous bolus of C-peptide.

The minimal model technique provides an insulin secretion profile during the IVGTT using a simple one-compartmental model approach (89). A combined model that employs both insulin and C-peptide data has also been proposed (90,91). This model allows estimation of both insulin and C-peptide kinetic parameters during the IVGTT. Evaluation of the initial phase of insulin secretion also can be obtained. Cobelli and Pacini expanded this procedure to model both C-peptide and insulin kinetics using two compartments (92), thus yielding information on both posthepatic appearance and prehepatic delivery, including both the first and second phases of insulin secretion.

Most of the procedures described above can also be adapted to measure insulin clearance. As reviewed by Castillo et al. (93), the most commonly used method involves the use of C-peptide/insulin molar ratios during steady-state conditions, or by integrating areas under the concentration-time curves or averaging plasma concentrations of both peptides. Because of its simplicity, the molar ratio has been used to measure insulin clearance in a number of studies, but the differences in kinetics of removal of the two peptides from the post-hepatic circulation necessitate mathematical modeling to allow calculation of rates of insulin clearance (94).

Mathematical analysis of plasma decay curves of insulin after an acute insulin input (either through a known amount of exogenously administered insulin or after a stimulus to increase the endogenous level) has been used to calculate estimates of the metabolic clearance rate of insulin. The decay curve is then analyzed using either a single-compartment model or by multicompartmental approaches. The more complex, compartmental modeling yields more complete and precise information on the insulin kinetics.

Use of radiolabeled insulin allows measurement of insulin clearance at concentrations of the hormone that do not lower plasma glucose and hence reduces measurement error. Tracer labeling procedures are useful only if the labeled hormone chosen is shown to behave similarly to unlabeled insulin. Use of methods where endogenous insulin secretion is stimulated requires a precise characterization of this secretion and hence is critically dependent upon the accuracy of measuring the plasma C-peptide concentrations. In addition, the kinetic parameters obtained under basal conditions may not be the same as those obtained after its secretion is stimulated. Indeed, the high concentrations attained may result in nonlinear clearance kinetics. Use of the modified, frequently sampled IVGTT also allows estimation of insulin clearance. This technique has been adapted to determine both posthepatic insulin clearance rate and hepatic insulin extraction. Fractional disappearance rate of insulin can be calculated using the combined minimal model described above (90).

Continuous insulin input at a constant rate results in stable plasma levels at steady state, where the rate of removal equals its rate of administration. This method obviates the need for analyzing multiexponential plasma decay curves following a single insulin input. Radiolabeled insulin may instead be infused if a bioactive form of tracer can be obtained. Cold insulin, however, has been used more commonly. During insulin infusion glucose must be given simultaneously to avoid hypoglycemia. Varying the infusion rate of the insulin allows determination of insulin kinetics at different steady-state insulin levels. Insulin metabolism may be assessed during the euglycemic insulin clamp or in the absence of glucose clamping, when insulin and glucose are given at prefixed rates (95). The above methodologies have been used to demonstrate that the insulin clearance mechanisms saturate at high plasma hormone levels. These approaches have also been adapted to the measurement of insulin clearance during basal steady state. Again, precise estimation of the endogenous secretion rate must be known. Using the two-compartment model of C-peptide kinetics (84), on the other hand, allows estimation of insulin secretion rates even under non-steady-state conditions (88), determining various fractional rate constants that describe the rates of irreversible removal as well as those that govern the passage of C-peptide from one compartment to another.

2. Adaptations in Splanchnic Insulin Dynamics in Abdominal Obesity

Mechanisms responsible for the compensatory hyperinsulinemia characteristic of abdominal obesity are complex. We have previously alluded to this issue and reviewed possible components involved (3). While a generalized excess of total body fat is associated with hypersecretion of insulin, a high level of abdominal adipose tissue specifically is associated with a reduced hepatic extraction of insulin (22,25). We have also proposed that the enlarged visceral fat depot, which is characterized by increased lipolysis, may contribute to this adaptation by exposing the liver to high FFA levels and consequently reducing hepatic insulin extraction (96,97). In addition, altered levels of sex steroids may be involved. The high free testosterone and reduced sex hormone–binding globulin seen in abdominally obese women could contribute to their insulin resistance, as well as the adaptations in insulin dynamics (97). Each of these factors may thus potentially regulate insulin production and its actions and clearance in abdominal obesity.

Increased secretion of insulin is a primary feature of obesity (9,98). Increased β-cell mass and islet hypertrophy have been reported (99,100). Compared with lean individuals, abdominally obese subjects have greater prehepatic insulin production and portal vein insulin levels, both in the fasting state and following oral or intravenous glucose stimulation (22). Portal concentrations of insulin and C-peptide are also increased, in both the basal state (101,102) and following stimulation with insulin secretagogues (103). This increase in insulin secretion is not correlated with the degree of peripheral insulin insensitivity (22,104,105). The hyperinsulinemia, which only partially compensates the decrease in insulin sensitivity, may thus represent one response to the insulin resistance of abdominal obesity.

The basis for the increased secretion is uncertain. During the past few years, an increasing body of evidence

indicates that the patten of insulin release may be important in detecting early dysfunction of the beta cell. It is generally agreed that fluctuations in plasma insulin levels reflect fluctuations in insulin release (106). Pancreatic insulin release is a highly dynamic process, exhibiting specific patterns of temporal variations. Weigle suggested that under certain conditions pulsatile insulin delivery might have greater biological effects than continuous delivery (107), and that fluctuations in plasma insulin concentration may be important in regulating islet cell function. It is also possible that the aberrant pulsatility might be secondary to SNS overactivity (108). Autonomic innervation of the islets controls insulin release during food intake and food digestion, along with the absorbed glucose and amino acids and gastrointestinal hormones, and absence of this parasympathetic influence leads to wider fluctuations of blood glucose. It also controls the availability of nutrients for the CNS and muscles during emotional and physical stress, occurring mainly by suppression of insulin and activation of glucagon. Abnormalities in insulin release pulsatilities may thus exacerbate the insulin resistance and contribute to the hyperglycemia of abdominal obesity.

Low-frequency insulin secretory pulses with a periodicity of 80–120 min occurring during the steady states of overnight rest and continuous enteric feeding have been observed (109). The periodicity of these pulses is similar to that of the hypothalamically driven ultradian hormone release. Pulse amplitudes during feeding are increased and are coupled with changes in plasma glucose levels. Similar pulsatilities have been observed during iv glucose infusion and meal intake. In abdominally obese subjects the mean insulin secretion rate (ISR) is increased two- to fourfold over that of normal subjects (23). Entrainment between this form of pulsatility and the concomitant pulsations in plasma glucose supports the contention that this pulsatility mode is part of the glucose/insulin feedback loop (110,111). In abdominally obese individuals ultradian pulsatilities exhibit high pulse nadirs and diminution of relative pulse amplitudes (23). Their coupling with pulsations in plasma glucose also appears to be disrupted. Although the number of pulsations does not differ significantly from normal, their amplitudes are abnormal. Ultradian pulses are also less regular and exhibit marked variability in pulse maximum, nadir, and amplitude consistent with the heterogeneity among individuals with this form of obesity (Fig. 7).

In addition to the low-frequency mode, high-frequency insulin secretory pulses with a periodicity of 8–16 min have also been reported (112–114). Their periodicity and amplitude are independent of intrapancreatic neuronal connections or local paracrine influences. These pulses are

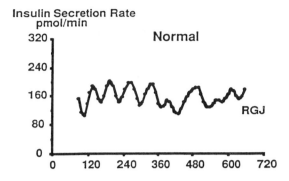

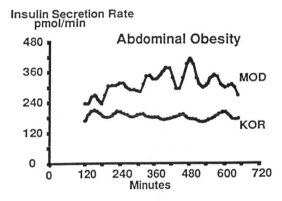

Figure 7 Ultradian insulin secretion pulsatilites during continous enteral feeding. Representative data from one normal subject and two individuals with abdominal obesity. (Adapted from Ref. 23.)

production rates being lower at each level of glycemia. Under these circumstances the islet mass engaged in hormone secretion is either reduced or else its secretory sensorship (response) has been impaired (Fig. 9).

That the increased insulin production cannot completely compensate for the insulin insensitivity suggests that in abdominal obesity the ability of the insulin secretory process to sense the marked increase in peripheral insulin demand may be limited or defective. A decline in insulin clearance is necessary to produce the systemic hyperinsulinemia found in the compensated abdominally obese women. Reduced hepatic insulin extraction in obesity has been demonstrated by several groups (116,117). This reduction is also apparent during the fed states (102), where high insulin levels are needed to overcome the defect in insulin-mediated peripheral glucose utilization. As discussed above, hepatic insulin extraction, evaluated by noninvasive techniques, has been shown to be reduced in the abdominally obese, both in the basal state and following stimulation of insulin secretion by intravenous or oral

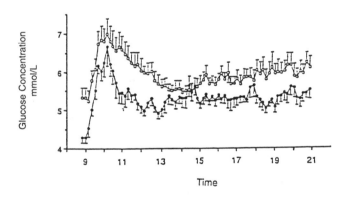

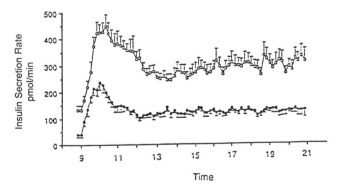

Figure 8 Insulin secretion profiles during continuous enteral feeding. Subjects received liquid formula at a constant rate through an enteric tube placed into the lower third of the duodenum. (●) Normals; (○) abdominally obese subjects. (Data from Ref. 23.)

superimposed on broader ultradian pulses, both in the fasting state (107) and during iv glucose infusion (115). Alterations in the patterns of this pulsatility may also represent another early beta-cell defect.

Despite the three- to fourfold increase in insulin secretion in abdominal obesity, the initial phase of insulin release in response to continuous enteral feeding shows proper rise and delayed fall with marked interindividual variability. Its duration is also prolonged, indicating the sluggishness of the beta-cell secretory apparatus (Fig. 8). Indeed, the beta-cell sensorships to stepped glucose infusions are consistent with disturbed secretory mechanisms in those individuals with impaired glucose tolerance. Thus in the obese subjects with normal glucose tolerance, stepped glucose infusions (between 4 and 14 mM) are accompanied by steeper-than-normal increases in insulin secretion in the islet mass engaged in the secretory process. In these individuals insulin secretion rate, at each level of glycemia, is higher than normal. In obese individuals with impaired glucose tolerance, on the other hand, the secretory curve is markedly shifted to the right, insulin

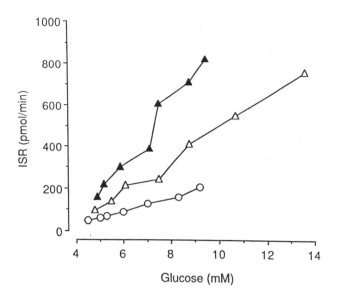

Figure 9 Insulin secretory response to glucose during stepped infusions of glucose. (▲) Obese with normal glucose tolerance; (△) obese with impaired glucose tolerance; (○) lean controls. (From G. E. Sonnenberg et al., unpublished.)

glucose (22) and during enteric feeding (23). The metabolic clearance rate (MCR) of exogenously administered insulin has also been determined during the insulin euglycemic clamp technique (25; Fig. 10). Increasing WHR is associated with decreasing MCR, with the MCR of the

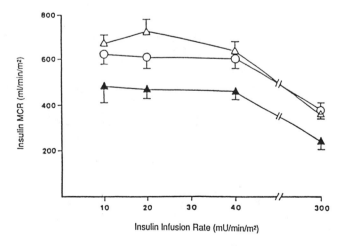

Figure 10 Insulin metabolic clearance rate (MCR) in relation to body fat distribution. Clearance rates are determined at four insulin infusion rates during euglycemic clamps in the upper-body obese (▲), the lower-body obese (△), and the nonobese (○). (Data from Ref. 78.)

upper-body obese significantly lower than that of the nonobese or the age- or weight-matched lower-body-obese subjects. No significant difference in insulin MCR was observed between the lower-body obese and the nonobese subjects, but the decline in MCR in the upper- as compared to the lower-body-obese subjects or the nonobese is demonstrable at all insulin levels tested. Within the obese group a positive correlation is found between insulin MCR and peripheral insulin sensitivity.

Some of the reduction in hepatic insulin extraction of abdominal obesity may be due to down-regulation of the insulin receptors and thus the decreased removal by the liver. In addition, it has long been known that plasma FFA concentration is elevated in obesity, particularly in abdominal obesity. An increase in the size of the visceral fat depot is a precursor to the increased lipolysis, elevated FFA flux, and subsequent overexposure of hepatic tissues to FFA, which may then promote changes in insulin dynamics (96,118). As reviewed previously (3), infusion of long-chain fatty acids in dogs increases both plasma FFA and insulin levels in parallel. Obesity induced by high-fat feeding in rats is associated with increased portal FFA levels and decreased hepatic insulin extraction. Furthermore, visceral obesity in the male SHHF/Mcc-fa^{cp} rat is associated with decreased hepatic insulin extraction and marked hyperinsulinemia (119). Additional, raising portal vein FFA levels in isolated rat livers decreases insulin clearance (120). We have therefore proposed that the increased FFA flux in visceral obesity might be responsible for the accompanying reductions in hepatic insulin extraction and clearance.

Exposure of isolated hepatocytes to physiological concentrations of albumin-bound palmitate induces a dose-dependent reduction in cell-surface insulin receptor binding (121–123). This is also associated with a proportionally diminished receptor-mediated internalization and decreased intracellular and total receptor-mediated insulin degradation. Moderate increases in FFA release, such as those that occur in abdominal obesity, could thus contribute to the reduced hepatic insulin extraction and peripheral hyperinsulinemia. As glucose also influences splanchnic insulin dynamics, relative contributions from FFA and glucose needed to be distinguished. To test these findings from in vitro and animal studies, we undertook studies raising plasma FFA levels in lean normal subjects, using Intralipid and heparin infusion, with or without concomitant hyperglycemia (124). Maintaining a high FFA flux while raising plasma glucose levels significantly increased plasma insulin concentrations, as a result of both increased pancreatic insulin secretion (Fig. 11) and decreased insulin clearance. The suppressive effects of glucose and FFA on endogenous insulin clearance were

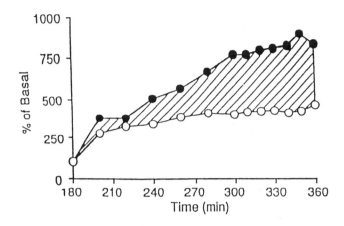

Figure 11 Insulin secretion rate (○) and plasma insulin concentration (●) in lean premenopausal women during hyperglycemia and elevated FFA flux. Plasma FFA flux was doubled by infusing Intralipid and heparin while plasma glucose was clamped at 11 mM. Data expressed as percentages of their best value. (Data from Ref. 124.)

independent and additive. One potential mechanism explaining the hyperinsulinemia of abdominal obesity might thus be the increased levels of FFA flux, particularly during hyperglycemia.

Synergistic effects have been described between obesity and gender on hepatic insulin binding and clearance (119), which could result from their interaction on hepatic insulin receptor expression. While neither gender nor obesity affects hepatic insulin receptor mRNA content in SHHF/Mcc-FA^{cp} rats, total hepatic insulin receptor content is decreased by more than 50% in animals of either gender (125). Obesity and sex steroids may thus affect hepatic insulin receptor protein content and cell surface binding via translational or posttranslational mechanisms.

These studies suggested a mechanism by which obesity might modify insulin receptor expression and compartmentalization in liver as a result of concomitant changes in sex hormone levels. As reviewed previously (3,29), insulin sensitivity is impaired in nonobese, hyperandrogenized, hirsute women. Giving derivatives of testosterone to women results in impaired glucose tolerance and hyperinsulinemia. Furthermore, administration of testosterone to female, ovariectomized rats reduces insulin sensitivity in skeletal muscle, produces capillary rarefaction, and changes muscle fiber morphology (126). The reduction of hepatic insulin uptake in abdominal obesity may also be associated with an increase in androgenic activity (24). Estradiol is known to increase insulin binding to hepatocytes from ovariectomized rats, while testosterone reduces binding and degradation (127). Another mechanism accounting for the association between upper-body fat localization and the aberrations in hepatic insulin extraction

and peripheral insulin sensitivity might thus be related to common events involving increased androgenic activity.

Such influences of FFA metabolism and steroid hormone levels could play roles in the insulin resistance of abdominal obesity. It is also clear that the pathway of potential linkages between abdominal obesity and the adverse metabolic profile involves complex interactions between genetics and neuroendocrine, as well as environmental, traits, influencing some aspects of insulin sensitivity, splanchnic insulin dynamics, and possibly the metabolic profile as well. These might act in concert to influence cellular, microvascular, and neurohumoral mechanisms to promote insulin resistance and splanchnic insulin dynamics and eventually create the adverse metabolic profile of central obesity.

In summary, lower-body obesity is associated with only a mild decline in peripheral insulin sensitivity, accompanied by an increase in pancreatic insulin production. Upper-body obesity, on the other hand, is characterized by a more severe form of insulin resistance, compensated by an additional decline in hepatic insulin removal, and consequently a much higher degree of peripheral hyperinsulinemia. These relationships are illustrated schematically in Figure 12.

IV. BIOLOGY OF THE CLINICAL COMPONENTS: ROLE OF BODY FAT TOPOGRAPHY

The predictive power of body fat distribution and major health morbidities is due in part to its association with

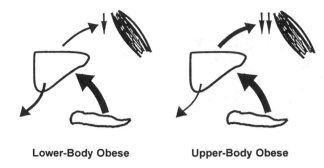

Lower-Body Obese   **Upper-Body Obese**

Figure 12 Representation of insulin sensitivity and splanchnic insulin dynamics in upper- and lower-body obese subjects. (Adapted from Ref. 29.)

aberrant insulin dynamics and, consequently, a cluster of adverse metabolic profiles, including glucose intolerance, dyslipidemia, and elevated blood pressure. The following section reviews mechanisms by which these associations, as well as other independent mechanisms, could lead to expression of clinical components of the metabolic syndrome and their morbidities.

A. Glucose Intolerance and NIDDM

As early as 1959, Yalow and Berson demonstrated wide variances in insulin levels among heterogeneous groups of diabetics (128). Whereas in some individuals insulin levels during oral glucose tolerance tests are markedly reduced, others exhibit moderate or even very high levels. Based upon measurements of plasma hormone concentrations, several studies documented both increased and decreased levels of insulin among NIDDM subjects. The most conclusive documentation of insulin resistance in NIDDM came from studies that employed the pancreatic suppression test (42) and the insulin clamp technique (46). With the development of procedures for noninvasive measurement of prehepatic insulin production, Polonsky's group demonstrated in subjects with NIDDM decreased production during a three-meal study protocol and during iv or oral glucose stimulation (105). Their studies, along with those of our group, have also demonstrated secretory disturbances, with the periodic fluctuations in ultradian pulses being irregular in frequency and the amplitudes markedly blunted (23,110). The normally entrained relationship between glucose and insulin secretion pulsatilities is severely disturbed. Finally, the sensorship for stepped doses of glucose infusion is markedly shifted to the right and blunted. These abnormalities could both be secondary to the severity of the insulin resistance, however, since the amplitude of impaired insulin-mediated glucose utiliza-

tion is equal to that observed in nondiabetic, abdominally obese subjects (Fig. 4). The expression of overt diabetes is thus contingent upon additional primary defect(s) in the secretory machinery of the islets. Inabilities to sense glucose levels and engineer appropriate secretory responses not only exacerbate a further decline in peripheral glucose utilization, but could also play an important role in the unsuppressed glucose production and evolution of overt hyperglycemia.

Abdominal obesity is associated with a moderate decline in hepatic insulin sensitivity, which is overcome by a sustained increase in portal vein insulin levels. This is accomplished both by an increased pancreatic insulin secretion rate and by a reduction in the hepatic removal of insulin. Hepatic insulin extraction is diminished after both oral and iv administration of glucose in upper- but not in lower-body-obese subjects; this is also seen after both the three-meal test and continuous enteral feeding. A significant reduction in the insulin clearance rate is also observed at all insulin levels, suggesting that postreceptor mechanisms may be responsible. The severity of hepatic insulin resistance in NIDDM exceeds that of abdominally obese, nondiabetic subjects, however, indicating that the more marked hepatic insulin resistance of NIDDM probably results from additional defect(s) in insulin action. Insulin controls glucose homeostasis by coordinating suppression of hepatic glucose production and stimulation of glucose uptake by splanchnic and peripheral tissues. Glucose uptake, in turn, depends on glucose oxidation and glucose storage. Defects in any of these processes, at the level of skeletal muscle or liver, may result in insulin resistance and glucose intolerance. The following sections describe mechanisms that may underlie the basis for the disturbances in insulin-glucose homeostasis of abdominal obesity that predispose to glucose intolerance and NIDDM.

1. Role of Free Fatty Acids

Randle et al. proposed that increased FFA levels are associated with a preferential FFA oxidation, which then interferes with such processes as insulin action, glucose oxidation, and glucose storage (129). This glucose–fatty acid hypothesis suggests that high levels of FFA, which are elevated in the portal circulation of the abdominally obese, may play a central role in the development of such metabolic diseases as NIDDM. Lipid infusion causes glucose intolerance and inhibits total glucose uptake in healthy individuals (130). For the glucose–fatty acid cycle to operate, the increase in FFA levels must result in an increase in lipid oxidation, since small elevations in plasma FFA levels do not decrease glucose oxidation (although increased FFA oxidation will decrease glucose oxidation). Increased basal lipolysis with no change in lipid oxidation relative to lean controls has been demonstrated in the abdominally obese (131), along with defects in glucose metabolism (73). This suggests a defect in lipid oxidation, since raising circulating levels of FFA in healthy, lean volunteers is associated with enhanced lipid oxidation (132). Similar observations have also been reported in abdominally obese individuals (133) and in NIDDM subjects. The ability of insulin to suppress lipid oxidation is also impaired in the abdominally obese, likely the cumulative effect of a failure to raise basal oxidation in the face of increased fatty acid flux and an impaired capacity of insulin to suppress fat oxidation (131).

Fatty acid oxidation may also influence the systemic delivery of insulin. Moderate increases in FFA release could contribute to the reduced hepatic insulin extraction, as discussed above, and, along with the enhanced insulin secretion, would augment the compensatory peripheral hyperinsulinemia. Under basal conditions, elevating FFA flux or raising plasma glucose to physiological postprandial levels increased both plasma insulin concentration and the insulin secretion rate (124). Maintaining a high FFA flux during the glucose clamp resulted in a significantly higher plasma insulin clearance due to the additive effects of increased pancreatic secretion and decreased insulin clearance (Fig. 11). Thus the hyperinsulinemia of abdominal obesity might be mediated in part by both increased FFA flux and levels of glycemia observed in this obesity phenotype.

Skeletal muscle, which is responsible for a substantial part of both whole-body glucose uptake and glucose oxidation, thereby represents a major site in the development of insulin resistance. Both skeletal muscle glucose oxidation and nonoxidative disposal (glycogen synthesis and anaerobic glycolysis) are impaired in the abdominally obese (73). The strong negative correlation between the rates of FFA flux and glucose oxidation at several levels of insulinemia is also consistent with the Randle hypothesis. Figure 13 shows the significantly negative correlations demonstrated in groups of lean and abdominally obese individuals between insulin-mediated glucose oxidation and lipid oxidation. On the other hand, there are no significant correlations between the rates of lipid oxidation and nonoxidative glucose disposal in the same groups. That there is no significant relationship between lipid oxidation and glucose storage suggests that mechanisms other than enhanced FFA are responsible for the abnormal glucose storage capacity, the major characteristic defect of the insulin resistance in abdominal obesity.

2. The Neuroendocrine Dysregulation Hypothesis

Björntorp proposed that stressful social, behavioral, and biological stimuli may initiate chronic neuroendocrine dysregulations that result over time in a more pronounced android profile of fat deposition. Individual differences in the amount and the nature of stress exposure and in the level of ensuing hypothalamic arousal are related to variations in hormonal responses that can influence body fat topography. The growing visceral fat depots have been proposed to act synergistically with the prevailing hormonal profile, leading progressively to metabolic disturbances and eventually to the complete metabolic profile (Fig. 14).

Multiple perturbations of glucocorticoid and steroid hormone concentrations and dynamics may be intimately involved in the pathogenesis of the insulin resistance of abdominal obesity (134). A high sensitivity of the CRF-ACTH-cortisol axis is characteristic of abdominal obesity. In addition, cortisol displays direct actions on insulin sensitivity and glucose tolerance, while perinatal and peripubertal sex hormones play major roles in influencing both insulin dynamics and fat deposition (3). The association in women between upper-body fat localization, the aberrations in hepatic insulin extraction and peripheral insulin sensitivity, and the resultant changes in glucose and lipid metabolism might be mediated by a common mechanism involving increased androgenic activity. Increasing androgenic activity (as measured by percent free testosterone) is negatively correlated with both insulin sensitivity and hepatic insulin extraction in premenopausal women (Fig. 15). A sex hormone imbalance causing regional differences in fat morphology and metabolic activity may also be directly exacerbated by hepatic and extrahepatic disturbances in insulin-glucose homeostasis, and this situation may further be adversely influenced by such environmentally related factors as physical and psychological stresses, diet, smoking, and alcohol.

3. Genetic Susceptibility to NIDDM

Defects leading to insulin resistance and disturbances in splanchnic insulin dynamics are caused by a combination of genetic and environmental factors, such as diet and activity. Ethnic and geographic variations in frequency of diabetes in certain populations suggest a genetic predisposition. Martin and co-workers (135) used the minimal model to study nondiabetic individuals who had two parents with NIDDM and examined familial clustering of insulin sensitivity (insulin-dependent glucose disposal). Some families were found to be made up primarily of individuals with high insulin sensitivity, whereas others

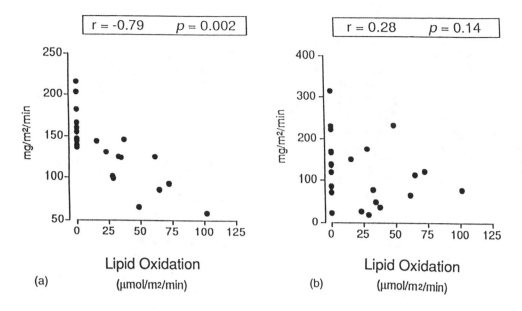

Figure 13   Relationships of lipid oxidation to glucose oxidative (a) and nonoxidative glucose disposal (b) in nonobese and abdominally obese subjects. (Data from M. M. I. Hennes et al., unpublished.)

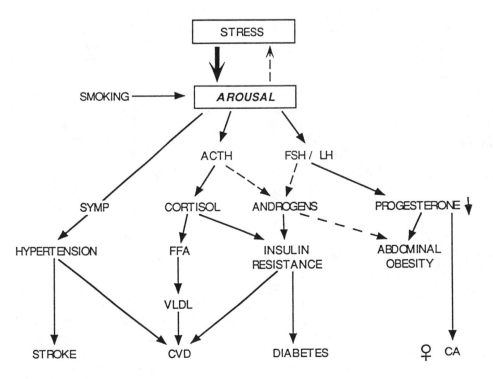

Figure 14   Neuroendocrine mechanisms in abdominal obesity and its metabolic sequelae: the hypothalamic-arousal hypothesis. (Adapted from Ref. 134.)

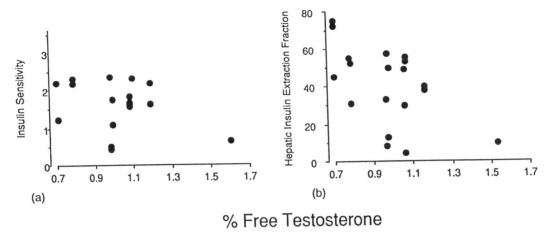

% Free Testosterone

Figure 15 Relationships of percent free testosterone levels to insulin-sensitive glucose utilization (a) (mg/min/m²/μU-ml) and hepatic insulin extraction fraction (% of total) in obese premenopausal women (b). (Data from Ref. 24.)

were mostly insulin insensitive. Such familial clustering was also observed in longitudinal and in cross-sectional studies (see Ref. 136 for review) in Pima Indians, where impaired glucose tolerance in obese subjects was due primarily to a reduction in insulin action, and in Mexican-Americans, where the glucose-tolerant offspring of two NIDDM parents were found to be characterized by hyperinsulinemia and demonstrated insulin resistance. The high prevalence of impaired glucose tolerance in African-Americans and in certain South Pacific island populations, with a high occurrence of NIDDM, also suggest a genetic component to insulin resistance.

The prevalence of both clinical diabetes and abnormal glucose tolerance is significantly greater among the close relatives of diabetics than among similar relatives of non-diabetic individuals. In addition, family and twin studies support the role of genetic factors in diabetes risk. Studies on monozygotic twins who share genes and gene variants have demonstrated that the concordance for NIDDM diagnosis within twin pairs exceeds 90% (137), even when the twins had not been living together for several years or did not display similar levels of body fat. Concordance for NIDDM decreases in first- and second-degree relatives, as the percentage of shared genes decreases. In addition, a number of animal species variants bred to develop syndromes that model human NIDDM bolster arguments that genetic risk factors are important in the etiology of NIDDM.

NIDDM is a polygenic, multifactorial disease that predisposes certain individuals to develop the disease (138). Life-style and nutritional habits also influence the clinical course of the disease. Family and epidemiological studies have shown that patients with NIDDM are more likely to have affected mothers than affected fathers. The disorder is also often inherited through multiple maternal generations. It may be possible that the diabetic environment *in utero* has a metabolic effect on the fetus that increases the risk for diabetes, although it is also possible that mitochondrial DNA (mtDNA) mutations predispose to diabetes (see Ref. 139 for review), since the inheritance of mtDNA is exclusively maternal. Such mutations, although rare, have been found in a few large pedigrees with maternally transmitted diabetes and in population screening of diabetic patients. Normal insulin secretion by the pancreatic islet cells is dependent on oxidative phosphorylation, and a defect in this process might play a role in NIDDM. One mutation, coding for the leucine tRNA, was associated with diminished insulin secretion, while another, coding for an amino acid change in a putative NADH dehydrogenase enzyme, was highly associated with NIDDM. More recently, a mutation in the tRNA for glutamic acid was also found to be associated with diabetes. Whether such defects occur and may influence or be influenced by abdominal fat remains to be demonstrated.

There are three basic approaches to locating genes that may play a role in the pathogenesis of insulin resistance, bearing in mind that some of these genes may be primary and actually cause the insulin resistance, whereas others may be secondary to this state. The first approach involves the hit-or-miss procedure of trying to identify candidate genes. Defects in enzymes and proteins involved in hepatic glucose production, glucose utilization and disposal, and insulin signal transduction are all possibilities. Some evidence of involvement has been produced in such diverse components of insulin action as metabolic factors (such as insulin receptor substrate-1, glycogen synthase, and the glucagon receptor; 140) and structural factors (such as skeletal muscle fiber types; 141), although their contributions are likely small and the most obvious candidate genes, those for insulin, the insulin receptor, and the glucose transporters, have been excluded as major diabetogenes. The second is the random gene approach, where marker genes are identified by positional cloning. This requires examining thousands of marker genes, however. A third approach is the limited random search, or subtraction cloning (142), which focuses on genes from one tissue (muscle, for example, which is the site of the earliest detectable insulin resistance in NIDDM). Subtraction libraries prepared from these tissues represent genes preferentially expressed in either the normal or insulin-resistant state. Kahn et al. have used this approach to screen thousands of muscle genes for possible changes in expression that might be specific for NIDDM and have identified a number of diabetes-associated changes in gene expression (140). These include genes that code for glycogen phosphorylase and several mitochondrial genes coding for proteins involved in oxidative phosphorylation. Clearly, the identification of other genes responsible for causing the insulin resistance associated with abdominal obesity and NIDDM will be a major focus for research.

B. Dyslipidemia and Coronary Heart Disease

Obesity, and abdominal obesity in particular, is strongly associated with an adverse dyslipidemic profile and an increased risk for coronary artery disease. Abdominal obesity, however, is itself a heterogeneous condition. Some abdominally obese individuals are resistant to NIDDM, related dyslipoproteinemias, and CHD, whereas others are at high risk for these metabolic disorders. Precisely what separates these groups is not known, although subtypes can easily be identified.

Lipid and lipoprotein metabolism is a complex series of events, which include proper coordination of apolipoproteins, receptors, modifying enzymes, substrate availability, and other factors involved in lipoprotein synthesis, secretion, modeling, and clearance (143,144). Understanding the basis of dyslipidemia in upper-body obesity is therefore a daunting task. Dyslipidemia associated with diminished levels of HDL in the plasma is commonly associated with abdominal obesity (145). This disorder, which is often associated with low levels of apoAI or with defective cholesterol esterification, is highly correlated with an increased susceptibility to atherosclerosis. On the other end of the spectrum is hyperapobetalipoproteinemia, a dyslipidemia associated with increased levels of VLDL and LDL. These may in some instances result from a defect in

the LDL receptor but could equally be due to the increased plasma FFA levels seen in abdominal obesity.

1. Mechanisms of the Abnormalities in Lipoprotein Metabolism

Visceral fat, because of its close anatomical proximity to the liver, facilitates a high exposure of the liver to FFA. The close relationship of plasma FFA flux with VLDL-TG and apoB production rates suggests that increased FFA flux might be important in the pathogenesis of the lipoprotein disorder in abdominal obesity (29). VLDL secretion is mainly regulated by the synthesis of TG for transport, which in turn depends on the availability of FFA. In this manner, FFA can likely regulate the synthesis and secretion of both VLDL and apoB, subsequently increasing serum LDL.

Increased delivery of FFA to tissues in abdominal obesity results in hyperinsulinemia, which has been implicated as a contributor to the hypertriglyceridemia and low HDL associated with upper-body obesity. WHR and insulin levels correlate positively with triglyceride levels and inversely with HDL-cholesterol levels (146). The relationship with triglycerides is not seen when corrected for insulin variation, implicating insulin levels as a potential mediator of the effect of abdominal adiposity on triglycerides. There is also evidence that hyperinsulinemia per se increases hepatic VLDL-TG production. Insulin levels correlate with production rates of VLDL-TG and VLDL-apoB, with a proportionally larger response of triglycerides, resulting in TG-rich particles. Strong correlations have been found between insulin resistance and insulin response, and between insulin response and VLDL-TG production rate, supporting a central role for hyperinsulinemia in the pathology of hypertriglyceridemia.

Insulin appears to play a number of potential regulatory roles in lipid and lipoprotein metabolism. Changes in triglyceride levels, such as those that might occur in abdominal obesity, radically alter HDL size and composition and LDL particle size distribution (147), and insulin is known to regulate enzymes involved in these pathways (145). Insulin increases peripheral catabolism of VLDL and triglyceride and subsequent uptake and storage of released FFA by adipose tissue via activation of lipoprotein lipase and its subsequent translocation to the functional site at the capillary endothelium. Insulin, which also regulates LDL binding, enhances the metabolic channeling of VLDL into LDL, determining both the rate of LDL synthesis and the fraction of VLDL reentering the plasma as remnant particles. Insulin could thus affect the transfer of cholesterol from chylomicrons and VLDL to HDL, and by influencing the activity of hepatic triglyceride lipase, insulin can also affect the catabolism of HDL constituents. The recently reported insulin-mediated regulation of the synthesis of apolipoprotein C-III (148), a protein whose overexpression is associated with hypertriglyceridemia, may further contribute to the hypertriglyceridemia of abdominal obesity. In addition, insulin may regulate the concentration of the potentially thrombogenic and atherogenic lipoprotein Lp(a) (149). The complex mechanisms relating abdominal obesity and the associated abnormalities in insulin dynamics to lipid disorders remain to be detailed.

Another important feature of abdominal obesity is the decreased HDL that results from a selective decline in the HDL$_2$ subspecies. A negative correlation has been observed between WHR and levels of HDL$_2$ (146). The mechanism responsible for the decrease in HDL cholesterol in these individuals is uncertain. The endogenous hyperinsulinemia of abdominal obesity may result in decreased adipose tissue lipoprotein lipase activity and increased hepatic triglyceride lipase, reducing conversion of HDL$_3$ to HDL$_2$ and diminishing total HDL cholesterol. Abdominal fat localization is also associated with increased HDL$_2$ fractional catabolic rate.

Since obesity and abdominal fat accumulation are associated with increased plasma VLDL concentration, and since apoE is essential in receptor-mediated lipoprotein uptake, several groups have sought to examine whether apoE polymorphism could alter the relationships between abdominal obesity and plasma lipids and lipoproteins. ApoE polymorphism appears to modulate obesity-lipoprotein relationships in children and adults alike (150,151). Individuals with the E2 isoform have body fatness variables that are lower than in those carrying the apoE3 isoform. Both VLDL and LDL components are positively correlated to body fatness variables in women with apoE3, while in those with apoE2, body fat variables are predominately associated with the VLDL components, and those with E4 correlate with LDL cholesterol and LDL-apo B (152). In women carrying the apoE ϵ2 allele and in those homozygous for the apoE ϵ3 allele, plasma insulin and glucose areas under the curve measured during OGTT are significantly associated with plasma triglyceride concentrations, while no such relationships are seen in women carrying the apoE ϵ4 allele. ApoE polymorphisms might thus modulate the relationship between insulinemia and plasma lipoprotein lipid levels (152).

One important aspect of the metabolic profile in abdominal obesity is the density profiles of LDL and VLDL in relation to body fat distribution (see Ref. 153 for review). In a large cohort study, WHR is significantly and positively correlated with dense LDL, IDL, and dense VLDL, and slightly negatively correlated with large HDL. Austin and co-workers have identified two distinct phenotypes of LDL subclasses (147). Phenotype A is characterized by a predominance of large, buoyant LDL particles, and phenotype B consists of a major peak of small, dense LDL particles. These phenotypes are closely associated with variations in plasma levels of lipids, lipoproteins, and apolipoproteins. Phenotype B is associated with a threefold increased risk for coronary artery disease, which may be due in part to the increased susceptibility of these small, dense LDL to oxidative modification (154).

Sex differences in total serum cholesterol and TG levels are well known. Cholesterol values are higher in females during childhood and after the mid-50s, but the sex difference in serum TG is more pronounced, being lower in women than men at all ages. Men have higher plasma VLDL-TG and cholesterol, while women have higher HDL cholesterol concentrations. That changes in lipoprotein concentrations vary during the course of pregnancy also suggests that the sex hormones play an important role in regulating lipoprotein kinetics. In estrogen-deficient women, estrogen increases VLDL and HDL levels and decreases LDL concentrations (155). Premenopausal women with upper-body fat localization exhibit increased androgenic activity, which is correlated with the increases in serum TG and decreased HDL cholesterol levels. Estrogens reversibly enhance both VLDL-TG and VLDL apoB production in a dose- and duration-dependent manner (144,156). Administration of estradiol to ovariectomized rats increases fatty acid synthesis and enhances hepatic FFA esterification and TG production. In addition, estradiol inhibits adipose tissue lipoprotein lipase, possibly by altering the compositional ratios of apoC and apoE in VLDL. Estradiol decreases VLDL removal, limiting formation of LDL from VLDL, and induces hepatic LDL receptor activity, thereby increasing hepatic LDL uptake. Production rates of HDL and apoAI are increased, along with HDL lipid constituents. These changes are associated with a significant decrease in hepatic triglyceride lipase activity. Progesterone, on the other hand, increases the efficiency of plasma triglyceride removal. Androgens increase hepatic VLDL-TG and apoB synthesis, but they also enhance channeling of VLDL into LDL and increase LDL production. Androgens appear to decrease the synthesis of HDL and apoA, thereby decreasing HDL levels (157). Freedman et al. examined adjusted sex differences in lipid and lipoprotein levels (158; Table 4). Adjusting for age, alcohol consumption, exercise, and cigarette smoking slightly increased the magnitude of the differences between men and women. Even after controlling for body

Table 28.4 Sex Differences in Lipid and Lipoprotein Levels After Adjustment for Selected Charactertistics

Characteristic controlled for	Male excess levels (mg/gl)				
	TG	HDL-chol	Total/HDL	ApoB	ApoAI
None	38*	−15*	1.2*	11*	−19*
Covariates[a]	42*	−17*	1.3*	12*	−23*
Covariates + BMI	37*	−16*	1.2*	11*	−22*
Covariates + WHR	−2	−10*	0.4**	0	−15*
Change in male/female difference[b] (%)	94	33	66	98	21
Multiple R^2	0.17	0.28	0.26	0.20	0.24

Unadjusted male/female differences in lipoprotein levels and the effect of controlling for various characteristics. Subjects were 20–69-year-old Caucasians (709 men and 415 women).
[a]Covariates: age, age^2, alcohol intake, exercise, and current smoking status.
[b](Unadjusted difference—adjusted difference)/unadjusted difference. Levels are adjusted for covariates and WHR.
*$p < 0.001$; **$p < 0.01$. p values are for equality of means between men and women.
Source: Data from Ref. 158.

mass index (BMI), large contrasts were still evident, although adjustment for age alone did not alter the adjusted values. Controlling for WHR reduced the male/female differences. Thus the disturbed ovarian function and the increased androgenic activity in women with abdominal obesity might play an additive role in the etiology of the lipid and lipoprotein abnormalities characteristic of the metabolic syndrome.

2. Relationship to Thrombosis

Elevated plasma fibrinogen level is a risk factor for the development of cardiovascular disease (159), and there is an association between the fibrinogen level and the severity of angiographically defined coronary artery disease. Activated coagulation and impaired fibrinolytic function are related to WHR (160) and may be responsible for increased cardiovascular disease in these study populations. Fibrinogen levels correlate with both WHR and insulin levels (161). Vague et al. proposed that hyperinsulinemia results in a change in fibrinolytic activity (162). Although no direct relationship between fibrinogen and insulin has been shown, increased plasminogen activator inhibitor, depressed fibrinolytic activity, and decreased left ventricular pump function have all been demonstrated in subjects with abdominal obesity, along with lower HDL levels and higher apoB and Lp(a) levels. A long duration of obesity is further correlated with WHR and factor VII antigen. Thus obese subjects with abdominal body fat distribution

are characterized by metabolic and hemostatic abnormalities associated with silent left ventricular dysfunction.

The development of the atherosclerotic lesion is a complex process. Injury to the endothelial lining of the artery appears to be the initial event in the development of the atherosclerotic plaque; this injury may be caused by hypertension, hyperglycemia, hyperlipidemia, or other means. This can lead to platelet aggregation, which leads to release of vasoconstrictor and aggregation-promoting prostaglandins and platelet-derived growth factors. These and circulating insulin stimulate smooth muscle and macrophage proliferation. Insulin also increases binding and local synthesis of lipoprotein by these cells.

Another process that may contribute to atherothrombosis is oxidative modification of LDL by free radicals. Oxidation of LDL and VLDL appears to be involved in lipid accumulation in the arterial wall and subsequent plaque formation (163). Van Gaal and co-workers have recently demonstrated that oxidizability of the non-HDL fraction increases with BMI (164). They have demonstrated further that the WHR is related to lipoprotein oxidation independent from total body fat or BMI. This may be related to the preponderance of small, dense LDL particles, which themselves are prone to increased oxidizability (154). Abnormal local lipoprotein dynamics, in combination with the abnormally atherogenic circulating lipoproteins seen in abdominal obesity, might thus facilitate lipid deposition within the arterial wall.

3. Genetic Susceptibility to Dyslipidemia

The significant variation observed in the response of plasma lipoproteins to chronic overfeeding or exercise regimens indicates significant heterogeneity of the abdominally obese. There is, however, a subset of individuals who are clearly susceptible to dyslipidemia and coronary heart disease (30), and this difference is likely to be accounted for by genetic variation. One area that is receiving a good deal of attention is LDL subclasses. Austin has reviewed the genetic influences on these phenotypes (166). Using a candidate gene approach to map the chromosomal location of the proposed locus controlling LDL subclass phenotypes, Austin and co-workers have found some indication of linkage between LDL subclass heterogeneity and the LDL receptor locus on chromosome 19 (167). Ironically, there is also some linkage with the insulin receptor locus on this same chromosome.

Defects in the gene coding for the LDL receptor are well-documented causes of premature atherosclerosis and coronary heart disease in humans (168). LDL receptor is responsible for clearing LDL from the circulation; mutations that abolish the function of this protein have dramatic effects on plasma LDL levels (see Ref. 169 for review), and a number of DNA polymorphisms of the gene encoding this protein have been reported. The variation in apoE isoproteins among abdominally obese women (150) supports the concept of heterogeneity among these women and strongly suggests that variation in genes relevant to lipoprotein metabolism may substantially alter the association between regional adipose tissue distribution and plasma lipoprotein levels.

The hydrolysis of core triglycerides and surface phospholipids of chylomicron remnants, HDL, and IDL is carried out by hepatic lipase. This enzyme also converts large LDL into small LDL in vitro and could thus be important in the derivation of the LDL subclass phenotypes (170). Individuals with heritable reduced hepatic lipase activity generally exhibit elevated levels of triglycerides and cholesterol and may be subject to premature atherosclerosis. Lipoprotein lipase also plays a critical role in the metabolism of lipoproteins by hydrolyzing the triglycerides in chylomicrons and VLDL, influencing the production of HDL. Polymorphisms of the lipoproteins lipase gene are associated with variability in plasma lipid concentrations (171). These enzymes thus represent candidate genes for disturbances in lipoprotein metabolic disorders and atherosclerosis.

C. Blood Pressure and Hypertension

Upper-body fat localization and increased visceral fat mass are associated with increased systolic and diastolic blood pressure. Elevated blood pressures and essential hypertension, like atherosclerosis, have a complex etiology. Normal blood pressures are regulated by several interacting systems that control cardiac output, peripheral resistance, blood volume, renal function, and sodium balance. The renin/angiotension system (RAS), one of these systems, is closely involved in the control of systemic and intrarenal blood pressures and sodium retention.

The search for a pathogenetic link with abdominal obesity has implicated resistance to insulin's glucoregulatory effects and consequently hyperinsulinemia as primary factors (19,172). Reaven and Hoffmann have reviewed the evidence for a role for insulin in hypertension (35). One potential pathway is through insulin's action on the sympathetic nervous system. Insulin infusion increases not only the concentration of norepinephrine but also pulse pressure and systolic blood pressure, independently of glucose level (172). Differences in the regulation of β- and α-adrenergic receptor activities may also contribute to altered arterial responsiveness. In addition, insulin-mediated elevations in plasma norepinephrine appearance rate and its ability to generate increased skeletal muscle blood flow might also be impaired. The hyperinsulinemia of abdominal obesity may result in increased stimulation of the heart, blood vessels, and kidneys, so small increases in plasma insulin levels at several sites may have important effects on blood pressure control. In addition to changes in sympathetic nervous system activity, alterations in cation transport across cell membranes may also represent a mechanism linking insulin with elevations in blood pressure (72).

1. Role of Free Fatty Acids

Increased FFA flux in abdominal obesity may also be involved in the development of the hypertension. FFA flux in normotensive, abdominally obese subjects is high basally but is suppressed by high concentrations of insulin. This insulin suppression is not seen, however, in abdominally obese hypertensives (73,131). Since elevations of FFA flux in turn increase plasma insulin levels by decreasing hepatic insulin extraction or clearance, FFA metabolism thus appears to play a role in the insulin resistance of abdominal obesity, with or without hypertension.

We have previously examined interactions between body fat distribution, hypertension, and the insulin resistance of stimulated peripheral glucose uptake. Both oxidative and nonoxidative glucose metabolism are significantly higher in the leans than in the obese groups, and there are no significant differences between the two obese groups (Fig. 16). The coexistence of hypertension with abdominal obesity did not worsen the defect in insulin-mediated glucose metabolism associated with abdominal obesity without hypertension. Figure 17 shows the insulin dose-response curves for suppression of FFA flux during euglycemic hyperinsulinemia. When plasma insulin was raised approximately 150 pmol/L above basal, FFA flux rates were decreased by 50% in normotensive lean and abdominally obese individuals, with only a 28% suppression in the abdominally obese hypertensive subjects. When plasma insulin was increased 600 pmol/L above basal, FFA flux rates were further suppressed in all three groups, and mean FFA flux rate remained significantly higher in the abdominally obese hypertensives than in the normotensive groups. Abdominally obese hypertensives are thus distinguished from lean and abdominally obese normotensive individuals by greater resistance to insulin's antilipolytic action. The marked differences in FFA concentrations and turnover suppressibility by insulin suggest that the link between insulin resistance and hypertension may be confined to the effects on FFA metabolism.

The potential mechanism by which FFA might raise blood pressure in abdominal obesity may include the hyperinsulinemia, which can contribute to sympathetic activation, increased renal Na^+/water reabsorption, increased mRNA for renin, aldosterone synthesis, vascular hypertrophy, or other actions that may raise blood pressure (see Ref. 35 for review). Raising local FFA concentrations by infusing a lipid emulsion (Intralipid) and heparin into normal subjects augments local vascular tone (173) and α-adrenergic responsiveness (174). The positive correlation between FFA flux and total systemic vascular resistance thus suggests that the high plasma FFA flux in abdominal obesity may contribute to the vascular abnormalities in hypertensive subjects. Levels of FFA may also

perpetuate a rise in blood pressure by inhibiting Na^+/K^+-ATPase activity, enhancing calcium influx, and by activation of protein kinase C. Fatty acids such as arachidonic acid are metabolized to such biologically active substances as prostaglandins, leukotrienes, and lipid hydroperoxides. These metabolites, which could alter vascular tone, capillary permeability, platelet aggregation, and leukocyte adhesion, are thought to be involved in hypertension, ischemic heart disease, and atherosclerosis.

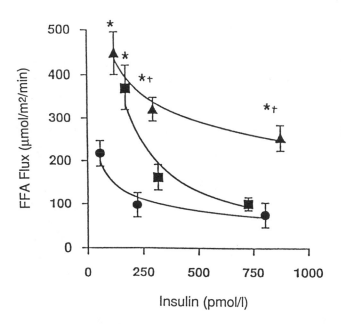

Figure 17 FFA flux during the euglycemic insulin clamp. (●) Lean normotensives (LN, NT); (■) abdominally obese normotensives (AO, NT); (▲) abdominally obese hypertensives (AO, HT). Values are expressed as percentage of baseline values for each subject group. *$p < 0.0001$ versus LN, NT; $^\dagger p < 0.005$ versus AO, NT. (Adapted from Ref. 131.)

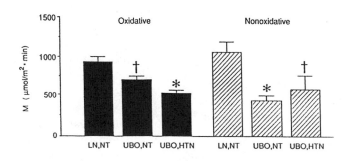

Figure 16 Oxidative and nonoxidative glucose metabolism during the euglycemic insulin clamp in upper-body obese hypertensives (UBO, HTN); upper-body obese normotensives (UBO, NT); and lean normotensives (LN, NT). *$p < 0.005$ versus LN, NT; $^\dagger p < 0.05$ versus LN, NT. (Data from Ref. 73.)

Abdominally obese subjects with cardiovascular risk factor clustering have greater activity of the components of the RAS (175). Since adipocytes possess local angiotensin-converting enzyme (ACE; 176), and since angiotensin modulates adipocyte function (177), the local release of RAS components could influence adipose tissue perfusion and hormonal exposure, with overactivity of this system playing a potential role in the predisposition to insulin-resistant lipolysis. Recent studies have demonstrated that inhibiting converting enzyme activity enhances insulin's actions on fatty acid turnover more than on glucose disposal (73,131). Subjects who received an ACE inhibitor, enalapril, have lower FFA concentrations and flux rates during the hyperinsulinemic euglycemic clamp than those subjects who received placebo. The ability of insulin to suppress FFA flux in abdominally obese hypertensive subjects during the 40 mU/m^2/min insulin clamp correlates positively with the magnitude of the reduction in mean blood pressure induced by the ACE inhibitor, enalapril. Unlike peripheral glucose utilization, the resistance of FFA turnover to suppression by insulin during insulin infusion is significantly improved by the drug. During euglycemic hyperinsulinemia at 40 mU/m^2/min, FFA flux is significantly lowered after enalapril treatment (10 mg b.i.d.). Peripheral glucose utilization is unaffected by enalapril administration. ACE inhibition enhances insulin's effects on fatty acid turnover more than on glucose disposal and raises the possibility that insulin sensitivity is augmented to a greater extent in adipocytes than in skeletal muscle, as a result of local metabolic and hemodynamic consequences of inhibiting angiotensinogen II production by adipocytes. A more active RAS may thus explain, in part, the insulin-resistant lipolysis in abdominal obesity (131). This, together with the high FFA concentrations and increased turnover, may account for some of the insulin resistance in abdominal obesity.

2. Role of Nitric Oxide

Nitric oxide (NO) is a small physiological messenger that can diffuse freely through the cell membrane (see Ref. 178 for review) and react with heme iron. Among its many putative physiological roles are increasing cGMP production, which acts to reduce platelet adhesion and to relax vascular smooth muscle, and increasing production of cyclic ADP-ribose, which has been reported to stimulate the release of calcium into the sarcoplasmic reticulum. In addition, NO can inhibit glycolysis (by stimulating ribosylation of glyceraldehyde-3-phosphate dehydrogenase). NO-stimulated ribosylation of G-proteins may inhibit their function and alter plasma membrane signal transduction.

A number of actions have been demonstrated for NO in vascular tissues, including endothelium-dependent vascular relaxation in response to kinins, resistance to vasoconstrictors, and inhibition of mitogenesis and proliferation of vascular smooth muscle cells. Recent studies have shown that NO also plays an important role in the cardiovascular regulatory center of the brain, decreasing sympathetic nerve traffic and blood pressure. Attenuation of the NO synthase activity of a cardiovascular regulatory center may contribute to arterial pressure elevation in the salt-sensitive hypertensive rat.

The role of NO in experimental hypertension and in promoting hypertension in abdominal obesity is unknown. Reports indicating that NO production in hypertension is depressed suggest that the elevated arterial pressure reflects diminished vasodilation, while publications describing excessive NO production in hypertension indicate that NO acts to compensate hypertension via vasodilation. Insulin itself acts to increase NO production and release via an unknown interaction with the endothelium, resulting in vasodilation, but most indications from clinical studies suggest that there is a deficiency in the release of NO by the endothelium in hypertension. That this was not seen in all studies may be indicative of subject heterogeneity.

3. Genetic Contributions

Familial aggregation, population, and twin studies all point to important genetic influences on the level of blood pressure in childhood and adolescence (see Ref. 179 for review). An increase in body weight is among the factors that have been reported to be related to familial aggregation of blood pressure, but the familial resemblance of body weight appears to be determined genetically as well. A family history of obesity might increase the risk of hypertension developing in obese subjects. A significant portion of the variability in systolic and diastolic blood pressure appears under genetic control. Four Mendelian forms of human hypertension are recognized in which mutation in a single gene leads to elevated blood pressure in a high proportion of affected subjects (180). Mutations resulting in loss of function of 11β-hydroxysteroid dehydrogenase, which converts cortisol to cortisone, for example, have recently been shown to cause one of these disorders, apparent mineralocorticoid excess (181).

That there are a dozen or more different intermediate phenotypes in hypertension highlights the probable contribution of an overlapping array of a variety of genetic variants to essential hypertension. One group of genes of great interest is the components of the RAS. While renin and angiotensin-converting enzyme have not demonstrated linkage with human essential hypertension, the angiotensinogen gene is a strong candidate (182,183), as indicated by population studies in Salt Lake City and Paris. In addition, other genes are rapidly being implicated in human hypertension. For example, a mutation truncating the epithelial sodium channel in the nephron results in constitutive activation of channel activity, leading to increased sodium reabsorption and hypertension (184).

Of the genes that have been identified or inferred in human hypertension, most appear to affect blood pressure by altering renal sodium reabsorption (180). A recent report, however, has identified a genetic locus near the lipoprotein lipase gene that contributes to the variation of systolic, but not diastolic, blood pressure levels in nondiabetic family members at high risk for insulin resistance and NIDDM (185). As these and other genetic loci are identified, their quantitative effects on blood pressure and their relationships to abdominal obesity and insulin dynamics can subsequently be assessed.

V.   SUMMARY AND PERSPECTIVES

We have proposed a unifying hypothesis of the causal factors leading to individual differences in body fat topography (3; Fig. 18). Regional adipose tissue growth and metabolism is influenced both by primary genes of as-yet-undetermined nature and by neuroendocrine and environmental traits (some of which may also be determined by other primary genes). These genetic factors may also act in concert with visceral fat to promote insulin resistance, which, through increased FFA flux, helps create the adverse metabolic profile and eventual morbidity. Among the environmental and neuroendocrine factors influencing regional adipose tissue growth and metabolism are stress, diet, smoking, alcohol, glucocorticoids, sex hormones,

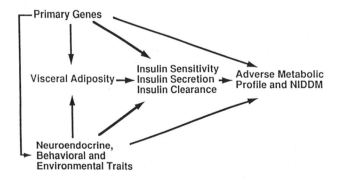

Figure 18   Potential causal mechanisms and pathways accounting for abdominal obesity and the associated adverse metabolic profile and morbidity. (Adapted from Ref. 3.)

and sexual dimorphism. This model favors the recognition of a panel of potential candidate genes that can be searched for by sophisticated genetic studies. In turn, identification of these genes and subsequent elucidation of their actions should lead to more meaningful understanding of pathophysiology of abdominal obesity and the metabolic syndrome.

Abdominal-visceral fat, a significant correlate of hyperinsulinemia, increased plasma triglyceride levels, decreased HDL levels, and elevated blood pressure, is a phenotypic companion for a cluster of metabolic abnormalities. Chief among these is decreased insulin sensitivity, which is compensated by increased insulin secretion and diminished hepatic insulin extraction, with resultant hyperinsulinemia. Hyperinsulinemia is the most significant metabolic variable in these associations. As stated above, abdominal obesity results from interactions between genetic, neuroendocrine, and environmental mechanisms, and each of these can affect insulin actions and dynamics independently. Abdominal obesity and its associated insulin resistance are predictive of a myriad of disorders, including glucose intolerance, dyslipidemia, and hypertension, and result in such morbidities as NIDDM, coronary heart disease, and stroke, and increased mortality rate. Again the etiology of these disorders is contingent upon genetic, neuroendocrine, and environmental factors, and it is possible that abdominal obesity and/or insulin resistance operates as a provocative or exacerbating event facilitating the expression of these disorders.

Clearly, addressing the molecular genetic basis of these relatively common and medically as well as economically serious disorders should be the focus of research of several laboratories. What are these genes? How are they transmitted and expressed? To what extent could they perpetuate or interact with each other? Are the neuroendocrine and environmental traits also genetically determined, and how might they influence the expression of the primary genes? And finally, could these genetic traits be modified and/or prevented by behavioral, dietary, or even therapeutic means? These are just a few of the questions that will be directing future research in this area.

The coexistence of hyperinsulinemia and impaired glucose tolerance in abdominal obesity implicates insulin resistance as the underlying abnormality, but the exact locus of this insulin resistance is unknown. Several cellular events are likely involved, although the contribution of each and which is primary or secondary remain unresolved. Indeed, attempts to implicate the insulin receptor, elements of the hormone signaling apparatus cascade, and/or rate-determining enzyme systems in either abdominal obesity per se or NIDDM have not yet been successful. The macrocirculation and abnormalities in blood flow regulation could contribute to the diminished glucose uptake, but these cannot explain the intensity of the insulin resistance encountered in these subjects. Microcirculatory redistribution of blood perfusion from shunt nonnutritive channels to regions of higher metabolic activity and greater capacity to metabolize and store glucose as glycogen, on the other hand, may also contribute to the insulin resistance. This notion raises the intriguing question of whether the insulin insensitivity of abdominal obesity could result from a primary neurohumoral dysregulation of this system. Could this dysregulation be intensified by either genetically and/or environmentally overactive "arousal systems"? How might these events influence skeletal muscle capillary rarefaction and fiber composition? In addition, could the resultant microcirculatory changes and metabolic events contribute to or accompany changes in regional and systemic hemodynamics, predisposing to increased blood pressure and eventually to hypertension?

Abdominal obesity is characterized by the preferential deposition of fat in the visceral region, and the overall activity of the adipose tissue mass favors enhanced lipolysis and increased FFA flux into the circulation. This increase appears to be linked to the occurrence of a specific form of dyslipidemia similar to that seen in individuals with the phenotype B lipoprotein profile, which in turn is linked to increased risk of cardiovascular disease. Could overexposure of the liver to high FFA flux be a primary factor in the expression of this lipoprotein phenotype? What is the role of concomitant hyperinsulinemia and possibly of hyperglycemia? How do these hormones and substrates interact at the level of the hepatocyte? Might some genetic elements be activated or even induced by this exposure? And finally, is there one specific fatty acid that initiates these interactions? What is the role of steroid hormones, and particularly of androgens, whose levels are altered in abdominal obesity?

Recent evidence indicates that adipose tissue also serves as an endocrine organ, with the capacity to synthesize and secrete hormones like leptin, which influences food intake as well as body weight regulation, and could potentially play a significant role in the neuroendocrine regulatory processes accompanying this obesity phenotype. Adipose tissue is also a site of several kinins and modulators of vasoreactivity, such as angiotensin, and of the angiotensin-converting enzyme. Lack of suppressibility of adipose tissue lipolysis by insulin is correlated with increased peripheral vascular resistance and could contribute to insulin resistance. By what mechanisms could FFA influence blood pressure? What organs are involved? Could these events be prevented by reducing the size of this fat depot, or at least might we be able to suppress its

activity through therapeutic intervention? Clearly, the biology of adipose tissue is another area for intense research.

Insulin resistance in abdominal obesity is compensated by an increase in the overall secretion of insulin, but the magnitude of this increase is not commensurate with the degree of insulin insensitivity. Diminished hepatic insulin extraction thus plays the important role of further enhancing the flow of insulin to the periphery, consequently augmenting this compensation. Part of this hepatic compensatory reaction appears to be mediated by increased FFA flux, although increased blood glucose seems to exert a synergistic role. Neurogenic and hormonal factors may also be involved. How might these factors elicit this response? And why is this not seen in overt NIDDM?

Although the total insulin secretion rate is increased in the nondiabetic abdominally obese, the dynamic modes of insulin release and their entrainment with glucose fluctuations are aberrant. Thus the first-phase insulin response to enteric feeding is delayed or blunted, and the ultradian pulsatilites are of low relative amplitude, exhibiting high variations in both amplitude and frequency, and in some individuals are completely disrupted. Furthermore, the sensorship of the process to stepped doses of glucose infusion is shifted to the right. These abnormalities are worsened in overt diabetics. Are these dynamic profiles early markers of a primary β-cell secretary dysfunction in abdominal obesity? Which of these components might be secondary to insulin resistance? How might these adaptations influence the expression of a primary genetic defect?

The anatomical location and a/β-adrenoceptor sensitivity of fat deposited around the waist suggest that FFA flux from this tissue may play a major role in suppressing hepatic insulin clearance and contributing to the peripheral insulin resistance. Along with its involvement in regulating glucose-insulin homeostasis, increased fatty acid flux resulting from visceral obesity may also influence lipoprotein metabolism and vascular events leading to such metabolic morbidities as glucose intolerance, dyslipidemia, and hypertension. Could differences in the regulation of β- and α-adrenergic receptor activities also contribute to altered arterial responsiveness? Furthermore, insulin-mediated elevations in plasma norepinephrine appearance rate and its ability to generate increased skeletal muscle blood flow might also be impaired. The ability of insulin to increase skeletal muscle blood flow is blunted in some obese individuals, correlating with the reductions in leg and total-body glucose utilization. Moreover, this response may be partially reversible. Might an increase in arterial tone be due to attenuation of the insulin-mediated vasodilator response, and could this be a significant factor contributing to the defect in peripheral glucose utilization?

Finally, in the past few years we have learned a great deal about the pathophysiology of abdominal obesity and the metabolic syndrome. But we have just commenced a careful examination of this complex trait. It is hoped that the answers to the questions at hand and to the many questions to come will eventually lead to a more meaningful understanding of the pillars of this very common and highly lethal syndrome and to the development of means for its prevention and/or treatment.

ACKNOWLEDGMENTS

This work was supported in part by National Institutes of Health Grants HL-34989 and DK-45949 and General Clinical Research Center Grant RR-00058. Gratitude is expressed to the TOPS organization for their continued support in these studies. Also greatly appreciated is the skillful assistance of the General Clinical Research Center nurses, nutrition, data management, and core laboratory staff, in addition to the investigators whose contributions have greatly advanced this knowledge.

REFERENCES

1. Reaven G. Role of insulin resistance in human disease: Banting Lecture 1988. Diabetes 1988; 37:1592–1607.
2. Kissebah AH, Freedman DS, Peiris AN. Health risks of obesity. Med Clin North Am 1989; 73:111–138.
3. Kissebah AH, Krakower GR. Regional adiposity and morbidity. Physiol Rev 1994; 74:761–811.
4. Morgagni GB. Adversaria anatomica omnia. Patavii: Josephus Cominus, 1719.
5. Paullin JE, Sauls HC. A study of the glucose tolerance test in the obese. Southern Med J 1922; 15:249–253.
6. John HJ. A summary of the findings in 1100 glucose tolerance tests. Endocrinology 1929; 13:388–392.
7. Joslin EP, Dublin LI, Marks HH. Studies in diabetes mellitus. IV. Etiology. Am J Med Sci 1936; 192:9–23.
8. Vague J. The degree of masculine differentiation with obesities: a factor determining predisposition to diabetes, atherosclerosis, gout, and uric calculous disease. Am J Clin Nutr 1956; 4:20–34.
9. Karam JH, Grodsky GM, Forsham PH. Excessive insulin response to glucose in obese subjects as measured by immuno-chemical assay. Diabetes 1963; 12:197–204.
10. Kissebah A, Vydelingum N, Murray R, Evans D, Hartz A, Kalkhoff RK, Adams PW. Relation of body fat distribution to metabolic complications of obesity. J Clin Endocrinol Metab 1982; 54:254–260.
11. Krotkiewski M, Björntorp P, Sjöström L, Smith U. Impact of obesity on metabolism in men and women: importance of regional adipose tissue distribution. J Clin Invest 1983; 72:1150–1162.
12. Lemieux S, Després JP. Metabolic complications of visceral obesity: contribution to the aetiology of type 2 diabetes and implications for prevention and treatment. Diabetes Metab 1994; 20:375–393.
13. Hartz AJ, Rupley DC, Kalkhoff RK, Rimm AA. Relationship of obesity to diabetes: influence of obesity level and body-fat distribution. Prev Med 1983; 12:351–357.
14. Morris RK, Rimm AA. Association of waist to hip ratio and family history with the prevalence of NIDDM among 25,272 adult, white females. Am J Public Health 1991; 81:507–509.
15. West KM, Kalbfleisch JM. Influence of nutritional status on prevalence of diabetes. Diabetes 1971; 20:99–108.
16. Evans DJ, Hoffmann RG, Kalkhoff RK, Kissebah AH. Relationship of body fat topography to insulin sensitivity and metabolic profiles in premenopausal women. Metabolism 1984; 33:68–75.
17. Lillioja S, Bogardus C. Obesity and insulin resistance: lessons learned from the Pima Indians. Diabetes Metab Rev 1988; 4:517–540.
18. Peiris AN, Hennes MI, Evans DJ, Wilson CR, Lee MB, Kissebah AH. Relationship of anthropometric measurements of body fat distribution to metabolic profile in premenopausal women. Acta Med Scand 1988; (Suppl 723): 179–188.
19. Peiris AN, Sothmann MS, Hoffmann RG, Hennes MI, Wilson CR, Gustafson AB, Kissebah A. Adiposity, fat distribution, and cardiovascular risk. Ann Intern Med 1989; 110:867–872.
20. Fujioka S, Matsuzawa Y, Tokunaga K, Tarui S. Contribution of intraabdominal fat accumulation to the impairment of glucose lipid metabolism in human obesity. Metabolism 1987; 36:54–59.
21. Sparrow D, Borkan GA, Gerzof SG, Wisniewski C, Silbert CK. Relationship of fat distribution to glucose intolerance. Results of computed tomography in male participants of the Normative Aging Study. Diabetes 1986; 35:411–415.
22. Peiris A, Mueller RA, Smith GA, Struve MF, Kissebah AH. Splanchnic insulin metabolism in obesity: Influence of body fat distribution. J Clin Invest 1986; 78:1648–1657.
23. Sonnenberg GE, Hoffmann RG, Mueller RA, Kissebah AH. Splanchnic insulin dynamics and secretion pulsatilites in abdominal obesity. Diabetes 1994; 43:468–477.
24. Peiris AN, Mueller RA, Struve MF, Smith GA, Kissebah AH. Relationship of androgenic activity to splanchnic insulin metabolism and peripheral glucose utilization in premenopausal women. J Clin Endocrinol Metab 1987; 64:162–169.
25. Peiris AN, Struve MF, Mueller RA, Lee MB, Kissebah AH. Glucose metabolism in obesity: influence of body fat distribution. J Clin Endocrinol Metab 1988; 67:760–767.
26. Jouve A, Vague J, Mongin M. La differenciation sexuelle en pathologie cardiovasculaire. Arch Mal Coeur 1951; 44: 893–900.
27. Lapidus L, Bengtsson C, Larsson B, Pennert K, Rybo E, Sjöström L. Distribution of adipose tissue and risk of car-

diovascular disease and death: a 12-year follow-up of participants in the population study of women in Gothenburg, Sweden. Br Med J 1984; 289:1257–1261.

28. Larsson B, Svärdsudd K, Welin L, Wilhelmsen L, Björntorp P, Tibblin G. Abdominal adipose tissue distribution, obesity, and risk of cardiovascular disease and death: a 13-year follow-up of participants in the study of men born in 1913. Br Med J 1984; 289:1401–1404.

29. Kissebah AH, Peiris AN. Biology of regional body fat distribution: relationship to non-insulin-dependent diabetes mellitus. Diabetes Metab Rev 1989; 5:83–109.

30. Després J-P, Moorjani S, Lupien PJ, Tremblay A, Nadeau A, Bouchard C. Genetic aspects of susceptibility to obesity and related dyslipidemias. Mol Cell Biochem 1992; 113:151–169.

31. Favier G. L'hypertension arterielle chez les obeses. Thesis, Med. Univ, Marseille, 1945.

32. MacMahon SW, Blacket RB, Macdonald GJ, Hall W. Obesity, alcohol consumption and blood pressure in Australian men and women: the National Heart Foundation of Australia Risk Factor Prevalence Study. J Hypertens 1984; 2:85–91.

33. Egan BM, Bassett DR, Block WD. Comparative effects of overweight on cardiovascular risk in younger versus older men. Am J Cardiol 1991; 67:248–252.

34. Fournier AM, Gadia MT, Kubrusly DB, Skyler JS, Sosenko JM. Blood pressure, insulin and glycemia in nondiabetic subjects. Am J Med 1986; 80:861–864.

35. Reaven G, Hoffmann BB. A role for insulin in the aetiology and course of hypertension. Lancet 1987; ii:435–437.

36. Voors AW, Radhakrishnamurthy B, Srinivasan SR, Webber LS, Berenson GS. Plasma glucose level related to blood pressure in 272 children, ages 7–15 years, sampled from a total biracial population. Am J Epidemiol 1981; 113:347–356.

37. Modan M, Halkin H, Almog S, Lusky A, Eshkol A, Shefi M, Shitrit A, Fuchs Z. Hyperinsulinemia: a link between hypertension obesity and glucose intolerance. J Clin Invest 1985; 75:809–817.

38. Himsworth H. Diabetes mellitus: a differentiation into insulin-sensitive and insulin-insensitive types. Lancet 1936; i:127–130.

39. Himsworth HP, Kerr RB. Insulin-sensitive and insulin-insensitive types of diabetes mellitus. Clin Sci 1939; 4:119–152.

40. Shen S-W, Reaven GM, Farquhar J. Comparison of impedance to insulin-mediated glucose uptake in normal subjects and in subjects with latent diabetes. J Clin Invest 1970; 49:2151–2160.

41. Ginsberg H, Kimmerling G, Olefsky JM, Reaven GM. Demonstration of insulin resistance in untreated adult onset diabetic subjects with fasting hyperglycemia. J Clin Invest 1975; 55:454–461.

42. Harano Y, Ohgaku S, Hidaka H, Haneda K, Kikkawa R, Shigeta Y, Abe H. Glucose, insulin, and somatostatin infusion for the determination of insulin sensitivity. J Clin Endocrinol Metab 1977; 45:1124–1127.

43. Nagulesparan M, Savage PJ, Unger RH, Bennett PH. A simplified method using somatostatin to assess in vivo insulin resistance over a range of obesity. Diabetes 1979; 28:980–983.

44. Ratzmann KP, Besch W, Witt S, Schulz B. Evaluation of insulin resistance during inhibition of endogenous insulin and glucagon secretion by somatostatin in non-obese subjects with impaired glucose tolerance. Diabetologia 1981; 21:192–197.

45. Sherwin RS, Kramer KJ, Tobin JD, Insel PA, Liljenquist JE, Berman M, Andres R. A model of the kinetics of insulin in man. J Clin Invest 1974; 53:1481–1492.

46. DeFronzo RA, Tobin TD, Andres R. Glucose clamp technique: a method for quantifying insulin secretion and resistance. Am J Physiol 1979; 237:E214–E223.

47. Best JD, Taborsky GJ Jr, Halter JB, Porte D Jr. Glucose disposal is not proportional to plasma glucose level in man. Diabetes 1981; 30:847–850.

48. deBodo RC, Steele R, Altszuler N, Dunn A, Bishop JS. On the hormonal regulation of carbohydrate metabolism: studies with C-14 glucose. Recent Prog Horm Res 1963; 19:445–482.

49. Steele R. Influences of glucose loading and injected insulin on hepatic glucose output. Ann NY Acad Sci 1959; 82:420–430.

50. Allsop JR, Wolfe RR, Burke JF. The reliability of rates of glucose appearance in vivo calculated from constant tracer infusions. Biochem J 1978; 172:407–416.

51. Radziuk J, Norwich KH, Vranic M. Experimental validation of measurements of glucose turnover in nonsteady state. Am J Physiol 1978; 234:E84–E93.

52. Norwich KH. Measuring rates of appearance in systems which are not in steady state. Can J Physiol Pharmacol 1973; 51:91–101.

53. Finegood DT, Bergman RN, Vranic M. Modeling error and apparent isotope discrimination confound estimation of endogenous glucose production during euglycemic glucose clamps. Diabetes 1988; 37:1025–1034.

54. Bradley DC, Poulin RA, Bergman RN. Dynamics of hepatic and peripheral insulin effects suggest common rate-limiting step in vivo. Diabetes 1993; 42:296–306.

55. Caumo A, Homan M, Katz H, Cobelli C, Rizza R. Glucose turnover in presence of changing glucose concentrations: error analysis for glucose disappearance. Am J Physiol 1995; 269:E557–E567.

56. Hother-Nielsen O, Henriksen JE, Holst JJ, Beck-Nielsen H. Effects of insulin on glucose turnover rates in vivo. Isotope dilution versus constant specific activity technique. Metabolism 1996; 45:82–91.

57. Schutz Y. The basis of direct and indirect calorimetry and their potentials. Diabetes/Metab Rev 1995; 11:383–408.

58. Heiling VJ, Miles JM, Jensen MD. How valid are isotopic measurements of fatty acid oxidation? Am J Physiol 1991; 261:E572–E577.

59. Lacroix M, Morosa F, Pontus M, Lefebre P, Luyckx A, Lopez-Habib G. Glucose naturally labelled with carbon-13: use for metabolic studies in man. Science 1973; 181: 445–446.

60. DeFronzo RA. The triumverate: β-cell, muscle, and liver. A collusion responsible for NIDDM. Diabetes 1988; 37: 667–687.

61. Kolterman OG, Insel J, Saekow M, Olefsky JM. Mechanisms of insulin resistance in human obesity: evidence for receptor and postreceptor defects. J Clin Invest 1980; 65: 1272–1284.

62. Landis EM, Pappenheimer JR. Exchange of substances through the capillary walls. In: Handbook of Physiology, Section 2. Circulation Vol II. Am Physiol Soc, Washington DC, 1963:961–1034.

63. Rabinowitz D, Zierler KL. Forearm metabolism in obesity and its response to intra-arterial insulin. Characterization of insulin resistance and evidence for adaptive hyperinsulinism. J Clin Invest 1962; 41:2173–2181.

64. Bergman RN, Ider YZ, Bowden CR, Cobelli C. Quantitative estimation of insulin sensitivity in vivo. Am J Physiol 1979; 236:E667–E677.

65. Pacini G, Bergman RN. A computer program to calculate insulin sensitivity and pancreatic responsivity from the frequently sampled intravenous glucose tolerance test. Computer Meth Prog Biomed 1986; 23:113–122.

66. Bergman RN, Prager R, Volund A, Olefsky JM. Equivalence of the insulin sensitivity index in man derived by the minimal model method and the euglycemic glucose clamp. J Clin Invest 1987; 79:790–800.

67. Yang Y, Youn J, Bergman RN. Modified protocols improve insulin sensitivity estimation using the minimal model. Am J Physiol (Endocrinol Metab) 1987; 16:E595–E602.

68. Finegood DT, Hramiak IM, Dupre J. A modified protocol for estimation of insulin sensitivity with the minimal model of glucose kinetics in patients with insulin-dependent diabetes. J Clin Endocrinol Metab 1990; 70: 1538–1549.

69. Welch S, Gebhart SS, Bergman RN, Phillips LS. Minimal model analysis of intravenous glucose tolerance test-derived insulin sensitivity in diabetic subjects. J Clin Endocrinol Metab 1990; 71:1508–1518.

70. Yki-Järvinen H, Koivisto VA. Effects of body composition on insulin sensitivity. Diabetes 1983; 32:965–969.

71. Evans DJ, Murray R, Kissebah AH. Relationship between skeletal muscle insulin resistance, insulin-mediated glucose disposal, and insulin binding: effects of obesity and body fat topography. J Clin Invest 1984; 74:1515–1525.

72. Baron AD. Hemodynamic actions of insulin. Am J Physiol (Endocrinol Metab) 1994; 30:E187–E202.

73. O'Shaughnessy IM, Myers TJ, Stepniakowski K, Nazzaro P, Kelly TM, Hoffmann RG, Egan BM, Kissebah AH. Glucose metabolism in abdominally obese hypertensive and normotensive subjects. Hypertension 1995; 26:186–192.

74. Laakso M, Edelman SV, Brechtel G, Baron AD. Decreased effect of insulin to stimulate skeletal muscle blood flow in obese men. A novel mechanism for insulin resistance. J Clin Invest 1990; 85:1844–1852.

75. Baron AD, Steinberg HO, Chaker H, Leaming R, Johnson A, Brechtel G. Insulin-mediated skeletal muscle vasodilation contributes to both insulin sensitivity and responsiveness in lean humans. J Clin Invest 1995; 96:786–792.

76. Saltin B, Henriksson J, Nygaard E, Jansson E, Andersen P. Fiber types and metabolic potential of skeletal muscles in sedentary men and endurance runners. Ann NY Acad Sci 1977; 301:3–29.

77. Duckworth WC. Insulin degradation: mechanisms, products, and significance. Endocr Rev 1988; 9:319–345.

78. Peiris AN, Struve MF, Kissebah AH. Relationship of body fat distribution to the metabolic clearance of insulin in premenopausal women. Int J Obes 1987; 11:581–589.

79. Hovorka R, Jones RH. How to measure insulin secretion. Diabetes/Metab Rev 1994; 10:91–117.

80. Waldhausl W, Bratusch-Marrain P, Gasic S, Korn A, Nowotny P. Insulin production rate following glucose ingestion estimated by splanchnic C-peptide output in normal man. Diabetologia 1979; 17:221–227.

81. Radziuk. J. The numerical solution from measurement data of linear integral equations of the first kind. Int J Num Meth Engin 1977; 11:729–735.

82. Meistas MT, Zadik Z, Margolis S, Kowarski AA. Correlation of urinary excretion of C-peptide with the integrated concentration and secretion rate of insulin. Diabetes 1981; 30:639–643.

83. Faber OK, Hagen C, Binder C, Markussen J, Naithani VK, Blix P, Kuzuya H, Horwitz DL, Rubenstein AH, Rossing N. Kinetics of human connecting peptide in normal and diabetic subjects. J Clin Invest 1978; 62:197–203.

84. Eaton RP, Allen RC, Schade DS, Erickson KM, Standefer J. Prehepatic insulin production in man: kinetic analysis using peripheral connecting peptide behavior. J Clin Endocrinol Metab 1980; 51:520–528.

85. Matthews DR, Rudenski AS, Burnett MA, Darling P, Turner RC. The half-life of endogenous insulin and C-peptide in man assessed by somatostatin suppression. Clin Endocrinol 1985; 23:71–79.

86. Kaneko T, Meinemura M, Oka H, Oda T, Suzuki H, Tasuda H, Tanaihara N, Nakagawa S, Makabe K. Demonstration of C-peptide immunoreactivity in various body fluids and clinical evaluation of the determination of urinary C-peptide immunoreactivity. Endocrinol Jpn 1975; 22:207–222.

87. Blix PM, Boddie WC, Landau RL, Rochman H, Rubenstein AH. Urinary C-peptide: an indicator of beta cell secretion under different metabolic conditions. J Clin Endocrinol Metab 1982; 54:574–580.

88. Polonsky KS, Licinio-Paixao S, Given BD, Pugh W, Rue P, Galloway J, Karrison T, Frank B. Use of biosynthetic human C-peptide in the measurement of insulin secretion rates in normal volunteers and type I diabetic patients. J Clin Invest 1986; 77:98–105.

89. Toffolo G, Bergman RN, Finegood DT, Bowden CR, Cobelli C. Quantitative estimation of beta cell sensitivity to glucose in the intact organism. A minimal model of insulin kinetics in the dog. Diabetes 1980; 29:979–990.

90. Volund A, Polonsky KS, Bergman RN. Calculated pattern of intraportal insulin appearance without independent assessment of C-peptide kinetics. Diabetes 1987; 36:1195–1202.

91. Watanabe RM, Volund A, Roy S, Bergman RN. Prehepatic β-cell secretion during the glucose tolerance test in humans: application of a combined model of insulin and C-peptide kinetics. J Clin Endocrinol Metab 1989; 69:790–797.

92. Cobelli C, Pacini G. Insulin secretion and hepatic extraction in humans by minimal modeling of C-peptide and insulin kinetics. Diabetes 1988; 37:223–231.

93. Castillo MJ, Scheen AJ, Letiexhe MR, Lefebvre PJ. How to measure insulin clearance. Diabetes/Metab Rev 1994; 10:119–150.

94. Polonsky KS, Rubenstein AH. C-peptide as a measure of the secretion and hepatic extraction of insulin. Pitfalls and limitations. Diabetes 1984; 33:486–494.

95. Heine RJ, Bilo HJG, Van der Meer J, Van der Veen EA. Sequential infusions of glucose and insulin at prefixed rates: a simple method for assessing insulin sensitivity and insulin responsiveness. Diabetes Res 1986; 3:453–461.

96. Kissebah AH, Peiris A, Evans DJ. Mechanisms associating body fat distribution to glucose intolerance and diabetes mellitus: window with a view. Acta Med Scand 1988; 723(Suppl):79–89.

97. Evans DJ, Hoffmann RG, Kalkhoff RK, Kissebah AH. Relationship of androgenic activity to body fat topography, fat cell morphology, and metabolic aberrations in premenopausal women. J Clin Endocrinol Metab 1983; 57:304–310.

98. Jeanrenaud B. Hyperinsulinemia in obesity syndromes: its metabolic consequences and possible etiology. Metab Clin Exp 1978; 27:1881–1892.

99. Ogilvie RF. The islands of Langerhans in 19 cases of obesity. J Pathol 1933; 37:473–481.

100. Mahler RJ. The pathogenesis of pancreatic islet cell hyperplasia and insulin insensitivity in obesity. Adv Metab Disord 1974; 7:213–241.

101. Savage PJ, Flock EV, Mako ME, Blix PM, Rubenstein AH, Bennett PH. C-peptide and insulin secretion in Pima Indians and Caucasians: constant fractional hepatic extraction over a wide range of insulin concentrations and in obesity. J Clin Endocrinol Metab 1979; 48:594–598.

102. Bonora E, Zavaroni I, Bruschi F, Alpi O, Pezzarossa A, Guerra L, D'Allaglio E, Coscelli C, Butturini U. Peripheral hyperinsulinemia of simple obesity: pancreatic hypersecretion or impaired insulin metabolism? J Clin Endocrinol Metab 1984; 59:1121–1127.

103. Walter RM, Gold EM, Michas CA. Portal and peripheral vein concentrations of insulin after glucose and arginine infusions in morbidly obese subjects. Life Sci 1980; 26:261–266.

104. Bogardus C, Lillioja S, Mott DM, Hollenbeck C, Reaven G. Relationship between degree of obesity and in vivo insulin action in man. Am J Physiol 1985; 248:E286–E291.

105. Polonsky KS, Given BD, Hirsch LJ, Tillil H, Shapiro ET, Beebe C, Frank BH, Galloway JA, Van Cauter E. Abnormal patterns of insulin secretion in non-insulin-dependent diabetes mellitus. N Engl J Med 1988; 318:1231–1239.

106. Lefebvre PJ, Paolisso G, Scheen AJ, Henquin JC. Pulsatility of insulin and glucagon release: physiological significance and pharmacological implications. Diabetologia 1987; 30:443–452.

107. Weigle DS. Pulsatile secretion of fuel-regulatory hormones. Diabetes 1987; 36:764–775.

108. Strubbe JH, Steffens AB. Neural control of insulin secretion. Horm Metab Res 1993; 25:507–512.

109. Sonnenberg GE, Hoffmann RG, Johnson CP, Kissebah AH. Low- and high-frequency insulin secretion pulses in normal subjects and pancreas transplant recipients. J Clin Invest 1992; 90:545–553.

110. Shapiro ET, Tillil H, Polonsky KD, Fang VS, Rubinstein AH, Van Cauter E. Oscillations in insulin secretion during constant glucose infusion in normal man: relationship to changes in plasma glucose. J Clin Endocrinol Metab 1988; 67:307–314.

111. Sturis J, Van Cauter E, Blackman JD, Polonsky KS. Entrainment of pulsatile insulin secretion by oscillatory glucose infusion. J Clin Invest 1991; 87:439–445.

112. Bergstrom RW, Fujimoto WY, Teller DC, De Haen C. Oscillatory insulin secretion in perifused isolated rat islets. Am J Physiol 1989; 257:E479–E485.

113. Chou H-F, Ipp E, Bowsher RR, Berman N, Ezrin C, Griffiths S. Sustained pulsatile insulin secretion from adenomatous human β-cells: synchronous cycling of insulin, C-peptide, and proinsulin. Diabetes 1991; 40:1453–1458.

114. Stagner JI, Samols E, Weir GC. Sustained oscillations of insulin, glucagon, and somatostatin from the isolated canine pancreas during exposure to a constant glucose concentration. J Clin Invest 1980; 65:939–942.

115. Simon C, Brandenberger G, Follenius M. Ultradian oscillations of plasma glucose, insulin, and C-peptide in man during continuous enteral nutrition. J Clin Endocrinol Metab 1987; 64:669–674.

116. Faber OK, Christensen K, Kehlet J, Madsbad S, Binder C. Decreased insulin removal contributes to hyperinsulinemia in obesity. J Clin Endocrinol Metab 1981; 53:618–621.

117. Rossell R, Gomis R, Casamitjana R, Segura R, Vilardell E, Rivera F. Reduced hepatic insulin extraction in obesity: relationship with plasma insulin levels. J Clin Endocrinol Metab 1983; 56:608–611.

118. Björntorp P. "Portal" adipose tissue as a generator of risk factors for cardiovascular disease and diabetes. Arteriosclerosis 1990; 10:493–496.

119. Hennes MMI, McCune SA, Shrago E, Kissebah AH. Synergistic effects of male sex and obesity on hepatic insulin dynamics in SHR/Mcc-cp rat. Diabetes 1990; 39: 789–795.

120. Svedberg J, Strömbland G, Wirth A, Smith U, Björntorp P. Fatty acids in the portal vein of the rat regulate hepatic insulin clearance. J Clin Invest 1991; 88:2054–2058.

121. Hennes MMI, Shrago E, Kissebah AH. Receptor and postreceptor effects of free fatty acids (FFA) on hepatocyte insulin dynamics. Int J Obes 1990; 14:831–841.

122. Hennes MMI, Shrago E, Kissebah AH. Divergent effects of free fatty acids (FFA) oxidation on hepatocyte insulin processing. In: Oomura Y, Tarui S, Inoue S, Shimazu T, eds. Progress in Obesity Research. London: John Libbey, 1992:277–284.

123. Svedberg J, Björntorp P, Smith U, Lönnroth P. Free-fatty acid inhibition of insulin binding, degradation, and action in isolated rat hepatocytes. Diabetes 1990; 39:570–574.

124. Hennes MMI, Dua A, Kissebah AH. Effects of free fatty acids and glucose on splanchnic insulin dynamics. Diabetes 1997; 46:57–62.

125. Meier DA, Hennes MMI, McCune SA, Kissebah AH. Effects of obesity and gender on insulin receptor expression in liver of SHHF/Mcc-FA^{cp} rats. Obes Res 1995; 3: 465–470.

126. Holmäng A, Svedberg J, Jennische E, Björntorp P. Effects of testosterone on muscle insulin sensitivity and morphology in female rats. Am J Physiol 1990; 259: E555–E560.

127. Krakower GR, Meier DA, Kissebah AH. Female sex hormones, perinatal, and peripubertal androgenization on hepatocyte insulin dynamics in rats. Am J Physiol 1993; 264:E342–E347.

128. Yalow RS, Berson SA. Assay of plasma insulin in human subjects by immunological methods. Nature 1959; 184: 1648–1649.

129. Randle PJ, Garland PB, Hales CH, Newsholme EA. The glucose fatty-acid cycle: its role in insulin sensitivity and the metabolic disturbances of diabetes mellitus. Lancet 1963; i:785–789.

130. Saloranta C, Groop L. Interactions between glucose and FFA metabolism in man. Diabetes/Metab Rev 1996; 12: 15–36.

131. Hennes MMI, O'Shaughnessy IM, Kelly TM, LaBelle P, Egan BM, Kissebah AH. Insulin-resistant lipolysis in abdominally-obese hypertensives. Role of the renin-angiotensin system. Hypertension 1996; 28:120–126.

132. Thiebaud D, DeFronzo RA, Jacot E, Golay A, Acheson K, Maeder E, Jéquier E, Felber J-P. Effect of long chain triglyceride infusion on glucose metabolism in man. Metabolism 1982; 31:1128–1136.

133. Kelly DE., Simoneau J-A. Impaired free fatty acid utilization by skeletal muscle in non-insulin-dependent diabetes mellitus. J Clin Invest 1992; 94:2349–2356.

134. Björntorp P. Metabolic implications of body fat distribution. Diabetes Care 1991; 14:1132–1143.

135. Martin BC, Warram JH, Rosner B, Rich SS, Soeldner JS, Krolewski AS. Familial clustering of insulin sensitivity. Diabetes 1992; 41:850–854.

136. Hamman RF. Genetic and environmental determinants of non-insulin-dependent diabetes mellitus (NIDDM). Diabetes/Metab Rev 1992; 8:287–338.

137. Pyke DA. Diabetes: the genetic connections. Diabetologia 1979; 17:333–343.

138. Poller W, Schatz H. Molecular genetic analysis of NIDDM. Exp Clin Endocrinol 1993; 101:58–68.

139. Gerbitz KD. Does the mitochondrial DNA play a role in the pathogenesis of diabetes? Diabetologia 1992; 35: 1181–1186.

140. Kahn CR, Vicent D, Doria A. Genetics of non-insulin-dependent (type-II) diabetes mellitus. Annu Rev Med 1996; 47:509–531.

141. Lillioja S, Young AA, Cutler CL, Ivy IL, Abbott GH, Zawadzki IK, Yki-Järvinen H, Christin L, Secomb TW, Bogardus C. Skeletal muscle capillary density and fiber type are possible determinants of in vivo insulin resistance in man. J Clin Invest 1987; 80:19–25.

142. Schweinfest CW, Henderson KW, Gu J-R. Subtraction hybridization of cDNA libraries from colon carcinoma and hepatic cancer. Gene Anal Technol 1990; 7:64–70.

143. Kissebah AH. Low density lipoprotein metabolism in non-insulin-dependent diabetes mellitus. Diabetes/Metab Rev 1987; 3:619–651.

144. Kissebah AH, Schectman G. Hormones and lipoprotein metabolism. Baillière's Clin Endocrinol Metab 1987; 1: 699–725.

145. The Expert Panel. Summary of the second report of the National Cholesterol Education Program (NCEP) Expert Panel on Detection, Evaluation, and Treatment of High Blood Cholesterol in Adults (Adult Treatment Panel II). JAMA 1993; 269:3015–3023.

146. Haffner SM, Fong D, Hazuda HP, Pugh JA, Patterson JK. Hyperinsulinemia, upper-body adiposity and cardiovascular risk factors in non-diabetics. Metabolism 1988; 37: 333–345.

147. Austin MA, King M-C, Vranizan KM, Krauss RM. Atherogenic lipoprotein phenotype. A proposed genetic marker for coronary heart disease risk. Circulation 1990; 82: 495–506.

148. Chen M, Breslow JL, Li W, Deff T. Transcriptional regulation of the apoC-III gene by insulin in diabetic mice: correlation with changes in plasma triglyceride levels. J Lipid Res 1994; 35:1918–1924.

149. Kuusi, T, Yki-Järvinen H, Kauppinen-Makelin R, Jauhiainen M, Ehnholm C, Kauppila M, Seppala P, Viikari J, Kujansuu E, Rajala S, Lahti J, Niskanen L, Marjanen T, Salo S, Ryysy L, Tulokas T, Taskinen M-R. Effect of insulin treatment on serum lipoprotein(a) in non-insulin-dependent diabetes. Eur J Clin Invest 1995; 25:194–200.

150. Pouliot M-C, Després J-P, Moorjani S, Lupien PJ, Tremblay A, Bouchard C. Apolipoprotein E polymorphism alters the

association between body fatness and plasma lipoproteins in women. J Lipid Res 1990; 31:1023–1029.

151. Srinivasan R, Ehnholm C, Wattigney WA, Berenson GS. Relationship between obesity and serum lipoproteins in children with different apolipoprotein E phenotypes: the Bogalusa Heart Study. Metabolism 1994; 43:470–475.

152. Després J-P, Verdon M-F, Moorjani S, Pouliot M, Nadeau A, Bouchard C, Tremblay A, Lupien PJ. Apolipoprotein E polymorphism modifies relation of hyperinsulinemia to hypertriglyceridemia. Diabetes 1993; 42:1474–1481.

153. Krauss RM. Dense low density lipoproteins and coronary artery disease. Am J Cardiol 1995; 75:53B–57B.

154. Degraaf J, Hak-Lemmers HLM, Hectors MPC, Demacker PNM, Hendriks JCM, Stalenhoef AFH. Enhanced susceptibility to in vitro oxidation of the dense low density lipoprotein subfraction in healthy subjects. Arterioscler Thromb 1991; 11:298–306.

155. Furman RH, Alaupovic R, Howard RP. Hormones and lipoproteins. Prog Biochem Pharm 1967; 2:215–249.

156. Glueck CJ, Fallat RW, Scheel D. Effects of estrogenic compounds on triglyceride kinetics. Metabolism 1975; 24:537–545.

157. Haffner SM, Kushwaha RS, Foster DM, Applebaum-Bowden D, Hazzard WR. Studies on the metabolic mechanism of reduced high density lipoproteins during anabolic steroid therapy. Metabolism 1983; 32:413–420.

158. Freedman DS, Jacobsen SJ, Barboriak JJ, Sobocinski KA, Andersen AJ, Kissebah AH, Sasse EA, Gruchow HW. Body fat distribution and male/female differences in lipids and lipoproteins. Circulation 1990; 81:1498–1506.

159. Stone MC, Thorp JM. Plasma fibrinogen—a major coronary risk factor. JR Coll Gen Pract 1985; 35:565–569.

160. Landin K, Stigendal L, Eriksson E, Krotkiewski M, Risberg B, Tengborn L, Smith U. Abdominal obesity is associated with an impaired fibrinolytic activity and elevated plasminogen activator inhibitor-1. Metabolism 1990; 39:1044–1048.

161. Ditschuneit HH, Flechtner-Mors M, Adler G. Fibrinogen in obesity before and after weight reduction. Obes Res 1995; 3:43–48.

162. Vague P, Juhan-Vague I, Aillaud MF, Badier C, Viard R, Alessi MC, Collen D. Correlation between blood fibrinolytic activity, plasminogen activator inhibitor level, plasma insulin level and relative body weight in normal and obese subjects. Metabolism 1986; 35:250–263.

163. Heinecke JW. Cellular mechanisms for the oxidative modification of lipoproteins: implications for atherogenesis. Coronary Artery Dis 1994; 5:205–210.

164. Van Gaal LF, Zhang A, Steijaert M, De Leeuw I. Human obesity: from lipid abnormalities to lipid oxidation. Int J Obes 1995; 19(Suppl 3):S21–S26.

166. Austin MA. Genetic epidemiology of low-density lipoprotein subclass phenotypes. Ann Med 1991; 24:477–481.

167. Nishina PM, Johnson JP, Naggert KJ, Krauss RM. Linkage of atherogenic lipoprotein phenotype to the low density

lipoprotein receptor locus on the short arm of chromosome 19. Proc Natl Acad Sci USA 1992; 89:708–712.

168. Brown MS, Goldstein JL. A receptor mediated pathway for cholesterol homeostasis. Science 1986; 232:34–47.

169. Lusis AJ. Genetic factors affecting blood lipoproteins: the candidate gene approach. J Lipid Res 1988; 29:397–429.

170. Krauss RM. Low-density lipoprotein subclasses and risk of coronary artery disease. Curr Opin Lipidol 1991; 2:248–252.

171. Mitchell RJ, Earl L, Bray P, Fripp YJ, Williams J. DNA polymorphisms at the lipoprotein lipase gene and their associations with quantitative variation in plasma high-density lipoproteins and triacylglycerides. Hum Biol 1994; 66:383–397.

172. Rowe JW, Young JB, Minaker KL, Stevens AL, Pallota J, Landsberg L. Effect of insulin and glucose infusions on sympathetic nervous system activity in normal man. Diabetes 1981; 30:219–225.

173. Stepniakowski KT, Egan BM. Additive effects of hypertension and obesity to limit venous distensibility: hemodynamic correlates and metabolic mechanism. Am J Physiol 1995; 268:R562–R568.

174. Stepniakowski KT, Goodfriend TL, Egan BM. Fatty acids enhance vascular α-adrenergic sensitivity. Hypertension 1995; 25:774–778.

175. Egan BM, Stepniakowski K, Goodfriend TL. Renin and aldosterone are higher and the hyperinsulinemic effects of salt restriction greater in subjects with risk factor clustering. Am J Hypertens 1994; 7:886–893.

176. Jonsson JR, Game PA, Head RJ, Frewin DB. The expression and localization of the angiotensin-converting enzyme mRNA in human adipose tissue. Blood Press 1994; 3:72–75.

177. Frederich RC, Kahn BB, Peach MJ, Flier JS. Tissue-specific nutritional regulation of angiotensinogen in adipose tissue. Hypertension 1992; 19:339–344.

178. Dominiczak AF, Bohr DF. Nitric oxide and its putative role in hypertension. Hypertension 1995; 25:1202–1211.

179. Morris BJ. Identification of essential hypertension genes. J Hypertens 1993; 11:115–120.

180. Lifton RP. Genetic determinants of human hypertension. Proc Natl Acad Sci USA 1995; 92:8545–8551.

181. Mune T, Rogerson FM, Nikkila H, Agarwal AK, White PC. Human hypertension caused by mutations in the kidney isozyme of 11 beta-hydroxysteroid dehydrogenase. Nat Genet 1995; 10:394–399.

182. Jeunemaitre X, Soubrier F, Kotelevtsev YV, Lifton RP, Williams CS, Charru A, Hunt SC, Hopkins PN, Williams RR, Lalouel JM, Corvol P. Molecular basis of human hypertension: role of angiotensinogen. Cell 1992; 71:169–180.

183. Hata A. Role of angiotensinogen in the genetics of essential hypertension. Life Sci 1995; 57:2385–2395.

184. Hansson JH, Nelson-Williams C, Suzuki H, Schild L, Shimkets R, Canessa C, Iwasaki T, Rossier B, Lifton RP. Hypertension caused by a truncated epithelial sodium chan-

nel gamma subunit: genetic heterogeneity of Liddle syndrome. Nat Genet 1995; 11:76–82.

185. Wu D-A, Bu X, Warden CH, Shen DDC, Jeng C-Y, Shue WHH, Fuh MMT, Katsuya T, Dzau VJ, Reaven GM, Lusis AJ, Rotter JI, and Chen Y-DI. Quantitative trait locus mapping of human blood pressure to a genetic region at or near the lipoprotein lipase gene locus on chromosome 8p22. J Clin Invest 1996; 97:2111–2118.

186. Terry RB, Wood PD, Haskell WL, Stefanick ML, Krauss RM. Regional adiposity patterns in relation to lipids, lipoprotein cholesterol, and lipoprotein subfraction mass in men. J Clin Endocrinol Metab 1989; 68:191–199.

187. Kanai H, Tokunaga K, Fujioka S, Yamashita S, Kameda-Takemura K, Matsuzawa Y. Decrease in intra-abdominal visceral fat may reduce blood pressure in obese hypertensive women. Hypertension 1996; 27:125–129.

29

The Effects of Obesity on the Cardiovascular System

Edward Saltzman
Tufts University School of Medicine, New England Medical Center and The Jean Mayer USDA Human Nutrition Research Center on Aging at Tufts University, Boston, Massachusetts

Peter N. Benotti
Englewood Hospital and Medical Center, Englewood, New Jersey and Mt. Sinai School of Medicine, New York, New York

I. INTRODUCTION

Cardiovascular disease is a major cause of premature morbidity and mortality in severe obesity (1). Obesity contributes to increased risk for ischemic heart disease, arrhythmia, sudden death, and congestive heart failure. Recognition of the adverse cardiovascular sequelae of the obese state, coupled with the increasing prevalence of obesity (2), has stimulated considerable research into the relationships between obesity and the cardiovascular system. Since obesity promotes several risk factors for cardiovascular disease, debate persists as to the role of excess weight per se in cardiovascular pathology. There can be no debate, however, that obesity, whether contributing directly or indirectly, is associated with deleterious effects on the heart and circulatory system.

In this chapter, we briefly review basic aspects of cardiovascular physiology and adaptation of the cardiovascular system to obesity, followed by a discussion of associated disease states. That some obese individuals are afflicted by cardiovascular disease while others are not warrants a discussion of interindividual, gender, and ethnic differences in obesity-related cardiovascular disease. Finally, the effects of weight loss on cardiovascular function and pathology are discussed.

II. BASIC ASPECTS OF CARDIOVASCULAR PHYSIOLOGY AND THE ADAPTATION TO OBESITY

Viewed simply, the function of the heart is to pump blood throughout the body via the circulatory system. The amount of blood pumped by the heart to the systemic circulation, termed cardiac output, is in general regulated by the metabolic needs of the body. Expressed in liters per minute, cardiac output is determined by the amount of blood ejected by the heart each time pumping occurs (stroke volume), and by the rate of pumping (heart rate). In states characterized by increased metabolic demands, the required increment in cardiac output can be achieved by increases in stroke volume and/or heart rate. Obesity is characterized by increased total body oxygen consumption, due to expanded lean mass and skin, as well as the oxidative demands of metabolically active adipose tissue (3,4). Absolute cardiac output in obesity is increased, but when it is normalized to body surface area (cardiac index), values remain in the normal range (5). Because blood flow per unit of adipose tissue and oxygen consumption requirements are lower for adipose tissue than those for lean tissue, oxygen consumption expressed per kilogram of body weight in obesity is less than that in lean subjects (4–7).

Pumping of blood to the systemic circulation is primarily effected by the left ventricle, and left ventricular function is determined by the characteristics of the ventricle itself as well as loading characteristics. Preload refers to the volume of ventricular filling and thus the extent to which the ventricle is stretched during filling (diastole). Afterload refers to the resistance against which blood is ejected during contraction (systole). According to Starling's law, preload is proportional to the end-diastolic volume of the left ventricle. As end-diastolic volume increases, contractile performance of the ventricle improves, increasing stroke volume; this relationship is defined by the Frank-Starling curve. Factors that increase end-diastolic volume, and thus preload, have in common increased venous return of blood to the heart, and include expanded blood volume, increase in venous tone, increased skeletal muscle pumping action, and negative thoracic pressure. Ejection fraction is the percentage of end-diastolic volume that is ejected with each contraction, and normal values approximate 65%. This is a valuable clinical index of ventricular function and can be measured by radionuclide imaging or by echocardiogram.

It has been observed that in obesity, the increased demand for cardiac output is achieved by increases in stroke volume, while heart rate remains comparatively unchanged (8–10). Obesity-related increases in stroke volume result from increases in diastolic filling of the left ventricle (6–8,11). Total blood volume in obese individuals is increased in proportion to body weight (8,12), such that obesity can be considered a volume-expanded state. Thus volume expansion of the circulatory system contributes to the increase in left ventricular preload, and the commonly observed increases in total blood and plasma volume in obesity are associated with increased resting cardiac output. Since arteriovenous extraction of oxygen from blood, another mechanism by which additional oxygen could be supplied to tissue, is little changed in obesity, increases in cardiac output correlate well with increases in total body oxygen consumption (6). Table 1 lists some hemodynamic alternations in severe obesity.

The volume expansion and increased cardiac output in obesity eventually lead to structural changes of the heart. Increased left ventricular filling in obesity serves to increase left ventricular cavity dimension and increases left ventricular wall stress. Over time, increased wall stress acts to stimulate hypertrophy of the ventricle, enlarging ventricular mass and thus normalizing wall stress. As left ventricular dilatation is accompanied by myocardial hypertrophy, the ratio between ventricular cavity radius and wall thickness is preserved. This process, called eccentric hypertrophy, is of importance in maintaining functional cardiovascular reserve (Fig. 1).

Table 1 Hemodynamic Alterations in Severe Obesity

Heart rate	↔ or ↑
Oxygen consumption	↑
Cardiac output	↑
Cardiac index	↔ or ↑
Blood pressure	↔ or ↑

Hypertrophy is manifest by increases in left ventricular mass and can be measured by echocardiogram or angiography. Ventricular mass increases directly in proportion to the body mass index or degree of overweight, as has been demonstrated in the Framingham Heart Study (13) and by others (14–17). The relationship between left ventricular mass and body mass index is also observed in children and adolescents, and overweight prior to adulthood may be associated with increased left ventricular mass beyond that predicted by linear growth (18,19).

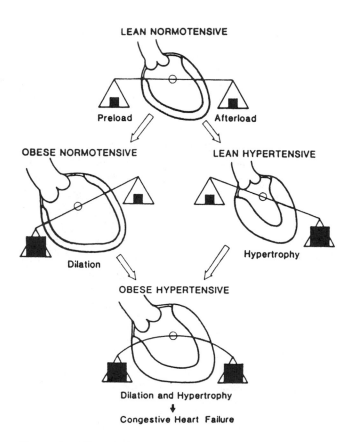

Figure 1 Effect of obesity and hypertension on cardiac structure. (Adapted from Messerli, FH, Cardiovascular effects of obesity, Lancet 1982;1:1165.)

Blood pressure is a function of cardiac output and the vascular resistance against which blood is pumped, or systemic vascular resistance. Given the elevations of cardiac output in obesity, a concomitant rise in blood pressure might be expected. Elevated cardiac output is common in mild and moderate obesity and is universal in severe obesity (6); that all these individuals are not hypertensive suggests that a compensatory mechanism exists. Indeed, in normotensive obesity, increases in blood pressure are prevented by commensurate drops in systemic vascular resistance (5,7,12). The hemodynamic state of normotensive obesity can be contrasted with that of hypertensive obesity (5). Hypertension in lean patients is in general characterized by increased cardiac output, elevated systemic vascular resistance, and a contracted intravascular volume. Like normotensive obesity, hypertension in obesity is characterized by increased cardiac output and volume expansion. However, hypertensive obesity reflects normal or increased levels of systemic vascular resistance. Proposed factors leading to normal or elevated vascular resistance in obesity include enhanced sympathetic activity (20), abnormal vascular responses to hyperinsulinemia (21), effects of hypoxia, and hypoventilation (6,22). Arterial hypertension, by increasing the force against which the left ventricle must pump, also increases wall tension and stimulates ventricular hypertrophy. Since intravascular volume is contracted in lean hypertensives, ventricular wall dimensions increase disproportionately to the chamber radius, resulting in concentric hypertrophy. Figure 1 demonstrates the respective effects of obesity and hypertension on the left ventricle. The effects of hypertension appear additive to those of excess weight in stimulating ventricular hypertrophy (23–25). The combination of hypertension and obesity causes significant increases in cardiac work, which is defined as the product of stroke volume and the left ventricular pressure generated. The hypertensive subject increases work by increasing systolic pressure, while obese patients increase work by increasing stroke volume. The combination of severe obesity and hypertension markedly increases cardiac work by conditions of overloaded pressure and volume (26).

Recent research efforts have focused on definition of those factors in the obese most likely to be associated with ventricular hypertrophy. Central adiposity in normotensive men has been reported to be an equal or stronger predictor of left ventricular mass than is body mass index (14,16) and may reflect an unfavorable hemodynamic profile associated with visceral obesity (27). Since visceral adiposity is associated with alterations in insulin metabolism (as discussed in other chapters), a link between insulin metabolism and ventricular hypertrophy has been suggested. Preliminary studies have reported associations between left ventricular hypertrophy and measures of insulin resistance or hyperinsulinemia, but the complex interactions between body weight or fatness, insulin, blood pressure and ventricular hypertrophy are not yet clearly defined (28–30).

III. OBESITY AND CARDIOVASCULAR PATHOLOGY

The observation that the structural adaptation of the heart to obesity is related to clinical disease is not a recent one. In 1933, Smith and Willius reported their findings from postmortem examinations of 136 obese patients who died of congestive heart failure, but were free of coronary artery or other heart disease (31). These authors noted a direct relationship between body weight and heart weight but, along with other investigators of that day, attributed increased mass and resultant disease to fatty infiltration (31,32).

In large part due to the pioneering efforts of J. K. Alexander and F. H. Messerli, the hemodynamic, clinical, and pathological basis of the cardiomyopathy of obesity has been elucidated. In a 1965 autopsy study, Amad et al. (33) examined the relationship between body weight and heart weight in 12 severely obese subjects without hypertension, coronary artery disease, or other heart disease. Heart weight was far in excess of that predicted for ideal body weight, gross ventricular hypertrophy was present, and on microscopic examination the cause was noted to be myocardial hypertrophy. Numerous additional studies have confirmed the presence of left ventricular hypertrophy in the setting of obesity (6), and as discussed below, numerous others have demonstrated that this hypertrophy is not an entirely benign adaptation to excess weight.

Fatty infiltration of the heart, defined as extension of epicardial fat into the myocardium and perivascular regions, has subsequently been observed in about 3% of obese subjects in autopsy studies (34). Since this condition has been found in many clinical settings apart from obesity, the role it plays in cardiovascular pathophysiology and dysfunction is unclear. There are several anecdotal reports of obese patients dying of presumed arrhythmia with subsequent findings of fatty infiltration of the conduction system, suggesting that fatty infiltration can be associated with significant morbidity and mortality.

Over the last several decades, multiple scenarios in which obesity contributes to cardiovascular disease have become evident. First, the physiological adaptation to obesity may be incomplete, and thus the expanded intravascular volume in obesity cannot be circulated effectively, leading to congestive heart failure. Second, physiological adaptation may itself be associated with risks for cardio-vascular disease. Also, the obese state is associated with or promotes other cardiovascular risk factors. Finally, obesity may promote cardiovascular disease, directly or indirectly, by processes yet to be elucidated. Compelling evidence exists for the former three scenarios, while current controversies in the link between cardiovascular disease and obesity leave much room for identification of new important factors.

A. Left Ventricular Hypertrophy and Congestive Heart Failure

Cardiovascular adaptation to the increased intravascular volume of obesity may not completely restore normal hemodynamic function. As a result, the heart may ineffectively circulate blood through the body and lungs, leading to circulatory congestion. Both systolic (pumping) and diastolic (filling) dysfunction contribute to congestive heart failure, and both are observed in obesity. Clinically, this ranges from diminished cardiovascular reserves (for example, as needed for exercise) to frank heart failure. Figure 2 illustrates the progression from cardiac adaptation and compensation to congestive heart failure.

Marked systolic dysfunction occurs as the ventricle can no longer adapt to volume overload, resulting in dilatation. With dilatation, the left ventricular cavity radius to wall thickness ratio increases and eventually ventricular contractility declines (6). Systolic dysfunction in obesity appears to be a function of the degree, as well as the duration, of overweight. Licata et al. (8) showed that left ventricular ejection fraction decreased in relationship to body mass index (BMI) and to duration of overweight (Fig. 3). Despite elevated cardiac output, obese individuals have been shown to have depressed myocardial contractility by load-dependent and -independent indexes, and that impairment in contractility is proportional to excess weight (7,35).

With left ventricular hypertrophy, reduced ventricular compliance may alter the ability of the chamber to accommodate increased volume during diastole. Such diastolic dysfunction accompanying obesity and eccentric hypertrophy has been demonstrated by echocardiography (9,15,16,25). Lavie et al. (25) showed that electrocardiographic evidence of left atrial abnormality correlated with impaired diastolic function in subjects who averaged 170% of ideal weight. Since electrocardiographic evidence of left ventricular hypertrophy in severe obesity may be obscured by chest wall thickness, the presence of atrial abnormality not only suggests diastolic dysfunction, but should also raise suspicion of underlying structural changes such as hypertrophy.

Alexander (6) has suggested that obese patients presenting with symptoms of congestive heart failure may represent two scenarios that are clinically indistinguishable. In one scenario, systolic function is well preserved by eccentric hypertrophy, and congestive symptoms arise from diastolic dysfunction. In the other, impaired systolic function is found. As Alexander notes, assessment of left ventricular function by echocardiography or angiography may be necessary to differentiate the underlying pathophysiology.

Systolic and diastolic dysfunction in obesity can progress to clinically significant heart failure. Body weight, independent of several traditional risk factors, was directly related to development of congestive heart failure in the Framingham Heart Study (36). When age groups and genders in that study are combined, those subjects who were greater than 130% of Metropolitan Relative Weight (MRW) had an incidence of congestive heart failure almost twice that of subjects less than 110% of MRW. Further evidence is provided by Kasper et al. (37) who performed endocardial biopsy on lean and overweight patients with clinically evident dilated cardiomyopathy to assess the etiology of heart failure. Specific pathological diagnoses were evident in 64% of the patients with BMI <30 kg/m^2, while in those patients with BMI >35 kg/m^2, no specific tissue diagnosis could be made in 77%, suggesting that obesity may have been the primary etiological factor. While further clinicopathological studies are needed, this work suggests that the dilated cardiomyopathy of obesity is a major cause of cardiac failure in the obese.

In addition to congestive heart failure, the presence of left ventricular hypertrophy has been associated with greater risk of morbidity and mortality from coronary heart disease and sudden death (38–42), as well as arrhythmia (reviewed in Ref. 41). One cautionary note, however, is that concentric and eccentric forms of left ventricular hypertrophy have not been differentiated in relation to adverse effects in several investigations. While both forms are likely to be associated with increased cardiovascular risk, better definition of the risks associated with eccentric or concentric hypertrophies is needed.

B. Coronary Artery Disease

The specific relationship between coronary artery disease (atherosclerotic disease of the arteries supplying the myocardium) and body weight remains controversial. It is ironic that while excess body weight is associated with or promotes multiple risk factors for coronary artery disease, clear definition of the role of obesity in coronary artery disease has proved elusive. Autopsy evidence for clinically significant or premature coronary artery disease in obese

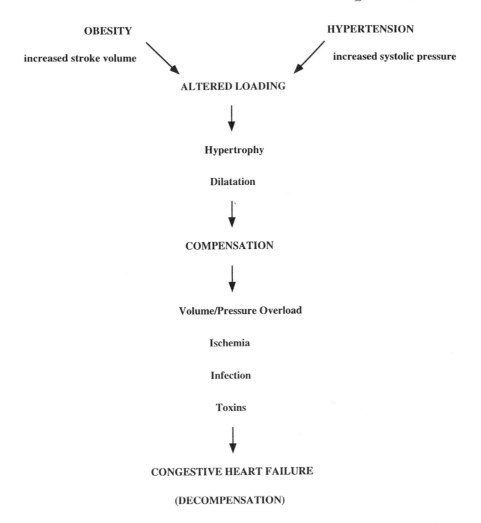

OBESITY

increased stroke volume

HYPERTENSION

increased systolic pressure

ALTERED LOADING

Hypertrophy

Dilatation

COMPENSATION

Volume/Pressure Overload

Ischemia

Infection

Toxins

CONGESTIVE HEART FAILURE

(DECOMPENSATION)

Figure 2 Progression from hemodynamic alterations in obesity to congestive heart failure.

patients has been inconsistent, and the burden of proof has rested on epidemiological studies (43–45). Many, but not all, epidemiological studies have shown significant relationships between body weight and coronary artery disease. The most consistent relationship observed between obesity and coronary artery disease is a univariate one, not incorporating control for other risk factors (46). In the Framingham Heart Study (36,47), the 26-year incidence of coronary heart disease in men and women related proportionately to excess weight as defined by percent of MRW. In that study, incidence of coronary disease increased by a factor of 2.4 in obese (MRW >130% vs. <110%) women and by a factor of 2 in obese men under the age of 50 years. Keys et al. (48) reported significant risks for coronary disease when BMI exceeded 27 kg/m^2 in American and Southern European men (but not Northern European men). The Nurses Health Study (49),

the Honolulu Heart Program (50), the U.S. National Health and Nutrition Examination Survey I Epidemiologic Follow-up Study (51), and the Whitehall Study (52) provide further epidemiological evidence for a univariate relationship between obesity and coronary artery disease.

When multivariate models are employed, less consistency for the role of obesity in coronary artery disease is found. For example, the contribution of obesity to coronary disease found by Keys et al. (48) was eliminated by controlling for traditional coronary risk factors. However, several recent prospective studies have demonstrated a persistent contribution of body weight to coronary artery disease and myocardial infarction when one or more confounding factors (such as blood pressure, hyperlipidemia, diabetes, smoking, and age) were incorporated into multivariate models (36,49,50,52,53). For example, in the Nurses Health Study the magnitude of elevated relative

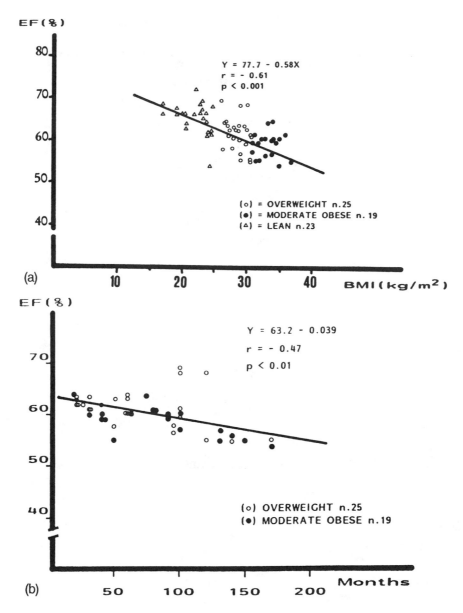

Figure 3 Effects of body mass index (a) and duration (b) of overweight on ejection fraction (EF). Reproduced from Licata (1991) [8], with permission.

risk of coronary disease between highest and lowest BMI quintiles was diminished, but not eliminated, by adjustment for several known risk factors (RR 3.4 vs. 1.9, unadjusted vs. adjusted) (49). The independent risk of coronary artery disease attributed to obesity in multivariate analysis may reflect either unmeasured or unrecognized mediators. Table 2 lists a number of these factors that have been proposed to predispose to coronary heart disease in the setting of excess weight.

As obesity is associated with multiple risk factors for coronary artery disease, many authors have suggested that, despite the absence of a consistent independent association between obesity and coronary artery disease, the univariate relationship carries with it important implications for prevention and treatment of obesity. Further, in the clinical setting it seems imprudent to dismiss or ignore the potential impact of obesity on cardiovascular disease even if associated risk factors are absent.

Table 2 Proposed Factors Contributing to Coronary Artery Disease in Obesity

---
Androgen excess
Antioxidant vitamin metabolism
Altered rheology and hemostasis
Homocysteinemia
Hyperinsulinemia/insulin resistance
Sleep apnea
Uric acid

Source: Refs. 22, 104–111.

In most epidemiological studies, degree of obesity is inferred by relative or actual body weight, BMI, or assessment of skinfolds. Since visceral obesity is most associated with adverse risk factor profiles for coronary heart disease (as discussed in other chapters), body fat distribution may better predict those obese patients who subsequently develop disease. Waist-to-hip ratio has been a predictor of coronary heart disease risk in the Health Professionals Follow-Up Study (54), in Swedish women (55), in U.S. military men followed for 23 years after discharge (56), and in black women (57). Waist-to-hip ratio has best predicted disease in individuals younger than 65 years, underscoring the contribution of visceral adiposity to *premature* morbidity and mortality.

C. Arrhythmia and Sudden Death

Obesity is also associated with increased risk of arrhythmia (abnormal heart rhythm) and sudden death (1,36,58). Messerli et al. found that ventricular ectopy, a marker of electrical instability thought to predispose to more serious rhythm disturbances, was dramatically increased in moderately obese patients with hypertension when compared to lean hypertensives (58). In that investigation, a 10-fold increase in ectopy was seen in obese hypertensives, and a 30-fold increase was found in obese hypertensives with left ventricular hypertrophy. Also noted was that the complexity, or potential dangerousness, of the ectopy correlated closely with left ventricular mass. The aforementioned direct relationship between left ventricular mass and body weight suggests that the most obese patients are at greatest risk of complex ectopy, although this association was not observed by Messerli et al. (58). Larger studies may be needed to confirm that this relationship does in fact exist.

Sudden death can result from arrhythmia, myocardial infarction, and other conditions. The exact proportion of sudden deaths attributable to arrhythmia is not known since these patients often experience fatal events in unmonitored settings or are not subject to postmortem examination, which could reveal other mechanisms of death. Left ventricular hypertrophy is a known risk factor for sudden death from arrhythmia (59), and suspicion remains high that arrhythmia is a major cause of sudden death in obesity. The first observation of increased risk of sudden death in obesity is attributed to Hippocrates, who over 2 millennia ago noted, "Sudden death is more common in those who are naturally fat than in the lean" (60). In the Framingham cohort, body weight was highly predictive of sudden death in men (the small number of deaths observed in women precluded significance), and risk for sudden death was independent of traditional cardiovascular risk factors (36). That study also revealed a fivefold increased risk of sudden death in those with congestive heart failure as compared to the general population (42). In a retrospective survey of U.S. surgeons treating severely obese patients, a total of 60 sudden deaths were noted; 52 of these patients died suddenly during weight loss after gastric surgery for obesity, whereas eight patients died while waiting for surgery (61). Although the eight sudden deaths in patients awaiting surgery suggests a dramatic increase in risk, no conclusions regarding relative risk can be made owing to the small number of events and the nature of the study. A major predictor of risk in this series included a prolongation of the Q-T interval on the electrocardiogram.

Mechanisms linking obesity to increased risk for arrhythmia remain unclear. Alterations in parasympathetic and sympathetic cardiac innervation have been observed in the obese (62,63) and in those gaining weight (64) by measurement of heart rate variability. It has been proposed that the resulting autonomic imbalance predisposes to arrhythmia (64,65). As reviewed by Fisler (66), severely obese individuals demonstrate increased rates of Q-T abnormalities on electrocardiograms, which may contribute to arrhythmia risk. Mechanisms secondary to structural changes in obesity have been proposed, including qualitative changes in myocyte electrophysiology, fatty infiltration, fibrosis, physical disruption of the conducting system by hypertrophy, and myocardial ischemia secondary to reduced coronary reserve and increased myocardial work (45,59). Autopsy results in persons dying of sudden death suggest that ventricular hypertrophy or dilated cardiomyopathy are the most common findings, whereas other causes to which death could be attributed appear variable. At autopsy, young (aged 6–32 years) obese individuals have been found to have hypertrophy and greater-than-expected rates of fatty and fibrotic infiltration of the cardiac conduction system, with a history of obstructive sleep apnea noted in several subjects (45). (Sleep apnea itself is associated with arrhythmia and is likely to exacerbate other cardiovascular pathology (22,67)). In contrast, a study of slightly older obese sudden death victims (average age midthirties) revealed a greater degree of dilated cardiomyopathy and nonfatal coronary artery disease (44).

There are also reports of sudden, unexplained deaths in patients undergoing weight loss by fasting and very-low-calorie diets, especially diets of poor nutritional quality (66,68). The exact incidence of this problem has not been established, but the suggestion in the literature is that it is probably quite low. Many theories have been advanced to explain these sudden cardiovascular catastrophes, including nutritionally inadequate protein (69,70), a sensitivity to sympathetic stimulation of the myocardium (66), and micronutrient or electrolyte abnormalities (68–70). Several risk factors for arrhythmia that have emerged from analyses of patients suffering these complications include a prolongation of the Q-T interval and a declining QRS voltage on the electrocardiogram (66,71, 72). Occurrence of these phenomena in a patient during weight loss demands close scrutiny and evaluation of the nutritional adequacy of the diet. While electrocardiographic changes of varying degrees may occur during weight loss, efforts have begun to delineate those changes that may be tolerated without undue risk of arrhythmia or other complication (73).

IV. THE OBESE AFFECTED WITH CARDIOVASCULAR DISEASE VERSUS THE UNAFFECTED; ETHNIC, GENDER, AND INTERINDIVIDUAL DIFFERENCES

That all obese individuals do not suffer cardiovascular problems leads to the question of what differentiates the affected from the unaffected. This issue can be examined from the perspective of ethnic, gender, and interindividual differences among obese patients with and without cardiovascular disease. Since it is beyond the scope of this chapter to explore each of these in detail, an overview is presented, with specific references and reviews noted.

A. Ethnicity

Recent U.S. National Health and Nutrition Examination Survey III (2) data show that the observed prevalence of obesity in black, white, and Hispanic populations does not necessarily predict the prevalence and ill effects of cardiovascular disease.

Population studies in blacks reveal earlier onset and equal (74) or greater (75–77) cardiovascular morbidity and mortality rates compared to whites and Hispanics. Associations between body weight and coronary artery disease among blacks have been even more difficult to demonstrate than in other ethnic groups (78), as has been reviewed by Kumanyika (77,79). The high prevalence of overweight and obesity-related risk factors for heart disease make the absence of the relationship between weight and heart disease surprising, but methodological issues may have impaired efforts to date (77).

Hispanics have a disproportionate amount of obesity, android obesity, diabetes, and hypertension in comparison to non-Hispanic whites. Yet in middle-aged and older Hispanics, mortality from cardiovascular disease has been less than or equal to that in non-Hispanic whites (80,81). Hispanic Americans are approximately two-thirds Mexican-American, and most studies reflect this subgroup; since other subgroups have differing levels of black and Native American admixture, generalization to all Hispanic subgroups may not be appropriate (81).

Of particular concern are secular patterns of cardiovascular disease in minority groups. Trends in cardiovascular morbidity and mortality reveal an overall decrease, but the rate of decline for blacks and Hispanics has been less than that for whites (75,77,81). The proposed reasons for these secular trends, as well as other particularly important issues, are discussed elsewhere (77,79,81).

American Indians, although a heterogeneous group, have a lower prevalence of cardiovascular disease compared to either U.S. whites or the total U.S. population, and yet are characterized by equal or greater degrees of obesity and hypertension. In the Strong Heart Study (76,82), three geographically diverse subgroups of American Indians were assessed for rates of coronary heart disease and associated risk factors. Obesity was a significant predictor of coronary heart disease independent of other known risk factors, although the overall occurrence of coronary heart disease was less than that reported in many studies of non-Hispanic whites and blacks. Among American Indian subgroups studied, Arizona Indians are characterized by a high degree of obesity and a high prevalence of diabetes, yet they have a comparatively low prevalence of coronary heart disease; suspected mitigating factors in this population include lower prevalence of lipid abnormalities and smoking (76).

Controversy exists regarding the need to adjust parameters of cardiovascular disease for ethnic differences. For example, when the left ventricular hypertrophic response to hypertension is assessed by echocardiography, differences between blacks and whites are found for particular structural changes. Electrocardiographic differences between ethnic groups have also been noted (83). This issue warrants further attention so that appropriate diagnostic criteria can be adopted to prevent bias in measurement and assessment of cardiovascular pathology between ethnic groups.

B. Gender

Although prevalence of cardiovascular disease is lower in women than men, the cardiovascular adaptation to obesity as well as the obesity-related risk of cardiovascular disease in women is similar to, or surpasses, that in men (13, 23,36,84). Associations between obesity, increased androgenicity, and cardiovascular risk (induced by both obesity and hormonal factors) are becoming evident. Recent attention has been directed toward the pathophysiological roles of central adiposity (51,57), hyperinsulinemia (85,86), alterations in sex steroid hormones and related binding proteins (80,85,86), and specific individual syndromes such as the polycystic ovary syndrome (85,87).

C. Interindividual Differences

Even after accounting for ethnic and gender effects on obesity-related cardiovascular disease, there remain substantial interindividual differences, as well as unspecified genetic contributions. The degree and duration of overweight have been shown to play important roles. The increase of childhood and adolescent obesity when coupled with the lifelong risks associated with childhood obesity (88), as well as observations in older populations, raise issues about the role of age in mediating cardiovascular disease. Obesity in older age appears less directly related to cardiovascular disease than in younger populations, which suggests that risks specifically need to be defined for those obese persons living into old age. Another factor likely to contribute to interindividual differences in risk is level of physical activity (89,90), although effects in severely obese patients are unclear. Weight cycling has been a topic of considerable research effort and controversy and is discussed at length in another chapter. Finally, factors such as those in Table 2 may account for some interindividual difference in risk for cardiovascular disease in obesity.

V. EFFECTS OF WEIGHT LOSS

The increasing prevalence of obesity and its influence on cardiovascular disease have stimulated tremendous interest in medical and surgical weight loss. Significant weight loss should result in physiological changes that favor an improvement in cardiovascular physiology. Body mass falls and, thus, circulatory demands will drop. Diuresis and normalization of blood pressure should be anticipated. Despite this, the balance between risks and benefits of major weight loss for the grossly obese remains somewhat controversial (91). Factors complicating this analysis include reports of sudden death and serious cardiovascular morbidity in the severely obese, often occurring during periods of rapid weight loss.

An emerging literature supports the favorable cardiovascular changes that occur with weight loss (92). Weight loss has been shown to favorably affect both blood pressure and the left ventricle. Since the consequences of hypertension and the hemodynamic and structural effects of obesity are additive, amelioration of both is especially important.

Many investigators have now documented a significant fall in blood pressure with weight loss in obese hypertensive subjects (93,94). Trials in severely obese hypertensive patients have demonstrated marked improvement in hypertension following gastric surgery (95,96). Importantly, maximum benefit in blood pressure control occurs well before a normal weight is achieved (93). Mechanisms may include diuresis, reduction in blood volume, as well as changes in sympathetic drive associated with weight loss or control, negative energy balance, and decreases in fat mass.

In addition, a number of recent trials suggest that both cardiac structure and function appear to improve after weight loss. McMahon and associates demonstrated reductions in left ventricular mass and septal thickness in moderately obese subjects as well as normalization of blood pressure following medical weight reduction of an average of 8.3 kg (97). Similar observations regarding improvement in blood pressure, ventricular mass, and chamber size have been made in several series of patients following weight reduction as a result of gastric surgery for obesity, pharmacological treatment, and hypocaloric diet with exercise (98–102). Improvement in systolic function has also been demonstrated following surgical and medical weight loss (98,102,103). While weight loss is accompanied by hemodynamic improvement, it remains unclear, however, if regression of left ventricular mass will translate to reduction in risk for associated disease such as arrhythmia and coronary artery disease (59).

The clinical evidence suggests that medically supervised weight reduction can be of great benefit for the grossly obese patient. However, medical supervision requires considerable attention to serial clinical, biochemical, and electrocardiographic data.

VI. CONCLUSION

Obesity is associated with significant risk for cardiovascular morbidity and mortality. The obese state is characterized by increased hemodynamic demands, which result in cardiovascular adaptation. Adaptive mechanisms are limited and are themselves associated with adverse health consequences. The exact role played by obesity in promoting cardiovascular disease is not yet defined, and the extent to which these diseases are reversible with weight loss is not yet clear. However, efforts to date provide encouraging evidence that the prevention and treatment of obesity will substantially reduce cardiovascular disease.

REFERENCES

1. Drenick E, Bale G, Seltzer F, Johnson D. Excessive mortality and causes of death in morbidly obese men. JAMA 1980; 243:443–445.
2. Kuczmarski RJ, Flegal KM, Campbell SM, Johnson CL. Increasing prevalence of overweight among US adults. JAMA 1994; 272:205–211.
3. Ravussin E. Energy expenditure and body weight, In: Brownell K, Fairburn C, eds. Eating Disorders and Obesity. New York: Guilford Press, 1995:32–37.
4. Frayn KN. Studies of human adipose tissue in vivo, In: Kinney JM, Tucker HN, eds. Energy Metabolism: Tissue Determinants and Cellular Corollaries. New York: Raven Press, 1992:267–291.
5. Messerli FH, Ventura HO, Reisin E, Dreslinski GR, Dunn FG, MacPhee AA, Frohlich ED. Borderline hypertension and obesity: two prehypertensive states with elevated cardiac output. Circulation 1982; 66:55–60.
6. Alexander JK. The cardiomyopathy of obesity. Prog Cardiovasc Dis 1985; 27:325–334.
7. De Divitiis O, Fazio S, Petitto M, Maddalena G, Contaldo F, Mancini M. Obesity and cardiac function. Circulation 1981; 64:477–482.
8. Licata G, Scaglione R, Barbagallo M, Pfarrinelo G, Capuana G, Lipari R, Merlino B, Ganguzza A. Effect of obesity on left ventricular function studied by radionuclide angiocardiography. Int J Obes 1991; 15:295–302.
9. Chakko S, Mayor M, Allison MD, Kessler KM, Materson BJ, Myerburg RJ. Abnormal left ventricular diastolic filling in eccentric left ventricular hypertrophy of obesity. Am J Cardiol 1991; 68:95–98.
10. Alexander JK. Obesity and the circulation. Mod Concepts Cardiovasc Dis 1963; 32:799–803.
11. Carabello BA, Gittens L. Cardiac mechanics and function in obese normotensive persons with normal coronary arteries. Am J Cardiol 1987; 59:469–473.
12. Messerli FH, Sundgaard-Riise K, Reisin E, Dreslinski G, Dunn FG, Frohlich E. Disparate cardiovascular effects of obesity and arterial hypertension. Am J Med 1983; 74: 808–812.
13. Lauer MS, Anderson KM, Kannel WB, Levy D. The impact of obesity on left ventricular mass and geometry. JAMA 1991; 266:231–236.
14. Rasooly R, Sasson Z, Gupta R. Relation between body fat distribution and left ventricular mass in men without structural heart disease or systemic hypertension. Am J Cardiol 1993; 71:1477–1479.
15. Alpert MA, Lambert CR, Terry BE, Cohen MV, Mukerji V, Massey CV, Hashimi MW, Panayiotou H. Interrelationship of left ventricular mass, systolic function and diastolic filling in normotensive morbidly obese patients. Int J Obes 1995; 19:550–557.
16. Wikstrand J, Petterson P, Björntorp P. Body fat distribution and left ventricular morphology and function in obese females. J Hypertens 1993; 11:1259–1266.
17. Gottdiener JS, Reda DJ, Materson BJ, Massie BM, Notargiacomo A, Hamburger RJ, Williams DW, Henderson WG. Importance of obesity, race and age to the cardiac structural and functional effects of hypertension. J Am Coll Cardiol 1994; 24:1492–1498.
18. Urbina EM, Gidding SS, Bao W, Pickoff AS, Berdusis L, Berenson GS. Effect of body size, ponderosity, and blood pressure on left ventricular growth in children and young adults in the Bogalusa heart study. Circulation 1995; 91: 2400–2406.
19. Yoshinaga M, Yuasa Y, Hatano H, Kono Y, Nomura Y, Oku S, Nakamura M, Kenekura S, Otsubo K, Akiba S, Miyata K. Effect of total adipose weight and systemic hypertension on left ventricular mass in children. Am J Cardiol 1995; 76:785–787.
20. Tuck ML. Obesity, the sympathetic nervous system, and essential hypertension. Hypertension 1992; 19(Suppl I): I-67–I-77.
21. Baron AD. Hemodynamic actions of insulin. Am J Physiol 1994; 267:E187–E202.
22. Bonsignore M, Marrone O, Insalaco G, Bonsignore G. The cardiovascular effects of obstructive sleep apnoeas: analysis of pathogenic mechanisms. Eur Respir J 1994; 7: 786–805.
23. de Simone G, Devereux RB, Roman MJ, Alderman MH, Laragh JH. Relation of obesity and gender to left ventricular hypertrophy in normotensive and hypertensive adults. Hypertension 1994; 23:600–606.
24. de la Maza M, Estevez A, Bunout D, Klenner C, Oyonarte M, Hirsch S. Ventricular mass in hypertensive and normotensive obese subjects. Int J Obes 1994; 18:193–197.
25. Lavie CJ, Amodeo C, Ventura HO, Messerli FH. Left atrial abnormalities indicating diastolic ventricular dysfunction in cardiopathy of obesity. Chest 1987; 92:1042–1046.
26. Messerli FH. Cardiopathy of obesity—a not-so-Victorian disease. N Engl J Med 1985; 314:378–379.
27. Jern S. Hemodynamics of the male fat distribution pattern. Blood Pressure 1992; 4(Suppl):21–28.

28. Sasson Z, Rasooly Y, Bhensania T, Rasooly I. Insulin resistance is an important determinant of left ventricular mass in the obese. Circulation 1993; 88:1431–1436.

29. Sharp SD, Williams RR. Fasting insulin and left ventricular mass in hypertensives and normotensive controls. Cardiology 1992; 81:207–212.

30. Flack JM, Sowers JR. Epidemiologic and clinical aspects of insulin resistance and hyperinsulinemia. Am J Med 1991; 91:115–215.

31. Smith HL, Willius FA. Adiposity of the heart: a clinical and pathologic study of one hundred and thirty-six obese patients. Ann Intern Med 1933; 52:930–931.

32. Saphir O, Corrigan M. Fatty infiltration of the myocardium. Ann Intern Med 1933; 52:911.

33. Amad KH, Brennan JC, Alexander JK. The cardiac pathology of chronic exogenous obesity. Circulation 1965; 32:740–745.

34. Carpenter HM. Myocardial fat infiltration. Am Heart J 1962; 63:491–496.

35. Garavaglia GE, Messerli FH, Nunez BD, Schmieder RE, Grossman E. Myocardial contractility and left ventricular function in obese patients with essential hypertension. Am J Cardiol 1988; 62:594–597.

36. Hubert HB, Feinleib M, McNamara PM, Castelli WP. Obesity as an independent risk factor for cardiovascular disease: a 26-year follow-up of participants in the Framingham Heart Study. Circulation 1983; 67(5):968–977.

37. Kasper EK, Hruban RH, Baughman KL. Cardiomyopathy of obesity: a clinicopathologic evaluation of 43 obese patients with heart failure. Am J Cardiol 1992; 70:921–924.

38. Casale PN, Devereux RB, Milner M, Zullo G, Harshfield GA. Value of echocardiographic measurement of left ventricular mass in predicting cardiovascular morbid events in hypertensive men. Ann Intern Med 1986; 105:173–178.

39. Levy D, Garrison RJ, Savage DD, Kannel WB, Castelli WP. Left ventricular mass and incidence of coronary heart disease in an elderly cohort. Ann Intern Med 1989; 110:101–107.

40. Ghali JK, Liao Y, Simmons B, Castaner A, Cao G, Cooper RS. The prognostic role of left ventricular hypertrophy in patients with or without coronary artery disease. Ann Intern Med 1992; 117:831–836.

41. Lavie CJ, Ventura HO, Messerli FH. Left ventricular hypertrophy: its relationship to obesity and hypertension. Postgrad Med 1992; 91:131–143.

42. Kannel WB, Plehn JF, Cupples LA. Cardiac failure and sudden death in the Framingham Study. Am Heart J 1988; 115(4):869–875.

43. Barrett-Connor E. Obesity, atherosclerosis, and coronary artery disease. Ann Intern Med 1985; 103:1010–1019.

44. Duflou J, Virmani R, Rabin I, Burke A, Farb A, Smialek J. Sudden death as a result of heart disease in morbid obesity. Am Heart J 1995; 130:306–313.

45. Bharati S, Lev M. Cardiac conduction system involvement in sudden death of obese young people. Am Heart J 1995; 129:273–281.

46. Stern M. Epidemiology of obesity and its link to heart disease. Metabolism Clin Exp 1995; 44:1–3.

47. Kannel W, D'Agostino R, Cobb J. Effect of weight on cardiovascular disease. Am J Clin Nutr 1996; 63(Suppl): 419S–422S.

48. Keys A, Aravanis C, Blackburn H, Van Buchem F, Buzina R, Djordjevic B, Fidanza F, Karvonen M, Menotti A, Puddu V, Taylor H. Coronary heart disease: overweight and obesity as risk factors. Ann Intern Med 1972; 77: 15–27.

49. Manson JE, Colditz GA, Stampfer MJ, Willett WC, Rosner B, Monson RR, Speizer FE, Hennekens CH. A prospective study of obesity and risk of coronary heart disease in women. N Engl J Med 1990; 322:882–889.

50. Reed D, Yano K. Predictors of arteriographically defined coronary stenosis in the Honolulu Heart Program. Am J Epidemiol 1991; 134:111–122.

51. Freedman DS, Williamson DF, Croft JB, Ballew C, Byers T. Relation of body fat distribution to ischemic disease: the National Health and Nutrition Examination Survey I (NHANES I) Epidemiologic Follow-up Study. Am J Epidemiol 1995; 142:53–63.

52. Fitzgerald AP, Jarrett RJ. Body weight and coronary heart disease mortality: an analysis in relation to age and smoking habit. 15 years follow-up data from the Whitehall Study. Int J Obes 1992; 16:119–129.

53. Coleman MP, Key TJA, Wang DY, Hermon C, Fentiman IS, Allen DS, Jarvis M, Pike MC, Sanders TAB. A prospective study of obesity, lipids, apolipoproteins and ischaemic disease in women. Atherosclerosis 1992; 92: 177–185.

54. Rimm EB, Stampfer MJ, Giovannucci E, Ascherio A, Spiegelman D, Colditz GA, Willett WC. Body size and fat distribution as predictors of coronary heart disease among middle-aged and older US men. Am J Epidemiol 1995; 141:1117–1127.

55. Lapidus L, Bengtsson C, Larson B, Pennert B, Rybo E, Sjostrom L. Distribution of adipose tissue and risk of cardiovascular disease and death: a 12 year follow up of participants in the population study of women in Gothenburg, Sweden. Br Med J 1984; 289:1257–1260.

56. Terry RB, Page WF, Haskell WL. Waist/hip ratio, body mass index and premature cardiovascular disease mortality in US Army veterans during a twenty-three year follow-up study. Int J Obes 1992; 16:417–423.

57. Clark L, Karve M, Rones K, Chang-DeMoranville B, Atluri S, Feldman J. Obesity, distribution of body fat and coronary artery disease in black women. Am J Cardiol 1994; 73:895–896.

58. Messerli FH, Nunez BD, Ventura HO, Synder DW. Overweight and sudden death: increased ventricular ectopy in cardiopathy of obesity. Arch Intern Med 1987; 147: 1725–1728.

59. Messerli F, Soria F. Ventricular dysrhythmias, left ventricular hypertrophy, and sudden death. Cardiovasc Drugs Ther 1994; 8:557–563.

60. Chadwick J, Mann, WN. The Medical Works of Hippocrates. Oxford: Blackwell Scientific Publications, 1950.

61. Drenick EJ, Fisler JS. Sudden cardiac arrest in morbidly obese surgical patients unexplained after autopsy. Am J Surg 1988; 155:720–726.

62. Gao YY, Lovejoy JC, Sparti A, Bray GA, Keys LK, Partington C. Autonomic activity assessed by heart rate spectral analysis varies with fat distribution in obese women. Obes Res 1996; 4:55–63.

63. Zahorska-Markiewicz B, Kuagowaska E, Kucio C, Klin M. Heart rate variability in obesity. Int J Obes 1993; 17:21–23.

64. Hirsch J, Leibel RL, Mackintosh R, Aguirre A. Heart rate variability as a measure of autonomic function during weight change in humans. Am J Physiol 1991; 261:R1418–R1423.

65. van Ravenswaaij-Arts CMA, Kollee LAA, Hopman JCW, Stoelinga GBA, van Geijn HP. Heart rate variability. Ann Intern Med 1993; 118:436–447.

66. Fisler JS. Cardiac effects of starvation and semistarvation diets: safety and mechanisms of action. Am J Nutr 1992; 56:230S–234S.

67. Noda A, Okada T, Yasuma F, Nakashima N, Yokota M. Cardiac hypertrophy in obstructive sleep apnea syndrome. Chest 1995; 107:1538–1544.

68. Lantiqua RA, Amatruda JM, Biddle TL, Forbes GB, Lockwood DH. Cardiac arrythmias associated with a liquid diet for the treatment of obesity. N Engl J Med 1980; 303:735–738.

69. Amatruda JM, Biddle TL, Patton MK, Lockwood DH. Vigorous supplementation of a hypocaloric diet prevents cardiac arrhythmias and mineral depletion. Am J Med 1983; 74:1016–1022.

70. Lowy SL, Fisler JS, Drenick EJ, Hunt IF, Swendseid ME. Zinc and copper nutriture in obese men receiving very low calorie diets of soy or collagen protein. Am J Clin Nutr 1986;43:272–287.

71. Rasmussen LH, Andersen T. The relationship between QTc changes and nutrition during weight loss after gastroplasty. Acta Med Scand 1985; 217:271–275.

72. Pringle T, Scobie T, Murray R, Kesson C, Maccuish A. Prolongation of the QT interval during therapeutic starvation: a substrate for malignant arrhythmias. Int J Obes 1983; 7:253–261.

73. Seim H, Mitchell J, Pomeroy C, de Zwaan M. Electrocardiographic findings associated with very low calorie dieting. Int J Obes 1995; 19:817–819.

74. Keil JE, Sutherland SE, Knapp RG, Lackland DT, Gazes PC, Tyroler H. Mortality rates and risk factors for coronary disease in black as compared with white men and women. N Engl J Med 1993; 329(2):73–78.

75. Clark LT, Emerole O. Coronary heart disease in African Americans: primary and secondary prevention. Cleveland Clin J Med 1995; 62:285–292.

76. Howard BV, Lee ET, Cowan LD, Fabsitz RR, Howard WJ, Oopik AJ, Robbins DC, Savage PJ, Yeh JL, Welty TK. Coronary heart disease prevalence and its relation to risk factors in American Indians: the Strong Heart Study. Am J Epidemiol 1995; 142:254–268.

77. Kumanyika S. Searching for the association of obesity with coronary artery disease. Obes Res 1995; 3:273–275.

78. Adams-Campbell LL, Peniston RL, Kim KS, Mensah E. Body mass index and coronary artery disease in African-Americans. Obes Res 1995; 3:215–219.

79. Kumanyika A. Special issues regarding obesity in minority populations. Ann Intern Med 1993; 119:650–654.

80. Stern M, Patterson J, Mitchell B, Haffner S, Hazuda H. Overweight and mortality in Mexican-Americans. Int J Obes 1990; 14:623–629.

81. Caralis PV. Coronary heart disease in Hispanic Americans: how does ethnic background affect risk factors and mortality rates? Postgrad Med 1992; 91:179–188.

82. Welty TK, Lee ET, Yeh J, Cowan LD, Go O, Fabsitz RR, Le NA, Oopik AJ, Robbins DC, Howard BV. Cardiovascular disease risk factors among American Indians: the Strong Heart Study. Am J Epidemiol 1995; 142:269–287.

83. Rautaharju PM, Zhou SH, Calhoun HP. Ethnic differences in ECG amplitudes in North American white, black, and Hispanic men and women. J Electrocardiol 1995; 27 (Suppl):20–31.

84. Selmer R, Tverdal A. Body mass index and cardiovascular mortality at different levels of blood pressure: a prospective study of Norwegian men and women. J Epidemiol Commun Health 1995; 49:265–270.

85. Conway G, Agrawal R, Betteridge D, Jacobs H. Risk factors for coronary artery disease in lean and obese women with the polycystic ovary syndrome. Clin Endocrinol 1992; 37:119–125.

86. Wild R. Obesity, lipids, cardiovascular risk, and androgen excess. Am J Med 1995; 98(Suppl 1A):1A-27S–1A-32S.

87. McKeigue P. Are women with polycystic ovary syndrome at special risk for coronary artery disease? Clin Endocrinol 1992; 37:117–118.

88. Must A, Jaques PF, Dallal GE, Bajema CJ, Dietz WH. Long-term morbidity and mortality of overweight adolescents: a follow-up of the Harvard Growth Study of 1922 to 1935. N Engl J Med 1992; 327:1350–1355.

89. Paffenbarger R, Wing A, Hyde R. Physical activity as an index of heart attack risk in college alumni. Am J Epidemiol 1978; 108:161–175.

90. Paffenbarger RSJ, Hyde PHR, Wing A, Hsieh CC. Physical activity, all-cause mortality, and longevity of college alumni. N Engl J Med 1986; 314:605–613.

91. Gallagher D, Hemsfield SB. Obesity is bad for the heart, but is weight loss always good? Obes Res 1994; 2:160–163.

92. Benotti PN, Bistrian B, Benotti JR, Blackburn G, Forse RA. Heart disease and hypertension in severe obesity: the benefits of weight reduction. Am J Clin Nutr 1992; 55: 586S–590S.

93. Reisin E, Frolich ED, Messerli FH, Dreslinski GR, Dunn FG, Jones MM, Batson HM Jr. Cardiovascular changes after weight reduction in obesity hypertension. Ann Intern Med 1983; 98:315–319.

94. Elaihou HE, Iaina A, Gaon T, Shochat J, Modan M. Body weight reduction necessary to attain normotension in the overweight hypertensive patient. Int J Obes 1981; 5(Suppl):157–163.

95. Foley EF, Benotti PN, Borlase BL, Hollingshead J, Blackburn GL. Impact of gastric restrictive surgery on hypertension in the morbidly obese. Am J Surg 1992; 163: 294–297.

96. Carson JL, Ruddy ME, Duff AE, Holmes NJ, Cody RP, Brolin RE. The effect of gastric bypass surgery on hypertension in morbidly obese patients. Arch Intern Med 1994; 154:193–200.

97. MacMahon SW, Wilcken D, MacDonald GJ. The effect of weight reduction on left ventricular mass. N Engl J Med 1986; 314:334–339.

98. Alaud-din A, Meterissan S, Lisbona R, MacLean LD, Forse RA. Assessment of cardiac function in patients who were morbidly obese. Surgery 1990; 108:809–820.

99. Alpert MA, Terry BE, Kelly DL. Effect of weight loss on cardiac chamber size and left ventricular function in morbid obesity. Am J Cardiol 1985; 55:783–786.

100. Alpert M, Lambert C, Terry B, Kelly D, Panayiotou H, Mukerji V, Massey C, Cohen M. Effect of weight loss on left ventricular mass in nonhypertensive morbidly obese patients. Am J Cardiol 1994; 73:918–921.

101. Jordan J, Messerli F, Lavie C, Aepfelbacher F, Soria F. Reduction of weight and left ventricular mass with serotonin uptake inhibition in obese patients with systemic hypertension. Am J Cardiol 1995; 75:743–744.

102. Wirth A, Kroger H. Improvement of left ventricular morphology and function in obese subjects following a diet and exercise program. Int J Obes 1995; 19:61–66.

103. Alpert M, Terry B, Lambert C, Kelly D, Panayiotou H, Mukerji V, Massey C, Cohen M. Factors influencing left ventricular systolic function in nonhypertensive morbidly obese patients, and effect of weight loss induced by gastroplasty. Am J Cardiol 1993; 71:733–737.

104. Grunstein RR, Stenlof K, Sjostrom L. Impact of obstructive sleep apnea and sleepiness on metabolic and cardiovascular risk factors in the Swedish Obese Subjects (SOS) Study. Int J Obes 1995; 19:410–418.

105. Vague P, Raccah D, Scelles V. Hypofibrinolysis and the insulin resistance syndrome. Int J Obes 1995; 19(Suppl 1):S11–S15.

106. Ohrvall M, Tengblad S, Vessby B. Lower tocopherol serum levels in subjects with abdominal adiposity. J Intern Med 1993; 234:53–60.

107. Lee G, Sparrow D, Vokonas PS, Landsberg L, Weiss ST. Uric acid and coronary heart disease risk: evidence for a role of uric acid in the obesity–insulin resistance syndrome. Am J Epidemiol 1995; 142:288–294.

108. Feskens EJM, Kromhout D. Hyperinsulinemia, risk factors, and coronary heart disease: the Zutphen Elderly Study. Arterioscler Thromb 1994; 14:1641–1647.

109. Bavenholm P, Proudler A, Tornvall P, Godsland I, Landou C, de Faire U, Hamsten A. Insulin, intact and split proinsulin, and coronary artery disease in young men. Circulation 1995; 92:1422–1429.

110. Wysocki M, Krotkiewski M, Braide M, Bagge U. Hemorheological disturbances, metabolic parameters and blood pressure in different types of obesity. Atherosclerosis 1991; 88:21–28.

111. Suter P, Locher R, Wetter W. Is abdominal obesity a risk factor for increased homocyteine levels? FASEB J 1994; 8: A16 (abstract).

30

Obesity and Lipoprotein Metabolism

Jean-Pierre Després
Laval University and Medical Research Center, Ste.-Foy, Quebec, Canada

Ronald M. Krauss
Ernest Orlando Lawrence Berkeley National Laboratory, University of California at Berkeley, Berkeley, California

I. DYSLIPIDEMIC PHENOTYPES IN CORONARY HEART DISEASE: BEYOND CHOLESTEROL

The measurement of plasma cholesterol levels is now commonly used to assess the risk of coronary heart disease. In fact, many epidemiological studies have shown that there is a significant positive relationship between blood cholesterol levels and deaths associated with coronary heart disease (1–3). The data obtained from the Multiple Risk Factor Intervention Trial (MRFIT) and published by Stamler et al. (4) showed that in a sample of 356,222 male subjects, the increased blood cholesterol levels were associated with a progressive increase in coronary heart disease mortality. However, despite the fact that numerous studies have shown this relationship, Genest et al. (5) have reported that nearly 50% of patients with ischemic heart disease had plasma cholesterol levels equal to or even lower than those of healthy subjects.

Accordingly, Sniderman and Silberberg (6) emphasized that although the mean blood cholesterol concentration in coronary heart disease patients is generally significantly higher than that of healthy subjects, there is a considerable overlap between coronary heart disease patients and healthy subjects. Thus, the clinical value of total cholesterol measurement alone is of limited use in distinguishing coronary heart disease patients from healthy subjects. It was therefore suggested that additional determinations of blood lipid variables were needed in order to more accurately assess risk.

Cholesterol is a hydrophobic compound and is transported in the blood by lipoproteins. Lipoproteins vary in size, composition, and density, and four main families can be identified: chylomicrons, very-low-density lipoproteins (VLDL), low-density lipoproteins (LDL), and high-density lipoproteins (HDL) (Fig. 1). Chylomicrons are large particles found after a meal that are responsible for the transport of alimentary lipids. They are generally absent from the fasting plasma of healthy subjects. Triglyceride and cholesterol molecules of hepatic origin are secreted in VLDL particles, which are converted to LDL following hydrolysis by the enzyme lipoprotein lipase (LPL). During the hydrolysis of chylomicrons and VLDL, excess surface component aggregates to form nascent HDL particles. Additional newly formed and immature HDL particles originate from the intestine and the liver.

Several prospective studies have shown that when low levels of cholesterol are transported by HDL, there is an increased risk of coronary heart disease and of related mortality. Austin (7) reviewed the literature on HDL cholesterol and coronary heart disease in 1991 and found 19 prospective studies having examined this relationship. Of these, 15 reported that HDL had a protective effect, three noted a tendency, and only one failed to observe a significant association between HDL-cholesterol levels and coronary heart disease. These data support the notion that

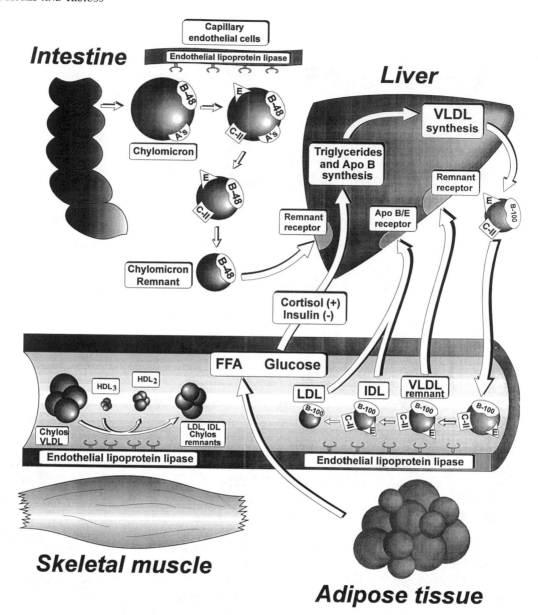

Figure 1 Simplified overview of lipoprotein metabolism. After hydrolysis of dietary triglycerides by intestinal lipase and their secretion in the lymph as chylomicrons (containing dietary cholesterol, triglycerides, phospholipids, apo B-48, and apo A-I, A-II, and A-IV, these nascent particles acquire apo C and E in the circulation. The chylomicron binds to the enzyme lipoprotein lipase located on the surface of the endothelial cells of several tissues, including adipose tissue and skeletal muscle. This process allows the transfer of excess surface components (apo A-I, A-II, and A-IV, of the C apolipoproteins and of phospholipids) to HDL. The chylomicron remnant particle is then cleared from the circulation via the hepatic apo E (remnant) receptor. The first step of chylomicron catabolism, which involves hydrolysis by endothelial lipoprotein lipase, appears to be modulated by numerous hormonal and metabolic factors. The second step, which involves the clearance of chylomicron remnants by hepatocytes, does not seem to be under close hormonal or metabolic control. Endogenous lipids are secreted by the liver as very-low-density lipoprotein (VLDL) particles. Availability of lipids appears to determine the fate of constitutively synthesized apo B-100 and will protect apo B against its degradation. Insulin and cortisol also seem to be important modulators of VLDL secretion via indirect (substrate availability) and direct (apo B synthesis) effects. Apo B is synthesized on ribosomes of the rough endoplasmic reticulum and associates with lipids in its smooth surface end. The nascent VLDL particle is then transported to the Golgi. Particles are packed in secretion vesicles and then secreted. VLDL particles will acquire additional apoproteins in the circulation. With the action of endothelial LPL, VLDL will be hydrolyzed into VLDL remnants, IDL, and finally, LDL. About 50% of the particles will be cleared as IDL by the apo B/E receptor, whereas the others will be eliminated by extrahepatic and hepatic apo B/E receptors as LDL particles. Nascent HDL particles have multiple origins (gut, liver, plasma). However, considerable evidence suggests that hydrolysis of TG-rich lipoproteins (chylomicrons and VLDL) is a major process by which excess surface components are transferred from TG-rich lipoproteins to nascent HDL particles. Thus, the more efficient is the hydrolysis of TG-rich lipoproteins, the higher is LPL activity in the postheparin plasma and the higher are plasma HDL concentrations, especially the HDL_2 subfraction.

low HDL-cholesterol levels increase coronary heart disease risk. It thus seems reasonable to assume that an intervention resulting in an increase in HDL-cholesterol levels could decrease the incidence of ischemic heart disease.

In this regard, it is appropriate to mention that patients who have low HDL-cholesterol levels also frequently have elevated triglyceride concentrations. Results of some, but not all, prospective epidemiological studies have indicated that an elevated triglyceride concentration did not constitute an independent risk factor for coronary heart disease when statistical corrections were made for other lipoprotein or lipid variables such as HDL cholesterol (7). In addition, results of the PROCAM study have shown that the presence of low HDL-cholesterol levels alone also increased the risk of coronary heart disease (8). Finally, it has been found that increased levels of apo AI and HDL in transgenic mice were sufficient to prevent the development of atherosclerosis (9). Consequently, a low plasma HDL-cholesterol concentration, with or without elevated triglyceride concentrations, must be given special attention by the clinician.

With this in mind, some mechanisms have been proposed to explain the protective effect of HDL in ischemic heart disease. HDL cholesterol has been suggested to be involved in the reverse cholesterol transport, a concept introduced by Glomset (10) in the late 1960s. According to this model, after a certain amount of free cholesterol is transferred from the cell membrane to the HDL particle, it is esterified and gradually migrates to the center of the lipoprotein by the action of the enzyme lecithin:cholesterol acyltransferase (LCAT).

Another model suggests that the presence of high plasma HDL-cholesterol levels could be indicative of a very effective catabolism of triglyceride-rich lipoproteins. As shown in Figure 2, the rapid breakdown of chylomicrons and VLDL by the action of the enzyme LPL could lead to an increase in the production of HDL, more specifically, the HDL$_2$ subfraction, which seems to be particularly abundant when LPL activity is high. Consequently, the role of LPL in the breakdown of triglyceride-rich lipoproteins and the production of HDL could contribute to explain the well-established inverse relationship between plasma triglyceride and HDL-cholesterol concentrations.

Moreover, lipid transfer proteins found in plasma allow the exchange of lipids between different lipoprotein fractions. In fact, one of these transfer proteins, cholesterol ester transfer protein (CETP), favors the exchange of the triglycerides found in triglyceride-rich lipoproteins for HDL-cholesterol esters, resulting in the depletion of cholesterol in HDL particles. In addition, and as mentioned previously, a low LPL activity contributes to a decreased production of HDL precursors originating from the aggre-

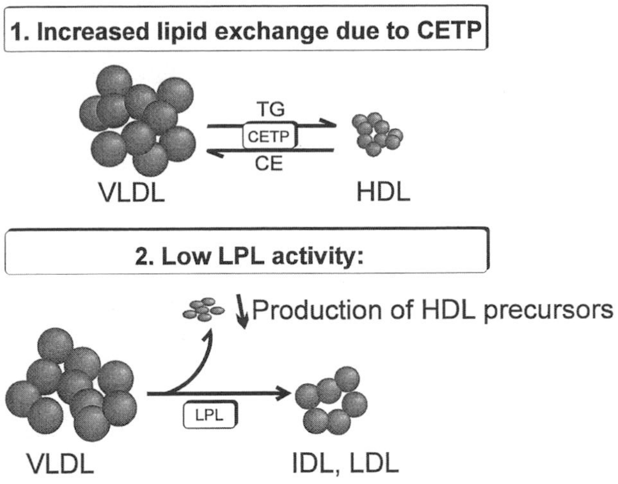

Figure 2 Lipid transfer proteins contribute to the exchange of lipids between the various lipoproteins. In this case, cholesterol ester transfer protein (CETP) allows the exchange of triglycerides in triglyceride-rich lipoproteins for cholesterol esters of the HDL fractions, which ultimately leads to a reduced cholesterol content of HDL particles.

gation of an excessive number of surface components released by the hydrolysis of VLDL and chylomicrons. In this regard, we further examined the metabolic heterogeneity underlying high triglyceride and low HDL-cholesterol levels (11).

We first studied the relationship between triglycerides and HDL-cholesterol levels and found the expected negative correlation between these two variables, as shown in Figure 3. However, although the correlation was highly significant, the shared variance was low (34%), which allowed us to study the following subgroups of subjects:

1. Subjects with normal triglyceride and HDL-cholesterol levels
2. Individuals with normal triglyceride but low HDL-cholesterol levels
3. Subjects with elevated triglyceride (>2.0 mM) and normal HDL-cholesterol levels (>0.9 mM)
4. Individuals with the combination of high triglyceride (>2.0 mM) and low HDL-cholesterol levels (<0.9 mM)

We then measured fasting insulin concentrations and insulin levels following a 75-g oral glucose load as the integrated response (11). We found that individuals with low HDL-cholesterol/normal triglyceride levels did not show elevated plasma insulin levels either in the fasting state or in response to the glucose challenge (Figure 4). Moreover, hypertriglyceridemia alone was not associated

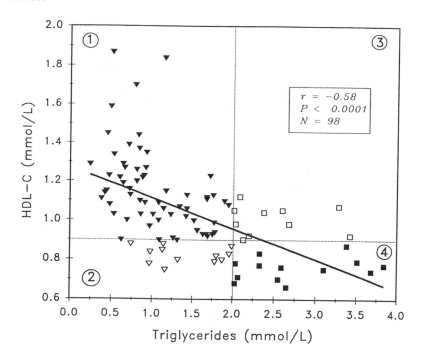

Figure 3 Scatterplot showing the relation of plasma triglyceride (TG) to high-density lipoprotein cholesterol (HDL-C) levels in a sample of 98 men. Cutoffs used to build the four subgroups are also identified. ▼, Normal HDL-C and TG levels; ▽, low HDL-C and normal TG levels; □, normal HDL-C and high TG levels; ■, low HDL-C and high TG levels. (From Ref. 11.)

with increased plasma insulin levels. The combination, however, of high triglyceride and low HDL-cholesterol concentrations was associated with a considerable and significant increase in plasma insulin concentrations measured in the fasting state and in response to the oral glucose load, thus suggesting that this dyslipidemia was particularly related to hyperinsulinemia stemming from resistance of tissues to insulin.

In the PROCAM Study conducted in Munster, Germany (9) and in the Helsinki Study (12), the combination of high triglyceride and low HDL-cholesterol levels was associated with a significant increase in the risk of coronary heart disease, and a high percentage of coronary events were specifically related to this dyslipidemia. Indeed, among individuals in the PROCAM study whose triglyceride and HDL-cholesterol levels were higher than 200 mg/dl and lower than 35 mg/dl, respectively, the incidence of coronary events observed over a 6-year period was 5.3-fold higher (128 cases per 1000 people) than among subjects with a normal lipid profile (24 cases per 1000 people) (9). Consequently, this dyslipidemic profile (including hypertriglyceridemia and hypoalphalipoproteinemia) associated with hyperinsulinemia secondary to insulin resistance significantly increases the risk of ischemic

heart disease among individuals with this cluster of metabolic abnormalities.

Reaven (13) was the first to suggest the term "insulin resistance syndrome" to describe a cluster of metabolic abnormalities that includes hypoalphalipoproteinemia, hypertriglyceridemia, hyperinsulinemia, and increased blood pressure. To measure the sensitivity to insulin, Reaven used the euglycemic hyperinsulinemic clamp in about 100 normal subjects as well as in glucose-intolerant and NIDDM patients (13). In this technique, a certain amount of insulin is infused to induce hyperinsulinemia to a predetermined level. Obviously, the rate at which blood sugar levels drop varies if there is no simultaneous infusion of glucose. The greater the sensitivity to insulin, the faster the blood glucose levels fall and the higher is the quantity of glucose needed to maintain euglycemia. Consequently, the sensitivity to insulin, or the M value, corresponds to the amount of glucose required to maintain a normal blood glucose level under a standardized hyperinsulinemic state; this value is expressed in milligrams of glucose infused per kilogram of body weight per minute.

Reaven and colleagues next subdivided the group of 100 nondiabetic subjects according to fasting insulin concentrations. The first quartile was comprised of individ-

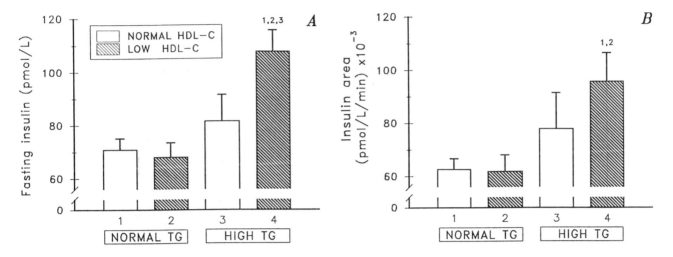

Figure 4 Bar graphs comparing plasma insulin concentrations measured in the fasting state (A) and following an oral glucose load (insulin area) (B) among four groups of men defined on the basis of plasma triglyceride and HDL-cholesterol levels. HDL-C, high-density lipoprotein cholesterol; TG, triglyceride. Values are means ± SEM. (For TG and HDL-cholesterol cut points, refer to Fig. 3). (From Ref. 11.)

uals with the highest blood insulin levels; the fourth, of individuals with the lowest. Within these four groups, considerable differences were observed in terms of in vivo sensitivity to insulin. Subjects of the lowest insulin quartile were very sensitive to insulin (M value >300) whereas subjects of the highest insulin quartile were clearly insulin resistant (M value barely above 100). Two critically important observations were made. First, considerable differences in terms of sensitivity to insulin were found even among individuals with normal glucose tolerance. Furthermore, in 25% of normal individuals, the magnitude of the insulin-resistant state was similar to that found among glucose-intolerant individuals or type II diabetic patients. Consequently, Reaven concluded that insulin resistance is prevalent in our population since 25% of nondiabetic subjects seem to have this characteristic.

There is now evidence indicating that insulin resistance is associated with a proatherogenic dyslipidemic state (14,15). Considering the high prevalence of insulin resistance, this condition probably represents the most common cause of dyslipidemic states found in coronary heart disease patients (16,17).

Cholesterol and LDL-cholesterol levels are frequently within the normal range in patients with high triglyceride and low HDL-cholesterol concentrations. However, other techniques have made it possible to conclude that this form of dyslipidemia related to insulin resistance is frequently associated with high levels of apo B (the apolipoprotein of LDL) in the presence of a relatively normal LDL-cholesterol value, suggesting the presence of a greater number of LDL particles relatively depleted in cholesterol esters. Indeed, additional techniques that use gradient gel electrophoresis to separate LDL on the basis of size have helped confirm the fact that the high triglyceride/low HDL-cholesterol dyslipidemia is associated with an increased proportion of small, dense LDL particles (16).

In this regard, Austin et al. have suggested that over 80% of individuals characterized by a low proportion of dense LDL (phenotype A) have triglyceride levels lower than 92 mg/dl (1.05 mM) (18). Consequently, it could be possible, on the basis of fasting triglyceride concentrations, to identify a fairly large percentage of individuals who have an increased proportion of dense LDL particles (phenotype B). Furthermore, their work has indicated that over 50% of patients with elevated apolipoprotein B levels could also be characterized by an atherogenic phenotype that would include hypertriglyceridemia, hypoalphalipoproteinemia, and an increased proportion of smaller and denser LDL particles. This atherogenic phenotype is frequently observed in coronary heart disease patients with almost normal plasma cholesterol or LDL-cholesterol concentrations (16).

Clinically, it is interesting that the atherogenic B phenotype is found in about 20–30% of the population (7,18). This figure is remarkably similar to the prevalence of the insulin resistance syndrome (about 25%) (13). Thus, the hypothesis has been put forward that most patients characterized by hyperapobetalipoproteinemia and the atherogenic phenotype B may have a metabolic disorder in common: insulin resistance.

The Québec Cardiovascular Study recently published 5-year prospective data that provided findings relevant to the present discussion (19). In this study, 2103 healthy men in their late fifties and initially free from clinical manifestations of ischemic heart disease (IHD) were followed for 5 years. During this period, 114 of them developed ischemic heart disease (effort angina, myocardial infarction, or coronary death). Although plasma cholesterol concentrations were higher (7%) in men who developed IHD than in men who remained healthy, the most substantial differences were noted for the total cholesterol/HDL-cholesterol ratio (16%) and apolipoprotein (apo) B levels (12%) (19). We used a simple algorithm to quantify the prevalence of dyslipidemic phenotypes (19). While we found that type II dyslipidemia (hypercholesterolemia) was more prevalent among IHD than in healthy men, hyperapolipoprotein B (with or without hypertriglyceridemia) was the most prevalent abnormality among men who developed IHD. Stepwise logistic regression analyses revealed that apo B concentration analyzed as a continuous variable was the best lipoprotein component predictive of IHD (20). However, in a model excluding apo B, the total cholesterol/HDL-cholesterol ratio was the best variable of the lipoprotein profile to predict IHD risk (20). It is important to point out that both apo B and the total cholesterol/HDL-cholesterol ratio are increased in an insulin-resistant state, a finding that provides further support that insulin resistance substantially increases the risk of IHD. In this regard, no prospective study has reported data on the risk of IHD associated with an impaired in vivo insulin action. Four prospective studies have, however, measured fasting plasma insulin concentrations as a crude index of insulin sensitivity. These studies reported that hyperinsulinemia was associated with an increased risk of IHD in men (21–24). As hyperinsulinemia resulting from in vivo insulin resistance is associated with a dyslipidemic state that includes hypertriglyceridemia, elevated apo B levels, and reduced HDL-cholesterol concentrations, it will still unclear whether the hyperinsulinemia-IHD relationship is independent from the concomitant alterations in plasma lipoprotein levels. Results from the Paris and Caerphilly prospective studies have suggested that the risk associated with hyperinsulinemia is no longer significant after control for plasma triglyceride levels (24–26).

Recent observations from the 5-year follow-up data of the Quebec Cardiovascular Study provided data applicable to this issue (27). Indeed, the 114 men who developed IHD during the 5-year follow-up period were matched for age, body mass index, smoking, and alcohol consumption with 114 men who remained healthy. After exclusion of diabetic patients and of IHD patients who could not be matched with controls due to extreme smoking habits, we were able to match 91 nondiabetic cases and 105 controls (27). Fasting insulin concentrations were initially 18% higher in men who developed IHD than in those who remained healthy. Furthermore, logistic regression analyses revealed that insulin level kept its association with IHD after adjustment for concomitant variation in plasma lipoproteins including apo B concentrations (27). Finally, subjects in the highest tertile of insulin concentrations and with elevated apo B levels (above the 50th percentile) were 11 times more at risk of IHD than men with both low insulin (first tertile) and low apo B (below the 50th percentile) concentrations (27). Hyperinsulinemia and elevated apo B levels are frequent metabolic abnormalities in an insulin-resistant state, and these aberrations are often found in the presence of almost normal cholesterol and LDL-cholesterol levels. Thus, the clinician dealing with type II diabetics or nondiabetics but insulin-resistant patients should not only focus on plasma cholesterol or LDL-cholesterol levels. Indeed, the simultaneous presence of hyperinsulinemia, hypertriglyceridemia, reduced HDL-cholesterol levels, elevated apo B, and an increased total cholesterol/HDL-cholesterol ratio is clearly predictive of an increased IHD risk. The prevalence of this cluster of metabolic abnormalities is such that it probably represents the main cause of IHD in our population, but it should be emphasized that it will frequently be found among subjects with "normal" cholesterol and LDL-cholesterol levels (16).

II. OBESITY, BODY FAT DISTRIBUTION, AND DYSLIPIDEMIA

Obesity is generally considered to be detrimental to cardiovascular health (3,28) and has long been associated with the presence of dyslipidemic states and coronary heart disease (28–30). Although some prospective studies have shown that obesity is a significant risk factor for CVD and related mortality in univariate analyses, it should be recognized that this association has generally been found to be rather weak, the relative risk ratio barely reaching 1.5 in overweight subjects in comparison with nonobese individuals (3,31–33). Indeed, multivariate analyses conducted in some studies failed to identify obesity as an independent risk factor for CVD (34,35). Thus, whether or not obesity per se is an independent predictor of CVD-related mortality has remained controversial and this issue is still a matter of some debate in the scientific community.

In this regard, three possibilities have been raised to explain the weak association between obesity and mortality (36). First, most epidemiological studies have used anthropometric correlates of total body fat, which only provide a crude assessment of total body fatness. In addition, in order to observe the detrimental effects of disturbances in carbohydrate and lipid metabolism on clinical manifestations of CVD, it is likely that a prolonged follow-up may be necessary. Prospective studies that have reported positive associations between relative weight and mortality had follow-up periods of 10–15 years and even more (37). Finally and most important, it has been shown that the health hazards of obesity are more closely related to the localization of excess body fat rather than to an elevated body weight per se.

Indeed, although obesity is highly prevalent among patients showing metabolic aberrations, the magnitude of the associations reported has been quite variable and clinicians have often been confronted with the metabolic heterogeneity of obesity. Therefore, it is important to adequately define obesity as a health hazard in order to develop measures aimed at the prevention and treatment of its complications (38).

Body weight expressed as a function of height has long been used to obtain a crude measurement of body fatness. More than a century ago, Quetelet (39) noted that body weight (kg) was proportional to height squared (m^2). More recently, Keys and colleagues (40) redefined the Quetelet index as the body mass index (BMI), which also divides the body weight (kg) by height squared (m^2). This measure is commonly used as a valuable index of relative weight and obesity (41). Some studies that have used the BMI to evaluate the body composition have reported significant associations with morbidity and mortality (28,32,37,42). The relationship between relative weight, expressed as BMI, and mortality rate is characterized by a J-shaped curve (42). Both extremities of the curve are associated with an exponential increase in the risk of mortality. Therefore, a BMI under 20 (underweight) and a BMI above 27 (overweight) are associated with an increased risk of death. Moreover, BMI values between 27 and 30 are associated with only a slight increase in mortality rate and there is a further progression of risk for values between 30 and 35, whereas BMI values above 35 are clearly associated with an increased mortality rate (42). Although very useful to estimate overall obesity, the BMI has limitations. Thus, individuals who do not have a large excess of body fat, such as those with large muscle masses, would be misclassified as having a high-risk body weight. Furthermore, the BMI does not provide information on the localization of body fat and additional anthropometric measurements such as the waist-to-hip ratio (WHR), and subcutaneous skinfolds have commonly been used to estimate regional adipose tissue distribution (42).

Anthropometric estimates such as WHR and skinfold measurements have generated considerable evidence to support the notion that the localization of adipose tissue rather than the accumulation of total body fat is a critical correlate of metabolic disturbances that are significant risk factors for CVD (28,29,33,43–45). Therefore, several epidemiological and metabolic studies published over the last decade have indicated that the regional distribution of body fat was indeed the main factor involved in the relation of obesity to dyslipoproteinemias and CVD (16,17,28–30,43–64).

In this regard, Professor Jean Vague, from the University of Marseille, first proposed, more than 40 years ago, that body fat topography was a better correlate of the complications of obesity (diabetes, hypertension, CVD) than excess fatness per se. Vague (47) defined the male type of fat distribution as "android obesity," mostly characterized by an accumulation of adipose tissue over the trunk, whereas he referred to the common fat pattern of women as "gynoid obesity," where adipose tissue accumulates mostly around the hips and thighs, this type of obesity seldom being associated with the common complications of excess fatness. However, it took more than four decades before these pioneering observations became widely accepted by the scientific community. During this period, the concept of adipose tissue distribution did not receive a lot of attention and only a few studies published in the sixties examined this issue. In 1964, Albrink and Meigs (48) reported stronger correlations between plasma triglyceride levels and trunk skinfolds than any other skinfold considered. Allard and Goulet (49) also reached similar conclusions in the late sixties. Although these studies showed associations between excess trunk fat and plasma triglyceride levels, the concept of regional adipose tissue distribution only received serious consideration when prospective studies published in the 1980s indicated that excess abdominal fat was associated with an increased mortality rate in a manner independent of concomitant variation in total fatness as estimated by the BMI (46,50–52). Indeed, these studies have shown that regional fat distribution, assessed by WHR or skinfolds, was associated with a higher incidence of diabetes and CVD, and with an increased mortality rate (50–53).

The related dyslipidemic state was an obvious possibility to explain the increased CVD risk associated with abdominal obesity, and several studies have examined the potential associations between abdominal fat accumulation and dyslipidemias. More specifically, it has been demonstrated that subjects characterized by a high accumulation of abdominal fat have elevated fasting plasma triglyceride levels (54–56) and reduced plasma HDL-cholesterol concentrations (43,54,57,58,59).

Studies for which HDL subfractions were measured revealed that the reduction in HDL-cholesterol observed with excess abdominal fat was mainly attributed to a decrease in the concentration of plasma HDL_2-cholesterol concentrations (57–61). In addition, it has been shown that in abdominal obesity, plasma HDL-cholesterol levels were reduced to a greater extent than plasma HDL-apoliprotein A-I levels and that HDL were triglyceride-enriched (62).

Additional work has revealed that LDL particle concentration, composition, and density are altered among subjects with a high WHR. Indeed, abdominal obesity has been associated with an increased proportion of small, dense, cholesterol ester–depleted LDL particles. The dense LDL phenotype has been associated with higher concentrations of TG and lower levels of HDL-cholesterol (18), alterations often found in CHD patients (63).

Abdominal obesity has also been reported to be related to alterations in indices of plasma glucose-insulin homeostasis. Indeed, prospective studies have shown that an excess of abdominal fat is associated with an increased risk of diabetes (53). Although the mechanisms linking abdominal obesity to type II diabetes are not fully understood, it appears that a preferential accumulation of adipose tissue in the abdominal region is associated with glucose intolerance, hyperinsulinemia, and insulin resistance, which are metabolic conditions predictive of an increased risk of NIDDM (44,45).

Using anthropometric measurements, several studies reported that upper body obesity is more prevalent in diabetic patients than in control subjects (64). Moreover, alterations in indices of plasma glucose-insulin homeostasis are frequently observed in abdominal obese patients (45,47,55,56). More specifically, the preferential accumulation of abdominal fat has been shown to be related to hyperinsulinemia in the fasting state as well as following a glucose load (44,45). Increased insulin secretion, insulin resistance, and decreased hepatic insulin extraction are common metabolic disturbances in abdominal obesity (45,65–67). These important metabolic events may explain the resulting hyperinsulinemia found in patients with an excess of abdominal fat. Furthermore, glucose intolerance, or at least an increased plasma glucose response to a glucose load, is frequently found in abdominal obese patients despite the presence of hyperinsulinemia confirming the presence of insulin resistance (44,45). These alterations in lipoprotein-lipid and insulin-glucose metabolism found in abdominal obese patients contribute to explain the high prevalence of CVD and NIDDM in these subjects (68).

III. BODY FAT DISTRIBUTION AND DYSLIPIDEMIA: IMPORTANCE OF VISCERAL ADIPOSE TISSUE

A. Measurement of Visceral Adipose Tissue

The recent development of imaging techniques such as computed tomography (CT) has allowed the precise assessment of adipose tissue distribution (69–71). Using CT, one can easily distinguish adipose from lean tissues. Indeed, the attenuation scores generated by CT vary from −1000 (air) to +1000 (bone) depending on the level of absorption of emitted X-ray beams (71,72). Studies that have examined the attenuation of tissues have established that the range of attenuation values [Hounsfield units (HU)] for adipose tissue varies between −190 and −30 HU (71,72).

CT is also quite useful to precisely assess the amount of abdominal adipose tissue and particularly helpful to distinguish the adipose tissue located in the abdominal cavity (the so-called intra-abdominal or visceral adipose tissue) from subcutaneous abdominal fat. When this procedure is performed, the subject is examined in the supine position with both arms stretched above the head (71,72). To measure subcutaneous and visceral abdominal adipose tissue areas, CT scans are usually performed between L4 and L5 vertebrae. Total adipose tissue areas are calculated by delineating the abdominal area with a graph pen and then computing total adipose tissue surface with an attenuation range of −190 to −30 HU (71,72). To measure the area of visceral adipose tissue, a line is drawn by passing through the muscle wall delineating the abdominal cavity (Fig. 5).

B. Metabolic Disturbances Associated with Excess Visceral Adipose Tissue

Studies that have used this technique have reported that the amount of visceral adipose tissue is a critical correlate of the common metabolic complications found in obese patients. Fujioka and colleagues (73) have studied a heterogeneous group of obese patients and assessed cross-sectional areas of adipose tissue located subcutaneously or in the abdominal cavity (visceral adipose tissue). They reported that individuals with a preferential accumulation of abdominal visceral fat showed higher plasma glucose responses following an oral glucose challenge and higher fasting plasma triglyceride levels than individuals with similar BMI values but characterized by an excess of subcutaneous abdominal fat (73–75). Several cross-sectional studies have also consistently found that an excess of abdominal visceral adipose tissue was associated with sub-

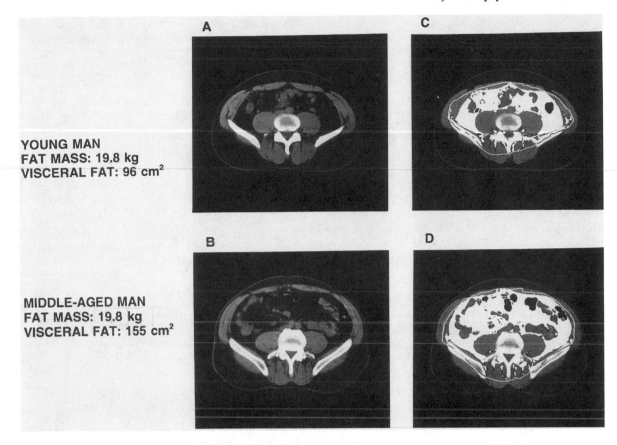

YOUNG MAN
FAT MASS: 19.8 kg
VISCERAL FAT: 96 cm²

MIDDLE-AGED MAN
FAT MASS: 19.8 kg
VISCERAL FAT: 155 cm²

Figure 5 Cross-sectional abdominal adipose tissue areas measured by computed tomography at L4–L5 in a middle-aged man and a young man with similar total body fat mass values. The visceral adipose tissue, delineated by drawing a line within the muscle wall surrounding the abdominal cavity, is highlighted. (From Ref. 113.)

stantial alterations in indices of plasma glucose-insulin homeostasis and in plasma lipoprotein-lipid levels (60,61,76–79).

We have examined the potential relationships between visceral adipose tissue accumulation and plasma lipoprotein levels in obese premenopausal women (60) and found that the level of visceral adipose tissue was the best correlate of lipoprotein variables that are commonly used to predict the risk of coronary heart disease. Indeed, excess visceral adipose tissue was associated with increased apolipoprotein B concentrations and low plasma HDL-cholesterol levels. Furthermore, the HDL cholesterol to LDL cholesterol and the HDL-apolipoprotein A1/LDL-apolipoprotein B ratios were negatively correlated with the level of abdominal visceral adipose tissue (60).

Furthermore, we have examined the independent contributions of obesity versus visceral adipose tissue accumulation by comparing obese individuals with either low or high levels of visceral adipose tissue to a group of lean subjects (Table 1 and Fig. 6). As shown in Figure 6, the

only significant difference noted between the obese subjects with low levels of visceral fat and lean individuals was a moderate increase in plasma triglyceride levels in the obese group whereas obese individuals with high levels of visceral fat showed important alterations in their plasma lipoprotein profile compared to lean controls. Consequently, obese individuals with a high level of visceral adipose tissue may represent the subgroup of obese individuals potentially at high risk for coronary heart disease (43,79).

We have also compared indices of plasma glucose-insulin homeostasis among these three groups of subjects (78–80) and found that obese subjects with high levels of visceral adipose tissue had a higher glycemic response to a glucose challenge in the presence of hyperinsulinemia, reflecting an insulin-resistant state (Fig. 7). In contrast, obese subjects with a low accumulation of visceral adipose tissue showed normal glucose tolerance and only a slight elevation in plasma insulin levels. These analyses and group comparisons were performed in both men and

Table 1 Metabolic Profile of Two Subgroups of Obese Men Matched for Age and Percentage Body Fat but Characterized by Either Low or High Levels of Visceral Adipose Tissue Measured by Computed Tomography (compared to a control sample of lean men)

	Lean men ($n = 29$)	Obese men	
		Low visceral AT ($n = 10$)	High visceral AT ($n = 10$)
Cholesterol (mmol/L)	4.7 ± 0.8	5.1 ± 0.6	5.1 ± 0.9
Triglycerides (mmol/L)	1.18 ± 0.60	1.79 ± 0.99	2.27 ± 1.14*
Apo B (mg/dl)	81.1 ± 20.5	89.9 ± 15.0	98.3 ± 20.7 *
LDL cholesterol (mmol/L)	3.2 ± 0.8	3.4 ± 0.6	3.3 ± 0.6
HDL cholesterol (mmol/L)	1.10 ± 0.22	1.00 ± 0.19	0.91 ± 0.17*
HDL_2 cholesterol (mmol/L)	0.43 ± 0.17	0.37 ± 0.12	0.27 ± 0.08*
HDL_3 cholesterol (mmol/L)	0.67 ± 0.13	0.62 ± 0.10	0.64 ± 0.13
HDL_2/HDL_3 cholesterol	0.67 ± 0.31	0.60 ± 0.18	0.43 ± 0.13*
HDL/total cholesterol	0.24 ± 0.07	0.20 ± 0.04	0.19 ± 0.05*
Fasting glucose (mmol/L)	4.9 ± 0.5	5.3 ± 0.6	5.4 ± 0.6 *
Fasting insulin (pmol/L)	66 ± 19	73 ± 23	120 ± 40 *†
Glucose area (mmol/L/min) $\times 10^{-3}$	1.08 ± 0.20	1.22 ± 0.23	1.38 ± 0.23*
Insulin area (pmol/L/min) $\times 10^{-3}$	51.7 ± 21.3	54.3 ± 21.3	125.9 ± 33.0 *†

Values are means ± SD. AT, adipose tissue; Apo B, apolipoprotein B: HDL, high-density lipoprotein; LDL, low-density lipoprotein.
*Significantly different from lean men, $p < 0.05$.
†Significantly different from obese men with low levels of visceral adipose tissue, $p < 0.05$.
Source: From Ref. 79.

women and similar conclusions were reached (78–80). Thus, these results indicate that obesity per se is associated with moderate metabolic alterations whereas excess visceral adipose tissue accumulation is related to substantial disturbances in indices of plasma glucose-insulin homeostasis that are predictive of an increased risk of non-insulin-dependent diabetes mellitus.

Using CT, it has been reported that marked gender differences exist regarding visceral adipose tissue accumulation. Indeed, men have almost twice the amount of abdominal visceral adipose tissue for a given body fat mass as premenopausal women (Fig. 8) (81). Furthermore, we have studied the potential contribution of gender differences in visceral adipose tissue accumulation to the sex dimorphism found in cardiovascular disease risk variables (82). After control for the gender dimorphism in visceral adipose tissue accumulation, it was found that most of the differences observed in indices of plasma glucose-insulin homeostasis and in plasma lipoprotein-lipid profile were no longer significantly different between men and women (82), suggesting that the greater CVD risk noted in men compared to premenopausal women may be partly due to the preferential accumulation of visceral adipose tissue in male subjects.

Finally, in an attempt to examine whether there could be a threshold of visceral adipose tissue accumulation above which complications may be found, several varia-

bles predictive of CVD and NIDDM risk were compared among samples of young adults and premenopausal women who were divided into quintiles formed on the basis of their cross-sectional visceral adipose tissue area measured by CT. Figure 9 shows that in both men and women, a value below 100 cm² was associated with a rather favorable risk profile (83). However, a cross-sectional visceral adipose tissue area of 130 cm² and above was associated with further deterioration in the cardiovascular risk profile (83).

Visceral abdominal obesity is therefore accompanied by several changes in the metabolic profile predictive of increased risk for metabolic complications. These alterations (state of insulin resistance, hyperinsulinemia, glucose intolerance) observed along with an excess of visceral adipose tissue are considered factors that increase the risk of NIDDM. Furthermore, several studies have shown that insulin resistance is associated with changes in plasma lipoprotein-lipid levels (increased triglyceride and apo B levels and reduced HDL-cholesterol concentrations) that contribute to substantially increase the risk of cardiovascular disease. As previously mentioned, this cluster of metabolic alterations has been described as syndrome "X" or insulin resistance syndrome (13). Our findings clearly suggest that visceral obesity is a frequent component of this syndrome.

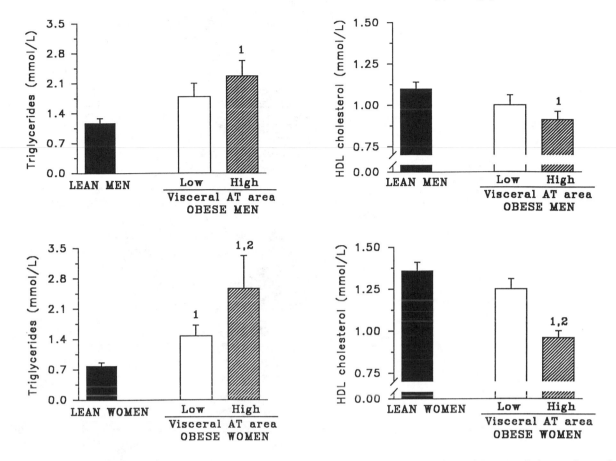

Figure 6 Plasma triglyceride and HDL-cholesterol concentrations in nonobese subjects and in subgroups of obese subjects (Upper panel, men; lower panel, women) matched for body composition but having either low or high levels of visceral adipose tissue (AT) determined by computed tomography. (1) Significantly different from nonobese subjects, $p < 0.05$. (2) Significantly different from obese subjects with low levels of visceral adipose tissue, $p < 0.05$. (From Ref. 79.)

IV. HYPERINSULINEMIA, INSULIN RESISTANCE, AND THE DYSLIPIDEMIC STATE OF VISCERAL OBESITY

As previously discussed, abdominal visceral obesity shows significant relations to both insulin resistance and dyslipoproteinemia. Furthermore, it has been shown that insulin sensitivity measured by the euglycemic hyperinsulinemic clamp technique is an important correlate of plasma lipoprotein levels (14,15). Indeed, it has been reported that a decreased insulin sensitivity is associated with high TG levels and low HDL-cholesterol concentrations (14) and with an increased proportion of dense LDL particles (15). Furthermore, results from five prospective studies have shown that hyperinsulinemia (a crude marker of insulin resistance in nondiabetic subjects) was associated with an increased mortality rate from coronary heart disease (21–24,27). It has also been shown in another prospective design that elevations in plasma insulin levels preceded the development of numerous metabolic complications (66) such as low HDL, high TG, and NIDDM. Furthermore, even after control for concomitant variation in body fatness and regional adipose tissue distribution, the same group also reported that fasting plasma insulin concentrations remained significantly related to the incidence of low high-density lipoprotein (HDL)-cholesterol concentrations and higher triglyceride levels as well as to the incidence of non-insulin-dependent diabetes mellitus (66). These results suggest that the hyperinsulinemic–insulin resistant state that is associated with visceral obesity is a relevant predictor of the future development of the high triglycerides/low HDL-cholesterol dyslipidemic state as summarized in Figure 10.

Ferrannini and colleagues (84) have studied the prevalence rates of obesity, NIDDM, IGT, hypertension, hy-

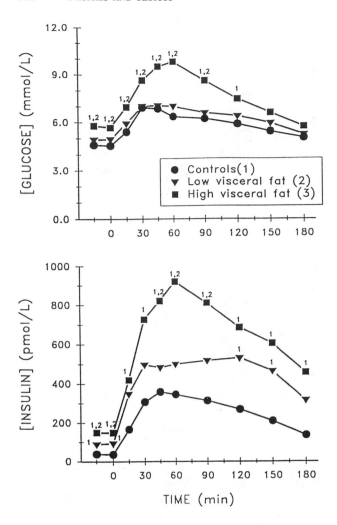

Figure 7 Plasma glucose and insulin concentrations in fasting state (−15 and 0 min) and during oral glucose tolerance test in obese women with high (■) or low (▼) levels of visceral adipose tissue (n = 10 subjects/group) and in a sample of lean women (n = 25). (1) Significantly different from (●); (2) significantly different from (▼), p < 0.05. (From Ref. 80.)

pertriglyceridemia, and hypercholesterolemia in a population-based survey of 2930 subjects. They calculated the prevalence for each condition and they quantified the prevalence of these disorders isolated from the others (free from the other five). They found that the prevalence of these metabolic complications in their isolated forms was significantly lower than in combined forms, supporting the notion that several metabolic risk factors for CVD are often simultaneously present in a given individual (84). In addition, these authors have shown that hyperinsulinemia was generally present in each metabolic disorder, suggesting that impaired insulin action is a common feature of these metabolic alterations (84).

As previously mentioned, insulin resistance is a condition found in 25% of the nondiabetic population (13) whereas the dense LDL (cholesterol ester depleted) phenotype has been estimated (18) to characterize about 30% of the population. We have estimated that almost 30% of nondiabetic men may be characterized by a high accumulation of visceral adipose tissue, insulin resistance, and disturbances in plasma lipoprotein concentrations (increased triglyceride and reduced HDL cholesterol levels, reduced HDL_2 cholesterol levels, reduced postheparin plasma LPL activity), which are consistent with the features of the insulin resistance syndrome (85). Thus, from these observations, it is suggested that visceral obesity is a component of a complex network of metabolic interactions that markedly increase CHD risk. The mechanisms proposed to explain these interrelationships are briefly discussed in the following section.

V. DOES THE DYSLIPIDEMIA OF VISCERAL OBESITY REFLECT A CAUSE-EFFECT RELATIONSHIP?

It has been suggested that enlarged omental adipocytes, which have been shown to display a high lipolytic activity, poorly inhibited by insulin (28,44,45,86), contribute to a greater flux of free fatty acids (FFA) toward the liver through the portal circulation. As shown in Figure 11, high portal FFA levels are associated with a reduced hepatic insulin extraction (87,88) and lead to an increased VLDL synthesis and apolipoprotein B production (29,86). Moreover, it has been suggested that an increased lipid oxidation is associated with impaired glycolysis (89,90) and with a decrease in glycogen synthase activity (91). Furthermore, this elevated lipid oxidation provides precursors for gluconeogenesis (92). Thus, the evidence available suggests that insulin action is impaired in subjects displaying high FFA levels and that compensatory hyperinsulinemia is thus required to regulate plasma glucose levels in insulin-resistant subjects (13).

Lipoprotein lipase is an enzyme responsible for the catabolism of TG-rich lipoproteins, and its activity has been found to be correlated with metabolic alterations associated with visceral obesity. Indeed, visceral obesity has been shown to be associated with decreased LPL and with increased HTGL (hepatic triglyceride lipase) activities (61). Such a decrease in LPL activity contributes to reduce the catabolic rate of TG-rich lipoproteins (43,93) whereas higher HTGL might enhance the degradation of HDL_2 particles or lead to an increase in their conversion to HDL_3 (43,61,93). Pollare et al. (94) have reported a reduced skeletal muscle LPL activity in insulin-resistant subjects

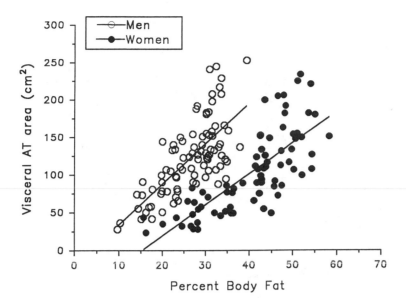

Figure 8 Relation of total body fat mass to abdominal visceral adipose tissue (AT) area measured by CT in 89 men and 75 premenopausal women. Both correlations were significant at *p* < 0.0001. (From Ref. 81.)

and that in vivo insulin sensitivity was positively correlated with skeletal muscle LPL activity.

The higher concentrations of TG-rich lipoproteins resulting from an increased hepatic VLDL production and decreased degradation (through reduced LPL activity) are associated with an increased transfer of TG from VLDL to LDL or HDL particles (61,62) in exchange for LDL and HDL-cholesterol esters, leading to the triglyceride enrichment of LDL and HDL. Such triglyceride enrichment is associated with a reduced cholesterol content of HDL. Furthermore, triglyceride-rich LDL particles represent a good substrate for the enzyme HTGL, ultimately generating atherogenic dense LDL particles (29). Thus, reciprocal changes in LPL and HTGL activities are important correlates of dyslipidemia found in an insulin-resistant state associated with visceral obesity.

The mechanisms leading to in vivo insulin resistance are not fully understood and it is also known that impaired insulin action can be present in both obese and nonobese subjects (13). These observations suggest that insulin resistance is a heterogeneous condition and provide further evidence that some genetic factors are likely to be involved. Studies conducted among insulin-resistant or NIDDM subjects have shown that the presence of a family history of diabetes may alter the relationship of abdominal fat accumulation to indices of plasma glucose-insulin homeostasis (95,96). Indeed, we have previously reported that in subjects with a similar level of deterioration in plasma glucose-insulin homeostasis, those who

displayed a positive family history of diabetes had lower levels of abdominal fat than subjects without a family history of diabetes (96). These results suggest that the presence of genetic susceptibility reduces the threshold of abdominal fat above which metabolic alterations predictive of an increased NIDDM risk are observed.

Thus, in abdominal visceral obese patients, high FFA concentrations (increased lipolysis of the visceral depot), decreased LPL activity, and reduced insulin sensitivity may lead to metabolic changes that are ultimately involved in the development of insulin resistance, glucose intolerance, hyperinsulinemia, dyslipoproteinemia, NIDDM, and CVD.

In addition to the impaired free fatty acid metabolism hypothesis briefly reviewed above, it has been suggested that abdominal obesity is associated with altered sex steroid levels. Indeed, results that have crudely assessed body fat distribution by the waist-to-hip ratio have reported low levels of sex hormone–binding globulin (SHBG) concentrations and high levels of free testosterone in women with excess abdominal fat (44,97–99). Moreover, the altered sex steroid concentrations observed in abdominal obese women have also been associated with variations of in vivo insulin sensitivity (44,99). Studies have also shown that the hyperinsulinemic state of abdominal obesity was partly attributed to a reduction in the hepatic extraction of insulin (97), the latter phenomenon being associated with lower SHBG concentrations. Furthermore, a reduced hepatic insulin extraction has also been related to high free testosterone levels in women (97). Thus, the associ-

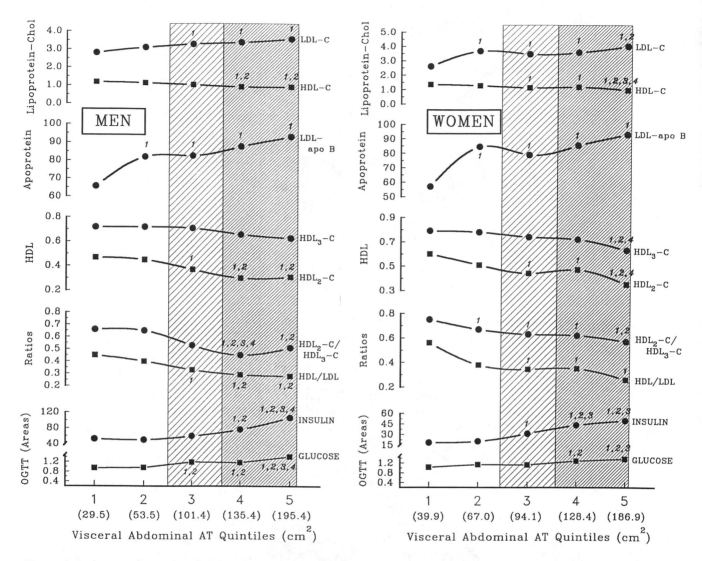

Figure 9 Relations of quintiles of abdominal visceral adipose tissue area to variables predictive of non-insulin-dependent diabetes mellitus (NIDDM) and cardiovascular disease (CVD) risk in samples of 115 men and 72 women, respectively. Visceral adipose tissue areas above 100 cm² are associated with moderate, but significant, metabolic changes whereas visceral adipose tissue areas greater than 135 cm² in men and 128 cm² in women are clearly associated with further metabolic deteriorations that suggest an increased risk of NIDDM and CVD. 1, 2, 3, and 4 are significantly different from quintiles 1, 2, 3, and 4, respectively ($p < 0.05$). (From Ref. 83.)

ations of steroid levels with metabolic disturbances have been shown to be partly independent of the concomitant variation in adipose tissue distribution. It has also been suggested that although there is clearly an independent association between visceral fat accumulation and metabolic alterations, the dyslipidemic state observed in abdominal obese women could also be due partly to the concomitant alterations in the sex steroid profile (44).

In men, however, the associations between sex steroids, visceral obesity, and the metabolic profile are quite different from those noted in women. Indeed, as opposed to abdominal obese women, visceral obesity in men is rather associated with a reduction of plasma testosterone levels (100,101). It is also not well established whether or not reduced levels of androgenic steroids are independently associated with an excess abdominal visceral fat accumulation after control for the concomitant variation in the amount of total body fat (101). Furthermore, the alterations found in steroid hormone levels have been found to be significantly correlated with glucose intolerance (102) and with the dyslipidemic state observed in visceral obesity (Tchernof et al., unpublished observations). It is also

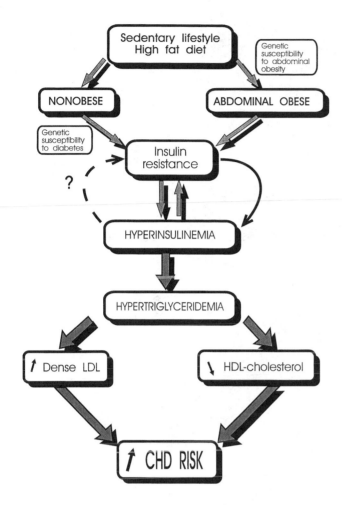

Figure 10 Working model for etiology of insulin resistance and related disorders in plasma lipid transport in nonobese and abdominally obese subjects. (From Ref. 85.)

relevant to note that, after controlling for variations in testosterone, the relationships between the amount of visceral adipose tissue to insulin resistance and to dyslipidemia remained significant (102).

In addition, the potential role of glucocorticoids on the regulation of lipid metabolism in visceral obesity must be considered (103–105). Indeed, it has been proposed that the insulin-resistant state observed in subjects with excess visceral adipose tissue is partly the consequence of altered glucocorticoid levels (103–105). In this regard, environmental stress can induce an activation of the hypothalamic-pituitary-adrenal axis thereby increasing cortisol production (106). Furthermore, visceral adipose cells have been reported to have the highest density of glucocorticoid receptors (107,108) in comparison to adipocytes from other fat depots and this could explain the greater sensitivity of visceral adipose tissue to stressor agents. Fur-

thermore, the metabolic effects of glucocorticoids (103) are in accordance with the alterations observed in visceral obesity (29,43,103). Indeed, glucocorticoids stimulate VLDL and apo B production, reduce the activity of LDL receptors, and induce insulin resistance (103).

In summary, the dyslipidemic state of visceral obesity results from complex metabolic and hormonal interactions that lead to insulin resistance and to an increased CVD risk (Fig. 11).

VI. FROM VISCERAL OBESITY TO DYSLIPIDEMIA AND CORONARY HEART DISEASE: CONTRIBUTION OF GENETIC SUSCEPTIBILITY

Genetic susceptibility is of paramount importance in the ultimate determination of NIDDM and CVD risk in visceral obese patients. In this regard, the investigation of family history of diabetes and early coronary heart disease is of great importance in the assessment of the health hazard associated with a given excess of abdominal adipose tissue. Thus, the magnitude of the dyslipidemic state found in a visceral obese patient will obviously be modulated by his/her genetic susceptibility to dyslipidemia. Thus, the dyslipidemic phenotype observed depends on the patient's genetic background. In this regard, several candidate genes could alter plasma lipoprotein levels in visceral obesity such as those coding for apolipoproteins, lipoprotein receptors, and enzymes involved in lipoprotein metabolism such as lipoprotein lipase (LPL), hepatic triglyceride lipase (HTGL), cholesterol ester transfer protein (CFTP), and lecithin cholesterol acyl transferase (LCAT) (109). Thus, individuals with similar levels of visceral adipose tissue and of insulin resistance may not necessarily be characterized by a comparable dyslipidemic state.

Apolipoprotein (apo) E polymorphism was the first of these modulators that we examined in visceral obesity. This apolipoprotein plays an important role in the clearance of triglyceride-rich lipoproteins. Apo E is polymorphic, and three main isoforms (E_2, E_3, E_4) can be identified by techniques such as isoelectric focusing (110,111). With the use of this method, we found that E_2 carriers and E_3 homozygotes showed the expected correlations between visceral adipose tissue accumulation, fasting plasma insulin levels, and triglyceride concentrations. Thus, visceral obesity and hyperinsulinemia were associated with hypertriglyceridemia in these subjects (110,111). Among E_4 carriers, however, these associations could not be found and hyperinsulinemia was not associated with hypertriglyceridemia in this group. Thus, these results pro-

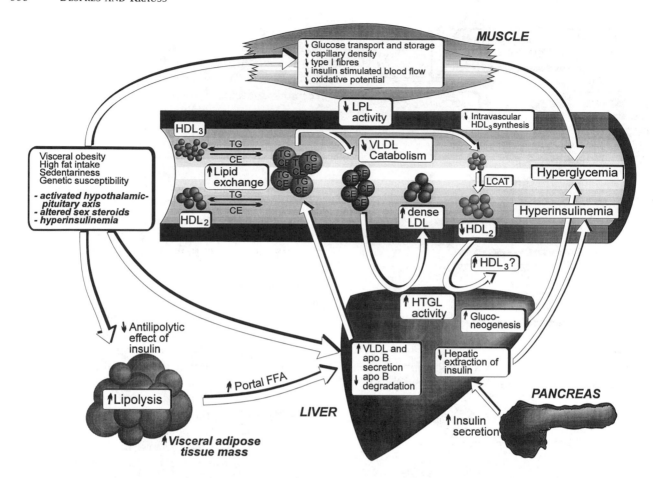

Figure 11 Complex metabolic interactions that presumably occur with the insulin resistance–dyslipidemic phenotype. In this case, insulin resistance is frequently accompanied by excess intra-abdominal (visceral) adipose tissue. The liver, via the portal circulation, becomes exposed to high levels of free fatty acids (FFA) as the compensatory hyperinsulinemia poorly inhibits the lipolysis of intra-abdominal fat cells. This phenomenon stimulates gluconeogenesis as well as VLDL synthesis and secretion. Moreover, the catabolism of triglyceride-rich lipoproteins appears to be slow, this being attributable to the fact that lipoprotein lipase (LPL) activity is reduced and the postprandial adipose tissue LPL response is inadequate. Impaired LPL activity may explain, at least to some degree, the low HDL-cholesterol levels of insulin-resistant individuals characterized by visceral obesity. The high activity of another enzyme, hepatic lipase, is a contributing factor in the further decrease of HDL-cholesterol level. The high triglyceride levels resulting from the increased production and slower catabolism of VLDL promote the transfer of triglycerides to LDL and HDL in exchange for their cholesterol esters. This phenomenon leads to an increase in VLDL cholesterol esters, a process considered atherogenic. Moreover, the triglyceride-enriched LDL and HDL fractions represent the substrate of choice for hepatic lipase, this process favoring the formation of dense LDL, the concentration of which is higher in coronary artery disease patients. These complex metabolic interactions increase not only the risk of diabetes but also the risk of coronary heart disease in insulin-resistant individuals. (From Ref. 17.)

vided the first simple example of a polymorphic apolipoprotein altering the relation expected between visceral obesity and hypertriglyceridemia.

We then examined the potential contribution of an Eco RI polymorphism in the apo B-100 gene in men (112). We found that among heterozygous subjects for the absence of the restriction site (+/−), visceral obesity was associated with elevated apo B concentrations. However, (+/+) homozygotes failed to show this significant relationship. Thus, apo B-100 gene Eco RI (+/−) men appeared to be more prone to hyperapolipoprotein B in the presence of visceral obesity than men who were homozygotes for the presence of this restriction site.

More recently, we have reported that a HindIII polymorphism in the LPL gene was also an important modulator of the susceptibility to hypertriglyceridemia in visceral obesity (113). We are currently examining other genes such as those coding for apo A-II and CETP and we are finding additional evidences of significant interactions (M. C. Vohl et al., unpublished observations).

Consequently, there is increasing evidence that genetic variation ultimately modulates the magnitude of the dyslipidemic state found in visceral obesity. An additional challenge will be to investigate gene-gene interactions but this issue will require the study of very large cohorts. Furthermore, gene-environment interactions will also have to be further examined in longitudinal designs (both observational and intervention studies). These approaches will contribute to a better understanding of genetic and lifestyle patterns ultimately involved in the development of the insulin-resistant dyslipidemic syndrome found in visceral obese patients.

VII. VISCERAL OBESITY, DYSLIPIDEMIA, AND CORONARY HEART DISEASE: CLINICAL IMPLICATIONS

From the evidence reviewed, the detection of the subgroup of obese patients at risk for complications associated with excess visceral adipose tissue is clinically important. Thus, an adequate estimation of visceral adipose tissue accumulation is of great relevance to better quantify the patient's risk of CVD. Although computed tomography (CT) is very accurate and reliable, it is not accessible to most clinicians and it was relevant to develop approaches to offer simple tools for the detection, prevention, and treatment of visceral obesity.

A. Is Anthropometry an Appropriate Alternative to CT?

Numerous studies have examined the correlations between anthropometric measurements and cross-sectional visceral adipose tissue areas measured by CT (114–117). Until recently, the WHR had generally been considered the most relevant variable in the assessment of visceral obesity (50–59), this ratio often being used in prospective and metabolic studies. Although the use of WHR has contributed to highlight the importance of body fat distribution, we have reported that visceral adipose tissue accumulation showed better correlations with the waist circumference alone than with the WHR (118). Figure 12 shows that the relation of visceral adipose tissue area to the waist girth was stronger than for the WHR, especially in women. Furthermore, the relationship between waist circumference and visceral adipose tissue was found to be similar in men and women. Moreover, waist circumference also appears to be a good correlate to total body fatness and therefore provides a better index of abdominal obesity

than the WHR alone, which is a weak correlate of total adiposity (18).

For example, a nonobese woman with small hips may have a WHR value that could be similar to the WHR of an obese woman with a large accumulation of abdominal fat but with also a substantial deposition of fat at the hip level. Thus, despite similar WHR values in these two subjects, the obese woman would have a much greater accumulation of visceral adipose tissue than the nonobese woman despite the fact that their WHR are similar. Consequently, the use of WHR alone can be quite misleading whereas a high waist girth obviously indicates that excess abdominal fat and obesity are simultaneously present. Indeed, the waist circumference is positively correlated with both an accumulation of total body fat and an elevated deposition of visceral adipose tissue (118). In this context, we have proposed that the waist circumference provides a valuable index of the absolute amount of abdominal fat as compared to the WHR, which rather reflects relative abdominal adipose tissue deposition, which is not always associated with a marked increase in the absolute accumulation of abdominal visceral adipose tissue (118).

These concepts have considerable public health implications. First, it appears that obesity is often a problem of abdominal adiposity rather than of excess body weight and that waist circumference alone may provide useful information on both total body fatness and abdominal adipose tissue deposition. Accordingly, it has been proposed that a waist circumference of 100 cm would represent an approximate threshold above which metabolic alterations may be observed (118,119). Since genetic susceptibility plays a significant role, it should be emphasized that this measure defines a gray zone rather than a well-defined cut point above which complications are likely to be found. It is also important to point out that subjects with a family history of diabetes or of premature coronary heart disease may show complications at lower levels of abdominal fat.

From the epidemiological and metabolic evidence available, there is no doubt that abdominal obesity is an important risk factor for the development of dyslipidemia and CVD. Several prospective studies have shown that abdominal obesity is associated with an increased mortality rate related to CVD (46,50–52,120–122). However, it is also important to acknowledge that no intervention study has shown that reducing obesity and the amount of abdominal fat would lead to a reduction in the incidence of diabetes and CVD-related mortality. To the best of our knowledge, the only ongoing project on this issue is the study of Swedish Obese Subjects (SOS study) (123). In this study, a sample of about 4000 obese individuals have been randomly assigned to a CVD risk factor management group or to a group where obesity is surgically treated via

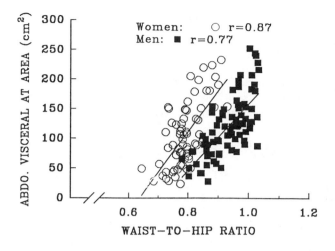
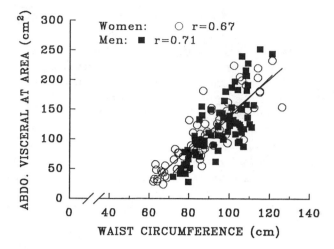

Figure 12 Relation of either waist circumference or WHR to abdominal (ABDO) visceral adipose tissue areas measured by computed tomography in men and women. (From Ref. 118.)

gastric stapling, vertical banded gastroplasty, or gastric bypass procedures (123). The incidence of morbidity and mortality will be followed over several years. Although this does not represent an approach where abdominal obesity is treated by life-style modification, this study will provide the first evidence that reducing the body weight may prevent the incidence of diabetes and coronary heart disease. However, a considerable amount of literature has indicated that reducing body weight and lowering the amount of abdominal fat lead to major improvements in CVD risk profile, which would include reduction in blood pressure, improvement in plasma lipoprotein-lipid levels, and improvement in insulin sensitivity leading to a reduction in plasma insulin levels and to an improvement of glucose tolerance (83).

Taken together, these results are consistent with the notion that body weight management, especially in the subgroup of abdominal obese individuals, is relevant for the prevention of CVD. Another important issue is that the prevalence of visceral obesity has been estimated to reach 25% of sedentary adult males (85). It has therefore been suggested that the insulin resistance state associated with visceral obesity and with high triglyceride and low HDL-cholesterol levels is likely to represent the most prevalent cause of CVD and related mortality in developed countries. Thus, the public health implications of identifying individuals with abdominal obesity and at risk for the complications related to an excess of visceral adipose tissue are of tremendous importance. Although no prospective study has shown that lowering body weight reduces the incidence of diabetes, CVD, and related mortality, approaches that have used either diet or exercise to

improve the CVD risk profile have reported substantial metabolic improvements in abdominal obese subjects (30,83,119,124).

B.   Dietary Treatment of Visceral Obesity

The positive correlation between total body fatness and visceral adipose tissue accumulation suggests that weight loss through dieting may induce a mobilization of visceral adipose tissue (83). It is also relevant to point out that some individuals are more susceptible to visceral adipose tissue accumulation than others and that susceptibility to visceral adipose tissue accumulation appears to be strongly genetically determined (125,126). Furthermore, it has also been shown that individuals with initially high levels of visceral adipose tissue are those showing the greatest loss of this depot in response to a reduced caloric intake (74,75,127). Thus, visceral obese patients are likely to represent the subgroup of obese individuals who would benefit the most from a low-fat diet. However, additional studies on the dietary treatment of insulin resistance and of the related dyslipidemia in visceral obesity are clearly warranted. Available evidence has, however, indicated that the magnitude of body fat loss induced by dieting is correlated with the magnitude of improvement in CVD risk variables such as glucose tolerance, plasma insulin, and lipoprotein-lipid levels (75,83,127). Furthermore, it does appear that normalization of body weight is not required to normalize the cardiovascular disease profile of abdominal obese patients (128). Indeed, as a preferential mobilization of visceral adipose tissue is observed when visceral obese patients are subjected to a low-fat diet and a reduced calorie intake, normalization of CVD risk profile may be observed even in the absence of normalization of body weight (83). These observations are consistent with the substantial metabolic improvements that are observed when a moderate loss of body weight is achieved (5–10% loss of body weight) (128). Furthermore, a substantial mobilization of visceral adipose tissue may be observed in the presence of a small loss of body weight (30,83). Therefore, we believe that preventive approaches should aim at reducing visceral adipose tissue mass rather than normalizing body weight in the overweight patient. Indeed, normalization of body weight is difficult to achieve and not always clinically justified.

C. Exercise

No studies have shown that a physically active life-style may reduce the risk of CVD-related mortality in overweight subjects or in individuals with abdominal obesity. However, it is well accepted that endurance exercise training induces favorable changes in body composition, insulin sensitivity, and plasma lipoprotein concentrations (3,83,124,129–131). Therefore, although no direct evidence is available, endurance exercise may be considered a valuable approach for the prevention of CVD and diabetes in the visceral obese patient. Studies that have examined the metabolic effect of endurance exercise training in abdominal obese patients have reported substantial metabolic improvements, which include improved insulin action, reduced triglyceride levels, increased HDL cholesterol concentration, and a reduction of the proportion of small dense LDL particles (83,124,129). It is also important to point out that these metabolic improvements were observed even in the absence of major changes in cardiorespiratory fitness and were rather dependent upon the magnitude of visceral adipose tissue and total body fat losses (124). Thus, it does not appear necessary to substantially improve cardiorespiratory fitness in overweight abdominal obese patients to reduce the risk of NIDDM and CVD, and it seems more relevant to focus on the duration of exercise rather than on its intensity (124).

Indeed, it has been suggested that prolonged endurance exercise training performed at moderate intensity, that is 45–50% of VO$_2$max (which corresponds to a brisk walking period performed on an almost daily basis for 40–45 min), may induce substantial metabolic improvements in abdominal obese patients even in the absence of major changes in body composition (124). Therefore, the traditional approach where exercise training is performed 3 times per week, 20 min per session at 70–75% of VO$_2$max (the most common exercise prescription to improve fitness) (124,132) will induce a trivial increase in

daily energy expenditure that is unlikely to lead to major improvements in CVD risk variables (124). Furthermore, it is once again important to emphasize that endurance exercise training may induce beneficial changes in the plasma lipoprotein-lipid profile, insulin sensitivity, and plasma insulin levels in the absence of any apparent change in body composition (133–142).

Thus, an abdominal obese individual who is physically active on a daily basis may have a lower risk of diabetes and CVD than a sedentary subject with the same excess of abdominal adipose tissue. It is therefore likely that the favorable CVD risk profile observed in the physically active individual may be related to the effect of endurance training on in vivo insulin action as insulin resistance appears to be a major correlate of the dyslipidemic profile observed in abdominal obesity.

Finally, some pharmacological approaches have been tested to reduce body fatness (143–146). However, very few long-term studies focusing on insulin sensitivity and plasma lipoprotein levels are available and the impact of the pharmacological treatment of obesity on the incidence of diabetes and CVD and relative mortality have never been tested. Although some approaches appear promising (30,147), randomized trials will be necessary and additional studies in this area are clearly warranted.

VIII. CONCLUSION

From the literature available, we believe that the evidence indicating that abdominal obesity is an important risk factor for CVD and related mortality is sound. However, no intervention studies have shown that reducing abdominal fat accumulation will lead to a lower incidence of diabetes and cardiovascular diseases. Nevertheless, studies that have used either diet or exercise to improve the metabolic condition of the visceral obese patient have reported substantial improvements in the plasma lipoprotein profile, which were proportionate to the magnitude of visceral adipose tissue loss. Finally, it is important to consider genetic susceptibility to dyslipidemia and coronary heart disease in the ultimate modulation of the health hazard of visceral obesity. No prospective study has examined the potential interaction of family history of diabetes and early coronary heart disease in the modulation of CVD mortality associated with excess abdominal fat, and additional studies on this topic are needed. In this context, it has been proposed that abdominal obesity is a permissive factor that exacerbates the individual's genetic susceptibility to dyslipidemia and premature coronary heart disease (30,43,109,119,147). From the literature available, it therefore appears important to emphasize that preventive measures aimed at primary and secondary prevention of cardiovascular disease via improvements in metabolic risk factors should focus on controlling visceral adipose tissue mass to a greater extent than normalizing body weight.

ACKNOWLEDGMENT

The work of the authors reviewed in this chapter has been supported by the Medical Research Council of Canada, the Canadian Diabetes Association, the Heart and Stroke Foundation of Canada, Warner-Lambert/Parke-Davis, Fournier Pharma/Jouveinal, and Servier Canada. The contribution of Marie Lesage and André Tchernof to the preparation of this document is also gratefully acknowledged.

REFERENCES

1. Keys A. Coronary heart disease in seven countries. Circulation 1970; 41(Suppl 1):I1–I211.

2. WHO Expert Committee on the Prevention of Coronary Heart Disease, World Health Organization Technical Reports Series 678. Geneva, Switzerland: World Health Organization, 1982.

3. NIH Consensus Conference: Lowering blood cholesterol to prevent heart disease. JAMA 1985; 253:2080–2086.

4. Stamler J, Wentworth D, Neaton JD. Is relationship between serum cholesterol and risk of premature death from coronary heart disease continuous or graded? Findings in 356,222 primary screenees of the Multiple Risk Factor Intervention Trial (MRFIT). JAMA 1986; 256:2823–2828.

5. Genest JJ, McNamara JR, Salem DN, Schaefer EJ. Prevalence of risk factors in men with premature coronary heart disease. Am J Cardiol 1991; 67:1185–1189.

6. Sniderman AJ, Silberberg J. Is it time to measure apolipoprotein B? Arteriosclerosis 1990; 10:665–667.

7. Austin MA. Plasma triglyceride and coronary heart disease. Arterioscler Thrombo 1991; 11:1–14.

8. Assmann G, Schulte H. Relation of high-density lipoprotein cholesterol and triglycerides to incidence of atherosclerotic coronary artery disease (the PROCAM Experience). Am J Cardiol 1992; 70:733–737.

9. Rubin EM, Krauss RM, Spangler E, Verstuyft S, Clift S. Inhibition of early atherogenesis in transgenic mice by human apolipoprotein A-I. Nature 1991; 353:265–267.

10. Glomset JA. The plasma lecithin:cholesterol acyltransferase reaction. J Lipid Res 1968; 9:155–167.

11. Lamarche B, Després JP, Pouliot MC, Prud'homme D, Moorjani S, Lupien PJ, Nadeau A, Tremblay A, Bouchard C. Metabolic heterogeneity associated with high plasma triglyceride or low HDL-cholesterol levels in men. Arterioscler Thrombo 1993; 13:33–40.

12. Manninen V, Tenkanen L, Koskinen P, Huttunen JK, Mäntärri M, Heinonen OP, Frick MH. Joint effects of serum triglyceride and LDL-cholesterol and HDL-cholesterol concentrations on coronary heart disease risk in the Helsinki Heart study. Implications for treatment. Circulation 1992; 85:37–45.

13. Reaven GM. Role of insulin resistance in human disease. Diabetes 1988; 37:1595–1607.

14. Laakso M, Sarlund H, Mykkänen L. Insulin resistance is associated with lipid and lipoprotein abnormalities in subjects with varying degrees of glucose tolerance. Arteriosclerosis 1990; 10:223–231.

15. Reaven GM, Chen YDI, Jeppesen J, Maheux P, Krauss RM. Insulin resistance and hyperinsulinemia in individuals with small, dense, low density lipoprotein particles. J Clin Invest 1993; 92:141–146.

16. Després JP. Visceral obesity: A component of the insulin resistance-dyslipidemic syndrome. Can J Cardiol 1994; 10:17B–22B.

17. Després JP & Marette A. Relation of components of insulin resistance syndrome to coronary disease risk. Curr Opin Lipid 1994; 5:274–289.

18. Austin MA, King MC, Vranizan KM, Krauss RM. Atherogenic lipoprotein phenotype: A proposed genetic marker for coronary heart disease. Circulation 1990; 82:495–506.

19. Lamarche B, Després JP, Moorjani S, Cantin B, Dagenais G, Lupien PJ. Prevalence of dyslipidemic phenotypes in ischemic heart disease (prospective results from the Québec Cardiovascular Study). Am J Cardiol 1995; 75:1189–1195.

20. Lamarche B, Moorjani S, Lupien PJ, Cantin B, Bernard PM, Dagenais G, Després JP. Apolipoprotein A-I and B levels and the risk of ischemic heart disease during a five-year follow-up of men in the Québec Cardiovascular Study. Circulation 1996 (in press).

21. Pyörälä K. Relationship of glucose tolerance and plasma insulin to the incidence of coronary heart disease: Results from the two population studies in Finland. Diabetes Care 1979; 2:131–141.

22. Welborn TA, Wearne K. Coronary heart disease incidence and cardiovascular mortality in Busselton with reference to glucose and insulin concentrations. Diabetes Care 1979; 2:154–160.

23. Eschwège E, Richard JL, Thibult N, Ducimetière P, Warnet JM, Rosselin G. Coronary heart disease mortality in relation with diabetes, blood glucose and plasma insulin levels: The Paris Prospective Study, ten years later. Horm Metab Res 1985; 15(Suppl):41–46.

24. Yarnell JWG, Sweetnam PM, Marks V, Teale JD, Bolton CH. Insulin in ischemic heart disease: Are associations explained by triglyceride concentrations? The Caerphilly Prospective Study. Br Heart J 1994; 171:293–296.

25. Fontbonne A, Eschwège E, Cambien F, Richard JL, Ducimetière P, Thibult N, Warnet JM, Claude JR. Hypertriglyceridemia as a risk factor of coronary heart disease mortality in subjects with impaired glucose tolerance or diabetes: results from the 11-year follow-up of the Paris Prospective Study. Diabetologia 1989; 32:300–304.

26. Fontbonne E, Charles MA, Thibult N, Richard JL, Claude JM, Warnet JM, Rosselin GE, Eschwège E. Hyperinsulinemia as a predictor of coronary heart disease mortality in a healthy population: the Paris Prospective Study. 15-year follow-up. Diabetologia 1991; 34:356–361.

27. Després JP, Lamarche B, Mauriège P, Cantin B, Dagenais GR, Moorjani S, Lupien PJ. Hyperinsulinemia as an independent risk factor for ischemic heart disease. N Engl J Med 1996; 334:952–957.

28. Kissebah AH, Freedman DS, Peiris AN. Health risks of obesity. Med Clin North Am 1989; 73:111–138.

29. Després JP. Obesity and lipid metabolism: Relevance of body fat distribution. Curr Opin Lipidol 1991; 2:5–15.

30. Després JP. Dyslipidemia and obesity. Ballière's Clin Endocrinol Metab 1994; 8:629–660.

31. Barrett-Connor E. Obesity, atherosclerosis, and coronary artery disease. Ann Intern Med 1985; 103:1010–1019.

32. Manson JE, Willett WC, Stampfer MJ, Colditz GA, Hunter DJ, Hankinson SE, Hennekens CH, Speizer FE. Body weight and mortality among women. N Engl J Med 1995; 333:677–685.

33. Bouchard C, Després JP. Variation in fat distribution with age and health implications. In: Eckert HM, Spirduso W, eds. Physical Activity and Aging. American Academy of Physical Education, 1989:78–106.

34. Bray GA, Davidson MB, Drenick EJ. Obesity: a serious symptom. Ann Intern Med 1972; 77:779.

35. The Pooling Project Research Group. Relationship of blood pressure, serum cholesterol, smoking habit, relative weight and ECG abnormalities to incidence of major coronary events: final report of the pooling project. J Chronic Dis 1978; 31:201.

36. Björntorp P. Hazards in subgroups of human obesity. Eur J Clin Invest 1984; 14:239–241.

37. Harrison GH. Height-weight tables. Ann Intern Med 1985; 103:989–994.

38. Després JP. Assessing obesity: beyond the BMI. Natl Inst Nutr Rev #19, Rapport NIN 1992; 7(Suppl):1–4.

39. Quetelet LAJ. Physique Sociale, vol 2. Brussels: C. Muquardt, 1869:92.

40. Keys A, Fidanza F, Karvonen MJ, et al. Indices of relative weight and obesity. J Chronic Dis 1972; 25:329–334.

41. Garrow J. Meta-analysis on the effect of exercise on the composition of weight loss. Int J Obes 1994; 18:517.

42. Bray GA, Gray DS. Treatment of obesity: an overview. Diabetes Metab Rev 1988; 4:653–679.

43. Després JP, Moorjani S, Lupien PJ, Tremblay A, Nadeau A, Bouchard C. Regional distribution of body fat, plasma lipoproteins, and cardiovascular disease. Arteriosclerosis 1990; 10:497–511.

44. Kissebah AH, Peiris AN. Biology of regional body fat distribution: relationship to non-insulin-dependent diabetes mellitus. Diabetes Metab Rev 1989; 5:83–109.

45. Björntorp P. Abdominal obesity and the development of non-insulin dependent diabetes mellitus. Diabetes Metab Rev 1988; 4:615–622.

46. Donahue RP, Abbott RD, Bloom E, Reed DM, Yano K. Central obesity and coronary heart disease in men. Lancet 1987; 1:822–824.

47. Vague J. La différenciation sexuelle, facteur déterminant des formes de l'obésité. Presse Méd 1947; 30:339–340.

48. Albrink MJ, Meigs JW. Interrelationship between skinfold thickness, serum lipids and blood sugar in normal men. Am J Clin Nutr 1964; 15:255–261.

49. Allard C, Goulet C. Serum lipids: an epidemiological study of an active Montreal population. Can Med Assoc J 1968; 98:627–637.

50. Lapidus L, Bengtsson C, Larsson B, Pennert K, Rybo E, Sjöström L. Distribution of adipose tissue and risk of cardiovascular disease and death: a 12 year follow-up of participants in the population study of women in Gothenburg, Sweden. Br Med J 1984; 289:1261–1263.

51. Larsson B, Svardsudd K, Welin L, Wilhemsen L, Björntorp P, Tibblin G. Abdominal adipose tissue distribution, obesity and risk of cardiovascular disease and death: 13 year follow-up of participants in the study of men born in 1913. Br Med J 1984; 288:1401–1404.

52. Ducimetière P, Richard J, Cambien F. The pattern of subcutaneous fat distribution in middle-aged men and the risk of coronary heart disease: the Paris Prospective Study. Int J Obes 1986; 10:229–240.

53. Ohlson LO, Larsson B, Svärdsudd K, Welin L, Eriksson H, Wilhelmsen L, Björntorp P, Tibblin G. The influence of body fat distribution on the incidence of diabetes mellitus—13.5 years of follow-up of the participants in the study of men born in 1913. Diabetes 1985; 34:1055–1058.

54. Anderson AJ, Sobocinski KA, Freedman DS, Barboriak JJ, Rimm AA, Gruchow HW. Body fat distribution, plasma lipids and lipoproteins. Arteriosclerosis 1988; 8:88–94.

55. Kissebah AH, Vydelingum N, Murray R, Evans DJ, Hartz AJ, Kalkhoff RK, Adams PW. Relation of body fat distribution to metabolic complications of obesity. J Clin Endocrinol Metab 1982; 54:254–260.

56. Krotkiewski M, Björntorp P, Sjöström L, Smith U. Impact of obesity on metabolism in men and women. Importance of regional adipose tissue distribution. J Clin Invest 1983; 72:1150–1162.

57. Albrink MJ, Krauss RM, Lindgren FT, von der Groeben J, Pam S, Wood PD. Intercorrelations among plasma high density lipoprotein, obesity and triglycerides in a normal population. Lipids 1980; 15:668–676.

58. Ostlund RE, Staten M, Kohrt WM, Schultz J, Malley M. The ratio of waist-to-hip circumferences, plasma insulin level, and glucose intolerance as independent predictors of the HDL$_2$-cholesterol level in older adults. N Engl J Med 1990; 322:229–234.

59. Terry RB, Wood PD, Haskell WL, Stefanick ML, Krauss RM. Regional adiposity pattern in relation to lipids, lipoprotein cholesterol, and lipoprotein subfraction mass in men. J Clin Endocrinol Metab 1989; 68:191–199.

60. Després JP, Moorjani S, Ferland M, Tremblay A, Lupien PJ, Nadeau A, Pinault S, Thériault G, Bouchard C. Adipose tissue distribution and plasma lipoprotein levels in obese women: importance of intra-abdominal fat. Arteriosclerosis 1989; 9:203–210.

61. Després JP, Ferland M, Moorjani S, Tremblay A, Lupien PJ, Thériault G, Bouchard C. Role of hepatic-triglyceride lipase activity in the association between intra-abdominal fat and plasma HDL-cholesterol in obese women. Arteriosclerosis 1989; 9:485–492.

62. Després JP, Moorjani S, Tremblay A, Ferland M, Lupien PJ, Nadeau A, Bouchard C. Relation of high plasma triglyceride levels associated with obesity and regional adipose tissue distribution to plasma lipoprotein-lipid composition in premenopausal women. Clin Invest Med 1989; 12:374–380.

63. Austin MA, Breslow JL, Hennekens CH, Buring JE, Willet WC, Krauss RM. Low density lipoprotein subclass patterns and risk of myocardial infarction. JAMA 1988; 260: 1917–1921.

64. Hartz AJ, Rupley DC, Kalkhoff RD, Rimm AA. Relationship of obesity to diabetes: influence of obesity and body fat distribution. Prevent Med 1983; 12:351–357.

65. Landin K, Lonnroth P, Krotkiewski G, Smith U. Increased insulin resistance and fat cell lipolysis in obese but not lean women with a high waist/hip ratio. Eur J Clin Invest 1990; 20:530–535.

66. Haffner SM, Stern MP, Mitchell BD, Hazuda HP, Patterson JK. Incidence of type II diabetes mellitus in Mexican Americans predicted by fasting insulin and glucose levels, obesity and body fat distribution. Diabetes 1990; 39: 283–289.

67. Peiris AN, Struve MF, Kissebah AH. Relationship of body fat distribution to the metabolic clearance of insulin in premenopausal women. Int J Obes 1987; 11:581–589.

68. Kannel WB, Gordon T, Castelli WP. Obesity, lipids and glucose intolerance. the Framingham Study. Am J Clin Nutr 1979; 32:1238–1245.

69. Borkan GA, Gerzof SG, Robbins AH, Hults DE, Silbert CK, Silbert JE. Assessment of abdominal fat content by computed tomography. Am J Clin Nutr 1982; 36: 172–177.

70. Tokunaga K, Matsuzawa Y, Ishikawa K, Tarui S. A novel technique for the determination of body fat by computed tomography. Int J Obes 1983; 7:437–445.

71. Sjöström L, Kvist H, Cederblad A, Tylen U. Determination of total adipose tissue and body fat in women by computed tomography, ^{40}K, and tritium. Am J Physiol (Endocrinol Metab) 1986; 250:E736–E745.

72. Kvist H, Chowdhury B, Grangard U, Tylén U, Sjöström L. Total and visceral adipose tissue volumes derived from measurements with computed tomography in adult men and women: predictive equations. Am J Clin Nutr 1988; 48:1351–1361.

73. Fujioka S, Matsuzawa Y, Tokunaga K, Tarui S. Contribution of intra-abdominal fat accumulation to the impair-

ment of glucose and lipid metabolism in human obesity. Metabolism 1987; 36:54–59.

74. Fujioka S, Matsuzawa Y, Tokunaga K, Kano Y, Kobatake T, Tarui S. Treatment of visceral obesity. Int J Obes 1991; 15:59–65.

75. Fujioka S, Matsuzawa Y, Tokunaga K, Kawamoto T, Kobatake T, Keno Y, Kotani K, Yoshida S, Tarui S. Improvement of glucose and lipid metabolism associated with selective reduction of intra-abdominal visceral fat in premenopausal with visceral fat obesity. Int J Obes 1991; 15:853–859.

76. Sparrow D, Borkan GA, Gerzof SG, Wisniewski CK. Relationship of body fat distribution to glucose tolerance. Results of computed tomography in male participants of the normative aging study. Diabetes 1986; 35:411–415.

77. Peiris AN, Sothmann MS, Hennes MI, Lee MB, Wilson CR, Gustafson AB, Kissebah AH. Relative contribution of obesity and body fat distribution to alterations in glucose insulin homeostasis: predictive values of selected indices in premenopausal women. Am J Clin Nutr 1989; 49: 758–764.

78. Després JP, Nadeau A, Tremblay A, Ferland M, Lupien PJ. Role of deep abdominal fat in the association between regional adipose tissue distribution and glucose tolerance in obese women. Diabetes 1989; 38:304–309.

79. Pouliot MC, Després JP, Nadeau A, Moorjani S, Prud'homme D, Lupien PJ, Tremblay A, Bouchard C. Visceral obesity in men. Associations with glucose tolerance, plasma insulin, and lipoprotein levels. Diabetes 1992; 41: 826–834.

80. Després JP. Visceral obesity, insulin resistance, and related dyslipoproteinemias. In: Rifkin H, Colwell JA, Taylor SI. eds. Diabetes 1991. Amsterdam: Elsevier Science Publ., 1991:95–99.

81. Lemieux S, Prud'homme D, Bouchard C, Tremblay A, Després JP. Sex differences in the relation of visceral adipose tissue accumulation to total body fatness. Am J Clin Nutr 1993; 58:463–467.

82. Lemieux S, Després JP, Moorjani S, Nadeau A, Thériault G, Prud'homme D, Tremblay A, Bouchard C, Lupien PJ. Are gender differences in cardiovascular disease risk factors explained by the level of visceral adipose tissue? Diabetologia 1994; 37:757–764.

83. Després JP, Lamarche B. Effects of diet and physical activity on adiposity and body fat distribution: implications for the prevention of cardiovascular disease. Nutr Res Rev 1993; 6:137–159.

84. Ferrannini E, Haffner SM, Mitchell BD, Stern MP. Hyperinsulinemia: the key feature of a cardiovascular and metabolic syndrome. Diabetologia 1991; 34:416–522.

85. Després JP. Abdominal obesity as an important component of insulin resistance syndrome. Nutrition 1993; 9: 452–459.

86. Björntorp P. "Portal" adipose tissue as a generator of risk factors for cardiovascular disease and diabetes. Arteriosclerosis 1990; 10:493–496.

87. Hennes M, Shrago E, Kissebah AH. Receptor and post receptor effects of FFA on hepatocyte insulin dynamics. Int J Obes 1990; 14:831.

88. Svedberg J, Björntorp P, Smith V, Lonnroth P. FFA inhibition of insulin binding, degradation, and action in isolated rat hepatocytes. Diabetes 1990; 39:570.

89. Randle PJ, Garland PB, Hales CN, Newsholme EA. The glucose fatty-acid cycle; its role in insulin sensitivity and the metabolic disturbances of diabetes mellitus. Lancet 1963; 1:785–789.

90. Taylor SI, Mukherjee C, Jungas RL. Regulation of pyruvate dehydrogenase in isolated rat liver mitochondria. J Biol Chem 1975; 250:2028–2035.

91. Felber JP. From obesity to diabetes. Pathophysiological considerations. Int J Obes 1972; 16:937–952.

92. Jahoor F, Klein S, Wolfe R. Mechanism of regulation of glucose production by lipolysis in humans. Am J Physiol 1992; 262(Endocrinol Metab 25):E353–E358.

93. Jackson RL, McLean LR, Demel RA. Mechanism of action of lipoprotein lipase and hepatic triglyceride lipase. Am Heart J 1987; 113:551–554.

94. Pollare T, Vessby B, Lithell H. Lipoprotein lipase activity in skeletal muscle is related to insulin sensitivity. Arterioscler Thrombo 1991; 11:1192.

95. Fujimoto WY, Leonetti DL, Newell-Morris L, Shuman WP, Wahl PW. Relationship of absence or presence of a family history of diabetes to body weight and body fat distribution in type 2 diabetes. Int J Obes 1990; 15:111–120.

96. Lemieux S, Després JP, Nadeau A, Prud'homme D, Tremblay A, Bouchard C. Heterogeneous glycaemic and insulinaemic responses to oral glucose in non-diabetic men: interactions between duration of obesity, body fat distribution and family history of diabetes mellitus. Diabetologia 1992; 35:653–659.

97. Peiris AN, Mueller RA, Struve MF, Smith GA, Kissebah AH. Relationship of androgenic activity to splanchnic insulin metabolism and peripheral glucose utilization in premenopausal women. J Clin Endocrinol Metab 64: 162–169.

98. Evans DJ, Hoffmann RG, Kalkhoff RK, Kissebah AH. Relationship of androgenic activity to body fat topography, fat cell morphology, and metabolic aberrations in premenopausal women. J Clin Endocrinol Metab 1983; 57: 304–310.

99 Kissebah AH, Evans DJ, Peiris A, Wilson CR. Endocrine characteristics in regional obesities: Role of sex steroids. In: Vague J, Björntorp P, Guy-Grand B, et al, eds. Metabolic Complications of Human Obesities. Amsterdam: Elsevier Science Publ, 1985:115–130.

100. Seidell JC, Björntorp P, Sjöström L, Kvist H, Sannerstedt R. Visceral fat accumulation is positively associated with insulin, glucose and C-peptide levels, but negatively with testosterone levels. Metabolism 1990; 39:897–901.

101. Tchernof A, Després JP, Bélanger A, Dupont A, Prud'homme D, Moorjani S, Lupien PJ, Labrie F. Reduced

102. Tchernof A, Després JP, Dupont A, Bélanger A, Nadeau A, Prud'homme D, Moorjani S, Lupien PJ, Labrie F. Importance of body fatness and adipose tissue distribution in the relation of steroid hormones to glucose tolerance and plasma insulin levels in men. Diabetes Care 1995; 18: 292–299.

103. Brindley DN, Rolland Y. Possible connections between stress, diabetes, obesity, hypertension, and altered metabolism that may result in atherosclerosis. Clin Sci 1989; 77:453–461.

104. Brindley DN. Metabolic approaches to atherosclerosis: effect of gliclazide. Metabolism 1992; 41(Suppl 1):20–24.

105. Brindley DN. Neuroendocrine regulation and obesity. Int J Obes 1992; 16:S73–S79.

106. Björntorp P. Visceral fat accumulation: the missing link between psychosocial factors and cardiovascular disease? J Intern Med 1991; 230:195–201.

107. Rebuffé-Scrive M, Lundholm K, Björntorp P. Glucocorticoid binding of human adipose tissue. Eur J Clin Invest 1985; 15:267–271.

108. Pedersen SB, Jonler M, Richelsen B. Characterization of regional and gender differences in glucocorticoid receptors and lipoprotein lipase activity in human adipose tissue. J Clin Endocrinol Metab 1994; 78:1354–1359.

109. Després JP, Moorjani S, Lupien PJ, Tremblay A, Nadeau A, Bouchard C. Genetic aspects of susceptibility to obesity and related dyslipidemias. Mol Cell Biochem 1992; 113: 151–169.

110. Pouliot MC, Després JP, Moorjani S, Lupien PJ, Tremblay A, Bouchard C. Apolipoprotein E polymorphism alters the association between body fatness and plasma lipoprotein in women. J Lipid Res 1990; 31:1023–1029.

111. Després JP, Verdon MF, Moorjani S, Pouliot MC, Nadeau A, Bouchard C, Tremblay A, Lupien PJ. Apolipoprotein E polymorphism modifies relation of hyperinsulinemia to hypertriglyceridemia. Diabetes 1993; 42:1474–1481.

112. Pouliot MC, Després JP, Dionne FT, Vohl MC, Moorjani S, Prud'homme D, Bouchard C, Lupien PJ. Apolipoprotein B-100 gene EcoRI polymorphism: relations to the plasma lipoprotein changes associated with abdominal visceral obesity. Arterioscler Thrombo 1994; 14:527–533.

113. Vohl MC, Lamarche B, Moorjani S, Prud'homme D, Nadeau A, Bouchard C, Lupien PJ, Després JP. The plasma lipoprotein lipase HindIII polymorphism modulates plasma triglyceride levels in visceral obesity. Arterioscler Thrombo Vasc Biol 1995; 15:714–720.

114. Seidell JC, Oosterlee A, Thijssen MAO, Burema J, Deurenberg P, Hautvast JGAJ, Ruijs JHJ. Assessment of intra-abdominal and subcutaneous abdominal fat: relation between anthropometry and computed tomography. Am J Clin Nutr 1987; 45:7–13.

115. Seidell JC, Oosterlee A, Deurenberg P, Hautvast JGAJ, Ruijs JHJ. Abdominal fat depots measured wth computed

tomography: effects of degree of obesity, sex and age. Eur J Clin Nutr 1988; 42:805–815.

116. Ferland M, Després JP, Tremblay A, Pinault S, Nadeau A, Moorjani S, Lupien PJ, Thériault G, Bouchard C. Assessment of adipose tissue distribution by computed axial tomography in obese women: Association with body density and anthropometric measurements. Br J Nutr 1989; 61:139–148.

117. Després JP, Prud'homme D, Pouliot MC, Tremblay A, Bouchard C. Estimation of deep abdominal fat accumulation from simple anthropometric measurements in men. Am J Clin Nutr 1991; 54:471–477.

118. Pouliot MC, Després JP, Lemieux S, Moorjani S, Bouchard C, Tremblay A, Nadeau A, Lupien PJ. Waist circumference and abdominal sagittal diameter: Best simple anthropometric indexes of abdominal visceral adipose tissue accumulation and related cardiovascular risk in men and women. Am J Cardiol 1994; 73:460–468.

119. Després JP. Lipoprotein metabolism in visceral obesity. Int J Obes 1991; 15:45–52.

120. Folsom AR, Kaye SA, Sellers TA, Hong CP, Cerhan JR, Potter JD, Prineas RJ. Body fat distribution and 5-year risk of death in older women. JAMA 1993; 269:483–487.

121. Stokes J III, Garrison RJ, Kannel WB. The independent contributions of various indices of obesity to the 22-year incidence of coronary heart disease: the Framingham Heart Study. In: Vague J, Björntorp P, Guy-Grand B, et al, eds. Metabolic Complications of Human Obesities. Amsterdam: Elsevier Science Publishers, 1985:49–57.

122. Terry RB, Page WF, Haskell WL. Waist/hip ratio, body mass index and premature cardiovascular disease mortality in US army veteran during a twenty-three year follow-up study. Int J Obes 1992; 16:417–23.

123. Sjöström L, Larsson B, Backman L, Bengtsson C, Bouchard C, Dahlgren S, et al. Swedish Obese Subjects (SOS). Recruitment for an intervention study and a selected description of the obese state. Int J Obes 1992; 16:465–479.

124. Després JP & Lamarche B. Low-intensity endurance exercise training, plasma lipoproteins and the risk of coronary heart disease. J Intern Med 1994; 236:7–22.

125. Bouchard C, Tremblay A, Després JP, Nadeau A, Lupien PJ, Thériault G, Dussault J, Moorjani S, Pinault S, Fournier G. The response to long-term overfeeding in identical twins. N Engl J Med 1990; 322:1477–1482.

126. Pérusse L, Després JP, Lemieux S, Rice T, Rao DC, Bouchard C. Familial aggregation of abdominal visceral fat level: results from the Québec Family Study. Metabolism 1996 (in press).

127. Leenen R, Van der Kooy K, Deurenberg P, Seidell JC, Weststrate JA, Schuten FJM, Hautvast JGAJ. Visceral fat accumulation in obese subjects: relation to energy expenditure and response to weight loss. Am J Physiol (Endocrinol Metab) 1992a; 263:E913–E919.

128. Goldstein DJ. Beneficial health effects of modest weight loss. Int J Obes 1992; 16:397–415.

129. Bouchard C, Després JP, Tremblay A. Exercise and obesity. Obes Res 1993; 1:40–54.

130. Wood PD, Stefanick ML, Dreon DM, Frey-Hewitt B, Garay SC, Williams PT, et al. Changes in plasma lipids and lipoproteins in overweight men during weight loss through dieting as compared with exercise. N Engl J Med 1988; 319:1173–1179.

131. Björntorp P, De Jounge K, Sjöström L, Sullivan L. The effect of physical training on insulin production in obesity. Metabolism 1970; 19:631–638.

132. American College of Sports Medicine. Position stand on The recommended quantity and quality of exercise for developing and maintaining cardiorespiratory and muscular fitness in healthy adults. Med Sci Sports Exerc 1990; 22:265–274.

133. Després JP, Pouliot MC, Moorjani S, Nadeau A, Tremblay A, Lupien PJ, Thériault G, Bouchard C. Loss of abdominal fat and metabolic response to exercise training in obese women. Am J Physiol (Endocrinol Metab) 1991; 261: E159–E167.

134. Nye ER, Carlson K, Kirstein P, Rossner S. Changes in high density lipoprotein subfractions and other lipoproteins induced by exercise. Clin Chim Acta 1981; 113:51–57.

135. Lamarche B, Després JP, Pouliot MC, Moorjani S, Lupien PJ, Thériault G, Tremblay A, Nadeau A, Bouchard C. Is body fat loss a determinant factor in the improvement of carbohydrate and lipid metabolism following aerobic exercise training in obese women? Metabolism 1992; 41: 1249–1256.

136. Lampman RM, Santiga JT, Savage PJ, Bassett DR, Hydrick CR, Flora JD, Block WD. Effect of exercise training on glucose tolerance, insulin sensitivity, lipid and lipoprotein concentration in middle-aged men with mild hypertriglyceridemia. Metabolism 1985; 34:205–211.

137. Raz I, Rozenbilt H, Kark JP. Effect of moderate exercise on serum lipids in young men with low high density lipoprotein cholesterol levels. Arteriosclerosis 1988; 8: 245–251.

138. Raz I, Israeli A, Rozenbilt H, Bar-On H. Influence of moderate exercise on glucose homeostasis and serum testosterone in young men with low HDL-cholesterol levels. Diabetes Res 1988; 9:31–35.

139. Després JP. Obesity, regional adipose tissue distribution and metabolism: effect of exercise. In: Romsos DR, Himms-Hagen J, Suzuki M, eds. Obesity: Dietary Factors and Control. Tokyo: Japan Scientific Societies, 1991: 251–259.

140. Krotkiewski M, Björntorp P. Muscle tissue in obesity with different distribution of adipose tissue: effects of physical training. Int J Obes 1986; 10:331–341.

141. Oshida Y, Yamamouchi K, Hayamizy S, Saton Y. Long-term mild jogging increases insulin action despite no influence on body mass index or Vo_2max. J Appl Physiol 1989; 66:2206–2210.

142. Williams PT, Krauss RM, Vranizan KM, Wood PD. Changes in lipoprotein subfractions during diet-induced

and exercise-induced weight loss in moderately over-weight men. Circulation 1990; 81:1293–1304.

143. Bray GA. Use and abuse of appetite-suppressant drugs in the treatment of obesity. Ann Intern Med 1992; 119: 707–713.

144. Levine LR, Rosenblatt S, Bosomworth J. Use of serotonin reuptake inhibitor, fluoxetine, in the treatment of obesity. Int J Obes 1987; 11:185–190.

145. Greenway FL, Bray GA. Human chorionic gonadotrophin (HCG) in the treatment of obesity—a critical assessment of the Simeons method. West J Med 1977; 127:461–463.

146. Guy-Grand B, Apfelbaum M, Crepaldi G, Gries A, Lefeb-vre P, Turner P. International trial of long-term dexfen-fluramine in obesity. Lancet 1989; 2:1142–1144.

147. Després JP, Lemieux S, Lamarche B. Prud'homme D, Moorjani S, Brun LD, Gagné C, Lupien PJ. The insulin-resistance syndrome: contribution of visceral obesity and therapeutic implications. Int J Obes 1995; 19(Supp): S76–S86.

31

Obesity and Blood Pressure Regulation

Albert P. Rocchini
Children's Memorial Hospital and Northwestern University, Chicago, Illinois

I. INTRODUCTION

One of the major public health implications of obesity is that it is an independent risk factor for the development of both hypertension and cardiovascular disease. This chapter summarizes techniques for measuring blood pressure in obese individuals and the effect of obesity on these measurements; the evidence that substantiates that obesity is an independent risk factor for the development of hypertension; an explanation of how obesity may result in the development of hypertension; a brief summary of other cardiovascular abnormalities associated with obesity; and finally, how to manage the hypertensive obese individual.

II. MEASUREMENT OF BLOOD PRESSURE IN OBESE INDIVIDUALS

For years, some physicians believed that the high blood pressure observed in many obese individuals was an artifact related to use of indirect methods for measuring blood pressure. The indirect method of measuring blood pressure usually results in an overestimation of both systolic and diastolic blood pressure. The overestimation of blood pressure is due, in part to, the fact that pressure measured by the cuff and sphygmomanometer is not just the force required to occlude the brachial artery, but also includes the force required to compress the soft tissues of the arm. In the case of obesity, the increased subcutaneous fat in the upper arm imposes a greater resistance to com-

pression and therefore a higher cuff inflation pressure. Most of the effects of obesity on the indirect measurement of blood pressure can be corrected by using an appropriate-size blood pressure cuff. Compared with intra-arterial measurements of blood pressure, the indirect method is less precise; nevertheless, when properly measured, elevated indirect blood pressure readings are a reliable method for diagnosing hypertension. The major determinants of errors in blood pressure measurement include cuff size, type of instrumentation for measuring blood pressure, and observer errors.

A. Cuff Size

The selection of an appropriate-size compression cuff is critical to obtaining an accurate reading. The cuff consists of an inflatable bladder with a cloth cover. The dimensions of the inner bladder, not the size of the cover, determine cuff size (Fig. 1). The bladder must be the correct width for the circumference at the midpoint of the upper arm. (Table 1) A bladder that is too small will give a falsely high pressure. The bladder should be wide enough to cover approximately 75% of the upper arm between the top of the shoulder and the olecranon. The length of the bladder also influences the accuracy of measurements. A bladder length that is roughly twice the width is ideal and should result in the cuff nearly encircling the arm. If a question arises as to which of two cuffs is appropriate, a cuff that is slightly wider and longer than needed should be chosen. It is unlikely that slightly too large a cuff will

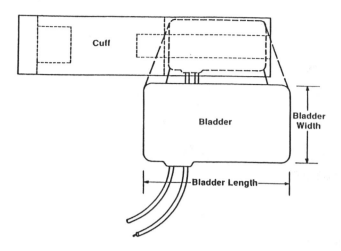

Figure 1 Schematic representation of a blood pressure cuff.

mask hypertension, but a cuff that is too small will lead to an overestimate of blood pressure.

B. Types of Equipment for Indirect Measurement of Blood Pressure

Physicians have taken reliable blood pressure measurements for nearly 90 years with a compression cuff, sphygmomanometer, and stethoscope. The major errors associated with use of the sphygmomanometer and stethoscope relate to calibration of the manometer, position of the arm (if the arm is below "heart level," due to hydrostatic pressure, a falsely elevated blood pressure will be recorded), and the experience and training of the observer.

To eliminate observer errors, automated blood pressure devices were developed. Most of these devices use the oscillometric technique, which involves analysis of arterial

Table 1 Recommended Bladder Dimensions for Blood Pressure Cuffs

Circumference of arm at midpoint[a] (cm)	Name of cuff	Bladder width (cm)	Bladder length (cm)
13–20	Child	8	13
17–26	Small adult	11	17
24–32	Adult	13	24
32–42	Large adult	17	32
42–50	Thigh	20	42

[a]Midpoint of arm is defined as half the distance from the acromion to the olecranon.

"flutter," the lower frequency oscillations that occur, with each heartbeat, under an occluding cuff between the systolic and diastolic pressures. A sensitive transducer attached to the cuff detects the flutter by selectively amplifying the oscillations and rejecting most artifacts. In general, these devices more reliably predict systolic than diastolic blood pressure.

C. Observer Errors

An observer may record the blood pressure inaccurately because of hearing impairment, inattention, carelessness, or subconscious bias. An example of such bias is "digit preference," a well-documented phenomenon resulting in recording pressures ending with zero or five (i.e., 120 or 125 systolic or 80 or 85 diastolic) more often than expected by chance. The observer should be taught that systolic pressure is the point at which initial Korotkoff sounds are audible for two consecutive heartbeats (phase I). Diastolic blood pressure should be measured at the pressure at which Korotkoff sounds disappear (phase V). With appropriate training, observer errors can be greatly reduced.

D. Summary

Although the indirect method of blood pressure measurement may be imprecise in the obese individual, if appropriate care is taken to use a trained observer, a large enough blood pressure cuff, and a calibrated measurement device reliable measurements of blood pressure can be made even in extremely obese individuals.

III. RELATIONSHIP BETWEEN OBESITY AND HIGH BLOOD PRESSURE

A. Epidemiological Studies Linking Obesity to Hypertension

The association between obesity and hypertension has been recognized since the early 1900s. Several large epidemiological studies documented the association between increasing body weight and an increase in blood pressure (1–12). Symonds (3) analyzed 150,419 policyholders in the Mutual Life Insurance Corporation and documented that systolic and diastolic blood pressure increased with both age and weight. In 1925, the Actuarial Society of America also documented a similar relationship in over 500,000 men (1). The Framingham Study (4) documented that the prevalence of hypertension in obese individuals was twice that of those individuals who were normal weight. This relationship held in all age groups of both women and men. In the National Heart Association of Australia Risk Factor Prevalence Study (12), body mass index was independently associated with blood pressure level in both men and women. In that study, obesity was felt be the cause of the hypertension in over 30% of the individuals. In a study of 1 million North American subjects, Stamler et al. (2) found that the odds of hypertension were significantly increased in obese compared to nonobese individuals (comparing obese with nonobese subjects the odds ratio for hypertension was 2.42:1 in subjects aged 20–39 years and 1.54:1 in subjects aged 40–64 years). Thus, a large number of population-based studies have documented a strong association between obesity and hypertension in both sexes, in all age groups, and for virtually every geographic and ethnic group.

B. Relationship of Weight Gain to Blood Pressure Level

There have been no studies in humans that have looked at the effect of weight gain on blood pressure. However, in the dog, it has been shown that weight gain is directly related to an increase in blood pressure. Cash and Wood in 1938 (13) demonstrated that weight gain caused dogs with renal vascular hypertension to further increase their blood pressure. More recently, Rocchini et al. (14,15) found that normal mongrel dogs fed a high-fat diet gained weight and developed hypertension (Fig. 2). In these dogs the hypertension was associated with sodium retention, hyperinsulinemia, and activation of the sympathetic nervous system. Hall et al. (16) have also observed that weight gain in the dog is directly associated with an increase in arterial blood pressure. Thus, in the dog, weight gain is directly associated with an increase in arterial pressure.

C. Effect of Weight Loss on Blood Pressure Level

Weight loss is associated with a lowering of blood pressure. Haynes (17) reviewed the literature up to the mid-1980s on the relationship of weight loss to reductions in arterial pressure. He used strict criteria to examine only well-conducted studies and noted that only six studies were available. Three of the six studies that met Haynes criteria demonstrated a clear effect of weight loss on lowering arterial pressure. Overall, many clinical trials that have been published since the late 1970s have clearly documented the blood-pressure-lowering effect of weight loss (17–31). However, one of the controversial aspects of these studies is whether the weight loss alone, independent of alterations in dietary sodium, was responsible for the observed reductions in blood pressure. Dahl et al. (27)

concluded that the reduced salt intake inherent in hypocaloric diets, rather than weight loss, is responsible for the lowering of blood pressure. Similarly, Fagerberg et al. (21) noted no decrease in blood pressure in individuals after weight loss using a 1230-calorie, unrestricted-sodium diet; however, in another group of individuals, similar caloric restriction combined with a low-sodium diet resulted in a significant blood pressure reduction. Reisen et al. (25) reported that hypertensive individuals placed on diets designed to cause weight loss, but without sodium restriction, resulted in a substantial reduction in blood pressure. Tuck et al. (28) reported that weight loss decreased blood pressure in individuals who received either a 40 mmol/day sodium diet or a 120 mmol/day sodium diet. Maxwell et al. (22) reported that in obese subjects, weight loss resulted in the same blood pressure reduction whether sodium intake was restricted to 40 mmol/day of sodium or maintained at 20 mmol/day. Gillum and co-workers (23) found that weight loss without significantly altered sodium intake resulted in blood pressure decreases. Rocchini et al. (29) demonstrated that prior to weight loss, the blood pressure of a group of obese adolescents was very sensitive to dietary sodium intake; however, after weight loss, the obese adolescents lost their blood pressure sensitivity to sodium. Finally, several large clinical trials have also documented that weight loss independent of sodium restriction results in blood pressure lowering. The Hypertension Prevention Trial (19) documented that in individuals with borderline elevations in blood pressure, a mean weight loss of 5 kg was associated with as much as 5/3 mm decrease in blood pressure. The TAIM study (18) also found a significant blood-pressure-lowering effect of weight loss.

A limitation with the use of studies documenting that weight loss is associated with a reduction in blood pressure is that most studies do not address the long-term effect of weight change on blood pressure in subjects who are again placed on unrestricted diets. Dornfield and co-workers (30) have clearly documented that the long-term changes in blood pressure correlate with changes in body weight. In obese subjects whose blood pressure fell during a very-low-calorie, protein-supplemented fast, when weight loss stopped and body weight was maintained for 1 month, blood pressure did not increase. In compliant patients who regained less than 15 lb, 6 months after discontinuation of the very-low-calorie, protein-supplemented fast by blood pressure increased minimally. Similarly, in another group of individuals, who were studied 21 months after being on unrestricted calorie and sodium intake but at a different body weight, Dornfield and associates also documented that differences in blood pressure correlated with differences in body weight. Reisen

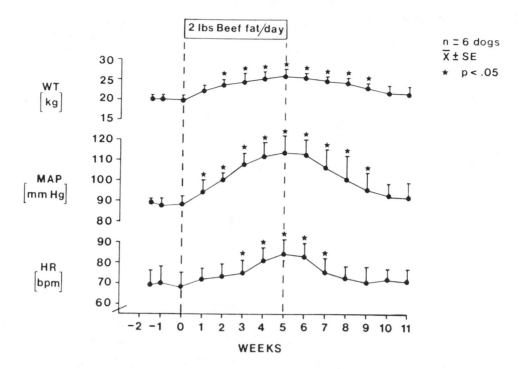

Figure 2   Weight, mean arterial pressure and heart rate of six dogs fed a high-fat diet. With weight gain there is a significant increase in heart rate and blood pressure and this is reversed with weight loss. Adapted from Rocchini AP, Moorehead C, Wentz E, Reremer S. Obesity-induced hypertension in the dog. (Adapted from Ref. 14.)

and Frohlich (31) also reported that blood pressure remained reduced in individual who maintained weight loss for 12–18 months. Finally, Davis et al. (20) reported that weight loss is an effective long-term therapy for maintaining blood pressure in the normal range when it is used as monotherapy or in combination with either thiazide diuretics or β-blockers. Thus, based on all of these weight loss studies, calorie restriction and weight loss are associated with a reduction in blood pressure. In addition, it is clear that even modest weight loss (i.e., 10% of body weight) improves blood pressure, and many individuals achieve normal blood pressure levels without attaining their calculated ideal weight.

D.   Effect of Body Fat Distribution on Blood Pressure

The definition of obesity also contributes to the controversy regarding the independence of obesity as an etiological determinant of hypertension. Obesity is defined not just as an increase in body weight, but rather as an increase in adipose tissue mass. Adipose tissue mass can be estimated by multiple techniques such as: skinfold thickness, body mass index [(weight in kg)/(height in meters)^2], hydrostatic weighing, bioelectrical impedance, and water dilution methods. In most clinical studies, body mass index is usually used as the index of adiposity. Obesity is generally defined as a body mass index of greater than 27 kg/m^2. In 1956, Jean Vague (32) reported that the cardiovascular and metabolic consequences of obesity were greatest in individuals whose fat distribution pattern favored the upper body segments. Since that observation, several population-based studies have demonstrated that upper body obesity is a more important cardiovascular risk factor than body mass index alone (33–39). The Normative Aging Study (33) has demonstrated that there is a significant relationship between abdominal circumference and diastolic blood pressure. In fact, the risk of developing hypertension was better predicted by upper body fat distribution than by either body weight or body mass index (Fig. 3). In the Bogalusa Heart Study (34), blood pressure correlated strongly with upper body fat pattern, but not with measures of global obesity. Therefore, since most published studies investigating the role of obesity in hypertension have used total body weight or body mass index, the true role of adiposity in blood pressure regulation may have been obscured.

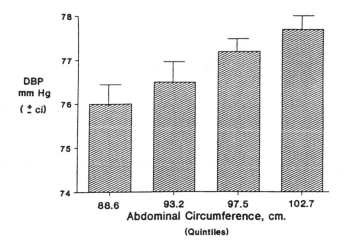

Figure 3 Relationship between diastolic blood pressure (DBP) and abdominal circumference by quintile. With increasing abdominal girth, DBP increases. DBP is shown with 95% confidence intervals for 1,972 subjects in Normative Aging Study. (Adapted from Ref. 33.)

E. Prevalence of Hypertension in Different Obese Populations

The final proof that obesity is an independent risk factor for hypertension, rather than a chance coexistence of two common clinical disorders, is that the prevalence of hypertension in obese individuals is much higher than in the general population. This increased prevalence of hypertension in obese individuals is even observed in populations with both a high (black Americans) (2) and low (Mexican Americans) (40) incidence of hypertension.

IV. MECHANISM WHEREBY OBESITY MIGHT CAUSE HYPERTENSION

The exact mechanism whereby obesity causes hypertension is still unknown. For years it has been recognized that hypertension is common in both obese and diabetic individuals. Glucose intolerance, independent of obesity, is also associated with hypertension (41). Analysis of data from the San Antonio Heart Study has demonstrated an impressive pattern of overlap among hypertension, diabetes, and obesity. It has been estimated that by the fifth decade of life 85% of diabetic individuals are hypertensive and obese, 80% of obese subjects have abnormal glucose tolerance and are hypertensive, and 67% of hypertensive subjects are both diabetic and obese (7,40). In 1985, Modan et al. (41) demonstrated in a large epidemiological study that a strong association exists between obesity, glu-

cose intolerance, and hypertension. A number of studies in both obese and nonobese humans demonstrate a strong relationship between insulin resistance and blood pressure (7,41–52). The relationship between insulin resistance and blood pressure has been observed in most populations (49–52). Preliminary results from the Insulin Resistance Atherosclerosis Study (53,54) suggest that after multivariate analysis, insulin resistance and body mass index, but not insulin level, predict hypertension. Therefore, insulin resistance has been suggested by many investigators to be the metabolic link that connects obesity to hypertension.

In support of the hypothesis that hyperinsulinemia may be causally linked to obesity hypertension, it has been demonstrated that in hypertensive obese subjects a 10-hr infusion of somatostatin, a hormone that suppresses pancreatic insulin release, causes a reduction in both plasma insulin and arterial pressure (55). Somatostatin has also been demonstrated to improve the hyperinsulinemia, hypertension, and dyslipemia associated with fructose-induced hypertension in the rat (56).

Factors known to improve insulin resistance are also associated with reductions in blood pressure. Weight loss has been documented to be associated with both a decrease in blood pressure and an improvement in insulin sensitivity (43,44). The decline in blood pressure associated with exercise training programs seems to be limited to individuals who are initially hyperinsulinemic and have the greatest fall in plasma insulin level as a result of the training program (44,57).

In addition to human data linking insulin and blood pressure, there are also animal data that suggest that insulin is an important regulator of blood pressure. Rocchini et al. (14,15) demonstrated that the weight gain associated with feeding dogs cooked beef fat is directly associated with an increase in blood pressure and insulin. Reaven and co-workers (58–61) demonstrated that normal Sprague-Dawley rats fed a fructose-enriched diet develop insulin resistance and hypertension. They have shown that the hypertension can be eliminated or attenuated by correcting the insulin resistance either with exercise training or by the administration of somatostatin. Kurtz et al. (62) have shown that the genetically obese, insulin-resistant Zucker rat has increased blood pressure compared to the genetically lean, non-insulin-resistant Zucker rat or Lewis rat. Several investigators have demonstrated that insulin resistance and hyperinsulinemia are also seen in spontaneously hypertensive rats (63–65). In addition, insulin-stimulated glucose uptake is lower in adipocytes isolated from these animals (64). Finally, Frands et al. (66) and Meehan et al. (67) have demonstrated that infusion of insulin into normal rats results in the development of hypertension. In both studies, a rise in arterial pressure occurred within 2 days of starting the insulin infusion.

Finally, there is evidence that in normal-weight individuals, hyperinsulinemia and insulin resistance precede the development of hypertension. Young black males with borderline high blood pressure have been reported to have higher insulin levels and more insulin resistance than normotensive black men (49,50). In the Tecumseh Study (68), individuals with borderline hypertension have higher plasma insulin levels and greater weight than normotensive individuals. Normotensive children with a family history of hypertension have higher insulin levels and more insulin resistance than children with no family history of hypertension (69).

However, in contrast to these and other reports (7,41–52) linking hyperinsulinemia to hypertension, there have been other studies that have been unable to establish a relationship between hyperinsulinemia and high blood pressure. There is at least one study of a group of hypertensive obese individuals (71) that did not find a correlation between hyperinsulinemia and hypertension. In normal dogs, a chronic infusion of insulin, with or without an infusion of norepinephrine, failed to increase blood pressure (21). In addition, even in those reports that have documented a relationship between insulin and blood pressure there is significant overlap in insulin resistance between those individuals who are hypertensive and those who are normotensive. For example, Pollare and coworkers (43) demonstrated a significant linear relationship between insulin resistance, measured during a euglycemic insulin clamp study, and blood pressure in a group of 143 hypertensive and 51 normotensive subjects; however, approximately 50% of the hypertensive subjects had insulin-mediated glucose uptake values that were within one standard deviation of the normotensive group (that is, at least one-half of the hypertensive subject were not insulin-resistant). No correlation has been found between blood pressure and plasma insulin or insulin sensitivity in Pima Indians (72) or obese Mexican American women (40). Thus, from all of these studies it is clear that not all hypertensive subjects are insulin-resistant and not all insulin-resistant subjects are hypertensive.

Based on available data in the literature, it appears that selective insulin resistance, not just hyperinsulinemia, is probably the metabolic link that is responsible for the observed epidemiological relationship between obesity and hypertension. The term "selective insulin resistance" implies that although an individual or animal may have an impaired ability of insulin to cause whole-body glucose uptake, some of the other physiological actions of insulin may be preserved. With respect to hypertension, one of the potentially important actions of insulin is the ability

to induce renal sodium retention. Obese adolescents have selective insulin resistance in that they are resistant with respect to insulin's ability to stimulate glucose uptake yet are still sensitive to the renal sodium-retaining effects of insulin (73) (Fig. 4). The spontaneously hypertensive rat has also been documented to have impaired insulin-mediated, whole-rat glucose uptake, yet normal insulin sensitivity to induce renal sodium retention (65). In non-obese essential hypertensives, insulin resistance has been demonstrated to involve glucose metabolism but not lipid or potassium metabolism and is limited to the nonoxidative pathways of intracellular glucose disposal (42,74).

Thus there is evidence that in obese hypertensive subjects, insulin resistance is *selective* (mostly involving glucose metabolism), *tissue specific* (predominantly effecting skeletal muscle), and *pathway specific* (insofar as only gly-

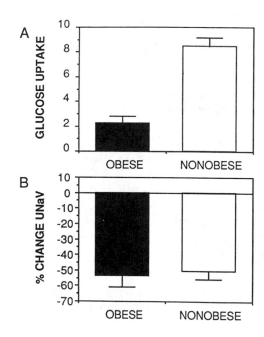

Figure 4   (A) Change in glucose uptake (M) (mg/kg/min) during euglycemic hyperinsulinemia in seven obese and five nonobese subjects. Compared to the nonobese individuals, a 40 mU/m²/min infusion of insulin resulted in a significant depression in whole-body glucose uptake in the obese subjects ($p <$ 0.001). The plasma insulin response to the insulin infusion was not significantly different between obese and nonobese subjects. (B) Percent change in urinary sodium excretion (% change UNaV) that occurred in the same seven obese and five nonobese subjects during water diuresis and euglycemic hyperinsulinemia. Insulin infusion resulted in a significant (~50%) decrease in urinary sodium excretion in both the obese and nonobese subjects. No significant difference in the response of urinary sodium excretion to hyperinsulinemia was observed between the two groups. (Adapted from Ref. 73.)

cogen synthesis is usually affected). Therefore, in any individual or animal the degree to which insulin resistance is tissue and/or pathway specific may determine whether or not hypertension will develop.

Selective insulin resistance may modulate the development of hypertension through the following physiological and tissue-specific sequence: enhanced renal sodium retention, changes in vascular structure and function, alterations in cation fux, activation of the renin-angiotensin aldosterone system, and activation of the sympathetic nervous system.

A. Enhanced Sodium Retention

Human and animal data suggests that insulin resistance and/or hyperinsulinemia can result in chronic sodium retention. Insulin can enhance renal sodium retention both directly, through its effects on renal tubules (73,75,76), and indirectly, through stimulation of the sympathetic nervous system and augmenting angiotensin II–mediated aldosterone secretion (77,78). There also are data to suggest that insulin resistance is directly related to sodium sensitivity in both obese and nonobese subjects. Rocchini et al. (29) have also shown in obese adolescents that insulin resistance and sodium sensitivity of blood pressure are directly related. They demonstrated that the blood pressure of obese adolescents is more dependent on dietary sodium intake than the blood pressure of nonobese adolescents and that hyperinsulinemia and increased sympathetic nervous system activity appear to be responsible for the observed sodium sensitivity and hypertension. In addition, in comparison with nonobese adolescents, the obese adolescents have a renal-function relation (plot of urinary sodium excretion as a function of arterial pressure) that has a shallower slope. The renal-function relationship is also normalized by weight loss (Fig. 5). The relationship between urinary sodium excretion and mean arterial pressure can be altered by intrinsic and extrinsic factors that are known to affect the ability of the kidney to excrete sodium. Some of the factors that produce alterations in the renal-function curves are constriction of the renal arteries and arterioles, changes in glomerular filtration coefficients, changes in the rate of tubular reabsorption, reduced renal mass, and changing levels of renin-angiotensin activation, aldosterone, vasopressin, insulin, sympathetic nervous system activation, and atrial natriuretic hormone. Finta et al. (79) demonstrated that the endogenous hyperinsulinemia that occurs in obese subjects following a glucose meal can result in urinary sodium retention. In that study, the investigators also demonstrated that the obese adolescents who were the most sodium sensitive had significantly higher fasting insulin concentrations, higher glucose-stimulated insulin levels, and greater urine sodium retention in response to the oral glucose load. Finally, in nonobese subjects with (80) or without (81) essential hypertension there is a direct relationship between sodium sensitivity and insulin resistance.

There are also animal data that suggest that insulin resistance may be responsible in part for the sodium retention associated with obesity hypertension. In a dog model of obesity-induced hypertension, Rocchini et al. (14,15) have demonstrated that during the first week of the high-fat diet, the increase in sodium retention appeared to best relate to an increase in plasma norepinephrine activity, whereas during the latter weeks of the high-fat diet, an increase in plasma insulin appeared to be the best predictor of sodium retention. Finally, Rocchini demonstrated that the hypertension associated with weight gain in the dog occurs only if adequate salt is present in the diet (80). Thus in both obese human and dog, insulin appears to play an important role in sodium retention.

B. Alterations in Vascular Structure and Function

The second method by which selective insulin resistance could cause hypertension is through alterations in vascular structure and function. Insulin and insulin-like growth factors are mitogens capable of stimulating smooth muscle proliferation (82). Hyperinsulinemia could result, therefore, in vascular smooth muscle hypertrophy, narrowing of the lumen of resistance vessels, and ultimately the development of hypertension (83). Vascular abnormalities are also known to exist in obese individuals. In normal, nonobese volunteers, insulin induces peripheral arterial vasodilation (85). In obese adolescents, Rocchini et al. (84) demonstrated that ischemic exercise results in a decreased maximum forearm blood flow and an increased minimum vascular resistance. These investigators demonstrated that the abnormal vascular responses to ischemic exercise directly correlate with fasting insulin and whole-body glucose uptake, and that the vascular and metabolic abnormalities improve with weight loss.

In addition to insulin resistance possibly being associated with the development of vascular changes, there are also data that suggest that abnormalities in skeletal muscle vascular regulation may be a cause of insulin resistance. In both the dog (71) and human (85) euglycemic hyperinsulinemia has been documented to result in vasodilation, not vasoconstriction. Even though the exact mechanism of how insulin induces vasodilation in non-insulin-resistant individuals is unknown, some investigators believe that this vasodilator response is, in part, due to stimulation of endothelial-dependent relaxing factor

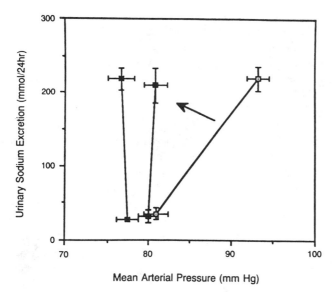

Figure 5 Renal-function relationship for 18 nonobese (X) and 60 obese adolescents before a weight loss program (□) and 36 obese adolescents who lost weight during a 20-week weight loss program (■). In comparison with the nonobese adolescents' renal-function relation, the obese adolescents' renal-function relation has a shallow slope ($p < 0.001$). In those who lost weight, the slope increased (arrow). This increase was due to a decrease in the mean arterial pressure during the 2 weeks of the high-salt diet. (From Ref. 29.)

(86,87). Type II, but not type I, diabetic subjects respond abnormally to acetylcholine, which induces vasodilation by stimulation of endothelial-dependent relaxing factor (88).

Insulin-mediated glucose uptake is determined both by insulin's ability to stimulate glucose extraction at the level of tissues/cells and by the rate of glucose and insulin delivery (blood flow). Thus, the relative contributions of tissue and blood flow actions of insulin will determine the overall rate of glucose uptake (i.e., degree of insulin resistance). In obese individuals with insulin resistance, an attenuated limb vasodilator response to hyperinsulinemia has been reported (89,90) (Fig. 6). Insulin's inability to produce vasodilation has led Baron et al. (91) to speculate that abnormalities of skeletal muscle vascular regulation may be a cause, not a result, of insulin resistance. This hypothesis is also supported by the fact that antihypertensive drugs that are vasodilators (i.e., captopril, calcium channel blockers, and prazosin) tend to improve insulin resistance, whereas other antihypertensive drugs, such as diuretic or beta blockers, do not (92–94).

Skeletal muscle characteristics are altered in obesity (95–98) and hypertension (99–102) and these alterations

may be involved in the etiology of these two diseases. Human muscle has three categories of fiber: type I, IIa, and IIb (103). Type I fibers have high aerobic capabilities and increased capillarization. Type II fibers tend to be better suited for anaerobic metabolism. Type IIa fibers have the same capillary supply as type I fibers, whereas type IIb fibers have a reduced capillary supply. Lithel et al. (96) reported that muscle fiber diameter and capillary density

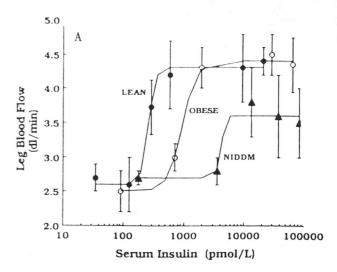

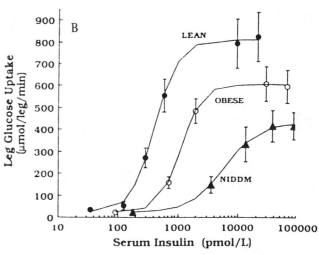

Figure 6 Rates of leg blood flow (A) and of leg glucose uptake (B) determined during euglycemic clamp studies over a wide range of steady-state serum insulin concentrations in lean (●) and obese nondiabetic subjects (○) and patients with non-insulin-dependent diabetes mellitus (NIDDM; ▲). The log scale is shown on the abscissa. To convert the insulin concentrations from pmol/L divide by 7.175. (Adapted from Laakso M, Edelman SV, Brechtel G, Baron AD. Impaired insulin-mediated skeletal muscle blood flow in patients with NIDDM. Diabetes 1992; 41:1076–1083.)

correlate with fasting insulin levels. These investigators also demonstrated that obese men have an increased fiber diameter with no increase in the number of capillaries per fiber (i.e., a reduced capillary density). Lillioja et al. (95) reported similar results in a group of Pima Indians. Wage et al. (98) and Staron et al. (97) reported a significant inverse correlation between the presence of type I fibers and body fatness. However, Simoneau and Bouchard (104) found no relationship between percent body fat and the percentage of type I fibers in a group of 126 women and 213 men. The only significant correlation between body fatness and fiber type observed in this study was that obese men appeared to have an increased percentage of type IIb fibers with low aerobic enzyme activities. Krotkiewski and Bjorntrop (105) observed that upper body obesity, increased waist-to-hip ratio, was associated with an increased percentage of type II fibers. Based on these observations, it has been speculated that the hypertension and insulin resistance observed in some obese individuals, especially those with upper body obesity, may be due to the high percentage of type IIb muscle fibers that have low capillary density and reduced aerobic enzyme activities. In support of this theory is the observation that endurance training in obese and nonobese individuals improves insulin resistance by increasing muscle oxidative capacity and increasing capillary density (106,107).

C. Alterations in Ion Transport

The third method by which insulin resistance could cause hypertension is through alterations in cation transport. Insulin has been shown to affect sodium and calcium transport, although controversy still exists regarding the molecular mechanism of this effect. A direct effect of insulin on sodium/hydrogen exchange has been demonstrated in vitro (108). Insulin has been reported to both increase and decrease Na, K-ATPase activity (109). Insulin has been linked to both Na-Li countertransport and Na-K cotransport (109). In a study of leukocyte sodium content and sodium pump activity in overweight and lean hypertensive subjects, it was observed that overweight hypertensive subjects accumulated intracellular sodium probably through abnormalities of sodium pump activity (110). In obese hypertensive men, the renin-angiotensin system and sympathetic nervous system activity are reported to influence the regulation of erythrocyte sodium turnover during sodium and energy restriction (111). Thus alteration in intracellular sodium concentration could lead to an increased intracellular calcium, an increase in vascular smooth muscle tone, and hypertension. Insulin alone has also been demonstrated to elevate cytosolic free calcium levels in adipocytes of normal subjects (112). In addition,

weight loss in obese individuals is reported to be accompanied by a significant decrease in platelet free calcium levels (113).

Insulin-mediated glucose transport is dependent on an intracellular calcium concentration of between 40 and 375 nm/L (114). Thus, increased intracellular calcium concentration might lead to insulin resistance, increased vascular resistance, and hypertension (44). In hypertensive type II diabetics a decrease in calcium adenosine triphosphate activity is associated with increased intracellular calcium concentration (115). Insulin has also been shown to stimulate plasma membrane calcium adenosine triphosphate activity (88) and sodium-potassium adenosine triphosphate activity (109). Insulin resistance may blunt these pump functions and could lead to chronic increases in intracellular calcium, increased peripheral vascular resistance, and hypertension. Finally, reduced intracellular levels of magnesium are also associated with increased vascular resistance and insulin resistance (116). Therefore, alterations in either intracellular calcium and/or magnesium could result in the development of both hypertension and insulin resistance.

D. Stimulation of the Renin-Angiotensin-Aldosterone System

The fourth method by which selective insulin resistance could cause hypertension is through insulin's ability to stimulate the renin-angiotensin-aldosterone system. Enhanced activity of the renin-angiotensin system has been reported in obese humans and dogs (28,78,117–122). Tuck et al. (28) demonstrated, in obese hypertensives, that with weight loss plasma renin activity decreases and that the decrease in plasma renin activity was statistically correlated with the weight loss–associated decrease in mean arterial pressure. Granger and co-workers (122) reported that plasma renin activity is 170% higher in obese dogs than in control dogs.

Obesity is also associated with abnormalities in the angiotensin-aldosterone system. In the dog, Rocchini et al. (14,15) demonstrated that the increase in blood pressure associated with weight gain is directly related to sodium retention and that this sodium retention is in part accompanied by an increase in plasma norepinephrine, insulin, and aldosterone concentrations. Tuck and associates (28) demonstrated in obese adults that weight loss lowered both plasma renin activity and aldosterone concentration. Hiramatsu et al. (118) documented in obese hypertensives that with increasing body weight, there is a progressive increase in the ratio of plasma aldosterone to plasma renin activity. Scavo et al. (119,120) reported that although obese adults have a normal plasma renin activity, they have an increased plasma aldosterone concentration and an increased aldosterone secretion rate. Spark and co-workers (121) reported, in obese patients, that during the early stages of fasting there is a dissociation between plasma renin activity and aldosterone. To determine the role of aldosterone in the regulation of blood pressure in obese adolescents, Rocchini et al. (117) measured supine and 2-hr upright plasma renin activity and aldosterone in 10 nonobese and 30 obese adolescents before and after a 20-week weight loss program. The obese adolescents had significantly higher supine and 2-hr upright aldosterone concentrations. Although plasma renin activity was not significantly different between the two groups of adolescents, these authors observed that a given increment in plasma renin activity produced a greater increment in aldosterone in the obese adolescents (Fig. 7). Compared with an obese control group, weight loss resulted in a significant decrease in plasma aldosterone. After weight loss there was also a significant decrease in the slope of the posture-induced relationship between plasma renin activity and aldosterone. In addition, after weight loss there was a significant correlation between the change in plasma aldosterone and the change in mean blood pressure. The authors speculated that increased plasma aldosterone concentration in some obese subjects is caused by increased adrenal sensitivity to angiotensin II.

Insulin has been shown to influence the renin-angiotensin-aldosterone system in normal subjects (77,123) and patients with diabetes (124). Since hyperinsulinemia is a characteristic feature of obesity, Rocchini et al. (78) hypothesize that increased aldosterone levels observed in obese individuals are caused by hyperinsulinemia and insulin's ability to augment angiotensin II–mediated aldosterone production. To determine whether hyperinsulinemia alters angiotensin II–mediated aldosterone secretion, Rocchini et al. (78) measured the increase in plasma aldosterone after intravenous angiotensin II (5, 10, and 20 ng/kg/min for 15 min each) before and after euglycemic hyperinsulinemia in seven chronically instrumented dogs. Euglycemic hyperinsulinemia (at insulin doses of 2, 4, or 8 mU/kg/min) resulted in a significantly greater ($p < 0.01$) change in the angiotensin II–stimulated increments of plasma aldosterone than was observed when angiotensin II was administered alone. However, there was no dose dependence of insulin's effect on angiotensin II–stimulated aldosterone. The effect of weight gain on the angiotensin II response was also evaluated in five dogs. Weight gain significantly increased angiotensin II–stimulated aldosterone; however, with hyperinsulinemia the response was not significantly different than that observed in the dogs prior to eight gain. The authors speculated that possible mechanisms whereby in-

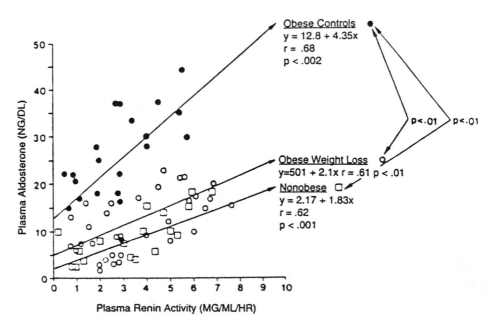

Figure 7   Regression relations between posture-induced changes in plasma renin activity and plasma aldosterone in 10 obese control subjects (dots), in 20 obese subjects after weight loss (circles), and in 10 nonobese subjects (squares). The two weight loss groups were combined. Compared to nonobese individuals, obese subjects (prior to weight loss) have a steeper relationship between posture-induced changes in plasma renin activity and aldosterone and this relationship normalizes with weight loss. (Adapted from Ref. 117.)

sulin could increase angiotensin II–stimulated aldosterone production include: increased intracellular potassium, reduced plasma free fatty acids, and a direct action of insulin to induce increased adrenal steroidogenesis.

E. Increased Activation of the Sympathetic Nervous System

The final method by which selective insulin resistance could cause hypertension is through insulin's ability to stimulate the sympathetic nervous system. For over 20 years it has been recognized that diet affects the sympathetic nervous system. Fasting suppresses sympathetic nervous system activity, whereas overfeeding with either a high-carbohydrate or high-fat diet simulates the sympathetic nervous system (125–128). Insulin is believed to be the signal that networks dietary intake and nutritional status to sympathetic activity. Glucose- and insulin-sensitive neurons in the ventromedial portion of the hypothalamus have been demonstrated to alter the activity of inhibitory pathways between the hypothalamus and brainstem (129). It is believed that the physiological role of the link between dietary intake and sympathetic nervous system activity is to regulate energy expenditure in the hope of maintaining weight homeostasis. Landsberg and Krieger (130) have suggested that in obese individuals the sympathetic nervous system is chronically activated in an attempt to prevent further weight gain and that hypertension is a by-product of the overactive sympathetic nervous system. They and their associates, as well as others, have clearly documented that euglycemic hyperinsulinemia in both normal and obese humans and animals causes activation of the sympathetic nervous system as documented by increases in heart rate, blood pressure, and plasma norepinephrine (26,78,130–133). More recently it has been shown that hyperinsulinemia in normal humans is associated not only with an increase in circulation catecholamines, but also with an increase in sympathetic nerve activity (85). Fisher rats fed a high-fat diet develop obesity, hypertension, and insulin resistance. When euglycemic insulin infusions are performed, increases in systolic blood pressure are observed in the fat-fed animals but not in controls. The blood pressure increase is reversible by combined α-blockade and β-blockade, thus suggesting a role for increased sympathetic activity (134). Although many studies in obese individuals have demonstrated increased sympathetic nervous system activity, this has not been a universal finding (135). Part of the controversy regarding the role of the sympathetic nervous system in obesity relates to relying on plasma levels of catecholamines as the index of sympathetic activity. Recent data from the Normative Aging

Study (33) strongly suggest that obesity is associated with increased sympathetic nervous system activity. This study demonstrated that sympathetic activity, assessed by measuring 24-hr urinary norepinephrine excretion, is directly related to abdominal girth, waist-to-hip ratio, and body mass index. In addition, norepinephrine excretion is also directly correlated with both glucose level and fasting insulin concentration (33,136). Other recent studies using the appearance rate of norepinephrine in the circulation (137) and the effects of somatostatin-induced suppression of insulin on plasma norepinephrine levels (138) provide additional corroborative data for an increase in sympathetic activity linked to obesity and driven by insulin.

Abnormalities in the sympathetic nervous system also may play role in the actual pathogenesis of some forms of obesity. The recent identification and cloning of the β_3-adrenergic receptor have spurred great interest in the potential role of this receptor in the regulation of energy expenditure and ultimately in the development of obesity. The β_3-adrenergic receptor is predominantly expressed in omental fat tissue and gall bladder, at low levels in ileum and colon, and absent in muscle, heart, liver, lung, kidney, thyroid, and lymphocytes (139). Mutations in the β_3-adrenergic receptor gene have been detected in Pima Indians and Mexican Americans, two populations with a high incidence of obesity and diabetes (140). Finally, preliminary studies in obese humans have demonstrated that the administration of an agent with high specificity for the β_3-adrenergic receptor results in increased energy expenditure that is accompanied by a marked improvement in insulin sensitivity and glucose tolerance (141).

F. Summary

Conclusive data suggest that obesity, especially upper-body fat distribution, is an independent risk factor for the development of hypertension. Calorie restriction and weight loss are associated with a reduction in blood pressure. In addition, it is clear that even modest weight loss (i.e., 10% of body weight) improves blood pressure, and many individuals achieve normal blood pressure levels without attaining their calculated ideal weight. Although controversy exists as to the role that insulin resistance and hyperinsulinemia play in the pathogenesis of obesity hypertension, ample data suggest that selective insulin resistance and hypertension are directly related. Finally, since insulin resistance is selective and both tissue and pathway specific, it is possible that in a given individual or animal the degree of selectivity and/or tissue specificity determines whether or not hypertension will develop. Further studies will be necessary not only to clarify the origin of defects in insulin action that are responsible for the development of insulin resistance, but also to more precisely define the exact role that insulin and insulin resistance play in blood pressure homeostasis.

V. OBESITY AS A CARDIOVASCULAR RISK FACTOR

The Framingham Heart Study (4) also identified obesity and hypertension as independent risk factors for the development of cardiovascular disease. Obese normotensive and hypertensive men have a higher rate of coronary heart disease than normal-weight men (39). Manson et al. (142) have also reported that, in women, the relative risk of fatal and nonfatal coronary heart disease increased from the lowest to the highest quartiles of obesity. However, other large studies (143,144) have reported an attenuated risk of cardiovascular mortality and morbidity among individuals who have both hypertension and obesity.

Long-standing obesity is associated with preclinical and clinical left ventricular dilation (145) and impaired systolic function (146,147), with heart failure frequently being the ultimate cause of death in morbidly overweight individuals (148).

A physiological change that may contribute to the development of left ventricular dilatation in association with obesity is sodium retention and a concomitant increase in blood volume and cardiac output. Although many investigators (149) have reported that obesity is associated with an increased cardiac output and blood volume, when cardiac output and blood volume are indexed for body surface area, the differences between lean and fat disappear. Since obese and nonobese hypertensive subjects do not differ in their hemodynamic and volume characteristics when normalized for surface area, some investigators (150) have concluded that obesity does not result in a unique alteration in the vascular system that would produce hypertension. However, normalization for surface area may not be appropriate in the obese subject. Since the increment in cardiac output associated with obesity cannot be explained by an increase in adipose tissue perfusion alone; some have suggested that blood flow to the nonadipose mass must also be increased in obese subjects (150a,151). Thus, obesity is characterized by a relative volume expansion in the presence of restricted vascular capacity.

Regional changes in organ blood flow and resistance have been studied in the dog (152). After 6 weeks of the high-fat diet, regional flows significantly increased in all measured organ beds, whereas in the control dogs, regional flows remained unchanged from baseline values. Weight gain was not associated with a change in vascular

resistance in the heart, kidney, or brain but was associated with a significant decrease in gastrointestinal tract resistance. In addition to these data in the dog, there are also human data to suggest that regional hemodynamic abnormalities are present in obesity. Both renal and splanchnic blood flow (150) have been reported to be increased in obese subjects. In the obese adolescent, regional forearm blood flow, measured by venous occlusion plethysmography, is increased and forearm vascular resistance is decreased (84). Both of these abnormalities are reversed with weight loss. Finally, Schmieder and Messerli (153) assessed systemic and renal hemodynamics and left ventricular function and structure in a group of 207 individuals. They noted that obese hypertensives had lower total peripheral resistance, a significantly higher stroke volume-pulse pressure index, and an elevated renal vascular resistance. They also noted that the degree of left ventricular hypertrophy was greater in the hypertensive than the normotensive individuals, and it progressively increased with obesity.

Since obesity is associated with an increased preload to the left ventricle, dilation and eccentric left ventricular hypertrophy (145,150,154) evolve. Hypertension increases afterload, and as a consequence, the left ventricle adapts with an increase in wall thickness. The combination of obesity and hypertension therefore creates a double burden on the heart, ultimately leading to the development of impaired ventricular function (146–148,155,156).

MacMahon et al. (145) reported that 50% of individuals who are more than 50% overweight have left ventricular hypertrophy. As with blood pressure, weight loss can result in a regression in the left ventricular hypertrophy (145,154,156). Unlike the universal finding of left ventricular hypertrophy in obese individuals, not all studies have demonstrated an impairment in left ventricular function. Schmeider and Messerli (153) reported that obese hypertensive individuals have normal global left ventricular systolic function as measured by left ventricular fractional shortening and velocity of circumferential fiber shortening. However, since both of these indices of left ventricular systolic function are dependent on ventricular preload and afterload, the results of Schmeider and Messerli's study do not document that left ventricular contractility is normal. In fact, Blake and co-workers (154) demonstrated that despite a normal left ventricular ejection fraction at rest, obese individuals have an impaired left ventricular ejection fraction in response to dynamic exercise. Guillermo et al. (155) reported that the end-systolic wall stress to end-systolic volume index, a load-independent index of left ventricular function, is also abnormal in even mildly or moderately obese individuals. These investigators also documented a significant inverse relationship between the index of end-systolic wall stress to end-systolic volume and body mass index, diastolic diameter, and left ventricular mass index.

Abnormalities in left ventricular filling have also been reported to occur in obese individuals (156), i.e., decreased peak filling rate, duration of peak filling, and left atrial emptying index (157), an increased isovolumic relaxation time, and an abnormal mitral valve Doppler filling pattern. The left ventricular hypertrophy, depressed myocardial contractility, and diastolic dysfunction can predispose individuals to excessive ventricular ectopy. Messerli et al. (158) reported that the prevalence of premature ventricular contractions was 30 times higher in obese individuals with eccentric left ventricular hypertrophy than in lean individuals.

The cardiovascular response to stress is also thought to relate to cardiovascular risk. Rockstroh and associates (159) demonstrated that obese hypertensive individuals respond abnormally to stress. In their study, they evaluated the hemodynamic responses to mental and isometric stress in obese and nonobese hypertensive individuals. They observed that obese hypertensive individuals responded to mental stress with vasoconstriction and to isometric stress with an exaggerated increase in arterial pressure.

Finally, as with hypertension, insulin resistance may also be related to both the cardiac hypertrophy and abnormal cardiac function that is observed in many obese individuals. Nakajima et al. (160) reported that there is a direct relationship between intra-abdominal fat accumulation and the cardiac abnormalities associated with obesity. Since increased upper-body and intra-abdominal fat accumulation relates to the presence of insulin resistance even without significant overall obesity, these investigators speculated that the cardiac dysfunction observed in obese individuals may be related to insulin resistance.

VI. MANAGEMENT OF THE OBESE INDIVIDUAL WITH HYPERTENSION

Weight loss is the cornerstone of hypertensive management in the obese individual. Weight loss in both adolescents and adults improves all of the cardiovascular abnormalities associated with obesity, including: hypertension, dyslipidemia, sodium retention, structural abnormalities in resistant vessels, and left ventricular hypertrophy and dysfunction. The method by which weight loss is accomplished is important. Although weight loss in general results in a drop in resting systolic/diastolic blood pressure and heart rate, when the weight loss is incorporated with physical conditioning, the greatest decrease

in resting systolic blood pressure, peak exercise diastolic pressure, and heart rate can be achieved (26). Similarly, a weight loss program that incorporates exercise along with caloric restriction produces the most favorable effects on insulin resistance (26,57), dyslipidemia (57,161), and vascular reactivity (26,84). Endurance training in obese and nonobese individuals improves insulin resistance, in part by increasing muscle oxidative capacity and increasing capillary density (106,107). Most investigators believe the additive effect of exercise to weight loss is related to the fact that exercise improves insulin resistance independent of weight loss.

Although weight loss and exercise are the cornerstones of blood pressure management in obese hypertensive individuals, most obese individuals are either unable or unwilling to lose weight or are unable to keep from regaining lost weight. Therefore, pharmacological therapy is frequently required in the hypertensive obese individual. When choosing an antihypertensive agent, it is important to remember, that depending on the antihypertensive agents used, insulin resistance has been reported to improve, worsen, or remain unchanged. In general, thiazide diuretics (48,92,162) and β-blockers (48,92) are known to impair insulin sensitivity and glucose tolerance; calcium blockers do not seem to adversely affect carbohydrate metabolism (163–165); indapaminde, potassium-sparing diuretics (166), and most central sympatholytic agents also do not influence glucose homeostasis; and finally, angiotensin-converting enzyme inhibitors (92) and α_1-blockers (93,167) may even improve glucose metabolism and insulin resistance. In addition to their unfavorable effect on insulin resistance, thiazide diuretics impair pancreatic insulin secretion (168,169) and increase LDL cholesterol and total cholesterol (92,170). β-Blockers are associated with a two- to threefold incidence of inducing diabetes mellitus (171) and are associated with a significant lowering of HDL cholesterol (172,173). However, despite the different pharmacological profiles of the antihypertensive drugs, there exists no clear recommendation for obese hypertensive individuals. Although β-blockers adversely effect the dyslipemia of obesity, Schmeider et al. (174) reported that in obese hypertensive individuals the β-blocker metoprolol decreases diastolic blood pressure to a greater extent than in those individuals receiving the calcium channel blocker isradipine. Conversely, these investigators found that isradipine was more effective than metoprolol in reducing blood pressure in lean hypertensives. Frohlich (175) randomly assigned obese and lean hypertensive subjects to receive either a β-blocker or a calcium channel blocker. This study clearly suggested that the probability of excellent blood pressure control was greater when metoprolol was given to obese individuals and isradipine to nonobese subjects. Thus, when deciding on the use of an antihypertensive in an obese individual, one must also take into account the lipid profile of the patient and the presence or risk of developing diabetes mellitus.

Finally, new pharmacological agents are currently in development that show promise in the treatment of hypertensive obese individuals. Drugs that alter central serotonin levels, dexfenfluramine and fenfluramine, induce weight loss. They also are associated with a reduction in sympathetic nervous system activity and a lowering of blood pressure (176). It is unknown whether these serotonergic drugs have any effect on blood pressure independent of weight loss. Two other classes of agents, biguandines (metformin) and thiazolidinediones (pioglitizone and troglitizone), also appear to reverse insulin resistance, hypertension, and dyslipidemia (177).

ACKNOWLEDGMENT

This work was supported in part by Grants 1R01 HL 52205, HL-18575, 2R01-HL-35743, and 2P60 AM 20572 from the National Institutes of Health.

REFERENCES

1. Dublin LI. Report of the Joint Committee on Mortality of the Association of Life Insurance Medical Directors. New York: The Actuarial Society of America, 1925.
2. Stamler R, Stamler J, Riedlinger WF, Algera G, Roberts R. Weight and blood pressure. Findings in hypertension screening of 1 million Americans. JAMA 1978; 240: 1607–1609.
3. Symonds B. Blood pressure of healthy men and women. JAMA 1923; 8:232.
4. Hubert HB, Feinleib M, McNamara PM, Castelli WP. Obesity as an independent risk factor for cardiovascular disease: a 26-year follow-up of participants in the Framingham Heart Study. Circulation 1983; 67:968–977.
5. McMahon SW, Blacket RB, McDonald GJ, Hall W. Obesity, alcohol consumption and blood pressure in Australian men and women: National Heart Foundation of Australia Risk Factor Prevalence Study. J Hypertens 1984; 2:85–91.
6. Bloom E, Swayne R, Yano K, MacLean C. Does obesity protect hypertensives against cardiovascular disease? JAMA 1986; 256:2972–2975.
7. Ferannini E, Haffner SM, Stern MP. Essential hypertension: an insulin-resistance state. J Cardiovasc Pharmacol 1990; 15(Suppl 5):S18–S25.
8. Manolio TA, Savage PJ, Burke GL, Liu KA, Wagenknecht LE, Sidney S, Jacobs DR Jr, Roseman JM, Donahue RP, Oberman A. Association of fasting insulin with blood pressure and lipids in young adults. The CARDIA Study. Atherosclerosis 1990; 10:430–436.
9. Larimore JW. A study of blood pressure in relation to type of bodily habitus. Arch Intern Med 1923; 31:567.
10. Levy RL, Troud WD, White PD. Transient hypertension: it significance in terms of later development of sustained hypertension and cardiovascular-renal diseases. JAMA 1944; 126:82.
11. Hypertension Detection and Follow-Up Program Cooperative Group. Race, education and prevalence of hypertension. Am J Epidemiol 1977; 106:351–361.
12. Kannel W, Brand N, Skinner J, et al. The relation of adiposity to blood pressure and development of hypertension. The Framingham study. Ann Intern Med 1967; 67: 48.
13. Cash JR, Wood JR. Observations upon the blood pressure of dogs following changes in body weight. South Med J 1938; 31:270–282.
14. Rocchini AP, Moorehead C, Wentz E, Deremer S. Obesity-induced hypertension in the dog. Hypertension 1987; 9(Suppl III):III64–68.
15. Rocchini AP, Moorehead CP, DeRemer S, Bondie D. Pathogenesis of weight-related changes in blood pressure in dogs. Hypertension 1989; 13;922–928.
16. Hall JE, Brands MW, Dixon WN, et al. Obesity-induced hypertension. Renal function and systemic hemodynamics. Hypertension 1993; 22:292–299.
17. Haynes R. Is weight loss an effective treatment for hypertension? Can J Physiol Pharmacol 1985; 64:825.
18. Langford H, David B, Blaufox D, et al. Effect of drug and diet treatment of mild hypertension on diastolic blood pressure. Hypertension 1991; 17:210.
19. Hypertension Prevention Treatment Group. The Hypertension Trial: three-year effects of dietary changes on blood pressure. Arch Intern Med 1990; 150:153.
20. Davis BR, Blaufox D, Oberman A, Wassertheil-Smoller S, Zimbaldi N, Cutler JA, Kirchner K, Langford HG. Reduction in long-term antihypertensive medication requirements: effects of weight reduction by dietary intervention in overweight persons with mild hypertension. Arch Intern Med 1993; 153:1773–1782.
21. Fagerberg B, Andersson O, Isaksson B, et al. Blood pressure control during weight reduction in obese hypertensive men: separate effects of sodium and energy restriction. Br Med J 1984; 288:11.
22. Maxwell M, Kushiro T, Dornfeld L, et al. BP changes in obese hypertensive subjects during rapid weight loss. Comparison of restricted v unchanged salt intake. Arch Intern Med 1984; 144:1581.
23. Gillum R, Prineas R, Jeffrey R, et al. Nonpharmacological therapy of hypertension: the independent effects of weight reduction and sodium restriction in overweight borderline hypertensive patients. Am Heart J 1983; 105:128.
24. Reisen E. Weight reduction in the management of hypertension: epidemiologic and mechanistic evidence. Can J Physiol Pharmacol 1985; 64:818.
25. Reisen E, Abel R, Modan M, et al. Effect of weight loss without salt restriction on the reduction of blood pressure

in overweight hypertensive patients. N Engl J Med 1978; 298:1.

25a. Reisen E, Fröhlich ED, Messerli FH, et al. Cardiovascular changes after weight reduction in obesity hypertension. Ann Intern Med 1983; 98:315–319.

26. Rocchini AP, Katch V, Anderson J, Hinderliter J, Becque D, Marti M, Marks C. Blood pressure and obese adolescents: effect of eight loss. Pediatrics 1988; 82; 116–123.

27. Dahl LK, Silver L, Christie RW. The role of salt in the fall of blood pressure accompanying reduction in obesity. N Engl J Med 1958; 258:1186–1192.

28. Tuck MI, Sowers J, Dornfield L, Kledzik G, Maxwell M. The effect of weight reduction on blood pressure plasma renin activity and plasma aldosterone level in obese patients. N Engl J Med 1981; 304:930–933.

29. Rocchini AP, Key J, Bondie D, Chico R, Moorehead C, Katch V, Martin M. The effect of weight loss on the sensitivity of blood pressure to sodium in obese adolescents. N Engl J Med 1989; 321:580–585.

30. Dornfield TP, Maxwell MH, Waks AU, Schroth P, Tuck ML. Obesity and hypertension: long-term effects of weight reduction on blood pressure. Int J Obes 1985; 9: 381–389.

31. Reisen E, Frohlich ED. Effects of weight reduction on arterial pressure. J Chronic Dis 1982; 33:887–891.

32. Vague J. The degree of masculine differentiation of obesities: a factor determining predisposition to diabetes, atherosclerosis, gout, and uric calculous disease. Am J Clin Nutr 1956; 4:20–34.

33. Landsberg L. Obesity and hypertension: experimental data. J Hypertens 1992; 10:S195–201.

34. Shear CL, Freedman DS, Burke GL, Harsha DW, Berenson GS. Body fat patterning and blood pressure in children and young adults: the Bogalusa Heart Study. Hypertension 1987; 9:236–244.

35. Itallie V. Health implications of overweight and obesity in the United States. Ann Intern Med 1985; 103:983.

36. Kalkoff R, Hartz A, Rupley D, et al. Relationship of body fat distribution to blood pressure, carbohydrate tolerance, and plasma lipids in healthy obese women. J Lab Clin Med 1983; 102:621.

37. Kissebah A, Vydelingum N, Murray R, et al. Relation of body fat distribution to metabolic complications of obesity. J Clin Endocrinol Metab 1982; 54:254.

38. Peiris A, Sothmann M, Hoffmann R, et al. Adiposity, fat distribution, and cardiovascular risk. Ann Intern Med 1989; 110:867.

39. Donahue RP, Abbot RD, Bloom E, Reed DM, Yano K. Central obesity and coronary heart disease in men. Lancet 1987; 1:882–884.

40. Haffner SM, Ferrannini E, Hazuda HP, et al. Clustering of cardiovascular risk factors in confirmed prehypertensive individuals: the San Antonio Heart Study. Diabetes 1992; 41:715–722.

41. Modan M, Halkin H, Almog S, et al. Hyperinsulinemia: a link between hypertension, obesity and glucose intolerance. J Clin Invest 1985; 75:809–817.

42. Ferrannini E, Buzzigoli G, Bonadonna R, et al. Insulin resistance in essential hypertension. N Engl J Med 1987; 317:350–357.

43. Pollare T, Lithell H, Berne C. Insulin resistance is a characteristic feature of primary hypertension independent of obesity. Metabolism 1990; 39:167–174.

44. Rocchini AP, Katch V, Schork A, Kelch RP. Insulin's role in blood pressure regulatin during weight loss in obese adolescents. Hypertension 1987; 10:267–273.

45. Welborn TA, Breckneridge A, Rubinstein HT, Dollery CT, Russel-Fraser T. Serum insulin in essential hypertension and in peripheral vascular disease. Lancet 1966; 2: 1336–1337.

46. Lucas CP, Estigarribia JA, Daraga LL, Reaven GM. Insulin and blood pressure in obesity. Hypertension 1985; 7: 702–706.

47. Sowers JR. Insulin resistance, hyperinsulinemia, dyslipidemia, hypertension, and accelerated atherosclerosis. J Clin Pharmacol 1992; 32:539–535.

48. Swislocki ALM, Hoffman BB, Reaven GM. Insulin resistance, glucose intolerance, and hyperinsulinemia in patients with hypertension. Am J Hypertens 1989; 2: 419–423.

49. Falkner B. Differences in blacks and whites with essential hypertension: biochemistry and endocrine. Hypertension 1990; 15:681–686.

50. Falkner B, Hulman S, Tannenbaum, et al. Insulin resistance and blood pressure in young black males. Hypertension 1988; 12:352–358.

51. Shen D-C, Shieh S-M, Fuh MM-T, et al. Resistance to insulin-stimulated-glucose uptake in patients with hypertension. J Clin Endocrinol Metab 1988; 66:580–583.

52. Darwin CH, Alpizar M, Buchanan TA, et al. Insulin resistance does not correlate with hypertension in Mexican American women. In: 75th Annual Meeting Abstracts. Bethesda, MD: Endocrine Society Press, 1989, p. 233.

53. Hsueh WA, Buchanan TA. Obesity hypertension. Endocrinol Metab Clin North Am 1994; 23:405–427.

54. Saad MF, Howard G, Rewers M, et al. Insulin resistance but not insulinemia is associated with hypertension: the insulin resistance atherosclerosis study. 34th Annual Conference on Cardiovascular Disease, Epidemiology, and Prevention, Tampa, FL, March 16–19, 1994 (abstract).

55. Carretta R, Fabris B, Fischetti F, Constantini M, DeBiasi F, Muiesan S, Bardelli M, Vran F, Campanacci L. Reduction of blood pressure in obese hyperinsulinemic hypertensive patients during somatostatin infusion. J Hypertens 1989; (6)Suppl 7:S196–197.

56. Reaven GM, Ho H, Hoffman BB. Somatostatin inhibition of fructose-induced hypertension. Hypertension 1989; 14:117–120.

57. Krotkorwski M, Mandroukas K, Sjostrom L, Sullivan L, Wetterquist H, Bjorntrop P. Effect of long-term physical

training on body fat, metabolism and blood pressure in obesity. Metabolism 1979; 28:650–658.

58. Zavaroni I, Sander S, Scott S, Reaven GM. Effect of fructose feeding of insulin secretion and insulin action in the rat. Metabolism 1980; 29:970–973.

59. Hwang IS, Ho H, Hoffman BB, Reaven GM. Fructise-induced insulin and hypertension in rats. Hypertension 1987; 10:512–516.

60. Reaven GM, Ho H, Hoffman BB. Attenuation of fructose-induces hypertension in rats by exercise drainage. Hypertension 1988; 12:129–132.

61. Reaven GM, Ho H, Hoffman BB. Somatostatin inhibition of fructose-induced hypertension. Hypertension 1989; 14:117–120.

62. Kurtz TW, Morris RC, Pershadsingh HA. The Zucker fatty rat as a genetic model of obesity and hypertension. Hypertension 1989; 13(6 pt 2):896–901.

63. Mondon CE, Reaven GM. Evidence of abnormalities of insulin-stimulated glucose uptake in adipocytes isolates from spontaneously hypertensive rats with spontaneous hypertension. Metabolism 1988; 37:303–305.

64. Reaven GM, Chang H, Hoffman BB, Azhar S. Resistance to insulin-stimulated glucose uptake in adipocytes isolates from spontaneously hypertensive rats. Diabetes 1989; 38:1155–1160.

65. Finch D, Davis G, Bower J, Kirchner K. Effect of insulin on renal sodium handling in hypertensive rats. Hypertensive rats. Hypertension 1990; 15:514–518.

66. Brands MW, Hildebrandt DA, Mizell HL, et al. Sustained hyperinsulenemia increases arterial pressure in conscious rats. Am J Physiol 1991; 260:R764–R768.

67. Meehan WP, Buchanan TA, Hsueh WA. Chronic insulin administration elevates blood pressure in rats. Hypertension 1994; 23:1012–1017.

68. Julius S, Jamerson K, Mejiia A, et al. The association of borderline hypertension with target organ changes and higher coronary risk. Techumseh Blood Pressure Study. JAMA 1990; 264:354–358.

69. Ferrari P, Weidmann P, Shaw S, et al. Altered insulin sensitivity, hyperinsulinemia, and dyslipidemia in individuals with a hypertensive parent. Am J Med 1991; 91:589–596.

70. Grugni G, Ardizzi A, Dubini A, Guzzaloni G, Sartorio A, Morabito F. No correlation between insulin levels and high blood pressure in obese subjects. Horm Metab Res 1990; 22(2):124–125.

71. Hall JE, Brands MW, Kivlighn SD, Mizelle HL, Hidebrandt DA, Gaillard CA. Chronic hyperinsulinemia and blood pressure: interaction with catecholamines? Hypertension 1990; 15:519–527.

72. Brechtold P, Jorgens V, Finke C, et al: Epidemiology and hypertension. Int J Obes 1981; 5(Suppl 1):1–7.

73. Rocchini AP, Katch V, Kveselis D, Moorehead C, Martin M, Lampman R, Gregory M. Insulin and renal retention in obese adolescents. Hypertension 1989; 14:367–374.

74. DeFronzo RA, Tobin JD, Andres R. Glucose clamp technique: a method for quantifying insulin secretion and resistance. Am J Physiol 1979; 237:214–223.

75. DeFronzo RA, Cooke CR, Andres R, Fabona GR, Davis PJ. The effect of insulin on renal handling of sodium, potassium, calcium and phosphate in man. J Clin Invest 1975; 55:845–855.

76. Baum M. Insulin stimulates volume absorption in the proximal convoluted tubule. J Clin Invest 1987; 79:1104–1109.

77. Vierhapper H, Waldhausl W, Nowontny P. The effect of insulin on the rise in blood pressure and plasma aldosterone after angiotensin II in normal man. Clin Sci 1983; 64:383–386.

78. Rocchini AP, Moorehead C, DeRemer S, Goodfriend TL, Ball DL. Hyperinsulinemia and the aldosterone and pressor responses to angiotensin II. Hypertension 1990; 15:861–866.

79. Finta KM, Rocchini AP, Moorehead C, Key J, Katch V. Sodium retention in response to an oral glucose tolerance test in obese and nonobese adolescents. Pediatrics 1992; 90:442–446.

80. Rocchini AP. Insulin resistance, obesity, and hypertension. J Nutr 1995; 126(Suppl 6):1718S–1724S.

81. Sharma AM, Spies KP, Ruland K, Distler A. Hyperinsulinemia response to oral glucose in normotensive salt-sensitive subjects. Am J Hypertens 1991; 4:13A.

82. King GL, Goodman D, Buzney S, Moses A, Kahn. Receptors and growth promoting effects of insulin and insulin like growth factors on cells from bovine retinal capillaries and aorta. J Clin Invest 1985; 75:1028–1036.

83. Folkow B. Cardiovascular structural adaptation: its role in the inhibition and maintenance of primary hypertension: Volhard lectur. Clin Sci 1978; 55:3s–22s.

84. Rocchini AP, Moorehead C, Katch V, Key J, Finta KM. Forearm resistance vessel abnormalities and insulin resistance in obese adolescents. Hypertension 1992; 19:615–620.

85. Anderson EA, Hoffman RP, Balon TW, Sinkey CA, Mark AL. Hyperinsulinemia produces both sympathetic neural activation and vasodilation in normal humans. J Clin Invest 1991; 87:2246–2252.

86. Wu H-Y, Jeng YY, Yue C-J, et al. Endothelial-dependent vascular effects of insulin and insulin-like growth factor-I in the rat perfused mesenteric artery and aortic rings. Diabetes 1994; 43:1027–1032.

87. Yagi S, Takata S, Kiyokawa H, et al. Effects of insulin on vasoconstrictive responses to norepinephrine and angiotensin II in rabbit femoral artery and vein. Diabetes 1988; 37:1064–1067.

88. Zemel MB, Sowers JR, Shehin S, et al. Impaired calcium metabolism associated with hypertension in Zucker obese rats. Metabolism 1990; 39:704–708.

89. Natali A, Buzzigoli G, Taddei S, Santoro D, Cerri M, Perdrinelli R, Ferrannini E. Effects of insulin on hemody-

namics and metabolism in human forearm. Diabetes 1990; 39:490–500.

90. Laakso M, Edelman SV, Brechtel G, Baron AD. Decreased effect of insulin to stimulate skeletal muscle blood flow in obese man. J Clin Invest 1990; 85:1844–1952.

91. Baron AD, Laasko M, Brechtel G, Edelman SV. Mechanism of insulin resistance in insulin-dependent diabetes mellitus: a major role for reduced skeletal muscle blood flow. J Clin Endocrinol Metab 1991; 73:637–643.

92. Pollare T, Lithell H, Berne C. A comparison of the effects of hydrochlorothiazide and captopril on glucose and lipid metabolism in patients with hypertension. N Engl J Med 1989; 321:868–873.

93. Swislocki AL, Hoffman BB, Sheu WH, Chen YD, Reaven GM. Effect of prazosin treatment on carbohydrate and lipoprotein metabolism in patients with hypertension. Am J Med 1989; 86:14–18.

94. Pollare T, Lithell H, Morlin C, Prantare H, Hvarfner A, Ljunghall S. Metabolic effects of diltiazem and atenolol: results from a randomized, double-blind study with parallel groups. J Hypertens 1989; 7:551–559.

95. Lillioja S, Young AA, Cultr CL, et al. Skeletal muscle capillary density and fiber type are possible determinants of in vivo insulin resistance in man. J Clin Invest 1987; 80: 415–424.

96. Lithel H, Lindegarde F, Hellsin K, Lundqvist G, Nygaard E, Vesby B, Saltin B. Body weight, skeletal muscle morphology, and enzyme activities in relation to fasting serum insulin concentration and glucose tolerance in 48-year-old-men. Diabetes 1981; 30:19–25.

97. Staron RS, Hikida RS, Hagerman FC, Dudley, GA Murray TF. Human muscle fibre type adaptability to various workloads. J Histochem Cytochem 1984; 32:146–152.

98. Wage AJ, Marbut MM, Round JM. Muscle fibre type and aetiolog of obesity. Lancet 1990; 335:805–808.

99. Juhlin-Dannfelt A, Frisk-Holmberg M, Karlsson J, Tesch P. Central and peripheral circulation in relation to muscle fibre composition in normo- and hypertensive man. Clin Sci 1979; 56:335–340.

100. Julius S, Gudbrandsson T, Jamderson K, Shahab ST, Andersson O. The hemodynamic link between insulin resistance and hypertension. J Hypertens 1991; 9:983–986.

101. Julius S, Gudbrandsson T, Jamerson K, Andersson O. The interconnection between sympathetics, microcirculation, and insulin resistance in hypertension. Blood Pressure 1992; 1:9–19.

102. Frisk-Holmberg M, Essen B, Fredrikson M, Strom G and Wibell L. Muscle fibre composition in relation to blood pressure response to isometric exercise in normotensive and hypertensive subjects. Acta Med Scand 1983; 213: 21–26.

103. Bergstrom J. Muscle electrolytes in man. Scand J Clin Lab Med 1962; 14:511–513.

104. Simoneau JA, Bouchard C. Skeletal muscle metabolism in normal weight and obese men and women. Int J Obes 1993; 17(Suppl 2):31.

105. Krotkiewski M, Björntorp P. Muscle tissue in obesity with different distribution of adipose tissue: effects of physical training. Int J Obes 1986; 10:331–341.

106. Anderson, P. and J. Henriksson. Capillary supply of the quadriceps femoris muscle of man: adaptive response to exercise. J Physiol 1977; 270:677–690.

107. Chi. MMY, Hintz CS, Henriksson J. Chronic stimulation of mammalia muscle: enzyme changes in individual fibers. Am J Physiol 1986; 251:c633–642.

108. Lagadie-Grossman D, Chesnais JM, Dewray D. Intracellular pH regulation in papillary muscle cells from streptozotocin dibetic rats: an ion-sensitive microelectrode study. Pflügers Arch 1988; 412:613–617.

109. Tedde R, Sechi LA, Marigliano A, Scano L, Pala A. In vitro action of insulin on erythrocyte sodium transport mechanisms: its possible role in the pathogenesis of arterial hypertension. Clin Exp Hypertens 1988; 10:545–559.

110. Ng LL, Harker M, Abel ED: Leucocyte sodium content and sodium pump activity in overweight and lean hypertensives. Clin Endocrinol (Oxf) 1989; 30(2):191–200.

111. Herlitz H, Fagerberg B, Jonsson O, Hedner T, Andersson OK, Aurell M: Effects of sodium restriction and energy reduction on erythrocyte sodium transport in obese hypertensive men. Ann Clin Res 1988; 48(20 Suppl):61–65.

112. Draznin B, Kao M, Sussman KE. Insulin and glyburide increase in cytosolic free calcium concentration in isolated rat adipocutes. Diabetes 1987; 36:174–178.

113. Jacobs DD, Sowers JR, Hmeidan A, Niyogi T, Simpson L. Standley PR. Effects of weight reduction on cellular cation metabolism and vascular resistance. Hypertension 1993; 21:308–314.

114. Dranzin B, Sussman K, Koa M, et al: The existence of an optimal range of cystolic free calcium for insulin-stimulated glucose transport in rat adipocytes. J Biol Chem 1987; 262:1485–1488.

115. Shaefer W, Prieben J, Mannhold R, et al: Ca^{2+}-Mg^{2+}-ATPase activity of human red blood cells in healthy and diabetic volunteers. Klin Wochenschr 1987; 65:17–21.

116. Resnick LM, Gupta RK, Gruenspan H, et al: intracellular free magnesium in hypertension: relation to peripheral insulin resistance. J Hypertens 1988; 6:S199–S201.

117. Rocchini AP, Katch VL, Grekin R, Moorehead C, Anderson J. Role for aldosterone in blood pressure regulation of obese adolescents. Am J Cardiol 1986; 57:613–618.

118. Hiramatsu K, Yamada T, Ichikawak T, Izumiyama T, Nagata H. Changes in endocrine activity to obesity in patients with essential hypertension. J Am Geriatr Soc 1981; 29:25–30.

119. Scavo D, Borgia C, Iacobelli A. Aspetti di funzione corticosurrenalica nell "obesita." Nota VI. Il coportamento della secrezione di aldosterone e della escrezione dei suoi metabolite nel corso di alcune prove dinamiche. Fol Endocrinol 1968; 21:591–602.

120. Scavo D, Iacobelli A, Borgia C. Aspetti fi funzione corticosurrenalica nell "obesita." Nota V. La secrezonia giornlieª lia di aldosterone. Fol Endocrinol 1968; 21:577–590.

121. Spark RF, Arky RA, Boulter RP, Saudek CD, Obrian JT. Renin, aldosterone and glucagon in the natriuresus of fasting. N Engl J Med 1975; 292:1335–1340.

122. Granger JP, West D, Scott J. Abnormal pressure natriuresis in the dog model of obesity-induced hypertension. Hypertension 1994; 23(Suppl I):I8–I11.

123. Trovati M, Massucco P, Anfossi G, Caralot F, Mularoni E, Mattiello L, Rocca G, Emaneulli G. Insulin influences the renin-angiotensin-aldersterone system in humans. Metabolism 1989; 38:501–503.

124. Farfel Z, Iania A, Eliahou HE. Presence of insulin-renin-aldosterone-potassium interrelationship in normal subjects, disrupted in chronic hemodialysis patients. Clin Endocrinol Metab 1978; 47:9–17.

125. Young JB. Landsberg L. Suppression of sympathetic nervous system during fasting. Science 1977; 196: 1473–≡475.

126. Young JB, Landsberg L. Stimulation of the sympathetic nervous system during sucrose feeding. Nature 1977; 269:615–617.

127. Landsberg L, Young JB. Fasting, feeding and regulation of the sympathetic nervous system. N Engl J Med 1978; 298: 1295–1301.

128. Young JB, Saville ME, Rothwell NJ, Stock MJ, Landsberg L. Effect of diet and cold exposure on norepinephrine turnover in brown adipose tissue in the rat. J Clin Invest 1982; 69:1061–1071.

129. Landsberg L, Young JB. Insulin-mediated glucose metabolism in the relationship between dietary intake and sympathetic nervous system activity. Int J Obes 1985; 9: 63–68.

130. Landsberg L, Krieger DR. Obesity, metabolism and the sympathetic nervous system. Am J Hypertens 1989; 2: 125s–132s.

131. Young JB, Kaufman LN, Saville ME, Landsberg L. Increased sympathetic nervous system activity in rats fed a low protein diet: evidence against a role for dietary tyrosine. Am J Physiol 1985; 248:r627–637.

132. Rowe JW, Young BY, Minaker KL, Stevens AL, Pallatta J, Landsberg L. Effect of insulin and glucose infusions on sympathetic nervous system activity in normal human man. Diabetes 1981; 30:219–225.

133. O'Hare JA, Minaker K, Young JB, Rowe JB, Rowe JW, Pallotta JA, Landberg L, Insulin increases plasma norepinephrine (NE) and lowers plasma potassium equally in lean and obese men. Clin Res 1985; 33:441a (abstract).

134. Assy W, Wan JM, Coyle S, Blackburn GL, Bistrain BR, Istfan NW: Fasting increases the sensitivity of blood pressure response to insulin in obese rats. Clin Res 1991; 39: a34.

135. Young JB, Macdonald IA: Sympathoadrenal activity in human obesity: heterogeneity of findings since 1980. Int J Obes 1992; 16:959–967.

136. Landsberg L, Troisi R, Parker D, Young JB, Weiss St. Obesity, blood pressure and the sympathetic nervous system. Ann Epidemiol 1991; 1:295–303.

137. Elahi D, Sclater A, Waksmonski C, et al. Insulin resistance, sympathetic activity and cardiovascular function in obesity. Clin Res 1991; 39:355a (abstract).

138. Elahi D, Krieger DR, Young JB, Landsberg L. Effects of somatostatin infusion on plasma or norepinephrine (NE) and cardiovascular function in men. Clin Res 1991; 39: 395a (abstract)

139. Krief S, Lonnquest F, Raimbault S. Tissue distribution of β_3-adrenergic receptor RNA in man. J Clin Invest 1993; 91:344–349.

140. Walston J, Silven K, Bogardus C, Knowler WC, Celi FS, Austen S, Manning B, Raben N. Time of onset of noninsulin dependent mellitus and genetic variation in β_3-adrenergic receptor gene. N Engl J Med 1995; 333: 343–347.

141. Wheeldon NM, McDevett DG, McFarlane LC, Lipworth BJ. β-Adrenoceptor subtypes mediatery the metabolic effects of BRL 35135 in man. Clin Sci 1994; 86:331–337.

142. Manson JE, Colditz GA, Stampfer MJ, Willnet WC, Rosner B, Monson RR, Speizer FE, Hennekens CH. A prospective study of obesity and risk of coronary heart disease in women. N Engl J Med 1990; 322:882–889.

143. Marrett-Connor E, Khaw KT. Is hypertension more benign when associated with obesity? Circulation 1985; 72: 53–60.

144. Chambien F, Chreitien JM, Docimetiere P, Guize L, Richard JL. Is the relationship between blood pressure and cardiovascular risk dependent on body mass index? Am J Epidemiol 1985; 122:434–442.

145. MacMahon SW, Wicken DEL, MacDonald GJ. Effect of weight loss on left ventricular mass, a randomized controlled trail in young overweight hypertensive patients. N Engl J Med 1985; 314:334–339.

146. Alpert MA, Singh A, Terry BE, Kelly DL, Villarreal D, Mukerji V. Effect of exercise on left ventricular systolic function and reserve in morbid obesity. Am J Cardiol 1989; 63:1478–1482.

147. De Divittis O, Fazio S, Petitto M, Maddalena G, Contaldo F, Mancini M. Obesity and cardiac function. Circulation 1981; 64:477–482.

148. Alexander JK, Pettigrove JR. Obesity and congestive heart failure. Geriatrics 1967; 22:101–108.

149. Raison HJ, Achimastos A, Bouthier J, London G, Safar M. Intravascular volume, extracellular fluid volume, and total body water in obese and non-obese hypertensive patients. Am J Cardiol 1983; 51:165–170.

150. Dustin HP, Tarazi RC, Mujais S. A comparison of hemodynamic and volume characteristics of obese and non-obese hypertensive patients. Int J Obes 1981; 5(Suppl 1): 19–25.

150a. Reisin E, Frohlich ED, Messerli FH, Dreslinski GR, Dunn FG, Jones MM, Batson HM. Cardiovascular changes after weight reduction in obesity hypertension. Ann Intern Med 1983; 98:315–319.

151. Lesser GT, Deutsch S. Measurement of adipose tissue blood flow and perfusion in man by uptake of 85-Kr. J Appl Physiol 1967; 23:621–631.

152. Roccluni AP. Cardiovascular regulation in obesity-induced hypertension. Hypertension 1992; 19:I56–I59.

153. Schmeider RE, Messerli FH: Does obesity influence early target organ damage in hypertensive patients? Circulation 1993; 87:1482–1488.

154. Blake J. Devereaux RB, Borer JS, Szulc M, Pappas TW, Laragh JH. Relation of obesity, high sodium intake, and eccentric left ventricular hypertrophy to left ventricular exercise dysfunction in essential hypertension. Am J Med 1990; 88:477–4785.

155. Guillermo E, Garavaglia E, Messerli FH, Nunez BD, Schmieder RE, Grossman E. Myocardial contractility and left ventricular function in obese patients with essential hypertension. Am J Cardiol 1988; 62:594–597.

156. Stoddard MF, Tseuda K, Thomas M, Dillon S, Kupersmith J. The influence of obesity on left ventricular filing and systolic function. Am Heart J 1992; 124:694.

157. Grossman E, Orren S, Messerli FH. Left ventricular filling in the systematic hypertension of obesity. Am J Cardiol 1991; 60:57–60.

158. Messerli FH, Nunez BD, Ventura HO, Snyder DW. Overweight and sudden death: increased ventricular ectopy in cardiopathy in obesity. Arch Intern Med 1987; 147:1725–1728.

159. Rockstroh JK, Schmieder RE, Schachinger H, Messerli FH. Stress response pattern in obesity and systematic hypertension. Am J Cardiol 1992; 70:1035–1039.

160. Nakajima T, Fugiola S, Tokunaga K, Matsuzawa Y, Tami S, Correlation of intraabdominal fat accumulation and left ventrical performance in obesity. Am J Cardiol 1989; 64:369–373.

161. Becque MD, Katch VL, Rocchioni AP, Marks CR, Moorehead C. Coronary risk incidence of obese adolescents: reductions of exercise plus diet intervention. Pediatrics 1988; 81:605–612.

162. Beardwood DM, Alden JS, Graham CA, et al. Evidence for a peripheral action of chlorothizide in normal man. Metabolism 1966; 15:88–93.

163. Gill JS, Al-Hussary N, Anderson DC. Effect of nifedipine on glucose tolerance, serum insuline, and serum fructosamine in diabetic patients. Clin Ther 1987; 9:304–310, 1987.

164. Klauser R, Ptager R, Gaube S, et al. Metabolic effects on isradipine versus hydrochlorothiazide in diabetes mellitus. Hypertension 1991; 17:15–21.

165. Pollare T, Lithell H, Morlin C, et al. Metabolic effects of detiazem and atenolol: Results from a randomized, double-blind study with parallel groups. J Hypertens 1989; 7:551–559, 1989.

166. Grunfeld CM, Chappell DA. Prevention of glucose intolerance of thiazide diuretics by maintenance of body potassium. Diabetes 1983; 32:106–111.

167. Pollare T, Lithell H, Selinus I, et al. Application of prazosin is associated with an increase of insulin sensitivity in obese patients with hypertension. Diabetologia 1988; 31:415–420.

168. Fajans SS, Floyd JC, Knopf RF, et al. Benthiadiazine suppression of insulin release from normal and abnormal islet cell tissue of a man. J Clin Invest 1966; 45:481–493.

169. Amery A, Birkenhager W, Brixo P. Glucose intolerance during diuretic therapy in elderly hypertensive patients. Postgrad Med J 1986; 62:919–925.

170. Morgan TO: Metabolic effects of various antihypertensive agents. J Cardiovascular Pharmacol 1990; 15(Suppl 5): s39–s45.

171. Bergtsson C, Blhme 6, Lapidus. Do antihypertensive drugs precipitate diabetes? Br Med J 1984; 289:1495–7.

172. Greenberg G, Brennan PJ, Miall WE. Effects of diuretic and β-Blocker therapy in the MRC trial. Am J Med 1984; 76:45–51.

173. Gemma G, Mantanari G, Suppe G, et al. Plasma lipid and lipoprotein changes in hypertensive patients treated with propranolol and prazosin. J Cardiovasc Pharmacol 1982; 4(Suppl 2):s233–237.

174. Schmieder RE, Gatzka C, Schachinger H, Schobel H, Ruddel H. Obesity as a determinant for the response to antihypertensive treatment. Br Med J 307:537–540.

175. Frohlich ED. Obesity hypertension: converting Enzyme inhibitors and calcium antagonists. Hypertension 1992; 19(Suppl 1):I119–I123.

176. Kolanowski J, Younis LT, Vanbutsele R, et al. Effect of dexfenfluramine treatment on body weight, blood pressure and noradrenergic activity in obese hypertensive patients. Eur J Clin Pharmacol 1992; 42:599–606.

177. Kobayashi M, Iwanishi M, Egawa K, et al. Pioglitizone increases insulin sensitivity by activation insulin receptor kinase. Diabetes 1992; 41:476–483.

32

Obesity and Diabetes

Jeanine Albu and F. Xavier Pi-Sunyer
St. Luke's–Roosevelt Hospital and Columbia University College of Physicians and Surgeons, New York, New York

I. ASSOCIATION BETWEEN OBESITY AND DIABETES

Obesity is rare in insulin-dependent type I diabetes (IDDM), but is common in type II non-insulin-dependent diabetes (NIDDM). About 85% of diabetics can be classified as type II, and of these 90% are obese.

An initial observation that obesity and diabetes mellitus are associated was made by John (1) in 1929. Also, early on, it was observed that weight loss improves glucose control (2). West and Kalbfleisch (3), in the 1960s, in a series of population studies including many geographic areas, races, and cultures, noted a strong association between the prevalence of diabetes and overweight. They proposed that the largest environmental influence on the prevalence of diabetes in a population group was the degree of obesity present in that community (4). In some of these populations, diabetes was found to be as much as threefold higher in females than in males. These sex differences were abolished by controlling for adiposity. In the National Health Examination Survey (NHANES) II data, the prevalence of reported diabetes was 2.9 times higher in overweight than in nonoverweight persons (5). Also, a study of over 15,000 American women showed that clinical diabetes was related directly not only to increasing obesity, but also to increasing central obesity. Women with both upper body fat predominance and severe obesity had a relative risk of diabetes 10.3 times as great as nonobese subjects with lower body fat predominance (6). In the Bedford diabetes survey of 1962, Fowler et al. (7) found

that whereas in individuals under 40 years of age there was no relation of weight to the prevalence of diabetes, in the 40–70-year-old age range the persons with diabetes were fatter. Feldman et al. (8), studying a group of over 7000 people at multiple sites, found that those with diabetes were fatter and also had a more central distribution of their fat. They suggested that in diabetes there is an abnormality in hormone balance that causes women to be more like men in central fat distribution and exaggerates this effect in men. Baird et al. (9) investigated siblings of diabetic patients and siblings of nondiabetic matched controls and found that siblings of diabetics had a threefold higher prevalence of diabetes, but those with the highest prevalence were the obese siblings of nonobese diabetic propositi.

More recently, Knowler et al. have shown that in the Pima Indian population, the likelihood of developing diabetes rises steeply with increasing fatness (see Fig. 1) (10). Cross-sectional studies have also shown that obese patients have an increased relative risk for diabetes. Prospective studies in a number of countries, including the United States (11), Norway (12), Sweden (13), and Israel (14), have shown that increasing weight increases the risk of diabetes. In the Nurses' Health Study, which has followed 114,824 women for 14 years, it has also been found that the risk of developing diabetes increases as body mass index (BMI) increases (15). It is important to note that this rise begins at levels of BMI of 22, considered generally to be a rather lean weight. These investigators observed that weight gain after the age of 18 years could be cor-

697

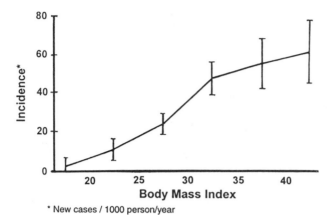

Figure 1   Age and sex-adjusted incidence of diabetes by body mass index with 95% confidence intervals. The data are adjusted by age and sex using the 1980 U.S. white population as a standard to give average incidence rates according to body mass index. (From Ref. 10.)

related to the increased incidence of diabetes, with a greater risk as the baseline of weight from which an individual started increased and also with a greater risk as weight gain increased (Fig. 2). Other studies have found a similar risk for diabetes with increasing weight gain (16,17).

II. INFLUENCE OF THE DISTRIBUTION OF BODY FAT

The possibility of a relationship between the distribution of body fat and diabetes was first raised by Vague (18),

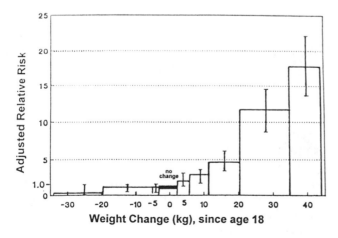

Figure 2   Age-adjusted relative risk for diabetes mellitus during 14 years of follow-up and weight change since age 18 years. (From Ref. 16.)

who clinically observed and reported in 1947 the occurrence of two kinds of "obesities": the android, "apple" shape, or predominantly upper body distribution of the adipose tissue, and the gynoid, "pear" shape, or predominantly lower body distribution of the adipose tissue. Subsequent cross-sectional and prospective studies have linked diabetes mellitus, dyslipidemia, and other cardiovascular risk factors to the distribution of body fat.

Distribution of body fat has been measured anthropometrically by three methods: the ratio of the waist circumference to the hip circumference (WHR), the "centrality index," i.e., the adipose tissue of the trunk versus that of the limbs expressed as the subscapular versus the triceps skinfold ratio (SSF/TSF), and the waist versus the thigh circumference ratio.

The first reports in large population samples prospectively linking fat distribution to diabetes came from Sweden. Ohlson et al. (19) reported that WHR was an independent risk factor for the development of diabetes in men followed for 13.5 years in Göteborg, Sweden, and Lundgren et al. (20) reported that diabetes mellitus and an increase in fasting blood glucose were independently predicted by the WHR measured 13 years earlier in women also in Göteborg.

In the United States, the influence of body fat distribution on the incidence and prevalence of NIDDM has been particularly studied in Mexican Americans. This population has the second highest incidence of diabetes in the United States after that found in the Pima Indians. Mexican Americans with diabetes were found to have a history of faster adult weight gain after the age of 18 than nondiabetics, to attain a higher weight at an earlier age than the nondiabetics, and to have more trunk fat as measured by subscapular skin fold, and less leg fat (21). The WHR was better associated with NIDDM than was the subscapular to the triceps skinfold ratio in the Mexican American population in the San Antonio Heart Study (22). However, cross-sectionally, both the WHR and the SSF/TSF were associated with the incidence of NIDDM in women (22). Prospectively, in the San Antonio heart study, men and women with an upper body fat distribution measured by the highest tertile of the ratio of the subscapular to the triceps skinfolds were more likely to get diabetes (23,24) than the other subjects. The relationship of the centrality index to conversion to diabetes was probably mediated by the relationship with insulin resistance since, in multivariate analysis, it no longer remained associated once fasting insulin and glucose were taken into account.

Results of Caucasian population studies in the United States, such as the non-Hispanic white cohort of the San Antonio Heart Study, are also consistent with a relationship between the WHR and the incidence of NIDDM (22).

In another study of a population of 41,837 women aged 55–69 years, followed over a 2-year period in Iowa, body fat distribution determined by self-measurement of the WHR was significantly and independently predictive of NIDDM development (25).

III. INSULIN RESISTANCE

The reason for the relationship of obesity to diabetes mellitus is not totally clear, but two facts are incontrovertible. The accretion of excess body fat is associated with increasing insulin resistance (26), and insulin resistance is a predisposing factor for diabetes (27).

The phenomenon of excessive blood insulin level in obesity, both basal and postprandial, is one manifestation of the fact that an insulin resistance or insensitivity is present. Studies of intra-arterial insulin infusions in the forearm have revealed insulin resistance in both adipose tissue and muscle (28). Also, the insulin insensitivity of muscle in obesity extends to amino acid metabolism. The amino acids usually most sensitive to the action of insulin are elevated, despite the hyperinsulinism (29). These elevated blood amino acids from skeletal muscle have been postulated as constituting a possible feedback stimulus for hyperinsulinemia in obesity (29).

There is experimental evidence that the liver in obese subjects also manifests insulin resistance. Obese subjects, when compared to lean subjects, have a higher splanchnic uptake of glucose precursors and have a smaller inhibition in splanchnic glucose output with equivalent insulin increases (31). If glucose is infused at rates causing comparable inhibition in splanchnic glucose output, a greater increase in insulin occurs (30). This is manifested in the liver by increased hepatic glucose output and in the periphery by a decreased glucose uptake by peripheral tissues, primarily muscle and adipose tissue. Insulin resistance is caused by both receptor and postreceptor defects in insulin action. Whether an individual with insulin resistance develops impaired glucose tolerance or frank diabetes depends on the ability of the beta cells of the pancreas to compensate for the insulin resistance by secreting more insulin. That individual whose beta cells can keep up remains euglycemic, though hyperinsulinemic (31).

IV. INSULIN RECEPTORS

In obese persons, there is a decrease in the number of insulin receptors on the cell membranes of insulin-sensitive target cells, such as adipocytes (32). This down-regulation of the number of insulin receptors is thought to occur as a result of the increased circulating insulin levels (32), although it might be a primary defect. It is likely that this occurs by increased receptor internalization (33). Insulin receptor binding is thus decreased.

V. POSTRECEPTOR EFFECTS

After insulin binds to its receptor, it activates messages within the cell, allowing the many functions of insulin to be carried out. The so-called "second messenger" for this is not clear and may actually be a multiplicity of signals. At least one is tyrosine kinase, an enzyme complex that is an integral part of the receptor itself (34). It is autophosphorylated, initiating the events that lead to the utilization of glucose, that is, glucose transport and glucose oxidation and storage.

Glucose transport in insulin-sensitive cells, which occurs via a carrier-mediated facilitated diffusion system, is greatly enhanced by insulin. This occurs by translocation of glucose transporters from the intracellular pool to the plasma membrane (35). With regard to these "postreceptor" effects, insulin receptor kinase activity is decreased in obesity, and even further decreased when diabetes occurs (36). In obesity, glucose transporters in muscle and adipose tissue are decreased (37). This may be due to pretranslational suppression of the glucose transporters, as has been shown in animal models of obesity. It has also been reported that in insulin resistance there is a diminished effect of insulin on the movement of glucose transporters to the cell membrane surface (38).

Experimental studies of skeletal muscle biopsies taken from morbidly obese persons have shown that the muscle is equally and severely resistant to the action of insulin in those obese patients without diabetes as in those with diabetes (36). On the other hand, adipose tissue is less insulin resistant in obesity than it is once diabetes has supervened (36).

Glucose disposal is impaired in obese persons (32,39). Use of indirect calorimetry during insulin clamp studies has allowed measurement of glucose uptake in human subjects. The difference between glucose oxidation and glucose disposal, that is, the nonoxidative glucose disposal, is used to measure glucose storage as glycogen (39,40), since there is little net glucose conversion to lipid and little of the glucose that is taken up by muscle is released as lactate. Both glucose oxidation and glucose storage are impaired in obesity, and more so in diabetes. However, the major defect of glucose metabolism is in glucose storage, since oxidation is less impaired (41). This is shown in Figure 3 taken from one of our studies (42). Glycogen synthase activity is a determinant of in vivo insulin-mediated glucose storage (43), and it is impaired in both obesity and NIDDM. In fact, the earliest detectable tissue defect responsible for insulin resistance in persons who are destined to develop NIDDM is an abnormality in the synthesis of glycogen (44).

VI.   FREE FATTY ACIDS

As a rule, patients with obesity, and particularly as they develop diabetes, have elevated levels of free fatty acids (FFA) (27). In insulin resistance, the ability of insulin to inhibit the release of FFA is impaired. The resulting increase in FFA availability causes the muscle tissue to switch to utilize more fat fuel, impairing the utilization of glucose (45). Also, the high levels of free fatty acids presented to the liver stimulate this organ to increase gluconeogenesis, thereby enhancing hepatic glucose output (46). The net effect of these two phenomena is to increase circulating glucose levels and stress the beta-cell insulin secretory system.

VII.   UPPER BODY FAT DISTRIBUTION AND VISCERAL ADIPOSITY ARE ASSOCIATED WITH INSULIN RESISTANCE AND GLUCOSE INTOLERANCE

The large population studies on fat distribution described earlier raise the question of the mechanisms linking body fat distribution to NIDDM. While a few of these mechanisms have been clarified, others are still unclear and are now being studied.

Kissebah and associates published several papers relating WHR to a decreased insulin action at the muscle (47), liver (48), and adipose tissue level (49), in obese nondiabetic women. They also found an association between increased WHR, hyperinsulinemia, and increased hepatic glucose output (48) and reported that the hyperinsulinemia was due both to increased insulin production and decreased hepatic insulin extraction (50). Evans et al (51) showed that the WHR was independently associated with insulin resistance, hyperinsulinemia, and higher insulin and glucose levels after ingestion of glucose. They (51) also showed that insulin binding in muscle and the sensitivity of the muscle to insulin action, as measured by the percentage of glycogen synthase present in the I form in muscle, decreases independently with obesity and with an increase in WHR. This can contribute to decreased glucose storage. In vivo it can be overcome by increasing insulin levels and maintenance of insulin responsiveness. If plasma insulin secretory response cannot increase appropriately, diabetes will develop. It was postulated that this

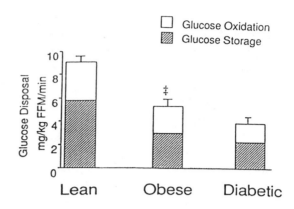

Figure 3   Total glucose disposal during euglycemic hyperinsulinemic clamp. Values are means ± SE partitioned into glucose oxidation (determined by indirect calorimetry) and nonoxidative glucose disposal (storage). **$p < 0.001$ for glucose oxidation, glucose storage, and total glucose disposal: lean > obese > diabetic men. (Adapted from Ref. 43.)

defect in muscle insulin binding could be due to decreased insulin receptor number, though we now know post-receptor effects are more important (36).

Björntorp postulated that the unfavorable effect of upper body fat distribution, as measured by the WHR, on insulin action and glucose tolerance is due to the accumulation particularly of visceral fat, increased free fatty acid flux to the liver, and subsequent hyperinsulinemia and insulin resistance in liver, muscle, and subcutaneous fat (52–54). Visceral fat accumulation measured by CT scan as well as the visceral to the subcutaneous adipose tissue ratio at the abdominal level were indeed found to be independently associated with glucose intolerance in males participating in the Normative Aging Study in the United States (55). Visceral fat accumulation was found to be associated with glucose intolerance in premenopausal women (56) and in men in Canada (57) and with glucose intolerance in Japanese men and women (58). These associations were independent of the overall degree of obesity.

In addition, in a cohort of Japanese Americans, increased visceral fat was shown to predict the prevalence of NIDDM after 30 months of follow-up. This association was no longer significant after adjusting for the initial C-peptide level (hyperinsulinemia). The role of visceral fat in NIDDM development was postulated to be linked to the degree of insulin resistance it produces (59). The mechanism by which visceral fat relates to NIDDM is being studied. Visceral fat has been associated with insulin resistance in women (60,61), but in men this relationship has recently been questioned (62).

VIII. TUMOR NECROSIS FACTOR-α

Recently, tumor necrosis-α (TNF-α) has emerged as possibly playing a key role in the insulin resistance of obesity and NIDDM (63,64). TNF-α expression is elevated in adipose tissue of multiple experimental models of obesity. TNF-α is a powerful inhibitor of insulin-stimulated tyrosine phosphorylations (65), and neutralization of TNF-α improves insulin sensitivity by increasing the activity of the insulin receptor tyrosine kinase in muscle and fat tissue of experimental animals (66). It could also be of importance in the development of insulin resistance in humans, but the importance of its role needs to be further investigated.

IX. INSULIN SECRETION

The response to the insulin resistance of obesity is an increased production of insulin by the beta cells of the pancreas. Thus, all obese persons are hyperinsulinemic (67,68). In general, the fatter an individual, the higher will be the basal or fasting insulin (69). This basal insulin is correlated to adiposity rather than overweight and is related to the increasing insulin resistance that occurs with increasing adiposity. The degree of the insulin response to glucose or other stimuli is related to basal insulin secretory levels and therefore can be correlated closely with the degree of obesity (70). This correlation between insulin response and obesity disappears if the response is expressed as a percentage of the basal value; i.e., the insulin response as a percentage of the basal value does not rise higher in the obese than in lean subjects. Also, there is an upper limit to this relation between adiposity and insulin secretory response. There is increasing insulin resistance as the percent of fat in the body increases up to about 35–40%; after that, insulin resistance does not increase further and insulin levels no longer rise (71).

In those obese individuals who begin to develop abnormal glucose metabolism, the postprandial increase of insulin over basal values is actually decreased in comparison to normal subjects. Thus, the impairment of glucose disposal can be correlated to an accompanying impairment of insulin secretion. This impairment is first observed as patients move from normal to impaired glucose tolerance to frank diabetes. Initially these is a reduction in overall insulin response (72). Subsequently, when fasting glucose begins to rise, the early phase of insulin response is lost (73), and as carbohydrate tolerance continues to deteriorate, all of the insulin response is further reduced. Even though an obese diabetic may be secreting a greater amount of insulin than a lean diabetic person, it

will not be enough to maintain normal glucose tolerance, and the insulin response will be less than that of an obese person with equal adiposity who has normal glucose tolerance.

The documented aberrations in insulin secretion in obese individuals, coupled with other hormonal abnormalities such as poor response to growth hormone and glucagon stimulation, made it unclear whether the hormonal defects seen in obesity were primary or a consequence of the obesity. The hormonal abnormalities have been shown to be a consequence of the obesity since they revert to normal with effective weight loss and are found to appear after prolonged overfeeding of normal volunteers to an obese state (74).

The cause of the hyperinsulinism associated with obesity is unclear. Although a compensatory response of the pancreatic beta cell to the insulin-resistant state is the most popular hypothesis, it has also been proposed that the hyperinsulinism may be a result, at least in part, of dietary factors rather than exclusively a consequence of insulin antagonism. Excess calories (75) and excess carbohydrate (76) may enhance insulin secretory response.

At some point, certain individuals cannot keep up with the required increased insulin levels and become relatively hypoinsulinemic. Most experimental data suggest that the first phase of insulin response is initially affected (77). However, there have been some studies suggesting an impairment of the second-phase response, or of both (78). At that point, hyperglycemia and frank diabetes supervene. The onset of hyperglycemia is not predictable in a particular individual and seems to be determined by genetic predisposition. However, studies have suggested that the duration of obesity rather than the degree of obesity can best be correlated with carbohydrate intolerance in both obese adults and obese children (79). The genetic abnormality is likely to be an intrinsic defect in the beta cell (32,80). In fact, there is probably a heterogeneity of defects. For example, the abnormality in maturity-onset diabetes of the young is in the glucokinase gene, leading to impaired insulin release (81).

X. THE EFFECT OF EXERCISE

Obese individuals tend to have a sedentary existence, and recent epidemiological evidence has reported that a sedentary life-style is a risk factor for the development of diabetes. The prevalence of both impaired glucose tolerance and NIDDM is higher in inactive than active persons (82). In a prospective study of University of Pennsylvania male alumni, followed over 14 years, the age-adjusted incidence rates of diabetes decreased as the reported activity increased (83). This was also found in the Nurses Health Study (84). Physical activity is inversely associated with obesity and central fat distribution, and physical training can reduce both of these conditions (85,86). In a prospective study of diabetes prevention in persons with impaired glucose tolerance, a 5-year trial of diet and exercise showed that those individuals taking part in the diet and exercise program had less than half the progression rate to diabetes than the controls for whom no intervention was planned (87). The data are thus very suggestive of a relationship between activity and the prevention or delay of onset of NIDDM. For this to be adequately confirmed, a randomized control trial would need to be done.

XI. HYPERTENSION: ITS LINK TO BOTH OBESITY AND DIABETES

Once diabetes manifests itself, however, the nature of the disease can be similar to that in nonobese individuals, and all types of complications can ensue. Obesity, even independent of diabetes, is a risk factor for hypertension (88) and for cardiovascular disease (89,90). When it is combined with diabetes, the risk of acquiring these illnesses is therefore greater, leading to a significantly increased morbidity and mortality (12).

The hyperinsulinemia that occurs in obesity and in NIDDM is likely to abet the hypertension. Insulin has been found to be abnormally high in patients with essential hypertension, many of whom manifest a degree of insulin resistance (91,92). Hypertension and glucose intolerance show a highly significant association from the mildest levels of both conditions (93). The hormone exerts a powerful effect on the kidney, increasing sodium reabsorption and thus expanding plasma volume (94).

XII. DYSLIPIDEMIA: ITS RELATIONSHIP TO OBESITY AND DIABETES

It is likely that the pathogenesis for the accelerated coronary artery disease (CAD) in diabetic patients are the high levels of LDL cholesterol and triglycerides and the low levels of HDL cholesterol that are common in diabetic patients (95). These abnormalities in circulating lipids are already present in obese individuals before the development of NIDDM and help to accelerate the morbidity from CAD. In addition, as mentioned above, obese patients tend to have higher levels of free fatty acids (FFA) (28). This is particularly true of those obese individuals with central obesity (96). The enhanced FFA flux, along with the hyperinsulinemia, and the ready availability of glycerol

phosphate greatly enhance the production of triglycerides in the liver. The triglycerides are packaged in the liver primarily as very-low-density lipoproteins (VLDL) and released into the circulation. Lipoprotein lipase, released from endothelial cells in capillaries of the adipose depot, helps to hydrolyze the VLDL, clear them from the circulation, and store them in the adipose tissue (97). In obesity and NIDDM, lipoprotein lipase activity is impaired and the clearance of VLDL is delayed (98). One result is hypertriglyceridemia.

These individuals also have a decreased HDL cholesterol (99). In the normal process of HDL production, mature HDL is made from nascent HDL interaction with triglyceride-rich lipoprotein and lipoprotein lipase. This is defective in obese, insulin-resistant persons.

The final abnormality in lipids in this group of patients is in the LDL cholesterol. There is a tendency to have an increased amount of small, dense LDL particles (100,101). In addition, the LDL cholesterol may be oxidized and/or glycated, again enhancing its atherogenicity (102). These glycated or oxidized particles are more atherogenic than larger particles and may be very important in the pathogenesis of the atherosclerosis that accompanies NIDDM. Correction of the insulin resistance of obesity and NIDDM by vigorous dietary and pharmacological means improves blood lipids and also hyperglycemia (103).

XIII. MACROVASCULAR DISEASE RISKS

Macrovascular disease is the leading cause of death in obese individuals with NIDDM. The improvement of glucose control does not in itself seem to have an effect in improving the morbidity and mortality from CAD. It has been suggested by numerous investigators that the prevailing elevated insulin levels in these individuals may predispose them to CAD. A recent study comparing cardiovascular risk factors in normoinsulinemic and hyperinsulinemic individuals found that the hyperinsulinemic persons manifest higher triglycerides, lower HDL cholesterol, higher total cholesterol, and higher mean blood pressure (104). In addition, there have been three large epidemiological studies that have shown an association between either fasting or stimulated insulin and CAD (105–107). Monitoring risk factors in a longitudinal design, all three found an independent effect of insulin on coronary heart disease. Stout (108) has discussed the potential mechanisms by which insulin may enhance the atherosclerotic process. These include increased growth factor activity leading to enhanced smooth muscle proliferation and connective tissue growth, formation of lipid plaques, and enhancing cholesterol uptake by plaque tissue.

Other factors that can enhance the progression of CAD in obese patients, which is abetted if they are diabetic also, are enhanced platelet aggregability, prolonged platelet survival time, and abnormal levels of plasminogen activator and plasminogen activator inhibitor 1 (109,110). These all enhance the risk of clotting in atherosclerotic blood vessels.

XIV. MANAGEMENT OF THE OBESE DIABETIC PATIENT

As previously mentioned, obesity is present in the great majority of patients with NIDDM. When present, obesity complicates the management of diabetes (111,112). Two issues arise in the management of the obese, insulin-resistant diabetic patient; first, glycemic control should be achieved but not at the expense of adipose tissue accumulation, especially in the visceral adipose depot with associated hyperinsulinemia and, consequently, in the long run, more insulin resistance; and second, weight control must be achieved without losing sight of the need for tight glycemic control.

In the obese diabetic patient, as in any other diabetic patient, microvascular disease is primarily related to the presence of hyperglycemia (113). Uncontrolled glycemia is also responsible for an unfavorable lipoprotein pattern, an increase in glycosylation end-products in all tissues, and an increased risk of thrombotic events (114). In obese diabetic patients, tight glycemic control is thus warranted. The majority of the NIDDM patients are treated with oral hypoglycemic agents, which increase insulin sensitivity and enhance the beta-cell response to glucose (115). Exogenous insulin is usually necessary to control blood glucose in the obese diabetic patient when other therapeutic measures have failed to normalize blood glucose (115). Edelman and Henry recently reviewed the use of insulin for the treatment of the type II diabetes (116). They concluded that obese diabetic patients could and should be evaluated for intensive insulin therapy. The candidates should be motivated, compliant, and should be able to do home glucose monitoring and insulin administration. Combination therapy with insulin and oral agents can be a tool to normalize glycemia if oral agents fail. The adverse effects of and potential risks of intensive insulin treatment include weight gain, which is directly associated with increased hyperinsulinemia (112,117–119). Hyperinsulinemia, as mentioned previously, has been associated with

atherosclerotic risk factors, although a cause-and-effect relationship has not been proven (120).

Weight control must therefore be an important part of diabetes management. It should be initiated early in the management of diabetes and it should continue throughout the duration of the treatment in the obese diabetic patient (121).

Caloric restriction and consequent weight loss in obese diabetic patients greatly improves their metabolic control because it results in improved insulin action in both liver and muscle and frequently also results in improved beta-cell response to insulin secretory stimuli (121). In addition, weight control favorably changes cardiovascular disease risk factors such as hypertension and dyslipidemia (121). Weight control can and must be achieved through a medically supervised, moderately restricted-calorie diet and an exercise program with long-term maintenance goals (122). Chronic use of appetite suppressant drugs such as fenfluramine and dexfenfluramine, alone or in combination with noradrenergic medications, has recently been proposed as a long-term treatment for weight control (123). Long-term studies as to the efficacy versus the safety of these treatments in diabetic patients are still to be done.

One has to question the effectiveness of weight-reducing programs for obese diabetics treated with large doses of insulin. In such instances, the danger of hypoglycemia must be recognized and there is need for close monitoring of blood glucose with frequent decreases in insulin as necessary. Some of the postulated reasons for weight gain with insulin therapy are decreased thermogenesis (124) and increased appetite (125), and thus, it may be impossible to achieve weight loss with caloric restriction unless insulin (or oral agents that increase insulin levels) are being adequately adjusted to the lower-calorie diet prescribed.

Recently, various classes of hypoglycemic agents have been identified which, when used to normalize blood glucose, do not produce weight gain or hyperinsulinemia (126). The approved oral agents metformin and acarbose and the still investigational oral agent troglitazone are such medications. It is our opinion that hypoglycemic agents that are not likely to produce weight gain should be used in the obese diabetic patient whenever possible, that is, when endogenous insulin secretion is adequate. If insulin secretagogues or exogenous insulin needs to be used, it would be very beneficial to combine them with insulin-sensitizing agents to minimize weight gain and the amount of insulin needed to achieve glycemic control.

In conclusion, the goal of the treatment for the obese diabetic patient is to achieve glycemic control, minimize weight gain, and minimize the amount of insulin required to achieve glycemic control.

REFERENCES

1. John HJ. Summary of findings in 100 glucose tolerance estimations. Endocrinology 1929; 13:388–392.
2. Newburgh LH. Control of hyperglycemia of obese "diabetics" by weight reduction. Ann Intern Med 1942; 17:935–942.
3. West KM, Kalbfleisch JM. Glucose tolerance, nutrition and diabetes in Uruguay, Venezuela, Malaya, and East Pakistan. Diabetes 1966; 15:9–18.
4. West KM, Kalbfleish JM. Influence of nutritional factors on prevalence of diabetes. Diabetes 1971; 20:99–108.
5. Health implications of obesity. National Institutes of Health Consensus Development Conference Statement. Ann Intern Med 1985; 103:1073–1077.
6. Hartz AJ, Rupley DC Jr, Kalkhoff RD, Rimm AA. Relationship of obesity to diabetes: influence of obesity level and body fat distribution. Prev Med 1983; 12:351–357.
7. Fowler G, Butterfield WJ, Acheson RM. Physique, glycosuria and blood glucose levels in Bedford. Guy's Hosp Rep 1970; 119(4):297–314.
8. Feldman R, Sener AJ, Siegelaub AB. Difference in diabetic and nondiabetic fat distribution patterns by skinfold measurements. Diabetes 1969; 18:478–486.
9. Baird JD. Diabetes mellitus and obesity. Proc Nutr Soc 1973; 32(3):199–203.
10. Knowler WC, Pettit PJ, Savage PJ, Bennett PH. Diabetes incidence in Pima Indians: contributions of obesity and parental diabetes. Am J Epidemiol 1981; 113:144–156.
11. Lew EA, Garfinkel L. Variations in mortality by weight among 750,000 men and women. J Chronic Dis 1979; 32:563–576.
12. Westlund K, Nicolaysen R. Ten-year mortality and morbidity related to serum cholesterol. Scand J Clin Lab Invest 1972; 30(127):1–24.
13. Larsson B, Björntorp P, Tibblin G. The health consequences of moderate obesity. Int J Obes 1981; 5:97–116.
14. Medalie JH, Herman JB, Goldbourt U, et al. Variations in the incidence of diabetes among 10,000 adult Israeli males and factors related to their development. In: Levine R, Luft R, eds.: Advances in Metabolic Disorders, Vol 9. New York: Academic Press, 1978:78.
15. Colditz GA, Willet WC, Stampfer MJ, Manson JE, Hennekens CH, Arky RA, Speizer. Weight as a risk factor for clinical diabetes in women. Am J Epidemiol 1990; 132:501–513.
16. Holbrook TL, Barrett-Connor E, Wingard DL. The association of lifetime weight and weight control patterns with diabetes among men and women in an adult community. Int J Obes 1989; 13:723–729.
17. Bray GA. Obesity increases the risk of diabetes. Int J Obes 1992; 16(Suppl 4):513–517.
18. Vague J. Les obésités: études biométriques. Presse Med 1947; 30:339.
19. Ohlson LO, Larsson B, Svardsudd K, et al. The influence of body fat distribution on the incidence of diabetes mellitus. Diabetes 1985; 34:1055–1058.
20. Lundgren H, Bengtsson C, Blohme G, Lapidus L, Sjöström L. Adiposity and adipose tissue distribution in relation to incidence of diabetes in women: results from a prospective population study in Gothenburg, Sweden. Int J Obes 1989; 13:413–423.
21. Joos SK, Mueller WH. Diabetes alert study: weight history and upper body obesity in diabetic and non-diabetic Mexican American adults. Ann Hum Biol 1984, 11; 2:167–171.
22. Haffner SM, Stern MP, Hazuda HP, Pugh J, Patterson JK. Do upper-body and centralized adiposity measure different aspects of regional body-fat distribution? Diabetes 1987; 36:43–51.
23. Haffner SM, Stern MP, Braxton DM, Hazuda HP, Patterson JK. Incidence of type II diabetes in Mexican Americans predicted by fasting insulin and glucose levels, obesity, and body-fat distribution. Diabetes 1990; 39:283–288.
24. Haffner SM, Braxton MD, Hazuda HP, Stern MP. Greater influence of central distribution of adipose tissue in women than men. Am J Clin Nutr 1991; 53:1312–1317.
25. Kaye SA, Folsom AR, Sprafka JM, Prineas RJ, Wallace RB. Increased incidence of diabetes mellitus in relation to abdominal adiposity in older women. J Clin Epidemiol 1991; 44:329–334.
26. Olefsky JM. Insulin resistance and insulin action: an in vitro and in vivo perspective. Diabetes 1981; 30:148–162.
27. Reaven GM. Role of insulin resistance in human disease. Diabetes 1988; 37:1595–1607.
28. Rabinowitz D, Zierler KL. Forearm metabolism in obesity and its response to intra-arterial insulin. Characterization of insulin resistance and evidence for adaptive hyperinsulinism. J Clin Invest 1962; 41:2173–2181.
29. Felig P, Marliss E, Cahill GF Jr. Plasma amino acid levels and insulin secretion in obesity. N Engl J Med 1969; 281:811–816.
30. Felig P, Wahren J, Hendler R, Brundin J. Splanchnic glucose and amino acid metabolism in obesity. J Clin Invest 1974; 53:582–590.
31. De Fronzo RA. The triumvirate; B cell, muscle, liver: a collusion responsible for NIDDM. Diabetes 1988; 37:644–667.
32. Kolterman OG, Insel J, Saekow M, Olefsky JM. Mechanisms of insulin resistance in human obesity: evidence for receptor and postreceptor defects. J Clin Invest 1980; 65:1272–1284.
33. Marshall S, Olefsky JM. Characterisation of insulin-induced receptor loss and evidence of internalisation of the insulin receptor. Diabetes 1981; 30:746–753, 1981.
34. Saltiel AR. Second messengers of insulin action. Diabetes Care 1990; 13:244–253.

35. Garvey WT, Huecksteadt TP, Birnbaum MJ. Pretranslational supression of an insulin-responsive glucose transporter in rats with diabetes mellitus. Science 1989; 245: 60–68.

36. Caro JF, Dohm LG, Pories WJ, Sinha MK. Cellular alterations in liver, skeletal muscle, and adipose tissue responsible for insulin resistance in obesity and type II diabetes. Diabetes/Metab Rev 1989; 5:665–689.

37. Hissin PJ, Foley JE, Wardzala LJ, Karnieli E, Simpson IA, Salans LB, Cushman SW. Mechanism of insulin-resistant glucose transport activity in the enlarged adipose cell of the aged, obese rat. J Clin Invest 1982; 70:780–790.

38. Hissin PJ, Karnieli E, Simpson IA, Salans LB, Cushman SW. A possible mechanism of insulin resistance in the rat adipose cell with high-fat/low-carbohydrate feeding. Diabetes 1982; 31:589–592.

39. DeFronzo RA, Jacot E, Jequier E, Maeder E, Wahren J, Felber JP. The effect of insulin on the disposal of intravenous glucose. Diabetes 1981; 30:1000–1007.

40. Bogardus C, Thuillez P, Ravussin E, Vasquez B, Narimiga M, Azhar S. Effect of muscle glycogen depletion on in vivo insulin action in man. J Clin Invest 1983; 72: 1605–1610.

41. Bogardus C, Lillioja S, Howard BV, Reaven G, Mott D. Relationships between insulin secretion, insulin action, and fasting glucose concentration in non-diabetic and non-insulin dependent diabetic subjects. J Clin Invest 1984; 74:1238–1246.

42. Segal KR, Edano A, Abalos A, Albu, Blando L, Tomas MB, Pi-Sunyer FX. Effect of exercise training on insulin sensitivity and glucose metabolism in lean, obese, and diabetic men. J Appl Physiol 1991; 71:2402–2411.

43. Bogardus C, Lillioja S, Stone K, et al. Correlation between muscle glycogen depletion and glycogen synthase activation on in vivo insulin action in man. J Clin Invest 1984; 73:1185–1190.

44. Eriksson J, Frassila-Kallunki A, Ekstrand A, Saloranta C, Widen E, Schalin C, Groop L. Early metabolic defects in persons at increased risk for non-insulin-dependent diabetes mellitus. N Engl J Med 1989; 321:337–343.

45. Randle PJ, Garland PB, Hales CN, Newsholme EA. The glucose fatty-acid cycle. Its role in insulin sensitivity and the metabolic disturbances of diabetes mellitus. Lancet 1963; 1:785–789.

46. Ferrannini E, Barrett EJ, Bevilacqua S, DeFronzo RA. Effect of fatty acids on glucose production and utilization in man. J Clin Invest 1983; 72:1737–1747.

47. Evans DJ, Hoffmann RG, Kalhoff RN, Kissebah AH. Relationship of body fat topography to insulin sensitivity and metabolic profiles in premenopausal women. Metabolism 1984; 3:68–75.

48. Peiris AN, Struve MF, Mueller RA, Lee MB, Kissebah AH. Glucose metabolism in obesity: influence of body fat distribution. J Clin Endocrinol Metab 1988; 67:760–767.

49. Kissebah AH, Vydelingum N, Murray R, Evans DJ, Hartz AJ, Kalkhoff RK, Adams PW. Relation of body fat distribution to metabolic complications of obesity. J Clin Endocrinol Metab 1982; 54:254–260.

50. Peiris AN, Muller RA, Smith GA, Struve MF, Kissebah AH. Splanchnic insulin metabolism in obesity. Influence of body fat. J Clin Invest 1986; 78:1648–1657.

51. Evans DJ, Murray R, Kissebah AH. Relationship between skeletal muscle insulin resistance, insulin-mediated glucose disposal and insulin binding. Effects of obesity and body fat topography. J Clin Invest 1984; 74:1515–1525.

52. Vague J. The degree of masculine differentiation of obesities determining predisposition to diabetes, gout and uric calculus disease. Am J Clin Nutr 1956; 4:20.

53. Vague J, Björntorp P, Guy-Grand B, et al. Metabolic Complications of Human Obesities. Amsterdam: Elsevier, 1985.

54. Björntorp P, Smith U, Lönnroth P. Health Implications of Regional Obesity. Acta Med Scand Sympser no. 4. Stockholm: Almqvist & Wiksell, 1988.

55. Sparrow D, Borkan GA, Gerzof SG, Wisniewski C, Silbert CK. Relationship of fat distribution to glucose tolerance. Diabetes 1986; 35:411–415.

56. Després JP, Nadeau A, Tremblay A, Ferland M, Moorjani S, Lupien PJ, Theriault G, Pinault S, Bouchard C. Role of deep abdominal fat in the association between regional adipost tissue distribution and glucose tolerance in obese women. Diabetes 1988; 38:304–309.

57. Pouliot MC, Després JP, Ndeau A, Moorjani S, Purd'-homme D, Lupien PJ, Tremblay A, Bouchard C. Viceral obesity in men. Diabetes 1992; 41:826–834.

58. Fujioka S, Matsuzawa Y, Tokunaga K, Tarui S. Contribution of intra-abdominal fat accumulation to the impairment of glucose and lipid metabolism in human obesity. Metabolis 1987; 36:54–59.

59. Bergstrom RW, Newell-Morris LL, Leonetti DL, Shuman WP, Wahl PW, Fujimoto WY. Association of elevated fasting c-peptide level and increased intra-abdominal fat distribution with development of NIDDM in Japanese-American men. Diabetes 1990; 39:104–111.

60. Bonora E, Del Prato S, Bonadonna RC, Gulli G, Solini A, Shank ML, Ghiatas AA, Lancaster JL, Kilcoyne RF, Alyassin AM, DeFronzo RA. Total body fat content and fat topography are associated differently with in vivo glucose metabolism in nonobese and obese nondiabetic women. Diabetes 1992; 41:1151–1159.

61. Carey DG, Jenkins AB, Campbell LV, Freund J, Chisholm DJ. Abdominal fat and insulin in normal and overweight women. Diabetes 1996; 45:633–638.

62. Abate N, Garg A, Peshock RM, Stray-Gundersen J, Grundy SM. Relationships of generalized and regional adiposity to insulin sensitivity in men. J Clin Invest 1995; 96:88–89.

63. Hotamisligil GS, Spiegelman BM. Tumor necrosis factor-α: a key component of the obesity-diabetes link. Diabetes 1994; 43:1271–1278.

64. Hotamisligil GS, Arner P, Caro JF, Atkinson RL, Spiegelman BM. Increased adipose tissue expression of tumor

necrosis factor-α in human obesity and insulin resistance. J Clin Invest 1995; 95:2409–2415.

65. Hofmann C, Lorenz K, Braithwaite SS, Colca JR, et al. Altered gene expression for tumor necrosis factor-α and its receptors during drug and dietary modulation of insulin resistance. Endocrinology 1994; 134:264–270.

66. Hotamisligil GS, Budavari A, Murray DL, Spiegelman BM. TNF-α inhibits signaling from insulin receptor. Proc Natl Acad Sci USA 1994; 91:4854–4858.

67. Karam JH, Grodsky GM, Forsham PH. Excessive insulin response to glucose in obese subjects as measured by immunochemical assay. Diabetes 1963; 12:197–204.

68. Kreisberg RA, Boshell BR, DiPlacido J, Roddam RF. Insulin secretion in obesity. N Engl J Med 1967; 276:314–319.

69. Bagdade JD, Bierman EL, Porte D, Jr. Significance of basal insulin levels in the evaluation of the insulin response to glucose in diabetic and nondiabetic subjects. J Clin Invest 1967; 46:1549.

70. Kreisberg RA, Boshell BR, DiPlacido J, Roddam RF. Insulin secretion in obesity. N Engl J Med 1967; 276:314–319.

71. Lillioja S, Bogardus C. Obesity and insulin resistance: lessons learned from the Pima Indians. Diabetes Metab Rev 1988; 4:517–540.

72. Lillioja S, Mott DM, Howard BV, Bennett PH, Yki-Jarvinen H, et al. Impaired glucose tolerance as a disorder of insulin action: longitudinal and cross-sectional studies in Pima Indians. N Engl J Med 1988; 318:1217–1225, 1988.

73. Efenic S, Grill V, Luft R, Wajngot A. Low insulin response: a marker of prediabetes. Adv Exp Med Biol 1988; 246:167–174.

74. Sims EAH, Goldman RF, Gluck CM, Horton ES, Kelleher PC, Rowe DW. Experimental obesity in man. Trans Assoc Am Physicians 1968; 81:153–170.

75. Jimenez J, Zuñiga-Guarjardo S, Zinman B, Angel A. Effects of weight loss in massive obesity on insulin and C-peptide dynamics: sequential changes in insulin production, clearance, and sensitivity. J Clin Endocrinol Metab 1987; 64:661–668.

76. Ogilvie RF. Sugar tolerance in obese subjects. Q J Med 1935; 4:345.

77. Simpson R, Benedetti A, Grodsky G, Karam J, Forsham P. Early phase of insulin release. Diabetes 1968; 17:684–692.

78. Hoker J, Rudenski A, Burnett M, Matthews D, et al. Similar reduction of first- and second-phase B-cell responses at three different glucose levels in type II diabetes and the effect of gliclazide therapy. Metabolism 1989; 38:707–772.

79. Martin MM, Martin ALA. Obesity, hyperinsulinism, and diabetes mellitus in childhood. Pediatrics 1973; 82:192–201.

80. Pimenta W, Korytkowski M, Mitrakou A, Jenssen T, et al. Pancreatic beta-cell dysfunction as the primary genetic lesion in NIDDM. JAMA 1995; 273:1855–1861.

81. Erikksson J, Franssila-Kallunki A, Ekstrand A, et al. Early metabolic defects in persons at increased risk for non-insulin-dependent diabetes mellitus. N Engl J Med 1989; 321:337–344.

82. Dowse GK, Gareeboo H, Simmet PZ, Alberti KGGM, Tuomilehto J, et al. Abdominal obesity and physical inactivity are risk factors for NIDDM and impaired glucose tolerance in Indian, Creole, and Chinese Mauritians. Diabletes Care 1991; 14:271–282.

83. Helmrich SP, Ragland DR, Leung RW, Paffenbarger RS. Physical activity and reduced occurrence of non-insulin-dependent diabetes mellitus. N Engl J Med 1991; 325:147–152.

84. Manson JE, Rimm EB, Stampfer MJ, Colditz GA, Willett WC, et al. Physical activity and incidence of non-insulin dependent diabetes mellitus in women. Lancet 1991; 338:774–778.

85. Després JP, Tremblay A, Nadeau A, Bouchard C. Physical training and changes in regional adipose tissue distribution. Acta Med Scand 1988; 723(Suppl):205–212.

86. Krotkiewski M. Can body fat patterning be changed? Acta Med Scand 1988; 723(Suppl):213–223.

87. Eriksson KF, Lindgarde F. Prevention of type 2 (non-insulin-dependent) diabetes mellitus by diet and physical exercise. Diabetologia 1991; 34:891–898.

88. Stamler R, Stamler J, Riedlinger WF, et al. Weight and blood pressure, findings in hypertension screening of 1 million Americans. JAMA 1978; 240:1607–1610.

89. Hubert HB, Feinleib M, McNamara PM, Castelli WP. Obesity as an independent risk factor for cardiovascular disease: a 26-year follow-up of participants in the Framingham Heart Study. Circulation 1983; 67:968–977.

90. Willett WC, Manson JE, Stampfer MJ, Colditz GA, Rosner B, Speizer FE, Hennekens CH. Weight, weight change, and coronary heart disease in women. JAMA 1995; 273(6):461–465.

91. Ferannini E, Buzzigoli G, Bonadonna R, et al. Insulin resistance in essential hypertension. N Engl J Med 1987; 317:350–357.

92. Welborn TA, Breckinridge A, Rubinstein AH, Dollery CT, Fraser TR. Serum-insulin in essential hypertension and in peripheral vascular disease. Lancet 1966; 1:1336–1337.

93. Modan M, Halkin H, Almog S, et al. Hyperinsulinemia, a link between hypertension, obesity and glucose intolerance. J Clin Invest 1985; 75:809–817.

94. Defronzo RA, Cooke CR, Andres R, Faloona GR, Davis PJ. The effect of insulin on renal handling of sodium potassium, calcium, and phosphate in man. J Clin Invest 1975; 55:845–855.

95. Eaton RP. Lipids and diabetes: the case for treatment of macrovascular disease. Diabetes Care 1979; 2:46–50.

96. Jensen MD, Haymond MW, Rizza RA, Cryer PE, Miles JM. Influence of body fat distribution on free fatty acid metabolism in obesity. J Clin Invest 1989; 83:1168–1173.

97. Eckel RH, Yost TJ. Weight reduction increases adipose tissue lipoprotein lipase responsiveness in obese women. J Clin Invest 1987; 80:992–997.

98. Eckel RH. Lipoprotein lipase: a multifunctional enzyme relevant to common metabolic diseases. N Engl J Med 1989; 320:1060–1068.

99. Howard B. Lipoprotein metabolism. I. Diabetes mellitus. J Lipid Res 1987; 28:613–628.

100. Austin MA, Breslow JL, Hennekens CH, Buring JE, Willett WC, Krauss RM. Low density lipoprotein subclass patterns and risk of myocardial infarction. JAMA 1988; 260: 1917–1921.

101. Trible DL, Hull LG, Wood PD, Krauss RM. Variations in oxidative susceptibility among six low density lipoprotein subfractions of different density and particle size. Atherosclerosis 1992; 93:189–1942.

102. Steinberg D, Parthasarathy S, Carew TE, Khoo JC, Witztum JL. Beyond cholesterol. Modifications of low density lipoprotein that increase its atherogenicity. N Engl J Med 1989; 320:915–924.

103. UKPDS Group. U.K. Prospective Diabetes Study 7: response of fasting plasma glucose to diet therapy in newly presenting type II diabetic patients. Metabolism 1990; 146:1749–1753.

104. Zavaroni I, Bonora E, Pagliara M, et al. Risk factors for coronary artery disease in healthy persons with hyperinsulinemia and normal glucose tolerance. N Engl J Med 1989; 320:702–706.

105. Pyorala K, Savolainen E, Kaukola S, Haapakoski J. Plasma insulin as coronary heart disease risk factor; relationship to other risk factors and predictive value during 9-year follow-up of the Helsinki Policemen Study population. Acta Med Scand 1985; 701(Suppl):38–52.

106. Fontbonne AM, Eschwege EM. Insulin and cardiovascular disease: Paris Prospective Study. Diabetes Care 1991; 14: 461–469.

107. Welborn TA, Wearne K. Coronary heart disease incidence and cardiovascular disease mortality in Busselton with reference to glucose and insulin concentrations. Diabetes Care 1979; 2:154–160.

108. Stout RW. Insulin and atheroma: a 20-yr perspective. Diabetes Care 1990; 13:631–654.

109. Vague P, Juhan-Vague I, Aillaud MF, et al. Correlation between blood fibrinolytic activity, plasminogen activator inhibitor level, plasma insulin level, and relative body weight in normal and obese subjects. Metabolism 1986; 2:250–253.

110. Vague P, Juhan-Vague I, Chabert V, Alessi MC, Atlan C. Fat distribution and plasminogen activator inhibitor activity in nondiabetic obese women. Metabolism 1989; 38: 913–915.

111. Galloway JA. Treatment of NIDDM with insulin agonists or substitutes. Diabetes Care 1990; 13:1209–1239.

112. Genuth JF. Insulin use in NIDDM. Diabetes Care 1990; 13:1240–1264.

113. Diabetes Control and Complications Trial Research Group: The effect of intensive treatment of diabetes on the development and progression of long-term complications in insulin-dependent diabetes mellitus. N Engl J Med 1993; 329:977–986.

114. Brownlee M. Glycation products and the pathogenesis of diabetic complications. Diabetes Care 1992; 15: 1835–1843.

115. American Diabetes Association: Clinical Practice Recommendations, American Diabetes Association 1992–1993. Diabetes Care 1993; 16(Suppl 2):1–118.

116. Edelman SV, Henry RR. Insulin therapy for normalizing glycosylated hemoglobin in type II diabetes. Application, benefits and risks. Diabetes Rev 1995; 3:308–334.

117. Henry RR, Gumbiner B, Ditzler T, Wallace P, Lyon R, Glauber HS. Intensive conventional insulin therapy for type II diabetes: metabolic effects during a 6-month outpatient trial. Diabetes Care 1993; 16:21–31.

118. Yki-Jarvinen H, Kauppila M, Kujansuu E, Lahti J, Marjanen T, Niskanen L, Rajala S, Leena R, Salo S, Seppala P, Tulokas T, Viikari J, Karjalainen J, Taskinen M-R. Comparison of insulin regimens in patients with non-insulin-dependent diabetes mellitus. N Engl J Med. 1992; 327: 1426–1433.

119. Kudlacek S, Schernthaner G. The effect of insulin treatment on HbA1c, body weight and lipids in type 2 diabetic patients with secondary failure to sulfonylureas: a five year follow up study. Horm Metab Res 1992; 24: 478–483.

120. Stolar MW. Atherosclerosis in diabetes: the role of hyperinsulinemia. Metabolism 1988; 37(Suppl 1):1–9.

121. Albu J, Konnarides C, Pi-Sunyer FX. Weight control. Metabolic and cardiovascular effects. Diabetes Rev 1995; 3: 335–347.

122. Beebe CA, Pastors JG, Powers MA, Wylie-Rosett J. Nutrition management for individuals with non-insulin-dependent diabetes mellitus in the 90-s: a review by the Diabetes Care and Education Dietetic Practice Group. J Am Diet Assoc 1991; 91:196–207.

123. Bray GA. Drug treatment of obesity. Am J Clin Nutr 1992; 55:538S–544S.

124. Bray GA. Basic mechanisms and very low calorie diets. In: Blackburn GL, Bray GA, eds. Management of Obesity by Severe Caloric Restriction. Littleton, MA: PSG, 1985: 129–169.

125. Flier JS. Obesity and lipoprotein disorders. In: Khan RC, Weir GC, eds. Joslin's Diabetes Mellitus. Philadelphia: Lea & Febiger, 1994:351–356.

126. Bressler R, Johnson D. New pharmacological approaches to therapy of NIDDM. Diabetes Care 1992; 15:792–805.

33

Obesity and Gallbladder Disease

Cynthia W. Ko and Sum P. Lee
University of Washington and Veterans Administration Puget Sound Health Care System, Seattle, Washington

I. INTRODUCTION

Gallbladder disease is a common problem in the general population and has an even higher prevalence in the obese and in those losing weight. Complications of gallstones include biliary colic, acute and chronic cholecystitis, and pancreatitis. Three conditions are necessary for cholesterol gallstone formation: supersaturation of bile with cholesterol, nucleation of cholesterol crystals, and gallbladder stasis. In obese subjects, these pathogenetic mechanisms may be modified, leading to a predisposition to gallstone formation. This chapter will review the pathogenesis of cholesterol gallstones and the effects of obesity and weight loss on gallbladder disease.

II. PATHOGENESIS OF CHOLESTEROL GALLSTONES

Bile is a complex substance composed of lipids, proteins, electrolytes, and water. There are three principal biliary lipids: cholesterol, bile acids, and phospholipids (primarily phosphatidylcholine). Many species of proteins are present, and they are derived from serum proteins, as well as hepatocyte, bile duct, and gallbladder epithelial secretion. Gallstone formation is determined by the physico-chemical interactions of all of these components present in bile (1).

A. Synthesis and Secretion of Biliary Lipids

1. Cholesterol

The liver is the site of primary site of cholesterol synthesis and lipoprotein metabolism in the body. Free cholesterol is synthesized in the endoplasmic reticulum of hepatocytes. The rate-limiting enzyme in cholesterol synthesis is HMG-CoA reductase (2). Each day, several grams of cholesterol derived from lipoproteins is taken up in the liver. Cholesterol enters the liver in esterified form, and is transported to the lysosomes where it is converted into its free form. It is then transported to the endoplasmic reticulum and reesterified for storage. Cholesterol esters in the endoplasmic reticulum are continually undergoing hydrolysis, thus providing a constant supply of free cholesterol. Free cholesterol in the endoplasmic reticulum constitutes the substrate pool for bile acid and lipoprotein synthesis and is the pool that is secreted into bile. The rate of biliary excretion from this pool varies with the rate of bile salt synthesis and secretion and with the rate of lipoprotein synthesis. Biliary cholesterol secretion is quantitatively correlated with bile salt secretion (2). However, relatively higher amounts of cholesterol are secreted at low rates of bile salt secretion, such that the ratio of cholesterol to bile salts secreted increases as bile salt secretion decreases. This in part explains the finding of more saturated bile (higher cholesterol to bile salt ratio) at low rates of bile flow. Currently, cholesterol is believed to be secreted from the liver in the form of phospholipid-cholesterol vesicles (3).

2. Bile Acids

Bile acids are synthesized from cholesterol through the rate-limiting enzyme cholesterol 7α-hydroxylase, a microsomal enzyme. Following cholesterol feeding and bile diversion, the activity of this enzyme can be rapidly regulated by the rate of its gene transcription, but the exact molecular mechanism of regulation is unclear. Bile acids, which are amphiphilic, solubilize and transport cholesterol. Two primary bile acids, chenodeoxycholic acid $(3\alpha,7\alpha)$ and cholic acid $(3\alpha,7\alpha,12\alpha)$ are synthesized in vivo. The relative proportions of these are regulated by the activity of the enzyme 12α-hydroxylase, which converts chenodeoxycholic into cholic acid. Cholic acid is less capable of solubilizing cholesterol than chenodeoxycholic acid, and more cholesterol per molecule of bile salt is secreted with cholic acid than with chenodeoxycholic acid. 12α-Hydroxylase can be induced by estrogens, resulting in higher proportions of cholic acid and more lithogenic bile (1,2).

After synthesis, bile acids bind to and are transported across membranous structures within the hepatocyte by carrier proteins. In the hepatocyte, bile acids are conjugated with glycine and taurine, increasing their water solubility. They are then actively secreted by bile acid transporters located in the canalicular surface of the hepatocyte into the biliary ductules and enter the intestine, where they are metabolized by intestinal bacteria. The glycine or taurine is first deconjugated, followed by dehydroxylation of the bile acid. Cholic acid is converted to deoxycholic acid, and chenodeoxycholic acid to lithocholic acid. Bile acids are reabsorbed in the terminal ileum and circulate via the portal vein to the liver. Here, they are reabsorbed, reamidated, and then resecreted into bile in a process known as the enterophepatic circulation. Bile acids are initially excreted as individual molecules. However, at the critical micellar concentration, they will aggregate to form micelles that are capable of solubilizing cholesterol and phospholipids (1,2,4). Patients with ileal disease, such as Crohn's disease, will have diminished bile salt absorption and a relatively reduced bile acid pool. These patients are predisposed to gallstone development. Bile acids, in part by their osmotic effect, enhance bile flow, a phenomenon known as choleresis. However, some bile acids, such as ursodeoxycholic acid, can also induce hypercholeresis, an increase in bile flow greater than that expected from the osmotic effect alone. Hypercholeresis is associated with a selective increase in biliary bicarbonate secretion (1,2).

3. Phospholipids

Phospholipids in bile are believed to be derived from membranous structures within the hepatocyte, such as the endoplasmic reticulum or lysosomes, or from the hepatocyte canalicular membrane. Over 95% of the phospholipids are phosphatidylcholines. The mechanism of phospholipid secretion is unclear at this time, but probably involves bile salt–induced formation of phospholipid-cholesterol vesicles derived from membranous structures in the hepatocyte (1). Phospholipids are amphiphilic molecules and, similarly to bile acids, can solubilize and transport cholesterol. It is believed that phospholipid is translocated across the canalicular lipid bilayer by a protein similar to the multidrug resistance gene protein (5,6), and cholesterol is then incorporated into the phospholipids and secreted as a vesicle. The secretory pathway of phospholipid and cholesterol is independent of that of the bile acid transporter pathway. However, vesicular secretion is quantitatively driven by bile acid secretion (1,2).

4. Proteins

Protein composes less than 5% of biliary solids. Proteins in bile are derived from plasma, the hepatocyte, and biliary ductular epithelium. Most biliary proteins, such as albumin, α_2-macroglobulin, and IgG, are derived from plasma, but are present in bile in much lower concentrations. These proteins may enter bile by simple diffusion from the plasma compartment through hepatocyte tight junctions or through the epithelium of periductular capillaries. Other proteins, such as apolipoproteins, secretory IgA, or hemoglobin-haptoglobin complex, are actively secreted into bile following nonspecific or receptor-mediated vesicular transport though the hepatocyte. The gallbladder adds to biliary proteins by secreting mucin, immunoglobulins, and other glycoproteins, which may have an important role in promoting gallstone formation (4,7).

B. Physical Chemistry of Biliary Lipids

Cholesterol is a hydrophobic molecule. To be transported in an aqueous environment such as bile, it must be solubilized by amphiphilic molecules such as bile acids or phospholipids. Cholesterol is transported in two forms, micellar and nonmicellar (vesicular), in bile (6). The thermodynamic stability of these two forms of transport differs. Since only a limited amount of cholesterol can be solubilized by bile acids and phospholipids, the relative concentrations of cholesterol, phospholipid, and bile acids may determine the gallstone-forming capability, or lithogenicity, of bile. Lithogenicity is expressed as the cholesterol saturation index (8,9). Bile with a cholesterol saturation index greater than one is, by definition, supersaturated. One prerequisite for gallstone formation is the presence of bile supersaturation.

I. Nonmicellar Cholesterol Transport

Recently, a vesicular mode of biliary cholesterol transport has been defined (3,10–13). These vesicles are unilamellar, 40–70 nm in diameter, consisting of a bilayer of phospholipid interdigitated with cholesterol. Vesicles contain very little or no bile acids. In bile with a higher concentration of bile acids, such as gallbladder bile, these vesicles may fuse and form larger, multilamellar vesicles up to 500–1000 nm in diameter (11–13). Vesicles are believed to be thermodynamically less stable than mixed micelles, and cholesterol in these vesicles may coalesce to form a metastable state (3,10,14–16). Lithogenicity correlates with a shorter nucleation time for cholesterol crystal formation (17). Cholesterol in vesicles is thus felt to be more prone to nucleate and precipitate (16–19), and gallstone patients may have a larger proportion of cholesterol transported in this form (18).

2. Micellar Cholesterol Transport

Cholesterol is also transported in the form of mixed micelles (2). These structures have diameters of 4–8 nm. In low bile salt concentration and a highly dilute solution, such as in canalicular or ductular bile, bile salt mixed micelles are probably rod-shaped aggregates. As bile is being concentrated, mixed disc or spherical aggregates form (20). Cholesterol can undergo dynamic exchange between the nonmicellar and micellar forms of transport (21,22), but only the micellar form is considered thermodynamically stable. Cholesterol equilibration between nonmicellar and micellar forms starts immediately after secretion. Transfer of both cholesterol and phospholipids from the nonmicellar to the micellar fraction is facilitated by increasing bile acid concentrations, such as may occur with gallbladder stasis. During this phase of "micellation," more phospholipid than cholesterol is transferred to the forming micelle (2). The residual vesicles are thus less stable due to higher cholesterol-to-phospholipid ratio. However, with lower rates of bile acid secretion, the relative concentration of bile acids is too low to solubilize all biliary cholesterol, and therefore most cholesterol is transported in vesicular, less stable, form (17). Under these circumstances, cholesterol crystals may form.

C. Role of the Gallbladder

Cholesterol gallstones occur rarely in patients who have undergone previous cholecystectomy. Therefore, the gallbladder is felt to play an important role in gallstone formation. The gallbladder has storage, concentrative, absorptive, secretory, and contractile properties that may contribute to development of gallstones.

I. Motor Function

Gallbladder motility is commonly assessed by measuring fasting volume, contracted or residual volume, and fractional emptying. Maximal contraction is seen after meals. Between meals, the gallbladder may undergo partial emptying and filling. During periods of fasting, gallbladder contraction is weak, and bile accumulates in the gallbladder, with sequestration of the circulating bile acid pool. As bile acid secretion rates fall, bile becomes progressively more saturated, with the potential for cholesterol crystallization and stone formation. Contractile function of the gallbladder is felt to be important to empty any saturated bile, sludge, or small stones before larger stones can form (23). Gallbladder contractility is controlled through the endocrine and nervous systems. The most important hormone regulating gallbladder contractility is cholecystokinin (CCK). This hormone is released by the duodenum after meals and causes gallbladder contraction and sphincter of Oddi relaxation (23). Other hormones with an effect on gallbladder motility include secretin, vasoactive intestinal peptide, and motilin (24,25). Neural control is mediated through both the vagus nerve and the sympathetic nervous system. Vagal activity enhances gallbladder contraction, while the role of sympathetic innervation is generally inhibitory (23).

Abnormalities of gallbladder motility have been noted in animals and in a subgroup of patients who form sludge and gallstones (26–28). These abnormalities include increased fasting volume, increased residual volume, and decreased fractional emptying (29–33). Fasting and residual volume may be correlated with overall body mass, unrelated to the level of obesity (32). Some studies also show a slower rate of contraction after a fatty meal in gallstone patients (28). In many conditions that predispose to sludge or gallstone formation, gallbladder emptying is markedly inhibited due to endocrine or neurological abnormalities (23). For example, patients who are fasting or receiving total parenteral nutrition will have markedly diminished CCK release and gallbladder hypomotility (34,35). Treatment with the CCK antagonist somatostatin, as in patients with acromegaly, can inhibit gallbladder contractility (36,37). The obese, who are also predisposed to sludge and stone formation, may have diminished responsiveness of the gallbladder wall to CCK (32). Progesterone levels similar to that found during pregnancy can also inhibit gallbladder contractility in vitro (38,39). In patients after gastrectomy, during which the vagal branch to the gallbladder may be cut, gallbladder motility is markedly diminished (23).

2. Mucosal Function

The gallbladder is generally thought of as a storage organ. However, several recent studies have demonstrated mucosal function in concentration of bile and alteration of its constituents. The gallbladder epithelium acidifies bile, actively transports sodium and chloride, and absorbs water by passive osmosis. During this process, initially dilute hepatic bile is concentrated, leading to higher concentrations of biliary lipids, a process important to bring about cholesterol nucleation. As bile concentration increases, concentrations of total lipids, cholesterol, phospholipid, and potassium also increase. Chloride concentration decreases. With concentration, bile pH decreases and carbonate concentration decreases (40–43). Although cholesterol concentration increases, molar percentage of cholesterol and the cholesterol saturation index decrease (9). The mathematically derived saturation index in this setting is misleading. It is calculated as the amount of cholesterol capable of being solubilized by bile salt mixed micelles. As bile is being concentrated, there are more mixed micelles, and in theory, gallbladder bile should be able to solubilize more cholesterol. However, the saturation index fails to account for the vesicular cholesterol that is now enriched as bile is being concentrated. Vesicular cholesterol is the cholesterol that eventually will end up in nucleation or precipitation (9). Nucleation times decrease with bile concentration (44). With acidification, calcium solubility increases, such that all bile will be unsaturated with respect to calcium when pH is less than 7 (43,45).

In addition to its concentrative and absorptive functions, gallbladder epithelium secretes mucin glycoprotein, another possible enhancing factor for cholesterol crystal nucleation (46). Mucin glycoprotein has extensive hydrophobic domains that can bind biliary lipids. In more concentrated bile, vesicles and micelles are entrapped in these binding sites and come into close and prolonged contact (47–51). Mucin hypersecretion has been shown to precede gallstone formation in prairie dog models and probably entraps cholesterol within its hydrophobic domains (51–53). The stimulus for mucin hypersecretion is not entirely clear, but may be lithogenic bile, hydrophobic bile salts, prostaglandins, or arachidonic acid (52–54). Gallbladder mucosal blood flow increases in prairie dogs fed a cholesterol-rich diet, and lithogenic bile in these animals is shown to induce increased mucosal blood flow, possibly due to an effect of substances in lithogenic bile that alter vascular tone (55).

3. Nucleation of Cholesterol Crystals

Nucleation is the first step in gallstone formation. Nucleation is initiated by aggregation and fusion of unilamellar vesicles to multilamellar vesicles, with subsequent aggregation of cholesterol molecules to form crystals. This initial aggregation is mediated at least in part by mucin binding of these lipids. Cholesterol that precipitates is derived primarily from biliary vesicles and precipitates using mucin glycoprotein as a nidus (16,47,56). Phosphatidylcholine in vesicles may bind preferentially to mucin, with the subsequent increase in the cholesterol/phosphatidylcholine ratio in vesicles leading to vesicle fusion and nucleation. Calcium ions are also felt to be important in gallstone formation, as they can promote fusion of phospholipid-cholesterol vesicles. Calcium salts can serve as a nidus for cholesterol precipitation and are usually found in the central core region of cholesterol stones (2). Proteins, including albumin and other calcium-binding proteins, are found in the matrix of cholesterol stones and thus may also serve as sites for nucleation (56–58). When cholesterol crystals reach a certain critical size, gallstone formation can occur with further deposition of cholesterol on the surface of the aggregate.

Experimental evidence exists that normal biliary proteins have pronucleating (59–65) and antinucleating (66,67) properties. In addition to mucin, the proteins with pronucleating properties include IgA, IgG, haptoglobin, phospholipase C, and aminopeptidase N (59–65). Proteins with antinucleating properties include apolipoprotein A-I and A-II (67) and some small acidic glycoproteins (66). It is felt that these proteins somehow interact with and stabilize biliary lipids and calcium. The existence of proteins with antinucleating properties may explain the prolonged stability of bile that is supersaturated with cholesterol. The presence of proteins with pronucleating properties may contribute to nucleation, as high biliary protein concentrations have been found in supersaturated bile with cholesterol crystals, relative to control groups and to supersaturated bile without cholesterol crystals (68). Besides the proteins already listed, many poorly characterized, nonmucin proteins are found as a small percentage of the core of cholesterol gallstones (56,57). The exact nature and role in gallstone pathogenesis of these proteins is unknown at this time.

4. Growth of Cholesterol Crystals into Stones

Once a crystal of adequate size has formed, cholesterol, calcium bilirubinate, and other biliary lipids can deposit on its surface, leading to formation of visible gallstones. One study has suggested that bile in obese patients promotes more rapid crystal growth than in the nonobese

(69). However, this process has not been as extensively studied as crystal nucleation, and little information is available on factors that may influence growth of stones.

III. EFFECTS OF OBESITY

As can be seen from the previous discussion, gallstone formation requires three conditions: secretion of supersaturated bile, nucleation of cholesterol crystals from supersaturated bile, and gallbladder stasis. Obesity has direct effects on bile composition and gallbladder motility. This section will review the epidemiology of gallbladder disease and the effects of obesity on bile composition and gallbladder motility that predispose to gallstone formation.

A. Epidemiology of Gallbladder Disease

Gallstones occur in populations throughout the world, but the prevalence varies substantially (70–73). In Western countries, the majority of gallstones are composed of cholesterol, whereas in Africa and Asia, pigment gallstones are most common. Gallstones in the obese are composed primarily of cholesterol. The prevalence of gallstones in females varies from 3.7% in Indians and Pakistanis to 62.2% in Pima Indians (71,72). In males, the prevalence varies from 2.9% in Thailand to 25.9% in Pima Indians (72,73). Both racial and genetic factors likely contribute to the wide variation in prevalence. Despite the high prevalence of gallstones, about two-thirds of patients with known gallstones do not have symptoms of biliary tract disease.

In all populations studied, the prevalence of gallstones increases with age (70–73). Between the age of 30 and 39, 2% of men and 6% of women have gallstones on ultrasound or cholecystography. The prevalence of gallbladder disease increases markedly in those over 40 years old, such that 10–15% of Caucasian men and 20–40% of Caucasian women over the age of 60 have gallstones ultrasonographically. In the Pima Indians, a group known to have a high prevalence of gallstones, 68% of men and 90% of women over the age of 65 had gallbladder disease by oral cholecystography (72). With aging, biliary cholesterol secretion becomes excessive through mechanisms that are not well understood (74).

At all ages, females have a higher prevalence of gallstones than males, but in older age groups, the female predominance of gallstone incidence is less marked. Other states with high estrogen stimulation, such as oral contraceptive use, high parity, and estrogen replacement therapy, also are associated with greater risk of gallstones (75–77). Multiple theories have been put forth to explain this gender difference. Females may have a higher level of the enzyme 12α-hydroxylase, with resulting higher biliary levels of cholic acid and more supersaturated bile (see above). Estrogens increase receptors for lipoproteins B and E, leading to increased hepatic cholesterol uptake (78). High levels of circulating estrogens have been shown to decrease the total bile acid pool and the pool of chenodeoxycholic acid, with resulting increases in the cholesterol-to-phospholipid ratio and cholesterol supersaturation (79).

Risk factors other than ethnicity, age, and gender are less well defined and understood. Patients with diabetes mellitus or glucose intolerance have a higher incidence of gallstones in some, but not all, studies, likely secondary to altered gallbladder motility and hepatic lipid metabolism (80–82). A weak negative association between total serum cholesterol or LDL levels and gallstone formation has been seen in some, but not all, studies (75,76,81,83–85). Gallstone patients have mean triglyceride levels 21–26% higher and HDL cholesterol levels 14–19% lower than matched control patients (75,83–85). There is no clear consensus on the effect of alcohol consumption, smoking, or occupation on the risk of gallbladder disease (78,81,86,87).

Dietary factors have been implicated in gallbladder disease, but there are currently no clear data on the potential effects or mechanisms. Evidence exists that higher total caloric intake correlates with cholesterol gallstone formation. In the Nurses' Health Study, a significant trend toward higher risk of gallstones was seen with increasing caloric intake (87). However, in a study of Japanese-American men, there was an inverse correlation between total caloric intake and gallstone incidence (86). No study has found a significant alteration in risk with total fat, protein, or carbohydrate intake. In a prairie dog model, an artificially high cholesterol intake has increased the risk of gallstone formation (88). Likewise, high dietary cholesterol intake in humans increases biliary cholesterol secretion and decreases hepatic synthesis of bile acids, changes that may predispose to formation of supersaturated bile, cholesterol crystals, and cholesterol gallstones (89).

B. Risk of Gallstones in the Obese

Many studies have shown that obese women are predisposed to gallbladder disease (Table 1). The relative risk seems to increase as body weight increases (75,76,80,86,87,90–93). Thus, the risk of gallstones relative to nonobese women is increased 2 times in women with a body mass index (BMI, defined as weight in kg divided by height in m^2) over 30 kg/m^2 and 7 times in women with a BMI over 45 kg/m^2 (87). However, there is not a defined threshhold effect, as the relative risk of

Table 1 Relative Risk of Gallstones with Obesity in Various Populations

Ref.	Study population	Diagnostic criteria	Normal population	Obese population	Relative risk
80	Japanese men aged 48–56	Screening by US	BMI < 22.5	BMI > 25	1.9
86	Japanese-American men	Screening by US	BMI < 21.65	BMI 21.6–23.8	1.1
				BMI 23.8–25.8	1.4
				BMI > 25.8	1.8
87	Nurses' Health Study	Previous cholecystectomy or symptoms	BMI < 24	BMI 30–35	3.69
				BMI 35–40	4.72
				BMI 40–45	5.11
				BMI > 45	7.36
91	Nurses' Health Study	US if symptomatic	BMI < 22	BMI 22–24.9	1.6
				BMI 25–31.9	3.3
				BMI > 32	6.3
131	Obese prior to bariatric surgery	Previous cholecystectomy and intraoperative US	BMI < 20 (Ref. 91)	BMI 35–40	5
				BMI 40–50	7
				BMI 50–60	8

US, ultrasound; BMI, body mass index.

gallstones increases with BMI, even within the "normal" range, commonly defined as 20–25 kg/m^2. Some have shown a linear and others an exponential increase in risk with increasing BMI (Table 1). These data may differ due to differences in study design: some studies have examined patients with symptomatic gallstones only, while some have studied all patients using ultrasonography looking for gallstones. Obesity seems to confer a greater relative risk in younger populations (93–95). In one study of obese adolescents, 55% of adolescent females undergoing cholecystectomy were obese, compared to 23% of adolescent females undergoing surgery for sinusitis or nasal septum deviation, a relative risk of 4.2 (95). This relationship between obesity and gallstones is less striking in men. Two large prospective studies have shown a relative risk of 1.6–2.0 of gallstones in men in the highest quartile of BMI relative to men in the lowest (81,96). In series of both men and women undergoing bariatric surgery, up to 43% have gallbladder disease, defined as prior cholecystectomy or gallstones, at the time of surgery. An additional 33% have supersaturated bile when analyzed at the time of surgery (97,98).

In addition to the effects of overall obesity, central or truncal adiposity, commonly measured by waist-hip circumference or truncal skinfold thickness ratio, is also correlated with the risk of gallstones in some studies in both men and women. In the San Antonio Heart Study of Mexican-American women, the risk for developing gallstone disease was 30% higher for women in the highest quartile of subscapular-triceps skinfold thickness ratio

when compared to those in the lowest quartile (99). An association with central adiposity and gallstones was not seen in Mexican-American men in the same study, although statistical power of this study was limited by the small numbers of men with gallstones (100). In the Zutphen Study, truncal skinfold thickness ratio was positively correlated with later symptomatic gallstone formation in men, with men in the highest quartile having risk 2.5 times greater than men in the lowest quartile. This association was not altered after adjusting for initial BMI (101). In a study limited to obese white women, Hartz et al. also found an association between central adiposity and the risk of gallbladder disease, with a risk of gallbladder disease 75% higher in women in the highest quartile of waist-hip circumference ratio when compared with those in the lowest quartile (102).

C.   Alterations in Serum Lipids

Excessive body weight correlates strongly with increased daily cholesterol synthesis and a larger total body cholesterol pool. Excessive body weight is also correlated to the metabolically active cholesterol pool in the body, including that found in adipose tissue. In addition, there is some impairment of hepatic conversion of cholesterol into bile acids in the obese. Although serum cholesterol levels do not correlate strongly with the rate of cholesterol production, higher serum levels of total cholesterol are found in the obese. Total serum cholesterol levels are a reflection of the balance between synthesis, uptake by the adipose storage pool, and hepatic metabolism. Equilibration occurs slowly between the serum pool and the adipose tissue pool. The obese therefore have dual mechanisms contributing to the higher total cholesterol pool: increased synthesis and decreased degradation (103–105). There are also alterations in lipid subfraction concentrations in serum, with decreased HDL cholesterol and higher LDL cholesterol levels. In the obese, serum triglycerides are elevated due to excess hepatic synthesis of VLDL and triglycerides, an effect of peripheral hyperinsulinemia and enhanced peripheral lipolysis. Lower lipoprotein lipase activity leads to decreased triglyceride clearance (106). As discussed previously, gallstone formation has also been correlated with higher serum triglyceride and lower serum HDL levels. However, it is not clear if altered serum lipids are a direct cause of gallstones, or if both disorders are a reflection of an underlying common metabolic derangement.

D. Alterations in Bile Composition

In the obese, biliary cholesterol secretion is increased relative to the nonobese with or without gallstones. When normalized to subject weight, cholesterol secretion appears normal in obese patients without gallstones. However, in obese patients with gallstones, cholesterol secretion remains markedly elevated, even when corrected for body weight (88,107–111). This marked cholesterol hypersecretion, with a resulting higher cholesterol saturation index, is felt to be the primary mechanism predisposing to gallbladder disease in the obese (107–111).

The pathophysiology of cholesterol hypersecretion in the obese is poorly understood. Putative mechanisms of cholesterol hypersecretion include increased cholesterol uptake from lipoproteins (78), increased cholesterol synthesis by HMG CoA reductase (105), decreased cholesterol catabolism by cholesterol 7α-hydroxylase (112), and decreased esterification of cholesterol within the hepatocyte (105). It seems likely that cholesterol hypersecretion is secondary to a combination of these effects.

In contrast to the consistent data showing cholesterol hypersecretion, the data on alterations in bile acid secretion are variable. The total pool and biliary secretion of bile acids are felt to be normal to increased in the obese. However, the relative percentage of bile acids is lower than in normals due to the marked increase in cholesterol secretion. In addition, when normalized for body weight, bile acid secretion is lower than in the nonobese (108–110,113–115). The data on phospholipid secretion are also variable, with different studies showing unchanged to elevated total phospholipid secretion (107–110). Evidence also conflicts on the relative percentage of biliary phospholipids, with studies showing either unchanged or increased molar ratios. These results are not altered after adjusting secretion rates for body weight. No change in the relative composition of biliary phospholipids is found with obesity (108).

From the previous evidence, if follows that markedly increased cholesterol secretion in the obese, coupled with an unchanged to mildly increased bile acid secretion, leads to an increase in the cholesterol/bile salt ratio (115). Cholesterol saturation index thus increases with BMI, independent of age, gender, or ethnicity (115). As a correlate, bile becomes more lithogenic and thus predisposes to gallstone formation. This is true for measurements of both hepatic and gallbladder bile. In contrast to nonobese individuals, where bile is supersaturated only with fasting, supersaturation of bile is not transient, but persists even after feeding. The obese thus have more supersaturated bile that persists for longer periods. In the nonobese, the presence of antinucleating proteins inhibits cholesterol crystal nucleation from supersaturated bile (66,67). Obese persons may have differences in antinucleating and pronucleating factors in bile, but this has not yet been extensively examined.

E. Alterations in Gallbladder Motility

Gallbladder stasis is an important factor in the nonobese that predisposes to formation of biliary sludge and stones. Obesity in itself is associated with gallbladder hypomotility and stasis. Documented abnormalities include increased fasting volume, increased residual volume, and decreased fractional emptying. There is a linear correlation between fasting gallbladder volume and total body weight, but the decreases in gallbladder contractility and the rate of gallbladder emptying do not clearly correlate with body surface area, BMI, or excess body weight (29–32). Multiple mechanisms may predispose to alterations in gallbladder motility in the obese. Alterations in peripheral CCK levels have been postulated, but not yet studied. Diminished gallbladder responsiveness to CCK has been proposed in one study (32). Another proposed mechanism is related to accelerated gastric emptying. Rapid emptying of a meal would diminish the amount of time that food or chyme is in the duodenum. There would then be a resulting decrease in release of CCK, with lesser stimulation of gallbladder emptying (31).

IV. EFFECTS OF WEIGHT LOSS

Obesity itself is associated with a marked increase in incidence of gallbladder disease. Paradoxically, weight loss, through either dieting or bariatric surgery, is also associated with a further increase in the incidence of gallstone formation (Table 2). This section will review the incidence, pathophysiology, and prevention of gallstone formation during weight loss.

A. Incidence of and Risk Factors for Gallstone Formation

1. Incidence

In follow-up of the Nurses' Health Study, women losing 4–10 kg had a 44% increase and those losing over 10 kg had a 94% increase in the risk of gallstones (91). The overall incidence of gallstones ranges up to 25% in the 8–16 weeks after initiation of a weight reduction diet. This association is also found in men, even after adjusting for factors such as initial body mass index (116–120). Liddle et al. found that over 25% of their patients developed gallstones after 8 weeks of a very-low-calorie diet (420 kcal, less than 1 g of fat per day), and another 6% developed biliary sludge, a precursor to gallstones (120). Cho-

lecystectomy became necessary in 6%. Some gallstones resolved spontaneously after the diet was discontinued. In contrast, only 4% of patients given a weight reduction diet containing 800–840 kcal and 13–23 g of fat per day developed gallstones after 10 weeks. Other studies have shown that patients given a diet containing over 10 g of fat per day are at lower risk of gallstone formation, perhaps due to maintenance of gallbladder motility (121–124).

Patients losing weight with either low-calorie diets or bariatric surgery (gastric exclusion or jejunoileal bypass) seem to be at risk (125). One study has shown a 37% incidence of gallstones ultrasonographically 6 months after bariatric surgery. However, the risk for patients after bariatric surgery (up to 38% developing gallstones in the first 6 months postoperatively) have been difficult to separate from the effects of major abdominal surgery, which in itself will inhibit gallbladder motility and induce biliary sludge formation (126–130). A high percentage of patients will also develop biliary sludge in the first postoperative year (126). The risk for gallstone formation is

Table 2 Risk of Gallstone Formation with Weight Reduction

Ref	Study population	Method of weight loss	Diagnostic test	Follow-up period	Percent with gallstones
116	Obese undergoing bariatric surgery	Jejunoileal bypass	US if symptomatic	24 months	Male 10% Female 90%
117	Obese undergoing bariatric surgery	Jejunoileal bypass	Oral Cholecystogram	36 months	10.3%
118	Obese undergoing bariatric surgery	Jejunoileal bypass	US if symptomatic	60 months	20%
120	Obese on low-calorie diet	540-kcal diet	US screening	4 weeks / 8 weeks	7.8% / 25.5%
126	Obese undergoing bariatric surgery	Gastric bypass	US screening	6 months	36%
132	Obese on low-calorie diet	520-kcal diet	US screening	16 weeks	10.9%
133	Obese on low-calorie diet	605-kcal diet	US if symptomatic	6 months	11%
138	Obese undergoing bariatric surgery	Gastric bypass	US screening	6 months / 12 months / 18 months	37% / 37% / 37%
148	Obese undergoing bariatric surgery	Gastric bypass	US screening	3 months	43%

US, ultrasound.

greatest in the first postoperative year, but may be increased for up to 3 years postoperatively, as weight loss continues. Although these periods are coincident with the periods of greatest weight loss and ongoing weight loss, respectively, the risk for gallstone formation does not correlate with any of these parameters. In addition, 90–95% of patients without gallstones on preoperative screening ultrasound will be seen to have gallbladder disease such as chronic cholecystitis or cholesterolosis if routine cholecystectomy is done at the time of surgery (97,98); 24–40% of those developing gallstones will be symptomatic, and about 28% may need repeat surgery for cholecystectomy (97,98,126). Asymptomatic gallstones will resolve in about 50% after 1–2 years. It is not be possible to predict who will develop gallstones on the basis of gallbladder bile acid, cholesterol, or phospholipid concentrations, or cholesterol saturation index, although some suggestion has been made that patients who form sludge have a lower percentage of cholesterol, a lower cholesterol-to-phospholipid ratio, and a lower cholesterol saturation index (117,125,129–132). Acute cholecystitis or pancreatitis has been reported as a consequence of these gallstones.

2. Risk Factors

Both initial BMI and the absolute rate of weight loss are predictors of gallstone development (132). The effect of initial BMI has only been proven in men. Higher relative weight loss also seems to be a risk factor. Absolute weight loss is more difficult to assess, as it is highly dependent on initial BMI (132). Likewise, the rapidity of weight loss has not been established as a definite risk factor due to confounding with absolute and relative amounts of weight lost. Higher rates of gallstone formation during weight loss are seen in men. However, this effect is removed when controlling for the higher initial BMI, relative BMI lost, and initial serum triglycerides seen in obese men as compared with obese women (132). High serum triglycerides are a risk factor in some, but not all, studies (132,133). Diets in which gallbladder motility is maintained, such as diets with higher caloric or fat contents, do not seem to be associated with as great a risk of gallstone formation (121,124). No studies have looked at effects of repeated weight loss or weight loss due to increases in physical activity in relation to gallstone formation.

3. Effects of Refeeding

Studies of cholesterol saturation after entering a weight maintenance phase have shown stabilization of the cholesterol saturation index (CSI) at a level lower than the initial value. Absolute output of cholesterol, bile acids, and phospholipids is lower than in the obese phase. The total bile acid pool again increases during weight maintenance. Again, the individual bile acid profile does not change (134).

B. Pathophysiology of Gallstone Formation During Weight Loss

Changes in bile composition that lead to increased lithogenicity are seen with very-low-calorie diets. CSI in bile increases on average during weight reduction (119,122,124,134–138). However, this effect is not seen in all subjects studied; some patients have large increases, and others large decreases in saturation index. CSI and nucleation time decrease in nearly all patients after a prolonged fast. It is felt that hepatic cholesterol secretion increases during weight loss and decreases again during weight maintenance. Similarly, the molar percentage of cholesterol increases during the weight loss phase and decreases in the weight maintenance phase (126,134–138). The excess excreted cholesterol during weight loss is mobilized from peripheral adipose tissue. Counteracting these factors is the fact that low caloric intake lowers cholesterol input and may reduce bile acid secretion and cholesterol synthesis. Biliary cholesterol secretion will reflect a balance of all these variables. In the weight stabilization phase after a low-calorie diet, CSI decreases to below the baseline value. Nucleation time decreases concurrently with these changes (136).

Bile acid and phospholipid secretion do not reliably change with weight loss, but generally are lower (113,137–139). The total bile acid pool decreases during weight reduction, but the individual bile acid profile does not change (113). If patients regain weight, the cholesterol saturation index and molar percentage of cholesterol will again increase (140). In weight loss induced after jejunoileal bypass, similar changes in bile composition and lithogenicity are noted. Bile salt pool is initially reduced, and saturation index increased. However, bile composition reverts to normal by about 1 year postoperatively (136,137). This suggests that these changes are not due entirely to ileal bypass.

Changes in bile composition also occur after bariatric surgery. Biliary bile salt concentration increases significantly, and cholesterol and phospholipid concentrations slightly. Molar percentage of cholesterol increases during weight loss and decreases again at weight stabilization. Marked increase in gallbladder mucin is seen postoperatively, then declining slowly back to baseline levels (137–140). Total and free biliary calcium also increase postoperatively, preceding gallstone formation (137,141).

In patients with jejunoileal bypass, absorption of bile salts is reduced as the effective length of the terminal ileum is reduced, with subsequent reduction in the circulating pool.

Alterations in gallbladder motility are seen with weight reduction. Decreases in gallbladder motility are seen after major abdominal surgery. With gastric bypass, gallbladder hypomotility may be induced because of intraoperative transection of the hepatic branch of the vagus nerve during mobilization of the liver (31,124,125,127–130). Many of these changes in bile composition that are seen in weight reduction could be a reflection of this gallbladder stasis, rather than a direct result of alterations in hepatic secretion or gallbladder mucosal function. With very-low-calorie diets, increased fasting and residual gallbladder volumes can be seen. This effect may be reversed by inclusion of adequate calories (over 800 kcal/day) or dietary fat (over 10g/day) to maximally stimulate gallbladder contractility (121–123).

C. Preventive Measures

1. Screening for Gallstones Prior to Weight Reduction

Patients undergoing bariatric surgery are routinely screened with preoperative ultrasound to determine the need for concomitant cholecystectomy. These studies have shown an incidence of gallstones up to 25% preoperatively (97,98). However, preoperative ultrasound has a low sensitivity for gallbladder disease in the obese and may not be the best test to determine need for cholecystectomy. Some have advocated screening for gallbladder disease prior to weight-reduction dieting and possibly dietary modification if gallstones are found. However, this approach has not been studied systematically (125). It is not known if patients with preexisting cholelithiasis are at higher risk of complications, such as acute cholecystitis or pancreatitis, with weight reduction.

2. Prophylactic Cholecystectomy

Some authors have advocated prophylactic cholecystectomy at the time of bariatric surgery, due to the greater than 30% incidence of gallstones in the initial period of rapid weight loss. Ten to twenty-five percent of patients who have not had a prior cholecystectomy will already have gallstones at the time of surgery, and 95% of patients undergoing cholecystectomy at bariatric surgery will have pathological evidence of gallbladder disease (97,98). Preoperative ultrasound has low sensitivity for a calculous cholecystitis, cholesterolosis, and gallstones in the obese, and thus has not been a reliable screening test in these

patients. Cholecystectomy adds only minimally to procedure time (30–45 min), and patients undergoing prophylactic cholecystectomy have not had a higher incidence of perioperative complications or a longer hospital stay. Many centers have moved to routinely performing cholecystectomy at the time of gastric bypass surgery (97,98). Prophylactic cholecystectomy before initiation of a weight reduction diet has not been advocated.

3. Bile Acid Supplementation During Weight Loss

Bile acid supplementation has been used as a nonsurgical treatment for gallstones. Certain bile acids, chenodeoxycholic acid (CDCA) and its stereoisomer ursodeoxycholic acid (UDCA), contribute to cholesterol solubilization and can decrease bile lithogenicity. Bile acid supplementation is generally well tolerated and without significant adverse effects.

In the nonobese, treatment with CDCA desaturates bile and prolongs nucleation times (16,142). However, this effect is not seen consistently in the obese, even with the same doses per kilogram being administered (113,14,143–146). Biliary cholesterol concentrations and saturation indexes reliably decrease to unsaturated ranges only with high-dose therapy (143–146). Rates of phospholipid and bile acid secretion do not change with treatment (113). HMG CoA reductase activity is reduced during CDCA therapy, with subsequent reduction in hepatic cholesterol synthesis and secretion (113). However, CDCA is a potent inhibitor of cholesterol 7α-hydroxylase and thus decreases cholesterol catabolism. With oral therapy, this bile acid can increase the total bile acid pool and the rate of bile acid secretion and, in fact, becomes the predominant circulating bile acid. Because higher doses per kilogram of CDCA are often needed to cause bile desaturation, some have recommended that duodenal bile composition be monitored in obese patients treated with bile acids to ensure adequate therapy (143,144). Although it has beneficial effects on bile composition, CDCA may increase gallbladder mucin secretion and potentially enhance cholesterol crystal nucleation (52–54).

Currently, the use of UDCA has superseded that of CDCA. UDCA is safe and effective. Treatment with UDCA prolongs nucleation times and decreases the concentration of cholesterol and phospholipid present in the vesicular phase, having a greater effect than CDCA (16,143–148). Gallbladder bile from patients treated with UDCA contains only a trace of cholesterol in vesicles, the more lithogenic form of transport (149). Similar to CDCA, UDCA decreases biliary cholesterol concentration by decreasing activity of hepatic HMG CoA reductase (113). It has no effect on the activity of cholesterol 7α-hydroxylase, the rate-limiting enzyme in bile acid synthesis. The molar percentage of bile acids is unchanged to slightly increased with UDCA, and UDCA becomes the predominant bile acid during therapy (113,147,148). All these factors combined indicate that UDCA may have a role in prophylaxis or treatment of gallstones in the obese. One study giving UDCA at 1200 mg/day during weight reduction dieting showed that bile significantly desaturates during therapy, and that 0 of 23 patients receiving UDCA developed gallstones, microstones, or crystals (148,150). UDCA has been more effective in gallstone dissolution than CDCA in nonobese and obese patients, probably because of the unreliable decline in bile saturation with CDCA. However, one study has shown that combination CDCA and UDCA therapy may be more effective than either alone in reducing cholesterol concentration and cholesterol saturation index (146).

4. Other Pharmacological Measures

One study looking at high-dose aspirin (1300 mg/day) showed that none of 22 patients receiving aspirin developed gallstones during weight-reducing diet. Three of these patients developed microstones or crystals (150). However, there was no change in the saturation index, cholesterol concentration, bile acid concentration, or biliary glycoprotein concentration. Other studies have shown a possible effect of nonsteroidal anti-inflammatory drugs in inhibiting gallstone recurrence after dissolution therapy (151). Although mucin secretion and prostaglandin metabolism may be modified by nonsteroidal anti-inflammatory drugs, the long-term clinical use of these compounds can be associated with substantial complications. The feasibility of this approach in clinical practice is far from established.

V. SUMMARY

Gallstones are a common clinical problem in the obese and the nonobese. Three separate conditions are required for gallstone formation: secretion of supersaturated bile, nucleation of cholesterol crystals, and gallbladder stasis. In obesity, bile is more saturated owing to cholesterol hypersecretion, and gallbladder motor function is impaired, predisposing to gallstone formation. Paradoxically, weight reduction either through dietary modification or through bariatric surgery also predisposes to gallstone formation. The mechanisms of gallstone formation during weight reduction are not entirely clear, but also involve altered bile composition and gallbladder motility. UDCA is the only medical therapy that has been studied for gallstones during weight reduction. Further research needs to be done

into the risk factors for and treatment of gallstone disease and its prevention in the obese and in those losing weight.

REFERENCES

1. Scharschmidt BF. Bilirubin metabolism, bile formation, and gallbladder and bile duct function. In: Sleisinger MH, Fordtran JS, eds. Gastrointestinal Disease: Pathophysiology, Diagnosis, Management. Philadelphia: WB Saunders, 1993:1730–1746.
2. Cooper AD. Epidemiology, pathogenesis, natural history, and medical therapy of gallstones. In: Sleisinger MH, Fordtran JS, eds. Gastrointestinal Disease: Pathophysiology, Diagnosis, Management. Philadelphia: WB Saunders, 1993:1788–1804.
3. Somjen GJ, Gilat T. A non-micellar mode of cholesterol transport in human bile. FEBS Lett 1983; 156:265–168.
4. Reuben A. Bile formation: sites and mechanisms. Hepatology 1984; 4:15S–24S.
5. Smit JJM, Schinkel AH, Oude Elferink RPJ, et al. Homozygous disruption of the murine mdr2 P-glycoprotein gene leads to a complete absence of phospholipid from bile and to liver disease. Cell 1993; 75:451–462.
6. Smith AJ, Timmermans-Hereijgers JL, Roelofsen B. The human MDR3 P-glycoprotein promotes translocation of phosphatidylcholine through the plasma membrane of fibroblasts from transgenic mice. FEBS Lett 1994; 354: 263–266.
7. Reuben A. Biliary proteins. Hepatology 1984; 4:46S–50S.
8. Admirand WH, Small DM. The physiochemical basis of cholesterol gallstone formation in man. J Clin Invest 1968; 47:1043–1052.
9. Carey MC, Small DM. The physical chemistry of cholesterol solubility in bile: relationship to gallstone formation and dissolution in man. J Clin Invest 1978; 61:998–1026.
10. Lee SP, Park HZ, Madani H, Kaler EW. Partial characterization of a nonmicellar system of cholesterol solubilization in bile. Am J Physiol 1987; 252:G374–383.
11. Halpern Z, Dudley MA, Kibe A, Lynn MP, Breuer AC, Holzbach RT. Rapid vesicle formation and aggregation in abnormal human biles. A time-lapse video-enhanced contrast microscopy study. Gastroenterology 1986; 90: 875–885.
12. Kibe A, Dudley MA, Halpern Z, Lynn MP, Breuer AC, Holzbach RT. Factors affecting cholesterol monohydrate crystal nucleation time in model systems of supersaturated bile. J Lipid Res 1985; 26:1102–1111.
13. Halpern Z, Dudley MA, Lynn MP, Nader JM, Breuer AC, Holzbach RT. Vesicle aggregation in model systems of supersaturated bile: relation to crystal nucleation and lipid composition of the vesicular phase. J Lipid Res 1986; 27: 295–306.
14. Somjen GJ, Marikovsky Y, Lekles P, Gilat T. Cholesterol-phospholipid vesicles in human bile: an ultrastructural study. Biochim Biophys Acta 1986; 879:14–21.

15. Carey MC, Conrad DE. Biliary transport of cholesterol in vesicles, micelles and liquid crystals. In: Paumgartner G, Stiehl A, Gerok W, eds. Bile Acids and the Liver. Lancaster: MTP Press, 1987:287–300.

16. Hirota I, Chijiiwa K, Noshiro H, Nakayama F. Effect of chenodeoxycholate and ursodeoxycholate on nucleation time in human gallbladder bile. Gastroenterology 1992; 102:1668–1674.

17. Zhao XT, Schoenfield LJ, Bonorris GG, VanDeVelde RL, Marks JW. Increased cholesterol in vesicles is associated with rapid nucleation of human gallbladder bile. Hepatology 1994; 20:117A (abstract).

18. Holzbach RT. Recent progress in understanding cholesterol crystal nucleation as a precursor to human gallstone formation. Hepatology 1986; 6:1403–1406.

19. Holzbach RT, Halpern Z, Dudley MA, et al. Biliary vesicle aggregation and cholesterol crystal nucleation: evidence for a coupled relationship. In: Paumgartner G, Stiehl A, Gerok W, eds. Bile Acids and the Liver. Lancaster: MTP, 1987:301–316.

20. Long MA, Kaler EW, Lee SP. Structural characterization of the micelle-vesicle transition in lecithin-bile salt solutions. Biophys J 1994; 67:1733–42.

21. Little TE, Lee SP, Madani H, Kaler EW, Chinn K. Inter-conversions of lipid aggregates in rat and model bile. Am J Physiol 1991; 260:G70–79.

22. Pattison NR, Chapman BA. Distribution of biliary cholesterol between mixed micelles and nonmicelles in relation to fasting and feeding in humans. Gastroenterology 1986; 91:697–702.

23. Tierney S, Pitt HA, Lillemoe KD. Physiology and pathophysiology of gallbladder motility. Surg Clin North Am 1993; 73:1276–1290.

24. Cameron AJ, Phillips SF, Summerskill WH. Effect of cholecystokinin, gastrin, secretin, and glucagon on human gallbladder in vitro. Proc Soc Exp Biol Med 1969; 131:149–154.

25. Kalfin R, Milenov K. The effect of vasoactive intestinal polypeptide (VIP) on the canine gallbladder motility. Comp Biochem Physiol 1991; 100:513–517.

26. Fridhandler TM, Davison JS, Shaffer EA. Defective gallbladder contractility in the ground squirrel and prairie dog during the early stages of cholesterol gallstone formation. Gastroenterology 1983; 85:830–836.

27. Behar J, Lee KY, Thompson WR, Biancani P. Gallbladder contraction in patients with pigment and cholesterol stones. Gastroenterology 1989; 97:1479–1484.

28. Pomeranz IS, Shaffer EA. Abnormal gallbladder emptying in a subgroup of patients with gallstones. Gastroenterology 1985; 88:797–791.

29. Palasciano G, Serio G, Portincasa P, et al. Gallbladder volume in adults, and relationship to age, sex, body mass index, and gallstones: a sonographic population study. Am J Gastroenterol 1992; 87:493–497.

30. Kucio C, Besser P, Jonderko K. Gallbladder motor function in obese versus lean females. Eur J Clin Nutr 1988; 42:121–124.

31. Marzio L, Capone F, Neri M, Mezzetti A, de Angelis C, Cuccurullo F. Gallbladder kinetics in obese patients. Effect of a regular meal and low-calorie meal. Dig Dis Sci 1988; 1:4–9.

32. Vezina WC, Paradis RL, Grace DM, et al. Increased volume and decreased emptying of the gallbladder in large (morbidly obese, tall normal, and muscular normal) people. Gastroenterology 1990; 98:1000–1007.

33. Glasbrenner G, Dominguez-Munoz J, Nelson DK, et al. Postprandial release of cholecystokinin and pancreatic polypeptide in health and in gallstone disease: relationships with gallbladder contraction. Am J Gastroenterol 1994; 89:404–410.

34. Cano N, Cicero F, Ranieri F, Martin J, di Costanzo J. Ultrasonographic study of gallbladder motility during total parenteral nutrition. Gastroenterology 1986; 91:313–317.

35. Messing B, Bories C, Kunstlinger F, Bernier JJ. Does total parenteral nutrition induce gallbladder sludge formation and lithiasis? Gastroenterology 1983; 84:1012–1019.

36. Fisher RS, Koch E, Levin G. Effects of somatostatin on gallbladder emptying. Gastroenterology 1987; 92:88–90.

37. Johansson C, Kollberg B, Efendic S, Uvnaswallenstein K. Effects of graded dose of somatostatin on gallbladder emptying and pancreatic enzyme output after oral glucose in man. Digestion 1981; 22:24–31.

38. Davis M, Ryan J. Influence of progesterone on guinea pig gallbladder motility in vivo. Dig Dis Sci 1986; 31:513–518.

39. Ryan J, Pellechia D. Effect of progesterone on guinea pig gallbladder motility in vitro. Gastroenterology 1982; 83:81–83.

40. Diamond JM. Transport of salt and water in rabbit and guinea pig gallbladder. J Gen Physiol 1964; 48:1–14.

41. Dietschy JM. Water and electrolyte movement across the wall of the everted rabbit gallbladder. Gastroenterology 1964; 47:395–408.

42. Wood JR, Svanvik J. Gall-bladder water and electrolyte transport and its regulation. Gut 1983; 24:579–593.

43. Schiffman ML, Sugerman HJ, Moore EW. Human gallbladder mucosal function. Effect of concentration and acidification of bile on cholesterol and calcium solubility. Gastroenterology 1990; 99:1452–1459.

44. van Erpecum KJ, van Berge Henegouwen GP, Stoelwinder B, Schmidt YMG, Willekens FLH. Bile concentration is a key factor for nucleation of cholesterol crystals and cholesterol saturation index in gallbladder bile of gallstone patients. Hepatology 1990; 11:1–6.

45. Gleeson D, Hood KA, Murphy GM, Dowling RH. Calcium and carbonate ion concentrations in gallbladder and hepatic bile. Gastroenterology 1992; 102:1707–1716.

46. Lee SP. The mechanism of mucus secretion by the gallbladder epithelium. Br J Exp Pathol 1980; 61:117–119.

47. Smith BF. Human gallbladder mucin binds biliary lipids and promotes cholesterol crystal nucleation in model bile. J Lipid Res 1987; 28:1088–1097.

48. Levy PF, Smith BF, LaMont JT. Human gallbladder mucin accelerates nucleation of cholesterol in artificial bile. Gastroenterology 1984; 87:270–275.

49. Gallinger S, Taylor RD, Harvey PRC, Petrunka CN, Strasberg SM. Effect of mucous glycoprotein on nucleation time of human bile. Gastroenterology 1985; 89:648–658.

50. Lee TJ, Smith BF. Bovine gallbladder mucin promotes cholesterol crystal nucleation from cholesterol-transporting vesicles in supersaturated bile. J Lipid Res 1989; 30: 491–498.

51. Doty JE, Pitt HA, Kuchenbecker SL, Porter-Fink V, DenBesten LW. Role of gallbladder mucus in the pathogenesis of cholesterol gallstones. Am J Surg 1983; 145: 54–61.

52. Lee SP. Hypersecretion of mucus glycoprotein by the gallbladder epithelium in experimental cholelithiasis. J Pathol 1981; 134:199–207.

53. Lee SP, LaMont JT, Carey MC. Role of gallbladder mucus hypersecretion in the evolution of cholesterol gallstones. J Clin Invest 1981; 67:1712–1733.

54. LaMont JT, Turner BS, DiBenedetto D, Handin R, Schafer S. Arachidonic acid stimulates mucin secretion in prairie dog gallbladder. Am J Physiol 1983; 235:G92–G98.

55. Conter RL, Washington JL, Liao CC, Kauffman GL. Gallbladder mucosal blood flow increases during early cholesterol gallstone formation. Gastroenterology 1992; 102: 1764–1770.

56. Smith BF, LaMont JT. Identification of gallbladder mucin-bilirubin complex in human cholesterol gallstone matrix. Effects of reducing agents on in vitro dissolution of matrix and intact gallstones. J Clin Invest 1985; 76:439–445.

57. Murray FE, Smith BF. Non-mucin proteins in the matrix of human cholesterol gallstones. Scand J Gastroenterol 1991; 26:717–723.

58. Shimizu S, Sabsay B, Veis A, Ostrow JD, Dawes LG, Rege RV. A 12 kDa protein from cholesterol gallstones inhibits precipitation of calcium carbonate and is present in human bile. Hepatology 1988; 8:1257A (abstract).

59. Afdal NH, Gong D, Niu N, Turner B, LaMont JT, Offner GD. Cholesterol cholelithiasis in the prairie dog: role of mucin and nonmucin glycoproteins. Hepatology 1993; 17:693–700.

60. Marks JW, Bonorris GG, Albers G, Schoenfield LJ. The sequence of biliary events preceding the formation of gallstones in humans. Gastroenterology 1992; 103:566–570.

61. Little TE, Madani H, Lee SP, Kaler EW. Lipid vesicle fusion induced by phospholipase C activity in model bile. J Lipid Res 1993; 34:211–217.

62. Luk AS, Kaler EW, Lee SP. Phospholipase C-induced aggregation and fusion of cholesterol-lecithin small unilamellar vesicles. Biochemistry 1993; 32:6965–6973.

63. Groen AK, Noordam C, Drapers JAG, Egbers P, Jansen PLM, Tytgat NJ. Isolation of a potent cholesterol nuclea-tion promoting activity from human gallbladder bile. Hepatology 1990; 11:523–533.

64. Groen AK, Stout JPJ, Drapers JAG, Hoek FJ, Grijm R, Tytgat NJ. Cholesterol-nucleation promoting activity in T-tube bile. Hepatology 1988; 8:347–352.

65. Harvey PRC, Uphadya GA, Strasberg SM. Immunoglobulins as nucleation proteins in the gallbladder bile of patients with cholesterol gallstones. J Biol Chem 1991; 266: 13996–14003.

66. Holzbach RT, Kibe A, Thiel E, Howell JH, Marsh M, Hermann RE. Biliary proteins. Unique inhibitors of cholesterol crystal nucleation in human gallbladder bile. J Clin Invest 1984; 73:35–45.

67. Kibe A, Holzbach RT, LaRusso NF, Mao SJT. Inhibition of cholesterol crystal formation by apolipoproteins in supersaturated model bile. Science 1984; 225:514–516.

68. Strasberg SM, Toth JL, Gallinger S, Harvey PRC. High protein and total lipid concentration are associated with reduced metastability of bile in an early stage of cholesterol gallstone formation. Gastroenterology 1990; 98: 739–746.

69. Whiting MJ, Watts JM. Supersaturated bile from obese patients without gallstones supports cholesterol crystal growth but not nucleation. Gastroenterology 1984; 86: 243–248.

70. GREPCO. The epidemiology of gallstone disease in Rome, Italy. Part I. Prevalence data in men. Hepatology 1988; 8: 904–906.

71. Huang WS. Cholelithiasis in Singapore. Gut 1970; 11: 141–147.

72. Sampliner RE, Bennett PH, Comess LJ, Rose FA, Burch TA. Gallbladder disease in Pima Indians: demonstration of high prevalence and early onset by cholecystography. N Engl J Med 1970; 283:1358–1364.

73. Stitnimankarn T. The necropsy incidence of gallstones in Thailand. Am J Med Sci 1960; 240:349–352.

74. Einarsson K, Nilsell K, Leijd B, Angelin B. Influence of age on secretion of cholesterol and synthesis of bile acids by the liver. N Engl J Med 1985; 313:277–282.

75. GREPCO. The epidemiology of gallstone disease in Rome, Italy. Part II. Factors associated with the disease. Hepatology 1988; 8:907–913.

76. Friedman GD, Kannel WB, Dawber TR. The epidemiology of gallbladder disease: observations in the Framingham Study. J Chronic Dis 1966; 19:273–292.

77. Sastic JW, Glassman GI. Gallbladder disease in young women. Surg Gynecol Obstet 1982; 155:209–211.

78. Everson GT, McKinley C, Kern F Jr. Mechanisms of gallstone formation in women. Effects of exogenous estrogen (Premarin) and dietary cholesterol on hepatic lipid metabolism. J Clin Invest 1991; 87:237–246.

79. Henriksson P, Einarsson K, Erikson A, Kelter U, Angelin B. Estrogen-induced gallstone formation in males. J Clin Invest 1989; 84:811–816.

80. Kono S, Shinchi K, Ikeda N, Yanai F, Imanishi K. Prevalence of gallstone disease in relation to smoking, alcohol

use, obesity, and glucose tolerance: a study of Self-Defense officials in Japan. Am J Epidemiol 1992; 136:787–94.

81. Kono S, Kochi S, Ohyama S, Wakisaka A. Gallstones, serum lipids, and glucose tolerance among male officials of Self-Defense Forces in Japan. Dig Dis Sci 1988; 33: 839–844.

82. Lu SN, Chang WY, Wang LY, et al. Risk factors for gallstones among Chinese in Taiwan: a community sonographic survey. J Clin Gastroenterol 1990; 12:542–546.

83. Thijs C, Knipschild P, Brombacher P. Serum lipids and gallstones: a case-control study. Gastroenterology 1990; 99:843–849.

84. Laakso M, Suhonen M, Julkunen R, Pyorala K. Plasma insulin, serum lipids and lipoproteins in gall stone disease in non-insulin dependent diabetic subjects: a case control study. Gut 1990; 31:344–347.

85. Halpern Z, Rubin M, Harach G, et al. Bile and plasma lipid composition in non-obese normolipidemic subjects with and without cholesterol gallstones. Liver 1993; 13: 246–252.

86. Kato I, Nomura A, Stemmerman GN, Chyou PH. Prospective study of clinical gallbladder disease and its association with obesity, physical activity, and other factors. Dig Dis Sci 1992; 37:784–790.

87. Stampfer MJ, Maclure KM, Colditz GA, Manson JE, Willett WC. Risk of symptomatic gallstones in women with severe obesity. Am J Clin Nutr 1992; 55:652–658.

88. Bennion LJ, Grundy SM. Effects of obesity and caloric intake on biliary lipid metabolism in man. J Clin Invest 1975; 56:996–1011.

89. Kern F Jr. Effects of dietary cholesterol on cholesterol and bile acid homeostasis in patients with cholesterol gallstones. J Clin Invest 1994; 93:1186–1194.

90. Tucker LE, Tangedahl TN, Newmark SR. Prevalence of gallstones in obese Caucasian American women. Int J Obes 1982; 6:247–251.

91. Maclure KM, Hayes KC, Colditz GA, Stampfer MJ, Speizer FE, Willett WC. Weight, diet, and the risk of symptomatic gallstones in middle-aged women. N Engl J Med 1989; 321:563–569.

92. Thijs C, Knipschild P, Leffers P. Is gallstone disease caused by obesity or by dieting? Am J Epidemiol 1992; 135: 274–280.

93. Palasciano G, Portincasa P, Vinciguerra V, et al. Gallstone prevalence and gallbladder volume in children and adolescents: an epidemiological ultrasonographic survey and relationship to body mass index. Am J Gastroenterol 1989; 84:1378–1382.

94. Pettiti DB, Sidney S. Obesity and cholecystectomy among women: implications for prevention. Am J Prev Med 1988; 4:327–330.

95. Honore LH. Cholesterol cholelithiasis in adolescent females. Arch Surg 1980; 115:62–64.

96. Weatherall R, Shaper AG. Overweight and obesity in middle-aged British men. Eur J Clin Nutr 1988; 42:221–231.

97. Amaral JF, Thompson WR. Gallbladder disease in the morbidly obese. Am J Surg 1985; 149:551–557.

98. Calhoun R, Willbanks O. Coexistence of gallbladder disease and morbid obesity. Am J Surg 1987; 154:655–658.

99. Haffner SM, Diehl AK, Stern MP, Hazuda HP. Central adiposity and gallbladder disease in Mexican Americans. Am J Epidemiol 1989; 129:587–595.

100. Samet JM, Coultas DB, Howard CA, Skipper BJ, Hanis CL. Diabetes, Gallbladder disease, obesity, and hypertension among Hispanics in New Mexico. Am J Epidemiol 1988; 128:1302–1311.

101. Moerman CJ, Berns MPH, Smeets FWM, Kromhout D. Regional fat distribution as risk factor for clinically diagnosed gallstones in middle-aged men: a 25-year follow-up study (the Zutphen Study). Int J Obes 1994; 18: 435–439.

102. Hartz AJ, Rupley DC, Rimm AA. The association of girth measurements with disease in 32,856 women. Am J Epidemiol 1984; 119:71–80.

103. Nestel PJ, Schreibman PH, Ahrens EH. Cholesterol metabolism in human obesity. J Clin Invest 1973; 52: 2389–2397.

104. Nestel J, Whyte HM, Goodman DWS. Distribution and turnover of cholesterol in humans. J Clin Invest 1969; 48:982–991.

105. Miettinen TA. Cholesterol production in obesity. Circulation 1971; 44:842–850.

106. Stamler J. Overweight, hypertension, hypercholesterolemia, and coronary heart disease. In: Mancini M, Lewis B, Contaldo F, eds. Medical Complications of Obesity. London: Academic Press, 1979:191–216.

107. Madura JA, Loomis RC, Harris RA, Grosfeld J, Tompkins RK. Relationship of obesity to bile lithogenicity in man. Ann Surg 1978; 189:106–111.

108. Angelin B, Einarsson K, Ewerth S, Leijd B. Biliary lipid composition in obesity. Scand J Gastroenterol 1981; 16: 1015–1019.

109. Mabee TM, Meyer P, DenBesten L, Mason EE. The mechanism of increased gallstone formation in obese human subjects. Surgery 1976; 79:460–468.

110. Reuben A, Maton PN, Murphy GM, Dowling RH. Bile lipid secretion in obese and non-obese individuals with and without gallstones. Clin Sci 1985; 69:71–79.

111. Salen GS, Nicolau G, Shefer S, Mosbach EH. Hepatic cholesterol metabolism in patients with gallstones. Gastroenterology 1975; 69:676–684.

112. Marcus SN, Heaton KW. Deoxycholic acid and the pathogenesis of gallstones. Gut 1988; 29:522–533.

113. Mok HYI, von Bergman K, Crouse JR, Grundy SM. Biliary lipid metabolism in obesity. Effects of bile acid feeding before and during weight reduction. Gastroenterology 1979; 76:556–567.

114. Einarsson K, Hellstrom K, Kallner M. Bile acid kinetics in relation to sex, serum lipids, body weights, and gallbladder disease in patients with various types of hyperlipoproteinemia. J Clin Invest 1974; 54:1301–1311.

115. Grundy SM, Duane WC, Adler RD, Aron JM, Metzger AL. Biliary lipid outputs in young women with cholesterol gallstones. Metabolism 1974; 23:67–73.

116. DeWind LT, Payne JH. Intestinal bypass surgery for morbid obesity. Long-term results. JAMA 1976; 236: 2298–2301.

117. Delaney AG, Duerson MC, O'Leary JP. The incidence of cholelithiasis after jejunoileal bypass. Int J Obes 1980; 4: 243–248.

118. Hocking MP, Duerson MC, O'Leary JP, Woodward ER. Jejunoileal bypass for morbid obesity. Late follow-up in 100 cases. N Engl J Med 1983; 308:995–999.

119. Wise L, Stein T. The effect of jejunoileal bypass on bile composition and the formation of biliary calculi. Ann Surg 1978; 187:57–62.

120. Liddle RA, Goldstein RB, Saxton J. Gallstone formation during weight reduction dieting. Arch Intern Med 1989; 149:1750–1753.

121. Hoy MK, Heshka S, Allison DB, et al. Reduced risk of liver-function-test abnormalities and new gallstone formation with weight loss on 3350-kJ (800-kcal) formula diets. Am J Clin Nutr 1994; 60:249–254.

122. Gebhard RL, Prigge WF, Ansel HJ, et al. Rapid weight loss, gallbladder function and cholesterol gallstones. Hepatology 1994; 20:267A (abstract).

123. Stone BG, Ansel HJ, Peterson FJ, Gebhard RL. Gallbladder emptying stimuli in obese and normal-weight subjects. Hepatology 1992; 15:795–798.

124. Festi D, Orsini M, Li Bassi S, et al. Risk of gallstone formation during rapid weight loss: protective role of gallbladder motility. Gastroenterology 193; 102:A311 (abstract).

125. Andersen T. Liver and gallbladder disease before and after very-low-calorie diets. Am J Clin Nutr 1992; 56:235S–239S.

126. Shiffman ML, Sugerman HJ, Kellum JM, Brewer WH, Moore EW. Gallstone formation after rapid weight loss: a prospective study in patients undergoing gastric bypass surgery for treatment of morbid obesity. Am J Gastroenterol 1991; 86:1000–1005.

127. Inoue K, Fuchigami A, Higashide S, et al. Gallbladder sludge and stone formation in relation to contractile function after gastrectomy. Ann Surg 1992; 215:19–26.

128. Little JM, Avramovic J. Gallstone formation after major abdominal surgery. Lancet 1991; 337:1135–1137.

129. Takahashi T, Yamamura T, Utsunomiya J. Pathogenesis of acute cholecystitis after gastrectomy. Br J Surg 1990; 77: 536–539.

130. Bolondi L, Gaiani S, Testa S, Labo G. Gallbladder sludge formation during prolonged fasting after gastrointestinal surgery. Gut 1985; 26:734–738.

131. Schiffman ML, Sugerman HJ, Kellum JH, Brewer WH, Moore EW. Gallstones in patients with morbid obesity. Relationship to body weight, weight loss and gallbladder bile cholesterol solubility. Int J Obes 1993; 17:153–158.

132. Yang H, Peterson GM, Roth MP, Schoenfield LJ, Marks JW. Risk factors for gallstone formation during rapid loss of weight. Dig Dis Sci 1992; 37:912–918.

133. Kamrath KO, Plummer LJ, Sadur CN, et al. Cholelithiasis in patients treated with a very low-caloric diet. Am J Clin Nutr 1992; 56:225S–227S.

134. Reuben A, Qureshi Y, Murphy GM, Dowling RH. Effect of obesity and weight reduction on biliary cholesterol saturation and the response to chenodeoxycholic acid. Eur J Clin Invest 1985; 16:133–142.

135. Schlierf G, Schellenberg B, Stiehl A, Czygan P, Oster P. Biliary cholesterol saturation and weight reduction—effects of fasting and low calorie diet. Digestion 1981; 21: 44–49.

136. Soorensen TIA, Bruusgaard A, Pederson LR, Krag E. Lithogenic index of bile after jejunoileal bypass operation for obesity. Scand J Gastroenterol 1977; 12:449–451.

137. Shiffman ML, Sugerman HJ, Kellum JM, Moore EW. Changes in gallbladder bile composition following gallstone formation and weight reduction. Gastroenterology 1992; 103:214–221.

138. Shiffman ML, Sugerman HJ, Kellum JM, Brewer WH, Engle K, Moore EW. Gallstone formation following rapid weight loss. I. Incidence of gallstone formation and relation to gallbladder (GB) bile lipid composition. Gastroenterology 1990; 90:A262 (abstract).

139. Shiffman ML, Shamburek RD, Schwartz CC, Sugerman HJ, Kellum JM, Moore EW. Gallbladder mucin, arachidonic acid, and bile lipids in patients who develop gallstones during weight reduction. Gastroenterology 1993; 105:1200–1208.

140. Freeman JB, Meyer PD, Printen KJ, Mason EE, DenBesten L. Analysis of gallbladder bile in morbid obesity. Am J Surg 1975; 129:163–166.

141. Shiffman ML, Kellum JM, Sugerman HJ, Moore EW. Gallstone (GS) formation following rapid weight loss. II. Free Ca^{++} ion in gallbladder (GB) increases prior to appearance. Gastroenterology 1990; 98:A262 (abstract).

142. Danzinger RG, Hofmann AF, Thistle JL, et al. Effect of oral chenodeoxycholic acid on bile acid kinetics and biliary lipid composition in women with cholelithiasis. J Clin Invest 1983; 52:2809–2821.

143. Mazzella G, Bazzoli F, Festi D, et al. Comparative evaluation of chenodeoxycholic and ursodeoxycholic acids in obese patients. Effects of biliary lipid metabolism during weight maintenance and weight reduction. Gastroenterology 1991; 101:490–496.

144. Iser JH, Maton PN, Murphy GM, Dowling RH. Resistance to chenodeoxycholic acid (CDCA) treatment in obese patients with gallstones. Br Med J 1978; 1:1509–1512.

145. Maton PN, Murphy GM, Dowling RH. Lack of response to chenodeoxycholic acid in obese and non-obese patients. Gut 1980; 21:1082–1086.

146. Whiting MJ, Hall JC, Iannos J, Roberts HG, Watts JM. The cholesterol saturation of bile and its reduction by

chenodeoxycholic acid in massively obese patients. Int J Obes 1984; 8:681–688.

147. Zuin M, Petroni ML, Grandinetti G, et al. Comparison of effects of chenodeoxycholic and ursodeoxycholic acid and their combination on biliary lipids in obese patients with gallstones. Scand J Gastroenterol 1991; 26:257–262.

148. Worobetz LJ, Inglis FG, Shaffer EA. The effect of ursodeoxycholic acid therapy on gallstone formation in the morbidly obese during rapid weight loss. Am J Gastroenterol 1993; 88:1705–1710.

149. Okamoto S, Nakano K, Kosahara K, et al. Effects of pravastatin and ursodeoxycholic acid on cholesterol and bile acid metabolism in patients with cholesterol gallstones. J Gastroenterol 1994; 29:47–55.

150. Broomfield PH, Chopra R, Sheinbaum RC, et al. Effects of ursodeoxycholic acid and aspirin on the formation of lithogenic bile and gallstones during loss of weight. N Engl J Med 1988; 319:1567–1572.

151. Hood K, Gleeson D, Ruppin DC, Dowling RH. Prevention of gallstone recurrence by non-steroidal anti-inflammatory drugs. Lancet 1988; 2:1223–1225.

34

Obesity and Pulmonary Function

Kingman P. Strohl
Case Western Reserve University, Cleveland, Ohio

Richard J. Strobel and Richard A. Parisi
University of Medicine and Dentistry of New Jersey and Robert Wood Johnson Medical School, New Brunswick, New Jersey

I. INTRODUCTION

Defined as an excess of adipose tissue, obesity is often expressed as the relationship of body weight to "ideal body weight" normalized for height and sex; body weights in excess of 110% or 120% of ideal body weight are often used to define the obese phenotype. Another variable used to define obesity is body mass index (BMI) >29 (men) or >27 (women). Using either definition, obesity is increasing at a rate of 7% per year in the United States, and approximately 300,000 deaths a year are attributed to "overnutrition" in the United States making it second only to smoking as an indirect cause of death (1–4).

The literature up to 1980 on the respiratory effects of obesity was reviewed by Luce (5); however, new evidence has emerged on the effects of obesity on gas exchange and respiratory muscle function. Also, there is better information showing that obese persons are at considerably higher risk than lean individuals for developing hypertension and other cardiovascular diseases such as hypertension, dyslipidemia, insulin resistance, and hyperinsulinemia and sleep disorders such as sleep apnea (5–8). These comorbid conditions may complicate assessment and impact upon respiratory morbidity independent of abnormalities of pulmonary function imposed by excess body fat (9).

In general, studies in the respiratory literature are cross-sectional, comparing lean and obese individuals, in-

volve small groups of subjects, and examine one or another physiological variable or set of measures. Assessments of medical illnesses such as sleep apnea or obesity-hypoventilation syndrome, or of symptoms of dyspnea, have been performed in patients identified from clinic populations rather than individuals in the general population who might be equally obese but do not seek medical advice or experience medical illness. Hence, the potential in the literature for ascertainment bias and for a lack of generality to either clinical practice or to population guidelines is considerable. Also, there are no longitudinal studies of respiratory impairment and obesity, i.e., a natural history approach. It might be assumed that there will be increasing respiratory morbidity from obesity with the passage of time (aging), as well as with the length of time in the obese state. Central patterns of fat deposition may impair and embarrass the respiratory system more than peripherally distributed fat stores (10). In the literature on sleep apnea, this effect of central obesity is emphasized (8), but in the studies of respiratory mechanics and control, it has not often been considered. Another design limitation of the respiratory studies on obesity is the lack of controls for cardiovascular and metabolic factors associated with obesity.

The importance of this chapter lies in the fact that impairment of respiratory function by obesity is potentially reversible and, therefore, should be a focus for therapeutic intervention. This review will be comprised of three major parts. First will be the description of the changes in respiratory mechanics, gas exchange, and control in obesity, as defined by physiological decrements that result in dyspnea, the increased work of breathing, and abnormalities in gas exchange that many obese individuals exhibit. The second part will include a discussion of staging of respiratory impairment in obesity, using as a basis a classification system proposed by Bates (11). The third part of this review will outline the emerging literature on obstructive sleep apnea, in which obesity is one of the more common comorbid traits.

II. PHYSIOLOGICAL DECREMENTS WITH OBESITY

A. Respiratory Compliance and the Work of Breathing

A threshold effect of obesity associated with respiratory compromise has not been defined. While most studies in this literature use a starting point of at least 120% of ideal body weight (IBW), some use different thresholds for entry—150% or 200% IBW, BMI values >30 (males) or >28 (females). The literature is too heterogeneous to combine studies or to examine the relationship of obesity to respiratory function using continuous variables for each condition. Therefore, we will discuss studies that examined categorical effects (obese vs. nonobese subjects).

Respiratory compliance is a measure that relates to the pressure changes that are required to increase lung volume and can be influenced by the mechanical properties of both the lungs and the chest wall (12). One major problem in obesity is that increased weight pressing on the thoracic cage and abdomen makes the chest wall stiff and noncompliant (13–16). Chest wall compliance may fall even more as obese subjects move from the sitting to the supine or even prone position (16,17). There is a relationship between chest wall compliance and CO_2 retention, independent of body fat; in those obese individuals with an increase in arterial P_{CO_2}, and therefore alveolar hypoventilation, chest wall compliance was one-third of normal, whereas in equally obese but eucapnic subjects, chest wall compliance was in the normal range (12). The mechanism for the differences in chest wall compliance in the two groups was not studied; the interpretation of the results only centered around the role of chest wall compliance in CO_2 retention.

The lung itself may be indirectly affected by chest wall mass loading, as lung compliance, in addition to chest wall compliance, is decreased in some obese individuals (16,18–20). Mechanisms for increased lung stiffness include a larger pulmonary blood volume and/or closure of

dependent airways. Experimental mass loading of the chest wall produces a closure of dependent bronchiolar-alveolar units with atelectasis, which increases further the work of breathing (21). Given both increased lung and chest wall stiffness in an obese individual, there is an increased mechanical work of breathing as well as an oxygen cost of breathing (15,22). Work of breathing can be increased two- to threefold even in obese eucapnic individuals.

B. Abnormalities in Pulmonary Function Tests

Obesity produces a restrictive ventilatory deficit that becomes more evident as an individual becomes progressively more obese. There are decreases in the functional residual capacity, the expiratory reserve volume, and total lung capacity (TLC) in those defined as obese (>120% of IBW) (11,12,14,23–27). Both the forced vital capacity (FVC) and the maximal ventilatory ventilation (MVV) are reduced proportional to the rise in body weight and the decrease in respiratory compliance (11,28,29). However, body weight and respiratory compliance appear to account for approximately 60–70% of the variance in values in obese individuals, indicating that other factors act to reduce FVC and MVV in this population.

C. Gas Exchange and Respiratory Control

Obesity exerts an increased demand to maintain normal arterial P_{CO_2} and P_{O_2} levels. The work involved in moving increased body weight results in a larger CO_2 production for height in obese than in nonobese subjects; this effect is present during rest but is more evident with exercise (14,15,22). Obese subjects with increased respiratory system compliance also must work harder to eliminate CO_2 (30). The majority of obese subjects exhibit an increased ventilatory drive and maintain a eucapnic state (12,16). Most reviews emphasize that with obesity-hypoventilation syndrome there is a marked decrease in hypercapnic ventilatory drive (31–33); however, other studies do not support this contention (34–36).

In moderately and severely obese individuals (>150% to >200% of IBW), arterial blood gases often show hypoxemia due to a widened alveolar-to-arterial (A-a) gradient (37). The increased A-a gradient arises from a mismatch of ventilation and perfusion, i.e., relating to increased relative perfusion at the lung basis where underventilation occurs due to airway closure and alveolar collapse (37–41).

Obese patients who have normal or slightly reduced levels of CO_2 have either increased or normal ventilatory drives arising from hypoxic responses. Those with obesity-hypoventilation syndrome, defined as obese individuals with a $PCO_2 > 50$ mmHg, can have significantly lower hypoxic ventilatory drive (36,42). Therefore, it appears that reduced chemoresponsiveness to hypercapnia and/or hypoxia can be a part of obesity-hypoventilation syndrome. While it is assumed that obesity or body fat explains this association, there are alternative explanations. These include genetic variations in ventilatory responses, interactions between the metabolic effects of obesity and respiratory control, or effects of comorbid cardiovascular or metabolic events also linked to obesity acting on respiratory control (8).

The respiratory control system includes not only activities in the brainstem but also the distribution of neuromuscular drive to the chest wall muscles such as the diaphragm and the intercostal muscles. Muscles can be compromised by fatty infiltration, and their mechanical action on ventilation influenced by abnormalities in chest wall compliance, i.e., the coupling between muscle activity and the generation of pressure for inspiration (11,12, 43). Furthermore, the respiratory control system determines ventilation by independent alterations in tidal volume and frequency (44), which must optimize ventilation in the face of challenges like exercise and sleep.

Lourenço measured respiratory drive as the increase in diaphragmatic electrical activity per unit increase in CO_2 in subjects who were morbidly obese and found that the respiratory drive needed for any change in CO_2 was three to four times that found in normal subjects (45). This high value of respiratory drive is a reflection of the need to sustain a high level of diaphragm energy expenditure to maintain adequate ventilation, a demand that must increase further with a change to the supine position (46). The reduction in this relationship is indicative of a diminished capacity to increase respiratory muscle activity to meet demands for ventilation. The morbidly obese patient will exhibit static inspiratory pressures 60–70% of normal in both upright and supine positions (13,16,43,46). Therefore, increasing EMG activity acts to move the massive chest wall rather than increase ventilation (35).

The direct effects of obesity on muscle size and function are not resolved. In a Zucker rat model of obesity in which respiratory function changes are similar to those found in human obesity, there is a greater size and number of muscle fibers in the diaphragm of obese than of nonobese siblings (47). In contrast, in the obese (*ob/ob*) mouse model the diaphragm is thinner in obese than in lean siblings (E. Schenker, personal communication). Systematic analyses of respiratory muscle thickness and fiber types in obese individuals are not currently available.

Studies of hypercapnic obese human subjects suggest that the degree of CO_2 retention correlates with decreases in inspiratory strength, reductions in vital capacity, and reductions in the ability to sustain a maximal voluntary ventilation (35,45). The latter finding, i.e., an inability to sustain a level of ventilation, may indicate a degree of respiratory muscle fatigue and may contribute to the development of a chronic hypoventilation syndrome (48,49).

Two other factors may contribute to inefficiencies in gas exchange. Obese individuals achieve a minute ventilation with a relatively smaller tidal volume and increased frequency, and while this pattern reduces the work of breathing, it increases the dead space and decreases alveolar ventilation at any given minute ventilation of breathing (44). A second factor is that in severely obese subjects the diaphragm may be overstretched in the supine position (46). Overstretching is a consequence of the mechanical loading by abdominal contents and places the diaphragm at a mechanical disadvantage that contributes to decreased inspiratory strength in the supine posture (46). This factor may be particularly important during sleep when postural muscle tone is decreased (28).

D. Dyspnea and Exercise

A common complaint in the obese individual is dyspnea, a sense of shortness of breath on exertion or at rest (1,9). The factors that appear to correlate with increased shortness of breath include the decrease in chest wall compliance and the inefficiency of the respiratory control system (see above). The moderately obese individual, though, can sustain a level of ventilation to maintain normal levels of arterial PCO_2 and increase ventilation appropriately with exercise (49). This indicates that the metaboreceptor response to exercise can be intact, at least in moderately obese individuals.

There are three somewhat unique aspects of exercise related to obesity. The first relates to the increased ventilatory demands imposed by the increased weight of the individual. This effect is seen clearly in that ventilation for a given work load on treadmill testing is much greater than that on bicycle testing (14,33,49,50). This is related to the weight borne while walking. A second effect relates to the observation that while ventilation is usually increased in relationship to oxygen consumption, in the moderately obese subject studied both at rest and with exercise, arterial oxygen levels increase on exercise with little change in $PaCO_2$. This can be attributed to improved ventilation-perfusion matching (49), indicating that gas exchange abnormalities at rest are functional rather than structural.

A third factor is the mechanical constraint on end-expiratory lung volume before and during exercise (51). The lower end-expiratory lung volume during resting breathing in the obese subject is principally due to the changes in mechanical properties of the chest wall (25). Even in simple obesity the pressure-volume curve, while displaced, is linear above end-expiratory lung volume but, unlike normal subjects, very nonlinear below FRC (12). Furthermore, in contrast to lean individuals, obese individuals do not decrease their end-expiratory lung volume during exercise (52). Mechanisms have not been extensively studied; however, it may be that the reduction in chest wall compliance makes the chest wall harder to displace inward or that, below FRC, expiratory muscles operate more inefficiently in expiration in the obese individual. The consequence of a failure to reduce end-expiratory lung volume during exercise is a failure to place the diaphragm at a better mechanical advantage and an inefficient partitioning of the work of breathing between the inspiratory and expiratory muscles (51). This impaired exercise response is seen even in mildly obese individuals and may explain dyspnea on exertion even in those with normal spirometry or gas exchange.

In summary, the metabolic consequences of obesity combined with abnormalities in motor outflow and muscle dysfunction contribute to the respiratory complaints at rest and to exercise intolerance in the obese individual. What is not known is how these develop over time and whether or not certain individuals are predisposed to abnormalities because of factors independent of the level of obesity or factors present as a consequence of the metabolic and cardiovascular syndromes associated with obesity.

III.   CATEGORIES OF RESPIRATORY COMPROMISE IN OBESITY

Bates (11) proposed that the respiratory effects of obesity be classified into three stages relating to the magnitude of obesity and clinical illness associated with obesity. This staging of dysfunction may have been derived from efforts to classify cardiovascular morbidity (10). We see a staging scheme as a convenient starting point to discuss the degrees of influence that obesity can have on respiratory pathophysiology and illness. What should be emphasized at the onset is that such a classification system serves merely to organize thinking about obesity and its effects on respiratory function and pathophysiology. Individuals will not fall neatly into each category, and the health outcome effects of an initial classification of individuals are not known, with the possible exception of those with morbid obesity. Also, despite its common use in study criteria, we suspect that the distinction between mild, moderate, and severe consequences of obesity may not

have, as a defining trait, a numerical value for obesity, expressed as percent of IBW or BMI. Rather, illness is the result of interactions between fat deposition sites, time, and other inherited or acquired traits of respiratory function or comorbid conditions, such as cardiovascular disease.

Patients in stage I (Table 1) include those who are mildly obese, with a ratio of weight to height (kilograms over centimeters) of less than 1 and body weight of approximately 120% of ideal body weight. In many of these individuals lung mechanics are usually normal, airway resistance is normal, and the subdivisions of the lung volume show only a small reduction in expiratory reserve. Arterial blood gases are usually normal at rest. This might be termed simple obesity, but even simple obesity increases the risk of breathing abnormalities during exercise and during sleep due to the mechanical effects of chest wall loading. Exercise tolerance may be reduced both by inactivity and/or by a failure to reduce end-expiratory lung volume. Recumbency with sleep results in inefficiencies in ventilation, in vascular perfusion, and in diaphragm function.

In stage II, patients are more severely obese with a ratio of weight to height of more than 1; these individuals are generally >150% of ideal body weight. In these individuals there are decreases in lung as well as chest wall compliance and hypoxemia due to an increasing A-a gradient. These changes are due to the increasingly small difference

Table 1   Classification of Obesity-Related[a] Respiratory Compromise

Stage I:	weight-to-height ratio[b] <1, normal FVC and FEV$_1$, reduction in end-expiratory reserve volume, Pa$_{CO_2}$ at the lower limit of normal (36–40 mmHg), decrements in exercise capacity related to weight and reserve volumes, independent of conditioning
Stage II:	weight-to-height ratio >1, impairments in lung volumes, dyspnea at exercise and at rest, increased A-a gradient, decrements in function in the supine posture, normal Pa$_{CO_2}$ (40–45 mmHg) or mild hypercapnia at rest may indicate sleep-disordered breathing
Stage III:	stage II compromise in the presence of illness: pulmonary hypertension and right heart failure, obesity-hypoventilation syndrome, obstructive sleep apnea syndrome, and morbid obesity syndrome

[a]>120% of ideal body weight.
[b]kilograms/centimeters
Source: After Bates (11).

between expiratory reserve volume and closing volume and to ventilation-perfusion mismatching. Gas exchange abnormalities can be reversed; the arterial PaO$_2$ may increase as much as 18 mmHg after deep breaths, indicating a functional rather than structural deficit related to atelectasis or ventilation-perfusion mismatching under conditions of quiet breathing. There is a restrictive defect with FVC and TLC below 80% of predicted, and the ratio of FRC to TLC falls to approximately 25%. In patients with moderate obesity there is a steady decline in ventilation-perfusion ratio from apex to base in the upright posture and airway closure is further enhanced in the supine posture. Polycythemia may be present and more severe blood gas changes can be demonstrated during sleep.

In this group of patients (stage II), respiratory frequency is increased at rest, tidal volume decreased, and the respiratory drive increased with an increased response to hypoxia but a decreased response to hypercapnia. The ventilatory response to exercise can be normal even in those whose hypercapnic response is depressed. Gas exchange during sleep is impaired by increased closure of lung units and by impairment of muscle function. Apneas during sleep are increased (53), and hypercapnia may occur during sleep secondary to hypoventilation. The presence of hypercapnia during the day may be a consequence of sleep-disordered breathing (54) or coexisting illness (55) or upper airway obstruction (56). However, sleep-disordered breathing is not accompanied by signs and symptoms of illness during the day; the degree of sleepiness resulting from sleep fragmentation is similar to that in the general population (8).

In this group of patients, weight loss achieved either through behavioral modification of through ileojejunoileal bypass can result in improvement in all these physiological abnormalities (5,7,23,29,57). But it must be noted that many of these good results were reported for younger subjects with moderate obesity. Respiratory complications of surgery for weight loss occur more commonly in older individuals, those who are hypercapnic (perhaps as a result of sleep-disordered breathing), and those who seem to have a reduced expiratory reserve volume prior to surgery (11,28). This impression should be confirmed in longitudinal and prospective studies of outcome assessment.

Stage III or illness-defined obesity impairment includes morbid obesity with edema and cor pulmonale, the obesity-hypoventilation syndrome, and sleep apnea (reviewed separately below). The colorful term "Pickwickian syndrome" (58) is, however, outdated. Patients in this category exhibit an increased predisposition to pulmonary emboli (55,59). Pulmonary hypertension, which can be present in these patients particularly during light exercise, may predispose these patients to inactivity, to dependent edema, and to subsequent risk for venous thrombosis (55). The effects of pulmonary emboli on the lung of an obese individual will be compounded by abnormalities in respiratory function imposed by increased weight alone (59).

In obesity-hypoventilation syndrome, respiratory control is impaired, and the following can be evident: a rapid, shallow breathing pattern, blunted responsiveness to both carbon dioxide and hypoxia, and impaired respiratory muscle function (60). It may be difficult to determine the relative influence of mechanical and control deficits that result in hypercapnia. Obesity and hypothyroidism (61) and obesity and upper airway pathology (56) can also coexist resulting in alveolar hypoventilation and severe morbidity.

Mortality among these obese individuals may be considerable and has been attributed to either pulmonary emboli or cardiopulmonary arrest (3,55,62). Patients in this category are more likely to have coexisting diseases of hypertension, coronary artery disease, gallstones, and arthritis, conditions that can complicate respiratory assessment (55).

The stages described above and presented in Table 1 are proposed for convenience to underscore the range of pulmonary abnormalities and morbidity present in an obese population. A limitation of this classification is a lack of stratification for comorbid conditions, length of obese condition, age, sex, or other independent risks that coexist with obesity. There may also be inherent or genetic determinants of ventilatory control or of diseases like diabetes with independent effects on lung mechanics as well as muscle function.

Another confounding factor in this classification is the relationship of respiratory morbidity to the circulatory physiology of obesity (55,63). Obesity is associated with an increased blood volume and cardiac output, and obesity is a hypervolemic and/or hyperdynamic state, which increases left ventricular work. Left ventricular muscle size can be related to the degree of obesity but also occurring is an increase in right ventricle thickness, epicardial fat, or fat infiltration of the myocardium. Left ventricular hypertrophy in obesity has been linked to left ventricular failure; even with moderate obesity, end-diastolic filling pressure is at the upper limits of normal and diastolic dysfunction is present with exercise. Elevations in end-diastolic filling pressure return to normal when weight is lost; however, central blood volume, pulmonary blood volume, and the impedance to left ventricular emptying (afterload) also fall and will contribute to the improvement in cardiac function (63). There is new evidence that hypertension and left ventricular mass are correlated more clearly with the presence of sleep-disordered breathing than with obesity per se (64), but an interaction between these two conditions may be present.

Another use of this classification scheme could be in the identification of risk in perioperative morbidity and mortality. Postoperative atelectasis, aspiration pneumonitis, and pulmonary embolism have been suggested to be more common in obesity (1,55,59), but as obesity becomes more common, risk stratification/classification and modification may need to become more selective. Aggressive supportive pulmonary care of the obese patient is currently suggested throughout all phases of the hospital course; however, with cost containment, hospital resources for such interventions may be limited and emphasis will shift to postoperative care at home or in less skilled facilities. Newer ways of reducing ventilatory impairment could include the use of nasal continuous positive airway pressure (CPAP) support before and after surgery to maintain lung volumes, reduce the presence of atelectasis, improve the respiratory disturbances during sleep, and possibly improve outcome in regard to a more rapid return to daily living or to work or to a reduction in established postoperative problems in obesity.

IV.   SLEEP-DISORDERED BREATHING AND OBESITY

Obstructive sleep apnea (OSA) syndrome is characterized by loud snoring, episodic partial or complete obstruction of the upper airway during sleep, and consequent sleep fragmentation leading to excessive daytime sleepiness. In addition to the morbidity associated with chronic sleepiness, patients with OSA are at increased risk for hypertension, myocardial infarction, and stroke (8). The diagnosis and treatment of OSA have been reviewed elsewhere (8,61,65,66), although a few key points are mentioned here. When OSA is suspected clinically, the diagnosis is conventionally confirmed via polysomnography, a test in which multiple physiological variables including the electroencephalogram, electrocardiogram, and several measures of respiratory function are recorded during sleep. The most common measure of OSA severity determined in this manner is the total number of apneas (cessation of airflow ≥10 sec) and hypopneas (partial obstructions) per hour of sleep (apnea + hypopnea index, AHI); however, other features in the presentation may indicate the need for a therapeutic intervention.

General population studies in the United States and several other countries suggest that the syndrome of obstructive apneas, daytime sleepiness, and cardiovascular illness is present in some 1–4% of working men and women (8,67). There are pockets of higher prevalence, for instance in minority populations and children with tonsillar hypertrophy; however, one of the best-characterized associations is between obesity and OSA. The correlation between body weight and sleep apnea was so strong as to dominate recognition strategies for almost two decades and link sleep apnea almost exclusively with obesity-hypoventilation or Pickwickian syndrome (61,66,68); however, in community studies the association of OSA with obesity is not as strong as in clinic-based case collections or reviews from referral centers (8,68). A brief review of this association follows, as does a more thorough account of the literature regarding mechanism and weight reduction.

A.   Association Between Obesity and Obstructive Sleep Apnea

In clinic populations, two-thirds are noted to be at least 130% of ideal body weight (8), and obesity (expressed as BMI in kg/m^2) is the strongest predictor of AHI in subjects >age 50. Compared to the other factors studied, BMI was twice as strong as gender, and fourfold stronger than age, in predicting AHI, even when subjects with the most severe disease (AHI > 60) were excluded from analysis (69). In a polysomnographic study of 250 obese patients without sleep complaints, only 40% of the men and 3% of the women were found to have sleep apnea severe enough to warrant treatment (70). The recent population-based study of Wisconsin state employees supports the findings of these clinic-based reports (67). In this cohort of over 600 men and women between 30 and 60 years of age, an increase in BMI of one standard deviation was associated with a fourfold increase in risk for OSA (defined as an AHI > 5/hr). After examining several measures of body composition and metrics related to fat deposition, neck circumference was the strongest predictor of AHI although all anthropomorphic variables were highly correlated. These and other observations suggest that an upper body fat deposition profile, rather than a more generalized distribution of body fat, may be important for the development of sleep apnea.

Given the strength of the association, defining the causal relationship between excess body weight and OSA remains surprisingly difficult. Studies of mechanisms can be grouped into one or more categories based on hypotheses involving alterations in upper airway (UA) structure or function or alterations in respiratory drive, particularly to muscles regulating nasopharyngeal and oropharyngeal patency.

B. Obesity and Upper Airway Function

The major theory is that obesity leads to a change in UA geometry, either through loading of the pharyngeal wall or by encroachment from periluminal fat deposits, placing it at increased risk of collapse due to physical forces acting on the pharyngeal segment during inspiration. Imaging studies indicate that obese patients with OSA have significant narrowing of the UA compared with nonobese controls while awake using computed tomography (71–73). These studies have demonstrated significant differences in cross-sectional area at naso-, oro-, and hypopharyngeal levels, with obese patients having smaller airways than controls. Although in some of these studies patients and controls were not matched for obesity, the finding of a small retropalatal airway in OSA patients compared to weight-matched controls has been shown in additional studies (74,75). Using magnetic resonance imaging to compare obese OSA patients with weight-matched controls, fat deposition was increased at sites removed from the periluminal space, primarily in areas posterior and lateral to the oropharynx at the level of the palate, as well as within the soft palate (76). Differences in pharyngeal shape have also been observed between obese OSA patients and normal-weight controls (73,77). Specifically, when the pharynx was viewed in coronal section, awake OSA patients had elliptically shaped airways, the long axes of which were oriented in the anteroposterior plane; normals had airways oriented transversely.

Obesity-related decreases in lung volume, as discussed earlier in this chapter, may also result in greater instability of the UA, as lung volume has been directly correlated with upper airway size (78,79). Moreover, pharyngeal distensibility, or "compliance," has been shown to be greater in both males and females with OSA than in obesity-matched controls using the acoustic reflection technique (80–82). Similar findings were obtained when lung volume was passively altered using continuous positive airway pressure (83). Both increases in lung volume and pharyngeal volume and decreases in this measure of UA distensibility in obese sleep apneics after weight loss have been observed (84,85). Together with a decrease in AHI, upper airway closing pressures during non-REM sleep declined from 3.1 to -2.4 cm H_2O after a 17% reduction in BMI in moderately obese subjects, indicating a specific beneficial effect of weight loss on improvement in pharyngeal function and sleep apnea (86). Taken together, it appears that weight loss in obese individuals is an appropriate and specific therapy for OSA; however, the anatomical mechanisms explaining how obesity impairs upper airway structure remain to be elucidated.

C. Alterations in Respiratory Drive

Ventilatory responses and load compensation can be altered in the obese individual and have a significant impact on breathing during sleep. A reduction in central respiratory drive coupled with increased respiratory system mechanical loading has been implicated in the pathogenesis of the obesity-hypoventilation syndrome (31–36,42, 65), and similar abnormalities have been sought in eucapnic patients with OSA (87,88). Although the data are not consistent across all studies, simple obesity (stage I) may be associated with reduced awake ventilatory chemoresponsiveness, although this is based on data from a limited number of subjects (89,90). Obesity accompanied by OSA may or may not be associated with a reduction in chemoresponsiveness. In an early study, ventilatory and mouth occlusion pressure responses to CO_2 rebreathing were reduced from normals in both eucapnic and hypercapnic OSA patients (91,92), and a relative decrease in the awake ventilatory response to CO_2 in eucapnic obese OSA patients has also been documented more recently (93). Abnormal load compensation must play a role in initiation or maintenance of obstructive apneas during sleep, given that obesity is accompanied by mechanical impairments in upper airway function. Both blunted chemoresponsiveness and load compensation might result from the sleep fragmentation and episodic hypoxemia that occur in OSA. Increases in the ventilatory response to added resistive loads (91) as well as a more brisk CO_2 response curve occur after treatment of OSA with nasal CPAP (94). This finding is interpreted to indicate that OSA may play a primary role in blunting the respiratory responses. We are not aware of studies that follow ventilatory and load compensation responses with weight loss alone.

D. Clinical Studies of Weight Loss and OSA

Further evidence for the role of obesity in obstructive sleep apnea comes from clinical studies of weight loss in patients with OSA. Approximately 15 studies have been reported to date, which have included a variety of weight loss methods, patient selection criteria, efficacy and outcome measures, and research designs. Surgical and nonsurgical approaches to weight reduction have been employed in patients with varying degrees of obesity and sleep apnea, and treatment follow-up has ranged from 2 to 24 months. Significant weight loss has been reported in most studies, which has been associated with varying degrees of improvement in sleep-disordered breathing, oxygen hemoglobin saturation, sleep fragmentation, and daytime performance. Related changes in UA function, and to a much more limited extent, airway structure, have also been evaluated.

Despite the strong support for the role of obesity as a causal factor in OSA, and the potential value of weight loss as a primary treatment intervention for obese patients with OSA, several key issues and concerns remain to be addressed. In particular, it is unclear from these studies whether a critical threshold level for weight loss exists, and which patients are most likely to benefit from treatment. Also lacking is information about the relative risks and benefits associated with dietary or surgical weight reduction procedures in patients with OSA and selection of optimal treatment approaches for specific subgroups of patients. The mechanisms of treatment efficacy are also uncertain at this point. Finally, the issue of long-term maintenance of weight loss and associated improvements in OSA has not been adequately addressed to date.

E.   Surgically Induced Weight Loss and OSA

Several studies have observed marked changes in AHI, nocturnal SaO_2, and sleep continuing and architecture following surgical weight loss interventions (see Table 2). The first study of this type (95) evaluated the effects of jejeunoileal bypass surgery in four morbidly obese individuals. Mean body weight prior to surgery was 231.0 kg, which decreased to 123 kg. A dramatic decrease in sleep-disordered breathing was observed following a 47% weight reduction at 2 years postsurgery with the mean AHI decreasing from 78 to 1.4 events/hr. Total sleep time was improved although low (4.1 hr/night) at follow-up. One subject died following surgery and was not included in the data analysis, and no long-term follow-up data were provided. Additionally, patient selection factors were not controlled for, nor were the effects of concomitant therapies evaluated.

Two other studies reported on changes in sleep-disordered breathing in morbidly obese patients receiving gastric bypass surgery (96,97). Moderately and morbidly obese patients reporting a combination of loud snoring, restless sleep, and daytime somnolence were scheduled for overnight sleep studies, which were performed prior to and at varying intervals (2–6 months) after surgery. Both studies reported similar changes, in both the amount of weight loss achieved and associated improvements in OSA and sleep architecture. Studies were lacking in a detailed description of postsurgical complications or longer-term assessment of treatment outcome.

Sugerman and co-workers (98) examined the role of gastric bypass surgery in the management of obesity complicated by obesity-hypoventilation. Those with significant OSA and apnea-induced arrhythmias also received tracheotomies at the time of gastric surgery. Based on preoperative polysomnography, 10 patients had obesity-hypoventilation syndrome, nine had OSA, and 19 had both. Of these, two died shortly after surgery and an additional four patients were lost to follow-up. Follow-up studies performed at 3–5 months postsurgery revealed significant weight loss (a 62% reduction in excess body weight) associated with improvements in both OSA and daytime somnolence, as reported subjectively. Percent apnea time (total duration of apneas/total sleep time $\times$ 100) declined from a baseline of 44% to 8% following surgery. Unfortunately, no data were provided regarding sleep architecture, AHI, or nocturnal SaO_2 before or after surgery. As in the previous studies, these authors also failed to provide long-term assessment of surgical weight loss or changes in OSA.

A final study describing the effects of vertical banded gastroplasty on OSA in morbidly obese patients (BMI $\geq$ 40 kg/m²) involved screening patients for OSA using clinical criteria in addition to the results of a 90-min daytime nap study (99). Of a total of 27 patients, 11 were thus identified as having sleep apnea and underwent full nocturnal polysomnography. The severity of OSA in these patients was highly variable; the oxygen desaturation index (episodic desaturations $\geq$4% lasting between 6 and 120 sec/hr) ranged from 14 to 99. Fourteen patients underwent gastroplasty, of whom three were diagnosed as having OSA; the remaining patients received dietary intervention. Methods of assigning patients to surgery versus conservative therapy were not specified. Among patients with OSA there was a 30–38% reduction in BMI postsurgery and a decline in respiratory events during sleep from 85 to 100%. In the eight OSA patients treated with dietary management alone, reductions in BMI were less dramatic; one patient with the greatest amount of weight loss (33% decrease in BMI) was cured of his OSA, and two additional patients showed improvement (i.e., $\geq$50% reduction) in sleep-disordered breathing. Duration of follow-up for either group was not specified.

Overall, impressive results have been observed in terms of both weight loss and associated changes in sleep quality and OSA; the studies suffer overall from a lack of rigorous design and, as a series of case reports, represent the lowest level of evidence (Sackett Level V) for a therapeutic intervention (100). Methodological difficulties have been noted in each of the studies reviewed, including lack of control for the effects of surgery or other forms of medical intervention, nor have the mechanisms of action been investigated. Insufficient data are provided regarding the risks and benefits associated with surgical weight loss for OSA, although a significant rate of postsurgical complications is

Table 2 Effects of Surgical Weight Loss on Obstructive Sleep Apnea Syndrome

Author	N	Length of follow-up (months)	Surgical procedure	Weight change (kg)	Change in AHI (events/hr)	Comments
Harman et al., 1982	4	4–24	Jejeunoileal bypass	−108.0 (−47%)	−76.6 (98%)	All subjects much improved
Charuzi et al., 1984	13	6	Gastric bypass	? (−72.5%)	−80.8 (91%)	Sleep architecture improved postsurgery
Peiser et al., 1984	15	4–8	Gastric bypass	−44.2 (−31%)	−74.3 (89%)	12 subjects much improved
Rajala et al., 1991	3	N/A	Gastroplasty	? (−34.3%)	−39.3 (−92.7%)	2 subjects with mild SDB cured (ODI <10)

to be expected (101). Finally, none of the studies to date has included assessment of waking performance following treatment, nor has adequate long-term assessment of treatment effects been conducted, in terms of either weight loss or improvements in sleep and sleep-disordered breathing (102,103).

F. Dietary Weight Loss and OSA

Several studies have been performed in the past decade on the effects of dietary weight loss in patients with OSA (Table 3). Despite differences in experimental design, methods used for achieving weight loss, and the duration of follow-up assessment, a consistent trend has been observed toward improvement in sleep and AHI following weight loss intervention. Results generally are not as dramatic as those observed with surgical weight loss, but clinically significant improvements are apparent in most studies. The major issues that have not been adequately addressed to date are: (1) the amount of weight loss needed to achieve significant improvement in both OSA and daytime somnolence; (2) associated structural or functional changes in the upper airway; and (3) maintenance of weight loss beyond the traditional 6–12-month observation period. Evidence from other sources suggests that relapse after 1 year is to be expected following dietary weight loss by most methods (102,103).

Two of the first studies of dietary weight loss in patients with OSA were reported by investigators at Johns Hopkins University. In the first study (86), 23 patients with moderate sleep apnea and obesity were randomly assigned to either weight loss (N = 15) or control (N = 8) groups. Weight loss treatment consisted solely of instructions to reduce caloric intake, and no special diets, medications, or behavior modification techniques were provided. Pa-

tients were followed until significant weight loss had occurred in the treatment group, or until stable weight was achieved in the control group. Patients were reassessed at 5 months after the baseline study in the weight loss group, and at just over 8 months after baseline in the control group. There was an approximate 10-kg weight loss in the treatment group, which was associated with a significant decline in mean AHI from 55 to 30 events/hr following treatment. Significant improvements were also noted in mean and maximum nocturnal SaO_2 following treatment. In contrast, no changes were observed in weight, AHI, or nocturnal arterial oxygen saturation in the controls. Improvements in sleep quality and daytime alertness were also observed following treatment. In this study a significant association was observed between the amount of weight loss achieved and improvement in mean fall in SaO_2 during sleep ($r = 0.69$, $p < 0.01$). A positive although nonsignificant correlation was observed between weight loss and improvement in mean apnea frequency following treatment. Of note, patients with relatively mild degrees of obesity (i.e., 110–115% of ideal body weight) and moderate sleep apnea also showed improvements following treatment. No evidence was provided of long-term maintenance of weight loss or sleep quality in this study.

In a subsequent study (104), the group evaluated the effects of weight loss on sleep apnea and UA critical closing pressure in 26 patients with moderate obesity and OSA. Following baseline evaluations, patients were assigned to either an intensive weight loss condition or usual care treatment. The weight loss intervention consisted of weekly dietary counseling sessions and behavior modification for 12–24 months. Among patients selecting this option, 13 of 23 subjects had at least a 5% reduction in body weight during treatment and were scheduled for follow-up evaluation. The usual care treatment group

Table 3 Effects of Dietary Weight Loss on Obstructive Sleep Apnea Syndrome

Author	Number of subjects	Length of follow-up (months)	Method of weight loss	Weight change (kg)	Change in AHI (events/hr)	Comment
Smith et al., 1985	Weight loss = 15 Controls = 8	5.3 ± 1.6 (treatment group); 8.5 ± 3.5 (controls)	Dietary instruction and follow-up	−9.6 (−9%) (treatment group); no change in controls	−25.8 (−47%)	Controls showed no change in weight or AHI
Rubinstein et al., 1988	12	13 (range = 8–18)	Dietary instruction /gastroplasty	−24.0 (−20%)	−43.0 (−75%)	Decreased pharyngeal collapsibility after weight loss
Pasquall et al., 1990	23	Unspecified	Very-low-calorie diet, no CPAP	−18.5 (−16%)	−33.5 (−49%)	SDB improved even with little (i.e., <10 kg) wt loss; unspecified follow-up time
Rajala et al., (1991) (see Table 1)	8	Unspecified	Dietary	? (−12%)	−14.1 (−33%)	Patient with greatest wt loss (−33% BMI) cured; 2 improved; 5 no change in SDB
Schwartz et al., 1991	26 Weight loss = 13 Controls = 13	4.5 16.9 + 10 (treatment group); 18.4 ± 9.5 (controls)	Dietary instruction /CPAP	−7.3 kg/m² (−17%)	−50.8 (−61%)	Significant decrease in upper airway critical pressure (P_{crit}) following weight loss
Suratt et al., 1992	8	24.0	Very-low-calorie diet (VLCD)	−20.6 (−13%)	−28.0 (−30%)	Full weight gain at 24 mo follow short-term decrease in AHI
Kiselak et al., 1993	14	4.5–5	Diet/behavioral therapy	−27.2 (?)	−16.6 (?)	Soft palate width decreased following treatment
Nahmias et al., 1993	28	10.7 (range = 4–17)	Dietary instruction, VLCD; CPAP	−22.1 (−18%)	−25.8 (74%)	No change in sleep architecture following weight loss

served as controls and consisted of 13 age-, sex-, and weight-matched patients not given dietary counseling; they were restudied approximately 18 months following baseline assessment. All patients were maintained on nasal CPAP throughout the trial. Weight loss was associated with a significant decrease in the frequency of non-REM apneas, although no changes were observed in either mean or minimum nocturnal SaO_2 following treatment. Of particular note, a significant change was observed in upper airway closing pressure in the weight loss group, which was highly correlated with changes in both BMI and sleep-disordered breathing.

The effects of very-low-calorie diets (VLCD) on weight loss and sleep-disordered breathing have been investigated in three studies to date. In a study of 23 Italian patients with sleep apnea and moderate obesity (105), significant weight loss was achieved by means of a combination of VLCD and dietary counseling. The average weight loss was 18 kg, and the follow-up period ranged from 3 to 14 months. Significant improvements in AHI and mean SaO_2 during sleep were observed following treatment, and a significant correlation was noted between the amount of weight lost and decrease in apnea frequency. Although OSA was improved in patients with relatively modest weight loss, these effects were mitigated by the presence of otorhinolaryngeal pathology (e.g., tonsillar hypertrophy, tongue enlargement). In additional studies of VLCD-induced weight loss, both Suratt et al. (106,107) and Nahmias et al. (108) observed significant weight loss and marked improvements in OSA following treatment, although these gains were not maintained at 2 years posttreatment. Unfortunately, none of these studies has systematically compared VLCD with more conventional forms of dietary weight loss in patients with OSA.

Finally, the effects of dietary intervention and cognitive-behavioral therapy on weight loss, sleep apnea, and hypertension were recently investigated by Kiselak and associates (109). Patients for this study were recruited from a hospital-based, obesity management program and were scheduled for polysmnographic assessment prior to and following treatment. The number of patients with clinically significant OSA was limited in this study ($N = 7$; mean AHI 24 events/hr in the five with hypertension); however, the results for both weight loss and associated sleep changes were significant. Following an intensive, 20-week program of dietary intervention, weekly exercise training, and cognitive-behavioral therapy, a mean weight loss of 27 kg was achieved. This was associated with a significant change in AHI (mean decrease = 17 events/hr) and improvements in blood pressure, vital capacity, and functional residual capacity. Additionally, a significant decrease in soft palate width was observed following

weight loss. Major weaknesses of the study were the absence of electroencephalographic monitoring of sleep and assessments of daytime alertness, the concomitant use of antihypertensive and other medications, and lack of follow-up evaluation.

G. Anorexiant Drugs

Given the potential role of fenfluramine and phentermine in the long-term treatment of obesity (110), the paucity of experience with anorexiants in obese OSA patients is surprising. In an uncontrolled pilot study using fenfluramine in 13 patients, a decrease in mean AHI from 82 to 51 events/hr, a reduction in therapeutic nasal CPAP from 12 to 7 cm H_2O, and an average weight loss of 14 kg after approximately 6 months of drug use were observed (111). Clearly, additional, controlled trials of anorexiants in patients with OSA are warranted. We await the opportunity to examine pharmacological agents derived from molecular observations on the pathogenesis of obesity.

V. SUMMARY AND CONCLUSIONS

Obesity impairs respiratory structure and function, leading to physiological and pathophysiological impairments. The degree to which increased fat deposition affects respiratory function may vary according to age, length of the obese condition, comorbidity, and other individual traits, including those related to chemoresponsiveness, load compensation, and sleep-induced alterations in respiratory drive. The influence of obesity on pharyngeal function and the appearance of OSA appears related not only to BMI, but to measures of central obesity and neck size. How neck size is determined and related to other well-studied obese phenotypes remains to be determined by longitudinal studies or by cross-sectional studies in established cohorts being examined for obesity or diabetes. Also needed are outcome-based studies of the impact on obesity on cardiorespiratory morbidity with surgery and with the development of OSA. The classification presented in this chapter is intended to encourage thought and debate in this area.

Obesity appears an important variable to examine in regard to respiratory health given that most studies involving weight loss show significant improvement or frank reversal of abnormalities in ventilatory control, respiratory mechanics, and illness like OSA and obesity-hypoventilation syndrome. Effective therapy for achieving weight loss would address perhaps half of the current patients diagnosed with obstructive sleep apnea syndrome and could play a role in prevention of OSA. The therapeutic avenues opened by molecular mechanisms for obesity and the obese phenotype will be particularly relevant to understanding sleep-disordered breathing in obesity.

There are gaps in our knowledge; some areas for further research are listed in Table 4. Studies have involved rather small groups of subjects and the relationships between obesity and respiratory function have been handled by categorical analyses, whereas it is our suspicion that examination of measures of obesity and measures of respiratory function during wakefulness and sleep as continuous variables might disclose new interactions, potentially important not only for therapy but also for public health.

Table 4 Areas of Needed Research

Epidemiology
  Sharply defined epidemiological work to capture the intermediate phenotypes for obesity that confer risk for ventilatory impairment and sleep-disordered breathing
  Examine interactions between risk factors for sleep apnea (craniofacial anatomy, hormonal status, ventilatory responsiveness, and family history) and obesity
  Identify population and clinical subgroups at greatest risk for adverse clinical outcomes from obesity, including those defined by race, gender, or age
  The genetic epidemiology of obesity and respiratory traits of lung function, ventilatory control, and gas exchange
Pathophysiology
  Determine if sleep and sleep interruption impact on performance, eating behavior, and growth, particularly in obese school-age children
  Describe the various outcomes and independence of interactions between obesity and sleep apnea on daytime performance and cardiovascular risk
  Determine the basis for interactions among obesity and age in regard to upper airway function in sleep apnea
Treatment
  Determine the impact of interventions for obesity on ventilatory function and breathing during sleep particularly during a preclinical phase (stage I)
  Compare effectiveness of behavioral interventions for obesity in nonapneic and apneic individuals
  Estimate the extent of medical care utilization, health care costs, and measures of quality of life associated with obesity with and without concomitant sleep disorders

REFERENCES

1. American Thoracic Society. Evaluation of impairment/disability secondary to respiratory disorders. Am Rev Respir Dis 1986; 133(6):1205–1209.

2. Council on Scientific Affairs of the American Medical Association. Treatment of obesity in adults. JAMA 1988; 260:2547–2551.

3. Pi-Sunyer FX. Health implications of obesity. Am J Clin Nutr 1991; 53:1595S–1603S.

4. Stunkard AJ. Current views on obesity. Am J Med 1996; 100:231–232.

5. Luce JM. Respiratory complications of obesity. Chest 1980; 78:626–631.

6. Sims EA. Mechanisms of hypertension in the syndromes of obesity. Int J Obes 1981; 5(Suppl 1):9–18.

7. Strohl KP, Boehm KD, Denko CW, Novak RD, Decker MJ. Biochemical morbidity in sleep apnea. ENT J 1993; 72(1): 34, 39–41.

8. Strohl KP, Redline SR. State-of-the-Art: Recognition of sleep apnea. AJRCCM 1996; 154:279–289.

9. American College of Sports Medicine. Guidelines for Exercise Testing and Prescription. Philadelphia: Lea & Febiger, 1986; 1–179.

10. Björntorp P. Classification of obese patients and complications related to the distribution of surplus fat. Am J Clin Nutr 1987; 45:1120–1125.

11. Bates D. Respiratory Function in Disease, 3rd ed. Philadelphia: WB Saunders, 1989.

12. Sharp JT. The chest wall and respiratory muscles in obesity, pregnancy, and ascites. In: Roussos C, ed. The Thorax, Part B. New York: Marcel Dekker, 1985:999–1021.

13. Naimark A, Cherniack RM. Compliance of the respiratory system in health and obesity. J Appl Physiol 1960; 15: 377–382.

14. Ray C, Sue D, Bray G, Hansen J, Wasserman K. Effects of obesity on respiratory function. Am Rev Respir Dis 128(3):501–506.

15. Dempsey J, Reddan W, Balke, B. Work capacity determinants and physiologic cost of weight-supported breathing in obesity. J Appl Physiol 1966; 21:1815–1820.

16. Sharp J, Barrocas M, Chokroverty S. The cardiorespiratory effects of obesity. Clin Chest Med 1980; 1:103–118.

17. Suratt P, Wilhoit S, Hsiao, H, Atkinson R, Rochester D. Compliance of chest wall in obese subjects. J Appl Physiol 1984; 57:403–407.

18. Bouhuys A, Beck GJ, Schoenberg JB. Lung function: normal values and risk factors. In: Sadoul P, Milic-Emili J, Simonsson BG, Clark TJH, eds. Small Airways in Health and Disease. Symposium, Copenhagen, March 1979. Amsterdam: Excerpta Medica, 1979.

19. Douglas FG, Chong PY. Influence of obesity on peripheral airways patency. J Appl Physiol 1972; 33:559–563.

20. Rochester D, Enson Y. Current concepts in the pathogenesis of the obesity-hypoventilation syndrome. Am J Med 1974; 57:402–420.

21. Sharp JT, Henry JP, Sweany SK, Meadows WR, Pietras RJ. Effects of mass loading the respiratory system in man. J Appl Physiol 1964; 19:959–966.

22. Sharp J, Henry J, Sweany S, Meadows W, Pietras R. The total work of breathing in normal and obese men. J Clin Invest 1964; 43:728–739.

23. Jacobsen E, Dano P, Skovsted P. Respiratory function before and after weight loss following intestinal shunt operation for obesity. Scand J Respir Dis 1974; 55:332–339.

24. Reichel G. Lung volumes, mechanics of breathing and changes in arterial blood gases in obese patients and in Pickwickian syndrome. Bull Physiopathol Respir 1972; 8: 1011–1020.

25. Barlett HL, Buskirk ER. Body composition and the expiratory reserve volume in lean and obese men and women. Int J Obes 1983; 7:339–343.

26. Stalnecker M, Suratt P, Chandler J. Changes in respiratory function following small bowel bypass for obesity. Surgery 1980; 87:645–651.

27. Chodoff P, Imbembo A, Knowles C, Margand P. Massive weight loss following jejunoileal bypass. I. Effects on pulmonary function. Surgery 1977; 81:399–403.

28. Rochester DF, Arora NJ. Respiratory failure from obesity. In: Mancini M, Lewis B, Contaldo F, eds. Medical Complications of Obesity. New York: Academic Press, 1980: 183–190.

29. Farebrother M, McHardy G, Munro J. Relation between pulmonary gas exchange and closing volume before and after substantial weight loss in obese subjects. Br Med J 1974; 3:391–393.

30. Sampson M, Grassino A. Load compensation in obese patients during quiet tidal breathing. J Appl Physiol 1983; 55:1269–1276.

31. Emirgil E, Sobol BJ. The effects of weight reduction on pulmonary function and the sensitivity of the respiratory center in obesity. Am Rev Respir Dis 1973; 108:831–842.

32. Hackney JD, Crane MG, Collier CC. Syndrome of extreme obesity and hypoventilation: studies of etiology. Ann Intern Med 1959; 51:541–552.

33. Burki N, Baker R. Ventilatory regulation in eucapnic morbid obesity. Am Rev Respir Dis 1984; 129:538–543.

34. Kronenberg RS, Gabel RA, Severinghaus JW. Normal chemoreceptor function in obesity before and after ileal bypass surgery to force weight reduction. Am J Med 1975; 59:349–353.

35. Lopata M, Freilich RA, Ona E, Pearle J, Lourenco RV. Ventilatory control and the obesity hypoventilations syndrome. Am Rev Respir Dis 1979; 119:165–168.

36. Kronenberg RS, Drage CW, Stevenson JE. Acute respiratory failure and obesity with normal ventilatory response to carbon dioxide and absent hypoxic ventilatory drive. Am J Med 1977; 62:772–776.

37. Rorvik S, Bo G. Lung volumes and arterial blood gases in obesity. Scand J Respir Dis 1976; 95(Suppl):60–64.

38. Holley HS, Milic-Emili J, Becklake MR, Bates DV. Regional distribution of pulmonary ventilation and perfusion in obesity. J Clin Invest 1967; 46:475–481.

39. Demedts M. Regional distribution of lung volumes and of gas inspired at residual volume: influence of age, body weight and posture. Bull Eur Physiopathol Respir 1980; 16:271–285.

40. Partridge MR, Ciofetta G, Hughes JMB. Topography of ventilation-perfusion ratios in obesity. Bull Eur Physiopathol Respir 1978; 14:765–773.

41. Hurewitz AN, Susskind H, Harold WH. Obesity alters regional ventilation in lateral decubitus position. J Appl Physiol 1985; 59:774–783.

42. Zwillich CW, Sutton FD, Pierson DJ, Creagh EM, Weil JV. Decreased hypoxic ventilatory drive in the obesity-hypoventilation syndrome. Am J Med 1975; 59:349–353.

43. Rochester DF. Tests of respiratory muscle function. Clin Chest Med 1988; 9:249–261.

44. Milic-Emili J, Gruenstein MM. Drive and timing components of ventilation. Chest 1976; 70:5131–5133.

45. Lourenço R. Diaphragm activity in obesity. J Clin Invest 1969; 438:1609–1614.

46. Sharp JT, Durz WS, Kondragunta VK. Diaphragmatic responses to body position changes in obese patients with obstructive sleep apnea. Am Rev Respir Dis 1986; 133: 32–37.

47. Farkas GA, Gosselin LE, Zhan W, Schlenker EH, Sieck GC. Histochemical and mechanical properties of diaphragm muscle in morbidly obese Zucker rats. J Appl Physiol 1994; 77:2250–2259.

48. Sampson MG, Grassino A. Diaphragmatic muscle fatigue in the massively obese. Am Rev Respir Dis 1981; 123 (Suppl):183.

49. Beck KC, Babb TG, Staats BA, Hyatt RE. Dynamics of breathing in exercise. In: Whipp BJ, Wasserman K, eds. Exercise: Pulmonary Physiology and Pathophysiology. New York: Marcel Dekker, 1991:67–97.

50. Freyschuss U, Melcher A. Exercise energy expenditure in extreme obesity: influence of ergometry type and weight loss. Scand J Clin Lab Invest 1978; 38:753–759.

51. Martin JG, DeTroyer A. The thorax and control of functional residual capacity. In: Roussos C, Macklem PT, eds. The Thorax, New York: Marcel Dekker, 1985:899–921.

52. Babb TG, Buskirk ER, Hodgson JL. Exercise end-expiratory lung volumes in lean and moderately obese women. Int J Obes 1989; 13:11–19.

53. Block A, Boysen P, Wynne J, Hunt L. Sleep apnea, hypopnea, and oxygen desaturation in normal subjects. N Engl J Med 1979; 300:513–517.

54. Harman E, Whynne J, Block A, Malloy-Fisher L. Sleep-disordered breathing and oxygen desaturation in obese patients. Chest 1981; 79:256–260.

55. Pi-Sunyer FX. Medical hazards of obesity. Ann Intern Med 1993; 119:655–660.

56. Licht JR, Smith WR, Glauser FL. Tonsillar hypertrophy in an adult with obesity-hypoventilation. Chest 1976; 70: 672–674.

57. Harman E, Wynne J, Block A. The effect of weight loss on sleep-disordered breathing and oxygen desaturation in morbidly obese men. Chest 1982; 82:291–294.

58. Comroe JH Jr. Retrospectroscope: Frankenstein, Pickwick, and Ondine. Am Rev Respir Dis 1975; 111:689–692.

59. Miller A, Granada M. In-hospital mortality in the Pickwickian syndrome. Am J Med 1974; 56:144–150.

60. Rochester D, Enson Y. Current concepts in the pathogenesis of the obesity-hypoventilation syndrome; mechanical and circulatory factors. Am J Med 1974; 57:402–420.

61. Gastaut H, Tassinari CA, Duron B. Polygraphic study of the episodic diurnal and nocturnal (hypnic and respiratory) manifestations of the Pickwick syndrome. Brain Res 1966; 2:167–186.

62. Lukomsky GI, Ovehinnikov AA, Bilal A. Complications of bronchoscopy. Chest 1981; 79:316–321.

63. Higgins M, D'Agostino R, Kannel W, Cobb J. Benefits and adverse effects of weight loss: observations from the Framingham Study. Ann Intern Med 1993; 119:758–763.

64. Carlson JT, Hedner JA, Ejnell H, Peterson L-E. High prevalence of hypertension in sleep apnea patients independent of obesity. Am J Respir Crit Care Med 1994; 150: 72–77.

65. Strohl KP, Cherniack NS, Gothe B. Physiological basis of therapy for sleep apnea. Am Rev Respir Dis 1986; 134: 791–802.

66. Strollo PJ Jr, Rogers RM. Current concepts: obstructive sleep apnea. N Engl J Med 1996; 334:99–104.

67. Young T, Palta M, Dempsey J, Skatrud J, Weber S, Badr S. The occurrence of sleep-disordered breathing among middle-aged adult. N Engl J Med 1993; 328:1230–1235.

68. Blondal T, Torebjork E. Hypersomnia and periodic breathing. Scand J Respir Dis 1977; 58:273–278.

69. Bliwise DL, Feldman DE, Bliwise NG, Carskadon MA, Kraemer HC, North CS, Petta DE, Seidel WF, Dement WC. Risk factors for sleep disordered breathing in heterogeneous geriatric populations. J Am Geriatr Soc 1987; 35:132–141.

70. Vgontzas AN, Tan TL, Bixler EO, Martin LF, Shubet D, Kales A. Sleep apnea and sleep disruption in obese patients. Arch Intern Med 1994; 154:1705–1711.

71. Haponick EF, Smith PL, Bohlman ME, Allen RP, Goldman SM, Bleecker ER. Computerized tomography in obstructive sleep apnea correlation of airway size with physiology during sleep and wakefulness. Am Rev Respir Dis 1983; 127(2):221–226.

72. Suratt P, Dee P, Atkinson RL, Armstrong P, Wilhoit SC. Fluoroscopic and computed tomographic features of the pharyngeal airway in obstructive sleep apnea. Am Rev Respir Dis 1983; 127:487–492.

73. Schwab RJ, Gefter WB, Hoffman EA, Gupta KB, Pack AI. Dynamic upper airway imaging during awake respiration in normal subjects and patients with sleep disordered breathing. Am Rev Respir Dis 1993; 148:1385–1400.

74. Kuna S, Bedi D, Ryckman C. Effect of nasal airway positive pressure on upper airway size and configuration. Am Rev Respir Dis 1988; 138:969–975.

75. Rivlin J, Hoffstein V, Kalbfleisch J, McNicholas W, Zamel N, Bryan AC. Upper airway morphology in patients with idiopathic obstructive sleep apnea. Am Rev Respir Dis 1984; 129(3):355–360.

76. Horner RL, Mohiaddin RH, Lowell DG, Shea SA, Burman ED, Longmore DB, Guz A. Sites and sizes of fat deposits around the pharynx in obese patients with obstructive sleep apnoea and weight matched controls. Eur Respir J 1989; 2:613–622.

77. Rodenstein DO, Dooms G, Thomas Y, Liistro G, Stanescu DC, Culee C, Aubert-Tulkens G. Pharyngeal shape and dimensions in healthy subjects, snorers, and patients with obstructive sleep apnea. Thorax 1990; 45(10):722–727.

78. Van de Graaff W. Thoracic influence on upper airway patency. J Appl Physiol 1988; 65:2125–2131.

79. Van De Graaff W. Thoracic traction on the trachea: mechanisms and magnitude. J Appl Physiol 1991; 70: 1328–1336.

80. Brown I, Bradley TD, Phillipson EA, Zamel N, Hoffstein V. Pharyngeal compliance in snoring subjects with and without obstructive sleep apnea. Am Rev Respir Dis 1985; 132:211–215.

81. Hoffstein V, Zamel N, Phillipsons E. Lung volume dependence of pharyngeal cross-sectional area in patients with obstructive sleep apnea. Am Rev Respir Dis 1984; 130:175–178.

82. Rubinstein I, Hoffstein V, Bradley T. Lung volume-related changes in the pharyngeal area of obese females with and without obstructive sleep apnea. Eur Respir J 1989; 2: 344–351.

83. Brown I, McClean PA, Boucher R, Zamel N, Hoffstein V. Changes in pharyngeal cross-sectional area with posture and application of continuous positive airway pressure in patients with obstructive sleep apnea. Am Rev Respir Dis 1987; 136:628–632.

84. Rubinstein I, Colapinto N, Rotstein LE, Brown IG, Hoffstein V. Improvement in upper airway function after weight loss in patients with obstructive sleep apnea. Am Rev Respir Dis 1988; 138(5):1192–1195.

85. Suratt P, McTier R, Wilhoit S. Collapsibility of the nasopharyngeal airway in obstructive sleep apnea. Am Rev Respir Dis 1985; 132:967–971.

86. Schwartz AR, Gold AR, Schubert N, Stryzak A, Wise RA, Permutt S, Smith PL. Effect of weight loss on upper airway collapsibility in obstructive sleep apnea. Am Rev Respir Dis 1991; 144(3 Pt 1):494–498.

87. Rajagopal K, Abbrecht P, Tellis C. Control of breathing in obstructive sleep apnea. Chest 1984; 85:174–180.

88. Onal E, Lopata M. Periodic breathing and the pathogenesis of occlusive sleep apneas. Am Rev Respir Dis 1982; 126:676–680.

89. Kunimoto F, Kimura H, Tatsumi K, Kuriyama T, Watanabe S, Honda Y. Sex differences in awake ventilatory drive and abnormal breathing during sleep in eucapnic obesity. Chest 1988; 93(5)968–976.

90. Burki N, R. Baker. Ventilatory regulation in eucapnic morbid obesity. Am Rev Respir Dis 1984; 129:538–543.

91. Greenberg H, Scharf S. Depressed ventilatory load compensation in sleep apnea; reversal by nasal CPAP. Am Rev Respir Dis 1993; 148:1610–1615.

92. Lopata M, Onal E. Mass loading, sleep apnea, and the pathogenesis of obesity hypoventilation. Am Rev Respir Dis 1982; 126:640–645.

93. Gold AR, Schwartz AR, Wise RA, Smith PL. Pulmonary function and respiratory chemosensitivity in moderately obese patients with sleep apnea. Chest 1993; 103(5):1325–1329.

94. Berton-Jones M, Sullivan C. Time course of change in ventilatory response to CO_2 with long-term CPAP therapy for obstructive sleep apnea. Am Rev Respir Dis 1987; 135:144–147.

95. Harman E, Wynne J, Block A. The effect of weight loss on sleep-disordered breathing and oxygen desaturation in morbidly obese men. Chest 1982; 82:291–294.

96. Peiser J, Lavie P, Ovnat A, Charuzi I. Sleep apnea syndrome in the morbidly obese as an indication for weight reduction surgery. Ann Surg 1984; 199:112–115.

97. Charuzi I, Ovnat A, Peiser J, Saltz H, Weitzman S, Lavie P. The effect of surgical weight reduction on sleep quality in obesity-related sleep apnea syndrome. Surgery 1985; 97(5):535–538.

98. Sugerman H, Fairman RP, Baron PL, Kwentus JA. Gastric surgery for respiratory insufficiency of obesity. Chest 1986; 90(1):81–86.

99. Rajala R, Partinen M, Sane T, Pelkonen R, Huikuri K, Seppalainen AM. Obstructive sleep apnea syndrome in morbidly obese patients. J Intern Med 1991; 230(2):125–129.

100. Cook DJ, Guyatt GH, Laupacis A, Sackett DL. Rules of evidence and clinical recommendations on the use of antithrombotic agents. Chest 1992; 102:305s–311s.

101. Mason E, Ito C. Gastric bypass. Ann Surg 1969; 170:329–339.

102. Garner D, Wooley S. Confronting the failure of behavioral and dietary treatments for obesity. Clin Psych Rev 1991; 11:729–780.

103. Wilson G. Behavioral treatment of obesity: thirty years and counting. Adv Behav Res Ther 1994; 16:31–75.

104. Smith P, Gold A, Meyers D, Haponik E, Bleecker E. Weight loss in mildly to moderately obese patients with obstructive sleep apnea. Ann Intern Med 1985; 103:850–855.

105. Pasquali R, Colella P, Cirignotta F, Mondini S, Gerardi R, Buratti P, Rinaldi Ceroni A, Tartari F, Schiavina M, Melchionda N. Treatment of obese patients with obstructive sleep apnea syndrome (OSAS): effect of weight loss and interference of otorhinolarygotiatro pathology. Int J Obes 1990; 14:207–217.

106. Suratt P, McTier RF, Findley LJ, Pohl SL, Wilhoit SC. Changes in breathing and the pharynx after weight loss in obstructive sleep apnea. Chest 1987; 92:631–637.

107. Suratt P, McTier RF, Findley LJ, Pohl SL, Wilhoit SC. Effect of very-low-calorie diets with weight loss on obstructive sleep apnea. Am J Clin Nutr 1992; 56:182S–184S.

108. Nahmias J, Kirschner M, Karetsky M. Weight loss and OSA and pulmonary. N J Med 1993; 90:48–53.

109. Kiselak J, Clark M, Pera V, Rosenberg C, Redline S. The association between hypertension and sleep apnea in obese patients. Chest 1993; 104(3):775–780.

110. Weintraub M, Bray G. Drug treatment of obesity. Med Clin North Am 1989; 73:238–249.

111. Strobel RJ, Lewin D, Rosen RC, Parisi RA. Fenfluramine hydrochloride-assisted weight loss in obstructive sleep apnea syndrome. Am J Respir Crit Care Med 1994; 149:A495.

35

Obesity, Arthritis, and Gout

Flavia M. Cicuttini
Monash University, Victoria, Australia

Tim D. Spector
St. Thomas' Hospital, Guys' and St. Thomas' Trust, London, England

I. OBESITY AND OSTEOARTHRITIS

Osteoarthritis (OA) is a disorder of movable joints characterized by deterioration and abrasion of the joint cartilage and formation of new bone at the joint surfaces. Obesity is likely to be the most important preventable risk factor for OA. Overall, results to date suggest that the link between obesity and OA is more consistent in women and is strongest in OA of the knees and less conclusive in other joints. This has important implications since OA is an enormous public health problem in developed countries as it is the commonest single cause of disability (1) and the major reason for hip and knee replacements (2). The combination of its effect on patients and the therapeutic procedures used produce a huge burden on society (3). Recently, efforts have been focused on potential risk factors for OA with a view to identifying possible preventive measures. The management of obesity is likely to be a key factor in the management of OA.

A. Association of Obesity and OA of the Knee

Cross-sectional epidemiological studies have consistently shown a relationship between obesity and knee OA, which has generally been stronger in women than in men. The reported increased risks have ranged from two- to sevenfold for women in the top tertile of body mass index (BMI) compared to women in the bottom tertile (4–10)

(Table 1). The earliest survey to mention this link was by Fletcher and Lewis-Faning in 1945 (4). In 1958 Kellgren and Lawrence found that knee OA was commoner in obese people and twice as common in females than males (5). Data from the large National Health and Nutrition Exam Survey (NHANES I) 1971–1975 found that the risk of OA increased with degree of obesity, and that long-term obesity was significantly associated with knee OA (9,10). Obesity was strongly related to bilateral knee disease (11).

A population-based, cross-sectional prevalence study of obesity and OA in middle-aged females confirmed obesity as a strong risk factor for OA knees in women (12). This study showed a nearly 18-fold increased risk for bilateral disease. This same effect was also seen in the subgroup of asymptomatic women. The proportion of OA estimated to be attributable to obesity in this group of middle-aged women was 63%.

B. Association of Obesity with OA in the Different Knee Compartments

Until recently, little consideration was given to the multicompartmental nature of the knee joint in epidemiological studies of OA. However, recent work has suggested that a significant proportion of symptomatic knee OA may be caused by patellofemoral disease (13–15), which is not visualized by conventional anteroposterior radiography. Consequently, little attention has been focused on whether

Table 1 Evidence of Association Between Knee OA and Obesity from Some Recent Population-Based Studies

Study	Comparison groups of body weight	Relative risk (95% CI)
Felson et al., 1988 (8)	Quintile 5 (MRW > = 129) vs Quintile 1 (MRW <105)	Men 1.51 (1.14, 1.98)
	Quintile 5 (MRW > =128) vs Quintile 1 (MRW <100)	Women 2.007 (1.67, 2.55)
Davis et al., 1990 (10)	BMI > 30 vs. BMI < = 30	3.64 (2.21, 6.02)
Hart and Spector, 1993 (12)	Tertiel 3 (BMI > 26.4) vs. Tertile 1 (BMI <23.4)	Women 6.17 (3.26–11.71)

MRW = Metropolitan relative weight, a measure of weight in pounds adjusted for height.

the risk factors for OA differ between the different knee compartments. A recent population-based, case-control study examined whether risk factors for OA differ between the different knee compartments (16). This study did not show a significant effect of obesity on the patellofemoral joint but showed an effect at the tibiofemoral joint. This case-control study, based on small numbers, was the first to consider the possibility that OA in different compartments may have different etiologies and that previously described risk factors such as obesity may have differential effects in the different compartments. In contrast, data from a population-based, cross-sectional study of middle-aged women showed it to be an important risk factor for both medial tibiofemoral and patellofemoral joint disease (17). This is an area where further work will be needed to clarify the role of obesity as a risk factor in OA in the different compartments of the knee. This is likely to have important implications for preventive strategies in OA of the knee and for our understanding of the pathogenesis of OA.

C. Evidence from Longitudinal Studies of the Association of Obesity with Knee OA

The Framingham Study examined the association between obesity and knee OA in a longitudinal study. At the time of this study, the group had been followed up for 35 years (18). Radiographs that were obtained on examination 18 (subject's mean age 73 years) were used, together with weights on the same subjects that had been obtained at the beginning of the Framingham Study when the mean age of participants was 37 years. No radiographs were available at the age of 37, but the assumption when analyzing the data was that the prevalence of OA at age 37 was low. This study was able to look at obesity prior to

the development of OA. A strong association between being overweight in 1948–1951 and having knee OA approximately 36 years later was found. This association was stronger for women than men after controlling for possible confounders such as age, uric acid level, and physical activity. Furthermore, this association was present for both symptomatic and asymptomatic disease. In addition, there was a stronger association with more severe, rather than mild, radiological disease.

These data are supported by other studies where, although data on actual weight preceding the onset of OA were not available, self-reported, recall weights were used. In the NHANES study, the effect of past obesity on the risk of developing OA was examined by using self-reported minimum adult weight as a proxy measure of long-term obesity (9). In this study, past obesity was found to be associated with OA. In the Chingford population study of 1003 middle-aged women, a similar association was observed between self-reported minimum weight at age 20 and OA in middle age (12). In this study it was argued that the recalled weight was probably quite accurate as it coincided with the approximate age at which many of the women got married, thus improving the likelihood of accurate recall of their weight at that time.

Further evidence suggesting that obesity precedes OA, rather than the converse, is that the association between OA and obesity is strong even for individuals with radiological evidence of knee OA who are asymptomatic (9,12,17). This is important as radiological disease has been shown to correlate with later disability (19,20). Furthermore, a strong dose-response effect has also been observed between obesity and OA. Those individuals who were obese [body mass index (BMI) > 30] were shown to have a markedly increased risk of knee OA relative to those who were only modestly overweight (BMI > 25 to ≤ 30) (9). This dose-response relationship provides additional evidence of a possible etiological effect.

D. Evidence from Twin Studies of the Role of Obesity in OA

A further method for examining the association between obesity and osteoarthritis is via twin studies that have been used to estimate the magnitude of the weight difference associated with the development of OA (17). Twin studies provide a special research methodology that, in addition to assessing the relative contributions of genetic and environmental factors to a disease, may also be used to examine environmental risk factors in twin pairs discordant for that disease trait. The twin model used in this study enabled close matching of the diseased and nondiseased twin for genetic similarity and many known or unknown environmental factors, thus providing a useful tool to quantify the magnitude of the difference in obesity between the twin with disease and the cotwin with no disease.

The twin study confirmed that obesity is a strong risk factor for OA of the knee, with twins with OA of the tibiofemoral and patellofemoral joints of the knee tending, on average, to be 3–5 kg heavier than their cotwin (Fig. 1). This weight difference was also observed in asymptomatic women, again suggesting that obesity is a cause of OA rather than the converse. After adjusting for other potential risk factors, the results showed that for every kilogram increase in weight, a twin had a 14% increased risk of developing tibiofemoral osteophytes and a 32% increased risk of developing patellofemoral osteophytes compared to the cotwin. These results were consistent with a previous population study, in a similar age group of women, that showed that the risk of knee OA increased

by 35% for every 5 kg of weight gain (12). This suggests that in middle-aged women even small increases in body weight are associated with significant increases in risk of developing OA. Risks in men, however, cannot be extrapolated from these results and separate studies are needed.

E. Association of Obesity and OA of the Hand

Results regarding the association of obesity with hand OA are conflicting. OA of the distal interphalangeal joints has been associated with obesity in some studies, although principally in men (5,21). Secondary analysis of data from the National Health Examination Survey showed a significant association of BMI with the presence of hand OA in men after adjustment for age, race, and skinfold thickening but not after adjustment for waist girth and seat breadth (22). An association between radiographic hand OA and BMI in men was also observed in the longitudinal, prospective study of 70-year-old people in Goteborg (23). An association between obesity and finger OA was observed in the New Haven Survey, with this association being stronger in women (6).

No association was observed between indices of obesity and hand OA in men in the Baltimore Longitudinal Study of Aging (24) or for women between BMI and hand OA in the National Health Examination Survey (22). However, an association was observed between BMI and the grade of hand OA for women in the Tecumseh Community Health Study (25). Obesity was also modestly associated with distal interphalangeal and carpometacarpal OA, but not but not with the proximal interphalangeal OA in the women in the Chingford Study (12).

Data from a twin study showed a mean weight difference (95% CI) within twin pairs discordant for carpometacarpal osteophytes of 3.06 (0.83, 5.28) kg (17). The results suggested that there was a 9% increase in risk of developing carpometacarpal osteophytes for every kilogram increase in body weight. However, there was no significant difference in weight within twin pairs discordant for osteophytes at the distal interphalangeal (distal interphalangeal) or proximal interphalangeal (proximal interphalangeal) joints.

F. Evidence from Longitudinal Studies of the Association of Obesity with Hand OA

Less information is available on the effect of long-term obesity and hand OA. One of the few studies to examine this was the Tecumseh Community Health Study, a longitudinal study that investigated the role of obesity in the etiology of hand OA (26). This study, conducted in Tecumseh, Michigan, began in 1962 with baseline exami-

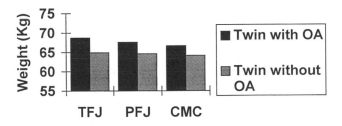

Figure 1 Body weight for twins with osteoarthritis in the tibiofemoral (TFJ) joint of the knee, the patellofemoral (PFJ) joint of the knee, and the carpometacarpal (CMC) joint of the hand. The weight differences between the twins with OA and the twins without OA were significant at all the above joints: TFJ (*p* < 0.001), PFJ (*p* < 0.001), CMC (*p* < 0.002).

nations of clinical, biochemical, and radiological characteristics. A 1985 reexamination of the cohort characterized OA status in 1276 participants (588 males and 688 females), who were aged 50–74 years at this follow-up. Baseline obesity, as measured by an index of relative weight, was found to be significantly associated with the 23-year incidence of osteoarthritis of the hands among subjects disease-free at baseline. Greater baseline relative weight was also associated with greater subsequent severity of OA of the hands. However, the difference between baseline and follow-up weight values was not significantly associated with the incidence of OA of the hands. Furthermore, there was no evidence that development of osteoarthritis subsequently led to increased incidence of obesity.

G. Association of Obesity and OA of the Hip

The available data suggest that there may be a modest association between hip OA and obesity (5,7,21). When data from 4225 persons from the National Health and Nutrition Examination Survey (HANES) were examined by dividing subjects into four groups on the basis of sex and race, relative weight was weakly associated with OA of the hips in white women and nonwhite men (7). A case-control study that examined BMI at age 20, 30, 40, and 50 years in 239 men who had just received a hip prosthesis because of osteoarthritis and in 302 controls randomly selected from the general population (27) showed that men with a BMI greater than one standard deviation above the mean had an increased relative risk of developing severe OA than men with a BMI less than one standard deviation below the mean. Those slightly obese at the age of 40 years had a relative risk of 2.5 for later surgery of the hip. In contrast, however, data from the First National Health and Nutrition Examination Survey (NHANES-I) did not support this (28). Obesity, and fat distribution were not associated with hip osteoarthritis.

H. Possible Mechanisms for Obesity in the Pathogenesis of OA

OA is a disease of cartilage in which cartilage breakdown and erosion are accompanied by bony changes such as osteophytes subchondral sclerosis, and bony cysts. Although the mechanisms by which obesity may lead to OA are unknown, three hypothesis have been proposed (10,11,29) (Table 2): (1) obesity increases the load across the knee joint resulting in increased or abnormal stress and resultant deterioration of the joint structures; (2) obesity acts indirectly by metabolic changes associated with

Table 2 Possible Mechanisms for Obesity in the Pathogenesis of OA

Mechanical
Increase in load across the joint
Abnormal stresses across a joint
Systemic
Association with raised serum glucose, hypertension, hypercholesterolemia, hyperuricemia, and insulin resistance
?Excess endogenous steroids
Dietary
High fat content resulting in abnormal joint structures

increased fatness such as glucose intolerance, hyperlipidemia, hyperoestogenemia or changes in bone density; and (3) elements of the diet that result in obesity, such as high fat content, adversely affect bone, cartilage, or other joint structures (Table 2). Obesity may initiate cartilage, breakdown or may promote joint destruction after the initial incipient lesion. Although obesity possibly leads to disease because it causes increased force on the cartilage, it also may produce disease by increasing subchondral bony stiffness (30) and by making subchondral bone less deformable to impact loads. This stiff bone would then transmit the increased force to underlying cartilage, making it more vulnerable.

A number of factors suggest a metabolic/systemic component to OA. These include the female preponderance, menopausal onset of generalized OA, the unequal effect of obesity on knee and hip OA, and the inverse relationship with osteoporosis. Furthermore, obesity is also linked to OA of the fingers and the base of the thumb, in which mechanical force is less likely to play an important role.

I. Evidence for Obesity Acting Via a Systemic Mechanism

I. Association Between OA and Other Metabolic Conditions

Hypertension. On analysis of the data from the 1960s survey in Leigh and Wensleydale, Lawrence found that hypertension was associated with generalized OA in men and with knee OA in hypertensive, nonobese females (31). The relationship was between diastolic blood pressure and knee OA, in both obese and nonobese females, and this association remained in each 5-year age group from 45 to 69. The association between hypertension and OA was also observed in the Chingford population study, which showed that "ever treated" hypertension was associated with the development of OA and that this association was strongest for those with bilateral knee disease (32). In contrast, some studies have failed to confirm an association between OA and blood pressure. No association was found in a study of 70-year-old people in Goteborg (23). In univariate analysis of NHANES-I data, an increase in recorded diastolic and systolic blood pressure was found in women with knee OA, but this association disappeared after adjusting for weight (33).

Cholesterol. A significant association was found with hand OA and above-average measured serum cholesterol in women in the 1960s survey in Leigh and Wensleydale (34). However, the association disappeared in those with very high serum cholesterol. Furthermore, Lawrence found that subjects with OA and hypertension in this same population did not have an association with high serum cholesterol or uric acid (31). In analyses of the data from NHANES-I and the data from the study of 70-year-old people in Goteborg (23), serum cholesterol was not significantly associated with either unilateral or bilateral knee OA (11). In contrast, the data from the Chingford population study suggested an association between bilateral knee disease and hypercholesterolemia (32).

Glucose. Few studies have examined the association between blood glucose and OA. Cimmino and Cutolo studied 1026 subjects with OA from clinics, compared them to 220 healthy population controls, and found slightly higher levels of plasma glucose in women in the OA group after adjusting for age (35). A study comparing 25 female diabetic patients with knee OA and 48 nondiabetic women who were matched for age, weight, symptoms, and duration of OA found an increased incidence of osteophytes on the radiographs of the diabetic patients while the joint space narrowing and sclerosis were equal between the two groups (36). An association between serum glucose and osteoarthritis was also observed in the Chingford population study (32). In this study, raised blood glucose was a significant factor in all forms of knee OA but the association was strongest for patients with bilateral knee disease (32). It has been speculated that the link between diabetes and OA may be through elevated growth hormone levels that alter cartilage metabolism and increase bone density (10,11). Increased bone density associated with obesity has been hypothesised to increase the forces acting on the cartilage, thus predisposing for the development of OA (10,11). However, these theories have not been well examined and not all epidemiological studies have shown an association between serum glucose and OA. In the analyses of the NHANES-I data, self-reported diabetes was not associated with either unilateral

or bilateral knee OA (11). Furthermore, no association was observed between blood glucose levels and OA in a study of 70-year-old people in Goteborg (23).

Uric Acid. Data from the New Haven population survey showed that a raised serum uric acid level was significantly associated with OA, with the association being stronger in women than men (6). In univariate analysis of NHANES-I data, hyperuricemia was found to be related to knee OA in women, but the association disappeared after adjusting for body weight (9). There was no significant association with either unilateral or bilateral knee OA (11). This is further supported by a study of 70-year-old people in Goteborg (23) where no association was observed between serum uric acid level and OA. In contrast, the data from the Chingford population study suggested a possible association between raised serum uric acid levels and bilateral knee disease (32).

Summary. The data suggesting a link between OA and raised serum glucose, cholesterol, uric acid, and hypertension remains inconclusive. However, one possible explanation for an association between hypertension, hyperlipidaemia, and OA is insulin resistance, or Reven's syndrome (37). This syndrome may be a distinct genetic trait, or alternatively, it may represent a physiological adaptation to chronic obesity (38).

2. Association Between OA and Body Fat Distribution

Adipose tissue distribution is associated with a number of metabolic complications, with a pattern of central central body fat (particularly abdominal fat) indicating increased risk of diabetes, cardiovascular disease, and mortality, independent of degree of obesity (39). Recent interest has focused on the distribution of body fat in OA in an effort to understand whether systemic factors are important in the development of OA. Analysis of the NHANES data showed that BMI correlated best with presence of OA using different anthropomorphic measurements, suggesting that body fat may be more important than the absolute weight (29). In this study there was a significant association between hand and feet OA and seat breadth in men, odds ratio 1.45 (1.03–2.06). Although this association was also observed in women, the confidence intervals included one. However, no association was found in this study between a centralized pattern of body fat distribution with hand or knee OA. In fact, this study found some evidence of an association of peripheral body fat pattern and combined hand and feet OA (10). Consistent with these observations, the Chingford population study of middle-aged women (32) and the Baltimore Longitudinal Study of Aging (40) of both women and men also failed to show an association between body fat distribution and OA, independent of body weight.

3. Summary

Together these data support a stronger contribution of mechanical as opposed to systemic factors to explain the association between obesity and OA. The results suggest that peripheral distribution of fat may act as a mechanical effect rather than a metabolic cause of OA. However, there is increasing evidence that OA is not a single disorder but a heterogeneous group of disorders. It is postulated that a complex interplay of several factors may result in a common pathway of joint damage. Therefore, it is possible that obesity has a mechanical effect on some joints and a metabolic effect on other joints. Several studies have shown an association of obesity with hand OA (5,6, 21,23). Thus, it may be that obesity causes knee OA because of an increase in mechanical stress across the joint but that the effect of obesity on the small joints of the hand is through metabolic consequences.

J. Role of Obesity in Progression of OA

The natural history of knee OA is poorly understood, and few studies have any detailed data on prognostic factors such as obesity, although the available data suggest that obesity is important. In a small group of clinical cases followed up for 11 years, there was no clear effect of obesity (41) However, in the EPOZ study Schouten et al. found that obesity, age, Heberden's nodes, and valgus deformity were all associated with cartilage loss over a 12-year period (42). Factors related to joint space progression in the multicenter French study were obesity and number of affected joints (43). A recent study that examined the rates of incident OA in the contralateral knee in a general population sample showed that in middle-aged women with early unilateral OA of the knee a high percentage (34%) develop OA in the contralateral knee within 2 years and 22.4% progress radiologically in the index joint. Obesity appeared to have a marked effect on the incidence rates, with nearly a fivefold increase in overweight women compared to thin women. This is supported by a further study that showed that the odds ratio for BMI was 11.1 (3.3–37.3) for the fourth versus the first quartile (42). BMI was also found to be related to loss of cartilage in those who had OA (42).

K. Association of Obesity with Symptoms and Disability in OA

Most nonfatal chronic conditions are strongly age-related (43,44), with their prevalence rising with increasing age of the population. Thus, as the total population continues to age due to the decrease in birth rate and to recent declines in mortality in the older age groups, the burden of nonfatal diseases and impairments will continue to increase. This has highlighted the need to examine prognostic factors for disability. Using the 1984 Supplement on Aging conducted by the National Center for Health Statistics, the risk factors for disability among US adults aged 55+ who had arthritis were compared to those who did not have arthritis (45). This study showed that obesity was strongly implicated in disability once arthritis was present. Thus, obesity is not only a risk factor for developing OA, but also contributes to the disability once it occurs. The contribution of obesity to symptom development in individuals who already have the pathological changes of OA is unclear. Studies that have assessed whether obese subjects with concurrent radiographic OA are more likely to have symptoms have yielded conflicting results (7,46). Furthermore, the role of eight loss in alleviating symptoms remains an unanswered, but very important, clinical question.

L. Is Weight Loss Effective in Reducing the Risk of OA?

Few studies have looked at the effect of weight loss in subjects who have established disease. Felson et al. (47), in the Framingham cohort, observed that weight loss in mid- and later adult life substantially reduced the risk of symptomatic OA of the knee. To evaluate the effect of weight loss in preventing symptomatic knee OA, women who participated in the Framingham Knee Osteoarthritis Study (1983–1985) were examined. Sixty-four of 796 women studied had recent-onset symptomatic knee OA (knee symptoms plus radiographically confirmed OA) and were compared with women without disease. Weight change significantly affected the risk for the development of knee OA. For example, a decrease in BMI of 2 units or more (weight loss, approximately 5 kg) over the 10 years before the current examination decreased the odds for developing OA by over 50% (odds ratio, 0.46; 95% Cl, 0.24–0.86). Among those women with a high risk for OA due to elevated baseline BMI (greater than or equal to 25), weight loss also decreased the risk (for 2 units of BMI, odds ratio, 0.41). Weight gain was associated with a slightly increased risk for OA, which was not statistically significant, while weight loss reduced the risk for symptomatic knee OA in women. Furthermore, extrapolating from cross-sectional data suggests that risk of knee OA increases by 35% for every 5 kg of weight gain (12).

The available data suggest that reduction or maintenance of weight may have an important role in the prevention of OA. There is also evidence that weight reduction is associated with a decrease in musculoskeletal symptoms (48,49). However, there is little data on whether weight loss affects the progression of OA, and this area needs further work.

II. OBESITY AND GOUT

There has been an increase in prevalence of gout since World War II (50). Although increased awareness of the disease may in part explain this, and milder cases are being identified, particular interest has focused on the role of changes in diet and weight over this time. The evidence from cross-sectional and prospective studies for an association between obesity and gout is presented in the following sections.

A. Evidence from Cross-Sectional Studies for Obesity as a Risk Factor for Gout

A large body of evidence exists to support an association between gout and obesity. The New Haven Survey showed that certain metabolic conditions, including hyperuricemia, were associated with obesity (6). In a cross-sectional study of 73,000 women aged 30–49, obesity was shown to be significantly associated with gout ($p < 0.001$) (51). In 460 apparently healthy Dutch men and women aged 65–79 years, serum uric acid level was found to be positively associated with body weight, BMI, body fatness, and lean body mass in men but not women (52). In a study of 7735 middle-aged men in 24 British towns, a positive association was observed between BMI and gout (53).

The association between obesity and hyperuricemia has also been observed in other ethnic groups. A survey of 115 Maori men of working age showed a strong relationship between hyperuricemia and obesity (54). In Melanesian and Asian Indians in Fiji, BMI was shown to have a significant and independent association with plasma uric acid levels in both nondiabetic and diabetic men and women (55). However, the most extreme example of an association between gout and obesity was seen in sumo wrestlers, who do not appear to have any underlying genetic predisposition to gout (56). In a study of 96 sumo wrestlers in Japan, mean serum levels of uric acid were

significantly higher than those of 89 age-matched healthy men. Weight correlated significantly with uric acid.

Some recent data have suggested that body fat and the distribution pattern of fat may be more important than total weight as a risk factor for gout (57). The association between fat distribution and gout was examined in 95 overweight adult men and 210 overweight adult women (57). It was found that, adjusted for age and BMI, a high waist-thigh circumference ratio was a risk factor for gout, particularly in women. The association of waist-hips circumference ratio with gout was less pronounced in men.

B. Evidence from Longitudinal Studies for Obesity as a Risk Factor for Gout

The association of obesity with hyperuricemia is also supported by longitudinal studies. A cohort study of medical students was performed recently with the aim of identifying potentially modifiable risk factors for the development of gout (58). A total of 1271 predominantly young (median age, 22 years), white, male students, received a standardized medical examination and questionnaire during medical school. The outcome measure was the development of gout. Sixty cases of gout (47 primary and 13 secondary) were identified among 1216 men; none occurred among 121 women. In this study, BMI at age 35 years and excessive weight gain between cohort entry and age 35 years were significant risk factors for gout in univariate analysis. Multivariate analyses confirmed the association of BMI at age 35 years and excessive weight gain as risk factors for gout.

Data from the Harvard Growth Study of 1922–1935 were used to examine the long-term effect of obesity in adolescence on morbidity, including the development of gout (59). A total of 508 lean or overweight adolescents 13–18 years old who participated in the Harvard Growth Study were included in this subanalysis. Overweight adolescents were defined as those with a BMI that on two occasions was greater than the 75th percentile in subjects of the same age and sex in a large national survey. Lean adolescents were defined as those with a BMI between the 25th and 50th percentiles. The risk of gout was increased among men who had been overweight in adolescence. Overweight in adolescence was a more powerful predictor of this risk than overweight in adulthood.

C. Association of Gout and Other Metabolic Disorders

Hyperuricemia has been shown to correlate with a cluster of metabolic and hemodynamic disorders closely associated with insulin resistance syndrome (IRS) in young, apparently healthy individuals (60). After adjustment for sex, serum uric acid concentration showed positive associations with BMI, waist/hip girth, waist/thigh girth, and subscapula/triceps skinfold ratios. Furthermore, serum uric acid was also positively correlated with fasting insulin, serum triglycerides, LDL cholesterol, and negatively with HDL/total cholesterol ratio. This has been confirmed in other studies (61). Furthermore, urinary uric acid clearance appears to decrease in proportion to increases in insulin resistance in normal volunteers, leading to an increase in serum uric acid concentration. Thus, it appears that modulation of serum uric concentration by insulin resistance is exerted at the level of the kidney (61).

Thus, obesity has a number of effects on unrate metabolism, which include decreasing urate clearance (61) and increasing urate production (62). It has been suggested that other factors, such as muscle mass, may also play a role in producing hyperuricemia (63). Weight reduction has been associated with a modest lowering of the serum urate concentration (64).

D. Diet

It is thought that the increase in the prevalence of gout this century may relate to the changing nutritional patterns associated with increasing industrialization (65). Genetic factors and nutrition combine in order that the disease may become manifest. Interest has largely focused on the more abundant diet, which is also richer in purines. For example, a study in the Ukraine showed that in the period from 1925–1928 to 1970–1971 there was an increase in the consumption of animal products (milk, meat, fish, eggs), of sugar, vegetables, and fruits, and a fall in the consumption of cereals (bakery products, grits, macaroni, beans) and potatoes (66). In parallel with these dietary changes, the incidence of diseases such as gout increased over the same time period (66).

Population-based studies have confirmed the association between diet and gout. A study of 460 apparently healthy Dutch elderly, aged 65–79 years, showed that serum uric acid correlated with alcohol intake (men) and consumption of meat and fish (women), and inversely with consumption of bread, margarine, and milk products (women), independent of confounders such as BMI (67). A community-based survey of 1738 registered residents over 30 years of age in Pu-Li Township, Taiwan, from 1987 to 1988, showed that organ meat consumption significantly correlated with hyperuricemia after simultaneously controlling for weight (68).

Migration studies have also suggested a role for a richer diet in gout. The incidence of hyperuricemia and gout has been well recognized to be higher among Filipinos in Hawaii, Alaska, and mainland United States than in their native country (69). It appears that Filipino hyperuricemia may become manifest because some Filipinos possess a renal defect that may lead to hyperuricemia due to renal inability to compensate for an increased purine intake, which may occur in the shift from a low-purine Filipino diet to a high-purine Western diet in the new environment (69).

To examine the effect of ingesting some purine-rich foods (beef, liver, haddock fillets, and soybeans) on uric acid metabolism, a crossover study was performed where three isoenergetic and isonitrogenous meals were fed to 18 male subjects with no history of gout or kidney disorder during a 3-week period (70). Only the content of uricogenic bases (adenine and hypoxanthine) varied among the test meals. Ingestion of all experimental meals caused an increase in serum uric acid levels at 120 min, and this increase was more marked (about twofold) with haddock and soybean ingestion. In all groups, the postprandial serum uric acid levels at 240 min were lower than those obtained at 120 min, but still remained elevated in comparison to the fasting level. As expected, 24-hr urinary uric acid excretion was similar for the three test meals due to the isonitrogenous load of proteins and purines. This study suggested that assessment of each purine base content rather than the total purine content of foods may be important in the management of hyperuricemic individuals.

E. Alcohol

Many studies with different study designs and in different populations have now shown a relationship between alcohol consumption and gout (71–77). For example, in a population-based study in Denmark, 5249 males aged between 40 and 59 were interviewed to identify a history of gout (77). A total of 104 men who had experienced gout were compared to 208 computer-selected, age-matched controls drawn at random from the entire sample. Alcohol consumption was higher in gout patients than controls. In a cohort of 2046 initially healthy men in the Normative Aging Study followed for 14.9 years with serial examinations and measurement of urate levels, alcohol intake was a strong predictor of gout when examined in a proportional hazards model (78).

Migration studies have also confirmed the association between alcohol and gout. In a study of the prevalence and 14-year incidence of clinical gout in the Polynesian population of Tokelauans living in the Pacific basin, nonmigrant Tokelauans living in their isolated atoll homeland were compared with migrant Tokelauans living in urban New Zealand (79). Self-reported alcohol consumption at entry to the study was a strong predictor of gout in men. Factors predisposing to acute gout were investigated in a case-control study (80) of 70 patients with acute gout and matched for age and sex controls. Gout was significantly associated with obesity (odds ratio 3.7, 95% confidence interval 1.4, 9.1) and high alcohol intake (odds ratio 3.3, 95% confidence interval 1.1, 9.8). In these patients, it was estimated that 23% of gout was attributable to obesity and 16% to high alcohol consumption.

To determine the contribution of alcohol to increased production and decreased excretion of uric acid, a study was performed where oral ethanol (1.8 g/kg of body weight every 24 hr) for 8 days or intravenous ethanol (0.25–0.35 g/kg/hr) for 2 hr was given to six patients with gout (81). The results of this study suggested that ethanol increases urate synthesis by enhancing the turnover of adenine nucleotides (81). A further study showed that chronic oral ethanol administration was associated with increased serum urate, urine uric acid excretion, urine uric acid clearance, and oxypurine excretion (82). The daily rate of uric acid turnover was significantly increased. Intravenous ethanol administration was associated with increased uric acid excretion, increased uric acid clearance, and significantly increased oxypurine excretion. Excretion of radioactivity derived from intravenously administered adenine increased significantly. It was concluded that hyperuricemia related to ethanol consumption at lower blood ethanol levels (less than 150 mg/dl) results from increased production of uric acid probably secondary to accelerated degradation of adenine nucleotides.

Although red wine and not beer drinking has traditionally been linked to gout, beer drinking may have an additional effect on the risk of gout. A recent study of 61 men with gout and 52 control subjects showed that the patients with gout drank significantly more alcohol while the average daily intake of most other nutrients, including total purine nitrogen, was similar (83). Beer was the most popular beverage, and 25 (41%) of those with gout consumed more than 60 g of alcohol daily (equivalent to 2.5 L of beer). The heavy drinkers had a significantly higher intake of purine nitrogen, half of which was derived from beer. Though the effect of ingested purine on the blood uric acid was difficult to estimate in this study, it probably was sufficient to have a clinical effect, augmenting the hyperuricemic effect of alcohol itself. A further study attempted to simulate the beer-drinking habits of gout patients and examine the effect on uric acid levels (84). Beer or squash was drunk over a 4-h period on two successive days by five gouty and five normouricemic men. Serum lactate increased with beer and squash, but elevation of plasma uric acid was confined to beer drinking. Urate clearance increased with both beverages, but 24-hr uric acid excretion was accentuated only by beer. The purine content of several beers was measured and the principal constituent found to be guanosine, which is probably the most readily absorbed dietary purine. It was concluded that the hyperuricemic effect of beer was mediated by the digestion of purines contained by the beer and by an effect of ethanol on uric acid synthesis. However there was no evidence that beer taken in usual quantities reduced the renal excretion of uric acid.

III. SUMMARY

Obesity is an important risk factor for OA and gout, which are two common, chronic diseases associated with significant morbidity and cost to the community. Preventive efforts to reduce obesity in the population are likely to have a major impact on these two conditions.

REFERENCES

1. Verbrugge LM. From sneezes to adieux: Stages of health for American men and women. In: Ward RA, Tobin SS Eds. Health in Aging: Sociological Issues and Policy Directions. New York: Springer, 1987:17–57.
2. Bulstrode C. Keeping up with orthopaedic epidemics. Br Med J 1987; 295:514 (editorial).
3. Dieppe PA. Osteoarthritis; the scale and scope of the clinical problem. In: Osteoarthritis: Current Research and Prospects for Pharmacological Intervention. IBC Technical Services Ltd, 1991.
4. Fletcher E, Lewis-Faning E. Chronic rheumatic diseases with special reference to chronic arthritis: a survey based on 1000 cases. Postgrad Med J 1945; 21:51–56.
5. Kellgren JH, Lawrence JS. Osteoarthritis and disk degeneration in an urban population. Ann Rheum Dis 1958; 17:388–396.
6. Acheson RM, Collart AB. New Haven Survey of joint disease: relationship between some systemic characteristics and osteoarthritis in a general population. Ann Rheum Dis 1975; 34:379–384.
7. Hartz AJ, Fischer ME, Bril G, Kelber S, Rupley D Jr, Oken B, Rimm AA. The association of obesity with joint pain and osteoarthritis in the HANES data. J Chronic Dis 1986; 39:311–319.
8. Felson DT, Anderson JJ, Naimark A, Walker AM, Meenan RF. Obesity and knee osteoarthritis. The Framingham Study. Ann Intern Med 1988; 109:18–24.
9. Anderson JJ, Felson DT. Factors associated with osteoarthritis of the knee in the first national health and nutrition

examination survey (NHANES I). Am J Epidemiol 1988; 128:179–189.

10. Davis MA, Ettinger WH, Neuhaus JM. Obesity and osteoarthritis of the knee: evidence from the national health and nutrition examination survey. Semin Arthritis Rheum 1990: 20; 34–41.

11. Davis MA, Ettinger WH, Neuhaus JM, Sangsook AC, Hauck WW. The association of knee injury and obesity with unilateral and bilateral osteoarthritis of the knee. Am J Epidemiol 1989; 137:278–288.

12. Hart DJ, Spector TD. The relationship of obesity, fat distribution and osteoarthritis in women in the general population: the Chingford Study. J Rheumatol 1993; 20: 331–335.

13. Cooper C, Cushnaghan J, Kirwan J, et al. Radiological assessment of the knee joint in osteoarthritis. Br J Rheum 1992; 51:80–82.

14. McAlindon TE, Snow S, Cooper C, Dieppe PA. Radiographic patterns of knee osteoarhtitis in the community: the important of the patellofemoral joint. Ann Rheum Dis 1993; 51:844–849.

15. Ledingham J, Regan M, Jones A, Doherty M. Radiographic patterns and associations of osteoarthritis of the knee in patients referred to hospital. Ann Rheum Dis 1993; 52: 520–526.

16. Cooper C, McAlindon T, Snow S, Vines K, Young P, Kirwan J, Dieppe P. Mechanical and constitutional factors for symptomatic knee osteoarthritis: differences between medail tibiofemoral and patellofemoral disease. J Rheumatol 1994; 21:307–313.

17. Cicuttini FM, Baker JR, Spector TD. The association of obesity with osteoarthritis of the hand and knee in women: a twin study. J Rheumatol 1996; 23:1221–1226.

18. Felson DT, Anderson JJ, Naimark A, Walker AM, Meenan RF. Obesity and knee osteoarthritis: the Framingham Study. Ann Intern Med 1992; 116:535–539.

19. Hochberg MC, Lawrence RC, Everett DF, Coroni-Huntley J. Epidemiological associations of pain in osteoarthritis of the knee: data from the National Health and Nutrition Examination Survey and the National Health and Nutrition Examination-I epidemiological follow-up survey. Semin Arthritis Rheum 1989; 18:4–9.

20. Acheson RM, Kelsey JL, Ginsburg GN. The New Haven Survey of joint diseases. XVI. Impairment, disability and arthritis. Br J Prev Med 1974; 27:168–176.

21. van Saase JLC, Vandenbruke JP, van Romunde LK, Valkenberg HA. Osteoarthritis and obesity in the general population. A relationship calling for an explanation. J Rheumatol 1988; 15:1152–1158.

22. Davis MA, Neuhaus JM, Ettinger WH, Muller WH. Body fat distribution and osteoarthritis. Am J Epidemiol 1990; 132:701–707.

23. Bagge E, Bjelle A, Eden S, Svanborg A. Factors associated with radiographic osteoarthritis: results from the population study 70-year-old people in Goteborg. J Rheumatol 1991; 18:1218–1222.

24. Hochberg MC, Lethbridge-Cejku M, Plato CC, Wigley FM, Tobin JD. Factors associated wth osteoarthritis of the hand in males: data from the Baltimore Longitudinal Study of Aging. Am J Epidemiol 1991; 132:1121–1127.

25. Sowers MF, Zobel D, Weissfeld L, Hawthorne VM, Carman W. Progression of osteoarthritis of the hand and metacarpal bone loss: a twenty-year followup of incident cases. Arthritis Rheum 1991; 34:36–42.

26. Carman WJ, Sowers M, Hawthorne VM, Weisfeld LA. Obesity as a risk factor for osteoarthritis of the hand and wrist: a prospective study. Am J Epidemiol 1994; 139:119–129.

27. Vingard E. Overweight predisposes to coxarthrosis. Body-mass index studied in 239 males with hip arthroplasty. Acta Orthop Scand 1991; 62:106–109.

28. Tepper S, Hochberg MC. Factors associated with hip osteoarthritis: data from the First National Health and Nutrition Examination Survey (NHANES-I). Am J Epidemiol 1993; 137(10):1081–1088.

29. Davis MA, Ettinger WH, Neuhaus JM, Hauck WW. Sex differences in osteoarthritis of the knee: the role of obesity. Am J Epidemiol 1988; 127:1019–1030.

30. Dequeker J, Goris P, Uytterhoeven R. Osteoporosis and osteoarthritis. JAMA 1983; 249:1448–1451.

31. Lawrence JS. Hypertension in relation to musculoskeletal disorders. Ann Rheum Dis 1975; 34:451–456.

32. Hart DJ, Doyle DV, Spector TD. The association between metabolic factors and knee osteoarthritis in women. J Rheumatol 1995; 22:1118–1123.

33. Davis MA, Ettinger WH, Neuhaus JM. The role of metabolic factors and blood pressure in the association of obesity with osteoarthritis of the knee. J Rheumatol 1988; 128: 179–189.

34. Kellgren JH. Osteoarthritis in patients and populations. Br Med J 1961; 1:1–6.

35. Cimmino MA, Cutolo M. Plasma glucose concentration in symptomatic osteoarthritis: a clinical an epidemiological survey. Clin Exp Rheumatol 1990; 8:251–257.

36. Horn CA, Bradley JD, Brandt KD, Kreipke DL, Slowman SD, Kalasinski LA. Impairment of osteophyte formation in hyperglycaemic patients with type II diabetes mellitus and knee osteoarthritis. Arthritis Rheum 1992; 35:336–334.

37. Reven GM. Banting Lecture 1988. Role of insulin resistance in human disease. Diabetes 1988; 37:1595–1607.

38. Eckel RH. Insulin resistance: an adaptation for weight maintenance. Lancet 1992; 340:1452–1453.

39. Joos SK, Mueller WH, Hanis Cl, et al. Diabetes Alert Study: weight history and upper body obesity in diabetic and non-diabetic Mexican American adults. Ann Hum Biol 1984; 11:1671–1677.

40. Hochberg MC, Lethbridge-Cejku M, Scott WW Jr, Reichle R, Plato CC, Tobin JD. The association of body weight, body fatness and body fat distribution with osteoarthritis of the knee: data from the Baltimore Longitudinal Study of Aging. J Rheumatol 1995; 22:488–493.

41. Spector TD, Dacre JE, Harris PA, Huskisson EC. The radiological progression of osteoarthritis; an eleven year

follow-up study of the knee. Ann Rheum Dis 1992, 51: 1107–1110.

42. Schouten JSAG, van den Ouweland FA, Valkenburg HA. A twelve year follow-up study in the general population on prognostic factors of cartilage loss in osteoarthritis of the knee. Ann Rheum Dis 1992; 51:932–937.

43. Dougados M, Gueguen A, Nguyen M, Thiesce A, et al. Longitudinal radiologic evaluation of osteoarthritis of the knee. J Rheumatol 1992; 19:378–384.

44. Chirikos TN. Accounting for the historical rise in work disability prevalence. Milbank Mem Fund Q/Health Soc 1986; 64:271–301.

45. Verbrugge LM, Gates DM, Ike RW. Risk factors for disability among US adults with arthritis. J Clin Epidemiol 1991; 44: 167–182.

46. Bremner JM, Bier F. Osteoarthrosis: prevalence in and relationship between symptomns and X-ray changes. Rheum Dis 1966; 25:1–24.

47. Felson DT, Zhang Y, Anthony JM, Naimark A, Anderson JJ. Weight loss reduces the risk for symptomatic knee osteoarthritis in women. The Framingham Study. Ann Intern Med 1992; 116:535–539.

48. Willims RA, Foulsham BM. Weight reduction in osteoarthritis using phentermine. Practitioner 1981; 22S: 231–232.

49. McGoey B, Deitel M, Saplys RJ, Kliman ME. Effect of weight loss on musculoskeletal pain in the morbidly obese. J Bone Joint Surg 1990; 72B:322–323.

50. Mertz DP, Babucke G. Epidemiology and clinical findings in primary gout. Observations between 1948 and 1968. Munchen Med Wochenschr 1971; 113:617–624.

51. Rimm AA, Werner LH, Yserloo BV, Bernstein RA. Relationship of obesity and disease in 73,532 weight-conscious women. Public Health Rep 1975; 90:44–54.

52. Loenen HM, Eshuis H, Lowik MR, Schouten EG, Hulshof KF, Odink J, Kok FJ. Serum uric acid correlates in elderly men and women with special reference to body composition and dietary intake (Dutch Nutrition Surveillance System). J Clin Epidemiol 1990; 43:1297–1303.

53. Weatherall R, Shaper AG. Overweight and obesity in middle-aged British men. Eur J Clin Nutr 1988; 42:221–231.

54. Gibson T, Waterworth R, Hatfield P, Robinson G, Bremner K. Hyperuricaemia, gout and kidney function in New Zealand Maori men. Br J Rheumatol 1984; 23:276–282.

55. Tuomilehto J, Zimmet P, Wolf E, Taylor R, Ram P, King H. Plasma uric acid level and its association with diabetes mellitus and some biologic parameters in a biracial population of Fiji. Am J Epidemiol 1988; 127:321–336.

56. Nishizawa T, Akaoka I., Nishida Y, Kawaguchi Y, Hayashi E. Some factors related to obesity in the Japanese sumo wrestler. Am J Clin Nutr 1976; 29:1167–1174.

57. Seidell JC, Bakx JC, De Boer E, Deurenberg P, Hautvast JG. Fat distribution of overweight persons in relation to morbidity and subjective health. Int J Obes 1985; 9:363–374.

58. Roubenoff R, Klag MJ, Mead LA, Liang KY, Seidler AJ, Hochberg MC. Incidence and risk factors for gout in white men. JAMA 1991; 266:3004–3007.

59. Must A, Jacques PF, Dallal GE, Bajema CJ, Dietz WH. Long-term morbidity and mortality of overweight adolescents. A follow-up of the Harvard Growth Study of 1922 to 1935. N Engl J Med 1992; 327:1350–1355.

60. Cigolini M, Targher G, Tonoli M, Manara F, Muggeo M, De Sandre G. Hyperuricaemia: relationships to body fat distribution and other components of the insulin resistance syndrome in 38-year-old healthy men and women. Int J Obes Relat Metab Disord 1995; 19:92–96.

61. Facchini F, Chen YD, Hollenbeck CB, Reaven GM. Relationship between resistance to insulin-mediated glucose uptake, urinary uric acid clearance, and plasma uric acid concentration. JAMA 1991; 66:3008–3011.

62. Emmerson BT. Alteration of uric acid metabolism by weight reduction. Aust NZ J Med 1973; 3:410–412.

63. Brauer GW, Prior IAM. A prospective study of gout in New Zealand maoris. Ann Rheum Dis 1978; 37:466–472.

64. Scott JT. Obesity and uricaemia. Clin Rheum Dis 1977; 3: 25–35.

65. Zollner N. Consequences of malnutrition in prosperous countries. Zentralbl Bakteriol Orig B 1976; 163:111–117.

66. Maistruk PN, Priputina LS, Rudenko AK, Smoliar VI. Nutrition and the state of health of the population of the UkrSSR. Vopr Pitan 1976; Jan-Feb(1):13–17.

67. Loenen HM, Eshuis H, Lowik MR, Schouten EG, Hulshof KF, Odink J, Kok FJ. Serum uric acid correlates in elderly men and women with special reference to body composition and dietary intake (Dutch Nutrition Surveilance System). J Clin Epidemiol 1990; 43:1297–1303.

68. Chou P, Soong LN, Lin HY. Community-based epidemiological study on hyperuricemia in Pu-Li, Taiwan. J Formos Med Assoc 1993; 92:597–602.

69. Torralba TP, Bayani Sioson PS. The Filipino and gout. Semin Arthritis Rheum 1975; 4:307–320.

70. Brule D, Sarwar G, Savoie L. Changes in serum and urinary uric acid levels in normal human subjects fed purine-rich foods containing different amounts of adenine and hypoxanthine. J Am Coll Nutr 1992; 11:353–358.

71. Takahashi S, Yamamoto T, Moriwaki Y, Tsutsumi Z, Higashino K. Impaired lipoprotein metabolism in patients with primary gout-influence of alcohol intake and body weight. Br J Rheumatol 1994; 33:731–734.

72. Lutalo SK, Mabonga N. A clinical assessment of the consequences of alcohol consumption in "communal" drinkers in the Zimbabwean Midlands. Cent Afr J Med 1992; 38: 380–384.

73. Al Jarallah KF, Shehab DK, Buchanan WW. Rheumatic complications of alcohol abuse. Semin Arthritis Rheum 1992; 22:162–171.

74. Cook DG, Shaper AG, Thelle DS, Whitehead TP. Serum uric acid, serum glucose and diabetes: relationships in a population study. Postgrad Med J 1986; 62:1001–1006.

75. Tofler OB, Woodings TL. A 13-year follow-up of social drinkers. Med J Aust 1981; 2:479–481.

76. Nishioka K, Mikanagi K. Hereditary and environmental factors influencing on the serum uric acid throughout ten years population study in Japan. Adv Exp Med Biol 1980; 122A:155–159.

77. De Muckadell OB, Gyntelberg F. Occurrence of gout in Copenhagen males aged 40–59. Int J Epidemiol 1976; 5:153–158.

78. Campion EW, Glynn RJ, DeLabry LO, Asymptomatic hyperuricemia. Risks and consequences in the Normative Aging Study. Am J Med 1987; 82:421–426.

79. Prior IA, Wellby TJ, Ostbye T, Salmond CE, Stokes YM. Migration and gout: the Tokelau Island migrant study. Br Med J Clin Res Ed 1987; 295:457–461.

80. Waller PC, Ramsay LE. Predicting acute gout in diuretic-treated hypertensive patients. J Hum Hypertens 1989; 3:457–461.

81. Faller J, Fox IH. Ethanol-induced hyperuricemia: evidence for increased urate production by activation of adenine nucleotide turnover. N Engl J Med 1982; 307:1598–1602.

82. Faller J, Fox IH. Ethanol induced alterations of uric acid metabolism. Adv Exp Med Boil 1984; 165Pt A:457–462.

83. Gibson T, Rodgers AV, Simmonds HA, Court-Brown F, Todd E, Meilton V. A controlled study of diet in patients with gout. Ann Rheum Dis 1983; 42:123–127.

84. Gibson T, Rodgers AV, Simmonds HA, Toseland P. Beer drinking and its effect on uric acid. Br J Rheumatol 1984; 23:203–209.

36

Effects of Obesity on Endocrine Function

Madeleine L. Drent
Free University Hospital, Amsterdam, The Netherlands

I. INTRODUCTION

The obese state is characterized by the presence of abnormalities in the endocrine systems. These changes can be important in the pathogenesis of obesity or only secondary to the obese state and therefore reversible after treatment. Some of the endocrine changes are related to the increased health risk attending obesity. Therapeutic strategies for obesity, like the use of diets or pharmacological agents leading to weight loss, also may influence endocrine systems. The use of hormones as therapeutic agents is still in the experimental phase. In this chapter these issues are discussed in relation to the endocrine system. Some parts of the text have been published before (1,2).

II. HYPOTHALAMIC-PITUITARY-ADRENOCORTICAL AXIS

A. Obesity

In obesity, normal basal plasma cortisol levels, basal plasma adrenocorticotropin (ACTH) levels, free urinary cortisol excretion, and a normal diurnal pattern of cortisol are shown both in adults and in children (3–8). Normal plasma cortisol levels are the result of both an increased cortisol production rate and increased cortisol metabolism in the obese state (9–11). The adrenocortical overactivity is reflected by the presence of elevated urinary 17-hydroxycorticosteroids, 17-ketogenic steroids, or 17-ketosteroids (11–14). Conflicting results are reported

Table 1 The Hypothalamic-Pituitary-Adrenocortical Axis in Obesity

Basal cortisol	N
Cortisol production	↑
Cortisol metabolism	↑
Diurnal cortisol rhythm	N
Stimulated cortisol	N/↓
Basal ACTH	N
Stimulated ACTH	N/↑/↓
Urinary 17-hydroxycorticosteroids	↑
Urinary 17-ketogenic steroids	↑
Urinary 17-ketosteroids	↑

N = normal; ↑ = increased; ↓ = decreased.

on whether the higher adrenal activity is due to real hypercorticism or is related to a changed body composition, i.e. hyperactivity in subjects with an abdominal fat distribution, or overnutrition (13,15–20). It has been suggested that the increased turnover of cortisol is a consequence of the obese state and is caused by enhanced cortisol metabolism in the adipocytes (15). On the other hand, it has been shown that in both lean and obese subjects cortisol production is correlated with lean body mass, suggesting that obese persons do not have an abnormally increased adrenocortical function, but have a greater lean body mass with a concomitantly greater cortisol production (12,21). Normal ACTH and cortisol responses, but also an impaired cortisol response or increased ACTH response to pituitary stimulation by insulin-induced hypoglycemia and a normal cortisol response by direct adrenal stimulation by synacthen, are reported (4,18,22). In prepubertal obese children the cortisol response to insulin-induced hypoglycemia is comparable to that in normal-weight controls, whereas the response is higher in obese adolescents (7,8). Both normal and impaired cortisol responses as well as normal and subnormal ACTH responses are reported to pituitary stimulation with corticotropin-releasing hormone (CRH) (4,23–25). Dexamethasone suppressibility of cortisol production seems to be normal (17).

The best way to differentiate between obesity and Cushing's syndrome is the measurement of urinary free cortisol levels, being normal in obesity. Urinary 17-hydroxycorticosteroids and 17-ketogenic steroids do not distinguish between the two states. The same is true for the 1-mg overnight dexamethasone suppression test.

B. Altered Energy Intake and Changes in Body Weight

Both in normal-weight volunteers and in obese subjects, conflicting results are reported on pituitary and adrenocortical responses to changes in energy intake and body weight. After 3 days of total fasting, normal-weight volunteers show an increase in plasma cortisol and plasma ACTH levels (26). In obese subjects after 1–2 weeks of total fasting, increases in 24-hr cortisol levels and urinary free cortisol levels as well as unchanged plasma cortisol levels are shown (27–30). Furthermore, a flattening of the diurnal cortisol rhythm and a decrease in the urinary 17-ketosteroids excretion are reported (27,29,30). The cortisol production rate seems to be unchanged, as is the responsiveness to suppression with dexamethasone and stimulation with ACTH (29). The ACTH and cortisol response to insulin-induced hypoglycemia diminishes after total fasting (30). After 2–12 months of energy restriction with a caloric intake of 400–1200 kcal/day (1672–5016 kJ/day), obese subjects show a decrease in plasma ACTH and cortisol levels (3,17,31). In normal-weight subjects cortisol production rate is reported to be elevated with overnutrition and subsequent weight gain, whereas the opposite is shown after decreased energy intake and weight loss (32). These changes are related to absolute body weight and the same has been reported in obese patients (17).

Not only the total energy content of the diet and changes in body weight, but also the amount of protein in the diet, leads to changes in cortisol metabolism. Increases and decreases in the protein content of the diet result, respectively, in elevated or diminished cortisol production rates and urinary free cortisol excretion (27).

C. Weight-Reducing Drugs

It has been shown that cortisol levels increase within an hour after the ingestion of a meal (33). In contrast, the ingestion of a sham meal fails to induce changes in cortisol levels (33). Ingestion of protein is more effective in inducing an increment of cortisol levels than ingestion of fat or carbohydrates. A direct signal from the gut to the brain in the form of cholecystokinin might explain this phenomenon. The essential amino acids tyrosine and tryptophan are effective in increasing cortisol levels in contrast to choline (33–35). Increments of ACTH are also shown after oral tryptophan (35). Increased plasma levels of these amino acids may lead to increased brain concentrations, leading to subsequent acceleration of the synthesis of serotonin, a neurotransmitter involved in the release of various hormones of the hypothalamopituitary axis.

Serotonin seems to stimulate the release of CRH in the paraventricular nucleus leading to diminished food intake, especially a reduction in fat and carbohydrate intake (36–38). Evidence exists that the use of serotonin agonists indeed leads to decreased intake of both carbohydrates and fat (39–43). Acute as well as chronic intraventricular administration of CRH in rats is followed by an increase in sympathetic activity and brown adipose tissue thermogenesis, an important contributary factor in total energy expenditure, whereas food intake is reduced (44–48). The subsequent weight loss is more pronounced in obese than in lean animals. Adrenalectomy leading to endogenous stimulation of CRH release also restores brown adipose tissue thermogenesis probably by increasing the sympathetic stimulation of the brown adipose tissue (47,49). Increases in corticosterone levels after intraventricular CRH are reported as well (47). In both lean and obese humans the intravenous administration of CRH acutely increases energy expenditure (25).

Acute administration of serotonin or the serotonin agonists dexfenfluramine or fluoxetine in rats induces a dose-dependent increase in CRH, ACTH, and corticosterone levels, whereas chronic administration has no effect (50–53). In most studies in humans, comparable results are obtained. Acute administration of serotonin, serotonin agonists, or the immediate precursor of serotonin, 5-hydroxytryptophan, will lead to increased levels of cortisol or ACTH, and these effects can be blunted by serotonin antagonists (51,54–58). Only one study, using the initial precursor of serotonin, tryptophan, demonstrated a decrease in cortisol levels (59). Chronic administration seems to have no effect on ACTH and cortisol levels (51,55,60,61). It has been hypothesized that the difference in effects of acute and chronic administration of serotonin may be explained by down-regulation of the serotonin receptors or the involvement of factors other than serotonin involved in the regulation of the pituitary-adrenocortical axis (51).

III. GROWTH HORMONE AND INSULIN-LIKE GROWTH FACTOR I

A. Obesity

Total 24-hr serum concentrations of growth hormone (GH) are lower in obese patients than in lean controls (62,63). This is caused by a decreased production rate of GH, as reflected by fewer GH pulses and prolonged pulse intervals, resulting in a production rate that is one-fourth of normal, as well as by increased metabolic clearance (62). The degree of these changes correlates with the body mass index or the percentage of body fat (62–64). However, this correlation disappears in older persons because GH declines with age, as in lean persons (63). The circadian rhythm of GH is normal, except for lower amplitudes of the pulses (62). The GH-binding protein concentration is normal (62). A positive correlation exists between the insulin-to-GH ratio and the body mass index, caused by both increased insulin levels and decreased GH levels, probably leading to facilitation of lipid storage (63). The GH response to various stimuli, like growth hormone–releasing hormone (GHRH), insulin-induced hypoglycemia, arginine, L-dopa, glucose, and exercise, is diminished in both adult and childhood obesity (8, 65–74). There is a negative correlation between percentage of ideal body weight and the GH response (66,75). The exact mechanism for the changes in basal GH levels or in GH responses to stimuli is unknown, but several hypotheses have been proposed: decreased pituitary stimulation by GHRH or decreased sensitivity of the pituitary to GHRH, increased somatostatin inhibitory tone, probably caused by decreased cholinergic tone or a diminished GH releasable pool in the pituitary (62, 65,76–78).

In contrast, in most studies insulin-like growth factor I (IGF-I) levels are reported to be normal in obesity, or even elevated in obese children, while normally, IGF-I levels reflect the GH status (9,10,62,67,69,79–81). It has been suggested that IGF-I is stimulated by the hyperinsulinism that often is present in the obese state (82). These stimulated IGF-I levels may be another explanation for the impairment in GH output because of the negative-feedback mechanism of IGF-I on the hypothalamus or pituitary, probably by stimulating somatostatin release (67,69,82,83).

B. Altered Energy Intake and Changes in Body Weight

It is likely that the disturbances in basal and stimulated GH levels are a consequence rather than a cause of the obese state. Healthy volunteers who participated in an overfeeding study to gain weight showed similar changes in GH to those observed in spontaneous obesity (11). Furthermore, the GH responsiveness to GHRH, insulin-induced hypoglycemia, or arginine restores, at least partially, after a weight-reducing program (66,67,73). However, this improvement is also observed after a short-term period of fasting before hardly any weight loss is obtained, suggesting that dietary intake per se also influences the system (67). The nutritional status, especially total energy intake and protein intake, is also an important determinant of the IGF-I concentration in the blood (82,84,85). Nutrition probably is one of the controlling factors of IGF-I release by the liver. Fasting leads to a lowering and refeeding to an increase of IGF-I levels (81,82,84,85). Insulin-like growth factor II (IGF-II), which is less dependent on GH levels than IGF-I, is not influenced by short-term changes in nutritional status (86). The IGF-binding protein IGFBP-3 also decreases during fasting and protein restriction, in this way regulating the amount of IGF-binding (87–89).

C. Weight-Reducing Drugs

Because of its anabolic and lipolytic properties, GH can be used in the treatment of obesity in addition to dietary restriction. A beneficial effect is seen on preservation of lean body mass as reflected by diminished urinary nitrogen loss or improved nitrogen balance (90–94). This effect seems to be dose-dependent (92,95). Fat loss itself is not significantly enhanced by GH therapy (91,92). Because

Table 2 Growth Hormone and Insulin-like Growth Factor I in Obesity

GH production	↓
GH metabolism	↑
Circadian GH rhythm	N
GH-binding protein	N
Stimulated GH	↓
IGF-I	N

N = normal; ↑ = increased; ↓ = decreased.

GH mediates its effects through IGF-I, the latter can also be used as additional therapeutic agent. The effect on nitrogen balance is comparable to the effect of GH, whereas IGF-I, in contrast to GH, also has a beneficial lowering effect on glucose, insulin, and C-peptide levels (90–92).

Some evidence exists that the serotoninergic system is involved in GH regulation. Inconsistent effects on basal and stimulated GH levels are seen after administration of the serotonin precursors tryptophane and 5-hydroxytryptophan or the serotoninergic drug fenfluramine. A single dose of the serotonin precursors results in increased GH levels in lean subjects, whereas after continuous administration GH levels return to normal (55,57,59). In obese patients a single dose of fenfluramine results in an improved GH response to arginine (96,97). Administration of fenfluramine for 7 days does not affect the GH response to arginine or GHRH in both obese and obese diabetic patients (98,99). Although in some studies opposite results are shown, it appears that the serotonergic effect on GH release, if of great importance, acts through sporadic, not continuous, release (61,100,101).

IV. HYPOTHALAMIC-PITUITARY-THYROID AXIS

A. Obesity

In general, thyroid function in obesity is normal. Most authors cannot find any relationship between thyroid hormones and body weight or body mass index, but others show a positive correlation between 3,3′,5-triiodothyronine (T3) levels and body weight (102–104). Normal 3,3′,5,5′-tetraiodothyronine or thyroxine (T4) levels and both normal and elevated T3 levels are reported, the latter probably caused by overfeeding and not by the obese state itself (102,104,105). Basal thyroid-stimulating hormone (TSH) levels are within the normal range and TSH levels after stimulation with thyrotropin-releasing hormone (TRH) are reported to be elevated, blunted, or within the normal range (102,106–108). In obese chil-

dren basal as well as stimulated thyroid parameters after insulin-induced hypoglycemia or TRH administration are in the normal range (6,8).

B. Altered Energy Intake and Changes in Body Weight

Reduction of energy intake leads to a decrease in T3 levels, an increase in 3,3′,5′-triiodothyronine, or reverse T3 (rT3) levels and normal T4 levels (26,109–117). Reduced absorption of nutrients in the gut that occurs after bypass surgery, used in the treatment of obesity or hypercholesterolemia, shows comparable effects (102,105). The decrease in T3 levels is dependent not only on the total amount of energy in the diet, but also on the amount of carbohydrates (106,111). The changes in rT3 levels are not affected by dietary carbohydrates, but only by total energy intake (106,111). In contrast, refeeding after fasting or overfeeding leads to an increase in T3 levels, a decrease in rT3 levels, and an increased TSH response to TRH (26,106,118–120). These changes can be explained by altered extrathyroidal conversion of T4, the biologically less active thyroid hormone, to T3, the active thyroid hormone, and rT3 (106,112). Decreased T3 levels during fasting are considered to act as a protective mechanism of the organism because of its sparing effects on lean body mass and its lowering effects on metabolic rate. During fasting, basal TSH levels and the TSH response after TRH are reported to be normal and lowered (106,109,113).

C. Weight-Reducing Drugs

In some studies T3 supplement is given in addition to fasting. This results in prevention of the decrease in metabolic rate, but also in a state of increased catabolism, leading to weight loss caused by a decrease in lean body mass instead of fat mass (106,121–123). Evaluating these results, T3 is not a suitable therapeutic agent in the treatment of obesity. Supplementation with T4 is less effective, because of the diminished peripheral conversion to T3 during fasting (112).

Involvement of serotonin in thyrotropin secretion is controversial. In rats serotonin seems to influence TSH release, both in vitro and in vivo, probably by changing TRH release (124–126). However, both increased and decreased TSH responses are shown. In humans, evidence for serotonergic control of TSH is less clear. In most studies administration of tryptophan, a precursor of serotonin, or the serotonin agonist fenfluramine has no effect on basal TSH levels or the TSH response to TRH (59, 127,128). However in some studies serotonin increases basal TSH levels or the TSH response, and some evidence

Table 3 The Hypothalamic-Pituitary-Thyroid Axis in Obesity

Basal T3	N/↑
Basal T4	N
Basal TSH	N
Stimulated TSH	N/↑/↓

N = normal; ↑ = increased; ↓ = decreased.

exists that serotonin may be involved in the diurnal rhythm of TSH secretion (55,129).

V.   HYPOTHALAMIC-PITUITARY-GONADAL AXIS

A.   Obesity

In obese children luteinizing hormone (LH) levels are reported to be normal, whereas follicle-stimulating hormone (FSH) levels are reported to be normal as well as elevated (6,8). In both obese prepubertal and pubertal boys and girls testosterone levels are comparable to the levels in normal-weight children (6,130). Estradiol levels are reported normal in obese boys and normal as well as lower in obese girls (6,130). Sex hormone–binding globulin (SHBG) levels are found to be lower already in obese children, leading to a higher free testosterone index (130). Both in men and in women obesity is associated with abnormalities concerning reproductive functions. In women an increased incidence of menstrual cycle disturbances, infertility, and hirsutism is present (131–135). Also an increased incidence of carcinomas of tissues responsive to estrogenic stimulation is found, especially carcinoma of the endometrium. In men impotence and decreased libido are frequently reported (10).

In obese postmenopausal women a clear increase in estrogens is demonstrated due to increased aromatase activity in the adipose tissue, leading to increased conversion of androgens into estrogens (136,137). In premenopausal eumenorrheic women this is less clear because of the dominant role of the ovarian estrogen production (138). In obese premenopausal oligomenorrheic women hormonal disturbances are more severe than in eumenorrheic women. In these women increased androgen levels are shown, probably leading to increased estrone and estradiol levels and decreased SHBG levels (134,136,139–141).

These disturbances are more clear in women with upper body obesity than in women with lower body obesity (142–144). A correlation exists between the changes in androgen status, the decreased SHBG levels, and the hyperinsulinemic state, which also frequently accompanies upper body obesity (145–151). There is some evidence that obesity and hyperandrogenism are independently associated with insulin resistance and also with dyslipidemia (152). Insulin resistance has also been induced by the administration of androgens to healthy females (153). These changes all taken together may lead to an unfavorable risk profile for macrovascular disease. LH and FSH levels are normal as are their responses to luteinizing hormone-releasing hormone (LHRH) (139,154). In patients with polycystic ovary disease the same hormonal disturbances are reported as in the obese oligomenorrheic women, including an abnormal response of LH and FSH to LHRH and a constantly elevated LH-to-FSH ratio (139,155).

In obese men elevated estrogen levels are demonstrated together with decreased LH and FSH levels and decreased androgen and SHBG levels (141,147,156–160). In general, feminization is not present in obese men, which may be explained by the low SHBG levels and therefore rather normal free testosterone levels. The LH and FSH responses to LHRH are normal in men (107,159). Only in severe obesity are disturbances in LH pulsatility found (161). A relationship seems to be present between the severity of hormonal disturbances and the degree of excess body weight (147,156). However, in some studies no relationship is found between the amount of visceral fat and sex hormone metabolism (162). Evidence is present that hyperestrogenemia in men is a risk factor for macrovascular disease (163). Again this may be explained by the development of insulin resistance (153).

B.   Altered Energy Intake and Changes in Body Weight

The changes in reproductive hormones like decreased SHBG levels, as well as the reproductive disorders like cycle disturbances, normalize after caloric restriction and weight loss (3,9,10,133,140,154,157,164–168). This suggests that the abnormalities are not the cause, but rather the consequence, of the obese state. On the other hand, undernutrition and weight loss can also lead to altered reproductive function probably due to alterations in the responses of LH and FSH to LHRH (169,170). Prolonged fasting leads to decreased LH secretion and increased LH and FSH secretion after stimulation with LHRH (154). Diet-related amenorrhea in adolescent girls and, more extreme, the development of the syndrome of anorexia nervosa both illustrate this problem (170). Reduced energy

Table 4   The Hypothalamic-Pituitary-Gonadal Axis in Obesity

	Women	Men
Estrogens	N/↑	↑
Androgens	↑	↓
SHBG	↓	↓
Basal LH	N	↓
Basal FSH	N	↓
Stimulated LH	N	N
Stimulated FSH	N	N

N = normal; ↑ = increased; ↓ = decreased.

intake leads to reduced LH pulse frequency and to increased LH pulse amplitude in lead female volunteers (171). Energy restriction in women with the polycystic ovary syndrome also improves SHBG levels, insulin levels, menstrual function, and fertility (172). In men reproductive function is not affected by energy restriction.

C.   Weight-Reducing Drugs

In laboratory animals some evidence is present for a regulatory role of serotonin on LH secretion (50,173–175). In healthy human volunteers, however, controversial results have been found after the administration of serotonin precursors on LH and FSH secretion (55,59,176,177).

VI.   SYMPATHETIC NERVOUS SYSTEM

A.   Obesity

The sympathetic nervous system consists of the sympathetic nerves releasing norepinephrine as a neurotransmitter and the adrenal medulla releasing epinephrine. Normal, elevated, and reduced basal levels of plasma catecholamines are reported in obesity (10,178–184). The response of catecholamines to exercise seems to be reduced in obesity (185,186). In some studies a negative correlation between the level of catecholamines and the percentage of body fat or the body mass index is shown (180). However, it is more likely that the level of nutrient intake is the most important determinant for sympathetic nervous system activity and that body weight itself is a more chronic factor.

Both an elevated and a reduced activity of the sympathetic nervous system can explain some of the pathophysiological aspects of obesity or its complications. Elevated sympathetic activity is associated with the prevalence of essential hypertension and other cardiovascular complications (182,184,187,188). It has been hypothesized that obesity-related hypertension may be an unfortunate byproduct of insulin resistance, an adaptive process to restore energy balance and to prevent further weight gain. Hyperinsulinemia stimulates sympathetic activity on the one hand, leading to an increase of energy expenditure by

enhancing thermogenesis, but on the other hand leads to increased vasoconstriction, cardiac output, and sodium reabsorption and thus hypertension (189–193). Decreased sympathetic activity or reduced sensitivity for catecholamines, probably caused by decreased expression of β_2-adrenoceptors in visceral fat cells, will lead to diminished energy expenditure, reduced lipolysis, and enhanced lipogenesis, in this way contributing to the development and maintenance of obesity (180,194–196). This can explain the weight gain during treatment with β-blockers (197).

In the central nervous system, norepinephrine has an inhibitory effect on CRH production in the paraventricular nucleus of the hypothalamus leading to stimulation of feeding (36,38).

B.   Altered Energy Intake and Changes in Body Weight

Reduced nutrient intake as well as weight loss leads to a decrease of sympathetic activity as reflected by lower levels of plasma catecholamines, lower urinary excretion of metabolites, and a decreased norepinephrine turnover in organ tissues both in humans and in animals (178,183,189,198–205). Overfeeding results in the opposite. However, there is evidence that a dissociation exists between the norepinephrine response and the adrenomedullary epinephrine response, suggesting that when the sympathetic nervous system is suppressed as in fasting, the adrenal medulla becomes more important as a source of circulating catecholamines (202).

Carbohydrates and fat stimulate sympathetic activity, even when total caloric intake is not increased, whereas protein has no effect (189,206–208). This effect depends on the absorption of these nutrients. Both carbohydrate malabsorption induced by acarbose, a disaccharidase inhibitor, and fat malabsorption induced by cholestyramine antagonize the stimulatory effect even when carbohydrate or fat intake is high (206,207). The decreased sympathetic activity during fasting, resulting in a decreased metabolic rate, is probably a protective mechanism against weight loss, whereas increased activity during overfeeding may reduce excess energy storage. A comparable mechanism is shown for thyroid hormone metabolism and the two systems may have a synergistic effect (198,209).

The decrease in glucose and insulin levels and the increase in glucagon levels and lipolysis that occur during early starvation do not seem to be caused by the changes in sympathetic activity, but probably by the reduced nutrient flow (198,210). Independent of sodium intake, due to the changes in the sympathetic nervous system, a de-

Table 5   Catecholamines in Obesity

Basal catecholamines	N/↑/↓
Stimulated catecholamines	↓

N = normal; ↑ = increased; ↓ = decreased.

crease in blood pressure occurs before a considerable amount of weight loss is achieved during fasting (182,184,203,211,212).

C. Weight-Reducing Drugs

In rats acute as well as chronic administration of serotonin and fenfluramine is able to enhance sympathetic activity leading to increased stimulation of brown adipose tissue and therefore to an increased thermogenic response (49,213,214). On the other hand, some studies in humans show a decrease in norepinephrine levels after chronic treatment with fenfluramine resulting in a beneficial effect on blood pressure (215,216).

β-Adrenergic agonists are being studied for their weight-reducing potential by stimulation of thermogenesis, but their therapeutic use is limited because of the appearance of cardiovascular side effects (217–219).

VII. PANCREAS AND GUT HORMONES

A. Insulin and C-Peptide

1. Obesity

Hyperinsulinemia, both basal and after a glucose load, is common in obesity, especially in upper body obesity (220–223). This is already found in obese children (8). Discussion is still going on as to whether this is due to increased insulin secretion by the β cells of the pancreas, diminished hepatic insulin clearance, or both (224–230). Evidence exists that insulin turnover is increased in the

Table 6 Pancreas and Gut Hormones in Obesity

Basal insulin	↑
Stimulated insulin	↑
Insulin secretion	↑
Insulin clearance	↓
Basal C-peptide	↑
Stimulated C-peptide	↑
Basal glucagon	N/↑
Stimulated glucagon	N/↑/↓
Basal GIP	N/↑
Stimulated GIP	N/↑
Basal PP	N/↓
Stimulated PP	N/↓
Basal CCK	N?
Stimulated CCK	N?

N = normal; ↑ = increased; ↓ = decreased.

obese state, because increased capacity of insulin cleavage in white adipose tissue is found (231). Because insulin and C-peptide are secreted by the β cells in equimolar concentrations and insulin is extracted from the plasma by the liver, whereas C-peptide is not, many authors have used C-peptide concentrations or the ratio between insulin and C-peptide to provide information on the secretion and clearance of insulin in obesity and type II diabetes mellitus (224,225,227–229, 232). However, this method is not yet validated and the results of these studies should be interpreted with caution (233). More information on insulin secretion patterns and insulin sensitivity can be obtained by the use of the hyper- and euglycemic insulin clamp technique (232,234).

The combination of hyperinsulinemia and normal glucose levels in obesity indicates the presence of insulin resistance. Hyperinsulinemia probably plays a role in the development of risk factors for cardiovascular disease, like hypertension, dyslipidemia (increased levels of plasma triglycerides and decreased levels of HDL cholesterol), and glucose intolerance (191,192,235,236).

2. Altered Energy Intake and Changes in Body Weight

During weight reduction in adults and children basal and stimulated plasma insulin levels and insulin sensitivity normalize, even when body weight is still above ideal (232,237–239). Again, it is not clear whether this amelioration of the insulin levels is due to reduced secretion, increased hepatic extraction of insulin, or both (232,238,240). The same is true for plasma C-peptide levels, especially after prolonged calorie restriction (232,238). The hyperinsulinemia probably is an adaptational process to the state of overnutrition, which is reversible after calorie restriction. Amelioration of the risk factors for cardiovascular disease is also demonstrated with weight loss (192,241). In obese children with impaired glucose tolerance achievement of normal body weight results in normalization of glucose tolerance without normalization of the hyperinsulinemia (242). In children who gain weight insulin responses to an oral glucose tolerance test decrease together with an increased 2-hr glucose level (242). This may be the first sign of pancreatic secretory deficiency.

3. Weight-Reducing Drugs

Evidence exists that serotonin receptor agonists like fenfluramine and dexfenfluramine are able to improve plasma glucose levels and insulin sensitivity independent of the weight-reducing effects of these drugs (99,243–249).

These effects have been demonstrated both in animals and in humans, especially in type II diabetic patients. Whether the amelioration of insulin sensitivity is the primary effect that subsequently leads to a better glycemic control or whether glycemic control improves by better dietary compliance leading to increased insulin sensitivity remains unclear.

B. Glucagon

I. Obesity

Glucagon has its function in maintaining fasting plasma glucose levels. Because insulin resistance is a common feature in obesity, it might affect glucagon levels. Glucagon is a catabolic hormone and, when administered exogenously, increases plasma free fatty acid levels and plasma β-hydroxybutyrate levels in normal-weight subjects. However, obese subjects are reported to be resistant to these catabolic actions (250). This effect is probably related to the hyperinsulinism present in the obese state. Fasting glucagon levels are reported to be normal or elevated in obese patients (251–256). After stimulation with arginine, increased, unchanged, and decreased glucagon responses have been demonstrated (251,252,257,258). In obese children both normal basal glucagon levels and normal peak levels after insulin-induced hypoglycemia are found (8). In one study the augmented response appeared to correlate with the degree of elevated triglyceride levels and the presence of a fatty liver (259). These differences in the metabolic state of the obese patients may be the explanation for the controversies in the literature and should be taken into account when α-cell function is evaluated. The glucagon response to other stimuli like a protein meal or a mixed meal remains unchanged compared to lean control subjects, and the same is true for the glucagon suppression after a glucose load (251,252,260). In obese patients with insulin resistance it has been demonstrated that the glucagon-suppressing effect of glucose is dependent on the degree of insulin sensitivity (253). However, in obese patients with impaired glucose tolerance a normal glucagon-suppressing effect of glucose was found (261).

2. Altered Energy Intake and Changes in Body Weight

In lean subjects basal plasma glucagon levels increase after a 3–4-day period of fasting (262,263). The glucagon response after an infusion with arginine or L-alanine also increases after starvation (262,263). In obese patients basal glucagon levels are reported to remain unchanged as well as to increase after a period of starvation (262,264,265). The increase found has been reported to

be caused by diminished clearance of glucagon and not by increased secretion (265). The glucagon responses after stimulation with arginine and L-alanine are reported to be increased as well as decreased after starvation or weight loss (252,262).

3. Weight-Reducing Drugs

Glucagon itself has been demonstrated to have anorectic properties both in animals and in humans (36,266,267). These effects can be blocked by pretreatment with glucagon antibodies. The anorectic effect seems to be mediated by the vagal nerve leading signals to the brain. Up to now, administration of glucagon in the treatment of human obesity has not yet been established.

C. Gastric Inhibitory Polypeptide

I. Obesity

The interaction between the gastrointestinal tract and the pancreatic islets is known as the enteroinsular axis, and substances with an insulinotropic action released from the gastrointestinal tract after meals containing glucose are known as incretins. One of these incretins is gastric inhibitory polypeptide (GIP), which refers to its capacity to inhibit gastric acid secretion and gastric motor activity. GIP also stands for glucose-dependent insulinotropic polypeptide, referring to the stimulatory effect of GIP on insulin synthesis and secretion, which depends on plasma glucose concentration. Furthermore, GIP has a metabolic effect on adipose and liver tissue by activating lipoprotein lipase, inhibiting glucagon-induced lipolysis and glycogenolysis, and increasing the incorporation of fatty acids into adipose tissue (268,269). In postobese subjects consumption of a high-fat meal leads to an increased response of GIP together with a decreased response of epinephrine compared to lean controls (270). This hormonal pattern will favor lipid storage. Considering these actions, GIP may play a role in the development of obesity. The ingestion of large amounts of nutrients leads not only to the availability of substrates for fat storage, but also to increased GIP secretion, which facilitates triglyceride synthesis in adipose tissue. In this way GIP may be important in the pathogenesis of obesity (269,271).

Another, even more potent, incretin is glucagon-like peptide-1 (GLP-1), a cleavage product of proglucagon (272–275).

Basal GIP levels are normal or elevated in obese patients compared to lean control subjects (271,276–281). GIP is released by stimulation with glucose and even more by the presence of fat in the meal (282–285). The responses of GIP after both mixed meals and oral or intravenous glucose loads are reported to be both normal and increased (271,276–281,286–288). Elevated GIP responses are found especially after high-calorie meals (280,287). Because insulin levels are reported to be elevated even in the absence of elevated GIP levels, it can be concluded that GIP is not responsible for the hyperinsulinemia of obesity (276,280,287,289). In obese non-insulin-dependent diabetic subjects GIP levels after stimulation with an oral glucose tolerance test are reported to be elevated, suggesting that insulin resistance is involved in GIP hypersecretion (288).

2. Altered Energy Intake and Changes in Body Weight

Basal GIP levels remain unchanged or increase after weight reduction (281,286). The GIP responses to mixed meals or glucose loads are found to be both unchanged and diminished after food restriction and weight reduction (281,286,290). Because insulin levels always decrease after weight reduction, it can be concluded again that GIP levels are not responsible for the hyperinsulinism in obesity.

D. Pancreatic Polypeptide

1. Obesity

Pancreatic polypeptide is released from the endocrine pancreas in a biphasic manner after stimulation with amino acids, a protein-rich meal, or a fat-rich meal (291–294). Other strong stimuli are hypoglycemia, vagal stimulation, and gastrointestinal hormones like cholecystokinin (291,293–299). The release of pancreatic polypeptide is under vagal control. Vagotomy or administration of atropine, resulting in cholinergic blockade, leads to abolished responses (294,297). Pancreatic polypeptide levels may therefore be used as an indicator of vagal tone. The levels increase with age (300,301). The physiological function of pancreatic polypeptide still remains uncertain. However, it seems that the hormone has an "anticholecystokinin" effect in the form of relaxation of the gallbladder and inhibition of pancreatic secretion both in humans and in animals (299,302–304). In obese patients basal plasma levels of pancreatic polypeptide are reported to be both lower, as found in most studies, and unchanged, as found in a minority of studies, compared to control subjects (292,296,305,306). The responses of pancreatic polypeptide after stimulation with insulin-induced hypoglycemia, protein-rich meals, or mixed meals are reported to be diminished compared to lean controls (260,292,296,306). In one study the response is found to be unchanged after stimulation with a mixed meal, but in this study the basal

levels were also comparable to the levels of lean controls (305). A possible explanation for the lower plasma levels is the presence of elevated free fatty acid and glucose levels in obesity, because these substrates are able to lower pancreatic polypeptide levels (291,293,294,307).

2. Altered Energy Intake and Changes in Body Weight

After a period of fasting, plasma pancreatic polypeptide levels increase in healthy females, which may be related to a decrease in plasma glucose levels (293).

E. Cholecystokinin

1. Obesity

Cholecystokinin is released by the presence of fat, protein, and amino acids in the duodenal and jejunal lumen and has a function in the stimulation of gallbladder contraction, exocrine pancreatic enzyme, and bicarbonate secretion, inhibition of gastric emptying, and possibly in stimulation of endocrine pancreatic hormone secretion and reduction of food intake (308). It has been suggested that cholecystokinin may also have an incretin effect, but this seems to be of little or no importance (309–311). Little is known about basal or stimulated cholecystokinin levels in obesity. In one study basal cholecystokinin levels are reported comparable in lean and obese subjects, whereas the postprandial levels after stimulation with a liquid test meal tended to be higher in the obese subjects (312). Exogenous administration of cholecystokinin in obese patients leads to a diminished response of pancreatic enzyme and bile acid secretion after vagal stimulation by sham feeding (313). These results give the impression that cholecystokinin secretion itself is normal in obesity, but that the sensitivity to cholecystokinin is decreased. Some data are published on cholecystokinin levels in patients suffering from bulimia nervosa. However, the pathogenesis of this type of obesity is supposed to be quite different from the pathogenesis of simple obesity. In patients with bulimia fasting cholecystokinin levels are reported to be comparable to those of healthy control subjects (314). The cholecystokinin levels in response to a liquid mixed meal were lower than in the control subjects. The same was true for the subjective satiety, suggesting a relationship between this type of hyperphagia and cholecystokinin levels. The hyperphagia present in patients suffering from seasonal affective disorder does not seem to be related to altered cholecystokinin levels (315). In one patient with melancholic depression, which is associated with appetite and weight loss, an increased cholecystokinin response to a liquid mixed meal seemed to be present (315).

2. Weight-Reducing Drugs

Because of its anorectic properties cholecystokinin per se may be of value as a weight-reducing compound. Both in rats and in humans evidence exists that exogenous administration as well as endogenous release of cholecystokinin can reduce food intake in a dose-dependent manner (36,316–319). These effects can be blocked by pretreatment with antagonists of cholecystokinin (320). The exact mechanism of action is unclear. It seems that cholecystokinin leads to a shorter period of food intake, which is named satiation, and this effect is not due to aversive reactions (321,322). The effect of satiation is probably caused by several mechanisms, like delayed gastric emptying, leading to gastric distension, small bowel distension, and signals to the brain via vagal nerve fibers (321–324). It has not been completely established whether this effect is induced by physiological or pharmacological doses of cholecystokinin (321,322).

One of the stimuli of cholecystokinin release is the presence of digested fat in the small intestine. The use of a lipase inhibitor, a new and promising concept in the treatment of obesity, leads to increased amounts of undigested and unabsorbed fat in the gut (325–327). This might influence cholecystokinin release and subsequently food intake (328,329). However, no effect of lipase inhibition is found on cholecystokinin levels after prolonged administration in obese subjects (330).

VIII. SUMMARY AND CONCLUSIONS

This chapter reviewed the relationship between obesity and its treatment, on the one hand, and changes in endocrine parameters, on the other. Most endocrine abnormalities, like changes in growth hormone or thyroid hormones, as found in obese patients seem to be secondary to the obese state or increased food intake and therefore can be normalized by weight loss or reducing energy intake. Some endocrine changes, like decreased insulin sensitivity or changes in levels of catecholamines, may play a role in the development of macrovascular complications of obesity. Pharmacological treatment for weight reduction, for example by the use of serotonin agonists or lipase inhibitors, although useful in weight reduction, does not seem to have clinically relevant effects on most endocrine changes in obesity. The use of hormones in the treatment of obesity is still in the experimental phase. The results of some compounds seem to be promising, like the use of growth hormone because of its capacity to preserve lean body mass or the use of cholecystokinin because of its anorectic properties.

REFERENCES

1. Drent ML, Van der Veen EA. Review. Endocrine aspects of obesity. Neth J Med 1995; 47:127–136.
2. Drent ML. Endocrine aspects and the treatment of obesity. Thesis, 1993. Free University, Amsterdam.
3. Grenman S, Rönnemaa T, Irjala K, Kaihola HL, Grönroos M. Sex steroid, gonadotropin, cortisol and prolactin levels in healthy, massively obese women: Correlation with abdominal fat cell size and effect of weight reduction. J Clin Endocrinol Metab 1986; 63:1257–1261.
4. Kopelman PG, Grossman A, Lavender P, Besser GM, Rees LH, Coy D. The cortisol response to corticotrophin-releasing factor is blunted in obesity. Clin Endocrinol 1988; 28:15–18.
5. Köbberling J, von zur Mühlen A. The circadian rhythm of free cortisol determined by urine sampling at two-hour intervals in normal subjects and in patients with severe obesity or Cushing's syndrome. J Clin Endocrinol Metab 1974; 38:313–319.
6. Genazzani AR, Pintor C, Corda R. Plasma levels of gonadotropins, prolactin, thyroxine, and adrenal and gonadal steroids in obese prepubertal girls. J Clin Endocrinol Metab 1978; 47:974–979.
7. Genazzani AR, Facchinetti F, Petraglia F, Pintor C, Corda R. Hyperendorphinemia in obese children and adolescents. J Clin Endocrinol Metab 1986; 62:36–40.
8. AvRuskin TW, Pillai S, Kasi K, Juan C, Kleinberg DL. Decreased prolactin secretion in childhood obesity. J Pediatr 1985; 106:373–378.
9. Glass AR. Endocrine aspects of obesity. Med Clin North Am 1989; 73:139–160.
10. Glass AR, Burman KD, Dahms WT, Boehm TM. Endocrine function in human obesity. Metabolism 1981; 30:89–104.
11. Sims E, Danforth E Jr, Horton E, Bray G, Glennon J, Salans L. Endocrine and metabolic effects of experimental obesity in man. Recent Prog Hormone Res 1973; 29:457–496.
12. Migeon CJ, Green OC, Eckert JP. Study of adrenocortical function in obesity. Metabolism 1963; 12:718–739.
13. Copinschi G, Cornil A, Leclercq R, Franckson JRM. Cortisol secretion rate and urinary corticoid excretion in normal and obese subjects. Acta Endocrinol (Copenh) 1966; 51:186–192.
14. Dunkelman SS, Fairhurst B, Plager J, Waterhouse C. Cortisol metabolism in obesity. J Clin Endocrinol Metab 1964; 24:832–841.
15. Schteingart DE, Gregerman RI, Conn JW. A comparison of the characteristics of increased adrenocortical function in obesity and in Cushing's syndrome. Metabolism 1963; 12:484–497.
16. Strain GW, Zumoff B, Kram J, Strain JJ, Levin J, Fukushima D. Sex difference in the influence of obesity on the 24-hour mean plasma concentration of cortisol. Metabolism 1982; 31:209–213.

17. Cohen MR, Pickar D, Cohen RM, Wise TN, Cooper JN. Plasma cortisol and β-endorphin immunoreactivity in human obesity. Psychosom Med 1984; 46:454–462.

18. Weaver JU, Kopelman PG, McLoughlin L, Forsling ML, Grossman A. Hyperactivity of the hypothalamo-pituitary-adrenal axis in obesity: a study of ACTH, AVP, β-lipotrophin and cortisol responses to insulin-induced hypoglycaemia. Clin Endocrinol 1993; 39:345–350.

19. Mårin P, Darin N, Amemiya T, Andersson B, Jern S, Björntorp P. Cortisol secretion in relation to body fat distribution in obese premenopausal women. Metabolism 1992; 41:882–886.

20. Pasquali R, Cantobelli S, Casimirri F, Capelli M, Bortoluzzi L, Flamia R, Labate AMM, Barbara L. The hypothalamic-pituitary-adrenal axis in obese women with different patterns of body fat distribution. J Clin Endocrinol Metab 1993; 77.341–346.

21. Strain GW, Zumoff B, Strain JJ, Levin J. Fukushima DK. Cortisol production in obesity. Metabolism 1980; 29:980–985.

22. Kopelman PG, Pilkington TRE, White N, Jeffcoate SL. Impaired hypothalamic control of prolactin secretion in massive obesity. Lancet 1979; i:747–749.

23. Grossman A, Howlett TA, Kopelman PG. The use of CRF-41 in the differential diagnosis of Cushings-syndrome and obesity. Horm Metab Res 1987; 16(Suppl):62–64.

24. Pijl H, Koppeschaar HPF, Willekens FLA, Frölich M, Meinders AE. The influence of serotonergic neurotransmission on pituitary hormone release in obese and non-obese females. Acta Endocrinol (Copenh) 1993; 128:319–324.

25. Chong PKK, Jung RT, Bartlett WA, Browning MCK. The acute effects of corticotropin-releasing factor on energy expenditure in lean and obese women. Int J Obes 1992; 16:529–534.

26. Beer SF, Bircham PMM, Bloom SR, Clark PM, Hales CN, Hughes CM, Jones CT, Marsh DR, Raggatt PR, Findlay ALR. The effect of a 72-h fast on plasma levels of pituitary, adrenal, thyroid, pancreatic and gastrointestinal hormones in healthy men and women. J Endocrinol 1989; 120:337–250.

27. Galvao-Tales A, Graves L, Burke CW, Fotherby K, Fraser R. Free cortisol in obesity: effect of fasting. Acta Endocrinol (Copenh) 1976; 81:321–329.

28. Copinschi G, de Laet M-H, Brion JP, Leclercq R, L'Hermite M, Robyn C, Virasoro E, van Cauter E. Simultaneous study of cortisol, growth hormone and prolactin nyctohemeral variations in normal and obese subjects: influence of prolonged fasting in obesity. Clin Endocrinol 1978; 9:15–26.

29. Sabeh G, Alley RA, Robbins TJ, Naruduzzi JV, Kenny FM, Danowski TS. Adrenocortical indices during fasting in obesity. J Clin Endocrinol Metab 1969; 29:373–376.

30. Bell JP, Donald RA, Espiner EA. Pituitary response to insulin-induced hypoglycemia in obese subjects before and after fasting. J Clin Endocrinol Metab 1970; 31:546–551.

31. Scavo D, Barletta C, Buzzetti R, Vagiri D. Effects of caloric restriction and exercise on β-endorphin, ACTH and cortisol circulating levels in obesity. Physiol Behav 1988; 42:65–68.

32. O'Connell M, Danforth E Jr, Horton ES, Salans L, Sims EAH. Experimental obesity in man III: adrenocortical function. J Clin Endocrinol Metab 1973; 36:323–329.

33. Ishizuka B, Quigley ME, Yen SSC. Pituitary hormone release in response to food ingestion: evidence for neuroendocrine signals from gut to brain. J Clin Endocrinol Metabol 1983; 57:1111–1116.

34. Modlinger RS, Schonmuller JM, Arora SP. Stimulation of aldosterone, renin and cortisol by tryptophan. J Clin Endocrinol Metab 1979; 48:599–603.

35. Modlinger RS, Schonmuller JM, Arora SP. Adrenocorticotropin release by tryptophan in man. J Clin Endocrinol Metab 1980; 50:360–363.

36. Morley JE. Neuropeptide regulation of appetite and weight. Endocr Rev 1987; 8:256–287.

37. Rothwell NJ. Central effects of CRF on metabolism and energy balance. Neurosci Biobehav Rev 1990; 14:263–271.

38. Morley JE. An approach to the development of drugs for appetite disorders. Neuropsychobiology 1989; 21:22–30.

39. Drent ML, Zelissen PMJ, Koppeschaar HPF, Nieuwenhuyzen Kruseman AC, Lutterman JA, Van der Veen EA. The effect of dexfenfluramine on eating habits in a dutch ambulatory android overweight population with an overconsumption of snacks. Int J Obes 1995; 19:299–304.

40. Lafreniere F, Lambert J, Rasio E, Serri O. Effects of dexfenfluramine treatment on body weight and postprandial thermogenesis in obese subjects. A double-blind placebo-controlled study. Int J Obes 1993; 17:25–30.

41. Hill AJ, Blundell JE. Model system for investigating the actions of anorectic drugs: effect of d-fenfluramine on food intake, nutrient selection, food preferences, meal patterns, hunger and satiety in healthy human subjects. Adv BioSci 1986; 60:377–389.

42. Cangiano C, Ceci F, Cascino A, Del Ben M, Laviano A, Muscaritoli M, Antonucci F, Rossi-Fanelli F. Eating behavior and adherence to dietary prescriptions in obese adult subjects treated with 5-hydroxytrytophan. Am J Clin Nutr 1992; 56:863–867.

43. Blundell JE, Hill AJ. Do serotoninergic drugs decrease energy intake by reducing fat or carbohydrate intake? Effect of d-fenfluramine with supplemented weight-increasing diets. Pharmacol Biochem Behav 1988; 31:773–778.

44. Arase K, Shargill NS, Bray GA. Effects of intraventricular infusion of corticotropin-releasing factor (CRF) on VMH-lesioned obese rats. Am J Physiol 1989; 256:R751–R756.

45. Arase K, York DA, Shimizu H, Shargill N, Bray GA. Effects of corticotropin-releasing factor on food intake and brown adipose tissue thermogenesis in rats. Am J Physiol 1988; 255:E255–E259.

46. Arase K, Shargill NS, Bray GA. Effects of corticotropin releasing factor on genetically obese (fatty) rats. Physiol Behav 1989; 45:565–570.

47. York DA. Corticosteroid inhibition of thermogenesis in obese animals. Proc Nutr Soc 1989; 48:231–235.

48. Rothwell NJ. Central activation of thermogenesis by prostaglandins: dependence on CRF. Horm Metab Res 1990; 22:616–618.

49. Arase K, York DA, Shargill NS, Bray GA. Interaction of adrenalectomy and fenfluramine treatment on body weight, food intake and brown adipose tissue. Physiol Behav 1989; 45:557–564.

50. Montange M, Calas A. Serotonin and endocrinology, the pituitary. In: Osborn NN, Hamon M, eds. Neuronal Serotonin. New York: Wiley, 1988:271–303.

51. Oliver C, Jezova D, Grino M, Guillaume V, Boudouresque F, Conte-Delvolx B, Pesce G, Dutour A, Becquet D. Differences in the effects of acute and chronic administration of dexfenfluramine on cortisol and prolactine secretion. Adv Exp Med Biol 1990; 274:427–443.

52. Serri O, Rasio E. The effect of d-fenfluramine on anterior pituitary hormone release in the rat: in vivo and in vitro studies. Can J Physiol Pharmacol 1987; 65:2449–2453.

53. Serri O, Rasio E. Temporal changes in prolactin and corticosterone response during chronic treatment with d-fenfluramine. Horm Res 1989; 31:180–183.

54. Jackson RV, Grice JE, Jackson AJ, Vella RD, Armour MB. Inhibition of serotonin-induced ACTH release in man by clonidine. Clin Exp Pharmacol Physiol 1988; 15:293–298.

55. Mashchak CA, Kletzky OA, Spencer C, Artal R. Transient effect of L-5-hydroxytryptophan on pituitary function in men and women. J Clin Endocrinol Metab 1983; 56:170–176.

56. Lewis DA, Sherman BM. Serotonergic stimulation of adrenocorticotropin secretion in man. J Clin Endocrinol Metab 1984; 58:458–462.

57. Imura H, Nakai Y, Yoshimi T. Effect of 5-hydroxytryptophan (5-HPT) on growth hormone and ACTH release in man. J Clin Endocrinol Metab 1973; 36:204–206.

58. Prescott RWG, Kendall-Taylor P, Weightman DR, Watson MJ, Ratcliffe WA. The effect of ketanserin, a specific serotonin antagonist on the PRL, GH, ACTH and cortisol responses to hypoglycemia in normal subjects. Clin Endocrinol 1984; 20:137–142.

59. Woolf PD, Lee L. Effects of the serotonin precursor, tryptophan, on pituitary hormone secretion. J Clin Endocrinol Metab 1977; 45:123–133.

60. Andersson B, Zimmerman ME, Hedner T, Björntorp P. Haemodynamic, metabolic and endocrine effects of short-term dexfenfluramine treatment in young obese women. Eur J Clin Pharmacol 1991; 40:249–254.

61. Drent ML, Adèr HJ, Van der Veen EA. The influence of chronic administration of the serotonin agonist dexfenfluramine on responsiveness to ACTH-releasing hormone (CRH) and growth hormone-releasing hormone (GHRH) in moderately obese people. J Endocrinol Invest 1995; 18:780–788.

62. Veldhuis JD, Iranmanesh A, Ho KKY, Waters MJ, Johnson ML, Lizarralde G. Dual defects in pulsatile growth hormone secretion and clearance subserve the hyposomatotropism of obesity in man. J Clin Endocrinol Metab 1991; 72:51–59.

63. Meistas MT, Foster GV, Margolis S, Kowarski AA. Integrated concentrations of growth hormone, insulin, C-peptide and prolactin in human obesity. Metabolism 1982; 31:1224–1228.

64. Weltman A, Weltman JY, Hartman ML, Abbott RD, Rogol AD, Evans WS, Veldhuis JD. Relationship between age, percentage body fat, fitness, and 24-hour growth hormone release in healthy young adults: effects of gender. J Clin Endocrinol Metab 1994; 78:543–548.

65. Csizmadi I, Brazeau P, Serri O. Effect of dietary restriction and repeated growth hormone-releasing factor injections on growth hormone response to growth hormone-releasing factor in obese subjects. Metabolism 1989; 38:1016–1021.

66. Williams T, Berelowitz M, Joffe SN, Thorner MO, Rivier J, Vale W, Frohman LA. Impaired growth hormone responses to growth hormone-releasing factor in obesity. N Engl J Med 1984; 311:1403–1407.

67. Kelijman M, Frohman LA. Enhanced growth hormone (GH) responsiveness to GH-releasing hormone after dietary manipulation in obese and nonobese subjects. J Clin Endocrinol Metab 1988; 66:489–494.

68. Kopelman PG, Noonan K, Goulton R, Forrest AJ. Impaired growth hormone response to growth hormone releasing factor and insulin-hypoglycemia in obesity. Clin Endocrinol 1985; 23:87–94.

69. Loche S, Cappa M, Borrelli P, Faededa A, Crinò A, Cella SG, Corda R, Müller EE, Pintor C. Reduced growth hormone response to growth hormone-releasing hormone in children with simple obesity: evidence for somatomedin-C mediated inhibition. Clin Endocrinol 1987; 27:145–153.

70. De Marinis L, Folli G, D'Amico C, Mancini A, Sambo P, Tofani A, Oradei A, Barbarino A. Differential effects of feeding on the ultradian variation of the growth hormone (GH) response to GH-releasing hormone in normal subjects and patients with obesity and anorexia nervosa. J Clin Endocrinol Metab 1988; 66:598–604.

71. Hansen AP. Serum growth hormone response to exercise in non-obese and obese normal subjects. Scand J Clin Lab Invest 1973; 31:175–178.

72. Fingerhut M, Krieger DT. Plasma growth hormone response to L-Dopa in obese subjects. Metabolism 1974; 23:267–271.

73. Londono JH, Gallagher TF, Bray GA. Effect of weight reduction, triiodothyronine and diethylstilbestrol on growth hormone in obesity. Metabolism 1969; 18:986–992.

74. Gama R, Teale JD, Marks V. The effect of synthetic very low calorie diets on the GH-IGF-1 axis in obese subjects. Clin Chim Acta 1990; 188:31–38.

75. Davies RR, Turner SJ, Cook D, Alberti KGMM, Johnston DG. The response of obese subjects to continuous infusion of human pancreatic growth hormone-releasing factor 1-44. Clin Endocrinol 1985; 23:521–525.

76. Cordido F, Casanueva FF, Dieguez C. Cholinergic receptor activation by pyridostigmine restores growth hormone (GH) responsiveness to GH-releasing hormone administration in obese subjects: evidence for hypothalamic somatostatinergic participation in the blunted GH-release of obesity. J Clin Endocrinol Metab 1989; 68:290–293.

77. Ghigo E, Mazza E, Corrias A, Imperiale E, Goffi S, Arvat E, Bellone J, De Sanctis C, Müller EE, Camanni F. Effect of cholinergic enhancement by pyridostigmine on growth hormone secretion in obese adults and children. Metabolism 1989; 38:631–633.

78. Lee EJ, Kim KR, Lee KM, Lim SK, Lee HC, Lee JH, Lee DJ, Huh KB. Reduced growth hormone response to L-dopa and pyridostigmine in obesity. Int J Obes 1994; 18:465–468.

79. Jung R. Endocrinological aspects of obesity. Clin Endocrinol Metab 1984; 13:597–612.

80. Kopelman PG. Neuroendocrine function in obesity. Clin Endocrinol 1988; 28:675–689.

81. Caufriez A, Golstein J, Lebrun P, Herchuelz A, Furlanetto R, Copinschi G. Relations between immunoreactive somatomedin C, insulin and T3 patterns during fasting in obese subjects. Clin Endocrinol 1984; 20:65–70.

82. Clemmons DR, Van Wyk JJ. Factors controlling blood concentration of somatomedin C. Clin Endocrinol Metab 1984; 13:113–143.

83. Berelowitz M, Szabo M, Frohman LA, Firestone S, Chu L. Somatomedin-C mediates growth hormone negative feedback by effects on both the hypothalamus and the pituitary. Science 1981; 212:1279–1281.

84. Phillips LS, Goldstein S, Gavin JR III. Nutrition and somatomedin XVI: Somatomedins and somatomedin inhibitors in fasted and refed rats. Metabolism 1988; 37:209–216.

85. Isley WL, Underwood LE, Clemmons DR. Dietary components that regulate serum somatomedin-C concentrations in humans. J Clin Invest 1983; 71:175–182.

86. Davenport ML, Svoboda ME, Koerber KL, Van Wijk JJ, Clemmons DR, Underwood LE. Serum concentrations of Insulin-Like Growth Factor II are not changed by short term fasting and refeeding. J Clin Endocrinol Metab 1988; 67:1231–1236.

87. Young SCJ, Underwood LE, Celniker A, Clemmons DR. Effects of recombinant insulin-like growth factor-I (IGF-I) and growth hormone on serum IGF-binding proteins in calorically restricted adults. J Clin Endocrinol Metab 1992; 75:603–608.

88. McCusker RH, Campion DR, Jones WK, Clemmons DR. The insulin-like growth factor-binding proteins of porcine serum: endocrine and nutritional regulation. Endocrinology 1989; 125:501–509.

89. Thissen J-P, Underwood LE, Maiter D, Maes M, Clemmons DR, Ketelslegers J-M. Failure of insulin-like growth factor-I (IGF-I) infusion to promote growth in protein-restricted rats despite normalization of serum IGF-I concentrations. Endocrinology 1991; 128:885–890.

90. Clemmons DR, Smith-Banks A, Underwood LE. Reversal of diet-induced catabolism by infusion of recombinant insulin-like growth factor-I in humans. J Clin Endocrinol Metab 1992; 75:234–238.

91. Clemmons DR, Snyder DK, Williams R, Underwood LE. Growth hormone administration conserves lean body mass during dietary restriction in obese subjects. J Clin Endocrinol Metab 1987; 64:878–883.

92. Snyder DK, Underwood Le, Clemmons DR. Anabolic effects of growth hormone in obese diet-restricted subjects are dose dependent. Am J Clin Nutr 1990; 52:431–437.

93. Snyder DK, Clemmons DR, Underwood LE. Treatment of obese, diet-restricted subjects with growth hormone for 11 weeks: effects on anabolism, lipolysis and body composition. J Clin Endocrinol Metab 1988; 67:54–61.

94. Drent ML, Wever LDV, Adèr HJ, Van der Veen EA. Growth hormone administration in addition to a very low calorie diet and an exercise program in obese subjects. Eur J Endocrinol 1995; 132:565–572.

95. Snyder DK, Clemmons DR, Underwood LE. Dietary carbohydrate content determines responsiveness to growth hormone in energy-restricted humans. J Clin Endocrinol Metab 1989; 69:745–752.

96. Altomonte L, Zoli A, Ghirlanda G, Manna R, Greco AV. Effect of fenfluramine on insulin/growth hormone ratio in obese subjects. Pharmacology 1988; 36:106–111.

97. Altomonte L, Zoli A, Alessi F, Ghirlanda G, Manna R, Greco AV. Effect of fenfluramine on growth hormone and prolactin secretion in obese subjects. Horm Res 1987; 27:190–194.

98. Argenio GF, Bernini GP, Sgró M, Vivaldi MS, Del Corso C, Santoni R, Franchi F. Blunted growth hormone (GH) responsiveness to GH-releasing hormone in obese patients: influence of prolonged administration of the serotoninergic drug fenfluramine. Metabolism 1991; 40:724–727.

99. Larsen S, Vejtorp L, Hornnes P, Bechgaard H, Sestoft L, Lyngsoe J. Metabolic effects of fenfluramine in obese diabetics. Br J Clin Pharm 1977; 4:529–533.

100. Bernini GP, Argenio GF, Vivaldi MS, Del Cirso C, Birindelli R, Luisi M, Franchi F. Impaired growth hormone response to insulin-induced hypoglycemia in obese patients: restoration blocked by ritanserin after fenfluramine administration. Clin Endocrinol 1990; 32:453–459.

101. Medeiros-Neto G, Lima N, Perozim L, Pedrinola F, Wajchenberg BL. The effect of hypocaloric diet with and without D-Fenfluramine treatment on growth hormone release after growth hormone-releasing factor stimulation in pa-

tients with android obesity. Metab Clin Exp 1994; 43: 969–973.

102. Wilcox RG. Triiodothyronine, TSH and prolactin in obese women. Lancet 1977; 1:1027–1029.

103. Bray GA, Fisher DA, Chopra IJ. Relation of thyroid hormones to body-weight. Lancet 1976; 1:1206–1208.

104. Chomard P, Vernhes G, Autissier N, Debry G. Serum concentrations of total T_4, T_3, reverse T_3, and free T_4, T_3 in moderately obese patients. Hum Nutr Clin Nutr 1985; 39c:371–378.

105. Faber J, Sorensen TIA, Lumholtz IB, Klein HC, Kirkegaard C, Blickert-Toft M. Serum levels of T4, T3, reverse T3, 3,3′-diiodothyronine and 3′,5′-diiodohyronine in obesity before and after jejunoileal bypass. Clin Endocrinol 1981; 14:119–124.

106. Azizi F. Effect of dietary composition on fasting-induced changes n serum thyroid hormones and thyrotropin. Metabolism 1978; 27:935–942.

107. Amatruda JM, Hochstein M, Hsu T-H, Lockwood DH. Hypothalamic and pituitary dysfunction in obese males. Int J Obes 1982; 6:183–189.

108. Donders SHJ, Pieters GFFM, Heevel JG, Ross HA, Smals AGH, Kloppenborg PWC. Disparity of thyrotropin (TSH) and prolactin responses to TSH-releasing hormone in obesity. J Clin Endocrinol Metab 1985; 61:56–59.

109. Vagenakis AG. Thyroid hormone metabolism in prolonged experimental starvation in man. In: Vigersky RA, ed. Anorexia Nervosa. New York: Raven Press, 1977: 243–253.

110. Vagenakis AG. Non thyroid diseases affecting the thyroid hormone metabolism. In: Hesch RD, ed. The Low T3 Syndrome. New York: Academic Press, 1981:127–139.

111. Spaulding SW, Chopra IJ, Sherwin RS, Lyall SS. Effect of caloric restriction and dietary composition on serum T_3 levels and reverse T_3 in man. J Clin Endocrinol Metab 1976; 42:197–200.

112. Merimee TJ, Fineberg ES. Starvation-induced alterations of circulating thyroid hormone concentrations in man. Metabolism 1976; 25:79–83.

113. Carlson HE, Drenick Ej, Chopra IJ, Hershman JL. Alterations in basal and TRH-stimulated serum levels of thyrotropin, prolactin and thyroid hormones in starved obese men. J Clin Endocrinol Metab 1977; 45:707–713.

114. Van Gaal LF, De Leeuw IH. Reverse T_3 changes during protein supplemented diets. Relation to nutrient combustion rates. J Endocrinol Invest 1989; 12:799–803.

115. Wadden TA, Mason G, Foster GD, Stunkard AJ, Prange AJ. Effects of a very low calorie diet on weight, thyroid hormones and mood. Int J Obes 1990; 14:249–258.

116. Croxson MS, Hall TD, Kletzky OA, Jaramillo JE, Nicoloff JT. Decreased serum thyrotropin induced by fasting. J Clin Endocrinol Metab 1977; 45:560–568.

117. Palmblad J, Levi L, Burger A, Melander A, Westgren U, von Schenk H, Skude G. Effects of total energy withdrawal (fasting) on the levels of growth hormone, thyro-

tropin, cortisol, adrenaline, noradrenaline, T_4, T_3, rT_3 in healthy males. Acta Med Scand 1977; 201:15–22.

118. Danforth E Jr, Horton ES, O'Connell M, Burger AG, Ingbar SH, Braverman L, Vagenakis AG. Dietary induced alterations in thyroid hormone metabolism during overnutrition. J Clin Invest 1979; 64:1336–1347.

119. Welle S, O'Connell M, Danforth E Jr, Campbell R. Decreased free fraction of serum thyroid hormones during carbohydrate overfeeding. Metabolism 1984; 33:837–839.

120. Oppert JM, Dussault JH, Tremblay A, Despres JP, Theriault G, Bouchard C. Thyroid hormones and thyrotropin variations during long term overfeeding in identical twins. J Clin Endocrinol Metab 1994; 79:547–553.

121. Gardner DF, Kaplan MM, Stanley CA, Utiger RD. Effect of tri-iodothyronine replacement on the metabolic and pituitary responses to starvation. N Engl J Med 1979; 300: 579–584.

122. Carter WJ, Shakir KM, Hodges S, Faas FH, Wynn JO. Effect of thyroid hormone on metabolic adaptation to fasting. Metabolism 1975; 24:1177–1183.

123. Nair KS, Halliday D, Ford GC, Garrow JS. Effect of triiodothyronine on leucine kinetics, metabolic rate, glucose concentration and insulin secretion rate during two weeks of fasting in obese women. Int J Obes 1989; 13:487–496.

124. Krulich L, Vijayan E, Coppings RJ, Giachetti A, McCann SM, Mayfield MA. On the role of the central serotoninergic system in the regulation of the secretion of thyrotropin and prolactin: thyrotropin-inhibiting and prolactin-releasing effects of 5-hydroxytryptamine and quipazine in the male rat. Endocrinology 1979; 105:276–283.

125. Chen YF, Ramirez VD. Serotonin stimulates thyrotropin-releasing hormone release from superfused rat hypothalami. Endocrinology 1981; 108:2359–2366.

126. Jordan D, Poncet C, Mornex R, Ponsin G. Participation of serotonin in thyrotropin release I. Evidence for the action of serotonin on thyrotropin releasing hormone release. Endocrinology 1978; 103:414–418.

127. Coccaro EF, Siever LJ, Kourides IA, Adan F, Campbell G, Davis KL. Central serotoninergic stimulation by fenfluramine challenge does not affect plasma thyrotropin-stimulating hormone levels in man. Neuroendocrinology 1988; 47:273–276.

128. Argenio GF, Bernini GP, Vivaldi MS, Del Corso C, Monzani F, Baschieri L, Bertolozzi G, Santoni R, Franchi F, Luisi M. Effects of fenfluramine on prolactin and thyroid stimulating hormone response to thyrotropin releasing hormone in obese and normal women. Eur J Clin Pharmacol 1990; 39:13–16.

129. Zelissen PMJ, Koppeschaar HPF, Thijssen JHH, Erkelens DW. TSH and prolactin secretion in obesity: influence of weight reduction and of treatment with the serotoninergic drug dexfenfuramine. Thesis, 1991. State University, Utrecht.

130. Dunkel L, Sorva R, Voutilainen R. Low levels of sex hormone-binding globulin in obese children. J Pediatr 1985; 17:95–97.

131. Rogers J, Mitchell GW Jr. The relation of obesity to menstrual disturbances. N Engl J Med 1952; 247:53–55.

132. Hosseinian AH, Kim MH, Rosenfield RL. Obesity and oligomenorrhea are associated with hyperandrogenism independent of hirsutism. J Clin Endocrinol Metab 1976; 42:765–769.

133. Glass AR, Dahms WT, Abraham G, Atkinson RL, Bray GA, Swerdloff RS. Secondary amenorrhea in obesity: etiologic role of weight-related androgen excess. Fertil Steril 1978; 30:243–244.

134. Zhang Y-W, Stern B, Rebar RW. Endocrine comparison of obese menstruating and amenorrheic women. J Clin Endocrinol Metab 1984; 58:1077–1083.

135. Hartz AJ, Barboriak PN, Wong A, Katayama KP, Rimm AA. The association of obesity with fertility and related menstrual abnormalities in women. Int J Obes 1979; 3:57–73.

136. Nimrod A, Ryan KJ. Aromatization of androgens by human abdominal and breast fat tissue. J Clin Endocrinol Metab 1975; 40:367–372.

137. Edman CD, MacDonald PC. Effect of obesity on conversion of plasma androstenedione to estrone in ovulatory and anovulatory young women. Am J Obstet Gynecol 1978; 130:456–461.

138. Zumoff B, Strain GW, Kream J, O'Connor J, Levin J, Fukushima DK. Obese young men have elevated plasma estrogen levels but obese premenopausal women do not. Metabolism 1981; 30:1011–1014.

139. Kopelman PG, Pilkington TRE, White N, Jeffcoate SL. Abnormal sex steroid secretion and binding in massively obese women. Clin Endocrinol 1980; 12:363–369.

140. Pasquali R, Antenucci D, Casimirri F, Venturoli S, Paradisi R, Fabbri R, Balestra V, Melchionda N, Barbara L. Clinical and hormonal characteristics of obese amenorrheic hyperandrogenic women before and after weight loss. J Clin Endocrinol Metab 1989; 68:173–179.

141. Friedman CI, Kim MH. Obesity and its effect on reproductive function. Clin Obstet Gynecol 1985; 28:645–663.

142. Kirschner MA, Samojlik E, Drejk M, Szmal E, Schneider G. Ertel N. Androgen-estrogen metabolism in women with upper body versus lower body obesity. J Clin Endocrinol Metab 1990; 70:473–479.

143. Van Gaal LF, Vanuytsel JL, Vansant GA, De Leeuw IH. Sex hormones, body fat distribution, resting metabolic rate and glucose-induced thermogenesis in premenopausal obese women. Int J Obes 1994; 18:333–338.

144. Evans DJ, Hoffmann RG, Kalkhoff RK, Kissebah AH. Relationship of androgenic activity to body fat topography, fat cell morphology, and metabolic aberrations in premenopausal women. J Clin Endocrinol Metab 1983; 57: 304–310.

145. Proetsky L. On the paradox of insulin-induced hyperandrogenism in insulin-resistant states. Endocr Rev 1991; 12:3–13.

146. van Gaal L, Vansant G, van Acker K, de Leeuw I. Decreased hepatic insulin extraction in upper body obesity: Relationship to unbound androgens and sex hormone binding globulin. Diabetes Res Clin Pract 1991; 12: 99–106.

147. Pasquali R, Casimirri F, Cantobelli S, Melchionda N, Labate AMM, Fabbri R, Capelli M, Bortoluzzi L. Effect of obesity and body fat distribution on sex hormones and insulin in men. Metabolism 1991; 40:101–104.

148. Nestler JE. Editorial: Sex hormone-binding globulin: a marker for hyperinsulinemia and/or insulin resistance. J Clin Endocrinol Metab 1993; 76:273–274.

149. Birkeland KI, Hansen KF, Torjesen PA, Vaaler S. Level of sex hormone-binding globulin is positively correlated with insulin sensitivity in men with type 2 Diabetes. J Clin Endocrinol Metab 1993; 76:275–278.

150. Peiris AN, Stagner JI, Plymate SR, Vogel RL, Heck M, Samols E. Relationship of insulin secretory pulses to sex hormone-binding globulin in normal men. J Clin Endocrinol Metab 1993; 76:279–282.

151. Preziosi P, Barrett-Connor E, Papoz L, Roger M. Saint-Paul M, Nahoul K, Simon D. Interrelation between plasma sex hormone-binding globulin and plasma insulin in healthy adult women: the telecom study. J Clin Endocrinol Metab 1993; 76:283–287.

152. Geisthövel F, Olbrich M, Frorath B, Thiemann M, Weitzell R. Obesity and hypertestosteronaemia are independently and synergistically associated with elevated insulin concentrations and dyslipidemia in pre-menopausal women. Hum Reprod 1994; 9:610–616.

153. Polderman KH, Gooren LJG, Asscheman H, Bakker A, Heine RJ. Induction of insulin resistance by androgens and estrogens. J Clin Endocrinol Metab 1994; 79: 265–271.

154. Newmark SR, Rossini AA, Naftolin Fl, Todd R, Rose LI, Cahill GF JR. Gonadotropin profiles in fed and fasted obese women. Am J Obstet Gynecol 1979; 133:75–80.

155. Insler V, Lunenfeld B. Pathophysiology of polycystic ovarian disease: new insights. Hum Reprod 1991; 6: 1025–1029.

156. Zumoff B, Strain GW, Miller LK, Rosner W, Senie R, Seres DS, Rosenfeld RS. Plasma free and non-sex-hormone-binding-globulin-bound testosterone are decreased in obese men in proportion to their degree of obesity. J Clin Endocrinol Metab 1990; 71:929–931.

157. Stanik S, Dornfeld LP, Maxwell MH, Viosca SP, Korenman SG. The effect of weight loss on reproductive hormones in obese men. J Clin Endocrinol Metab 1981; 53: 828–832.

158. Schneider G, Kirschner MA, Berkowitz R, Ertel NH. Increased estrogen production in obese men. J Clin Endocrinol Metab 1979; 48:633–638.

159. Glass AR, Swerdloff RS, Bray GA, Dahms WT, Atkinson RL. Low serum testosterone and sex-hormone-binding-globulin in massively obese men. J Clin Endocrinol Metab 1977; 45:1211–1219.

160. Strain GW, Zumoff B, Kream J, Strain JJ, Deucher R, Rosenfeld RS, Levin J, Fukushima DK. Mild hypogonado-

tropic hypogonadism in obese men. Metabolism 1982; 31:871–875.

161. Giagulli VA, Kaufman JM, Vermeulen A. Pathogenesis of the decreased androgen levels in obese men. J Clin Endocrinol Metab 1994; 79:997–1000.

162. Leenen R, Van der Kooy K, Seidell JC, Deurenberg P, Koppeschaar HPF. Visceral fat accumulation in relation to sex hormones in obese men and women undergoing weight loss therapy. J Clin Endocrinol Metab 1994; 78: 1515–1520.

163. Phillips GB. Evidence for hyperestrogenaemia as a risk factor for myocardial infarction in men. Lancet 1976; ii: 14–18.

164. Pirke KM, Schweiger U, Strowitzki T, Tuschl RJ, Laessle RG, Broocks A, Huber B, Middendorf R. Dieting causes menstrual irregularities in normal weight young women through impairment of episodic luteinizing hormone secretion. Fertil Steril 1989; 51:263–268.

165. O'Dea JPK, Wieland RG, Hallberg MC, Llerena LA, Zorn EM, Genuth SM. Effect of dietary weight loss on sex steroid binding, sex steroids and gonadotropins in obese postmenopausal women. J Lab Clin Med 1979; 93: 1004–1008.

166. Tegelman R, Lindeskog P, Carlström K, Pousette A, Blomstrand R. Peripheral hormone levels in healthy subjects during controlled fasting. Acta Endocrinol (Copenh) 1986; 113:457–462.

167. Kopelman PG, White N, Pilkington TRE, Jeffcoate SL. The effect of weight loss on sex steroid secretion and binding in massively obese women. Clin Endocrinol 1981; 14: 113–116.

168. Strain G, Zumoff B, Rosner W, Pi-Sunyer X. The relationship between serum levels of insulin and sex hormone-binding globulin in men: the effect of weight loss. J Clin Endocrinol Metab 1994; 79:1173–1176.

169. Warren M, Jewelewicz R, Dyrenfurth I, Ans R, Khalaf S, Van De Wiele RL. The significance of weight loss in the evaluation of pituitary response to LH-RH in women with secondary amenorrhea. J Clin Endocrinol Metab 1975; 40:601–611.

170. Warren MP. Effects of undernutrition on reproductive function in the human. Endocr Rev 1983; 4:363–377.

171. Loucks AB, Heath EM, Law T, Verdun M, Watts JR. Dietary restriction reduces luteinizing hormone (LH) pulse frequency during waking hours and increases LH pulse amplitude during sleep in young menstruating women. J Clin Endocrinol Metab 1994; 78:910–915.

172. Kiddy DS, Hamilton-Fairley D, Bush A, Short F, Anyaoku V, Reed MJ, Franks S. Improvement in endocrine and ovarian function during dietary treatment of obese women with polycystic ovary syndrome. Clin Endocrinol 1992; 36:105–111.

173. Kamberi IA, Mical RS, Porter JC. Effect of anterior pituitary perfusion and intraventricular injection of catecholamines and indoleamines on LH release. Endocrinology 1970; 87:1–12.

174. Leonardelli J, Dubois MP, Poulain P. Effect of exogenous serotonin on LH-RH secreting neurons in the guinea pig hypothalamus as revealed by immunofluorescence. Neuroendocrinology 1974; 15:69–72.

175. Kamberi IA, Mical RS, Porter JC. Effects of melantonin and serotonin on the release of FSH and prolactin. Endocrinology 1971; 88:1288–1293.

176. Feldman JM, Plonk JW, Bivens CE. Alterations of pituitary-gonadal function in the carcinoid syndrome. Am J Med Sci 1974; 268:215–226.

177. MacIndoe JH, Turkington RW. Stimulation of human prolactin secretion by intravenous infusion of L-tryptophan. J Clin Invest 1973; 52:1972–1978.

178. Jung RT, Shetty PS, James WPT, Barrand MA, Callingham BA. Plasma catecholamines and autonomic responsiveness in obesity. Int J Obes 1982; 6:131–141.

179. Peiris A, Kissebah A. Endocrine abnormalities in morbid obesity. Gastroenterol Clin North Am 1987; 16:389–398.

180. Peterson HR, Rothschild M, Weinberg CR, Fell RD, McLeish KR, Pfeifer MA. Body fat and the activity of the autonomic nervous system. N Engl J Med 1988; 318: 1077–1083.

181. Leibel RL, Berry EM, Hirsch J. Metabolic and hemodynamic responses to endogenous and exogenous catecholamines in formerly obese subjects. Am J Physiol 1991; 260:R785–R791.

182. Tuck ML. Obesity, the sympathetic nervous system and essential hypertension. Hypertension 1992; 19 (Suppl 1): 67–77.

183. Astrup A, Andersen T, Christensen NJ, Bülow J, Madsen J, Breum L, Quaade F. Impaired glucose-induced thermogenesis and arterial norepinephrine response persist after weight reduction in obese humans. Am J Clin Nutr 1990; 51:331–337.

184. Sowers JR, Whitfield LA, Beck FWJ, Catania RA, Tuck ML, Dornfeld L, Maxwell M. Role of enhanced sympathetic nervous system activity and reduced Na$^+$, K$^+$-dependent adenosine triphosphatase activity in maintenance of elevated blood pressure in obesity: effects of weight loss. Clin Sci 1982; 63:121–124.

185. Gustafson AB, Kalkhoff RK. Influence of sex and obesity on plasma catecholamine response to isometric exercise. J Clin Endocrinol Metab 1982; 55:703–708.

186. Gustafson AB, Farell PA, Kalkhoff RK. Impaired plasma catecholamine response to submaximal treadmill exercise in obese women. Metabolism 1990; 39:410–417.

187. Schwartz RS, Jaeger LF, Veith RC, Lakshminarayan S. The effect of diet or exercise on plasma norepinephrine kinetics in moderately obese young men. Int J Obes 1990; 14:1–11.

188. Sowers JR, Nyby M, Stern N, Beck F, Baron S, Catania R, Vlachis N. Blood pressure and hormone changes associated with weight reduction in the obese. Hypertension 1982; 4:686–691.

189. Landsberg L, Krieger DR. Obesity, metabolism and the sympathetic nervous system. Am J Hypertens 1989; 2: 125–132.

190. Landsberg L. Insulin resistance, energy balance and sympathetic nervous system activity. Clin Exp Hypertens 1990; 12:817–830.

191. Daly PA, Landsberg L. Hypertension in obesity and NIDDM. Role of insulin and sympathetic nervous system. Diabetes Care 1991; 14:240–248.

192. DeFronzo RA, Ferrannini E. Insulin resistance. A multifaceted syndrome responsible for NIDDM, obesity, hypertension, dyslipidemia, and atherosclerotic cardiovascular disease. Diabetes Care 1991; 14:173–194.

193. Landsberg L. Pathophysiology of obesity-related hypertension: role of insulin and the sympathetic nervous system. J Cardiovasc Pharmacol 1994; 23 (Suppl 1):S1–S8.

194. Connacher AA, Jung RT, Mitchell PEG, Ford RP, Leslie P, Illingworth P. Heterogeneity of noradrenergic thermic responses in obese and lean humans. Int J Obes 1988; 12: 267–276.

195. Schwartz RS, Halter JB, Bierman EL. Reduced thermic effect of feeding in obesity: role of norepinephrine. Metabolism 1983; 32:114–117.

196. Reynisdottir S, Wahrenberg H, Carlström K, Rössner S, Arner P. Catecholamine resistance in fat cells of women with upper-body obesity due to decreased expression of beta₂-adrenoceptors. Diabetologia 1994; 37:428–435.

197. Astrup AV, Christensen NJ, Simonsen L, Bulow J. Effects of nutrient intake on sympathoadrenal activity and thermogenic mechanisms. J Neurosci Methods 1990; 34:187–192.

198. Jung RT, Shetty PS, James WPT. Nutritional effects on thyroid and catecholamine metabolism. Clin Sci 1980; 58: 183–191.

199. Young JB, Landsberg L. Suppression of sympathetic nervous system during fasting. Science 1977; 196:1473–1475.

200. Grossman E, Eshkol A, Rosenthal T. Diet and weight loss: their effect on norepinephrine, renin and aldosterone levels. Int J Obes 1985; 9:107–114.

201. DeHaven J, Sherwin R, Hendler R, Felig P. Nitrogen and sodium balance and sympathetic-nervous-system activity in obese subjects treated with a low-calorie protein or mixed diet. N Engl J Med 1980; 302:477–482.

202. Young JB, Rosa RM, Landsberg L. Dissociation of sympathetic nervous system and adrenal medullary responses. Am J Physiol 1984; 247:E35–E40.

203. Jung RT, Shetty PS, Barrand M, Callingham BA, James WPT. Role of catecholamines in hypotensive response to dieting. Br Med J 1979; 1:12–13.

204. O'Dea K, Esler M, Leonard P, Stockigt JR, Nestel P. Noradrenaline turnover during under- and over-eating in normal weight subjects. Metabolism 1982; 31:896–899.

205. Andersen HB, Raben A, Astrup A, Christensen NJ. Plasma adrenaline concentration is lower in post-obese than in never-obese women in the basal state, in response to

206. sham-feeding and after food intake. Clin Sci 1994; 87: 69–74.

206. Schwartz JH, Young JB, Landsberg L. Effect of dietary fat on sympathetic nervous system activity in the rat. J Clin Invest 1983; 72:361–370.

207. Walgren MC, Young JB, Kaufman LN, Landsberg L. The effects of various carbohydrates on sympathetic activity in heart and interscapular brown adipose tissue of the rat. Metabolism 1987; 36:585–594.

208. Welle S, Lilavivathana U, Campbell RG. Increased plasma norepinephrine concentrations and metabolic rates following glucose ingestion in man. Metabolism 1980; 29: 806–809.

209. Rothwell NJ, Saville ME, Stock MJ. Sympathetic and thyroid influences on metabolic rate in fed, fasted, and refed rats. Am J Physiol 1982; 243:R339–R346.

210. Brodows RG, Campbell RG, Al-Aziz AJ, Pi-Sunyer FX. Lack of central autonomic regulation of substrate during early fasting in man. Metabolism 1976; 25:803–807.

211. Cignarelli M, De Pergola G, Garutti G, Corso M, Cospite MR, Paternostro A, Romanazzi V, Giorgino R. Changes in overall plasma norepinephrine turnover and lymfomonocyte beta-adrenoreceptor number during combined caloric and sodium restriction in normotensive obese subjects. Int J Obes 1990; 14:429–437.

212. Maxwell MH, Heber D, Waks AU, Tuck ML. Role of insulin and norepinephrine in the hypertension of obesity. Am J Hypertens 1994; 7:402–408.

213. Rothwell NJ, Stock MJ. Effect of diet and fenfluramine on thermogenesis in the rat: possible involvement of serotonergic mechanisms. Int J Obes 1987; 11:319–324.

214. Arase K, Sakaguchi T, Bray GA. Effect of fenfluramine on sympathetic firing rate. Pharmacol Biochem Behav 1988; 29:675–680.

215. Lake CR, Coleman MD, Ziegler MG, Murphy DL. Fenfluramine and its effect on the sympathetic nervous system in man. Curr Med Res Opin 1979; 6(Suppl 1): 63–72.

216. De la Vega CE, Slater S, Ziegler MG, Lake CR, Murphy DL. Reduction in plasma norepinephrine during fenfluramine treatment. Clin Pharmacol Ther 1977; 21:216–221.

217. Himms-Hagen J. Brown adipose tissue thermogenesis and obesity. Prog Lipid Res 1989; 28:67–115.

218. Landsberg L, Young JB. Sympathoadrenal activity and obesity: physiological rationale for the use of adrenergic thermogenic drugs. Int J Obes 1993; 17(Suppl 1): S29–S34.

219. Nisoli E, Tonello C, Carruba MO. SR 58611A: a novel thermogenetic β-adrenoceptor agonist. Eur J Pharmacol 1994; 259:181–186.

220. Peiris AN, Struve MF, Mueller RA, Lee MB, Kissebah AH. Glucose metabolism in obesity: influence of body fat distribution. J Clin Endocrinol Metab 1988; 67:760–767.

221. Peiris AN, Stagner JI, Vogel RL. Nakagawa A, Samols E. Body fat distribution and peripheral insulin sensitivity in

healthy men: role of insulin pulsatility. J Clin Endocrinol Metab 1992; 75:290–294.

222. Walton C, Godsland IF, Proudler AJ, Felton CV, Wynn V. Effect of body mass index and fat distribution on insulin sensitivity, secretion, and clearance in nonobese healthy men. J Clin Endocrinol Metab 1992; 75:170–175.

223. Pouliot M-C, Després J-P, Nadeau A, Moorjani S, Prud'homme D, Lupien PJ, Tremblay A, Bouchard C. Visceral obesity in men. Associations with glucose tolerance, plasma insulin and lipoprotein levels. Diabetes 1992; 41:826–834.

224. Faber OK, Christensen K, Kehlet H, Madsbad S, Binder C. Decreased insulin removal contributes to hyperinsulinemia in obesity. J Clin Endocrinol Metab 1981; 53:618–621.

225. Savage PJ, Flock EV, Mako ME, Blix PM, Rubenstein AH, Bennett PH. C-peptide and insulin secretin in Pima indians and Caucasians: constant fractional hepatic extraction over a wide range of insulin concentrations and in obesity. J Clin Endocrinol Metab 1979; 48:594–598.

226. Peiris AN, Mueller RA, Smith GA, Struve MF, Kissebah AH. Splanchnic insulin metabolism in obesity: influence of body fat distribution. J Clin Invest 1986; 78:1648–1657.

227. Bonora E, Zavaroni I, Bruschi F, Alpi O, Pezzarossa A, Guerra L, Dall'Aglio E, Coscelli C, Butturini U. Peripheral hyperinsulinemia of simple obesity: pancreatic hypersecretion or impaired insulin metabolism? J Clin Endocrinol Metab 1984; 59:1121–1127.

228. Rossell R, Gomis R, Casamitjana R, Segura R, Vilardell E, Rivera F. Reduced hepatic insulin extraction in obesity: relationship with plasma insulin levels. J Clin Endocrinol Metab 1983; 56:608–611.

229. Meistas MT, Margolis S, Kowarski AA. Hyperinsulinemia of obesity is due to decreased clearance of insulin. Am J Physiol 1983; 245:E155–E159.

230. Polonsky KS, Given BD, HIrsch L, Shapiro ET, Tillil H, Beebe C, Galloway JA, Frank BH, Karrison T, Van Cauter E. Quantitative study of insulin secretion and clearance in normal and obese subjects. J Clin Invest 1988; 81:435–441.

231. Rafecas I, Fernández-López JA, Salinas I, Formiguera X, Remesar X, Foz M, Alemany M. Insulin degradation by adipose tissue is increased in human obesity. J Clin Endocrinol Metab 1995; 80:693–695.

232. Jimenez J, Zuniga-Guajardo S, Zinman B, Angel A. Effects of weight loss in massive obesity on insulin and C-peptide dynamics: sequential changes in insulin production, clearance and sensitivity. J Clin Endocrinol Metab 1987; 64:661–668.

233. Polonsky KS, Rubenstein AH. C-peptide as a measure of the secretion and hepatic extraction of insulin. Pitfalls and limitations. Diabetes 1984; 33:486–494.

234. DeFronzo RA, Tobin JD, Andres R. Glucose clamp technique: a method for quantifying insulin secretion and resistance. Am J Physiol 1979; 237:E214–E223.

235. Reaven GM. Role of insulin resistance in human disease (Banting lecture 1988). Diabetes 1988; 37:1595–1607.

236. Reaven GM. Insulin resistance, hyperinsulinemia, hypertriglyceridemia and hypertension. Parallels between human disease and rodent models. Diabetes Care 1991; 14:195–202.

237. Fink G. Gutman RA, Cresto JC, Selawry H, Lavine R, Recant L. Glucose-induced insulin release patterns: effect of starvation. Diabetologia 1974; 10:421–425.

238. Gama R, Marks V. The reduction of peripheral insulin concentrations in obese subjects following a hypocaloric diet: reduced pancreatic secretion or increased hepatic extraction? Ann Clin Biochem 1989; 26:388–392.

239. Boden G, Baile CA, McLaughlin CL, Matschinsky FM. Effects of starvation and obesity on somatostatin, insulin and glucagon release from an isolated perfused organ system. Am J Physiol 1981; 241:E215–E220.

240. Letiexhe MR, Scheen AJ, Gerard PL, Desaive C, Lefèbvre. Postgastroplasty recovery of ideal body weight normalizes glucose and insulin metabolism in obese women. J Clin Endocrinol Metab 1995; 80:364–369.

241. Olefsky J, Reaven GM, Farquhar JW. Effects of weight reduction on obesity. Studies of lipid and carbohydrate metabolism in normal and hyperlipoproteinemic subjects. J Clin Invest 1974; 53:64–76.

242. Malecka-Tendera E, Koehler B, Wiciak B, Ramos A. Impaired glucose tolerance in obese children—a long-term prospective study. In: Ditschuneit H, Gries FA, Hauner H, Schusdziarra V, Wechsler JG, eds. Obesity in Europe 93. Proceedings of the 5th European Congress on Obesity. London: John Libbey, 1994:153–158.

243. Scheen AJ, Paolisso G, Salvatore T, Lefèbvre PJ. Improvement of insulin-induced glucose disposal in obese patients with NIDDM after 1-wk treatment with d-fenfluramine. Diabetes Care 1991; 14:325–332.

244. Storlien LH, Thornburn AW, Smythe GA, Jenkins AB, Chisholm DJ, Kraegen EW. Effect of d-fenfluramine on basal glucose turnover and fat-feeding-induced insulin resistance in rats. Diabetes 1989; 38:499–503.

245. Brindley DN. Metabolic and hormonal effects of dexfenfluramine on stress situations. Clin Neuropharmacol 1988; 11(Suppl 1):S86–S89.

246. Brindley DN. Neuroendorine regulation and obesity. Int J Obes 1992; 16:S73–S79.

247. Pestell RG, Crock PA, Ward GM, Alford FP, Best JD. Fenfluramine increases insulin action in patients with NIDDM. Diabetes Care 1989; 12:252–258.

248. Verdy M, Charbonneau L, Verdy I, Belanger R. Bolte E, Chiasson JL. Fenfluramine in the treatment of non-insulin dependent diabetics: hypoglycemic versus anorectic effect. Int J Obes 1983; 7:289–297.

249. Pestell RG, Crock RA, Ward GM, Alford FP, Best JD. Fenfluramne increases insulin action in patients with NIDDM. Diabetes Care 1989; 12:252–258.

250. Schade DS, Eaton PR. Modulation of the catabolic activity of glucagon by endogenous insulin secretion in obese man. Acta Diabetol Lat 1977; 14:62–72.

251. Gossain VV, Matute ML, Kalkhoff RK. Relative influence of obesity and diabetes on plasma alpha-cell glucagon. J Clin Endocrinol Metab 1974; 38:238–243.

252. Kalkhoff RK, Gossain VV, Matute ML. Plasma glucagon in obesity. Response to arginine, glucose and protein administration. N Engl J Med 1973; 289:465–467.

253. Borghi VC, Wajchenberg BL, Cesar FP. Plasma glucagon suppressibiity after oral glucose in obese subjects with normal and impaired glucose tolerance. Metabolism 1984; 33:1068–1074.

254. Bonora E, Moghetti P, Cacciatori V, Zenere M, Tosi F, Travia D, Zoppini G, Perobelli L, Muggeo M. Plasma concentrations of glucagon during hyperglycemic clamp with or without somatostatin infusion in obese subjects. Acta Diabetol Lat 1990; 27:309–314.

255. Starke AAR, Erhardt G, Berger M, Zimmerman H. Elevated pancreatic glucagon in obesity. Diabetes 1984; 33: 277–280.

256. Golland IM, Vaughan Williams CA, Shalet SM, Laing I, Elstein M. Glucagon in women with polycystic ovary syndrome (PCO): relationship to abnormalities of insulin and androgens. Clin Endocrinol 1990; 33:645–651.

257. Schade DS, Eaton RP. Role of insulin and glucagon in obesity. Diabetes 1974; 23:657–661.

258. Santiago JV, Haymond MW, Clarke WL, Pagliara AS. Glucagon, insulin and glucose responses to physiologic testing in normal and massively obese adults. Metabolism 1977; 26:1115–1122.

259. Inokuchi T, Kameyama HK, Orita M, Kasai T, Isogai S. Elevated pancreatic glucagon in moderately obese patients: relationship of fatty liver and hypertriglyceridemia. Jpn J Med 1989; 28:355–361.

260. Holst JJ, Schwartz TW, Lovgreen NA, Pedersen O, Beck-Nielsen H. Diurnal profile of pancreatic polypeptide, pancreatic glucagon, gut glucagon and insulin in human morbid obesity. Int J Obes 1983; 7:529–538.

261. Ratzmann KP, Schulz B, Witt S, Ziegler M. Pancreatic glucagon response to glucose in obesity with normal and impaired carbohydrate tolerance. Int J Obes 1981; 5: 163–169.

262. Wise JK, Hendler R, Felig P. Evaluation of alpha-cell function by infusion of alanine in normal, diabetic and obese subjects. N Engl J Med 1973; 288:487–490.

263. Aguilar-Parada E, Eisentraut AM, Unger RH. Effects of starvation on plasma pancreatic glucagon in normal man. Diabetes 1969; 18:717–723.

264. Marliss EB, Aoki TT, Unger RH, Soeldner JS, Cahill GF. Glucagon levels and metabolic effects in fasting man. J Clin Invest 1970; 49:2256–2270.

265. Fisher M, Sherwin RS, Hendler R, Felig P. Kinetics of glucagon in man: effects of starvation. Proc Natl Acad Sci USA 1976; 73:1735–1739.

266. Smith GP, Gibbs J. Brain-gut peptides and the control of food intake. In: Martin JB, Reichlin S, Bick KL, eds. Neurosecretion and Brain Peptides. New York: Raven Press, 1981:389–395.

267. Geary N. Pancreatic glucagon signals postprandial satiety. Neurosci Biobehav Rev 1990; 14:323–338.

268. Eckel RH, Fjuimoto WY, Brunzell JD. Gastric inhibitory polypeptide enhanced lipoprotein lipase activity in cultured preadipocytes. Diabetes 1979; 28:1141–1142.

269. Beck B. Gastric inhibitory polypeptide: a gut hormone with anabolic functions. J Mol Endocrinol 1989; 2: 169–174.

270. Raben A, Andersen HB, Christensen NJ, Madsen J, Holst JJ, Astrup A. Evidence for an abnormal postprandial response to a high-fat meal in women predisposed to obesity. Am J Physiol Endocrinol Metab 1994; 267: E549–E559.

271. Mazzaferri EL, Starich GH, Lardinois CK, Bowen GD. Gastric inhibitory polypeptide responses to nutrients in caucasians and american indians with obesity and non-insulin-dependent Diabetes Mellitus. J Clin Endocrinol Metab 1985; 61:313–321.

272. Gutniak M, Orskov C, Holst JJ, Ahrén B, Efendic S. Antidiabetogenic effect of glucagon-like peptide-1 (7-36)amide in normal subjects and patients with diabetes mellitus. N Engl J Med 1992; 326:1316–1322.

273. Ensinck JW, D'Alessio DA. The enteroinsular axis revisited: a novel role for an incretin. N Engl J Med 1992; 326.1352–1353.

274. Orskov C. Glucagon-like peptide-1, a new hormone of the entero-insular axis. Diabetologia 1992; 35:701–711.

275. Kreymann B, Ghatei MA, Williams G, Bloom SR. Glucagon-like peptide-1 7-36: a physiological incretin in man. Lancet 1987; 2:1300–1303.

276. Jorde R, Amland PF, Burhol PG, Giercksky K-E, Ebert R. GIP and insulin responses to a test meal in healthy and obese subjects. Scand J Gastroenterol 1983; 18:1115–1119.

277. Service FJ, Rizza RA, Westland RE, Hall LD, Gerich JE, Go VLW. Gastric inhibitory polypeptide in obesity and diabetes mellitus. J Clin Endocrinol Metab 1984; 58: 1133–1140.

278. Salera M, Giacomoni P, Pironi L, Cornia G, Capelli M, Marini A, Benfenati F, Miglioli M, Barbara L. Gastric inhibitory polypeptide release after oral glucose: relationship to glucose intolerance, diabetes mellitus and obesity. J Clin Endocrinol Metab 1982; 55:329–336.

279. Sarson DL, Kopelman PG, Besterman HS, Pilkington TRE, Bloom SR. Disparity between glucose dependent insulinotropic polypeptide and insulin responses in obese man. Diabetologia 1983; 25:386–391.

280. Krarup T. Immunoreactive gastric inhibitory polypeptide. Endocr Rev 1988; 9:122–134.

281. Jones IR, Owens DR, Luzio SD, Hayes TM. Obesity is associated with increased post-prandial GIP-levels which

are not reduced by dietary restriction and weight loss. Diabetes Metab 1989; 15:11–22.

282. Ebert R, Creutzfeldt W. Decreased GIP secretion through impairment of absorption. In: Creutzfeldt W, ed. The Entero Insular Axis. Frontiers of Hormone Research, Vol. 7: Basel: S Karger, 1980:192–201.

283. Collier G, O'Dea K. The effect of congestion of fat on the glucose, insulin and gastric inhibitory polypeptide responses to carbohydrate and protein. Am J Clin Nutr 1983; 37:941–944.

284. Creutzfeldt W, Ebert R, Willms B, Frerichs H, Brown JC. Gastric inhibitory polypeptide (GIP) and insulin in obesity: increased response to stimulation and defective feedback control of serum levels. Diabetologia 1978; 14: 15–24.

285. Krarup T, Holst JJ, Lindorf Larsen K. Responses and molecular heterogeneity of IR-GIP after intraduodenal glucose and fat. Am J Physiol 1985; 249:E195–E200.

286. Willms B, Ebert R. Creutzfeldt W. Gastric inhibitory polypeptide (GIP) and insulin in obesity II. Reversal of increased response to stimulation by starvation or food restriction. Diabetologia 1978; 14:379–387.

287. Ebert R. Creutzfeldt W. Gastric inhibitory polypeptide (GIP) hypersecretion in obesity depends on meal size and is not related to hyperinsulinemia. Acta Diabetol Lat 1989; 26:1–15.

288. Fukase N, Igarashi M, Takahashi H, Manaka H, Yamatani K, Daimon M, Tominaga M, Sasaki H. Hypersecretion of truncated glucagon-like peptuide-1 and gastric inhibitory polypeptide in obese patients. Diabet Med 1993; 10: 44–49.

289. Groop P-H. The influence of body-weight, age and glucose tolerance on the relationship between GIP-secretion and beta-cell function in man. Scand J Clin Lab Invest 1989; 49:367–379.

290. Jones IR, Owens DR, Moyle C, Gicheru K, Luzio S, Birtwell AJ, Hayes TM, Sarsons D, Bloom SR. The role of the entero-insular axis in the hyperinsulinaemia of obesity. Diabetologia 1982; 23:469 (abstract).

291. Schwartz TW. Pancreatic polypeptide: a hormone under vagal control. Gastroenterology 1983; 85:1411–1425.

292. Marco J, Zulueta MA, Correas I, Villanueva ML. Reduced pancreatic polypeptide secretion in obese subjects. J Clin Endocrinol Metab 1980; 50:744–747.

293. Floyd JC Jr, Fajans SS, Pek S, Chance RE. A newly recognized pancreatic polypeptide: plasma levels in health and disease. Recent Prog Horm Res 1977; 33:519–570.

294. Floyd JC Jr. Human pancreatic polypeptide. J Clin Endocrinol Metab 1979; 8:379–399.

295. Marco J, Hedo JA Villanueva ML. Control of pancreatic polypeptide secretion by glucose in man. J Clin Endocrinol Metab 1978; 46:140–145.

296. Lassmann V, Garcia LC, Vialettes B, Vague P. Impaired pancreatic polypeptide response to insulin hypoglycemia in obese subjects. Horm Metab Res 1985; 17:663–666.

297. Adrian TE, Besterman HS, Bloom SR. The importance of cholinergic tone in the release of pancreatic polypeptide by gut hormones in man. Life Sci 1979; 24:1989–1994.

298. Lonovics J, Guzman S, Devitt P, Hejtmancik KE, Suddith RL, Rayford PL, Thompson JC. Release of pancreatic polypeptide in humans by infusion of cholecystokinin. Gastroenterology 1980; 79:817–822.

299. Lonovics J, Guzman S, Devitt PG, Hejtmancik KE, Suddith RL, Rayford PL, Thompson JC. Action of pancreatic polypeptide on exocrine pancreas and on release of cholecystokinin and secretin. Endocrinology 1981; 108: 1925–1930.

300. Hanukoglu A, Chalew S, Kowarski AA. Human pancreatic polypeptide in children and young adults. Horm Metab Res 1990; 22:41–43.

301. Berger D, Crowther RC, Floyd JC Jr, Pek S, Fajans SS. Effect of age on fasting plasma levels of pancreatic hormones in man. J Clin Endocrinol Metab 1978; 47: 1183–1189.

302. Adrian TE, Besterman HS, Mallinson CN, Greenberg GR, Bloom SR. Inhibition of secretin stimulated pancreatic secretion by pancreatic polypeptide. Gut 1978; 20:37–40.

303. Greenberg GR, McCloy RF, Adrian TE, Chadwick VS, Baron JH, Bloom SR. Inhibition of pancreas and galbladder by pancreatic polypeptide. Lancet 1978; 2:1280–1282.

304. Beglinger C, Taylor IL, Grosman MI, Solomon TE. Pancreatic polypeptide inhibits exocrine pancreatic responses to six stimulants. Am J Physiol 1984; 246:G286–G291.

305. Pieramico O, Malfertheiner P, Nelson DK, Glasbrenner B, Ditschuneit H. Interdigestive cycling and post-prandial release of pancreatic polypeptide in severe obesity. Int J Obes 1990; 14:1005–1011.

306. Lassmann V, Vague P, Vialettes B, Simon M-C. Low plasma levels of pancreatic polypeptide in obesity. Diabetes 1980; 29:428–430.

307. Hedo JA, Villanueva ML, Marco J. Influence of plasma free fatty acids on pancreatic polypeptide secretion in man. J Clin Endocrinol Metab 1979; 49:73–77.

308. Cantor P. Cholecystokinin in plasma. Digestion 1989; 42: 181–201.

309. Reimers J, Nauck M, Creutzfeldt W, Strietzel J, Ebert R, Cantor P, Hoffmann G. Lack of insulinotropic effect of endogenous and exogenous cholecystokinin in man. Diabetologia 1988; 14:271–280.

310. Ebert R. Gut signals for islet hormone release. Eur J Clin Invest 1990; 20(Suppl 1):S20–S26.

311. Hildebrand P, Ensinck JW, Ketterer S. Delco F, Mossi S, Bangerter U, Beglinger C. Effect of a cholecystokinin antagonist on meal-stimulated insulin and pancreatic polypeptide release in humans. J Clin Endocrinol Metab 1991; 72:1123–1129.

312. Burhol PG, Jenssen TG, Jorde R, Lygren I, Johnson JA. Plasma cholecystokinin (CCK) before and after a jejunoileal bypass operation in obese patients with reference to appetite regulation. Int J Obes 1984; 8:233–236.

213. Wisén O, Rössner S, Johansson C. Ipaired pancreaticob-iliary response to vagal stimulation and to cholecystokinin in human obesity. Metabolism 1988; 37:436–441.

314. Geracioti TD Jr, Liddle RA. Impaired cholecystokinin se-cretion in bulimia nervosa. N Engl J Med 1988; 319:683–688.

315. Geracioti TD Jr, Kling MA, Joseph-Vanderpool JR, Kan-ayama S, Rosenthal NE, Gold PW, Liddle RA. Meal-related cholecystokinin secretion in eating and affective disorders. Psychopharmacol Bull 1989; 25:444–449.

316. Garlicki J, Konturek PK, Majka J, Kwiecien N, Konturek SJ. Cholecystokinin receptors and vagal nerves in control of food intake in rats. Am J Physiol 1990; 258:40–45.

317. Kissileff HR, Pi-Sunyer FX, Thornton J, Smith GP. C-terminal octapeptide of cholecystokinin decreases food intake in man. Am J Clin Nutr 1981; 34:154–160.

318. Welleer A, Smith GP, Gibbs J. Endogenous cholecystoki-nin reduces feeding in young rats. Science 1990; 247:1589–1591.

319. Mueller K, Hsiao S, Current status of cholecystokinin as a short-term satiety hormone. Neurosci Biobehav Rev 1978; 2:79–88.

320. Dourish CT, Rycroft W, Iversen SD. Postponement of sa-tiety by blockade of brain cholecystokinin (CCK-B) re-ceptors. Science 1989; 245:1509–1511.

321. Peikin SR. Role of cholecystokinin in the control of food intake. Gastroenterol Clin North Am 1989; 18:757–775.

322. Lieverse RJ, Jansen JBMJ, Lamers CBHW. Cholecystokinin and satiation. Neth J Med 1993; 42:146–152.

323. Liddle RA, Morita ET, Conrad CK, Williams JA. Regula-tion of gastric emptying in humans by cholecystokinin. J Clin Invest 1986; 77:992–996.

324. Fried M, Erlacher U, Schwizer W, Löchner C, Koerfer J, Beglinger C, Jansen JB, Lamers CB, Harder F, Bischof-Delaloye A, Stalder GA, Rovati L. Role of cholecystokinin in the regulation of gastric emptying and pancreatic en-zyme secretion in humans. Studies with the cholecysto-kinin-receptor antagonist loxiglumide. Gastroenterology 1991; 101:503–511.

325. Drent ML, Van der Veen EA. Lipase inhibition: a novel concept in the treatment of obesity. Int J Obes 1993; 17:241–244.

326. Drent ML, Larsson I, William-Olsson T, Quaade F, Czu-bayko F, Von Bergmann K, Strobel W, Sjöström L, Van der Veen EA. Orlistat (RO 18-0647), a lipase inhibitor, in the treatment of human obesity: a multiple dose study. Int J Obes 1995; 19:221–226.

327. Drent ML, Van der Veen EA. First clinical studies with Orlistat: a short review. Obes Res 1995; 3(Suppl 4):623S–625S.

328. Fried M, Schwizer W, Froehlich F, Güzelhan C, Jansen J, Lamers C, Gonvers J, Blum AL, Hartmann D. Role of lip-ase in the regulation of upper gastro-intestinal functions in man. Studies with THL-a new highly specific lipase inhibitor. Gastroenterology 1991; 100:A272 (abstract).

329. Fried M, Schwizer W, Asal K, Güzelhan C, Jansen J, La-mers C, Blum A, Gonvers J, Hartmann D. Role of lipase in the regulation of upper gastrointestinal funtions in man: nutrient specific effects—studies with THL, a new highly specific lipase inhibitor. Gastroenterology 1992; 102:A266 (abstract).

330. Drent ML, Popp-Snijders C, Adèr HJ, Jansen JBMJ, Van der Veen EA. Lipase inhibition and hormonal status, body composition and gastrointestinal processing of a liquid high-fat mixed meal in moderately obese subjects. Obes Res 1995; 3:573–581.

37

Obesity and Pregnancy

Stephan Rössner
Karolinska Institute, Stockholm, Sweden

I. GENERAL HORMONAL BACKGROUND

By definition, obesity implies an excess of adipose tissue, which is not an inert storage area for triglycerides but an organ that is hormonally very active (1). Fat cells are known to convert androstenedione to estrone (2,3). Increased concentrations of estrone in obesity may interfere with the feedback system to the hypothalamohypophysial axis, increasing the levels of gonadotropins and androgens (4). As a consequence, anovulation may occur. Furthermore, in obesity a reduction in sex hormone–binding globulin (SHBG) concentrations is seen and the end result is an increased concentration of biologically active free androgens.

Menstrual disturbances are frequent in obesity and may be normalized after weight reduction (5–7). Several studies have demonstrated that with weight reduction various characteristics of the hormonal profile can be normalized. The relationship between obesity and menstrual disorders was reported as early as 1953 (8). Although the relationship between obesity and anovulatory cycles has been established, few supporting studies have been carried out. In some such studies, endocrine characteristics of the subjects have not been reported, which has made it difficult to compare fertile and infertile obese women with regard to their androgen, insulin, or gonadotropin levels. Weight loss in obese anovulatory women is often associated with normalization of the menstrual cycle and associated changes in the hormonal pattern. A particular clinical syndrome associated with obesity and anovulation is the polycystic ovarian syndrome (PCOS), characterized by anovulation, hyperandrogenism, insulin resistance, and altered gonadotropin secretion (9,10). Several investigations have analyzed the relationship between weight loss and menstrual function in PCOS, but often these designs have had clinical and methodological limitations. In some situations, appropriate endocrine characteristics have not been available and in others no proper control group has been included.

In the study of Guzick et al., on the other hand (11), a group of obese hyperandrogenic anovulatory women were studied in a prospective, randomized, controlled fashion before and after a weight loss of 16.2 kg. This weight loss resulted in a significant increase in SHBG, a significant reduction in non-SHBG testosterone, and resumed ovulation in two-thirds of these subjects. These changes occurred in spite of nonsignificant reductions in fasting insulin concentrations and luteinizing hormone and follicle-stimulating hormone characteristics.

The positive effects of weight reduction in obese women with PCOS are underscored by a study of Hamilton-Fairley et al. (12) in which 100 women with clomiphene resistance were treated with standard low-dose gonadotropin therapy. The women were divided into a normal-weight group and a moderately overweight group, and the rates of ovulation, pregnancy, and miscarriage were compared. After gonadotropin treatment, significantly more ovulatory cycles were observed in the lean group. The obese women needed larger doses of gonadotropin to achieve ovulation. Although the proportion of women who became pregnant was similar in both groups, miscarriage was more frequent in the obese group. These authors suggest that overweight women—whether with PCOS or not—should be advised to lose weight before attempted conception in order to improve their chances of a successful outcome and, furthermore, that PCOS women requiring gonadotropin treatment should consider weight loss before treatment to improve their chances of a successful pregnancy outcome.

II.   OBESITY AFTER PREGNANCY

At the Obesity Unit of the Karolinska Hospital, about 40–50% of our female patients reported that pregnancies had been important trigger events that led to development of obesity to the extent that they requested professional support. Pregnancy can in fact be viewed as an example of weight cycling; increased interest has been focused on the behavioral and metabolic consequences of such repeated body weight cycling (13). Generally, weight cycles have been caused by initial weight loss during dieting programs with subsequent regain after relapse. The weight increase and subsequent fall during pregnancy constitutes an interesting biological and "normal" cause of such weight cycling.

Recently, interest has been focused on the possible role of repeated changes in body weight as a risk factor for coronary heart disease and all-cause mortality (14). Some authors have discussed pregnancy-associated weight changes in terms of weight cycling and risk, but mainly in normal-weight women and in relation to the fat distribution pattern (13).

As part of the Stockholm Pregnancy and Weight Development Study a retrospective pilot study to obtain an impression of the role of pregnancy on body weight development in severely obese women was carried out (15). Self-reported data on body weight before each pregnancy, year of each delivery, and body weight 1 year after delivery were recorded. The present weight and height were measured according to the unit routine in connection with the regular visits. These women, who were in maintenance programs at the Obesity Unit, were also questioned in connection with their regular visits to the unit. The data are representative of the typical female patients at the Obesity Unit with a mean age of 47.8 ± 10.7 years (SD) and a body mass index (BMI) of 37.8 ± 5.5 kg/m² (mean weight 104.4 ± 16.6 kg, mean height 166 ± 6 cm). The mean age of the women at the birth of their first child was 24.1 ± 5.1 years. The pregnancies resulted in considerable weight increases retained 1 year postpartum.

Seventy-three percent of these women (83/113) retained more than 10 kg in association with the pregnancy period and up to 1 year after delivery. In the questionnaire, one question referred to weight cycling of more than 10 kg apart from that associated with pregnancy. All women but three reported such weight-cycling episodes, and many of them had undergone numerous such weight-cycling events.

Although it has been well documented that the body weight of women increases with parity and that many women have a higher body weight at the beginning of a subsequent pregnancy compared to the previous one (16), there is little information concerning the importance of pregnancies in the development of obesity.

Several methodological questions may be raised regarding the validity of the self-reported data and the retrospective design of the study. For some women, their pregnancies had occurred many years earlier and it can be argued that memory must have been uncertain. However, it is a common clinical experience that many women do remember their pregnancy-associated weight changes quite well. From these data it seems reasonable to assume that for many women, pregnancy has resulted in pronounced and sustained weight gain.

III.   WEIGHT DEVELOPMENT AND PREGNANCY—BACKGROUND FROM THE LITERATURE

Maternal weight development can vary to a very great extent and still be compatible with healthy pregnancy outcome, which makes rigid recommendations meaningless. As reviewed by Johnston (17), weight loss during pregnancy as well as increases up to more than 23 kg may result in quite normal birth outcomes. Some factors affecting variation in weight gain are maternal characteristics such as age, prepregnancy weight, parity, multiple pregnancies, ethnic origin, various aspects of socioeconomic status, drug abuse, and physical activity levels, but minor variance (less than 5% of variance in weight gain) is also explained by additional factors such as height, smoking, education, and alcohol consumption. Some of the factors will be addressed below.

A.   Pregnancy, Weight, and Age

Numerous studies indicate that the mean body weight and the prevalence of obesity increase with pregnancy. Some of these studies are reviewed in Table 1, partly based on the initial report by Rookus et al. (18). Since body weight

Table 1 Longitudinal Studies of the Effect of Pregnancy on Body Weight

Ref.	Cases	Age correction	Prepregnancy weight	Time of weight postpartum	Pregnancy-associated weight change mean (kg)
McKeown & Record (78)	110 women; population-based sample: $n = 383$ $n = 289$	Yes	Estimated: measures /estimated at 124 days gestation—2.3 kg	12 months 24 months	2.4 2.3
Abitoll (79)	700 clinic patients	No	Self-reported	6 weeks	1.8
Billewicz & Thomson (16)	5830 women; population-based sample	Yes	Measured at 20th week of gestation	[a]	0.5–1.0
Garn et al. (80)	223 smoking women; 254 nonsmoking women	No	Not indicated	[a]	0.5–1.3 1.4–1.5
Beazley & Swinhoe (81)	50 clinic patients	No	20 weeks' gestation	[a]	1.0
Gormican et al. (42)	600 clinic records	No	Measured when first seen at clinic	4–8 weeks	2.1
Newcombe (82)	35,556 deliveries; population-based sample	Yes	Estimated: (weight measured at 20 weeks' gestation)—4 kg	[a]	0.7
Rookus & al. (18)	49 pregnant women; 400 controls	Yes	Measured, expressed as BMI units	9 months	0.34 kg/m²
Öhlin & Rössner (31)	1423 deliveries	Yes	Estimated	12 months	1.5
Brown & al. (83)	41,184 retrospectively	Yes	Questionnaires	18–50 year change[a]	0.55

[a]Pregnancy-associated weight change based on changes in body weight between consecutive pregnancies.
Source: Partly based on data from Ref. 18.

also increases with age in the fertile age groups, it has been necessary to analyze weight increase, parity, and age separately. Such studies demonstrate that the weight increase associated with pregnancy is age-independent. The relationship between body weight development and parity is illustrated in Figure 1, derived from a Finnish study (19).

Body weight increases with age, whether women have children or not. Figure 2, from Wolk and Rössner (20) and based on a representative sample of the entire Swedish adult population, demonstrates, although cross-sectionally, that there is an marked increase in BMI with age, more pronounced in women than in men, and that a further steep increase can be observed during onset of the menopause. It should be kept in mind that the basal metabolic rate normally decreases by about 1% per year. For an individual who maintains an identical life-style

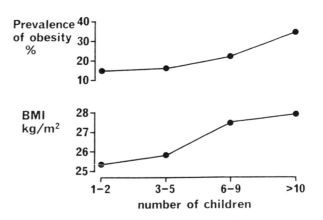

Figure 1 Relationship between body weight and parity (From Ref. 19.)

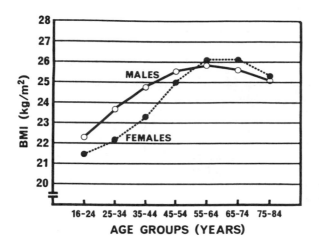

Figure 2 Mean BMI in different Swedish age groups. [Derived from Statistics Sweden 1980–1981 by Kuskowska-Wolk and Rössner (20).]

with regard to eating habits and exercise, this implies a weight increase of about 4 kg per 10 years.

The average reported weight increase with pregnancy ranges from 0.4 to 3.8 kg compared with prepregnancy weight. However, as many authors point out, there are several methodological complications that have to be taken into account when these data are evaluated.

Women generally do not have recorded weight data at the time of conception. Initial body weight figures are therefore uncertain.

Weight increase during pregnancy consists of several components such as the weight of the fetus, the weight of the placenta, amniotic fluid, and enlarged uterus, the whole-body water retention caused by the pregnancy, and finally the adipose tissue increase of the mother (21) (Table 2). For obvious technical and ethical reasons, it is not always possible to analyze all of these factors in larger studies.

There is the methodological question of when to determine postpregnancy body weight. Many women may change their weight over a considerable period of time after delivery. If the weight measurement is taken soon after delivery, this figure may not be representative of the entire weight development associated with the pregnancy as such. If, on the other hand, the weight after delivery is recorded at a later stage, numerous other life changes may have taken place in addition to the pregnancy and delivery. In women in the active childbearing ages, some will be pregnant again if the measurement is taken about 1 year after delivery.

B. Weight Increase During Pregnancy

Generally a mean weight increase of about 12.5 kg is considered normal during an entire pregnancy. In studies reported by Ash et al., the mean increase has ranged from 10.7 kg to 15.2 kg (22). In developing countries, the weight increase is, for obvious reasons, generally considerably lower. Of the total weight increase a certain proportion consists of maternal adipose tissue. This increase ranges from 3 to 6 kg in different studies. This adipose tissue storage occurs mainly during the first two trimesters. From a nutritional point of view, it seems reasonable to assume that the adipose tissue storage during pregnancy provides energy for the child during the lactation period.

C. Menopause and Weight Development

In women a marked weight increase occurs at the time of menopause (Fig. 2). However, it is not clear whether this is related to the loss of the regular menstruations or whether aging itself has these effects on body weight development. Weight increase to the degree of overweight and even obesity at the time of menopause may have important health implications, since this is one of the risk factors associated with atherosclerotic manifestations. It has been demonstrated that with menopause there is an increase in the atherogenic lipoprotein profile (23,24).

In an analysis of the Healthy Women Study (25), weight changes and the effect of weight change on coronary heart disease risk factors were analyzed prospectively. A population-based sample of 485 women was studied when they were premenopausal and aged 42–50 years

Table 2 Weight Increase (Including Fluid Retention) in Various Tissues at Full Term

	Weight (g)	Fluid weight (g)
Fetus	3,300	2340
Placenta	650	540
Amniotic fluid	800	790
Uterus	900	740
Mammary glands	400	300
Blood	1,300	1100
Extracellular fluid	1,200	1200
Other tissues (mainly fat)	3,950	1000
Total	12,500	8010

Source: From Ref. 28.

and then restudied 3 years later. During this period the average weight gain was 2.3 ± 4.2 kg, but there were no significant differences in weight gain of women who remained premenopausal and those who had a natural menopause. The weight gain observed was significantly associated with increases in conventional risk factors for coronary heart disease. However, it was not possible to predict who would gain weight based on the variables at entry to the study. Table 3 demonstrates that the correlation of baseline behaviors and changes in behavior with weight change overall exhibited low *r* values without any distinctive pattern distinguishing women who remained premenopausal from those who had undergone a natural menopause.

During the perimenopausal transition there is not only an increase in body weight, but also a redistribution of adipose tissue with an increase in waist circumference and upper body fat (26). This shift is also related to the change in carbohydrate metabolism (25). The data from the Healthy Women Study underscore the fact that much more information is needed concerning the effects of menopause on body weight development. Of particular interest for future development are studies that are longitudinal and include various populations, since most previous work has almost exclusively been done in Caucasians. It

Table 3 Characteristics of Weight Development After Pregnancy

Statistically significant risk factors for sustained weight	
Weight increase during pregnancy	$r = .36$***
Lactation	$r = .09$**
Age	$r = .06$*
Irregular eating habits after delivery	$r = .07$*
Leisure time physical activity after delivery	$r = .05$*
Factors with major effects on weight retention (weight increase 1 year after delivery)	
Smoke cessation	+3.4 kg**
Marked weight changes (±6 kg) previous pregnancy	+2.5 kg*
Factors *not* significantly affecting body weight 1 year after delivery	
Initial body weight	
Parity	
Previous contraceptive pill	
Social class	
Occupation	
Marital status	
Nationality	
Dietary advice during pregnancy	

*$p < 0.05$; **$p < 0.01$; ***$p < 0.001$.
Source: Data from the Stockholm Pregnancy and Weight Development Study (31).

is of interest that a prospective study of Pima Indian women at the time of menopause found no changes in body weight with menopause and also no changes in lipoprotein levels (27).

D. Energy Metabolism During Pregnancy and Lactation

It is obvious that, to ensure an optimal outcome of a pregnancy, nutrient and energy intake should match maternal and fetal requirements. Maternal weight gain has been used as an indicator for nutritional status, and several studies have demonstrated that the weight gain is positively correlated with birth weight up to a certain weight level. Excessive weight gain during pregnancy is a clear risk for future development of obesity, and high weight gain during pregnancy is furthermore a risk factor associated with toxemia although it is likely that the toxemia of pregnancy in this case is rather the cause than the effect.

As mentioned above (Table 2), the body weight increase of the pregnant woman constitutes the sum of several tissues (28). To determine the true energy costs of a pregnancy longitudinal studies are essential, since inter-individual variations are marked. During recent years several longitudinal studies have been published. In general, they describe a similar pattern: In developing countries the energy costs of the pregnancy are low but increase in countries in the Western world. In all studies, however, the observed changes in energy intake over the entire pregnancy seem insufficient to meet the energy costs of the total pregnancy. This has led several researchers to speculate that substantial energy savings must occur during pregnancy.

The recommended weight gain in well-nourished, overweight, and obese women has been a matter of much debate, and it has been suggested that the recommended weight allowance has been unnecessarily generous, possibly triggering the development of obesity in a risk group of obesity-prone women. The weakening of the relationship between gestational weight gain and birth weight with increasing BMI of the woman suggests that in heavy women the energy supplies are generally sufficient, whereas in undernourished women the development of the fetus is more dependent on the state of the maternal nutrition. Thus different recommendations for suggested weight increase throughout a pregnancy may be appropriate in thin women. Energy balance is less of a problem in overweight women, and recommendations in this group would be adjusted accordingly.

After delivery and during pregnancy, the role of maternal body fat mobilization could theoretically be a matter of conflicting interests. Excessive maternal body fat mobilization during lactation could increase the concentration of fat-soluble contaminants in the breast milk, which theoretically could have adverse health effects for a baby relying entirely on breast feeding. This is a research area that should be addressed in future studies. A target group for such research would be older mothers, for several reasons. For example, body weight increases with age and parity and such mothers could be more inclined to try to use complete breast feeding as a help to revert to pre-pregnancy body weight levels. On the other hand, since environmental contaminants accumulate with time in adipose tissue, the fat stores of these older mothers might contain a higher concentration of such toxins and thus pose a larger risk for the infant.

Energy requirements for an entire pregnancy are about 80,000 kcal or about 300 calories per day, covering the needs for fetal growth and adipose tissue storage. Lactation has been assumed to facilitate weight loss, in particular if the period of lactation exceeds 2 months. Lactation has been calculated to increase the energy requirements by about 500 kcal/day, which also takes into account that production of milk is an energy-requiring process.

Studies by Rebuffé-Scrive and associates have demonstrated that the characteristics of the adipose tissue change dramatically during pregnancy (29). Adipose tissue lipolysis in the femoral region is limited during pregnancy, but can easily be stimulated hormonally during lactation. This seems to be a functional adaptation of the adipose tissue to the needs of the mother and the child.

However, the relationships between lactation, energy needs, and energy balance are not fully clarified. In some studies no difference in energy intake was found between lactating and nonlactating women. Other studies suggests that lactation plays a minor roll in weight reduction after delivery (18,30). In the Stockholm Pregnancy and Weight Development Study a minor role of lactation on body weight regulation was demonstrated (31,32).

From a theoretical point of view, weight changes after delivery could also depend on changes in basal metabolic rate. Prentice and Prentice (33) identify three hypothetical mechanisms that could explain the lack of weight loss after delivery:

1. Reduced basal metabolism
2. Impaired thermogenesis
3. Reduced physical activity

These mechanisms could account for reduction in energy requirements of up to about 240 calories per day. Thus it is possible that the energy need during lactation can be provided from different sources, such as a combination of an increased energy intake, utilization of adipose tissue in storage, and a metabolic adaptation.

These hypotheses were, however, not supported by a recent Dutch study. Spaaij et al. studied prospectively various aspect of energy metabolism in 27 women, who were monitored repeatedly before pregnancy, during each trimester, and during lactation (34–36). Three different aspects of such energy savings were analyzed: the possibility that the thermic effect of meal is reduced during pregnancy, the possibility that work efficiency improves during pregnancy, and the possibility that during lactation the metabolic efficiency is altered.

No changes were observed in any of these three factors, possibly explaining the discrepancy between energy intake and the energy costs of a pregnancy. Therefore, the Dutch group reassessed the extra energy needs during pregnancy and concluded that such extra needs may be met by an increase in energy intake but also by substantial behavioral adaptations. As an example, energy savings by reduced physical activity seem to be higher than earlier estimates. The large variations between subjects regarding both energy intake and energy expenditure led the Dutch group to suggest that energy intake recommendations for well-nourished pregnant women have little value. Since no metabolic adaptations seemed to appear, Spaaij et al. conclude that underestimation of the energy savings by reduced physical activity probably explains the imbalance between energy input and output.

In a similar design, a Swedish group has monitored energy expenditure of healthy women during pregnancy and lactation (37). In these studies, 23 healthy, normal-weight women were monitored before a planned pregnancy, and then immediately after delivery and 2 months and 6 months postpartum as regards body composition and energy metabolism. Only minor changes were found, with a slight increase in resting metabolic rate during lactation and a small energy intake increase during the lactation period of 280 ± 440 calories per day. In this group the main fat gain during pregnancy was 5.8 ± 4.2 kg, which was not lost during the first 2 months of lactation but disappeared partly between 2 and 6 months after delivery. These authors underscore the importance of methodological problems in estimating body composition and suggest that a lack of correlation between changes in body weight and body fat during early pregnancy might be explained by changes in the degree of hydration of the body. As regards physical activity, the Swedish study suggests that there was a tendency to increased physical activity during early pregnancy (38). The Swedish study supports previous work that lactation does not affect the metabolic efficiency but proposes that with methods that are extremely accurate it might still be possible to detect minor differences.

IV. THE STOCKHOLM PREGNANCY AND WEIGHT DEVELOPMENT STUDY

To further analyze the relationships between body weight, weight development, pregnancy, lactation, sociodemographic factors, and weight retention, the Stockholm Pregnancy and Weight Development Study was begun in the mid-1980s (31,32,39). The overall aim of the study was to monitor weight changes up to 1 year after delivery and to identify risk factors for sustained weight retention. The study design was both retrospective and prospective. Subjects represented a mixture of the southern Stockholm metropolitan area, Stockholm suburbs, and countryside. A total of 2342 women agreed to participate in this study. There were 47 exclusions for reasons such as twin pregnancy, insulin-dependent diabetes mellitus, severe nutritional problems, or lack of prepregnancy weight reports. Of the 2295 women who agreed to participate in the study at the maternity unit checkup, 872 dropped out during the following year. This corresponded to an overall dropout rate of 38%. A total of 1423 women completed the entire study. Detailed analyses failed to reveal that the salient results of the study could be explained by a selective dropout mechanism.

From the obstetric records and the questionnaires administered at follow-up, data were computed regarding: body weight, age, parity, nationality, occupation, living site, marital status, smoking habits, contraceptive practices, duration of lactation and lactation intensity, weight-losing practices, return to salaried work, eating, and exercise. The prepregnancy weight was accepted from the women's own reports. All ensuing weights were recorded in a standardized way in each of the 14 participating maternity clinics. Height was self-reported, and initial BMI calculated from the self-reported data.

The validity of the prepregnancy reported weight constitutes an important methodological problem. We compared the data with results obtained from a subgroup of 49 women, who were excluded from the 12-month follow-up because of a new pregnancy. This gave us an unforeseen opportunity to compare their reported weight with the weight that was recorded as the starting level for their next pregnancy. The reported mean weight was 0.92 kg lower at the onset of pregnancy than the latest recorded weight obtained under our study conditions. The mean weight loss between 6 and 12 months after delivery was calculated as 0.12 kg from data from the entire study. If

we subtract this weight from 0.92 kg, we can estimate that these women have reported an initial body weight at onset of the new pregnancy that was on average 0.8 kg lower than their true body weight.

These results fit reasonably well with studies of a group of Swedish women where true prepregnancy weight data could be obtained since these women were studied and weighed at a time when their intrauterine device was removed before a planned pregnancy (40).

A. Weight Development

In Figure 3 the overall body weight development in the 1423 women from conception to 12 months after delivery is summarized. The mean weight increase 1 year after delivery compared to the reported weight at the time of conception was 1.5 kg. When we corrected for the estimated underreporting of the weight at conception from our parallel studies (0.8 kg plus the estimated mean weight increase with time of 0.2 kg), the net mean weight increase induced by a pregnancy was calculated to be 0.5 kg. However, the range was very wide: 1.5% of the women had a mean weight increase of at least 10 kg and 13% had a weight increase between 5 and 10 kg. The majority (56%) had a weight increase of up to 5 kg. Of these women 30% lost weight. The weight change distribution 1 year after delivery is shown in Figure 4.

Women with more than 5 kg of weight retention differed from the other women in several respects. Whereas women with a small net increase in weight lost a mean of 2.3 kg between 2.5 and 12 months after delivery, women with larger weight retention increased 0.4 kg during the

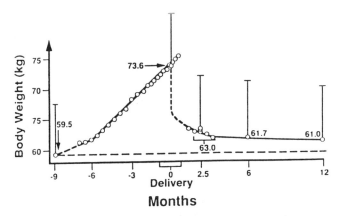

Figure 3 Body weight changes in 1423 Swedish women from conception until 12 months postpartum (kg ± SD). Dashed line shows mean prepregnancy weight. (From Ref. 31.)

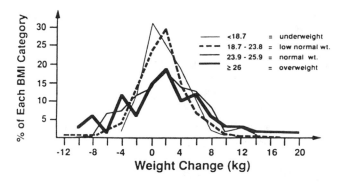

Figure 4 Distribution of weight changes from conception until 12 months postpartum in 1423 Swedish women with different prepregnancy BMI values. (From Ref. 31.)

same time period. Those who retained more weight had a larger initial body weight, increased more during pregnancy, were slightly less lactating, and stopped smoking during pregnancy to a larger extent. We also found a less well-structured eating pattern of dietary habits before, during, and after pregnancy (32). Those women who increased in body weight reported that their energy intake had increased after delivery, since they ate larger portions and snacked more frequently. They had less regular eating habits and did not eat breakfast and lunch as regularly as women who put on less weight. Age and parity did not differ between women who retained more than 5 kg and those who retained less.

B. Life-Style Trends

In the Stockholm study a number of different trend patterns were constructed to demonstrate to what extent various predetermined types of behaviors as regards life-style questions affected weight change. An example of one such trend pattern is shown in Figure 5 and illustrates various ways to adapt physical activity habits to pregnancy and the postpartum period. The analysis demonstrates that the most common pattern was a modest physical activity maintained throughout the entire 21-month period, followed by a group that was more active before pregnancy, slowed down during pregnancy, but resumed the previous high activity level after delivery. In general, higher overall physical activity was associated with less weight retention.

Factors explaining the net weight increase after pregnancy are summarized in Table 3. Weight increase during pregnancy was the most important factor explaining weight retention, and here the weight increase during the first trimester was the most important explanatory variable. Figure 6 demonstrates that the weight increase dur-

ing the first trimester is predictive of future overall weight increase. This could have preventive implications and suggests that life-style recommendations concerning optimal weight increase should start early during pregnancy. In the Stockholm study, weight retention increased only slightly with age and not with parity. Women who gave up smoking when they became pregnant increased more than others; 45% of these women retained more than 5 kg.

Interestingly, lactation played a small role in weight control after delivery. Although there was a significant relationship between the lactation score and weight retention, the r value was low ($r = 0.05$, $p < 0.01$) (Fig. 7). However, there was a difference with time, in that women with a high lactation score lost more weight during the first half year after delivery. Toward the end of the year, the differences between the groups were limited. Only in a small subset of subjects, who had been lactating for a whole year, a reduction of body weight compared to prepregnancy weight was found.

The slight importance of lactation for weight loss after delivery may seem surprising, but has been reported previously by Rookus et al. (18) and was also described by others, as cited in their review.

In clinical practice, women are often instructed to try to breast-feed as much as possible to revert to normal weight after delivery. This seems logical, since a full lactation requires about 500 calories per day, which may constitute about 20–25% of the daily energy requirement of women in this age group. However, it is possible that the changes in eating behavior and in life-style affect women in such a way that they only use their adipose tissue storage when food is not readily available, as has been suggested by Prentice and Prentice (33).

In the analyses of social factors affecting weight development after delivery, social class had little importance but women in suburban areas increased slightly more in weight. Questions regarding eating habits, physical activity, and life-style revealed that there was a tendency for women who retain more weight to develop a more sedentary and irregular life-style. This can, of course, be explained by the new social situation and the lack of opportunities to engage in outdoor activities, when the care of the newborn has became a first priority. Women who had received dietary guidance during pregnancy did not have a more favorable weight outcome than those who did not receive such support. It is likely that the weight retention after delivery can be better explained by changes in life-style associated with the arrival of a new family member than by metabolic, anthropometric, and social factors before pregnancy.

In summary, the metabolic cost of an entire pregnancy seems to be extremely flexible and is influenced by several

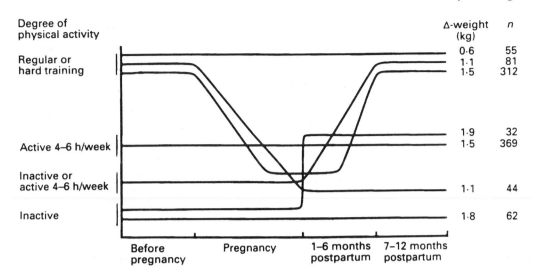

Figure 5 Different trend patterns in physical activity and effects on postpartum body weight development. (From Ref. 32.)

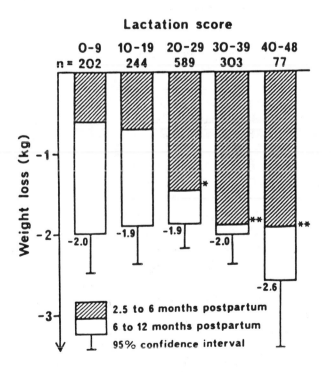

Figure 6 Stockholm Pregnancy and Weight Development Study. Weight loss in kg from 2.5 to 12 months postpartum in groups with different lactation scores. Statistically significant differences from score 0–9 and 10–19 shown as $*p < 0.05$ and $**p < 0.01$. (From Ref. 31.)

factors, such as maternal prepregnancy nutritional status, energy intake during pregnancy, fetal size, and a combination of these factors. Metabolic adaption may possibly occur to spare some energy for fetal growth, should this be insufficient.

C. Maternal Body Weight and Birth Weight

The definition of optimal weight gain during pregnancy remains controversial. The old saying is that a pregnant woman should "eat for two." On the other hand, in affluent societies where overweight is more of a problem than starvation, it is important that the dietary recommendations given do not expose pregnant vulnerable women to the risk of subsequently developing an excess of fat that they may later have great difficulty in losing. The safety of the newborn is one basic concern, and a low birth weight constitutes a well-known risk, but must be balanced against the adverse effects of overweight and obesity.

A linear relationship has been reported by some authors between birth weight and maternal pregnancy weight gain at all levels of pregnancy weight (41–43). Others suggest that as maternal weight increases, the infant's birth weight will increase proportionately less (44–47). As part of the data analyses of the Stockholm Pregnancy and Weight Development Study, the relation-

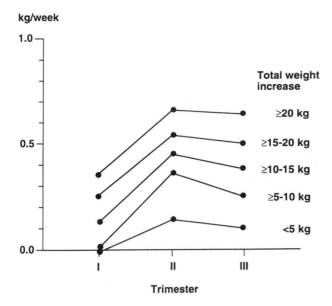

Figure 7 Trimester-related mean weight increase in women with different total weight increase. (From Öhlin A and Rössner S, Ref. 84.)

ships between initial maternal body weight, weight development during pregnancy, and birth weights were studied (48). The linear regression analyses gave the following overall r values for birth weight versus maternal body weight variables: birth weight − maternal initial BMI $r = 0.13$ ($p < 0.001$), birth weight − maternal initial weight (kg) $r = 0.20$ ($p < 0.001$), birth weight − (maternal weight gain − birth weight) (kg) $r = 0.18$ ($p < 0.001$), and birth weight − maternal weight retention at 12 months of follow-up, $r = 0.04$ (n.s.).

In women with initial BMI below 20.0 kg/m^2 there was a significant correlation between birth weight and BMI ($r = 0.12$, $p < 0.01$). In the BMI 20.0–23.9 kg/m^2 interval there was also a low but significant correlation between birth weight and BMI ($r = 0.08$, $p < 0.01$). In the two highest prepregnancy weight classes there were no significant BMI correlations with the corresponding mean birth weights ($r = 0.03$ and −0.02, respectively).

The birth weight increased significantly with maternal pregnancy weight gain minus birth weight in each group, as shown by analysis of variance, where children of mothers in the two groups with the highest net weight increase were significantly heavier than those of the two groups that increased <10 kg. However, in the three groups of women who had a net weight gain exceeding 10 kg, no further significant birth weight increase was found. For the total group the correlation between net maternal

weight gain and birth weight was $r = 0.17$ ($p < 0.001$). In a multiple regression analysis, factors explaining the birth weight were further detailed. Net weight increase (defined as maternal weight increase minus birth weight) explained only 3.0% of the variation in birth weight. When initial body weight was added, these two factors together explained 5.0% of the variation in birth weight. Numerous factors, such as paternal and maternal heredity, maternal prepregnancy weight, nutrition, and several hormonal factors, ultimately determine the infant's birth weight (49). The Stockholm study is confined to total maternal body weight, but it should be borne in mind that lean body mass rather than adipose tissue seems to be the important determinant of birth weight.

In this analysis a commonly used BMI range recommendation for normal body weight of 20–24 kg/m^2 for women was applied, and the overweight women were then divided into two groups. For lean and normal-weight women we found a correlation between the birth weight of the child and initial maternal body weight, but not for women above the upper normal BMI level. On the other hand, there was a consistent increase in birth weight with maternal net pregnancy weight gain. Our data support the concept that birth weight increases with maternal weight up to a certain level, and then levels off.

V. PREGNANCY, WEIGHT, AND SMOKING

Is is well known that smoking affects body weight. Generally, smoking increases the basal metabolic rate by about 10% (50). The weight development pattern in pregnancy is confounded by the fact that many smoking women give up this habit when they learn of their pregnancy. In this situation the weight gain thus is influenced by an additional factor apart from the growth of the fetus.

The relationship between smoking in general and body weight is well established, smokers being leaner (51,52). In pregnancy, early work showed that smoking mothers gained about 13% less per week than nonsmokers (53). In this study from Australia, "reformed smokers," who decided to quit when they learned of their pregnancy, had the highest weekly weight gain in the group. Our Stockholm data show similar results, both with a high pregnancy weight gain and with higher weight retention than in those who never smoked or who continued to smoke (31). However, these results are not in agreement with all other studies. For example, in the large Ontario Perinatal Mortality Study of 31,788 women smoking habits were unrelated to maternal weight gain distribution (54).

VI. OBESITY, WEIGHT GAIN, AND PREGNANCY COMPLICATIONS

Obesity is considered a risk factor in pregnancy but knowledge of the relationship of the degree of maternal obesity to risk for specific complications and pregnancy outcome remains unclear (55–59). Several methodological factors explain the lack of precise knowledge about these interrelationships, such as exact definitions of obesity and adequate control groups. In a study from Chile, a group of obese pregnant women were compared with a group matched for age and parity but with normal weight (60). Differences between the two groups were found with regard to gestational hypertension, inadequate pregnancy weight gain, cesarean section frequency, postpartum infections, and large-for-gestational-age infants, but no significant increase in the incidence of diabetes, toxemia, breech presentation, postpartum hemorrhage, infant morbidity, or lactational failure was noted in the obese women. The authors conclude that although obesity is an important risk factor, methodological aspects of previous studies may have magnified the severity of the problem.

This view is also supported by later studies. In a case-control study from California with a similar design, it was shown that massively obese pregnant women were significantly more likely to have a multitude of adverse effects (61). The frequency of cesarean section was doubled, and child malformation or growth retardation was much more prevalent. However, when obese women with diabetes and/or hypertension antedating pregnancy were excluded from the analyses, no statistically significant differences in perinatal outcome persisted. These authors thus conclude that although massively obese pregnant women are at high risk for adverse perinatal outcome, these risks are more closely related to preexisting morbid conditions than to obesity itself.

In the Stockholm study the overall frequency of cesarean sections was 12%. There was a tendency, although statistically nonsignificant ($\chi^2 = 2.62$, n.s.), toward a higher frequency of sections in mothers with higher initial BMI values. The mean initial BMI for vaginal deliveries was 21.46 versus 21.80 kg/m^2 for cesarean sections.

The design of the Stockholm Pregnancy and Weight Development Study, where for logistic reasons women were recruited after delivery, implies that women with pregnancies necessitating cesarean section may have been underrepresented, when these pregnancies resulted in the delivery of a newborn with complications. On the other hand, the frequency of cesarean sections in all women in this study is close to the available Swedish average figure of 12.4%, reported from the early 1980s. The reason for an increased need for cesarean sections in obese mothers is not clear (62). Our data suggest, however, that in the moderately obese women who were studied here, cesarean sections were not performed more often than in the women with normal body weights.

VII. DIABETES, OBESITY, AND PREGNANCY

Maternal obesity represents a significant risk factor for the development of gestational diabetes mellitus and subsequent adult-onset diabetes. Obesity in itself is associated with major alterations in carbohydrate metabolism such as insulin resistance and hyperinsulinemia, eventually developing into hyperglycemia (63). Not only is the degree of overweight important for the likelihood to develop diabetes, but body fat distribution is also significant, with upper body obesity being a more important risk factor than generalized increase in body fat (64). In a study of pregnant women with various types of fat distribution, repeated oral glucose tolerance tests were carried out during each trimester and postpartum (65). This study demonstrates that pathological carbohydrate metabolism became apparent in upper body obese women already during the second trimester and that a significant relationship between waist/hip ratio and glucose levels, as well as insulin areas, was found in late pregnancy in all obese subjects.

VIII. BODY FAT DISTRIBUTION AND CONCEPTION CAPACITY

Although obesity is common among multiparous women, it is possible that this weight increase is the result of multiple pregnancies rather than a prerequisite for conception. From ancient history the obese female has been considered a symbol of fertility. In some cultures it has even been believed that obese women are more likely to bear twins. Although it is well known that underweight women have an impaired capacity to conceive, the effects of overweight and obesity on female fecundity have been less studied. A shift of the hormonal balance toward increased androgenicity in association with abdominal obesity has been found to lead to menstrual disorders (5,66).

A. Weight and Infertility

Even a moderate degree of overweight may affect reproductive capacity significantly. In a case-control study of BMI and ovulatory infertility, 597 white infertile women with ovulatory dysfunction were compared with 1695 primiparous control women (67). The study demonstrated an increased risk for primary ovulatory infertility in women with a BMI of 27 kg/m² or greater. Above BMI 25 kg/m² the risk of ovulatory infertility had almost doubled.

Women admitted to an in vitro fertilization unit provide a unique opportunity to study determinants of fecundity while controlling for several other confounders related to the conception. In a Dutch study the probability of conception after insemination was studied in 500 women (68). The main reasons for artificial insemination were infertility or subfertility of the partner with azoospermia or oligospermia, respectively. The youngest woman was 20 years old; only a few women were above age 40. A total of 260 women reported regular smoking habits. As expected, the women were less likely to conceive at higher ages ($p < 0.05$). The study demonstrated that a 0.1-unit increase in waist-hip ratio was associated with a 30% decrease in probability of conception per cycle. These data were adjusted for age, overall fatness, clinical indication for insemination, cycle characteristics, smoking habits, and parity. The main finding of this study is that an increase in waist-hip ratio suggesting increased androgenicity was associated with a reduced fecundity. In obese women weight loss often normalizes the regular menstrual cycles as well as sex hormone concentrations (8,69). This indicates that obesity itself, rather than a primary endocrine dysfunction, is the cause of the reproductive insufficiency.

B. Diabetes, Weight, and Fertility

Non-insulin-dependent diabetes (NIDDM) is associated with obesity as well as with pregnancy. The association between parity and NIDDM has been studied in several populations where either no relationship or a positive association generally has been described. On the other hand, infertility has been associated with a high risk for NIDDM. The complex interrelationship between these factors has recently been studied among Pima Indian women (70). In a longitudinal epidemiological study of diabetes, the role of parity and obesity was analyzed after control for age. This study demonstrates that Pima women who have never been pregnant had a higher prevalence of NIDDM but also a higher BMI than women who had been pregnant. To a certain extent, this difference could thus be accounted for by a higher degree of obesity. One explanation put forward is the fact that obesity is associated with an increased conversion of androgens to estrogens in the adipose tissue (71). Thus high estrogen concentrations could explain the oligomenorrhea or amenorrhea and thus

the decreased fertility through a negative feedback mechanism at the hypothalamopituitary level.

The fact that there is no consistent relationship between parity and NIDDM may be due to a combination of two effects counteracting each other. On one hand, pregnancy may be diabetogenic by leading to an accelerated and sustained weight gain that could precipitate a clinically manifest form of NIDDM. On the other hand, it is possible that women of low fertility run a higher risk of developing NIDDM because of a common factor or several factors contributing to both conditions.

IX. SOCIOECONOMIC AND ETHNIC ASPECTS OF PREGNANCY-RELATED WEIGHT GAIN

Women with low education and low income are at increased risk of gaining weight and becoming overweight. Furthermore, there seem to be differences in race. Over a 10-year period the overall mean weight gain for black women was 36% higher than for white women (72). Parker and Abrams have analyzed the 1988 National Maternal and Infant Health Survey to study whether this additional increase in body weight among black women could be explained by factors relating to pregnancy (73). They found that black mothers were twice as likely to retain at least 20 lb as white mothers (adjusted odds ratio 2.20, 95% confidence interval 1.50–3.22), but that this black-white difference could not be explained by differences in socioeconomic status. There were other differences in the weight increase pattern. Weight retention was more likely to occur in white women who were unmarried whereas weight retention in black mothers was more often associated with high parity. These data suggest that it may be necessary to develop population-specific strategies in helping mothers return to their prepregnancy body weight.

X. WEIGHT DEVELOPMENT IN PREGNANT ADOLESCENTS

Since maternal weight gain is an important and manageable determinant of infant birth weight among adolescents, some studies have addressed factors related to weight gain in young women. Generally, the women studied have been poor and with numerous psychosocial problems including drug abuse. Stevens-Simon and McAnarney studied 141 pregnant black teenagers (74). The group was divided into three different weight gain subgroups. Slow weight gain was associated with a lower quality of food intake. Teenagers who gained more weight during their pregnancies were more compliant with prenatal visits but also reported more depressive symptoms and alcohol consumption. An important finding was the substantial variability in the amount of weight gain, ranging from 1.8 to 27.9 kg with a mean weight increase of 14.3 ± 6.0 kg (SD). This study suggests that proper nutritional care in this group of young women may be an effective method to promote optimal gestational weight gain.

Apart from the nutritional aspect of optimal weight gain for a successful pregnancy outcome, the attitudes of the young women may affect their weight development during pregnancy. In an analysis of 99 pregnant young women registered in a maternity program in Denver, Colorado, most were poor but an ethnic variability was noted (75). The authors had anticipated that negative attitudes toward pregnancy weight gain would be more common among these young women and that such attitudes would adversely affect an optimal adolescent maternal weight gain. These teenagers were studied by means of a weight gain attitude scale as well as several other determinants of nutritional status, dietary and health habits, and social history. Surprisingly, the authors demonstrated that these young women were not more concerned about staying slim than older pregnant adolescents and adults. Negative weight gain attitudes were more commonly found among heavy and depressed adolescents and those who did not have family support.

The examples of weight gain–related factors in adolescents given above relate to the problems in the United States. It is reasonable to believe that the situation will be quite different in other cultures, where, e.g., pregnancy early in the life of a young woman is considered a normal life event or in societies where the attitude toward abortion in pregnant teenagers is different. It is possible that for this special group of women appropriate food supplies may be one simple method to ensure optimal weight gain and good pregnancy outcome.

XI. WEIGHT GAIN DURING TWIN PREGNANCIES

Few data are available concerning the optimal weight development during twin gestation. A study by Pederson et al. (76) has addressed this question in a retrospective evaluation of the outcome of 217 twin pregnancies. The optimal outcome was associated with a mean weight gain of 20 kg. These authors were able to construct a weight gain curve for twin gestation, which was compared with the standard weight development curve for singleton pregnancies. During the first half of the pregnancy, curves for

singleton and twin pregnancies were similar, after which a more marked increase was seen in twin pregnancies during the second trimester and until term. It is still unknown whether multiple pregnancies require different nutritional needs, but until such data are available it seems practical to use weight gain as a proxy measure of the nutritional status of the mother and her twin fetuses.

XII. VARIA

Finally, a different approach to the subject of pregnancy and weight-related matters: Deeply entrenched in obstetric and midwifery folklore is the hypothesis that the weight of candy gifts is proportional to the birth weight. So far this hypothesis has never been scientifically tested. However, recently Nordin conducted a prospective study of postpartum candy gift net weight and its correlation with birth weight (77). Thirty-nine chocolate gifts were recorded during the study period at the Musgrove Park Hospital in Somerset, United Kingdom during a period when 1491 infants were delivered. The box candy net weights ranged from 200 to 1200 g, the birth weights from 2260 to 4926 g. However, the coefficient of correlation between candy and birth weights was only 0.15 ($p = 0.2$). The author assumes that socioeconomic and prematurity-related factors were responsible for the poor candy giving. Possibly parents of high-birth-weight infants are themselves overweight or obese and find it impossible to express their gratitude with a chocolate box of correspondingly significant proportions. It is also possible that the design of this study was flawed by the fact that rumors spread in the hospital that the same data would be used retrospectively to test the separate hypothesis that midwife waist measurement would be directly proportional to the net weight of the boxed candy. This was expected to result in severe underreporting.

REFERENCES

1. Kumar A, Mittal S, Buchshee K, Farooq A. Reproductive functions in obese women. Prog Food Nutr Sci 1993; 17: 89–98.
2. Siiteri PK, MacDonald PC. Role of extraglandular estrogen in human endocrinology. In: Green PO, Astwood E, eds. Handbook of Physiology, Vol 2. Washington, DC: American Physiological Society, 1973:615–629.
3. MacDonald PC, Edman CD, Hemsell DL, Porter JC, Siiteri PK. Effect of obesity on conversion of plasma androstenedione to estrone in postmenopausal women with and without endometrial cancer. Am J Obstet Gynecol 1978; 130: 448–455.

4. Loughlin T, Cunningham SK, Culliton M, Smyth PPA, Meagher DJ, Mckenna TJ. Altered androstenedione and estrone dynamics associated with abnormal hormonal profile in amenorrheic subjects with weight loss or obesity. Fertil Steril 1985; 43:720–725.

5. Rogers J, Mitchell GWJR. The relation of obesity to menstrual disturbances. N Engl J Med 1952; 257:53–55.

6. Kopelman PG, White N, Pilkington TRE, Jeffcoate SL. The effect of weight loss on sex steroid secretion and binding in massively obese women. Clin Endocrinol 1981; 14:113–116.

7. Glass AR, Dahms WT, Abraham G, Atkinson RL, Bray GA, Swerdloff RS. Secondary amenorrhea in obesity: etiologic role of weight related androgen excess. Fertil Steril 1978; 30:243–244.

8. Mitchell GW, Rogers J. The influence of weight reduction on amenorrhea in obese women. N Engl J Med 1953; 249:835–837.

9. Barbieri RL, Smith S, Ryan KJ. The role of hyperinsulinemia in the pathogenesis of ovarian hyperandrogenism. Fertil Steril 1988; 50:197–212.

10. Yen SS, Vela P, Rankin J. Inappropriate secretion of follicle-stimulating hormone and luteinizing hormone in polycystic ovarian disease. J Clin Endocrinol Metab 1970; 30:435–442.

11. Guzick DS, Wing R, Smith D, Berga SL, Winters SJ. Endocrine consequences of weight loss in obese, hyperandrogenic, anovulatory women. Fertil Steril 1994; 61:598–604.

12. Hamilton-Fairley D, Kiddy D, Watson H, Paterson C, Franks S. Association of moderate obesity with a poor pregnancy outcome in women with polycystic ovary syndrome treated with low dose gonadotrophin. Br J Obstet Gynaecol 1992; 99:128–131.

13. Rodin J, Radke-Sharpe N, Rebuffé-Scrive M, Greenwood MRC. Weight cycling and fat distribution. Int J Obes 1990; 14:303–310.

14. Lissner L, Odell R, D'Agostino R, et al. Health implications of weight cycling in the Framingham population. Am J Epidemiol 1988; 128:1180–1184.

15. Rössner S. Pregnancy, weight cycling and weight gain. Int J Obes 1992; 16:145–147.

16. Billewicz WZ, Thomson AM. Body weight in parous women. Br J Prev Soc Med 1970; 24:97–104.

17. Johnston EM. Weight changes during pregnancy and the postpartum period. Prog Food Nutr Sci 1991; 15:117–157.

18. Rookus MA, Rokebrand P, Burema J, Deurenberg P. The effect of pregnancy on the body mass index 9 months postpartum in 49 women. Int J Obes 1987; 11:609–618.

19. Heliövaara M, Aromaa A. Parity and obesity. J Epidemiol Commun Health 1981; 35:197–199.

20. Kuskowski-Wolk A, Rössner S. Prevalence of obesity in Sweden: Cross-sectional study of a representative adult sample. J Intern Med 1990; 227:241–246.

21. Hytten FE, Leitch I. The Physiology of Human Pregnancy. Oxford: Blackwell Scientific Publications, 1971.

22. Ash S, Fischer CC, Truswell AS, Allen JR, Irwing L. Maternal weight gain, smoking, and other factors in pregnancy as predictors of infant birth-weight in Sydney women. Aust NZ J Obstet Gynaecol 1989; 29:212–219.

23. Hjortland MC, McNamara, Kannel WB. Some atherogenic concomitants of menopause: the Framingham Study. Am J Epidemiol 1976; 103:304–311.

24. Lindquist O, Bengtsson C. Serum lipids, arterial blood pressure and body weight in relation to the menopause: results from a population study of women in Goteborg, Sweden. Scand J Clin Lab Invest 1980; 40:629–636.

25. Wing RR, Matthews KA, Kuller LH, Meilahn EN, Plantinga PL. Weight gain at the time of menopause. Arch Intern Med 1991; 151:97–102.

26. Kuller LH, Meilahn EN, Cauley JA, Gutai JP, Matthews KA. Epidemiologic studies of menopause: changes in risk factors and disease. Exp Gerontol 1994; 29:495–509.

27. Hamman RF, Bennett PH, Miller M. The effect of menopause on serum cholesterol in American (Pima) Indian women. Am J Epidemiol 1975; 102:164–169.

28. Hytten FE, Leitch I. The Physiology of Human Pregnancy. Oxford: Blackwell Scientific Publications, 1971.

29. Rebuffé-Scrive M, Enk L, Crona P, et al. Fat cell metabolism in different regions in women. Effects of menstrual cycle, pregnancy and lactation. J Clin Invest 1985; 75:1973–1976.

30. Illingworth PJ, Jung RT, Howie PW, Isles TE. Reduction in postprandial energy expenditure during lactation. Br Med J 1987; 294:1573–1576.

31. Öhlin A, Rössner S. Maternal weight development after pregnancy. Int J Obes 1990; 14:159–173.

32. Öhlin A, Rössner S. Trends in eating patterns, physical activity and sociodemographic factors in relation to postpartum body weight development. Br J Nutr 1994; 71:457–470.

33. Prentice AM, Prentice A. Energy costs of lactation. Ann Rev Nutr 1988; 8:63–79.

34. Spaaij CJK, van Raaij JMA, van der Heijden LJM, et al. No substantial reduction of the thermic effect of a meal in pregnancy in well-nourished Dutch women. Br J Nutr 1994; 71:335–344.

35. Spaaij CJK, van Raaij JMA, van der Heijden LJM, de Groot CPGM, Boekholt HA, Hautvast JGAJ. No changes during pregnancy in the net cost of cycling exercise. Eur J Clin Nutr 1994; 48:513–521.

36. Spaaij CJK, van Raaij JMA, de Groot CPGM, van der Heijden LJM, Boekholt HA, Hautvast JGAJ. Effect of lactation of resting metabolic rate and on diet- and work-induced thermogenesis. Am J Clin Nutr 1994; 59:42–47.

37. Forsum E, Sadurskis A, J. W. Estimation of body fat in healthy Swedish women during pregnancy and lactation. Am J Clin Nutr 1989; 50:465–473.

38. Forsum E, Kabir N, Sadurskis A, Westerterp K. Total energy expenditure of healthy Swedish women during pregnancy and lactation. Am J Clin Nutr 1992; 56:334–342.

39. Öhlin A. Pregnancy and overweight (in Swedish). Thesis, Karolinska Institute, Stockholm, 1991.

40. Sadurskis A, Kabir N, Wager J, Forsum E. Energy metabolism, body composition and milk production in healthy Swedish women during lactation. Am J Clin Nutr 1988; 48:44–49.

41. Harrison GG, Udall JN, Morrow G. Maternal obesity, weight gain in pregnancy, and infant birth weight. Am J Obstet Gynecol 1980; 136:411–412.

42. Gormican A, Valentine J, Satter E. Relationships of maternal weight gain, prepregnancy weight, and infant birth weight. J Am Diet Assoc 1980; 77:662–667.

43. Luke B, Dickinson C, Petrie RH. Intrauterine growth: Correlations of maternal nutritional status and rate of gestational weight gain. Eur J Obstet Gynecol Reprod Biol 1981; 12:113–121.

44. Eastman NJ, Jackson E. Weight relationships in pregnancy. Obstet Gynecol Surv 1968; 23:1003–1024.

45. Niswander KR, Singer J, Westphal M, Weiss W. Weight gain during pregnancy and prepregnancy weight gain. Obstet Gynecol 1969; 33:482–491.

46. Winikoff B, Debrovner CH. Anthropometric determinants of birth weight. Obstet Gynecol 1981; 58:678–684.

47. Abrams BF, Laros RK. Pregnancy weight, weight gain, and birth weight. Am J Obstet Gynecol 1986; 154:503–509.

48. Rössner S, Öhlin A. Maternal body weight and relation to birth weight. Acta Obstet Gynecol Scand 1990; 69: 475–478.

49. Langhoff-Roos J. Determinants of infant birth weight at term. Thesis, Uppsala University, 1987.

50. Rössner S. Cessation of cigarette smoking and body weight increase. Acta Med Scand 1986; 219:1–2.

51. Lincoln JE, Morris P. Weight gain after cessation of smoking. JAMA 1969; 210:1765.

52. Dallosso HM, James WPT. The role of smoking in the regulation of energy balance. Int J Obes 1984; 8:365–375.

53. Newnham JP, Patterson L, James I, Reid SE. Effects of maternal cigarette smoking on ultrasonic measurement of fetal growth and on Doppler flow velocity waveforms. Early Hum Dev 1990; 24:23–26.

54. Meyer MB. How does maternal smoking affect birth weight and maternal weight gain? Evidence from the Ontario Perinatal Mortality Study. Am J Obstet Gynecol 1978; 131: 888–893.

55. Gross T, Sokol RJ, King K. Obesity in pregnancy: risks and outcome. Obstet Gynecol 1980; 56:446–450.

56. Garbaciak JA Jr, Richter M, Miller S, Barton JJ. Maternal weight and pregnancy complications. Am J Obstet Gynecol 1985; 152:238–245.

57. Mitchell MC, Lerner E. A comparison of pregnancy outcome in overweight and normal weight women. J Am Coll Nutr 1989; 8:617–624.

58. Johnson SR, Kolberg BH, Warner MW, Railsback LD. Maternal obesity and pregnancy. Surg Gynecol Obstet 1987; 164:431–437.

59. Naeye RL. Maternal body weight and pregnancy outcome. Am J Cin Nutr 1990; 52:273–279.

60. Tilton Z, Hodgson MI, Donoso E, Arteaga A, Rosso P. Complications and outcome of pregnancy in obese women. Nutrition 1989; 5:95–99.

61. Perlow JH, Morgan MA, Montgomery D, Towers CV, Porto M. Perinatal outcome in pregnancy complicated by massive obesity. Am J Obstet Gynecol 1992; 167:958–962.

62. Gross TL. Operative considerations in the obese pregnant patient. Clin Perinatol 1983; 10:411–421.

63. Reaven GM. Role of insulin resistance in human disease [Banting Lecture 1988]. Diabetes 1988; 37:593–607.

64. Kissebah AH, Vydelingum N, Murray R. Relation of body fat distribution to metabolic complications of obesity. J Clin Endocrinol Metab 1982; 54:254–260.

65. Landon MB, Osei K, Platt M, O'Dorisio T, Samuels P, Gabbe SG. The differential effects of body fat distribution on insulin and glucose metabolism during pregnancy. Am J Obstet Gynecol 1994; 171:875–884.

66. Hartz AJ, Rupley DC, Rimm AA. The association of girth measurements with disease in 32856 women. Am J Epidemiol 1984; 119:71–80.

67. Grodstein F, Goldman MB, Cramer DW. Body mass index and ovulatory infertility. Epidemiology 1994; 5:247–250.

68. Zaadstra BM, Seidell JC, Van Noord PAH, et al. Fat and female fecundity: prospective study of effect of body fat distribution on conception rates. Br Med J 1993; 306: 484–487.

69. Grenman S, Ronnema T, Irisia K, Kaihola HL, Gross M. Sex steroid, gonadotrophin, cortisol and prolactin levels in healthy, massively obese women: correlation with abdominal fat cell size and effect of weight reduction. J Clin Endocrinol Metab 1986; 63:1257.

70. Charles MA, Pettitt DJ, MCance DR, Hanson RL, Bennett PH, Knowler WC. Gravidity, obesity and non-insulin-dependent diabetes among Pima Indian women. Am J Med 1994; 97:250–255.

71. Edman CD, MacDonald PC. Effect of obesity on conversion of plasma androstenedione to estrone in ovulatory and anovulatory young women. Am J Obstet Gynecol 1978; 130: 456–461.

72. Kahn HS, Williamson DF, Stevens JA. Race and weight change in US women: The roles of socioeconomic and marital status. Am J Public Health 1991; 81:319–323.

73. Parker JD, Abrams B. Differences in postpartum weight retention between black and white mothers. Obstet Gynecol 1993; 81:768–774.

74. Stevens-Simon C, McAnarney ER. Determinants of weight gain in pregnant adolescents. J Am Diet Assoc 1992; 92: 1348–1351.

75. Stevens-Simon C, Nakashima I, Andrews D. Weight gain attitudes among pregnant adolescents. J Adolesc Health 1993; 14:369–372.

76. Pederson AL, Worthington-Roberts B, Hickok DE. Weight gain patterns during twin gestation. J Am Diet Assoc 1989; 89:642–646.

77. Nordin AJ. A prospective study of postpartum candy gift net weight: correlation with birth weight. Obstet Gynecol 1993; 82:156–158.

78. McKeown T, Record RG. The influence of reproduction on body weight in women. J Endoncrinol 1957; 15:393–409.

79. Abitol MM. Weight gain in pregnancy. Am J Obstet Gynecol 1969; 104:140–157.

80. Garn SM, Shaw HA, McCabe KD. Effect of maternal smoking on weight and weight gain between pregnancies. Am J Clin Nutr 1978; 31:1302–1303.

81. Beazley JM, Swinhoe JR. Body weight in parous women: is there any alteration between successive pregnancies? Acta Obstet Gynecol Scand 1979; 5:45–47.

82. Newcombe RG. Development of obesity in parous women. J Epidemiol Commun Health 1982; 36:306–309.

83. Brown JE, Kaye SA, Folsom AR. Parity-related weight change in women. Int J Obes 1992; 16:627–631.

84. Rössner S, Öhlin A. Pregnancy as a Risk Factor for Obesity: Lessons from the Stockholm Pregnancy and Weight Development Study. Obesity Research. 1995; September. Vol 3. Suppl. 2. 267–275.

38

Weight Cycling

Definitions, Mechanisms, and Problems with Interpretation

Richard L. Atkinson
University of Wisconsin–Madison, Madison, Wisconsin

Judith S. Stern
University of California at Davis, Davis, California

I. INTRODUCTION

Few subjects in the field of obesity have generated as much publicity and controversy as the topic of weight cycling. Many articles in the lay press accept as dogma that weight cycling, "yoyo dieting," or repeated weight loss and regain is dangerous. Some authors writing in the popular press have suggested that it is healthier to remain obese than to risk the hazards of weight cycling (14,77). These sentiments have been advanced in scientific publications as well (28,102,103). A number of epidemiological studies suggest that weight loss or weight cycling is associated with a higher rate of morbidity and mortality (9,37,38,56,57,68). However, several recent critical reviews have concluded that the balance of studies suggest that there are minimal or no short-term adverse effects of weight cycling, and that there are potential alternate explanations for the negative health effects described in some epidemiological studies (74,100,104). This chapter will discuss definitions of weight cycling, potential mechanisms of harm, and problems with interpretation of the data in the context of a review of the relevant data from experimental animals and humans.

II. DEFINITIONS OF WEIGHT CYCLING

There is no single accepted definition of weight cycling, and the different methods of defining or assessing weight cycling have fueled the controversy in the literature. A valuable and comprehensive review, assembled primarily by Yanovski with assistance by members of the National Task Force on Prevention and Treatment (NIDDK, National Institutes of Health), deftly summarized definitions used as well as a large number of factors that might be considered in defining weight cycling (104). One factor is the *number of times* a person has lost and regained weight. As few as one cycle (89) or as many as four or more cycles have been used in different analyses (62,63). A second factor used to define weight cycling is *weight change*. This has been expressed as kilograms lost, as a percentage of initial body weight lost, or as intraindividual variability of body weight about the slope of weight over a period of years (4,8,9,37,43,44,55–66,71,72,76,79,82–84,88,93). A third factor to define weight cycling is the actual *amount of weight lost and regained* in one or more cycles. This figure varied from as little as 2.3 kg to as much as 10 kg or more (104). One study defined a cycle as regain of at least 30% of lost weight (89). A fourth factor, *the length of time over which a cycle occurred*, was used in some studies, but not in others. Periods between cycles varied from a few days in some of the weight-cycling wrestlers (83) to as long as 7 years in an outpatient obesity treatment program (8).

Yanovski et al. (104) raised a series of questions about the definition, characteristics, and outcomes of weight cycling that have not been satisfactorily answered. These questions and/or variables, plus others listed below, are critical when attempting to define a weight cycle. For most of these questions there is insufficient information to draw any conclusion at this time. Some of the important considerations are:

1. Is the magnitude of weight change in each cycle important?
2. Is a loss followed by a gain similar in effect to a gain followed by a loss?
3. Does the number of cycles matter?
4. Does the pattern of weight cycling make a difference? For example, are several small cycles more or less detrimental than one or two large cycles and is the rate of weight loss and regain important?
5. Does the duration of the cycle make a difference?
6. Does the time maintenance of weight loss affect the benefit?
7. What is the time frame of deleterious effects of weight cycling? Specifically, are there long-term effects not seen in the initial evaluations?
8. Does the initial body weight make a difference?
9. Are there subgroups for whom cycling is more dangerous than others? For example, are women more susceptible to the effects of weight cycling than are men?

III. POTENTIAL MECHANISMS OF HARM WITH WEIGHT CYCLING

For most of the time that life has been on Earth, there have been periods of insufficient quantities of food. These periodic famines certainly must have caused greater or lesser degrees of weight loss, followed by weight gain in times of plenty. It seems reasonable to conclude that evolution would have favored individuals who could withstand periodic famine with little or no adverse consequences on health or performance. Studies by Prentice et al. (71) of Gambians who annually experience periods of surfeit and famine show no apparent adverse consequences. However, it also seems reasonable to conclude that any such evolutionary trends would apply only to short-term adverse events. The average life expectancy during most of mankind's development was 40 years or less, and only in relatively recent times has a significant

percentage of humans survived into old age when longer-term adverse effects of earlier famines and weight cycling might present themselves.

Natural selection in primitive humans may have favored individuals who could withstand periods of famine and consequent weight cycling without detriment. It is possible that the situation is different in the 20th century in many industrialized societies where food is relatively plentiful and good tasting, and where most people do not have to expend a lot of energy to obtain food.

Many people eat a diet high in fat and refined carbohydrates and low in fiber, and are very inactive. In primitive humans the necessity for large amounts of physical activity, coupled with the primitive diet, which was low in fats and high in fiber, could have been protective against any potentially negative effects of weight cycling. The modern human life-style would not provide these protections against adverse effects of weight cycling.

Weight fluctuations occur often in both obese and lean humans (97,98). A number of harmful effects have been postulated to occur with weight cycling (Table 1). Even though several critical reviews have concluded that many of these harmful effects do not appear to occur (74, 100,104), we cannot dismiss concerns about the dangers of weight cycling. As noted in questions 8 and 9 above, there may be subgroups for whom weight cycling is dangerous, while other subgroups would suffer no ill effects. Also, there may be long-term effects for which no studies have been designed or completed. Thus, while the consensus may be that weight cycling is not dangerous for the short term, our present state of knowledge is sufficiently incomplete that we cannot draw definitive conclusions about either short- or long-term consequences, and more research is needed.

Table 1 Postulated Harmful Effects of Weight Cycling[a]

1. Rebound weight gain leading to obesity
2. Reduced effectiveness of subsequent weight loss efforts
3. Changes in energy metabolism
4. Changes in body composition
5. Increases in visceral adipose depots
6. Alterations in food intake and food preferences
7. Increased risk of insulin resistance, hyperinsulinemia, and/or diabetes
8. Increase in risk factors for cardiovascular disease
9. Adverse psychological effects (e.g., depression, anxiety)
10. Onset of binge eating or other eating disorders
11. Increased frequency of alcohol and drug abuse

[a]Although the adverse effects of weight cycling have been postulated here, almost all have been demonstrated not to occur.

Alterations in food intake and dietary preferences including increased calorie intake during weight regain and an increased preference for dietary fat have been described in some studies in both humans and experimental animals (26). There is evidence that good-tasting foods are preferred after deprivation (49–51). Early studies by Brownell et al. (15), suggested that weight cycling may increase food efficiency.

These alterations in food intake, food preferences, and food efficiency were postulated to lead to increasing body weight and changes in body composition, including an increased percent body fat and altered fat distribution reflecting a shift to increased visceral fat. Obesity, and particularly increased visceral fat, is a risk factor for a number of chronic diseases including hypertension, diabetes, hyperlipoproteinemia, cardiac disease, cerebrovascular disease, some cancers, and even death (6,7,30,36,48,61, 67,70). Increasing obesity, particularly visceral obesity, has been advanced as one explanation for the results of epidemiological studies that show a correlation of weight loss or weight cycling with cardiac disease and overall mortality (9,37,38,56,58,68).

Finally, repeated weight loss and regain has been postulated to lead to adverse psychological events. Specifically, there is concern that weight cycling leads to binge eating, bulimia, and perhaps anorexia nervosa. Since the classic studies by Keys et al. (47) on starvation in healthy young men, it has been known that significant weight loss followed by regain may alter patterns of dietary intake and may produce episodes of binge eating. Krahn et al. (49–51) noted that binge eating and other eating disorders are associated with the presence and severity of dieting and weight loss efforts in college age women. Rats and monkeys that are food-deprived self-administer increased amounts of drugs and alcohol (49–51) compared to ad libitum–fed animals. These drugs include cocaine, heroin, amphetamine, pentobarbital, and nicotine (51). In the semistarvation studies of Keys et al. (47), chronically food-deprived young men markedly increased consumption of the two drugs available to them, nicotine and caffeine. Women who were not alcohol abusers at the beginning of their freshman year in college had a greater chance of becoming abusers of alcohol if they were dieters as compared to nondieters (49). Krahn et al. (49–51) postulate that deprivation alters the neurochemistry of the brain, perhaps in the nucleus acumbens, and leads not only to an increased tendency to binge eating, but to the increased potential for abuse of alcohol and drugs (49).

IV. PROBLEMS WITH DATA INTERPRETATION

Before reviewing the experimental animal and human literature, it is useful to consider the problems of interpretation of the data. As noted above, definitions of weight cycling have not been standardized, and caution must be taken when comparing results from different studies. In a review of studies using experimental animals, Reed and Hill (74) defined weight cycling as "one or more cycles of weight loss (produced by fasting or food restriction) followed by weight regain." They differentiated "weight cycling" from "diet cycling," which was defined as "altering diet composition (usually from a high to a low fat diet and back)." Changes in diet composition can alter body weight and body composition (10,11). This is a critical point because many of the studies of "weight cycling" also involve alterations not only of calorie intake, but of the percentages of fat and carbohydrate (CHO) in the diet. Conclusions may not be drawn about the effects of weight cycling without appropriate control groups (74,104). However, there is some concern about eliminating experimental animal studies that combine weight and diet cycling. In humans, weight loss programs often combine energy and fat restriction, whereas weight regain may be accompanied by increased energy, fat, and simple sugar intake.

The tendency to regain above baseline weight after a bout of weight loss is a highly negative experience and has fostered the belief among the lay public that weight cycling "causes" obesity. In studies with experimental animals, body weight may be steadily higher after each weight cycle. However, many people and experimental animals experience a steady weight gain during adulthood. Bray has noted that after an episode of weight loss, body weight rises to the level that would have been predicted by the slope of the curve of long-term weight gain (13). Wadden et al. (93) provide an excellent graph demonstrating this phenomenon in 50 women over a period of about 25 years. This steadily increasing body weight and body fatness must be factored into the interpretation of studies of weight cycling, and without appropriate control groups, this phenomenon cannot be taken as evidence for an adverse effect of weight cycling.

Changes in body composition in experimental animals and humans after weight cycling must be interpreted with caution. Some studies have shown that during and immediately after weight regain, body composition may be altered, with an increased fat mass compared to baseline (18,74,76). This phenomenon may be short term, and body composition returns to baseline within a short period after weight regain. Similarly, a preference for dietary fat may be a temporary phenomenon. These cautions and explanations do not address the problem of continuous or frequent brief intervals of dietary restriction on diet preference and body composition. The studies of Krahn et al. (49–51) suggest that women who repeatedly diet may weigh more and be more likely to have eating disorders and abuse alcohol and drugs.

Lissner et al. (56) describe four cautions that must be considered when interpreting epidemiological studies, many of which suggest that weight loss and/or weight cycling is associated with an increase in morbidity and mortality (9,37,38,56,58,68). The first is the absence of data on volitional weight loss. Numerous epidemiological studies and studies of longevity in experimental animals have shown that unintentional weight loss is an ominous sign. Disease as diverse as cancer, infection including tuberculosis, gastrointestinal diseases, and depression, all of which cause weight loss, are associated with a significantly increased mortality rate. Most studies have not been designed to assess whether subjects are trying to lose weight, and in the few in which any information has been obtained, the methodology has been very simplistic. Even if intent to lose weight is documented, the very poor long-term success rate of voluntary weight loss (1,93) should promote caution in interpretation of the data. Individuals who report that they successfully lose weight may have an underlying illness that is responsible.

Second, an individual who successfully loses weight may have a personal or family history of risk factors that provides a higher degree of motivation than the general population. Risk factors such as hypertension, hyperlipidemia, diabetes, or family history of early death may overwhelm the beneficial effects of the modest weight loss achieved by most people.

Third, there may be subgroups in the population of a given study that confound the data. For example, in the MRFIT study (9), the negative consequences of weight loss were seen only in smokers. Since smokers often try to quit smoking, and this often leads to weight gain, there may be repeated cycles of weight loss and regain, but the negative long-term health outcomes may be related to the smoking behavior. Other potential factors that distinguish subgroups who may be at greater or lesser risk from weight cycling than the general population include age, sex, presence of other underlying medical conditions, and genetic factors that influence metabolism or disease risk.

The final interpretation of the epidemiological studies advanced by Lissner et al. (56) is that weight cycling might actually cause long-term negative health outcomes. The consensus of critical reviews (74,100,101,104) suggests that this is incorrect, but all who have addressed this issue recommend caution and additional research.

V.   REVIEW OF THE LITERATURE: EXPERIMENTAL ANIMAL STUDIES

The study of Brownell et al. (15) showing that rats had an increased food efficiency after several bouts of weight cycling provided much of the impetus for the hypothesis that weight cycling adversely affects health. Brownell et al. (15) postulated that the clinical observations of rapid weight regain, difficulty with subsequent weight loss efforts, and the tendency to gain beyond the starting weight might be explained by changes in metabolism due to weight cycling. Reed and Hill (74) critically reviewed the experimental animal literature to address these questions. The authors noted that weight cycling had not been adequately defined and discussed many of the points noted above.

Reed and Hill (74) noted that three studies suggested that weight cycling has an effect on subsequent body weight and ability to lose weight in subsequent cycles (2,15,32). Two of these studies lacked a maturity control group (15,32). The third study was confounded because the cycle was defined differently and was produced by feeding a different diet (2). Mice were fed a high-CHO diet, which caused weight gain. Then they were food-restricted. The weight gain before food restriction was compared to the "catch-up" weight gain after food restriction. It was concluded that weight cycling produced the same amount of weight gain in a shorter period. This set of comparisons may not be analogous to the usual form of weight cycling.

A number of studies have not found any independent effect of weight cycling on weight loss or regain (24,35,73). Reed et al. (73) found an increase in body weight with three weight cycles, but a maturity control group did not differ, showing the importance of such control groups. Desautels and Dulos (24) found no effects of cycled versus noncycled mice in 14 weight cycles.

Some studies show that during the regain phase of weight cycling, rats increase their preference for dietary fat when given access to three dishes containing fat, CHO, or protein (35,74,75). Reed et al. (75) found that rats ate about 43–48% of kcal as fat, whereas Gerardo-Gettens et al. (32) noted increases to as high as 74%. Both weight cyclers and diet cyclers increased consumption of dietary kcal as fat, showing that weight cycling was not required to produce an increased fat preference (75). In rats that previously had been weight-cycled, Graham et al. (34) did not find an increased preference for dietary fat.

Enhanced food efficiency with progressive weight cycles was found in three studies (2,15,22) that did not use a maturity control group. Two studies that used a maturity control group (35,73) and several other studies (19,20,

75,87) found no overall increased food efficiency. Graham et al. (34) followed rats for 50 days after the last of three weight cycles and found no difference in food efficiency in cycled versus control rats.

Weight cycling has been postulated to decrease energy expenditure. Indirect calorimetry is the best measure of energy expenditure, but the usual equations on which energy expenditure is calculated assume a steady state. Therefore, measurements cannot be easily interpreted during the weight loss phase or the weight regain phase of a weight cycle because the animals are not in a stable situation with respect to weight. Three studies that measured energy expenditure in an indirect calorimeter have not confirmed the hypothesis that weight cycling alters energy expenditure (24,32,34). Gerardo-Gettens et al. (32) measured resting metabolic rate (RMR) for a 3-hr period at the end of the refeeding phase and found no differences between cycled rats and controls. Desautels and Dulos (24) also measured short periods of oxygen consumption in mice after 14 weight cycles. In contrast to the above hypothesis on weight cycling, the cycled rats had an *increased* oxygen consumption compared to controls. It is possible the difference was due to increased activity levels or to other errors of short-term measurements of energy expenditure. Finally, Graham et al. (34) measured 24-hr energy expenditure in weight-cycled versus control rats, but only long after weight regain at the last cycle. The weight-cycled rats had a lower total energy expenditure, but similar expenditures adjusted for lean body mass.

If weight cycling were to increase food efficiency and decrease energy expenditure, it is reasonable to assume that there would be changes in body composition, that is, increased body fat and obesity. Increased obesity after weight cycling has been postulated, but the majority of the studies that evaluated the effects of weight and/or fat gain after weight cycling concluded that there is no increase in obesity with weight cycling (5,18,34,39,40,96). Hill et al. (34,39,40,96) evaluated this question in several experiments and could not find any differences in body weight or body composition in cycled rats. Turk (87), Hill et al. (39,40,96), and Szepesi and Epstein (86) performed multiple cycles of restriction and refeeding on rats and found no differences in body weight or body composition with one, two, four, or eight cycles as compared to control or to a lower number of weight cycles. In some of the studies that found a difference in body fat, total body fat was not measured, and only specific depots were measured (21,22,28). These studies also had inappropriate control groups, with differences in diet composition during refeeding. Two studies evaluated visceral fat depots in

weight-cycled rats and found no increase with weight cycling (34,75). In several of the studies in which rats were weight-cycled, the final amounts of adipose tissue in the body were *less* in the cycled rats than in the controls (34,73).

An increased mortality from cardiovascular disease with weight cycling should be preceded by an increase in the risk factors associated with heart disease, including increased insulin resistance, hyperinsulinemia, hyperlipidemia, and hypertension. The majority of studies suggest that weight cycling does not increase risk factors in experimental animals. Several investigators have found no difference in fasting insulin levels between weight-cycled animals and controls (15,19–22). Reed et al. (75) found increased insulin levels in both weight-cycled and diet-cycled rats, but this presumably was a diet effect. Lu et al. (59) found that three cycles of weight loss and regain increased insulin levels and insulin resistance. Ernsberger and Nelson (27) noted that weight-cycled rats had a higher systolic blood pressure than controls, but this was not confirmed by Contreras et al. (21,22) or by Lu et al. (59).

In summarizing the experimental animal data, there is little support for an adverse effect of weight cycling. Specifically, there appears to be minimal or no increase in body weight, body fat, dietary preferences, or energy expenditure, and minimal change in cardiovascular risk factors in weight-cycled animals versus controls.

VI. REVIEW OF THE LITERATURE: HUMAN STUDIES

Similar to the situation in the experimental animal literature, there is little evidence in the human literature that weight cycling actually causes the potentially harmful effects listed in Table 1. Two excellent reviews of the literature have concluded that few or no short-term adverse effects may be attributed to weight cycling. While reassuring, the studies available do not exclude the possibility that some subgroups may suffer adverse health consequences from weight cycling. For example, weight cycling could have different consequences in obese versus lean individuals. The reviews of this topic are focused on metabolic consequences of weight cycling (100,104), and only modest attention has been paid to psychological and/or neuropsychiatric consequences. Finally, prospective long-term studies on weight cycling are lacking. This section will review the evidence for each of the potentially harmful effects of weight cycling in the human literature.

A. Effects of Prior Weight Cycling on Subsequent Weight Loss

Several studies in humans show that obese humans who have undertaken a weight loss program and regained their lost weight are not as successful with subsequent weight loss efforts (104). Blackburn et al. (8) reported that patients who repeated a very-low-calorie diet (VLCD) did not lose as much weight the second time. There was a highly variable period between the first and second episode of dieting, and changes associated with aging may have contributed to the results. In addition, patients may not have adhered to the diet as carefully during the second VLCD. However, 14 subjects were studied as inpatients on VLCD, and despite similar caloric restriction, weight losses were less during the second period. Other studies have not confirmed these observations (4,46,65,88,93). For many of these studies (45,46,82) weight loss was less in subsequent episodes of VLCD, but this would be expected as compliance was not as good. The poorer weight loss in some of these studies was due in major part to the fact that patients dropped out of the programs earlier in the second or subsequent treatment periods than they did in the first. Beeson et al. (4) studied four patients on a formula diet with a markedly restricted calorie intake and found weight losses were similar with two episodes of dieting. Wadden et al. (93) studied 50 patients and correlated self-reports of previous weight loss by dieting from one to 11 times. There was no correlation of weight loss in prior weight loss programs with the weight loss on a VLCD over 12 weeks in their study. Most of these studies have elements of study design that limit the conclusions that may be drawn. The studies of Smith and Wing (82), van Dale and Saris (88), and Wadden et al. (93) relied on retrospective recall of prior weight loss efforts. It is likely that most patients can reliably recall the amounts of weight lost on prior programs (93), but there is no way to verify such reports, and actual measurements would be preferable. The studies of Kaplan et al. (46) and of Kamrath et al. (45) had measurements of prior weight loss, but both report poorer adherence to the dietary regimen on subsequent weight loss efforts. Also, not all of the patients in each study had returned to baseline weight. Smith and Wing (82) had a similar problem of starting at different baseline weights. Even if subjects were selected from patients who had regained all of their starting weight, the problem of increased body weight with aging would confound the conclusions to some degree. In summary, there are sufficient problems with study design, sample size, and differences in adherence that it is not possible to conclude with certainty that weight cycling makes subsequent weight loss more difficult, but most studies suggest that this is not so.

B. Rebound Weight Gain Leading to Obesity

Weight regain to a level above baseline weight after a period of weight loss has been noted commonly in experimental animals and humans. There are two potential explanations for this phenomenon. As noted above, some animals and humans gain weight each year in a regular pattern. If this gain is interrupted by a period of weight reduction, body weight rises above baseline to the "programmed" weight, giving the appearance that the weight loss contributed to the excessive weight gain. The second possibility is that weight cycling changes the level at which body weight is regulated and there is a negative effect of weight cycling.

There is no evidence that weight cycling leads to excessive weight regain and obesity in humans because the appropriate controlled studies have not been done. Wadden et al. (93) demonstrate a steadily increasing body weight over a 25-year period punctuated by weight loss efforts in 50 women, but they do not have a control for aging noncycling women. Prentice et al. (71) report more than 20,000 body weight observations over 10 years in a population of rural Gambian women, with a dramatic fluctuation in weight each year due to the annual famine. Body weight returns to almost exactly the same level each year.

C. Changes in Energy Metabolism

One mechanism by which body weight or body fat might increase due to weight cycling is that energy metabolism may become more efficient with cycling. Leibel et al. (54) demonstrated that in both lean and obese subjects, weight loss resulted in a decrease in energy expenditure per kilogram of lean body mass and weight gain resulted in an increase in energy expenditure per kilogram of lean body mass. Changes in energy expenditure were greater during the process of weight loss or weight gain, but were also present at stable weight after the perturbations. Return to initial weight after weight gain resulted in a return to initial energy expenditure, but the authors did not report the results in subjects who had lost weight and then regained to the initial level. These data suggest that body weight is regulated and that attempts at alteration of weight by dietary means produce chronic changes in metabolic rate. However, this study does not answer the question of whether such changes in energy expenditure are persistent in people who lose weight and then regain it.

Studies by Steen et al. (83) and by Manore et al. (60) suggested that weight cycling enhanced energy efficiency, but the majority of the studies that have studied humans after weight cycling demonstrate no evidence for enhanced efficiency (43,55,62–66,71,78,79,88,93). Steen et al. (83) studied wrestlers who dieted frequently to reduce their weight to a lower competitive category. Wrestlers who weight-cycled had a lower metabolic rate than those who did not. Several other studies also looked at weight-cycling wrestlers and did not confirm these observations (62–66,79). Manore et al. (60) reported a lower metabolic rate per kilogram of body mass during exercise in weight cyclers versus noncyclers, but the weight-cycling subjects were heavier and fatter. Since adipose tissue is less metabolically active than lean tissue, fatter subjects will have a lower energy expenditure compared to leaner subjects if the data are expressed as per kilogram of body mass. This method of expressing the results severely limits the conclusions that may be drawn from the study of Manore et al. (60). In contrast to this paper, van Dale and Saris (88) assessed resting metabolic rate (RMR) and maximal aerobic power (VO_2 max) in 23 women who were divided into groups based on a history of weight cycling. From a previous study (23), a fourth group of dieting subjects with a history of weight cycling was used for comparison. These authors concluded that there were no effects of previous history of weight cycling on RMR or on VO_2 max.

Two papers, by Jebb et al. (43) and Prentice et al. (71), compare the changes in metabolic rate in a group of 11 moderately obese young women who underwent three cycles of VLCD for 2 weeks each, with a 4-week ad libitum period between each episode of dieting. Weight loss was successively less with each cycle, but the subjects did not regain to initial weight with any of the ad libitum feeding periods and were still about 6 kg below baseline weight at the end of the last refeeding cycle. Basal metabolic rate dropped with weight loss, but there were no differences in energy expenditure expressed per kilogram of lean body mass or in absolute energy expenditure.

Lissner et al (55) evaluated data from 846 men in the Baltimore Longitudinal Study on Aging and did not find any reduction in metabolic rate with fluctuation in body weight. Indeed, individuals with the greatest fluctuations in body weight had the smallest decreases in metabolic rate with aging. As noted above, fluctuation in weight as a measure of weight cycling is subject to problems of interpretation. However, the findings of this study go in the opposite direction to that expected if weight cycling were reducing metabolic rate.

D. Changes in Body Composition and Visceral Adipose Depots

There has been concern that weight cycling produces changes in body composition. Even if body weight did not change following weight cycling, a change in body composition toward a higher percentage of fat or a greater amount of fat in visceral depots might increase the risk of morbidity and mortality. Increased visceral fat is a known risk factor for hypertension, diabetes, hyperlipoproteinemia, cardiac disease, cerebrovascular disease, some cancers, and death (6,7,25,30,48,70). The possibility of increased visceral fat deposition after weight cycling, with or without weight gain, is of great concern.

The studies of Keys et al. (47) suggested that following an episode of severe dieting, during which subjects lost about 25% of initial body weight, weight regain during ad libitum feeding consisted of a higher proportion of fat than lean body mass. With the exception of the study by Manore et al. (60), no studies have shown an increase in body fat with weight cycling (43,55,62–66,88–90,93). For several studies, there was a negative correlation of weight cycling and increase in body fat. In other words, body fat of weight cyclers either was less or increased at a slower rate than in the noncycling individuals (44, 55,62–64,70).

There are fewer data on the possibility that weight cycling increases the proportion of upper body obesity. Rodin et al. (76) evaluated 87 premenopausal women and noted a correlation of weight cycling with waist-hip ratio (WHR). Also, there was a significant association of WHR with body mass index (BMI) only in subjects defined as weight cyclers. However, the patient population in this study was somewhat unusual, as there was no correlation of BMI with age and no correlation of age and WHR. The mean BMI was 22.7 and only about 10% of patients had a WHR greater than 0.80. The measure of weight cycling was an index computed by factoring the number of prior episodes of weight loss and the median of the range of weight loss on a grid. Since the subjects on average were of normal weight, they would likely not have lost a great deal of weight in a weight cycle. It is likely that anyone with a high score might not be representative of the general population of women. In their analysis of this study, Yanovski et al. (104) pointed out that it was surprising that WHR was not correlated with BMI in noncyclers and speculated that this might be due to a twofold increase in variance of BMI in the weight cyclers. Thus, the expected correlation was more likely to be apparent in cyclers than in the noncyclers, in whom the range of BMI was more narrow. Wadden et al. (93) and van Dale and Saris (88) assessed WHR in subjects who reported a history of weight cycling, but found no increase as compared to noncyclers.

Lissner et al. (55) noted tht body weight variability, a somewhat problematic surrogate for weight cycling as noted above, correlated with an increased ratio of subscapular to triceps skinfold thickness. Since truncal obesity versus extremity obesity has a higher correlation with morbidity and mortality, this might suggest increased upper body obesity in a higher-risk pattern. However, there was no increase in WHR, suggesting that there was deposition on both upper and lower body.

Perhaps the most elegant study was that of van der Kooy et al. (90,91), who evaluated visceral and subcutaneous adipose tissue deposition using magnetic resonance imaging (MRI) in a series of 32 subjects. The subjects had an MRI at baseline, after weight loss that averaged 12.9 kg, and 67 weeks later when the subjects had gained about 90% of their lost weight. The weight regain did not result in increased body fatness or in increased deposition of visceral fat. In fact, there was a decrease in total body fat of 1.5 kg, a decrease in visceral fat area of 10 cm^2 120 $\pm$ 41 vs. 110 $\pm$ 48 cm^2), and a slight tendency to reaccumulate subcutaneous fat at the expense of visceral fat. A potential confounding factor in the analysis of these data is that the subjects did not regain all of the weight that they had lost.

Taken together, these studies do not suggest that weight cycling increases visceral fat stores or results in an increased body fat.

E. Alterations in Food Intake and Food Preferences

As noted above, the success rate of weight loss efforts after a previous period of weight loss and regain is lower than initial attempts. This is due in many cases to a poorer compliance with the dietary regimen and, by definition, a higher calorie intake on subsequent weight loss efforts. There have been no studies that have tried to analyze whether calorie intake is higher during the weight regain phase in two or more cycles of weight loss and regain. The major reason for this lack of data is that patients drop out of the program and are lost to follow-up. Likewise, there are few data on the changes in dietary preferences during refeeding, at least in obese patients. Jeffrey et al. (4) divided 202 obese men and women into quartiles of frequency of weight cycling and evaluated dietary preference with food frequency questionnaires. There were no differences in preference for dietary fat among the four quartiles, suggesting that preference for dietary fat does not increase with weight cycling as shown in some experimental animal studies. However, these data were all

self-reported rather than measured and the times from last weight loss and/or regain were not standardized. Since preference for dietary fat is said to be temporary, it is possible that similar preferences in humans were missed due to the variable times after dieting.

Drewnowski and Holden-Wiltse (26) evaluated preferences for sweet and fat solutions and found that obese subjects with a history of weight cycling preferred higher concentrations of both sugar and fat. Since diary products with differing amounts of fat and sugar were used in these studies, the relationship to other foods is not clear.

Krahn (51) assessed food intakes in female college freshman and noted that individuals who reported frequent dieting tended to eat higher-fat foods when given access to test meals. Although it is likely that many of these individuals may have been weight cyclers, other variables, such as differences in body weight among subject groups, may have contributed to the findings.

In summary, there are insufficient data to draw conclusions about changes in taste preferences after weight cycling.

F. Increase in Risk Factors, Morbidity, and Mortality

Epidemiological studies suggest that weight loss and/or weight cycling is associated with an increase in morbidity and mortality (9,37,38,56,58,68). However, as noted above, it is difficult to interpret most of the papers that have reported on the effects of weight cycling on morbidity and mortality because they are not prospective or were not designed to evaluate the effects of weight cycling. The most bothersome reports come from several epidemiological studies that suggest that weight loss or fluctuations in body weight increase cardiovascular events such as myocardial infarctions and thereby increase mortality.

Lissner et al. (56) analyzed data from 1462 women and 855 men in the Gothenberg Prospective Studies and noted that men had a positive association of cardiovascular disease and mortality with weight fluctuation. In women, mortality was significantly correlated with weight fluctuation. The women's study was one of the few that actually attempted to study eating behavior, and adherence to weight loss diets was documented. This study found an association of dieting history and fluctuation in weight, as expected. However, a history of voluntary dieting did not predict mortality. Finally, association does not prove causality. It is possible that repeated weight loss associated with insufficient intake of one or more nutrients may place the subject at increased risk. For example, the process of weight loss results in calcium loss from the body. There is evidence that high calcium intake is associated with a reduced risk of hypertension and a lower all-cause mortality (17).

The Western Electric Study by Hamm et al. (37) evaluated 2107 men aged 40–56 years and requested they recall their weights at 5-year intervals from ages 20 to 40. These investigators found a positive correlation of self-reported weight fluctuation, defined as a 10% loss or a 10% gain, with cardiovascular mortality, but the increase in all-cause mortality was not significant.

A total of 5127 inhabitants of Framingham, Massachusetts were weighed every 2 years starting in 1948, when subjects were 30–62 years of age (58). Subjects were followed for 32 years and mortality from heart disease, cancer, and total mortality were correlated with fluctuations in weight. To eliminate the possibility that preexisting illness was responsible for the findings, the endpoints were assessed only if they occurred more than 4 years after the last body weight measurement. The analyses were adjusted to eliminate a number of confounding variables, including smoking status, serum cholesterol, systolic blood pressure, glucose tolerance, level of physical activity, age, mean BMI, annual change in BMI, and coefficient of variation about the mean BMI. The authors found that cardiovascular and all-cause mortality were increased in subjects with the greatest weight fluctuations. Men had increased total and cardiovascular mortality and women had increased cardiovascular mortality. These associations held true even when the data were adjusted for obesity, and the authors concluded that the risks of obesity did not necessarily outweigh the risks of weight cycling.

In an accompanying editorial to this article, Bouchard (12) pointed out that this study had considerable strength, but there are a number of limitations. Age at entry was quite variable. Body weight increases with age, predominantly through addition of adipose tissue, and a disproportionate amount of this adipose tissue is deposited in the visceral depots. Since visceral obesity is a major predictor of long-term mortality, it could have been a confounding factor that may have contributed to the apparent outcome, but was not measured.

The Multiple Risk Factor Intervention Trial (MRFIT) evaluated the effects of multiple interventions on cardiac and all-cause mortality in a randomized study design in 12,866 men aged 35–57 years who were at high risk for coronary vascular disease (9). Half of the subjects underwent training in diet and exercise techniques, and the other half received standard care. Blair et al. (9) analyzed the data and showed a positive correlation of weight fluctuation with cardiovascular disease and with all-cause mortality. However, these correlations were significant only in smokers. Smokers usually have weight fluctuations with attempts at ceasing smoking or, conversely, starting again. The results on cardiovascular disease and all-cause mortality are confounded by the correlation of weight fluctuations and episodes of smoking cessation. In addition, leaner individuals had the most negative outcomes of weight fluctuation, giving further credence to the hypothesis that smoking and its consequences may have played a role in the results.

Although the above studies suggested that weight fluctuations were associated with a higher risk of cardiovascular and/or all-cause mortality, other epidemiological studies have come to different conclusions. The Zutphen Study, Baltimore Longitudinal Aging Study, and Charleston Heart Study are smaller epidemiological studies that found no increased risks of weight fluctuation (56,57,84). The Zutphen Study is a population-based prospective study in 40–59-year-old Dutch men with 100% follow-up 25 years later (41,57). Residual fluctuation in BMI was used as the measure of weight cycling and there was no correlation after adjustment for smoking and age. The Baltimore Study, also a prospective study, followed 846 males, aged 20–92 years at baseline, every 12–24 months (58). Weight cycling was defined as the intraindividual variability in body weight about a time-dependent regression slope as compared to calculation of variability about an individual's mean. The Charleston Heart Study, another prospective study, examined 2182 individuals in Charleston County, South Carolina, of whom about one-third were black (84). Subjects were weighed at baseline in 1960 and again in 1963–1964 and 1973–1974. Outcomes of over 95% of the subjects were known in 1986. Body weight variability was calculated as the coefficient of variation of body weights over three points in time.

Several studies have shown that weight loss, not necessarily associated with weight cycling, is associated with increased mortality (38,53,68). Although controlled for smoking and corrected for preexisting illness by excluding early observation periods, these studies are perhaps most flawed by not being designed to evaluate intentionality of weight loss. A more recent study by Williamson et al. (99), in which limited information was obtained on the voluntary nature of weight loss, came to the opposite conclusion: weight loss in obese patients was protective if the weight loss was intentional. Unintentional weight loss was an ominous sign that carried a very poor prognosis. In this paper, as well as in studies of Pamuk et al. (68) and of Blair et al. (9), initial body weight was an important factor determining risk. Leaner individuals who lost weight had a poorer prognosis than those who were obese. Conversely, obese individuals benefited more from weight loss than did lean people.

There is no substitute for prospective trials that evaluate long-term hard outcomes of weight fluctuation such as mortality or disease-specific morbidity. However, such trials are difficult to carry out and it would take years to obtain results. Some clues to the potential results may be gleaned from trials that have evaluated the risk factors associated with morbidity and mortality. The overwhelming majority of studies suggest that weight cycling does not increase the major risk factors and complications of obesity that are associated with morbidity and mortality, including hypertension (44,55,65,66,72,83), glucose intolerance and insulin resistance (44,62–64,72,80), and hyperlipidemia (44,57,66,72,104). In contrast, there is no doubt that weight loss reduces risk factors associated with long-term morbidity and mortality, and in some studies, improvements in these risk factors persist even if weight is regained.

The report by Lissner et al. (55) is an exception because it found glucose intolerance to be increased with increases in the variability of body weight. However, this was a modest effect. Each kilogram of weight deviation about the slope was associated with a 1 mg/dl increase in serum glucose. This is about half of the effect noted with weight gain across time. Also, Holbrook et al. (42) noted an increased risk for diabetes in older adults with weight gain or weight fluctuations. They did not note any increased risk due to dieting. In contrast to these studies, Jeffrey et al. (44) evaluated 202 subjects with a spectrum of weight-cycling episodes in the past and found that weight cycling was associated with a decrease in blood glucose. These authors noted that of 88 associations examined, only seven showed correlations with weight cycling and six of the seven suggested that weight cycling was not harmful.

Some perspective should be included on patients who have major obesity. These patients have a high incidence of the complications and risk factors noted above (36, 61,69,70). Also, they often attempt to lose weight and thus may be at risk of weight cycling, since the long-term success rate of diet, exercise, and behavior modification is poor (1,92). Even modest weight loss has been shown to be beneficial (33). Recent advances in obesity surgery and obesity drugs suggest that if these obese patients are able to lose weight and maintain their loss, they enjoy significant long-term improvements in risk factors and even in specific diseases. Sugerman et al. (85) reported disappearance of sleep apnea and dramatic improvements in pulmonary function in massively obese patients who lose large amounts of weight and keep it off. The Swedish Obesity Study (SOS) is a large-scale, prospective comparison of medical and surgical treatments in massively obese patients ranging in age from 37 to 59 years (81). Preliminary data show that over a 2-year period, standard medical treatments do not result in a significant decrease in body weight (−0.6 kg). In contrast, surgery produced significant weight loss (−38 kg) that persisted for at least 2 years. Also, there was a dramatic decrease in the appearance of non-insulin-dependent diabetes mellitus (NIDDM) in the surgical group (0.5%) as compared to the medical group (7.8%) over 2 years of follow-up (81).

Weintraub et al. (94,95) administered phentermine and fenfluramine to patients for up to 3.5 years and noted persistent weight loss as long as drugs were given, although the magnitude of weight loss was much less than reported above with obesity surgery. Elevated serum lipids continued to be lowered at 210 weeks of drug treatment (95). These results have been confirmed in preliminary studies by Atkinson et al. (3), who found that at 1 year on drugs, blood pressure and blood lipids were markedly improved.

It appears that treatment approaches that are continuously effective reduce cardiovascular risk factors. Presumably risk reduction will result in reductions in long-term morbidity and mortality, but more research is needed to confirm this hypothesis. Such studies should be built into large-scale, long-term, prospective studies, such as the Women's Health Initiative.

G. Adverse Psychological Effects

Brownell and Rodin (16) and Yanovski et al. (104) reviewed the studies of effects of weight cycling on psychological factors and found that few studies are available and little evidence exists that weight cycling has major effects on psychological status (29,52). Brownell and Rodin (16) cited in press or unpublished data suggesting that individuals with a history of weight cycling showed significantly greater pathological findings than those with stable weights, independent of body weight. Also, weight cycling was associated with lower levels of life satisfaction in females, but not males. It is difficult to attribute causation in cross-sectional studies because the increase in weight cycling, psychopathology, and decreased life satisfaction may be concomitants of an underlying disorder.

Krahn et al. (49–51) evaluated female college freshmen and reported several disturbing findings. The prevalence of eating disorders increased with the prevalence of dieting efforts. Of more concern, there was a correlation of eating disorders and abuse of drugs and alcohol. Of most concern was the finding that in women who at baseline were not alcohol abusers, but had an eating disorder or strict dieting, the frequency of alcohol abuse increased significantly over the freshman year. Coupled with the findings in experimental animals that food deprivation leads to increased intake of alcohol and drugs such as cocaine, heroin, and amphetamine (51), these findings suggest that clinicians should take a careful history of dieting and weight-cycling efforts, especially from female patients. Patients who admit to strict dieting or to eating disorders should be carefully questioned about possible alcohol and drug abuse, and such patients should be followed carefully across time with their weight loss efforts to intervene early if signs or symptoms of alcohol or drug abuse appear.

VII. CONCLUSIONS

The bulk of the evidence suggests that weight cycling is well tolerated by humans and that there are few or no short-term adverse consequences, including changes in body weight, body composition, body fat distribution, energy metabolism, and cardiovascular risk factors. This perhaps should be expected since the evolutionary pressures of frequent famines would select for individuals who could tolerate wide swings in food intake without impairment. There is less assurance that long-term adverse consequences of weight cycling do not occur, since there are few or no long-term prospective studies that address the question and epidemiological studies may not be suitable to answer the question. The life-style of Western civilization represents a significant change from that of primitive mankind. Our diets are higher in fat and simple carbohydrates, lower in dietary fiber, and our daily activity is markedly lower. Also, there may be subgroups for whom weight cycling is dangerous. However, to put the problem into perspective, the long-term risks of continued obesity are so great that it is likely that any increased risk of single or repeated weight loss attempts would be lost on a population basis if adequate treatments of obesity existed. The studies of obesity surgery and long-term use of antiobesity drugs in subjects with medically significant obesity suggest that risk factors and even disease are markedly reduced. These findings apply to obese people, but the picture is less clear for lean individuals. Several studies show decreases in morbidity or mortality only for the obese. Conversely, weight loss in lean individuals does not appear to improve prognosis and may be associated with long-term adverse outcomes. The current mania for thinness, especially on the part of the female population, may be counterproductive. There is some evidence that strict dieting may lead to an increased prevalence of eating disorders in a small percentage of individuals and perhaps to substance abuse. Clinicians should make every effort to educate patients on the concepts of "healthy weights" even if these weights are above the "socially acceptable" levels. A paradigm shift in public perception may be needed to reorient society as to appropriate standards for body weight.

ACKNOWLEDGMENTS

We thank Virginia Schmidt for secretarial assistance and manuscript typing. This study was supported with funds from the Beers-Murphy Clinical Nutrition Center at the University of Wisconsin, Madison.

REFERENCES

1. Andersen T, Stokholm KH, Backer OG, Quaade F. Long term (5 year) results after either horizontal gastroplasty or very-low-calorie diet for morbid obesity. Int J Obes 1988; 12:277–284.
2. Archambault CM, Czyzewski D, Cordua y Cruz GD, Foreyt JP, Marlotto MJ. Effects of weight cycling in female rats. Physiol Behav 1989; 46:417–421.
3. Atkinson RL, Blank RC, Loper JF, Schumacher D, Lutes RA. Combined drug treatment of obesity. Obes Res 1995; 3(Suppl 4):497S–500S.
4. Beeson V, Ray C, Coxon RA, Kreitzman S. The myth of the yo-yo: consistent rate of weight loss with successive dieting by VLCD. Int J Obes 1989; 13(Suppl 2):135–139.
5. Bell RR, McGill TJ. Body composition in mice maintained with cyclic periods of food restriction and refeeding. Nutr Res 1987; 7:173–182.
6. Björntorp P. Abdominal fat distribution and disease: an overview of epidemiological data. Ann Med 1992; 24: 15–18.
7. Björntorp P. The associations between obesity, adipose tissue distribution and disease. Acta Med Scand 1988; (Suppl 723):121–134.
8. Blackburn GL, Wilson GT, Kanders BS, et al. Weight cycling: the experience of human dieters. Am J Clin Nutr 1989; 49:1105–1109.
9. Blair SN, Shaten J, Brownell K, Collins G, Lissner L. Body weight change, all-cause mortality, and cause-specific mortality in the Multiple Risk Factor Intervention Trial. Ann Intern Med 1993; 119:749–757.
10. Boozer CN, Atkinson RL. Dietary fat and adiposity: a dose-response relationship in adult rats fed isocalorically. Am J Physiol 1995; 268:E546–550.
11. Boozer CN, Brasseur A, Elhady AH, Atkinson RL. High fat diet promotes retention of body fat and increased LPL during food restriction. Am J Clin Nutr 1993; 58: 846–852.
12. Bouchard C. Is weight fluctuation a risk factor? N Engl J Med 1991; 324:1887–1889.
13. Bray GA. The Obese Patient. Philadelphia: WB Saunders, 1976.
14. Brody JE. For most trying to lose weight, dieting only makes things worse. New York Times, November 23, 1992; A1.
15. Brownell KD, Greenwood MRC, Stellar E, Shrager EE. The effects of repeated cycles of weight loss and regain in rats. Physiol Behav 1986; 38:459–464.

16. Brownell KD, Rodin J. Medical, metabolic and psychological effects on weight cycling. Arch Intern Med 1994; 154: 1325–1330.

17. Browner WS, Seeley DG, Vogt TM, Cummings SR. Non-trauma mortality in elderly women with low bone mineral density. Study of Osteoporosis Fractures Research Group. Lancet 1991; 338:355–358.

18. Chen Z, Cunnane SC. Weight cycling does affect body composition. Am J Clin Nutr 1993; 58:242.

19. Cleary MP. Consequences of restricted feeding/refeeding cycles in lean and obese female Zucker rats. J Nutr 1986; 116:290–303.

20. Cleary MP. Response of adult lean and obese female Zucker rats to intermittent food restriction/refeeding. J Nutr 1986; 116:1489–1499.

21. Contreras RJ, King S, Rives L, Williams A, Wattleton T. Dietary obesity and weight cycling in rats: a model of stress-induced hypertension? Am J Physiol 1991; 262: R848–R857.

22. Contreras RJ, Williams A. High fat/sucrose feeding attenuates the hypertension of spontaneously hypertensive rats. Physiol Behav 1989; 46:285–291.

23. Van Dale D, Saris WHM, Schoffelen PFM, Ten Hoor F. Does exercise give an additional effect in weight reduction regimens? Int J Obes 1987; 11:367–375.

24. Desautels M, Dulos RA. Effects of repeated cycles of fasting-refeeding on brown adipose tissue composition in mice. Am J Physiol 1988; 255:E120–E128.

25. Despres JP. Abdominal obesity and the risk of coronary artery disease. Can J Cardiol 1992; 8(6):561–562.

26. Drewnowski A, Holden-Wiltse J. Taste responses and food preferences in obese women: effects of weight cycling. Int J Obes 1992; 16:639–648.

27. Ernsberger P, Nelson DO. Refeeding hypertension in dietary obesity. Am J Physiol 1988; 254:R47–R55.

28. Ernsberger P, Koletsky RJ. Weight cycling and mortality: support from animal studies. JAMA 1993; 269:116.

29. Foreyt JP, Brunner RL, Goodrick GK, Cutter G, Brownell KD, St Jeor ST. Psychological correlates of weight fluctuation. Int J Eating Disord 1995; 17:263–275.

30. Fujimoto WY, Newell-Morris LL, Grote M, Bergstrom RW, Shuman WP. Visceral fat obesity and morbidity: NIDDM and atherogenic risk in Japanese American men and women. Int J Obes 1991; 15(Suppl 2):41–44.

31. Garner DM, Wooley SC. Confronting the failure of behavioral and dietary treatments for obesity. Clin Psychol Rev 1991; 11:729–780.

32. Gerado-Gettens T, Miller GD, Horwitz BA, McDonald RB, Brownell KD, Greenwood MRC, Rodin J, Stern JS. Exercise decreases fat selection in female rats during weight cycling. Am J Physiol 1991; 260:R518–524.

33. Goldstein DJ. Beneficial health effects of modest weight loss. Int J Obes 1992; 16:379–415.

34. Graham B, Chang S, Yakubu F, Lin D, Peters JC, Hill JO. Effect of weight cycling on susceptibility to dietary obesity. Am J Physiol 1990; 259:R1103–R1110.

35. Gray DS, Fisler JS, Bray GA. Effects of repeated weight loss and regain on body composition in obese rats. Am J Clin Nutr 1988; 47:393–399.

36. Grundy SM, Barnett JP. Metabolic and health complications of obesity. Dis Mon 199-; 36(12):641–731.

37. Hamm P, Shekelle RB, Stamler J. Large fluctuations in body weight during young adulthood and twenty-five year risk of coronary death in men. Am J Epidemiol 1989; 129:312–318.

38. Higgins M, D'Agostino R, Kannel W, Cobb J. Benefits and adverse effects of weight loss: observations from the Framingham Study. Ann Intern Med 1993; 119:758–763.

39. Hill JO, Thacker S, Newby D, Nickel M, DiGirolamo M. A comparison of constant feeding with bouts of fasting-refeeding at three levels of nutrition in the rat. Int J Obes 1987; 11:201–212.

40. Hill JO, Newby D, Thacker S, Sykes MN, DiGirolamo M. Influence of food restriction coupled with weight cycling on carcass energy restoration during ad libitum refeeding. Int J Obes 1988; 12:547–555.

41. Hoffmans MDAF, Kromhout D. Changes in body mass index in relation to myocardial infarction incidence and mortality. Int J Obes 1989; 13:25.

42. Holbrook TL, Barrett-Connor E, Wingard DL. The association of lifetime weight and weight control patterns with diabetes among men and women in an adult community. Int J Obes 1989; 13:723–729.

43. Jebb SA, Goldberg GR, Coward WA, Murgatroyd PR, Prentice AM. Effects of weight cycling caused by intermittent dieting on metabolic rate and body composition in obese women. Int J Obes 1991; 15:367–374.

44. Jeffrey RW, Wing RR, French SA. Weight cycling and cardiovascular risk factors in obese men and women. Am J Clin Nutr 1992; 5:641–644.

45. Kamrath RO, Diner RG, Plummer LJ, Sadur CN, Weinstein RL. Repeated use of the very-low-calorie diet in a structured multidisciplinary weight-management program Am J Clin Nutr 1992; 56:288S–289S.

46. Kaplan GD, Miller KC, Anderson JW. Comparative weight loss in obese patients restarting a supplemented very-low-calorie diet. Am J Clin Nutr 1992; 56:290S–291S.

47. Keys A, Brozek J, Henschel A, et al. The Biology of Human Starvation, Vol 1 and 2. Minneapolis: University of Minnesota Press, 1950.

48. Kissebah AH, Vydelingum N, Murray R, Evans DJ, Hartz AJ, Kalkoff RK, Adams PW. Relation of body fat distribution to metabolic complications of obesity. J Clin Endocrinol Metab 1982; 54:254–260.

49. Krahn DD, Gosnell B, Kurth C. Dieting and alcohol use in women. Drug Alcohol Abuse Rev 1994; 5:177–192.

50. Krahn DD, Kurth C, Demitrack M, Drewnowski A. The relationship of dieting severity and bulimic behaviors to alcohol and other drug use in women. J Substance Abuse 1992; 4:341–353.

51. Krahn DD. The relationship of eating disorders and substance abuse. J Substance Abuse 1991; 3:239–253.

52. Kuehnel RH, Wadden TA. Binge eating disorder, weight cycling, and psychopathology Int J Eating Disord 1994; 15:321–329.

53. Lee IM, Paffenbarger RS. Changes in body weight and longevity. JAMA 1992; 268:2045–2049.

54. Leibel RL, Rosenbaum M, Hirsch J. Changes in energy expenditure resulting from altered body weight. N Engl J Med 1995; 332:621–628.

55. Lissner L, Andres R, Muller DC, Shimokata H. Body weight variability in men: metabolic rate, health and longevity. Int J Obes 1990; 14:373–383.

56. Lissner L, Bengtsson C, Lapidus L, Larsson B, Bengtsson B, Brownell K. Body weight variability and mortality in the Gothenberg Prospective Studies of men and women. In: Björntorp P, Rossner S, eds. Obesity in Europe 88: Proceedings of the First European Congress on Obesity. London: John Libbey, 1989:55–60.

57. Lissner L. Brownell KD. Weight cycling, mortality, and cardiovascular disease: a review of epidemiologic findings. In: Björntorp P, Brodoff BN, eds. Obesity. Philadelphia: JB Lippincott, 1992:653–661.

58. Lissner L, Odell PM, D'Agostino RB, et al. Variability of body weight and health outcomes in the Framingham population. N Engl J Med 1991; 324:1839–1844.

59. Lu H, Buison A, Uhley V, Jen KLC. Long-term weight cycling in female Wistar rats: effects on metabolism. Obes Res 1995; 3:521–530.

60. Manore MM, Berry TE, Skinner JS, Carroll SS. Energy expenditure at rest and during exercise in nonobese female cyclical dieters and in nondieting control subjects. Am J Clin Nutr 1991; 54:41–46.

61. Manson JE, Colditz GA, Stampfer MJ, et al. A prospective study of obesity and risk of coronary heart disease in women. N Engl J Med 1990; 322:882–889.

62. McCargar L, Taunton J, Birmingham CL, Pare S, Simmons D. Metabolic and anthropometric changes in female weight cyclers and controls over a one year period. J Am Dietet Assoc 1993; 93:1025–1030.

63. McCargar LJ, Crawford SM. Metabolic and anthropometric changes with weight cycling in wrestlers. Med Sci Sports Exerc 1992; 24:1270–1275.

64. McCargar LJ, Simmons D, Craton N, Tauton JE, Birmingham CL. Physiological effects of weight cycling in female lightweight rowers. Can J Appl Physiol 1993; 18: 291–303.

65. Melby CL, Syliaasen S, Rhodes T. Diet-induced weight loss and metabolic changes in obese women with high versus low prior weight loss/regain. Nutr Res 1991; 11: 971–978.

66. Melby CL, Schmidt WD, Corrigan D. Resting metabolic rate in weight-cycling collegiate wrestlers compared with physically active noncycling control subjects. Am J Clin Nutr 1990; 52:409–414.

67. Must A, Jacques PF, Dallal GE, Bajema CJ, Dietz WH. Long-term morbidity and mortality of overweight adolescents: a follow-up of the Harvard growth study of 1922–1935. N Engl J Med 1992; 327:1350–1355.

68. Pamuk ER, Williamson DF, Serdula MK, Madans J, Byers TE. Weight loss and subsequent death in a cohort of US adults. Ann Intern Med 1993; 119:744–748.

69. Phinney SD. Weight cycling and cardiovascular risk in obese men and women. Am J Clin Nutr 1992; 56:781.

70. Pi-Sunyer FX. Health implications of obesity. Am J Clin Nutr 1991; 53:1595S–1603S.

71. Prentice AM, Jebb SA, Goldberg GR, Coward WA, Murgatroyd PR, Poppitt SD, Cole TJ. Effects of weight cycling on body composition. Am J Clin Nutr 1992; 56: 209S–216S.

72. Rebuffe-Scrive M, Hendler R, Bracero N, Cummings N, McCarthy S, Rodin J. Biobehavioral effects of weight cycling. Int J Obes 1994; 18:651–658.

73. Reed GW, Cox G, Yakubu F, Ding L, Hill JO. Effects of weight cycling in rats allowed a choice of diet. Am J Physiol 1993; 264:R35–R40.

74. Reed GW, Hill JO. Weight cycling: a critical review of the animal literature. Obes Res 1993; 1:392–402.

75. Reed DR, Contreras RJ, Maggio C, Greenwood MRC, Rodin J. Weight cycling in female rats increases dietary fat selection and adiposity. Physiol Behav 1988; 42:389–395.

76. Rodin J, Radke-Sharpe N, Rebuffe-Scrive M, Greenwood MRC. Weight cycling and fat distribution. Int J Obes 1990; 14:303–310.

77. Rovney S. Yo-yo dieting: worse than being overweight. Washington Post, December 13, 1988; health section:16.

78. Saris WHM. Physiological aspects of exercise in weight cycling. Am J Clin Nutr 1989; 49:1099–1104.

79. Schmidt WD, Corrigan D, Melby CL. Two seasons of weight-cycling does not lower resting metabolic rate in college wrestlers. Med Sci Sports Exerc 1993; 25: 613–619.

80. Schotte DE, Cohen E, Singh SP. Effects of weight cycling on metabolic control in male outpatients with non-insulin dependent diabetes mellitus. Health Psychol 1990; 9: 599–605.

81. Sjostrom CD, Hakangard AC, Lissner L, Sjostrom L. 1994. Relationships between cardiovascular risk factors and visceral and subcutaneous adipose tissue distribution. Int J Obes 1994; 18(Suppl 2):15.

82. Smith DE, Wing RR. Diminished weight loss and behavioral compliance during repeated diets. Health Psychol 1991; 10:378–383.

83. Steen SN, Oppliger RA, Brownell KD. Metabolic effects of repeated weight loss and regain in adolescent wrestlers. JAMA 1988; 260:47–50.

84. Stevens J, Lissner L. Body weight variability and mortality in the Charleston Heart Study. Int J Obes 1990; 14: 385–386.

85. Sugerman HJ, Fairman RP, Baron PL, Qwentus JA. Gastric surgery for respiratory insufficiency of obesity. Chest 1986; 90:81–86.

86. Szepesi B, Epstein MG. Effect of repeated food restriction-refeeding on growth rate and weight. Am J Clin Nutr 1977; 30:1692–1702.

87. Turk DE. Effect of cyclic fasting on young adult rats. Nutr Rep Intern 1988; 37:165–172.

88. Van Dale D, Saris WHM. Repetitive weight loss and weight regain: effects on weight reduction, resting metabolic rate, and lipolytic activity before and after exercise and/or diet treatment. Am J Clin Nutr 1989; 49: 409–416.

89. Van der Kooy K, Leenen R, Seidell J, Deurenberg P, Hautvast JG. Effect of a weight cycle on visceral fat accumulation. Am J Clin Nutr 1993; 58:853–857.

90. Van der Kooy K, Leenen R, Seidell JC, Deurenberg P, Visser M. Abdominal diameters as indicators of visceral fat: comparison between magnetic resonance imaging and anthropometry. Br J Nutr 1993; 70:47–58.

91. Van der Kooy K, Leenen R, Seidell JC, Deurenberg P, Droop A, Bakker CJG. Waist-hip ratio is a poor predictor of changes in visceral fat. Am J Clin Nutr 1993; 57: 327–333.

92. Wadden TA, Sternberg JA, Letizia KA, Stunkard AJ, Foster GD. Treatment of obesity by very low calorie diet, behavior therapy, and their combination: a five year perspective. Int J Obes 1989; 13(Suppl 2):39–46.

93. Wadden TA, Bartlett S, Letizia KA, Foster GD, Stunkard AJ. Relationship of dieting history to resting metabolic rate, body composition, eating behavior, and subsequent weight loss. Am J Clin Nutr 1992; 56:203–208.

94. Weintraub M, Sundaresan PR, Schuster B. Long-term weight control study VII (weeks 0 to 210): serum lipid changes. Clin Pharmacol Ther 1992; 51:634–641.

95. Weintraub M. Long term weight control: the National Heart, Lung, and Blood Institute funded multimodal intervention study. Clin Pharmacol Ther 1992; 51:581–646.

96. Wheeler J, Martin R, Yakubu F, Lin D, Hill JO. Weight cycling in female rats subjected to varying meal patterns. Am J Physiol 1990; 258:R124–R139.

97. Williamson PS, Levy BT. Long-term body weight fluctuation in an overweight population. Int J Obes 1988; 12: 579–583.

98. Williamson DF, Serdula MK, Anda RF, Levy A, Byers T. Weight loss attempts in adults: goals, duration, and rate of weight loss. Am J Public Health 1992; 82:1251–1257.

99. Williamson DF, Pamuk E, Thun M, Flanders D, Byers T, Heath C. Prospective study of intentional weight loss and mortality in never-smoking overweight US white women aged 40–64 years. Am J Epidemiol 1995; 141: 1128–1141.

100. Wing RR. Weight cycling in humans: a review of the literature. Ann Behav Med 1992; 14:113–119.

101. Wing RR, Jeffrey RW, Hellerstedt WL. A prospective study of effects of weight cycling on cardiovascular risk factors. Arch Intern Med 1995; 155:1416–1422.

102. Wooley SC, Wooley OW. Should obesity be treated at all? In: Stunkard AJ, Stellar E, eds. Eating and Its Disorders. New York: Raven Press, 1984:185–192.

103. Wooley SC, Garner DM. Obesity treatment: the high cost of false hope. J Am Dietet Assoc 1991; 91:1248–1251.

104. Yanovski SZ, Atkinson RL, Dietz WH, et al., National Task Force on the Prevention and Treatment of Obesity. Weight cycling. JAMA 1994; 272:1196–1202.

39

Weight Loss and Risk of Mortality

Steven N. Blair
The Cooper Institute for Aerobic Research, Dallas, Texas

I-Min Lee
Brigham and Women's Hospital and Harvard Medical School, Boston, Massachusetts

I. INTRODUCTION

Obesity is a major public health problem in the United States and in many other industrialized countries. The problem receives considerable attention from public health authorities and is a major preoccupation of millions of overweight men and women. It is estimated that as much as 33 billion dollars is spent each year in the United States on weight loss efforts (1). In spite of this attention and effort, the prevalence of obesity in the United States continues to increase, with current estimates of approximately one-third of the adult population classified as obese (2).

The health hazards of obesity are well documented and are reviewed elsewhere in this volume. It is sufficient to note here that risk of diseases and conditions as diverse as coronary heart disease, osteoarthritis of the knee, job and social discrimination, gall bladder disease, and functional limitations are known to be associated with excess body weight. These relations appear to be causal, with many biological mechanisms described that link obesity with poor health outcome.

It also is clear that weight loss produces improvements in many clinical conditions and risk factors. Improvements in glucose tolerance, lipoprotein profile, blood pressure, and mobility result from weight loss, and these benefits have been documented repeatedly in well-controlled, randomized clinical trials, as well as in observational stud-

ies. Benefits of weight loss on these and other clinical conditions are thoroughly reviewed in other chapters.

In view of the apparently beneficial physiological adaptations consequent to weight loss, it is logical to conclude that weight loss should be encouraged in overweight and obese individuals, with the expectation that it will improve their health. It seems reasonable to assume that obese persons who lose weight should experience increased longevity when compared with their obese peers who remain heavy. In fact, if the benefits of weight reduction are as beneficial as most lay persons and clinicians appear to believe, it should be relatively easy to demonstrate convincingly that weight loss does reduce morbid events and mortal outcomes. Unfortunately, such evidence is sparse. Most of the large population observational studies that provide data on weight loss fail to show a clear benefit, and most in fact suggest an increased risk for mortality in the group that loses weight. The increased risk in these studies associated with weight reduction should not necessarily be interpreted as directly resulting from the weight loss. There are numerous possible biases and confounding variables that could explain these paradoxical findings. The purpose of this chapter is to critically evaluate existing evidence on weight loss and health, examine possible alternative explanations of the findings, reach a conclusion about the advisability of recommending weight loss to overweight individuals, and recommend crucial research questions that need to be addressed.

II. WEIGHT LOSS AND MORTALITY STUDIES

Several studies over the past 40 years investigated the association of weight loss in large populations to subsequent all-cause mortality. In the next section we describe some of the features of these studies, discuss their limitations, and present some of the specific details and findings of the studies. We include studies in which there were at least two determinations of body weight so weight change could be calculated. Only studies of adults are included. There are important issues about the possible benefits and risks, such as growth impairment, of weight loss in children and adolescents, but we do not address this question here. The list of studies may not include all possible reports, but most of the better-known epidemiological studies are included.

All of the studies reviewed here are observational rather than experimental. Most of the study subjects were of normal weight or only moderately obese; thus, these studies do not adequately address the benefit of weight loss in severely obese individuals. Many of the studies are limited in the ability to control for potentially confounding variables such as dietary composition, physical activity, alcohol intake, health status, psychological variables, and other environmental or clinical characteristics. Only one of the studies reviewed included information on whether the weight loss was voluntary or involuntary; thus, one of the major possible biases is nonfatal disease. A serious illness that occurred between the first and subsequent weight measurement could likely produce a weight loss, and also be the cause of death. Many of these observational studies could well have missed detecting serious illness in study participants due to inadequate disease surveillance systems. Few of the studies included more than two weight measurements. This could introduce misclassification bias if weight loss was temporary, perhaps due to a relatively minor acute illness. None of the studies included extensive measurements of body composition. Most relied on some combination of height and weight, usually body mass index (BMI). This measurement is a valid estimate of overall body fatness in population studies, but it cannot provide detailed information on items known to be clinically important, such as body fat distribution.

III. EPIDEMIOLOGICAL STUDIES ON WEIGHT LOSS AND RISK OF MORTALITY

In this section, we review the findings from 19 studies where investigators have examined the association between weight change, including weight loss and subsequent all-cause mortality. (The effect of weight loss on nonfatal morbid conditions has been discussed in other chapters.) Table 1 summarizes the salient design features of each of the 19 studies, arranged in chronological order by date of publication, as well as the main results.

A. The Metropolitan Life Insurance Company Study (3,4)

This study represents one of the earliest epidemiological investigations of the effect of weight loss on mortality. Using life insurance data, Dublin and Marks compared the mortality experience of individuals who are overweight, but subsequently lost weight, with the mortality experience of all insured individuals belonging to the same height and original weight class (including those overweight who went on to lose weight). Overweight persons who lost weight were identified as those initially charged an extra premium on their life insurance rates because of overweight (degree of overweight was not explicitly defined), but who subsequently reduced their weight sufficiently to qualify for lower rates or standard rates. Weight loss appeared beneficial, with up to 39% reduction in mortality observed.

One strength of this study is that subjects with an adverse medical history were excluded. Thus, bias arising from subjects who already were unhealthy at baseline and who continued to lose weight was unlikely. Investigators conducted additional analyses that included a lag period. This further minimizes the impact of such a bias because subjects who were unhealthy at baseline would likely die early during follow-up. One limitation of the study, though, is the lack of information on whether weight loss was intentional. Involuntary weight loss, even among individuals who appear healthy at baseline, is a concern because this may be a harbinger of serious illness. Had this been considered, the reduction in mortality might have been more marked. Another potential limitation is that overweight persons who lost weight had to undergo a second medical examination to qualify for reduced insurance rates. It is unclear whether those found to be unhealthy at this second examination were excluded from further study. Had this been the case, the observed reduction in mortality might have been overestimated, since overweight persons who lost weight then might have been a healthier group than all insured persons. Finally, confounding as a result of differences in smoking habits (5) or alcohol consumption (6) may have occurred, as adjustments were not made for these factors.

B. The Build and Blood Pressure Study (7)

Like the preceding study, the Build and Blood Pressure Study also was based on life insurance data and utilized a similar study design. In this study, the unit of observation was not an individual, but rather an insurance policy. Although the study was large, involving almost five million policies, only 225 policies terminated by death occurred among overweight men (again, degree of overweight was not explicitly defined) who lost weight. Investigators were unable to analyze the data for overweight women who lost weight, since the number of policies terminated by death among such women was 21. Overweight men who lost weight fared favorably, experiencing up to 36% reduction in mortality rates.

Because of the similar study design, this study possesses the same strengths and suffers from the same potential limitations as the Metropolitan Life Insurance Company Study. The major limitations are bias due to involuntary weight loss, screening that might have resulted in overweight men who lost weight being a healthier group, and confounding by cigarette smoking and alcohol intake.

C. The American Cancer Society Study (8,9)

In the first analysis of this study published in 1969, all-cause mortality was not investigated (8). Only deaths from coronary heart disease and stroke were assessed. Investigators classified subjects according to their self-reported weight loss in the 5 years prior to follow-up. There was no clear evidence of survival benefit from either disease among overweight subjects (≥110% of mean weight for height) who lost 4.5–8.9 kg or ≥9 kg.

As with the two previous studies, one strength of this study is that investigators made an effort to exclude unhealthy individuals at the start of follow-up. The American Cancer Society Study represents the only study where investigators did assess whether weight loss was voluntary. Unfortunately, the data were not presented according to volition of weight loss in this analysis. Investigators merely remarked that findings were similar for both unintentional and intentional weight loss; thus, bias from involuntary weight loss may have accounted for the findings. However, another group of investigators subsequently reanalyzed the data, presented below, according to whether weight loss was intentional. A second limitation of the

present analysis is that investigators did not adjust for differences in cigarette smoking or alcohol consumption.

A subsequent analysis of the American Cancer Society Study data, using a longer follow-up period, has been conducted by Williamson et al. (9). In this analysis, investigators focused on overweight (BMI ≥ 27 units, before weight change), white women aged 40–64 years who had never smoked. Women reported on questionnaires in 1959–1960 regarding whether they had experienced a change in weight, whether a loss or gain, the amount of change, the time interval over which this occurred, and whether they had tried to bring about this change (i.e., whether intentional or not). Based on the weight change information, investigators classified women into one of seven groups: unintentional weight loss, intentional weight loss of 0.5–9.0 kg, intentional weight loss of ≥9.1 kg, no change, unintentional weight gain, intentional weight gain, or unknown weight change status. Because very few women reported intentional weight gain, the data for this group were not presented. Investigators then followed women for mortality until 1972. Findings were presented separately for two groups of women: those with no preexisting illnesses and those with obesity-related health conditions. Discounting women with unknown weight change information in the former group, lowest mortality occurred among women who intentionally lost ≥9.1 kg (especially if this occurred over a period of less than 1 year), and highest mortality among those who lost weight unintentionally. For women with obesity-related health conditions, lowest mortality occurred among women who lost 0.5–9.0 kg intentionally (again, especially in the space of a year), while equally high mortality rates were observed among those with unintentional weight loss and among those with no weight change.

The major advantage of this second analysis is the ascertainment of the volition of weight loss. Other strengths included the exclusion of unhealthy subjects, the inclusion of a lag period in analyses, and the adjustment for differences in smoking and alcohol intake. The most serious drawback is the relatively large proportion of women with unknown information regarding weight loss: 23% of those with no preexisting illnesses and 11% of those with obesity-related health conditions. In both groups of women, mortality rates among women in the "unknown" category ranked highest among the six categories of weight change (data for intentional weight gain were sparse and, thus, not provided). The distribution of women with unknown weight change, had their weight change information been known, into the known weight change categories may alter the mortality rates for these known weight change categories.

Table 1 Epidemiological Studies of Weight Change and Mortality

Study (ref.)	No. of subjects and sex	Age at baseline[a] (years)	Weight change interval (years)	Follow-up period for mortality[b] (years)	Assessment of whether weight loss was voluntary
Metropolitan Life Insurance Company (3,4)	1700 M 600F	20–64	Not given	Up to 25	No
Build and Blood Pressure Study (7)	4,900,000[c] M+F	15–69	Not given	Mean, 7.8	No
American Cancer Society Study (8)	358,534 M 445,875 F	35–74	5	6	Yes, but data not presented according to volition of weight loss
American Cancer Society Study (9)	43,457 F	40–64	Not given	12	Yes
Build Study (10)	4,200,000[c] M+F	15–69	Not given	Mean, 6.6	No
Glostrup Study (11)			25	10	No
Honolulu Heart Study (12,13)	7,643 M	25	20–43	10	No
Paris Prospective Study (14)	7,591 M	20	23–33	Mean, 10	No
Kaiser Permanente (15)	2,125 M 2,314 F	Not given; 40–79 at end of weight change interval	(1) Change from greatest adult weight; (2) mean, 3.67	8–16	No
Framingham Heart Study (16)	597 M 1,126 F	55	10	1–23	No
Framingham Heart Study (17)	1,367 M 1,804 F	25	19–51	18	No
Framingham Heart Study (18)	1,114 M 1,386 F	35–54	10	20	No
Western Electric Study (19)	2,107 M	40–56	20	25	No
Gothenburg Study (20)	698 M 1,268 F	50 (M) 33–55 (F)	10 (M) 11 (F)	11 (M) 12 (F)	No
Baltimore Longitudinal Study of Aging (21)	761 M	17–101	Not given	2–27	No
British Regional Heart Study (22)	7,275 M	40–59	5	Mean, 4	No
Dutch Longitudinal Study among the Elderly (23)	275 M 237 F	65–99	5	22	No
Lipid Research Clinics Follow-up Study (24)	3,260 M 1,691 F	18	≥12	Mean, 8.4	No
Harvard Alumni Health Study (25)	11,703 M	30–79	11–15	12	No
MRFIT (26)	10,529 M	35–57	6–7	Mean, 3.8	No
NHANES I Epidemiologic Follow-up Study (27)	2,453 M 2,739 F	Not given; 45–74 at end of weight change interval	Not given	12–16	No
Nurses' Health Study (28)	115,195 F	18	12–37	12	No

Exclusion of unhealthy subjects at baseline	Elimination of early mortality	Control for smoking	Findings for weight change–all-cause mortality[b] association
Yes	Yes	No	20–39% reduction in mortality among men who lost weight 16–37% reduction in mortality among women who lost weight
Yes	Yes	No	15–36% reduction in mortality among men who lost weight. Insufficient data for women
Yes	No	No	Men: 11% reduction to 31% excess CHD deaths, 6% reduction to 46% excess stroke deaths among those losing ≥4.5 kg Women: 1% reduction to 22% excess CHD deaths, 25% reduction to 102% excess stroke deaths among those losing ≥4.5 kg
Yes	Yes	Yes (never-smokers)	Women with no preexisting diseases: lowest mortality among those with intentional weight loss of ≥9.1 kg, highest mortality among those with unintentional weight loss Women with obesity-related diseases: lowest mortality among those with intentional weight loss of 0.5–9 kg, highest mortality both among those with unintentional weight loss and those with no weight change
Yes	Yes	No	"Quite favorable" for men Insufficient data for women
Yes	No	Yes	No association
No	Yes	Yes	Generally reverse J-shaped curve, nadir at BMI change of −1.13–1.12 units
No	No	No	Reverse J-shaped curve, nadir at BMI change of 2.5–4.4 units
Yes	No	No	(1) Men: direct association, lowest mortality at 0–1.9 kg loss. Women, thin: findings as in men Women, average: lowest mortality at ≥12 kg loss (2) Men: lowest mortality at ≥2 kg loss Women, thin: lowest mortality at 1.9 kg loss to 1.9 kg gain. Women, average: findings as in men.
No	No	Yes (nonsmokers)	Both sexes: reverse J-shaped curve, nadir at BMI gain of 0–9%
Yes	Yes	Yes	Inverse
No	Yes	Yes	Men: inverse, nadir at weight gain Women: reverse J-shaped curve, nadir at stable weight
Yes	No	Yes	Lowest mortality among no change group
No (M) Yes (F)	Yes	Unclear (M) Yes (F)	Both sexes: inverse
No	No	No	Inverse
No	No	Yes	J-shaped curve; nadir at stable weight
No	Yes	Yes	Generally U-shaped Lowest quartile of BMI, nadir at BMI gain of 0.5–<2.5 units. Quartiles 2 and 3 of BMI, nadir at BMI loss of 0.5–<2.5 units. Highest quartile of BMI, nadir at BMI loss of 0.5–<2.5 units
Yes	No	Yes	Men: inverse Women: no association
Yes	Yes	Yes	Reverse J-shaped curve, nadir at stable weight
Yes	No	Yes	J-shaped; lowest mortality at stable weight
Yes	Yes	Yes	Men, BMI < 29: inverse; lowest mortality at <5% of maximum weight lost Men, BMI ≥ 29; lowest mortality at 5 to 14% of maximum weight lost Women, all: inverse; lowest mortality at <5% of maximum weight lost
Yes	No	Yes	Lowest mortality among women losing ≥10 kg Highest mortality among women gaining ≥20 kg

[a]That is, beginning of weight change interval.
[b]All-cause mortality was the endpoint of interest, except where otherwise indicated in the findings.
[c]Number of insurance policies.

D. The Build Study (10)

This large-scale insurance study is similar to the Build and Blood Pressure Study, but covered a later period. As in the earlier study, the data on overweight (definition of overweight not given) persons who reduced their weight were sparse: 1900 policies with 35 terminated by death in men, and fewer than 100 policies in women. Detailed data were not provided; investigators merely reported that in men, mortality experience among those overweight who reduced their weight was "quite favorable." The limited data in women precluded analysis. Inherent in this insurance study are the same strengths and potential limitations as the Build and Blood Pressure Study.

E. The Glostrup Study (11)

The main focus of this study was the association of body weight at different ages with subsequent mortality. Among other data, investigators collected information on self-reported body weight at age 25 years and measured weight at age 50 years. In analyzing the data on body weight at these two ages, investigators included a term for weight change between the ages of 25 and 50 years in regression models. Although the coefficient for this term was positive (i.e., indicating greater mortality with greater weight gain), this was not statistically significant.

One strength of this study is that investigators did exclude unhealthy subjects from analyses and controlled for smoking and alcohol intake. A potential limitation is bias due to involuntary weight loss.

F. The Honolulu Heart Study (12,13)

In this study, weight change was determined as the difference between self-reported weight at age 25 years and measured weight at the start of follow-up, when men had aged to 45–68 years (12). Investigators then classified men into four categories of change in BMI: <-1.13; -1.13 to $+1.12$; 1.13–3.75; and >3.75 units. Findings were presented according to quartile of BMI at age 25 years. In all but the second quartile, minimum mortality occurred among men falling in the category of BMI change of -1.13 to $+1.12$ units. Men in the second quartile of BMI at age 25 years experienced minimum mortality if they had gained 1.13–3.75 BMI units from age 25 to 45–68 years.

A strength of this study is the adjustment in analyses for differences in cigarette smoking habit; however, investigators did not control for differences in alcohol intake. As with all but one of the other studies, another potential

limitation is bias resulting from involuntary weight loss. This may have been compounded further by the nonexclusion of unhealthy men, such as those with cancer, from the study. In fact, the authors attributed the excess mortality observed among thin men to be likely due to occult antecedent disease.

A follow-up report on weight loss and mortality in men enrolled in the Honolulu Heart Study was published in 1995 (13). The investigators examined the relation of weight loss 6 years after baseline, during which time weight was determined at three clinical examinations. Mortality follow-up occurred over the next 16 years. Men who lost >4.5 kg had an adjusted (for age, average weight, smoking status, cigarettes/day, alcohol consumption, physical activity, total caloric intake, job classification, and preexisting disease) relative risk for all-cause mortality of 1.21 (95% confidence interval = 1.02–1.43) when compared with men who had stable weights. Men who gained >4.5 kg had no increased mortality risk. The association of increased risk in those who lost weight was not seen in the subgroup of healthy men who had never smoked.

G. The Paris Prospective Study (14)

Investigators categorized men in this study into five groups of BMI change: <0.5; 0.5–2.4; 2.5–4.4; 4.5–6.4; and ≥6.5 units. Body weight change was calculated from age 20 years, using measured weight during military service, to age 43–53 years using measured weight at a medical examination. Minimum mortality during follow-up occurred among men gaining 2.5–4.4 units, maximum mortality among those gaining <0.5 units. Potential limitations of this study include bias from unintentional weight loss and nonexclusion of unhealthy subjects, as well as confounding by smoking and alcohol.

H. The Kaiser Permanente Study (15)

Subjects enrolled into this study were healthy individuals belonging to a health maintenance organization. Investigators classified men and women into several categories of weight change, using two different definitions. First, men and women had their weight measured at a multiphasic health examination, during which they also reported their maximum adult weight. Based on these data, investigators grouped subjects into four categories of weight loss from maximum adult weight: 0–1.9; 2.0–6.9; 7.0–11.9; and ≥12.0 kg. In both thin (decile 1 of BMI, after weight loss) and average-weight (deciles 4 and 5 of BMI) men, mortality during follow-up increased steadily with increasing weight loss. The same was true for thin (decile 1 of BMI) women. In average-weight (deciles 4 and 5) women, minimum mortality occurred at a weight loss of ≥12.0 kg, maximum mortality at 2.0–6.9 kg loss. Second, investigators classified subjects according to their measured weight change between two multiphasic health examinations held, on average, 3.67 years apart. Three categories were defined: ≥2.0 kg weight loss, 1.9 kg loss to 1.9 kg gain, and ≥2.0 kg gain. In both thin and average men, as well as average-weight women, minimum mortality was observed among those losing ≥2.0 kg. In thin women, minimum mortality was experienced by those with 1.9 kg weight loss to 1.9 kg weight gain.

The limitations to consider in this study are, first, the potential for involuntary weight loss to bias the findings. Also, when investigators asked women to report their greatest adult weight, they did not differentiate between pregnant and nonpregnant weights. Finally, confounding by smoking and alcohol intake may have occurred.

I. The Framingham Heart Study (16–18)

The Framingham Heart Study is an ongoing prospective cohort study established in 1948. As part of the study protocol, subjects are brought in for a medical examination every 2 years. Based on these data, three different analyses of weight change and its association with mortality have been published. In the first analysis (16), investigators enrolled nonsmoking men and women aged 55 years. Subjects were followed over the next 10 years for BMI change and categorized thus: loss of ≥10%, loss of 0–9%, gain of 0–9%, or gain of ≥10%. Investigators then followed subjects over the ensuing 1–23 years (mean 9.5 years) for mortality. In both sexes, after accounting for BMI level at the start of mortality follow-up, minimum mortality occurred at a BMI gain of 0–9%, maximum mortality at a BMI loss of ≥10%. In the second analysis (17), the primary hypothesis tested was that weight fluctuation increases mortality. In the course of their analysis, investigators ran regression models that included a term for BMI change per year between ages 25 and 44–76 years and adjusted for average BMI level over the period of weight change. BMI change per year was estimated from the regression of measured weights at biennial examinations against time. The coefficient for BMI change, associated with mortality over 14 years of subsequent follow-up, was negative and statistically significant. This indicated that with BMI loss, mortality increased; conversely, with BMI gain, mortality decreased. In the last analysis (18), subjects aged 35–54 years were grouped according to their BMI change over the next 10 years.

Investigators estimated BMI change per year in the same fashion as in the second analysis. Three categories, "loss," "no change," and "gain," were defined. These corresponded to mean weight changes per year of −0.52, 0.05, and 0.60 kg, respectively, in men and −0.39, 0.16, and 0.71 kg, respectively, in women. Findings were presented separately by tertile of BMI at baseline. In men, for all BMI tertiles, minimum mortality occurred among the "gain" group, maximum mortality among the "loss" group. In women, however, minimum mortality occurred among the "no change" group, with higher mortality experienced by those losing or gaining BMI.

A strength of this study is that smoking was taken into account in all analyses; however, alcohol intake was not. Another limitation of all analyses is potential bias from involuntary weight loss. Further, in the first and third analyses, investigators did not exclude unhealthy subjects from study.

J. The Western Electric Study (19)

The primary aim of this study was to test the hypothesis that persons with large weight fluctuations are associated with higher risk of coronary heart disease than those with more stable weights. Subjects for the Western Electric Study were men aged 40–56 years in 1957, who had been employed for at least 2 years at a Western Electric Company plant. At the initial examination held between 1957 and 1958, body weight was measured. At the same time, men were asked to recall their weights at ages 20, 25, 30, 35, and 40 years. Investigators then calculated percent weight change from ages 20 to 25, 25 to 30, 30 to 35, and 35 to 40 years in order to identify the maximum percentage loss and gain for each subject. Subjects were classified into four groups of weight change: no change (maximum loss <5% and maximum gain <5% and weight at initial examination <5% different from weight at age 20 years), gain only (maximum gain ≥10% and weight progressively increased from age 20 to 40 years), gain and loss (maximum loss ≥10% and maximum gain ≥10%), and "all others." Vital status was determined at the 25th anniversary of each subject's initial examination. Investigators reported that lowest mortality was experienced by men in the no-change group, highest mortality by men in the gain and loss group.

The advantages of this study are the exclusion of unhealthy subjects and the adjustment in analyses for differences in smoking and alcohol consumption patterns; however, a potential limitation is the lack of determination of the volition of weight loss. Further, because investigators primarily were concerned about weight fluctuation, they did not identify a group of men who only lost weight; thus, we are unable to make direct inferences regarding weight loss alone.

K. The Gothenburg Study (20)

In this study, investigators also were interested primarily in the relationship of weight fluctuation with mortality. When analyzing their data, they included a term for weight change in regression models. Weight change was calculated over 10 years in men, 11 years in women. In men, both weights were measured but, in women, the initial weight was self-reported. For both sexes, the coefficient for weight change was negative and statistically significant. That is, with greater weight loss, higher mortality ensued. These analyses took into account the average BMI level over the period of weight change.

One strength of this study is that, in women, investigators did consider the potential for confounding by cigarette smoking; however, it is unclear whether smoking was accounted for in men. Moreover, unhealthy women were excluded from analyses, but unhealthy men were not excluded from analyses. Finally, there exists the potential for bias due to involuntary weight loss.

L. The Baltimore Longitudinal Study of Aging (21)

This represents yet another study where the primary concern was the association of weight fluctuation with mortality. In this study protocol, investigators brought men in to be examined periodically. Measured weights in men were available from 3 to 16 examinations. Investigators estimated change in BMI over time by regressing BMI against time period to obtain a slope. A negative slope, therefore, implies weight loss; a positive slope, weight gain. After adjusting for weight variability and average level of BMI over the period of weight change, BMI change was inversely associated with mortality during follow-up. That is, with increasing weight loss, mortality rate increased, but with increasing weight gain, mortality decreased. This finding was of borderline statistical significance.

Alternative explanations for these observations include bias resulting from unintentional weight loss, nonexclusion of unhealthy subjects at the start of follow-up for mortality, and potential confounding by cigarette smoking and alcohol intake.

M. The British Regional Heart Study (22)

For this study, subjects had their body weight measured initially; 5 years later, men were asked to self-report their weight. Investigators then categorized men thus: loss of >10% body weight, loss of 4–10%, stable weight (i.e., loss or gain of <4%), gain of 4–10%, gain of 10–15%, or gain of >15%. In the ensuing 4 years, on average, of follow-up, men with stable weight experienced lowest mortality. The weight change–mortality curve was J-shaped, with highest mortality observed among those gaining the most weight.

A strength of this study is the adjustment for differences in smoking habit; however, investigators did not adjust for differences in alcohol habit. A second potential limitation is that involuntary weight loss may have biased findings. Moreover, unhealthy men were not excluded from study. This limitation is compounded by the relatively short period of follow-up because mortality among unhealthy men, who may have lost weight, would likely occur early in follow-up.

N. Dutch Longitudinal Study Among the Elderly (23)

Investigators examined men and women aged 65–99 years once at the start of this study and again 5 years later. Based on their measured body weights, subjects were classified into five groups of BMI change: loss of ≥2.5 units, loss of 0.5–<2.5 units, stable weight (loss or gain of <0.5 units), gain of 0.5–<2.5 units, and gain of ≥2.5 units. Findings were presented by quartile of BMI at the start of the weight change interval. For all quartiles of initial BMI, the curve assessing the relation between weight change and mortality generally was U-shaped; however, the nadir of the curve varied. Among subjects in the lowest BMI quartile, lowest mortality was experienced by those who gained 0.5–<2.5 units. For the middle two quartiles combined, lowest mortality occurred among those who lost 0.5–<2.5 units. A similar finding was seen for subjects at the initial examination. U-shaped curves with the nadir at BMI loss of 0.5–<2.5 units were observed for those aged 65–74 years, as well as for those older. Next, investigators stratified their findings by sex and reported a U-shaped curve with lowest mortality at a BMI loss of 0.5–<2.5 units in men. In women, although mortality generally increased with increasing weight gain, lowest mortality also was experienced by those losing 0.5–<2.5 units of BMI.

A strength of this study is that investigators did consider the potential for confounding by cigarette smoking; however, no adjustment was made for alcohol consumption. Another limitation is that investigators did not determine whether weight loss was voluntary or not. Moreover, unhealthy subjects were not excluded from study; thus, the lag period of 2 years used in some analyses may have been insufficient to remove bias from illness-related weight loss.

O. The Lipid Research Clinics Follow-up Study (24)

Here, investigators took advantage of data from the Lipid Research Clinics Program to examine the association between weight change during adulthood and later mortality. At the start of follow-up for mortality, men and women aged ≥30 years had their body weight measured. At that time, subjects also were asked to self-report their weight at age 18 years. Investigators then calculated percent change in weight, using data from these two time points, and entered this variable as a single term in regression models. After adjusting for BMI at the start of follow-up for mortality, smoking habit, alcohol consumption, and other cardiovascular risk factors, percent weight change in men was inversely related to all-cause mortality. That is, with increasing weight gain, mortality decreased. In women, however, weight change did not predict mortality.

The strengths of this study include the elimination of unhealthy subjects from study, as well as the adjustment in analyses for differences in smoking and alcohol habits. Investigators did not possess information on whether weight loss was intentional or unintentional; thus, bias from unintentional weight loss cannot be excluded.

P. The Harvard Alumni Health Study (25)

The Harvard Alumni Health Study represents another long-term, prospective cohort study, ongoing since 1962. Subjects periodically are contacted and asked to self-report on questionnaires their sociodemographic characteristics, health habits, and medical history. In this particular analysis, middle-aged Harvard alumni self-reported their weight on two questionnaires, separated in time by 11–15 years. Investigators then grouped men into five categories of weight change: loss of >5 kg, loss of >1–5 kg, stable weight (i.e., loss or gain of ≤1 kg), gain of >1–5 kg, or gain of >5 kg. After adjustment for height, BMI before weight change, and smoking habit, they observed that men with stable weight experienced lowest mortality. As weight was lost or gained, mortality increased. The weight change–mortality curve was reverse J-shaped. A similar reverse J-shaped curve was seen when investigators examined nonsmokers separately. Next, investigators proceeded to examine the effect of weight change in less obese (BMI < 25 units) and more obese men (BMI ≥ 25 units), separately. In both groups of men, investigators continued to note minimum mortality among men of sta-

ble weight and higher mortality among those losing or gaining weight.

The increased mortality with weight gain was expected; however, the decreased longevity also observed among men losing weight was not expected. One alternative explanation was that weight loss may have been involuntary and that the findings reflected increased mortality among unhealthy men or those with occult disease who lost weight. Investigators tried to minimize this bias by excluding men with cardiovascular disease or cancer from study. Moreover, in additional analyses that allowed for a lag period of 6 years, findings did not change. Since weight loss from occult illnesses would likely be due to cancer, investigators further analyzed cause-specific mortality. They found no association between weight change and cancer mortality, but noted instead a marked U-shaped curve for coronary heart disease mortality. One limitation that investigators did not address, however, is the potential for confounding by alcohol intake.

Q. The Multiple Risk Factor Intervention Trial (MRFIT) (26)

The aim of this randomized, primary prevention trial was to test whether intensive intervention could reduce mortality from coronary heart disease among men at high risk. Investigators measured body weight of participants at every visit. For men in the intervention group, visits occurred every 4 months; for those in the usual care group, annually. Men were categorized into three weight change groups: steady loss (i.e., ≥5% loss from a previous visit that was not regained), no change (i.e., <5% change from baseline at every visit), or steady gain (i.e., ≥5% gain from a previous visit that was not lost). In addition, two other categories of weight cycling patterns were defined. We will discuss only the weight change categories. Investigators observed a reverse J-shaped curve, with lowest all-cause and cardiovascular disease mortality occurring among "no change" men. When they analyzed never-smokers only, again a reverse J-shaped curve was seen. Investigators then repeated the analyses, separately, by tertiles of baseline BMI. In the thinnest men, an inverse, graded relationship was found, with lowest mortality among men gaining weight and highest mortality in those losing weight. However, for the middle tertile, as well as among the heaviest men, investigators observed reverse J-shaped curves, with highest mortality rates in men who lost weight.

Strengths of this study include the exclusion of unhealthy men from study and the adjustment in analyses for smoking habit and alcohol intake; however, bias from unintentional weight loss could potentially explain these findings.

R. The First National Health and Nutrition Examination Survey (NHANES I) Epidemiologic Follow-up Study (27)

In this study, investigators calculated change in body weight from self-reported maximum lifetime weight and measured weight at the start of follow-up for mortality. Men and women were grouped into three categories of weight loss from maximum body weight: ≥15% loss, 5–14% loss, or <5% loss. Analyses were adjusted for maximum body weight and smoking habit and stratified by maximum BMI. In men with BMI < 26 units, as well as those with BMI 26–<29 units, the association of weight change and mortality was inverse. That is, mortality was greatest among those losing the most weight. For the heaviest men with BMI ≥ 29 units, the curve was U-shaped, with minimum mortality occurring among those losing 5–14% of maximum body weight. In women, however, the inverse association was observed for all three categories of BMI. When never-smokers were examined separately, findings were similar.

Although unhealthy subjects were not excluded, investigators attempted to account for this by adjustment in analysis for the presence of illness. No data were available as to whether weight loss was voluntary; thus, bias may have occurred from involuntary weight loss. Finally, confounding by alcohol intake represents another limitation.

S. The Nurses' Health Study (28)

The primary focus of this paper was to examine the association between BMI, assessed in 1976, and mortality among 115,195 women who were aged 30–55 years and free of cardiovascular disease and cancer at that time. Investigators used data from the Nurses' Health Study, another ongoing, long-term, prospective cohort study. Since 1976, the nurses in this study have been contacted every 2 years via questionnaires and asked about their health habits and medical history.

In their analyses, investigators also provided findings on the relationship between weight change and mortality. Women reported their current weight and height on the 1976 questionnaire; additionally, recalled weight at age 18 was reported on the 1980 questionnaire. Investigators then divided women into six categories of weight change between age 18 and 30–55 years: loss of ≥10 kg, loss of 4–9 kg, stable weight (i.e., loss or gain of <4 kg), gain of 4–9kg, gain of 10–19kg, or gain of ≥20 kg. Among women who were never-smokers and who were free of cardiovascular disease and cancer, 1059 deaths occurred between 1980 and 1992. After adjustment for age and BMI at age 18, the lowest mortality risk was observed

among those losing ≥10 kg, with highest mortality among those gaining ≥20 kg. There was a significant trend of increasing risk of mortality with increasing weight gain.

One strength of this study is the exclusion of unhealthy subjects from the study. Further, by analyzing only never-smokers, confounding by cigarette habit could not have occurred. Investigators did not assess whether weight loss was intentional.

IV. COMMENT ON EPIDEMIOLOGICAL DATA

From a noncritical perspective, the epidemiological data collectively indicate that weight loss appears hazardous, being linked to higher mortality rates in most studies. Only eight of the studies discussed provided any suggestion that weight loss is associated with lower mortality: the Metropolitan Life Insurance Company Study (3,4), the Build and Blood Pressure Study (7), the American Cancer Society Study (8), the Build Study (investigators merely reported that weight loss was "quite favorable"; actual data were not provided) (10), the Kaiser Permanente Study (only among persons of average weight, but not among thin persons) (15), the Dutch Longitudinal Study (only among persons in the upper three quartiles of BMI, but not among persons in the lowest quartile of BMI) (23), the NHANES I Epidemiologic Follow-up Study (only among men with BMI of ≥29 units, but not among men of lighter weight nor among women) (27), and the Nurses' Health Study (28). Conversely, men in the MRFIT study who were in the highest tertile of baseline BMI (>28.82) and lost ≥5% of their baseline weight had an 11% increased risk for cardiovascular disease mortality and a 62% increased risk for all-cause mortality when compared with weight-stable men (26). In fact, most of the studies reviewed noted that individuals faring best (i.e., enjoying lowest mortality) were those who gained weight or who maintained stable weight, regardless of their starting body weight.

Another finding that deserves comment is the failure to observe increased mortality in some studies for groups who gained weight. For example, the overweight (BMI ≥ 27) women in the American Cancer Society Study who had an unintentional weight *gain* had death rates comparable to the women who did not gain weight (9). If overweight is hazardous, why did these women, who were already overweight, not have an increase in mortality risk after they gained even more weight? In contrast, the Nurses' Health Study (28) reported significantly increased risks of all-cause mortality among women gaining >10 kg since age 18. It may be that the associations between weight, weight gain, and health risks are more complicated than most appreciate.

These epidemiological data seem paradoxical because they run counter to the physiological benefits known to be associated with weight loss. Before we conclude that weight loss indeed is detrimental to longevity, we need to consider the limitations of the studies from which these data derive. The most crucial limitation is the lack of differentiation between unintentional and intentional weight loss. As discussed previously, involuntary weight loss, even in a seemingly healthy individual, may be ominous because it may signal hidden pathology. Because almost all studies did not possess information on the volition of weight loss, investigators have tried to minimize this bias in a variety of ways. These include:

1. Eliminating unhealthy persons (usually those with cardiovascular disease and cancer, as these two conditions account for a large proportion of chronic diseases) from study
2. Including a lag period in analysis (since those unhealthy and who lose weight would likely die early during follow-up)
3. Analyzing cause-specific mortality (since weight loss in an ostentatiously healthy person is likely to be associated with occult cancer).

However, even with these measures, the bias from unintentional weight loss may not be completely eliminated.

Only one group of investigators (9) was able to analyze their data according to whether weight loss was intentional or not. Findings from the second analysis of the American Cancer Society Study suggest that the implications of involuntary and voluntary weight loss are completely different: Involuntary weight loss was associated with highest mortality, while voluntary weight loss was associated with lowest mortality in this study. Unfortunately, the American Cancer Society Study cannot be considered definitive. In this study, there was a fairly large category of women with unknown information on their weight change. This group of women experienced the highest mortality rates; thus, had their weight change been known and had these women been redistributed into the other weight change categories, the findings from this study might have been different. Further, it is unclear whether the results of this study may be applicable to other than white women with a BMI $\geq$ 27 units. A related issue, for which no data are available, is whether voluntary weight loss using physical activity is associated with better health outcomes since physical activity is associated with lower risks of chronic diseases and increased longevity.

A second limitation of the studies discussed is the potential for confounding due to differences in cigarette smoking and/or alcohol consumption. These two factors are strong predictors of mortality; thus, failure to consider differences in these two characteristics among persons belonging to various weight change categories also may lead to biased findings.

Many of the studies relied on self-reported weight to assess weight change; however, self-reports are unlikely to have biased findings, since they appear to deviate little from actual measurements (29–31). Moreover, all the studies described were prospective, with weight ascertained at the start of follow-up for mortality. Any misclassification is likely to be nondifferential and would not explain the increased mortality observed among those losing weight.

Finally, because the studies were population-based, investigators enrolled few subjects with morbid obesity. Other studies have shown that surgical treatment of such obesity is associated with decreased morbidity and mortality (32).

V. RECOMMENDATIONS

Despite the preponderance of evidence indicating increased mortality risk with weight loss, it is premature to declare that weight loss is hazardous. The available data are from observational studies, and their limitations are discussed in previous sections. The health risks of obesity and the clear benefit of weight loss on variables such as blood pressure and glucose tolerance encourage appropriate weight loss in selected individuals; however, it is puzzling that some studies show no increase in mortality risk in overweight persons who gain more weight. There is a clear lack of definitive data showing that weight loss in nonmorbidly obese individuals prevents major morbidity such as heart attack or stroke, or extends longevity. Furthermore, questions about limited benefits of weight loss on longevity and of possible harmful effects of weight loss require that recommendations must be carefully stated, constantly reviewed, and revised as appropriate.

A. Research

Much research is needed to clarify possible benefit or harm resulting from weight loss. The overall issue is to confirm or refute the hypothesis that weight loss increases mortality risk. Perhaps the central unanswered question relates to voluntary or involuntary weight loss, and whether effects are different for these two exposures. Although most studies do not have data on whether weight loss is voluntary or not, data from the National Health Interview Survey suggest that approximately 60% of individuals who report weight loss were trying to lose weight, and the data were consistent for both men and women (33). Thus, it seems that much of the weight loss observed in the population must be intentional.

The association of weight loss in various subgroups needs to be evaluated. Several related questions remain unanswered. None of the studies above stated explicitly that extremely overweight subjects were enrolled. It is likely that of those overweight, most were moderately overweight only. We are unclear whether the association between weight loss and mortality differs among persons who are thin, of normal weight, moderately overweight, or severely obese. Data from the Kaiser Permanente Study (15) and the Dutch Longitudinal Study (23) indicate that weight loss appears to have different implications for those who are thin and for those who are of at least normal weight, while data from the NHANES I Epidemiologic Follow-up Study (27) suggest that findings differ between men with BMI of <29 units and heavier men. However, data from the MRFIT (26) suggest that there may be increased mortality risk with weight loss even in men with a baseline BMI of ≥28.8. Meanwhile, weight loss among the morbidly obese has been shown to be associated with decreased morbidity and mortality (32).

Next, is the pattern of weight change over time important? This is difficult to investigate because characterizing the nature of body weight change over time can be extremely complicated. In most of the studies reviewed, investigators obtained information on weight at two points in time to determine weight loss or gain, and in some cases there were up to a few decades between measurements. Alternatively, investigators documented a series of weights for an individual and fitted a straight line to these data to describe weight change over time. In the former situation, weights at other times were not considered. In the latter situation, a simplistic model is assumed for the character of the weight loss. Patterns of weight loss over time may have bearing for longevity; for example, the data from some studies suggest that weight fluctuation may be associated with higher mortality (17,19,20,25,26). Studies fo weight fluctuation are discussed in more detail in another chapter.

Finally, other unanswered questions include: Is the composition of weight loss (e.g., fat vs. muscle loss) relevant? Does the anatomical distribution of weight loss (e.g., predominantly central vs. peripheral loss) have any health implications? In the studies described above, no data are available on these parameters. These factors may be important; for example, the pattern of fat distribution itself has health implications. We know that central obesity increases risk of cardiovascular disease, hypertension, and diabetes mellitus (34,35).

If additional studies continue to suggest weight loss is hazardous, at least in some subgroups, a better understanding of possible biological mechanisms must be developed. There is evidence that dieting may lead to electrocardiographic changes that could increase risk of sudden death (36). Other possible mechanisms, such as dieting leading to deficiencies of some critical nutrients or psychological disturbances, should be studied.

B. Public Health Policy

Representative population surveys indicate a high prevalence of weight loss attempts, with 44 million adults 25 years of age or older reporting trying to lose weight in 1990 (37). Individuals report using a wide variety of methods to lose weight, although caloric restriction and increased exercise are most common (37,38). In addition, most attempts at weight loss are not successful over the long term (1). Given that we cannot conclusively refute the current data that severe dieting leading to weight loss among normal-weight or moderately obese is harmful to health, public health policies must be carefully formulated and stated to avoid adding to the already considerable emphasis on weight loss in countries such as the United States. However, among those morbidly obese, weight loss produced by surgical intervention is associated with decreased morbidity and mortality (32). Since there is a possibility of harm from weight loss and long-term success is unlikely for many overweight individuals, public health policies perhaps should focus on the prevention of overweight rather than treatment. Public health education and intervention recommendations should focus on promoting eating a healthy diet and obtaining regular physical activity. There is ample evidence that these two recommendations lead to improved health and reduction in mortality risk.

C. Clinical Practice

What should a clinician do when counseling an overweight patient? Should weight loss be recommended automatically? Or, should fear of possible hazards of weight loss lead to ignoring the overweight? There are no easy answers to these questions. We think there is at least a possibility that weight loss is contraindicated for at least some individuals. A report from the Food and Nutrition Board of the National Academy of Medicine presents suggestions for a stepped-care approach to weight reduction (1). We believe this strategy has benefits. We encourage physicians and other health care professionals to avoid an automatic recommendation to lose weight to every person with a few extra pounds. Weight loss recommendations should be reserved for those more severely overweight and persons with other obesity-related diseases such as hypertension or diabetes, or with significant risk factors for these diseases.

Weight loss, when recommended, should be encouraged by long-term life-style changes. Regular physical activity is a critical factor. Maintenance of weight loss is much more likely in persons who become physically active (26), and exercise may induce metabolic normality without producing weight loss (39). Furthermore, men with a BMI $\geq$ 30 who were physically fit had no higher all-cause death rates during an 8-year follow-up than fit men with a BMI < 27 (40). In fact, the obese men who were at least moderately physically fit had a lower all-cause death rate than normal-weight men who were unfit. These findings suggest there are important health benefits from physical activity, even if the activity does not make you lean. We believe there should be a shift in emphasis from one solely on weight to one that focuses on a healthy diet and regular physical activity.

VI. CONCLUSION

Observational studies on weight loss and mortality are paradoxical. Although obesity is directly associated with mortality risk, most population-based studies show higher mortality rates in men and women who lose weight. Bias and confounding cannot be excluded as alternate explanations for these results, but there also is the possibility that weight loss is hazardous, at least for some subgroups of the population. Additional research is clearly needed to resolve this question, and public health and clinical recommendations must be considered tentative until more definitive data are available. In summary, despite the majority of epidemiological studies showing that weight loss in the general population is associated with greater mortality, it is not at all clear that weight loss is hazardous. Such data may reflect bias due to unintentional weight loss. The one study where voluntary weight loss could be investigated, unfortunately, was not free from other limitations. We need further studies designed to simultaneously address all the limitations discussed, not only to clarify the health effects of intentional weight loss, but to answer other outstanding research questions.

ACKNOWLEDGMENTS

This work was supported in part by Public Health Service Research Grant AG06945 from the National Institute on Aging, Bethesda, Maryland. We thank Melba Morrow, M.A., for editorial assistance and Stephanie Parker for secretarial support. Part of this report was presented at "Nutrition and Physical Activity to Optimize Performance and Well-Being," a conference sponsored by International Life Sciences Institute in Atlanta, Georgia, April 5–7, 1995.

REFERENCES

1. Weighing the Options. Washington, DC: National Academy Press, 1995.
2. Kuczmarski RS, Flegal KM, Campbell SM, Johnson CL. Increasing prevalence of overweight among U.S. adults: the National Health and Nutrition Examination Surveys, 1960 to 1991. JAMA 1994; 272:205–211.
3. Dublin LI. Relation of obesity to longevity. N Engl J Med 1951; 248:971–974.
4. Dublin LI, Marks HH. Mortality among insured overweights in recent years. Transactions of the Association of Life Insurance Medical Directors of America 1951; 35: 235–263.
5. Manson JE, Stampfer MJ, Hennekens CH, Willett WC. Body weight and longevity: a reassessment. JAMA 1987; 257:353–358.
6. Liu S, Serdula MK, Williamson DF, Mokdad AH, Byers T. A prospective study of alcohol intake and change in body weight among US adults. Am J Epidemiol 1994; 140: 912–920.
7. Build and Blood Pressure Study. Chicago, IL: Society of Actuaries. 1959.
8. Hammond EC, Garfinkel L. Coronary heart disease, stroke and aortic aneurysm: factors in the etiology. Arch Environ Health 1969; 19:167–182.
9. Williamson DF, Pamuk E, Thun M, Flanders D, Byers T, Heath C. A prospective study of intentional weight loss and mortality in never smoking overweight white women aged 40 to 64 years. Am J Epidemiol 1995; 141:1128–1141.
10. Build Study. Chicago, IL: Society of Actuaries and Association of Life Insurance Medical Directors of America. 1979.
11. Schroll M. A longitudinal epidemiological survey of relative weight at age 25, 50, and 60 in the Glostrup population of men and women born in 1914. Danish Med Bull 1981; 28:106–116.
12. Rhoads GG, Kagan A. The relation of coronary disease, stroke, and mortality to weight in youth and in middle age. Lancet 1983; 1:492–495.
13. Iribarren C, Sharp DS, Burchfiel CM, Petrovitch H. Association of weight loss and weight fluctuation with mortality among Japanese American men. N Engl J Med 1995; 333: 686–692.
14. Avons P, Ducimetiere P, Rakotovao R. Weight and mortality. Lancet 1983; 1:1104.
15. Sidney S, Friedman GD, Siegelaub AB. Thinness and mortality. Am J Public Health 1987; 77:317–322.
16. Harris T, Cook EF, Garrison R, Higgins M, Kannel W, Goldman L. Body mass index and mortality among nonsmoking

older persons: the Framingham Heart Study. JAMA 1988; 259:1520–1524.

17. Lissner L, Odell PM, D'Agostino RB, et al. Variability of body weight and health outcomes in the Framingham population. N Engl J Med 1991; 324:1839–1844.

18. Higgins M, D'Agostino R, Kannel W, Cobb J. Benefits and adverse effects of weight loss: observations from the Framingham Study. Ann Intern Med 1993; 119:758–763.

19. Hamm P, Shekelle RB, Stamler J. Large fluctuations in body weight during young adulthood and twenty-five-year risk of coronary death in men. Arch Environ Health 1989; 19:167–182.

20. Lissner L, Bengtsson C, Lapidus L, Larsson B, Bengtsson B, Brownell K. Body weight variability and mortality in the Gothenburg Prospective Studies of men and women. In: Björntorp P, Rossner S, eds. Obesity in Europe 88: Proceedings of the First European Congress on Obesity. London: John Libbey, 1989:55–60.

21. Lissner L, Andres R, Muller DC, Shimokata H. Body weight variability in men: metabolic rate, health and longevity. Int J Obes 1990; 14:373–383.

22. Wannamethee G, Shaper AG. Weight change in middle-aged British men: implications for health. Eur J Clin Nutr 1990; 44:133–142.

23. Deeg DJH, Miles TP, Van Zonneveld RJ, Curb JD. Weight change, survival time and cause of death in Dutch elderly. Arch Gerontol Geriatr 1990; 10:97–111.

24. Wilcosky T, Hyde J, Anderson JJB, Bangdiwala S, Duncan B. Obesity and mortality in the Lipid Research Clinics Program Follow-up Study. J Clin Epidemiol 1990; 43:743–752.

25. Lee IM, Paffenbarger RS, Jr. Change in body weight and longevity. JAMA 1992; 268:2045–2049.

26. Blair SN, Shaten J, Brownell K, Collins G, Lissner L. Body weight change, all-cause mortality, and cause-specific mortality in the Multiple Risk Factor Intervention Trial. Ann Intern Med 1993; 119:749–757.

27. Pamuk ER, Williamson DF, Serdula MK, Madans J, Byers TE. Weight loss and subsequent death in a cohort of US adults. Ann Intern Med 1993; 119:744–748.

28. Manson JE, Willett WC, Stampfer MJ, et al. The nurses' health study: body weight and mortality among women. N Engl J Med 1995; 333:677–685.

29. Palta M, Prineas RJ, Berman R, Hannan P. Comparison of self-reported and measured height and weight. Am J Epidemiol 1982; 115:223–230.

30. Stewart AW, Jackson RT, Ford MA, Beaglehole R. Underestimation of relative weight by use of self-reported height and weight. Am J Epidemiol 1987; 125:122–126.

31. Stunkard AJ, Albaum JM. The accuracy of self-reported weights. Am J Clin Nutr 1981; 34:1593–1599.

32. Buchwald H, Varco RL, Matts JP, et al. Effect of partial ileal bypass surgery on mortality and morbidity from coronary heart disease in patients with hypercholesterolemia: report of the Program on the Surgical Control of the Hyperlipidemias (POSCH). N Engl J Med 1990; 323:946–955.

33. Meltzer AA, Everhart JE. Unintentional weight loss in the United States. Am J Epidemiol 1995; 142:1039–1046.

34. Folsom AR, Prineas RJ, Kaye SA, et al. Body fat distribution and self-reported prevalence of hypertension, heart attack, and other heart disease in older women. Int J Epidemiol 1989; 18:361–367.

35. Ohlson LO, Larsson B, Svardsudd K, et al. The influence of body fat distribution on the incidence of diabetes mellitus: 13.5 years of follow-up of the participants in the study of men born in 1913. Diabetes 1985; 34:1055–1058.

36. Greenway FL, Raum WJ, Atkinson RL. Higher calorie content preserves myocardial electrical activity during very-low-calorie dieting. Obes Res 1994; 2:95–99.

37. Horm J, Anderson K. Who in America is trying to lose weight? Ann Intern Med 1993; 119:672–676.

38. Levy AS. Weight control practices of U.S. adults trying to lose weight. Ann Intern Med 1993; 119:661–666.

39. Tremblay A, Despres JP, Maheux J, et al. Normalization of the metabolic profile in obese women by exercise and a low fat diet. Med Sci Sports Exerc 1991; 23:1326–1331.

40. Barlow CE, Kohl HW, III, Gibbons LW, Blair SN. Physical fitness, mortality and obesity. Int J Obes 1995; 19(Suppl 4):S41–S44.

40

Prevention of Obesity

Robert W. Jeffery
University of Minnesota School of Public Health, Minneapolis, Minnesota

I. INTRODUCTION

Prevention is a new area of focus in obesity research that has attracted recent attention because of dramatic increases in obesity prevalence and the persistent failure of most obesity treatments to achieve long-term success. This chapter reviews research done on this topic to date, considering the problem from both individual and population perspectives. Susceptibility to obesity in individuals is most striking in those with a family history of the disorder and in those showing signs of it at an early age (e.g., in childhood). In populations affluence, and the life-styles it affords, is the strongest predictor of obesity, though the strong inverse association between social class and obesity in developed societies suggests that affluence can have a protective effect under some circumstances. Research on obesity prevention among those at high risk is perhaps best exemplified in studies of obesity interventions for children. In preadolescent age groups such treatments show considerable promise. Substantial reductions in obesity risk have been demonstrated for as long as 10 years. Only one study to date has examined obesity prevention efforts in adults. Although it was successful for 1 year, more research is needed in this area. Public health or population-oriented strategies for obesity prevention have included school-based programs targeting youth and work-site-based and community-wide strategies targeting adults. These efforts, which have been largely educational in orientation, have been successful in engaging large numbers of people, some overweight and some not. For the most part, however, they have not been able to demonstrate the ability to favorably modify obesity prevalence or upward trends in body weight over time. It is suggested that a broader environmental perspective on factors that encourage an imbalance between energy intake and expenditure may be needed if the public health problem of obesity is to be successfully addressed. An environment that exposes its human population to a diet that is high in energy, palatability, and variety, but low in cost, and that provides little or no inducement to be physically active can be expected to produce high rates of obesity. Changes in the environment that reduce the attractiveness of energy intake and increase the attractiveness of physical activity might be more helpful than educational approaches in reversing the direction of recent trends in obesity prevalence.

This chapter reviews what is known about obesity prevention. Prevention is a relatively unstudied aspect of the problem of obesity, but one that has attracted recent attention for several reasons. Despite ample evidence for individual differences in susceptibility to obesity, obesity is not innate, but rather develops over time. A reasonable question, therefore, is whether and how this developmental process can be stopped or delayed. Interest in obesity prevention is also heightened by the fact that, once obesity had developed, it is very difficult to treat. No treatment, short of surgery, has an excellent long-term prognosis. Might it not be easier, less expensive, and more effective to change behavior so as to prevent weight gain or to reverse small gains, than to treat obesity after it has fully developed? Finally, many of the health consequences of obesity are the result of the cumulative stress of excess weight over a long period of time and are not fully reversible by weight loss. Thus, obesity prevention may also be the best way to address the health problems it causes.

Prevention will be considered here at two levels, that of the individual and that of the population as a whole. At the individual level the question is whether and how the accumulation of body fat in susceptible persons over time can be reduced. In the population as a whole, the question is whether and how the proportion of people who fall victim to obesity over time can be reduced. The causes of obesity in individuals and of increasing obesity prevalence in populations are not necessarily the same. Thus, preventive approaches in individuals and in populations may also be different.

II.   THE NATURAL HISTORY OF OBESITY

A.   Individuals

Obesity can develop at any time between early childhood and old age, and once it develops, it tends to persist. The most common time in the life cycle for obesity development is during adulthood. Approximately 10–15% of people in the United States become obese during childhood and adolescence. An additional 30–40% develop the problem between early adulthood and middle age (1). Gradual accumulation of body fat over long periods is the typical pattern. Between age 20 and age 50, both men and women gain an average of 1–2 lb of body fat per year. Men's weights tend to stabilize and then slowly decrease after age 50, whereas women experience continuing increases in body weight through age 60–65 and then experience weight declines (1). Interpreting decreases in weight at older ages in regard to obesity is somewhat difficult. Because older adults tend to lose lean body mass as they age, many may actually increase in fatness in old age despite stable or decreasing body weights (2).

In the overall context of gradual weight gain with age, there are a variety of individual patterns (3). Natural history studies suggest that stable body weight across the life span (weight gain prevention) is an unusual weight pattern. Using recalled weights in middle-aged males, Hamm et al. found that only 9% reported stable weight between ages 20 and 40 (4). French et al. found that only 2% of elderly women reported stable weight between ages 20 and 60 (5). Weight losses greater than 10% of body weight that are maintained over periods of 10 years or more are even rarer (6), although sizable weight fluctuation is common. It is not known whether some patterns of weight fluctuation are more conducive to the development of

obesity than others. Increases in weight are usually not reversed, however, regardless of the route by which they are arrived at.

In sum, virtually all individuals are at risk for fatness gain throughout their lives. If obesity is to be prevented across the board, prevention efforts must clearly begin at an early age. Weight gain prevention efforts throughout the adult years, however, are warranted.

B.   Populations

At a population level, obesity in the United States and many other industrialized nations has reached epidemic proportions. Most recent data from the National Center of Health Statistics indicates that approximately 34% of U.S. adults are obese, an increase of nearly 31% in the last decade alone (1). Although historical data on obesity rates are incomplete, it is fairly clear that obesity was relatively rare in the early part of the century and has increased steadily ever since. Cross-cultural comparisons of obesity rates reveal an interesting pattern that may be informative about the causes and potential treatments of the problem at this level (7). Obesity rates in countries with relatively low levels of affluence are generally low, whereas those in affluent societies are high. The distribution of obesity within these populations also differs (8). In poor populations obesity is confined almost exclusively to the wealthier social classes. In affluent populations, on the other hand, obesity is most problematic in lower social classes as well as within ethnic groups suffering most economic hardship. The inverse social class gradient of obesity is particularly striking in women.

Population studies of obesity provide some reason for optimism about the potential for obesity prevention. A phenomenon that has developed over a period of one or two generations in response to changing social and economic conditions might plausibly be reversed if the causal conditions could be identified and remedied. Population studies also suggest that in terms of maximum impact of prevention efforts, targeting of groups of lower socioeconomic status, and particularly women, may be needed.

III.   RISK FACTORS FOR THE DEVELOPMENT OF OBESITY

A.   Individuals

Not all individuals are equally susceptible to the development of obesity. The single strongest predisposing factor appears to be family history, probably mediated by genetic predisposition rather than shared environment. Genetic predisposition has been estimated by some to account for as much as 50% of body fatness under environmental conditions present in affluent societies (9).

Another important risk factor for the development of obesity is early development of lesser degrees of fatness. Individuals who are at the upper end of the weight distribution in childhood, adolescence, or young adulthood are at a much increased risk of becoming truly obese later in life compared to those who are leaner (10). Individuals who develop the most extreme forms of obesity are almost always those who suffer earliest in life. In targeting obesity prevention efforts, particular attention needs to be given to individuals with a family history and to those showing early signs of developing the condition.

Data on the relationship between diet and exercise behaviors and risk for obesity development are mixed. Overall, cross-sectional associations between total energy intake and obesity are weak or even inverse (11). Heavier individuals report eating less than those with less body weight. These results have been questioned on the grounds that they are biologically implausible, and it has been documented that the overweight individuals may underreport their energy intake to a greater extent than do the lean (12). Nevertheless, abnormally high habitual energy intake is clearly not a uniform characteristic of the obese, although the possibility that episodic bouts of excess eating might contribute has not been ruled out. Some have suggested that it is fat intake rather than total energy intake that is the risk-conferring behavior of obesity (13). Again, however, data on this issue are at best inconsistent (11). A finding difficult to explain with this hypothesis is the fact that increasing rates of obesity in the United States over the last decade have occurred at the same time that fat intake as a percentage of total energy has decreased. Lack of exercise is also not a behavior pattern unique to obesity. The obese are indeed less active than the nonobese (14), but in analyses of this relationship that adjust for body mass, total energy expenditure in physical activity is similar in the two groups (15). Part of the problem with trying to identify diet and exercise habits that are prognostic of obesity development is imprecision in the instruments for measuring these behaviors (i.e., the error in measurement may often be as great as or greater than the differences in diet and exercise needed to sustain substantial differences in fat mass). Somewhat better predictive power has been obtained in a few studies that have looked at specific dietary and exercise markers rather than attempting to characterize total intake or expenditure. Frequency of consumption of high-fat meats and French fries, for example, may predict obesity and change in obesity better than estimates of total energy intake or fat intake (16,17). Similarly, frequency of engaging in well-specified aerobic activities may predict obesity better than global

measures of habitual physical activity. In any event, not much progress has been made in identifying unique eating or exercise behaviors that would be useful in targeting individuals for obesity prevention efforts.

A final area of possible interest in regard to predicting obesity development is critical life periods or life events. There is some evidence that marriage, at least for women, is a risk factor for weight gain, although the magnitude of the risk is fairly small (18). It has also been suggested, largely based on retrospective reports of obese persons themselves, that stressful life events are risk factors for development of obesity. Women, for example, often cite childbirth as a critical life event. Prospective data to support these reports, however, are largely lacking. On average, pregnancy is associated with quite small net gains in body weight and these are primarily confined to the first pregnancy (19).

A potentially interesting dimension of the critical-periods concept is whether there are times in people's lives when they would be more receptive to obesity prevention efforts (i.e., when they are more susceptible to positive behavior change). Unfortunately, although there is some research on the association between negative life events and weight loss (e.g., illness and stress) (20), there is little or none at present on positive life events that might facilitate such an outcome.

B. Population Factors

As noted above, the most striking correlate of population obesity prevalence overall is population affluence. It may be inferred, therefore, that changes in social and economic conditions that typically accompany population affluence contribute to population obesity. Likely factors are those that increase availability and affordability of a highly palatable diet and those that decrease requirements for physical exertion and increase the attractiveness of inactivity. The dramatic increases in obesity rates that have occurred in the last decade, for example, have been accompanied by equally dramatic trends in the availability of fast foods and of inactive forms of entertainment. The percentage of food dollars spent away from home increased by about 40% between 1980 and 1990 (21). Access to sedentary forms of entertainment through VCRs and cable television increased even more dramatically (22).

Substantial differences in obesity prevalence between relatively affluent populations may indicate that cultural influences may mediate or moderate the effects of affluence on obesity rates. Among developed societies, the United States has the highest obesity rates, Japan the lowest, with Western European countries in between. Comparisons of the diet and exercise habits in these countries suggest that Americans eat the least in total energy, exercise the least, and have the highest-fat diet. Differences in cultural values or traditions among these different countries may contribute to differing obesity rates. At present, the characterization and measurement of "culture" is not well developed.

IV. PREVENTION OF OBESITY IN CHILDREN

A. Treatment of High-Risk Youth

In many respects, treatment of obesity in children is always a form of obesity prevention. Overweight among children is one of the major risk factors for development of severe obesity in adulthood. Thus, treating obesity in children may prevent or delay adult obesity. The goal of obesity treatment in children is also different from that in adults. Whereas adult treatment focuses on weight loss, childhood treatment often targets the prevention of weight gain. Since children will experience increase in lean body mass as they age, keeping fat mass constant will often result in a normalization of body weight.

A search of the research literature on childhood obesity treatments for this chapter identified 20 controlled research studies that experimentally evaluated treatments for obesity in children or adolescents that had follow-ups of at least 6 months (23–42). Twelve of these were roughly in the preadolescent age group, ages 2–12, while the remainder were in adolescents, ages 12 and above.

All of the studies reviewed employed behavior modification methods to treat obesity. Treatment was typically conducted in groups that met weekly to receive education on diet and exercise behaviors. It also included training in behavioral techniques, such as goal setting, stimulus control, self-monitoring, and reinforcement of behavior changes. Most of the studies involved treatments in which parent involvement was required, especially in the preadolescent age group. With rare exception, program efficacy was evaluated in terms of changes in relative weight in relation to age, sex, and height-adjusted normative standards.

Short- and medium-term results of studies focusing on the preadolescent age group provide, as a whole, an optimistic perspective on the possibility of producing and sustaining reduction in relative weight in children. Percent reductions in relative body weight at 6–12 months following the initiation of the treatment ranged from 8 to 64%. The mean reduction in percent overweight across studies was 30%. Although untreated comparison groups were usually not followed for 6 months or more, the few studies

providing such data indicate that failure to treat results in either no change or an increase in percent overweight.

Results of weight loss studies in adolescents were also positive, although not as strongly so as those in young children. Two of the seven studies reviewed reported no significant treatment effect at 6 months or more. The remaining five reported modest reductions in relative weight at 6+ months. Possibly noteworthy is the observation that in treatment studies with adolescents weight regains between the end of treatment and 6–12 months appear similar in magnitude to those reported in adults (i.e., substantial regain is common). Many of the studies in preadolescents, by contrast, have observed relatively stable maintenance of reduced relative weight following the end of treatment.

It is difficult to arrive at clear recommendations about the optimal content of obesity treatment programs for children based on the heterogeneous research available to date. Two generalizations are ventured, however. First, on the basis of several studies that have explicitly tested variations on parental involvement, it appears that actively involving parents in treatment is important and beneficial. For preadolescents the preferred involvement mode seems to be as an active participant in all aspects of treatment of the child. For adolescents, a more distant support role may be more appropriate. Second, programs comparing treatment using behavioral methods (e.g., self-monitoring, goal setting, problem solving, and contingency management) have done better than those using a purely nutrition education format. Whether these better results are due to the skills being taught or to less specific factors, such as intensity or performance expectancy, is not as clear.

Epstein and colleagues have provided the only data bearing on the question of whether treatment of obesity in children reduces the burden of obesity in these children when they become adults (43). In an outstanding example of programmatic research, Epstein has followed up 158 children from four studies 10 years after their initial treatment. At the time of the initial treatment the children were 6–12 years of age, averaged 40–50% overweight, and had at least one obese parent. Thus, they were at high risk for significant obesity as adults. The studies involved different treatment conditions, but all involved group behavior modification presented intensively over an 8–12-week period, followed by monthly maintenance sessions over a 6–12-month period. Long-term results of these studies are quite encouraging. In six of nine actively treated groups, net change in percent overweight was between 10 and 20 percentage points. The three treatment groups that did not succeed long-term were one in which the children were treated without their parents, a second that employed a weak exercise program, and a third in which the children had a particularly strong family history of obesity. The only negative finding in Epstein's studies was a fairly high percent of children developing psychiatric disorders, although since treated and untreated subjects developed problems at similar rates, it seems unlikely that the treatment program contributed.

It is premature to make broad generalizations about the efficacy of obesity treatment in children. Nevertheless, the studies reviewed above give reason for optimism about the potential for comprehensive behavioral treatments to offer enduring benefits to obese children. A much needed research step would seem to be to conduct a longitudinal trial that evaluates whether results like those achieved by Epstein and colleagues can be replicated at other sites and in other populations, and whether tangible health benefits, in both health and social domains, can be demonstrated. Such a trial would be an important step in establishing a standard of care for prevention of adult obesity in a population at particularly high risk.

B. Population Approaches

Preventing obesity in children at the population level requires at least two elements that are absent in the clinical intervention studies reviewed above: (1) the ability to reach large numbers of both obese children and nonobese children at high risk, and (2) the ability to do so in a cost-effective manner. A logical setting for pursuing such objectives, and indeed the only one that has received research attention, is through the school system. In preparing this chapter, three published studies were located that specifically addressed treatment of high-risk (obese) children in the school systems, and three others were identified that addressed multiple health behaviors in schools and could, at least broadly, be considered as targeting obesity prevention. Each of these studies merits a brief description.

The earliest school-based obesity intervention study is one reported by Seltzer and Mayer (44). Between 1964 and 1967, 350 elementary and junior high school-aged children (ages 8–14) in a public school were identified as obese based on age- and sex-specific norms for tricep skinfold thickness and invited to participate in a school-based obesity intervention program over a period of 5–6 months. A total of 189 children chose to do so and 161 declined. The program was conducted during school hours and consisted of an intensive exercise and nutrition education program delivered over a 5–6-month period. Program efficacy was evaluated using a quasi-experimental design, comparing the rate of change in weight and skin-fold thickness among those who chose to participate in the program and those who declined. Outcome data were presented separately for elementary aged boys and girls and junior high school–aged girls. Statistically significant differences were observed as a function of the intervention in the elementary school boys and the junior high school girls. Increases in weight were lower in the treated than the untreated group. The elementary aged girls receiving the program also experienced weight changes in the desired direction compared to controls, but the difference is not statistically significant.

Christakis and colleagues also reported the results of a school-based program for obese adolescent boys, but with a stronger experimental design (45). A total of 390 high school freshmen, aged 13–14 years, were screened for obesity and 90 met entry criteria defined by height/weight standards. These adolescents were distributed across 10 classes. Six of the classes were assigned to a treatment condition ($n = 55$) and four classes were assigned to a no-treatment control group ($n = 35$). The intervention program was delivered after school over the entire school year and was comprised of biweekly nutrition education classes lasting about 15 min and an after-school exercise program and basketball league. Over 18 months of observation, subjects in the experimental condition reduced their percent overweight from 41% to 30%, whereas those in the no-intervention control condition changed from 40% at baseline to 37% at follow-up.

The third published report on interventions for obese school children was reported by Foster et al. (46). Eighty-nine children in grades 2–5 were identified as obese. Those in the experimental school were given a 12-week obesity management program comprised of counseling sessions three times per week and weekly nutrition education and exercise classes. After 30 weeks, the percent overweight of subjects from the treatment schools dropped from 32% to 28% and in the control school from 29% to 28%.

These three studies demonstrate that in-school intervention programs targeting high-risk children and adolescents can be successfully implemented and can reach substantial proportions of children in need of obesity prevention. Results over periods of 6–18 months are modestly encouraging and would seem to justify additional research in this area.

The strategy of obesity prevention addressed by previous studies was to target children who are at high risk of adult obesity. An alternative approach would be to provide obesity prevention interventions to all children, independent of their risk status. The rationale for this broader approach is that even though obese children represent a high-risk group, most people who will eventually become obese are not overweight as children. To date no research studies have evaluated interventions that are specifically targeted in this way. However, at least three have been conducted in the context of heart disease risk reduction and deserve attention because the behaviors they targeted are similar to those one would target in obesity prevention. Walter and colleagues recently reported the results of a multiple-risk-factor, school-based intervention involving 22 elementary schools in the Bronx, New York (47). Over a 1-year period an educational intervention was introduced into the school health curriculum that targeted prevention of smoking onset, increasing physical activity, and improving quality of diet. Evaluation data were derived from a population survey of schoolchildren before and after the intervention (n = 805 in education schools and 310 in control schools). Indices of obesity were sum of skinfold thickness and pounderosity index. Neither of these indices changed significantly between treated and untreated schools at 1 year, although the direction of the mean changes was in the hypothesized direction.

A second similar study involving children in grades 4–6 in nine schools in the Washington, D.C. area was recently published by Bush and colleagues (48). The intervention program was based on the same model as that in the New York study (the "Know Your Body Program"). Measures of obesity used in the study were skinfold thickness; relative body weight for age, sex, and height norms; and pounderosity index. The study was evaluated in a cohort of children over a 2-year period. Unfortunately, in this case the changes in all the measures of obesity showed greater weight gain in the treated than in the untreated children. The magnitude of the difference approached statistical significance (p = .07).

The largest and most comprehensive study of health risk behavior intervention in school children is that very recently completed under the title "Child and Adolescent Trial for Cardiovascular Health" (CATCH) (49). A total of 96 schools participated in this study beginning in the fall of 1991 and continuing to the spring of 1994. They were located in California, Louisiana, Minnesota, and Texas. Fifty-six schools were in the intervention condition and 40 in a usual care control condition. A comprehensive intervention for multiple-risk-factor reduction was conducted in the intervention schools for 3 years in grades 3–5. The intervention included modifying the school food service, enhancing the physical education curriculum to encourage activities involving greater energy expenditure, and an enhanced classroom health curriculum. In addition, half of the experimental schools had a family education component. The program targeted tobacco use, dietary fat, and physical activity. Obesity measures included body mass index (BMI), tricep skinfold, and subscapular skinfold. A total of 5106 children, in third grade at the beginning of the study, were tracked for 3 years. No significant differences between intervention and control conditions were observed for any of the obesity measures.

In summary, population-based efforts to prevent obesity in children have to date focus primarily on schools. These studies have shown that such interventions can reach large numbers of children in the schools at a reasonable cost. Those interventions that have been specifically obesity-focused and targeted obese children have shown positive short-term effects over periods of as long as 18 months. Broad-based programs of school health education that target multiple health behaviors, however, have so far not proved effective in reducing obesity in children. Further research in this area is clearly needed.

V. PREVENTION OF OBESITY IN ADULTS

A. Individual Intervention

Reviewing the success of intervention programs to prevent obesity in adults is relatively easy since to date there has been only one study published on this issue (50). Forster and colleagues sent invitation letters to 3000 normal-weight adults (relative weight ≤ 1.15) who had previously participated in a community health risk screening. Among those who could be reached, 25% expressed interest in participating in a study of weight gain prevention by completing and returning an invitation postcard. Of those returning postcards, 87% agreed to make personal appointments to consider study enrollment, and 60% of these actually enrolled (an overall response rate of 13%). The final sample was 29% male and averaged 46 years of age. Total enrollment was 219.

Study participants were randomized to a weight gain prevention treatment or to a no-contact control condition and followed for 1 year. The treatment was comprised of three elements. First, an informational newsletter about weight control practices was sent to study participants monthly. Second, a short course on weight control consisting of four nutrition education sessions was made available 6 months after enrollment. Third, subjects participated in an incentive program involving deduction of $10.00 from their bank account each month which could be redeemed by weighing in at the clinic (a State Health Department site) and verifying that they had not gained weight since study enrollment. Participation levels were reasonably high. Seventy-five percent returned postcards attached to each newsletter, 28% weighed in at the Health Department each month, and 29% attended the midyear short course on weight control. After 1 year, those in the treated group were found to have lost weight (about 1 kg), while the weights of control participants remained unchanged. The difference between these two was statistically significant ($p = .03$). Further subgroup analysis showed that the greatest treatment impact was among men, individuals over the age of 50, nonsmokers, and those with little prior experience with formal weight loss services. Results of this study suggest that low-intensity programs for preventing weight gain may be reasonably attractive to nonobese individuals, and that they may have a positive impact on body weight. The special nature of this population and the relatively short duration of this study, however, clearly indicate a need for more extensive research in this area.

B. Population Level Interventions

The U.S. government has been active in providing public health recommendations for weight control over many years, periodically publishing normative standards for weight in relation to height that are thought to promote optimal health and including prevention of obesity among recommendations for a healthy life-style. Although no formal evaluation of these efforts has been conducted, it is clear that the vast majority of the U.S. population recognizes that obesity is a health risk and that most who are overweight have done or are trying to do something about it (51). The net result of these efforts has, of course, not been very successful since the prevalence of obesity has risen. However, it is certainly conceivable that the situation might be worse without these educational messages. The social class gradient in obesity might also reflect, in part, the impact of these messages (i.e., those with higher levels of education and, thus, more access to health messages about obesity have been gaining weight at a lower rate than the less educated).

There have been no population-based research studies evaluating methods for specifically reducing the population burden of obesity. However, research in two areas bears to some extent on this issue. The first is worksite health promotion. Providing health education interventions in worksites has gained in popularity in recent years and attracted research attention. Although most studies in this area have been narrowly focused and of short duration, two published reports have provided information on the effects of these programs on body weight in entire working populations, including both those that are obese and those not obese. Rose and colleagues, as part of a large World Health Organization–sponsored study of heart disease risk reduction, conducted a worksite study among middle-aged men in 24 factories in Great Britain

(52). The study included 18,210 men, aged 40–59. The factories were matched in pairs on the basis of size, industry type, and region and randomized to receive intervention or no intervention for a period of 5 or 6 years. The intervention consisted of risk factor screening and personal physician follow-up for individuals at high risk for coronary disease as estimated from serum cholesterol, blood pressure, and smoking habits. Over 6 years of follow-up, changes in body weight were negligible in intervention and control worksites.

The second worksite study was conducted by Jeffery and colleagues in the United States between 1988 and 1990 (53). Thirty-two worksites, with a combined population of about 20,000, were randomized either to an intervention program that focused on both cigarette smoking and obesity or to a no-treatment control group. Weight loss classes were offered at intervention worksites on four occasions during a 2-year time span and were open to all employees independent of their initial body weight. About 20% of the employees overall and 40% of obese employees enrolled. Average weight losses of program participants were about 2 kg in the 6 months following enrollment. After 2 years, however, no differences were seen between treated and untreated worksites in the mean BMI or change in BMI over time of random samples of all employees.

In addition to these worksite studies, three large community-wide studies of heart disease risk reduction have also been completed recently in the United States that also speak to the issue of obesity prevention (54–56). These studies, one in California, one in Minnesota, and one in Rhode Island, used total communities as their population base and delivered sustained cardiovascular risk factor reduction education messages through multiple channels (e.g., news media, direct mail, public schools, worksites, health professional education, etc.) for periods ranging from 4 to 7 years. Primary emphasis was on cholesterol, blood pressure, and smoking, but obesity receives considerable attention because of its effects on the first two of these risk factors. An interesting aspect of these studies is that all were conducted during the 1980s, a time during which obesity prevalence rose dramatically across the country. All three programs were evaluated by population surveys that included both cross-sectional and cohort samples. All also used mean population BMI as their primary index of obesity. A brief summary of the results of these programs follows. In the Rhode Island community program the residents of the intervention community had significantly lower BMIs at baseline than those in the comparison community. Over a 6-year period, significantly less increase in BMI was observed in the treated community compared to the control community in cross-sectional analysis. No differences were seen in the cohort samples, however. The California study obtained a similar result. Both treated and control communities gained in obesity prevalence over time. The rate of gain was larger in the control than in the treated communities in cross-sectional analysis, but not in the cohort analysis. The Minnesota study observed substantial gains in obesity over 7 years of observation in treated as well as untreated communities. Between-community differences were not statistically significant.

In sum, evaluation of worksite and community-wide intervention efforts in adults provide little reason for optimism about the potential for public health education to reduce or reverse recent upward trends in obesity prevalence in the United States. Intervention effects have been inconsistent and small in magnitude, considerably smaller than would be needed to successfully counter recent secular trends. On the basis of these studies, it is tempting to conclude that educational approaches to preventing obesity at the population level are not likely to be effective. It should be kept in mind, however, that none of these efforts focused on obesity alone, which may have limited their impact on this outcome.

VI. ALTERNATIVE PUBLIC HEALTH PERSPECTIVES

The review of obesity prevention efforts presented above presents a fairly discouraging picture of the possibilities for successfully addressing this important public health problem. Before giving up on population approaches, however, it is well to keep in mind that virtually all population-based efforts to address obesity to date have proceeded from the premise that the problem stems from faults in people (i.e., their inability because of innate susceptibility and lack of knowledge or skill to deal effectively with an environment in which there are plentiful inducements to engage in behaviors that lead to a chronic positive energy imbalance). An alternative view is that the problem is not in people, but rather is in the environment. If modern environments promote the development of obesity, it may well be that changing the environment may be a more effective approach to obesity prevention than trying to improve human nature. The remainder of this chapter will address this issue.

Historically many of our most successful efforts to improve the health of the population have come from environmental strategies. One prime example is water sanitation to reduce population exposure to water-borne disease agents. Another is motor vehicle and roadway design standards that reduce the likelihood that human error will result in automobile accidents and mitigate the consequence of those that do occur. It is believed that similar approaches to environmental factors that encourage overeating and underexercise might make an important contribution to obesity prevention as well.

Outlined below are a range of public health intervention strategies that might be applied to the problem of obesity. Five general environmental protection strategies will be considered: improving the quality of food supply, improving access to physical activity, controlling advertising practices, economic incentives, and education.

1. *Improving the quality of the food supply.* It is widely recognized that the food supply available to people in industrialized societies has much abuse potential. Food products widely available at low cost are energy-dense, diverse, and highly palatable. Food environments, like those that humans are exposed to constantly, have been described by animal researchers as the "supermarket diet." The diet is obesity-promoting when presented to other species, an effect that is reversible by replacing the "supermarket diet" environment with a "lab chow" environment (57). Based on animal models, it is logical to assume that if obesity-promoting features of the human food supply were removed, the prevalence of obesity in human populations might also be reduced. The most direct method of improving food is collective regulation (i.e., by law) of commercially marketed foods. Such regulation could specify calorie density, fat content, sugar content, or other characteristics depending on which factors are most conducive to excess ad lib consumption. Research on this question is much needed.

2. *Improving access to physical activity.* Among the most widely cited reasons for people not to engage in regular physical activity is inconvenience. Transportation on foot or by bicycle is considered unsafe because our transportation systems are predominantly designed for automobiles, there are few inexpensive facilities to which people can go to pursue leisure-time physical activity, and the ability to make healthful choices, like taking stairs instead of elevators, is hampered because environmental engineers have designed structures that assume that sedentary choices will be preferred. Systematic public policies to address these access issues might facilitate increases in voluntary physical activity. Construction of more safe walking and bicycling areas, including perhaps banning motor vehicles entirely from some streets, might help; as might improving lighting at night, increasing security patrols, building more community recreation centers, and adopting construction standards for public buildings that take the desirability of having people take short flights of stairs (one or two stories) as a given rather than treating stairways as emergency exits only.

3. *Controlling advertising.* Most of the food and energy-saving devices purchased and consumed in the United States are actively promoted by those who produce them. Indeed, one of the obstacles faced by those who promote healthy eating and exercise through education is that a great deal more money is being spent to promote consumption of food products of questionable nutritional value and use of sedentary devices, such as TVs and VCRs, than is being spent to educate consumers about their potential hazards. Concern has frequently been raised about advertising practices, particularly those aimed at children (e.g., of high-sugar breakfast cereals). Public regulation of promotional practices for products that impact population energy balance is another potential environmental strategy to reduce population obesity. Specific regulatory strategies might include improved labeling of food products, limits on advertising to vulnerable audiences (e.g., children), and perhaps nutrition warning labels. Promotion of sedentary activities like watching television might also be limited, analogous to restrictions placed on advertising tobacco products.

4. *Economic incentives.* Taxation policies have a history of use to discourage the consumption of dangerous products. Tobacco and alcohol are currently subject to substantial excise taxes, which have been demonstrated to influence consumption. In the area of food, it is well known that food consumption patterns are highly sensitive to price. Thus, excise taxes on foods with high abuse potential would seem to be a logical way to address population dietary patterns. One way to think about taxation policy with regard to food would be to focus on nutrient constituents that increase palatability and/or energy content (i.e., fat and sugar). Taxing food products in proportion to their fat and sugar content would have the effect of discouraging their use. Similar strategies could also be applied to encourage energy expenditure. A general increase in taxation rates on energy (e.g., on gasoline and electricity) might encourage changes in transportation and recreation patterns that use more human energy. Taxing specific uses of energy that contribute to sedentariness might also be feasible (e.g., making TV access entirely fee-for-service and taxing the service at rates that would encourage more selective usage). Revenues generated by taxation policies on undesirable habits could also be used to reduce the cost of desirable ones.

5. *Education.* Education has been, and always will be, an important public health strategy. In connection with environmental policy, it is suggested that public health education needs not only to inform people about what behaviors are good for them as individuals, but also about what they might do collectively to make it easier for them to engage in those behaviors. Obesity is clearly a problem that has lent itself to victim blaming. It is important that the public recognize that even though the behaviors necessary to prevent or correct obesity are known, there are individual differences in susceptibility to poorer behavioral choices and that the expression of this susceptibility depends on an environment that potentiates it. The food and exercise opportunities present in our environment are a collective responsibility and collective action is critical to determining the degree of exposure to obesity-promoting conditions. The relationship between the population exposure and obesity prevalence needs to be understood in the same way that infectious disease rates and population exposure to infectious pathogens are understood.

VII. SUMMATION

Prevention of obesity as a relatively new area of exploration. However, as the population prevalence of obesity rises and we better recognize the limitations of clinical treatment options, the idea of obesity prevention becomes more attractive. Early work on prevention strategies has used educational approaches. Results have been most promising in young children (i.e., treating obesity in preadolescents as a means of reducing obesity as adults). Prevention of weight gain in adults is an area that needs more attention. The effect of environmental conditions on population obesity rates is a little-studied aspect of the overall problem. More serious attention needs to be given to this area if a broad understanding of the causes of and preventive strategies for obesity is to be achieved.

ACKNOWLEDGMENT

Preparation of this chapter was supported by NIH Grants DK45361, HL41332, and DK50456.

REFERENCES

1. Kuczmarski RJ, Flegal KM, Campbell SM, Johnson CL. Increasing prevalence of overweight among US adults: the National Health and Nutrition Examination Surveys, 1960 to 1991. JAMA 1994; 272(3):205–211.
2. Forbes GB, Retina JC. Adult lean body mass declines with age: some longitudinal observations. Metabolism 1970; 19: 653–663.
3. Hartz AJ, Rimm AA. Natural history of obesity in 6,946 women between 50 and 59 years of age. Am J Public Health 1980; 70(4):385–388.
4. Hamm P, Shekell RB, Stamler J. Large fluctuations in body weight during young adulthood and twenty-five-year risk

of coronary death in men. Am J Epidemiol 1989; 129(2): 312–318.

5. French SA, Jeffery RW, Folsom AR, Williamson DF, Byers T. Weight variability in a population-based sample of older women: reliability and intercorrelation of measures. Int J Obes 1995; 19:22–29.

6. French SA, Jeffery RW, Folsom AR, McGovern P, Williamson DF. Weight loss maintenance in young adulthood: prevalence and correlations with health behavior and disease in a population-based sample of women aged 30–69 years. Int J Obes 1996; 20:303–310.

7. West KM. Epidemiology of adiposity. In: Vague J, Boyer J, eds. The Regulation of the Adipose Tissue Mass. New York: American Elevier, 1973:201–207.

8. Sobal J, Stunkard AJ. Socioeconomic status and obesity: a review of the literature. Psychol Bull 1989; 105(2):260–275.

9. Bouchard C, Perusse L. Heredity and body fat. Annu Rev Nutr 1988; 8:259–277.

10. Williamson DF, Kahn HS, Byers T. The 10-y incidence of obesity and major weight gain in black and white US women aged 30–55 y. Am J Clin Nutr 1991; 53: 1515S–1518S.

11. Shah M, Jeffery RW. Is obesity due to overeating and inactivity, or to a defective metabolic rate? A review. Ann Behav Med 1991; 13(2):73–81.

12. Prentice AM, Black AE, Coward WA, et al. High levels of energy expenditure in obese women. Br Med J 1986; 292: 983–987.

13. Romieu I, Willett WC, Stampfer MJ, Colditz GA, Sampson L, Rosner B, Hennekens CH, Speizer FE. Energy intake and other determinants of relative weight. Am J Clin Nutr 1988; 47:406–412.

14. Wing RR, Kuller LH, Bunker C, Matthews K, Caggiula A, Meihlan E, Kelsey S. Obesity, obesity-related behaviors and coronary heart disease risk factors in black and white premenopausal women. Int J Obes 1989; 13:511–519.

15. Waxman M, Stunkard AJ. Caloric intake and expenditure of obese boys. J Pediatr 1980; 96(2):187–193.

16. French SA, Jeffery RW, Forster JL, McGovern PG, Kelder SH, Baxter JE. Predictors of weight change over two years among a population of working adults: the Healthy Worker Project. Int J Obes 1994; 18:145–154.

17. Harris JK, French SA, Jeffery RW, McGovern PG, Wing RR. Dietary and physical activity correlates of long-term weight loss. Obes Res 1994; 2(4):307–313.

18. Rauschenbach B, Sobal J, Frongillo Jr. EA. The influence of change in marital status on weight change over one year. Obes Res 1995; 3(4):319–327.

19. Smith DE, Lewis CE, Careny JL, Perkins LL, Burke GL, Bild DE. Longitudinal changes in adiposity associated with pregnancy: the CARDIA Study. JAMA 1994; 271:1747–1751.

20. Greeno CG, Wing RR. Stress-induced eating. Psychol Bull 1994; 115(3):444–464.

21. Kinsey JD. Food and families socioeconomic status. J Nutr 1994; 124:1878S–1885S.

22. Salvaggio JL, Bryant J, eds. Media Use in the Information Age: Emerging Patterns of Adoption and Consumer Use. Hillsdale, NJ: Lawerence Erlbaum Associates, 1989.

23. Aragona J, Cassady J, Brabman RS. Treating of obese children through parental training and contingency contracting. J Appl Behav Anal 1975; 8(3):269–278.

24. Brownell KD, Kelman JH, Stunkard AJ. Treatment of obese children with and without their mothers: changes in weight and blood pressure. Pediatrics 1983; 71(4):515–523.

25. Coates TJ, Jeffery RW, Slinkard LA, Killen JD, Danaher BG. Frequency of contact and monetary reward in weight loss, lipid change, and blood pressure reduction with adolescents. Behav Ther 1982; 13:175–185.

26. Coates TJ, Killen JD, Slinkard. Parent participation in a treatment program for overweight adolescents. Int J Eating Disord 1982; 1(3):37–48.

27. Epstein LH, Wing RR, Koeske R, Andrasik F, Ossip DJ. Child and parent weight loss in family-based behavior modification programs. J Consult Clin Psychol 1981; 49(5):674–685.

28. Epstein LH, Wing RR, Koeske R, Ossip D, Beck S. A comparison of lifestyle change and programmed aerobic exercise on weight and fitness changes in obese children. Behav Ther 1982; 13:651–665.

29. Epstein LH, Wing RR, Koeske R, Valoski A. A comparison of lifestyle exercise, aerobic exercise, and calisthenics on weight loss in obese children. Behav Ther 1985; 16: 345–356.

30. Epstein LH, Wing RR, Koeske R, Valoski A. Effects of diet plus exercise on weight change in parents and children. J Consult Clin Psychol 1984; 52(2):429–437.

31. Epstein LH, Wing RR, Penner BC, Kress MJ. Effect of diet and controlled exercise on weight loss in obese children. J Pediatr 1985; 107(3):358–361.

32. Epstein LH, Wing RR, Woodall K, Penner BC, Kress MJ, Koeske R. Effects of family-based behavioral treatment on obese 5-to-8-year-old children. Behav Ther 1985; 16: 205–212.

33. Graves T, Meyers AW, Clark L. An evaluation of parental problem-solving training in the behavioral treatment of childhood obesity. J Consult Clin Psychol 1988; 56(2): 246–250.

34. Israel AC, Solotar LC, Zimand E. An investigation of two parental involvement roles in the treatment of obese children. Int J Eating Disord 1990; 9(5):557–564.

35. Israel AC, Stolmaker L, Andrian CAG. The effects of training parents in general child management skills on a behavioral weight loss program for children. Behav Ther 1985; 16:169–180.

36. Israel AC, Stolmaker L, Sharp JP, Silverman WK, Simon LG. An evaluation of two methods of parental involvement in treating obese children. Behav Ther 1984; 15:266–272.

37. Kingsley RG, Shapiro J. A comparison of three behavioral programs for the control of obesity in children. Behav Ther 1977; 8:30–36.

38. Mellin LM, Slinkard LA, Irwin CE. Adolescent obesity intervention: validation of the SHAPEDOWN program. J Am Diet Assoc 1987; 87(3):333–338.

39. Mendonca PJ, Brehm SS. Effects of choice on behavioral treatment of overweight children. J Soc Clin Psychol 1983; 1(4):343–358.

40. Wadden TA, Stunkard AJ, Rich L, Rubin CJ, Sweidel G, McKinney S. Obesity in black adolescent girls: a controlled clinical trial of treatment by diet, behavior modification, and parental support. Pediatrics 1990; 85(3):345–352.

41. Weiss AR. A behavioral approach to the treatment of adolescent obesity. Behav Ther 1977; 8:720–726.

42. Wheeler ME, Hess KW. Treatment of juvenile obesity by successive approximation control of eating. J Behav Ther Exp Psychiatry 1976; 7:235–241.

43. Epstein LH, Valoski A, Wing RR, McCurley J. Ten-year outcomes of behavioral family-based treatment for childhood obesity. Health Psychol 1994; 13(5):373–383.

44. Seltzer CC, Mayer J. An effective weight control program in a public school system. Am J Public Health 1970; 60(4): 679–689.

45. Christakis G, Sajecki S, Hillman RW, Miller E, Blumenthal S, Archer M. Effect of a combined nutrition education and physical fitness program on the weight status of obese high school boys. Fed Proc 1966; 25:15–19.

46. Foster GD, Wadden TA, Brownell KD. Peer-led program for the treatment and prevention of obesity in schools. J Consult Clin Psychol 1985; 53(4):538–540.

47. Walter HJ, Hofman A, Connelly PA, Barrett LT, Kost KL. Primary prevention of chronic disease in childhood: changes in risk factors after one year of intervention. Am J Epidemiol 1985; 122(5):772–781.

48. Bush PJ, Zuckerman AE, Theiss PK, Taggart VS, Horowitz C, Sheridan MJ, Walter HJ. Cardiovascular risk factor prevention in black schoolchildren: two-year results of the "Know Your Body" Program. Am J Epidemiol 1989; 129(3): 466–482.

49. Luepker RV, Perry CL, McKinlay SM, Nader PR, Parcel GS, Stone EJ, Webber LS, Elder JP, Feldman HA, Johnson CC, Kelder SH, Wu M. Outcomes of a field trial to improve children's dietary patterns and physical activity: the Child and Adolescent Trial for Cardiovascular Health (CATCH). JAMA 1996; 275:768–776.

50. Forster JL, Jeffery RW, Schmid TL, Kramer FM. Preventing weight gain in adults: a pound of prevention. Health Psychol 1988; 7(6):515–525.

51. French SA, Jeffery RW. Consequences of dieting to lose weight: effects on physical and mental health. Health Psychol 1994; 13(3):195–212.

52. Rose G, Heller RF, Pedoe HT, Christie DGS. Heart disease prevention project: a randomised controlled trial in industry. Br Med J 1980; 1:747–749.

53. Jeffery RW, Forster JL, French SA, Kelder SH, Lando HA, McGovern PG, Jacobs DR, Baxter JE. The Healthy Worker Project: a work-site intervention for weight control and smoking cessation. Am J Public Health 1993; 83(3): 395–401.

54. Taylor CB, Fortmann SP, Flora J, Kayman S, Barrett DC, Jatulis D, Farquhar JW. Effect of long-term community health education on body mass index. Am J Epidemiol 1991; 134(3):235–249.

55. Jeffery RW. Community programs for obesity prevention: the Minnesota Heart Health Program. Obes Res 1995; 3(Suppl 2):283s–288s.

56. Carleton RA, Lasater TM, Assaf AR, Feldman HA, McKinlay S, and the Pawtucket Heart Health Program Writing Group. The Pawtucket Heart Health Program: community changes in cardiovascular risk factors and projected disease risk. Am J Public Health 1995; 85(6):777–785.

57. Danforth E. Diet and obesity. Am J Clin Nutr 1985; 41: 1132–1145.

41

Classification and Evaluation of the Overweight Patient

George A. Bray

Pennington Biomedical Research Center, Louisiana State University, Baton Rouge, Louisiana

I. CLINICAL CLASSIFICATION OF OVERWEIGHT

Overweight and obesity are frequently used interchangeably. However, overweight refers to weight above some standard and obesity to excess body fat. One of the most widely used ways of assessing overweight is the body mass index (BMI) (kg/m²), which will be used throughout this chapter. The criteria for evaluating body fat are not as well established as for overweight. When overweight is sufficiently great, however, i.e., a BMI above 30 kg/m², obesity and overweight are almost always congruent. In this chapter, obesity will be categorized in several ways and guidelines for its evaluation will be outlined.

A. Historical Approaches to Classifying Obesity

Table 1 summarizes some of the approaches that have been proposed as ways of classifying obesity during the 20th century. Several themes run through these classifications. Some classifications are largely anatomical or deal with fat distribution (1–5). Others emphasize etiological or pathophysiological considerations (6–16). The classification used in the present discussion is a combination of these approaches but also extends them to include the associated risks.

B. Proposed Classification

The classification that will be used in this chapter has four components:

1. The anatomical characteristics of adipose tissue and fat distribution
2. The age at onset of obesity
3. Etiological factors in the development of obesity
4. Associated risks

Each component will be considered in more detail below.

II. ANATOMICAL CHARACTERISTICS OF ADIPOSE TISSUE AND FAT DISTRIBUTION

An anatomical classification of obesity can be based on the number of adipocytes, on the regional distribution of body fat, or on the characteristics of localized fat deposits.

A. Number of Fat Cells

The number of fat cells can be estimated when there is a measure of total body fat and an estimate of average fat cell size (17,18). Because fat cells differ in size from one region to another (19,20), a reliable estimate of the total number of fat cells should be based on the average of fat cell sizes from more than one location. In adults, the upper limit of normal fat cell number ranges from 40 to 60×10^9 cells (21). The number of fat cells increases most rapidly during late childhood and puberty but may increase even in adult life (22). The number of fat cells can increase by 3–5 times normal when obesity occurs in childhood or adolescence. Hypercellular obesity shows

Table 1 Historical Classifications of Obesity

Author	Year	Ref.	Proposed classification
Noorden	1900	1	Exogenous
			Endogenous
Bauer	1923	2	Rubens' type
			Breeches' type
			Fat over upper half of body
			Fat over lower half of body
Zondek	1926	3	Alimentary (gluttony)
			Endocrine (thyroid, pituitary, genital, pineal, pancreatic
			Localized (lipomatosis)
Jarlov	1932	4	Hypertrophic–diffuse
			Plethoric
			Myxematoid
			Lipomatoid
Rony	1940	5	Specific forms (hypothalamic, pituitary, adrenal)
			Essential
			Mixed
Vague	1947	6	Gynoid
			Android
Bruch	1957	7	Developmental
			Reactive
			Normal obesity
Stunkard	1955	8	Binge eating
	1959	9	Night eating
Mayer	1960	10	Genetic
			Metabolic
			Regulatory
Kemp	1966	11	Childhood
			Early adult life
			Pregnancy
			Middle life
Hirsch and Knittle	1970	12	Hypercellular
			Hyperplastic
Bray and York	1971	13	Genetic
			Hypothalamic
			Dietary
			Physical inactivity
			Endocrine
Garrow	1982	14	Grade 1: BMI < 25
			Grade 2: BMI 25–29.9
			Grade 3: BMI 30–39.9
			Grade 4: BMI > 40

varying degrees of enlargement of fat cells. This type of obesity usually begins in early or middle childhood, but may also occur in adult life. An increased total number of fat cells is usually present in individuals who are more than 75% above their desirable weight (21). Hypertrophic obesity tends to correlate with an android or truncal fat distribution and is often associated with metabolic disorders such as glucose intolerance, hyperlipidemia, hypertension, and coronary artery disease (23–26).

B. Fat Distribution

Fat distribution can be estimated by a variety of techniques including skinfold, circumference, or sophisticated methods employing ultrasound, computed tomography (CT), or magnetic resonance imaging (MRI). The ratio of the waist circumference to the circumference of the hips was the technique used in the pioneering studies of Kissebah et al. (27), Lapidus et al. (28), and Larsson et al. (29), which brought international recognition to a relationship originally suggested by Vague (25). The subscapular skinfold has also served as a valuable tool to estimate central fat in epidemiological studies (30,31). A more sophisticated technique to evaluate skinfold uses principal-component analysis of skinfold at several sites on the body (32,33). The principal-components analysis groups together those skinfolds that are best correlated and gives an estimate of total fat, central fat, and peripheral fat. More recent data have shown that the most reliable estimates of visceral fat can only be made by CT or MRI scans (34,35). Using CT scan data in relation to lipids, Pouliot et al. (34) have shown that the waist circumference alone is as good as either the sagittal diameter or the ratio of the waist circumference to the hip circumference. Waist

Table 1 Continued

Author	Year	Ref.	Proposed classification
Bouchard	1995	15	Excess body mass or percent fat
			Excess subcutaneous truncal-abdominal fat (android
			Excess abdominal visceral fat
			Exceel gluteo-femoral fat (gynoid)
Bray		16	Anatomical
			Age at onset
			Etiological
			Associated risks

circumference alone and waist circumference divided by hip circumference will be used later in this chapter.

C. Localized Deposits of Fat

There are several kinds of localized fat accumulations, including single lipomas, multiple lipomas, liposarcomas, and idiopathic accumulations of fat. The lipomas vary in size from 1 cm to more than 15 cm. They can occur in any region of the body and represent encapsulated accumulations of fat. Multiple lipomatosis is an inherited disease transmitted as a dominant trait. von Recklinghausen's syndrome, the Mafucci syndrome, and Madelung's disease are examples.

Liposarcomas are relatively rare, representing less than 1% of the lipomas. They have a predilection for the lower extremities and consist of four types: well-differentiated myxoid type; poorly differentiated myxoid type; round cell or adenoid type; and mixed type.

Weber-Christian disease and Dercum's disease are both idiopathic accumulations of fat. Dercum's disease, also called adiposis dolorosa, is named after the painful nodules in the subcutaneous fat of middle-aged women. Weber-Christian disease, on the other hand, is a relapsing febrile disease occurring in younger women. All of these forms of localized fat deposits are relatively rare (36).

III. AGE AT ONSET OF OBESITY

Obesity can begin at any age. Birth weight of children who will become obese later in life has nearly the same frequency distribution as birth weight of those who will maintain normal weight in later life (36,37). The first appearance of obesity is in infancy, when body fat rises rapidly. During the first year of life the size of fat cells increases nearly twofold, but there is no measurable increase in the number of fat cells (38,39). Birth weight has a low, but significant, correlation with weight at ages 6–11 (40) and at age 14 (41).

A second period during which childhood obesity begins is between the ages of 4 to 11 years (42). When obesity appears in this age group, there can be a progressive deviation of body weight from the upper limits of normal for height. I call this progressive obesity (36). This type of obesity is usually lifelong and is associated with an increase in the number of fat cells.

A. Childhood Onset of Obesity

Obesity in childhood and adolescence may be related to subsequent obesity and risks of ill health. A prospective British study has followed individuals for over 36 years (43). At age 36, 3322 individuals from the cohort of 5362 individuals born in March 1946 were interviewed and subdivided into weight categories, using the BMI: 5.3% of the men and 8.4% of the women were severely overweight (BMI greater than 30 kg/m^2) and 38.0% of the men and 24.2% of the women were overweight (BMI of 25–29.9 kg/m^2). The correlation between BMI at age 26 and 36 was $r = 0.64$ for men and $r = 066$ for women. From these studies, the authors draw several important conclusions. First, there is a subgroup of about 25% of individuals who were obese in both childhood and adult life. Second, the remaining 75% of obese 36-year-olds first became obese in adult life and could not be predicted from weight before age 20. Those individuals who became obese between age 11 and 36 were often not the most overweight in childhood. Only 50–60% of men and women in the top decile for weight at age 36 could be correctly predicted at age 26 using all the socioeconomic, demographic, and weight data available. Several studies suggest that childhood weight status predicts risk for cardiovascular disease later in life (44–46). In a 55-year follow-up of adolescents into late adult life, Must et al. (46) found that the weight status in adolescence predicted later adverse health risks.

B. Adult-Onset Obesity

1. Females

Most obesity in females develops after the end of puberty. Estimates from several sources have suggested that less than one-third of the obese adults were obese in childhood (36). For women, the central event is pregnancy. The woman who becomes pregnant will be heavier 2 years after the pregnancy than the woman who was not pregnant (47), but this effect is variable. Williamson et al. (48) conclude that the risk of weight gain associated with childbearing after age 25 is quite modest for American women. However, there are a few women for whom pregnancy is a time of major weight gain, with reports of weight increasing more than 50 kg (48,49). For fetal outcome, the optimal weight gain for normal weight women is 10–12 kg. As the body weight increases, the optimal weight gain to minimize fetal loss declines; for women who are more than 50 kg above desirable weight, a weight gain of 6–8 kg is optimal for fetal survival (50). Weight loss during pregnancy is never desirable.

A second event that may trigger obesity in some women is the use of estrogen/progesterone containing oral contraceptives. As the dose of estrogen/progesterone in these preparations has declined, this may be less of a problem.

A third period of weight gain and change in fat distribution in women is menopause. At this time the decline in estrogens and progesterone alters fat cell biology to increase central fat deposition (51).

2. Males

For many men, the transition from the active lifestyle associated with the teenage years to a more sedentary lifestyle in early adult years is associated with weight gain. There is clear evidence from the Framingham study and from the physical examinations done by the military that men have become progressively heavier for height during this century (52). A rise in body weight continues through adult years until the sixth decade. After age 55–64, relative weight remains stable, and then begins to decline in both sexes.

IV. ETIOLOGICAL FACTORS IN OBESITY

There are a number of etiological causes for obesity (53). Table 2 lists the forms of obesity that are primarily environmental at the top and those that are primarily genetic at the bottom. There is, of course, some overlap.

A. Iatrogenic Causes

1. Medications

Several drugs can lead to an increase in body weight (Table 3) (54). Phenothiazines are among the most common drugs that increase body fat. One study found that on admission to a mental institution men averaged 5 lb less than "desirable" weight for their height. They gained 7 lb during an average stay of 35 months. The use of phenothiazines played a particularly important role in this weight gain. Amitriptyline is a tricyclic antidepressant that is especially likely to produce weight gain. Cyproheptadinee (Periactin) has been shown to increase food intake in human subjects, without an alteration in metabolism. Glucocorticoids are widely used in treating chronic immunological diseases, and one of the side effects of this treatment is weight gain, similar to that seen in Cushing's syndrome (55). Estrogens alone or in birth control pills have been reported to produce weight gain (56). Progestins are more likely than estrogens to increase weight. Megestrol acetate (Megase) is a progestational agent used in women with breast cancer to increase appetite and induce weight gain (57). Valproate is an antiepileptic drug that acts on the NMDA (GABA) receptor (58). It produces weight gain in more than half of the subjects who receive it. Lithium, which is used in treating depression, has also

Table 2 An Etiological Classification of Obesity

A. Iatrogenic causes
  1. Medications
  2. Hypothalamic surgery (neuroendocrine)
B. Sedentary life-style
  1. Enforced inactivity (postoperative)
  2. Aging
C. Dietary obesity
  1. Infant feeding practices
  2. Progressive hyperphagic obesity
  3. Frequency of eating
  4. High fat
  5. Overeating
  6. Tube feeding
  7. Night eating syndrome
  8. Binge eating
D. Neuroendocrine obesities
  1. Hypothalamic syndrome
  2. Cushing's syndrome
  3. Hypothyroidism
  4. Polycystic ovary (Stein-Leventhal) syndrome
  5. Pseudohypoparathyroidism
  6. Hypogonadism
  7. Growth hormone deficiency
  8. Insulinoma and hyperinsulinism
E. Social and behavioral factors
  1. Socioeconomic factors
  2. Ethnicity
  3. Psychological factors
  4. Restraint and disinhibition
  5. Seasonal affective disorder
F. Genetic (dysmorphic) obesities
  1. Autosomal recessive traits
  2. Autosomal dominant traits
  3. X-linked traits
  4. Chromosomal abnormalities

Table 3 Drugs Associated with Weight Gain

1. Phenothiazines (chlorpromazine)
2. Tricyclic antidepressants (amitriptylline)
3. Cypropeptadine (Periactin)
4. Glucocorticoids
5. Progestagens (megestrol acetate)
6. Valproate
7. Lithium
8. Insulin
9. Sulfonylureas

been implicated in weight gain. Finally, insulin and sulfonylureas can also increase body weight (59).

There is a large body of data about weight gain, increased food intake, and hunger following cessation of cigarette smoking, suggesting that nicotine may reduce food intake (60).

2. Hypothalamic Surgery

Surgery in the posterior fossa may be associated with obesity postoperatively if there is damage to critical regions in the ventromedial hypothalamus. This is discussed in more detail below.

B. Sedentary Life-Style

Obesity in rats can be produced by restriction of activity. In the modern affluent society, energy-sparing devices also reduce energy expenditure and may enhance the tendency to become fat. In one clinical study the onset of obesity was associated with inactivity in 67.5% of the patients. In epidemiological studies the highest frequency of overweight men was found in the groups with sedentary occupations. Recent estimates of energy intake and energy expenditure in Great Britain by Prentice and Jebb (61) suggest that reduced energy expenditure is more important than increased food intake since both have been declining but at different rates. Likewise, Dutch data showed that in middle-aged men the decline in food intake was not as fast as the decline in energy expenditure accounting for almost all of their weight gain (62). In the Surgeons General's report of Physical Activity, the percent of adult Americans participating in physical activity decreases steadily with age (63). Reduced energy expenditure in adults (64) and children (65,66) is predictive of weight gain. These observations suggest the importance of shifting patterns of physical activity in the regulatory systems controlling the storage, distribution, and utilization of calories.

C. Diet and Obesity

The composition of the diet is another etiological factor in obesity. This is particularly prominent in experimental animals (53) but may also play a role in the development of human obesity. When rodents eat a high-fat diet (67), drink sucrose containing solutions (68), or eat a cafeteria type of diet (69), most strains are unable to regulate energy balance appropriately and ingest more energy than is needed for weight maintenance. The excess energy is accumulated as fat and the animals become obese to variable degrees.

1. Infant Feeding Practices

Infant feeding practices have also been related to obesity. Infants fed an artificial formula were significantly heavier than expected from height and weight tables, whereas breast-fed infants showed a smaller weight gain. Studies on the weight gain and milk intake of infants during the first 112 days of life (70) showed that the bottle-fed infants at the 10th percentile for birth weight were similar in weight to breast-fed infants at all ages up to 112 days. However, infants at the 90th percentile for birth weight who were fed by bottle were heavier and longer at 112 days of age than those who were breast-fed. When bottle-fed infants were divided into two groups, one fed formula that contained 67 kcal/100 ml and another fed formula that provided 133 kcal/100 ml, the infants receiving the more concentrated formula drank less than the other group. Of particular interest was the gain in body weight. During the first 6 weeks the infants receiving the more concentrated formula ingested more calories each day and gained more weight. It is this same period of life that some authors think is predictive of obesity in children at age 6. However, other researchers cannot find any relation between the rate of weight gain in children and whether as infants they received early nutrition from a bottle or from the breast.

2. Progressive Hyperphagic Obesity

In a small number of people whose obesity begins in childhood, the progressive weight gain is unrelenting. In my experience these individuals have usually surpassed 150 kg (330 lb) by age 30. They show a remarkably consistent pattern of weight gain year after year. Once calculated, this increment provides a good prognostic yardstick. One man I saw first at age 44 weighed 200 kg (440 lb). He had gained 4.5 kg (10 lb) almost every year of his life. Since his energy requirements were rising year by year, so must his intake of nutrient energy rise year by year. This is a clear case of hyperphagic progressive obesity.

3. Frequency of Eating and Obesity

The relationship of the frequency of eating to the development of human obesity remains unsettled. It has been observed clinically that obese individuals frequently eat fewer meals than normal-weight people, but this is a difficult point to document. Direct evidence on the relationship of obesity to the frequency of food intake was obtained in a survey of 379 men aged 60–64 (71). The men who ate one or two meals per day were heavier, had thicker skinfolds, had higher levels of cholesterol, and frequently had impaired glucose tolerance as compared to men who ate three or more meals per day. This finding was confirmed in a study of schoolchildren: those children who were fed only three meals per day tended to gain more weight than the children eating five to seven meals per day.

The frequency of eating also changes the metabolism of glucose and the concentration of cholesterol. When normal volunteers ate several small meals a day, they had lower concentrations of cholesterol than when the same total intake was eaten in a few large meals (72,73). This reduction of cholesterol with frequent ingestion of small meals has been confirmed many times. Glucose tolerance curves are also improved when eating three or more meals as compared with one or two large meals. In one laboratory study (74) six severely obese patients were fed a 5000-calorie diet for 8 weeks. During one 4-week period the calories were divided into 20 small meals, and during the other 4 weeks they were eaten as one large meal. The period with one large meal was associated with more rapid formation of fat as measured by incorporation of carbon from glucose into fatty acids in adipose tissue (74). Of the enzymatic changes that were studied, the only one that showed a significant alteration during the rapid food ingestion was the cytoplasmic glycerol-3-phosphate dehydrogenase. This contrasts with the numerous enzymatic changes that have been observed in the adipose tissue of rats trained to eat large meals rather than to nibble.

4. Dietary Fat and Obesity

Several types of studies have examined the relationship of dietary fat in humans to the development of obesity (75). Many, but not all, population studies have found associations (76) (Table 4). Intervention studies, on the other hand, have suggested that reducing dietary fat intake can have modest effects on weight loss (Table 5). The rising prevalence of obesity in different countries is unlikely due to an increase in fat intake since total fat, if anything, has decreased.

5. Overeating and Tube Feeding

Voluntary overeating, i.e., repeated ingestion of energy in excess of daily energy needs, has been seen in a variety of settings. When healthy volunteers consciously overeat to gain weight, they have invariably lost the excess weight when the study is over (77–79). This contrasts with the Japanese sumo wrestlers. These men eat large quantities of food twice a day for many years along with a very active training schedule. Their visceral fat is remarkably low for their total weight. When their active career ends, they rarely lose weight but tend to remain heavy but with in-

creased percent fat and a high probability of developing diabetes.

In animals, excess quantities of energy provided by tube feeding will produce weight gain. This technique has been used in rodents (80–82) and in dogs (83) to evaluate the consequences of obesity and study its mechanisms.

6. Night-Eating Syndrome

The night-eating syndrome was described by Stunkard et al. (10) and is present in individuals who consume at least 25% and more usually 50% of their energy intake after the evening meal. The problem is related to sleep disturbances and may be a component of sleep apnea where daytime somnolence and nocturnal wakefulness are common.

7. Binge-Eating Disorder

The binge-eating disorder is included in the 4th edition of the *Diagnostic and Statistical Manual of Mental Disorders* (DSM-IV). It refers to the uncontrolled episodes of eating that usually occur in the evening. Binge-eating disorder may respond well to treatment with drugs that modulate serotonin release or reuptake.

D. Neuroendocrine Obesities

1. Hypothalamic Obesity

Hypothalamic obesity is a rare syndrome in humans (84) but can be regularly produced in animals by injury to the ventromedial or paraventricular region of the hypothalamus or the amygdala (53). These regions of the brain are responsible for integrating metabolic information about nutrient stores with afferent sensory information about availability of food. When the ventromedial hypothalamus is damaged, hyperphagia develops and obesity follows. Two syndromes can be identified in animals; one is due to damage of the paraventricular nucleus (PVN), which results in hyperphagia. Food restriction prevents this obesity (85). The second syndrome, due to damage of the ventromedial nucleus (VMN), occurs without hyperphagia but is associated with altered activity in both parts of the autonomic nervous system (53). The increased secretion of insulin associated with the change in hypothalamic function and autonomic balance may be one pathogenetic link in its development (86). Experimental animals with this syndrome have enlarged islets of Langerhans and hyperinsulinemia. The rise of plasma insulin occurs immediately after injury to the ventromedial hypothalamus and precedes any fall in glucose. If the rise in insulin is prevented by destroying the beta cells of the pancreas,

Table 4 Associations Between Obesity and Fat Intake

Ref.	Subjects	Method of measurement		Association of fat intake with obesity
		For obesity	For fat intake	
Lissner (1987)	4583 males	% body fat calculated from skinfold	24-hr recall	+
	4703 females (NHANES2)			+
Dreon et al (1988)	155 males	BMI	7-day food record	+
		% body fat (densitometry)		+
Romieu et al. (1988)	141 females	BMI	Four 1-week weighed food records at 3-month intervals	+
Tremblay et al. (1989)	244 males	Weight	3-day food record	n.s.
	244 males	Trunk skinfold		+
	244 males	Extremity skinfold		n.s.
	133 males	Fat mass (densitometry)		+
George et al. (1990)	344 males	BMI	3-day food record	+
	335 females			+
	191 males	% body fat (densitometry)		n.s.
	169 females			n.s.
Miller et al. (1990)	107 males	% body fat (densitometry)	Dietary history plus 2-day food record	+
	109 females			+
Colditz et al. (1990)	31,940 females	BMI	Food frequency questionnaire (Harvard Willett instrument)	+
Tucker and Kano (1992)	205 females	BMI	NCI food questionnaire (Block)	+
		Skinfolds		+
Slattery et al. (1992)	5115	BMI	Diet-history questionnaire (CARDIA)	n.s
	Males			n.s.
	White			
	Black			—
	Females			n.s.
	White			
	Black			
Pudel and Westenhoefer (1992)	$n = 20,6415$ overweight males and females	BMI	7-day food diary	+
Klesges et al. (1992)	142 males, yr 1	BMI	Food frequency questionnaire (Harvard Willett instrument)	+
				+
				+
	yr 2			n.s.
				+
	yr 3			+
	152 females, yr 1			
	yr 2			
	yr 3			
Lissner and Lindroos (1994)	412 women	BMI	24-hr recall + diet history	n.s.
Lindroos, Lissner, and Sjostrom (unpublished)	138 nonobese vs. 181 severely obese women	BMI <28 vs. >32	SOS dietary questionnaire	+

BMI = body mass index (kg/m^2); n.s. not significant.
Source: From Ref. 75.

Table 5   Randomized Dietary Fat Intervention Studies Without Energy Restriction

Investigators	Intervention group (n)	Change in % fat	Intervention period	Weight loss kg	Weight loss g/day
Puska et al. (1983)	35	39 → 23	6 weeks	0.7	17
Sheppard et al. (1991)	184	39.2 → 20.9	9 months	3.2	18
Hunninghake et al. (1993)	97	41 → 26	9 weeks	1.4	22
Kazim et al. (1993)	34	36 → 18	3 months	3.4	38
Levitsky and Strupp (1994)	28	37 → 27	6 weeks	0.9	22
Shah et al. (1994)	47	33.8 → 21.0	6 months	4.4	24

Source: From Ref. 75.

thereby making animals diabetic, hyperphagia is markedly reduced and the animals do not become obese (87). The connection between the ventromedial hypothalamus and the secretion of insulin appears to be through both the vagus and the sympathetic nerves (87). Transection of the vagus nerves prevents the hyperphagia and obesity that usually occur after injury to the ventromedial hypothalamic nuclei (88). Further demonstration of this mechanism comes from studies that showed an increased firing rate of the vagus nerve (89). Conversely, the firing rate of sympathetic nerves is decreased (90). These disturbances in the function of the autonomic nervous system may play an important etiological role in this syndrome (53).

Hypothalamic obesity is produced in human beings by trauma, malignancy, inflammatory disease, or increased intracranial pressure with pseudo tumor cerebri producing pressure on the ventromedial hypothalamus (84). The clinical features that accompany this syndrome are listed in Table 6. These symptoms can be divided into three groups. The first are related to changes in intracranial pressure and include headache and diminished vision due to papilledema. The second group of symptoms are manifestations of endocrine alterations and include impaired reproductive function with amenorrhea or impotence, diabetes insipidus, and thyroid or adrenal insufficiency. The third group of symptoms are a variety of neurological and physiological derangements including convulsions, coma, somnolence, and hypothermia or hyperthermia. Treatment of the syndrome requires treating the underlying disease and giving appropriate endocrine support (84).

2. Cushing's Disease

Cushing's syndrome is the endocrine disease most often associated with obesity. This syndrome includes weight gain, hypertension, glucose intolerance, hirsutism, amenorrhea, plethora, and fullness of the face (91). It can result from hyperplasia of the adrenal glands when they are stimulated by excess ACTH from the pituitary, from an ACTH-secreting or CRH-secreting tumor, or from injections of ACTH. Excess corticosteroids may also be produced by an adenoma or carcinoma of the adrenal or may be given as treatment for other diseases. The pattern of weight gain in Cushing's syndrome is characteristic (92). Fat is accumulated on the trunk, in the supraclavicular fossa, and over the dorsal posterior cervical region. The arms and legs are usually spared. The development of obesity as a manifestation of Cushing's syndrome is most striking in children. In this age group linear growth stops and fat accumulates rapidly. In one obese child, with adrenal hyperplasia, removal of the adrenals was followed by return of body weight to normal. Because Cushing's

Table 6   Clinical Features Among 77 Patients with Hypothalamic Obesity Due to Tumors

Feature	Number[a] (%)
Pressure symptoms	50 (65%)
Headache	
Impaired vision	49 (64%)
Endocrine symptoms	39 (52%)
Impaired reproductive function	
Diabetes insipidus polyuria or polydipsia	24 (31%)
Impaired growth	7 (9%)
Neurological and physiological symptoms	5 (6%)
Convulsions	
Somnolence	28 (36%)
Behavioral changes	15 (19%)

[a]Number of patients with each symptom (85).

disease is a curable form of obesity, its differential diagnosis requires careful attention. Effective treatment of Cushing's disease lowers cortisol and body fat is redistributed (92).

3. Hypothyroidism

Hypothyroid patients frequently gain weight and some of this is fat. Conversely, hyperthyroidism enhances catabolism and leads to loss of fat and lean body mass.

4. Polycystic Ovary Syndrome

The syndrome of polycystic ovaries, originally described by Stein and Leventhal, may be a combination of hypothalamic and endocrine obesity. The complex consists of reduced or absent menses and of moderate hirsuitism and weight gain, which usually develops in young women shortly after menarche (93). These women are often infertile and markedly insulin-resistant. Menstruation and fertility can frequently be restored by wedge resection of the ovary. The anovulatory state is associated with increased LH relative to FSH. Increased testosterone production is common and may be a response to IGF-1, which acts on the ovary because its binding protein IGFBP-1 is low. Hypersecretion of adrenal steroids, which is often observed in these patients, may be caused by several factors. The complex of hyerphagia, hypofunction of the gonads, and hyperfunctioning of the pituitary-adrenal system is reminiscent of some of the defects observed in experimental animals with obesity, particularly the yellow obese mouse in which obesity, mild hyperglycemia, and enlarged adrenal glands develop at or just after puberty.

5. Pseudohypoparathyroidism

Patients with pseudohypoparathyroidism have round facies and are overweight. The adipose tissue from these patients has reduced activity of the G-α form, which may be involved in their mild obesity (94).

6. Hypogonadism

Castration in males removes the primary source of testosterone and body fat increases. Testosterone treatment reduces body fat and increases protein and lean tissue (95).

7. Growth Hormone and Prolactin

Growth hormone affects body fat and fat distribution (96). Its deficiency is associated with increased body fat, and replacement doses of growth hormone significantly reduce body fat and decrease visceral fat. Conversely, removal of a growth hormone-secreting adenoma is followed by a fall in growth hormone levels and a decrease in total body fat, with a large amount being visceral.

Impaired prolactin secretion has been reported in up to 15% of obese individuals and may provide one basis for classifying obese patients. Prolactin is an important hormone for fat metabolism in birds and may be involved to a minor degree in humans.

8. Hyperinsulinism

Shortly after the discovery of insulin it was noted that its use could lead to increased body weight and body fat. This was quantitated most recently when type I diabetics were tightly controlled with insulin (59). The spontaneous hypersecretion of insulin that occurs in insulinoma can also increase body weight, but the effect is usually small.

E. Social and Behavioral Factors

1. Socioeconomic Factors

Obesity in the United States, as well as elsewhere, is more prevalent in the lower socioeconomic groups. Using a scale of 12 to divide socioeconomic groups, Goldblatt et al. (97) were the first to show that among the highest socioeconomic groups (i.e., the most educated and affluent) only 4% were overweight, whereas in the lowest socioeconomic groups 36% were overweight. These effects are most prominent in women. Similar conclusions have been drawn from data gathered by the National Center for Health Statistics (98). There was significantly more obesity, as assessed by skinfold thickness, in the lower socioeconomic groups. The importance of social factors can also be seen in children. Overweight children were detected among first graders from the lower socioeconomic groups but there were no overweight children from the highest socioeconomic groups at this age. When overweight did appear, it was less prevalent in children from the higher social classes than in those from the lower classes.

2. Ethnicity

Ethnicity influences obesity (98). Black males were consistently less obese than white males, whereas black women showed a consistently higher prevalence of obesity at all ages than white women. Both black and white males in the lower income levels had a higher prevalence of obesity than black or white males in the higher income levels. The effects of income levels in women produced a more complex picture. Among older women, both black and white, lower income was associated with a lower prevalence of obesity. For younger women, the relationship was not clear-cut. In some age groups obesity was more prevalent in women from the lower income groups, but not in all. Hispanics in most categories had higher prevalence rates than Caucasians.

3. Psychological Factors

Psychological factors in the development of obesity are widely recognized, but attempts to define a specific personality type in association with obesity have been unsuccessful. Much of the early work on the psychological factors of obesity came from studies of single patients who had undergone intensive psychiatric analysis. Formulations based on these cases were tantalizing and tended to focus on the oral features of the obese patient as an important variable in the development of this syndrome. A review of psychological factors in obesity indicates several different approaches to the problem. One of them comes from the extensive studies of Bruch (99). She identifies three types of obesity. The first she called "reactive obesity." It results from ingestion of excess food as an emotional reaction to situations in the environment. According to Bruch (99), this abnormality is a reflection of inappropriate responses to the feeding situation during growth and development of the child. The second type of obesity she calls "developmental obesity." In these individuals, emotional problems are minimal. The third type she labels "normal" obesity. From an analysis of profiles on the Minnesota Multiphasic Personality Inventory (MMPI) and the Thematic Apperception Test (TAT), certain features stood out forming what has been labeled the obese trait. Depression was common but not severe. Ingestion of food had frequently been used to reduce the feelings of emotional deprivation that had been present since early childhood and were historically associated with unstable marriages in the family of many of these patients. Such characteristics as stubbornness, defiance, the need for autonomy, and wariness of entangling relationships, as well as conflicts over exhibitionism, were prominent features in the personality structures of these patients. These characteristics contribute to the traditional reputation of the obese as "difficult" patients.

4. Restraint and Disinhibition

Restrained eating is an important feature in many normal-weight women. It indicates that a level of "cerebral" control can be exercised to control the wishes for food. Stunkard and Messick have modified the questionnaire of Herman and Polivy to provide a 3 Factor Eating Questionnaire. In addition to restraint, this questionnaire identifies eating due to hunger and to "disinhibition." Disinhibition is loss of control. In our clinic most older women

showed some element of restraint (100). The presence or absence of restraint may account for some of the differences in prevalence rates for obesity associated with socioeconomic status. Almost all of the obese women in our clinic showed low disinhibition or loss of control over their eating.

5. Seasonal Affective Disorder

Seasonal affective disorder (SAD) is identified among some individuals living above the 45th parallel. It is seasonal depression that occurs during the "winter" season and can be treated by exposure to light during this time of year. Individuals who have SAD tend to have a seasonal fluctuation in body weight, which can be effectively treated with drugs that modulate serotonin release or reuptake.

F. Genetic Causes of Obesity

Genetic factors play a role in the onset of obesity. This influence is of two types. The first are genes or chromosomal abnormalities that are primary factors in the development of obesities. I have called these conditions "dysmorphic obesity." The second type of effect is through genes that modulate the interaction with environmental factors such as diet, exercise, and drugs.

1. Rare Genetic Syndromes or Dysmorphic Obesities

There are a group of rare diseases, often with associated dysmorphic features, in which genetic factors are of primary importance. A comparison of several of these syndromes is shown in Table 7.

Prader-Willi Syndrome. The Prader-Willi Syndrome (PWS) is among the most common of the dysmorphic forms of human obesity. It is characterized by obesity, hypotonic musculature, mental retardation, hypogonadism, short stature, and small hands and feet (101).

Reduced intrauterine fetal movements, hypotonia at birth, and typical facies raised the possibility that this syndrome might be genetic. The Prader-Willi syndrome has been concordant in two sets of monozygotic twins and discordant in several sets of dizygotic twins. It has also been reported in siblings on several occasions as well as in first cousins, but consanguinity has been rare (101). Deletions or translocations involving the short arm (q1.2) region of chromosome 15 have been reported in 50% or more of these individuals. Transmission of PWS occurs from the male due to a chromosomal defect. When this defect is transmitted on maternal chromosome 15, Angle-

Table 7 A Comparison of Syndromes of Obesity—Hypogonadism and Mental Retardation

Feature	Syndrome				
	Prader-Willi	Bardet-Biedl	Ahlstrom	Cohen	Carpenter
Inheritance	Chromosomal defect from father with imprinting	Autosomal recessive	Autosomal recessive	Probably autosomal recessive	Autosomal recessive
Stature	Short	Normal; infrequently short	Normal; infrequently short	Short or fall	Normal
Obesity	Generalized Moderate to severe Onset 1–3 years	Generalized Early onset, 1–2 years	Truncal Early onset, 2–5 years	Truncal Midchildhood, age 5	Truncal Gluteal
Cranofacies	Narrow bifrontal diameter Almond-shaped eyes Strabismus V-shaped mouth High arched palate	Not distinctive	Not distinctive	High nasal bridge Arched palate Open mouth Short philtrum	Acrocephaly Flat nasal bridge High arched palate
Limbs	Small hands and feet Hypotonia	Polydactyly	No abnormalities	Hypotonia Narrow hands and feet	Polydactyly Syndactyly Genu valgum
Reproductive status	1° hypogonadism	1° hypogonadism	Hypogonadism in males but not in females	Normal gonadal function or hypogonadotropic hypogonadism	2° hypogonadism
Other features	Enamel hypoplasia Hyperphagia Temper tantrums Nasal speech	Congenital heart disease; nephropathy	Acanthosis nigricans; baldness	Dysplastic ears Delayed puberty	
Mental retardation	Mild to moderate		Normal IQ	Mild	Slight

man's syndrome, is the result. This syndrome includes more severe mental retardation, but no obesity. This gender effect is attributed to imprinting that differentially inactivates one of the chromosomes (102). The prevalence of PWS is between 1 per 10,000 and 1 per 30,000 births. The likelihood of the sibling of a proband having PWS is between 1.4 and 1.6%. Miscarriages may also be increased and the syndrome occurs in all races.

The cardinal clinical features of PWS are summarized in Table 8 (101). Most patients with PWS are short and have an adult height that averages 150 cm (59 in.) in girls and 155 cm (61 in.) in boys. Body weight is increased to a mean of 80 kg in girls and 98 kg in boys. Affected individuals are mentally retarded but the degree of this retardation is highly variable. Emotional problems including temper tantrums are well known (103). Scoliosis has been observed in many patients, but bone age is usually the same as the chronological age or only slightly retarded.

Advanced dental caries and hypoplastic enamel have been observed, as has dysplasia of the hip. The profound hypotonia present at birth usually improves somewhat during the first 2 or 3 years of life.

Diabetes mellitus has been described in a number of patients with PWS (101). Two deaths from diabetes in patients with PWS have been reported. The diabetes is of the non-insulin-dependent type (type II), but at least one individual has developed ketoacidosis. Diabetes has appeared as early as 2 1/2 years of age, and the development of microaneurysms has been reported. It thus seems clear that there is an increased incidence of diabetes mellitus in individuals with PWS but that a major part of this results from their obesity.

Hypogonadism and cryptorchidism are characteristic features of PWS (101). The penis is usually small and other components of the male reproductive system are also small but present. Histological examination of the testis shows immaturity without germinal cells, but with Sertoli cells and diminutive tubules. Menarche and menstruation have both been reported and precocious puberty has been noted in several clinics (101). These reports of precocious pubertal development may represent a variant of PWS in which the hypothalamic-pituitary-gonadal axis functions normally with premature onset of menarche; however, there is an alternative explanation for this phenomenon. The initial phases of sexual development are produced by adrenal steroids and thus are called the "adrenarche." Among these changes are development of pubic hair, budding of the breasts, and the beginnings of axillary hair. This is normally followed by production of ovarian estrogen and completion of the sequence. In patients with PWS, adrenal function is adequate to permit the adrenarche to appear. Production of estrogen by aromatization in adipose tissue of androstenedione may be increased due to the increased amount of fat. It is conceivable that breakthrough bleeding, occurring in a partially estrogenized uterus, might be interpreted as menstruation. It would be more likely to occur in the more obese girls with PWS. The hyperphagia, hypogonadism, and short stature have suggested a hypothalamic problem, but careful histological examination of the brain by routine methods has failed to show any lesions. Attempts to treat these patients by blockade of opioid receptors with naloxone (104) or pancreatic polypeptide (105) have been unsuccessful.

Several reports of autopsy findings provide a little insight into the nature of the problem in PWS. However, great strides have been made in the identification of the genetic defect (102). Two imprinted genes have been identified. One is the SNRPN gene, which encodes the SmN protein involved in mRNA splicing. The second is a novel zinc finger protein encoded by the gene ZNF127. The expression of these genes in the paternal chromosome is associated with DNA methylation.

The Bardet-Biedl Syndrome. The Lawrence-Moon and Bardet-Biedl syndromes are often considered together, but represent distinct entities (106–108) (see Table 7). In 1866, Lawrence and Moon described four patients with retinal degeneration of the pigment cells, mental retardation, hypogenitalism, and a neurological defect characterized as spastic paraplegia (109). Obesity was present in two, spastic paraplegia in one, and ataxia in two but digital anomalies were absent. Nearly 60 years later, Bardet, in his doctoral thesis, described a syndrome consisting of retinitis pigmentosa, obesity, and polydactyly (110). Two years later, Biedl independently described two patients with additional findings of genital hypoplasia, mental retardation, and anal atresia (111). Although often grouped together, the Bardet-Biedl and Lawrence-Moon syndromes

Table 8 Clinical Findings in the Prader-Willi Syndrome

Gestation	Poor fetal vigor	84%
	Breech presentation	38%
	Nonterm delivery	33%
Neonatal and infancy	Low birth weight	100%
	(<5 lb)	90%
	Hypotonia	90%
Central nervous system	Mental retardation	100%
	Seizures	20%
	Personality problems	71%
Growth	Obesity	100%
	Short stature	90%
	Delayed bone age	90%
Facies	Strabismus	95%
Limbs	Small hands and feet	100%
Sexual development	Cryptorchidism (males)	100%
	Hypogenitalism (males)	100%
	Menstruation	33%

Source: From Ref. 102.

differ in a number of important ways and are considered as separate entities. Both are inherited as autosomal recessive traits and the defect has been associated with chromosomes 3, 11, 15, and 16 (112,113). Pigmentary retinopathy is present in the Lawrence-Moon syndrome and tapetoretinal degeneration in the Bardet-Biedl syndrome. Spastic paraplegia is present in the Lawrence-Moon syndrome but does not occur in the Bardet-Biedl syndrome. Obesity occurs earlier in persons with the chromosome 15 variant and those with chromosome 16 variant are the leanest (113). Croft et al. (114) have suggested that carriers of the BB gene may be more susceptible to obesity. Polydactyly is rare in the Lawrence-Moon syndrome. In addition, the Bardet-Biedl syndrome may be associated with congenital heart disease and nephropathy, which has been reported to be as high as 71% in one autopsy series (115).

Alstrom-Hallgren Syndrome. Obesity, blindness in childhood, sensory nerve deafness, and diabetes mellitus characterize the Alstrom-Hallgren syndrome, which has some similarities to the Bardet-Biedl syndrome (116) (see Table 7). The absence of polydactyly and mental retardation and the presence of nerve deafness and diabetes mellitus help separate these conditions. The obesity usually begins between ages 2 and 10 years and body weight ranges between 116% and 230% of "ideal." The obesity subsided in 3 of 10 patients in one report when they reached adult-

Table 9 Form for Recording Clinical and Laboratory Data

Identifying number:	_____
Today's date:	_____
Name:	_____
Age:	_____
D.O.B.	_____
Height (in or cm)	_____
Weight (lb or kg)	_____
BMI (kg/m²)	_____
Waist circumference (in or cm)	_____
Hip circumference (in or cm)	_____
$\frac{\text{Waist circumference}}{\text{Hip circumference}}$ (WHR)	_____
Weight gain since 18 (lb or kg)	_____
Duration of obesity	_____
Age at onset	_____
Blood pressure (mmHg)	_____
Triglycerides (mg/dL or mM)	_____
HDL cholesterol (mg/dL or mM)	_____
Fasting glucose (mg/dL or mM)	yes/no
Sleep apnea	_____
Etiological factor (if known)	_____

hood. Acanthosis nigricans, baldness, hypogonadism, and growth deficiency may also be features (117).

Cohen Syndrome. The cardinal features in cases of the Cohen syndrome are hypotonia, truncal obesity, mental retardation, and a characteristic craniofacial appearance, characterized by a high nasal bridge, high arched palate, short philtrum, small jaw, and a characteristic open mouth (118–121) (see Table 7). The obesity is truncal and begins in midchildhood, i.e., approximately 5 years of age. Delayed puberty is present but there is normal gonadal function or in some cases hypogonadotropic hypogonadism. Mental retardation is only mild. This syndrome is probably inherited as an autosomal recessive trait and may involve a chromosomal translocation between chromosomes 5 and 7 (122). Friedman and Sack have raised the possibility that it may have a higher prevalence among Ashkenazi Jews (120).

Carpenter Syndrome. The Carpenter syndrome belongs to the wider entity known as acrocephalopolysyndactyly. It is rare and transmitted as an autosomal recessive trait (123) (see Table 7). The characteristics of this syndrome include craniosynostosis with peculiar facies and apparent exophthalmos. Dysmorphic features include a flat nasal ridge, low-set ears, retrognathism, a high arched palate, and partial syndactyly with brachymesophalangy (124).

X-Linked Obesity. Several reports have documented cases of X-linked obesity usually in association with severe degrees of mental retardation (125–129). Borjeson et al. (125) reported an X-linked, recessively inherited form of obesity, with severe mental retardation, hypogonadism with low or normal levels of gonadotropin, and short stature. Most of these patients have coarse facial features with large ears and microcephaly. In 1979 Vasquez et al. reported an X-linked type of obesity with profound mental retardation, true gynecomastia, and short stature with many other features similar to PWS, except for the mode of inheritance and the normal size of the hands and feet (126). Subsequently Young and Hughs reported four patients with X-linked mental retardation with short stature, obesity, and hypogonadism in one family (127). Seizures were present in three of the four individuals and mental tests revealed an IQ of approximately 25. Gonadotropins were high in these individuals and testosterone, measured in one case, was low. Persons with these X-linked forms associated with obesity seem to have more severe mental retardation than reported in the other forms of dysmorphic obesity.

V. CLINICAL EVALUATION OF THE OBESE PATIENT

Assessment of the obese patient requires both clinical and laboratory techniques. The information collected can be used to characterize the type of obesity and to provide a basis for making recommendations about treatment. It can also aid in understanding the natural history and prognosis of obesity. This section is intended to provide the framework in which to collect the desired information and a rationale for its collection. The approach is predicated on the assumption that there are many types of obesity with differing degrees of associated risk (130). Some types of obesity can be separated from one another and the relative risks identified. The importance of guidelines for evaluating the obese patient has increased as the number of potential treatments has increased. Several reports have been prepared to help give guidelines for this evaluation. These reports come from the American Obesity Association (131), the American Association of Clinical Endocrinologists (132), the International Obesity Task Force (133), and the Scottish Intercollegiate Guideline Network (134).

A. Overweight and Obesity

A form to record some important clinical and laboratory data is presented in Table 9. Accurate measurement of

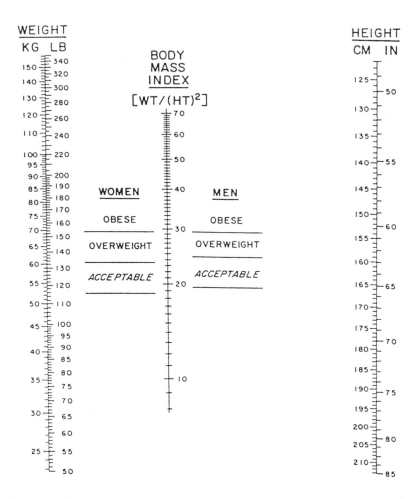

Figure 1 Nomogram for determining body mass index. To use this nomogram, place a ruler or other straight edge between the body weight in kilograms or pounds (without clothes) located on the left-hand line and the height in centimeters or in inches (without shoes) located on the right-hand line. The body mass index is read from the middle of the scale and is in metric units. (Copyright 1978, George A. Bray. Used by permission.)

height and weight is currently the initial step in the clinical assessment of overweight. The most practical way to evaluate the degree of "overweight" is with the BMI (Table 9). This index is calculated as the body weight (kg) divided by the stature [height (m)) squared (wt/(ht)²] and can be obtained from the nomogram in Figure 1 or Table 10. The BMI is correlated with body fat and is relatively unaffected by height. Overweight is defined as a BMI between 25 and 30 kg/m², and obesity as a BMI above 30 kg/m². The BMI shows a curvilinear relation to risk (Fig. 2). From this figure several levels of risk can be identified. These cutpoints are largely derived from data collected on Caucasians. The extent to which they apply to other ethnic groups is not yet clear. Data on Hispanic and African-Americans suggest that increased body fat produces a

greater risk of diabetes, but less impact on heart disease or hypertension.

B.   Regional Fat Distribution

Visceral fat and central fatness can be evaluated by several methods. The most accurate are the CT or MRI scan but these are expensive and are used primarily in research settings. A simple waist circumference and the ratio of waist circumference divided by the hip circumference (WHR) are good clinical alternatives. The waist circumference is measured with a flexible tap placed in a horizontal plane at the level of the natural waistline or narrowest part of the torso as seen from the anterior view. The hip circumference is measured in the horizontal plane

Table 10 A Table of Body Mass Index (BMI) Values

BMI ▶ Height	Good weights								Increasing risk					
	19	20	21	22	23	24	25	26	27	28	29	30	35	40
							Weight (pounds)							
4'10"	91	96	100	105	110	115	119	124	129	134	138	143	167	191
4'11"	94	96	104	109	114	119	124	128	133	138	143	148	173	198
5'	97	102	107	112	118	123	128	133	138	143	148	153	179	204
5'1"	100	106	111	116	122	127	132	137	143	148	153	158	185	211
5'2"	104	109	115	120	126	131	136	142	147	153	158	164	191	218
5'3"	107	113	118	124	130	135	141	146	152	158	163	169	197	225
5'4"	110	116	122	128	134	140	145	151	157	163	169	174	204	232
5'5"	114	120	126	132	138	144	150	156	162	168	174	180	210	240
5'6"	118	124	130	136	142	148	155	161	167	173	179	186	216	247
5'7"	121	127	134	140	146	153	159	166	172	178	185	191	223	255
5'8"	125	131	138	144	151	158	164	171	177	184	190	197	230	262
5'9"	128	135	142	149	155	162	169	176	182	189	196	203	236	270
5'10"	132	139	146	153	160	167	174	181	188	195	202	209	243	278
5'11"	136	143	150	157	165	172	179	186	193	200	208	215	250	286
6'	140	147	154	162	169	177	184	191	199	206	213	221	258	294
6'1"	144	151	159	166	174	182	189	197	204	212	219	227	265	302
6'2"	148	155	163	171	179	186	194	202	210	218	225	233	272	311
6'3"	152	160	168	176	184	192	200	208	216	224	232	240	279	319
6'4"	156	164	172	180	189	197	205	213	221	230	238	246	287	328

The health risk from any level of BMI is increased if you have gained more than 11 lb since age 25 or if you have a waist circumference above 40 in. (100 cm) due to central fatness.
Source: Adapted from Ref. 16.

at the level of maximal circumference including the maximum extension of the buttocks posteriorly. A nomogram is shown in Figure 3 and the risk range in Figure 4.

Table 11 indicates how to establish risk from waist circumference and WHR, along with the way to adjust BMI (134). The waist circumferences for men and women that are equivalent to waist-hip ratio values for low, moderate, and high risk are presented. As with BMI, the relationship of central fat to risk factors for health varies between populations as well as within them. The Japanese-Americans and Indians from South Asia living in London have more visceral factors and are at higher risk than Caucasians living in the same region. Thus, the risk assigned to the waist circumference or WHR in Table 11 must be tempered by the group to which it will be applied. Even though the BMI is below 25, central fat may be increased, and thus, adjustment of BMI for central fat is particularly important in the BMI range 22–29.

C. Etiological Factors and Age of Onset

The presence of etiological factors and the age at which obesity began should be identified if possible. These have

been described in detail above and should be recorded if they can be identified.

D. Associated Risks

1. Age

A patient's age is important in determining the risk from obesity. In my view, age 40 is the dividing line. The risk for a given degree of obesity seems to be greater in people below 40 years of age than in those above 40 years of age, probably because of the longer time period over which it can act.

2. Weight Gain Since Age 18

Weight gain since age 18 increases risk at all levels of BMI (135). A weight gain of >5 kg is of concern and a weight gain of more than 15 kg adds significantly to risk. A way to adjust the BMI is also shown in Table 12.

3. Duration of Obesity

Duration of obesity may also be important and may influence the associated risks.

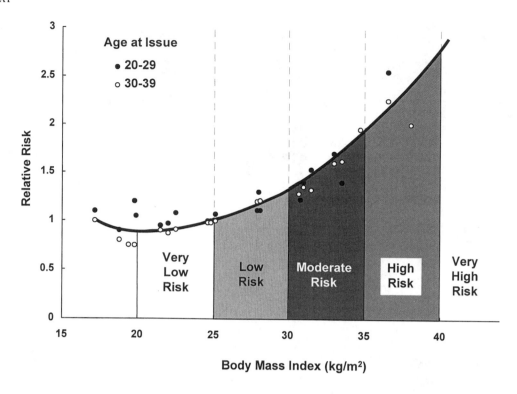

Figure 2 Mortality ratio and body mass index. Data from the Life Insurance Study have been plotted for men and women to show relationship of body mass index to overall mortality. At a body mass index below 20 kg/m² and above 25 kg/m² there is an increase in relative mortality. The major causes for this increased mortality are listed along with division of body mass index groupings into various levels of risk. (Copyright 1987, George A. Bray. Used by permission.)

4. Metabolic Risks

Evaluation of the metabolic risks associated with obesity is important from both a clinical and prognostic point of view. It is well established that the obese have an increased frequency of high blood pressure, diabetes mellitus, and coronary artery disease. This highlights the importance of delineating the presence of any cardiac risk factors such as hypertension, hyperlipidemia, glucose intolerance, and history of cigarette smoking. Menstrual disorders, including irregular bleeding and amenorrhea, are common among obese females. From puberty onward, women are fatter than men, and women tend to gain more fat during adult life than men. Yet women have a lower risk associated with any degree of extra body fat (26). This may be explained partly by differences in fat distribution. In one study an extra 20 kg of fat was needed for women to show the same impairment in glucose tolerance as in men (26). Moreover, men and women with similar fat distribution have similar risk (136). Obesity is associated with osteoarthritis but the role of excess body weight in its etiology remains controversial. Morbid obesity can compromise pulmonary function and cause sleep apnea. The sleep ap-

nea syndrome (Pickwickian syndrome) is often associated with obesity and is improved by weight loss. Therefore, it is important to find out about these functional impairments and to measure blood pressure, HDL cholesterol and triglyceride levels, and blood glucose. If history warrants, evaluation of the gall bladder by ultrasound and measurement of pulmonary function may be performed. Finally, obese people have been found to suffer from psychological and social problems and these should be identified. Body image may be severely distorted in people with childhood-onset obesity and obese people may be discriminated against in school and the workplace. A prospective study from Denmark showed that obese military recruits had attained a much lower social class status than lean recruits after an average 12.5 years of follow-up.

E. Algorithms

To evaluate an obese patient, three algorithms have been developed. The first algorithm will help identify etiological factors (Fig. 5). Use of the algorithm is straightforward. Questions begin in the upper left hand corner and proceed via the appropriate arrows. At each point a positive answer to the question leads to suggestions for workup. For example, once the presence of overweight has been established, the possibility of hypertension is addressed. If hypertension is present, the physician is directed to search for clinical signs of Cushing's syndrome. If these are present, a urinary free cortisol test is recommended to be followed by dexamethasone suppression if indicated; if they are not, a hypertension workup is suggested. In turn, the algorithm directs the physician to search for clinical clues of hypothyroidism, glucose intolerance, hyperlipidemia, hypoventilation syndrome, CNS lesions, polycystic ovarian syndrome, and congestive heart failure. Acanthosis nigricans deserves a brief comment. This is a clinical condition with increased pigmentation in the folds of the neck, along the exterior surface of the distal extremities, and over the knuckles. It may signify increased insulin resistance, and this should be evaluated. At each point, suggestions for further workup are given when appropriate.

Once the workup for etiological and complicating factors is complete and BMI, body fat distribution, sex, and age are recorded, the physician is referred to Figure 6 for risk classification. The algorithm shown in Figure 6 is used to determine the degree of risk associated with a given BMI. Body mass is divided into five unit intervals beginning at 25 kg/m². As BMI increases, the level of risk increases. Because any given level of BMI provides only one assessment of risk, the BMI needs to be adjusted up or down based on the presence or absence of associated risks.

A method for adjusting the BMI for other risk is shown in Tables 11 and 12 and the strategy for treatment based on this adjustment is shown in the algorithm in Figure 7. Table 11 provides the adjustment scores for central fat distribution using either waist circumference or waist/hip circumference ratio and the comments about ethnic variability cited above. Using either waist circumference or WHR, identify BMI adjustment and note it on the appropriate line on Table 12. Table 12 also provides the basis for adjusting BMI for each of several other metabolic and clinical variables related to obesity. The scores for each are recorded on the right hand side and added to the patient's BMI at the bottom to obtain the adjusted BMI.

When the adjusted BMI is determined, the overall risk assessment and treatment goals can be obtained from Figure 7. This algorithm divides adjusted BMI into five unit intervals. The risk, goals, and potential strategies for treatment are noted opposite each of these intervals. Low levels of the comorbid risks reduce the impact of any level of BMI whereas high levels of comorbid risk factors augment the effect of the BMI. With the adjusted BMI it is then

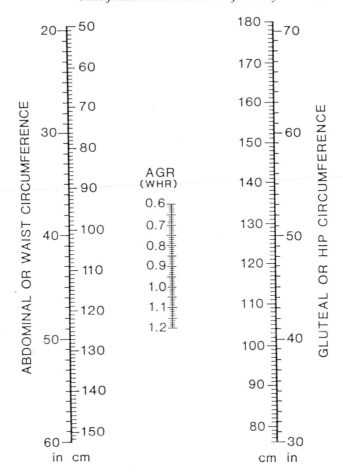

Figure 3 Nomogram for determining abdominal (waist) to gluteal (hips) ratio. Place a straight edge between the column for waist circumference and the column for hip circumference and read the ratio from the point where this straight edge crosses the AGR or WHR line. The waist or abdominal circumference is the smallest circumference below the rib cage and above the umbilicus, and the hips or gluteal circumference is taken as the largest circumference at posterior extension of the buttocks. (Copyright 1987, George A. Bray. Used by permission.)

possible to select or rank-order the treatments that are available.

Before initiating any treatment, it is important to establish that the patient is ready to make changes. When using these guidelines for the patient who is ready to lose weight, it is essential to accommodate individual variations and ethnic age and other differences. Guidance of this sort is not rigid and must be used to help guide clinical decision making, and not serve as an alternative to considering individual factors in making a treatment plan. Because of increasing complications from obesity, more aggressive efforts at therapy should be directed at people in each of the successively higher risk classifications.

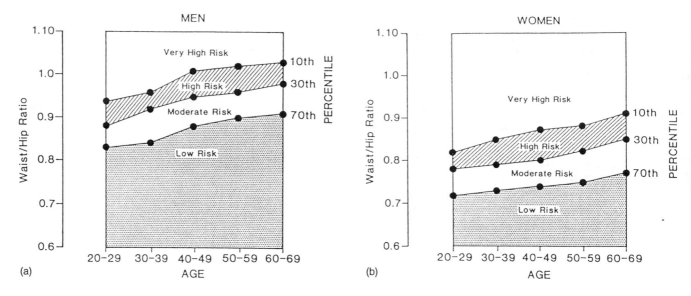

Figure 4 Percentiles for fat distribution. The percentiles for the ratio of abdominal circumference to gluteal circumference (ratio of waist to hips) are depicted for men (a) and women (b) by age groups. The relative risk for these percentiles is indicated based on the available information. (From tabular data in the Canadian Standardized Test of Fitness Third Edition 1986. Copyright 1987 George A. Bray.)

Table 11   Risk Associated with Central Fat

			Risk		
			Low	Moderate	High
BMI adjustment if initial BMI is between 22 and 29			0	+2	+4
Men	Waist circumference	in.	<37	37–40;	>40
		cm	<94	94–102	>102
	WHR		<.90	.90–1.00	>1.00
Women	Waist circumference	in.	<32	32–35	>35
		cm	<80	80–88	>88
	WHR		<.75	.75–.85	>.85

This evaluation and adjustment of BMI for the added risk of central fat is done for individuals with a BMI below 30 kg/m².

Table 12   Table for Adjusting Body Mass Index for Metabolic Variables

Score	Adjustment score			BMI adjustment score
	0	+1	+3	
Weight gain since age 18 (kg)	<5	5–15	>15	_____
Triglyceride/HDL cholesterol	<5	5–8	>8	_____
Blood pressure (mMHg)	<140/<90	140–160/90–100	>160/>100	_____
Fasting glucose (mg/dl)	<100	100–40	>140	_____
Sleep apnea	Absent	—	Present	_____
Osteoarthritis	Absent	Present	—	_____
		Adjustment to BMI for central fat (Table 11)		_____
		Calculated BMI		_____
		Adjusted BMI		[_____]

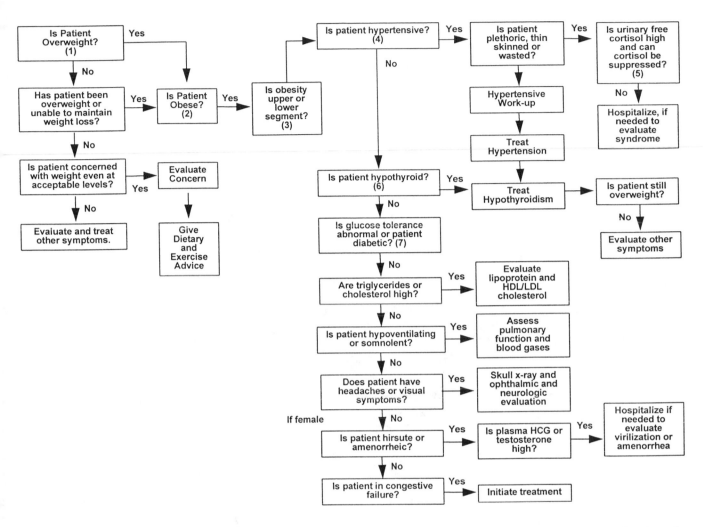

Figure 5 Algorithm for evaluating the obese individual. (1) Overweight is defined as body mass index between >25 and 30 kg/m² (see Table 10). Obesity is defined as body mass index >30 kg/m². (3) Fat distribution is defined by waist circumference or the ratio of waist circumference divided by hip circumference. (4) Blood pressure readings taken with a large cuff that encircles 75% of the arm. (5) Dexamethasone suppression test: cortisol less than 3 μg/dl (80 nmol/L) at 8:00 A.M., 9 hr after 1 mg of dexamethasone orally. (6) Thyroid function:

	Serum thyroxine (corrected) (μg/dl)(nmol/L)	Serum thyrotropin (μU/ml = mU/L)
High	12(154)	7
Normal	5.5–12.0 (71–154)	7
Borderline low	4.0–5.5 (51–71)	7–10
Low	4.0 (51)	10

In the presence of severe illness, a low serum thyroxine must be interpreted cautiously; it may be a bad prognostic sign, but not indicative of hypothyroidism unless TSH is elevated. (7) The diagnosis of diabetes in nonpregnant adults is based on the following: (a) Unequivocal hyperglycemia and classic symptoms of diabetes mellitus. (b) Fasting venous plasma glucose above 140 mg/dl (7.8 mmol/L) on more than one occasion. (c) Fasting plasma glucose above 140 mg/dl (7.8 mmol/L) at some point between 0 and 2 hr, and at 2 hr after an oral glucose tolerance test with 75 g glucose (or for children 1.75 g/kg of ideal body weight, not to exceed 75 g).

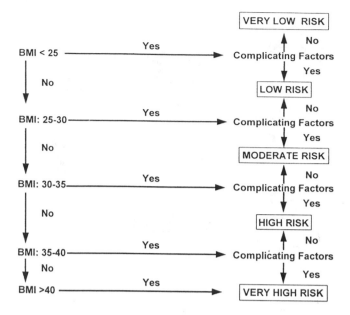

Figure 6 Risk classification algorithm. The patient is first placed into a category based on initial body mass index. Associated risks are defined in Tables 2 and 9. (Copyright 1987, George A. Bray. Used by permission.)

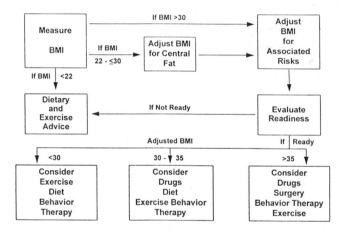

Figure 7 Algorithm for adjusting body mass index for other comorbid risk factors and obtaining an overall assessment off risk and a goal for weight loss and a rank order for potential treatments.

REFERENCES

1. Bauer J. Constitution and disease. 2nd ed. New York: 1945.
2. Jarlov E. The clinical types of abnormal obesity. Acta Med Scand 1932; S42:1–70.
3. Vague, J. The degree of masculine differentiation of obesities: a factor in determining predisposition to diabetes atherosclerosis, gout and uric calculus disease. Am J Clin Nutr 1956; 4:20.
4. Hirsch J, Knittle JL. Cellularity of obese and nonobese human adipose tissue. Fed Proc 1970; 29:1516–1521.
5. Bouchard C (ed). The Genetics of Obesity. Boca Raton, FL: CRC Press, 1994; 17–33.
6. Noorden, K. Von. Die Fettsucht. Nothnagel Spec Pathol 1900; 7:1–156.
7. Zondek B. Die Krankheiten der endokrinen Drusen. In: Berlin: 1926.
8. Rony HR. Obesity and Leanness. Philadelphia: Lea & Febiger, 1940.
9. Bruch H. The importance of overweight. New York: WW Norton, 1957.
10. Stunkard AJ, Grace WJ, Wolff HG. The night-eating syndrome. A pattern of food intake among certain obese patients. Am J Med 1955; 19:78–86.
11. Stunkard AJ. Eating pattern and obesity. Psychiatr Q 1959; 33:284–295.
12. Mayer J. Genetic, traumatic and environmental factors in the etiology of obesity. Physiol Rev 1953; 33:472–508.
13. Kemp R. The overall picture of obesity. Practitioner 1972; 209:654–660.
14. Bray GA, York DA. Genetically transmitted obesity in rodents. Physiol Rev 1971; 51:598–646.
15. Garrow JS. Treat Obesity Seriously. Philadelphia: WB Saunders, 1980.
16. Bray GA, Gray DS. Obesity. Part I. Pathogenesis. West J Med 1988; 149:429–441.
17. Björntorp P, Sjostrom L. Fat cell size and number in adipose tissue in relation to metabolism. Isr J Med Sci 1972; 8(3):320–324.
18. Hirsch J, Gallian E. Methods for the determination of adipose cell size in man and animals. J Lipid Res 1968; 9: 110–119.
19. Björntorp P. Adipose tissue in obesity (Willendorf lecture). In: Hirsch J, Van Itallie TB, eds. Recent Advances in Obesity Research, 4th ed. London: John Libbey, 1985: 163–170.
20. Salans LB, Cushman SW, Weismann RE. Studies of human adipose tissue. Adipose cell size and number in nonobese and obese patients. J Clin Invest 1973; 52(4):929–941.
21. Hirsch J, Batchelor B. Adipose tissue cellularity in human obesity. J Clin Endocrinol Metab 1976; 5:299–311.
22. Knittle JL, Timmers K, Ginsberg-Fellner F, Brown RE, Katz DP. The growth of adipose tissue in children and adolescents: cross-sectional and longitudinal studies of adipose cell number and size. J Clin Invest 1979; 63:239–246.
23. Kissebah AH, Vydelingum N, Murray R, et al. Relation of body fat distribution to metabolism complications of obesity. J Clin Endocrinol Metab 1982; 54:254–260.
24. Feldman R, Sender AJ, Sieglaub AB. Difference in diabetic and non diabetic fat distribution patterns by skin fold measurements. Diabetics 1969; 18:478–486.
25. Vague J. Degree of masculine differentiation of obesities: factor determining predisposition to diabetes, atheroscle-

rosis, gout, and uric calculous disease. Am J Clin Nutr 1956; 4:20–34.

26. Krotkiewski M, Björntorp P, Sjostrom L, Smith U. Impact of obesity on metabolism in men and women. Importance of regional adipose tissue distribution. J Clin Invest 1983; 72:1150–1162.

27. Kissebah AH, Vydelingum N, Murray R, et al. Relation of body fat distribution to metabolism complications of obesity. J Clin Endocrinol Metab 1982; 54:252–260.

28. Lapidus L, Bengtsson C, Larsson B, et al. Distribution of adipose tissue and risk of cardiovascular disease and death: a 12 year follow-up of participants in the population study of women in Gothenburg, Sweden. Br Med J 1984; 289:1257–1261.

29. Larsson B, Svardsudd K, Welin L, Wilhelmsen L, Björntorp P, Tibblin G. Abdominal adipose tissue distribution, obesity, and risk of cardiovascular disease and death: 13 year follow-up of participants in the study of men born in 1913. Br Med J 1984; 288:1401–1404.

30. Stokes J, III, Garrison RJ, Kannel WB. The independent contributions of various indices of obesity to the 22-year incidence of coronary heart disease: the Framingham Heart Study. In: Vague J, Björntorp P, Guy-Grand B, Rebuffe-Scrive M, Vague P, eds. Metabolic Complications of Human Obesities. Amsterdam: Excerpta Medica, 1985: 49–57.

31. Donahue RP, Abbott RD, Bloom E, Reed DM, Yano K. Central obesity and coronary heart disease in men. Lancet 1987; 1:821–824.

32. Mueller WH. The genetics of human fatness. Yearbook Phys Anthropol 1983; 26:215–230.

33. Ducimetiere P, Richard J, Cambien F. The pattern of subcutaneous fat distribution in middle-aged men and the risk of coronary heart disease: the Paris Prospective Study. Int J Obes 1986; 10:229–240.

34. Pouliot MC, Després JP, Lemieux S, et al. Waist circumference and abdominal sagittal diameter: best simple anthropometric indexes of abdominal visceral adipose tissue accumulation and related cardiovascular risk in men and women. Am J Cardiol 1994; 73:460–468.

35. Kvist H, Chowdhury B, Grangard U, Tylen U, Sjostrom L. Total and visceral adipose-tissue volumes derived from measurements with computed tomography in adult men and women: predictive equations. Am J Clin Nutr 1988; 48:1351–1361.

36. Bray GA. The Obese Patient: Major Problems in Internal Medicine, 9th ed. Philadelphia: WB Saunders, 1976.

37. Serdula MK, Ivery D, Coates RJ, Freedman DS, Williamson DF, Byers T. Do obese children become obese adults? A review of the literature. Prev Med 1993; 22:167–177.

38. Bray GA. Obesity. In: Current Concepts, A Scope Publication. Kalamazoo: Upjohn Company, 1982: 4–52.

39. Hager A, Sjostrom L, Arvidsson B, Björntorp P, Smith U. Body fat and adipose tissue cellularity in infants: a longitudinal study. Metabolism 1977; 26(6):607–610.

40. Brody DJ, Flegal KM, Gergen PJ. Birth-weight and childhood size in a national sample of 6-year-old to 11-year old children. Am J Hum Biol 1995; 7:293–301.

41. Gofin R, Adler B, Maddela R. Birth weight and weight, stature, and body mass index at ages 6 and 14 years. Am J Hum Biol 1993; 5:559–564.

42. Mossberg H. 40-year follow-up of overweight children. Lancet 1989; 2(8661):491–493.

43. Braddon FEM, Rodgers B, Wadsworth MEJ, Davies JMC. Onset of obesity in a 36 year birth control cohort study. Br Med J 1986; 293:299–303.20.

44. Abraham S, Collins G, Nordsieck M. Relationship of childhood weight status to morbidity in adults. Public Health Rep 1971; 86:273–284.

45. Webber LS, Srinivasan SR, Wattigney WA, Berenson GS. Tracking of serum lipids and lipoproteins from childhood to adulthood: the Bogalusa Heart Study. Am J Epidemiol 1991; 133:884–899.

46. Must A, Jacques PF, Dallal GE, Bajema CJ, Dietz WH. Long-term morbidity and mortality of overweight adolescents. A follow-up of the Harvard Growth Study of 1922 to 1935. N Engl J Med 1992; 327:1355.46.

47. McKeown T, Record RG. The influence of reproduction on body weight in women. J Endocrinol 1957; 15: 393–409.

48. Williamson DF, Madans J, Pamuk E. Flegal KM, Kendrick JS, Serdula MK. A prospective study of childbearing and 10-year weight gain in US white women 25 to 45 years of age. Int J Obes Metab Disord 1994; 18:561–569.

49. Ohlin A, Rossner S. Maternal body weight development after pregnancy. Int J Obes 1990; 14:159–173.

50. Naeye RL. Weight gain and the outcome of pregnancy. Am J Obstet Gynecol 1979; 135:3–9.

51. Rebuffe-Scrive M, Anderson B, Olbe L, Björntorp P. Metabolism of adipose tissue in intraabdominal depots in severely obese men and women. Metabolism 1990; 39(10):1021–1025.

52. Kannel WB, Gordon T. Physiological and medical concomittants of obesity: the Framingham study. In: Bray GA, ed. Obesity in America. Washington, DC: DHEW #79-249, 1979:125–153.

53. Bray GA, Fisler JS, York DA. Neuroendocrine control of the development of obesity: understanding gained from studies of experimental animal models. Front Neuroendocrinol 1990; 11(2):128–181.

54. Fernstrom MH. Drugs that cause weight gain. Obes Res 1995; 3(Suppl 4):435S–439S.

55. Glass AR. Endocrine aspects of obesity. Med Clin North Am 1989; 73:139–160.

56. Haarbo J, Christiansen C. Treatment-induced cyclic variations in serum lipids, lipoproteins, and apolipoproteins after 2 years of combined hormone replacement therapy: exaggerated cyclic variations in smokers. Obstet Gynecol 1992; 80(4):639–644.

57. Aisner J, Parnes H, Tait N, et al. Appetite stimulation and weight gain with megestrol acetate. Semin Oncol 1990; 17(6):2–7.

58. Breum L, Astrup A, Gram L, et al. Metabolic changes during treatment with valproate in humans: implication for untoward weight gain. Metabolism 1992; 41:666–670.

59. The DCCT Research Group. Weight gain associated with intensive therapy in the Diabetes Control and Complications Trial. Diabetes Care 1988; 11(7):567–573.

60. Williamson DF, Madans J, Anda RF, Kleinman JC, Giovino GA, Byers T. Smoking cessation and severity of weight gain in national cohort. N Engl J Med 1991; 324: 739–745.

61. Prentice AM, Jebb SA. Obesity in Britain: gluttony or sloth? Br Med J 1995; 311:437–439.64

62. Kromhout D. Changes in energy and macronutrients in 871 middle-aged men during 10 years of follow-up (the Zutphen Study). Am J Clin Nutr 1983; 37:287–294.

63. Physical Activity and Health: A Report of the Surgeon General. Atlanta, GA: US Department of Health and Human Services, Centers for Disease Control and Prevention, National Center for Chronic Disease Prevention and Health Promotion, 1996.

64. Ravussin E, Lillioja S, Knowler WC, et al. Reduced rate of energy expenditure as a risk factor for body-weight gain. N Engl J Med 1988; 318:467–472.

65. Roberts SB, Savage J, Coward WA, Chew B, Lucas A. Energy expenditure and intake in infants born to lean and overweight mothers. N Engl J Med 1988; 318:461–466.

66. Griffiths M, Payne PR, Stunkard AJ, Rivers JPW, Cox M. Metabolic-rate and physical development in children at risk of obesity. Lancet 1990; 336(8707):76–78.

67. Schemmel R, Mickelson O, Motawi P. Conversion of dietary to body energy in rats as affected by strains, sex and ration. J Nutr 1972; 102:1187–1197.

68. Kanarek RB, Hirsch E. Dietary-induced overeating in experimental animals. Fed Proc 1977; 36:154–158.

69. Rothwell NJ, Stock MJ. The development of obesity in animals: the role of dietary factors. Clin Endocrinol Metab 1984; 13:437–463.

70. Fomon SJ, Filer LJ, Thomas LN, Roger RR, Proksch AM. Relationship between formula concentration and rate of growth of normal infants. J Nutr 1969; 98:241–254.

71. Fabry P, Fodor J, Hejl Z, Braun T, Zvolankova K. The frequency of meals: its relationship to overweight, hypercholesterolemia, and decreased glucose-tolerance. Lancet 1964; 2:614–615.

72. Young CM, Hutter LF, Scanlan SS. Metabolic effects of meal frequency in normal young men. J Am Diet Assoc 1972; 61:391–398.

73. Jenkins DJ, Wolever TM, Vuksan V. Nibbling versus gorging: metabolic advantages of increased meal frequency. N Engl J Med 1989; 321(14):929–934.

74. Bray GA. Lipogenesis in human adipose tissue: some effects of nibbling and gorging. J Clin Invest 1972; 51: 537–548.

75. Lissner L, Heitmann BL. Dietary fat and obesity: evidence from epidemiology. Eur J Clin Nutr 1995; 49:79–90.

76. Romieu I, Willett WC, Stampfer MJ, et al. Energy intake and other determinants of relative weight. Am J Clin Nutr 1988; 47:406–412.

77. Sims EA, Danforth E, Horton ES, Bray GA, Glennon JA, Salans LB. Endocrine and metabolic effects of experimental obesity in man. Recent Prog Horm Res 1973; 29: 457–487.

78. Bouchard C, Tremblay A, Despres JP, et al. The response to long-term overfeeding in identical twins. N Engl J Med 1990; 322:1477–1482.

79. Forbes GB, Brown MR, Welle SL, Lipinski BA. Deliberate overfeeding in women and men: energy cost and composition of the weight gain. Br J Nutr 1986; 56:1–9.

80. Rothwell NJ, Stock MJ. Regulation of energy balance in two models of reversible obesity in the rat. J Comp Physiol Psychol 1979; 93:1024–1034.

81. Nishizawa Y, Bray GA. Evidence of a circulating ergostatic factor: studies on parabiotic rats. Am J Physiol 1980; 239: R344–R351.

82. Wahlgren MC, Powley TL. Effects of intragastric hyperalimentation on pair fed rats with ventromedial hypothalamic lesions. Am J Physiol 1985; 248(2 Pt 2):R172–180.

83. West DB, Wehberg KE, Kieswetter K, Granger JP. Blunted natriuretic response to an acute sodium load in obese hypertensive dogs. Hyptertension 19; S1:I96–I100, 1992.

84. Bray GA. Syndromes of hypothalamic obesity in man. Pediatr Ann 1984; 13(7):525–536.

85. Parkinson WL, Weingarten HP. Dissociative analysis of ventromedial hypothalamic obesity syndrome. Am J Physiol 1990; 259:R829–R835.

86. York DA, Bray GA. Dependence of hypothalamic obesity on insulin, the pituitary and the adrenal gland. Endocrinology 1972; 90:885–894.

87. Inoue S, Bray GA, Mullen Y. Transplantation of pancreatic beta cells prevents the development of hypothalamic obesity in rats. Am J Physiol 1978; 235(9):E226–E271.

88. Powley TL, Opsahl CA. Ventromedial hypothalamic obesity abolished by subdiaphragmatic vagotomy. Am J Physiol 1974; 226:25–33.

89. Sauter JF, Niijima A, Berthoud HR, Jeanrenaud B. Vagal neurons and pathways to the rat's lower viscera: an electrophysiological study. Brain Res Bull 1983; 11:487–491.

90. Sakaguchi T, Bray GA. Ventromedial hypothalamic lesions attenuate responses of sympathetic nerves to carotid arterial infusions of glucose and insulin. Int J Obes Metab Disord 1990; 14:127–134.

91. Orth DN. Cushing's syndrome. N Engl J Med 1995; 332: 791–803.

92. Lonn L, Kvist H, Ernest I, Sjostrom L. Changes in body composition and adipose tissue distribution after treatment of women with Cushing's syndrome. Metabolism 1994; 43:1517–1522.

93. Dunaif A, Segal KR, Futterweit W, Dobrjansky A. Profound peripheral insulin resistance, independent of obe-

sity, in polycystic ovary syndrome. Diabetes 1989; 38: 1165–1174.

94. Kaartinen JM, Kaar ML, Ohisalo JJ. Defective stimulation of adipocyte adenylate cyclase, blunted lipolysis, and obesity in pseudohypoparathyroidism. Pediatr Res 1994; 35(5):594–597.

95. Forbes GB, Porta CR, Herr BE, Griggs RC. Sequence of changes in body composition induced by testosterone and reversal of changes after drug is stopped. JAMA 1992; 267:397–399.

96. Bengtsson BA, Eden S, Lonn L, Kvist H, Stokland A, Lindstedt G, Bosaeus I, Tolli J, Sjostrom L, Isaksson OG. Treatment of adults with growth hormone (GH) deficiency with recombinant human GH. J Clin Endocrinol Metab 1993; 76:309–317.

97. Goldblatt PB, Moore E, Stunkard AJ. Social factors in obesity. JAMA 1965; 192:1930–1944.

98. Kuczmarski RJ, Flegal KM, Campbell SM, Johnson, CL. Increasing prevalence of overweight among US adults: the National Health and Nutrition Examination Surveys, 1960 to 1992. JAMA 1994; 272:205–211.

99. Bruch H. Eating Disorders; Obesity, Anorexia Nervosa and the Person Within. New York: Basic Books, 1973.

100. Williamson DA, Lawson OJ, Brooks ER, Wozniak PJ, Ryan DH, Bray GA. Duchmann EG. Association of body mass with dietary restraint and disinhibition. Appetite 1995; 25:31–41.

101. Bray GA, Dahms WT, Swerdloff RS, Fiser RH, Atkinson RL, Carrel RE. The Prader-Willi syndrome: a study of 40 patients and a review of the literature. Medicine 1983; 62(2):59–80.

102. Nicholls RD, Glenn CC, Jong MTC, Saitoh S, Mascari MJ, Driscoll DJ. Molecular pathogenesis of Prader-Willi Syndrome. In: Bray GA, Ryan DH, eds. Molecular and Genetic Aspects of Obesity. Baton Rouge: Louisiana State University Press, 1995.

103. Holland AJ, Treasure J, Coskeran P, Dallow J, Milton N, Hilhouse E. Measurement of excessive appetite and metabolic changes in Prader-Willi syndrome. Int J Obes Relat Metab Disord 1993; 17:527–532.

104. Zipf WB, Berntson GG. Characteristics of abnormal food-intake patterns in children with Prader-Willi Syndrome and study of effects of naloxone. Am J Clin Nutr 1987; 46:277–281.

105. Zipf WB, O'Dorisio TM, Bernstson GG. Short-term infusion of pancreatic polypeptide: effect on children with Prader-Willi syndrome. Am J Clin Nutr 1990; 51(2): 162–166.

106. Klein D, Ammann F. The syndrome of Laurence-Moon-Bardet-Biedl and allied diseases in Switzerland. Clinical, genetic and epidemiologic studies. J Neurol Sci 1969; 9: 479–513.

107. Schachat AP, Maumenee IH. Bardet-Biedl syndrome and related disorders. Arch Ophthalmol 1980; 100:285–288.

108. Stiggelbout W. The Bardet-Biedl syndrome, including Hutchinson-Laurence-Moon syndrome. In: Vinkin PK, Bruyn GW, eds. Handbook of Clinical Neurology. New York: Elsevier North Holland, 1972:380–412.

109. Laurence JZ, Moon RC. Four cases of 'retinitis pigmentosa' occurring in the same family, and accompanied by general imperfections of developments. Ophthalmol Rev 1866; 2:32–41.

110. Bardet G. Sur un syndrome d'obesité congenitale avec polydactylie et retinite pigmentaire (contribution a l'edude des formes clinique de l'obesité hypophysaire). Paris 1920 Thesis.

111. Biedl A. Ein Geschwisterpaar mit adipose-genitaler dystrophie. Dtsch Med Wochenschr 1922; 48:1630.

112. Carmi R, Rokhlina T, Kwitek-Black AE, et al. Use of a DNA pooling strategy to identify a human obesity syndrom locus on chromosome-15. Hum Mol Genet 1995; 4:9–13.

113. Carmi R, Elbedour K, Sone EM, Sheffield VC. Phenotypic differences among patients with Bardet-Biedl syndrome linked to three different chromosome loci. Am J Med Genet 1995; 59:199–203.

114. Croft JB, Morrell D, Chase CL, Swift M. Obesity in heterozygous carriers of the gene for Bardet Biedl syndrome. Am J Med Genet 1995; 55:12–15.

115. Nadjimi B, Flanagan MJ, Christian JR. Laurence-Moon Biedl syndrome associated with multiple genitourinary tract abnormalities. Am J Dis Child 1968; 117:352–355.

116. Goldstein JL, Fialkow PJ. The Alstrom syndrome. Report of three cases with further delineation of the clinical, pathophysiological, and genetic aspects of the disorder. Medicine 1973; 52:53–71.

117. Alter CA, Moshang T. Growth hormone deficiency in two siblings with Alstrom syndrome. Am J Dis Child 1993; 147:97–99.

118. Cohen MM, Hall BD, Smith DW, Graham CB, Lampert KL. A new syndrome with hypotonia, obesity, mental deficiency, and facial, oral, ocular, and limb anomalies. J Pediatr 1973; 83:280–284.

119. Carey JC, Hall BD. Confirmation of the Cohen syndrome. J Pediatr 1978; 93:239–244.

120. Friedman E, Sack J. The Cohen syndrome: report of five new cases and a review of the literature. J Craniofac Genet Dev Biol 1982; 2:193–200.

121. Goecke T, Majewski F, Kauther KD, Sterzel U. Mental retardation, hypotonia, obesity, ocular, facial, dental, and limb abnormalities (Cohen syndrome). Report of three patients. Eur J Pediatr 1982; 138:338–340.

122. Fryns JP, Kleczkowska A, Smeets E, Thiry P, Geutjens J, Van Den Berghe H. Cohen syndrome and de novo reciprocal translocation t(5;7)(33.1;p15.1). Am J Med Genet 1990; 37:546–547.

123. Temtamy SA. Carpenters syndrome: acrocephalopolysyndactyly. An autosomal recessive syndrome. J Pediatr 1966; 69:111–120.

124. Pfeiffer RA. Acrocephalo(poly)syndactylies. In: Anonymous Syndromes with Neurological and Neuromuscular Involvement, 43th ed. 1992:317–328.

125. Borjeson M, Forssman H, Lehman O. An X-linked, recessively inherited syndrome characterized by grave mental deficiency, epilepsy, and endocrine disorder. Acta Med Scand 1962; 171:13–21.

126. Vasquez SB, Hurst DJ, Sotos JR. X-linked hypogonadism, gynecomastia, mental retardation, short stature and obesity—a new syndrome. J Pediatr 1979; 94:52–56.

127. Young ID, Hughes HE. X-linked mental retardation, short stature, obesity and hypogonadism: report of a family. J Ment Defic Res 1982; 25:153–162.

128. Wilson M, Mulley J, Gedeon A, Robinson H, Turner G. New X-linked syndrome of mental retardation, gynecomastia and obesity is linked to DXS255. Am J Med Genet 1991; 40:406–413.

129. Baraiter M, Reardon W, Vijeratnam S. Nonspecific X-linked mental retardation with acrocephaly and obesity: a further family. Am J Med Genet 1995; 57:380–384.

130. Itallie TB. Health implications of overweight and obesity in the United States. Ann Intern Med 1985; 103: 983–988.

131. Shape Up America, American Obesity Association. Guidance for treatment of adult obesity, 1996.

132. American Association of Clinical Endocrinology, AACE/ACE Obesity Task Force. AACE/ACE Position Statement on the Prevention, Diagnosis, and Treatment of Obesity. Endocrine Practice 1997; May–June.

133. International Obesity Task Force (IOTF). 6th meeting of the IOTF Council. 1997; Feb.

134. Scottish Intercollegiate Guidelines Network. Obesity in Scotland—Integrating prevention with weight management. Piloted. Edinburgh: Scottish Intercollegiate Guidelines Network (SIGN), 1996.

135. Willett WC, Manson JE, Stampfer MJ, et al. Weight, weight change and coronary heart disease in women: risk within the normal weight range. JAMA 1995; 273: 461–465.

136. Larsson B, Bengtsson C, Björntorp P, et al. Is abdominal body fat distribution a major explanation for the sex difference in the incidence of myocardial infarction? The study of men born in 1913 and the study of women, Goteborg, Sweden. Am J Epidemiol 1992; 135:266–273.

42

Behavioral Approaches to the Treatment of Obesity

Rena R. Wing

University of Pittsburgh School of Medicine, Pittsburgh, Pennsylvania

I. THE BEHAVIORAL APPROACH TO OBESITY: A THEORETICAL OVERVIEW

The behavioral approach to obesity grew out of learning theory (1,2) and was first applied to the treatment of obesity between 1960 and 1970 (3,4). The primary assumptions of the behavioral approach are that (1) eating and exercise behaviors affect body weight; by changing eating and exercise behaviors it is possible to change body weight; (2) eating and exercise patterns are learned behaviors and, like other learned behaviors, can be modified; and (3) to modify these behaviors long term, it is necessary to change the environment that influences them.

The behavioral approach does not deny the fact that an individual's genetic background may have a strong influence on his or her body weight. However, despite a predisposition to be a certain weight, changes in energy balance (i.e., decreases in energy intake and/or increases in energy expenditure) will produce weight loss.

Likewise, the behavioral approach recognizes the importance of an individual's past history. The individual's family and cultural background influence body weight by determining food preferences, food choices, and the preferred level of physical activity. However, while accepting the importance of historical antecedents, the focus of a behavioral approach is on current behaviors and the environmental factors controlling these current behaviors.

The essence of the behavioral approach to obesity is the functional analysis of behavior, delineating the association between eating and exercise behaviors and environmental events such as time of day, presence of other people, mood, and other activities (5,6). Patients are asked to self-monitor their eating and exercise behaviors to determine specific problem areas that should be targeted in treatment. The environment controlling these behaviors is then restructured to modify these problem behaviors.

A key technique in behavioral approaches is self-monitoring (7), which involves writing down exactly what is eaten and what type of physical activity is performed. This record allows the patient and therapist to identify problem behaviors that might be changed. For example, the self-monitoring record may reveal that a large percentage of an individual's calories are consumed in the form of desserts, that between-meal eating constitutes a major problem, or that an individual's portion sizes are unusually large. Alternatively, the individual may consume relatively few calories but lead a very sedentary life-style. These different behavior patterns would lead to different targets for the behavior change intervention.

Often in changing overall behavior, it is necessary to break the target behavior into several components, and then to work on each part in turn (i.e., "shape" the behavior). For example, to lower calorie intake in an overweight individual, a therapist might work first on reducing calories consumed at breakfast, and later move to lunch and dinner, or focus initially on decreasing the quantity of food consumed (i.e., portion sizes) and later work on changing the quality of the diet.

After the behavior to be changed has been defined, the next step is to change the environment that controls the behavior. The behavioral approach assumes that behavior is controlled by *antecedents*, or cues in the environment that set the stage for the behavior, and by *consequences*, or reinforcers that come after the behavior and lead to its recurrence (8). This A-B-C model is shown schematically in Figure 1. For example, the sight of food on a buffet table may lead a person to overeat, or the cue of seeing someone else eating may arouse feelings of hunger. Likewise, the positive consequences that come from the good taste of food or from reduction in feelings of hunger may lead to continued selection of these food items.

In the behavioral approach to weight control, patients are taught to restructure their home environment so that it will elicit the desired behaviors. These techniques are called stimulus control strategies (3,4). For example, patients are encouraged to refrain from purchasing high-calorie desserts, and to store all high-calorie foods in difficult-to-reach places; simultaneously they are taught to buy more fruits and vegetables and to keep them readily accessible. Patients are also taught strategies for changing thoughts and emotions, which can serve as powerful cues for overeating, and strategies for dealing with social cues and social pressure to overeat.

Patients in weight control programs often observe that they do not have the necessary "willpower" to avoid unhealthy foods. The behavioral approach is designed to restructure the environment to minimize the need for willpower. For example, if a patient opens the refrigerator and finds only low-calorie food items available, the chances are good that the patient will select a low-calorie item (even if the person lacks willpower). Likewise, if the patient plans ahead to meet a friend at the park for a walk after work, the chances are increased that the patient will actually take a walk. Planning ahead and developing a structure at a point in time when willpower is not required increase the likelihood that the desirable behavior will occur.

Finally, since environmental consequences are believed to play an important role in influencing behavior, behavioral programs attempt to develop new reinforcement contingencies. Behavior therapists use reinforcers, such as praise and positive feedback, to encourage patients to adopt new, healthier eating and exercise behaviors and teach patients to reinforce themselves for appropriate behavior change. Some behavioral programs also include more formal reinforcement systems, such as contingency procedures where patients deposit money with the therapist and earn back portions of their money contingent on behavior change (9,10).

II. HISTORY OF BEHAVIORAL APPROACHES TO OBESITY: 1970–1995

A. The Development of Treatments from 1970 to 1990

The earliest report of a behavioral treatment program for obesity was by Stuart, who successfully treated eight overweight women (4). These women experienced an average weight loss of 17 kg (range 12–21 kg) over a 12-month period. Stuart (an eminent behavior therapist) conducted the treatment program himself, selecting each patient individually and tailoring the program to fit the needs of the individual patient. At the start of therapy, the treatment sessions were scheduled frequently (several times per week), and then gradually less frequently. Eating and exercise behaviors were targeted, and patients weighed themselves four times each day. The program included cognitive interventions, as patients were taught to deal with their weight-related fears, and the patients were helped to develop new hobbies as alternative sources of reinforcement.

Stuart's successful report led to a flood of behavioral research studies. These studies in the early 1970s typically involved 10 weeks of group treatment with mildly overweight subjects and were often conducted as part of a student's doctoral dissertation (5,11). Thus, in many ways these studies represented an abrupt departure from Stuart's landmark treatment. The emphasis in these programs was on changing eating patterns (where and when foods were eaten), but the nutritional aspects of the diet (number of calories, macronutrient distribution) were ignored, in part to distinguish behavioral treatment from traditional dietary interventions. These early studies showed that behavior modification was more effective than nutrition education (12) or psychotherapy (13). On average, participants lost 3.8 kg over an 8.4 week treatment interval (5). When followed up an average of 15.5 weeks later, participants had maintained a weight loss of 4.0 kg.

The evolution of behavioral treatments from 1974 to 1990 is shown clearly in Table 1, a summary table reprinted from Wadden (14). As seen in this table, behavioral treatments gradually evolved over this period (1974–1990) to include heavier participants (from 73 to 92 kg at entry), longer treatment intervals (from 8.4 to

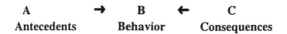

A → B ← C
Antecedents   Behavior   Consequences

Figure 1   A-B-C model of the behavioral approach to the treatment of obesity.

Table 1 Summary Analysis of Selected Studies from 1974 to 1990 Providing Treatment by Behavior Therapy and Conventional Reducing Diet

	1974	1978	1984	1985–1987	1988–1990
No. of studies included	15	17	15	13	5
Sample size	53.1	54.0	71.3	71.6	21.2
Initial weight (kg)	73.4	87.3	88.7	87.2	91.9
Initial % overweight	49.4	48.6	48.1	56.2	59.8
Length of treatment (weeks)	8.4	10.5	13.2	15.6	21.3
Weight loss (kg)	3.8	4.2	6.9	8.4	8.5
Loss per week (kg)	0.5	0.4	0.5	0.5	0.4
Attrition (%)	11.4	12.9	10.6	13.8	21.8
Length of follow-up (weeks)	15.5	30.3	58.4	48.3	53
Loss at follow-up	4.0	4.1	4.4	5.3	5.6

Source: Reprinted from Ref. 14.

21.3 weeks in length), and longer follow-up durations (increasing to a year-long follow-up). The program itself changed as well, placing far greater emphasis on nutrition (14). Patients in behavioral programs were now given calorie goals (usually 1200–1500 kcal/day) and self-monitored not only the events surrounding eating but also exactly what they ate (8,15). Calorie goals for exercise were also prescribed. Cognitive behavioral strategies were given greater emphasis (2), and financial incentives were often utilized. Thus, behavioral programs evolved from teaching strictly behavioral strategies to focusing equally on diet, exercise, and behavior modification. With this longer, more inclusive intervention, average weight losses increased to 8.5 kg in 1990. At 1 year follow-up, subjects maintained an average weight loss of 5.6 kg (66% of their initial weight loss).

B. Overview of Recent Behavioral Studies: 1990–1995

Table 2 presents the results of the randomized studies evaluating behavioral weight control strategies that were published between 1990 and 1995. To identify these studies, the *Journal of Consulting and Clinical Psychology, International Journal of Obesity, Obesity Research, American Journal of Clinical Nutrition, Behavior Therapy*, and *Addictive Behaviors* were reviewed. Other studies published outside these journals, but clearly behavioral, were included if identified. One of the clear trends in the behavioral weight control field has been to publish the results of these studies outside of the standard behavioral journals, making the task of identifying all published studies far more difficult.

The studies presented in Table 2 will be discussed in detail in the subsequent sections of this chapter. However, several things are apparent from Table 2. First, these re-

cent studies have utilized relatively large samples, often including 30 or more subjects per treatment condition. The heaviest patients (106 kg) are in year-long studies that include very-low-calorie diets (VLCDs) (16,17), but typically patients weigh 85–100 kg. Many of the studies involve only women or predominantly women, but a few recent studies (18,19) have specifically recruited equal numbers of men and women.

The length of the initial treatment program has varied widely (from 12 to 52 weeks of weekly treatment meetings). Likewise, the length of follow-up and the intensity of contact during follow-up have varied; some studies have provided no treatment meetings over 9–12 months of follow-up (17,20,21) whereas others have continued to see patients monthly or even biweekly (16,22).

The weight losses achieved initially in these behavioral programs also differ greatly across studies and treatment condition. One behavioral program (23), involving only slightly overweight females [body mass index (BMI) 25–35] and focusing on the use of computers, produced an average weight loss of only 1.8 kg over 12 weeks in the behavioral treatment condition. On the other hand, studies by Andersen et al. (24), Wadden et al. (16), and Wing et al. (17) produced weight losses of 10–18 kg in year-long programs with low-calorie diets, and slightly better results when a VLCD was included (16,17). Other studies (19,25) produced weight losses of similar magnitude (10–12 kg) at 24 weeks.

Although, given this variability, averaging across studies is somewhat questionable, the averages (excluding no-treatment control groups, computer treatment groups, and exercise-only conditions) are presented in Table 3. On average, subjects entering behavioral weight loss programs in 1990–1995 weighed 92 kg. They lost an average of 9.7 kg over 27 weeks (or 0.39 kg/week). Weight loss averaged

Table 2 Randomized Studies of Behavioral Treatment of Obesity 1990–1995

	Sample			Treatment			Follow-up[a]		
Topic/study	n	Wt (kg)	Characteristic	Duration (weeks)	n	Wt loss (kg)	Duration (weeks)	n	Wt loss (kg)
Evaluation of VLCDs									
Wing (46)									
BT + LCD (1000–1500 kcal)	19	103	NIDDM	20	16	10.1[b]	72	16	6.8
BT + VLCD (8 wk)	17		10 M/26 F		17	18.6[c]	4 contacts	17	8.6
Wadden (16)									
BT + LCD (1200 kcal)	21	106	All female	52	17	14.4	78	16	12.2
BT + VLCD (16 wk)	28				23	17.3	Biweekly	21	10.9
Wing (17)									
BT + LCD (1000–1200 kcal)	48	106	NIDDM	50	41	10.5[b]	102	37	5.7
BT + VLCD (2 12-wk bouts)	45		33 M/60 F		38	14.2[c]	No contact	36	7.2
Evaluations of low-fat diets									
Schlundt (20)									
Fat restriction	30	90	52F/8M	20	25	4.6[b]	36–52	17	2.6[b]
Fat + calorie restriction	30				24	8.8[c]	No contact	18	5.5[c]
Jeffery (56)									
Calorie restriction	61	80	All female 25–45 yrs 120–140% ideal wt	24 (weekly for 6 wks; then biweekly)	35	3.7	52 (78)	35	.5 (+1.8)
Fat restriction	61		All female		39	4.6	Monthly	39	2.1 (+.4)
Pascale (21)									
Calorie restriction	22	95	NIDDM FH+	16	16	4.6[b]	52	16	1.0[b]
	23				13	6.9		13	3.2
Fat + calorie restriction	22		NIDDM FH+		15	7.7[c]	4 meetings	15	5.2[b]
	23				16	7.5		16	3.1
Viegener (22)									
Low calorie	43	96	All female	24	32	8.9	52	30	9.0
Low fat (alternating)	42				31	10.2	Biweekly	30	9.0
Food provision									
Jeffery (19)									
No Tx control[d]	40	90	101 M/101 F 25–45 years	24	28	1.0[b]	76	28	0[b]
BT	40				26	7.7[c]	Monthly meetings;	26	4.1[c]
BT + food	40				36	10.1[d]	Weekly	36	6.4[d]
BT + $	41				35	7.7[c]	weigh-ins	35	4.1[c]
BT + food + $	41				34	12.0[d]		34	6.4[d]

Study	N	Completed (%)	Sample	Duration (wk)	Weight loss	Follow-up (wk)	Contact	N at follow-up	Follow-up weight loss
Wing (25)									
BT	40	86	All female	24	8.0[b]	76	Varied	32	3.3[b]
BT + menus	41				12.0[c]			37	6.9[c]
BT + food (cost shared)	41				11.7[c]			37	7.5[c]
BT + food (free)	41				11.4[c]			38	6.6[c]
Exercise									
Foreyt (18)									
Control[d]	38	97	Age 25–35	12	1.0	52	Monthly	—	—
Diet	42		85 M/80 F		7.0			29	6.3
Exercise[d]	43				0.3			30	2.6
Diet + exercise	42				6.9			27	8.1
Andersen (24)									
Diet only	16	95	All female	48	12.9				
Diet + aerobic exercise	16				13.4				
Diet + resistance training	18				17.9				
Diet + aerobics + resistance	16				15.3				
Jakicic (63)									
Short Bout Exercise	28	91	All female	20	8.9				
Long Bout Exercise	28				6.4				
Computer therapy									
Agras (23)									
Computer Tx[d]	30	78	All female	12	2.3	52	No contact	29	0.3
Computer + 4 group[d]	30		BMI 25–35		2.6			29	1.9
Behavior therapy	30				1.8			30	1.0
Taylor (71)									
Computer[d]	28	76	All female	12	3.1[b]	38	No contact	21	0.9[b]
1200-kcal diet + computer	28		BMI 25–35		5.3[c]			25	3.8[c]

[a] Duration and weight loss are calculated from start of study.

[b,c] Weight losses indicated with different superscripts differed significantly from each other.

[d] Excluded from averages computed for Table 3.

BT = Behavioral Treatment; LCD = low calorie diet; VLCD = very low calorie diet.

Table 3 Summary of Results of 14 Behavioral Treatment Studies 1990–1995[a] (mean ± SD)

	Total	LCD	VLCD
# of studies	14	14	3
# of treatment groups	34	31	3
Subjects/group at entry	33 ± 12	33 ± 12	30 ± 14
Initial wt (kg)	92.8 ± 7.9	91.6 ± 7.2	105 ± 1.7
Duration of treatment (weeks)	27 ± 13	26 ± 12	41 ± 18
% completing treatment	83 ± 13	82 ± 13	89 ± 10
Weight loss during treatment (kg)	9.7 ± 4.1	9.0 ± 3.6	16.7 ± 2.3
Rate of weight loss (kg/week)	0.39 ± 0.15	0.37 ± 0.12	0.51 ± 0.36
Duration of follow-up (from baseline) (weeks)	64 ± 17	62 ± 16	84 ± 16
Duration of follow-up from posttreatment (weeks)	40 ± 11	40 ± 11	43 ± 15
# of contacts during follow-up	6.3 ± 5.0	6.4 ± 4.9	5.7 ± 6.6
% completing follow-up	76 ± 13	75 ± 13	85 ± 13
Weight loss (pre to follow-up) (kg)	5.6 ± 3.0	5.2 ± 2.8	8.9 ± 1.9
% of initial weight loss retained	60.3 ± 21.7	61.1 ± 22.7	53.3 ± 8.7

[a]Excluding no-treatment control groups, computer-only treatment programs, and exercise-only conditions.

across the 34 treatment conditions was significantly related to both baseline weight ($r = .60$, $p < .0002$) and duration of treatment ($r = .71$, $p < .0001$). For the purpose of comparison with Table 1 (which did not include any programs with VLCDs), results for the three groups with VLCDs are presented separately. The three VLCD groups lost 16.7 ± 2.3 kg at the end of 41 weeks (.51 kg/week), whereas the other 31 groups, which did not utilize a VLCD, lost 9.0 ± 3.6 kg at 26 weeks.

The average time of follow-up (in the 28 treatment conditions with follow-up) was 64 weeks after treatment entry or 40 weeks after the end of the initial treatment phase. Patients maintained a weight loss of 5.6 kg at this time, or 60% of their initial weight loss. The three VLCD groups maintained a weight loss of 8.9 kg, or 53% of their initial weight loss; the low-calorie diet (LCD) conditions maintained a weight loss of 5.2 kg, or 61% of their initial weight loss. Those treatment groups that had the largest initial weight losses also had the largest weight losses at follow-up ($r = .82$, $p < .0001$), but there was a nonsignificant association ($r = .25$, $p > .10$) between initial weight loss and percent of weight loss maintained. In addition, time to follow-up (baseline to follow-up) was positively related to total weight loss ($r = .40$, $p < .05$) but the length of time between posttreatment and follow-up was unrelated to total weight loss. Number of treatment contacts during follow-up was also positively related to the magnitude of weight loss at follow-up ($r = .51$, $p < .01$). None of the other variables in Table 3 were related to percent of weight maintained. Thus, these data suggest that longer programs, larger initial weight losses, and more

frequent posttreatment contact are related to long-term weight loss results.

III. DESCRIPTION OF CURRENT BEHAVIORAL TREATMENT PROGRAMS

Before discussing the studies in Table 2 in more detail and the new directions being pursued by behavioral researchers, a more extensive description of a typical behavioral program is provided. Since, over time, behavioral programs have become fairly standardized, it is possible to describe a "typical" program. As will be noted, current programs differ quite markedly both from Stuart's early intervention and from the theoretical description of a behavioral program provided at the beginning of this chapter.

Currently almost all behavioral programs are delivered in groups of 10–20 patients (8,14). With this many patients in a group, it is difficult to conduct an individualized functional analysis of behavior. The program is offered as a series of lessons, and the entire group of participants receives lesson 1 on week 1, lesson 2 on week 2, and so forth. There is no assessment of whether the lessons relate to the individual participant's problem areas or whether the participant has mastered the skill before moving on to the next skill. However, individualization of treatment occurs through lessons on problem solving, allowing participants the opportunity to focus on their specific problem areas. Therapists for behavioral programs are likewise quite different. Some programs use one therapist throughout, but many use a team of therapists (including a behavior therapist, an exercise physiologist, and a nutritionist) and rotate therapists by the topic. Treatment usually involves weekly meetings for 16–24 weeks (with some programs now using year-long programs) and then less frequent contact.

Key strategies in current behavioral program include the following:

A. Self-Monitoring

Patients in behavioral programs are taught to write down everything they eat and the calories in these foods. Recently, many programs have begun to teach patients to also self-monitor the grams of fat in each food. After a few weeks in the program, self-monitoring of physical activity is added (with activity monitored either in minutes or in calories expended). Self-monitoring is prescribed daily throughout the initial 20–24-week program and periodically (or daily) during maintenance. Self-monitoring is often considered the *sine qua non* of behavioral programs and continued adherence to self-monitoring predicts long-term maintenance of weight loss (26,27).

B. Goal Setting

The goal in behavioral programs is to achieve a weight loss of 1–2 lb/week (.5–1 kg). To accomplish this, patients are given goals for total calories (usually 1000–1500 kcal/day), for grams of fat (usually given in grams of fat per day and set at a level to achieve a 20–30% fat diet), and for physical activity (gradually increased from 250 kcal/week to 1000 kcal/week). Patients may also set specific behavioral goals to achieve during various weeks of the project. Short-term goals that the participant can reasonably be expected to achieve are emphasized (28).

C. Nutrition

The nutritional aspects of weight loss are now given far more attention in behavioral weight loss programs (8,15). Virtually all programs ask participants to record what they are eating and the calorie and/or fat content of those foods. Lessons on healthy eating, which emphasize increasing intake of complex carbohydrates and fiber and decreasing dietary fat, are usually included. Moreover, the specific skills required to be able to consume a low-fat diet are taught during the course of the program, with lessons on topics such as recipe modification, label reading, restaurant eating, and demonstration of special cooking skills such as stir-fry cooking. Thus nutrition is taught both through educational classes designed to increase knowledge of what should be consumed and through demonstrations of how to accomplish the complex task of going from a high-calorie, high-fat diet to a lower-calorie, lower-fat regimen.

D. Exercise

Exercise is given a great deal of attention in behavioral weight loss programs because exercise is the single best predictor of long-term weight maintenance (29). Correlational studies comparing successful and unsuccessful weight losers consistently show that successful weight losers are best distinguished by their self-reported exercise behavior (30–32). The association between exercise and long-term weight loss has been observed in men, women, children, and adolescents and is seen in programs involving LCDs and VLCDs (29). In addition, randomized controlled trials, in which diet alone, exercise alone, and diet plus exercise are compared, consistently show that the combination of diet plus exercise produces the best results (33–35).

To increase exercise, participants in behavioral programs are given goals for exercise, and these goals are gradually increased over time to "shape" an exercise routine. Most programs encourage patients to gradually work up to 1000 calories/week of exercise, which can be accomplished by walking 10 miles/week (e.g., 2 miles on 5 days each week).

Behavioral treatment programs often distinguish between *life-style exercise*, such as using stairs instead of elevators or parking farther from the store, and *programmed exercise*, in which a specific time is set aside for the purpose of exercise. Both types of exercise are strongly encouraged in behavioral treatment programs. Moreover, based on Epstein et al.'s recent findings that decreasing sedentary activities such as TV watching is very effective in promoting weight loss (36), many programs now include lessons on this topic as well.

Again, as in discussing nutrition, behavioral programs help patients learn the specific skills required to become more active, such as learning to monitor their heart rate to determine the intensity of exercise, learning how to dress for exercise in cold or hot weather, and learning how to deal with barriers that make exercise difficult. Some behavioral programs include supervised exercise sessions to model these skills and help provide participants with social support for exercise (37).

E. Stimulus Control

Stimulus control techniques remain the hallmark of behavioral treatment programs (3,4). Based on the assumption that behaviors are controlled by environmental antecedents, participants in weight control programs are taught to change the environment they live in, so that there are an increased number of cues for appropriate diet and exercise behaviors and fewer cues for inappropriate behaviors. Specifically, participants in behavioral weight control programs are taught to increase their purchase of fruits and vegetables, to wash and prepare these foods for easy eating, and to place these foods prominently in the refrigerator. In contrast, high-fat/high-calorie products are to be decreased. If it is necessary to purchase these foods at all, they are to be stored in opaque containers or high cupboards, since "out-of-sight is out-of-mind." Some programs also encourage participants to select a designated eating place, to restrict all eating to that place, and to separate eating from other activities (such as watching television or reading). In this way, behavioral programs seek to limit the cues associated with eating.

F. Problem Solving

The problem-solving approach of D'Zurilla and Goldfried (38) is taught to participants in weight control programs. Participants learn to identify situations that pose a problem for their eating and exercise behaviors, to use brainstorming to generate possible solutions to the problem, to select one solution to try, and then to evaluate the success of their attempt. Through training in problem solving, behavioral programs are able to individualize the group-based weight control program and to teach patients strategies for dealing with their own personal problem areas.

G. Cognitive Restructuring

The cues for overeating and underexercising include not only physical cues such as the sight and smell of food, but also cognitive cues. A person's thoughts, such as the thought "I've had a bad day. I deserve a treat. I'll go for some ice cream," can lead to inappropriate behavior. Dividing the world into good and bad foods, developing excuses or rationalizations for inappropriate behavior, and making comparisons with others can all serve as negative thoughts. Behavioral programs teach participants to recognize that they are having these negative thoughts, to understand the function these thoughts serve for the participant, and then to counter these negative thoughts with more positive self-statements (39,40).

H. Relapse Prevention

Based on Marlatt and Gordon's theory of the relapse process (41,42), behavioral weight control programs now emphasize that lapses (or slips) are a natural part of the weight loss process. Patients are taught to anticipate the types of situations that might cause them to lapse and to plan strategies for coping with these situations. The goal is to keep lapses from becoming relapses.

IV. RECENT EFFORTS TO IMPROVE TREATMENT OUTCOME

In an effort to improve treatment outcome, behavioral researchers have focused their attention on strengthening the dietary component of the weight loss program, strengthening the exercise component, and/or strengthening the manner in which the behavioral strategies are implemented. Each of these areas of research will be discussed in turn. Recent clinical trials listed in Table 2 will be described in detail, along with a general description of ongoing research related to each of these strategies.

A. Strengthening the Dietary Component

1. Combining Behavior Modification and VLCD

One approach to improving weight loss in behavioral treatment programs has been to improve initial weight loss by using stricter dietary approaches, such as VLCD. VLCDs are diets of <800 kcal/day, usually consumed as liquid formula or as lean meat, fish, and fowl (43). These diets have been shown to produce excellent weight losses (9 kg in 12 weeks) (43,44) and appear to be safe when used with carefully selected patients and appropriate medical monitoring (43). By using VLCDs to produce large initial weight losses and behavioral training to improve maintenance, it was hoped that a more successful treatment approach could be developed.

In one of the earliest studies of the combination of behavior modification and a VLCD, Wadden and Stunkard (45) randomly assigned 59 overweight subjects to one of three conditions: an 8-week VLCD administered in a physician's office with no behavioral counseling (VLCD alone), a 20-week group behavioral weight loss program that used a balanced LCD throughout (BT + LCD), or a 20-week group behavioral program that included an 8-week period of VLCD (BT + VLCD). Subjects in the VLCD alone group lost 14.1 kg during the 8-week diet, but then rapidly regained their weight, maintaining a weight loss of 4.1 kg at 1-year follow-up (i.e., maintaining only 29% of their initial weight loss). Better results were obtained by subjects in the BT + VLCD condition, who lost 19.3 kg initially and maintained a weight loss of 12.9 kg at 1 year. However, while the initial weight losses in the BT + VLCD condition were better than those in the

BT + LCD (19.3 vs. 14.3 kg, respectively), at 1-year follow-up weight losses were no longer significantly different (12.9 vs. 9.5 kg in BT + VLCD vs. BT + LCD conditions, respectively). Thus, the greater initial weight losses in the VLCD were not successful in producing significantly better long-term results.

A similar finding occurred in the Wing et al. (46) study with a sample of 36 obese patients with non-insulin-dependent diabetes mellitus (NIDDM) (Table 2). At the end of a 20-week behavioral program that included an 8-week period of VLCD, weight losses averaged 18.6 kg and were significantly greater than those obtained when a 1000–1500-kcal LCD was used throughout (10.1 kg). At 1-year follow-up, subjects in the BT + VLCD condition had regained 54% of their initial weight loss, compared to only 33% in the BT + LCD group; consequently the overall weight losses (8.6 for BT + VLCD vs. 6.8 kg for BT + LCD) no longer differed significantly between the two treatment groups.

These studies of VLCDs were indeed successful in improving initial weight loss, as researchers had anticipated; however, increasing initial weight loss did not improve long-term outcome; rather, it simply increased the magnitude of weight regained. To try to better maintain these larger initial weight losses, several investigators have recently used VLCDs in combination with year-long behavioral programs (see Table 2). Wadden and colleagues (16) randomly assigned 49 overweight women to a behavioral treatment program that involved 52 weekly meetings and either used a balanced LCD throughout (1200 kcal/day) or included 16 weeks of VLCD. All subjects were then seen biweekly from week 52 to week 72. Subjects in the BT + VLCD condition had their maximum weight loss at 6 months (21.1 kg) and then gradually regained (17.3 kg at 12 months and 10.9 kg at 18 months). The BT + LCD group lost significantly less weight initially (11.86 kg at 26 weeks), but then continued to lose weight between 26 and 52 weeks (14.4 kg at 52 weeks). Consequently by week 52, differences between the VLCD and LCD condition were no longer significant. After week 52, subjects in the BT + LCD group regained weight despite continued contact, achieving a final weight loss of 12.2 kg at 18 months. The regain experienced by subjects in the LCD condition was much less than that of the VLCD subjects, so that at the end of the study, overall weight losses in the BT + LCD condition had exceeded but did not differ significantly from that of the BT + VLCD condition (12.2 kg vs. 10.9 kg).

Wing and colleagues (17) also examined the possibility of using the VLCD in the context of a year-long behavioral treatment program. These investigators studied 93 patients with NIDDM and randomly assigned them to either a balanced LCD (1000–1200 kcal) throughout the 52 weeks or to a program that included two 12-week periods of VLCD. Subjects in the BT + VLCD condition consumed 400 kcal/day for weeks 1–12 and 24–36 and then gradually increased their intake after these periods until they were eating 1000–1200 kcal/day. After 24 weeks of treatment, subjects in the BT + VLCD condition had lost 16.4 kg, while those in the BT + LCD condition had lost only 12.3 kg. Despite continued weekly contact and the use of a second 12-week interval of the VLCD, both groups regained approximately 2 kg over the next 6 months. At the end of the year-long program, the BT + VLCD group had lost 14.2 kg versus 10.5 kg in the BT + LCD conditions. This difference approached statistical significance ($p = .057$), but is of questionable clinical significance. Treatment was then terminated, and subjects were recontacted 1 year later. At that time, the VLCD group maintained a weight loss of 7.2 kg versus 5.7 kg in the LCD group.

VLCDs pose an interesting dilemma for behavior therapists. These regimens have been successful in accomplishing what they are designed to accomplish, namely, increasing the magnitude of initial weight loss. The diets are well tolerated by patients, and most patients find them easier to follow than balanced LCDs. However, to date it has not been possible to maintain the larger initial weight losses obtained with VLCDs. Wing et al. (17) showed that the greater the amount of weight lost initially, the greater the weight regain. This phenomenon was true for LCD and VLCD, and there was no evidence of greater regain following VLCDs after adjusting for differences in initial weight loss. Thus, the basic premise that overall weight losses can be improved by increasing initial weight loss may not be accurate.

Another issue that has been raised about VLCDs is whether the rigid rules of these diets and the fact that calories are restricted so severely may increase the tendency toward dietary lapses and/or be poorly tolerated by those individuals who have problems with binge eating. Wing and colleagues (47) compared the dietary lapses reported by subjects in the BT + VLCD condition and the BT + LCD condition in the study described above. The subjects' self-monitoring diaries and periodic telephone interviews were used to assess lapses. Both types of data indicated that lapses were reported with equal frequency by subjects on the VLCD and LCD. Lapses occurred rarely during months 1–3 of either program and then increased during months 4 and 5. While this increase would seem to be associated with refeeding in the VLCD, it occurred at the same point in time and to the same extent in the LCD condition, suggesting that length of time in the program rather than the type of diet (or the magnitude of weight loss) was related to the occurrence of lapses. The situations associated with lapses differed for the two diet regimens, with food and cravings triggering lapses in the VLCD condition and emotions triggering them in the LCD condition. There was no evidence that subjects in the VLCD condition had more negative psychological reactions to their lapses than subjects in the LCD conditions.

Binge eating has been shown to be a serious problem for approximately 30% of individuals in behavioral weight loss programs (48–50) and for these individuals, VLCDs might be questioned. Wadden et al. (51) studied 225 females in a behavioral program that included use of a VLCD and compared binge eaters ($n = 29$), episodic overeaters (defined as individuals who binged but did not lose control over their eating; $n = 26$), and nonbingers ($n = 180$). No significant difference between these three groups was observed for attrition, end of treatment weight loss, or subsequent weight maintenance.

Focusing more on the reports of binge eating, Telch and Agras (52) also examined binge eaters ($n = 20$) and nonbingers ($n = 71$) who participated in a treatment program involving behavior modification and a VLCD. Treatment began with a 12-week VLCD followed by gradual refeeding and 9 months of behavioral treatment (weekly meetings for 3 months, biweekly meetings for 3 months, and then monthly meetings for 3 months). Subjects self-reported their binge eating throughout this program by periodically reporting the number of binge days that had occurred in the prior week. Bingers reported 2.25 binge episodes per week at baseline, whereas the nonbingers had no binge episodes. Both groups had virtually no binges during the VLCD, but then both groups— nonbingers as well as bingers—reported an increase in binge eating during the behavioral program. At 9 months, both the bingers and nonbingers were reporting approximately 2 binges per week. By month 15 both bingers and nonbingers had returned to their baseline level of binge eating, with nonbingers reporting 0.5 binges per week and binge eaters reporting 2 binges per week. These data suggest that VLCD could cause a temporary period of binge eating in nonbingers. However, these data must be interpreted with caution because subjects may have temporarily changed their criteria for a binge episode after the VLCD. At this point in time, even small episodes of overeating may have been considered binges by nonbingers. The weight losses of the bingers and nonbingers were comparable, with a weight loss of approximately 14 kg at 3 months and maintenance of a 9.7-kg weight loss at 15 months (3 months after the end of the program).

The studies described above showed similar weight losses for bingers and nonbingers on a BT + VLCD regimen, a finding confirmed by Yanovski and colleagues (53). These investigators observed, however, that the bingers were more likely to regain their weight quickly after the VLCD. Bingers ($n = 21$) and nonbingers ($n = 17$) also had similar proportion of subjects who adhered perfectly to the VLCD, but bingers had fewer small lapses and more large lapses than nonbingers.

Taken as a whole, these studies indicate little difficulty in using VLCDs in the treatment of obese patients in general or obese bingers in particular. The concern that seems most appropriate to raise about these diets is not whether there are negative effects on lapses or binges, but rather whether these diets really lead to any improvement in long-term weight loss.

2. Low-Fat Diets

Another approach to improving weight loss in behavioral treatment programs has been to emphasize decreasing dietary fat intake, instead of or in addition to decreasing total calories. This approach is based on studies suggesting that subjects who are allowed to consume as much low-fat, high-carbohydrate food as they desire will decrease their calorie intake and lose weight (54,55).

Four recent behavioral studies have addressed the effects of restricting fat intake (Table 2). Jeffery and colleagues (56) compared the effectiveness of the usual behavioral approach of restricting calorie intake with a program based on restricting only the intake of dietary fat. Moderately overweight women ($n = 122$) were recruited; half of the women were given a fat goal (20 g of fat/day), but no calorie goal; the other half were given a calorie goal (1000–1200 kcal/day), but no dietary fat goal. Both groups were seen weekly for 6 weeks, biweekly for 20 weeks, and then monthly through 18 months. Weight losses at the end of 6 months were comparable in the two conditions; 4.6 kg for fat restriction and 3.7 kg for calorie restriction. Likewise no differences between conditions were seen at 12 or 18 months. By 18 months, both treatment groups had returned to their baseline weights. The weight losses of the calorie restriction condition are modest compared to most recent behavioral weight control studies, a finding that is not readily explained but may have been due to the fact that only six weekly meetings were held before turning to biweekly sessions.

Another group of investigators compared a low-fat, unrestricted-carbohydrate diet to the combination of calorie plus fat restriction. Schlundt et al. (20) randomly assigned 60 overweight subjects to a low-fat dietary intervention (20 g of fat) either with ad libitum carbohydrate intake or with calories restricted to 1200 kcal/day for women and 1500 for men. Forty-nine of the 60 subjects completed the 20-week treatment program. At the end of the 20 weeks, subjects in the low-fat, ad libitum carbohydrate condition had lost less weight than those who had both calorie and fat restriction (4.6 kg vs. 8.8 kg). Follow-up occurred after 9–12 months but included only 58% of the initial cohort. In these participants, follow-up weight losses averaged 2.6 kg for the ad libitum carbohydrate diet and 5.5 kg for the calorie-restricted subjects.

A calorie plus fat restriction condition similar to that used by Schlundt et al. (20) was also used by Pascale and colleagues (21), but compared in this study to the standard behavior approach of calorie restriction. Ninety subjects, half with non-insulin dependent diabetes (NIDDM) and half with a family history of diabetes, were studied. Subjects in the calorie restriction condition were instructed to consume 1000–1500 kcal/day, depending on initial body weight, and monitored the calories in each food they consumed. Those in the calorie plus fat restriction group were given a similar calorie goal, but in addition were given a fat gram goal corresponding to a fat intake of ≤20% of calories. These individuals recorded the calories and the grams of fat in each food they consumed. In the sample of NIDDMs, significant differences were seen between the two diet interventions, with greater weight loss in the calorie plus fat restriction condition both at the end of the 16-week treatment program (7.7 kg vs. 4.6 kg) and at 1-year follow-up (5.2 kg vs. 1.0 kg). There were no significant differences between the diet groups in the cohort of individuals at risk for diabetes. The data in Table 2 suggest that weight losses in the calorie restriction alone condition in the diabetic patients were poorer than would be expected given other similar studies.

All three of the above studies have somewhat poorer results than the majority of studies in Table 2. It might be speculated that emphasizing the diet, as was done in these three studies, decreases from the overall effectiveness of a behavioral program or that the shorter programs used in these studies were related to their poorer outcomes.

The best overall results in a dietary comparison study were reported by Viegener et al. (22). Eighty-five obese women were randomly assigned either to follow a 1200-kcal/day diet throughout or to alternate between an 800-kcal/day low-fat diet used 4 days per week and the 1200-kcal regimen. In this alternating condition, subjects were taught to restrict their fat intake to <25% of total calories on the 1200-kcal days and to <15% on the 800-kcal days. The goal of achieving "fat free" days was also introduced during this program and subjects were gradually encouraged to develop 4 fat-free days per week.

The dropout rate from this study was quite high (26%), but in the subjects who completed the 6-month behavioral program, there was a tendency toward greater weight losses in the alternating low-fat diet condition at months 1–4 of the program. At the end of the 6-month treatment, weight losses were comparable (8.9 kg in standard low calorie and 10.2 kg in alternating low fat). Subjects were then offered a chance to participate in a maintenance program with meetings held every two weeks for 6 months. Weight losses at the end of this 6-month maintenance program remained excellent in both groups (9.0 kg in both standard and alternating low fat).

Thus, taken as a whole, these studies suggest some potential benefit to a low calorie–low fat regimen, versus the traditional calorie-focused approach. However, the differences are not substantial. Moreover, the fact that several of the studies had a significant dropout rate makes conclusions from these studies more difficult. Additional evidence suggesting the importance of reducing dietary fat in behavioral weight control studies comes from a correlational analysis by Harris and colleagues (57) analyzing predictors of weight loss over an 18-month program in 82 men and 75 women. Changes in BMI were more strongly associated with changes in dietary fat intake than with changes in total calories. Moreover, decreases in consumption of certain specific foods—beef, hot dogs, and sweets—were associated with weight losses, as were increases in consumption of vegetables and increases in physical activity.

3. Providing More Structure Regarding Dietary Intake

As noted in the overview of the behavioral approach to obesity, teaching patients to rearrange their home environment is a key behavioral treatment strategy. Typically participants in behavioral weight control programs are encouraged to remove the high-calorie, high-fat foods from their home and to replace these items with healthier alternatives. Jeffery and colleagues (19) argued that better weight losses might be obtained if therapists intervened more directly on the home environment, by actually providing patients with the food they should eat in appropriate portion sizes. To test this hypothesis, these investigators recruited 202 overweight patients (half at the University of Minnesota and half at the University of Pittsburgh) and randomly assigned these participants to one of five groups. Group 1 was a no-treatment control group that received no weight control intervention and was simply followed over time. Group 2 received a standard behavioral treatment program (BT) with weekly meetings for 20 weeks and then monthly meetings and weekly weigh-ins through an 18-month treatment program. These participants were given a daily calorie goal of 1000 or 1500 kcal (depending on their initial weight) and encouraged to restrict their intake of dietary fat. In group 3, the standard behavioral program was supplemented by actual food provision. The calorie goals remained at 1000–1500 kcal/day, but subjects in group 3 were given a box of food each week that contained exactly what should be eaten for five breakfasts and five dinners each week. Patients selected their own lunches and all three meals on the other 2 days each week. Group 4 was designed to test the hypothesis that more direct reinforcement for weight loss might improve treatment outcome. The subjects in this group received BT, and in addition could earn up to $25.00 each week for losing weight and maintaining weight loss. Group 5 included BT, food provision, and payment for weight loss.

The main finding in this study was that food provision significantly increased weight loss. Weight losses with BT averaged 7.7, 4.5, and 4.1 kg at 6, 12, and 18 months, respectively, compared to 10.1, 9.1, and 6.4 with addition of food. Provision of incentives had no effect on weight loss.

After the 18-month program, all intervention was terminated and subjects were recontacted at 30 months to assess weight maintenance (58). Unfortunately, subjects in all four of the active treatment groups maintained weight losses of only 1.4–2.2 kg. These weight losses at 30 months were better than in the no-treatment control group, but did not differ among the four active treatment groups.

Since the use of food provision improved weight losses during the initial treatment program, actually doubling the results at month 12, a subsequent study was designed to determine which component of food provision was responsible for its success (25). Food provision includes actual food, which is provided free to subjects, and a meal plan specifying which foods should be eaten at which times. To determine which of these components is necessary, a cohort of 163 overweight women was recruited and the women were randomly assigned to either a standard behavioral program (BT), BT plus meal plans and grocery lists, BT plus meal plans plus food provided on a cost-sharing basis, or BT plus meal plans plus food provided free. Results at the end of the 6-month study showed that subjects in the BT condition had lost 8.0 kg. Weight losses in the other three groups, which were given meal plans or meal plans plus food, were all significantly better than those achieved by the BT condition and did not differ from each other (12.0, 11.7, and 11.4 kg, for groups 2–4, respectively). From these results, it appears that the most important component of food provision is the provision of structured meal plans and grocery lists; no further benefit was seen by actually giving food to the patients.

The meal plan and grocery lists appear to improve weight loss by changing the foods available in the home and creating a more regular meal pattern. Interestingly, the meal plans and grocery lists exerted as much of an effect on these variables as actual food provision.

Subjects in the treatment groups that were given either meal plans or actual food reported an increase in the number of days/week that they ate breakfast, an increase in the number of days that they ate lunch, and a decrease in the frequency of snacks. Likewise, when asked to survey their homes and to indicate what foods were currently stored in their homes, subjects given meal plans and those who were given the food reported greater increases than subjects in the BT condition in the number of fruits/vegetables, low-fat meats, medium-fat meats, breads/cereals, and low-calorie frozen entrees. Subjects in these conditions also reported less difficulty having appropriate foods available, estimating portion sizes, finding time to plan meals, and controlling eating when not hungry. On all these measures, the patients who were given the meal plans and grocery lists reported changes that were comparable to those of subjects who were actually given the food.

These data suggest that providing structure to participants on the type of foods they might consume for a low-calorie/low-fat eating plan is helpful to them. It remains unclear how long during treatment these meal plans should be continued and how best to help patients maintain their weight losses after the meal plans are terminated. However, these data do not suggest that patients should simply be handed a diet plan to use on their own. Rather, the meal plans and grocery lists were used as just one aspect of a far more extensive behavioral treatment program.

B. Exercise

As noted above, exercise is a key component of a behavioral weight loss program and has been strongly associated with the long-term maintenance of weight loss. However, despite the importance of exercise in the weight loss literature, there was little behavioral research on exercise conducted between 1990 and 1995. Previous to 1990, there were a number of behavioral treatment studies showing that the combination of diet plus exercise was more effective for long-term weight control than diet or exercise alone (33–35,59). Recently, Foreyt and colleagues (18) replicated this finding in a study of 165 mildly overweight adults who were randomly assigned to exercise only, diet only, diet plus exercise, or a waiting list control. Each group attended 12 weekly meetings, followed by three biweekly meetings and eight monthly meetings. The goal for the exercise groups was to complete three to five aerobic exercise sessions per week with each session lasting 45 min. The diet program focused on reducing fat to <30% of calories and utilized the Help Your Heart Eating Plan. At the end of 12 weeks, the two diet groups had lost significantly more weight (7.1 kg for diet only and 6.9 kg for diet plus exercise) than the exercise alone condition (0.32 kg) or the waiting list control (0.98 kg). Approximately 75% of participants completed the 1-year study. At that time, the diet plus exercise group maintained a weight loss of 8.1 kg, which was significantly greater than the exercise alone condition (2.7 kg), but not different from diet alone (6.3 kg).

Rather than simply addressing the issue of whether exercise is important to include in the behavioral treatment of obesity, some investigators have now begun to ask what type of exercise is best to prescribe (i.e., what type of exercise will produce the greatest adherence and best long-term weight loss?) and how best to prescribe exercise to promote adherence.

For example, Andersen and colleagues (24) compared a diet-only intervention, with a program that included either aerobic exercise, resistance training, or the combination of aerobic exercise and resistance training. One of the unique features of this study was that all of the treatments were conducted over a year-long period. Subjects in the exercise conditions attended supervised exercise sessions three times per week for the first 26 weeks of the study and then two times per week for the latter half of the program. For weeks 2–17 of the program, all groups followed a 925 kcal/day diet consisting of liquid meal replacements for two meals and a frozen entree for dinner.

Results at the end of the year-long program showed that all treatment groups had excellent weight losses but there were no significant differences between treatment groups. The diet-only group lost 12.9 kg over the year-long program, the diet plus aerobic exercise group lost 13.4 kg, the diet plus resistance training group lost 17.1 kg, and the diet plus both types of exercise group lost 15.3 kg. Thus, the diet-only group did not do more poorly than the groups given exercise interventions, as is usually seen. This difference may be due to the fact that all groups in this study consumed a diet of only 925 kcal/day for 16 weeks and continued to be seen for treatment interventions throughout a full year.

In his research with overweight children, Epstein has compared life-style exercise, aerobic exercise, and a calisthenics control condition (60,61). Subjects in the life-style condition could select any type of exercise and could exercise at the time of day they chose. In contrast, the aerobic exercise group was asked to commit themselves to a type of exercise and a specific time of day for exercise.

The life-style exercise condition produced somewhat greater reductions in obesity than the aerobic exercise condition at 5- and 10-year follow-up, but the major finding was that children in both these conditions maintained their weight losses far better than those in the calisthenics control conditions. Further research on life-style exercise is needed to test the effects of life-style exercise (such as using stairs instead of elevators) versus more structured or programmed exercise.

Epstein and colleagues also recently reported the results of a treatment program for overweight children that focused on increasing physical activity versus a program that focused on decreasing sedentary activities or the combination (36). In the decreased sedentary activity condition, the amount of time that the children could spend watching television or playing computer games was gradually reduced. At 1-year follow-up, the group that was taught to decrease sedentary activities had greater decreases in percent overweight than the group that was taught to increase aerobic exercise or the combination group. All groups increased in fitness, suggesting that the decreased sedentary activity group had used their extra time for more physical activities. In addition, children in the decreased sedentary activity group increased their liking of high-intensity physical activities more than the exercise conditions. These results suggest an interesting new approach that could be used to change activity level in overweight adults.

Several studies have tried to improve adherence to the exercise prescription by utilizing supervised exercise sessions (37), lottery or incentive systems (62), or by encouraging subjects to divide their exercise into several short bouts (e.g., four 10-min bouts each day rather than one 40-min bout). To test the effectiveness of prescribing exercise in multiple short bouts, Jakicic et al. (63) randomly assigned 56 overweight women to one of two treatments—a long-bout or a short-bout exercise condition. Both groups met weekly for 24 weeks and were provided with standard behavioral lessons and calorie and dietary fat monitoring. In addition, both groups were given comparable exercise goals, which gradually increased to a prescription of 40 min of exercise (brisk walking) 5 days/week. The long-bout exercise group was encouraged to set aside a time each day to accomplish this 40-min exercise. In contrast, the short-bout group was encouraged to divide their exercise into four 10-min episodes. Exercise adherence was determined by self-report diaries and by Tri-Trac accelerometers. The main findings of the study were that the short-bout group performed significantly more minutes of exercise over the 20-week program than the long-bout group and performed at least some exercise on more days/week. In addition, the short-bout group lost somewhat more weight than the long-bout group.

Another way to improve exercise adherence may be to use stronger antecedents to prompt exercise and stronger reinforcers. This approach was tested in a pilot study by Wing, Jeffery, and associates. To increase the cues for exercise, personal trainers were used; these trainers called the subjects regularly and met the participants at their office or house at the time scheduled for each walk. Financial incentives were used as a means of increasing reinforcement for exercise. Although neither the personal trainer nor the financial incentives produced statistically significant differences in exercise adherence or weight loss, the small sample size used in these studies limited the power to detect anything except large effects. Further research is needed to examine these approaches and other behavioral strategies that can be used to improve long-term adherence to exercise.

C. Strengthening the Behavioral Component

The research by Jeffery et al. (19) and Wing et al. (25) described above represents one approach to strengthening the behavioral component of weight loss programs by more directly modifying the home environment. Other recent approaches to improving behavioral programs have included lengthening the program, providing training in relapse prevention, and targeting specific subgroups of the obese population, most notably obese binge eaters. Each of these approaches will be discussed below.

1. Lengthening Treatment

Over the period 1970–1990, behavioral weight loss programs gradually succeeded in producing larger initial weight losses. Part of this improvement appeared to be due to lengthening of the treatment program. Whereas in 1974, the average treatment lasted 8 weeks and weight loss averaged 3.8 kg (0.5 kg weight loss/week), by 1990, the program had been increased to 21 weeks, and the weight loss had increased to 8.5 kg (0.4 kg weight loss/ week).

To more systematically investigate the effect of treatment length on outcome, Perri and colleagues compared a standard 20-week program to a 40-week program (64). The material presented was identical in the two conditions, but the 40-week program covered the lessons more gradually. At week 20, weight losses were comparable (8.9 kg in the standard 20-week program and 10.1 kg in the extended program). However, when treatment was terminated, subjects in the 20-week program began to regain weight, whereas those in extended treatment (who con-

tinued to participate in weekly therapy) increased their weight loss, thus producing significant differences between conditions at week 40 (6.4 kg in the standard program vs. 13.6 kg in the extended program). Between weeks 40 and 72, both groups regained weight, but at week 72, the extended condition maintained a significantly greater weight loss (9.8 kg vs. 4.6 kg).

While these data clearly show that lengthening treatment improves weight loss, it has been suggested that such continued contact merely delays the point at which weight regain occurs. The standard condition group regained 28% of their initial weight loss in the 20 weeks following cessation of therapy; the extended condition group regained the identical percent of their weight loss in the 32 weeks following the end of their treatment. Although it would thus appear that extended treatment is not helping participants learn the behavioral skills to a greater extent, the fact that relapse can be delayed is an important step forward—especially if by continuing to lengthen programs, relapse can be pushed further and further back in time.

Based on these findings, several recent treatment studies have evaluated year-long behavioral programs (16,17, 24). These studies were presented in detail in the sections on VLCD and exercise. As noted above, subjects in the Wadden et al. study (16) continued to lose weight over time, with weight losses averaging 11.9 kg at 26 weeks and 14.4 kg at 1 year. Wing et al. (17) found that the weight losses were best at 6 months (12.3 kg) and then subjects regained weight, maintaining a weight loss of 10.5 kg at 1 year. The changes between weeks 24 and 48 varied by treatment condition in the Andersen et al. study (24). From these results, it would appear that lengthening treatments to 1 year may be warranted. However, as noted by several of these investigators, attendance declines tremendously over time, and the cost:benefit ratio of extending treatment from 24 to 52 weeks is questionable.

Continuing to have regular contact with patients after the initial treatment program has also been shown to be beneficial for long-term maintenance of weight loss. Perri and colleagues (65) treated 123 women in a standard 20-week behavioral weight loss program, followed by different types of maintenance interventions over the subsequent year. One group of women received no further treatment contact over the year of follow-up; the others received 26 biweekly treatment contacts focusing on problem solving, problem solving plus aerobic exercise, problem solving plus social support, or problem solving plus aerobic exercise and social support. All four of the groups that received continued contact maintained their weight losses better than the no-contact condition, with no significant differences among the four conditions. Other studies have shown benefit to phone contact during the maintenance period (66,67). Thus, based on these studies, providing some form of ongoing contact with participants seems helpful, a conclusion also supported by the studies listed in Table 2.

2. Relapse Prevention

In 1985, Marlatt and Gordon developed a highly influential theory of relapse (42). Their writings stressed that relapse was a process, that it started with a lapse (or slip), and that depending on how the individual responded to the lapse, the situation might or might not develop into a full-blown relapse. This theory led behavioral researchers in two new directions: one focusing on the situation and events that might commonly trigger lapses, and the second focusing on the manner in which the individual coped with the lapse. Rosenthal and Marx (68) noted that approximately half of the lapses in dieters occurred during negative-affect situations, when the individual was alone, and the other half occurred in the company of others, usually due to enhancement of positive emotional states. Grilo et al. (69) extended this taxonomy and identified three clusters of situations that frequently caused temptations to lapse or actually precipitated lapses. One cluster, accounting for 48% of the crisis situations, involved mealtime situations and frequently occurred in restaurants or bars, during times of eating and socializing. A second cluster involved low arousal. This cluster accounted for 41% of the crises and most commonly occurred when the individual was at home, alone, during periods of relaxation. The third cluster accounted for only 11% of the crises but almost all of these crises resulted in overeating (i.e., the individual was not able to cope with the temptation to overeat and actually went on to overeat). These situations involved negative affect as the trigger or precipitant.

These authors also compared temptations and actual lapses and found that the factor that discriminated between these two was whether or not the individual reported any type of behavioral or cognitive coping. When no coping was reported, 100% of the episodes resulted in a lapse. In contrast, when either behavioral or cognitive coping was reported, approximately half of the episodes resulted in a lapse, and when both cognitive and behavioral coping were employed, only 15% of episodes resulted in a lapse.

Findings from the Grilo study (69) were used by Drapkin, Wing, and Shiffman (1995) to develop a hypothetical high-risk situation task. Ninety-three subjects who were about to enter a behavioral weight control program were asked to listen to four scenarios describing typical high-risk situations (family celebration, watching TV, tension at work, argument). These subjects were asked how they would cope with each of the high-risk situations and they indicated how difficult that particular situation would be for them. Telephone interviews were then conducted during the weight loss program to determine the situations in which dietary lapses actually occurred. Participants who rated the negative-affect situations (tension and anger) as most difficult were more likely to later lapse in situations involving negative affect. Moreover, those subjects who were able to generate more coping responses to these hypothetical high-risk situations later lost more weight. These data suggest that it might be possible to identify, at the start of the treatment program, those situations that will be most difficult for an individual participant and then to train these participants to handle such situations more effectively. Providing general training in coping also appears to be indicated.

While research stemming from Marlatt and Gordon's theory has provided insights into the relapse process, these insights have had limited impact on treatment outcome in the weight loss field. Perri and colleagues (66) supplemented a standard behavioral weight control program with six sessions devoted to individualized relapse prevention training. Participants were taught to identify situations posing high risk for overeating, to approach these situations with problem-solving skills, and to cognitively interpret these situations as learning experiences rather than as instances of failure. The participants also practiced their relapse prevention skills in two actual high-risk situations. This relapse prevention training was tested in a study involving three treatment groups (nonbehavior therapy, behavior therapy, or behavior therapy plus relapse prevention training) crossed with two maintenance strategies (posttreatment contact by mail and phone or no contact.) The only group that maintained its posttreatment weight loss through 12-month follow-up was the group given behavior therapy plus relapse prevention training and the posttreatment contact, suggesting some benefits from this relapse prevention training.

3. Programs for Binge Eaters

Approximately 30% of participants in behavioral weight control programs report significant problems with binge eating (48–50). These participants may do better in programs that focus not only on weight loss but also on their binge eating problems. To test this, Porzelius et al. (70) evaluated the effectiveness of a treatment program specifically designed for obese binge eaters. This program included training in coping skills to help patients deal with depression and binge eating, provided a socially supportive environment to improve social skills, and reduced overly restrictive dieting patterns that might contribute to binge eating. This binge eating program was compared to a standard behavioral treatment in a sample of 54 overweight women, who were classified by the Binge Eating Scale into those with no binge problems ($n = 16$), moderate problems ($n = 18$), and severe binge eating problems ($n = 20$). There was a significant interaction between binge status and treatment group for weight losses over the 17-week program.* Women with severe binge eating problems lost somewhat more weight when treated in the binge eating program rather than in the standard program (approximately 4.5 kg vs. 3.0 kg). In contrast, subjects with moderate and no binge problems lost more weight in the standard treatment condition than in the binge program (8.5 kg and 5 kg, respectively). At 12-month follow-up, all groups of women in the standard behavioral weight control program had regained most of their weight loss. In contrast, the severe binge eaters treated in the binge eating program continued to lose weight, reaching an overall weight loss of 8 kg at 1-year follow-up. This pattern of continued weight loss is very unusual and suggests that this treatment should be given further study. However, it should be noted that this result is based on a very small sample (11 women at pretreatment, nine of whom completed the 17-week program and seven of whom completed the follow-up.

4. Computerized Instruction

Finally, another approach to treatment is to use hand-held computers to provide more individualized and immediate feedback to participants. Two studies by Agras et al. (23,71) evaluated the effects of computerized instruction on weight control. The goal of these studies was to decrease the cost of behavioral treatment by substituting a hand-held computer for the large number of therapy sessions, and to allow more individualized and immediate feedback by having patients enter their foods and exercise on the computer, which then provided immediate feedback on the participants' progress. In the Agras et al. study (23), one group of subjects was given the computer plus one introductory session; another group was given the computer plus group meetings at weeks 2, 4, 6, and 8; and the third group was given 10 behavioral sessions over 12 weeks (with no computer). There were no significant

---

*The study by Porzelius was not included in Table 2 because it represents an effort to develop a behavioral program for a subset of obese patients, not for all obese patients, with the hypothesis and the observed result of an interaction between treatment condition and binge status.

differences in weight loss between groups, but what was most surprising about this study was the poor performance in the "standard" behavioral group. These subjects lost only 1.8 kg over 12 weeks, which, as seen in Table 2, is quite different from the majority of treatment studies.

Taylor et al. (71) attempted to improve the effectiveness of the computer by developing more sophisticated computer software and also using the computer along with a 1200-kcal diet based on consumption of frozen entrees. Group 1 used the computer and received four classes in behavioral treatment; they were encouraged to use the frozen foods as desired. Group 2, in contrast, used the frozen foods first, until achieving a 4–5-kg weight loss, and then used the computer. This latter strategy improved the 12-week weight loss outcome (5.3 kg vs. 3.1 kg). However, rather than supporting the effectiveness of the computer, this study suggests the effectiveness of a more structured eating plan, a strategy discussed above in more detail.

Thus, based on these two studies, there is little evidence that computer-assisted instruction is an appropriate alternative to group behavioral treatment programs.

V. CONCLUSIONS

Behavioral treatment programs focus on teaching participants to change their diet (calories and percent of fat consumed) and their exercise behaviors. It appears that there has been a fair amount of standardization in the way in which participants are helped to make these life-style changes. However, despite the seeming standardization, weight losses at the end of treatment have varied from 1.8 kg to 17 kg. Averaging across studies, participants in current (1990–1995) behavioral programs lose 9.7 kg, a slight improvement over results obtained in 1990. Reviewing the current studies, it appears that the best initial results are obtained in longer programs, i.e., those lasting 6–12 months. In addition, programs with VLCD produce better initial weight losses, with some evidence that structured meal plans, food provision, and alternating regimens (low calorie/low fat to very low calorie/very low fat) also improve initial outcome. In several studies with these characteristics (i.e., longer treatment intervals and more structured diets), weight losses have consistently been 10–17 kg at the end of the initial treatment (16,17,19,22,24,25). This ability to consistently produce weight losses of 10 kg or more represents a significant improvement in the effectiveness of behavioral treatment programs.

It is more difficult to draw conclusions about the variables associated with the long-term maintenance of weight loss. In current studies (1990–1995), participants maintain 60% of their initial weight loss, and the average weight loss at follow-up (5.6 kg) is no different than that obtained in 1990. Further research is clearly needed to determine how to produce better maintenance of initial weight losses. Evidence supporting the effectiveness of exercise as a maintenance strategy is compelling, but it is unclear what kind of exercise to include or how to achieve long-term performance of exercise. At present, the only other approach to improving maintenance of weight loss is to improve initial weight loss. Perhaps better long-term results could be obtained by returning to the initial premises of behavior modification and focusing more directly on a functional analysis of behaviors in individual participants. Alternatively, a better understanding of why participants have so much difficulty maintaining their weight loss might help us to develop more effective long-term approaches.

ACKNOWLEDGMENT

Preparation of this chapter was supported by NIH Grants HL41330, DK29757, DK46204.

REFERENCES

1. Skinner BF. The Behavior of Organisms: An Experimental Analysis. New York: Appleton-Century-Crofts, 1938.
2. Bandura A. Social Learning Theory. Englewood Cliffs, NJ: Prentice-Hall, 1977.
3. Ferster CB, Nurnberger JI, Levitt EB. The control of eating. J Mathetics 1962; 1:87–109.
4. Stuart RB. Behavioral control of overeating. Behav Res Ther 1967; 5:357–365.
5. Brownell KD, Wadden TA. Behavior therapy for obesity: modern approaches and better results. In: Brownell KB, Foreyt JP, eds. Handbook of Eating Disorders: Physiology, Psychology, and Treatment of Obesity, Anorexia and Bulimia. New York: Basic Books, 1986:180–198.
6. Wadden TA, Bell ST. Obesity. In: Bellack AS, Hersen M, Kazdin A, eds. International Handbook of Behavior Modification and Therapy, Vol II. New York: Plenum Press, 1990:449–472.
7. Kazdin AE. Self-monitoring and behavior change. In: Mahoney MJ, Thoresen CF, eds. Self-Control: Power to the Person. Monterey, CA: Brooks/Cole, 1974.
8. Wing RR. Behavioral strategies for weight reduction in obese type II diabetic patients. Diabetes Care 1989; 12: 139–144.
9. Jeffery RW, Thompson PD, Wing RR. Effects on weight reduction of strong monetary contracts for calorie restriction or weight loss. Behav Res Ther 1978; 16:363–369.
10. Jeffery RW, Gerber WM, Rosenthal BS, Lindquist RA. Monetary contracts in weight control: effectiveness of group and individual contracts of varying size. J Consult Clin Psychol 1983; 51(2):242–248.
11. Jeffery RW, Wing RR, Stunkard AJ. Behavioral treatment of obesity: the state of the art. Behav Ther 1978; 9:189–199.
12. McReynolds WT, Lutz RN, Paulsen BK, Kohrs MB. Weight loss resulting from two behavior modification procedures with nutritionists as therapists. Behav Ther 1976; 7: 283–291.
13. Penick Sb, Filion R, Fox S, Stunkard AJ. Behavior modification in the treatment of obesity. Psychosom Med 1971; 33:49–55.
14. Wadden TA. The treatment of obesity: an overview. In: Stunkard AJ, Wadden TA, eds. Obesity Theory and Therapy. New York: Raven Press, 1993:197–218.
15. Brownell KD. The LEARN Program for Weight Control. Dallas, TX: American Health Publishing Company, 1991.
16. Wadden TA, Foster GD, Letizia KA. One-year behavioral treatment of obesity: comparison of moderate and severe caloric restriction and the effects of weight maintenance therapy. J Consult Clin Psychol 1994; 62:165–171.
17. Wing RR, Blair E, Marcus M, Epstein LH, Harvey J. Year-long weight loss treatment for obese patients with type II diabetes: does inclusion of an intermittent very low calorie diet improve outcome? Am J Med 1994; 97:354–362.
18. Foreyt JP, Goodrick GK, Reeves RS, Raynaud AS, Darnell L, Brown AH, Gotto AM. Response of free-living adults to behavioral treatment of obesity: attrition and compliance to exercise. Behav Ther 1993; 24:659–669.
19. Jeffery RW, Wing RR, Thorson C, Burton LR, Raether C, Harvey J, Mullen M. Strengthening behavioral interventions for weight loss: a randomized trial of food provision and monetary incentives. J Consult Clin Psychol 1993; 61: 1038–1045.
20. Schlundt DG, Hill JO, Pope-Cordle J, Arnold D, Virts KL, Katahn M. Randomized evaluation of a low fat ad libitum carbohydrate diet for weight reduction. Int J Obes 1993; 17:623–629.
21. Pascale RW, Wing RR, Butler BA, Mullen M, Bononi P. Effects of a behavioral weight loss program stressing calorie restriction versus calorie plus fat restriction in obese individuals with NIDDM or a family history of diabetes. Diabetes Care 1995; 18(9):1241–1248.
22. Viegener BJ, Perri MG, Nezu AM, Renjilian DA, McKelvey WF, Schein RL. Effects of an intermittent, low-fat, low-calorie diet in the behavioral treatment of obesity. Behav Ther 1990; 21:499–509.
23. Agras WS, Taylor CB, Feldman DE, Losch M, Burnett KF. Developing computer-assisted therapy for the treatment of obesity. Behav Ther 1995; 21:99–109.
24. Andersen RE, Wadden TA, Bartlett SJ, Vogt RA, Weinstock RS. Relation of weight loss to changes in serum lipids and lipoproteins in obese women. Am J Clin Nutr 1995; 62: 350–357.
25. Wing RR, Jeffery RW, Burton LR, Thorson C, Sperber Nissinoff K, Baxter JE. Food provision vs. structured meal

plans in the behavioral treatment of obesity. Int J Obes 1996; 20:56–62.

26. Wadden TA, Letizia KA. Predictors of attrition and weight loss in patients treated by moderate and severe caloric restriction. In: Wadden TA, VanItallie TB, eds. Treatment of the Seriously Obese Patient. New York: Guilford Press, 1992:383–410.

27. Guare JC, Wing RR, Marcus M, Epstein LH, Burton LR, Gooding WE. Analysis of changes in eating behavior and weight loss in type II diabetic patients. Diabetes Care 1989; 12:500–503.

28. Bandura A, Simon KM. The role of proximal intentions in self-regulation of refractory behavior. Cognit Ther Res 1977; 1:177–193.

29. Pronk NP, Wing RR. Physical activity and long-term maintenance of weight loss. Obes Res 1994; 2:587–599.

30. Kayman S, Bruvold W, Stern JS. Maintenance and relapse after weight loss in women: behavioral aspects. Am J Clin Nutr 1990; 52:800–807.

31. Jeffery RW, Bjornson-Benson WM, Rosenthal BS, Lindquist RA, Kurth CL, Johnson SL. Correlates of weight loss and its maintenance over two years of follow-up among middle-aged men. Prev Med 1984; 13:155–168.

32. Colvin RH, Olson SB. Winners revisited: an 18-month follow-up of our successful weight losers. Addict Behav 1984; 9:305–306.

33. Dahlkoetter J, Callahan EJ, Linton J. Obesity and the unbalanced energy equation: exercise versus eating habit change. J Consult Clin Psychol 1979; 47:898–905.

34. Stalonas PM, Johnson WG, Christ M. Behavior modification for obesity: the evaluation of exercise, contingency management, and program adherence. J Consult Clin Psychol 1978; 46:463–469.

35. Wing RR, Epstein LH, Paternostro-Bayles M, Kriska A, Nowalk MP, Gooding W. Exercise in a behavioural weight control programme for obese patients with type 2 (non-insulin-dependent) diabetes. Diabetologia 1988; 31: 902–909.

36. Epstein LH, Valoski AM, Vara LS, McCurley J, Wisniewski L, Kalarchian MA, Klein KR, Shrager LR. Effects of decreasing sedentary behavior and increasing activity on weight change in obese children. Health Psychol 1995; 14: 109–115.

37. Craighead LW, Blum MD. Supervised exercise in behavioral treatment for moderate obesity. Behav Ther 1989; 20: 49–59.

38. D'Zurilla TJ, Goldfried MR. Problem solving and behavior modification. J Abnorm Psychol 1971; 78:107–126.

39. Beck AT. Cognitive Therapy and the Emotional Disorders. New York: International Universities Press, 1976.

40. Mahoney MJ, Mahoney K. Permanent Weight Control: A Total Solution to the Dieter's Dilemma. New York: WW Norton, 1976.

41. Marlatt GA, Gordon JR. Determinants of relapse: implications for the maintenance of behavior change. In: Davidson PO, Davidson SM, eds. Behavioral Medicine: Changing Health Lifestyles. New York: Brunner/Mazel, 1979:410–452.

42. Marlatt GA, Gordon JR. Relapse Prevention: Maintenance Strategies in Addictive Behavior Change. New York: Guilford Press, 1985.

43. National Task Force on the prevention and treatment of obesity. Very low-calorie diets. JAMA 1993; 270(8): 967–974.

44. Wadden TA, Stunkard AJ, Brownell KD. Very low calorie diets: their efficacy, safety, and future. Ann Intern Med 1983; 99:675–684.

45. Wadden TA, Stunkard AJ. Controlled trial of very low calorie diet, behavior therapy, and their combination in the treatment of obesity. J Consult Clin Psychol 1986; 54: 482–488.

46. Wing RR, Marcus MD, Salata R, Epstein LH, Miaskiewicz S, Blair EH. Effects of a very-low-calorie diet on long-term glycemic control in obese type 2 diabetic subjects. Arch Intern Med 1991; 151:1334–1340.

47. Wing RR, Shiffman S, Drapkin RG, Grilo CM, McDermont M. Moderate versus restrictive diets: implications for relapse. Behav Ther 1995; 26:5–24.

48. Yanovski SZ. Binge eating disorder: current knowledge and future directions. Obes Res 1993; 1(4):306–324.

49. Marcus MD, Wing RR, Hopkins J. Obese binge eaters: affect, cognitions, and response to behavioral weight control. J Consult Clin Psychol 1988; 56:433–439.

50. Marcus MD. Binge eating in obesity. In: Fairburn CG, Wilson GT, eds. Binge Eating. Nature, Assessment, and Treatment. New York: Guilford Press, 1993:77–96.

51. Wadden TA, Foster GD, Letizia KA. Response of obese binge eaters to treatment by behavior therapy combined with very low calorie diet. J Consult Clin Psychol 1992; 60:808–811.

52. Telch CF, Agras WS. The effects of a very low calorie diet on binge eating. Behav Ther 1993; 24:177–193.

53. Yanovski SZ, Gormally JF, Leser MS, Gwirtsman HE, Yanovski JA. Binge eating disorder affects outcome of comprehensive very-low-calorie diet treatment. Obes Res 1994; 2:205–212.

54. Insull W, Henderson MM, Prentice RL, Thompson DJ, Clifford C, Goldman S, Gorbach S, Moskowitz M, Thompson R, Woods M. Results of a randomized feasibility study of a low-fat diet. Arch Intern Med 1990; 150:421–427.

55. Kendall A, Levitsky DA, Strupp BJ, Lissner L. Weight loss on a low-fat diet: consequence of the impression of the control of food intake in humans. Am J Clin Nutr 1991; 53:1124–1129.

56. Jeffery RW, Hellerstedt WL, French SA, Baxter JE. A randomized trial of counseling for fat restriction versus calorie restriction in the treatment of obesity. Int J Obes 1995; 19: 132–137.

57. Harris JK, French SA, Jeffery RW, McGovern PG, Wing RR. Dietary and physical activity correlates of long-term weight loss. Obes Res 1994; 2(4):307–313.

58. Jeffery RW, Wing RR. Long-term effects of interventions for weight loss using food provision and monetary incentives. J Consult Clin Psychol 1995; 63:793–796.

59. Pavlou KN, Krey S, Steffee WP. Exercise as an adjunct to weight loss and maintenance in moderately obese subjects. Am J Clin Nutr 1989; 49:1115–1123.

60. Epstein LH, Wing RR, Koeske R, Valoski A. A comparison of lifestyle exercise, aerobic exercise, and calisthenics on weight loss in obese children. Behav Ther 1985; 16:345–356.

61. Epstein LH, Valoski A, Wing RR, McCurley J. Ten year outcomes of behavioral family based treatment for childhood obesity. Health Psychol 1994; 13:373–383.

62. Epstein LH, Wing RR, Thompson JK, Griffin W. Attendance and fitness in aerobics exercise: the effects of contract and lottery procedures. Behav Mod 1980; 4:465–479.

63. Jakicic JM, Wing RR, Butler BA, Robertson RJ. Prescribing exercise in multiple short bouts versus one continuous bout: effects on adherence, cardiorespiratory fitness, and weight loss in overweight women. Int J Obes 1995; 19:893–901.

64. Perri MG, Nezu AM, Patti ET, McCann KL. Effect of length of treatment on weight loss. J Consult Clin Psychol 1989; 57(3):450–452.

65. Perri MG, McAllister DA, Gange JJ, Jordan RC, McAdoo WG, Nezu AM. Effects of four maintenance programs on the long-term management of obesity. J Consult Clin Psychol 1988; 56:529–534.

66. Perri MG, Shapiro RM, Ludwig WW, Twentyman CT, McAdoo WG. Maintenance strategies for the treatment of obesity: an evaluation of relapse prevention training and post-treatment contact by mail and telephone. J Consult Clin Psychol 1984; 52:404–413.

67. King AC, Frey-Hewitt B, Dreon DM, Wood PD. The effects of minimal intervention strategies on long-term outcomes in men. Arch Intern Med 1989; 149:2741–2746.

68. Rosenthal BS, Marx RD. Determinants of initial relapse episodes among dieters. Obes Bariatr Med 1981; 10:94–97.

69. Grilo CM, Shiffman S, Wing RR. Relapse crises and coping among dieters. J Consult Clin Psychol 1989; 57(4):488–495.

70. Porzelius LK, Houston C, Smith M, Arfkin C, Fisher E, Jr. Comparison of a standard behavioral weight loss treatment and a binge eating weight loss treatment. Behav Ther 1995; 26:119–134.

71. Taylor CB, Agras WS, Losch M, Plante TG, Burnett K. Improving the effectiveness of computer-assisted weight loss. Behav Ther 1991; 22:229–236.

43

Dietary Treatment of Obesity

Luc F. Van Gaal
University of Antwerp, Antwerp, Belgium

I. REFLECTIONS ON DIET AND NUTRITION IN OBESITY

Despite recent advances in understanding the genetic basis of obesity (1,2), overeating and/or unbalanced food intake (3–5) remains a major element in the origin and the maintenance of overweight and obesity (6). Both total calorie intake and fat consumption (6,7) have been shown, together with abnormalities in energy expenditure, to be responsible for the development or maintenance of obesity. In addition, the self-perception of such unbalanced food intake is very low; this became clear from reports that obese individuals are underreporting not only total calorie intake (6), but also the intake of specific food items (8).

Many diets on the worldwide bestseller lists range from the sublime to the ridiculous; the rapid turnover of these popular diets can be considered a reflection of their sometimes rather limited scientific value. The proliferation and seemingly endless concern with diets for the treatment of obesity suggests that this search is sometimes more motivated by financial rewards for the promoters rather than by an honest desire to provide healthy and safe nutrition. However, a series of reports have shown that even modest weight reduction by diet modification can improve cardiovascular risk factors and reduce cardiovascular morbidity and mortality (9,10).

The most logical and complete approach to the treatment of obesity focuses not only on dietary regimens but also on life-style modification. Behavioral approaches include an emphasis on daily physical activity, as well as on overeating (11), impulsive (binge) or unplanned eating (12), and the macronutrient composition of the diet (13,14).

Dietary therapy remains the cornerstone of treatment, and the reduction of energy intake continues to be the basis of successful weight reduction programs (15). Over the years it became clear that long-term changes in food habits and dietary choices are needed, rather than a temporary restriction of calories (16). Absolute weight loss, per se, as expressed in kilograms of weight or fat loss, is not the only therapeutic target: one of the first steps in a clinical approach to any obese subject should be focused on the reduction and/or normalization of any potential or existing metabolic abnormality (glucose intolerance, dyslipidemia, hyperinsulinism, or hemostatic abnormalities), or complications such as diabetes, hypertension, or sleep apnea syndrome (17–20).

Changes in body composition mainly present in obesity involve storage of excess material, which is approximately 75% of fat but also 25% of nonfat tissue (21). It is therefore of extreme importance that a safe treatment for obesity should focus on loss of weight that is of similar magnitude and composition to that of excess weight. There is, however, no single dietary strategy for all obese individuals. The treatment of each individual should therefore meet the needs of that individual.

In a recent paper about the controversial issue of the treatment of obesity, Wooley and Garner express surprise that the debate about the effectiveness of dietary treatment still continues. They describe the well-known phenomenon that 90–95% of those who lose weight during a dietary program will regain it within several years (22). "Such a poor outcome has led to charges that a traditional treatment for obesity, should be abandoned and counter-charges that it is even irresponsible to withhold treatment for such a serious problem" (22).

Losing weight is relatively easy, but the maintenance of weight loss may be more distressing if the patient is not adequately informed on the correct ways and means of weight control. The failure of long-term dietary treatment is ascribable not only to the patient but to the method, which does not always take into account the biology of weight regulation, the heritability, and the patient-specific physiology of energy metabolism. In view of that "proper method"—correct ways and means of weight control—Garrow points out that failures of badly conducted therapies result in a worsening of the psychological condition (23). The maintenance of the weight loss may also be more difficult if the patient is not adequately informed on the correct way to control body weight. The author proposes a wide-scale educational program informing the general population about the threshold for morbid obesity and the consequences necessitating adequate therapy (23).

To the Shakespearian dilemma whether obesity should be treated or not, it is our own feeling that weight reduction appears desirable, even by dietary regimens, despite the fact that results are known to be poor and not long-lasting. Dietary approaches and outcome perspectives should be worked out in relation to the individual patient and the associated comorbidity. The treatment of obesity should concentrate on patients rather than on their weight.

In a recent review of treatments for obesity, Wadden showed rather optimistic results, reporting on studies that incorporated behavior modification, in addition to moderate and severe caloric restriction (24).

A review of 24 papers with almost 4000 subjects that included follow-up information of at least 3 years yielded a median percentage of 19% for subjects who maintained all their lost weight (25). The improvement in long-term results of weight loss programs has been shown to be related to the increased length of programs and to the development of maintenance sessions (26). Many papers have produced scientific knowledge over the last few years suggesting that prudent weight-reducing diets are capable of producing a reduction or "near-normalization" of atherosclerosis-linked risk factors, despite a limited reduction in fat (10,27).

In fact, a previous attitude of aggressive treatments with drastic caloric restriction and large pharmacological support is still widespread. This approach does not teach the patient a "normal" healthy eating behavior and, for psychological and biological reasons, sets the basis for weight cycling (28) and its possible negative health consequences (29). By contrast, a policy of small sacrifices for small benefits is often rewarding. In this respect, a partial result needs to be considered as beneficial and hence it may be a reasonable goal (30). The chances of achieving worthwhile weight loss in severe obesity are poor. We should recall that obesity is never severe when it begins (23); thus, we should also pay special attention to moderately overweight patients, in particular those with an unfavorable risk profile and visceral fat accumulation, in order to stop the progression of their condition. We should capitalize on the therapeutic options available today, although still largely imperfect, with the goal of improving the clinical condition of these patients.

II. GENERAL DIETARY ASPECTS AND OBJECTIVES

Although researchers have not yet arrived at a consensus on the definition of "successful weight loss," the general objective is to lose 0.5–1.0 kg/week by a combination of restricted energy intake and increased energy output (23). My personal experience has proven that it is often better to focus on limited weight loss, with reasonable perspectives of maintaining it, instead of unreasonable regimens with enormous and unpredictable psychological consequences.

Although most dieters strive to achieve "ideal" body weight, clinical and laboratory evidence supports the value of modest weight loss (9). It is known, that initial weight loss can be achieved relatively easily in therapy-naïve patients. Whenever a diet is not successful, patients often choose a modified fast as a strategy to lose weight, which will lead to a certain degree of desired weight loss. Unfortunately, for most individuals pursuing such a strategy, weight relapse is usual.

Among conventional reducing diets a variety of approaches have been proposed. These diets supply 800–1200 kcal daily, based on a selection of normal foods. Although this approach supplies less energy than the patient's maintenance requirements, the great disadvantage for inexperienced people is the difficulty of calculating the weight of each food item and the total energy content (21). They often underestimate energy intake not only outside the scope of treatment programs, but even the total energy of a prescribed diet.

It is theoretically possible to construct a diet by reducing the quantities of each food item, but this approach would also reduce the content of all other nutrients. It seems more logical, therefore, to make reductions in those food items that contain so-called "empty calories," such as fat, alcohol, and refined sugars (21). Moderate restriction of carbohydrates may have real calorie-reducing properties; limitation of bread, the most likely carbohydrate-containing item in an average Caucasian population, may lead to a reduction of items that are usually eaten on bread such as butter, jam, and other fat-containing "mixtures." In contrast to the possible advantages of a moderate carbohydrate restriction are the potential risks of carbohydrate avoidance as described in *Dr. Atkins Diet Revolution* (31). From a clinical point of view, severe carbohydrate restriction (<20 g daily) may lead to ketosis, water loss due to the depletion of body glycogen stores, possible electrolyte imbalances, and increased bile lithogenicity.

Another important phenomenon is the omission of dietary fiber in patients who severely restrict their carbohydrate intake. In addition, no real fat-mobilizing properties have been described with these diets. If both carbohydrate and fat are restricted, the only other source of energy is protein. The label 'high-protein diet' may mislead people to believe that high protein intake by itself may reduce weight. Protein-enriched diets are discussed in detail in the section on very low calorie diets (VLCDs).

A large number of exotic, nonsense, charlatan diets exist, including: the Beverly Hills diet; specific fruit diets; the "fabulous fructose diet"; the sherry diet; and the more recent Montignac diet. By following such diets, the nutritionally untrained "victims" run the risk of serious nutritional deficiencies, without having the guarantee of safe and successful weight reduction.

Other dietary approaches have been studied, a few of which will be mentioned. Lactovegetarian diets seem to be as effective as regular, traditional weight-reducing diets.

Treatment of obesity may affect many more than those taking part in the program itself. A positive effect on obese family members may be considered beneficial and has generally resulted in additional weight loss.

Caution should be given about the potential harm of commercially run weight groups. The best known are Weight Watchers International and Take Off Pounds Sensibly (TOPS). Data on the long-term effectiveness of these groups are limited. In a comprehensive survey of weight losses in Weight Watchers groups, it was found that, on average, patients lost approximately 13–14 kg in 30 weeks (32). Despite the fact that these results do not seem superior to results of outpatient clinics and the absence of medical supervision, their methodology may be better than many uncontrolled over-the-counter programs. It would seem worthwhile for commercial clinics to publish

their results in a scientific way in order to have correct information about the compliance, success, and impact of their program (33).

III. LOW-FAT VERSUS LOW-CALORIES

Clinical and experimental evidence stresses the importance of distinguishing between rapid versus slow weight loss, weight loss per se and weight stabilization. Several studies have shown that high-fat foods are among favorites for obese men and women (34,35), and that high fat foods are related to obesity (36), which suggests that fat-restricted diets may be beneficial. Low-fat, low-calorie diets have recently been compared against a low-fat, ad libitum carbohydrate diet. The former is suitable for achieving rapid weight loss (due to the larger energy deficit) and the latter for achieving a small weight loss (per time unit) or weight stabilization (35).

In an overweight person eating a low-fat, ad libitum carbohydrate diet, weight loss usually occurs gradually over a long period. The larger and the faster the weight loss, the larger the risk for weight relapse. Traditional low-fat, low-calorie diets should be monitored with the aid of food diaries, to identify patient compliance, and with the collaboration with skilled dieticians and/or an organized health education system.

According to recent research, diet composition may play an important role in the regulation of food intake and adipose stores (8,13). Fat, not carbohydrate, is the macronutrient associated with overeating and obesity (35). A diet that is high in fat while low in carbohydrate, especially when combined with a sedentary life-style, promotes the development and maintenance of large adipose stores (13). Studies of nutrient dilution have suggested that humans are unable to increase energy intake to compensate for removal of a substantial amount of fat from their daily food intake. Some have suggested that fat intake is not biologically well regulated while it stimulates overconsumption because of its palatability (37). Since dietary fat intake, as opposed to total energy intake, has attracted more attention in both the etiology and treatment of obesity, one of the recent challenging options in treating overweight patients is to use dietary fat reduction only, rather than total caloric restriction.

Information derived from population studies has suggested that the prevalence of obesity has increased over time in those groups where a concurrent increase in fat consumption was found (38). It was recently shown that with increasing fat content (30–50% of energy), there is a significant increase in the CHO/fat oxidation ratio (7).

Studies of dietary predictors of weight change have also reported that changes in the consumption of specific food items, rich in fat content, can predict the outcome of weight loss better than do changes in total energy intake (39). In the context of these findings it may be that the use of fat substitutes to reduce fat intake may be a particularly useful strategy for weight control (40).

Different studies have shown that weight loss can be obtained more easily in individuals on a low-fat diet, even when total energy intake is maintained at the predietary trial level. When comparing a low-fat, ad libitum carbohydrate diet with a low-fat, low-calorie diet, both interventions are known to lead to a decrease in body weight, despite the fact that the latter strategy induces nearly twice as much weight loss as the former (41). A beneficial effect was found regarding the loss of lean body mass with the low-fat, ad libitum carbohydrate diet, although the decrease in percentage fat mass was clearly larger with the low-calorie regimen. Restriction of fat and total energy intake seems a more efficient strategy for weight reduction than the restriction of fat alone. This is not surprising, since the amount of weight loss is principally determined by the amount of energy restriction.

The micronutrient composition, especially of vitamins, in an ad libitum carbohydrate diet is more favorable than that of a low-fat, low-carbohydrate diet. In view of the potentially important role of vitamins and micronutrients in disease prevention (antioxidant potential and prevention of cardiovascular disease risk), such a diet should be promoted in obese subjects, particularly in those at risk for heart disease (42).

Among a large group of moderately overweight, premenopausal women, fat restriction (20 g/day) was compared to caloric restriction (1000–1200 kcal). Although the weight losses after 6 months of the low-fat versus the low-caloric group were not significantly different (4.6 vs. 3.7 kg, respectively), women in the low-fat group showed a better long-term adherence and compliance with treatment guidelines, which may be expected to lead to better maintenance of weight loss. Fat intake predicted weight change better than total energy intake (43). Similar findings were previously reported (44) indicating that weight loss is possible in active life style women and more strongly associated with changes in percent energy from fat than with changes in total energy intake. In postmenopausal women receiving a low-fat diet as a part of therapy for early breast cancer, similar findings were reported (45).

More drastic weight-loss regimens may be more successful in the short term (43), but a large number of these subjects regain their weight after several months. Counseling women to eat a low-fat diet led to ratings of the diet as more palatable than a traditional energy-restricted diet, which could contribute to the greater reduction in binge eating scores found in that study, and to better long-term maintenance. A series of observations suggest that this approach to weight control may deserve further study, despite the fact that low-fat diets are shown not to be consistent in producing long-term weight change (43).

Several studies have emphasized the importance, of not only consuming low-fat foods, but also avoiding particular high-fat foods. In one recent study, the change in frequency for consumption of specific foods (beef, hot dogs, and sweets) accounted for a larger percentage of the variance in body mass index change than did change in macronutrient consumption (46).

IV. VERY-LOW-CALORIE DIETS

In an attempt to obtain as rapid weight loss as possible, total starvation and very-low-calorie diets (VLCD) have been proposed for many years (47). Therapeutic starvation is the ultimate low-caloric diet. This was an accepted form of inpatient treatment for morbid obesity in 1950s and the early 1960s. Numerous medical problems were associated with prolonged starvation, which led to its almost complete disappearance from the clinical scene (47). Not only medical complications (ventricular fibrillation, lactic acidosis, small bowel disease, vitamin and electrolyte deficiencies), but the poor maintenance of weight losses (50–80% of patients regained their initial weight), were important factors in its abandonment (47).

Starvation has been replaced by the VLCD (alternatively called the protein-sparing modified fast) as a safe alternative to the risks of severe negative nitrogen balance and electrolyte imbalances associated with starvation (47–50). VLCDs are used to achieve significant weight loss while supplying the minimum of energy and enough essential nutrients to avoid side effects. Introduced as a supplementation of proteins to prevent nitrogen loss, the initial diets contained between 200 and 400 kcal (850–1650 kJ) daily, predominantly as protein (51). Starting from 40–60 g protein per day, the daily amount was increased to 70–100 g in the 1970s (52). Using turnover studies with ^{15}N-glycine, it was suggested that 70 g of protein should be the minimal quantity of protein when energy intake was restricted to 1100 kcal/day (53). Current VLCDs consist of 0.8–1.0 g of protein per kg of desirable body weight, a minimum of 45–50 g of carbohydrate to minimize ketosis and nitrogen losses, and a small amount of essential fatty acids (10 g). Following the catastrophe using collagen or gelatin, which are of low biological quality, that led to heart rhythm disturbances, other starvation-related complications, and sudden death, the formula diets usually contain a wide range of high-biological-quality proteins such as lactalbumin, ovalbumin, casein, or soy protein (47,49). Despite the marked improvement in the quality of VLCD nutrients, VLCDs remain perhaps the most controversial among currently used diets. The reason is related to their safety and their long-term efficacy.

The modern VLCD containing adequate quantities of carbohydrate and other nutrients, especially potassium, magnesium, and minerals, are considered a well-established method for inducing rapid weight loss, in obese subjects with a BMI > 30 kg/m^2, even in those with refractory and morbid obesity, without important immediate risks (54). Usually the protein-sparing effects of this type of treatment have been documented using nitrogen balance studies in ambulatory and metabolic ward conditions (55). Using indirect calorimetry and by knowing the exact amount of nutrient intake in metabolic wards conditions, it was shown that under comparable degrees of energy expenditure, there was an absolute increase of fat catabolism and a decrease of carbohydrate catabolism, while the protein turnover remained constant (49). When comparing intake and combustion of the three nutrients, a combustion of approximately ± 150 g of fat per day could be obtained under VLCD conditions. Although these estimates of 24-hr substrate oxidation rates were extrapolated from only a 20-min period of observation by indirect calorimetry, the oxidation of 150 g fat per day was in accordance with similar results shown by Apfelbaum et al. years before using conventional methods (51).

Weight loss with VLCD can improve cardiovascular and other risk factors of obesity. VLCD also improve glucose tolerance and insulin insensitivity (56), primarily by enhancing insulin-stimulated glucose oxidation, whereas the effect of nonoxidative glucose metabolism is less pronounced (57). In addition, reduced lipid oxidation has been found, leading to a shift in fuel oxidation by enhancing glucose metabolism and insulin sensitivity. VLCDs were shown to cause significant reduction of fasting serum insulin, mainly because of enhanced hepatic insulin extraction as shown by a marked increase in the C-peptide/insulin molar ratio (58).

In subjects with established NIDDM, carefully monitored VLCD prescriptions led to an improvement of both parameters of metabolic control (glucose values and glycosylated hemoglobin) and indices of insulin sensitivity improve markedly (59). Clinical studies have shown that in at-risk patients low-energy diets can lead to substantial weight reduction without the cardiac arrythmias previously described. Antidiabetic drugs or insulin should usually be reduced drastically or even stopped in patients

adhering to VLCDs, and this decrease should begin shortly after the start of the therapy (60,61). Important effects on cardiovascular risk factors have been described during treatment with VLCD in NIDDM subjects (62).

Similar improvements have been shown on hypertension. The role of the sympathetic nervous system seems important in this phenomenon, since VLCD will markedly reduce plasma norepinephrine concentrations in hypertensive and nonhypertensive obese adults (63). The decrease in blood pressure during VLCD appears to be due to the effect of low-calorie intake on metabolic pathways affecting the sympathic nervous system, rather than on body weight reduction per se (63).

Special therapeutic attention should be given to subjects with obstructive sleep apnea, which is one of the most dangerous and life-threatening complications of morbid obesity (20,64). Obstructive sleep apnea can be considered a condition for which rapid weight loss may be necessary (65,66).

A VLCD is clearly only an initial step in the management of obesity, and dietary and behavioral reeducation of the slimmed patient is necessary to prevent relapse and weight regain. Liquid VLCD should therefore be regarded as a "stopgap" solution prior to a detailed attempt to a reorganized life-style (67). Nutritional education is a sine qua non for long-term life-style adaptation (54). An appropriate increase in physical activity will be necessary to prevent weight regain. It seems that, despite the positive effects of a VLCD program, unless the patient is committed to fullfill these elements in a modified fasting protocol, the success will be transient. Although combining behavior modifications with a VLCD improves successful maintenance of weight loss at 1 year from 5 to 32%, such combined treatment still remains disappointing, in respect to the time-consuming and costly efforts. Previous publications (61,68–70), including descriptive reports and controlled trials evaluating these regimens, have indicated that VLCD are relatively safe when used with carefully selected patients and appropriate medical management, and that they produce excellent short-term weight loss. However, the long-term results are disappointing (71). Four controlled trials (61,68–70) have compared the weight losses of patients who were randomly assigned to behavior modifications programs that either included a VLCD period or utilized a balanced, low-calorie diet (LCD) of 1000–1500 kcal/day throughout. All four studies found greater initial weight losses with the VLCD program than with the LCD program, but only one found a benefit for VLCD in terms of weight loss at 1-year follow-up.

Wadden and colleagues attempted to improve long-term results of the VLCD by increasing the period of use of VLCD from 8 to 16 weeks and by providing an extensive maintenance program following the VLCD (69). However, even with such an extensive and adapted maintenance program, subjects regained weight following the VLCD so that at the end of the intervention, there were no significant differences in success for the VLCD period compared with a more moderate dietary intervention (69). Also, when an intermittent VLCD was evaluated in a year-long behavioral weight control program in NIDDM subjects with marked obesity, there was improved weight loss and glycemic control with the intermittent program compared to a balanced 1000–1200-kcal diet. However, these effects were quite modest and, according to the authors, do not provide enough support to justify the clinical use of an intermittent VLCD in the context of a long-term behavioral program (71). The limited extra weight loss, often observed during the long-term VLCD programs, can probably be explained by the poor adherence observed.

One of the crucial points in safe VLCD weight reduction is the effect on lean body mass. Among many hypotheses, additional exercise training has been postulated as a way to overcome the loss of fat-free mass. During VLCD the initial degree of obesity does not seem to be a predictor of the loss of fat-free mass (FFM). Rapid and major weight reduction is usually associated with a reduction in resting metabolic rate; during a severe hypocaloric diet, fat mass decreases but FFM also declines, with a reduction in resting metabolic rate. We previously demonstrated, that after 6 months of therapy with a VLCD, a significant reduction in resting metabolic rate was found, although not so extreme as in other forms of caloric restriction without protein supplementation (72). Among the factors that contribute to the reduction in energy expenditure are the decrease not only in total fat mass and FFM but also in sex hormones, insulin levels, and fat distribution (72).

A new clinical challenge is the use of appetite-suppressing drugs to maintain and improve upon the initial VLCD success. VLCD followed by pharmacological support with serotonin agonists has been shown to be effective. A double-blind trial showed that patients begun on dexfenfluramine after 8 weeks on the VLCD lost substantially more weight in contrast to weight regain in the placebo-treated subjects (73).

Three studies (74–76) found that approximately 25% of obese subjects who consumed a 500 (or lower) kcal/day diet developed gall stones, which were sometimes asymptomatic. A recent report (77) indicated that this increased risk of gall stones is not limited to VLCD but that a 13% incidence of gall stone formation can also occur in subjects consuming popular over-the-counter meal replacement preparations containing approximately 925

Table 1 Contraindications to VLCD

Systemic infection or disease causing protein wasting
Renal and/or hepatic disease
Unstable angina pectoris and/or recent myocardial infarction
Malignant cardiac arrhythmias and prolonged Q-T interval
History of recent or recurrent transient ischemic attack or cerebrovascular accident
Pregnancy and lactation
Malignant hypertension
Malignancies
Type I insulin-dependent diabetes
Psychiatric disorders (including history of anorexia nervosa)
Intake of major antidepressants (e.g., lithium)
Very young and elderly patients
BMI < 25 kg/m^2

kcal/day, confirming previous reports that rapid weight loss can influence gall bladder emptying and lead to stone formation (78). Gall stones have also been shown to develop during the first 4 weeks of caloric restriction (75). Higher cholesterol and elevated triglyceride levels (77,79) are known to be risk factors, which predict the formation of gall stones during rapid weight loss. Subjects with a medical history of rapid weight loss (>1–1.5 kg/week during the initial treatment period) together with other risk factors would need a higher caloric intake or therapy with ursodeoxycholic acid, which has been shown to be effective in preventing stone formation during VLCD (74).

Based on a recent literature survey, it appears that the risk of gall stone formation increases with weight loss that averages 1.5 kg/week or more (80). If substantial or rapid weight loss increases the risk of developing gall stones, more gradual weight loss would seem to lessen such risk. Since VLCD may not contain enough fat to cause the gall bladder to contract enough to empty its bile, a recent National Institutes of Health publication suggests that a snack containing approximately 10 g of fat should be used (80,81). With less drastic calorie restriction (800-kcal formula diets) the risks of liver function abnormalities and formation of new gall stones with weight loss were reduced (82). In this era of enthusiasm for formula feeding it is necessary to show that ordinary food, based on the same principles of protein-enriched, low-fat items, is a valuable alternative, acceptable to the patient (67). Such a diet is based on natural foodstuffs: lean meat, egg albumin, fish, and seafood, all containing protein of high biological value. The emphasis is on readily available food and palatability for long-term use. Total energy ranges from 680 to 715 kcal/day, with 1.5 g protein per kg ideal body weight providing ~50% of the calories. Total fat intake is approximately 32 g, including at least 10 g of polyunsaturated fatty acids as vegetable oil. Carbohydrate intake varies from 30 to 40 g daily, derived from fresh food containing fiber, as vegetables and legumes. Cholesterol content does not exceed 300 mg/day, and intake of 2.5–3 g of potassium and 2 g of sodium per day is usual.

Noncaloric fluid should be taken ad libitum, with a minimum of 2 L/day. Artificial sweeteners are permitted and frequent feedings are advised. Daily vitamin and mineral supplementation is advocated to supply the Recommended Daily Allowance (RDA). Such kitchen-prepared regimens are usually well tolerated by most patients. The initial slight ketosis, which prevents hunger and gives a sense of mild euphoria, contributes to the good compliance. Compliance is comparable to that of earlier reports (83,84), reaching 38% after 6 months and 14% after 2 years. Figure 1 shows the percentage of men and women who lost ≥20 kg after 6 months of therapy. Acceptability of the diet and scoring of hunger feeling are comparable to data of Wadden et al. (85). Orthostatic hypotension and constipation are the most frequent side effects of long-term treatment. Transient hair loss occurs only in patients who use the diet more than 12 months. The results of such an approach demonstrate that, except for the initial period, commercial very-low-calorie preparations are not absolutely necessary and that the same long-term effect can be obtained with kitchen-prepared low-calorie, low-carbohydrate, high-protein foods (67).

The overall status of body minerals during very-low-calorie dieting has been investigated by Fisler and Drenick

(86). Deficiency of minerals, including calcium, magnesium, phosphate, and selenium, may influence cardiac conductivity and result in cardiac lesions. Neither calcium, albumin, nor protein changes were observed after VLCD treatment; an increase in serum phosphate levels even indicated a reduced myocardial instability, a phenomenon seen only with feeding protein of high biological quality. Results showed that a protein-supplemented hypocaloric diet does not cause negative magnesium balance, nor are there significant renal losses of magnesium, in contrast to total fasting (87). We cannot exclude fecal loss of magnesium but it is probably minimal, because stool volume decreases in semistarvation. Magnesium levels in serum and erythrocytes are usually similar, before, during, and after therapy.

VLCD can be considered a valuable stopgap in the short term but should be associated with other approaches to increase the rate of long-term success: incorporation of behavioral therapy and physical activity and possibly pharmacotherapy in VLCD treatment programs seems to improve maintenance (54). When well balanced in macro- and micronutrients, prescribed in well-selected patients under proper and careful medical supervision, with a duration adapted to the individual needs of the patient, VLCDs are usually safe and effective in promoting significant short-term weight loss, with concomitant improvement in comorbid conditions.

V. WEIGHT LOSS AND PREDICTIVE VARIABLES

It is well documented that the long-term results of dietary treatment for obesity are very poor. Successful weight loss in diet-conscious persons is common, but success in maintaining weight loss for an extended time is very limited (88). The prognosis for maintaining weight loss is not so pessimistic for all patients (89), since some obese subjects lose weight rather easily. For obvious reasons, it would be of great value to be able to predict the results of treatment in individual cases. In many recent studies, long-term results of treatment have been evaluated in relation to a series of baseline metabolic and hormonal parameters, such as gender and age, body fat distribution, energy expenditure, and sex hormones, to examine whether these variables could be used to predict success.

A. Weight Loss and Fat Distribution

The role of body fat distribution, particularly visceral adiposity, is an important determinant of metabolic and cardiovascular complications of overweight and obesity

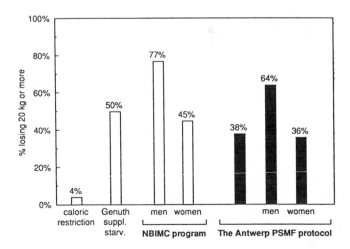

Figure 1 Percent of patients losing 20 kg or more over a 6-month period of VLCD/PSMF, as compared to general caloric restriction and the Genuth and NBIMC studies. (Adapted and redrawn from Refs. 67 and 83, with permission.)

(90,91). Assessment of the topography of body fat is therefore helpful in targeting patients at risk who are most likely to benefit from treatment (16). There is some older evidence suggesting that subjects with a predominantly abdominal fat distribution benefit more from weight reduction. It has been claimed (88) that individuals with gluteal (gynoid) obesity (mostly women) lose weight less easily than those with abdominal (android) obesity (mostly men) and that the increased susceptibility of visceral compared with subcutaneous adipose tissue to lipolytic stimuli may explain this difference.

Adipose tissue cellularity has been related to the prognosis for weight reduction by a series of authors. Recent observations using techniques that accurately describe abdominal or visceral fat accumulation have indicated that the distribution of body fat is not a predictor of the ability to lose weight. In a prospective study, Lanska et al. showed no significant differences in weight reduction between android and gynoid women (92). This was confirmed by Vansant et al. (93) and Wadden et al. (94), although the former study revealed that on a 4.2-mJ caloric diet, a weight loss of approximately 10% (about 10 kg) coincided with greater decreases in blood glucose and serum lipids in obese women with abdominal fat, when compared to women with gluteal-femoral fat.

In postmenopausal women, a recent report clearly shows that women with an android and gynoid fat distribution respond similarly to treatment of their obesity (95). There is therefore probably no difference in the weight loss achieved by individuals with android versus gynoid fat distribution when conditions are carefully controlled (94,96), though preferential mobilization of fat from the visceral regions may occur.

Some studies show clearly that it is possible to influence body fat distribution accompanying weight loss in obese men and women. Wadden et al. found a greater percentage reduction in waist than hip circumference in android obese patients while there was an identical reduction in both circumferences with the same weight loss in the gynoid obese group (94). We have also demonstrated a more pronounced decrease in waist circumference in women with upper versus lower body obesity (88). In view of the recent reports that the waist circumference more precisely reflects the amount of visceral fat than the waist-to-hip ratio (WHR), this might indicate that long-term weight reduction will result in a substantial decrease of visceral fat mass, confirming the recent findings by Stallone et al. in a study where comparable amounts of weight loss were reported (97). Previously it was shown that the WHR decreases with loss of fat mass but to a greater extent in the android obese subject and this effect may be greater when weight loss is achieved by a com-

bination of calorie restriction and regular aerobic exercise (98).

As subjects with android obesity are at increased risk of metabolic and vascular complications, there is greater potential for risk reduction with weight loss than in gynoid obesity. There are no intervention studies demonstrating benefit in terms of morbidity or mortality due to reduction in visceral fat, but reductions in serum cholesterol (99) and an increase in HDL cholesterol have been observed in individuals with abdominal obesity. Significant improvement of glucose parameters (88) and glucose tolerance (100) have also been reported in this specific group. The results of a recent study suggest, however, that a reduction of the WHR may not be the best indicator of improved fat distribution since changes in WHR underestimate changes in visceral fat. Using magnetic resonance imaging, the authors showed that the rate of fat loss was greater from visceral than from subcutaneous sites. Therefore, the reduction in risk due to loss of visceral fat may be greater than the reduction in WHR achieved.

When women with a preponderance of abdominal fat lose on average more than women with more peripheral fat, it is clear that this phenomenon can have an important influence on patient motivation and compliance. In this view, the results of these studies seem important because lack of motivation during dieting is a well-known phenomenon. Indices of abdominal body fat are not a prognostic indicator for the ability to lose weight. We have shown similar results, pointing out that android obesity cannot be used as a predictor for weight loss, but rather it is a predictor of risk normalization (88). Important gender differences seem to exist in relation to weight loss and the associated comorbidities.

Dietary-induced changes in body weight and body fat distribution, however, would produce favorable changes in risk factors for atherosclerosis, including reduction in serum lipid and lipoprotein levels. Some data indicate that the cardiovascular risk profile is improved in all groups, but is most pronounced in women with visceral fat excess. This gender difference deserves attention although it has not yet been reported in detail; it confirms previous findings about the changes in blood pressure, which were recently described (101). The WHR (but not BMI) before weight loss predicted a reduction of blood pressure in response to weight loss in women, but not in men (101). A recent study by Astrup and colleagues clearly showed that besides 24-hr energy expenditure and fat oxidation, initial high levels of dihydrotestosterone and plasma norepinephrine were associated with better weight loss at follow-up. This indicates that hormonal factors (102), probably related to visceral fat accumulation, may be prognostic markers for weight reduction in obese women.

B. Weight Cycling

Repeated periods of weight loss and regain, known as weight cycling or yo-yo dieting, frequently occur in both obese and nonobese humans. Weight cycling has been hypothesized to be a causative factor for obesity and to have deleterious metabolic, behavioral, and health consequences (103). In addition, weight cycling may make subsequent weight loss more difficult as it may affect body composition, metabolic efficiency, or fat mobilization from adipocytes. Weight cycling has been suggested to be a negative predictor of the ability to lose weight.

It has been suggested that women who were resistant to weight loss were characterized by a long previous history of dieting (104). Prior experience in formal weight loss programs has been suggested to be a negative predictor of subsequent weight loss in middle-aged obese subjects (105). However, weight loss maintenance was not related to the number of previous weight program enrollments, but regainers reported a significantly higher number of prior weight cycles. From the majority of studies, it is clear that weight cycling per se does not influence the success of subsequent weight loss efforts.

Among other recommendations that can help to avoid relapse of weight gain after weight loss is an emphasis on the possible role of dietary fat in the mechanisms of weight regain. The reduction of refined sugars and the enhancement of fiber intake are other general nutritional principles that, in a varied, nutritionally adequate and bulky diet, may help to limit the amount of energy ingested (106). There is in addition some suggestion that smaller, regular meals and snacks may have benefits over the same energy intake in large meals. Dietary approaches favoring dietary thermogenesis in postobese subjects also seem reasonable (106,107).

VI. EFFECTS OF MODEST WEIGHT REDUCTION

A number of physiological parameters affect cardiovascular morbidity and mortality. These include lipid abnormalities, the oxidizability of lipoproteins, arterial blood pressure, perturbations of the hemostatic system, and fibrinolytic abnormalities. Most of these risk factors are related to obesity, particularly to visceral obesity, and to insulin resistance (108,109). The cluster of risk factors linked to insulin resistance is referred to as syndrome X or the metabolic syndrome. Many investigators have reported that reductions in body weight of as little as 10% are sufficient to ameliorate the common complications of obesity, and an even more limited weight loss was re-

ported to reduce risk factors in non-insulin-dependent diabetes mellitus (NIDDM) (110).

In 1988, Wood et al., found that a modest weight loss of approximately 3.5–7.5 kg, over a 7-month period, using moderate caloric restriction to reduce baseline body fat by one-third, was associated with an increase in HDL cholesterol (111). Significant decreases in triglyceride levels were also found in this study. Fat loss through diet or exercise was associated with marked improvement. The same authors went on to investigate the effects of weight loss on HDL cholesterol in a prospective study, which included both men and women (27). A decrease in body weight of 5 kg, or a 5% weight reduction, achieved with diet alone reduced triglycerides but did not increase HDL cholesterol. When diet based on the step one hypocaloric NCEP Program (112) was combined with an exercise program, a significant decrease in triglycerides and a significant increase in HDL cholesterol and HDL_2 cholesterol were observed. There was a marked gender difference in the effects of weight loss. In women, the LDL:HDL cholesterol ratio decreased significantly only when diet was combined with exercise. In men, the decreases were much larger and were also seen in those receiving diet alone. These data suggest that the optimal prescription for successful weight loss, associated with the reduction of coronary heart disease risk factors in moderately overweight men and women, must include promotion of physical fitness and a reduction in saturated fat intake.

The effects of moderate weight loss on HDL-cholesterol have also been investigated by Wing et al., in a study involving overweight patients with type II diabetes (113). Weight loss in the range 2.4–6.8 kg, over a 1-year period, was associated with a significant decrease in triglycerides. A significant increase in HDL cholesterol, however, was observed only when weight loss was greater than 6.9 kg.

A preliminary 6-month study has recently evaluated the effects of weight loss on the oxidizability of lipids in obese individuals. A hypocaloric diet was associated with significant reductions in the in vitro oxidizability of lipids in patients with a moderate weight loss (10). A weight decrease of only 2.5 kg led to a decrease in indices of oxidizability. Although the number of patients in this preliminary trial was small, the results suggest that obese individuals who achieve moderate weight loss can improve their lipid oxidizability status and increase their resistance to lipid particle oxidation. This may be important when evaluating cardiovascular risk and may indicate a preserved antioxidant status by weight reduction.

Hemostatic factors are known to have an important role in the development of cardiovascular disease. Prospective epidemiological data have shown that elevated fibrinogen is an important risk factor for cardiovascular disease (114). In contrast to an important reduction of fibrinogen levels of up to 20% after a major weight reduction, the net change in fibrinogen levels by a more modest weight loss is more limited (115). This finding is important, since it has been shown that fibrinogen levels and blood viscosity are related to body mass index and to insulin resistance (116) and can be substantially reduced by weight reduction.

A study of the possible effects of weight loss on hemostatic factors, which are strong predictors of ischemic heart disease (117), found that a mean weight loss of 9.4 kg in men and 7.4 kg in women over a 6-month period significantly decreased factor VII levels by ±11% (115). Plasminogen activator inhibitor (PAI), of which PAI-1 is the most important, is involved in the fibrinolytic mechanisms and in the pathogenesis of coronary heart disease and atherosclerosis (118).

Velthuis-te Wierik et al. investigated the effects of a 10-week program of moderate (20%) energy restriction in nonobese middle-aged men (1990). This was associated with a significant decrease in PAI activity, primarily in subjects with high baseline PAI values. The 6-month TRIM study by Folsom et al. (115) also found that PAI activity decreased with increasing weight loss. This effect was greater in men than women. These findings suggest that even moderate weight loss can improve abnormalities in hemostatic and fibrinolytic factors, of about the same magnitude as reported for the occurrence of ischemic heart disease.

A. Clinical Outcomes

Can beneficial effects related to weight changes be translated into outcome data? Several studies have investigated whether modest weight reduction results in improved cardiovascular morbidity and mortality. The 1990 Lifestyle Heart Trial by Ornish et al. reported the results of a randomized prospective trial that aimed to determine whether 1 year of comprehensive life-style modification would affect the progression of coronary atherosclerosis (120). The study used computed tomography and quantitative angiography to evaluate changes in progression and regression of stenotic lesions. Of the group who were prescribed a low-fat vegetarian diet (approximately 10% of calories as fat, 15–20% protein, and 70–75% predominantly as complex carbohydrates), and lost approximately 10 kg, 82% showed an average regression of coronary arterial lesions. Individuals with the greatest adherence to the diet had the highest percentage of regression. In the control group, however, regression of the lesions was not observed (120).

A study published by Singh et al. in 1992 also gave promising results for the effects of moderate weight loss (121). A fat-reduced diet, with the addition of soluble dietary fiber and vitamins, was prescribed to individuals with a history of previous myocardial infarction. Data analysis found that when weight loss reached 7.1 kg over a 1-year study period, there was a significant reduction of cardiac events, total cardiac mortality, and total mortality. Of the subjects who lost at least 0.5 kg of weight, 17% died due to cardiac events or other causes. In comparison, of those who did not lose this minimal amount of weight, 36% died (121).

Although it cannot be proven that weight loss per se is the most important trigger of the reduced mortality, these studies prove that dietary manipulation can modulate risk factors and overall mortality. Although reductions in risk factors do not automatically reflect changes in the development of arteriosclerosis, based on the results of the Northwick Park Study (117), a significant reduction of risk factors such as factor VII might translate to a 29% lower risk for ischemic heart disease over 5 years. Intentional versus unintentional weight loss has to be distinguished. A recent paper convincingly showed that females with obesity-related health conditions who lose weight intentionally have a survival advantage. Females with obesity-related health conditions losing weight unintentionally and those without preexisting illnesses did not benefit from weight reduction (122).

VII. SPECIAL MEASURES

A. Antioxidants

In view of the recent findings that obesity, and especially android obesity, is characterized by an increased oxidizability of LDL and VLDL particles, eating foods naturally rich in dietary antioxidants, such as tocopherols, carotenoids, vitamin C, and flavonoids, should be encouraged. The disturbed equilibrium between pro- and antioxidants, potentially present in obese subjects under different kinds of dietary changes, and the evidence that increased oxidative stress increases cardiovascular risk provide the justification for this recommendation. We realize that no clear comparative studies have yet been performed in this field (42,123). These considerations are of particular interest during ketogenic diets, where different fatty acids are mobilized from the labile visceral body fat department. All commercial dietary preparations used as protein sparing modified fast (PSMF) and VLCD should be supplemented with the RDA of vitamins and minerals.

Natural antioxidants vary according to dietary habits in different populations. An inverse association between natural flavonoid intake and mortality from CHD has been reported (124). Available data suggest that these natural antioxidants are absorbed and may have some protective effects with respect to cardiovascular diseases. Among natural food items rich in flavonoids the non- or low-calorie selected foods include onion, celery, and broccoli (125).

Pharmacological doses of vitamin E have been shown to influence some metabolic risk factors, but present evidence does not justify the routine use of vitamin E in pharmacological quantities. For most minerals there are no grounds for making recommendations that differ from those for the general population. As for sodium, people with obesity and insulin resistance should be advised to restrict salt intake under 6 g/day with more marked reductions in those whose blood pressure levels show any degree of persistent elevation.

Recent papers have identified magnesium depletion in subjects with insulin resistance, especially in obese NIDDM (126). Although some papers have indicated that magnesium deficiency might exist in obesity, we do not advocate the routine use of magnesium supplements for the obese individual. During hypocaloric diets and VLCD, magnesium-rich foods should be encouraged in order to reach the normal recommended allowances.

B. Fiber

Obesity is frequently associated with insulin insensitivity, hyperinsulinemia, and abnormalities of glucose and lipid metabolism (127). Hypocaloric diets should therefore not only reduce weight, the first strategic approach to ameliorate metabolic and endocrine abnormalities, but should also target the different elements of the metabolic syndrome, of which insulin resistance is one of the key features. Piatti and colleagues recently reported a comparative study of three low-caloric diets with different complex and simple carbohydrate content on insulin sensitivity (128). Surprisingly, in this study a high complex/high starch and fiber diet (60% carbohydrate, 20% fat, 20% protein) induced an increase of peripheral insulin resistance, accompanied by an elevation of fasting free fatty acids (FFA) levels and a decreased suppression of FFA during a hyperglycemic clamp (128). Previous studies have also shown that diets rich in starch can increase insulin levels and decrease insulin sensitivity (129). This suggests that starch per se might induce, at least during hypocaloric dieting, a deleterious effect on insulin sensitivity, independently of fiber (130).

Although a RDA does not exist for dietary fiber, 20–40 g of fiber per day is usually recommended for most people. Obese women usually consume less. Older studies suggest that diets high in fiber may assist in weight loss.

The mechanism behind the effect of dietary fiber on adiposity may be the effect of fiber on intestinal transit time, increased postprandial satiety, and/or rate of glucose absorption.

C. Ethanol

There is controversy about the role of alcohol on body weight. It is questionable whether alcohol should be completely eliminated during a diet. This controversy stems from cross-sectional epidemiological results relating alcohol intake to body weight (131,132). Alcohol is considered as "empty" calories since, in contrast to other macronutrients, it is not essential to the body and does not carry any associated nutrient (vitamins, trace elements) and may even promote the utilization of some vitamins such as vitamin B_1 (133). In relation to the development or maintenance of overweight by ethanol use, its role on energy consumption needs to be considered.

In experimental conditions, a single dose of alcohol produces a thermic effect of food of approximately 12.5%, ranging from 8 to 17% of the ingested alcohol energy (134,135), which is better than the thermogenic response of carbohydrates and fat. Alcohol in a mixed meal is also able to displace fat and carbohydrate oxidation (136). From this perspective it can be concluded that alcohol calories count the same as other calories. When alcohol is coingested with high-fat diets, this combination may favor overfeeding and fat accumulation, even after control for energy density (137).

Previous studies indicating the negative association of alcohol intake and body weight did not take into account body composition. Weight loss after alcohol intake could be explained by an unfavorable loss of fat-free mass (138). Taking into account the difficulties of estimating the exact amount alcohol intake, most surveys have shown that ethanol calories may be added to or substituted for nonalcohol calories in light drinkers without significantly changing body weight (139). In squirrel monkeys binge drinking in contrast to regular daily consumption of limited amounts of alcohol gave rise to different changes in anthropometric indices.

Despite the fact that in animal and human studies, moderate alcohol intake seems to reduce body weight and body fat, it often is associated with hypertriglyceridemia and alcoholic fatty liver (140), particularly in subjects with abdominal adiposity in whom liver steatosis is a common finding. Binge drinking should be eliminated from a healthy diet since binge drinking may cause an increase in the atherogenic LDL particles with possible serious arterial wall injury and arterial occlusion as a consequence (141).

For many reasons precautions regarding alcohol intake that apply to the general public also apply to obese subjects. General recommendations regarding alcohol use are complicated by the fact that alcohol may have both untoward and beneficial effects. Alcohol may be an important energy source in overweight people since it spares fat from oxidation (135). It can also be associated with raised levels of blood pressure, increased triglycerides, an increased risk of hypoglycemia and it favors body fat deposition. On the other hand, moderate intake (equivalent to approximately one or two glasses of wine per day) may confer benefit by elevating levels of high-density lipoproteins, reducing coagulability, and decreasing lipid oxidation through the antioxidant nutrients present in wine. Therefore, a minimal amount of alcohol in the diet of an obese individual may be appropriate.

VIII. CRITERIA FOR A SAFE AND SUCCESSFUL WEIGHT LOSS PROGRAM

A responsible and safe weight loss program should be able to document the following guiding principles and characteristics (adapted from Refs. 21,142,143).

The diet should be safe. It should include all of the RDAs for vitamins, minerals, and protein. The weight loss diet should supply less energy than the patient's maintenance requirements, which means it should be low in energy, but not in essential nutrients. If possible, the diet should provide adequate quantities of dietary fiber.

The weight loss program should be directed toward a *slow, steady* weight loss unless the health condition of the patient requires more rapid weight loss.

The diet must be (as far as possible) palatable and acceptable to the patient, to endorse as high patient compliance as possible.

The program should include a strategy for *weight maintenance* after the weight loss phase. It is of little benefit to lose a large amount of weight only to regain it. The dietary strategy should therefore be associated with behavior modification help and physical exercise.

A medical assessment of the general health of the patient and medical conditions that might be affected by dieting and weight loss is a sine qua non prior to each dietary strategy. Also, medical advice on the appropriateness of weight loss is of utmost importance and a sensible goal of weight loss for each individual.

REFERENCES

1. Zhang Y, Proenca R, Maffei M, et al. Positional cloning of the mouse *obese* gene and its human homologue. Nature 1994; 372:425–432.
2. Pellymounter MA, Cullen MJ, Baker MB, et al. Effects of the obese gene product on body weight regulation in *ob/ob* mice. Science 1995; 269:540–543.
3. Shah M, Jeffery RW. Is obesity due to overeating and inactivity, or to a defective metabolic rate? A review. Ann Behav Med 1991; 13:73–81.
4. Miller WC, Niederpruem MG, Wallace JP, Lindeman AK. Dietary fat, sugar, and fiber predict body fat content. J Am Dietet Assoc 1994; 94:612–615.
5. Raben A, Andersen HB, Christensen NJ, et al. Evidence for an abnormal postprandial response to a high-fat meal in women predisposed to obesity. Am J Physiol (Endocrinol Metab) 1994; 267:E549–559.
6. Lichtman SW, Pisarska K, Berman ER, Pestone M, Dowling H, Offenbacher E, Weisel H, Heshka S, Matthews DE, Heymsfield SB. Discrepancy between self-reported and actual caloric intake and exercise in obese subjects. N Engl J Med 1992; 327:1893–1898.
7. Astrup A, Buemann B, Christensen NJ, et al. Failure to increase lipid oxidation in response to increasing dietary fat content in formerly obese women. Am J Physiol 1994; 266:E592–599.
8. Heitmann BL, Lissner L. Dietary underreporting by obese individuals—is it specific or non-specific? Br Med J 1995; 311:986–989.
9. Blackburn GL. How much weight loss? In: Angel A, et al, eds. Progress in Obesity Research VII. London: John Libbey, 1996:621–625.
10. Van Gaal LF, Wauters MA, De Leeuw IH. The beneficial effects of modest weight loss on cardiovascular risk factors. Int J Obes 1997; 27, in press.
11. Wadden TA, Bell ST. Obesity. In: Bellack AS, Hersen M, Kazdin A, eds. International Handbook of Behaviour Modification and Therapy, Vol II. New York: Plenum Press, 1990:449–472.
12. Devlin MJ, Walsh BT, Spitzer RL, Hasin D. Is there another binge eating disorder? A review of the literature on overeating in the absence of bulimia nervosa. Int J Eating Disord 1992; 11:333–340.
13. Flatt JP. Dietary fat, carbohydrate balance and weight maintenance: effects of exercise. Am J Clin Nutr 1987; 45:296–306.
14. Pi-Sunyer FX. Effects of the composition of the diet on energy intake. Nutr Rev 1990; 48:94–105.
15. Garrow JS. The safety of dieting. Proc Nutr Soc 1991; 50: 493–499.
16. Dyer RG. Traditional treatment of obesity: does it work? Ballière's Clin Endocrinol Metab 1994; 8:661–688.
17. Van Itallie TB. Health implications of overweight and obesity in the US. Ann Intern Med 1985; 103:983–988.

18. Van Gaal L, Rillaerts E, Creten W, De Leeuw I. Relationship of body fat distribution pattern to atherogenic risk factors in NIDDM. Diabetes Care 1988; 11:103–106.

19. Després JP. Dyslipidemia and obesity. Ballière's Clin Endocrinol Metab 1994; 8:629–660.

20. Grunstein RR, Wilcox I. Sleep disordered breathing and obesity. Ballière's Clin Endocrinol Metab 1994; 8:601–628.

21. Garrow JS. Dietary methods: an overview. In: Beuder A, Brookes LJ, eds. Body Weight Control. New York: Churchill Livingstone, 1987:109–116.

22. Wooley SC, Garner DM. Dietary treatments of obesity are ineffective. Br Med J 1994; 309:655–656.

23. Garrow JS. Should obesity be treated? Treatment is necessary. Br Med J 1994; 309:654–655.

24. Wadden TA. Treatment of obesity by moderate and severe caloric restriction. Results of clinical research trials. Ann Intern Med 1993; 119:688–693.

25. Ayyad C, Andersen T. A comprehensive literature study of long term efficacy of dietary treatment of obesity. Int J Obes 1994; 18(Suppl C):78 (abstract).

26. Brownell KD. Relapse and the treatment of obesity. In: Wadden TA, Van Itallie TB, eds. Treatment of the Seriously Obese Patient. New York: Guilford Press, 1992:437–455.

27. Wood PD, Stefanick ML, Williams PT, et al. The effect on plasma lipoproteins of a prudent weight reducing diet, with or without exercise, in overweight men and women. N Engl J Med 1991; 325:461–466.

28. Whing RR. Weight cycling in humans: a review of the literature. Ann Behav Med 1992; 14:113–119.

29. Blair SN, Shaten J, Brownell K, Collins G, Lissner L. Body weight change, all-cause and cause-specific mortality in the Multiple Risk Factor Intervention Trial. Ann Intern Med 1993; 119(part 2):749–757.

30. Cavagnini F. Obesity—to treat or not to treat? Eating Patterns Weight Control 1995; 4:20–22.

31. Atkins R. Dr. Atkins Diet Revolution. New York: David McKay, 1972.

32. Ashwell MA, Garrow J. A survey of three slimming and weight control organisations in the U.K. Nutrition 1975; 29:347–356.

33. Scheen A, Desaive C, Lefèbvre P. Therapy for obesity-today and tomorrow. Ballière's Clin Endocrinol Metabol 1994; 8:705–727.

34. Drewnowski A, Kurth C, Holden-Wiltse J, et al. Food preferences in human obesity: carbohydrates versus fats. Appetite 1992; 18:207–221.

35. Rolls BJ. Carbohydrates, fats and satiety. Am J Clin Nutr 1995; 61(Suppl):960S–967S.

36. Astrup A, Buemann B, Western P, et al. Obesity as an adaptation to a high-fat diet: evidence from a cross-sectional study. Am J Clin Nutr 1994; 59:350–355.

37. Booth DA. Sensory influences on food intake. Nutr Rev 1990; 48:71–77.

38. Dreon DM, Frey-Hewitt B, Ellsworth N et al. Dietary fat: carbohydrate ratio and obesity in middle-aged men. Am J Clin Nutr 1988; 47:995–1000.

39. French SA, Jeffery RW, Forster JL, et al. Predictors of weight change over two years among a population of working adults: the healthy worker project. Int J Obes 1994; 18:145–154.

40. Rolls BJ, Pirraglia PA, Jones MB, Peters JC. Effects of olestra, a noncaloric fat substitute, on daily energy and fat intake in lean men. Am J Clin Nutr 1992; 56:84–92.

41. Schlundt DG, Hill JO, Pope-Cordle J, et al. Randomized evaluation of a low fat "ad libitum" carbohydrate diet for weight reduction. Int J Obes 1993; 17:623–629.

42. Van Gaal LF, Zhang A, Steijaert M, et al. Human obesity, from lipid abnormalities to lipid oxidation. Int J Obes 1995; 19(Suppl 3):S21–S26.

43. Jeffery RW, Hellerstedt WL, French SA. A randomized trial of counseling for fat restriction versus calorie restriction in the treatment of obesity. Int J Obes 1995; 19:132–137.

44. Sheppard L, Kristal AR, Kushi LH. Weight loss in women participating in a randomized trial of low-fat diets. Am J Clin Nutr 1991; 54:821–828.

45. Chlebowski RT, Blackburn GL, Buzzard IM, Rose DP, Martino S, Khandekar JD, York RM, Jeffery RW, Elashoff RM, Wynder EL. Adherence to a dietary fat intake reduction program in postmenopausal women receiving therapy for early breast cancer. J Clin Oncol 1993; 11:2072–2080.

46. Harris JK, French SA, Jeffery RW, et al. Dietary and physical activity correlates of long-term weight loss. Obes Res 1994; 2:307–313.

47. Wadden TA, Stunkard AJ, Brownell KD. Very low calorie diets; their efficacy, safety and future. Ann Intern Med 1983; 99:675–684.

48. Apfelbaum M. The effects of very restrictive high protein diets. Clin Endocrinol Metab 1976; 5:417–429.

49. Van Gaal L, Snyders D, De Leeuw I, Bekaert J. Anthropometric and calorimetric evidence for the protein sparing effects of a new protein supplemented low calorie preparation. Am J Clin Nutr 1985; 41:540–544.

50. Foster GD, Wadden TA, Peterson FJ et al. A controlled comparison of three very-low-calorie diets: effects on weight, body composition and symptoms. Am J Clin Nutr 1992; 55:811–817.

51. Apfelbaum M, Fricker J, Igoin-Apfelbaum L. Low-and very-low-calorie diets. Am J Clin Nutr 1987; 45:1126–1134.

52. Blackburn GL, Bistrian RW, Flatt JP. Role of protein sparing fast in a comprehensive weight reduction programme. In: Howard AN, ed. Recent Advances in Obesity Research I. London: Newman, 1975:279–281.

53. Oi Y, Okuda T, Koishi H, et al. Effects of low energy diets on protein metabolism studies with (^{15}N) glycine in obese patients. J Nutr Sci Vitaminol 1987; 33:227–237.

54. National Task Force on the prevention and treatment of obesity. Very low caloric diets. JAMA 1993; 270:967–974.

55. Contaldo F, Di Biase G, Fischetti A, et al. Evaluation of the safety of very-low-calorie diets in the treatment of severely obese patients in a metabolic ward. Int J Obes 1981; 5:221–226.

56. Fukuda M, Tahara Y, Yamamoto, et al. Effects of very-low-calorie diet weight reduction on glucose tolerance, insulin secretion, and insulin resistance in obese non-insulin dependent diabetics. Diabetes Res Clin Pract 1989; 7:61–67.

57. Nakai Y, Taniguchi A, Fukushima M, et al. Insulin sensitivity during very-low-calorie diets assessed by minimal modeling. Am J Clin Nutr 1992; 56(Suppl I):179S–181S.

58. Van Gaal L, Vansant G, Van Acker K, De Leeuw I. Effect of a long term very low calorie diet on glucose/insulin metabolism in obesity. Influence of fat distribution on hepatic insulin extraction. Int J Obes 1989; 13(Suppl 2): 47–49.

59. Amatruda JM, Richeson JF, Welle SL, et al. The safety and efficacy of a controlled low-energy diet in the treatment of non-insulin-dependent diabetes and obesity. Arch Intern Med 1988; 148:873–877.

60. Bauman WA, Schwartz E, Rose HG, Eisenstein HN, Johnson DW. Early and long-term effects of acute caloric deprivation in obese diabetic patients. Am J Med 1988; 85: 38–46.

61. Wing RR, Marcus MD, Salata R. Effects of a very-low-calorie diet on long-term glycemic control in obese type II diabetics. Arch Intern Med 1991; 151:1334–1340.

62. Uusitupa MI, Laakso M, Sarlund H, et al. Effects of a very-low-calorie diet on metabolic control and cardiovascular risk factors in the treatment of obese non-insulin-dependent diabetics. Am J Clin Nutr 1990; 51:768–773.

63. Eliahou HE, Laufer J, Blau A, Shulman L. Effect of low-calorie diets on the sympathetic nervous system, body weight, and plasma insulin in overweight hypertension. Am J Clin Nutr 1992; 56(Suppl I):175S–178S.

64. Pasquali R, Collella P, Cirignotta F, et al. Treatment of obese patients with obstructive sleep apnea syndrome (OSAS): effect of weight loss and interference of otorhinolaryngologic pathology. Int J Obes 1990; 14:207–217.

65. Smith PL, Gola AR, Meyers DA, et al. Weight loss in mild to moderately obese patients with obstructive sleep apnea. Ann Intern Med 1985; 103:850–855.

66. Suratt PM, McTier RF, Findley L. Effect of very-low-calorie diets with weight loss on obstructive sleep apnea. Am J Clin Nutr 1992; 56:182S–184S.

67. Van Gaal L, De Leeuw I. Short and long-term effects of protein sparing very low calorie diets. In: Eds Berry E, Blondheim S, et al. Recent Advances in Obesity Research V. London; John Libbey, 1987:332–336.

68. Wadden TA, Stunkard AJ. Controlled trial of very low calorie diet, behavior therapy, and their combination in the treatment of obesity. J Consult Clin Psychol 1986; 54: 482–488.

69. Wadden TA, Foster GD, Letizia KA. One-year behavioral treatment of obesity: comparison of moderate and severe caloric restriction and the effects o of weight maintenance therapy. J Consult Clin Psychol 1994; 62:165–171.

70. Miura J, Arai K, Tsukahara S, et al. The long term effectiveness of combined therapy by behavior modification and very low calorie diet: 2 years-follow-up. Int J Obes 1989; 13:73–77.

71. Wing RR, Blair E, Marcus M, et al. Year-long weight loss treatment for obese patients with type II diabetes: does including an intermittent very-low-calorie diet improve outcome? Am J Med 1994; 97:354–362.

72. Van Gaal L, Vansant G, De Leeuw I. Factors determining energy expenditure during VLCD. Am J Clin Nutr 1992; 56:224S–229S.

73. Finer N, Finer S, Naoumova RP. Drug therapy after very-low-calorie diets. Am J Clin Nutr 1992; 56:195S–198S.

74. Broomfield PH, Chopra R, Sheinbaum RC, et al. Effects of ursodeoxycholic acid and aspirin on the formation of lithogenic bile and gallstone during loss of weight. N Engl J Med 1988; 319:1567–1572.

75. Liddle RA, Goldstein RB, Saxton J. Gallstone formation during weight reduction dieting. Arch Intern Med 1989; 149:1750–1753.

76. Weinsier RL, Ullman DO. Gallstone formation and weight loss. Obes Res 1993; 1:51–56.

77. Spirt BA, Graves LW, Weinstock R, Bartlett SJ, Wadden TA. Gallstone formation in obese women treated by a low-calorie diet. Int J Obes 1995; 19:593–595.

78. Stone BG, Ansel HJ, Peterson FJ, Gebhard RL. Gallbladder emptying stimuli in obese and normal weight subjects. Hepatology 1992; 15:795–798.

79. Yang HY, et al. Risk factors for gallstone formation during rapid weight loss. Dig Dis Sci 1992; 37:912–918.

80. Weinsier R, Wilson LJ, Lee J. Medically safe rate of weight loss: a guideline based on risk of gallstone formation. Am J Med 1995; 98:115–117.

81. US Public Health Service, NIH Publication 94-3677, 1993:1–4.

82. Hoy MK, Heshka S, Allison DB. Reduced risk of liver function rest abnormalities and new gallstone formation with weight loss on 800 calorie formula diets. Am J Clin Nutr 1994; 60:249–254.

83. Genuth SM, Castro JH, Vertes V. Weight reduction in obesity by outpatient semistarvation. 1974; 230:987–991.

84. Kirschner MA, Schneider G, Ertel N, Cortes G. Supplemented starvation: a successful method for control of major obesity. J Med Soc New Jersey 1979; 76:175–179.

85. Wadden TA, Stunkard AJ, Brownell K, Day SC. A comparison of two very-low-calorie diets: protein-sparing-modified fast versus protein-formulaliquid diet. Am J Clin Nutr 1985; 41:533–539.

86. Fisler JS, Drenick EJ. Calcium, magnesium and phosphate balances during very low calorie diets of soy or collagen protein in obese men: comparison to total fasting. Am J Clin Nutr 1984; 40:14–25.

87. Van Roelen W, Van Rooy P, Van Gaal L, et al. Magnesium status during dietary treatment of obesity. In: Halpern M,

Durlach J, eds. Magnesium Deficiency. Basel: Karger, 1985:224–226.

88. Van Gaal L, Vansant G, Moeremans M, De Leeuw I. Lipid and lipoprotein changes after long-term weight reduction: the influence of gender and body fat distribution. J Am Coll Nutr 1995; 14:382–386.

89. Bray GA: The myth of diet in the management of obesity. Am J Clin Nutr 1970; 23:1141–1148.

90. Björntorp P. Adipose tissue in obesity (Willendorf lecture). In: Hirsch J, Van Ittalie T, eds. Recent Advances in Obesity Research IV. London: John Libbey, 1985:163–170.

91. Larsson B, Svärdsudd K, Welin L, et al. Abdominal adipose tissue distribution, obesity and risk of cardiovascular disease and death: 13 year follow-up of participants in the study of men born in 1913. Br Med J 1984; 228: 1401–1404.

92. Lanska DJ, Lanska MJ, Hartz AJ, et al. A prospective study of body fat distribution and weight loss. Int J Obes 1985; 9:241–246.

93. Vansant G, Den Besten C, Weststrate J, Deurenberg P. Body fat distribution and the prognosis for weight reduction: preliminary results. Int J Obes 1988; 12:133–140.

94. Wadden TA, Stunkard AJ, Johnston FE, Wang J, Pierson RN. Body fat deposition in adult obese women. II. Changes in fat distribution accompanying weight reduction. Am J Clin Nutr 1988; 47:229–234.

95. Svendsen OL, Hasssage C, Christianssen C. The response to treatment of overweight in postmenopausal women is not related to fat distribution. Int J Obes 1995; 19: 496–502.

96. den Besten C, Vansant G, Weststrate JA, Deurenberg P. Resting metabolic rate and diet-induced thermogenesis in abdominal and gluteal-femoral obese women before and after weight reduction. Am J Clin Nutr 1988; 47: 840–847.

97. Stallone DDD, Stunkard AJ, Wadden TA, Foster GD, Boorstein J, Arger P. Weight loss and body fat distribution: a feasibility study using computed tomography. Int J Obes 1991; 15:775–780.

98. Després JP, Tremblay A, Nadeau A, Bouchard. Physical training and changes in regional adipose tissue distribution. Acta Med Scand 1988; 723:205–212.

99. Kanaley JA, Andresen-Reid ML, Oenning L, Kottke BA, Jensen MD. Differential benefits of weight loss in upper-body and lower-body obese women. Am J Clin Nutr 1993; 57:20–26.

100. Fujioka S. Matsuzawa K. Tokungaga T, et al. Improvement of glucose and lipid metabolism associated with selective reduction of visceral fat in premenopausal women with visceral fat obesity. Int J Obes 1991; 15:853–859.

101. Kotchen JM, Cox-Ganser J, Wright C, Kotchen TA. Gender differences in obesity-related cardiovascular disease risk factors among participants in a weight loss programme. Int J Obes 1993; 17:145–151.

102. Astrup A, Buemann B, Glund C, et al. Prognostic markers for diet-induced weight loss in obese women. Int J Obes 1995; 19:275–278.

103. Muls E, Kempen K, Vansant G et al. Is weight cycling detrimental to health? Int J Obes 1995; 19(Suppl 3): S46–S50.

104. Miller DS, Parsonage S. Resistance to slimming. Adaptation or illusion? Lancet 1975; 1:773–775.

105. Jeffery R, Rosenthal B, Lindquist R, et al. Correlates of weight loss and its maintenance over 2 years of follow-up. Prev Med 1984; 13:155–168.

106. James WP, Lean ME, McNeill G. Dietary recommendations after weight loss: how to avoid relapse of obesity. Am J Clin Nutr 1987; 45:1135–1141.

107. Schwarz JM, Schutz Y, Piolino V, et al. Thermogenesis in obese women: effect of fructose versus glucose added to a meal. Am J Physiol 1992; 262:E394–E401.

108. Pi-Sunyer MK. Medical hazards of obesity. Ann Intern Med 1993; 119:655–660.

109. Kluthe R. Schubert A. Obesity in Europe. Ann Intern Med 1995; 103:1037–1042.

110. Kaplan RM, Wilson DK, Hartwell SL, et al. Prospective evaluation of HDL cholesterol after diet and physical conditioning programs for patients with type II diabete mellitus. Diabetes Care 1985; 8:343–348.

111. Wood PD, Stefanick ML, Dreon DM, et al. Changes in plasma lipids and lipoproteins in overweight men during weight loss through dieting as compared with exercise. N Engl J Med 1988; 319:1173–1179.

112. National Cholesterol Education Program. Report of the Expert Panel on Detection, Evaluation and treatment of high blood cholesterol in adults. Bethesda, MD: NIH, 1989 (DHHS publication 89-2925).

113. Wing R, Koeske R, Epstein LH, et al. Long term effects of modest weight loss in type 2 diabetic patients. Arch Intern Med 1987; 147:1749–1753.

114. Kannel WB Wolf PA, Castelli WP, Agostino R. Fibrinogen and risks of cardiovascular disease: the Framingham Study. JAMA 1987; 258:1183–1186.

115. Folsom AR, Quamhich HT, Wing RR, et al. Impact of weight loss on plasminogen activator inhibition (PAI-1), factor VII and other hemostatic factors in moderately overweight adults. Arterioscler Thromb 1993; 13:162–169.

116. Rillaerts E, Van Gaal L, Xiang D, et al. Blood viscosity in human obesity. Relation to glucose tolerance and insulin status. Int J Obes 1989; 13:739–745.

117. Meade JW, Mellows, Brozovic M, Miller GJ, et al. Haemostatic function and ischemic heart disease: principal results of the Northwick Park Study. Lancet 1986; 2: 533–537

118. Hamsten A., Wiman B, De Faire U, Blomback M. Increased plasma levels of a rapid inhibitor of tissue plasminogen activator in young survivors of myocardial infarction. N Engl J Med 1985; 313:1557–1563.

119. Velthuis-te Wierik, et al. Beneficial effect of a moderately energy-restriction diet on fibrinolytic factors in non-obese men. Metabolism 1995; 44:1548–1552.

120. Ornish O, Brown S, Scherwitz LW, et al. Can lifestyle changes reverse coronary heart disease? Lancet 1990: 336: 129–133.

121. Singh R, Rasogi S, Verma R, et al. Randomised controlled trial of cardioprotective diet in patients with recent acute myocardial infarction: results of one yearup. Br Med J 1992; 304:1015–1019.

122. Williamson DF, Pamuk E, Thun M, et al. Prospective study of intentional weight loss and mortality in never-smoking overweight US white women aged 40–64 years. Am J Epidemiol 1995; 141:1128–1141.

123. Witzum JL. Susceptibility of low-density lipoprotein to oxidative modification. Am J Med 1993; 94:347–349.

124. Hertog ML, Faskens EJ, Katan MB, et al. Dietary antioxidant flavonoids and risk of coronary heart disease. the Zutphen Elderly Study. Lancet 1993; 342:1007–1011.

125. Hertog MG, Kromhout D, Aravanis, et al. Flavonoid intake and long-term risk of coronary heart disease and cancer in the Seven Countries Study. Arch Intern Med 1995; 155:381–386.

126. Paolisso G, Ravussin E. Intracellular magnesium and insulin resistance: results in Pima Indians and Caucasians. J Clin Endocrinol Metab 1995; 80:1382–1385.

127. Scheen AJ, Paquot N, Letiexhe MR, et al. Glucose metabolism in obesity: lessons from OGTT, IVGTT and clamp studies. Int J Obes 1995; 19(Suppl 3):S14–S20.

128. Piatti PM, Pontiroli AE, Saibeni A, et al. Insulin sensitivity and lipid levels in obese subjects after slimming diets with different complex and simple carbohydrate content. Int J Obes 1993; 17:375–381.

129. Anderson JW, Abayoni OA. Dietary fiber. An overview. Diabetes Care 1991; 14:1126–1131.

130. Karlstrom B, Vessly B, Asp NG, et al. Effect of an increased content of cereal fiber in the diet of type 2 NIDDM diabetic patients. Diabetologia 1984; 26:272–274.

131. Hellerstedt WL, Jeffrey RW, Murray DM. The association between alcohol intake and adiposity in the general population. Am J Epidemiol 1990; 132:594–611.

132. Tremblay A, Wouters E, Wenker M, et al. Alcohol and a high-fat diet: a combination favoring overfeeding. Am J Clin Nutr 1995; 62:639–644.

133. Mitchell MC and Herlong HF. Alcohol and nutrition; caloric value, bioenergetics, and relationship to liver damage. Annu Rev Nutr 1986; 6:457.

134. Weststrate J, Wunnink I, Deurenberg P, Hautvast JGAJ. Alcohol and its acute effects on resting metabolic rate and diet induced thermogenesis. Br J Nutr 1990; 64:413–425.

135. Suter MP, Schutz Y, Jéquier E. The effect of ethanol on fat storage in healthy subjects. N Engl J Med 1992; 326: 983–987.

136. Suter PM, Jéquier E, Schutz Y. Effect of alcohol on energy expenditure. Am J Physiol 1994; 266:R1204–R1212.

137. Tremblay A, St-Pierre S. The hyperphagic effect of a high-fat diet and alcohol intake persists after control for energy density. Am J Clin Nutr 1996; 63:479–482.

138. McDonald JT, Margen S. Wine versus ethanol in human nutrition I. Nitrogen and calorie balance. Am J Clin Nutr 1976; 29:1093–1103.

139. Gruchow HW, Sobocinski KA, Barboriak JJ, Scheller JG. Alcohol consumption, nutrient intake and relative body weight among U.S. adults. Am J Clin Nutr 1985; 42:289.

140. Lieber CS. The metabolism of alcohol. Sci Am 1976; 243: 25.

141. Gruchow HW, Hoffman RG, Anderson AJ, Barboriak. Coronary artery occlusion and alcohol consumption: effects of binge drinking. Am J Epidemiol 1981; 114:432.

142. Garrow JS. In: Obesity and related disorders. New York: Churchill Livingstone, 1988:145–183.

143. Choosing a Safe and Successful Weight-Loss Program. U.S. Department of Health. NIH Publication No. 94-3700, 1993.

44

Exercise as a Treatment for Obesity

Douglas L. Ballor
Tacoma, Washington

Eric P. Poehlman and Michael J. Toth
University of Vermont, Burlington, Vermont

I. INTRODUCTION

Obesity is a result of energy intake exceeding energy expenditure. When this phenomenon occurs, body weight will rise until the energy expenditure associated with the elevated body weight is equal to energy intake, at which point body weight stabilizes (1). Thus, since exercise increases energy expenditure, it has long been advocated as one treatment for obesity. There are many potential mechanisms by which exercise may facilitate maintenance of body weight at lower levels, including increased fat-free mass (2), elevated resting metabolic rate (for review see Ref. 3), increased concentrations of metabolic hormones (4), decreased preference for high-fat foods (5), energy expenditure associated with recovery processes (6), increased cycling of substrates (7), and psychological "facilitation" (8).

Therefore, it is not surprising that numerous studies, beginning with the classic work of Mayer et al. (9), have noted an inverse relationship between physical activity and body weight. Consistent with this, Williamson et al. (10) recently reported that the relative risk for weight gain over a 10-year period was 3 times higher in those who reported their activity levels as low at follow-up compared to those reporting high levels of activity. Specifically, during the 10-year period, the low-activity group gained 13 kg more than the high-activity group. Television viewing, a pseudo-index of inactivity, is likewise related to obesity.

For example, Tucker and Bagwell (11) report that adult females who watch 3–4 hr of television per day are twice as likely to be obese as those who watch less than 1 hr per day. Gortmaker et al. (12) report that adolescents watching more than 21 hr/week of television have 4 times the prevalence of obesity as those who watch less than 6 hr/week.

While available evidence does suggest a linkage between physical activity levels and body weight, it must be reconciled with data showing a genetic predisposition for obesity (8) and active defense of body weights at levels higher than some would consider desirable (13,14). Furthermore, as Flatt (1) has so eloquently noted, maintenance of body weight at a given level requires that in addition to being in energy balance, one must also be in fat balance where fat intake and fat oxidation are equal.

Since one can easily consume, at one sitting, one's daily energy needs, intake can easily overwhelm expenditure. Therefore, to interpret the results of exercise training on body weight, on must do so within a regulatory model. Thus, one's age, gender, eating habits, level of obesity, distribution of body fat, and number and type of fat cells all likely contribute to how one responds to exercise training. The extent to which exercise training can elicit reductions in body weight among the obese depends on where they lie within this regulatory paradigm especially as it relates to dietary compensation that may occur as a consequence of exercise training.

The dilemma one faces when examining the effect of exercise training on body weight is illustrated in Figure 1, which shows the effect of treadmill running exercise on body weight in Sprague-Dawley rats. Included are data from three separate studies (15–17) in which normal-weight males, normal-weight females, and obese males (high-fat diet) undergo 9–11 weeks of 5 days/week of treadmill exercise training. Compared to their respective sedentary counterparts, the body mass of the obese males, normal-weight males, and normal-weight females was reduced by 15% (95 g), 9% (39 g), and 1% (3 g), respectively. The daily energy intake for the exercise-trained groups declined by 11% in the obese males, by 6% in the normal-weight males, and increased by 2% in the normal-weight females. Thus, the different body weights between groups following exercise training are due in part to the varying degrees of dietary compensation that occur following increased physical activity. In addition, consistent with a desire to reduce weight, resting metabolic rate for the exercise-trained obese and normal-weight males increased significantly whereas that of the normal-weight exercise-trained females remained unchanged. These data suggest that both level of obesity and gender may effect how body weight adapts to exercise training.

In addition, the type of obesity (fat distribution, fat cell type and number) also effects how body weight responds to exercise training. Since types of obesity fall across a broad spectrum, a wide variety of responses are likely to occur in response to the same exercise training regimen. For example, den Besten et al. (18) examined the effects of weight loss on resting metabolic rate (RMR) and diet-induced thermogenesis in abdominal and gluteal-femoral obese women. They noted that weight loss resulted in a reduction in RMR of 10% and 2.5%, respectively, for the abdominal and gluteal-femoral obesity groups. Bouchard et al. (19) compared weight gain among monozygotic twins following 84 days of overfeeding (+1000 kcal/day). Weight gain ranged from 4.3 to 13.3 kg (mean = 8.1 kg). The similarity of the response within pairs of twins was significant ($p < 0.05$) with respect to gain of body weight and fat mass, and the variance among pairs was three times greater than that found within pairs. Després and Bouchard (20) report data examining how 20 weeks of aerobic endurance training affected epinephrine-maximal-stimulated lipolysis in eight pairs of monozygotic twins. Overall, suprailiac fat cell epinephrine-stimulated lipolysis increased by 55%. However, although there was a great deal of variability between pairs (i.e., high and low responders to training), there was a high degree of concordance ($r = 0.90$) as to how twins within a twin pair responded.

One mechanism by which exercise training promotes weight loss is by increasing total daily energy expenditure. There are a number of ways in which it could do this, including increased substrate flux, elevated rates of resting metabolism, repair/recovery associated with the exercise

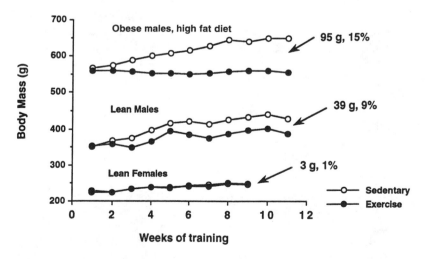

Figure 1 Effect of treadmill training on body weight in obese male, lean male, and lean female Sprague-Dawley rats. Rats became obese by eating a high-fat diet and continued this diet during the exercise training regimen. Other rats ate low-fat chow ad lib. Compared to sedentary rats, exercise training has a much greater effect in obese animals. Lean males and females also differed in their response to exercise training with females affected to a much lesser degree (exercise-trained and sedentary female groups actually overlap). (Data drawn from Refs. 15–17.)

training, and the energy cost of the activity itself. While these processes should lead to increased rates of daily energy expenditure, the overall effect may vary depending on the extent to which alterations in nonexercising time physical activity occur. However, while these processes provide a mechanism for increasing daily total energy expenditure, as noted by Mayer et al. (9), body weight will only drop until it reaches a nadir, at which point dietary intake will be increased so that a stable body weight is maintained.

Taken collectively, these data suggest that adaptations to exercise training may be quite variable and must be considered within the context of one's relative level and type of obesity, genetic disposition, gender, and dietary habits. Since our knowledge of how type of obesity and genetic disposition affect responses to exercise training is limited at best, it is problematic as to whether we can predict how a given individual will respond to an exercise training program. Previous research has generally selected subjects without regard to the above variables, thereby reducing the utility of these data.

The ability of exercise training to facilitate reductions in body weight depends in part on the extent to which body weight is regulated and compensatory adaptations in dietary intake take place with increases in energy expenditure. Keesey (13) has proposed that body weight is regulated and that resting metabolism is altered as required to maintain a stable body weight. In contrast, Flatt (1) suggests that body weight is driven by total energy and fat intake. Body weight rises or falls until daily energy intake and expenditure are equal. He further proposes that since fat intakes do not result in increased rates of fat oxidation (as happens with carbohydrate intake), high levels of fat intake will result in body weight gain until fat oxidation and fat intake are also equal. Ample evidence exists to support both theories (1,13) and these theories are not necessarily mutually exclusive.

The use of exercise training as a treatment for obesity should be viewed within the context and responses of individual fat cells. The rationale for this approach is that on a whole-body basis, the level of fat mass seems to be regulated. For example, when the body contains more fat than desired, insulin receptors on a fat cell will "downregulate" (21). When fat mass is below a desirable level, lipoprotein lipase activity increases to facilitate entry of fatty acids into fat cells (22). In addition, alpha- and beta-mediated fat cells respond differently to adrenergic stimulation (2) and the ratio of alpha- to beta-cell receptors on a fat cell can be affected by dietary status (23). Thus, how exercise training affects one's fat mass would depend, in part, on the volume of individual fat cells, with larger

reductions in fat mass occurring for fat cells containing greater amounts of fat.

Data from Krotkiewski et al. (24) and Björntorp (25) are consistent with this premise. Krotkiewski et al. (24) reported a correlation of $r = -0.48$ between body weight change and fat cell number following 6 months of exercise training, with those having larger numbers of fat cells losing less weight in response to exercise training. Björntorp (25) reported that following extended exercise training and stabilization of body weight, fat cell volumes were constrained within a fairly narrow range even though fat mass varied greatly among individuals. Further confirmation is provided by Tremblay et al. (26). They compared the effects of 20 weeks of exercise training in males and females who initially had relatively high or low fat cell volumes at the beginning of an exercise training program. Males with high fat cell weights lost an average of 4.4 kg of fat mass while males with low fat cell weights lost 0.7 kg. In contrast, exercise training did not affect fat mass of females with either relatively high or low fat cell weights.

Figure 2 illustrates a model that may help account for the varying responses that may occur following exercise intervention. From left to right across the figure the total number of fat cells in an organism increases. The effect of

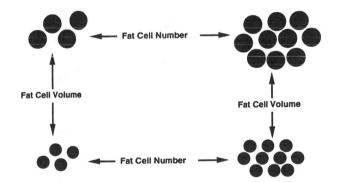

Figure 2 Theoretical model showing how variety of reductions in body weight can occur with manipulations of either the percentage of fat in one's diet or one's level of exercise training. As the percentage of fat in one's diet is decreased or the level of exercise energy expenditure increases, fat cell volumes will be reduced proportionally until they reach a critical volume at which point body weight stabilizes. As one goes from left to right and the number of fat cells increases, so does the total amount of body fat and hence the level of obesity. Thus, a variety of adaptations are possible to various diet and exercise manipulations.

exercise training (and/or switching to a low-fat diet) is shown as one goes from top to bottom during which fat cell volume decreases until a nadir is reached. One can then be obese by having a normal volume of fat in each fat cell but an abnormally large number of fat cells (hyperplastic obesity), by having a relatively normal number of fat cells with large fat cell volumes (hypertrophic obesity), or a combination of the two. If one assumes that exercise training (or dietary modifications) result in fat cell volumes being reduced to a critical level beyond which it is difficult to progress, one can explain why exercise training can result in substantial changes in fat mass for one individual (large fat cell volumes, relatively low number of fat cells) and limited effects in another (normal fat cell volumes, many fat cells) even though they may have the same total fat mass. Thus, Figure 2 suggests that exercise training will have little effect on body fat when fat cell volumes are near or at desirable levels (even though one may still be considered obese). It further suggests that those with hypertrophic obesity are more likely to lose body fat in response to exercise training than are those with hyperplastic obesity.

Following is a discussion of how exercise training may affect daily energy metabolism, body weight, and the ability to maintain weight at reduced levels. One must always view the information presented from a regulatory perspective and with the knowledge that a variety of responses to exercise training are possible depending on where one is within their regulatory paradigm.

II. VALIDITY OF COMMONLY USED TECHNIQUES USED TO ASSESS CHANGES IN BODY COMPOSITION

Underwater weighing (densitometry), bioelectrical impedance, and skinfold thickness are currently the three most commonly used methods for estimating body composition. While the three measures intercorrelate relatively well with respect to their ability to estimate percent body fat in individuals (27), serious flaws exist in each of these methods with respect to their ability to accurately assess body composition changes following exercise training. As such, there is a growing consensus against using two-compartment models of underwater weighing (28), bioelectrical impedance (29), and skinfold thickness (30) to measure exercise training–induced changes in body composition. Because of this we will limit our discussion on the effects of exercise training on body constituents as much as possible and focus instead on body weight.

III. EXERCISE AND RESTING METABOLIC RATE

We now consider recent studies that have advanced our understanding of the influence of exercise training on energy expenditure. In particular, the application of doubly labeled water methodology and room calorimeters have generated new questions regarding adaptations of total daily energy expenditure and its components to chronic exercise in obese and lean individuals. An understanding of the role of exercise and its impact on energy expenditure is important to the understanding of how exercise can be most appropriately prescribed to generate a significant energy deficit, induce fat loss, and preserve fat-free mass.

Whereas previous work has focused primarily on the effects of endurance exercise on energy expenditure (31–33), the use of resistance training has recently gained greater appeal as an intervention to increase muscular strength, preserve fat-free mass, and increase daily energy expenditure. Thus, we will also briefly examine studies that focused on the effects of resistance training on energy expenditure.

A. Effects of Exercise on Total Daily Energy Expenditure

Exercise is commonly prescribed alone or in combination with dietary restriction to promote body weight loss (see Ref. 32). Theoretically, exercise reduces body weight by increasing total daily energy expenditure without corresponding alterations in energy intake. The increase in total daily energy expenditure by participation in exercise results from several sources: (1) the direct energy cost of the exercise bout, (2) an elevated postexercise energy expenditure (34), (3) an increase in resting metabolic rate (4), and/or (4) increased energy expenditure associated with nonexercising physical activity.

A review of the effects of endurance exercise on resting and postexercise energy expenditure has previously been considered (31–33) and will not be considered in this review. In carefully performed studies, when volunteers are maintained in energy balance and/or when weight loss is not great (<5 kg), aerobic exercise has been shown to increase resting metabolic rate. On the other hand, when severe caloric restriction is combined with endurance exercise, it does not appear that exercise can reverse the dietary-induced depression of resting metabolic rate (35,36). With respect to the acute effects of exercise, it appears that exercise of greater intensity and duration results in a more prolonged increase in energy expenditure following exercise cessation (37).

Of greater interest, however, is the effects of exercise on daily energy expenditure, since it is ultimately the net difference between energy intake and energy expenditure that determines body energy reserves. Historically, methodological constraints have, until recently, limited the accurate assessment of the effect of exercise on total daily energy expenditure and free-living physical activity (38). During the past decade, the refinement and increased availability of two methods of measuring total daily energy expenditure, whole room indirect calorimetry and the doubly labeled water technique, have allowed investigators to explore the impact of exercise on total daily energy expenditure and its relationship to weight loss. Cross-sectional and intervention studies that have used these techniques to determine the influence of endurance exercise on total daily energy expenditure are summarized in Table 1. There is much disparity between studies regarding the effects of endurance exercise on total daily energy expenditure, with some studies finding elevated total daily energy expenditure associated with endurance training and others finding no effect. the following section will briefly review the findings of these studies and their implications for exercise prescription and weight loss.

B. Measurement of Total Daily Energy Expenditure

At present, two techniques are commonly used to measure total daily energy expenditure in humans: whole room indirect calorimetry and the doubly labeled water technique. The whole room calorimeter is an open-circuit, indirect calorimeter in which the subject resides for a period of approximately 24 hr. Energy expenditure is calculated from continuous measurements of oxygen and carbon dioxide concentrations and flow rates. Whole room calorimetry significantly advanced energy metabolism research by providing an accurate measure of total daily energy expenditure, its components, and substrate oxidation.

The doubly labeled water technique, first conceived by Lifson and colleagues (39) and later adapted for use in humans (40), allows for the measurement of energy expenditure in subjects in their free-living environment. In this method, the elimination rates of an oral dose of two stable isotopes of water, ^2H_2O and $H_2^{18}O)$, are used to measure total daily energy expenditure. A more detailed methodological discussion of these techniques is beyond the scope of this review and has been provided elsewhere (41,42).

Although both methods provide measures of total daily energy expenditure, the conditions under which these measures are derived are very different. Whole room indirect calorimetry provides a measurement of total daily energy expenditure in a controlled and confined environment. Because the subject's physical activity is confined to the room calorimeter (and likely reduced) for the measurement period, total energy expenditure will be underestimated (43,44). Research has shown that this underestimation can be as little as 20% in sedentary individuals (43) and as much as 68% in highly trained athletes (44).

In contrast, the doubly labeled water technique measures total daily energy expenditure in the subject's free-living environment. Therefore, this technique allows for a more accurate measurement of total daily energy expenditure compared to whole room indirect calorimetry. However, the doubly labeled water technique is limited in that it does not provide a measure of substrate utilization and cannot measure temporal changes in total daily energy expenditure. Furthermore, the cost of the isotope and its complicated analysis hamper widespread application of this method. Both measurement techniques provide unique, but possibly different, information regarding the effects of exercise training programs on total daily energy expenditure.

C. Cross-Sectional Studies and Daily Energy Expenditure

Schulz et al. (45) measured total daily energy expenditure by whole room indirect calorimetry in 20 endurance-trained and 43 untrained younger male volunteers. During the 23-hr measurement period, endurance-trained volunteers were prohibited from performing their normal exercise training routine. Furthermore, energy intake was reduced in athletes to compensate for the lower energy expenditure due to the absence of training. This approach permitted the subjects to be studied in a state of energy balance. No difference in total daily energy expenditure was noted between groups (trained: 2126 ± 186 kcal/day vs. untrained: 2154 ± 245 kcal/day) after controlling for difference in body composition.

Horton and colleagues (46) measured total daily energy expenditure in five female cyclists and five age- and weight-matched sedentary female controls in a room calorimeter. When the trained subjects were restricted from performing their exercise training program, no difference in total daily energy expenditure was found between groups (trained: 2264 ± 265 kcal/day vs. untrained: 2144 ± 249 kcal/day). However, total daily energy expenditure was higher in cyclists (3137 ± 419 kcal/day)

Table 1 Summary of Studies Examining Changes in Total Energy Expenditure (TEE) in Response to Training

Cross-sectional studies

Study	Method	Subject size	Training type	Difference in TEE[a]
Schulz et al., 1991 (45)	Whole room calorimeter	$n = 63$ young males, 20 trained, 43 untrained	Endurance trained	−28 kcal/day NS
Horton et al., 1994 (46)	Whole room calorimeter	$n = 10$ young females, 5 trained, 5 untrained	Endurance trained	+120 kcal/day NS

Intervention studies

Study	Method	Subject size and gender	Training type and duration	Change in TEE
Bingham et al., 1989 (49)	DLW	$n = 5$ young, 3 male, 2 female	Endurance training 9 weeks	Men: +956 kcal/day $p < 0.05$ Women: +244 kcal/day NS
Meiher et al., 1991 (51)	DLW	$n = 32$ young, 4 male, 4 female	Endurance training 20 weeks	Men: +788 kcal/day $p < 0.05$ Women: +311 kcal/day NS
Racette et al., 1995 (52)	DLW	$n = 23$ young, female	Endurance training 12 weeks	+17 kcal/day NS
Buemann et al., 1992 (53)	Whole room calorimeter	$n = 7$ young, postobese female	Endurance training 12 weeks	−11 kcal/day NS
Blaak et al., 1992 (54)	DLW	$n = 10$ young, male	Endurance training 4 weeks	+301 kcal/day $p < 0.05$
Goran and Poehlman, 1992 (55)	DLW	$n = 11$ elderly, 6 male, 5 female	Endurance training 8 weeks	+66 kcal/day NS

[a]Difference in trained compared to untrained subjects.

compared to controls (2206 ± 323 kcal/day; $p < 0.01$) when athletes were allowed to perform their daily exercise program due to the energetic cost of the exercise training. From these results, investigators of both studies concluded that an elevation in total daily energy expenditure in trained individuals was due to the direct energy cost of training and postexercise energy expenditure. However, the removal of trained individuals from their free-living environment with concomitant reductions in both energy intake and energy expenditure render conclusions regarding adaptive changes in energy expenditure in trained individuals questionable.

D. Intervention Studies and Daily Energy Expenditure

A question of significant interest is the impact of exercise training on daily energy expenditure and, in particular, the energy expenditure during nonexercising time. This component of total daily energy expenditure is highly variable among individuals (47,48) and may be influenced by endurance training. Although one assumes that exercise increases total daily energy expenditure, the inability to assess energy expenditure in free-living individuals outside a laboratory setting has not permitted a rigorous examination of this question. From an energetic and cardiovascular standpoint, the goal is to prescribe exercise that significantly enhances physical activity during the nonexercising time of the day. Exercise that results in significant increases in total daily energy expenditure would ultimately be most beneficial in the regulation of body weight.

Bingham and co-workers (49) found a significant increase in total daily energy expenditure in three young men (+956 kcal/day), but no change in two young women (+244 kcal/day) following 9 weeks of endurance training, as measured by the doubly labeled water technique. Because no changes in basal metabolic rate, overnight metabolic rate, or sleeping metabolic rate were noted following the training program, the increase in total daily energy expenditure in men was largely attributable to the increase in physical activity. The magnitude of the increase in energy expenditure of physical activity attributable to increase in nonexercising energy expenditure could not be calculated since the energy cost of each exercise session was not reported. However, considering that male participants were performing 1 hr of jogging by the end of the program at approximately 12.5 kcal/min (energy cost of a typical 65-kg man running 9 min/mile; see Ref. 50), the direct energetic cost of the exercise would be approximately 750 kcal/day. This suggests that training induced an increase in nonexercising energy expenditure of approximately 200 kcal/day. Although subjects were in negative energy imbalance throughout the study, no change in basal or sleeping metabolic rate was noted. The small sample size in the aforementioned study, however, should be kept in mind when interpreting these results.

Meijer and colleagues (51) investigated changes in total daily energy expenditure, using doubly labeled water, in four young male volunteers and four young female volunteers following 20 weeks of endurance training. Although a significant increase in total daily energy expenditure was found in males (+788 kcal/day; $p < 0.05$), no significant change was found in females (+311 kcal/day). The significant increase in total daily energy expenditure in men was attributable to an increase in nonexercising energy expenditure of approximately 215 kcal/day. Thus, together with the findings of Bingham et al. (49), these results underscore the need to properly measure the energy expenditure of the physical activity component of total daily energy expenditure. Although small sample sizes may have prohibited the detection of an effect of endurance training on total daily energy expenditure in women, the studies by Meijer et al. (51) and Bingham et al. (49) suggest that women may not increase their daily energy expenditure as much as men in response to endurance training even when corrections are made for differences in body weight.

Racette and colleagues (52) recently examined the effects of 12 weeks of endurance exercise training and dietary restriction on total daily energy expenditure, as measured by doubly labeled water. Twenty-three obese women were randomly assigned to either aerobic exercise or no exercise and to a high- or low-carbohydrate reducing diet. Similar to the study by Bingham and colleagues (49), subjects were in negative energy balance throughout the exercise program. In contrast, however, a reduction in resting metabolic rate and the thermic effect of a meal were found, suggesting that endurance exercise does not preserve these components of total daily energy expenditure when dietary intake is greatly reduced. Despite the reductions in RMR and the thermic effect of a meal, total daily energy expenditure remained unchanged due to the energy expenditure of physical activity (≈ 180 kcal/day). This finding suggests that endurance training may preserve total daily energy expenditure during dietary restriction by increasing the energy expenditure of physical activity.

Buemann and co-workers (53) also showed that endurance training did not affect total daily energy expenditure in women, as measured in a room calorimeter. They found no change in total daily energy expenditure (≥ 11 kcal/day), in seven young, postobese, weight-stable female volunteers following a 12-week endurance training program. Again, these findings may relate to the blunting of spontaneous physical activity when measurements are performed in a room calorimeter.

Two recent studies examining the effects of exercise on total daily energy expenditure were performed in children and older volunteers using the doubly labeled water technique. Blaak and colleagues (54) found an increase in total daily energy expenditure following 4 weeks of endurance training in 10 obese, preadolescent boys (+301 kcal/day). This increase in total daily energy expenditure was attributable to an increase in the energy expenditure of physical activity. Approximately 50% of this increase in physical activity energy expenditure was associated with the direct energetic cost of the exercise program, whereas the remainder was associated with increased nonexercising physical activity. Although no change in body composition was noted over the study period, these findings suggest that long-term exercise training may be a suitable intervention to treat obesity in adolescents due to its enhancing effects on nonexercising physical activity.

Our laboratory examined changes in total daily energy expenditure in response to 8 weeks of high-intensity ($\approx$85% of VO_2 max) endurance training in 11 elderly men and women (55). Although an 11% increase in RMR was noted, total daily energy expenditure did not change in response to training due to a reduction in activity during nonexercising times. This preliminary study suggests that high-intensity exercise in elderly patients may not be an ideal prescription to enhance daily energy expenditure due to a compensatory reduction in nonexercising physical activity. It can be argued, however, that the depression in nonexercising physical activity may subside following an exercise program of longer duration. Regardless, it is clear that further investigation into which combination of exercise intensity and duration of endurance exercise best stimulates total daily energy expenditure is needed.

E. Effects of Resistance Training on Energy Expenditure

Resistance training may influence energy expenditure through its trophic effects on fat-free tissue, particularly muscle mass, which in turn is related to RMR. For this reason, several studies have examined the effects of resistance training on RMR.

1. Cross-Sectional Studies: Resistance Training and Energy Expenditure

Our laboratory has completed a series of cross-sectional studies that examined the influence of aerobic and resistance training on RMR in young and middle-aged populations of men and women. All RMR values and differences in RMR between the training groups in the studies discussed below represent values adjusted for differences in fat-free mass.

Poehlman et al. (55a) examined RMR in young aerobic-trained ($n = 36$), resistance-trained ($n = 18$), and sedentary males ($n = 42$). RMR was 5% higher in resistance-trained compared to untrained men, whereas aerobic-trained individuals had a 10% higher RMR compared to untrained young men, respectively (Fig. 3). These differences correspond to a 187 and 86 kcal/day greater

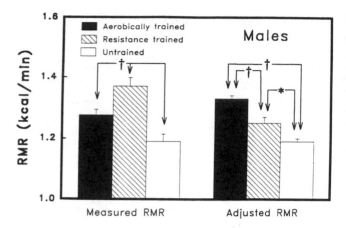

Figure 3 Mean measured RMR and adjusted RMR in untrained aerobically trained, and resistance-trained young men. RMR was adjusted for fat-free mass and compared between groups using analysis of covariance. Values are mean $\pm$ SE. *$p < 0.05$; †$p < 0.01$. (From Ref. 55a.)

resting energy expenditure in aerobic- and resistance-trained young men, respectively. In a similar study in young women, Ballor and Poehlman (56) found no differences in RMR between resistance-trained ($n = 13$) and untrained ($n = 48$) younger women, whereas aerobic-trained ($n = 21$) women showed a 6% higher RMR compared to both groups. The reason for the sex difference in the relationship between resistance training and RMR is unknown, although it may be a function of difference in training intensity and/or volume.

In middle-aged men, Toth and Poehlman (57) found no differences in RMR between 19 resistance-trained and 30 sedentary volunteers. Similar to younger men and women, however, aerobic-trained middle-aged men ($n = 37$) had a higher RMR compared to untrained volunteers (86 kcal/day). It is unclear why resistance training was not associated with an elevated RMR (per kilogram fat-free mass). In middle-aged women, RMR was 16% higher in resistance-trained compared to untrained volunteers, but similar to the aerobic-trained group (57). The elevated RMR in the resistance- and aerobic-trained middle-aged women translates to a 160 and 150 kcal/day increase in daily resting energy requirements, respectively. This finding suggests that both aerobic and resistance training may serve as effective interventions for blunting the age-related decline in RMR that occurs in women.

Bosselaers and co-workers (58) examined 24-hr energy expenditure in 10 resistance-trained subjects (nine men, one woman) and 10 healthy controls matched for age, sex, and percent body fat. They found a greater 24-hr energy expenditure in resistance-trained subjects compared to sedentary controls (+354 kcal/day), although there were no differences between groups when expressed on a kilogram per fat-free mass basis. Thus, the elevated energy expenditure in resistance-trained subjects is attributable, in part, to a greater quantity of fat-free mass. The disparity between these cross-sectional studies may be a result of exercise selection bias as well as genetic predisposition (59).

2. Intervention Studies: Resistance Training and Energy Expenditure

Limited information is available on the effects of resistance exercise training on RMR in younger individuals. Broeder et al. (60) found no change in RMR in 13 young male volunteers following 12 weeks of high-intensity training. Interestingly, RMR did not change, despite a 2-kg increase in fat-free mass. Similarly, Van Etten et al. (61) found no change in sleeping metabolic rate, despite a 1.1-kg increase in fat-free mass, after 12 weeks of resistance training in 21 young male subjects.

Most research examining resistance training and RMR has used older populations. Pratley and colleagues (62) examined changes in RMR following 16 weeks of resistance training in 13 older men. RMR increased by approximately 8% (120 kcal/day). Although fat-free mass increased during the training program (+1.6 kg), the increase in RMR persisted after controlling for changes in fat-free mass. This finding suggests that the elevation in RMR was due to both the increased amount and metabolic activity of fat-free mass. However, the investigators could not rule out the possibility that the elevated RMR was due to the residual effect of the last bout of exercise since the RMR measurement was performed only 24 hr following the last training session.

Campbell and co-workers (63) found a 6.8% increase in RMR in 12 older men and women following a 12-week resistance training program. Fat-free mass increased following training (1.4 kg) due to an increase in total body water. Thus, changes in RMR were not attributable to alterations in respiring tissue. These findings suggest that resistance training stimulates RMR in older individuals through a mechanism that is independent of changes in fat-free mass. Furthermore, RMR was measured ≈45 hr after the last training session and thus is unlikely to contain the residual effects from the last exercise bout.

Treuth et al. (64) found a 9% increase in RMR in 13 elderly women after a 16-week resistance training program. However, total daily energy expenditure was unchanged, as measured by whole room calorimetry. Since there were no significant changes in fat-free mass during the training program, these results suggest that the increase in RMR was independent of increases in fat-free mass. It should be noted that changes in fat-free mass in the aforementioned studies are small and frequently within the error of the measurement technique. Resistance training programs that are longer in duration and that result in larger increases in fat-free mass may help resolve the controversy regarding whether there is an increase in RMR above that which can be accounted for by changes in body composition.

Although the above studies do not outline the mechanisms by which resistance training affects RMR, they do suggest that it may be an effective intervention to increase total daily energy expenditure. Although findings have been mixed (see below), resistance training may be used as an adjunct with programs of caloric restriction to prevent the decline in fat-free mass and preserve RMR in obese individuals.

IV. EXERCISE TRAINING IN COMBINATION WITH DIETARY RESTRICTION

Exercise training is a logical adjunct to dietary restriction programs. In addition to its ability to enhance total energy expenditure and increase fat-free mass, exercise training may reduce the percentage of weight lost as fat-free mass.

A recently completed meta-analysis examined how aerobic exercise training in combination with dietary restriction affected the composition of diet-induced weight loss (65). Meta-analysis (66) is a technique that combines mean results from various studies, treats them as individual data points, and subjects them to parametric analysis. Analyses of this type allow one to draw inferences that would be difficult to make using traditional intervention paradigms. The results of 46 different studies were coded, entered into a database, and subjected to parametric statistical analyses. Exercise training included various types and intensities of aerobic exercise including walking and running. Sedentary weight loss groups lost an average of ≈11 kg and weight loss plus exercise training groups an average of ≈9 kg. Figure 4 depicts our findings with respect to the percentage of weight lost as fat-free mass. As can be seen, weight lost as fat-free mass decreased from ≈25% of total weight for the dietary restriction only group to ≈12% for the dietary restriction plus exercise group. In addition, men and women responded similarly to the interventions. There was, however, still a great deal of variability between studies. In addition, it is likely that

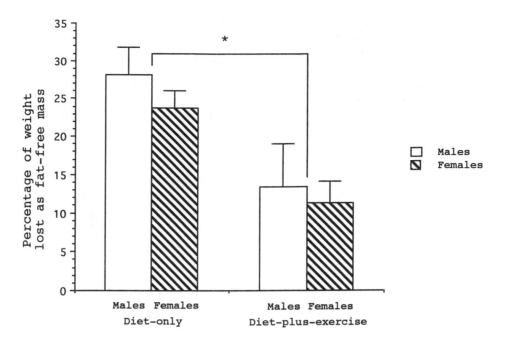

Figure 4 Percentage of weight lost as fat-free mass during weight loss with or without aerobic exercise training. *Exercise-trained groups significantly different from sedentary groups, $p < 0.05$. Males and females did not respond differently, $p > 0.05$. (Data from Ref. 65.)

the conservation of fat-free mass shown here actually reflects increased fat losses rather than conservation of protein-based fat-free mass.

Weight training exercise has been used much less frequently in combination with dietary restriction programs. Ballor et al. (67) reported that resistance weight training in combination with a modest weight loss program (≈ 4 kg) resulted in preservation of fat-free mass in comparison to a weight loss group that did not exercise. In contrast, Donnelly et al. (68) found that the addition of weight training exercise did not result in conservation of fat-free mass following a relatively large weight reduction (≈ 20 kg). Interestingly, they noted that aerobic exercise training also failed to elicit conservation of fat-free mass compared to dietary restriction alone. As we have noted previously (15–17,69), this may be due to the magnitude of the energy deficit.

Many recommend low-intensity exercise for inclusion in weight loss regimens since the likelihood of injury is lower and the percentage of energy derived from fat during exercise is higher compared to more rigorous forms of exercise (70). It is also theorized that increasing the percentage of energy derived from fat during exercise will result in additional losses of fat mass. From the limited research that has been done this does not seem to be the case. Ballor et al. (70) examined the effects of expending ≈ 275 kcal per session via cycling exercise at either high (80–90% of V_{O_2} max) or low (40–50% of V_{O_2} max) work rates three times per week on young women undergoing an 8-week weight loss program. While fat substrates provided $\approx 26\%$ and 67% of the energy for metabolism during exercise for the high- and low-intensity exercise groups, respectively, the percentage of total weight lost as fat did not differ between groups. A follow-up study was done (69) using treadmill running at 75% or 37.5% of V_{O_2} maximum in Sprague-Dawley male rats. The duration (90 or 45 min) and frequency (5 day/week) of exercise were greater, the severity of weight loss more pronounced (to 66% of body weight), and the method of body composition assessment more precise (ether fat extraction, nitrogen assays). Again the percentages of weight lost as fat and fat-free mass in the two groups were quite similar.

While the data presented earlier (65) suggest that exercise training in combination with dietary restriction results in a reduction in the percentage of weight lost as fat-free mass, one should be prudent in how one interprets these data as they are based on changes in body density (see Ref. 28) determined via underwater weighing. It is likely that these differences between sedentary and exercise-trained weight loss groups reflects increased fat mass loss coupled with gains in water mass for the exercise-trained groups rather than conservation of protein-based tissue. This is especially true since nitrogen balance data generally do not support the premise that exercise training reduces losses in protein mass during weight loss (36,71).

Data from animal experiments (15,17) can help illustrate this point and indicate on which body constituents exercise training is most likely to exert its effects during weight loss. In two separate experiments, obese and normal-weight male Sprague-Dawley rats underwent dietary manipulations intended to induce moderate or severe weight losses while simultaneously exercising on a treadmill or remaining sedentary. In addition, food allotments were altered as necessary such that the weight losses in the respective exercise-trained and sedentary groups remained equal. In essence, one is then examining the effects of exercise training when weight losses are equal.

As shown in Table 2, for both rats that were obese or of normal weight at the start of the weight loss regimen, as the level of weight loss increased, protein losses increased. At each level of restriction for both obese and normal-weight groups, exercise training did not differentially affect protein losses. In contrast, an exercise effect is noted on fat mass for obese but not normal-weight rats.

Table 2 Effects of Exercise Training on Protein and Fat Mass in Normal-Weight and Obese Sedentary and Exercise-Trained Sprague-Dawley Rats Subjected to Moderate and Severe Weight Loss Regimens

Group	Protein mass (g)		Fat mass (g)	
	Sedentary	Exercise	Sedentary	Exercise
Obese 77% of control wt.	103.6 ±3.2	107.9 ±2.7	72.5[a] ±7.7	45.4[a] ±4.7
Obese 63% of control wt.	93.4 ±1.9	94.3 ±1.7	28.4 ±2.1	20.5 ±1.8
Normal weight 86% of control wt.	80.4 ±2.1	80.9 ±1.2	33.9 ±2.3	28.6 ±2.8
Normal weight 67% of control wt.	63.9 ±0.7	63.4 ±0.7	14.5 ±1.9	10.4 ±1.4

Data are mean ± SE.
[a]Sedentary group is significantly different from respective exercise-trained group, $p < 0.05$. Mean weights at the end of each experiment are expressed as a percentage of the sedentary control groups weight.
Source: Data are drawn from Refs. 15–17.

Furthermore, this effect is limited to the moderate restriction group. As the level of weight loss becomes more severe, the size of the effect of exercise training on fat mass is greatly diminished.

Our research on weight loss and exercise using Sprague-Dawley rat models (15–17,69,72) has led to the following conclusions. (1) In males, as the level of dietary restriction increases, the ability of exercise training to exert an effect on fat mass and resting metabolic rate is greatly diminished and/or extinguished; (2) in females (16), while exercise training has a rather pronounced effect on total fat mass in ad lib fed animals, exercise training did not differentially effect changes in fat mass, protein mass, or resting metabolism. Taken collectively, these data suggest that exercise training may differentially affect males and females during weight loss and that as the weight loss becomes more pronounced, the effects of exercise training are greatly attenuated.

V. EXERCISE AND BODY WEIGHT

As noted earlier, a relationship appears to exist between body weight and physical activity (9). For sedentary individuals, increases in physical activity can result in reductions in body weight as well as concomitant reductions in dietary intake (9,17,72). With continued increases in activity, body weight will decrease until it eventually reaches a nadir and stabilizes with further increases in physical activity counterbalanced by increases in dietary intake. This section will examine how different types of exercise interventions may affect body weight. In addition, we will examine the extent to which age, gender, and level of obesity may affect responses to exercise training. It should be noted, however, that a majority of these studies used young normal-weight individuals as subjects, which likely understates the effect of exercise training on body weight. Furthermore, most studies are of a relatively short duration, which likely results in an overstatement of the rate at which weight is lost and an understatement of the magnitude of the weight loss that may occur.

A. Energy Expenditure and Body Weight

The energy balance equation requires that when energy expenditures exceeds energy intake, body weight must decrease. As body weight declines, overall energy expenditure decreases due to a reduced metabolic mass and the diminished energy expenditure associated with moving one's body. Body weight will continue to decline until expenditure and intake are again equal. Thus one would assume that any time physical activity is increased, there would be a corresponding reduction in body weight as long as compensatory adaptations in either energy intake or other portions of one's metabolism do not occur. But, as noted by Mayer et al. (9) and others (see Ref. 73 for review), dietary compensation following increases in physical activity varies greatly.

It is also possible that total daily energy expenditure may not rise if increases in physical activity are matched by decreases in activity in other areas. For example, Poehlman (74) measured total energy expenditure via doubly labeled water in older adults before and after an 8-week aerobic training program. Although resting metabolic rate increased by 11%, total daily energy expenditure remained unchanged. A reduction of 62% in the nonexercise energy expenditure accounted for the lack of an increase in total energy expenditure. These data suggest that participation in rigorous training programs may elicit adaptations in one's life-style that result in total daily energy expenditure increasing by less than one would predict from the physical activity alone. These data further support the premise that moderate low-intensity daily exercise might be better suited for facilitating increases in total daily energy expenditure. However, it should be noted that this study was of relatively short duration and it is possible that, over time, adaptations to the rigors of the exercise program would occur and that energy expenditure during nonexercise times would increase.

Within the constraints above, it appears that as the number of kilocalories one expends during exercise increases, so does the magnitude of the weight loss. Ballor and Keesey (2) completed a meta-analysis that examined how exercise training affected body weight and composition in adult males and females.

They located 64 different means (48 M, 16 F) for relatively normal-fat (M ≈ 20%, F ≈ 28%), generally young adults who participated in cycling or run/walk exercise training. Males trained for ≈17 weeks compared to 12 for females. As different studies (i.e., means) exercised at different intensities, durations, and frequencies and hence had different levels of energy expenditure, it is possible to do correlational analyses to examine the relationship between energy expenditure and change in body weight. For males, correlations of $r = -0.59$, -0.61, and -0.64 ($p < 0.05$) were found between reductions in body weight and energy expenditure on a per session, per week, and overall basis, respectively. In contrast, for females, the correlations were much lower and nonsignificant ranging from $r = 0.11$ to $r = -0.18$.

Leon et al. (75) examined the effects of 16 weeks of walking 90 min, 5 days/week at 5.1 kph (3.2 mph) on a 10% grade on body weight and body composition in six

obese (99.1 kg, 23.5% fat) young men. The energy expenditure was estimated at 4600 kJ (1100 kcal) per session. By the end of the intervention, body weight had dropped by almost 6 kg with all of the weight loss being as fat. Furthermore, the rate of weight loss was consistent throughout the study. Dietary intake increased slightly (≈180–200 kcal) during the first 12 weeks of the study and was slightly below (≈130 kcal) baseline at week 16. Leisure activity remained unchanged during the study.

Marti and Howald (76) examined the relationship between current activity levels and 15-year changes in body composition and body weight in 27 former elite runners. The subjects were divided into highly active ($n = 5$, run ≥ 90 km/week), active ($n = 13$, run 50–65 km/week), and formerly active ($n = 9$, run ≤30 km/week) groups based on their current training regimens. Over the 15-year period, the weights of the highly active, active, and formerly active groups changed by -0.4, 1.1, and 8.8 kg, respectively. These data illustrate the following. (1) Continued high levels of physical activity can block the weight gain that commonly occurs with age. (2) A threshold exists above which increases in physical activity are not matched with concomitant decreases in body weight (i.e., weight changes of highly active and active groups are not substantially different from each other).

B. Aerobic Exercise Adaptations and Level of Obesity

Ballor and Keesey (2) in their meta-analysis found correlations of $r = -0.33$ ($p < 0.05$) and -0.59 ($p < 0.05$), respectively, for males and females between initial percent body fat and weight loss during the exercise regimen. While these correlations are not particularly high, they are impressive nonetheless given the relatively low initial percent body fat of the groups.

Lee et al. (77) present data that classically illustrate the relationship between level of obesity and body weight changes with physical activity. They studied the effects of 20 weeks of intense military training on 197 male recruits divided into three tertiles (24–30% fat, 30–35% fat, 35+% fat). During the 20-week period the subjects participated in 554 hr (28 hr/week) of rigorous physical training. In addition, while the subjects underwent dietary counseling as to how best to reduce weight, they were allowed to feed ad lib.

The results of the 20 weeks of training are shown in Figure 5. Data are reported as the cumulative weight loss present at the end of each month of training. They demonstrate quite clearly that as the level of obesity increases, so does the magnitude of the weight loss. At the conclusion of the 20-week training period, the 24–30% fat group

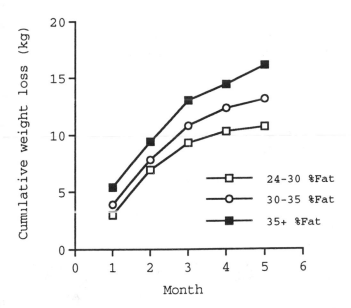

Figure 5 Effect of 5 months of military training on body weight in individuals with varying degrees of obesity. The greater the level of obesity, the greater the cumulative weight loss, i.e., the total weight loss that had been achieved at any given measurement period. Note that while weight loss had attenuated for the 24–30% fat group, weight loss was still continuing in the 35+% fat group. (Data from Ref. 77.)

had lost 10.7 kg, the 30–35% fat group 13.1 kg, and the 35+% fat group 16.1 kg. It is also apparent that the rate of weight loss was plateauing for the 24–30% fat group while that of the 35+% fat group was still continuing. These data demonstrate that weight stabilization may occur at different time points for different groups of individuals and that weight loss induced via exercise training can continue for extended periods of time. In addition, the fatter one is, the easier it is to lose weight.

Boileau et al. (78) conducted an interesting experiment in which lean (68 kg) and obese (122 kg) young (≈18 years old) sedentary men increased their daily energy expenditure by 600 kcal/day, 5 days/week for 8 weeks. Body weight declined by −1.0 and −3.2 kg for the lean and obese groups, respectively. Again, the same energy expenditure can elicit different reductions in body weight and suggest variable compensations in dietary and/or metabolic parameters.

C. Intensity of Aerobic Exercise and Body Weight Adaptations

Many assume that, for a given level of energy expenditure, as the intensity at which one exercises increases so do the

reductions in body weight and fat. This likely stems in part from the American College of Sports Medicine's position statement (79) on recommended levels of exercise training to elicit changes in body composition (i.e., 70–90% of maximum heart rate) and our implicit belief that harder is better. For this to occur, however, it would seem that high-intensity exercise would have to induce compensatory adjustments in either resting/recovery metabolism or dietary intake. Furthermore, these adjustments would have to also overcome any reductions in activity that may occur during other parts of the day (74).

At present it is unclear the extent to which dietary intake and the intensity at which one exercises is related. Resting metabolic rate and postexercise oxygen uptake are two mechanisms by which rigorous exercise training could theoretically facilitate greater weight loss. It has been suggested that the degree to which resting metabolic rate is elevated via exercise training is related to the intensity at which one exercises, although the literature is equivocal with regard to this matter (32). Postexercise oxygen uptakes have been shown to be higher following more rigorous types of exercise training (80). Thus to the extent the intensity at which one exercises affects resting/recovery metabolism, exercising at higher work rates could result in greater weight losses even when the levels of caloric expenditure during the exercise sessions are similar.

In contrast, advocates of low-intensity exercise note the increased emphasis on fat for fuel and believe this should translate into increased losses of body weight and fat. Further support for this premise comes from Flatt's fat balance hypothesis, which suggests that body weight will rise or lower until fat oxidation and fat intake are equal (1). However, while fat oxidized during exercise is likely to be higher during low-intensity exercise, higher-intensity exercise may well compensate for this deficit during the recovery processes associated with the exercise. In addition, it is important to note that, for most people, exercise training expenditures represent less than 5% of their weekly energy expenditure. Within this framework, the difference in the total amount of fat oxidized via one form of exercise or another compared to total fat oxidation may be too small to be meaningful. Generally, as shown below, the intensity at which one exercises and level of reduction in body weight do not seem strongly related.

Tremblay et al. (81) compared body weights of 2600 Canadian men and women separated into quartiles based on the work rate at which they exercised (<5, 5–7, 7–9, and >9 METS; 1 MET = 3.5 ML O_2/kg body weight/min). Body weights among the four groups were quite similar with the weights varying from 75.8 to 76.8 kg for men and from 59.2 to 60.3 for women. It should be noted, however, that there was a tendency for the sum of five skinfold thicknesses to decrease as the intensity at which one exercised increased, with skinfold thicknesses being ≈10% lower in the highest quartile compared to the lowest quartile.

Duncan et al. (82) compared the effects of walking 4.8 km/day, 5 days/week for 24 weeks at three different work rates (8.0 km/hr, 6.4 km/hr, 4.8 km/hr) on body weight and body composition in 59 normal-fat (≈27–28%), sedentary, premenopausal women 20–40 years of age. As one might suspect, as the speed at which these subjects walked increased so did the magnitude of their increase in maximal oxygen uptake (1.4, 3.0, and 5.0 ml/kg/min, respectively). However, neither body weight (low-intensity = +0.8 kg, moderate-intensity = +0.1 kg, high-intensity = +1.1 kg) nor percent body fat (low-intensity = −1.7% fat, moderate-intensity = −1.4% fat, high-intensity = −1.1% fat) was differentially affected by the intensity at which one exercised.

In contrast, Tremblay et al. (83) have recently presented data that suggest that high-intensity interval training in combination with endurance training may elicit greater reductions in fat mass than do relatively rigorous forms of endurance training alone. Seventeen young adults (8 M, 9 F) underwent a 20-week endurance training program during which the duration and intensity of cycle ergometry exercise was progressively increased until they were exercising for 45 min/session, 5 days/week at 85% of their maximal heart rate reserve. The high-intensity group (5 M, 5 F) exercised for 15 weeks during which they completed 25 30-min sessions of continuous aerobic exercise at 70% of maximal heart rate reserve. In addition, they completed 19 short- and 16 long-interval training sessions (a mixture of exercise and rest periods). The short bouts were of 30 sec duration (15 bouts/session) and the long bouts of 90 sec duration (5 bouts/session) and the work rate at a relatively high percentage of an individual's maximal work capacity.

The endurance training (ET) and high-intensity and endurance training (HI) groups did not differ with respect changes in body weight (ET = −0.5 kg, HI = −0.1 kg). However, substantial differences were present with respect to changes in the sum of six skinfold thicknesses (ET = −4.5 mm, HI = −13.9 mm). A muscle biopsy and subsequent biochemical analysis revealed that the change in muscle 3-hydroxyacyl coenzyme A dehydrogenase (HADH) enzyme activity was much greater for the high-intensity and endurance exercise group (ET = 0.65, HI = 2.1 U/g wet weight). Since HADH is a marker of β-oxidation activity, these data suggest that high-intensity interval training may promote lipid oxidation to a greater degree than that which occurs with less rigorous forms of

exercise training. It is unlikely, however, that the high-intensity and endurance training protocol that Tremblay et al. employed could be safely used with older and/or obese adults, which limits the applicability of their reported finding.

D. Gender and Age-Specific Adaptations to Exercise Training

There is ample evidence in the animal literature that suggests that males and females respond differently to exercise training with respect to changes in body weight. As shown in Figure 1, a common finding is that male rodents will decrease dietary intake and lose weight with the initiation of an exercise training regimen while female rodents will increase dietary intake and/or adjust activity during other parts of the day to keep body weight constant. A plausible rationale for this gender-based difference is that females need to conserve body fat for reproductive purposes and thus are more likely to make regulatory adjustments to buffer weight loss. In addition, women are more likely than men to store fat in alpha-mediated fat cells, which are less likely to release their constituents during adrenergic stimulation (20). To the extent that this is true, one would expect that postmenopausal women (who presumably would have no need to protect fat supplies) and women whose fat cells are fuller than normal would still respond to exercise training by losing weight. The literature is difficult to interpret with respect to this issue since men and women often initiate an exercise program with the intention of losing weight and as such are likely to modify their dietary habits at the same time.

There is, however, strong evidence supporting the existence of gender differences with respect to how physical activity affects body weight. Ballor and Keesey (2), as noted earlier, used meta-analysis to examine how exercise training, body weight, and body fat are related. While the average weight reduction for the 48 male means studied was −1.2 kg, females averaged only −0.2 kg of weight loss. For fat mass, males lost an average of 1.7 kg and females 1.0 kg.

Andersson et al. (84) compared responses in the following three groups who underwent aerobic exercise training 3 times per week for 3 months: slightly obese men (26% fat), slightly obese women (36% fat), and more obese women (42% fat). The men reduced their body weight and body fat by −2.0 and −2.9 kg, respectively. The slightly obese women reduced their body weight and body fat by −0.5 and −1.8 kg, respectively. The more obese women reduced their body weight and body fat by

−1.1 and −4.6 kg, respectively. Dietary intake did not increase for any of the groups and actually decreased for the more obese women. Thus, while the threshold body weight/fat level at which women seem to lose body weight and fat in response to an exercise program is higher than in men, when sufficient excess weight is present, reductions in body mass with exercise training do occur.

Kohrt et al. have recently completed two studies that illustrate not only gender differences in response to exercise training, but age effects as well. They compared body weight and composition among ≈370 young (mean ≈ 26 years) and older (mean ≈ 60 years) sedentary or endurance-trained adults (85). As one might expect, the younger sedentary males (% fat = 17) and females (% fat = 24) were much leaner than the older males (% fat = 29) and females (% fat = 38). The body weights of the exercise-trained young men and women were 6.9 and 2.5 kg less, respectively, than those of their respective sedentary counterparts. In contrast, the older exercise-trained males and females weighed 16.0 and 10.3 kg less, respectively, than their sedentary counterparts. Note that these are cross-sectional data and selection bias may influence the results. However, the results are still striking. The effect of exercise training on body weight change is 2 times and 4 times as great in older adults as is it in younger adults. If one assumes that the older adults trained throughout their life, this illustrates what the effect of long-term training can be. It is also consistent with the premise that truly overweight individuals will lose weight with increases in physical activity.

Kohrt et al. (86) examined in a prospective fashion the effects of 12 months of endurance exercise training in 100 men and women aged 60–70 years. The subjects exercised ≈46 min/session, 4 days/week at a work rate that elicited a heart rate ≈ 80% of maximum. Men lost −3.4 kg, or −3.7% of their body weight, and women lost −2.7 kg, or −2.9% of their body weight. While different on an absolute basis, when compared on a percentage of initial weight, older men and women did not differ with respect to the percentage of weight lost.

Thus the data presented herein suggest that gender differences likely exist with respect to how men and women respond to exercise training. However, older women and/or those with more fat are more likely to lose body weight in response to exercise training than are younger or more lean women. In addition, recent studies have documented that older adults respond to exercise training in a fashion quite similar to younger adults (87). The greater tendency to lose weight with exercise training for older adults would seem to be a function of their increased adiposity.

E. Duration and Frequency of Aerobic Exercise Training and Changes in Body Weight and Body Fat

As the duration and/or frequency of exercise increases, so does the level of energy expenditure. Thus, one would expect that to the extent that increases in energy expenditure lead to increased losses of weight or fat, so would increases in exercise frequency and duration. In their meta-analysis (2) Ballor and Keesey report, for men, a correlation of $r = -0.32$ and -0.47 ($p < 0.05$) between frequency of exercise and changes in body weight and fat and correlations of $r = -0.37$ and -0.43 ($p < 0.05$) between duration of exercise and changes in body weight and fat. For women, statistically significant correlations were not present for either duration or frequency of exercise and body weight. Statistically significant ($p < 0.05$) correlations of $r = -0.56$ and $r = -0.62$ were present between changes in fat mass and frequency and duration of exercise, respectively.

Pollock et al. (88) combined data from 10 experiments to examine how body weight, fat weight, and days per week of training are related for ≈100 moderately obese (% fat ≈ 22%) men (≈41 years old). Subjects ran 30–45 min, 2, 3, or 4 days/week for 20 weeks. As one went from 2 to 3 to 4 days/week of training, weight loss increased from −0.5 to −1.3 to −1.8 kg, respectively. Likewise, the sum of six skinfold fat measures declined by −6.7 (4.8%), −14.3 (10.5%), and −20.4 (15.6%) mm, respectively.

VI. EXERCISE AND WEIGHT RECIDIVISM

Just as level of activity is a predictor of becoming obese (10,12,89,90), it is also a predictor of which subjects will be successful in maintaining weights at reduced levels (91–94). The relationships are quite impressive. Kayman et al. (91) reported that 90% of obese women who successfully maintained reduced weights exercised regularly while only 34% of those who relapsed did so. Hartman et al. (93) examined ≈100 obese men and women 2–3 years after they had lost ≈27 kg on a very-low-energy diet. They divided the subjects into those who exercised at high levels, exercised moderately, and did not exercise. While all subjects regained some weight, the weight loss maintained at follow-up for those exercising at high levels (−18 kg) was substantially higher than for those exercising either moderately (−9 kg) or not at all (−6 kg).

There are several reasons why exercise training may facilitate maintenance of weight at reduced levels. Certainly, physical activity can increase daily energy expenditure via either the exercise itself or by facilitating increases in either resting or postexercise metabolism. Exercise training may also reduce one's preference for high-fat foods (5). Finally, exercise training may exert "psychological effects" (8). For example, Lavery and Loewy (94) have noted that "feeling in control of eating habits" is a significant predictor of being able to maintain a reduced body weight. To the extent that exercise training may facilitate "being in control" one is likely better able to resist eating foods that would promote weight regain.

VII. TO DIET OR NOT TO DIET

Ample evidence exists that the recent dramatic increase in obesity in modern industrialized societies is life-style driven. For example, when one compares regions where physical activity is more prevalent and diets are low in fat and refined sugars to those where the reverse is true, levels of obesity are quite different. Furthermore, recent studies indicate that both inactivity (10,12,90) and the percentage of fat in one's diet (95–97) are major predictors of the likelihood of whether one will become obese. Thus as one either becomes less active or increases the percentage of fat in one's diet, weight gain is often a consequence.

For an obese individual, current treatment involves a restriction of energy intake, initiation of exercise training and, in the best programs, counseling in how to modify one's life-style to avoid weight regain. When the patient has lost the desired amount of weight or weight loss plateaus, the patient is then put on a maintenance program that continues the exercise training and limits dietary intake to what is appropriate for the reduced body weight. The patient's body weight will remain at this level for as long as he or she adheres to the program. However, adherence seems problematic as most eventually regain lost weight (8).

We suggest that life-style modifications rather than dietary restrictions may be more advantageous for treating obesity. Counting calories or conscientiously attempting to monitor and control energy intake seem to doom one to failure and the high rates of recidivism following weight loss seem to confirm this. Figure 6 illustrates some of the important points in this argument. It theoretically compares two identical hypertrophic obese individuals. The first person initiates a severe reduction in dietary intake and loses a substantial amount of weight over a short period of time. Following this, he or she begins an exercise training regimen and is assigned an energy intake consistent with the reduced weight. The second person follows one of two programs. In the first, he or she skips the

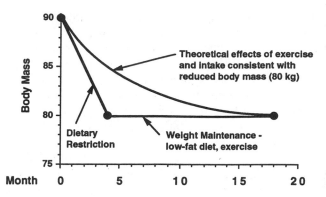

Figure 6 Theoretical model comparing traditional weight loss modalities with merely reducing intake to the level appropriated for a reduced body weight or adopting a life-style with regular exercise and a diet low in fat and refined sugars. A diet that is low in fat and refined sugars in combination with regular exercise should result in a reduction in body weight to the lowest maintainable level possible.

dietary restriction program and follows the same maintenance program as the above diet-restricted individual. After an extended period, his or her weight will plateau at the same point as that of the person who went on the weight loss regimen. The only difference is the length of time that it takes for body weight to reach its nadir. The reason for this is that the energy balance equation requires that when one reduces intake and/or increases physical activity, body weight must drop until energy expenditure and intake are again equal.

In the second case, the person begins an exercise training regimen and switches to a low-fat, complex-carbohydrate diet (limited refined sugars) and is allowed to eat ad lib. Recent evidence suggests that this individual will spontaneously reduce energy intake and that weight loss will occur until energy (and fat) intake and energy (and fat) expenditure are in balance. The level at which this person's weight would plateau depends on many factors, including the level of increase in physical activity, percentage reduction of dietary fats, degree of dietary compensation, and amount of weight one is above lower threshold levels. For the sake of simplicity, we would assume that it yielded the same result as the person in case 2. The maximum weight one could lose under this scenario (i.e., increased activity, decreased fat intake) would be the point at which energy intake reaches it nadir with reductions in the percentage of fat in the diet and/or the point at which increases in physical activity are matched by corresponding increases in dietary intake to keep weight stable. Neither of these points is known with any degree of confidence. However, the weight would be the lowest one could maintain without initiating physiological adjustments.

Currently many physicians recommend 20–25% of total energy intake as fat as a reasonable sustainable level for dietary fat (98). No such consensus exists for physical activity. The American College of Sports Medicine recommends 300 kcal (1260 kJ) per session 3–5 times/week (900–1500 kcal/week, 3800–6300 kJ/week) as the minimum level to induce changes in body composition (79). We suggest that the level of physical activity at which plateaus in body weight occur is somewhat higher than this. As many of the rationales for reducing levels of obesity in our society are health-related, a brief examination of the relationship between energy expenditure and the relative risk of death may be illustrative in this regard. The work of Paffenbarger et al. (99) suggests that the reduction in relative risk of death that occurs with increasing levels of physical activity plateaus around 8400 kJ (2000 kcal) per week of energy expenditure. It would not be unreasonable to assume that the plateauing in relative risk of death occurs in part because body weight has stabilized at reduced levels. Furthermore, recent evidence suggests that even though these individuals may weigh more than they desire, the excess fat is not particularly hazardous (100).

This is also a reasonable goal since it represents an individual walking about 8 km (3 miles) per day. The exercise need not be continuous and could be incorporated into one's life-style in a variety of ways. It is also consistent with recently recommended exercise guidelines (101). However, the challenge remains as to how to induce people to adopt a life-style that would reduce the level of obesity currently so prevalent in modern society.

ACKNOWLEDGMENTS

Dr. Poehlman is supported by a grant from the National Institute of Aging (RO1 AG07857) and a Research Career and Development Award from the National Institute of Aging (K04 AG00564). The work was partially supported by the Geriatric Research Education and Clinical Center (GRECC) and the University of Maryland Claude Pepper Older Americans Independence Center. Mr. Toth is supported by a predoctoral training grant from the National Institute of Aging (T32-AG00219).

REFERENCES

1. Flatt JP. Dietary fat, carbohydrate balance, and weight maintenance. Ann New York Acad Sci 1993; 683: 122–139.
2. Ballor DL, Keesey RE. A meta-analysis of the factors affecting exercise-induced changes in body mass, fat mass and fat-free mass in males and females. Int J Obes 1991; 15:717–726.
3. Poehlman ET, Melby CL, Badylak SF, Calles J. Aerobic fitness and resting energy expenditure in young adult males. Metabolism 1989; 38:85–90.
4. Poehlman ET, Danforth E Jr. Endurance training increases metabolic rate and norepinephrine appearance rate in older individuals. Am J Physiol 1991; 261:E233–E239.
5. Miller GD, Dimond AG, Stern JS. Exercise reduces fat selection in female Sprague-Dawley rats. Med Sci Sports Exerc 1994; 26:1466–1472.
6. Hermansen L, Grandmontagne M, Moehlum S. Ingnes I. Postexercise elevation of resting oxygen uptake: possible mechanisms and physiological significance. Med Sport Sci 1984; 17:119–129.
7. Bahr R, Hansson P, Sejersted OM. Triglyceride/fatty acid cycling is increased after exercise. Metabolism 1990; 39: 993–999.
8. Brownell KD, Wadden TA. Etiology and treatment of obesity: understanding a serious, prevalent, and refractory disorder. J Consult Clin Psychol 1992; 60:505–517.
9. Mayer J, Purnima R, Mitra KP. Relation between caloric intake, body weight and physical work: studies in an industrial male population in West Bengal. Am J Clin Nutr 1956; 4:169–175.
10. Williamson DF, Madans J, Anda RF, Kleinman JC, Kahn H, Byers T. Recreational physical activity and ten-year weight change in a US national cohort. Int J Obes 1993; 17:279–286.
11. Tucker LA, Bagwell M. Television viewing and obesity in adult females. Am J Public Health 1991; 81:908–911.
12. Gortmaker SL, Dietz WH, Cheung LWY. Inactivity, diet, and the fattening of America. J Am Diet Assoc 1990; 90: 1247–1252.
13. Keesey RE. Physiological regulation of body energy: implications for obesity. In: Stunkard AJ, Wadden TA, eds. Obesity: Theory and Therapy, 2nd ed. New York: Raven Press, 1993:77–96.
14. Leibel RL, Hirsch J. Diminished energy requirements in reduced-obese patients. Metabolism 1984; 33:164–170.
15. Ballor DL, Tommerup LJ, Smith DB, Thomas DP. Body composition, muscle and fat pad changes following two levels of dietary restriction and/or exercise training in male rats. Int J Obes 1990; 14:711–722.
16. Ballor DL. Effect of dietary restriction and/or exercise on 23-h metabolic rate and body composition in female rats. J Appl Physiol 1991; 71:801–806.
17. Ballor DL. Exercise training elevates RMR during moderate but not severe dietary restriction in obese male rats. J Appl Physiol 1991; 70:2303–2310.
18. den Besten C, Vansant G, Weststrate JA, Deurenberg P. Resting metabolic rate and diet-induced thermogenesis in abdominal and gluteal-femoral obese women before and

after weight reduction. Am J Clin Nutr 1988; 47:840–847.

19. Bouchard C, Tremblay A, Després JP, Nadeau A, Lupien PJ, Thériault G, Dussault J, Moorjani S, Pinault S, Fournier G. The response to long-term overfeeding in identical twins. N Engl J Med 1990; 322:1477–1482.

20. Després JP, Bouchard C. Effects of aerobic training and heredity on body fatness and adipocyte lipolysis in humans. J Obes Weight Regul 1984; 3:219–235.

21. Craig BW, Garthwaite SM, Holloszy JO. Adipocyte insulin resistance: effects of aging, obesity, exercise, and food restriction. J Appl Physiol 1987; 62:95–100.

22. Schwartz RS, Brunzell JD. Increase of adipose tissue lipoprotein lipase with weight loss. J Clin Invest 1981; 67:1425–1430.

23. Berlan M, Dang-tran L, Lafontan M, Denard Y. Influence of hypocaloric diet on alpha-adrenergic responsiveness of obese human subcutaneous adipocytes. Int J Obes 1981; 5:145–153.

24. Krotkiewski M, Mandoukas K, Sjöström L, Sullivan L, Wetterqvist H, Björntorp P. Effects of long-term physical training on body fat, metabolism, and blood pressure in obesity. Metabolism 1979; 28:650–658.

25. Björntorp P. Exercise in the treatment of obesity. Clin Endocrinol Metab 1976; 5:431–453.

26. Tremblay A, Després JP, Leblanc C, Bouchard C. Six dimorphism in fat loss in response to exercise-training. J Obes Weight Regul 1984; 3:193–203.

27. Pierson RN, Wang J, Heymsfield SB, Russell-Aulet M, Mazariegos M, Tierney M, Smith R, Thornton JC, Kehayias J, Weber DA, Dilmanian FA. Measuring body fat: calibrating the rulers. Intermethod comparisons in 389 normal Caucasian subjects. Am J Physiol 1991; 261:E103–E108.

28. Lohman TG. Research progress in validation of laboratory methods of assessing body composition. Med Sci Sports Exerc 1984; 16:595–603.

29. Baumgartner RN, Chumlea WE, Roche AF. Bioelectric impedance for body composition. Exerc Sport Sci Rev 1990; 18:193–224.

30. Ballor DL, Katch VL. Validity of anthropometric regression equations for predicting changes in body fat of obese females. Am J Hum Biol 1989; 1:97–101.

31. Poehlman ET, Arciero PJ, Goran MI. Endurance exercise in aging humans: effects on energy metabolism. In: Holloszy JO, ed. Exercise and Sports Science Reviews. Baltimore, MD: Williams & Wilkins, 1994:250–284.

32. Poehlman ET, Melby CL, Goran MI. The impact of exercise and diet restriction on daily energy expenditure. Sports Med 1991; 11:78–101.

33. Poehlman ET. A review: exercise and its influence on resting energy metabolism in man. Med Sci Sports Exerc 1989; 21:515–525.

34. Hermansen L, Grandmontagne M, Maehlum S, Ingnes I. Postexercise elevation of resting oxygen uptake: possible mechanisms and physiological significance. Med Sport Sci 1984; 17:119–129.

35. Henson LC, Poole DC, Donahoe CP. Effects of exercise training on energy expenditure during caloric restriction. Am J Clin Nutr 1987; 46:893–899.

36. Phinney SD, LaGrange BM, O'Connell M, Danforth E Jr. Effects of aerobic exercise on energy expenditure and nitrogen balance during very low calorie dieting. Metabolism 1988; 37:758–765.

37. Bahr R, Sejersted OM. Effect of intensity of exercise on excess postexercise O_2 consumption. Metabolism 1991; 40:836–841.

38. Lamb KL, Brodie DA. The assessment of physical activity by leisure-time physical activity questionnaires. Sports Med 1990; 10:159–180.

39. Lifson N, Gordon GB, McClintock R. Measurement of total carbon dioxide production by means of $D_2^{18}O$. J Appl Physiol 1955; 7:704–710.

40. Schoeller DA, Ravussin E, Schutz Y, Acheson KJ, Baertschi P, Jequier E. Energy expenditure by doubly labeled water: validation in humans and proposed calculation. Am J Physiol 1986; 250:R823–R830.

41. Schoeller DA. Measurement of Energy expenditure in free-living humans by using doubly labeled water. J Nutr 1988; 118:1278–1289.

42. Jequier E, Schutz Y. Long-term measurements of energy expenditure in humans using a respiration chamber. Am J Clin Nutr 1983; 38:989–998.

43. Leibel RL, Rosenbaum M, Hirsch J. Changes in energy expenditure resulting from altered body weight in men. N Engl J Med 1995; 332:621–628.

44. Schulz LO, Alger S, Harper I, Wilmore JH, Ravussin E. Energy expenditure of elite female runners measured by respiratory chamber and doubly labeled water. J Appl Physiol 1992; 72:28–38.

45. Schulz LO, Nyomba BL, Alger S, Andersen TE, Ravussin E. Effect of endurance training on sedentary energy expenditure measured in a respiratory chamber. Am J Physiol 1991; 260:E257–E261.

46. Horton TJ, Drougas HJ, Sharp TA, Martinez LR, Reed GW, Hill JO. Energy balance in endurance-trained female cyclists and untrained controls. J Appl Physiol 1994; 76:1937–1945.

47. Goran MI, Beer W, Wolfe RR, Poehlman ET, Young VR. Variation in total energy expenditure in young healthy free-living young men. Metabolism 1993; 42:487–496.

48. Goran MI, Poehlman ET. Total energy expenditure and energy requirements in healthy elderly persons. Metabolism 1992; 41:744–753.

49. Bingham SA, Goldberg GR, Coward WA, Prentice AM, Cummings JH. The effect of exercise and improved physical fitness on basal metabolic rate. Br J Nutr 1989; 61:155–173.

50. McArdle WD, Katch FI, Katch VL. Physique, performance, and physical activity. In: Exercise Physiology: En-

ergy, Nutrition, and Human Performance, 2nd ed. Philadelphia: Lea & Febiger, 1986:646.

51. Meijer GAL, Janssen GME, Westerterp KR, Verhoeven, Saris EHM, ten Hoor F. The effect of a 5-month endurance training programme on physical activity: evidence for a sex-difference in the metabolic response to exercise. Eur J Appl Physiol 1991; 62:11–17.

52. Racette SB, Schoeller DA, Kushner RF, Neil KM, Herling-Iaffaldano K. Effects of aerobic exercise and dietary carbohydrate on energy expenditure and body composition during weight reduction in obese women. Am J Clin Nutr 1995; 61:486–494.

53. Buemann B, Astrup A, Christensen NJ. Three months aerobic training fails to affect 24-hour energy expenditure in weight-stable, post-obese women. Int J Obes 1992; 16: 809–816.

54. Blaak EE, Westerterp KR, Bar-Or O, Wouters LJM, Saris WHM. Total energy expenditure and spontaneous activity in relation to training in obese boys. Am J Clin Nutr 1992; 55:777–782.

55. Goran MI, Poehlman ET. Endurance training does not enhance total energy expenditure in healthy elderly persons. Am J Physiol 1992; 263:E950–E957.

55a. Poehlman ET, Gardner AW, Ades Pa, Katzman-Rooks SM, Montgomery Sm, Atlas O, Ballor DL, Tyzbir RS. Resting energy metabolism and cardiovascular disease risk in resistance- and aerobically trained males. Metabolism 1992; 41:1351–1360.

56. Ballor DL, Poehlman ET. Resting metabolic rate and coronary-heart-disease risk factors in aerobically and resistance-trained women. Am J Clin Nutr 1992; 56: 968–974.

57. Toth MJ, Poehlman ET. Resting metabolic rate and cardiovascular disease risk in resistance and aerobic trained middle aged women. Int J Obes 1995; 19(supp4): S93–96.

58. Bosselaers I, Buemann B, Victor OJ, Astrup A. Twenty-four-hour energy expenditure and substrate utilization in body builders. Am J Clin Nutr 1994; 59:10–12.

59. Poehlman ET, Tremblay A, Nadeau A, Dussault J, Theriault G, Bouchard C. Heredity and changes in hormones and metabolic rates with short-term training. Am J Physiol 1986; 350:E711–717.

60. Broeder CE, Burrhus KA, Svanevik LS, Wilmore JH. The effects of either high-intensity resistance or endurance training on resting metabolic rate. Am J Clin Nutr 1992; 55:802–810.

61. Van Etten LMLA, Westerterp KR, Verstappen FTJ. Effect of weight-training on energy expenditure and substrate utilization during sleep. Med Sci Sports Exerc 1995; 28: 188–193.

62. Pratley R, Nicklas B, Rubin M, Miller J, Smith A, Hurley B, Goldberg AP. Strength training increases resting metabolic rate and norepinephrine levels in healthy 50- to 65-yr-old men. J Appl Physiol 1994; 76:133–137.

63. Campbell WW, Crim MC, Young VR, Evans WJ. Increased energy requirements and changes in body composition with resistance training in older adults. Am J Clin Nutr 1994; 60:167–175.

64. Treuth MS, Hunter GR, Weinsier KL, Kell S. Energy expenditure and substrate utilization in older women after strength training: results from a 24 hour metabolic chamber. J. Appl Physiol 1995; 78:2140–46.

65. Ballor DL, Poehlman ET. Exercise training enhances fat-free mass preservation during diet-induced weight loss: a meta-analytical finding. Int J Obes 1994; 18:35–40.

66. McGaw B. Meta-analysis. In: Keeves JP, ed. Educational Research, Methodology, Measurement: An International Handbook. New York: Pergamon Press. 1988:678–685.

67. Ballor DL, Katch VL, Becque MD, Marks CR. Resistance weight training during caloric restriction enhances lean body weight maintenance. Am J Clin Nutr 1988; 47: 19–25.

68. Donnelly JE, Pronk NP, Jacobsen DJ, Pronk SJ, Jakicic JM. Effects of a very-low-calorie diet and physical-training regimens on body composition and resting metabolic rate in obese females. Am J Clin Nutr 1991; 54:56–61.

69. Ballor DL, Smith DB, Tommerup LJ, Thomas DP. Neither high- nor low-intensity exercise promotes whole-body conservation of protein during severe dietary restrictions. Int J Obes 1990; 14:279–287.

70. Ballor DL, McCarthy JP, Wilterdink EJ. Exercise intensity does not affect the composition of diet- and exercise-induced body mass loss. Am J Clin Nutr 1990; 51: 142–146.

71. Warwick PM, Garrow JS. The effect of addition of exercise to a regime of dietary restriction on weight loss, nitrogen balance, resting metabolic rate and spontaneous physical activity in three obese women in a metabolic ward. Int J Obes 1981; 5:25–32.

72. Ballor DL, Tommerup LJ, Thomas DP, Smith DB, Keesey RE. Exercise training attenuates diet-induced reduction in metabolic rate. J Appl Physiol 1990; 68:2612–2617.

73. Pi-Sunyer FX, Woo R. Effect of exercise on food intake in human subjects. Am J Clin Nutr 1985; 42:983–990.

74. Poehlman ET. Energy expenditure and requirements in aging humans. J Nutr 1992; 122:2057–2065.

75. Leon AS, Conrad J, Hunninghake DB, Serfass R. Effects of a vigorous walking program on body composition, and carbohydrate and lipid metabolism of obese young men. Am J Clin Nutr 1979; 33:1776–1787.

76. Marti B, Howald H. Long-term effects of physical training on aerobic capacity: controlled study of former elite athletes. J Appl Physiol 1990; 69:1451–1459.

77. Lee L, Kumar S, Leong LC. The impact of five-month basic military training on the body weight and body fat of 197 moderately to severely obese Singaporean males aged 17 to 19 years. Int J Obes 1994; 18:105–109.

78. Boileau RA, Buskirk ER, Horstman DH, Mendez J, Nicholas WC. Body composition changes in obese and lean

men during physical conditioning. Med Sci Sports 1971; 3:183–189.

79. American College of Sports Medicine. Position stand: the recommended quantity and quality of exercise for developing and maintaining cardiorespiratory and muscular fitness in healthy adults. Med Sci Sports Exerc 1990; 22: 265–274.

80. Sedlock DA, Fissinger JA, Melby CL. Effect of exercise intensity and duration on postexercise energy expenditure. Med Sci Sports Exerc 1989; 21:662–666.

81. Tremblay A, Després JP, Leblanc C, Craig CL, Ferris B, Stephens T, Bouchard C. Effect of intensity of physical activity on body fatness and fat distribution. Am J Clin Nutr 1990; 51:153–157.

82. Duncan JJ, Gordon NF, Scott CB. Women walking for health and fitness: how much is enough? JAMA 1991; 266:3295–3299.

83. Tremblay A, Simoneau JA, Bouchard C. Impact of exercise intensity on body fatness and skeletal muscle metabolism. Metabolism 1994; 43:814–818.

84. Andersson B, Xu X, Rebuffé-Scrive M, Terning K, Krotkiewski, Björntorp P. The effects of exercise training on body composition and metabolism in men and women. Int J Obes 1991; 15:75–81.

85. Kohrt WM, Malley MT, Dalsky GP, Holloszy JO. Body composition of healthy sedentary and trained, young and older men and women. Med Sci Sports Exerc 1992; 24: 832–837.

86. Kohrt WM, Obert KA, Holloszy JO. Exercise training improves fat distribution patterns in 60- to 70-year-old men and women. J Gerontol 1992; 47:M99–M105.

87. Hagberg JM, Graves JE, Limacher M, Woods DR, Leggett SH, Cononie C, Gruber JJ, Pollock ML. Cardiovascular responses of 70–79-yr-old men and women to exercise training. J Appl Physiol 1989; 66:2589–2594.

88. Pollock ML, Miller HS, Linnerud AC, Cooper KH. Frequency of training as a determinant for improvement in cardiovascular function and body composition of middle-aged men. Arch Phys Med Rehabil 1975; 56:141–144.

89. French SA, Jeffery RW, Forster JL, McGovern PG, Kelder SH, Baxter JE. Predictors of weight change over two years among a population of working adults: the Healthy Worker Project. Int J Obes 1994; 18:145–154.

90. Ravussin E, Swinburn BA. Metabolic predictors of obesity: cross-sectional versus longitudinal data. Int J Obes 1993; 17:S28–S31.

91. Kayman S, Bruvold W, Stern JS. Maintenance and relapse after weight loss in women: behavioral aspects. Am J Clin Nutr 1990; 52:800–807.

92. Marston AR, Criss J. Maintenance of successful weight loss: incidence and prediction. Int J Obes 1984; 8: 435–439.

93. Hartman WM, Stroud M, Sweet DM, Saxton J. Long-term maintenance of weight loss following supplemented fasting. Int J Eating Disord 1993; 14:87–93.

94. Lavery MA, Loewy JW. Identifying predictive variables for long-term weight change after participation in a weight loss program. J Am Diet Assoc 1993; 93:1017–1024.

95. Miller WC, Lindeman AK, Wallace J, Niederpruem M. Diet composition, energy intake, and exercise in relation to body fat in men and women. Am J Clin Nutr 1990; 52:426–430.

96. Klesges RC, Klesges LM, Haddock CK, Eck LH. A longitudinal analysis of the dietary impact of dietary intake and physical activity on weight change in adults. Am J Clin Nutr 1992; 55:818–822.

97. Astrup A, Buemann B, Wester P, Toubro S, Raben A, Christensen NJ. Obesity as an adaptation to a high-fat diet: evidence from a cross-sectional study. Am J Clin Nutr 1994; 59:350–355.

98. Kendall A, Levitsky DA, Strupp BJ, Lissner L. Weight loss on a low-fat diet: consequences of the imprecision of the control of food intake in humans. Am J Clin Nutr 1991; 53:1124–1129.

99. Paffenbarger RS, Hyde RT, Wing AL, Hsieh C. Physical activity, all-cause mortality, and longevity of college alumni. N. Engl J. Med. 1986; 314:605–613.

100. Björntorp P. Visceral obesity: a "civilization syndrome." Obes Res 1993; 1:206–222.

101. Pate RR, Pratt M, Blair SN, Haskell WL, Macera CA, Bouchard C, et al. Physical activity and public health. A recommendation from the Centers for Disease Control and Prevention and the American College of Sports Medicine. JAMA 1995; 273:402–407.

45

Treatment of Overweight NIDDM Patients

Ian D. Caterson
University of Sydney, Sydney, New South Wales, Australia

Paul Zimmet
Monash University and International Diabetes Institute, Melbourne, Australia

I. INTRODUCTION

Non-insulin-dependent diabetes mellitus (NIDDM) is becoming more common throughout the world and it is often associated with central adiposity, overweight, and obesity (1). The increased incidence and prevalence are discussed below as are the possible theories of causation and association between NIDDM and adiposity. While many of the individuals who have NIDDM have been diagnosed, there is still a significant proportion of those who are overweight, have NIDDM, but are unaware of their problems. This is because overweight and obesity are not recognized as significant health problems, particularly by men, and because they have few symptoms or signs of their raised blood glucose levels. Even if diagnosed, NIDDM is often seen as a "mild" form of diabetes and treatment as being simple. Both these beliefs are untrue. NIDDM does cause complications and many have some or many of the complications of diabetes (in contrast to the situation in IDDM) at the time of diagnosis (2).

One of the major complications and the cause of most mortality in NIDDM is macrovascular disease (1,3). Treatment of NIDDM is not easy. Control is difficult to achieve, as is long-term weight loss. One of the theoretical problems is that many of the treatments utilized act to increase insulin secretion, and hyperinsulinemia may be both inappropriate and deleterious. This is relevant in the context of the metabolic syndrome as many subjects with NIDDM also have hypertension, central (upper body) obesity, and dyslipidemia (4). This group of patients is at very high risk of coronary artery, cerebrovascular (CVD), and peripheral vascular disease because each of this cluster is an important CVD risk factor (1). They contribute cumulatively to macrovascular disease.

It has been suggested that insulin resistance and hyperinsulinemia are involved in the etiology and natural history of three chronic diseases—NIDDM, hypertension, and coronary artery disease (CAD) (5,6). The cluster of related variables known as "syndrome X" was described by Reaven (5) and includes resistance to insulin-stimulated glucose uptake, glucose intolerance, hyperinsulinemia, increased VLDL triglyceride, decreased HDL cholesterol, and hypertension. Sufficient evidence exists to include central obesity as part of this more appropriately named metabolic syndrome (6). Hyperinsulinemia has been reported as a predictor of both NIDDM and CAD in a number of epidemiological studies (6). In this context, it has been suggested that insulin resistance and/or hyperinsulinemia was the central etiological factor for the components of the metabolic syndrome (5,6). Therefore, any therapeutic strategy that lessened insulin resistance and/or hyperinsulinemia should be beneficial for all of the CVD risk factors in the cluster.

However, as a number of studies have now demonstrated (6–9), the relationship of circulating insulin concentration with hypertension and CAD is inconsistent between ethnic groups and studies. As discussed below, hyperleptinemia/leptin resistance may play an important role, and perhaps the most important part of the metabolic syndrome, and may be the missing link in the epidemiological association between insulin and the endpoints of CAD and hypertension (10). Thus, the various components may need to be widened to include this along the lines of Table 1.

As two-thirds of NIDDM patients die from cardiovascular disease (3), the clustering of NIDDM, a well-documented risk factor for CVD, with the other well-established risk factors that constitute the metabolic syndrome seems the most likely explanation of the increased mortality due to CVD in persons with NIDDM. Thus, the management of NIDDM should focus not only on tight blood glucose control, but also on strategies for reduction of the other CVD risk factors as well as cessation of cigarette smoking.

This chapter will describe the epidemiology and etiology of NIDDM, current therapeutic practice, and the problem of diabetic complications and will attempt to present a logical approach to better therapy.

II. EPIDEMIOLOGY OF NIDDM

A. Prevalence

The term "epidemic," used so frequently in public health during the era of infectious diseases, is equally applicable to describe the dramatic rise in prevalence of NIDDM and obesity in many countries, both long developed and developed in recent times (1,11). Obesity is now epidemic in developed nations including Australia and the United States and is rapidly becoming so in many developing and disadvantaged populations, particularly American Indians, Pacific Islanders, Mexican Americans, and Afro-Americans as a penalty of modernization (12,13). The epidemiology of obesity is described in greater detail elsewhere in this book, so this section concentrates on the epidemiology of NIDDM.

Changes in life-style have led to major alterations in the profile of diseases that account for the morbidity and mortality in developing countries with the trends mirroring those in developed nations (1,14). Death from infectious causes has been replaced by the major killers, CAD, NIDDM, strokes, hypertension, and obesity. Diabetes is among the five leading causes of death by disease in most countries, yet mortality statistics greatly underestimate the true diabetes-related mortality, diabetes often being under-reported on death certificates (15). This is a great handicap when it comes to awareness of diabetes for setting public health priorities.

Table 1   Components of the Revised Metabolic Syndrome Including Hyperleptinemia

Glucose intolerance
Hyperinsulinemia
Insulin resistance
Increased VLDL triglycerides
Decreased HDL cholesterol
Hypertension
Upper body obesity
Hyperleptinemia
Leptin resistance
Microalbuminuria

Intense activity in studies of the epidemiology of NIDDM has taken place over the last two decades. Just under 20 years ago, Kelly West highlighted the potential for a future diabetes epidemic in his landmark book *Epidemiology of Diabetes and Its Vascular Lesions* (16). That prediction has been shown to be correct wih NIDDM now reaching epidemic proportions in many developing populations (11). Over the next decade, the epidemic of NIDDM will certainly escalate.

NIDDM constitutes about 85% of all cases of diabetes in developed countries (17). The diagnosis is usually made after the age of 50 years in persons of European extraction. However, NIDDM is seen at a younger age in high-prevalence populations such as the Pacific Islanders (18). In some developing countries, especially those with a high prevalence of diabetes, the majority of persons with diabetes fall in the 20–50-year category.

Large variations in NIDDM prevalence exist between populations (19). Currently, the prevalence of NIDDM varies dramatically from <2% in rural Bantu in Tanzania and Chinese in mainland China to the very high rates documented in populations who have changed from a traditional to a modern lifestyle, e.g., American Pima Indians, Micronesians, and other Pacific Islanders (up to 40% of adults), and about 20% in Australian aborigines, migrant Asian Indians and Chinese, and Mexican-Americans (1,14,19) (Fig. 1).

Populations previously free of NIDDM are showing rates that are extraordinarily high when compared to developed countries. A recent example is the urbanized Wanigela people of the Koki settlement in Papua New Guinea (20), who have recently been shown to have one of the world's highest community prevalences of glucose intolerance, comparable to that of the Micronesian Nauruans and American Pima Indians. The Canadian natives are also now showing NIDDM prevalence of the same order (B. Zinman, personal communication).

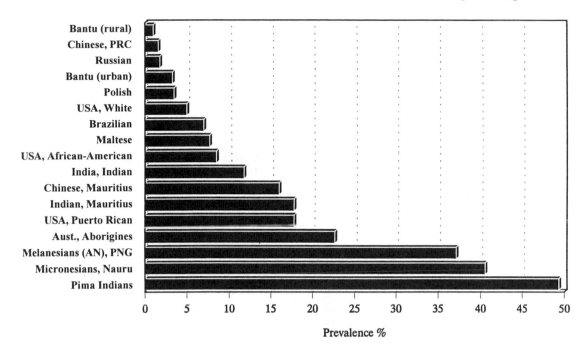

Figure 1 Prevalence of non-insulin-dependent diabetes mellitus in selected populations (aged 30–64 years) worldwide. Age standardized against Segi's world population. (Adapted from Ref. 19.)

Prevalence and incidence studies have shown marked variation in the prevalence and incidence of NIDDM within and between ethnic groups and countries (1,21). For example, in Europids, in Wadena, USA, the prevalence of diabetes in adults is 8.1%, and this is consistent with the national estimates for the United States. The prevalence in the United States overall is over twice that reported in Australia and Sweden (21,22).

Mauritius, a multiethnic island in the Indian Ocean, illustrates dramatically the potential public health disaster as a result of NIDDM that may soon affect many parts of the world (22,23). This country has among the highest diabetes prevalence and diabetes-related mortality in the world with the age- and gender-standardized prevalence of NIDDM very similar across ethnic groups—12.4% in Hindu Indians, 13.3% in Muslim Indians, 10.4% in Creoles, and 11.9% in Chinese. The high prevalence found in Asian Indians has also been reported from the United Kingdom, Singapore, South Africa, Fiji, and Tanzania and NIDDM is already common in some Indian subcontinent communities (23,24). The implications for public health, with modernization in India, from the expected NIDDM epidemic are enormous.

The Mauritius findings also provide devastating projections for the People's Republic of China and the African continent with respect to the NIDDM epidemic (22). In most parts of China, the prevalence of NIDDM is less than

1% (19), and the Mauritius data, coupled with evidence that prevalence is already high in other Chinese populations such as Singapore and Taiwan, set an alarming scenario (22). For example, between 1984 and 1992, the prevalence of NIDDM in Singaporean Chinese doubled from 4% to 8% (7). This highlights the prospect of an NIDDM epidemic in China, the world's most populated nation, with increasing socioeconomic development.

While genetic susceptibility to NIDDM is clearly important, there is strong evidence that the disease is unmasked by environmental factors (1,7,21). Several environmental risk determinants are associated with an increased risk of NIDDM including nutritional factors, sedentary life-style, obesity (particularly central), and intrauterine development (7). Extensive review of the genetic and environmental determinants can be found elsewhere (1,7,21).

III. INSULIN RESISTANCE AND INSULIN DEFICIENCY IN NIDDM

A. Insulin Resistance

Insulin resistance is defined as a situation in which a normal amount of insulin produces a subnormal biological response (6). The various causes are listed in Table 2 and

Table 2 Insulin Resistance Seen in a Clinical Setting

Obesity
NIDDM
Stress (e.g., infections, trauma, surgery)
Pregnancy
Insulin receptor defects (genetic) (e.g., leprechaunism)
Immune-mediated (e.g., insulin or insulin receptor antibodies)
Endocrine disorders (e.g., Cushing's syndrome, acromegaly)
Drug therapy (e.g., glucocorticoids)
Lipodystrophy

include obesity, physical inactivity, certain therapeutic agents, and pregnancy.

The accumulated evidence strongly supports the fact that resistance to the effect of insulin is a fundamental feature of NIDDM and obesity (5,6,25). It also occurs in people with normal glucose tolerance, there are now convincing data that it is a predictor of subsequent development of NIDDM and it has been suggested that it has a genetic basis (7).

When hyperinsulinemia is coupled with insulin resistance, what may happen from a metabolic viewpoint? In brief, when insulin secretion is stimulated by glucose ingestion, the combination of hyperglycemia and hyperinsulinemia promotes glucose uptake by splanchnic (liver and gut) and peripheral (mainly muscle) tissues and suppresses hepatic glucose production (7).

The debate as to which comes first in NIDDM—hyperinsulinemia or insulin resistance—still rages and the dilemma is not easily resolved. If the primary defect is in tissue sensitivity of muscle or liver, hyperinsulinemia would be a secondary and compensatory response. On the other hand, evidence exists that suggests hyperinsulinemia may be the primary defect and insulin resistance is secondary. It is quite feasible that these are two independent, genetically determined mechanisms for the development of NIDDM with the former being more evident in nonobese subjects and the latter in the obese. However, whatever the sequence, the primary event leads to the emergence of the other and the subsequent metabolic derangement would be similar. Quite apart from this, there is now the important question as to what role leptin may play in these metabolic events.

With insulin resistance in the peripheral tissues, the plasma glucose rises and the pancreas responds by increasing circulating insulin. This results in downregulation of the insulin receptors and may exacerbate insulin resistance in tissues. A vicious cycle ensues with a progressive rise in plasma glucose up to a point, the apex

of the "Starling curve of the pancreas," at which time the beta cell decompensates, insulin secretion falls, and this further exacerbates hyperglycemia (7). It seems quite possible that hyperglycemia per se plays a role in causing reduced insulin secretion, a phenomenon labeled "glucotoxicity" (26).

Why the beta cell decompensates at this point is still the subject of debate. It is possible that a lower beta-cell reserve or a defect in insulin synthesis or secretion may be present. Any of these could result from a genetically determined molecular abnormality in the pancreatic beta cell, as discussed in the next section.

B. Insulin Deficiency

Decreased insulin secretion (hypoinsulinemia) in NIDDM does occur (14), and the majority of patients with NIDDM with hypoinsulinemia are nonobese. Some of this group are clearly cases of NIDDM where hyperinsulinemia was present at an earlier stage and they have now traversed the "Starling curve of the pancreas" (14,26) and represent secondary forms of an insulin secretory defect as the result of beta-cell exhaustion. There are other forms that are associated with mutations of insulin, the insulin receptor, glucokinase genes, and mitochondrial DNA (14), while other cases are actually slow-onset IDDM masquerading as NIDDM (27). This latter group, which we have called latent autoimmune diabetes in adults (LADA), have been well described elsewhere and show a high prevalence of antibodies to glutamic acid decarboxylase (GAD) (27,28). They may constitute as many as 10–15% of all cases of adult-onset diabetes (14).

IV. COMPLICATIONS OF NIDDM

Not all the complications of diabetes will be described in this section, but rather those that have a major impact on the overweight individual with NIDDM. It should be remembered that, unlike the situation in insulin-dependent diabetes mellitus (IDDM), where complications develop after several years of known diabetes, there is a high likelihood of individuals with NIDDM having complications of diabetes at presentation. Diabetic retinopathy has been reported as present at the time of diabetes diagnosis in over 20% of cases (2). The reason for this is the insidious nature of onset of the disease and the probability that blood glucose concentrations have been elevated for some years prior to diagnosis. In fact, some individuals may present with one of the complications of diabetes.

A. Macrovascular Disease

This is common problem in those with NIDDM and in fact is the major cause of death in the disorder (1,3). For example, in a recent survey of the aging in rural New South Wales, a postmenopausal woman with diabetes has 14 times the risk of dying from CVD than women of the same age without diabetes and there is an increased risk for elderly men with NIDDM (29). Ischemic (coronary) heart disease, CVD, and peripheral vascular disease are all complications of this disorder and should be screened for at presentation. In addition to careful clinical examination, it is possible to visualize the carotid arteries with ultrasound to examine the state of the endothelium as well as plaques. An electrocardiogram (ECG) or an exercise stress test may be appropriate depending on age, sex, and symptoms. Newer diagnostic procedures include vascular (endothelial) reaction, which may be able to give earlier indication of vascular disease and may become part of the standard complications screen in the future.

Dyslipidemia, usually hypertriglyceridemia and a low HDL cholesterol, is a further complicating factor of NIDDM and macrovascular disease. Elevated LDL-cholesterol levels may also be found. While this dyslipidemia may be due in part to poor control of diabetes and tends to improve as NIDDM is treated, there are other causative mechanisms including the presence of abdominal adiposity (discussed elsewhere in this chapter and volume) and possibly hyperinsulinemia itself. Both these factors may remain even if blood glucose levels are low. The combination of hypertriglyceridemia with low-HDL cholesterol is a potent cardiovascular risk factor, and vascular risk factor generally, in those with diabetes and this form of dyslipidaema needs to be treated and not just accepted "as part of diabetes." The specific treatment of dyslipidemia depends on the major lipid abnormality in the individual with NIDDM; treatment with HMG CoA reductase ("statin") or fibric acid derivative (e.g., gemfibrozil) should be considered where appropriate.

Hypertension is another major problem in those with NIDDM. In addition to the usual causes, e.g., renovascular disease, essential hypertension, it should be remembered that hypertension is associated with insulin resistance (this does not necessarily imply causation) and the underlying cause may be the same as for NIDDM and the other features of the metabolic syndrome. Hypertension in NIDDM, as in IDDM, should be treated aggressively, as elevated blood pressure speeds the progression of other complications of diabetes (e.g., renal disease) as well as its usual detrimental effects on coronary and cerebrovascular disease. The aim of therapy, and to maintain health,

should be blood pressure less than 140/90. There is evidence to suggest the ACE inhibitors may be drugs of first choice in controlling the hypertension of those with NIDDM (30,31). This class of drugs has some effect on peripheral insulin resistance (32), alters renal vascular flow to assist compromised renal function, and does not have the suggested adverse coronary vascular events that may be present with calcium channel blockers.

B. Microvascular Disease

Microvascular complications of diabetes are also present and common in NIDDM. While microvascular disease may play a part in diabetic neuropathy (which will not be discussed in this chapter), the major complications to be considered are diabetic renal disease and retinopathy.

Diabetic renal disease does occur in those with NIDDM, the prevalence of end-stage renal disease being identical in IDDM and NIDDM (33). At the time of diagnosis some 8% of patients will have persistent proteinuria. It is not appropriate to discuss the various pathological changes in the kidney in this chapter; it suffices to say that once established, diabetic renal disease is slowly progressive to renal failure. In many developed countries, diabetic renal disease is one of the major problems leading to renal transplant programs. In Australia 12–15% of renal transplants are for diabetic renal disease, and in the United States this figure is higher still, of the order of 25–30%.

In the early phase of diabetic renal disease hyperfiltration occurs, and creatinine clearance may be higher than normal, and serum creatinine slightly lower than might be expected. The earliest sign of renal problems is microalbuminuria. The optimum collection for this is a timed collection (results given as μg/min); a 24-hr urine, or a shorter timed collection at rest. Spot urine samples can be used (results as mg/L). While the sample can be measured with a dipstick, in some cases the level of detection can be too high. There are several patterns of microalbuminuria: normal excretion, elevated but stable excretion, and progressive elevation. It is this latter pattern that requires intervention. Normal excretion is <30 μg/min, increased excretion 30–70 μg/min, and in this region better control of diabetes may reverse the problem. When excretion is greater than this, renal disease is likely. Once proteinuria (measured by dipstick) has been established, i.e., protein present on two occasions at least 1 month apart, there is inexorable progression to renal failure. This progression may be slowed by better control of NIDDM, strict treatment of hypertension (see above), and, where necessary, the use of a low-protein diet (approximately 40 g protein per day).

Retinopathy also occurs in NIDDM and may be present in 20% of patients on presentation (2). All types of retinopathy may occur, including background, proliferative, and macular exudates, with the latter two types requiring laser therapy. Regular screening of the eyes for retinopathy is necessary after diagnosis of NIDDM (unlike the situation in IDDM). While there is a correlation between the development of retinopathy and the presence of diabetic renal disease in patients with IDDM, no equivalent data are available for NIDDM

C.   The Diabetic Foot

Because of the conjunction of peripheral vascular disease (macro- and microvascular), peripheral neuropathy, and an increased tendency for infections (particularly with poor circulation), problems with the feet are common in NIDDM. In the overweight diabetic patient, these will be exacerbated by the increased pressure due to mass and peripheral edema due to hydrostatic factors, particularly abdominal and groin compression by fat. Lymphedema and local blistering may be added to the other diabetic problems. Problems range from small areas of dry gangrene (black spots) through pressure ulcers, gangrene, collapse of the foot, and osteomyelitis. Amputations commonly result (34).

The simplest and most effective preventive measure is to inspect the feet at every visit. Attention must be paid to circulation, sensation, presence of ankle jerks, pressure areas, the toes, and local infections. Advice on appropriate footwear, education in foot care, prompt institution of therapy for infections and ulcers, identification of pressure areas (assessed on pedobarograph if one is available, or by corns, calluses, and redness if not), and an aggressive approach to therapy reduce amputations and reduce time in hospital. The use of orthotics in shoes, to distribute pressure, casts to protect any pressure area and ulcer, dressings, and antibiotic therapy are all essential adjuncts and should be available for all those with "diabetic feet."

V.   STANDARD THERAPY

A.   Components of Therapy

Therapy for the overweight or obese individual with NIDDM commences with a "diet." This approach is based on broad general principles, the need to lose weight, the need to distribute the carbohydrate load throughout the day, and the need to reduce blood glucose and lipid levels. A number of types of diet are prescribed ranging from the older portion control through reduced-fat, high-

carbohydrate diets to newer approaches utilizing the glycemic index of foods (35). Diets vary from country to country depending on local foods and preference. The underlying principles have been well stated in the recommendations of the American Diabetes Association: "There is no one 'diabetic' diet. The recommended diet can only be defined as a dietary prescription based on nutritional assessment and treatment goals." This means that eating plans need to be individualized; unfortunately, with the overweight NIDDM patient such an approach is not always available or taken. However, with dietary therapy in the United Kingdom Prospective Diabetes Study (UKPDS) (36) some 17% of patients manage to attain normoglycemia with diet alone. Not all these patients are overweight, most have only mild hyperglycemia initially, and the majority do not lose much weight at all.

Most patients will require pharmacological therapy. There are two major groups of drugs, the sulfonylureas and the biguanide, metformin. This latter drug, though used successfully throughout the world for many years, is only just becoming available in the United States. While it is a mild hypoglycemic, it does permit weight loss and does not worsen hyperinsulinemia; so it is the drug treatment of first choice in many places. Again, not many overweight individuals lose weight satisfactorily, so this, coupled with the natural history of NIDDM, means that many patients must be treated with both classes of drugs. The sulfonylureas stimulate insulin secretion. Most NIDDM patients need insulin within 5–10 years after initial diagnosis. This can be given combined with oral hypoglycemics or therapy can be changed to insulin alone. Although it helps control blood sugar levels, insulin does promote weight gain.

In addition to control of blood sugar, the need to control blood lipid levels has been recognized increasingly. The most common dyslipidemia of NIDDM is hypertriglyceridemia associated with low HDL cholesterol and hyperinsulinemia. Therapy usually begins with a fibric acid derivative, though some individuals may have predominant hypercholesterolemia and may need to be treated with an HMG CoA reductase inhibitor (a "statin").

B.   Results of Therapy

Despite dietary therapy, potent drugs, and insulin, very few overweight patients with diabetes attain good metabolic control. As a broad general principle, those who manage to lose weight do maintain better control. The final results of the UKPDS are awaited with interest, particularly because this study will report on the relationship between control (or lack of it) and complications.

VI. LOGICAL THERAPY

Given the physiological and nutrition knowledge we have and the drugs that are available, it should be possible to design logical, effective treatment for overweight individuals with NIDDM. Health and medical resources will vary from area to area, country to country, but a logical approach aiming to reduce insulin resistance and provide appropriate insulin levels should be possible in most places. Such an approach must be individualized for each patient to attain maximum benefit, so patients will get some therapies from each grouping with the emphasis being different in each individual patient. Some will be concentrated on weight loss, others on glucose control, others on the management of complications. In this regard, all should have regular checks for the complications of diabetes. NIDDM is not a benign disease.

A. Changing Insulin Resistance

1. Eating Plans

Inappropriate eating can cause many of the problems underlying NIDDM. A high level of energy consumed will cause weight gain, adiposity, and insulin resistance; a high proportion of fat in the diet will do the same. The aim of the eating plan in NIDDM should be to reduce insulin resi. . .ce and to reduce weight. Despite the fact that a wide variety of dietary plans are available for diabetes in the overweight NIDDM individual, it is best to opt for a low-fat eating plan. An intake of <40 g fat per day will assist in weight reduction, and this level of fat requires an increase in carbohydrate, particularly complex carbohydrate, to maintain required daily energy intake and an appropriate bulk in the diet. Such a dietary intake is consistent with diets recommended for diabetes, is consistent with many traditional non-Western diets, and is easy to explain and implement. While individual, specialized nutritional advice and prescription is optimal, in many parts of the world nutritionists are not available, or their services are too expensive for the general population. As many of those with NIDDM come from developing countries, an eating plan concentrating on reducing fat can easily be implemented. In many parts of the world small books giving fat content of common foods are readily available.

A low-fat diet will assist in weight loss theoretically (37), as has also been shown in obese women undergoing a training program (38). In rodents a high-fat diet produces insulin resistance within days (39). This insulin resistance can be reversed by returning to a normal high-carbohydrate chow. In humans it is more difficult to demonstrate changes in insulin resistance to short-term (1 month) changes in diet composition without changes in adiposity, but this may reflect the time of the diet in a human's life span (40). Low-fat diets, as distinct from calorie counting, appear to have a benefit in maintaining weight loss (41). They are also of use in lowering blood lipids. Low-fat diets are easy to explain and prescribe but they do have limitations. Weight loss does not continue forever with a low-fat diet. As explained by Flatt (42), a plateau or new equilibrium is reached when the body has reduced its adiposity to a level where the body's 24-hr respiratory quotient is equal to the food quotient of the low-fat diet consumed. Other modalities of treatment must be instituted.

Traditional diabetic diets emphasize high-carbohydrate, low-fat intakes and also spread carbohydrate through the day. In the overweight NIDDM patient, not treated with insulin, the carbohydrate distribution is not as important as attaining some weight loss. So, as initial treatment a low-fat eating plan is a good starting point. Later in the course of NIDDM it may be necessary to discuss wider aspects of dietary management including carbohydrate distribution, calorie (energy) reduction, or more specific nutrition education. A time for such broader nutritional intervention should be planned as part of the ongoing management of the overweight individual with NIDDM, but from the above discussion, it is evident that a low-fat eating plan will assist early in the course of NIDDM by promoting weight loss, by reducing insulin resistance (possibly directly and certainly by the reduction in adiposity), by beneficial effects on serum glucose and lipids, and by ease of implementation and adherence. Calorie (energy) restriction itself can improve glycemic control. This has been shown in a study where subjects on a 400-calorie diet followed by a 1000-calorie intake were compared to those who had been treated with a 1000-calorie diet throughout. After the 400-calorie diet and weight loss equal to the 1000-kcal diet, the subjects in the lower-calorie diet had lower fasting glucose levels and better insulin sensitivity. When they were switched to a 1000-calorie diet, their glucose control worsened without weight gain (43). There is also evidence that by replacing fats in the diet with monounsaturated fatty acids, additional metabolic benefit may be gained in NIDDM (44).

2. Weight Reduction

Weight or rather adipose tissue reduction is an important means of altering the metabolic derangement of NIDDM (45). Permanent reduction in weight may obviate the need for pharmacotherapy and weight loss has been shown to reverse secondary failure of oral hypoglycemic agents (46). Initially a low-fat eating plan should be implemented (see above). To this should be added regular exercise. Though there remains some disagreement about the place of exercise in controlling blood sugar in NIDDM, regular exercise will reduce abdominal adiposity (for review see Ref. 47). This exercise should be regular but need not be excessive; indeed it is not necessary to get fit to see benefits such as a reduction in fasting serum insulin, reduction in insulin resistance, and reduction in serum lipid levels. Metformin is also useful. It does not prevent weight loss and in fact may help weight loss (48) and increase insulin sensitivity. Recent studies prior to metformin's introduction to the United States have reinforced the suggestion that it inhibits hepatic glucose output by inhibiting gluconeogenesis (49). Another agent that can help promote weight loss and is useful in NIDDM is dexfenfluramine (50–52).

Gastric bypass surgery can be very effective in producing weight loss in those with NIDDM, and postoperatively most patients were able to maintain normal fasting glucose and glycated hemoglobin at varying periods of follow-up (53). There is also some evidence to suggest that treatment with VLCDs (see below) together with intensive behavioral modification can improve long-term outcome (54).

All these treatment modalities can be combined, together with the usual behavior modification techniques, to produce weight loss. A continuing program for weight maintenance must then be commended.

3. Exercise

There is no clear evidence that exercise improves diabetic control in NIDDM. However, all authorities stress the importance of regular exercise. There are several reasons for this. Exercise improves insulin sensitivity; in particular, it promotes non-insulin-mediated glucose uptake into muscles. Regular exercise is important for weight loss and is one of the factors that has been shown to reduce abdominal (visceral) fat. As such, it improves insulin sensitivity, reduces hyperinsulinemia, and has beneficial effects on the serum lipid profile and other risk factors (55). Després (91) has found the weight loss produced by exercise is of the order of 5 kg in obese women in a training study. A reduction of the percentage of fat in their usual intake, with no change in energy, will then produce a further 11-kg loss while they continue to exercise. There have been suggestions that those with NIDDM lose less weight than nondiabetic obese individuals, and this may be because of the former require insulin or sulfonylureas. Exercise has been used as a treatment modality to prevent NIDDM in those found to be in the early stages of diabetes (56).

4. Metformin

Metformin is a mild hypoglycemic drug that acts by inhibiting hepatic glucose production and by altering peripheral insulin sensitivity and lipid oxidation (57). Although it is used extensively elsewhere in the world (58), it has only recently become available in the United States. It does not produce hypoglycemia, and it permits or perhaps promotes weight loss (49). In one of the recent American studies (59), patients on metformin lost a small amount of weight (mean 3.8 ± 0.2 kg) over the period of treatment (29 weeks) and those on combination therapy with a sulfonylurea gained slightly (0.4 ± 0.2 kg). In a second study (49), those on active treatment lost about 3 kg over 16 weeks. This was without any change in resting energy expenditure or physical activity (the latter self-reported) and was a loss of adipose tissue, lean body mass being maintained.

Metformin may have a beneficial effect on lipid profile directly (lowering total and LDL cholesterol and triglycerides), or through its actions on weight or control of diabetes. Its side effects include nausea and diarrhea, which may be alleviated by giving the drug immediately before or with a meal. The reason for the delay in introduction in the United States has been the association of lactic acidosis with the earlier biguanide phenformin. This does occur rarely with metformin, 3 cases per 100,000 patient-years, and it occurs when the levels of metformin (which is excreted unchanged) build up (60). Care should be taken with its use in those with poor renal function. The usual dose range is 250–3000 mg/day in two or three divided doses. Recent studies suggest it is as effective as glyburide and a hypoglycemic (59) and has an additive effect to the sulfonylurea when used in combination. In those who are overweight or obese with NIDDM, this is a useful first-line drug to help control diabetes and permit weight loss.

5. Appetite Suppressants/Regulators

Both major groups of appetite suppressants, the sympathomimetic amines and the serotonergic or serotonin reuptake inhibitors, will produce weight loss in those with NIDDM. Such weight loss will produce metabolic benefits in terms of control, but unfortunately, as with its use in "simple" obesity, there is weight regain on cessation of the drug.

Dexfenfluramine, a serotonin reuptake inhibitor, may convey additional benefits in the overweight individual in NIDDM. There is evidence from animal studies that this drug and a derivative, benfluorex, will improve insulin sensitivity when given acutely. Benfluorex ameliorates the insulin resistance produced by high-fat diets (61). Similarly in human studies, dexfenfluramine improves insulin sensitivity when given acutely and has been reported to cause both reduced hepatic glucose production and improved peripheral glucose uptake (62). When given to those with NIDDM for a period of weeks or months, dexfenfluramine, as well as producing some weight loss, improves metabolic control, can reduce insulin requirements, and reduces other risk factors (50,63). This, coupled with the possibility that dexfenfluramine preferentially reduces abdominal fat (64), suggests that this drug has potential in the treatment of the metabolic syndrome. Studies in NIDDM have used dexfenfluramine over a period of months and achieved benefit, but the optimal length of time for therapy with this drug in the overweight individual with NIDDM remains to be determined. Side effects reported include dry mouth, sleepiness, and some gastrointestinal tract disturbance. These tend to be transitory. Other side effects reported are rare mood disturbance and idiopathic primary pulmonary hypertension. This latter side effect is extremely rare, but serious.

Another possibility for use of appetite suppressants is "low-dose combined" therapy with dexfenfluramine (or fenfluramine) and phentermine. This therapy has been used successfully in overweight and obese individuals and weight losses of 15.6 kg after 60 weeks of therapy are reported (65). Side effects with this low-dose therapy are reduced. Such weight loss would be of great benefit to those with NIDDM, reducing insulin resistance and possibly the need for other pharmacotherapy.

6. Very-Low-Calorie Diets (VLCDs)

VLCDs are an effective treatment for insulin resistance. They improve diabetic control, reduce the need for medication, and improve associated risk factors (66,67). These facts have been known for a decade (68,69), but treatment with VLCDs should not be considered as standard dietary or weight loss therapy. It is not absolutely necessary to employ liquid formulas; similar results can be obtained with food-containing diets (70). This overall approach allows the very obese to lose weight quickly and to regain diabetic control. Both the calorie restriction and the weight loss attained appear to improve glycemic control and insulin sensitivity (43). Such treatment is effective for those with secondary failure of oral hypoglycemics and may mean that these individuals can return to oral medications and cease insulin or even in some cases return to diet control alone. Unfortunately, after this short-term therapy weight is regained and it is imperative to have a program in place to help weight maintenance. Appetite suppressants may play a role in this secondary phase (65). Despite the problem of weight regain, individuals do benefit from this therapy, there is some evidence that there may be some long-term benefit (71), and repeated courses every few years may be appropriate therapy in some selected individuals.

7. Angiotensin-Converting Enzyme (ACE) Inhibitors

The importance of controlling hypertension in NIDDM has been stressed. In this regard and for logical treatment, the ACE inhibitors are practical and have the theoretical advantage of reducing insulin resistance. This class of drugs is effective in reducing blood pressure and has been shown to be helpful in diabetic renal disease. The effects upon insulin resistance have been shown in acute and in vivo studies (72,73), and there are no indications that this class of drugs improves glycemic control.

B. Insulin Deficiency

When, despite the above measures, blood sugar levels cannot be controlled, then insulin deficiency has become the major problem. A number of treatments can be employed. Unfortunately, these treatments tend to promote weight gain and it is unusual for a patient with NIDDM to lose further weight once sulfonylureas or insulin are commenced. There is also the theoretical objection that these treatments increase hyperinsulinemia, itself a risk factor for cardiovascular disease (71,74,75,90). While this may occur initially, with better control and lower blood sugars it has been suggested that insulin levels may actually fall with time.

1. Sulfonylureas

The pharmacology of sulfonylurea drugs has been reviewed elsewhere (76). This family of drugs stimulates insulin secretion acutely by binding to receptors on B cells. It is possible that the receptor itself may be part of a K^+ channel. These islet cells are then stimulated directly by the sulfonylureas and are sensitized to nutrients. Subsequent to receptor binding K^+ channels close and Ca^{2+} channels open, and the resultant increase in intracellular Ca^{2+} stimulates insulin secretion.

Many sulfonylureas are available; these vary in dosage used and in time of action. There is some variation in disposal, some being excreted by the kidney, others undergoing hepatic degradation. Drugs available (and their recommended dosage range) include glibenclamide (2.5–20 mg), gliclazide (40–320 mg/day in divided dosage), glipizide (2.5–15 mg as single dose, dose above 15 mg should be given as divided doses, daily maximum in divided doses 40 mg), tolbutamide (500 mg–2 g/day in divided doses), glyburide (5–20 mg daily in divided doses), and chlorpropramide (100–500 mg as single dose). These drugs, particularly those with the longer duration of action such as glibenclamide, can cause hypoglycemia. They should therefore be used with greater caution in those with either impaired renal or hepatic function. There is also some rationale for using drugs with shorter duration of action (given in divided doses) in the elderly. Using more than the maximum dosage of sulfonylureas recommended by the manufacturers rarely adds greatly to their therapeutic effect (77). Except in the rare instance of primary failure (which is highly unlikely in an overweight or obese individual with NIDDM and indicates severe insulin deficiency), these drugs will be effective in lowering blood sugar levels. With extremely high blood sugar levels, the islets may not be able to secrete insulin due to glucose toxicity, and a short period of insulin therapy (see below), lowering the blood glucose level, may restore islet sensitivity and oral agents will again be effective.

While these drugs can be used alone in the obese or overweight individual with NIDDM, they can be used in combination with metformin and there is some indication that such a combination is more effective (59). In the logical scheme of treatment being presented here, if, despite maximum dosage of metformin, adequate control is not achieved, then a sulfonylurea would be added. Conversely, if an overweight individual with NIDDM has been started on a sulfonylurea, then metformin can be added to the regime. It is most likely that those on sulfonylureas will gain weight (78). It is the natural history of NIDDM to progress over the initial few years (36), and dosage titration of the drug chosen may be necessary, as well as addition of a second agent.

Again, the natural history of NIDDM is that after 5–10 years normoglycemia cannot be maintained by oral hypoglycemics and diet alone. This is sometimes called "secondary failure." By this stage, insulin is required to maintain normal blood sugar levels and insulin therapy should be commenced unless the general prognosis of the patient is poor.

2. Insulin

It is not the place of this discussion to give exact details of insulin types, regimens, and plans for follow-up. It suffices to say that there are two major approaches to this situation. In the first, a single evening injection of intermediate-acting (NPH or isophane) or long-acting (ultralente) insulin is added to the oral hypoglycemic therapy (79,80). This insulin is started at low dose (say 18 units) and increased gradually until appropriate glucose control is attained. With time, it may be possible to reduce the oral hypoglycemics. In the second approach, the overweight individual's oral medications are ceased and the patient is placed on a twice-daily insulin regime. Again, dosage adjustments are made until glucose control is achieved. Insulin resistance of NIDDM may be improved by this type of insulin therapy (81). There is no evidence that one approach is better than the other, though the advantage of combining oral hypoglycemic and insulin treatment may be greater in those who are overweight and who have a relatively short duration of NIDDM.

Prior to initiation of insulin therapy, the patient should have at least one formal dietetic consultation. Once insulin is started, as well as the dietary approach described above, there needs to be regularity of mealtimes and carbohydrate content so diabetes control can be optimized and the risk of severe hypoglycemia minimized.

With insulin therapy the chance of achieving weight loss is significantly reduced; more usually there is weight gain (82). Such gain must be balanced against diabetic control and prevention of complications.

C. Other Therapies

1. Diabetes Education

Diabetes education must be part of the management of the overweight individual with diabetes. Such education includes nutritional and dietetic education, awareness of the need for screening for diabetes complications, home glucose monitoring, the meaning of blood sugar readings, and other aspects of living with diabetes. There is no evidence that diabetes education improves diabetes control, but it provides an environment for the early recognition of problems and complications. In the specific case of the overweight NIDDM patient, this environment should provide the support and services for the patient to learn to eat and exercise properly, lose weight, and reduce insulin resistance.

2. Screening

It cannot be stressed too much that, unlike the situation with IDDM, the overweight or obese patient with NIDDM may present with the complications of diabetes and should be screened for these complications at presentation and then at regular intervals, at least yearly. In addition to formal ophthalmological checks of the fundus through dilated pupils, there should be checks of lipids and macrovascular disease (presence of pulses, ECG, and vascular reactivity—this latter technique may allow much earlier diagnosis of vascular disease) (83). A timed urine collection for microalbumin should be performed and there should be screening for neuropathy both peripheral and autonomic. The feet should be formally examined and possible pressure areas noted. It is important that adequate records be kept and abnormalities be acted upon.

3. Aggressive Therapy

When early complications are detected, there should be aggressive therapy. Any pressure area on the feet should have proper care and shoes may need to be changed. Special orthotic devices may be needed. Any infections or ulcers should be treated. These can be protected with a cast while antibiotic therapy is instituted. Hospital admission is rare and can be prevented, as can the frequency and need for amputations.

To prevent the progression of renal and macrovascular disease, blood pressure above 140/90 should be treated. Currently ACE inhibitors are the class of drugs utilized. They may reduce insulin resistance, improve renal blood flow, and prevent disease progression.

Dyslipidemia is common in NIDDM. It may be secondary to poor control of diabetes or to excess adiposity, but if after diabetes control and/or weight loss there remains an elevation in LDL cholesterol or triglycerides, then these abnormalities should be treated with an HMG CoA reductase inhibitor (statin) or fibric acid derivative, respectively. In those with NIDDM, elevation of triglycerides is an additional macrovascular risk factor, and the Helsinki Heart Study has shown that reduction of triglycerides in those with NIDDM will reduce cardiac events (84).

D. Proper Management

The management of NIDDM, like that of IDDM, is based on the team approach with the patient playing the key and central role. The process, which involves shared care (involvement of local or family physicians as well as specialized diabetes centers and ambulatory centers), is well described in detail elsewhere [for example, the *International Textbook of Diabetes Mellitus* (24)]. Such therapy must involve the specialist, the family physician, the dietitian, and the nurse educator. Whether the results of the Diabetes Control and Complications Trial (DCCT) (88) showing excellent control in reducing the impact of complications can be extrapolated to NIDDM is still to be determined. However, until it is, the goal of the team must be to aim for excellent metabolic control of glucose, lipids, and other key risk factors for both macro- and microvascular complications.

VII. COSTS OF NIDDM

NIDDM and its complications emerge as major threats to future public health throughout the world at a huge economic and social cost, particularly in developing countries (85,86). Apart from the health impact, the economic cost of diabetes and its complications is enormous, both for health care and for loss of productivity to society (17). While diabetes cost the United States $20.4 billion in 1987, the most recent estimate is $90 billion for 1994 (87).

Few reliable data exist on the economic costs of diabetes (85,86), which can be divided into direct and indirect costs (86). Direct costs include management of complications such as hospitalization, medical, surgical, and ambulatory care and rehabilitation. Indirect costs include premature morbidity and mortality, loss of productivity, and the consequences of disability.

Many of these expenses can be averted by adequate prevention programs (22). The recent landmark Diabetes Control and Complications Trial Research Group report (88) showed that the risk of all of the microvascular complications of IDDM can be reduced substantially (as much as 76%) by good metabolic control resulting from intensive therapy. Several studies have examined the costs of the specific complications of diabetes and the potential benefits of prevention (87,88). Screening for and prompt treatment of diabetic retinopathy could save $60 to $100 million annually (due to prevented or delayed blindness) in the United States (89). Foot care programs offer major potential savings in hospital costs for amputation and rehabilitation (34). In 1985, 56,000 below-knee amputations were attributable to diabetes in the United States (34), and half of them could have been prevented (17).

While NIDDM is now epidemic in many newly industrialized and westernized, developing countries, death certification practices leave much to be desired and the true impact of NIDDM on mortality is not available from most of these countries (10,15,34). As a result, prevention activities for diabetes and its complications do not get the priority they deserve or, indeed demand.

NIDDM and many of its complications may be preventable. Therefore, standardization of study design, death certification coding and recording, and data analysis for mortality are urgently required (15,16). Then, the risk factors for NIDDM mortality can be delineated consistently within and between populations. Until then, the gaps in our knowledge will handicap the rational design of prevention programs, and the disease will continue to be an economic burden on many countries that can ill afford it.

VIII.   CONCLUSIONS

NIDDM is likely to remain a huge threat to public health in the years to come. In the absence of effective interventions for NIDDM, the frequency will escalate worldwide with the main impact being seen in developing nations. Thus prevention of diabetes and its microvascular and macrovascular complications is an essential component of future public health strategies for all nations.

REFERENCES

1. Zimmet P. Challenges in diabetes epidemiology—from West to the rest. Diabetes Care 1992; 15:232–252.
2. Harris MI, Klein R, Welborn TA, Knuiman MW. Onset of NIDDM occurs at least 4–7 years before clinical diagnosis. Diabetes Care 1992; 15:815–819
3. Panzaram G. Mortality and survival in type 2 (non-insulin-dependent) diabetes mellitus. Diabetologia 1987; 30: 123–131.
4. Zimmet P. Non-insulin-dependent (type 2) diabetes mellitus—does it really exist? Diabet Med 1989; 6:728–735.
5. Reaven GM. Role of insulin resistance in human disease. Diabetes 1988; 37:1595–1607.
6. Zimmet P. Hyperinsulinaemia—how innocent a bystander? Diabetes Care 1993; 16:56–70.
7. Humphrey ARG, Zimmet PZ, Hamman RF. The epidemiology of diabetes mellitus. Diabetes Annu 1995; 9:1–31.
8. Collins VR, Dowse GK, Finch CF, Zimmet PZ. An inconsistent relationship between insulin and blood pressure in three Pacific Island populations. J Clin Epidemiol 1990; 43: 1369–1378.
9. Donahue RP, Skyler JS, Schneiderman N, Prineas R. Hyperinsulinemia and elevated blood pressure: cause, confounder or coincidence? Am J Epidemiol 1990; 132:827–836.
10. Zimmet P, McCarty D, Courten MD. The global epidemiology of non-insulin dependent diabetes mellitus and the metabolic syndrome. J Diabet Compl 1997 (in press).
11. McCarty D, Zimmet P. Diabetes 1994 to 2010: Global Estimates of Projections. Melbourne: International Diabetes Institute, 1994.
12. Dowse GK, Zimmet P, Collins VR, Finch CF. Obesity in Pacific populations. In: Björntorp P, Brodoff B, eds. Obesity. Philadelphia: JB Lippincott, 1992:619–639.
13. Zimmet PZ, Collier GR. Of mice and (wo)men: the obesity (*ob*) gene, its product leptin, and obesity. Med J Aust 1996; 164:393–394.
14. Zimmet P. The pathogenesis and prevention of diabetes in adults: genes, autoimmunity and demography. Diabetes Care 1995; 18:1050–1064.
15. Finch CF, Zimmet PZ. Mortality from diabetes. In: Alberti KGMM, Krall LP, eds. Diabetes Annual, Vol 4. Amsterdam: Elsevier, 1988:1–16.
16. West KM. Epidemiology of Diabetes and Its Vascular Lesions. New York: Elsevier, 1978.
17. Prevention of Diabetes Mellitus. World Health Organisation, Geneva, 1994.
18. Zimmet P, Dowse G, Serjeantson S, Finch C, King H. The epidemiology and natural history of NIDDM—lessons from the South Pacific. Diabetes Metab Rev 1990; 6:91–124.
19. King H, Rewer M. WHO Ad Hoc Diabetes Reporting Group. Global estimates for prevalence of diabetes mellitus and impaired glucose tolerance in adults. Diabetes Care 1993; 16:157–177.
20. Dowse GK, Spark RA, Mavo B, et al. Extraordinary prevalence of non-insulin-dependent diabetes mellitus and bimodal plasma glucose distribution in the Wanigela people of Papua New Guinea. Med J Aust 1994; 160:767–774.
21. Harris MI, Hadden WC, Knowler WC, Bennett PH. Prevalence of diabetes and impaired glucose tolerance and plasma glucose levels in US population aged 20–74 yr. Diabetes 1987; 36:523–534.
22. Zimmet P. Diabetes care and prevention—around the world in 80 days. In: Rifkin H, Colwell JA, Taylor SI, eds. Diabetes 1991. New York: Elsevier, 1991:721–729.
23. Dowse GK, Gareeboo H, Zimmet PZ, et al. High prevalence of NIDDM and impaired glucose tolerance in Indian, Creole and Chinese Mauritians. Diabetes 1990; 39:390–396.
24. Bennett PH, Bogardus C, Tuomilehto J, Zimmet P. Epidemiology and natural history of NIDDM: non-obese and obese. In: Alberti KGMM, DeFronzo RA, Keen H, Zimmet P, eds. International Textbook of Diabetes Mellitus, Vol 1. London: Wiley, 1992:147–176.
25. DeFronzo RA. Lilly Lecture 1987: The triumverate: B-cell, muscle, liver: a collusion responsible for NIDDM. Diabetes 1988; 37:667–687.
26. DeFronzo RA, Ferrannini E. Insulin resistance. A multifaceted syndrome responsible for NIDDM, obesity, hypertension, dyslipidemia and atherosclerotic cardiovascular disease. Diabetes Care 1991; 14:173–194.
27. Tuomi T, Groop LC, Zimmet PZ, Rowley MJ, Knowles W, Mackay IR. Antibodies to glutamic acid decarboxylase reveal latent autoimmune diabetes mellitus in adults with a non-insulin dependent onset of disease. Diabetes 1993; 42:359–362.
28. Zimmet PZ, Tuomi T, Mackay IR, et al. Latent autoimmune diabetes mellitus in adults (LADA)—the role of antibodies to glutamic acid decarboxylase in diagnosis and prediction of insulin dependency. Diabet Med 1994; 11:299–303.
29. Simons LA, McCallum J, Friedlander Y, Simons J, Powell I, Heller R. Dubbo Study of the Elderly: sociological and cardiovascular risk factors at entry. Aust NZ J Med 1991; 21:701–709.

30. Kasiske BL, Kalil RSN, Ma JZ, Liao M, Keane WF. Effect of antihypertensive therapy in patients with diabetes: a meta-regression analysis. Ann Intern Med 1993; 118:129–138.

31. Lewis EJ, Hunsicker LG, Bain RP, Rohde RD, Group ftCS. The effect of angiotensin-converting-enzyme inhibition on diabetic nephropathy. N Engl J Med 1993; 329:1456–1462.

32. Lithell HO, Pollare T, Berne C. Insulin sensitivity in newly detected hypertensive patients: influence of captopril and other antihypertensive agents on insulin sensitivity and related biological parameters. J Cardiovasc Pharmacol 1990; 15(Suppl 5):S46–S52.

33. Borch-Johnsen K. The costs of nephropathy in type II diabetes. PharmacoEconomics 1995; 8(Suppl 1):40–45.

34. Sussman KE, Reiber G, Albert SF. The diabetic foot problem—a failed system for health care? Diabetes Res Clin Prac 1992; 17:1–8.

35. Association AD. Nutrition recommendations and principles for people with diabetes mellitus. Diabetes Care 1996; 19(Suppl 1):S16–S19.

36. Group. TUPDS. UK Prospective Diabetes Study (UKPDS). VIII. Study design, progress and performance. Diabetologia 1991; 34:877.

37. Swinburn BA, Ravussin E. Energy and macronutrient metabolism. Clin Endocrinol Metab 1994; 8(3):527–548.

38. Despres JP, Lamarche B. Effects of diet and physical activity on adiposity and body fat distribution: implications for the prevention of cardiovascular disease. Nutr Res Rev 1993; 6:137–159.

39. Kraegen EW, Clark PW, Jenkins AB, Daley EA, Chisholm DJ, Storlien LH. Development of muscle insulin resistance after liver insulin resistance in high-fat-fed rats. Diabetes 1991; 40:1397–1403.

40. Borkman M, Campbell LV, Chisholm DJ, Storlien LH. Comparison of the effects on insulin sensitivity of high carbohydrate and high fat diets in normal subjects. J Clin Endocrinol Metab 1991; 72:432–437.

41. Toubro S, Astrup A. Ramdomized comparison of diets for maintaining obese subjects' weight after major weight loss: ad lib, low fat, high carbohydrate diet & fixed energy intake. Brit Med J 1997; 314:29–34.

42. Flatt J-P. The importance of nutrient balance in body weight regulation. Diabetes Metab Rev 1988; 6:571–581.

43. Wing RR, Blair EH, Bononi P, Marcus MD, Watanabe R, Bergman RN. Caloric restriction per se is a significant factor in improvements in glycaemic control and insulin sensitivity during weight loss in obese NIDDM patients. Diabetes Care 1994; 17:30–36.

44. Campbell LV, Marmot PE, Dyer JA, Borkman M, Storlien LH. The high-monounsaturated fat diet as a practical alternative for NIDDM. Diabetes Care 1994; 17:177–182.

45. Friedman JE, Dohm GL, Leggett-Frazier N, et al. Restoration of insulin responsiveness in skeletal muscle of morbidly obese patients after weight loss. Effect on muscle glucose transport and glucose transporter GLUT4. J Clin Invest 1992; 89:701–705.

46. Pontiroli AE, Calderara A, Pacchioni M, Cassisa C, Pozza G. Weight loss reverses secondary failure of oral hypoglycaemic agents in obese non-insulin-dependent diabetic patients independenty of the duration of the disease. Diabetes Metab 1993;19:30–35.

47. Despres J-P. Dyslipidaemia and obesity. Clin Endocrinol Metab 1994; 8(3):629–660.

48. Bailey CJ. Biguanides and NIDDM. Diabetes Care 1992; 15: 755–772.

49. Stumvoll M, Nurjhan N, Perriello G, Dailey G, Gerich JE. Metabolic effects of metformin in non-insulin-dependent diabetes mellitus. N Engl J Med 1995; 333:550–554.

50. Willey KA, Molyneaux LM, Overland JE, Yue DK. The effects of dexfenfluramine on blood glucose control in patients with type 2 diabetes. Diabet Med 1992; 9:341–343.

51. O'Connor HT, Richman RM, Steinbeck KS, Caterson ID. Dexfenfluramine treatment of obesity: a double blind trial with post trial follow up. Int J Obes 1995; 19:181–189.

52. Guy-Grand B, Crepaldi G, Lefebvre P, et al. International trial of long-term dexfenfluramine in obesity. Lancet 1989; 334:1142–1145.

53. Pories WJ, Swanson MS, MacDonald KG, et al. Who would have thought it? An operation proves to be the most effective therapy for adult-onset diabetes mellitus. Ann Surg 1995; 222:339–350.

54. Wing RR. Behavioral treatment of obesity. Its application to type II diabetes. Diabetes Care 1993; 16:193–199.

55. Barnard RJ, Ugianskis EJ, Martin DA, Inkeles SB. Role of diet and exercise in the management of hyperinsulinaemia and associated atherosclerotic risk factors. Am J Cardiol 1992; 69:440–444.

56. Eriksson KF, Lindgarde F. Prevention of type 2 (non-insulin-dependent) diabetes mellitus by diet and physical exercise. The 6 year Malmo Feasibility Study. Diabetologia 1991; 34:891–898.

57. Perriello G, Misericordia P, Volpi E, et al. Acute antihyperglycemic mechanisms of metformin in NIDDM. Evidence for suppression of lipid oxidation and hepatic glucose production. Diabetes 1994; 43:920–928.

58. Hermann LS, Melander A. Biguanides: basic aspects and clinical uses. In: Alberti KGMM, DeFronzo RA, Keen H, Zimmet P, eds. International Textbook of Diabetes Mellitus, Vol 1. Chicester: Wiley, 1992:773–795.

59. DeFronzo RA, Goodman AM, Group MMS. Efficacy of metformin in patients with non-insulin-dependent diabetes mellitus. N Engl J Med 1995; 333:541–549.

60. Lalau JD, Lacroix C, Coumhaguoy P. Role of metformin accumulation in metformin associated lactic acidosis. Diabetes Care 1995; 18:799–784.

61. Storlien LH, Oakes ND, Pan DA, Kusunoki M, Jenkins AB. Syndromes of insulin resistance in the rat. Inducement by diet and amelioration with benfluorex. Diabetes 1993; 42: 457–462.

62. Proietto J, Thorburn AW, Fabris S, Harrison LC. Effects of dexfenfluramine on glucose turnover in non-insulin-

dependent diabetes mellitus. Diabetes Res Clin Pract 1994; 23:127–134.

63. Willey KA, Molyneaux LM, Yue DK. Obese patients type 2 diabetes poorly controlled by insulin and metformin: effects of adjunctive dexfenfluramine therapy on glycemic control. Diabet Med 1992; 11:701.

64. Marks SJ, Moore NR, Clark ML, Strauss BJG, Hockaday TDR. Reduction of visceral adipose tissue and improvement of metabolic indices: effect of dexfenfluramine in NIDDM. Obes Res 1996; 4:1–7.

65. Atkinson RL, Blank RC, Loper JF, Schumacher D, Lutes RA. Combined drug treatment of obesity. Obes Res 1995; 3(Suppl 4):S497–S500.

66. Anderson JW, Hamilton CC, Brinkman-Kaplan V. Benefits and risks of an intensive very-low-calorie diet program for severe obesity. Am J Gastroenterol 1992; 87:6–15.

67. Wing RR. Use of very-low-calorie diets in the treatment of obese persons with non-insulin-dependent diabetes mellitus. J Am Diet Assoc 1995; 95:569–572.

68. Henry RR, Schaeffer L, Olefsky JM. Glycemic effects of intensive calorie restriction and isocaloric refeeding in non-insulin-dependent diabetes mellitus. J Clin Invest 1985; 61:917.

69. Henry RR, Wiest-Kent TA, Schaeffer L, al. e. Metabolic consequences of very-low-calorie diet therapy in obese non-insulin-dependent diabetic and non-diabetic subjects. Diabetes 1986; 35:155.

70. Anderson JW, Brinkman-Kaplan V, Hamilton CC, Logan JE, Collins RW, Gustafson NJ. Food-containing hypocaloric diets are as effective as liquid-supplement diets for obese individuals with NIDDM. Diabetes Care 1994; 17:602–604.

71. Henry RR, Gumbiner B. Benefits and limitations of very-low-calorie diet therapy in obese NIDDM. Diabetes Care 1991; 14:802–823.

72. Paolisso G, Gambardella A, Verza M, D'Amore A, Sgambato S, Varricchio M. ACE inhibition improves insulin-sensitivity in aged insulin-resistant hypertensive patients. J Hum Hypertens 1992; 6:175–179.

73. Henriksen EJ, Jacob S. Effects of captopril on glucose transport activity in skeletal muscle of obese Zucker rats. Metabolism 1995; 44:267–272.

74. Fontbonne A, Charles MA, Thibult N, et al. Hyperinsulinaemia as a predictor of coronary heart disease mortality in a healthy population: the Paris Prospective Study, 15 year follow-up. Diabetologia 1991; 34:356–361.

75. Fontbonne AM, Eschwege EM. Insulin and cardiovascular disease. Paris Prospective Study. Diabetes Care 1991; 14:461–469.

76. Lebovitz HE, Melander A. Sulphonylureas: basic aspects and clinical uses. In: Alberti KGMM, DeFronzo RA, Keen H, Zimmet P, eds. International Textbook of Diabetes Mellitus, Vol 1. Chichester: Wiley, 1992:745–772.

77. Stenman S, Melander A, Groop P-H, Groop LC. What is the benefit of increasing the sulfonylurea dose? Ann Intern Med 1993; 118:169–172.

78. Marsiaj HI, Catalano C, Sum CF, Home PD, Alberti KGMM. Management of newly diagnosed non-insulin-dependent (type 2) diabetes mellitus: a retrospective audit. Diabetes Res Clin Pract 1991; 12:129–136.

79. Holman RR, Steemson J, Turner RC. Sulphonylurea failure in type 2 diabetes: treatment with basal insulin supplement. Diabet Med 1987; 4:457–462.

80. Riddle MC, Hart JS, Bouma DJ, Phillipson BE, Youker G. Efficacy of bedtime NPH insulin with daytme sulfonylurea for subpopulation of type II diabetic subjects. Diabetes Care 1989; 12:623–629.

81. Scarlett JA, Gray RS, Griffin J, Olefsky JM, Kolterman OG. Insulin treatment reverses the insulin resistance of type II diabetes mellitus. Diabetes Care 1982; 5:353–363.

82. Heine RJ. Insulin treatment of non-insulin-dependent diabetes mellitus. Bailliere's Clin Endocrinol Metab 1988; 2:477–492.

83. Clarkson P, Celermajer DS, Donald AE, et al. Impaired vascular reactivity in insulin dependent diabetes mellitus is related to disease duration and LDL cholesterol levels. J Am Coll Cardiol 1996; 28:573–579.

84. Koskinen P, Manttari M, Manninen V, Huttunen JK, Heinonen OP, Frick MH. Coronary heart disease incidence in NIDDM patients in the Helsinki Heart Study. Diabetes Care 1992; 15:820–825.

85. Vaughan P, Gilson L, Mills A. Diabetes in developing countries: its importance for public health. Health Policy Planning 1989; 4:97–137.

86. Songer T. The economic costs of NIDDM. Diabetes Metab Rev 1992; 8:389–404.

87. Diabetes 1993 Vital Statistics. Alexandria, VA: American Diabetes Association, 1993.

88. Diabetes Control and Complications Trial Research Group. The effect of intensive treatment of diabetes on the development and progression of long-term complications in insulin-dependent diabetes mellitus. N Engl J Med 1993; 329:977–986.

89. Javitt JC, Canner JK, Sommer A. Cost-effectiveness of current approaches to the control of retinopathy in type I diabetes. Ophthalmology 1989; 96:253–262.

90. Despres J-P, Lamarche B, Mauriege P, et al. Hyperinsulinemia as an independent risk factor for ischaemic heart disease. N Engl J Med 1996; 334:952–957.

91. Després J-P, Pouliot M-C, Moorjani S et al. Loss of abdominal fat and metabolic response to exercise training in obese women. Am. J Physiol 1991; 261:E159–E167.

46

Treatment of the Obese Hypertensive

Ehud Grossman
The Chaim Sheba Medical Center, Tel-Hashomer, Israel

Franz H. Messerli
Alton Ochsner Medical Foundation, New Orleans, Louisiana

I. INTRODUCTION

The strong association between obesity and hypertension extends across age, race, and gender. The risk of becoming hypertensive increases with increasing weight, especially in those individuals with a high waist/hip ratio (upper body obesity). Controlling blood pressure in obese hypertensive patients is a great challenge for the physician, since these patients are more resistant to antihypertensive treatment (1–4) and usually have concomitant risk factors. Weight reduction effectively lowers blood pressure and may improve other risk factors (5–10); however, most obese patients are unable to maintain an adequately reduced caloric intake for a prolonged period of time. Therefore, antihypertensive medications are most often necessary to control blood pressure. This chapter will focus on the treatment of the obese hypertensive patient.

II. PATHOPHYSIOLOGY OF OBESITY HYPERTENSION

Understanding the pathogenesis of hypertension in obesity may be helpful when selecting the ideal antihypertensive treatment. However, although the association of obesity and hypertension is well recognized, the mechanism (5) involved in the pathogenesis of increased blood pressure in the obese is poorly understood. Several mechanisms have been proposed to explain this association.

A. Insulin Resistance

Obesity and hypertension are associated with insulin resistance and hyperinsulinemia (11). The degree of these alterations is greater in those whose obesity is predominantly located in the upper body or abdomen. Evidence supporting the concept that insulin resistance and hyperinsulinemia may lead to increased blood pressure derives mainly from epidemiological studies showing a correlation between insulin resistance, hyperinsulinemia, and blood pressure (12). The link between hyperinsulinemia and hypertension is explained by the effects of insulin to enhance renal sodium reabsorption in the distal tubule with consequent water retention, or through stimulation of the sympathetic nervous system (13,14). Insulin may also increase both the pressor response to angiotensin II and angiotensin II–mediated aldosterone production (15). Insulin also increases sodium sensitivity and may stimulate smooth muscle proliferation and increase intracellular calcium, which increases vascular peripheral resistance (16).

B. Overactivity of the Sympathetic Nervous System

There is evidence that the sympathetic nervous system participates in the hypertension of obesity (13). Increased sympathetic activity may cause elevated vascular resistance and sodium retention and thereby cause hypertension.

Sympathetic overactivity, as reflected by elevated plasma and urinary norepinephrine levels, faster heart rate, and increased vascular α-adrenergic tone and reactivity, has been reported in obesity hypertension (17–21). In a recent study, Kassab et al. (22) showed in dogs that renal sympathetic denervation attenuated the sodium retention and hypertension associated with obesity. Moreover, weight loss in obese hypertensives lowers blood pressure and reduces markers for excess sympathetic drive (19,23).

C.   Overactivity of the Renin-Angiotensin Cascade

The renin-angiotensin-aldosterone system may also contribute to hypertension of obesity. Some investigators found inappropriately increased renin and aldosterone levels in obese hypertensive patients (24,25), while Maxwell et al. (17) found no difference in plasma renin activity and aldosterone levels in obese and nonobese patients. Activation of the renin-angiotensin-aldosterone system may trigger sodium and water retention and produce hypervolemia that increases cardiac output in obese hypertensive patients (24).

D.   Reduced Na⁺, K⁺-ATPase Activity

Another mechanism that may contribute to hypertension of obesity is reduced Na^+, K^+-ATPase activity in red blood cells. This alteration has been described in obesity hypertension (26,27) and may produce an increase in intracellular calcium concentration that will in turn increase smooth muscle tone and vascular resistance.

III.   HEMODYNAMICS OF OBESITY HYPERTENSION (FIG. I)

Obese hypertensive patients are characterized by elevated absolute values of plasma and total blood volumes (28). Intravascular volume is not uniformly distributed throughout the body. As total body fat increases, the ratio of intravascular volume of body weight markedly falls from about 95 to 45 ml/kg (29). These data indicate that compared with lean tissue, adipose tissue seems to be underperfused (29). In a study of the extracellular fluid volume in obese hypertensive subjects, Raison et al. found an increased ratio of intracellular body water/interstitial fluid volume that may be related to either an elevated intracellular body water or a decreased interstitial fluid volume (30). In obese hypertensive patients, absolute values of cardiac output are increased due mainly to increased stroke volume, while the heart rate is usually unchanged (29). The elevated cardiac output means that the

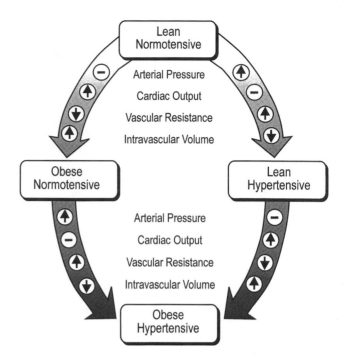

Figure 1   Effects of obesity and hypertension, separate and in combination, on systemic hemodynamics and intravascular volume. (Adapted with permission from Ref. 28.)

heart pumped a higher blood volume per unit time and is burdened by a higher workload for obese patients. Adipose tissue has low vascular resistance relative to muscle (31). The abundant fat tissue in obese hypertensives may therefore limit the increases in total peripheral resistance that are observed in lean hypertensives. Indeed, unlike lean hypertensive patients, who are characterized by increased peripheral resistance, obese hypertensive patients may have normal peripheral resistance (28). Raison et al. (32) studied the forearm hemodynamics in obese normotensive and hypertensive subjects. They found that obese hypertensives, when compared with nonobese hypertensives, were characterized by a hyperkinetic forearm circulation; i.e., they had higher values of blood flow velocity and blood flow and lower values of vascular resistance, whether absolute or normalized values were used. Thus, from a hemodynamic point of view, obesity hypertension may be the result of an inappropriately raised cardiac output in the presence of normal peripheral resistance.

IV.   NONPHARMACOLOGICAL APPROACH

Several life-style modifications, such as weight reduction, salt restriction, alcohol moderation, exercise, and reduced smoking, are recommended in the treatment of hypertension (33). Some of these interventions may be particularly promising in obesity hypertension. The Trials of Hypertension Prevention (TOHP-I) compared the effects of most of the individual nonpharmacological modalities on blood pressure (34). Patients with diastolic blood pressure of 80–89 mmHg were randomly assigned to one of three lifestyle changes (weight reduction, sodium restriction, or stress management) for 18 months or to one of four nutritional supplements (calcium, magnesium, potassium, or fish oil) for 6 months, with placebo controls for both groups. The results documented a significant antihypertensive effect of weight loss (average of 3.9 kg) and sodium restriction (average of 44 mmol/day) but no effect of the other modalities.

A. Weight Reduction

Weight reduction is effective in lowering blood pressure and offers several other metabolic benefits (5–10). A high-protein, low-carbohydrate, calorie-restricted diet for 6 months (35) normalized blood pressure in all hypertensive patients and reduced fasting and postprandial glucose and insulin plasma levels. More recent studies, using 24-hr ambulatory blood pressure monitoring, have further documented the efficacy of weight reduction in lowering blood pressure throughout the day and night (7,36). The blood pressure decrease with weight reduction can be maintained for long periods (34,37). Weight reduction lowers blood pressure independently of changes in salt intake. Reisin et al. (6) showed that weight reduction alone of 10 kg normalized blood pressure in 75% of obese hypertensive patients. Even modest weight reduction can lower blood pressure and improve lipid profile and glycemic control (38). The most dramatic fall in blood pressure is observed in the first phase of a calorie-restricted diet, and the amount of weight loss is not necessarily related to the antihypertensive effect.

There is a degree of weight loss beyond which further reductions in blood pressure would not occur (39). In obese rats undergoing a supplemented fast, blood pressure fell almost immediately but then stabilized despite continuing weight loss (40,41). The antihypertensive effect of fasting was reversed within 2 days of refeeding. It seems that nutritional state (fed, fasted, refed), but not body weight, has important effects on blood pressure (40,41). Several studies compared the effects of low-calorie diets and conventional drug treatment in obese hypertensive patients (42–44). Dietary treatment was inferior to conventional drug treatment in controlling blood pressure but superior in lowering serum concentrations of lipids. Moreover, antihypertensive treatment can be reduced significantly when an efficient hypocaloric diet is prescribed simultaneously (44). Caution is advised, however, in the use of sympathomimetic agents to reduce the appetite as they may raise the blood pressure (45), but either serotonin reuptake inhibitors, e.g., fluoxetine (46) or sertraline hydrochloride (47), or serotoninergic compounds, e.g., dexfenfluramine (48), seem to be safe and helpful in reducing weight and, in fact, may further the lowering of the blood pressure.

The precise mechanism by which weight reduction results in a decrease in blood pressure is unknown. In obese hypertensives caloric restriction improves insulin resistance and reduces plasma insulin levels (49). Insulin resistance and sodium sensitivity of blood pressure are directly related. Rocchini et al. (50) showed that obese adolescents are more salt-sensitive than nonobese adolescents and that this salt sensitivity is attenuated after weight loss. Antishin et al. (51) have demonstrated that the endogenous hyperinsulinemia that occurs in obese subjects after a glucose meal can result in urinary sodium retention. They also showed that those who were the most sodium-sensitive had higher fasting insulin concentrations, higher glucose-stimulated insulin levels, and greater urinary sodium retention in response to an oral glucose load.

Fasting or caloric deprivation is known to reduce sympathetic nervous system activity that may be mediated through the decrease in insulin levels (17,52,53). Several studies demonstrated that weight loss reduces plasma norepinephrine levels (54,55) with a concomitant decrease in blood pressure, and that the decrease in plasma norepinephrine levels parallels the fall in blood pressure (56). Suppression of the activity of the renin-angiotensin-aldosterone system has also been reported during weight reduction. Tuck et al. (57) found that weight reduction decreased levels of plasma renin activity and plasma aldosterone possibly due to a decrease in sympathetic activity. Eggena et al. (58) showed that the reduction in the activity of the renin-angiotensin-aldosterone system was mediated not only by changes in plasma norepinephrine levels, but also by changes in plasma renin substrate. Weight loss is also associated with changes in atrial natriuretic peptide (59), a decrease in plasma endothelin-1 levels (60), and a reduction in free cytosolic platelet calcium (36).

B. Salt Restriction

A low-salt diet is regarded as effective in lowering blood pressure, and several longitudinal studies have provided evidence of a relationship between salt intake and blood pressure (61–65). Modest restriction of dietary sodium intake, by about one-third of the usual intake down to a level of around 100 mmol/day, has been shown to lower blood pressure an average of 4.9 ± 1.3 mmHg systolic and 2.6 ± 0.08 mmHg diastolic (66). Weight reduction and salt restriction may have additive effects on the fall in blood pressure (67). Salt restriction is more beneficial in women and in older hypertensive patients (62,68,69). The blood pressure response to salt restriction is heterogeneous, and mainly salt-sensitive patients will respond to this manipulation. It has been claimed that obese subjects are more salt-sensitive than lean hypertensives and therefore should favorably respond to a low-salt diet (70). However, Davis et al. (71) demonstrated lack of effectiveness of a low-sodium/high-potassium diet in reducing antihypertensive medication requirements in overweight persons with mild hypertension. Moreover, even if a low-salt diet were effective in lowering blood pressure, adherence to such a diet is often difficult. Poor dietary compliance has been described by investigators who attempted to decrease salt intake by altering food habits (71–73). Most people find a low-salt diet tasteless and unacceptable, and the poor compliance can be attributed in part to lack of obvious feedback such as weight reduction. Thus, it is questionable whether a low-salt diet is a practical therapeutic strategy for long-term blood pressure management.

C.   Physical Activity

Higher levels of physical activity have been associated with a lower rate of cardiovascular morbidity and mortality (74). Aerobic exercise of moderate intensity reduces blood pressure in patients with mild-to-moderate essential hypertension, independent of weight loss (75). The positive effect of physical activity on blood pressure is further supported by the significant correlation between the degree of fall in systolic blood pressure and the increment in exercise capacity (76). Recently Kokkinos et al. (77) showed that the combined regimen of regular, moderately intense aerobic exercise and antihypertensive drug therapy reduced blood pressure and left ventricular mass in African-American men with severe hypertension. Moreover, the antihypertensive effects of exercise substantially reduced the amount of medication required to control blood pressure. Thus, increased physical activity should be encouraged in everyone, but one should remember that obese patients often experience difficulties engaging in prolonged, intense physical activity.

D.   Other Nonpharmacological Treatment

Epidemiological evidence supports an inverse relationship between potassium intake and blood pressure (78); several studies documented the efficacy of oral potassium supplementation in lowering blood pressure (79,80). Increased calcium intake may reduce the incidence of hypertension (81), and calcium supplements may lower the blood pressure of some hypertensive patients (82,83), but data from 10 trials involving hypertensive patients demonstrated the lack of significant effects (76). Other dietary manipulations include supplements of magnesium and fish oil and moderation of alcohol intake. However, the effects of these dietary manipulations have not been tested in obese hypertensive patients and therefore cannot be recommended as the sole antihypertensive treatment.

V.   DRUG THERAPY

When the nonpharmacological approach is inadequate to control blood pressure or when the initial blood pressure is very high, drug treatment is necessary. All the available antihypertensive agents are almost equally effective in lowering blood pressure (84), but diuretics are the only class of drugs so far that have been tested and shown to reduce overall cardiovascular morbidity and mortality (33).

The response of individual patients to different drugs may vary considerably (85). Obese hypertensive individuals are less responsive to antihypertensive treatment than lean individuals, perhaps as a manifestation of insulin resistance and hyperinsulinemia (4). Moreover, many obese hypertensive patients have concomitant disease that increases their risk for cardiovascular morbidity and mortality. Therefore, to initiate the appropriate antihypertensive agent, physicians should take into consideration the clinical pathophysiology, hemodynamic findings, and concomitant disease of their patient.

A.   Diuretics

Diuretics, used for more than 30 years, are still the most frequent agents prescribed to treat hypertension. This group includes thiazide or thiazide-like diuretics, loop diuretics, and potassium-sparing agents. Diuretics act by causing diuresis and natriuresis, which reduce plasma and extracellular fluid volume and thereby reduce cardiac output and blood pressure. With chronic use of thiazides, plasma volume returns partially toward normal, but at the same time, peripheral resistance decreases (86). Treatment is usually initiated with a thiazide-type diuretic that also includes chlorthalidone and indapamide. To reduce the likelihood of hypokalemia and the risk of primary cardiac arrest, a potassium-sparing agent may be added to thiazide diuretic drugs (87). A loop diuretic or metolazone is reserved mainly for patients with renal insufficiency (creatinine > 2.5 mg/dl). Diuretic therapy may cause hypokalemia, hypomagnesemia, hyponatremia, hyperuricemia, and hyperlipidemia. In addition, it may reduce insulin sensitivity and therefore impair glucose tolerance and worsen diabetic control. However, in a recent meta-analysis Gurwitz et al. (88) found that the risk of developing diabetes mellitus was not greater with diuretics than with other drugs. Most of the side effects described with diuretics were related to the high dose of the drugs, but a high dose of thiazides is usually unnecessary because the antihypertensive effect can be obtained with as little as 6.25–12.5 mg/day of hydrochlorothiazide with less hypokalemia and other side effects (89). The efficacy of diuretics in obesity hypertension is controversial. Modan et al. (4) showed that obesity, as well as glucose intolerance and hyperinsulinemia, is associated with decreased responsiveness to diuretics and that obese patients require a higher dose of diuretics to control their blood pressure, whereas Reisin and Weed (90) showed that obese hypertensive black women responded better to chlorthalidone than to the alpha-adrenergic agonist clonidine. Indeed, the study of Reisin and Weed (90) was a short one and included only a few patients, but since obesity hypertension is characterized by increased blood volume and cardiac output, it seems reasonable to choose low-dose diuretic for these patients.

B. Beta-Blockers

Beta-blockers have been used to treat hypertension for almost 30 years. They are generally well tolerated, provide secondary cardioprotection after an acute myocardial infarction, and offer the special advantage of relieving a number of concomitant diseases. This group includes a large series of similar drugs that differ mainly in their lipid solubility, cardioselectivity, and intrinsic sympathomimetic activity (86). Beta-blockers lower blood pressure by reducing cardiac output, suppression of renin release, perhaps a decrease in central sympathetic nervous outflow, a presynaptic blockade that inhibits catecholamine release, and a probable decrease in peripheral vascular resistance (86).

Beta-blockers are particularly recommended in patients with hyperkinetic circulation or in those with marked anxiety and stress, and in hypertensive patients with coexisting ischemic heart disease. They may be useful in patients with migraine headache, intention tremor, or glaucoma. Beta-blockers are contraindicated in bronchial asthma and obstructive pulmonary disease, in most patients with congestive heart failure, and in bradyarrhythmia. They are relatively contraindicated in patients with intermittent claudication, depression, and diabetes mellitus (86). The effect of beta-blockers in obesity hypertension is controversial. Obesity hypertension is characterized by sympathetic overactivity and increased cardiac output, and, therefore, beta-blockade may be very effective in lowering blood pressure (91). However, beta-blockade reduces insulin sensitivity, impairs glucose tolerance, raises serum triglycerides, lowers HDL cholesterol, and possibly counteracts weight loss by preventing the action of catecholamines on fatty acid mobilization. Modan et al. (4) showed that obese patients require a higher dose of beta-blockers to control their blood pressure. MacMahon et al. (92) also found that metoprolol was not effective in the control of blood pressure of obese hypertensive patients. However, Fagerberg et al. (93) showed that atenolol was superior to a dietetic regimen in controlling blood pressure in obese hypertensive patients, and Schmieder et al. (94) showed that metoprolol lowered blood pressure more effectively than the calcium blocker isradipine in obese patients, while the opposite was true in lean patients. Of note, metoprolol, a lipophilic beta-blocker, reduced blood pressure in obese patients despite interference with its kinetics and reduced plasma concentrations (95). Thus, it seems that in obese patients plasma concentrations are not reliable predictors of the therapeutic effects, and even when the plasma levels are low, beta-blockers may be effective in lowering blood pressure. Whether the metabolic adverse effects of these drugs may negate the benefits of the hypotensive effect is still unknown.

C. Calcium Antagonists

Calcium antagonists are very popular in the treatment of hypertension. Their use has increased dramatically because they are effective in lowering blood pressure and are tolerated well with relatively few side effects. This heterogeneous group includes three main classes, phenylalkylamines, benzothiazepines, and dihydropyridines. The best-known drug in each group is verapamil, diltiazem, and nifedipine, respectively. The three major classes of calcium antagonists differ in their molecular structure, their sites and modes of action on the slow calcium channel, and their effects on various other cardiovascular functions. They lower blood pressure mainly by reducing peripheral vascular resistance (86). Calcium antagonists also have the intrinsic ability to promote natriuresis (96) and therefore may work well in the obese hypertensive patient who has, at least relatively, intravascular volume expansion.

The efficacy of calcium antagonists in obese hypertensive patients has been evaluated by several investigators. Indeed, in a previously mentioned study Schmieder et al. (94) showed that isradipine, a dihydropyridine calcium antagonist, was less effective than metoprolol in reducing blood pressure in obese hypertensive patients. However, several other studies showed that calcium antagonists are very effective in obese hypertensive patients. Andronico et al. (97) showed that nifedipine was as effective as enalapril in reducing blood pressure in obese hypertensive patients but was superior to enalapril in regard to the metabolic effects. In another study that included a large number of obese hypertensive patients, treatment with nifedipine showed a 70–80% rate of efficacy (98). Raccah et al. (99) found, in a large group of obese hypertensive patients, that nicardipine was as effective as captopril in reducing blood pressure. Since obese hypertensives usually have insulin resistance and hyperinsulinemia and associated dyslipidemia, a reasonable therapeutic approach should include agents that do not further enhance the preexisting metabolic perturbations in these patients.

In most studies, calcium antagonists had no effect on glucose uptake. Diltiazem 90–180 mg/daily and verapamil 240 mg twice daily did not change the insulin sensitivity index (100). The results regarding nifedipine are less conclusive. While in one study nifedipine 20 mg twice daily decreased insulin sensitivity by 21% (100), in another study Sheu et al. (101) showed an increase in insulin sensitivity index following 4 months of treatment with nifedipine gastrointestinal therapeutic system up to 150 mg daily. Unlike diuretics and beta-blockers, which adversely affect lipid profile, calcium antagonists have little effect on blood lipids (102). Thus, calcium antagonists have theoretical advantages over diuretics and beta-blockers, but only results from ongoing longitudinal studies will indicate whether they are superior to these antihypertensive agents.

D. Angiotensin-Converting Enzyme (ACE) Inhibitors

Many agents in this class are available clinically. These agents inhibit the conversion of the inactive angiotensin I to the active vasoconstrictor angiotensin II and inhibit the breakdown of the vasodilator peptide bradykinin. Although there may be differences among these agents in their ability to penetrate different tissues and in their routes of elimination, all ACE inhibitors reduce blood pressure by decreasing peripheral resistance (86). In addition to lowering blood pressure, ACE inhibitors protect the function of the heart and the kidney. For the heart, ACE inhibitors provide multiple benefits. They seem to reduce left ventricular mass more effectively than other classes of drugs (103). They improve congestive heart failure by altering remodeling and reduction in preload and afterload, and they reduce recurrent myocardial infarction, congestive heart failure, and cardiac mortality in patients with low ejection fraction, without (104) or with (105) recent acute myocardial infarction.

In the kidney, ACE inhibitors preferentially vasodilate the efferent arterioles by reduction of angiotensin II, thereby increasing renal blood flow and decreasing intraglomerular hydrostatic pressure (86). This action explains the unique renal protective effect that ACE inhibitors provide in patients with diabetic nephropathy (106,107). Therefore, ACE inhibitors are recommended in patients with congestive heart failure, in patients after acute myocardial infarction with low ejection fraction, and in patients with diabetic nephropathy.

ACE inhibitors have no detrimental effect on blood lipids and have been shown to increase sensitivity to insulin and to lower plasma insulin levels (86). In view of the role of insulin resistance/hyperinsulinemia in the pathogenesis of obesity hypertension, ACE inhibitors may be the ideal therapeutic choice for these patients.

Obese hypertensive patients are usually salt-sensitive, and salt sensitivity is also associated with the inability to modulate the adrenal and renal responses to volume and angiotensin II in a normal manner (nonmodulating hypertension) (108). Since ACE inhibitors may correct nonmodulation (109), it is expected that they will also be more effective in salt-sensitive patients, and therefore in obesity hypertension.

Only a few studies have evaluated the efficacy of ACE inhibitors in obesity hypertension. Robles et al. (110) evaluated the effects of captopril in a model of obesity-induced hypertension in dogs. During 12 weeks of follow-up, animals were divided into two groups, either with or without oral captopril treatment. The captopril group presented significantly lower values of mean arterial pressure, plasma norepinephrine, and fasting glucose and cholesterol levels than those attained in the nontreated group. Furthermore, aorta samples from untreated animals showed profuse staining for fat content at the intima and adventitia layers, while this reaction was restricted to the outer layer in treated dogs. In previously mentioned studies, Andronico et al. (97) showed that enalapril was as effective as nifedipine in reducing blood pressure in obese hypertensive patients, and Raccah et al. (99) found that captopril improved insulin sensitivity and was as effective as nicardipine in reducing blood pressure. Thus, ACE inhibitors may be a prudent therapeutic choice for obese hypertensive patients, but further studies on the efficacy of these agents in obesity hypertension are required before they can become the recommended agent in these patients.

E. Alpha-1 Adrenoceptor Blockers

Selective alpha-1 blocking drugs block the activation of postsynaptic alpha-1 receptors by circulating or neurally released catecholamines, thereby causing dilatation of the resistance and capacitance vessels. Thus, these agents reduce blood pressure by reducing peripheral resistance without changing cardiac output (86). Until 1987, prazosin, a short-acting alpha-blocker, was the only one available of this group, but now long-acting agents, such as terazosin and doxazosin, that exert a uniform antihypertensive effect are available. These agents are equipotent to diuretics, beta-blockers, ACE inhibitors, and calcium antagonists in lowering blood pressure (85), and they can be effectively combined with a diuretic, beta-blocker, and calcium antagonist.

The main side effect of alpha-1 blockers is postural hypotension, seen particularly in volume-depleted patients given the shorter-acting agent prazosin. Alphablockers have favorable effects on blood lipid levels with a decrease in total and LDL cholesterol and triglycerides and a rise in HDL cholesterol (111). They also do not alter glucose tolerance in diabetics (111). In obese normoglycemic hypertensives, prazosin improved the disappearance rate of glucose during an intravenous glucose tolerance test and reduced both the peak and the total insulin response (112). Lithell (113) has reported an improvement in insulin sensitivity with both prazosin and doxazosin. These characteristics suggest that alphablockers may be advantageous in the control of blood pressure in obese patients, but further evidence is necessary to prove their efficacy.

F. Alpha- and Beta-Receptor Blockers

Modification of the conventional beta-blocker structure has provided agents with combined alpha- and beta-blocking properties. Labetalol, the prototype of this group, is a nonselective $beta_1$- and $beta_2$-receptor blocker and is, like prazosin, highly selective for $alpha_1$ receptors. The ratio of alpha- to beta-blocking action has been estimated as between 1:3 and 1:7. Labetalol lowers blood pressure via a fall in vascular resistance with little effect on cardiac output (114). In keeping with its alpha-blocking effect, labetalol does not adversely alter blood lipids. Its efficacy in obesity hypertension has not been studied.

G. Central-Acting Agonists

Central-acting agonists are sympatholytic agents because they suppress sympathetic outflow as reflected by a decrease in plasma norepinephrine levels. The main agents of this class are methyldopa and clonidine. They reduce blood pressure by a modest decrease in both peripheral resistance and cardiac output. In addition, they reduce the ability of the baroreceptor reflex to compensate for a decrease in blood pressure, causing a relative bradycardia and enhanced hypotensive action upon standing (86). Sympatholytic agents may be useful in obese hypertensive patients since these patients are characterized by sympathetic overactivity. However, Reisin and Weed (90) found that clonidine was less effective than diuretics in controlling blood pressure in this group. The use of central alpha-agonists has been limited by concern over a withdrawal syndrome, and they should be used only in patients who cannot tolerate beta-blockers.

H. Vasodilators

This class includes drugs that act directly to relax the smooth muscle in the walls of peripheral arterioles, thereby decreasing peripheral resistance and blood pressure (86). The main oral agents of this group are hydralazine and minoxidil. Unlike the indirect vasodilators, such as calcium antagonists, ACE inhibitors, and alpha-blockers, direct vasodilators activate the sympathetic nervous system and cause sodium and water retention. Thus, despite their ability to lower lipid levels, these agents are not recommended for obese hypertensive patients.

I. Angiotensin II Receptor Antagonists

The first of these agents, saralasin, was limited by the need for intravenous administration and by its partial agonistic effect. Recently losartan potassium, an orally active nonpeptide angiotensin II antagonist, has been introduced for clinical use in hypertension (115–117). This novel agent blocks the angiotensin II–induced physiological effects and lacks partial agonistic activity. This agent has been well tolerated in clinical trials and produces two- to threefold lower drug-related cough than the ACE inhibitors (117). Adverse metabolic effects have not been documented during losartan potassium therapy, and the drug does not activate the sympathetic nervous system (116). Thus, losartan potassium may be a good choice for obesity hypertension, but its efficacy in this subgroup of patients has yet to be tested.

VI. INDIVIDUALIZED TREATMENT IN OBESITY HYPERTENSION

As was shown above, several classes of antihypertensive drugs may be suitable for the obese hypertensive patient.

Therapy should be initiated with a single agent that would be the most appropriate for the individual patient (118). The first choice can be based on the presence of concomitant diseases and risk factors. If the first drug does not work or if side effects ensue, it should be stopped and a drug from another class should be tried. If a moderate dose of the first choice is well tolerated, but the blood pressure response is not sufficient, a second drug can be added, or the dose of the first drug can be increased (33). In the next section we will discuss how to start antihypertensive therapy and the specific combinations suggested in the individual obese hypertensive patient (Table 1).

VII. PATIENTS WITHOUT CONCOMITANT DISEASES OR RISK FACTORS

In obese hypertensive patients without concomitant diseases or risk factors, the initial therapy can be based on age, gender, race, and renin profile if available. Since elderly patients may have sluggish baroreceptor and sympathetic nervous responsiveness, as well as impaired cerebral autoregulation, therapy should be gentle and gradual. In these patients low doses of diuretic (e.g., 12.5 mg/day of hydrochlorothiazide, probably with a potassium-sparing agent) can be a first-line therapy (85).

Table 1 Individualization of Antihypertensive Treatment in the Obese Hypertensive Patient

Condition	First choice	Alternative	Contraindicated
Elderly	Thiazide + potassium-sparing agent, calcium antagonist	Beta-blocker, ACE inhibitors A II antagonist, alpha-blocker	
Young	Beta-blocker, ACE inhibitors A II antagonist	Calcium antagonist, alpha-blocker Thiazide + potassium-sparing agent	
Black	Thiazide + potassium-sparing agent, calcium antagonist	Beta-blocker, ACE inhibitors A II antagonist, alpha-blocker	
Low renin	Thiazide + potassium-sparing agent, calcium antagonist	Alpha-blocker, beta-blocker, ACE inhibitors, A II antagonist	
High renin	Beta-blocker, ACE inhibitor, A II antagonist	Thiazide, calcium antagonist, alpha-blocker	
Congestive heart failure	Diuretic, ACE inhibitor, A II antagonist	Alpha-blocker, dihydropyridine, calcium antagonist	Beta-blocker Verapamil Diltiazem[a]
Ischemic heart disease	Beta-blocker, calcium antagonist	Thiazide + potassium-sparing agent	
Post MI	Beta-blocker, ACE inhibitor	Verapamil, Diltiazem, ACE inhibitors Thiazide + potassium-sparing agent	High-dose nifedipine
LVH	ACE inhibitor, Verapamil Thiazide + potassium-sparing agent	Calcium antagonist, beta-blocker, alpha-blocker	
Renal failure	Loop diuretics, calcium antagonists	Beta-blocker, alpha-blocker, Minoxidil	Potassium-sparing agent
Diabetes mellitus	ACE inhibitor, calcium antagonist, alpha-blocker, A II antagonist	Low-dose diuretics	
Dyslipidemia	Alpha-blocker, ACE inhibitor Calcium antagonist	Diuretic, beta-blocker	
Bronchial asthma	Calcium antagonist Diuretic, alpha-blocker A II antagonist	ACE inhibitors	Beta-blocker

ACE = Angiotensin converting enzyme; Post MI = post myocardial infarction; LVH = Left ventricular hypertrophy.
[a]Low-dose beta-blocker with vasodilatory effect may be beneficial in dilated cardiomyopathy. Beta-blockers and calcium antagonists may be beneficial in diastolic dysfunction.

Diuretics may also protect elderly patients who are susceptible to developing osteoporosis (119). It is noteworthy that the full antihypertensive effect may not become apparent in 4 weeks (89), so patience is advised when low doses are prescribed. Young obese hypertensive patients, of both sexes, have increased sympathetic activity with hyperkinetic circulation, and therefore, a beta-blocker can be the first-line therapy (120). Blacks respond somewhat less well to beta-blockers and ACE inhibitors, and equally well to diuretics, calcium antagonists, and alpha-blockers (85). Thus, low-dose diuretics and/or calcium antagonists can be the first-line therapy in these patients. Levels of plasma renin activity may help to guide the choice of initial therapy. Those with lower renin levels respond somewhat better to diuretics and calcium antagonists (121,122), whereas those with higher renin levels respond better to beta-blockers, ACE inhibitors, and angiotensin II antagonists (116,123). However, the renin profile is not available in most patients treated in outpatient clinics. Moreover, as attractive as the concept is, in practice it often does not work.

VIII. PATIENTS WITH CARDIAC DISEASE

A. Coronary Disease

In obese hypertensive patients, of any age or race, with angina, beta-blockers or calcium antagonists are preferred. When the blood pressure is not well controlled with a single agent, calcium antagonists of the slow-release dihydropyridine group can be combined with beta-blockers. Patients who remain hypertensive after acute myocardial infarction can be treated with a beta-blocker or, in the presence of a low ejection fraction, with an ACE inhibitor (105,124). If beta-blockers are contraindicated, verapamil or diltiazem can be used (125,126). Short-acting nifedipine, in moderate to high dose, is not recommended in patients with coronary heart disease (127).

B. Congestive Heart Failure

Obese hypertensive patients are at particularly high risk of congestive heart failure (28). For those with congestive heart failure, diuretics and ACE inhibitors should be the drugs of choice (128). Generally beta-blockers and some calcium antagonists are contraindicated in these patients, unless the heart failure is due to either hypertrophic cardiomyopathy or diastolic dysfunction (129). Low doses of beta-blockers with vasodilatory effects such as carvedilol

may improve heart failure in patients with dilated cardiomyopathy (130).

C. Left Ventricular Hypertrophy

Left ventricular hypertrophy (LVH) is more common in obese hypertensives and is considered to be an independent risk factor for cardiovascular morbidity and mortality (131). Antihypertensive agents are capable of regressing LVH, but not all agents are equipotent in this regard (132). Dahlöf et al. (103) showed by meta-analysis that ACE inhibitors are the best in reducing left ventricular mass. However, recent data from the Treatment of Mild Hypertension Study showed that nutritional-hygienic intervention (mainly weight loss and sodium restriction) is as effective as nutrition-hygienic intervention plus pharmacological treatment in reducing left ventricular mass (133). The pharmacological treatment included agents from five classes of antihypertensive therapy, and only a diuretic (chlorthalidone) had a modest additional effect on reducing left ventricular mass. Whether reduction of LVH improves morbidity and mortality has to be documented, but indirect evidence suggests that it may be beneficial (134). In the meantime, it seems reasonable to prescribe ACE inhibitors and diuretics for obese hypertensives with LVH.

IX. PATIENTS WITH RENAL DISEASE

In patients with renal failure, volume excess plays a major role in the pathogenesis of hypertension; therefore, adequate diuretic therapy is required. If renal function is severely impaired (i.e., serum creatinine above 2.5 mg/dl), a loop diuretic or metolazone is recommended (86). A potassium-sparing diuretic should be avoided in most patients with severe chronic renal failure since hyperkalemia may be induced, particularly in diabetics who cannot secrete extra insulin to enhance transfer of potassium into cells and who may have low renin and low aldosterone levels. ACE inhibitors preferentially vasodilate the efferent arteriole, thereby reducing the capillary intraglomerular pressure, and provide protection against progressive sclerosis (106,107). Indeed, recent studies demonstrated that the ACE inhibitors reduce urinary albuminuria and attenuate renal deterioration in diabetic patients more effectively than other classes of antihypertensive drugs (106, 107,135). In a recent meta-analysis Kasiske et al. (136) showed that ACE inhibitors have beneficial effects on renal function above and beyond those simply due to blood pressure control. However, care must be exercised when using ACE inhibitors because they may infrequently accelerate renal insufficiency, particularly in patients with bilateral renal artery stenosis, and they may also provoke hyperkalemia (137). Since the excretion of most ACE inhibitors is decreased in chronic renal failure, a lower dose should be prescribed to these patients. The only exception is fosinopril, which can be excreted by the liver in the presence of renal failure (138).

Calcium antagonists are safe and effective in controlling blood pressure and in preserving already impaired renal function. Calcium antagonists preferentially vasodilate the afferent arterioles and increase glomerular hyperfiltration. Thus, calcium antagonists are less effective than ACE inhibitors in reducing albuminuria and retarding renal deterioration in diabetic nephropathy (86). A combination of an ACE inhibitor and a nondihydropyridine calcium antagonist may be particularly effective (139).

Beta-blockers can be used in patients with renal failure, but it should be remembered that these patients are more susceptible to developing hyperkalemia with beta-blockers (140). Those with refractory hypertension and renal failure may be successfully treated with the direct vasodilator minoxidil, but this drug should be given with an adrenergic blocker to prevent tachycardia, and with a diuretic to prevent fluid retention (86).

X. PATIENTS WITH ASTHMA AND CHRONIC OBSTRUCTIVE PULMONARY DISEASE

Patients with bronchospasm should not be given beta-blockers. In young obese hypertensive patients with bronchial asthma, a calcium antagonist, ACE inhibitor, or alpha-blocker may be used. If the patient has a hyperkinetic circulation, the nondihydropyridine calcium antagonist is preferred, but a central-acting agonist agent can also be used.

XI. PATIENTS WITH DIABETES

Hypertension accelerates target organ damage in diabetic patients (141). Therefore, a more aggressive reduction of blood pressure to a level of 130/85 mmHg is recommended in these patients (137). As noted above, ACE inhibitors are the best choice in the presence of diabetic nephropathy (106,107,135,136). Calcium antagonists and alpha-blockers are also recommended because of their efficacy and lack of adverse effects on glucose or insulin metabolism (137). Thiazide diuretics in small doses can

be used, particularly in elderly diabetic patients (137). If the dose is low, adverse effects on carbohydrate metabolism are uncommon. Diuretics are also very useful antihypertensive agents when combined with ACE inhibitors. This combination is often synergistic in lowering blood pressure and minimizing the metabolic side effects of diuretics (142). Beta-blockers are not recommended in diabetic patients unless they are given for ischemic heart disease (anginal syndrome or post myocardial infarction). Beta-blockers are not recommended because they have adverse effects on glucose and lipid metabolism, and they may mask the signs and prolong the recovery from hypoglycemia. When beta-blockers are added to diuretics, an aggravation of the hyperglycemic effect of the latter may occur (137).

XII. HYPERTENSION AND DYSLIPIDEMIA

Obese hypertensives have a higher prevalence of hyperlipidemia. Since diuretics and beta-blockers adversely affect lipid profile, total and HDL cholesterol and triglycerides should be closely monitored if these agents are used (86). Thus, the use of diuretics and beta-blockers should be reserved as a second-line therapy in these patients. Calcium antagonists and ACE inhibitors are neutral and alpha-blockers even improve lipid profile, and therefore should be considered as a first choice in obese hypertensive patients with hyperlipidemia.

XIII. COMBINATION THERAPY

Antihypertensive therapy in obesity hypertension should be initiated with a single agent that would be the most appropriate for the individual patient. The first choice can be based on the characteristic of the patient and the presence of concomitant diseases and risk factors. As obese hypertensive patients are more resistant to antihypertensive therapy (4), more than one-half of patients will require combination therapy. The choice of a second drug depends largely on the nature of the first one. If a diuretic is the first drug, the addition of an ACE inhibitor or an adrenergic inhibitor will usually provide a significant additional antihypertensive effect. If a nondiuretic agent is the first choice, a diuretic can be used as a second choice. However, if a diuretic is to be avoided, combinations of beta-blocker and a dihydropyridine calcium antagonist or of calcium antagonist and ACE inhibitor are usually effective (Table 2).

Table 2 Combination Therapy in Obese Hypertensive Patients

	Diuretics	β-blocker	ACE I	Verapamil	Diltiazem	Nifedipine	α-blocker
Diuretics		+	+++	++	++	+	++
β-blocker	+		+	—	—	++	++
ACE I	+++	+		++	++	++	+
Verapamil	++	—	++		—	—	++
Diltiazem	++	—	++	—		—	++
Nifedipine	+	++	++	—	—		++
α-blocker	++	++	+	++	++	++	

—, not recommended; +, possible; ++, recommended; +++, highly recommended.

XIV. CONCLUSIONS

Patients with upper body obesity usually have insulin resistance and hyperinsulinemia and tend to develop hypertension. Controlling blood pressure in obese hypertensive patients is a great challenge for the physician, since these patients are more resistant to antihypertensive treatment (1–4) and usually have concomitant risk factors. It is also clear that the optimal form of therapy is weight reduction that will normalize the pathophysiological alterations and will improve other risk factors. However, this type of behavioral modification is most difficult and does not normalize blood pressure in all patients. In those in whom weight reduction is not possible, pharmacotherapy is necessary. Diuretics and beta-blockers are effective in obesity hypertension, but they reduce insulin sensitivity and adversely affect lipid profile, especially when they are combined. Calcium antagonists, ACE inhibitors, and alpha-blockers are available for rational therapy. These agents lower blood pressure without aggravating preexisting metabolic alterations associated with the two diseases. However, whether the theoretical advantage of these agents over diuretics and beta-blockers, in obese hypertensive patients, can lead to a reduced morbidity and mortality has to be proven. Until solid evidence in favor of using one agent is available, the individualized approach that takes into consideration other risk factors and concomitant diseases should be used.

REFERENCES

1. Isaksson H, Ostergren J. Prognosis in therapy-resistant hypertension. J Intern Med 1994; 236(6):643–649.
2. Kaplan NM. Resistant hypertension: what to do after trying "the usual." Geriatrics 1995; 50:24–25, 29–30, 33 passim
3. Isaksson H, Cederholm T, Jansson E, Nygren A, Ostergren J. Therapy-resistant hypertension associated with central obesity, insulin resistance, and large muscle fibre area. Blood Pressure 1993; 2:46–52.
4. Modan M, Almog S, Fuchs Z, Chetrit A, Lusky A, Halkin H. Obesity, glucose intolerance, hyperinsulinemia, and response to antihypertensive drugs. Hypertension 1991; 17: 565–573.
5. Schotte DE, Stunkard AJ. The effects of weight reduction on blood pressure in 301 obese patients. Arch Intern Med 1990; 150:1701–1704.
6. Reisin E, Abel R, Modan M, Silverberg DS, Eliahou HE, Modan B. Effect of weight loss without salt restriction in the reduction of blood pressure in overweight hypertensive patients. N Engl J Med 19978; 298:1–6.
7. DasGupta P, Brigden G, Ramhamdany E, Lahiri A, Baird IM, Raftery EB. Circadian variation and blood pressure: response to rapid weight loss by hypocaloric hyponatraemic diet in obesity. J Hypertens 1991; 9:441–447.
8. Jalkanen L. The effect of a weight reduction program on cardiovascular risk factors among overweight hypertensives in primary health care. Scand J Soc Med 1991; 19: 66–71.
9. Singh RB, Niaz MA, Bishnoi I, Singh U, Begum R, Rastogi SS. Effect of low energy diet and weight loss on major risk factors, central obesity and associated disturbances in patients with essential hypertension. J Hum Hypertens 1995; 9:355–362.
10. Foster C, Rotimi C, Fraser H, Sundarum C, Liao Y, Gibson E, Holder Y, Hoyos M, Mellanson-King R. Hypertension, diabetes, and obesity in Barbados: findings from a recent population-based survey. Ethn Dis 1993; 3:404–412.
11. Krotkiewski M, Björntorp P, Sjostrom L, Smith U. Impact of obesity on metabolism in men and women. Importance of regional adipose tissue distribution. J Clin Invest 1983; 72:1150–1162.
12. Modan M, Halkin H, Almog S, et al. Hyperinsulinemia: A link between hypertension obesity and glucose intolerance. J Clin Invest 1985; 75:809–817.
13. Tuck ML. Obesity, the sympathetic nervous system, and essential hypertension. Hypertension 1992; 19(Suppl I): 167–177.

14. DeFronzo RA, Cooke CR, Andres R, Faloona GR, Davis PJ. The effect of insulin on renal handling of sodium, potassium, calcium, and phosphate in man. J Clin Invest 1975; 55:845–855.

15. Rocchini AP, Moorehead C, DeRemer S, Goodfriend TL, Ball DL. Hyperinsulinemia and the aldosterone and pressor responses to angiotensin II. Hypertension 1990; 15:861–866.

16. Tuck ML. Metabolic considerations in hypertension. Am J Hypertens 1990;3:355S–365S.

17. Maxwell MH, Heber D, Waks AU, Tuck ML. Role of insulin and norepinephrine in the hypertension of obesity. Am J Hypertens 1994; 7:402–408.

18. Landsberg L. Obesity and hypertension: experimental data. J Hypertens 1992; 10:195S–201S.

19. Sowers JR, Whitfield LA, Catania RA, et al. Role of sympathetic nervous system in blood pressure maintenance in obesity. J Clin Endocrinol Metab 1982; 54:1181–1186.

20. Egan BM, Schork NJ, Weder AB. Regional hemodynamic abnormalities in overweight men. Focus on alpha-adrenergic vascular responses. Am J Hypertens 1989; 2:428–434.

21. Troisi RJ, Weiss ST, Parker DR, Sparrow D, Young JB, Landsberg L. Relation of obesity and diet to sympathetic nervous system activity. Hypertension 1991; 17:669–677.

22. Kassab S, Kato T, Wilkins FC, Chen R, Hall JE, Granger JP. Renal denervation attenuates the sodium retention and hypertension associated with obesity. Hypertension 1995; 25(4 Pt 2):893–897.

23. Andersson B, Elam M, Wallin BG, Björntorp P, Andersson OK. Effect of energy-restricted diet on sympathetic muscle nerve activity in obese women. Hypertension 1991; 18:783–789.

24. Hiramatsu K, Yamada T, Ichikawa K, Izumiyama T, Nagata H. Changes in endocrine activities relative to obesity in patients with essential hypertension. J Am Geriatr Soc 1981; 29:25–30.

25. Rocchini AP, Katch VL, Grekin R, Moorehead C, Anderson J. Role for aldosterone in blood pressure regulation of obese adolescents. Am J Cardiol 1986; 57:613–618.

26. De Luise M, Blackburn GL, Flier JS. Reduced activity of the red-cell sodium-potassium pump in human obesity. N Engl J Med 1980; 303:1071–1022.

27. Klimes I, Nagulesparan M, Unger RH, Aronoff SL, Mott DM. Reduced Na⁺K⁺-ATPase activity in intact red cells and isolated membranes from obese man. J Clin endocrinol 1982; 54:721–724.

28. Messerli FH. Cardiovascular effects of obesity and hypertension. Lancet 1982; 1(8282):1165–1168.

29. Licata G, Scaglione R, Capuana G, Parrinello G, Di Vincenzo D, Mazzola G. Hypertension in obese subjects: distinct hypertensive subgroup. J Hum Hypertens 1990; 4:37–41.

30. Raison J, Achimastos A, Bouthier J, London G, Safar M. Intravascular volume, extracellular fluid volume, and total body water in obese and nonobese hypertensive patients. Am J Cardiol 1983; 51:165–170.

31. Ferrannini E. The haemodynamics of obesity: a theoretical analysis. J Hypertens 1992; 10:1417–1423.

32. Raison JM, Safar ME, Cambien FA, London GM. Forearm haemodynamics in obese normotensive and hypertensive subjects. J Hypertens 1988; 6:299–303.

33. Joint National Committee on the Detection, Evaluation, and Treatment of Blood Pressure: The 1992 Report of the Joint National Committee on the Detection, Evaluation, and Treatment of Blood Pressure (JNC-V). Arch Intern Med 1993; 153:154–183.

34. The Trials of Hypertension Prevention Collaborative Research Group. The effects of nonpharmacologic interventions on blood pressure of persons with high normal levels: results of the Trials of Hypertension Prevention, Phase 1. JAMA 1992; 267:1213–1220.

35. Nobels F, van Gaal L, de Leeuw I. Weight reduction with a high protein, low carbohydrate, calorie-restricted diet: effects on blood pressure, glucose and insulin levels. Neth J Med 1989; 35:295–302.

36. Scherrer U, Nussberger J, Torriani S, Waeber B, Darioli R, Hofstetter JR, Brunner HR. Effect of weight reduction in moderately overweight patients on recorded ambulatory blood pressure and free cytosolic platelet calcium. Circulation 1991; 83:552–558.

37. Reisin E, Frohlich ED. Effects of weight reduction on arterial pressure. J Chronic Dis 1982; 35:887–891.

38. Goldstein DJ. Beneficial health effects of modest weight loss. Int J Obes Relat Metab Disord 1992; 16:397–415.

39. Cohen N, Flamenbaum W. Obesity and hypertension. Demonstration of a "floor effect." Am J Med 1986; 80:177–181.

40. Ernsberger P, Nelson DO. Effects of fasting and refeeding on blood pressure are determined by nutritional state, not by body weight change. Am J Hypertens 1988; 1(3 Pt 3):153S–157S.

41. Ernsberger P, Nelson DO. Refeeding hypertension in dietary obesity. Am J Physiol 1988; 254(1 Pt 2):R47–55.

42. Berglund A, Andersson OK, Berglund G, Fagerberg B. Antihypertensive effect of diet compared with drug treatment in obese men with mild hypertension. Br Med J 1989; 299(6697):480–485.

43. Darne B, Nivarong M, Tugaye A, Safar M, Plouin PF, Guillanneuf MT, Cubeau J, Pannier B, Pequignot F, Cambien F. Hypocaloric diet and antihypertensive drug treatment. A randomized controlled clinical trial. Blood Press 1993; 2:130–135.

44. Davis BR, Blaufox MD, Oberman A, Wassertheil-Smoller S, Zimbaldi N, Cutler JA, Kirchner K, Langford HG. Reduction in long-term antihypertensive medication requirements. Effects of weight reduction by dietary intervention in overweight persons with mild hypertension. Arch Inter Med 1993; 153:1773–1782.

45. Grossman E, Messerli FH. High blood pressure: a side effect of drugs, poisons and food. Arch Intern Med 1995; 155:450–460.

46. Gray DS, Fujioka K, Devine W, Bray GA. Fluoxetine treatment of the obese diabetic. Int J Obes Relat Metab Disord 1992; 16:193–198.

47. Jordan J, Messerli FH, Lavie CJ, Aepfelbacher FC, Soria F. Reduction of weight and left ventricular mass with serotonin uptake inhibition in obese patients with systemic hypertension. Am J Cardiol 1995; 75:743–744.

48. Kolanowski J, Younis LT, Vanbutsele R, Detry JM. Effect of dexfenfluramine treatment on body weight, blood pressure and noradrenergic activity in obese hypertensive patients. Eur J Clin Pharmacol 1992; 42:599–605.

49. Grey N, Kipinis DM. Effect of diet composition on the hyperinsulinemia of obesity. N Engl J Med 1971; 285:827–831.

50. Rocchini AP, Key J, Bondie D, Chico R, Moorehead C, Katch V, Martin M. The effect of weight loss on the sensitivity of blood pressure to sodium in obese adolescents. N Engl J Med 1989; 321:580–585.

51. Antishin K, Rocchini AP, Moorehead C, Brown C. Sodium retention in response to an oral glucose load. Circulation 1990; 82(Suppl III):111–120 (absract).

52. Landsberg L, Young JB. Fasting, feeding and regulation of the sympathetic nervous system. N Engl J Med 1978; 298:1295–1301.

53. Landsberg L. Pathophysiology of obesity-related hypertension: role of insulin and the sympathetic nervous system. J Cardiovasc Pharmacol 1994; 23(Suppl 1):S1–8.

54. Sowers JR, Nyby M, Stern N, Beck F, Baron S, Catania R, Vlachis N. Blood pressure and hormone changes associated with weight reduction in the obese. Hypertension 1982; 686–691.

55. Grossman E, Eshkol A, Rosenthal T. Diet and weight loss: their effect on norepinephrine, renin and aldosterone levels. Int J Obes 1985; 9:107–114.

56. Kushiro T, Kobayashi F, Osada H, Tomiyama H, Satoh K, Otsuka Y, Kurumatani H, Kajiwara N. Role of sympathetic activity in blood pressure reduction with low calorie regimen. Hypertension 1991; 17(6 Pt 2):965–968.

57. Tuck ML, Sowers J, Dornfeld L, Kledzik G, Maxwell M. The effect of weight reduction on blood pressure, plasma renin activity and plasma aldosterone levels in obese patients. N Engl J Med 1981; 304:930–933.

58. Eggena P, Sowers JR, Maxwell MH, Barrett JD, Golub MS. Hormonal correlates of weight loss associated with blood pressure reduction. Clin Exp Hypertens 1991; A13:1447–1456.

59. Maoz E, Shamiss A, Peleg E, Salzberg M, Rosenthal T. The role of atrial natriuretic peptide in natriuresis of fasting. J Hypertens 1992; 10:1041–1044.

60. Ferri C, Bellini C, Desideri G, Di Francesco L, Baldoncini R, Santucci A, De Mattia G. Plasma endothelin-1 levels in obese hypertensive and normotensive men. Diabetes 1995; 44:431–436.

61. Muntzel M, Drueke T. A comprehensive review of the salt and blood pressure relationship. Am J Hypertens 1992; 5:1S–42S.

62. Law MR, Frost CD, Wald NJ. By how much does dietary salt reduction lower blood pressure? I. Analysis of observational data among populations. Br Med J 1991; 302(6780):811–815.

63. Intersalt Cooperative Research Group. Intersalt: An international study of electrolyte and blood pressure. Results for 24-hour urinary sodium and potassium excretion. Br Med J 1988; 297:319–328.

64. Elliott P. Observational studies of salt and blood pressure. Hypertension 1991; 17(Suppl 1):13–18.

65. Stamler R. Implications of the INTERSALT Study. Hypertension 1991; 17(Suppl 1):I16–I20.

66. Cutler JA, Follmann D, Elliott P, Suh I. An overview of randomized trials of sodium reduction and blood pressure. Hypertension 1991; 17(Suppl 1):I27–I33.

67. Gillum RF, Prineas RJ, Jeffery RW, Jacobs DR, Elmer PJ, Gomez O, Blackburn H. Nonpharmacologic therapy of hypertension: the independent effects of weight reduction and sodium restriction in overweight borderline hypertensive patients. Am Heart J 1983; 105:128–133.

68. Geleijnse JM, Witteman JC, Bak AA, den Breeijen JH, Grobbee DE. Reduction in blood pressure with a low sodium, high potassium, high magnesium salt in older subjects with mild to moderate hypertension. Br Med J 1994; 309(6952):436–440.

69. Nestel PJ, Clifton PM, Noakes M, McArthur R, Howe PR. Enhanced blood pressure response to dietary salt in elderly women, especially those with small waist:hip ratio. J Hypertens 1993; 11:1387–1394.

70. Rocchini AP. Cardiovascular regulation in obesity-induced hypertension. Hypertension 1992; 19(Suppl 1):156–160.

71. Davis BR, Oberman A, Blaufox MD, Wassertheil-Smoller S, Zimbaldi N, Kirchner K, Wylie-Rosett J, Langford HG. Lack of effectiveness of a low-sodium/high-potassium diet in reducing antihypertensive medication requirements in overweight persons with mild hypertension. TAIM Research Group. Trial of Antihypertensive Interventions and Management. Am J Hypertens 1994; 7:926–932.

72. Kumanyika S. Behavioral aspects of intervention strategies to reduce dietary sodium. Hypertension 1991; 17(Suppl I):I190–I195.

73. Wylie-Rosett J, Wassertheil-Smoller S, Blaufox MD, Davis BR, Langford HG, Oberman A, Jennings S, Hataway H, Stern J, Zimbaldi N. Trial of antihypertensive intervention and management: greater efficacy with weight reduction than with a sodium-potassium intervention. J Am Diet Assoc 1993; 93:408–415.

74. Paffenbarger RS Jr, Hyde RT, Wing AL, Lee IM, Jung DL, Kampert JB. The association of changes in physical-activity level and other lifestyle characteristics with mortality among men. N Engl J Med 1993; 328:538–545.

75. Arroll B, Beaglehole R. Does physical activity lower blood pressure: a critical review of the clinical trials. J Clin Epidemiol 1992; 45:439–447.

76. Kaplan NM. Treatment of hypertension: nondrug therapy. In: Kaplan NM, ed. Clinical Hypertension. Philadelphia: Williams & Wilkins, 1994:171–189.

77. Kokkinos PF, Narayan P, Colleran JA, Pittaras A, Notargiacomo A, Reda D, Papademetriou V. Effects of regular exercise on blood pressure and left ventricular hypertrophy in African-American men with severe hypertension. N Engl J Med 1995; 333:1462–1467.

78. Linas SL. The role of potassium in the pathogenesis and treatment of hypertension [Clinical conference]. Kidney Int 1991; 39:771–786.

79. Smith SR, Klotman PE, Svetkey LP. Potassium chloride lowers blood pressure and causes natriuresis in older patients with hypertension. J Am Soc Nephrol 1992; 2:1302–1309.

80. Cappuccio FP, MacGregor GA. Does potassium supplementation lower blood pressure? A meta-analysis of published trials. J Hypertens 1991; 9:465–473.

81. Dwyer JH, Curtin LR, Davis IJ, Dwyer KM, Feinleib M. Dietary calcium and 10 year incidence of treated hypertension in the NHANES I epidemiologic follow-up. Circulation 1992; 86(Suppl 1):678 (abstract).

82. Saito K, Sano H, Furuta Y, Yamanishi J, Omatsu T, Ito Y, Fukuzaki H. Calcium supplementation in salt-dependent hypertension. Contrib Nephrol 1991; 90:25–35.

83. Weinberger MH, Wagner UL, Fineberg NS. The blood pressure effects of calcium supplementation in humans of known sodium responsiveness. Am J Hypertens 1993; 6:799–805.

84. Neaton JD, Grimm RH Jr, Prineas RJ, et al. and Treatment of Mild Hypertension Study Research Group. Treatment of mild hypertension study: final results. JAMA 1993; 270:713–724.

85. Materson BJ, Reda DJ, Cushman WC, et al. Single-drug therapy for hypertension in men. The Department of Veterans Affairs Cooperative Study Group on Antihypertensive Agents. A comparison of six antihypertensive agents with placebo. N Engl J Med 1993; 328:914–921.

86. Kaplan NM. Treatment of hypertension: drug therapy. In: Kaplan NM, ed. Clinical Hypertension. Philadelphia: Williams & Wilkins, 1994:191–280.

87. Siscovick DS, Raghunathan TE, Psaty BM, et al. Diuretic therapy for hypertension and the risk of primary cardiac arrest. N Engl J Med 1994; 330:1852–1857.

88. Gurwitz JH, Bohn RL, Glynn RJ, Monane M, Mogun H, Avorn J. Antihypertensive drug therapy and the initiation of treatment for diabetes mellitus. Ann Intern Med 1993; 118:273–278.

89. Carlsen JE, Kober L, Torp-Pedersen C, Johansen P. Relation between dose of bendrofluazide, antihypertensive effect, and adverse biochemical effects. Br Med J 1990; 300:975–978.

90. Reisin E, Weed SG. The treatment of obese hypertensive black women: a comparative study of chlorthalidone versus clonidine. J Hypertens 1992; 10:489–493.

91. Kendall MJ, Lewis H, Griffith M, Barnett AH. Drug treatment of the hypertensive diabetic. J Hum Hypertens 1988; 1:249–258.

92. MacMahon SW, Macdonald GJ, Bernstein L, Andrews G, Blacket RB. Comparison of weight reduction with metroprolol in treatment of hypertension in young overweight patients. Lancet 1985; 1(8440):1233–1236.

93. Fagerberg B, Berglund A, Andersson OK, Berglund G, Wikstrand J. Cardiovascular effects of weight reduction versus antihypertensive drug treatment: a comparative, randomized, 1-year study of obese men with mild hypertension. J Hypertens 1991; 9:431–439.

94. Schmieder RE, Gatzka C, Schachinger H, Schobel H, Ruddel H. Obesity as a determinant for response to antihypertensive treatment. Br Med J 1993; 307(6903):537–540.

95. Galletti F, Fasano ML, Ferrara LA, Groppi A, Montagna M, Mancini M. Obesity and beta-blockers: influence of body fat on their kinetics and cardiovascular effects. J Clin Pharmacol 1989; 29:212–216.

96. Krishna GG, Riley LJ Jr, Deuter G, Kapoor SC, Narins RG. Natriuretic effect of calcium-channel blockers in hypertensives. Am J Kidney Dis 1991; 18:566–572.

97. Andronico G, Piazza G, Mangano MT, Mule G, Carone MB, Cerasola G. Nifedipine vs. enalapril in treatment of hypertensive patients with glucose intolerance. J Cardiovasc Pharmacol 1991; 18(Suppl 10):S52–54.

98. Bravo EL, Krakoff LR, Tuck ML, Friedman CP and the Modern Approach to The Treatment of Hypertension (MATH) Study Group. Antihypertensive effectiveness of nifedipine gastrointestinal therapeutic system in the elderly. Am J Hypertens 1990; 3:S327–S332.

99. Raccah D, Pettenuzzo-Mollo M, Provendier O, Boucher L, Cozic JA, Gorlier R, Huin P, Sicard J, Vague P. Comparison of the effects of captopril and nicardipine on insulin sensitivity and thrombotic profile in patients with hypertension and android obesity. CaptISM Study Group. Captopril Insulin Sensitivity Multicenter Study Group. Am J Hypertens 1994; 7:731–738.

100. Prisant LM, Carr AA. Antihypertensive drug therapy and insulin resistance. Am J Hypertens 1992; 5:775–777 (editorial).

101. Sheu WH, Swislocki AL, Hoffman B, Chen YD, Reaven GM. Comparison of the effects of atenolol and nifedipine on glucose, insulin, and lipid metabolism in patients with hypertension. Am J Hypertens 1991; 4:199–205.

102. Kasiske BL, Ma JZ, Kalil RSN, Louis TA. Effects of antihypertensive therapy on serum lipids. Ann Intern Med 1995; 122:133–141.

103. Dahlöf B, Pennert K, Hansson L. Regression of left ventricular hypertrophy—a meta-analysis. Clin Exp Hypertens A 1992; 14:173–180.

104. Yusuf S, Pepine CJ, Garces C, et al. Effect of enalapril on myocardial infarction and unstable angina in patients with low ejection fractions. Lancet 1992; 340:1173–1178.

105. Pfeffer MA, Braunwald E, Moye LA, et al. Effect of captopril on mortality and morbidity in patients with left ventricular dysfunction after myocardial infarction. Results of the survival and ventricular enlargement trial. The SAVE Investigators. N Engl J Med 1992; 327:669–677.

106. Lewis EJ, Hunsicker LG, Bain RP, Rohde RD. The effect of angiotensin-converting-enzyme inhibition on diabetic nephropathy. The Collaborative Study Group. N Engl J Med 1993; 329:1456–1462.

107. Viberti G, Mogensen CE, Groop LC, Pauls JF. Effect of captopril on progression to clinical proteinuria in patients with insulin dependent diabetes mellitus and micro-albuminuria. The European Microalbuminuria Captopril Study Group. JAMA 1994; 271:275–279.

108. Hollenberg NK, Williams GH. The renal response to converting enzyme inhibition and the treatment of sodium-sensitive hypertension. Clin Exp Hypertens A 1987; 9: 531–541.

109. Dluhy RG, Smith K, Taylor T, Hollenberg NK, Williams GH. Prolonged converting enzyme inhibition in non-modulating hypertension. Hypertension 1989; 13:371–377.

110. Robles RG, Villa E, Santirso R, Martinez J, Ruilope LM, Cuesta C, Sancho JM. Effects of captopril on sympathetic activity, lipid and carbohydrate metabolism in a model of obesity-induced hypertension in dogs. Am J Hypertens 1993; 6:1009–1015.

111. Giordano M, Matsuda M, Sanders L, Canessa ML, De-Fronzo RA. Effects of angiotensin-converting enzyme inhibitors, Ca^{2+} channel antagonists, and alpha-adrenergic blockers on glucose and lipid metabolism in NIDDM patients with hypertension. Diabetes 1995; 44:665–671.

112. Pollare T, Lithell H, Selinus I, Berne C. Application of prazosin is associated with an increase of insulin sensitivity in obese patients with hypertension. Diabetologia 1988; 31:415–420.

113. Lithell HO. Effect of antihypertensive drugs on insulin, glucose, and lipid metabolism. Diabetes Care 1991; 14: 203–209.

114. Opie LH. Role of vasodilation in the antihypertensive and antianginal effects of labetalol: implications for therapy of combined hypertension and angina. Cardiovasc Drugs Ther 1988; 2:369–376.

115. Siegl PK. Discovery of losartan, the first specific non-peptide angiotensin II receptor antagonist. J Hypertens 1993; 11(Suppl):S19–S22.

116. Grossman E, Peleg E, Carroll J, Shamiss A, Rosenthal T. Hemodynamic and humoral effects of angiotensin II antagonist losartan in essential hypertension. Am J Hypertens 1994; 7:1041–1044.

117. Goa KL, Wagstaff AJ. Losartan potassium: a review of its pharmacology, clinical efficacy and tolerability in the management of hypertension. Drugs 1996; 51:820–845.

118. Alderman MH. Blood pressure management: individualized treatment based on absolute risk and the potential for benefit. Ann Intern Med 1993; 119:329–335.

119. Felson DT, Sloutskis D, Anderson JJ, Anthony JM, Kiel DP. Thiazide diuretics and the risk of hip fracture. Results from the Framingham Study. JAMA 1991; 265:370–373.

120. Kaplan NM. The treatment of hypertension in women. Arch Intern Med 1995; 155:563–567.

121. Niarchos AP, Weinstein DL, Laragh JH. Comparison of the effects of diuretic therapy and low sodium intake in isolated systolic hypertension. Am J Med 1984; 77: 1061–1068.

122. Bühler FR. Antihypertensive care with calcium antagonists. In Laragh JH, Brenner BM, eds. Hypertension: Pathophysiology, Diagnosis, and management. New York: Raven Press, 1995:2801–2814.

123. Niutta E, Cusi D, Colombo R, et al. Predicting interindividual variations in antihypertensive therapy: the role of sodium transport systems and renin. J Hypertens 1990; 8(Suppl):S53–S58.

124. Hampton JR. Secondary prevention of acute myocardial infarction with beta-blocking agents and calcium antagonists. Am J Cardiol 1990; 66:3C–8C.

125. The Multicenter Diltiazem Postinfarction Trial Research Group. The effect of diltiazem on mortality and reinfarction after myocardial infarction. N Engl J Med 1988; 319: 385–392.

126. Effect of verapamil on mortality and major events after acute myocardial infarction (the Danish Verapamil Infarction Trial II—DAVIT II). Am J Cardiol 1990; 66:779–785.

127. Furberg CD, Psaty BM, Meyer JV. Nifedipine. Dose-related increase in mortality in patients with coronary heart disease. Circulation 1995; 92:1326–1331.

128. Groden DL. Vasodilator therapy for congestive heart failure. Lessons from mortality trials. Arch Intern Med 1993; 153:445–454.

129. Setaro JF, Zaret BL, Schulman DS, Black HR, Soufer R. Usefulness of verapamil for congestive heart failure associated with abnormal left ventricular diastolic filling and normal left ventricular systolic performance. Am J Cardiol 1990; 66:981–986.

130. Persson H, Erhardt L. Beta receptor antagonists in the treatment of heart failure. Cardiovasc Drugs Ther 1991; 5:589–604.

131. Levy D, Garrison RJ, Savage DD, Kannel WB, Castelli WP. Prognostic implications of echocardiographically determined left ventricular mass in the Framingham Heart Study. N Engl J Med 1990; 322:1561–1566.

132. Messerli FH, Oren S, Grossman E. Left ventricular hypertrophy and antihypertensive therapy. Drugs 1988; 35(Suppl 5):27–33.

133. Liebson PR, Grandits GA, Dianzumba S, Prineas RJ, Grimm RH Jr, Neaton JD, Stamler J. Comparison of five antihypertensive monotherapies and placebo for change in left ventricular mass in patients receiving nutritional-

hygienic therapy in the Treatment of Mild Hypertension Study (TOMHS). Circulation 1995; 91:698–706.

134. Messerli FH, Soria F. Does a reduction in left ventricular hypertrophy reduce cardiovascular morbidity and mortality? Drugs 1992; 44(Suppl 1):141–146.

135. Lebovitz HE, Wiegmann TB, Cnaan A, et al. Renal protective effects of enalapril in hypertensive NIDDM: role of baseline albuminuria. Kidney Int 1994; 45(Suppl): S150–S155.

136. Kasiske BL, Kalil RS, Ma JZ, Liao M, Keane WF. Effect of antihypertensive therapy on the kidney in patients with diabetes: a meta-regression analysis. Ann Intern Med 1993; 118:129–138.

137. The National High Blood Pressure Education Program Working Group. National High Blood Pressure Education Program Working Group report on hypertension in diabetes. Hypertension 1994; 23:145–158; discussion 159–160.

138. Murdoch D, McTavish D. Fosinopril. A review of its pharmacodynamic and pharmacokinetic properties, and therapeutic potential in essential hypertension. Drugs 1992; 43:123–140.

139. Bakris GL, Barnhill BW, Sadler R. Treatment of arterial hypertension in diabetic humans: importance of therapeutic selection. Kidney Int 1992; 41:912–919.

140. Mitch WE, Wilcox CS. Disorders of body fluids, sodium and potassium in chronic renal failure. Am J Med 1982; 72:536–550.

141. Sowers JR, Epstein M. Diabetes mellitus and associated hypertension, vascular disease, and nephropathy. An update. Hypertension 1995; 26:869–879.

142. Shamiss A, Carroll J, Peleg E, Grossman E, Rosenthal T. The effect of enalapril with and without hydrochlorothiazide on insulin sensitivity and other metabolic abnormalities of hypertensive patients with NIDDM. Am J Hypertens 1995; 8:276–281.

47

Treatment of Obese Patients with Dyslipoproteinemia

Yuji Matsuzawa, Kaoru Kameda-Takemura, and Shizuya Yamashita
Osaka University Medical School, Suita, Osaka, Japan

I. DYSLIPIDEMIA IN OBESITY

One of the most common complications of obesity is the disturbance of lipoprotein metabolism (1–4). Lipoprotein disorders observed in obesity show a wide variety of features. Some obese people have predominant hypertriglyceridemia, whereas others have mainly hypercholesterolemia. In other individuals, obesity induces mixed hyperlipidemia. In addition, not only does obesity raise serum lipids, it also reduces high-density lipoprotein (HDL) cholesterol. The increments in serum cholesterol and triglyceride levels are attributed to the increase in both very-low-density lipoprotein (VLDL) and low-density lipoprotein (LDL), although the extent of the increase in each lipoprotein is different among individuals probably depending on their genetic background. In some patients who have a genetic predisposition for type IV hyperlipidemia, a slight weight gain may induce hyperchylomicronemia or type V hyperlipoproteinemia. The mechanism for the rise in both VLDL and LDL is an overproduction of apolipoprotein (apo) B–containing lipoproteins by the liver. The decrease in HDL cholesterol has been shown to be attributed to the disturbance of triglyceride (TG)-rich lipoprotein catabolism due to low lipoprotein lipase (LPL) activity. Our recent study indicates that the increase in cholesteryl ester transfer protein (CETP) produced by adipose tissues may be one of the major causes of the reduction of HDL-cholesterol levels in obese subjects (5).

These lipoprotein disorders are not correlated to the extent of obesity, but a number of recent studies have suggested that visceral fat accumulation is one of the major causes of lipoprotein disorders in obesity. Visceral fat has been shown to be a very active adipose tissue with respect to lipogenesis and lipolysis. The accumulation of this adipose tissue may induce a high content of free fatty acids (FFAs) in portal circulation, which flow directly into the liver. Increased influx of FFAs into the liver may cause an enhancement of lipid synthesis. Visceral fat accumulation induces not only lipoprotein disorders (6), but also other complications such as hypertension (7) and impairment of glucose metabolism (6). Obesity can be the major nutritional problem promoting the development of cardiovascular diseases (8), when unfavorable effects of obesity on the lipoprotein metabolism are added to the other undesirable complications such as hypertension, hyperglycemia, or insulin resistance.

II. TREATMENT OF DYSLIPIDEMIA IN OBESITY: GENERAL TREATMENT

Since the major cause of raised serum lipid levels is fat accumulation due to excess dietary calorie intake, the reduction of body weight is, needless to say, the first and main form of therapy needed for dyslipidemia in obesity. In patients with mild hyperlipidemia induced by obesity, even a small weight reduction may cause a substantial decrease in serum lipids, even if body weight does not reach the ideal level. If a substantial weight reduction is achieved, a reduction in total cholesterol level by 10–15 mg/dl should be obtained. However, a moderate or severe hyperlipidemia accompanied by obesity may often remain even after conventional treatment for weight reduction. In such cases, specific dietary control and drug treatment should be considered for each type of dyslipidemia.

III. TREATMENT OF PREDOMINANT HYPERCHOLESTEROLEMIA IN OBESITY

Hypercholesterolemia is one of the major risk factors for cardiovascular diseases. Therefore, the management of serum cholesterol is the most important measure in treatment of these patients. Hypercholesterolemia observed in obese patients is mostly mild or moderate. All patients should have maximal dietary support in an attempt to achieve the goals outlined by the National Cholesterol Education Program (NCEP) (9). If these goals are not achieved, drug therapy should then be considered (Table 1). As suggested by the NCEP, patients with other risk factors are those who are the most in need of drug treatment, and serum total cholesterol and LDL-cholesterol levels in these patients should be maintained at lower levels than in those without any risk factors. Since obese patients, especially those with visceral fat obesity, frequently have multiple risk factors such as hypertension and diabetes mellitus, cholesterol-lowering treatment is very important even if hypercholesterolemia is mild or moderate.

A. Dietary Factors to Be Assessed in Treatment of Obese Patients with Hypercholesterolemia

In addition to the reduction of calorie intake as a dietary measure to reduce serum cholesterol, the curtailment of dietary cholesterol and certain fatty acids should be considered. The relative contributions of these two factors to the regulation of serum cholesterol levels depend on many variables, and one dietary factor cannot be called more hypercholesterolemic than the other. Dietary cholesterol, for example, has been considered to raise serum cholesterol levels more in younger adults than in older subjects. In contrast, fatty acids in the diet have apparently similar effects on cholesterol levels at all ages. In the following sections, the effect of these two dietary factors on serum cholesterol level is reviewed.

1. Dietary Cholesterol

High-cholesterol diet induces hypercholesterolemia in animals such as rabbits and monkeys. In humans, several epidemiological studies have demonstrated that the amount of dietary cholesterol is correlated with the incidence of cardiovascular diseases probably through the elevation of serum cholesterol. The extent of this rise is illustrated by human studies carried out by three different groups (10–12). The relationship between cholesterol intake and the increase in serum cholesterol was similar in humans, although not identical. Other studies in humans, however, showed that there are marked differences between individuals in the response of serum cholesterol to dietary cholesterol. The response of serum cholesterol to dietary cholesterol depends at least partly upon the extent of cholesterol absorption from the intestines. Limiting enzymes for cholesterol absorption are considered to be acyl-CoA:cholesterol acyltransferase (ACAT) and cholesterol esterase in the intestinal mucosa. An animal study (13) using streptozotocin-induced diabetic rats, a model of insulin-dependent diabetes mellitus (IDDM), showed that plasma cholesterol levels were slightly but significantly increased in diabetic rats compared with control animals, whereas a far more remarkable increase in plasma cholesterol was observed in diabetic rats fed a high-cholesterol diet. The intestinal ACAT activity was markedly enhanced

Table 1 Treatment Decisions Based on LDL Cholesterol Level

Patient category	Initiation level	LDL goal
Dietary Therapy		
Without CHD and with fewer than two risk factors	≥160 mg/dL	<160 mg/dL
Without CHD and with two or more risk factors	≥130 mg/dL	<130 mg/dL
With CHD	>100 mg/dL	≤100 mg/dL
Drug Treatment		
Without CHD and with fewer than two risk factors	≥190 mg/dL	<160 mg/dL
Without CHD and with two or more risk factors	≥160 mg/dL	<130 mg/dL
With CHD	≥130 mg/dL	≤100 mg/dL

LDL, low-density lipoprotein; CHD, coronary heart disease.
Source: Ref. 9.

in diabetic rats than in control rats. However, no significant difference in ACAT activity was noted between diabetic rats fed control chow and those fed a high-cholesterol diet. Insulin supplementation given to diabetic rats caused a reduction of ACAT activity to the levels found in control animals. These data suggest that enhancement of ACAT activity in the intestines might be one of the major factors responsible for hypercholesterolemia in diabetes.

Cell biology experiments using Caco-2 cells also suggest that ACAT activity is decreased by insulin supplementation (14). Furthermore, intestinal ACAT activity was also enhanced in Wistar fatty rats, an obese animal model of non-insulin-dependent diabetes mellitus (NIDDM) (15). Therefore, in obese patients with disturbances of glucose metabolism, cholesterol absorption may be increased through the enhancement of intestinal ACAT activity. We should be much more careful about the dietary cholesterol content in obese patients than in the general population. When we combine the data from the major studies, we find that the serum total cholesterol increases about 8–10 mg/dl for every 100 mg of dietary cholesterol/1000 calories on the average. The risk for coronary heart disease (CHD) rises about 1% for every 1 mg/dl increase in total cholesterol; therefore, the effect of cholesterol intake, especially in obese patients with glucose intolerance, is not trivial on an overall CHD risk. The increase in serum total cholesterol due to an increment in dietary cholesterol occurs mostly in the LDL fraction. This increase primarily results from a suppression of LDL receptor activity. The suppression of LDL receptor activity is attributed to the decrease in LDL receptor synthesis by the liver, which is regulated in part by an increased hepatic cholesterol content. Moreover, newly absorbed cholesterol associated with chylomicron and chylomicron remnants could be atherogenic. The average intake of cholesterol for adult American men is reportedly about 450 mg/day, and for women about 300 mg/day.

2. Dietary Fatty Acids

Saturated Fatty Acids.   The saturated fatty acids in general have been shown to increase serum total cholesterol levels. Epidemiological studies, such as the Seven Countries Study (16), indicate that serum cholesterol level is raised by dietary saturated fatty acids. A variety of saturated fatty acids of different chain lengths are usually contained in the diet. Saturated fatty acids come mainly from animal fats, although some tropical plant oils are also enriched with these fatty acids. Palmitic acid (16:0) is the major saturated fatty acids in foods, but various sources of dietary fat are different from each other in their patterns of

saturated fatty acids. All saturated fatty acids have been generally considered to be hypercholesterolemic (17–19); however, recent studies have indicated that some saturated fatty acids, such as caprylic acid (8:0), caproic acid (10:0) (20,21) and stearic acid (18:0), are not hypercholesterolemic (22–24). Therefore, palmitic acid, myristic acid (14:0), and lauric acid (12:0) are major cholesterol-raising saturated fatty acids.

The mechanisms by which these saturated fatty acids increase the serum cholesterol have not been fully elucidated. Previous studies suggest that they reduce the clearance rate of apo B–containing lipoproteins through LDL-receptor pathway (25). Although the responsiveness to dietary saturated fatty acids varies among individuals, the serum cholesterol level rises by approximately 2.7 mg/dl (18,19) on the average for every 1% of total calories of saturated fatty acids substituted for other nutrients. In the American diet the major sources of saturated fatty acids are milk products (28%), meats and meat products (33%), baked goods (9%), and miscellaneous foods (30%) (26). Milk fat contained in butter, cheese, and ice cream is the most hypercholesterolemic of fats owing to its high content of palmitic and myristic acids. Although beef fat is the largest source of saturated fat in the American diet, its high content of stearic acid makes it less hypercholesterolemic than milk fat. Miscellaneous foods containing saturated fatty acids include various cooking fats and oils, snack foods, mixed dishes, and fried foods.

Recently *trans*-monounsaturated fatty acids (27,28) have been identified as hypercholesterolemic fat. The major fatty acid of this category is elaidic acid. This has 18 carbon atoms and one double bond located at the omega 9 position. The double bond in this fatty acid is in the *trans*-configuration. *Trans*-fatty acids are found in various margarines and shortenings. The *trans*-double bond gives them a rigid structure, similar to that of saturated fatty acids, which may account for their ability to raise the serum cholesterol level.

Unsaturated Fatty Acids.   Unsaturated fatty acids include monounsaturated and polyunsaturated fatty acids (Table 2). Monounsaturated fatty acids have one double bond, while polyunsaturated fatty acids have two or more. The major monounsaturated fatty acid is oleic acid. It has 18 carbon atoms and one double bond located at the omega 9 position, namely nine carbon atoms from the terminal end of the molecule. The double bond is in the *cis*-configuration. The major polyunsaturated fatty acid in the diet is linoleic acid (18:2 omega 6). Another important group is the omega 3 polyunsaturated fatty acids. These include linoleic acid (18:3 omega 3), eicosapentaenoic acid (20:5 omega 3) (EPA), and docosahexaenoic acid

Table 2   Unsaturated Fatty Acids in Foods

Fatty acid	Designation	Food (representative)
Oleic acid	18:1 w9	Olive oil
Linoleic acid	18:2 w6	Vegetable oil
		Soybeans
		Sesame
Linoleic acid	18:3 w3	Some plant oil
Eicosapentaenoic acid	20:5 w3	Fish
Docosahexaenoic acid	22:6 w3	Fish

(DHA) (22:6 omega 3). Each type of polyunsaturated fatty acids has different effects on lipoprotein metabolism.

Recent studies have revealed that oleic acid, one of the monounsaturated fatty acids, may have similar ability to reduce serum LDL levels to the polyunsaturated fatty acids (29,30). It is noteworthy that large quantities of oleic acid have been consumed for a long time in Mediterranean countries where the incidence of CHD is relatively low. Interestingly, olive oil is the major source of oleic acid in these countries.

Dietary linoleic acid, a common constituent of vegetable oils, has been considered to lower LDL-cholesterol level, and therefore it has been widely recommended for cholesterol-lowering diets. However, based on recent reports (29,30), it appears that the effect of linoleic acid on the reduction of serum cholesterol is not so remarkable. Notably, a high intake of linoleic acid moderately lowers serum HDL-cholesterol levels (29,31–33). Moreover, linoleic acid may suppress the immune system and promote the development of tumors in animals. Clinically, linoleic acid may increase the risk for cholesterol gall stones in some patients and promote the oxidation of LDL, which plays a crucial role in atherogenesis. Therefore, it is now recommended that we should limit the intake of linoleic acid to less than 10% of total calories (34). Vegetable oils from beans and plant seeds are the major sources of linoleic acid.

The very-long-chain omega 3 fatty acids such as EPA and DHA are contained mainly in fish oil. Although their cholesterol-lowering effect may be trivial, they may have other beneficial effects for CHD prevention; they have been shown to inhibit coronary thrombosis because of their ability to prevent the aggregation of platelets.

3. Other Dietary Factors

A variety of carbohydrates are present in the diet. These are simple sugars and complex carbohydrates such as starches, cellulose, and soluble fibers. The sources of di-

etary carbohydrates are fruits, vegetables including rice and wheat, legumes, cereals, and processed foods. In the regular American diet, which is relatively enriched with fat, carbohydrate intake averages approximately 45% of total calories. In contrast, in other countries such as Japan where dietary fat intake is low, carbohydrates provide between 50% and 70% of total calories. In these countries, the incidence of CHD is very low, suggesting that a low-fat, high-carbohydrate diet will protect against CHD. Moreover, a low-fat, high-carbohydrate diet may also be an appropriate means to maintain desirable cholesterol levels and decrease the prevalence of obesity. As recommended by the American Heart Association (35) and the NCEP, a major part of the reduction in saturated fatty acids should be replaced by carbohydrates (9).

In countries such as Japan where a high-carbohydrate diet is already the regular diet, a high-carbohydrate diet by itself is not beneficial, but low-fat and lower calorie intake may be more important to decrease serum cholesterol. A high-carbohydrate diet stimulates the synthesis of VLDL triglycerides (36,37) and may reduce LPL activity (38,39), leading to high levels of VLDL triglycerides and low levels of HDL cholesterol. From animal experiments, sucrose feeding increases visceral adiposity, which may cause multiple metabolic disorders including hyperlipidemia (40). Therefore, the intake of sucrose needs to be limited in the treatment of hyperlipidemia in patients with visceral fat obesity.

On the other hand, nondigestible carbohydrates include the insoluble fibers (for example, cellulose) and soluble fibers (gums, pectins, and psylliums). Although the insoluble fibers have almost no effect on serum cholesterol level, the soluble fibers have been reported to lower LDL-cholesterol concentrations. When relatively high amounts of the soluble fibers are consumed, the serum cholesterol level is lowered by about 3–5%, although the mechanism is unknown.

B. Physical Exercise

Physical exercise is recommended in the general treatment of obesity, mainly for the purpose of increasing energy expenditure. For the treatment of dyslipidemia, however, physical exercise may have additional actions in lipoprotein metabolism. It may increase LPL activity, and recent studies suggest that physical exercise can also protect against visceral fat accumulation, which may prevent the elevation of serum lipids even in obese subjects (7). A unique example may be the case of Japanese Sumo wrestlers, a model of massive obesity. They consume more than 7000 kcal/day to gain body weight, but simultaneously they exercise rigorously every day. They have low serum cholesterol levels probably due to a markedly low ratio of visceral fat to subcutaneous fat (V/S ratio) that is related to the rigorous physical exercise.

C. Drug Treatment

Significant advances have been made in the past two decades in the use of drugs for the treatment of hyperlipidemia. Some of these drugs indeed have been shown to reduce the risk of CHD. In the treatment of obesity with dyslipidemia, drug treatment should be recommended when serum levels cannot be normalized by diet and physical exercise. In the following sections, currently available cholesterol-lowering drugs will be reviewed.

1. HMG-CoA Reductase Inhibitors

These drugs are a relatively novel class of agents that have been widely used very effectively for the treatment of hyperlipidemia (Fig. 1). Their pharmacological action is the selective inhibition of the conversion of 3-hydroxy-3-methylglutaryl (HMG) coenzyme A (CoA) to mevalonic acid. This conversion is catabolized by the enzyme HMG-CoA reductase and is a rate-limiting step in cholesterol biosynthesis. The prototype drug of HMG-CoA reductase inhibitors is compactin (mevastatin), which was developed from *Penicillium citrinum* by Endo in Japan (41,42) in 1976. Compactin was demonstrated to reduce serum total cholesterol in animals and humans. The first derivative to reach the market was lovastatin (43), developed in the United States. Pravastatin and simvastatin subsequently became available. Many other agents, such as fluvastatin and atorvastatin, are under investigation. The target of HMG-CoA reductase inhibitors is mainly the liver. Inhibition of cholesterol synthesis reduces the cholesterol content of hepatocytes, which stimulates LDL-receptor synthesis (44,45). This action accelerates LDL clearance, thus lowering serum LDL levels. Lovastatin is usually given once or twice a day in three doses such as 20, 40, and 80 mg/day. At 20 mg/day, the LDL-cholesterol level is lowered by about 25%, at 40 mg/day by approximately 30%, and at 80 mg/day by 35%. Pravastatin has a potency similar to that of lovastatin. Simvastatin has about twice the potency. Recent clinical trials using HMG-CoA reductase inhibitors have demonstrated their efficacy in preventing CHD with respect to both primary prevention and secondary prevention.

The HMG-CoA reductase inhibitors have been shown to have few side effects for most patients, but a few patients have gastrointestinal symptoms, hepatotoxicity, and myopathy. Three grades of myopathy can occur: (1) a mild to moderate increase in creatine kinase without symp-

toms, (2) mild muscle symptoms such as myalgia, and (3) severe myopathy with myoglobinemia and acute tubular necrosis. These nonhepatic organ toxicities may occur when serum levels of HMG-CoA reductase inhibitors become high. High blood levels can occur in association with liver or renal diseases. Combination of the drug with cyclosporine or fibric acids may increase the incidence of myopathy.

2. Bile Acid Sequestrants

Cholestyramine and colestipol are two bile acid sequestrants currently available. Their action is totally confined to the intestinal tract; these drugs inhibit the reabsorption of bile acids, thereby interrupting their entry into the hepatic circulation. The reduction of bile acid return to the liver induces the conversion of cholesterol into bile acids, thereby lowering the hepatic content of cholesterol. The synthesis of LDL receptors is then increased, leading to the reduced concentration of serum LDL. By a moderate intake of bile acid sequestrants such as 8 g/day or 12 g/day of cholestyramine, LDL cholesterol is reduced by 15–25%. Bile acid sequestrant therapy may increase serum triglycerides by stimulating VLDL triglyceride synthesis. The effectiveness of bile acid sequentrants for reducing the risk of CHD has been demonstrated in the Lipid Research Clinics Coronary Primary Prevention Trial (46).

The major side effects of bile acid sequestrants include mainly constipation and gastrointestinal symptoms. These drugs can interfere with the absorption of certain drugs such as warfarin, thyroxine, lipid-soluble vitamins, digitalis derivatives, β-adrenergic agents, and thiazide diuretics.

3. Probucol

Probucol is a unique cholesterol-lowering drug and the mechanism of cholesterol reduction by this drug is unknown. However, it was shown to promote the LDL clearance via LDL receptor-independent pathway (47). One of the characteristic features of probucol is that it also decreases serum HDL cholesterol. Despite the reduction of serum HDL cholesterol by probucol, a number of reports have indicated that it remarkably reduces xanthoma in patients with homozygous familial hypercholesterolemia (48). It also prevents the development of atherosclerotic lesions in cholesterol-fed rabbits and in Watanabe heritable hyperlipidemic rabbits (WHHL) with genetic hypercholesterolemia due to an LDL-receptor defect. Probucol is a potent antioxidant, and it interferes with the LDL oxidation in vitro induced by active oxygens (49–51). In addition to its action as an antioxidant, probucol may en-

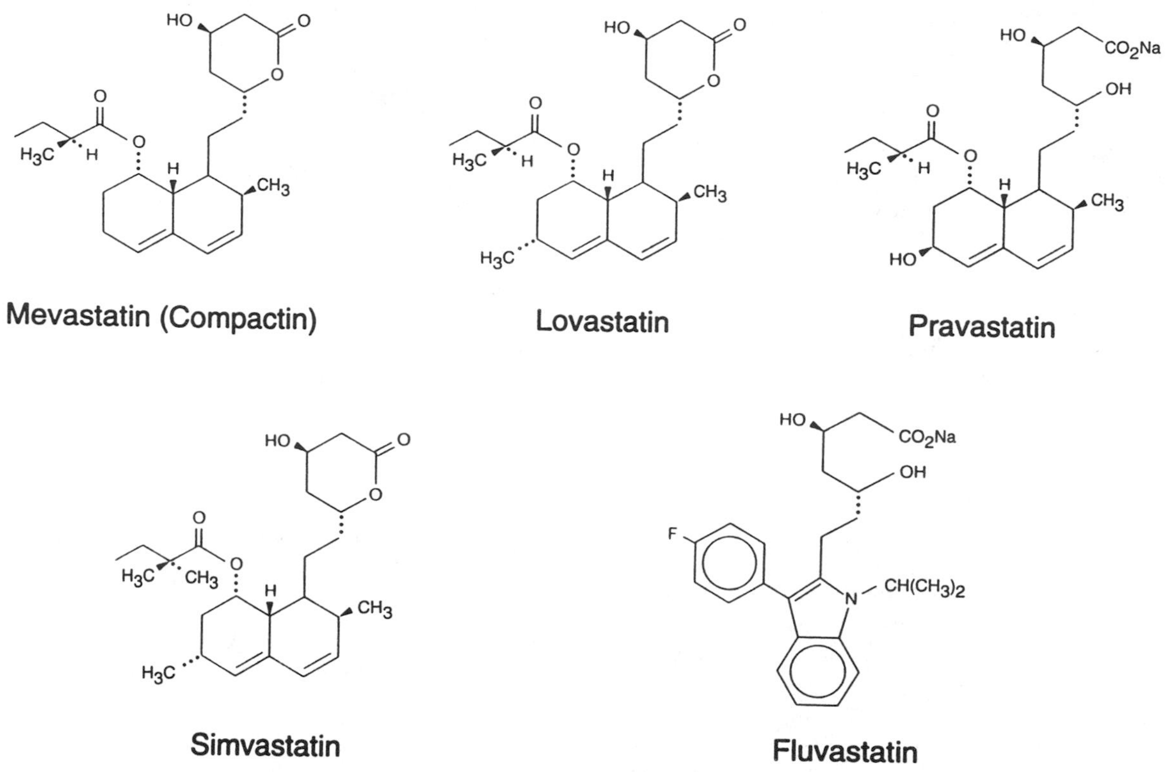

Figure 1   Structure formulas of HMG-CoA reductase inhibitors.

hance the reverse cholesterol transport that protects against cholesterol accumulation in peripheral tissues such as vascular walls. Probucol increases the activity and protein mass of plasma CETP (52,53) and it diminishes the particle size of HDL (52). Small HDL particles are known to facilitate cholesterol efflux from lipid-laden macrophages more markedly than large HDL particles, and recent evidence suggests that large apo E- and cholesteryl ester-rich HDL particles in CETP-deficient subjects are defective in terms of their antiatherosclerotic capacity (54). Furthermore, the addition of exogenous CETP to CETP-deficient plasma accelerates the formation of small very-high-density lipoprotein (VHDL)-like particles that are very active in removing cholesterol from macrophages (55). These findings raise the possibility that the HDL-lowering effect of probucol is not dangerous but rather advantageous. In any case, it is necessary to further examine the potential of probucol for preventing CHD in humans.

4.   Fibric Acids Derivatives

Figure 2 illustrates the chemical structure of fibric acid derivatives. These drugs have been used for a long time

for the treatment of hyperlipidemia (especially hypertriglyceridemia) (56). Although the mechanisms of the drug action have not been well clarified, some possible pharmacological actions have been suggested from clinical and animal studies. These include (1) the stimulation of LPL activity (57–59); (2) inhibition of cholesterol and bile acid synthesis (60–62); (3) acceleration of cholesterol secretion into bile; (4) induction of LDL-receptor activity (56), and so on. However, it still remains unknown whether these actions of fibric acid derivatives are direct or indirect. Fibric acid derivatives, one of the peroxisome proliferators, were shown to enhance the catabolism of plasma TG-rich lipoproteins. A recent report (63) has suggested that they work through suppression of apo C-III gene expression, which is due to transcriptional suppression of hepatic nuclear factor (HNF)-4 as well as displacement of HNF-4 from the apo C-III promoter. HNF-4 displacement exerted by peroxisome proliferators is mediated by peroxisome proliferators activated receptor (PPAR). Furthermore, Schoonjans et al. have recently demonstrated that fibrates and fatty acids induce LPL gene expression via PPAR (64).

Fibric acid derivatives in general reduce both serum cholesterol and triglycerides, but they are more effective

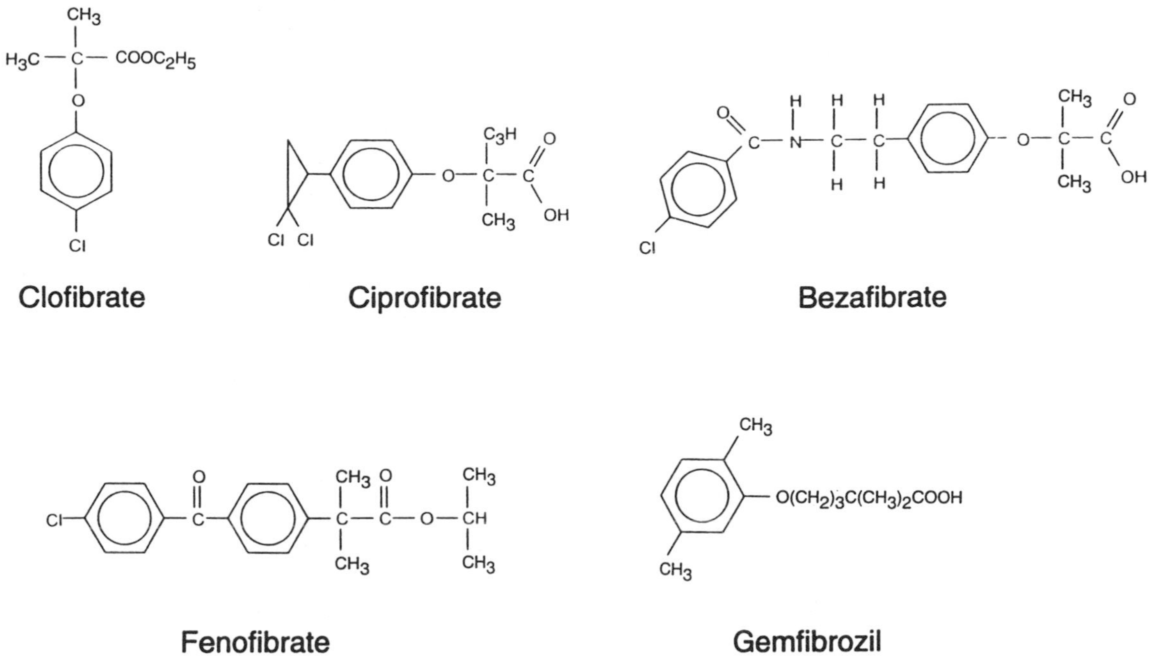

Figure 2 Structure formulas of fibric acid derivatives.

for the treatment of hypertriglyceridemia than hypercholesterolemia. Moreover, these drugs usually raise serum HDL-cholesterol levels. The currently available fibric acid derivatives throughout the world are clofibrate, clinofibrate, bezafibrate, gemfibrozil, and fenofibrate. The potency of pharmacological actions may differ among these agents, but there have been no reports that directly compare these drugs in terms of their efficacy and safety. As reported in the famous Helsinki Heart Study (65,66), gemfibrozil caused a reduction in the risk of CHD. In this study, the increase in HDL cholesterol was assumed to be partly responsible for this favorable result.

Regarding the side effects of fibric acid derivatives, these drugs can increase the risk for formation of cholesterol gall stones, which may be due to an enhanced secretion of cholesterol into bile. Since obese patients with hypertriglyceridemia already have a risk for gall stones, the use of these agents in obese subjects should be monitored cautiously. In some patients, myopathy or asymptomatic increase in creatine kinase can be observed. The risk for serious myopathy is seen only in patients with chronic renal failure. This is due to the elevation of drug concentrations in serum. An increase in liver enzymes can also be seen in some patients, although the elevation is mostly mild. Most of these adverse effects are usually not serious.

5. Nicotinic Acids

The mechanism of cholesterol-lowering effect of nicotinic acids has not been well elucidated. Some reports suggested that nicotinic acids reduce the secretion of VLDL particles by the liver. The drug may inhibit the release of free fatty acids from adipose tissues and stimulate LPl activity, resulting in a reduction of VLDL and LDL, and secondarily in an increase in serum HDL cholesterol.

Reductions of serum lipids after treatment with nicotinic acids are correlated to their dose. When a large dose, such as 4.5 g/day, is required, some patients cannot tolerate cutaneous responses such as flushing and itching and gastrointestinal irritation symptoms. Hepatotoxicity is also reported during treatment with nicotinic acids.

IV. TREATMENT OF PREDOMINANT HYPERTRIGLYCERIDEMIA IN OBESITY

A. Severe Hypertriglyceridemia

Obesity may cause severe hypertriglyceridemia, such as type V hyperlipidemia, in those who have genetic hypertriglyceridemia type IV. In patients who have serum triglyceride levels exceeding 1000 mg/dl, acute pancreatitis may occur. Therefore, the primary goal of dietary and drug therapy is to avoid the occurrence of acute pancreatitis. The most important goal of therapy of obese patients with type V hyperlipoproteinemia is to decrease the levels of circulating chylomicrons and VLDL. Multiple factors, such as genetic predisposition, glucose intolerance, and excess alcohol intake, often combine to produce type V hyperlipoproteinemia in obesity. In these patients, dietary therapy, of course, should be the first choice. In addition to weight reduction therapy such as calorie restriction, the intake of dietary fat needs to be limited. If the serum triglyceride level is not decreased below 1000 mg/dl with diet therapy alone, drug therapy must be considered. Fibric acid derivatives or nicotinic acid can be utilized.

B. Moderate Hypertriglyceridemia

A moderate hypertriglyceridemia means values in the range of 250–500 mg/dl in western countries and 150–500 mg/dl in Japan. The increase in serum triglycerides is attributed to its increment mainly in VLDL and partly in intermediate-density lipoprotein (IDL) or remnant lipoproteins in some patients. It is not established yet whether a mild hypertriglyceridemia by itself is atherogenic, but hypertriglyceridemia with a low-HDL-cholesterol level and an increase in remnant lipoproteins is atherogenic and should be treated. When obese patients have hypertriglyceridemia as one symptom of a multiple risk factor–clustering syndrome, classified as syndrome X or visceral fat obesity, it should be treated to reduce the coronary risk. In addition to weight reduction by calorie restriction, other secondary factors such as alcohol or excess dietary carbohydrate, especially sucrose, intake should be avoided in such a case. Several alternate drugs such as nicotinic acid and fibric acid derivatives can be used. If serum cholesterol level is also high, an HMG-CoA reductase inhibitor may be used. Fibric acids have been shown to raise serum HDL-cholesterol levels and also to reduce remnant lipoproteins, which may decrease the coronary risk.

V. IMPORTANCE OF THE REDUCTION OF VISCERAL FAT IN THE TREATMENT OF DYSLIPIDEMIA IN OBESITY

As already mentioned, visceral fat accumulation is one of the major causes of dyslipidemia in obesity. Visceral fat, including mesenteric fat and omental fat, has been known to be highly lipogenic and lipolytic. Therefore, its accumulation causes an increase in free fatty acid (FFA) release

into the portal circulation, which goes directly into the liver. FFA is a precursor of triglycerides and cholesterol. In addition, recent studies indicate that some FFAs may induce microsomal triglyceride transfer protein (MTP) (67), which is a limiting protein for lipoprotein assembly and secretion. An enhanced lipoprotein secretion from the liver to plasma may result in an increase in LDL particles and probably in the formation of small, dense LDL, which is one of the major risk factors of atherosclerosis. Therefore, it is essential to reduce visceral fat for the treatment of dyslipidemia in obese patients (68).

Accumulation of visceral fat may be induced by several factors including aging, menopause in females (69), over-intake of sucrose (70), physical inactivity (68), and so on. Among these factors, physical inactivity and undesirable dietary intake can be improved by appropriate instruction. Physical exercise and the reduction of sugar intake, in addition to the reduction of total energy intake, should be recommended for the purpose of visceral fat reduction. We have demonstrated, by examination of the interrelationship between the changes in body weight, body mass index (BMI), total and regional fat volume, and the changes in glucose and lipid metabolism, that the decrease in visceral fat/subcutaneous fat ratio (V/S ratio) as well as visceral fat volume was more strongly correlated with the improvement of plasma glucose and lipid metabolism compared to the decrease in body weight, BMI, total fat volume, and abdominal subcutaneous fat volume. Furthermore, a partial correlation analysis demonstrated that the metabolic improvements were associated with changes in visceral fat after control for changes in total adipose tissue volume (68).

Although no drug treatment for visceral fat accumulation has been developed yet, preliminary studies from our laboratory show that α-glucosidase inhibitor may reduce visceral fat accumulation, resulting in a decrease in serum lipids as well as improvement of glucose intolerance (71). The structure of AO-128, a new α-glucosidase inhibitor specific for intestinal maltose and sucrose, is shown in

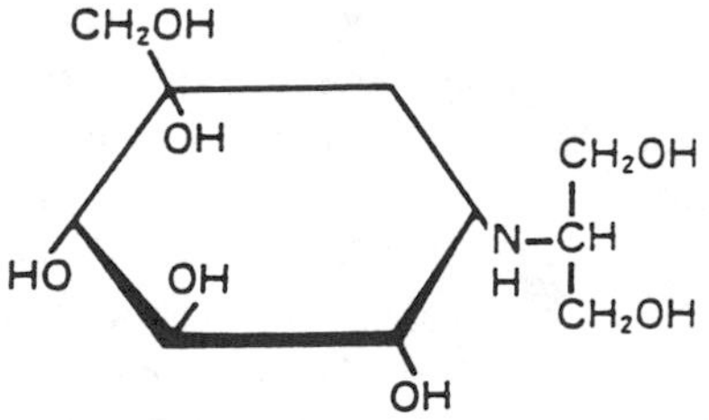

Figure 3 Structure formula of α-glucosidase inhibitor, AO-128.

Table 3 Changes of Clinical Features After Treatment with AO-128 (n = 9)

	Before	After
BMI (kg/m²)	31.8 ± 0.8	30.9 ± 0.7**
V/S ratio	0.44 ± 0.11	0.31 ± 0.05*
Glucose area (mg · hr/dl)	331 ± 57	247 ± 33*
Insulin area (μU · hr/ml)	120 ± 30	74 ± 15
Total cholesterol (mg/dl)	224 ± 14	212 ± 14
Triglyceride (mg/dl)	230 ± 68	115 ± 23
HDL cholesterol (mg/dl)	49 ± 3	48 ± 4

Mean ± SE.
*p < 0.05; **p < 0.01.
Source: Ref. 71.

Figure 3. Obese patients were given AO-128 three times daily (3 mg/day) before meals for 2 weeks, and changes in metabolic features and fat distribution were monitored after treatment with this drug. Although weight reduction was not remarkable, the plasma glucose area on an oral glucose tolerance test (O-GTT) significantly decreased and insulin area and plasma triglyceride tended to decrease with a substantial reduction in the V/S ratio (Table 3). Visceral fat accumulation is well known to correlate to the disturbance of glucose metabolism and hypertension in addition to dyslipidemia. Recent studies have revealed that the clustering of these risk factors may be an important and common background for the development of atherosclerosis. Therefore, treating dyslipidemia and visceral fat obesity should improve glucose metabolism and blood pressure as well (72).

Another approach for the treatment of hyperlipidemia associated with obesity may be insulin sensitizers such as troglitazone, pioglitazone, and BRL-49653. These drugs are thiazolidine derivatives that improve insulin resistance. They have been demonstrated in both animal models and humans to lower plasma glucose and insulin levels in an oral glucose tolerance test. Furthermore, they have been shown to reduce serum triglyceride levels (73,74), although no significant changes in serum total cholesterol or HDL cholesterol were observed. Therefore, these insulin sensitizers may be useful in the future for the treatment of both hyperlipidemia and diabetes mellitus in obese subjects.

VI. CONCLUSION

Profiles of lipoprotein abnormalities in obesity shows a wide variety of features, because a number of molecules related to lipid metabolism are involved. Basically, a common feature of metabolic abnormality of lipid in obesity may be overproduction of VLDL, due to overnutrition. In addition, genetic background in the disturbances of lipid metabolism may modify the phenotype of serum lipid and lipoprotein profiles. Therefore, the basic principle of the treatment of dyslipidemia in obesity is to reduce the energy intake for weight reduction. If lipid and lipoprotein abnormalities do not reach normal level, specific treatments for each lipoprotein disorder should be planned. Comments on the mechanism and the effect of lipid-lowering drugs were given in the text. Finally, the importance of the reduction of visceral fat to manage dyslipidemia in obesity was mentioned, which may improve not only dyslipidemia but also glucose intolerance and hypertension, and possibly prevent the development of atherosclerosis.

REFERENCES

1. Kannel WB, Gordon T, Castelli WP. Obesity, lipids, and glucose intolerance: the Framingham Study. Am J Clin Nutr 1979; 32:1238.
2. Garrison RJ, Wilson PW, Castelli WP, Feinleib M, Kannel WB, McNamara PM. Obesity and lipoprotein cholesterol in the Framingham Offspring Study. Metabolism 1980; 29:1053.
3. Shekelle RB, Shryock AM, Paul O, Lepper M, Stamler J, Liu S, Raynor WJ Jr: Diet, serum cholesterol, and death from coronary heart disease: the Western Electric Study. N Engl J Med 1981; 304:65.
4. Stamler J. Overweight, hypertension, hypercholesterolemia and coronary heart disease. In: Mananni M, Lewis B, Contaldo F, eds. Medical Complications of Obesity. London: Academic Press, 1979:191.
5. Arai T, Yamashita S, Hirano K, Sakai N, Kotani K, Nozaki S, Yamane M, Shinohara E, Islam AHMW, Ishigami M, Nakamura T, Takemura K, Tokunaga K, Matsuzawa Y. Marked increase of plasma cholesteryl ester transfer protein (CETP) in obese subjects—correlation between plasma CETP activity, high density lipoprotein-cholesterol levels and body fat distribution. Arterioscler Thromb 1994; 14:1129.
6. Fujioka S, Matsuzawa Y, Tokunaga K, Kawamoto T, Kobatake T, Keno Y, Kotani K, Yoshida S, Tarui S. Improvement of glucose and lipid metabolism associated with selective reduction of intra-abdominal visceral fat in premenopausal women with visceral fat obesity. Int J Obes 1991; 15:853.
7. Kanai H, Matsuzawa Y, Kotani K, Keno Y, Kobatake T, Nagai Y, Fujioka S, Tokunaga K, Tarui S. Close correlation of intra-abdominal fat accumulation to hypertension in obese women. Hypertension 1990; 16:484.

8. Nakamura T, Tokunaga K, Shimomura I, Nishida M, Yoshida S, Kotani K, Islam AHMW, Keno Y, Kobatake T, Nagai Y, Fujioka S, Tarui S, Matsuzawa Y. Contribution of visceral fat accumulation to the development of coronary artery disease in non-obese men. Atherosclerosis 1994; 107:239.

9. Expert Panel on Detection, Evaluation and Treatment of High Blood Cholesterol in Adults. Summary of the second report of the National Cholesterol Education Program (NCEP) Expert Panel on Detection, Evaluation and Treatment of High Blood Cholesterol in Adults (Adult Treatment Panel II). JAMA 1993; 269:3015.

10. Keys A, Anderson JT, Grande F. Serum cholesterol response to changes in the diet. II. The effect of cholesterol in the diet. Metabolism 1965; 14:759.

11. Hegsted DM. Serum cholesterol response to dietary cholesterol; a reevaluation. Am J Clin Nutr 1986; 44:299.

12. Mattson FH, Erickson BA, Klingman AM. Effect of dietary cholesterol on serum cholesterol in man. Am J Clin Nutr 1972; 25:589.

13. Jiao S, Matsuzawa Y, Matsubara K, Kihara S, Nakamura T, Tokunaga K, Kubo M, Tarui S. Increased activity of intestinal acyl-CoA: cholesterol acyltransferase in rats with streptozotocin-induced diabetes and restoration by insulin supplementation. Diabetes 1988; 37:342.

14. Jiao S, Moberly JB, Cole TG, Schonfeld G. Decreased activity of acyl-CoA: cholesterol acyltransferase by insulin in human intestinal cell line Caco-2. Diabetes 1989; 38:604.

15. Jiao S, Matsuzawa Y, Matsubara K, Kubo M, Tokunaga K, Odaka H, Ikeda H, Matsuo T, Tarui S. Abnormalities of plasma lipoprotein in a new genetically obese rat with non-insulin dependent diabetes mellitus (Wistar fatty rat). Int J Obes 1991; 15:487.

16. Keys A: Coronary heart disease in seven countries. Circulation 1970; 41(Suppl 1):1.

17. Ahrens EH, Hirsch J, Insull W, et al. The influence of dietary fats on serum-lipid levels in man. Lancet 1957; 1:943.

18. Keys A, Anderson JT, Grande F. Serum cholesterol response to changes in the diet. IV. Particular saturated fatty acids in the diet. Metabolism 1965; 14:776.

19. Hegsted DM, McGandy RB, Meyers ML, et al. Quantitative effects of dietary fat on serum cholesterol in man. Am J Clin Nutr 1965; 17:281.

20. Grande F. Dog serum lipid responses to dietary fats differing in the chain length of the saturated fatty acids. J Nutr 1962; 76:255.

21. Hashim SA, Arteaga A, van Itallie TB. Effect of a saturated medium chain triglyceride on serum-lipids in man. Lancet 1960; 1:1105.

22. Horlick L, Craig BM. Effect of long-chain polyunsaturated and saturated fatty acids'on the serum lipids of man. Lancet 1957; 2:566.

23. Grande F, Anderson JT, Keys A. Comparison of effects of palmitic and stearic acids in the diet on serum cholesterol in man. Am J Clin Nutr 1970; 23:1184.

24. Bonanome A, Grundy SM. Effect of dietary stearic acid on plasma cholesterol and lipoprotein levels. N Engl J Med 1988; 318:1244.

25. Spady DK, Dietschy JM. Dietary saturated triglycerides suppress hepatic low density lipoprotein receptors in the hamster. Proc Natl Acad Sci USA 1985; 82:4526.

26. Committee on Technological Options to Improve the Nutritional Attributes of Animal Products Board on Agriculture, National Research Council Designing Foods. Animal Product Options in the Marketplace. Washington, DC: National Academy Press, 1988.

27. Wilson JD. The quantification of cholesterol extension and degradation in the isotopic steady rate in the rat: the influence of dietary cholesterol. J Lipid Res 1964; 5:409.

28. Grundy SM. Trans monounsaturated fatty acids and serum cholesterol levels. N Engl J Med 1990; 323:480.

29. Mattson FH, Grundy SM. Comparison of effects of dietary saturated, monounsaturated, and polyunsaturated fatty acids on plasma lipids and lipoproteins in man. J Lipid Res 1985; 26:194.

30. Mensink RP, Katan MB. Effect of a diet enriched with monounsaturated or polyunsaturated fatty acids on levels of low-density and high-density lipoprotein cholesterol in healthy women and men. N Engl J Med 1989; 321:436.

31. Vega GL, Groszek E, Wolf R, Grundy SM. Influence of polyunsaturated fats on composition of plasma lipoproteins and apolipoproteins. J Lipid Res 1982; 23:811.

32. Shepherd J, Packard CJ, Patsch JR, Gotto AM Jr, Taunton OD. Effects of dietary polyunsaturated and saturated fat on the properties of high density lipoproteins and the metabolism of apolipoprotein A-I. J Clin Invest 1978; 61:1582.

33. Jackson RL, Kashyap ML, Barnhart RL, Allen C, Hogg E, Glueck CJ. Influence of polyunsaturated and saturated fats on plasma lipids and lipoproteins in man. Am J Clin Nutr 1984; 39:589.

34. Committee on Diet and Health Food and Nutrition Board, Commission on Life Sciences, National Research Council: Diet and Health. Implications for Reducing Chronic Disease Risk. Washington, DC; National Academy Press, 1989.

35. Grundy SM, Bilheimer D, Blackburn H, Brown WV, Kwiterovich PO Jr, Mattson F, Schonfeld G, Weidman WH. Rationale of the diet-heart statement of the American Heart Association. Report of Nutrition Committee. Circulation 1982; 65:839A.

36. Nestel PJ, Hirsch EZ. Triglyceride turnover after diets rich in carbohydrate or animal fat. Asian Ann Med 1965; 14:265.

37. Quarfordt SH, Frank A, Shames DM, Berman M, Steinberg D. Very low density lipoprotein triglyceride transport in type IV hyperlipoproteinemia and the effects of carbohydrate-rich diets. J Clin Invest 1970; 49:2281.

38. Nestel PJ, Carroll KF, Havenstein N. Plasma triglyceride response to carbohydrates, fats and caloric intake. Metabolism 1970; 19:1.

39. Fredrickson DS, Ono K, Davis LL. Lipolytic activity of post-heparin plasma in hypertriglyceridemia. J Lipid Res 1963; 4:24.

40. Kobatake T, Watanabe Y, Matsuzawa Y, Tokunaga K, Fujioka S, Kawamoto T, Keno Y, Tarui S, Yoshida H. Age-related changes in adrenergic $\alpha1$, $\alpha2$ and β receptors of rat white fat cell membranes: an analysis using (^{3}H) bunazosin as a novel ligand for the $\alpha1$ adrenoreceptor. J Lipid Res 1991; 32:191.

41. Endo A, Kuroda M, Tsujita Y. ML-236A, ML-236B, and ML-236C, new inhibitors of cholesterogenesis produced by *Penicillium citrinum*. J Antibiot (Tokyo) 1976; 29:1346.

42. Endo A, Kuroda M, Tanzawa K. Competitive inhibition of 3-hydroxy-3-methylglutaryl coenzyme A reductase by ML-236A and ML-236B fungal metabolites, having hypocholesterolemic activity. FEBS Lett 1976; 72:323.

43. Alberts AW, Chen J, Kuron G, Hunt V, Huff J, Hoffman C, Rothrock J, Lopez M, Joshua H, Harris E, Patchett A, Monaghan R, Currie S, Stapley E, Albers-Schonberg G, Hensens O, Hirshfield J, Hoogsteen K, Liesch J, Springer J. Mevinolin: a highly potent competitive inhibitor of hydroxymethylglutaryl-coenzyme A reductase and a cholesterol-lowering agent. Proc Natl Acad Sci USA 1980; 77:3957.

44. Kovanen PT, Bilheimer DW, Goldstein JL, et al. Regulatory role for hepatic low density lipoprotein receptors in vivo in the dog. Proc Natl Acad Sci USA 1981; 78:1194.

45. Bilheimer DW, Grundy SM, Brown MS, Goldstein JL. Mevinolin and colestipol stimulate receptor-mediated clearance of low density lipoprotein from plasma in familial hypercholesterolemia heterozygotes. Proc Natl Acad Sci USA 1983; 80:4124.

46. Lipid Research Clinics Program. The Lipid Research Clinics Coronary Primary Prevention Trial results. II. The relationship of reduction in incidence of coronary heart disease to cholesterol lowering. JAMA 1984; 251:351.

47. Kesaniemi YA, Grundy SM. Influence of probucol on cholesterol and lipoprotein metabolism in man. J Lipid Res 1984; 25:780.

48. Yamamoto A, Matsuzawa Y, Kishino B, Hayashi R, Hirobe K, Kikkawa T. Effects of probucol on homozygous cases of familial hypercholesterolemia. Atherosclerosis 1983; 48:157.

49. Parthasarathy S, Young S, Witztum JL, Pittman RC, Steinberg D. Probucol inhibits oxidative modification of low density lipoprotein. J Clin Invest 1986; 77:641.

50. Jialal I, Vega GL, Grundy SM. Physiologic levels of ascorbate inhibit the oxidative modification of low density lipoprotein. Atherosclerosis 1990; 82:185.

51. Jialal I, Grundy SM. Preservation of the endogenous antioxidants in low density lipoprotein by ascorbate but not probucol during oxidative modification. J Clin Invest 1991; 87:597.

52. Matsuzawa Y, Yamashita S, Funahashi T, Yamamoto A, Tarui S. Selective reduction of cholesterol in HDL2 fraction by probucol in familial hypercholesterolemia and hyperHDL2 cholesterolemia with abnormal cholesteryl ester transfer. Am J Cardiol 1988; 62:66B.

53. McPherson R, Hogue M, Milne RW, Tall AR, Marcel YL. Increase in plasma cholesteryl ester transfer protein during probucol treatment; relation to changes in high density lipoprotein composition. Arterioscler Thromb 1991; 11:476.

54. Ishigami M, Yamashita S, Sakai N, Hirano K, Hiraoka H, Kameda-Takemura K, Matsuzawa Y. Large and cholesteryl ester-rich high density lipoproteins in cholesteryl ester transfer protein (CETP) deficiency can not protect macrophages from cholesterol accumulation induced by acetylated low density lipoproteins. J Biochem 1994; 116:257.

55. Yamashita S, Ishigami M, Arai T, Sakai N, Hirano K, Kameda-Takemura K, Tokunaga K, Matsuzawa Y. Very high density lipoproteins induced by plasma cholesteryl ester transfer protein (CETP) have a potent antiatherogenic function. Ann NY Acad Sci 1995; 748:606.

56. Shepherd J, Packard CL. An overview of the effects of *p*-chlorophenoxyisobutyric acid derivatives on lipoprotein metabolism. In: Fears R, Prous JR, eds. Pharmacological Control of Hyperlipidemia. Barcelona, Spain: Science Publications, 1986:135.

57. Boberg J, Boberg M, Gross R, Grundy S, Augustin J, Brown V. The effect of treatment with clofibrate on hepatic triglyceride and lipoprotein lipase activities of postheparin plasma in male patients with hyperlipoproteinemia. Atherosclerosis 1977; 27:499.

58. Taylor KG, Holdsworth G, Dalton DJ. Clofibrate increases lipoprotein lipase activity in adipose tissue of hypertriglyceridaemic patients. Lancet 1977; 2:1106.

59. Nikkila EA, Huttunen JK, Ehnholm C. Effect of clofibrate on postheparin plasma triglyceride lipase activities in patients with hypertriglyceridemia. Metabolism 1977; 26:179.

60. Grundy SM, Ahrens EGJ, Salen G, Schreibman PH, Nestel PJ. Mechanism of action of clofibrate on cholesterol metabolism in patients with hyperlipidemia. J Lipid Res 1972; 13:531.

61. von Bergmann K, Leiss O. Effect of short-term treatment with bezafibrate and fenofibrate on biliary lipid metabolism in patients with hyperlipoproteinemia. Eur J Clin Invest 1984; 14:150.

62. Palmer RH. Effects of fenofibrate on bile lipid composition. Arteriosclerosis 1985; 5:631.

63. Hertz, R, Bishara-Shieban J, Bar-Tana J. Mode of action of peroxisome proliferators as hypolipidemic drugs; suppression of apolipoprotein C-III. J Biol Chem 1995; 270:13470.

64. Schoonjans K, Staels B, Deeb S, Auwerx J. Fibrates and fatty acids induce lipoprotein lipase gene expression via the peroxisome proliferator activated receptor. Circulation 1995; 92(Suppl):I-495 (abstract).

65. Frick MH, Elo O, Haapa K, Heinonen OP, Heinsalmi P, Helo P, Huttunen JK, Kaitaniemi P, Koskinen P, Manninen V, et al. Helsinki Heart Study: primary prevention trial with gemfibrozil in middle-aged men with dyslipidemia: safety

of treatment, changes in risk factors and incidence of coronary heart disease. N Engl J Med 1987; 317:1237.

66. Shimomura I, Tokunaga K, Kotani K, Keno Y, Yanase-Fujiwara M, Kanosue K, Jiao S, Funahashi T, Kobatake T, Yamamoto T, Matsuzawa Y. Marked reduction of acyl-CoA synthetase activity and mRNA in intra-abdominal visceral fat by physical exercise. Am J Physiol 1993; 265:E44.

67. Bennett AJ, Billett MA, Salter AM, White DA. Regulation of hamster hepatic microsomal triglyceride transfer protein mRNA levels by dietary fats. Biochem Biophys Res Commun 1995; 212:473.

68. Fujioka S, Matsuzawa Y, Tokunaga K, Kawamoto T, Kobatake T, Keno Y, Kotani K, Yoshida S, Tarui S. Improvement of glucose and lipid metabolism associated with selective reduction on intra-abdominal visceral fat in premenopausal women with visceral fat obesity. Int J Obes 1992; 15:853.

69. Kotani K, Tokunaga K, Fujioka S, Matsuzawa Y. Sexual dimorphism of age-related change in whole body fat distribution in the obese. Int J Obes 1994; 18:207.

70. Keno Y, Matsuzawa Y, Tokunaga K, Fujioka S, Kawamoto T, Kobatake T, Tarui S. High sucrose diet increases visceral fat accumulation in VMH-lesioned rats. Int J Obes 1991; 15:205.

71. Fujioka S, Matsuzawa Y, Tokunaga K, Keno Y, Kobatake T, Tarui S. Treatment of visceral fat obesity. Int J Obes 1991; 15:59.

72. Fujiwara T, Yoshioka S, Yoshioka T, Ushiyama I, Horikoshi H. Characterization of new oral antidiabetic agent CS-045; studies in KK and ob/ob mice and Zucker fatty rats. Diabetes 1988; 37:1549.

73. Ikeda H, Taketomi S, Sugiyama Y, et al. Effects of pioglitazone on glucose and lipid metabolism in normal and insulin resistant animals. Drug Res 1990; 40:156.

74. Suter SL, Nolan JJ, Wallace P, Gumbiner B, Olefsky JM. Metabolic effects of new oral hypoglycemic agent CS-045 in NIDDM subjects. Diabetes Care 1992; 15:193.

48

Pharmacological Treatment of Obesity

George A. Bray
Pennington Biomedical Research Center, Louisiana State University, Baton Rouge, Louisiana

I. INTRODUCTION

This chapter provides an up-to-date guide to the use of currently available medications for obesity and to new developments on the horizon for use in treatment of this problem. Following a brief historical review, the evolution of drug treatment will be briefly described, followed by a discussion of the drugs currently in use and those in development. The final section will focus on the clinical settings in which use of these agents may be indicated and the criteria for selecting appropriate treatment for an obese patient. First, a warning: Most available drugs for treatment of obesity are "scheduled" by the Drug Enforcement Agency. These "schedules" and Food and Drug Administration (FDA) guidelines are used by state medical licensing boards to develop regulations for medical practice that have the force of law. Use of any scheduled drug in a manner different from these regulations, regardless of whether that is reasonable medical practice or in the best interest of the patient, can result in criminal prosecution for a felony violation. Whether or not the regulations are based on truth, you can go to jail or have your license suspended. If you intend to use these drugs, check the regulations of your state licensing board.

II. EVOLUTION OF DRUG TREATMENT

A. Historical Review

Thyroid extract was the first drug used for the treatment of obesity (see Ref. 1), and its use has continued for nearly 75 years. However, thyroid hormones are not indicated for the treatment of obesity unless the patient is hypothyroid. Dinitrophenol (see Ref. 1) was the second drug introduced for the treatment of obesity after it was noted that textile workers lost weight when exposed to this drug. Dinitrophenol uncouples oxidative phosphorylation. Its use was discontinued because of serious side effects including neuropathies and cataracts. In 1937, dextroamphetamine (α-methyl phenethylamine) was introduced for the treatment of obesity (2). Over the next 30 years, a variety of drugs, including amphetamine, thyroid hormone, and digitalis, were used individually and in combination in a variety of different-colored pills for which the name "rainbow pills" was coined. These combinations were discontinued following the report of several deaths associated with their use in the United States (3). This mayhem, accompanied by the significant abuse potential for dextroamphetamine, led to a marked decrease in the use of drugs in the treatment of obesity and a "negative" amphetamine halo, which adumbrates all drugs for obesity. One goal of this chapter is to put the current use of these and related medications as a treatment for obesity into a modern perspective.

B. Mechanisms for Treatment of Obesity

1. Models

The past 25 years have been substantial strides in unraveling the mechanisms by which obesity might be treated. Several models have helped to provide a framework for understanding obesity and its treatment (4,5). In the pres-

---

Note added in second printing: On September 15, 1997, the U.S. Food and Drug Administration withdrew fenfluramine and dexfenfluramine from the market.

ent discussion, a feedback model for control of nutrient intake and metabolism will be used. This model consists of a controlled system (the body), which includes digestion, absorption, storage, and metabolism of carbohydrate, fat, and protein; a central control system in the brain; the afferent neural, hormonal, and nutrient signals that tell the brain about the state of the body; and finally, the efferent controls including the motor nervous system, the autonomic nervous system, and hormonal controls that regulate food intake and the "metabolic state" of the body (6). A more detailed discussion of this and other models may be found elsewhere (4–7).

2. Mechanisms

Food Intake. Three different mechanisms can be used to classify drug treatments for obesity. They are: (1) drugs that reduce food intake, (2) drugs that affect metabolism, and (3) drugs that increase energy expenditure. The first mechanism is to reduce food intake. Any agent that can reduce food intake has potential for treatment of obesity. Table 1 lists a number of receptor systems in the central nervous system that are known to reduce food intake or body weight.

Adrenergic Receptors. Stimulation of α_1-adrenergic receptors decreases food intake (8). Conversely, α_1-adrenergic antagonists can increase food intake and body weight (9). Stimulation of α_2-adrenergic receptors in the paraventricular nucleus of animals by clonidine or norepinephrine will increase food intake, particularly the intake of carbohydrate (10). Yohimbine, an α_2-adrenergic antagonist, blocks this effect of clonidine and in one clinical trial has been shown to reduce weight gain in women (11).

Stimulation of β_2-adrenergic receptors in the perifornical area decreases food intake. The increase in norepinephrine in the intraneuronal cleft by inhibition of norepinephrine reuptake and release of norepinephrine from nerve endings are two mechanisms by which the β_2-adrenergic receptors are activated by appetite-suppressing drugs. If β-adrenergic receptors are involved in feeding, blockade of these receptors with β-adrenergic blocking drugs might increase food intake and weight gain. This has been shown in patients treated with propranolol following a myocardial infarction (12).

Serotonin Receptors. Serotonin receptors also have significant effects on food intake (13). Cyproheptadine, a serotonin (5-HT) antagonist, significantly increases food intake and body weight. Stimulation of the 5-HT_{1A} receptors increases food intake (14). In contrast, drugs acting on the 5-HT_{1B} or 5-HT_{2C} serotonin receptors (MCPP,

CIN57493, quipazine, and MK212) decrease food intake (13). The racemic mixture of fenfluramine (rac-fenfluramine = Pondimin), a clinically available appetite suppressant drug (see below), acts to enhance serotonin release, which accounts for a significant part of its appetite suppressant effect. Partial blockade of serotonin reuptake by fenfluramine and a more complete blockade by fluoxetine (Prozac; Lovan) and sertraline (Zoloft) may account for the appetite suppressant effects of these agents (13). Some drugs that increase food intake, such as amitriptyline, may act by blocking serotonin receptors.

Dopamine Receptors. Dopaminergic receptors may also be involved in modulation of food intake as shown by the fact that sulpiride, an antagonist to dopamine D-1 receptors, can increase food intake. The dopaminergic receptors may also be involved in hedonic responses to food, and this may account for the abuse potential of some appetite-suppressing drugs that block reuptake of dopamine (15).

Histamine Receptors. Experimentally, histamine H_1 receptors in the central nervous system have been implicated in the feeding system (16). Destruction of histidine decarboxylase with α-fluoromethylhistidine or blockade of histamine receptors with clorpheniramine or meperamine can decrease food intake. Some of the weak neuroleptics such as chlorpromazine, thioridazine, and mesoridazine may increase body weight by acting on histamine receptors as well as on serotonin receptors.

GABA Receptors. Receptors for gamma aminobutyric acid (GABA) may increase or decrease food intake depending on the site of action in the brain (17). When GABA agonists are injected into the ventromedial hypothalamus, food intake is increased. In contrast, injection of GABA agonists into the lateral hypothalamus decreases food intake. Bicucculine, a drug that blocks GABA receptors, can also decrease food intake, providing further evidence that these receptors may play a physiological role in modulating food intake.

Peptides. A number of neurotransmitter peptides affect food intake by acting on specific receptors. Endogenous and exogenous opioids are potent stimulators of feeding (18). Dynorphin, acting primarily through kappa receptors, stimulates food intake when injected directly into the hypothalamus. Naloxone, an opioid antagonist, has been shown to decrease food intake in humans and animals (19).

Neuropeptide-Y (NPY) and galanin (GAL) both increase food intake, but their effect on the intake of macronutrients is very different (20). When animals are given a choice of individual macronutrients, NPY increases carbohydrate intake with little effect on the intake of other

Table 1 Mechanisms that Reduce Food Intake

System	Mechanism	Examples
Noradrenergic	α_1 Agonist	Phenylpropanolamine
	α_2 Antagonist	Yohimbine
	β_2 Agonist	Clenbuterol
	Stimulate NE release	Phentermine
	Block NE reuptake	Mazindol
Serotonergic	5-HT 1B or 1C agonist	Metergoline
	Stimulate 5-HT release	Fenfluramine
	Block reuptake	Fluoxetine
Dopaminergic	D-2 agonist	Apomorphine
Histaminergic	H-1 antagonist	Chlorpheniramine

macronutrients. Galanin, on the other hand, primarily increases the intake of fat in fat-preferring animals and carbohydrate in those with an innate preference for carbohydrate. A number of other peptides listed in Table 2 also affect intake of specific nutrients (21).

Nutrient Partitioning. A second major mechanism for modulating body fat stores is through control of "nutrient partitioning" (22). Nutrient partitioning refers to channeling or guiding dietary nutrients toward protein accretion and growth, toward milk synthesis and lactation, or toward fat storage. During the process of growth, ingested nutrients, particularly protein, are shunted toward linear growth rather than storage. As growth plateaus, nutrient partitioning into protein versus fat stores shifts toward fat storage. The degree of nutrient partitioning differs between

Table 2 Peptides that Stimulate or Suppress Feeding

Increase food intake	Decrease food intake
Dynorphin	Anorectin
β-Endorphin	Bombesin
Galanin	Calcitonin
Growth hormone-releasing hormone (low dose)	Cholecystokinin (CCK)
Neuropeptide Y (NPY)	Corticotropin-releasing hormone (CRH)
Somatostatin (low dose)	Cyclo-His-Pro
	Enterostatin
	Glucagon
	Insulin
	Neurotensin
	Oxytocin
	Thyrotropin-releasing hormone
	Vasopressin

individuals who are overfed (23), suggesting that drugs and techniques that modify nutrient partitioning have potential value in the treatment of obesity. Growth hormone directs nutrients toward linear growth and milk production. In adults, growth hormone shifts the partitioning of nutrients toward protein and away from fat. Gonadal hormones, particularly testosterone, are potent nutrient partitioning agents enhancing protein storage and decreasing fat storage, as is most evident at the onset of puberty. Adrenal glucocorticoids may also affect nutrient partitioning and fat distribution by enhancing protein catabolism and leading to increased fat storage particularly in the central or abdominal region. Finally, β-adrenergic drugs, particularly β_2- and/or β_3-adrenergic agonists, can enhance protein synthesis and reduce fat storage (24).

Thermogenesis. Thermogenesis is a third mechanism for modulating fat stores. There are three components to thermogenesis: (1) Resting metabolic rate, (2) facultative and nonfacultative thermogenesis in response to nutrients, and (3) physical activity.

Thyroid hormone represents the original thermogenic drugs (1). Deficiency of thyroid hormone reduces metabolic rate and hyperthyroidism increases metabolic rate. Because thyroid hormones can increase the loss of protein and calcium from the body (25), they should not be used to treat obesity per se.

Several other hormones are also thermogenic. Growth hormone is a nutrient-partitioning agent that is calorigenic in normal and obese humans and produces a shift in nutrient storage from fat to protein (26). Androgenic and anabolic steroids are also thermogenic, enhance nitrogen retention, and affect the depots in which fat is stored.

Some adrenergic agonists are also thermogenic. Norepinephrine and epinephrine have long been known to increase metabolic rate. Ephedrine, a synthetic noradrenergic drug, is thermogenic in normal and obese subjects and has been used therapeutically to treat obesity (27). Terbutaline is a β_2-adrenergic agonist that was developed for treatment of respiratory symptoms, but that is also thermogenic and induces weight loss (28). Several synthetic, thermogenic drugs have recently been developed (see below). Whether the shift from fat to protein storage and the thermogenic effects of these compounds are separable is unclear from the present literature.

III.   DRUGS APPROVED BY THE FDA FOR CLINICAL USE IN THE TREATMENT OF OBESITY

A.   Drugs Affecting Food Intake

1.   Noradrenergic Drugs that Release Norepinephrine or Block Its Reuptake into Neurons

Chemistry.   The chemical structure of the currently marketed drugs approved for the treatment of obesity is shown in Figure 1. They include two compounds in schedule III and four compounds in schedule IV. All of the currently available drugs, except mazindol, are derivatives of β-phenethylamine. Four types of chemical modification have been used to reduce the abuse potential and yet retain the appetite-suppressing effect. Most of these drugs probably act by releasing norepinephrine (NE) from stores in presynaptic vesicles. The NE in turn reduces food intake by acting on β-adrenergic receptors in the perifornical hypothalamus. As such, they have chemical similarities with NE and epinephrine. Mazindol, on the other hand, is a tricyclic compound and not a derivative of β-phenethylamine. It probably acts by blocking the reuptake of NE into presynaptic terminals, thus, increasing the interneuronal concentration of NE that acts on β-adrenergic receptors. However, its basic effects are similar to those of the β-phenethylamine derivatives (1).

Pharmacology.   Appetite suppressant drugs bind to hypothalamic receptors, and the potency of this binding is highly correlated with the degree of their suppression of appetite (29). The primary pharmacological effects of these drugs are on the CNS, on the cardiovascular system,

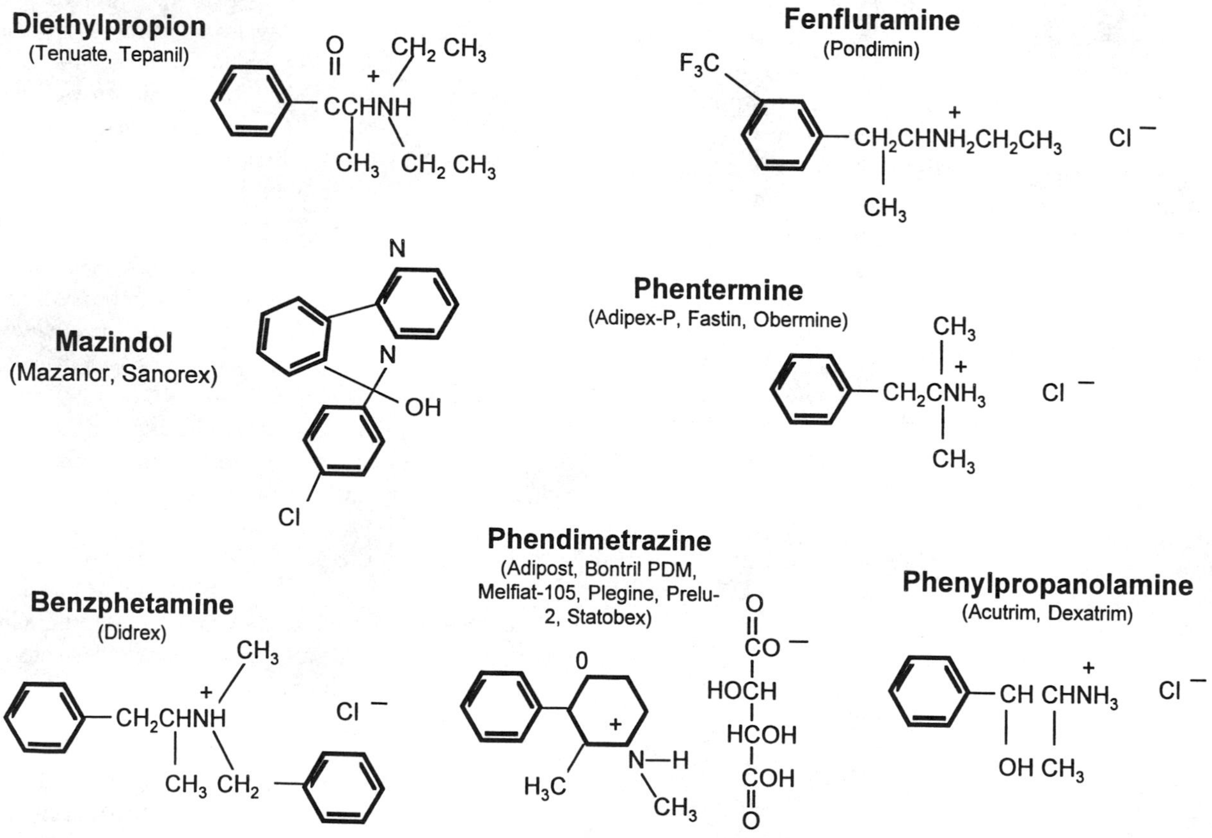

Figure 1   Formulas for drugs approved for the treatment of obesity.

and on peripheral metabolism. All of these drugs produce central excitation, manifested clinically as difficulty in sleeping and in some individuals as nervousness. This effect is most obvious shortly after the drug is started and wanes substantially with continued use. To a variable extent, these drugs may also increase heart rate and blood pressure. A slight elevation in blood pressure is seen mainly with amphetamine. This effect is usually short-lived and not clinically significant. Metabolic effects have also been observed with some of these drugs (when given systemically), including increased lipid mobilization in vitro and enhanced glucose uptake (1). The properties of the available appetite suppressants are shown in Table 3.

Efficacy. The largest review of effectiveness for noradrenergic appetite-suppressing drugs was conducted by the FDA in the early 1970s (30). There were 210 double-blind studies, which included 4543 patients treated with active drug and 3180 patients treated with placebo in trials lasting from 4 to 20 weeks. In over 90% of the studies, the active drug produced more weight loss than placebo. In 40% of the 160 trials comparing placebo and active drugs, the patients receiving the active drug lost significantly more weight than those receiving placebo. After 4 weeks of therapy, the dropout rate for patients on active drugs was 24.3% compared to 18.5% for those receiving placebo. Forty-four percent of patients on active drugs were able to lose 0.45 kg/week (1 lb/week) compared with only 26% of patients receiving placebo. In this study, 2% of patients receiving active drugs lost more than 1.4 kg/week (3 lb/week) compared to 1% with placebo. Average weight loss for patients taking the drug was 0.25 kg/week (0.56 lb/week) more than those receiving placebo at the end of 4 weeks of therapy (30). Studies comparing one active drug to another failed to show any significant advantage of one compound over another. From his study, "Scoville concluded that because drugs do not provide complete cures, . . . is no reason to reject them out of hand; partial success is clearly better than failure" (30).

Trials with noradrenergic appetite-suppressing drugs have been carried out for up to 60 weeks (Table 4). Several points are obvious in examining this table. First, there was considerable variation between studies in the amount of weight loss that occurred during the treatment with active drugs. Second, regardless of the length of study, which lasted up to 60 weeks, the drug-treated patients in

Table 3 Approved Appetite-Suppressing Drugs

	DEA schedule	Trade names	$t_{1/2}$ (hr)	Tablet size	Daily dose range (mg)
Noradrenergic agents					
Benzphetamine	III	Didrex	en12	25 or 50 mg before breakfast	25–150
Phendimetrazine	III	Anorex; Adipost; Bontril; Melfat −105; Obalan; Prelu-2; Plegine; Statobex; Wehless; and others	5–12	35 mg before meals or 105 mg (slow release)	70–210
Diethylpropion (Amfepramone)	IV	Tenuate; Tepanil; Generic	4–6	25 tab before meals 75 mg in A.M. (slow release)	75 75
Mazindol	IV	Mazanor Sanorex	10	1 mg before meals 2 mg before meals	1–3
Phentermine hydrochloride	IV	Fastin; Ionamin Phentrol; Adipex-P Obermine and generic	12–24	8, 15, 18.75, 30, and 37.5 mg	15–375
Phentermine resin	Not scheduled	Ionamin and generic	7–24	15 and 30 mg	25–75
Phenylpropanolamine		Dexatrim		25 and 75 mg	
Serotonergic agents					
Fenfluramine	IV	Pondimin	11–30	20 mg	60–120
Dexfenfluramine	IV	Redux	18–30	15 mg	30

Schedule II drugs have not been included because they are not approved by the FDA.

Table 4 Drug Treatment of Obesity

Drug	Dose (mg)	Duration (wk)	Patients (n) Drug	Patients (n) Placebo	Mean wt. loss (kg) Drug	Mean wt. loss (kg) Placebo	Net Wt. loss (kg)	Diet restriction	Ref.	Year
Schedule IV										
Diethylpropion	75 (slow release)	6	28	28	1.9	0.9	1.0	1200–1500 kcal	43	1971
	75 (slow release)	12	21	20	6.6	4.5	2.6	Restricted	10	1974
	25 thrice daily	12	41	33	9.1	4.5	4.6	1000 kcal	7	1975
	75 (slow release)	25	9	4	11.7	1.6	10.1	"Strict"	37	1975
	25 thrice daily	12	22	18	4.4	1.6	2.8	1000 kcal	38	1975
	25 thrice daily	12	20	17	6.8	4.4	2.4	1000 kcal	45	1975
	25 thrice daily	14	30	30	3.1	6.1	+3.0	—	14	1978
Mazindol	2	—	17		6	4.4	1.6	—	14	1978
	1 thrice daily	12	50	43	8.6	5.4	3.2	600 kcal	53	1973
	1 thrice daily	6	18	21	2.3	0.5	1.8	1000 kcal	16	1973
	1 thrice daily	6	15	12	5.1	1.2	3.9	None	32	1973
	1 thrice daily	12	14	12	8.5	2.4	6.1	None	32	1973
	1 thrice daily	12	32	33	6.4	2.6	3.8	1000 kcal	59	1974
	1 thrice daily	6	15	15	5.2	2.3	2.9	None	29‖	1975‖
	1 thrice daily	6	15	15	4.0	1.0	3.0	None	29‖	1975
	2	12	20	20	6.9	1.6	5.3	1200 kcal	30	1975
	2	12	40	20	8.4	1.1	7.3	1000 kcal	50	1975
	2	12	27	24	8.4	6.6	1.8	1000 kcal	51	1975
	2	12	19	23	1.4	0.3	1.1	Restricted	54	1975
	1 thrice daily	8	13	13	5.2	3.8	1.4	1200 kcal	58	1975
	2	12	19	23	5.0	3.6	1.4	2.3–4.5 kcal/kg	9	1975
	1	64	11	10	14.8	10.5	4.3	800–1200 kcal	19	1976
	4	20	28	28	1.9	+0.7	2.6	1000–1200 kcal	40	1976
	1	6	15	15	2.6	1	3.6	None	48	1976
	2	8	21	21	15.7	11.6	4.1	260 kcal	38	1977
	2	9	20	20	5.0	4.5	0.5	Behavior Mod.	8	1977
	2	9	20		3.4	4.5	+1.1	Behavior Mod.	8	1977
	1 thrice daily	14	30	30	3.8	2.7	1.1	Behavior Mod	14	1978
	2	6	72	28	3	0.77	3	None	60	1977
	2.11	12	114	114	4.2	1.2	3	None	33	1985
Phentermine	30 (resin complex)	16	21	16	9.2	5.2	4	9–10.2 kcal/lb	58	1972
	30 (resin complex)	16	19		8.8	5.2	3.6	9–12.2 kcal/lb	58	1972
	30	14	30	29	7.3	1.8	5.5	1000	24	1974
	30	6	78	77	3.8	1.5	2.3	1000	65,66	1975
	30	24	34		5.3	1.5	3.8	None	12	1977
	30	24	20	32	10.0	4.4	5.6	Individual diet	62	1977
	30	36	19	20	12.2	4.8	7.4	1000	42	1968
	30	36	14	11	13	4.8	8.2	1000	42	1968

Drug	Dose	Duration (wk)	No.		Drug wt loss	Placebo wt loss	Net wt loss	Diet	Ref.	Year
Schedule III										
Benzphetamine	97	8	50	50	1.9	0.9	1.0	1200–1500 kcal	43	1971
Chlorphentermine	20 twice daily	6	78		6.6	4.5	2.6	Restricted	10	1974
	20 twice daily to	6	76		9.1	4.5	4.6	1000 kcal	7	1975
	40 twice daily				11.7	1.6	10.1	"Strict"	37	1975
	20–40	6	38		4.4	1.6	2.8	1000 kcal	38	1975
	40	6	39		6.8	4.4	2.4	1000 kcal	45	1975
Clortermine	50	4	7 studies		3.1	6.1	+3.0	—	14	1978
	50	4	18 studies		3	4.4	1.6	—	14	1978
Phendimetrazine	105	12	36		8.6	5.4	3.2	600 kcal	53	1973
					2.3	0.5	1.8	1000 kcal	16	1973
Schedule II[a]										
Amphetamine	5 thrice daily	12	14		5.1	1.2	3.9	None	32	1973
	5 thrice daily	6	20		8.5	2.4	6.1	None	32	1973
	5 thrice daily	12	32		6.4	2.6	3.8	1000 kcal	59	1974
Phenmetrazine	75 (slow release)	6	53		5.2	2.3	2.9	None	29[b]	1975‖
	25 thrice daily	6	14		4.0	1.0	3.0	None	29[b]	1975
Unscheduled										
PPA	20 (fast acting) plus 55 (slow-acting)	12	53		6.9	1.6	5.3	1200 kcal	30	1975
					8.4	1.1	7.3	1000 kcal	50	1975
					8.4	6.6	1.8	1000 kcal	51	1975
					1.4	0.3	1.1	Restricted	54	1975
		4	33		5.2	3.8	1.4	1200 kcal	58	1975
	25 thrice daily with caffeine	2	70		5.0	3.6	1.4	2.3–4.5 kcal/kg	9	1975
					14.8	10.5	4.3	800–1200 kcal	19	1976
	25 thrice daily	2	51,36		1.9	+0.7	2.6	1000–1200 kcal	40	1976
Fluoxetine[b]	65		50		2.6	1		None	48	1976
	60	8	24		15.7	11.6		260 kcal	38	1977
	10	8	131		5.0	4.5	4.1	Behavior Mod.	8	1977
	20	8	131		3.4	4.5	0.5	Behavior Mod.	8	1977
	40	8	131		3.8	2.7	+1.1	Behavior Mod	14	1978
	60	8	131		3	0.77	1.1	None	60	1977
	60	52	14		4.2	1.2	3	None	33	1985
					9.2	5.2	3	9–10.2 kcal/lb	58	1972
	60	52			8.8	5.2	4	9–12.2 kcal/lb	58	1972
					7.3	1.8	3.6	1000	24	1974
	60	52	11		3.8	1.5	5.5	1000	65,66	1975
	60	6	11		5.3	1.5	2.3	None	12	1977
					10.0	4.4	3.8	Individual diet	62	1977
					12.2	4.8	5.6	1000	42	1968
					13	4.8	7.4	1000	42	1968
							8.2			

[a] Schedule categories provided by the Drug Enforcement Agency.
[b] Crossover study: same 15 patients first received drug and then received placebo.

almost all instances lost more weight than the placebo-treated patients. Third, there was no obvious advantage in terms of weight loss per week between drugs when studies lasting up to 20 weeks were separated from those beyond 20 weeks. Fourth, there is no obvious difference between medications and their relative effectiveness. A meta-analysis has been done on 40 of these randomized, placebo-controlled clinical trials using phentermine, dexfenfluramine, fenfluramine, mazindol, phenylpropanolamine, and ephedrine with and without caffeine in promoting weight loss (31). Phentermine, dexfenfluramine, and mazindol were identified as having effects significantly greater than that of phenylpropanolamine or ephedrine and its combinations. Effect size decreased significantly as the percentage of dropouts increased. This meta-analysis shows that combining literature data reveals significant differences in the outcome after treatment with different weight loss drugs.

Safety of Appetite Suppressants.   The safety of appetite suppressant drugs has been the subject of considerable discussion. Griffiths et al. (32), using baboons as subjects, have examined the reinforcing properties of intravenous preparations of several appetite-suppressing drugs and compared these effects to the potency of each drug to reduce food intake. The ratio of anorexiant dose to reinforcing dose, a measure of abuse potential, is shown for several drugs in Figure 3. At one extreme are diethylpropion and amphetamine. At the other extreme are fenflur-amine and phenylpropanolamine, which have no abuse potential. Although the ratio of appetite suppressant dose to reinforcing dose is of some utility in predicting abuse potential, it does not always correlate with clinical experience. For example, diethylpropion has been widely used as an appetite-suppressing drug, yet episodes of misuse are few. However, its appetite suppressant to reinforcing ratio in baboons is greater than that of amphetamine or phenmetrazine, both of which are readily abused. There is no indication for use of drugs in schedule II for treatment of obesity. Drugs in schedule IV are obviously preferred, but drugs in schedule III also have a low abuse potential.

Appetite-suppressing drugs have a number of side effects, which are summarized relative to placebo in Table 5 (33). Among the noradrenergic drugs, insomnia and dry mouth are among the most common side effects. Other responses tend to be less common, and none are serious.

2. Noradrenergic Drugs that Act as α_1-Adrenergic Agonists (There is only one approved drug in this class.)

Chemistry.   Phenylpropanolamine (Propadrine or PPA) is a series of isomers of pseudo- and norpseudo-ephedrine (34). The name phenylpropanolamine in the United States and the same name in Europe or Australia may represent different chemical isomers. This difference introduces confusion in interpreting some of the clinical literature, since

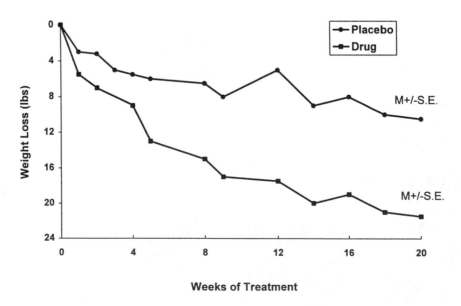

Figure 2   Effect of biphetamine or placebo on body weight. There were 30 patients in the drug-treated group and 15 in the placebo-treated group all of whom remained in treatment for the entire 20 weeks. (Adapted from 1.)

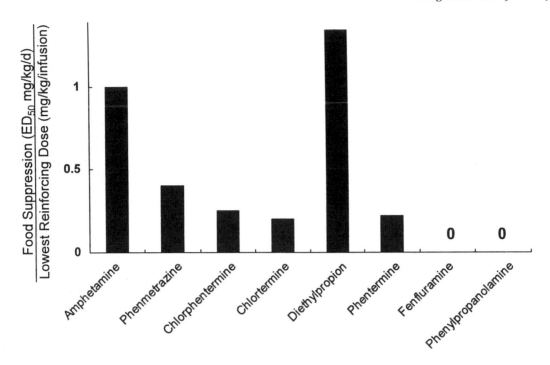

Figure 3 Effect of various anorexiant drugs on food intake and reinforcing potential. The lower the number, the smaller the reinforcing potential relative to food intake. (Adapted from Ref. 32.)

some of the isomers of phenylpropanolamine are considerably more effective in suppressing appetite than others (34).

Pharmacology. In animal studies, phenylpropanolamine has been shown to reduce food intake by acting on α_1-adrenergic receptors located in the paraventricular nucleus

(8). It is also a vasoconstrictor and this is its principal use in decongestants.

Efficacy. Phenylpropanolamine is used as both a nasal decongestant and a weight control drug (34). A summary by Weintraub of five trials of phenylpropanolamine versus placebo for weight loss is shown in Table 6 (35). The

Table 5 Side Effects of Various Anorexiant Drugs Compared with Those of Placebo

Drug[a]	Headache	Insomnia	Nervousness	Dizziness	Weakness or fatigue	Depression	Tremor	Anxiety	Rise in blood pressure	Tachycardia
Amphetamine/ Methamphetamine	2.2	6.9	2.1	6.3	0.9	1.2			38	30
Phenmetrazine	0.9	6.5	5.5	5.6	1.3	0.4			5	1.7
Phendimetrazine	0	4.6	1.4	6.6	—	0.9			—	—
Benzphetamine	—	2.1	7.4	2.2	0	0			—	—
Phentermine	—	3.2	—	1.6	—	1.0			—	—
Chlorphentermine	1.6	6.2	0.9	3.1	0.8	—			—	—
Clortermine	1.7	7.8	1.1	1.2	0.8	—			—	—
Diethylpropion	1.2	0.9	1.2	0.7	0.8	—			—	—
Mazindol	0.8	4.8	1.3	3.1	0.9	0.4			0	—
Fenfluramine	1.15	1.4	0.7	1.0	1.0	3.2			—	—
Placebo[c]	3.4	1.8	3.6	1.0	2.8	1.1			0.1	0.3
Fluoxetine 60 mg	0.6	2.7	1.3	1.6	n.o.	—	2.8	2.2	—	—

Table 5 (*Continued.*)

	Palpitations	Dry mouth	Nausea	Abdominal discomfort	Constipation	Diarrhea	Edema	Polyuria or frequency	Drowsiness	Sweating
Amphetamine/ methamphetamine	25	1.6	1.8	0.9	2.7	—	—	1.8[b]		
Phenmetrazine	20	3.8	3.3	0.4	1.6	—	2.3[b]	0		
Phendimetrazine	—	4.6	—	2.5	1.8	—	—	9.5[b]		
Benzphetamine	0.7	1.7	2.0	3.0	—	—	—	—		
Phentermine	—	0	2.7	—	—	—	—	—		
Chlorphentermine	—	3.7	2.3	—	2.5	—	5.0[b]	—		
Clortermine	—	3.4	1.1	—	2.5	—	2.6[b]	—		
Diethylpropion	—	1.2	3.2	1.3	1.8	—	—	—		
Mazindol	16	3.5	3.4	0.6	0.9	—	—	3.3[b]		
Fenfluramine	—	3.0	1.1	—	—	7.2	—	1.5[b]		
Placebo[c]	0.1	3.1	1.4	2.7	3.7	0	1.8	0		
Fluoxetine 60 mg	—	0.8	2.9	—	1.8	2.0	—	—	4.2	1.4

—, Data were not sufficient to make comparisons possible.

[a]The data given for each drug are expressed as the ratios of the percentage of drug subjects compared to the percentage of placebo subjects reporting each side effect. The placebo data represent the percentage of placebo subjects reporting each side effect (Br J Psychiatry 153:77–86).

[b]Percentage of patients reporting the symptom.

[c]Placebo-treated patients also experienced dysuria (0.3%) and chills (0.1%).

Source: Compiled by the author. Data derived from publications referenced in Bray GA. The Obese Patient. Major Problems in Internal Medicine, Vol 9. Philadelphia: WB Saunders, 1976:1–450.

mean weight loss for relatively short-term drug trials with PPA is 0.23 kg/week. Phenylpropanolamine thus produces significantly more weight loss than placebo, but the magnitude of this weight loss is smaller than with the noradrenergic drugs discussed above.

Safety. Two major concerns have been raised about phenylpropanolamine. The first is the potential for this drug, when combined with caffeine, to serve as a "look alike" drug in illicit trade. For this reason, the combination of phenylpropanolamine and caffeine is no longer allowed

Table 6 Clinical Trials of Phenylpropanolamine Alone

Study (date)	Study design	Comparison agent	Daily dosage (mg) Single	Total	Study length (weeks)	Number of subjects (dropouts) PPA	Placebo	Weight loss (gain) (kg/week) PPA	Placebo
Hoebel et al. (1975)	Crossover	Placebo	25	75	2	70 total completed		0.46 0.32	0.28 (0.05)
Sebok (1977)	Parallel	Placebo	50	100	6	36 (6)	36 (12)	0.47	0.27
Noble and Kalkhof (1981)	Parallel	Placebo	75	75	6	120 (1)	123 (8)	0.73	0.45
Noble and Respess (1981)	Crossover[a]	Placebo	50	50	6/-[a]	173 (68)	88 (36)	0.67	0.47
Settel (1965)	Crossover	Placebo	25	75	3/3	42 (12)	total	0.67	0.32
Schteingart (1992)	Parallel	Placebo	75	75	6	51 (15)	50 (23)	0.43	0.18
Greenway (1989)	Parallel	Placebo	75	75	12	50 (5)	48 (8)	0.23	0.10

[a]First 6 weeks only of study analyzed (as parallel group study).

Source: Compiled by the author from data in Alfschuler and Frazer, Curr Ther Res 1986; 40:211–217. Greenway, Clin Ther 1989; 11:584–589. Weintraub, Clin Pharm 1986; 39:501–509.

Alfschuler, Int J Obes 1982; 6:549–556.

in legitimate commerce in the United States. The second concern is that phenylpropanolamine may raise blood pressure. The literature is conflicting but suggests that high doses (above 75 mg) of the drug can raise blood pressure, but if the drug is used according to directions, this is a minor problem (36).

3. Serotonergic Drugs (*d,l*-Fenfluramine)

Chemistry. Fenfluramine is a β-phenethylamine (Fig. 1). Pharmacologically, however, the substitution of a trifluromethane group in the meta position on the phenyl ring completely alters the function of this drug (14).

Pharmacology. Fenfluramine is metabolized in the liver to norfenfluramine, which is also active. The half-life in the circulation of *d*-fenfluramine is 18 hr and of *d*-norfenfluramine 30 hr. The *d*-norfenfluramine enhances serotonin release from the neuron and acts as an agonist for $5-HT_{2c}$ receptors, which decrease food intake. *d*-Fenfluramine acts to block reuptake of serotonin into the neuron. The increased serotonin in the neuronal cleft along with *d*-norfenfluramine is believed to reduce food intake. Of the two isomers in the racemic mixture of fenfluramine, the *d*-isomer (dexfenfluramine) appears to be the anorectic compound (13). The L-isomer blocks dopamine reuptake, but not serotonin.

Efficacy. The clinical efficacy of *d,l*,-fenfluramine has been demonstrated in trials of short and long duration conducted over the past 30 years (Table 7). More than a dozen trials have been conducted with fenfluramine or dexfenfluramine (37). The largest is the double-blind, randomized, placebo-controlled, multicenter International Dexfenfluramine (INDEX) Trial, which enrolled 527 placebo-treated and 418 drug-treated patients (38). The INDEX Trial showed that the patients treated with dexfenfluramine lost 10.3% of initial weight at 12 months compared to 7.2% in the placebo group. Weight loss plateaued at approximately 6 months and was better maintained for the remaining 6 months in the drug-treated patients than in those receiving placebo. The placebo-treated patients in this trial also lost significant amounts of weight. Weight loss in placebo-treated groups in various trials varies considerably (39). At one extreme, weight loss in placebo-treated patients is not different from baseline. At the other extreme, rapid weight loss is reported in placebo-treated patients using very-low-calorie diets. This is accounted for by the use of very-low-calorie diets in at least two centers when the addition of drug did not produce any incremental weight loss (40,41).

Data from a number of trials are available with fluoxetine (Prozac, Lovan), a drug approved for treatment of depression, but not obesity. In a clinical trial lasting up to 8 weeks, fluoxetine, 10, 20, 40, 60, or 80 mg/day, produced a dose-dependent weight loss (42). In longer-term trials, fluoxetine has been shown to be significantly better than placebo in a number of trials. In a study by Darga et al. (43), weight loss with fluoxetine reached its nadir at 12–16 weeks and was significantly greater in drug-treated than in placebo-treated patients. After 16 weeks, the drug-treated regained weight even though continuing to take the medication. This weight gain was accompanied by an increased variance in body weight, indicating that some patients regained more weight while others maintained their weight loss.

Safety. Both *d,l*-fenfluramine and dexfenfluramine have a wide margin of safety. The profile of side effects for this compound versus the noradrenergic compounds is shown in Table 5. Dry mouth and insomnia occur with both groups. The diarrhea seen with fenfluramine is replaced by constipation with the noradrenergic drugs. There have been several reports of pulmonary hypertension, which is a rare but serious problem (44). A number of side effects have been reported with fluoxetine. In general, they are minor and tend to subside with continued treatment (Table 5).

4. Stepped or Combination Therapy

From the previous discussion, it is obvious that at least two mechanisms mediate the clinically effective appetite-suppressing drugs, one involving noradrenergic receptors and a second involving serotonergic receptors. Since a plateau in weight loss is observed with both drugs, the potential for achieving a greater weight loss or reduced side effects by using a combination of noradrenergic and serotonergic drugs has been evaluated by Weintraub and his colleagues (45). Their first trial showed that a combination of phentermine and *d,l*-fenfluramine used at half-maximal doses produced as much weight loss as either drug at maximal dose, but was accompanied by fewer side effects (45). With this positive result, they conducted a 4-year trial using a combination of phentermine and *d,l*-fenfluramine (46). Figure 6 shows the weight loss during the first double-blind phase of this trial (47). During the first 6-week run-in period, all patients were treated with a combination of behavior modification, exercise, and individual nutritional counseling. Subjects were randomized into drug or placebo treatment groups at the end of the 6-week run-in period, using minimization techniques to

Table 7   Drug Treatment of Obesity

Drug	Dose (mg)	Duration (weeks)	Patients (n)		Mean wt. loss (kg)		Net wt. loss (kg)	Diet restriction	Ref.	Year
			Drug	Placebo	Drug	Placebo				
d,l-Fenfluramine	20 twice daily	6	44	43	2.4	0.3	2.1	None	17	1975
	40	6	23	43	1.7	0.3	4.1	None	17	1975
	20 thrice daily	12	56	58	6.6	2.5	4.1	None	57	1976
	60 (extentabs)	12	60		4.7	2.5	2.2	None	57	1976
	60 twice daily	16	11	11	5.8	9.4	3.6	1000–1800 kcal	46	1976
	60 (pacaps)	12	18	22	3.0	0.0	3.0	None	11	1988
	60 (pacaps)	24	25	10	14.5	6.0	8.5	1000–1200 kcal	13	1981
	60 (pacaps)		32 (behavior mod.)		10.9	6.0	4.9	1000–1200 kcal	13	1981
	60 (pacaps)		23 (combined)		15.3	6.0	9.3	100–1200 kcal	13	1981
		52	21							
	60 (pacaps)	10	26	21	0	3.0	3.0	Dietary advice	18	1983
	60	36	16	25	5.9	3.3	2.6	18–20 kcal	61	1983
	20	36	8	13	11.9	9.5	2.4	1200 kcal	52	1985
	40	36	9		12.7	9.5	3.2	1200 kcal	52	1985
	60				10.6	9.5	1.1	1200 kcal	52	1985
Fenfluramine plus phentermine	60, 15	28	62	59	14.3	4.6	9.7		64	1992
Dexfenfluramine	15 twice daily	12	19 (hospital)	20 (hospital)	2.8 / 5.3	1.7	4.5	Counseling	22	1985
	15 twice daily	12	GP26	GP24	8.1	1.4	3.9	Counseling	22	1985
	30 twice daily	12	64	69	9.8	3.5	4.6	16 kcal/kg	20	1988
	15 twice daily	52	295	268	6.2	7.2	2.6	>400 kcal/day	26	1989
	15 twice daily	24	19	23	5.8	2.6	3.6	1200–1500 kg	44	1990
		26				2.9	8.7	Calories by 24–40%	23	1988

Schedule categories provided by the Drug Enforcement Agency.

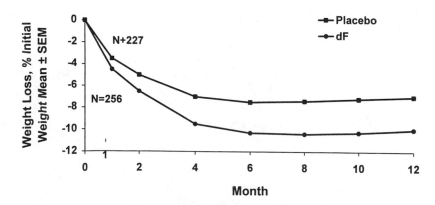

Figure 4   Effect of treatment with dexfenfluramine or placebo on body weight. This year-long trial was conducted in seven centers. Approximately half of the patients who began the trial remained in treatment at the end of the year, and drug-treated patients lost significantly more weight. (Redrawn from Ref. 38.)

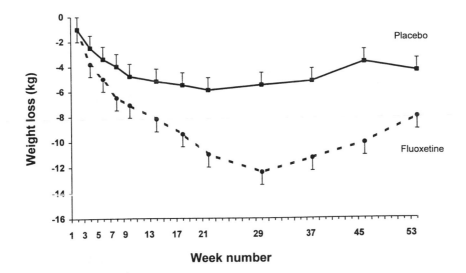

Figure 5 Effect of treatment with fluoxetine or placebo on body weight. The weight loss of the drug-treated group reached a nadir 29 weeks after beginning the drug and tended to regain weight thereafter. (From Ref. 43.)

make the groups as comparable as possible. Thus, at the beginning of the first double-blind drug trial, the placebo- and drug-treated patients had similar weights. Little additional weight was lost by the placebo-treated group during the ensuing 28 weeks. The mean overall weight loss in the placebo-treated group from the beginning of the run-in period to week 32 was 4.6 ± 0.8 kg (4.9 ± 0.9%)

of initial weight. In contrast, the fenfluramine-treated group continued to lose weight with an average weight loss of 14.2 ± 0.9 kg (15.9 ± 0.9% from baseline) over 32 weeks. Nearly half of the patients in this drug trial had an initial and sustained therapeutic benefit (46). Continuous therapy was more effective than intermittent therapy. Patients receiving active drugs continued to respond over

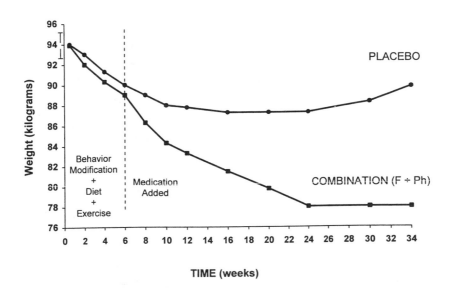

Figure 6 Effect of combination treatment with fenfluramine and phentermine. During the 6-week run-in period both groups were treated with diet, exercise, and behavior modification. Patients were randomized using minimization techniques to assure a close match at the start of the double-blind period. during the double-blind period the placebo-treated patients lost almost no additional weight, whereas the drug-treated patients plateaued at a significantly lower weight. (From Ref. 46.)

the entire 3½ years. When the drugs were withdrawn after 3½ years, patients regained weight, proving that drugs do not work when not taken. No serious untoward side effects were observed in this trial. Additional studies using combined therapy in different doses are clearly indicated.

IV. POTENTIAL AREAS FOR NEW DRUG DEVELOPMENTS

A. Drugs that Suppress Food Intake

1. Sibutramine: An Amine Reuptake Inhibitor

Reuptake of monoamines by nerve terminals is a major mechanism for terminating the action of neurotransmitters. A number of drugs that affect the monoamine reuptake systems reduce body weight (see Section III). In addition to mazindol and fenfluramine which work by this mechanism, a new drug, sibutramine, is in clinical trial for treatment of obesity. It inhibits the reuptake of both serotonin and norepinephrine. In a dose-ranging study, Weintraub et al. (47) found that during an 8-week trial, placebo-treated patients ($n = 19$) lost 1.4 ± 2.1 kg compared to 2.9 ± 2.3 kg for patients treated with 5 mg/day of sibutramine ($n = 18$) and 5.0 ± 2.7 kg for patients treated with 20 mg/day of sibutramine ($n = 18$). Weight loss with sibutramine has been reported from one site of a large multicenter trial that has recently been completed (48). The dose response to sibutramine was again evident. Weight loss was 0.96 ± 0.72 kg ($0.8 \pm 0.96\%$) for placebo and 12.25 ± 0.69 kg ($8.3 \pm 0.94\%$) for the 30 mg/day dose.

2. Antagonists of Opioid Receptors

Naloxone and naltrexone are opioid receptor antagonists and both acutely reduce food intake in human subjects (18). However, three clinical trials with naltrexone, a long-acting derivative of naloxone, showed that doses ranging from 50 to 300 mg/day administered for 8 weeks did not have a significant effect on body weight except for the female cohort in one of the three studies (49–52).

3. Biguanides

Metformin has recently been approved by the FDA to treat non-insulin-dependent (type II) diabetes mellitus. In contrast to sulfonylureas, which usually increase weight, metformin produces weight losses ranging from 2.3 kg (5 lb) in 7 months to 6.0 kg (13.2 lb) at the end of the period of observation, which lasted in some cases, up to 2 years (53).

4. α₂-Adrenergic Antagonists

Clonidine is an α_2-adrenergic agonist that stimulates food intake in experimental animals (54). Thus, blockade of α_2-adrenergic receptors might reduce food intake. Yohimbine, an α_2-adrenergic blocking drug, showed no effect in two studies with males (55,56), but in one study with females, there was a significant weight loss in the yohimbine-treated subjects (11). Yohimbine has also been reported to reduce local fat deposits when applied topically in a cream (57).

5. Peptides

Cholecystokinin. A number of neuropeptides are known to decrease or increase food intake (see Table 2). Agonists to the peptides that decrease food intake and antagonists to those that increase food intake offer viable strategies to develop new drugs. Cholecystokinin suppresses food intake when administered peripherally. In clinical studies the infusion of cholecystokinin prior to ingestion of a meal reduces food intake by producing early satiety in both lean and obese subjects (58,59). Antagonists to the CCK receptors (Devazepide and L-365; 260) increase food intake in experimental animals, suggesting a functional role for CCK (60). Cholecystokinin agonists are being developed for potential clinical use in treatment of obesity (61). None of the other anorectic peptides have yet spawned potentially viable drugs.

Neuropeptide Y. Neuropeptide Y is one of the most potent stimulators of food intake and it strongly stimulates carbohydrate intake. Antagonists to neuropeptide Y may thus be particularly interesting because they might affect the intake of specific macronutrients. The nutrient specificity of these peptides makes them good candidates for future research (21).

Bombesin. Gastrin-releasing peptide (GRP) isolated from the gut has been shown to decrease food intake. In clinical studies, peripheral administration of bombesin has been shown to produce a dose-dependent reduction in food intake. Studies in experimental animals suggest that the bombesin receptors may be the neuromedin-B receptors, since a combination of neuromedin-B and GRP can reduce food intake (62).

Enterostatin. Enterostatin is the signal pentapeptide produced when procolipase, a pancreatic acinar cell proenzyme, is secreted into the intestine. This pentapeptide has one of two structures in most mammalian species: Val-Pro-Asp-Pro-Arg (VPDPR) or Ala-Pro-Gly-Pro-Arg

(APGPR). In a variety of experimental animals, enterostatin has been shown to selectively reduce fat intake without influencing either carbohydrate or protein intake (63). In one clinical study, enterostatin at doses of 4 and 16 mg given intravenously to obese healthy volunteers was without effect on food intake (64).

Amylin and Glucagon. Amylin is a 37-amino-acid pancreatic peptide that reduces food intake in experimental animals. No clinical data are available. In contrast, pancreatic glucagon has been shown to reduce food intake in experimental animals and human beings (65). Glucagon-like peptide-1 (GLP-1) has been shown to reduce food intake when given centrally in animals, and an antagonist to the peptide will increase food intake, suggesting a possible physiological role for this peptide (66).

Leptin (ob protein). Although not yet tried clinically (67), the gene product whose defect produces obesity in the *ob/ob* (obese) mouse has been shown to reduce food intake in these animals and in animals that became obese eating a high-fat diet. This peptide, which contains 167 amino acids, reduces food intake when injected into obese animals and is increased in relation to body fat in humans (68).

6. Sugar Acids

A number of small sugar acids and lactones have been reported to either increase or decrease food intake in experimental animals. No clinical studies with these derivatives have yet been reported (69).

B. Nutrient Partitioning

1. Preabsorptive Nutrient Partitioning (Nutrient Availability)

Several approaches have been used to alter nutrient availability by altering digestion and absorption in the gastrointestinal tract, which will lead to nutrient partitioning of ingested food between absorption and fecal excretion.

Inhibitors of Gastric Emptying. A delay in gastric emptying might reduce food intake by increasing stomach volume and signaling early satiety. (—)-Threo-chlorocitric acid was found to reduce body weight experimentally in association with delayed gastric emptying (70). Clinical trials on this compound are suggestive but the development of this drug may have been terminated since no recent studies have been published.

Inhibitors of Carbohydrate Digestion. Amylase inhibitors from natural sources (jack beans), as well as α-glucosidase inhibitors and disaccharidase inhibitors, such as acarbose, miglitol, and AO128 (71), have been shown to reduce the digestion of starch and disaccharides such as maltose, lactose, and sucrose. Of these compounds the disaccharidase and sucrase inhibitors will reduce digestion of disaccharides to their monosaccharides and thus reduce absorption. The effect is dose-dependent, and at higher doses large quantities of carbohydrates reach the colon where they serve as substrates for bacteria with resultant bloating and intestinal discomfort. Excessive flatulence is a clinical side effect. Below these doses, the digestion curve is flattened, making these drugs potentially useful in treatment of diabetics. Clinical studies have yet to indicate any significant effect of these drugs on body weight.

2. Inhibition of Fat Digestion or Absorption

Cholestyramine. Cholestyramine is a bile acid–sequestering drug that provides one approach to inhibiting triglyceride digestion. It binds bile acids and thus disrupts micelle formation. At high doses it leads to increased fecal fat loss. Two older clinical trials with cholestyramine failed to show any significant effect on weight loss at nearly maximal tolerated doses (see Ref. 1), and no recent trials have been reported. The antibiotic neomycin reduces fat absorption but has deleterious effects on the intestinal mucosa (see Ref. 1). A third agent in this group is perfluorooctyl bromide, a contrast medium for gastrointestinal X-rays, which blocks absorption of all macronutrient classes in experimental animals. No clinical trials with this agent have been published.

Orlistat. Fat digestion can also be inhibited by blocking pancreatic lipase (72). In experimental studies orlistat (tetrahydrolipstatin) has been shown to be a potent inhibitor of lipase activity, which decreases intestinal triglyceride hydrolysis (73). Both European and American double-blind, randomized, placebo-controlled, multicenter trials have been conducted. The drug also has a dose-related effect on weight loss (74). Fecal fat loss on 30%-fat diets is dose-related (72). In one European multicenter trial, patients treated with 360 mg/day of orlistat lost 4.76 $\pm$ 0.38 kg in 12 weeks compared to 2.98 $\pm$ 0.38 kg in placebo group ($p < 0.001$) (75).

Pseudo-nutrients. Artificial sweeteners, indigestible fibers, and fat substitutes all fall in this group. Saccharin, cyclamates, aspartame, and acesulfame are the currently available artificial sweeteners. One trial with aspartame (76) showed that substitution of aspartame for sucrose led to weight loss in women but not men. The use of various fibers such as guar, mucilage, and pectin to treat obesity is based on the hypothesis that nondigestible bulking agents would reduce food intake and/or absorption. Results of clinical trials with fiber are variable.

Microparticulate protein. Two fat substitutes are available. One of these is a microparticulate protein that has the feel of fat on the tongue. Since it is a protein, it cannot replace fats in cooking but has been used as a fat substitute in foods such as ice cream. It has 4 kcal/g as compared to 9 kcal/g for fat. No trials have been reported with it in obese subjects.

Olestra. Olestra is a second pseudo-nutrient. It is a mixture of penta-, hexa-, and hepta-esters of sucrose, which cannot be hydrolyzed by pancreatic lipase. Depending on the nature of the free fatty acids incorporated into this molecule, its melting point and "taste feel" can be altered. Substitution of olestra for triglyceride in the diet decreases the digestible fats and thus has potential use for reducing caloric intake. Studies in normal-weight men fed olestra in the breakfast meal showed complete caloric composition within 24 hr when olestra is covertly substituted for a single meal. In a 2-week trial in which 25% of the total fat was replaced by olestra, there was no change in energy expenditure and no dietary compensation. A small weight loss occurred as the subjects continued to eat the same amount of carbohydrate, protein, and weight of food. All available data indicate that olestra is safe (77).

3. Postabsorptive Effectors of Nutrient Partitioning

Growth Hormone. Growth hormone is thermogenic in humans (26). Treatment with growth hormone will increase the amount of lean tissue and decrease the amount of fat in hypopituitary human subjects, particularly in the visceral area. Several clinical studies have been conducted with growth hormone in obesity (1,78,79), but its potential role is unclear since it produces acromegaly as a side effect.

Testosterone. The increase in upper abdominal obesity and visceral fat in women is associated with an increased level of free testosterone and a decreased level of sex hormone–binding globulin (SHBG) (80). In males, on the other hand, there is an inverse relationship between testosterone and central fat (81). Noting this relationship, Marin, Björntorp, and their colleagues have carried out two studies looking at the effects of replacement with testosterone on regional fat distribution in men (82,83). The first study used testosterone undecanoate, which is pack-

aged in chylomicrons by the intestine and is absorbed via the lymphatic system (82). In subsequent studies, they have used testosterone delivered via a transdermal patch (83). In both double-blind, randomized clinical trials, Marin et al. demonstrated that testosterone significantly decreased visceral fat in males whose circulating testosterone was at the lower limits of normal. Dihydrotestosterone, an androgenic metabolite of testosterone that is involved in gonadal development in males, was without effect on visceral fat.

Glucocorticoids. An increase in central fat deposition and an increase in catabolism of skin, muscle, and bone are characteristic of adrenal hyperfunction (Cushing's syndrome) and treatment with high doses of glucocorticoids. Treatment with glucocorticoids produces a central form of fat storage and enhanced protein breakdown. Addison's disease (adrenal insufficiency) is associated with loss of body fat. Moreover, glucocorticoids are essential for the development of obesity in animals (84), and blockade of glucocorticoids with RU-486 will reverse one type of experimental obesity (85). The possibility that blockade of glucocorticoid receptors could be exploited to treat obesity remains to be tested.

Other Steroids. Megestrol acetate (Megase) increased food intake in experimental animals and increases food intake possibly through effects on neuropeptide Y. In women with breast cancer it increases fat storage (86,87). Recently, dehydroepiandrosterone (DHEA), a major secretory steroid from the adrenal gland, has been shown to decrease body fat in several models of obesity (88). However, clinical trials have not shown a decrease in body fat in obese patients treated with DHEA (89). A metabolic derivative of DHEA, etocholandione, has also been tested in a small clinical trial with promising results.

Lipid Modulators. Several mechanisms might be probed to induce metabolic alteration of nutrient partitioning. Modulation of fat storage and breakdown offers the possibility of modifying nutrient flux. Since α_2-adrenergic receptors reduce lipolysis, α_2-adrenergic antagonists might enhance lipolysis (54). Modulation of the adenosine receptors is a second potential approach for enhancing lipolysis. Metformin, discussed above, might be put in this category since its mechanism of action is through channeling peripheral utilization of glucose.

4. Thermogenic Drugs

Adrenergic Drugs. β_2- and/or β_3-adrenergic drugs are thermogenic and also increase body protein and decrease body fat content in mice, rats, pigs, sheep, and cattle experimentally (90). Three β_2/β_3-adrenergic drugs have gone through early clinical trials. A Smith Kline Beecham compound, BRL-26830A, has had the most clinical study (91,92). In two trials published only in abstract, there was no significant effect of this drug on weight loss. In one long-term clinical trial, the drug was shown to be significantly more effective than placebo (91). Its major side effect was the development of mild tremors due to β_2-adrenergic effect of this compound on muscle (92). Three other compounds, one from the Imperical Chemical Industries (ICI D-7114), one from Hoffman LaRoche (Ro16-8714), and one from Lederle (CL 316,243), have also had clinical trials. The Roche compound increased energy expenditure in lean and obese subjects, but possibly because of a rise in heart rate, has not been studied further. The ICI compound, although effective in increasing thermogenesis in animals, was apparently without effect when administered to human volunteers (Astrup, personal communication). The Lederle compound has been tried clinically, but the data have not been published. Terbutaline, a β_2-adrenergic drug used to treat asthma, has been found to be thermogenic and to produce weight loss (28). Cloning of the rat and human β_3-receptor has shown that compounds directed against the rat receptor may not act on the human receptor. This may explain why no effective compounds have yet been identified.

V. DRUGS PREVIOUSLY USED BUT NOT APPROVED

A. Thyroid Hormone

Thyroid hormone, first used for the treatment of obesity in 1893 (see Ref. 1), has no place in the treatment of obesity unless hypothyroidism is present.

B. Dextroamphetamine, Methamphetamine and Phenmetrazine

These schedule II appetite suppressant drugs have significant potential for drug abuse. None of these three drugs should be used in the treatment of obesity.

C. Human Chorionic Gonadotropin (HCG)

Nearly 40 years ago, injections of HCG were tried in human subjects when it was observed that HCG treatment of adolescents with "Frohlich's syndrome" led to altered fat deposition. Four double-blind, randomized clinical trials with HCG injections compared to placebo showed no significant differences (93). There is thus no evidence that HCG injections are effective in treatment of obesity.

D. Dinitrophenol

Dinitrophenol uncouples oxidative phosphorylation, raises body temperature, and is thermogenic. Because of severe side effects including neuropathy, hepatic damage, and cataracts, the drug should not be used to treat obesity (see Ref. 1).

E. Digitalis

Anorexia and nausea are side effects of treatment with digitalis. This drug had a temporary use in the treatment of obesity (3), but because of the narrow range between therapeutic and toxic doses, digitalis has no place other than in treating disease (see Ref. 1).

VI. USE OF DRUGS IN THE CLINICAL TREATMENT OF OBESITY

A. Realities of Treatment

There are a number of realities about the treatment of obesity with drugs or any other modality. First, obesity is a chronic relapsing disease that has many causes. In most patients presenting with obesity, a clear etiological diagnosis is not possible. There are genetic factors: cases of neurological disorders with obesity as a consequence, cases of endocrine disease that produce obesity, and cases in which drug treatment leads to obesity. Because of its chronic nature and unknown cause, cure of obesity is rare, but palliation is a realistic goal. Weight loss occurs with most treatment, and except with the most drastic, it is usually slow, 0.5–1.0 kg/week. Recidivism, or regain of body weight, is common after a weight loss program is terminated. In contrast to the relatively slow rate of weight loss, weight regain may be rapid. A regain in weight after termination of treatment with the drugs is often ascribed to a failure of the drugs. A more appropriate interpretation is that medications do not work if not taken. This is true of medications for the treatment of obesity just as it is for medications used in the treatment of hypertension, diabetes, heart disease, asthma, and other chronic diseases (91).

B. Evaluation of the Obese Patient

1. Classification

The classification I propose for evaluating the patient with obesity is adapted from a classification used for heart disease. It involves three components: (1) an anatomical classification, 2) an etiological classification, and 3) a functional classification (Table 8).

An anatomical classification can be based either on the number of adipocytes or on the distribution of body fat. Both have been used, but the major empohasis should be on distribution of body fat. In many of the obese whose problem begins in childhood, the number of adipocytes may be increased by two- to fourfold, with the normal range being $20–60 \times 10^9$ fat cells. Individuals with increased numbers of fat cells have hyperplastic obesity,

Table 8   Classification of Obesity

I. Anatomical classification
  A. Microscopic
    1. Fat cell size
    2. Fat cell number
  B. Macroscopic
    1. Total body fat
    2. Subcutaneous fat distribution
    3. Visceral fat
    4. Abnormal or unusual fat deposits
II. Etiological classification
  A. Hypothalamic
  B. Endocrine
  C. Dietary
  D. Physical inactivity
  E. Genetic
  F. Drug-induced
  G. Unknown
III. Functional classification
  A. Degree of risk estimated from body mass index and fat distribution

Class	Grade	BMI	Circumference of waist (cm)		
			M <80	81–100	>100
			F <70	71–90	>90
1	0	20–<25	VL	L	M
2	1	25–<30	L	M	H
3	2	30–<35	M	H	VH
4	2	35–<40	H	VH	VH
4	3	>40	VH	VH	VH
5					

  B. Associated risks
    1. High blood pressure (systolic > 140; diastolic > 90 mmHg)
    2. Insulin resistance or diabetes [glucose (mg/dl) ÷ insulin (μU/ml)(G/I0 > 6]
    3. Total cholesterol ÷ HDL − chol (females > 5.0; males > 6.0)
    4. LVH by ECG
    5. Sleep apnea or high $PaCO_2$
    6. Hirutism or high LH/FSH ratio
    7. Smoking
    8. Restrained eaters
    9. Low physical activity

VL = very low; L = low; M = moderate; H = high; VH = very high.

which is to be distinguished from the hypertrophic form of obesity in which the total number of adipocytes is normal but the size of individual fat cells is increased. In general, all obesity is associated with an increase in the size of adipocytes, but only the markedly obese individual has an increase in the total number of fat cells. Individuals who are 75% or more overweight almost always have an increase in the number of fat cells. Thus, markedly overweight individuals have hypercellular obesity whereas those with modest degrees of obesity may have hypercellular obesity, but are more likely to have hypertrophic obesity. The duration of weight loss that follows successful dietary treatment of obesity is shorter and the rate at which weight is regained is more rapid in individuals with hypercellular obesity as compared to those with hypertrophic obesity.

The distribution of adipose tissue or body fat can be divided into three components. The first is the percentage of body fat. The second is the distribution of fat into either upper segment, android, or male-type obesity, where fat is primarily on the trunk and shoulders, as opposed to lower body, gynoid, or female-type obesity, in which the primary fat deposits are located on the thighs or hips. In women with upper segment body fat distribution, compared to women with lower body fat distribution but of total similar body fat levels, there is impairment of glucose tolerance and substantially increased insulin secretion following an oral glucose load. Women with upper body obesity also show an increased circulating level of free testosterone, reduced levels of SHBG, sex hormone binding globulin = SHBG increased insulin resistance, and reduced hepatic clearance of pancreatic insulin. Men with upper body obesity often have lower levels of testosterone, which has prompted studies using testosterone to reduce upper body fat in men. The third component of fat is visceral fat. This intra-abdominal depot increases with age and carries the highest risk for developing cardiovascular and other disease consequences.

2. Measurement

Obesity or fatness can be measured by a number of techniques. A summary of these methods is shown in Table 9, which lists the various methods and provides an estimate of cost and difficulty, as well as whether the method can measure body fat distribution. For epidemiological studies, fat is usually estimated using skinfold measurements. When the body mass index is above 30 kg/m², skinfold measurements and body mass index (BMI) are almost superimposable. The sum of the triceps plus subscapular skinfold greater than 45 mm in males and 65 mm in females can be used to define obesity. Where mea-

surements of body fat are available, a body fat above 25% for males and above 33% for females can also define obesity.

In addition to measurements of body fatness, regional fat distribution plays an important role in predicting health risks. Regional fat distribution can be estimated by several techniques. A computed tomographic CT scan or a magnetic resonance imaging scan, at the level of the L-4/L-5 intervertebral space, is the most accurate but also the most expensive. The ratio of the circumference of the waist to the circumference of the hips has been widely used in epidemiological studies. Ratios above 0.80 in women and above 0.95 in men put individuals in the high-risk category. The ratio of skinfolds on the trunk to that on the limbs and the sagittal diameter are two other techniques. Widely accepted standards for fat distribution do not exist.

3. Clinical Evaluation of the Obese Patient

Since all treatments for obesity entail some risk, it is important to decide whether drug treatment is appropriate for the risks involved (94). To do this requires an assessment of the risk associated with total fat and fat distribution in relation to the risks of treatment. Two variables can be used to make this assessment. The first is the BMI, and the second is the distribution of body fat.

There is a curvilinear relationship between BMI and mortality, which is often described as "J" or "U" shaped. Underweight individuals may have an increased risk for respiratory disease, tuberculosis, digestive disease, and some cancers. For overweight individuals, the risks are cardiovascular disease, gall bladder disease, high blood pressure, and diabetes. Body weights associated with a BMI of 20–25 kg/m² are good weights for most people. When BMI is below 18 kg/m² or above 27 kg/m², risk increases in a curvilinear fashion. Individuals with a BMI between 25 kg/m² and 30 kg/m² in men of any age and between 25 and 30 kg/m² in women under 35 or between 27 and 30 kg/m² in women over 35 may be described as having low risk. Individuals with a BMI between 30 kg/m² and 35 kg/m² have moderate risk, whereas those with a BMI between 35 kg/m² and 40 kg/m² are at high risk and those with a BMI above 40 kg/m² have very high risk from their obesity. The relative risk is shifted by a number of factors including smoking, hypertension, elevated total or LDL cholesterol, and reduced HDL cholesterol.

From epidemiological data, it is clear that increased abdominal and particularly visceral fat carries increased risks. The top tertile in abdominal fat distribution nearly doubles the risk of mortality and morbidity from heart disease, diabetes, and hypertension. This extra risk is ob-

Table 9 Methods of Estimating Body Fat and Its Distribution

Method	Cost	Ease of use	Accuracy	Measures regional fat
Height and weight	$	Easy	High	No
Skinfold	$	Easy	Low	Yes
Circumference	$	Easy	Moderate	Yes
Ultrasound	$$	Moderate	Moderate	Yes
Density				
Immersion	$	Moderate	High	No
Plethysmograph	$$$	Difficult	High	No
Heavy water				
Tritiated	$$	Moderate	High	No
Deuterium oxide, or heavy oxygen	$$$	Moderate	High	No
Potassium isotope (^{40}K)	$$$$	Difficult	High	No
Total body electrical conductivity (TOBEC)	$$$	Moderate	High	No
Bioelectric impedance (BIA)	$$	Easy	High	No
Fat-soluble gas	$$	Difficult	High	No
Absorptiometry (Dual-energy X-ray absorptiometry, DEXA; dual-photon absorptiometry, DPA)	$$$	Easy	High	No
Computed tomography (CT)	$$$$	Difficult	High	Yes
Magnetic resonance imaging (MRI)	$$$$	Difficult	High	Yes
Neutron activation	$$$$	Difficult	High	No

$ = low cost; $$ = moderate cost; $$$ = high cost; $$$$ = very high cost.

served in men and women and rises sharply for the top 10th percentile of abdominal fat distribution. When the difference in fat distribution is corrected, the excess mortality observed between men and women is largely, if not completely, eliminated. The risk associated with excess central accumulation of fat probably reflects the increase in visceral fat. Abnormal glucose tolerance, hypertension, and hyperlipidemia are more closely associated with the amount of visceral fat than with total body fat. The sagittal diameter has been proposed as a way to estimate visceral fat, but at the present time the only reliable way to determine visceral fat is with a CT or MRI scan. When newer, less expensive methods become available, this will be an important clinical advance.

VIII. SUMMARY

This review has dealt with an evaluation of currently available medications used in the treatment of obesity and the new areas in which agents are being developed. For a variety of reasons, the currently available drugs are probably not used effectively in treatment of obesity. This is suggested particularly by the long-term trial recently published by Weintraub and colleagues (46). The use of drugs

should be combined with an effective treatment program, and if they are to be used for "more than a few weeks" (FDA wording), an outline of the treatment plan should be prepared, informed consent by the patient should be obtained, and the local licensing authority should be notified of the intent to use drugs for long-term treatment.

REFERENCES

1. Bray GA. The Obese Patient, 9th ed. Philadelphia: WB Saunders, 1976.
2. Lesses MF, Myerson A. Human autonomic pharmacology. XVI. Benzedrine sulfate as an aid in the treatment of obesity. N Engl J Med 1938; 218(3):119–124.
3. United States Senate. Committee on the Judiciary. Diet Pill Industry Hearings. Washington, DC: U.S. GPO, 1968.
4. Booth DA. Hunger Models. Computable Theory of Feeding Control. London: Academic Press, 1978.
5. Bray GA. Obesity, a disorder of nutrient partitioning: The Mona Lisa Hypothesis. J Nutr 1991; 121:1146–1162.
6. Flatt JP. McCollum Award Lecture, 1995: Diet, lifestyle, and weight maintenance[1–4] Am J Clin Nutr 1995; 62:820–36.
7. Bouchard, C, GA Bray (eds). Regulation of body weight; Biological and behavioral mechanisms. Dahlem Workshop

Report LS 57. Chichester: John Wiley & Sons, Ltd., 1996; 1–323.

8. Wellman PJ, Davies BT. Reversal of cirazoline-induced and phenylpropanolamine-induced anorexia by the alpha-1-receptor antagonist prazosin. Pharm Bio B 1992; 42(1): 97–100.

9. Physicians' Desk Reference to Pharmaceutical Specialties and Biologicals, 46th ed. Oradell, NJ: Medical Economics, 1992:529.

10. Leibowitz SF. Reciprocal huger-regulating circuits involving alpha- and beta-adrenergic receptors located, respectively, in the ventromedial and lateral hypothalamus. Proc Natl Acad Sci USA 1970; 67(2):1063–1070.

11. Kucio C, Jonderko K, Piskorska D. Does yohimbine act as a slimming drug? Isr J Med Sci 1991; 27:550–556.

12. Rossner S, Taylor CL, Byington RP, Furberg CD. Long-term Propranolol treatment and changes in body-weight after myocardial-infarction. Br Med J 1990; 300(6729):902–903.

13. Garattini S, Bizzi A, Codegoni AM, Caccia S, Mennini T. Progress report on the anorexia induced by drugs believed to mimic some of the effects of serotonin on the central nervous system. Am J Clin Nutr 1992; 55:160S–166S.

14. Ebenezer IS. Effects on the 5-HT1A agonist 8-OH-DPAT on food-intake in food deprived rats. Neuroreport 1992; 3(11):1019–1022.

15. Capuano CA, Leibowitz SF, Barr GA. The pharmaco-ontogeny of the perifornical lateral hypothalamic beta 2-adrenergic and dopaminergic receptor systems mediating epinephrine- and dopamine-induced suppression of feeding in the rat. Brain Res Dev Brain Res 1992; 70(1):1–7.

16. Sakata T, Ookuma K, Fujimoto K, Fukagawa K, Yoshimat H. Histaminergic control of energy-balance in rats. Brain Res B 1991; 27(3–4):371–375.

17. Paredes RG, Agmo A. GABA and behavor: the role of receptor subtypes. Neurosci Biobehav Rev 1992; 16:145–170.

18. Morley JE. Neuropeptide regulation of appetite and weight. Endocrinol Rev 1987; 8:256–287.

19. Atkinson RL. Naloxone decreases food intake in obese humans. J Clin Endocrinol Metab 1982; 55(1):196–198.

20. Leibowitz SF. Hypothalamic neuropeptide Y, galanin, and amines. Concepts of coexistence in relation to feeding behavior. Ann NY Acad Sci 1989; 575:221–233.

21. Bray GA. Peptides affect the intake of specific nutrients and the sympathetic nervous system. Am J Clin Nutr 1992; 55: 265S–271S.

22. Reeds PJ, Mersmann HJ. Protein and energy-requirements of animals treated with beta-adrenergic agonists—a discussion. J Anim Sci 1991; 69(4):1532–1550.

23. Bouchard C, Tremblay A, Despres JP, et al. The response to long-term overfeeding in identical twins. N Engl J Med 1990; 322(21):1477–1482.

24. Eadara JK, Dalrymple RH, DeLay RL, Ricks CA, Romsos DR. Effects of cimaterol, a β-adrenergic agonist, on protein metabolism in rats. Metabolism 1989; 38(9):883–890.

25. Bray GA, Melvin KEW, Chopra IJ. Effect of triiodothyronine on some metabolic responses of obese patients. Am J Clin Nutr 1973; 26:715–721.

26. Bray GA, Raben MS, Londono J, Gallagher TF Jr. Effects of triiodothyronine, growth hormone and anabolic steroids on nitrogen excretion and oxygen consumption of obese patients. J Clin Endocrinol 1971; 33:293–300.

27. Stock MJ, Dulloo AG. Ephedrine, xanthines, aspirin and other thermogenic drugs to assist the dietary management of obesity. Int J Obes Relat Metabol Disord 1993; 17(Suppl 1):1S–83S.

28. Scheidegger K, O'Connell M, Robbins DC, Danforth E Jr. Effects of chronic beta-receptor stimulation on sympathetic nervous system activity, energy expenditure, and thyroid hormones. J Clin Endocrinol Metab 1984; 58(5):895–903.

29. Hauger R, Hulihan-Giblin B, Angel A, et al. Glucose regulates (^{3}H)(+)-amphetamine binding and Na$^+$K$^+$ATPase activity in the hypothalamus: a proposed mechanism for the glucostatic control of feeding and satiety. Brain Res Bull 1986; 16:281–288.

30. Scoville BA. Review of Amphetamine-like Drugs by the Food and Drug Administration: Clinical Data and Value Judgements. Obesity in Perspective. DHEW Publ No (NIH) 75-708 1975:441–443.

31. Wozniak P, Cutshall LC, Ryan DH, Bray GA. A meta-analysis of some anorexiant drugs. JAMA 1997 (in press).

32. Griffiths RR, Brady JV, Bradford LD. Predicting the abuse liability of drugs with animal drug self-administration procedures: psychomotor stimulants and hallucinogens. Adv Behav Pharmacol 1979; 2:163–208.

33. Bray GA. Current status of drug therapy in obesity. Morgan JP, Kagan DV, Brody JS, eds. Phenylpropanolamine: Risks, Benefits and Controversies. New York: Praeger, 1985: 94–131.

34. Lasagna L. Phenylpropanolamine—A Review. New York: Wiley, 1988.

35. Weintraub M. Phenylpropanolamine as an anorexiant agent in weight control: a review of published and unpublished studies. In: Morgan JP, Kagan DV, Brody JS, eds. Phenyl-propanolamine: Risks, Benefits and Controversies. New York: Praeger, 1985:53–79.

36. Morgan JP, Funderburk FR. Phenylpropanolamine and blood pressure: a review of prospective studies. Am J Clin Nutr 1992; 55:206S–210S.

37. Bray GA. Use and abuse of appetite-suppressant drugs in the treatment of obesity. Ann Intern Med 1993; 119: 707–713.

38. Guy-Grand B, Apfelbaum M, Crepaldi G, Gries A, Lefebvre P, Turner P. International trial of long-term dexfenfluramine in obesity. Lancet 1989; 2:1142–1144.

39. Bray GA, Ryan DH, Gordon D, Heidingsfelder S, Cerise F, Wilson K. A double-blind randomized placebo-controlled trial of sibutramine. Obes Res 1996; 4:263–270.

40. Mathus-Vliegen EMH, Van de Woord K, Kak AM, Res AM. Dexfenfluramine in the treatment of severe obesity: a placebo controlled investigation of the effects on weight loss,

cardiovascular risk factors, food intake and eating behavior. J Intern Med 1992; 232:119–127.

41. Andersen PH, Richelsen B, Bak J, et al. Influence of short-term dexfenfluramine therapy on glucose and lipid metabolism in obese non diabetic patients. Acta Endocrinol 1993; 128:251–258.

42. Levine LR, Enas GG, Thompson WL, et al. Use of fluoxetine, a selective serotonin-uptake inhibitor, in the treatment of obesity—a dose response study. Int J Obes 1989; 13(5): 635–645.

43. Darga LL, Carroll-Michals L, Botsford SJ, Lucas CP. Fluoxetine's effect on weight loss in obese subjects 1–3. Am J Clin Nutr 1991; 54(2):321–325.

44. Abenhaim L, Moride, Y, Brenot F, et al. For the International Primary Pulmonary Hypertension Study Group. N Engl J Med 1996; 335:609–616.

45. Weintraub M, Hasday JD, Mushlin AI, Lockwood DH. A double-bind clinical trial in weight control. Use of fenfluramine and phentermine alone and in combination. Arch Intern Med 1984; 144(6):1143–1148.

46. Weintraub M. Long-term weight control (parts 1–7)—the National-Heart-Lung-and-Blood-Institute funded multimodal intervention study. Clin Pharm 1992; 51(5):581–641.

47. Weintraub M, Rubio A, Golik A, Byrne L. Sibutramine dose ranging, efficacy study. Clin Pharm 1991; 50(3):330–337.

48. Bray GA, Ryan DH, Gordon D, Heidingsfelder H, Cerise F, Wilson K. A double-blind randomized placebo-controlled trial of sibutramine. Obes Res 1996; 4(3) (in press).

49. de Zwaan M, Mitchell JE. Opiate antagonists and eating behavior in humans: a review. J Clin Pharmacol 1992; 32: 1060–1072.

50. Maggio CA, Presta E, Bracco EF, Vasselli JR, Kissileff HR, Pfohl DN, Hashim SA. Naltrexone and human eating behavior: a dose-ranging inpatient trial in moderately obese men. Brain Res Bull 1985; 14:657–661.

51. Mitchell JE, Morley JE, Levine AS, Hatsukami D, Gannon M, Pfohl D. High-dose naltrexone therapy and dietary counseling for obesity. Biol Psychiatry 1987; 22:35–42.

52. Novi RF, Lamberto M, Mantovan M, Porta M, Molinatti GM. The role of an opioid antagonist in the treatment of obesity: results of a randomized, placebo-controlled, double-blind trial. Curr Ther Res 1992; 51(4):576–581.

53. Bailey CJ. Biguanides and NIDDM. Diabet Care 1992; 15(6):755–772. (review).

54. Angel I, Schoemaker H, Arbilla S, et al. SI 84.0418: a novel, potent and selective alpha-2 adrenoceptor antagonist: in vitro pharmacological profile. J Pharmacol Exp Ther 1992; 263(3):1327–1333.

55. Galitzky J, Riviere D, Tran MA, Montastruc JL, Berlan M. Pharmacodynamic effects of chronic yohimbine treatment in healthy volunteers. Eur J Clin Pharmacol 1990; 39: 447–451.

56. Sax, L. Yohimbine does not affect fat distribution in men. Int J Obes 1991; 15:561–565.

57. Greenway FL, Bray GA, Heber D. Topical fat reduction. Obes. Res. 1995; 3(Suppl 4):561S–568S.

58. Kissileff HR, Pi-Sunyer FX, Thorton J, Smith GP. C-terminal octapeptide of cholecystokinin decreases food intake in man. Am J Clin Nutr 1981; 34(2):154–160.

59. Pi-Sunyer X, Kissileff HR, Thornton J, Smith GP. C-terminal octapeptide of cholecystokinin decreases food intake in obese men. Physiol Behav 1982; 29(4):627–630.

60. Cooper SJ, Dourish CT, Clifton PG. CCK antagonists and CCK-monoamine interactions in the control of satiety. Am J Clin Nutr 1992; 55:291S–295S.

61. Asin KE, Bednarz L, Nikkel AL, Gore PA, Nadzan AM. A-71623, a selective CCK-A receptor agonist, suppresses food-intake in the mouse, dog, and monkey. Pharm Bio B 1992; 42(4):699–704.

62. Liverse RJ, Jansen JBMJ, van de Zwan A, et al. Bombesin reduces food intake in lean man by a cholecystokinin-independent mechanism. J Clin Endocrinol Metab 1993; 76:1495–1498.

63. Okada S, York DA, Bray GA, Erlanson-Albertsson C. Enterostatin, (Val-Pro-Asp-Pro-Arg), the activation peptide of procolipase selectivity reduces fat intake. Physiol Behav 1991; 49(6):1185–1189.

64. Rossner S, Barkeling B, Erlanson-Albertsson C, Larsson P, Wahlin-Boll E. Intravenous enterostatin does not affect single meal food-intake in man. Appetite 1995; 24(1):37–42.

65. Geary N. Pancreatic glucagon signals postprandial satiety. Neurosci Biobehav Rev 1990; 14:323–338.

66. Turton MD, O'Shea D, Gunn I, et al. A role for glucagon-like peptide-1 in the central regulation of feeding. Nature 1996; 379:69–72, 1996.

67. Zhang YY, Proenca R, Maffei M, Barone M, Leopold L, Friedman JM. Positional cloning of the mouse obese gene and its human homolog. Nature 1994; 372:425–432.

68. Considine RV, Sinha MK, Heiman ML, et al. Serum immunoreactive-leptin concentrations in normal-weight and obese humans. N Engl J Med 1996; 334:292–295.

69. Ono T, Nakamura K, Fukuda M, Kobayashi T. Central action of endogenous sugar acid (2-buten-4-olide): comparison with local anesthesia in hypothalamus. Brain Res Bull 1990; 24:793–802.

70. Triscari J, Sullivan AC. Studies on the mechanism of action of a novel anorectic agent, (—)-threo-chlorocitric acid. Pharmacol Biochem Behav 1981; 15(2):311–318.

71. Matsuo T, Odaka H, Ikeda H. Effect of an intestinal disaccharidase inhibitor (AO-128) on obesity and diabetes. Am J Clin Nutr 1992; 55:314S–317S.

72. Hauptman JB, Jeunet FS, Hartmann D. Initial studies in humans with the novel gastrointestinal lipase inhibitor Ro 18-0647 (tetrahydrolipstatin)1,2. Am J Clin Nutr 1992; 55: 309S–313S.

73. Tonstad S, Pometta D, Erkelens DW, et al. The effects of gastrointestinal lipase inhibitor, orlistat, on serum lipids and lipoproteins in patients with primary hyperlipidaemia. Eur J Clin Pharmacol 1994; 46:405–410.

74. Zhi J, Melia AT, Guerciolini R, et al. Retrospective population-based analysis of the dose-response (fecal fat excre-

tion) relationship of orlistat in normal and obese volunteers. Clin Pharmacol Ther 1994; 56:82–85.

75. Drent ML, Larsson I, Williamo T, et al. Orlistat (RO-18-0647), a lipase inhibitor, in the treatment of human obesity: a multiple dose study. Int J Obes 1995; 19:221–226.

76. Kanders BS, Lavin PT, Kowalchuk MB, Greenberg I, Blackburn GL. An evaluation of the effect of aspartame on weight loss. Appetite 1988; 11(Suppl 1):73–84.

77. Bergholtz CM. Safety evaluation of olestra, a nonabsorbed, fatlike fat replacement. Crit Rev Food Sci Nutr 1992; 32(2): 141–146.

78. Snyder DK, Clemmons DR, Underwood LE. Dietary carbohydrate content determines responsiveness to growth hormone in energy-restricted humans. J Clin Endocrinol Metab 1989; 69:745–752.

79. Snyder DK, Underwood LE, Clemmons DR. Anabolic effects of growth-hormone in obese diet-restricted subjects are dose dependent. Am J Clin Nutr 1990; 52:431–437.

80. Evans DJ, Hoffman RG, Kalkoff RK, Kissebah AH. Relationship of androgenic activity to body fat topography, fat cell morphology, and metabolic aberrations in premenopausal women. J Clin Endocrinol Metab 1983; 57:304.

81. Seidell JC, Björntorp P, Sjorstrom L, Kvist H, Sannerst R. Visceral fat accumulation in men is positively associated with insulin, glucose, and C-peptide levels, but negatively with testosterone levels. Metabolism 1990; 39(9):897–901.

82. Marin P, Kvist H, Lindstedt G, Sjostrom L, Björntorp P. Low concentrations of insulin-like growth factor-I in abdominal obesity. Int J Obes 1993; 17:83–89.

83. Marin P, Holmang S, Gustafsson C, et al. Androgen treatment of abdominally obese men. Obes Res 1993; 1(4): 245–251.

84. Bray GA, Fisler JS, York DA. Neuroendocrine control of the development of obesity: understanding gained from studies of experimental animal models. Frontiers Neuroendocrinol 1990; 11(2):128–181.

85. Okada S, York DA, Bray GA. Mifepristone (RU-486), a blocker of type II glucocorticoid and progestin receptors, reverses a dietary form of obesity. Am J Physiol 1992; 262(6 pt2):R1106–1110.

86. Aisner J, Parnes H, Tait N, Hickman M, Forrest A, Greco FA, Tchekmedyian NS. Appetite stimulation and weight reduction with magistral acetate. Semin Oncol 1990; 17 (6(Suppl 9)):2–7.

87. Aisner J, Tchekmedyian NS, Tait N, Parnes H, Novak M. Studies of high-dose megestrol acetate: potential application in cachexia. Semin Oncol 1988; 15(2 pt 1):68–75.

88. MacEwen EG, Kurzman ID. Obesity in the dog: role of the adrenal steroid dehydroepiandrosterone (DHEA). J Nutr 1991; 121:S51–S55.

89. Usiskin KS, Butterworth S, Clore JN, et al. Lack of effect of dehydroepiandrosterone in obese men. Int J Obes 1990; 14(5):457–463.

90. Arch JRS, Ainsworth AT, Cawthorne MA, et al. Atypical beta-adrenoceptor on brown adipocytes as target for antiobesity drugs. Nature 1984; 309(5964):163–165.

91. Connacher AA, Bennet WM, Jung RT. Clinical studies with the β-adrenoceptor agonist BRL 26830A. Am J Clin Nutr 1992; 55:258S–261S.

92. Connacher AA, Mitchell PEG, Jung RT. Weight loss in obese subjects on a restricted diet given BRL 26830A, a new atypical β-adrenoceptor agonist. Br Med J 1988; 26: 1217–20.

93. Greeway FL, Bray GA. Human chorionic gonadotropin (HCG) in the treatment of obesity: a clinical assessment of the Simeons method. West J Med 1977; 127(11):461–463.

94. Weintraub M, Bray GA. Drug treatment of obesity. Med Clin North Am 1989; 73:237–250.

49

Surgical Treatment of Obesity

John G. Kral
State University of New York Health Science Center at Brooklyn, Brooklyn, New York

I. INTRODUCTION

A. Justification

Unfortunately, with severe disease, physicians must first harm to then heal. If the treatment is perceived as more harmful than the disease, neither patient nor physician will choose the treatment. Education without intimidation is required to reconcile differences in perceptions of disease severity and side effects of treatment, but sometimes this is not enough.

Progress in educating the public as well as the medical profession about obesity, or even having it accepted as a disease, has been very slow, but is accelerating. Inability or even unwillingness to recognize obesity as a serious chronic disease that deeply compromises quality of life is the major obstacle to acceptance of surgical treatment, to resource allocation, to the study of obesity, and to realistic drug treatment.

The health consequences of obesity and their influence on public health have been well exposed. Analysis of tangible costs of obesity and its comorbidity have demonstrated the extraordinary costs to society even without accounting for impaired quality of life, regardless of how suffering is defined. Cost-benefit analyses of all forms of treatment of obesity are conspicuously absent, possibly because of the lack of effective treatment alternatives.

Surgical treatment can achieve sustained, substantial weight loss in the majority of eligible patients. This fact alone is sufficient to convince severely obese patients that to undergo a gastrointestinal operation for weight loss is worth the cost, the discomfort, and the risk taking if for no other reason than improving quality of life, i.e., regardless of any life-prolonging or comorbidity-reducing effects, whether proven or not. The absence of alternative methods capable of sustaining medically meaningful weight reduction further justifies surgical treatment of severe obesity.

B. Indications

The least controversial indication for antiobesity surgery is a body weight twice or 100% in excess of the weight associated with minimum mortality at a given height. These weight standards, most frequently based on life insurance statistics, are customarily not adjusted for age, though some surgeons operate on patients aged 70 years (1). Another, more "liberal" weight criterion often used is an excess weight of 45.5 kg (100 lb), corresponding to 78% excess in a woman 160 cm (5 ft 3 in.) tall and 66% in a man whose height is 175 cm (5 ft 9 in.). The body mass index (BMI) standard accepted by a National Institutes of Health Consensus Development conference on gastrointestinal surgery was BMI = 40 kg/m^2, also without adjusting for age. BMI $\geq$ 35 kg/m^2 was considered an indication in the presence of severe comorbidity (2).

Manifest comorbidity indicating surgical intervention at weight levels below BMI = 40 kg/m^2 commonly includes hypertension, diabetes, heart failure, history of thromboembolism, sleep apnea and vertebral disk herniation among others.

With significant improvements in antiobesity surgery and recent development of minimally invasive techniques, a reduction in weight criteria is expected. It is likely that a cost-benefit analysis of surgical treatment compared to chronic drug treatment will come out in favor of surgery as is the case with peptic ulcer disease. Indeed, one study has demonstrated that the cost per pound of maintained weight loss is less for operative treatment after 4 years of treatment (3).

II. METHODS

A. Mechanisms

Surgical methods are physical (mechanical), regulatory, i.e., influencing appetite regulation, or combinations of physical and regulatory. Table 1 presents the chronology of development of antiobesity operations. The main surgical principles are bypass of the intestinal tract resulting in malabsorption or maldigestion, restriction or obstruction of transit, and neuroregulation, not disrupting gastrointestinal continuity.

The simplest form of restriction is dental splinting or intermaxillary fixation, popularly called "jaw wiring" (4). It can only be used temporarily and as such is effective in reducing weight for short-term purposes in patients with-

Table 1 Operations for Obesity in Humans[a,b]

1918	Lipectomy
1952	Small bowel resection (malabsorption)
1954	Small bowel bypass = jejunoileal
1963	Jejunocolic bypass
1967	Gastric bypass (restriction and maldigestion)
1971	Gastroplasty (restriction)
1974	Hypothalamic electrocoagulation (regulatory)
1978	Gastric banding
1978	Gastric wrapping
1978	Truncal vagotomy
1979	Biliopancreatic bypass (restriction, maldigestion, and malabsorption)
1981	Vertical-banded gastroplasty
1981	Biliointestinal bypass
1982	Ileogastrostomy
1983	Intestinal interposition
1986	Esophageal banding
1986	Adjustable gastric banding

[a]Approximate year of introduction or publication in English. New physiological principles in parentheses.
[b]This is not a complete list of all published procedures, modifications, or combinations, which at last reckoning exceeded 30 in number.

out oronasal or respiratory problems. However, weight regain is immediate after removal of the wires. The more common restrictive or obstructive procedures function by creating an early sense of satiety or, more likely, aversive nimiety. Clearly, overdistention of the proximal stomach and distal esophagus elicits nausea or even vomiting if the patient disregards signals of fullness. Patients learn to "eat around" these procedures by selecting high-calorie soft or liquid foods to a void the aversive effects (soft-calorie syndrome) (5). Endoscopic insertion of balloons was an attempt at reducing functional gastric volume, at the same time obstructing flow. After a period of extensive marketing in the mid-1980s, intragastric balloons for obesity fell into disrepute (6).

Bypass procedures cause aversive reactions through overstimulation of the small intestine, unprotected by the "pyloric brake." Gastric bypass causes "dumping," which elicits release of gastrointestinal polypeptides that affect the central nervous system (Table 2). This is much more difficult to circumvent and may account for the superior weight loss following bypass procedures.

B. Lipectomy/Liposuction

Simply removing adipose tissue (lipectomy) cannot be considered a method for treating obesity, but rather addresses abnormal accumulations of fat, which may be a sequel of the obesity. Only in rare exceptions is lipectomy performed as a primary treatment for obesity: when a large pannus or panniculus causes secondary problems such as intertrigo or interferes with activities of daily living including mobility and personal hygiene (7).

Liposuction (introduced in 1972) (8) is currently the most frequently performed *cosmetic* operation in industrialized nations. It has few strict medical indications even though it can significantly enhance the quality of life of people troubled by localized collections of adipose tissue such as "love handles," "spare tires," or "riding britches" deformities.

There are no long-term clinical follow-up studies of liposuction or lipectomy to resolve the controversy over regrowth or compensation after surgical removal of fat. There is no evidence that extensive lipectomy influences energy balance in humans. Anecdotally, patients having reduced weight by dieting with subsequent lipectomy are not spared from weight (re)gain.

As suction lipectomy increased dramatically in the 1980s, it was generally accepted that amounts larger than 2000 ml could not be safely removed even with provision of blood products and fluid replacement. Recently techniques have been developed with reports in Europe of removal of more than 10 kg of fat. It is not known whether such extensive removal of adipose tissue has any metabolic effects, beneficial or detrimental, nor whether it influences energy balance over the long term. In animal studies, excising around 25% of body fat does not prevent continued weight gain (9).

Lipectomy and liposuction remove only a marginal percentage of total body fat and are thus unable to achieve medically significant weight loss (7). However, they may play an important psychological role in motivating patients to lose and maintain weight loss by other means.

C. Bypass of the Gastrointestinal Tract (Diversionary Procedures)

The first operation performed expressly to cause weight loss was *resection of small bowel* sufficient to achieve reduction in the absorption of calories (10). This was performed in three women who did remarkably well, living into their eighties without medical supervision! For reasons not known, the surgeon in question did not perform any more such operations, and there do not seem to be any published reports of small bowel resection as a primary procedure for obesity.

I. Intestinal Bypass Operations

To obviate the irreversibility of resections, *small intestinal bypass*, connecting 90 cm of jejunum to 45 cm of ileum, was performed in one patient in 1954 after a series of dog experiments (11). The patient developed recurring ulcers prompting the surgeon to discontinue such operations. Others performed extensive clinical studies of connecting the jejunum to the colon with planned reanastomosis of the bowel after "sufficient" weight loss had been achieved. Because of extraordinary complications from the operations and weight regain after reanastomosis, *jejunocolic bypass* was abandoned around 1966.

Remarkably, jejunocolic bypass was reintroduced in a series of eight patients with mean BMI = 63 kg/m^2 described in 1994 (12). Patients were supported with home infusion therapy for 11–18 months before takedown of the jejunocolostomy and construction of a vertical-banded gastroplasty. Follow-up after gastroplasty was 0.1–3.5 years in seven of the patients; thus no long-term ($\geq$5 years) evaluation is available.

By 1966 jejunocolic bypass had been replaced by end-to-side *jejunoileostomy* [14 in. (35.6 cm) of jejunum anastomosed to 4 in. (10.2 cm) of ileum]. Jejunoileal bypass (JIB) with modifications was the predominant antiobesity operation until around 1980 (13). Though large numbers

Table 2 Mechanisms of Weight Loss of Gastrointestinal Antiobesity Operations

I. Decreased energy intake via satiety or aversive nimiety
 A. Stimulation of esophagus/upper stomach
  1. Distention
   a. Small gastric pouch
   b. Narrow outlet of pouch
   c. Delayed emptying of stomach ("barostat")
 B. Stimulation of small intestine
  1. Distention
  2. Nutrients
 C. Central effects
  1. Peptides released by:
   a. Distention
   b. Nutrients
  2. Toxins
   a. Bacterial overgrowth
   b. Toxic bile acids
  3. Substrate
   a. FFA mobilization
   b. Hepatic gluconeogenesis
II. Increased output via malabsorption/maldigestion
 A. Rapid small intestinal transit
 B. Diversion of digestive juices
 C. Increased thermogenesis

of patients did well and still have intact jejunoileal bypass without recognized complications, too many had severe and irreversible complications, some of which were fatal. Great variations in the prevalence of complications after intestinal bypass are due to important differences in postoperative management including the vigilance and knowledge of the treating physician as well as the cooperation of the patient with recommended treatment plans and follow-up. Most complications can be prevented by appropriate management instituted immediately after the operation and maintained for life (14).

Modifications of jejunoileal bypass have been aimed at circumventing the adverse effects of the bypassed or "blind" loop, the cause of most complications. Strategies such as creating antireflux anastomoses, diverting bile into the blind loop (*biliointestinal bypass*), draining the blind loop into the less colonized stomach (*ileogastrostomy*), or creating a longer distal or ileal loop (50 cm vs. the "standard" 10.2 cm = "duodenoileal" bypass) have all been demonstrated to reduce complication rates. However, these series have often been smaller and thus more easily monitored and receiving superior care.

Currently intestinal bypass operations are seldom performed except under special circumstances in centers with interest in and knowledge of their management. Strictly malabsorptive operations have a role mainly in patients with failure of gastric restriction. In fact, the "brake" imposed, even by a failed gastroplasty, helps to decrease the complications of intestinal bypass operations (15). This implies that a high eating rate contributes to creating some bypass complications, ostensibly caused by rapid transit leading to diarrhea.

2. Gastric Bypass Operations

Though the first gastric antiobesity operations were reported in 1967, it took 15 years before they became more widely adopted. Widespread use of stapling instruments, making the gastric bypass less technically demanding, ushered in the new era of antiobesity surgery concomitant with the increased recognition of adverse effects of intestinal bypass operations.

Gastric bypass for obesity was modeled on gastric resections performed for cancer and ulcers and was introduced by Mason and Ito in 1967 (16) after extensive laboratory studies on dogs. Various configurations of gastric bypass, starting with resection and loop gastrojejunostomy and evolving to in-continuity cross-stapling to create a proximal pouch drained by a Roux-en-Y (side-end) gastrojejunostomy, were used by Mason until around 1981 when he abandoned gastric bypass. Gastric bypass (Fig. 1) has been adopted by many other groups and is the leading antiobesity operation performed in academic centers with a special interest in surgical treatment of obesity.

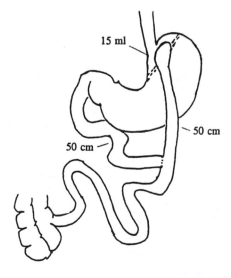

Figure 1 Gastric bypass excluding most of the stomach, the duodenum, and a 40–50-cm segment of proximal jejunum.

While much of the 1970s had been a period of experimenting with intestinal lengths and anastomoses in jejunoileal bypass the 1980s became a period of determining sizes of stomach pouches and outlets in gastric procedures. More recently, variations in lengths of incontinuity small bowel have (again) become the focus of interest.

The most extreme variant of gastric and malabsorptive procedures is *biliopancreatic diversion* (BPD), reported in English in 1979 after operations in dogs (17). In its original version it consisted in resecting a portion of the stomach (irreversible), closing the duodenum, and creating a bypass of 50% of the small bowel. Thus this operation has a gastric restrictive component (at least initially), as well as maldigestive (reduced gastric acid and pepsin and diverted bile and pancreatic enzymes) and malabsorptive components (17a).

On introduction in the United States BPD was modified to a bypass of the stomach rather than resection, much as the gastric bypass operation had evolved. This led to development of gastric bypass procedures with varying lengths of small bowel in continuity. In general, these more malabsorptive, "*long-limb*" gastric bypass operations (18) have been reserved for heavier patients (the "superobese" with BMI $\geq$ 50 kg/m²).

A further development of gastric bypass has focused on the gastric restrictive component. These variants employ different types and placements of bands to restrict the outflow of nutrients from the proximal gastric pouch (19,20). As was the case with modifications of intestinal bypass operations, where small and well-controlled series managed by zealous investigators performed well, this has been the case with modifications of gastric bypass. Longterm follow-up in large series in different centers will be required to ascertain whether the modifications are superior to conventional bypass.

The latest method in this group of operations is a variant of biliopancreatic diversion called "*duodenal switch*" (21). It consists in dividing the proximal duodenum just distal to the pylorus and connecting divided jejunum at this level. The distal end of the divided duodenum (above the entry of bile and pancreatic juice) is closed as a stump (as in BPD). This loop of duodenum and jejunum is attached further downstream emptying into the ileum, thus diverting the bile. This operation was developed in dogs to find a cure for bile reflux without causing ulcers (21) and was incidentally found to reduce weight.

D. Obstruction Procedures

While performing gastric bypass procedures in 1971, Mason tested the hypothesis that obstruction or restriction alone by partitioning the stomach horizontally was sufficient to achieve and maintain weight loss (22). He later attributed the failure of these first *gastroplasty* operations to the large size of the pouch and outlet. In 1976 a "new, improved" gastroplasty using horizontal stapling to create a small (30–50 ml) proximal pouch with a small outlet on the greater curvature side of the horizontal staple line was introduced. In time it became obvious that these operations only afforded temporary weight loss because of distention of the pouch and dilatation of the poorly reinforced stoma. During 1976–1980 attempts had been made to create external reinforcement of the stoma using bands of nylon or polypropylene mesh or strips of autologous fascia. Also, operations had been devised configuring the partition vertically instead of horizontally, thus making use of the more muscular and thicker stomach wall on the lesser curvature.

Vertical-banded gastroplasty (VBG) and *Silastic ring gastroplasty* incorporate the two principles of a vertical lesser curve pouch and external banding (Fig. 2) (23,24). VBG has been the dominant antiobesity procedure for the last 10 years because of its relative simplicity and absence of severe side effects. However, it is less effective than gastric bypass in achieving and sustaining large weight losses.

Just as gastroplasty was an attempt at simplifying gastric bypass, *circumgastric banding* is an attempt at simplifying gastroplasty. It was originally attempted in 1978 but quickly abandoned by its inventor because he understood that the proximal gastric pouch would expand, ultimately defeating the purpose of the operation. This led him to

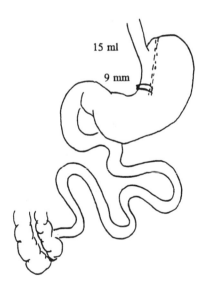

Figure 2 Vertical-stapled gastroplasty with a banded outlet from the 15-ml pouch.

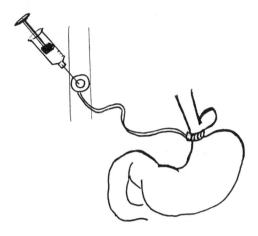

Figure 3. Adjustable gastric band attached to a subcutaneous port accessible via injection. This procedure has been adapted for laparoscopic surgery.

develop plication with external *wrapping* of the whole stomach with a Silastic jacket (25). Difficulties in performing this operation and reversing it when the need arises have limited the use of this form of gastric restriction.

Another form of banding was performed in eight pigs before a human trial was undertaken: *esophageal banding*, creating a stricture or narrowing of the cervical esophagus (26). The rationale was much the same as that of the Japanese fishermen of the Nagara River who use snares around the necks of cormorants to prevent them from swallowing any large fish they catch.

Only one patient among the seven reported had a sustained weight loss comparable to that of other surgical techniques in the literature. This patient had stricture and dilatation on esophagogram 42 months postoperatively. No studies were done to rule out microaspiration. This dangerous technique for treating obese people fortunately seems to have been abandoned.

Gastric banding was reintroduced around 1980. In its original version it proved to be less effective than vertical banded gastroplasty but it has had the appeal of greater simplicity. Kuzmak improved on gastric banding by standardizing the size and tension of the band (27). He later introduced an innovation that has paved the way for the latest development in this field. In 1986 he patented an *adjustable Silastic band* (28) attached to a subcutaneous port through which the band can be inflated or deflated as needed simply by injecting or withdrawing saline (Fig. 3).

Laparoscopic or minimally invasive surgical techniques have had a dramatic effect on most types of surgery and are being used more and more in the 1990s. With increasing proficiency, all types of antiobesity procedures have been attempted laparoscopically though it is not clear that laparoscopic performance of the more complex procedures is cost-efficient. *Laparoscopic adjustable banding*, on the other hand, is a logical and attractive improvement over the open procedure, though long-term results are as yet lacking (29). However, it is a mistake to believe that this operation will be any more effective in long-term weight control than any other gastric restrictive procedures—the limitations are the same.

E. Other Surgical Methods

Although the physical methods described above may affect appetite regulation and food intake through many different mechanisms as diverse as satiety signals from gastric distention (as in gastroplasty) and metabolic feedback from shunted nutrients (intestinal bypass), these techniques were primarily designed for their physical effects on the movement of gastrointestinal contents. The remaining class of antiobesity operations was designed for immediate effects on appetite regulation.

Animal experiments identifying hypothalamic centers stimulating and inhibiting food intake prompted Danish neurosurgeons to attempt *stereotactic electrocoagulation* of the hypothalamic hunger centers in obese patients, reported in 1974 (30). The effect was transitory and no further attempts at this approach have been published.

A different, though less extreme, neuroregulatory approach, also based on animal studies, is *truncal vagotomy*, severing the abdominal branches of the vagus nerve (31). This did achieve weight loss in the majority of patients, though the effects were moderate and insufficient in the opinion of the patients. Vagotomy in conjunction with gastric restriction has been demonstrated to potentiate the weight loss induced by restriction alone and seems to be a viable adjunctive surgical approach (32) awaiting trial in larger series of patients in different centers.

Clinical studies on patients with intestinal bypass and careful animal experiments revealed that JIB causes reductions in food intake that are reported to be more important than the loss of calories in the stools as an explanation for weight loss after intestinal bypass. These findings led to the hypothesis that food or undigested chyme appearing in the lower small intestine (terminal ileum) elicited satiety signals (33). Thus interposition of a segment of terminal ileum more proximal in the gastrointestinal tract was performed, first in rats and then in a small number of obese patients. *Intestinal interposition* had only a moderate and transitory effect in severely obese humans, though the results were dramatic in dogs (34). Further experimental work combining intestinal interposition with vagotomy is in progress and does not seem to have been attempted in humans. Interestingly, one of the patients who had intestinal interposition had concomitant vagotomy, which did not seem to potentiate the effects on weight loss.

F. Staged Surgery

The ideal of a single operation providing long duration (indefinite?) of reduced weight for a significant majority of obese patients (≥80%) with minimal risk of operative complications or long-term side effects is not yet available. In the absence of such an ideal single operation, a staged strategy is proposed (15). A step-care approach is a logical extension of prior treatment plans that start with conventional diets and progress to very-low-calorie diets (VLCD), exercise, medications, and combinations of these. Advancing to more mechanical and invasive methods might include belting or girdles, jaw wiring (unacceptable to many patients), intragastric balloons, and finally, laparoscopic adjustable banding (LAB).

A staged approach to surgical treatment (Fig. 4), starting with LAB, will identify a subgroup of patients who will only need the most benign operation, with minimal complications and side effects and no further operation. Depending on characteristics of the population, this might include up to 30% of candidates for antiobesity surgery. Some will self-select exclusion from any further operations, especially if they believe that repeat gastric restriction is the only option available to them.

The step-care strategy allows for continued education and behavioral treatment as well as assessment of patient cooperation (e.g., appointment-keeping behavior, adherence to medication). Since the patient is aware of further treatment options, she/he will be more likely to cooperate with follow-up care. "Failures," however they are defined, can be assigned more accurately to different types of operations as the second operation: revisional gastric restriction versus more or less aggressive malabsorption. Thus the LAB can be seen as a behavioral test for subsequent operations, analyzing such parameters as speed of relapse, soft-calorie syndrome, and pouch enlargement. Reoperations after silicone LAB are technically much easier than after other antiobesity operations because the band is nonreactive and the procedure itself is much less traumatic to tissues.

Added benefits of using a relatively benign operation are the reduced need for as extensive and rigorous preoperative evaluation or as meticulous follow-up as after the more aggressive operations with their greater potential for side effects. Indeed, the poor compliance of obese patients with follow-up is one argument against performing

Severe Obesity

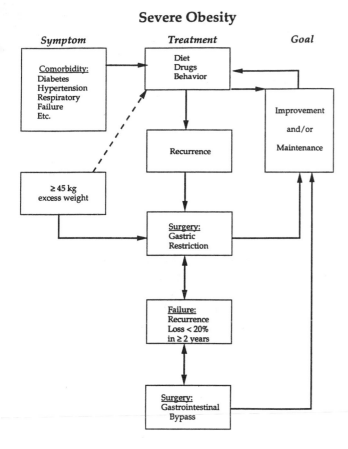

Figure 4   Algorithm for treatment of severe obesity. "Failure" means recurrence of comorbidity, weight regain, or loss of <20% of preoperative weight after 2 years.

malabsorptive operations because of the risk of causing clinically significant malnutrition.

There are numerous reasons for patients not returning for office visits. Unless they perceive tangible benefits such as assistance in developing coping strategies (often provided by surgeon-led support groups) or methods for potentiating or maintaining weight loss, patients drop out from follow-up. Among negative factors, shame over failure, reminder of perceived inadequacy, and being scolded are more often important than the cost of the visit in terms of time or money. Nevertheless, a staged approach will pose fewer risks for patients dropping out from follow-up.

III.   RESULTS

A.   Definition of "Success"

Weight loss is the simple outcome measure used by most investigators treating obesity. Its use is justified by the high and exponential relationship between body weight and the prevalence and severity of complications of obesity. However, it does not reflect reduction in morbidity or improvement in quality of life associated with treatment of obesity.

Excess weight is accompanied by a host of comorbidities that can be corrected by weight losses of undetermined magnitude. Tractability is related to duration of obesity, and it is not known whether there are thresholds for duration of exposure beyond which some conditions become irreversible. If there is a dose-response type of relationship between duration of excess weight and morbidity (as with pack-years and smoking), it is reasonable to expect that greater amounts of weight loss are required for correction of the condition the longer it has lasted. In general, surgeons have tried to achieve as great a reduction of excess weight as possible driven by the patients' cosmetic ambitions rather than a reasoned approach to the problem of medically optimal weight loss.

All students of nonsurgical treatment of obesity have been content to demonstrate the responsiveness of comorbidity to weight loss without ever providing follow-up data. This is understandable because those methods invariably fail to maintain weight loss or any of its salutary effects. It is true that the various surgical procedures are also encumbered by weight regain, usually in the 3–5 year period after an operation. For this reason it is suggested to withhold evaluation of any antiobesity operation until at least 5 years of follow-up data are available. The following review is limited to studies providing at least 5 years of follow-up.

By definition all comorbidities of obesity are ameliorated, if not cured, by weight loss. On purely medical grounds, "success" can be defined as improvement or cure of complications of obesity. From the patients' perspective, improvement in quality of life is the main criterion of success and this can only be determined by the individual patient. Mortality might appear to be a simple end-point in terms of success, but significant numbers of severely obese patients claim to prefer death to continuing a life of morbid obesity (35). Instead of enumerating the many conditions that have been demonstrated to be improved by surgical weight loss or the preventive potential of achieving significant prolonged weight loss, the following summarizes the quantitatively and qualitatively most important conditions improved or cured by antiobesity surgery.

B.   Mortality Reduction

Mortality is a simple and "hard" or unequivocal end-point for evaluating any therapy but it has several inherent methodological limitations in regard to severe obesity. Because of bias and ignorance that obesity truly is a disease, a listing of obesity is frequently omitted from hospital discharge summaries. In fact, there is no diagnosis-related grouping compensation for obesity, and the Centers for Disease Control and Prevention do not classify it in their mortality statistics. For these reasons it does not appear in the table of annual U.S. leading causes of death. Severe or "morbid" obesity does not have any separate World Health Organization classification, though some may argue that disease severity should not receive separate coding. Nevertheless, most large prospective studies have clearly demonstrated striking increases in mortality from severe obesity alone or in conjunction with diabetes, stroke, myocardial infarction, and cancer (for review see Ref. 36).

The natural history of severe obesity is also difficult to study. Characteristically the severely obese are infrequently sampled in national nutritional or other surveys. They frequently do not have access to scales sufficient to record weights above 90–115 kg (200–250 lb). Also, many physician's offices do not have such scales. Obese people have difficulties with transportation and ambulation and are often ashamed to be seen in public. In intervention studies their dropout rates are generally high, and extraordinary measures may be required to assure sufficient follow-up to allow statistically reliable conclusions. Furthermore, there is selection bias (37), which may be particularly significant among candidates for antiobesity surgery (38,39).

In spite of these limitations there is evidence that surgical treatment of severe obesity reduces mortality rates compared to reasonably adequate control subjects. In a convenience sample of severely obese subjects awaiting surgical treatment, there were relatively more victims of sudden unexplained death than among patients having undergone surgical treatment (40). In a retrospective study of patients who had various types of gastric surgery for obesity, mortality rates were no different than actuarial standards for the general population in the region (41). In a study of 154 severely obese patients with non-insulin-dependent diabetes mellitus (NIDDM) having gastric bypass compared to 72 matched NIDDM patients choosing not to be operated on, the probability of death was 4.6 times higher in the nonoperated patients (chi square: $p <$ 0.0001) (42). Data accruing from the Swedish prospective population study, Swedish Obese Subjects (39), seem to provide strong supportive evidence that surgical intervention clearly reduces the mortality of severe obesity.

C. Comorbidity Reduction

1. Non-Insulin-Dependent Diabetes Mellitus

One of the first comorbidities to be studied systematically after antiobesity surgery was impaired glucose tolerance (IGT), ameliorated by intestinal bypass (43). NIDDM has been the subject of numerous studies not only because of its prevalence and seriousness, but also because its dramatic response to surgical treatment was thought to provide insights into the pathogenesis of insulin resistance. Interestingly, there is an immediate correction of NIDDM postoperatively, even before any weight loss (44), demonstrating that primary defects in adipocyte, hepatocyte, or muscle sensitivity to insulin do not play a significant role in the etiology of obesity-related NIDDM.

There has been some controversy over whether the diversion of oral carbohydrate by gastric or intestinal bypass is responsible for the correction of IGT through interference with the enteroinsular axis or incretin effect. However, gastric restrictive procedures, as is the case with fasting or very-low-calorie diets, are equally effective as gastrointestinal bypass in normalizing glucose and insulin (45), implying that caloric intake is more important than insulin resistance for the syndrome of obesity-related NIDDM.

The best published data with respect to length (14 years) and completeness (97%) of follow-up, consistency of the operative procedure, and thoroughness of evaluation are presented in a series from Greenville, North Carolina of 608 severely obese patients, 165 of whom (27%) had NIDDM and 165 (27%) IGT (44). Average follow-up of 7.6 years after gastric bypass revealed that 83% of NIDDM patients maintained normal blood glucose and glycosylated hemoglobin, while 99% of IGT patients reverted to euglycemia. In an earlier study the authors calculated that weight loss from gastric bypass *prevented* the progression of IGT to diabetes more than 30-fold (46). In a more recent follow-up by these authors referred to above comparing 154 NIDDM patients having gastric bypass to 72 matched NIDDM patients choosing not to be operated on, mortality was reduced 4.6 times (42). Among these 226 patients, 81.5% of the 72 nonoperated patients versus 7.1% of the 154 operated patients required treatment for NIDDM.

2. Hypertension

The prevalence of hypertension preoperatively in the severely obese varies between 25 and 60% in the literature and depends on definitions and population characteristics. Among the 608 gastric bypass patients in Greenville, North Carolina followed 1–14 years, 58% were hypertensive preoperatively. After surgery the rate of hypertension was reduced to 14% representing an overall cure of 76% of the hypertensive population (44). Similar results varying between two-thirds and three-quarters of hypertensive patients resolving or improving after gastrointestinal operations for obesity have been reported (47,48).

As with dietary treatment of obesity-related hypertension, the greatest drop in blood pressure occurs early after surgery and does not require normalization of body weight. There is some controversy over the magnitude of weight loss necessary to improve blood pressure. Relationships between final weight at stabilization and the amount of weight loss and blood pressure reduction have been described. It is noteworthy that an initial reduction in diastolic pressure in *normotensive* patients at 12 months had disappeared by 48 months postoperatively in one study (48).

The rapidity of reduction of blood pressure postoperatively implies that reductions in nutrient-related sympathetic drive may be more important than decrease in blood volume, diuresis, resolution of hypoventilation, or reduced intra-abdominal pressure as contributing factors. As with NIDDM, caloric intake may be of primary importance in the pathogenesis of obesity-related hypertension.

3. Respiratory Insufficiency

Sleep apnea (SA) and obesity hypoventilation syndrome (OHS) are prevalent among the severely obese though full evaluations of pulmonary function are not performed routinely because they are not considered cost-effective. Among 1010 severely obese patients operated on at a center with a special interest in respiratory function, 12.5% ($n = 126$) had sleep apnea alone, hypoventilation alone, or both prior to undergoing gastroplasty or gastric bypass (49).

Surgically induced weight loss significantly reduces the apnea index in SA patients and increases PaO_2 and decreases $PaCO_2$ in patients with OHS. Approximately two-thirds of patients with sleep apnea and three-quarters of OHS patients were asymptomatic around 5 years postoperatively. Though immediate effects of antiobesity surgery on respiratory insufficiency are often quite dramatic, occasionally obviating a need for tracheostomy, with continued improvement during weight loss, it is remarkable that objective measures of hypoventilation reappear with relatively small regain of weight (50). Nevertheless, patients' subjective assessments are predominantly positive.

4. Dyslipidemia

The prevalence of dyslipidemia in severely obese patients varies between 15 and 25% and is mainly in the form of hypertriglyceridemia and low-HDL cholesterol. Intestinal bypass operations were early recognized to cause significant changes in serum lipids. Indeed, a modification of jejunoileal bypass designed to lower lipids without weight loss (partial ileal bypsss) remains the most effective and probably most cost-efficient means of treating hyperlipoproteinemia (51).

Unfortunately, most studies of gastric bypass operations do not present data on dyslipidemic patients separately instead electing to present conglomerate results of unselected patients followed over the long term. This is problematic because experience with intestinal bypass demonstrated significantly greater reductions in serum cholesterol and triglycerides in patients with elevated levels preoperatively than in normolipidemic patients. Indeed, the only study of dyslipidemic patients studied for a sufficiently long period after gastric bypass to avoid the confounding effects of dynamic weight loss clearly demonstrated a decrease in total cholesterol in patients maintaining this weight loss (52).

In other studies after gastric bypass without stratification for initial lipid levels there have not been effects on total cholesterol or apoprotein levels. The most consistent effects of all antiobesity operations on serum lipids are lowering of triglycerides and long-term increases in HDL cholesterol, both of which may be secondary to the improvements in insulin resistance. In aggregate there are significant modifications of the coronary risk factor profile in most patients after antiobesity operations (53).

5. Miscellaneous

Table 3 lists conditions that have been demonstrated to improve after antiobesity surgery according to published reports. It is reasonable to expect considerably more benefits derived from reductions in complications of these conditions, such as myocardial infarction, stroke, amputations, thromboembolism, and uremia to name a few. Furthermore, though more difficult to demonstrate in the absence of sufficiently large population studies, antiobesity surgery has extraordinary *preventive* potential mainly with respect to the obesity-related cancers: breast, colon, endometrial, and prostate, but also for infection proneness, hernia, and varicose veins.

6. Quality of Life

Impaired quality of life is probably the most difficult aspect for most obese patients to endure regardless of health

Table 3 Conditions Demonstrated To
Be Improved by Antiobesity Surgery

Cardiopulmonary
  Hypertension
  Heart Failure
  Edema
  Respiratory insufficiency
  Asthma
Diabetes
Dyslipidemia
Esophagitis
Gynecological
  Infertility
  Delivery
  Urinary incontinence
Liver cirrhosis and fibrosis
Operative risk
Osteoarthritis
Pseudotumor cerebri
Quality of life
Sleep disorder
Thromboembolism

status. Therefore, it should be an important outcome to measure. It is only recently that patient satisfaction and quality-adjusted life-years (QUALYs) have entered the arena of outcome assessment (54). Interestingly, this is occurring simultaneously with the almost universal trend toward cutting medical costs mainly through introduction of practice parameters and managed care.

There are very few studies of changes in non-health-related quality of life with any type of treatment of obesity. It is true that the results of such studies after surgical treatment agree in demonstrating increased employability and improved wages (work-performance domain), improved physical functioning (physical domain), and less psychological distress and increased sense of well-being (psychological domain), but there is some confusion because of the temporal and adaptive changes intrinsic in subjective quality-of-life assessment. Thus one of the long-term studies questions whether emotional and social changes are only temporary because self-assessment scores deteriorated with time, not considering that the subjects' level of ambition increased as their recollection of past impairment faded (55). This is in agreement with another short-term study demonstrating more depression in patients with "better" results of bariatric surgery (56). However, in aggregate the preponderance of long-term studies of quality of life after surgically induced weight loss unequivocally demonstrate substantial improvements. This is the most important factor driving patients to request sur-

gical treatment of obesity and is testimony to the tragic perceived liability of severe obesity (35).

D. Complications and Side Effects

Operative mortality is currently below 0.5% in centers specializing in antiobesity surgery (for review see Ref. 57) and is likely to decrease further because of the development of less invasive surgical techniques. The mortality rates of antiobesity operations are significantly lower than corresponding figures in severely obese patients having other operations. This may reflect selection bias or the inexperience of surgeons not routinely operating on the severely obese, in that only seriously ill obese patients are given other operations (58).

The difference between side effects and complications is that the former are expected if not desired and can usually be controlled, while the latter are neither expected nor controllable and are never desired. The most prevalent side effect of gastric restriction is intolerance of solid food and it is highly dependent on the preoperative education of the patient. Most vomiting after gastric restriction is behavioral. However, it is important to rule out stricture or stenosis or other complications that can cause vomiting. Endoscopy has the dual benefit of being diagnostic and also allowing treatment by dilatation of the stoma.

The most common side effect of gastric bypass is the "dumping syndrome" recognized from gastric resections for ulcers or cancer. Ingestion of calorically dense high osmotic food, rapidly emptied ("dumped") into the small intestine, causes release of vasoactive gastrointestinal polypeptides (59), which elicit tachycardia, palpitations, diaphoresis, light-headedness, and nausea. These autonomic physiological side-effects may well explain the superiority of gastric bypass operations over restrictive operations in achieving and maintaining weight loss, though patients without dumping lose similar amounts of weight.

Table 4 enumerates complications of antiobesity operations. The rates are strongly influenced by demographics and case mix including recognized risk factors such as smoking, hypertension, and diabetes and less studied psychological factors and selection criteria. The number and severity of complications associated with intestinal bypass operations have appropriately led to abandonment of these procedures except in selected patients in centers with a special interest in and knowledge of their management. Complications of intestinal bypass operations can be prevented and treated if recognized in time. This requires meticulous surveillance and the full cooperation of the patient. A recent review provides detailed instructions for managing complications and monitoring progress (60). Occasionally take-down of intestinal bypass is mandated,

Table 4 Procedure-Related Complications of Antiobesity Surgery

Malabsorptive operations	Gastric operations
Operative	Operative
Wound Infection	Leaks
Uncontrolled diarrhea	Splenectomy
Deficiencies	Uncontrolled vomiting
Fat-soluble vitamins	Deficiencies
Electrolytes: potassium,	Thiamine deficiency
magnesium, calcium	Alkalosis
Blind-loop syndrome	Inadequate diet
Enteritis	Iron
Arthropathy	Calcium
Liver cirrhosis	Vitamin B_{12}
Metabolic problems	Erosions or ulcers
Gall stones	Strictures
Urolithiasis	Weight loss failure
Encephalopathy	

though it must be understood that previously obese patients are very reluctant to undergo reversal, even in the face of life-threatening complications. Over the very long term (12–15 years or more) reversal operations have been described in approximately one-third of patients in published series. At the same time there is late mortality, but the absence of control groups with other treatment for comparison does not permit interpretation of whether the mortality figures are excessive considering the severity of the disease being treated.

Complications of gastric antiobesity operations are mechanical, nutritional, or behavioral, though both mechanical and nutritional sequelae may be secondary to behavioral problems. For obvious reasons, the frequency of nutritional complications is directly related to the efficacy of an operation. Gastric bypass has a greater risk of deficiencies with failure of the patient to take supplements and return for postoperative monitoring of serum levels than gastric restriction.

As mentioned earlier, the most prevalent side effect of gastric restrictive or obstructive operations is vomiting. In general, the mechanical complications such as esophagitis, ulcers, stricture, or perforation are secondary to behavioral problems, which may derive from inadequate preoperative teaching or from environmental stressors.

The side effects and complications of gastric bypass listed in Table 5 vary significantly between series depending on population factors, as mentioned, but also on the quality of the preoperative instruction and follow-up care as well as the zeal of the clinical team. A voluntary registry of data provided by mainly privately practicing surgeons

in the United States (National Bariatric Surgery Registry, NBSR) is prospectively compiling results on all patients entered into the data bank. This registry is providing a wealth of data through its multicenter approach. It will permit evaluation of complications and results of different types of procedures.

E. Failure of Antiobesity Surgery

1. Definition of "Failure"

Just as "success" is difficult to define in terms of weight loss, so is "failure." Surgeons often express weight loss results as reduction in excess weight, where "excess" means the weight exceeding actuarial weight-for-height standards. The reduction of excess weight is thus expressed as a percentage of excess weight. Unfortunately, the premise that any finite residual excess weight continues to exert (substantial) risk is untested and thus unfounded. In fact, there is evidence that even a modest loss of weight is beneficial albeit the patient continues to be moderately (BMI > 30 kg/m²) or even severely (BMI > 35 kg/m²) obese. Thus expressing failure in terms of weight loss is inappropriate on strictly medical grounds. There are no data on "desirable" or "ideal" body weight for height of subjects who have undergone weight reduction.

As indicated earlier, patients' criteria, whether based on perceived cosmetic standards or other goals, may be significantly more ambitious than those of physicians. Quality-of-life assessments are necessary to reconcile these disparate goals. In this context it is important to consider the patients' prior weight loss experiences as well as patients' changing needs as they get accustomed to a reduced weight. From a purely physical health-related standpoint, failure can readily be defined as inability to ameliorate manifest comorbidity or prevent recurrence of such comorbidity. According to this criterion, there is a 20% failure

Table 5 Side Effects and Complications of Gastric Bypass Compiled From Large Published Series

		Side effects	
Dumping	70%	Headache	40%
Dairy intolerance	50%	Hair loss	33%
Constipation	40%	Depression	15%
		Complications	
B_{12} deficiency	25%	Incisional hernia	15%
Abdominal pain	15%	Anemia	15%
Vomiting	15%	Arrhythmia	10%
Diarrhea	15%	Vitamin deficiency (non-B_{12})	10%

rate of standard gastric bypass operations over the long term in the Greenville experience (44). This criterion is easy to measure and should not be controversial. Any standard simply based on weight must be arbitrary, and as such debatable, until statistics on minimum mortality for reduced obese subjects become available. This may be an insurmountable task since it will require stratification for initial relative weight as well as duration of exposure.

Currently nonsurgical treatment can rarely provide more than a 10% reduction in pretreatment weight observed even for 1 year (61). Against the background of numerous published studies on results of different surgical techniques followed for 5 years or more and the empirical finding that long-term weight regain to within 20% of pretreatment weight is associated with reappearance of comorbidity and patient dissatisfaction (62), it seems reasonable to suggest this 20% level as an arbitrary definition of weight loss "failure" (Fig. 4).

According to this definition, a weight loss of less than 21 kg (46 lb) in a woman 160 cm (5 ft 3 in.) tall and weighing 103.7 kg (228 lb) (BMI = 40.5 kg/m^2), which is 45.5 kg (100 lb) above the life insurance standard of 58.2 kg (128 lb) (BMI = 22.7), is a failure of surgical treatment after 2 years when nadir should have been reached after most primary operations. Obviously at a weight of 82.7 kg (182 lb) this patient is still obese with a BMI = 32.3 kg/m^2. Similar calculations for a 175-cm (5 ft 9 in.) man weighing 114.5 kg (252 lb) (BMI = 37.4 kg/m^2) places weight loss failure at a loss of less than 22.7 kg (50 lb). The resultant weight of 91.8 kg (202 lb) after losing 22.7 kg corresponds to a BMI = 30 kg/m^2. Some investigators have suggested that any result, regardless of the patient's weight level preoperatively, that fails to reduce weight below an excess weight of 100% of ideal body weight should be regarded as failure, though there are no mortality or morbidity data to support this. The overall long-term experience with antiobesity surgery demonstrates losses between 25 and 40% of preoperative weight.

2. Reasons for Failure

Weight loss failure can be viewed as one of the most serious complications of antiobesity surgery because the operation has added its own morbidity to an already sick patient and because any further gastrointestinal operations are rendered more difficult (63). Surgical failure can result from surgical technical flaws, behavioral problems, or a combination of the two. The behavioral component must not be underestimated. Aggressive overeating can lead to technical failure of a perfectly executed operation, for example, by overdistention of a gastric pouch with subsequent breakdown of the staple line, perforation of the

pouch, or erosion and ulceration by the band. Some surgeons evaluate operations by their rate of reoperations though such data are very reliant on the completeness of follow-up. Unfortunately, there are no known methods for identifying patients prone to aggressive overeating preoperatively, so it is difficult to fault the patient selection process for such failure.

Gastric restrictive operations fail because the patient eats to the mechanical limit of the pouch, causing distention, which gradually enlarges pouch capacity. A more common reason is maladaptive eating or the soft-calorie syndrome, in which patients select calorically dense low-bulk liquid or melting foods that easily pass through the pouch outlet (5). The initial restrictive component of gastric bypass operations has the same limitations as the purely restrictive operations.

Gastric bypass procedures fail over the long term because of gradual adaptation of intestinal mucosa in the proximal small bowel conduit leading to reduction of the aversive effect of the "dumping syndrome" described earlier. It is also possible that there is down-regulation of central or peripheral receptors participating in the "satiety cascade." Another contributing factor may be behavioral adaptation of food selection to avoid the aversive effects of the bypass. Similar behavioral modifications have been reported by patients with intestinal bypass operations.

3. Reoperations for Failures of Antiobesity Surgery

There are no published standards for reoperative antiobesity surgery: indications have not been defined and criteria for choosing secondary procedures have not been developed. Reoperations are usually more difficult than primary operations and thus have a higher perioperative complication rate (63). Laparoscopic adjustable banding may be an exception, as outlined above. It might seem logical to reoperate for a technical flaw by simply correcting the problem, as in staple line disruption, enlarged pouch, or stomal problems. New technical modifications to prevent staple line disruption include dividing between staple lines to get better and stronger healing and introduction of more rows of staples. However, it is extremely important to try to rule out a behavioral cause of a presumed technical problem, which might instead indicate that the principle of the operation is inappropriate. Gastric restrictive operations are more prone to be conceptually flawed in this manner because many patients are simply unable to adapt to the requirements of the "gastroplasty diet" (60).

Strategies for reoperation of gastric restrictive procedures are either correction of the problem by restapling to shrink an enlarged pouch or to replace a disrupted staple line or conversion to a bypass operation to introduce appetitive effects of the small bowel. Failed gastric bypass procedures may be revised by shortening the digestive segment of small intestine thus creating malabsorption. Revisions of intestinal bypass operations for weight regain are unrewarding because of the inability to balance further weight loss against the risk of debilitating malnutrition. In patients requiring take-down of intestinal bypass because of complications, concomitant construction of a gastric restrictive operation usually is followed by some weight gain. However, most severely obese patients who have experienced weight loss after an operation are extremely unwilling to accept reversal, even in the face of life-threatening complications. This attests to the serious perceived liability of being severely obese (35).

IV. DISCUSSION

Surgical treatment has evolved as the only realistic option for safely and cost-efficiently achieving sustained, medically significant weight loss in patients with BMI 35 kg/m² or greater. With the exception of lipectomy (which does not have a role in the primary treatment of obesity because of the marginal amount of fat and skin removed), the surgical techniques have been developed over a period of 30–40 years and more than 30 different operations have been used clinically. It is true that many have been discarded, and some should never have been attempted in the absence of careful clinical evaluation, but the risks of currently perfected techniques are so low and the benefits, whether in terms of morbidity reduction, quality-of-life improvement, patient satisfaction, or mortality reduction, are so convincingly positive that surgical treatment of obesity must be considered an established and legitimate form of treatment.

Though opinions differ, there is no single procedure of choice or "gold standard" and never will be because of large variations in weight, duration of obesity, amount and severity of comorbidity, nature and magnitude of the eating disorder, and psychosocial background of severely obese patients. The largest unsolved problem in this field is identifying outcome predictors, whether they are metabolic, anthropometric, or behavioral (Table 6). The goal of individualizing therapy is elusive in the absence of predictors. For this reason alone, it is appropriate to have a staged or "step-care" approach to surgical treatment progressing to more aggressive methods (15).

Operations for obesity exist out of default, in the absence of any nonsurgical methods for palliating the severely obese. The standard requirement of evidence-based medicine for demonstration of superiority of one

Table 6 Influences on Outcome of Antiobesity Surgery

Proven	Probable
Age	Addictions
Diet	Anthropometry
Eating rate	Binge eating disorder
Economic status	Body composition
Metabolic rate	Diabetes
Psychiatric history	Domestic partner
Race	Secondary gain
Sex	Weight loss experience

treatment over another is the prospective, randomized, controlled trial. With severe obesity there are several obstacles to such studies, scientific as well as ethical. Patients selecting or agreeing to undergo surgery have different characteristics than those who do not. It is likely that those who agree to being randomized represent a subgroup that is quite different than the general population of severely obese (38). Since there is no evidence to demonstrate efficacy of any nonsurgical treatment, a fact that ethically must be disclosed in the consent process, it is not possible to portray different treatment arms as reasonably equivalent. Not offering any treatment (as a control) is also not ethical in the presence of serious disease. Most attempts at prospective, randomized, controlled trials have failed simply because the nonsurgical arm could neither be completed nor restudied.

The absence of effective treatments for obesity has also limited the ability to clarify the importance of obesity as an independent or secondary risk factor for major related diseases. In this regard too, surgical treatment, by achieving sustained significant weight loss, is uniquely suited to test the hypothesis that weight loss will improve longevity, morbidity, and quality of life. The ongoing Swedish Obese Subjects trial is addressing precisely this issue (39). By entering a large, nationwide, random sample of severely obese subjects receiving standard general practice "treatment" for obesity into the study, it will be possible to finally obtain data on the natural history of individuals with BMI ≥ 35 kg/m². Comparison with the surgical treatment arm will demonstrate the preventive potential of such treatment, as has already been done for NIDDM (42). Over the very long term it is possible that the SOS study will be able to clarify the optimum amount of weight loss conferring morbidity and mortality reduction ("ideal" or "desirable" reduced weight).

Last, but not least important: through its effectiveness, surgical treatment provides a tool to elucidate the pathogenesis of leading causes of death in industrialized nations, including atherosclerotic large- and small-vessel disease, hypertension, diabetes mellitus, and their complications. Just as the "cholesterol hypothesis" of atherosclerosis was proven by demonstrating that cholesterol lowering led to reduction of atherosclerotic plaque size and less disease progression (51), so it may be with the hypothesis that obesity has an independent role in the pathogenesis of these conditions: weight reduction achieved through surgery can provide the necessary proof. So far diabetes with insulin resistance is the best-studied example. Normalization of glucose and insulin immediately postoperatively, before any weight reduction (44), implies that tissue "resistance" is less important for impaired glucose tolerance or NIDDM than previously believed. Clearly, surgical treatment of severe obesity provides important methodology for significant advances in clinical research.

The strongest impediment to progress in the treatment of severe obesity is the prejudice of the lay public and legislators against all obesity and the even stronger biases of the medical community, surgeons in particular, against antiobesity surgery (35). The self-serving interests of the diet-exercise-drug coalition jealously protecting their finances operate in consort with the food industry in perpetuating this difficult problem.

V. SUMMARY

The history of systematic use of surgical methods to treat obesity spans a period of 30–40 years. In this time numerous variants have been briefly tested and enthusiastically promoted only to be abandoned when sufficient information accrued for adequate evaluation. Five predominant areas of investigation have characterized the evolution of antiobesity operations: 1) determination of lengths and proportions of jejunum and ileum in continuity in malabsorptive procedures ("Length titration"), 2) methods for preventing bacterial overgrowth of defunctionalized segments of intestines ("Blind loop modification"), 3) configurations for reducing stomach capacity including volume of reservoir and diameter of outlet ("Pouch and stoma construction"), 4) combinations of stomach reduction and varying lengths and proportions of jejunum and ileum ("Permutations"), and 5) manipulations influencing neurohumoral mechanisms involved in appetite regulation ("Regulatory methods"). Out of these efforts two safe and effective established surgical methods have evolved: 1) gastric restriction by gastroplasty and banding and 2) gastric bypass. Others are still being evaluated. Because of the diversity of obese patients there is no single method of choice.

These two surgical methods are no longer investigational or experimental but rather represent the only documented effective treatment for palliation of obesity complicated by serious, life-threatening morbidity. They function by aversive conditioning and are effective for periods exceeding 10 years in 50–80% of cases with perioperative mortality of <50%. The more effective operations require life-long supplementation and monitoring because of the potential for nutritional deficiencies in 30% of patients. Antiobesity operations are the most effective means of treating diabetes mellitus (NIDDM), hypertension, sleep apnea, pseudotumor cerebri, and a host of conditions related to obesity. Recent data provide conclusive evidence that mortality from obesity-related diabetes is reduced and progression of impaired glucose tolerance or development of frank diabetes is prevented by these operations.

Introduction of laparoscopic or minimally invasive surgical techniques such as the laparoscopic adjustable band (LAB) is increasing the margin of safety of antiobesity surgery and will allow expansion of the indications for such treatment to patients with BMI <35 kg/m^2. Furthermore, laparoscopic surgery has a logical place in a step-care strategy for treating the majority of severely obese patients with BMI exceeding 35–40 kg/m^2 before progressing to more aggressive malabsorptive techniques.

The most important problems remaining in this field pertain to refining patient selection for primary and remedial procedures and accruing longitudinal epidemiological data to define the natural history of severe obesity and increasing the data base of intervention studies to further demonstrate the cost-effectiveness of surgical intervention. The absence of outcome predictors justifies the use of a staged approach to treatment. The largest obstacle to progress in treating severe obesity remains the prejudice of large sectors of the medical establishment.

Improvement in the quality of life and patient satisfaction after antiobesity surgery exceed those of most other medical endeavors and are in themselves sufficient reward for undertaking the frequently daunting experience of treating these challenging and most unhappy human beings. Furthermore, surgical intervention in patients with BMI > 40 kg/m^2 substantially reduces mortality compared to a general population of severely obese subjects. Surgical treatment has evolved as the only realistic option for safely and cost-efficiently achieving sustained medically significant weight loss in the majority of patients with Body Mass Index 35 kg/m^2 or greater.

VI. CONCLUSIONS

Two main types of antiobesity surgery—gastric restriction and gastric bypass—are safe and effective over the long term.

Because of the heterogeneity of the severely obese population, there is no operation of choice.

Operative mortality <0.5% is less than actuarial mortality of severely obese subjects.

Diabetes, hypertension, respiratory insufficiency, dyslipidemia, and other serious conditions are significantly improved after antiobesity surgery.

Surgical treatment prevents diabetes and other co-morbidity as well as disease progression.

Longitudinal epidemiological data on effects of weight loss can only be provided through surgical intervention.

Prospective, randomized, controlled trials comparing antiobesity surgery to other treatment are not feasible scientifically or ethically.

Outcome predictors and "optimal" weight loss are not known. Criteria for reoperation are lacking.

Minimally invasive surgical techniques will allow widening of indications to weight levels below BMI of 35 kg/m^2.

A staged or step-care strategy is recommended for surgical treatment of severe obesity.

General and health-related quality of life is dramatically improved after antiobesity surgery.

REFERENCES

1. Macgregor AMC, Rand CSW. Gastric surgery in morbid obesity: outcome in patients aged 55 years and older. Arch Surg 1993; 128:1153–1157.

2. National Institutes of Health Consensus Development Conference. Gastrointestinal surgery for severe obesity. Am J Clin Nutr 1992; 55(Suppl):487S–619S.

3. Martin LF, Tan T-L, Horn JR, Bixler EO, Kauffman GL, Becker DA, Huner SM. Comparison of the costs associated with medical and surgical treatment of obesity. Surgery 1995; 118:599–607.

4. Kark AE. Jaw wiring. Am J Clin Nutr 1980; 33:420–424.

5. Kral JG, Kissileff HR. Surgical approaches to the treatment of obesity. Ann Behav Med 1987; 9:15–19.

6. Kral JG. Gastric balloons: a plea for sanity in the midst of baloonacy. Gastroenterology 1988; 95:213–215.

7. Kral JG. Surgical treatment of regional adiposity: lipectomy versus surgically induced weight loss. Acta Med Scand 1988; (Suppl 723):225–231.

8. Schrudde J. Lipexheresis in the correction of local adiposity. Int J Aesth Plast Surg 1972.

9. Kral JG. Surgical reduction of adipose tissue in the male Sprague-Dawley rat. Am J Physiol 1976; 231:1090–1096.

10. Henriksson V. [Is small bowel resection justified as treatment for obesity?] Nordisk Med 1952; 47:744.

11. Kremen AJ, Linner JH, Nelson CH. An experimental evaluation of the nutritional importance of proximal and distal small intestine. Ann Surg 1954; 140:439.

12. Grant JP. Duke procedure for super obesity: preliminary report with 3.5-year follow-up. Surgery 1994: 115:718–726.

13. NIH Consensus Development Conference: Surgical treatment of morbid obesity. Am J Clin Nutr 1980; 33:(Suppl 2):353–530.

14. Kral JG. Malabsorptive procedures in surgical treatment of morbid obesity. Clin Gastroenterol 1987: 16:293–305.

15. Kral JG. Surgical treatment of obesity. Med Clin North Am 1989; 73:251–264.

16. Mason EE, Ito C. Gastric bypass and obesity. Surg Clin North Am 1967; 47:1345–1352.

17. Scopinaro N, Gianetta E, Civalleri D, Bonalumi U, Bachi V. Biliopancreatic bypass for obesity. II. Initial experience in man. Br J Surg 1979; 66:618–620.

17a. Scopinaro N, Gianetta E, Adami GF, Friedman D, Traverso E, Marinari GM, Cuneo S, Vitale B, Ballari F, Colombini M, Baschieri G, Bachi V: Biliopancreatic diversion for obesity at eighteen years. Surgery 1996; 119:261–268.

18. Brolin RE, Kenler HA, Gorman JH, Cody RP. Long-limb gastric bypass in the superobese. Ann Surg 1992; 215:387–395.

19. Linner JH. Overview of surgical techniques for the treatment of morbid obesity. Clin Gastroenterol 1987; 16:253–272.

20. Salmon PA. Gastroplasty with distal gastric bypass: a new and more successful weight loss operation for the morbidly obese. Can J Surg 1988; 31:111–113.

21. DeMeester TR, Fuchs KH, Ball CS, Albertucci M, Smyrk TC, Marcus JN. Experimental and clinical results with proximal end-to-end duodenojejunostomy for pathologic duodenogastric reflux. Ann Surg 1987; 206:414–426.

22. Mason EE. Surgical treatment of obesity. Major Probl Gen Surg 1981; 26:1–493.

23. Mason EE. Vertical banded gastroplasty. Arch Surg 1982; 117:701–706.

24. Eckhout GV, Willbanks OL, Moore JT. Vertical-ring gastroplasty for morbid obesity: five-year experience with 1463 patients. Am J Surg 1986; 152:713–716.

25. Curley SA, Weaver W, Wilkinson LH, Demarest GB. Late complications after gastric reservoir reduction with external wrap. Arch Surg 1987; 122:781–783.

26. Peitersen E, Quaade F, Breum L, Olesen HP: Esophageal banding: pilot study of a new operation for obesity. Surg Res Commun 1990; 9:177–182.

27. Kuzmak LI. Gastric banding. In: Deitel M, ed. Surgery for the Morbidly Obese Patient. Philadelphia: Lea & Febiger, 1989:225–259.

28. Kuzmak LI. Stoma adjustable silicone gastric banding. Probl Gen Surg 1992; 9:298–317.

29. Belachew M, Monami B. Laparoscopic adjustable silicone gastric banding: technique and preliminary results. Obes Surg 1995; 5:258.

30. Quaade F, Vaernet K, Larsson S. Stereotaxic stimulation and electrocoagulation of the lateral hypothalamus in obese humans. Acta Neurochir 1974; 30:111–117.

31. Kral JG. Vagotomy as a treatment for severe obesity. Lancet 1978; I:307–308.

32. Kral JG, Görtz L, Hermanson G, Wallin GS. Gastroplasty for obesity: long-term weight loss improved by vagotomy. World J Surg. 1993; 17:75–79.

33. Koopmans HS, Sclafani A. Control of body weight by lower gut signals. Int J Obes 1981; 5:491.

34. Smithy WB, Cuadros CL, Johnson H, Kral JG. Effects of ileal interposition on body weight and intestinal morphology in dogs. Int J Obes 1986; 10:453–460.

35. Rand CSW, Macgregor A. Successful weight loss following surgery and the perceived liability of morbid obesity. Int J Obes 1991; 15:577–579.

36. Sjöström LV. Mortality of severely obese subjects. Am J Clin Nutr 1992; 55(Suppl):516S–523S.

37. Fitzgibbon ML, Stolley MR, Kirschenbaum DS. Obese people who seek treatment have different characteristics than those who do not seek treatment. Health Psychol 1993; 12:342–345.

38. Kral JG. Limitations of epidemiologic studies of the morbidly obese. Integrat Psychiatry 1983; 1:131

39. Sjöström L, Larsson B, Backman L, Bengtsson C, Bouchard C, Dahlgren S, Hallgren P, Jonsson E, Karlsson J, Lapidus L, Lindroos AK, Lindstedt S, Lissner L, Narbro K, Näslund I, Olbe L, Sullivan M, Sylvan A, Wedel H, Agren G. Swedish Obese Subjects (SOS): recruitment for an intervention study and a selected description of the obese state. Int J Obes 1992; 16:465–479.

40. Drenick EJ, Fisler JS. Sudden cardiac arrest in morbidly obese patients unexplained after autopsy. Am J Surg 1988; 155:720–726.

41. Mason EE, Kao C, Woolson RF, Scott DH, Maher JW. Impact of vertical banded gastroplasty on mortality from obesity. Obes Surg 1991; 1:115.

42. Long S, MacDonald KG, Swanson M, Brown B, Morris P, Dohm GL, Pories WJ. The gastric bypass operation reduces the progression and mortality of non-insulin dependent diabetes mellitus. Gastroenterology 1996; 110:A1400.

43. Rehfeld JF, Juhl E, Quaade F. Effect of jejunoileostomy on glucose and insulin metabolism in ten obese patients. Metabolism 1970; 19:529–538.

44. Pories WJ, Swanson MS, MacDonald KG, Long SB, Morris PG, Brown BM, Barakat HA, deRamon RA, Israel G, Dolezal JM, Dohm L. Who would have thought it? An operation proves to be the most effective therapy for adult-onset diabetes mellitus. Ann Surg 1995; 222:339–352.

45. Letiexhe MR, Scheen AJ, Gérard PL, Desaive C, Lefèbvre PJ. Insulin secretion, clearance and action before and after gastroplasty in severely obese subjects. Int J Obes 1994; 19:295–300.

46. Long SD, O'Brien K, MacDonald KG, Leggett-Frazier N, Swanson MS, Pories WJ, Caro JF. Weight loss in severely obese subjects prevents the progression of impaired glucose tolerance to type II diabetes. Diabetes Care 1994; 17:372–375.

47. Foley EF, Benotti 3PN, Borlase BC, Hollingshead J, Blackburn GL. Impact of gastric restrictive surgery on hypertension in the morbidly obese. Am J Surg 1992; 163:294–297.

48. Carson JL, Ruddy ME, Duff AE, Holmes NJ, Cody RP, Brolin RE. The effect of gastric bypass surgery on hypertension in morbidly obese patients. Arch Intern Med 1994; 154:193–200.

49. Sugerman HJ, Fairman RP, Sood RK, Engle K, Wolfe L, Kellum JM. Long-term effects of gastric surgery for treating respiratory insufficiency of obesity. Am J Clin Nutr 1992; 55(Suppl):597S–601S.

50. Charuzi I, Lavie P, Peiser J, Peled R. Bariatric surgery in morbidly obese sleep-apnea patients: short- and long-term follow-up. Am J Clin Nutr 1992; 55(Suppl):594S–596S.

51. Buchwald H, Varco RL, Matts JP, et al. Effect of partial ileal bypass surgery on mortality and morbidity from coronary heart disease in patients with hypercholesterolemia: report of the Program on the Surgical Control of the Hyperlipidemias (POSCH). N Engl J Med 1990; 323:946–955.

52. Brolin RE, Kenler HA, Wilson AC, Kuo PT, Cody RP. Serum lipids after gastric bypass surgery for morbid obesity. Int J Obes 1990; 14:939–950.

53. Gleysteen JJ, Barboriak JJ, Sasse EA. Sustained coronary-risk-factor reduction after gastric bypass for morbid obesity. Am J Clin Nutr 1990; 51:774–778.

54. Testa MA, Simonson DC. Assessment of quality-of-life outcomes. N Engl J Med 1996; 334:835–840.

55. Waters GS, Pories WJ, Swanson MS, Meelheim HD, Flickinger EG, May HJ. Long-term studies of mental health after the Greenville gastric bypass operation for morbid obesity. Am J Surg 1991; 161:154–158.

56. Ryden O, Olsson S-A, Danielsson A et al. Weight loss after gastroplasty: psychological sequelae in relation to clinical and metabolic observations. J Am Coll Nutr 1989; 9:15.

57. Kral JG. Side-effects, complications and problems in anti-obesity surgery: introduction of the obesity severity index. In: Angel A, Anderson H, Bouchard C, Lau D, Leiter L, Mendelson R, eds. Progress in Obesity Research 7. London: John Libbey, 1996:655–661.

58. Kral JG. Surgical risks in obese patients. In: Schettler G, Gotto AM Middelhoff G, Habenicht AJR, Jurutka KR, eds. Atherosclerosis VI. Berlin: Springer-Verlag, 1983:955–959.

59. Kellum JM, Kuemmerle JF, O'Dorisio TM, Rayford P, Martin D, Engle K, Wolf L, Sugerman HJ. Gastrointestinal hormone responses to meals before and after gastric bypass and vertical banded gastroplasty. Ann Surg 1990; 211:763–771.

60. Kral JG. Therapy of severe obesity. In: Haubrich W, Schaffner F, Berk JE, eds. Bockus Gastroenterology, 5th ed. Philadelphia: WB Saunders, 1994:3231–3239.

61. Bennett W. Dietary treatments of obesity. Ann NY Acad Sci 1981; 499:350–363.

62. Sugerman HJ, Kellum JM, DeMaria EJ: Conversion to distal gastric bypass for failed standard gastric bypass for morbid obesity. Gastroenterology 1996; 110:A1421.

63. Linner JH, Drew RL. Reoperative surgery—indications, efficacy, and long-term follow-up. Am J Clin Nutr 1992; 55(Suppl):606S–610S.

Index

Trumbauer M.

R804-152

979